CECIL ESSENTIALS OF
MEDICINE

TENTH EDITION 10

CECIL ESSENTIALS OF
MEDICINE

EDITORS

Edward J. Wing, MD, FACP, FIDSA
Former Dean of Medicine and Biological Sciences
Professor of Medicine
Warren Alpert Medical School
Brown University
Providence, Rhode Island

Fred J. Schiffman, MD, MACP
Sigal Family Professor of Humanistic Medicine
Vice Chair, Department of Medicine
Warren Alpert Medical School
Brown University
Providence, Rhode Island

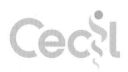

Elsevier
1600 John F. Kennedy Blvd.
Ste 1800
Philadelphia, PA 19103-2899

CECIL ESSENTIALS OF MEDICINE, TENTH EDITION

ISBN: 978-0-323-72271-1

Notice

Practitioners and researchers must always rely on their own experience and knowledge in evaluating and using any information, methods, compounds or experiments described herein. Because of rapid advances in the medical sciences, in particular, independent verification of diagnoses and drug dosages should be made. To the fullest extent of the law, no responsibility is assumed by Elsevier, authors, editors or contributors for any injury and/or damage to persons or property as a matter of products liability, negligence or otherwise, or from any use or operation of any methods, products, instructions, or ideas contained in the material herein.

Previous editions copyrighted 2016, 2010, 2007, 2004, 2001, 1997, 1993, 1990, and 1986.

Library of Congress Control Number: 2021932451

Content Strategist: Marybeth Thiel
Senior Content Development Specialist: Jennifer Ehlers
Publishing Services Manager: Catherine Jackson
Senior Project Manager: Daniel Fitzgerald
Designer: Maggie Reid

Printed in the United States of America.

Last digit is the print number: 9   8   7   6   5   4   3   2   1

Working together
to grow libraries in
developing countries

www.elsevier.com • www.bookaid.org

In Memoriam

Thomas E. Andreoli, MD

Dr. Thomas Andreoli, along with Drs. Lloyd Hollingsworth (Holly) Smith, Jr., Fred Plum, and Charles C.J. Carpenter, was one of the four founding editors of *Cecil Essentials of Medicine.* He served as editor for editions one through eight before he passed away on April 14, 2009. Dr. Andreoli was born in the Bronx, New York, in 1935, attended Catholic primary and high schools, and graduated from St. Vincent College and the Georgetown School of Medicine. He trained as a resident at Duke University under legendary Chair of Medicine Dr. Eugene Stead, who recognized him as a brilliant physician and scientist and encouraged his research career. Dr. Andreoli received his research training at the NIH and then in the laboratory of Dr. Tosteson at Duke. His research focused on the biochemical and biophysical properties of renal tubular cell membranes and their role in water and electrolyte transport. He made fundamental discoveries on the normal renal physiology, illuminating the way to subsequent work by many others on renal health and disease. His research was recognized with numerous awards and election to honorific societies both in the United States and in Europe. Dr. Andreoli also served as editor of *The American Journal of Physiology: Renal Physiology* and Editor in Chief of *Kidney International.*

Tom's national prominence and leadership qualities were recognized early in his career when he became head of Nephrology at the University of Alabama in Birmingham. There he helped faculty and trainees develop outstanding research, organized clinical services, and created a hemodialysis program to build one of the outstanding Divisions of Nephrology in the country. In 1979, Dr. Andreoli was appointed Chair of the Department of Internal Medicine at the University of Texas, Houston, where he assembled an outstanding faculty focused on research, clinical care, and teaching. In 1988, he accepted the position as Chairman of Internal Medicine at the University of Arkansas School of Medicine, a position he held until his death. There he again assembled a distinguished faculty who were outstanding researchers but also dedicated to outstanding clinical care and teaching. Morning report and clinical rounds with Dr. Andreoli were rigorous and riveting, focusing on the individual patient, not only their diagnoses and treatment but also on each patient's personal concerns and well-being. Dr. Andreoli was revered by medical students, his house staff, faculty, and colleagues, and I (EJW) personally can attest to what he regarded as his most cherished role—the mentorship and education of the next generation of physicians.

One of Dr. Andreoli's great interests was *Cecil Essentials of Medicine,* for which he was the editor/chief editor for eight of its ten editions, an interest that reflected his commitment to the education of students, house staff, and other physicians in the "essentials" of Internal Medicine.

Dr. Andreoli was devoted to his family. He was married to Elizabeth Berglund Andreoli from 1987 until his death. He was previously married to Dr. Kathleen Gainor Andreoli, mother of his three children and their ten grandchildren. Being of Italian ancestry and from Bronx, New York, it is not surprising that Dr. Andreoli was a passionate fan of the New York Yankees, Italian opera, which he could sing in Italian, and Frank Sinatra.

Dr. Andreoli's legacy lives on in his numerous previous students, house staff, colleagues, and in this book.

Charles C.J. Carpenter, MD

Dr. Charles C.J. Carpenter joined Drs. Thomas Andreoli, Lloyd Hollingsworth Smith, Jr., and Fred Plum as a founder of *Cecil Essentials of Medicine.* He served as editor for seven editions and was followed in that role by Dr. Ivor Benjamin and then Dr. Edward Wing. Sadly, Chuck passed away on March 19, 2020, surrounded by his wife and children. He was Professor Emeritus of Medicine at The Warren Alpert Medical School of Brown University and Physician-in-Chief Emeritus at The Miriam Hospital.

Chuck was born in Savannah, Georgia, on January 5, 1931. He attended college at Princeton and medical school at Johns Hopkins where he also did his house staff training, including chief residency, and then joined the Johns Hopkins faculty. With his young family, he travelled to Calcutta, India, where he carried out landmark studies for the treatment of cholera.

Before coming to Brown in 1986, he was Chair of Medicine at Baltimore City Hospital and Case Western Reserve University.

His contributions to medical science and clinical care were many. While in Calcutta, using basic scientific evidence coupled with practical approaches, Dr. Carpenter developed "oral rehydration therapy" to address the cholera epidemic there. This treatment has saved millions of lives. While at Case, one of his innovations was to develop the nation's first Division of Geographic Medicine because of his strong belief that all physicians should be medical citizens of the world. In 1987, as he became deeply involved in the clinical management of persons living with HIV, he initiated a unique program in which Brown University faculty and trainees assumed responsibility for all HIV care in the Rhode Island State prison system.

Dr. Carpenter served as Chairman of the American Board of Internal Medicine and President of the Association of American Physicians. He has been a member of the NIH AIDS Executive Committee, the National Advisory Allergy and Infectious Diseases Council, and the USPHS AIDS Task Force. He was Chair of the Antiretroviral Treatment Panel of the International AIDS Society-USA and authored their recommendations on antiretroviral treatment. He also served as Chair of the Treatment Committee to evaluate the President's Emergency Plan for HIV/AIDS Relief. He became the director of the Brown University International Health Institute and the director of the Lifespan/Brown Center for AIDS Research with several Boston hospitals.

Throughout his career, Dr. Carpenter was the recipient of many international, national, and regional awards, accepting each with characteristic humility. With both small and large groups of learners, Chuck made certain that every member of his team was well educated, and each felt that they contributed to the well-being of their patients. His ability to sit calmly at the bedside, hold the patient's hand, comfort them, and listen in a genuinely focused way, influenced so many physicians. He was truly grateful for the opportunity to care for those less fortunate than he, and the feeling of being privileged to do so was clearly transmitted to all. Dr. Carpenter was a wonderful blend of profound compassion combined with the adherence to scholarship and teaching. Sir William Osler wrote that physicians should "Do the kind thing and do it first." Chuck lived by this precept. Vigor and insight characterized his approach to clinical and ethical challenges, always with younger colleagues at his side. In a recent tribute to him, many emphasized that Dr. Carpenter dedicated his life to his patients, many of whom were the most vulnerable members of society. We hope that we will have some of his strength and use his example as our compass as we are challenged to reduce suffering and improve the health of all for whom we are responsible.

He is survived by his wife of 61 years, Sally; three sons, Charles, Murray, and Andrew; and seven grandchildren.

Dr. Edward J. Wing was an editor of *Cecil Essentials of Medicine,* editions 8 and 9, and is the lead editor of edition 10. He graduated from Williams College in 1967 and from the Harvard Medical School in 1971. He was a resident in Internal Medicine at the Peter Bent Brigham and completed an Infectious Diseases Fellowship at Stanford University. Joining the faculty at the University of Pittsburgh in 1975, he focused his NIH-funded research on mechanisms of cell-mediated immunity as well as various clinical aspects of Infectious Diseases. From 1990 to 1998, the University and UPMC appointed him as Physician-in-Chief at Montefiore Hospital, then Chief of Infectious Diseases, and finally Interim Chair of Medicine.

In 1998, Dr. Wing became Chair of Medicine at Brown University (1998–2008) where he consolidated the department across hospitals, practice plans, and training programs. As Dean of Medicine and Biological Sciences at Brown University (2008–2013) he strengthened ties with affiliated hospitals (Lifespan and Care New England), increased research, and oversaw the construction of a new medical school building. International exchange programs with medical schools in Kenya, the Dominican Republic, and Haiti were established during his years as chairman and dean. Dr. Wing has cared for patients with HIV since the beginning of the epidemic in outpatient clinics. He continues to be active in research, clinical care, and teaching.

Dr. Fred J. Schiffman, who along with Dr. Edward Wing is editor of *Cecil Essentials of Medicine,* 10th edition, attended Wagner College and then the New York University School of Medicine, from which he graduated in 1973. He performed his early house staff training at Yale–New Haven Hospital and then spent two years at the National Cancer Institute. He returned to Yale as Chief Medical Resident followed by a hematology fellowship. He became Medical Director of Yale's Primary Care Center before coming to Brown University in 1983, where he has been a leader in the medical residency program as well as Associate Physician-in-Chief at The Miriam Hospital.

Dr. Schiffman holds The Sigal Family Professorship in Humanistic Medicine at The Warren Alpert Medical School of Brown University. His scholarly interests include the structure and function of the human spleen and the intersection of the arts and medical care. He has directed or championed many projects and programs, including those that encourage and reinforce wellness and resilience in patients, families, and caregivers. He began a novel program that places medical students and physicians with other nonmedical professionals as they share in the viewing of works of art in the Museum of the Rhode Island School of Design. Dr. Schiffman recently led a Brown University edX course entitled, "Artful Medicine: Art's Power to Enrich Patient Care," with worldwide participation. Dr. Schiffman has also edited texts on hematologic pathophysiology, consultative hematology, and the anemias.

Jinnette Dawn Abbott, MD
Professor of Medicine
Director
Interventional Cardiology Fellowship
Cardiology
Brown Medical School
Associate Chief
Faculty Development and Academic
    Advancement
Cardiovascular Institute
Lifespan
Providence, Rhode Island

Rajiv Agarwal, MD
Professor of Medicine
Indiana University
Indianapolis, Indiana

Marwa Al-Badri, MD
Clinical Research Fellow
Clinical, Behavioral, and Outcome
Research
Joslin Diabetes Center
Boston, Massachusetts

Hyeon-Ju Ryoo Ali, MD
Cardiology Fellow
Houston Methodist Hospital
Houston, Texas

Jason M. Aliotta, MD
Associate Professor of Medicine
Division of Pulmonary, Critical Care and
    Sleep Medicine
Warren Alpert Medical School
Brown University
Providence, Rhode Island

Khaldoun Almhanna, MD, MPH
Associate Professor
Hematology and Oncology
Warren Alpert Medical School
Brown University
Providence, Rhode Island

Mohanad T. Al-Qaisi, MD
Gastroenterology and Hepatology
University of Arizona College of Medicine
Banner University Medical Center–Phoenix
Phoenix VA Medical Center
Phoenix, Arizona

Zuhal Arzomand, MD
Rheumatologist
Northern Virginia Arthritis and
    Rheumatology
Alexandria, Virginia

Akwi W. Asombang, MD, MPH
Assistant Professor of Medicine
Division of Gastroenterology and
    Hepatology
Warren Alpert Medical School
Brown University
Providence, Rhode Island

Su N. Aung, MD, MPH
Assistant Professor
Division of Infectious Diseases
University of California San Francisco
San Francisco, California

Christopher G. Azzoli, MD
Associate Professor of Medicine
Warren Alpert Medical School
Brown University
Providence, Rhode Island

Christina Bandera, MD
Chief
Obstetrics and Gynecology
Director of The Center for Gynecologic
    Cancers
Rhode Island Hospital and The Miriam
    Hospital
Clinical Assistant Professor of Surgery
Warren Alpert Medical School
Brown University
Providence, Rhode Island

Debasree Banerjee, MD
Assistant Professor
Warren Alpert Medical School
Brown University
Pulmonary, Critical Care and Sleep
    Medicine Staff Physician
Rhode Island Hospital and Miriam Hospital
Providence, Rhode Island

Mashal Batheja, MD
Chief of Hepatology
Gastroenterology and Hepatology
Phoenix VA Medical Center
Clinical Assistant Professor
University of Arizona–Phoenix
Phoenix, Arizona

Jeffrey J. Bazarian, MD, MPH
Professor of Emergency Medicine
University of Rochester, School of Medicine
    and Dentistry
Rochester, New York

Selim R. Benbadis, MD
Professor Neurology
University of South Florida
Tampa, Florida

Ivor J. Benjamin, MD, FAHA, FACC
Professor of Medicine
Medical College of Wisconsin
Milwaukee, Wisconsin

Eric Benoit, MD
Assistant Professor of Surgery
Tufts University School of Medicine
Division of Trauma & Acute Care Surgery
Lahey Hospital & Medical Center
Burlington, Massachusetts

Marcie G. Berger, MD
Professor
Cardiovascular Medicine
Medical College of Wisconsin
Milwaukee, Wisconsin

Clemens Bergwitz, MD
Associate Professor of Medicine
Section Endocrinology and Metabolism
Department of Medicine
Yale School of Medicine
New Haven, Connecticut

Nancy Berliner, MD
Chief
Division of Hematology
Medicine
Brigham and Women's Hospital
H. Franklin Bunn Professor
Medicine
Harvard Medical School
Boston, Massachusetts

Jeffrey S. Berns, MD
Professor of Medicine and Pediatrics
Renal, Electrolyte and Hypertension
    Division
Perelman School of Medicine at the
    University of Pennsylvania
Philadelphia, Pennsylvania

Pooja Bhadbhade, DO
Assistant Professor
Department of Internal Medicine
Division of Allergy, Clinical Immunology
    and Rheumatology
University of Kansas Medical Center
Kansas City, Kansas

Ratna Bhavaraju-Sanka, MD
Associate Professor of Neurology
Department of Neurology
University of Texas Health Science Center at
    San Antonio
San Antonio, Texas

Tanmayee Bichile, MD
Rheumatologist
Lupus Center of Excellence
Allegheny Health Network
Pittsburgh, Pennsylvania
Assistant Professor
Drexel University College of Medicine
Philadelphia, Pennsylvania

Ariel E. Birnbaum, MD
Assistant Professor of Medicine
Warren Alpert Medical School
Brown University
Providence, Rhode Island

Charles M. Bliss, Jr., MD
Clinical Assistant Professor of Medicine
Section of Gastroenterology
Department of Medicine
Boston University School of Medicine
Boston, Massachusetts

Andrew S. Blum, MD, PhD
Professor
Neurology
Warren Alpert Medical School
Brown University
Director
Comprehensive Epilepsy Program
Rhode Island Hospital
Providence, Rhode Island

Bryan J. Bonder, MD
Hematology and Oncology
University Hospitals Cleveland Medical
    Center
Cleveland, Ohio

Russell Bratman, MD
Assistant Professor of Medicine
Department of Medicine
Division of Endocrinology
Warren Alpert Medical School
Brown University
Providence, Rhode Island

Glenn D. Braunstein, MD
Professor of Medicine
Cedars-Sinai Medical Center
Professor of Medicine Emeritus
The David Geffen School of Medicine at
    UCLA
Los Angeles, California

Alma M. Guerrero Bready, MD
Attending Physician
Division of Hospital Medicine
Rhode Island Hospital
Providence, Rhode Island

Richard Bungiro, PhD
Senior Lecturer
Molecular Microbiology & Immunology
Brown University
Providence, Rhode Island

Anna Marie Burgner, MD, MEHP
Assistant Professor of Medicine
Vanderbilt University Medical Center
Nashville, Tennessee

Jonathan Cahill, MD
Associate Professor
Neurology
Warren Alpert Medical School
Brown University
Providence, Rhode Island

Andrew Canakis, DO
Resident Physician
Department of Medicine
Boston University School of Medicine
Boston, Massachusetts

Benedito A. Carneiro, MD, MS
Associate Director
Division of Hematology Oncology
Department of Medicine
Warren Alpert Medical School
Brown University
Providence, Rhode Island

Brian Casserly, MD
Respiratory Physician
Pulmonary, Critical Care and Sleep Medicine
University Hospital Limerick
Limerick, Ireland

Abdullah Chahin, MD, MA, MSc
Assistant Professor in Medicine
Department of Internal Medicine
Warren Alpert Medical School
Brown University
Providence, Rhode Island

Philip A. Chan, MD
Associate Professor of Medicine
Brown University
Providence, Rhode Island

Kimberle Chapin, MD
Director of Microbiology
Department of Pathology
Rhode Island Hospital
Professor of Medicine
Professor of Pathology
Warren Alpert Medical School
Brown University
Providence, Rhode Island

William P. Cheshire, Jr., MD
Professor of Neurology
Mayo Clinic
Jacksonville, Florida

Waihong Chung, MD, PhD
Fellow
Gastroenterology
Rhode Island Hospital
Providence, Rhode Island

Emma Ciafaloni, MD
Professor of Neurology and Pediatrics
University of Rochester
Rochester, New York

Joaquin E. Cigarroa, MD
Division Head of Cardiology
Professor of Medicine
Knight Cardiovascular Institute
Oregon Health and Sciences University
Portland, Oregon

Michael P. Cinquegrani, MD
Professor of Medicine
Cardiovascular Medicine
Medical College of Wisconsin
Milwaukee, Wisconsin

Andreea Coca, MD, MPH
Associate Professor of Medicine
Rheumatology
University of Pittsburgh
Pittsburgh, Pennsylvania

Harvey Jay Cohen, MD
Walter Kempner Professor of Medicine
Center for the Study of Aging and Human
    Development
Duke University School of Medicine
Durham, North Carolina

Scott Cohen, MD, MPH
Medical Director
Wisconsin Adult Congenital Heart Disease
    Program
Associate Professor of Internal Medicine and
    Pediatrics
Sections of Cardiovascular Medicine and
    Pediatric Cardiology
Medical College of Wisconsin
Milwaukee, Wisconsin

Beatrice P. Concepcion, MD, MS
Assistant Professor of Medicine
Vanderbilt University Medical Center
Nashville, Tennessee

Nathan T. Connell, MD, MPH
Associate Physician
Hematology Division
Brigham and Women's Hospital
Assistant Professor of Medicine
Harvard Medical School
Boston, Massachusetts

Maria Constantinou, MD
Assistant Professor of Medicine
Warren Alpert Medical School
Brown University
Providence, Rhode Island

Roberto Cortez, MD
Senior Resident
Surgery
Rhode Island Hospital/Warren Alpert
    Medical School
Brown University
Providence, Rhode Island

Timothy J. Counihan, MD, FRCPI
Hon. Professor in Medicine
School of Medicine
National University of Ireland Galway
Galway, Ireland

Anne Haney Cross, MD
Professor
Neurology
Washington University
St. Louis, Missouri

Cheston B. Cunha, MD, FACP
Associate Professor of Medicine
Medical Director, Antimicrobial
    Stewardship
Infectious Disease Division
Warren Alpert Medical School
Brown University
Providence, Rhode Island

Joanne S. Cunha, MD
Assistant Professor of Medicine
Warren Alpert Medical School
Brown University
Director
Rheumatology Fellowship Program at
    Brown University
Providence, Rhode Island

Susan Cu-Uvin, MD
Professor of Obstetrics and Gynecology
Professor of Medicine
Brown University
Providence, Rhode Island

Noura M. Dabbouseh, MD
Amita Health Heart and Vascular
Hinsdale, Illinois

Kwame Dapaah-Afriyie, MD, MBA
Professor of Medicine (Clinician Educator)
Brown University—Miriam Hospital
Providence, Rhode Island

Erin M. Denney-Koelsch, MD
Associate Professor of Medicine & Pediatrics
Medicine
University of Rochester
Rochester, New York

Andre De Souza, MD
Assistant Professor of Medicine
Division of Hematology Oncology
Department of Medicine
Warren Alpert Medical School
Brown University
Providence, Rhode Island

An S. De Vriese, MD, PhD
Division of Nephrology and Infectious
    Diseases
AZ Sint-Jan Brugge, Brugge, and Ghent
    University
Ghent, Belgium

Neal D. Dharmadhikari, MD
Fellow
Gastroenterology
Boston Medical Center
Boston, Massachusetts

Leah Dickstein, MD
Fellow in Neurocritical Care
Department of Neurosurgery
Division of Neurocritical Care
David Geffen School of Medicine at UCLA
Los Angeles, California

Don Dizon, MD, FACP, FASCO
Director of Womens' Cancers
Lifespan Cancer Institute
Director of Medical Oncology
Rhode Island Hospital
Professor of Medicine
Warren Alpert Medical School
Brown University
Providence, Rhode Island

Robyn T. Domsic, MD, MPH
Associate Professor of Medicine
Division of Rheumatology and Clinical
    Immunology
University of Pittsburgh
Pittsburgh, Pennsylvania

Kim A. Eagle, MD
Albion Walter Hewlett Professor of Internal
    Medicine
Department of Internal Medicine
University of Michigan
Ann Arbor, Michigan

Michael G. Earing, MD
Director
University of Chicago Adult Congenital
    Heart Disease Program
Professor
Internal Medicine and Pediatrics
Sections of Adult Cardiovascular Medicine
    and Pediatric Cardiology
University of Chicago
Chicago, Illinois

Pamela Egan, MD
Assistant Professor of Medicine
Department of Medicine
Warren Alpert Medical School
Brown University
Hematologist
Division of Hematology and Oncology
Rhode Island Hospital
Providence, Rhode Island

Wafik S. El-Deiry, MD, PhD, FACP
American Cancer Society Research Professor
Director of the Cancer Center at Brown
    University and Joint Program in Cancer
    Biology
Mencoff Family University Professor of
    Medical Science
Professor of Pathology and Laboratory
    Medicine
Warren Alpert Medical School
Brown University
Providence, Rhode Island

Mitchell S. V. Elkind, MD, MS
Professor
Neurology
Vagelos College of Physicians and Surgeons
Professor
Epidemiology
Mailman School of Public Health
Columbia University
New York, New York

Tarra B. Evans, MD
Gynecologic Oncologist
The Center for Gynecologic Cancers
Rhode Island Hospital
Clinical Assistant Professor of Surgery
Warren Alpert Medical School
Brown University
Providence, Rhode Island

Michael B. Fallon, MD
Professor of Medicine
Gastroenterology, Hepatology and Nutrition
Chair
Department of Internal Medicine
University of Arizona–Phoenix
Phoenix, Arizona

Dimitrios Farmakiotis, MD
Assistant Professor of Medicine
Internal Medicine, Infectious Diseases
Warren Alpert Medical School
Brown University
Providence, Rhode Island

Francis A. Farraye, MD
Director
Professor of Medicine
Inflammatory Bowel Disease Center
Mayo Clinic
Jacksonville, Florida

Ronan Farrell, MD
Fellow
Gastroenterology
Brown University
Providence, Rhode Island

Mary Anne Fenton, MD
Clinical Associate Professor
Department of Medicine
Warren Alpert Medical School
Brown University
Providence, Rhode Island

Fernando C. Fervenza, MD, PhD
Professor of Medicine
Nephrology and Hypertension
Mayo Clinic
Rochester, Minnesota

Sean Fine, MD
Assistant Professor
Gastroenterology
Brown University
Providence, Rhode Island

Arkadiy Finn, MD
Assistant Professor of Medicine
Clinician Educator
Warren Alpert Medical School
Brown University
Division of Hospital Medicine
The Miriam Hospital
Providence, Rhode Island

Timothy Flanigan, MD
Professor of Medicine
Warren Alpert Medical School
Brown University
Providence, Rhode Island

Brisas M. Flores, MD
Fellow
Gastroenterology
Boston Medical Center
Boston, Massachusetts

Andrew E. Foderaro, MD
Assistant Professor in Medicine
Clinician Educator
Pulmonary, Critical Care and Sleep
    Medicine
Brown University
Providence, Rhode Island

Theodore C. Friedman, MD, PhD
Chairman
Department of Internal Medicine
Chief of the Division of Endocrinology,
    Metabolism and Molecular Medicine
Endowed Professor of Cardio-Metabolic
    Medicine
Charles R. Drew University of Medicine &
    Science
Professor of Medicine
UCLA
Los Angeles, California

**Joseph Metmowlee Garland, MD,
AAHIVM**
Associate Professor of Medicine
Warren Alpert Medical School
Brown University
Providence, Rhode Island

Eric J. Gartman, MD
Associate Professor of Medicine
Division of Pulmonary, Critical Care, and
    Sleep Medicine
Warren Alpert Medical School
Brown University
Staff Physician
Division of Pulmonary, Critical Care, and
    Sleep Medicine
Providence VA Medical Center
Providence, Rhode Island

Abdallah Geara, MD
Assistant Professor of Clinical Medicine
Renal-Electrolyte and Hypertension
University of Pennsylvania
Philadelphia, Pennsylvania

Raul Macias Gil, MD
Infectious Disease Fellow
Division of Infectious Diseases
Brown University
Providence, Rhode Island

Timothy Gilligan, MD, FASCO
Associate Professor of Medicine
Vice-Chair for Education
Hematology and Medical Oncology
    Department
Cleveland Clinic Taussig Cancer Institute
Cleveland, Ohio

**Michael Raymond Goggins, MB BCh
BAO, MRCPI**
Medicine
University Hospital Limerick
Limerick, Ireland

Geetha Gopalakrishnan, MD
Associate Professor
Department of Medicine
Division of Endocrinology
Warren Alpert Medical School
Brown University
Providence, Rhode Island

Vidya Gopinath, MD
Assistant Professor of Medicine, Clinician-
    Educator
Warren Alpert Medical School
Brown University
Providence, Rhode Island

Susan L. Greenspan, MD, FACP
Division of Geriatric Medicine
University of Pittsburgh School of Medicine
Pittsburgh, Pennsylvania

Osama Hamdy, MD, PhD
Medical Director
Obesity Clinical Program
Endocrinology
Joslin Diabetes Center
Associate Professor of Medicine
Harvard Medical School
Boston, Massachusetts

Johanna Hamel, MD
Assistant Professor of Neurology, Pathology
    and Laboratory Medicine
University of Rochester Medical Center
Rochester, New York

Sajeev Handa, MD, SFHM
Assistant Professor of Medicine
Chief
Hospital Medicine
Rhode Island/Miriam & Newport Hospitals
Providence, Rhode Island

Mitchell T. Heflin, MD, MHS
Professor of Medicine
Professor in the School of Nursing
Associate Dean for Interprofessional
    Education and Care (IPEC)
Duke University School of Medicine
Durham, North Carolina

Robert G. Holloway, MD, MPH
Professor
Department of Neurology
University of Rochester Medical Center
Rochester, New York

Christopher S. Huang, MD
Clinical Associate Professor of Medicine
Department of Medicine
Section of Gastroenterology
Boston University School of Medicine
Boston, Massachusetts

Zilla Hussain, MD
Assistant Professor of Medicine and Medical
 Sciences
Warren Alpert Medical School
Brown University
Esophageal Disorders
Gastroenterology
Lifespan Physicians Group
Providence, Rhode Island

T. Alp Ikizler, MD
Catherine McLaughlin-Hakim Chair
Professor of Medicine
Vanderbilt University Medical Center
Nashville, Tennessee

Iris Isufi, MD
Assistant Professor of Medicine
 (Hematology)
Internal Medicine
Yale University
New Haven, Connecticut

Carlayne E. Jackson, MD
Professor of Neurology and Otolaryngology
Department of Neurology
University of Texas Health Science Center
San Antonio, Texas

Paul G. Jacob, MD, MPH
Assistant Professor
Division of Infectious Diseases
Vanderbilt University Medical Center
Nashville, Tennessee

Matthew D. Jankowich, MD
Associate Professor of Medicine
Pulmonary, Critical Care and Sleep
 Medicine
Warren Alpert Medical School
Brown University
Providence VA Medical Center
Providence, Rhode Island

Niels V. Johnsen, MD, MPH
Assistant Professor
Department of Urology
Vanderbilt University Medical Center
Nashville, Tennessee

Jessica E. Johnson, MD
Infectious Diseases
West Virginia University School of Medicine
Morgantown, West Virginia

Rayford R. June, MD
Assistant Professor of Medicine
Division of Rheumatology
Department of Medicine
Penn State College of Medicine
Hershey, Pennsylvania

Tareq Kheirbek, MD, ScM, FACS
Assistant Professor of Surgery
Clinical Educator
Surgery
Brown University
Providence, Rhode Island

Alok A. Khorana, MD, FACP, FASCO
Sondra and Stephen Hardis Endowed Chair
 in Oncology Research
Taussig Cancer Institute
Cleveland Clinic
Cleveland, Ohio

Sena Kilic, MD
Clinical Associate
Division of Cardiology
Knight Cardiovascular Institute
Oregon Health & Science University
Portland, Oregon

David Kim, MD
Chief Resident
Surgery
Rhode Island Hospital/Warren Alpert
 Medical School
Brown University
Providence, Rhode Island

James Kleczka, MD
Associate Professor
Department of Medicine
Medical College of Wisconsin
Milwaukee, Wisconsin

James R. Klinger, MD
Professor of Medicine
Pulmonary, Critical Care, and Sleep
 Medicine
Warren Alpert Medical School
Brown University
Providence, Rhode Island

Patrick Koo, MD, ScM
Associate Professor of Medicine (Affiliate)
University of Tennessee Health Science
 Center College of Medicine
Erlanger Hospital
Department of Medicine
Chattanooga, Tennessee

Pooja Koolwal, MD
Assistant Professor
Department of Internal Medicine
Division of Nephrology
UT Southwestern Medical Center
Dallas, Texas

Mary P. Kotlarczyk, PhD
Assistant Professor of Medicine
Division of Geriatric Medicine
University of Pittsburgh School of Medicine
Pittsburgh, Pennsylvania

Nicole M. Kuderer, MD
Chief Medical Officer
Medicine
Advanced Cancer Research Group
Seattle, Washington

Awewura Kwara, MD
Professor
Department of Medicine
University of Florida College of Medicine
Gainesville, Florida

Jennifer M. Kwon, MD, MPH
Professor
Neurology
University of Wisconsin School of Medicine
 and Public Health
Madison, Wisconsin

Richard A. Lange, MD, MBA
President
Texas Tech University Health Sciences
 Center El Paso
Dean
Paul L. Foster School of Medicine
El Paso, Texas

Jerome Larkin, MD
Associate Professor of Medicine
Infectious Diseases
Warren Alpert Medical School
Brown University
Providence, Rhode Island

Alfred I. Lee, MD, PhD
Associate Professor of Medicine
Hematology/Oncology Division
Yale School of Medicine
New Haven, Connecticut

Daniel J. Levine, MD
Director
Advanced Heart Failure
Cardiology
Brown University
Providence, Rhode Island

David E. Lewandowski, MD
Cardiology Fellow
Cardiology
Medical College of Wisconsin
Milwaukee, Wisconsin

Kelly V. Liang, MD, MS
Assistant Professor of Medicine
Renal-Electrolyte Division
University of Pittsburgh
Pittsburgh, Pennsylvania

Kimberly P. Liang, MD, MS
Assistant Professor of Medicine
Rheumatology and Clinical Immunology
University of Pittsburgh
Pittsburgh, Pennsylvania

David R. Lichtenstein, MD
Director of Endoscopy
Gastroenterology
Boston University Medical Center
Associate Professor of Medicine
Gastroenterology
Boston Medical Center
Boston, Massachusetts

Douglas W. Lienesch, MD
Chief
Rheumatology Division
Christiana Care Health System
Newark, Delaware

Geoffrey S.F. Ling, MD, PhD
Professor of Neurology
Johns Hopkins
Baltimore, Maryland

Ester Little, MD, FACP
Assistant Professor of Medicine
Department of Medicine
University of Arizona
Hepatologist
Banner Advanced Liver Disease and
    Transplant Institute
Banner University Medical Center Phoenix
Phoenix, Arizona

Yi Liu, MD
Resident Physician
Medicine
Beth Israel Lahey Health
Burlington, Massachusetts

Nicole L. Lohr, MD, PhD
Associate Professor
Medicine
Medical College of Wisconsin
Milwaukee, Wisconsin

**John R. Lonks, MD, FACP, FIDSA,
FSHEA**
Associate Professor of Medicine
Department of Medicine
Warren Alpert Medical School
Brown University
Providence, Rhode Island

Gary H. Lyman, MD, MPH
Professor
Public Health Sciences
Fred Hutchinson Cancer Research Center
Professor
Medicine
University of Washington
Seattle, Washington

Jeffrey M. Lyness, MD
Senior Associate Dean for Academic Affairs
    and Professor of Psychiatry & Neurology
Office of Academic Affairs
University of Rochester School of Medicine
    & Dentistry
Rochester, New York

Shane Lyons, MD, MRCPI, MRCP(UK)
Specialist Registrar in Neurology
Department of Neurology
St James's Hospital
Dublin, Ireland

Diana Maas, MD
Associate Professor of Medicine
Division of Endocrinology
Medical College of Wisconsin
Milwaukee, Wisconsin

Talha A. Malik, MD, MSPH
Assistant Professor of Medicine
Gastroenterology and Hepatology
Mayo Clinic Arizona
Scottsdale, Arizona

Sonia Manocha, MD
Rheumatologist
Lupus Center of Excellence
Allegheny Health Network
Pittsburgh, Pennsylvania
Assistant Professor
Drexel University College of Medicine
Philadelphia, Pennsylvania

Susan Manzi, MD, MPH
Chair
Medicine Institute
Director
Lupus Center of Excellence
Allegheny Health Network
Professor of Medicine
Temple University School of Medicine
Philadelphia, Pennsylvania

Frederick J. Marshall, MD
Professor
Neurology
University of Rochester
Rochester, New York

F. Dennis McCool, MD
Professor of Medicine
Division of Pulmonary and Critical Care
    Medicine
Warren Alpert Medical School
Brown University
Providence, Rhode Island

Russell J. McCulloh, MD
Associate Professor
Pediatrics
University of Nebraska College of Medicine
Division Chief
Pediatric Hospital Medicine
University of Nebraska Medical Center
Omaha, Nebraska

Kelly McGarry, MD, FACP
Professor of Medicine
Warren Alpert Medical School
Brown University
Providence, Rhode Island

Eavan Mc Govern, MD, PhD
Consultant Neurologist
Senior Clinical Lecturer
Beaumont Hospital
Royal College of Surgeons in Ireland
Ireland

Robin L. McKinney, MD
Assistant Professor of Pediatrics
Pediatric Critical Care Medicine
Warren Alpert Medical School
Brown University
Providence, Rhode Island

Anthony Mega, MD
Associate Professor of Medicine
Program Director Hematology/Oncology
    Fellowship
Division Hematology/Oncology
Warren Alpert Medical School
Brown University
Lifespan Cancer Institute
Providence, Rhode Island

Shivang Mehta, MD
Assistant Professor of Medicine
Gastroenterology, Hepatology, and
    Nutrition
Department of Internal Medicine
University of Arizona–Phoenix
Phoenix, Arizona

Douglas F. Milam, MD
Associate Professor
Department of Urology
Vanderbilt University Medical Center
Nashville, Tennessee

Maria D. Mileno, MD
Associate Professor of Medicine
Division of Infectious Diseases
Warren Alpert Medical School
Brown University
Attending Physician, Infectious Disease
    Consultant
Brown Medicine
The Miriam Hospital
Former Director of Travel Medicine Services
Providence, Rhode Island

Abhinav Kumar Misra, MBBS, MD
Assistant Professor of Medicine
Pulmonary, Critical Care and Sleep
    Medicine
Warren Alpert Medical School
Brown University
Providence, Rhode Island

Orson W. Moe, MD
Professor
Internal Medicine and Physiology
Division of Nephrology
Director
Charles and Jane Pak Center for Mineral
    Metabolism and Clinical Research
Chief
Division of Nephrology
UT Southwestern Medical Center
Dallas, Texas

Niveditha Mohan, MBBS
Associate Professor
Department of Medicine
Division of Rheumatology and Clinical
    Immunology
University of Pittsburgh
Pittsburgh, Pennsylvania

Larry W. Moreland, MD
Margaret J. Miller Endowed Professor of
    Arthritis Research
Division of Rheumatology and Clinical
    Immunology
Professor of Medicine, Immunology,
    Clinical and Translational Science
Chief
Division of Rheumatology and Clinical
    Immunology
University of Pittsburgh
Pittsburgh, Pennsylvania

Alan R. Morrison, MD, PhD
Assistant Professor of Medicine
Medicine (Cardiology)
Warren Alpert Medical School
Brown University
Providence, Rhode Island

Steven F. Moss, MD
Professor of Medicine
Division of Gastroenterology and
    Hepatology
Warren Alpert Medical School
Brown University
Providence, Rhode Island

Christopher J. Mullin, MD, MHS
Assistant Professor of Medicine, Clinician
    Educator
Pulmonary, Critical Care, and Sleep
    Medicine
Warren Alpert Medical School
Brown University
Providence, Rhode Island

**Sinéad M. Murphy, MB, BCh, MD,
FRCPI**
Consultant Neurologist
Neurology
Tallaght University Hospital
Clinical Associate Professor
Medicine
University of Dublin, Trinity College
Dublin, Ireland

**Sagarika Nallu, MD, FAAP, FAAN,
FAASM**
Director of Pediatric Sleep Medicine
Department of Pediatrics
University of South Florida
Tampa, Florida

Javier A. Neyra, MD, MSCS
Assistant Professor of Medicine
Director
Critical Care Nephrology
Division of Nephrology, Bone and Mineral
    Metabolism
University of Kentucky Medical Center
Lexington, Kentucky

Ghaith Noaiseh, MD
Associate Professor
Department of Internal Medicine
Division of Allergy, Clinical Immunology
    and Rheumatology
University of Kansas
Kansas City, Kansas

Thomas A. Ollila, MD
Assistant Professor of Medicine
Warren Alpert Medical School
Brown University
Providence, Rhode Island

Steven M. Opal, MD
Clinical Professor of Medicine
Infectious Diseases Division
Department of Medicine
Warren Alpert Medical School
Brown University
Rhode Island Hospital
Providence, Rhode Island

Biff F. Palmer, MD
Professor of Internal Medicine
Internal Medicine
University of Texas Southwestern Medical
    Center
Dallas, Texas

Jen Jung Pan, MD, PhD
Associate Professor of Medicine
Gastroenterology and Hepatology
Department of Internal Medicine
University of Arizona–Phoenix
Phoenix, Arizona

Anna Papazoglou, MD
Clinical Instructor
Postdoctoral Research Scholar
Division of Rheumatology and Clinical
    Immunology
University of Pittsburgh
Pittsburgh, Pennsylvania

Aric Parnes, MD
Attending Hematologist
Medicine
Brigham and Women's Hospital
Assistant Professor
Harvard Medical School
Boston, Massachusetts

Nayan M. Patel, DO, MPH
Assistant Professor of Medicine
Gastroenterology and Hepatology
Department of Internal Medicine
University of Arizona–Phoenix
Phoenix, Arizona

Ari Pelcovits, MD
Department of Medicine
Division of Hematology and Oncology
Warren Alpert Medical School
Brown University
Providence, Rhode Island

Mark A. Perazella, MD
Medical Director
Yale Physician Associate Program
Department of Medicine
Professor of Medicine
Section of Nephrology
Yale University School of Medicine
Director
Acute Dialysis Services
Yale-New Haven Hospital
New Haven, Connecticut

Michael F. Picco, MD, PhD
Director
Division of Gastroenterology and
    Hepatology
Mayo Clinic
Jacksonville, Florida

Kate E. Powers, DO
Pediatric Pulmonologist and Associate
    Director of the Cystic Fibrosis Pediatric
    Program
Pediatrics
Hasbro Children's Hospital
Assistant Professor of Pediatrics
Pediatrics
Warren Alpert Medical School
Brown University
Providence, Rhode Island

Laura A. Previll, MD, MPH
Assistant Professor
Duke University School of Medicine
Durham VAMC
Durham, North Carolina

Nilum Rajora, MD
Associate Professor
Department of Internal Medicine
Division of Nephrology
UT Southwestern Medical Center
Dallas, Texas

Adolfo Ramirez-Zamora, MD
Associate Professor of Neurology
Neurology
University of Florida
Gainesville, Florida

John Reagan, MD
Department of Medicine
Division of Hematology and Oncology
Warren Alpert Medical School
Brown University
Providence, Rhode Island

Rebecca Reece, MD
Assistant Professor of Medicine
Infectious Diseases
West Virginia University School of Medicine
Morgantown, West Virginia

Harlan Rich, MD, AGAF, FACP
Associate Professor of Medicine and Medical
    Science
Warren Alpert Medical School
Brown University
Clinical Director
Division of Gastroenterology
Brown Medicine/Brown Physicians, Inc.
Providence, Rhode Island
Medical Director
Brown Medicine Endoscopy Center
Riverside, Rhode Island

Jennifer H. Richman, MD
Associate Professor
Psychiatry
University of Rochester School of Medicine
    and Dentistry
Rochester, New York

Lisa R. Rogers, DO
Senior Staff
Department of Neurosurgery
Henry Ford Hospital
Detroit, Michigan

Ralph Rogers, MD
Assistant Professor
Internal Medicine, Infectious Diseases
Warren Alpert Medical School
Brown University
Providence, Rhode Island

Michal G. Rose, MD
Professor of Medicine
Medicine (Medical Oncology)
Yale School of Medicine
New Haven, Connecticut
Director
Cancer Center
VA Connecticut Healthcare System
West Haven, Connecticut

James A. Roth, MD
Associate Professor
Cardiovascular Medicine
Medical College of Wisconsin
Milwaukee, Wisconsin

Sharon Rounds, MD
Professor
Warren Alpert Medical School
Brown University
Pulmonary/Critical Care Staff Physician
Providence VA Medical Center
Providence, Rhode Island

Jason C. Rubenstein, MD
Associate Professor
Cardiovascular Medicine
Medical College of Wisconsin
Milwaukee, Wisconsin

Abbas Rupawala, MD
Assistant Professor of Medicine
Internal Medicine
Brown University
Co-Director
IBD Center
Internal Medicine
Brown Medicine/Brown Physicians' Inc.
Providence, Rhode Island

Jenna Sarvaideo, DO
Assistant Professor of Medicine
Division of Endocrinology
Medical College of Wisconsin
Milwaukee, Wisconsin

Ramesh Saxena, MD, PhD
Professor
Internal Medicine/Division of Nephrology
UT Southwestern Medical Center
Dallas, Texas

Fred J. Schiffman, MD, MACP
Sigal Family Professor of Humanistic
    Medicine
Vice Chair, Department of Medicine
Warren Alpert Medical School
Brown University
Providence, Rhode Island

Ruth B. Schneider, MD
Assistant Professor
Neurology
University of Rochester
Rochester, New York

Kristin A. Seaborg, MD
Assistant Professor
Pediatric Neurology
University of Wisconsin School of Medicine
    and Public Health
Madison, Wisconsin

Anil Seetharam, MD
Clinical Associate Professor of Medicine
Gastroenterology/Transplant Hepatology
University of Arizona College of Medicine
Phoenix, Arizona

Stuart Seropian, MD
Professor of Clinical Medicine (Hematology)
Internal Medicine
Yale University
New Haven, Connecticut

Jigme Michael Sethi, MD
Professor of Medicine (Affiliate)
University of Tennessee Health Science
    Center College of Medicine
Erlanger Hospital
Department of Medicine
Chattanooga, Tennessee

Sanjeev Sethi, MD, PhD
Professor
Laboratory Medicine and Pathology
Mayo Clinic
Rochester, Minnesota

Elizabeth Shane, MD
Professor
Medicine
Columbia University
Associate Dean
Medical Education
College of Physicians & Surgeons
New York, New York

Esseim Sharma, MD
Cardiovascular Disease Fellow
Cardiology
Brown University
Providence, Rhode Island

Shani Shastri, MD, MPH
Assistant Professor
Department of Internal Medicine
Division of Nephrology
UT Southwestern Medical Center
Dallas, Texas

Barry S. Shea, MD
Assistant Professor of Medicine
Pulmonary, Critical Care and Sleep
    Medicine
Warren Alpert Medical School
Brown University
Providence, Rhode Island

Lauren Shevell, MD, MPH
Fellow
Hematology/Oncology
University of Michigan
Ann Arbor, Michigan

Joseph A. Smith, Jr., MD
Professor
Department of Urology
Vanderbilt University Medical Center
Nashville, Tennessee

Robert J. Smith, MD
Professor of Medicine Emeritus
Warren Alpert Medical School
Brown University
Providence, Rhode Island

Davendra P.S. Sohal, MD, MPH
Associate Professor of Medicine
Director of Experimental Therapeutics
Clinic Medical Director
Division of Hematology/Oncology
University of Cincinnati
Cincinnati, Ohio

Christopher Song, MD, FACC
Assistant Professor of Medicine
Clinician Educator
Warren Alpert Medical School
Brown University
Providence, Rhode Island

Thomas Sperry, MD
Cardiology Fellow
Hypertension Section, Cardiology Division
University of Texas Southwestern Medical
    Center
Dallas, Texas

Jeffrey M. Statland, MD
Associate Professor of Neurology
University of Kansas Medical Center
Kansas City, Kansas

Emily M. Stein, MD
Director of Research
Metabolic Bone Service
Division of Endocrinology
Hospital for Special Surgery
Associate Professor of Medicine
Weill Cornell Medical College
New York, New York

Jennifer L. Strande, MD, PhD
Adjunct Professor
Department of Medicine
Medical College of Wisconsin
Milwaukee, Wisconsin

Rochelle Strenger, MD
Clinical Associate Professor
Department of Medicine
Warren Alpert Medical School
Brown University
Providence, Rhode Island

Thomas R. Talbot, MD, MPH
Professor
Department of Medicine
Vanderbilt University School of Medicine
Chief Hospital Epidemiologist
Vanderbilt University Medical Center
Nashville, Tennessee

Christopher G. Tarolli, MD, MSEd
Assistant Professor
Neurology
University of Rochester Medical Center
Rochester, New York

Yael Tarshish, MD
Resident Physician
Warren Alpert Medical School
Brown University
Providence, Rhode Island

Pushpak Taunk, MD
Assistant Professor
Division of Digestive Diseases and Nutrition
University of South Florida Morsani College
    of Medicine
Tampa, Florida

Philip Tsoukas, MD
Clinical Fellow, Rheumatology
Temple University Hospital
Philadelphia, Pennsylvania

Allan R. Tunkel, MD, PhD
Professor of Medicine and Medical Science
Senior Associate Dean for Medical
    Education
Warren Alpert Medical School
Brown University
Providence, Rhode Island

Jeffrey M. Turner, MD
Associate Professor of Medicine
Section of Nephrology
Yale University School of Medicine
New Haven, Connecticut

Zoe G.S. Vazquez, MD
Fellow
Division Pulmonary, Critical Care and Sleep
    Medicine
Warren Alpert Medical School
Brown University
Providence, Rhode Island

Stacie A. F. Vela, MD
Section Chief
Gastroenterology
Phoenix VA Health Care System
Clinical Associate Professor
Medicine
University of Arizona–Phoenix
Phoenix, Arizona

**Paul M. Vespa, MD, FCCM, FAAN,
FANA, FNCS**
Assistant Dean for Research in Critical Care
    Medicine
Gary L. Brinderson Family Chair in
    Neurocritical Care
Director of Neurocritical Care
Professor of Neurology and Neurosurgery
University of California–Los Angeles
David Geffen School of Medicine at UCLA
Los Angeles, California

Wanpen Vongpatanasin, MD
Professor of Medicine
Hypertension Section/Cardiology Division
Internal Medicine
University of Texas Southwestern Medical
    Center
Dallas, Texas

Marcella D. Walker, MD
Associate Professor of Medicine
Internal Medicine, Division of
    Endocrinology
Columbia University, College of Physicians
    and Surgeons
New York, New York

Eunice S. Wang, MD
Professor of Oncology
Medicine
Roswell Park Comprehensive Cancer Center
Buffalo, New York

Sharmeel K. Wasan, MD
Assistant Professor of Medicine
Medicine
Section of Gastroenterology
Boston University School of Medicine
Program Director
Gastroenterology
Boston Medical Center
Boston, Massachusetts

Thomas J. Weber, MD
Associate Professor
Medicine/Endocrinology
Duke University
Durham, North Carolina

Brandon J. Wilcoxson, MD
Senior Instructor of Medicine
Palliative Care
University of Rochester Medical Center
Rochester, New York

Edward J. Wing, MD, FACP, FIDSA
Former Dean of Medicine and Biological
    Sciences
Professor of Medicine
Warren Alpert Medical School
Brown University
Providence, Rhode Island

Ellice Wong, MD
Assistant Professor
Medicine (Medical Oncology)
Yale School of Medicine
New Haven, Connecticut
Attending
Internal Medicine, Hematology/Oncology
VA Connecticut Healthcare System
West Haven, Connecticut

John J. Wysolmerski, MD
Professor of Medicine
Section of Endocrinology and Metabolism
Department of Internal Medicine
Yale School of Medicine
New Haven, Connecticut

Rayan Yousefzai, MD
Heart Failure Cardiologist
Cardiology
Houston Methodist Hospital
Houston, Texas

Thomas R. Ziegler, MD
Professor of Medicine and Co-Director
Emory University Hospital Nutrition and
    Metabolic Support Service
Emory University School of Medicine
Atlanta, Georgia

Rebecca Zon, MD
Resident
Internal Medicine
Brigham and Women's Hospital
Boston, Massachusetts

ACKNOWLEDGMENTS

Dr. Schiffman and I wish to thank first of all, the authors of the 128 chapters that make up the tenth edition of *Cecil Essentials of Medicine*. They have worked diligently to compose the material for each chapter and apply their mastery as they added the newest information, in clear language, to the text. Their efforts are apparent in the excellence of the book, and we are immensely grateful for their work. We wish to also thank Marybeth Thiel, Jennifer Ehlers, and Dan Fitzgerald from Elsevier who guided and supported our work as editors and whose expertise has made this volume possible. Finally, we are always thankful to our wives, Dr. Rena Wing and Ms. Gerri Schiffman, without whose love, support, and especially humor, this book would not have happened.

CONTENTS

VIDEO CONTENTS

Introduction to Medicine

1

Introduction to Medicine

Edward J. Wing, Fred J. Schiffman

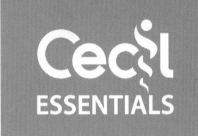

Cecil Essentials of Medicine presents a core of internal medicine and neurology information that every physician should know. This book provides an essential framework so physicians can appropriately assemble the key elements of history, physical examination, and laboratory data to understand their patient's illness and develop an appropriate diagnostic and therapeutic strategy. Furthermore, in order to understand advances in medicine, physicians must have a strong background for the acquisition and categorization of new medical knowledge.

Cecil Essentials of Medicine is designed for medical students as well as physicians in training, and we hope it will be an appropriate vehicle for course and examination review. We also believe, however, that physicians at all stages in their careers will find it to be a valuable resource for review and reference. This book also serves as a companion to the 26th edition of *Goldman-Cecil Medicine,* which is more comprehensive in scope and detailed in its content.

Cecil Essentials of Medicine is organized into sections, most often representing organ systems, with introductory and then organ-specific, disease-based chapters. The chapters themselves are subdivided. For example, the cardiovascular disease chapter is divided into Epidemiology, Anatomy, Pathophysiology, Clinical Diagnosis, and Treatment. The Suggested Readings sections at the end of each chapter include selected critical reviews, guidelines, and important randomized controlled trials. They are not meant to be an exhaustive reference list, but rather to highlight the essential information that physicians should know.

We believe that the information in *Cecil Essentials of Medicine* will encourage evidence-based diagnostic and therapeutic decision making. Importantly, the rational approach to medical problem-solving must be interwoven with the attentive presence of the physician at the bedside, clinic or office, undistracted by electronic devices (particularly the computer), displaying mindful humanistic patient care. Humanistic practice includes integrity, compassion, altruism, respect, service, and empathy, but also excellence. Both the art and the science of medicine must be part of the approach to any patient encounter. The editors believe that these concepts have been best expressed by Frances Peabody, who famously stated that "the significance of the intimate personal relationship between physician and patient cannot be too strongly emphasized, for in an extraordinary large number of cases both the diagnosis and treatment directly depend upon it. One of the essential qualities of the clinician is interest in humanity for the secret of the care of the patient is in caring for the patient," and by Sir William Osler, who said, "The practice of medicine is an art not a trade; a calling not a business; a calling in which your heart will be exercised equally with your head."

We believe that the fundamentally important bond between caregiver and patient is the starting point to the care of the patient. This is followed by a thorough history and a directed physical examination, which allow a diagnosis in the great majority of encounters. Laboratory data and imaging are supplementary. The focus of the diagnostic process should be on diseases that are common and treatable. Common presentations of common diseases account for the vast majority of cases; next in frequency are unusual presentations of common diseases; less common are typical presentations of rare diseases. Concentrate on common diseases, but know the rare ones as well.

We sincerely hope that *Cecil Essentials of Medicine* will be used to provide the basic and clinical data that are essential for us to practice medicine in a manner informed by both compassion and evidence, so that we may truly heal those with whose care we are entrusted.

SECTION II

Cardiovascular Disease

Structure and Function of the Normal Heart and Blood Vessels

Nicole L. Lohr, Ivor J. Benjamin

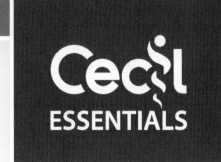

DEFINITION

The circulatory system comprises the heart, which is connected in series to the arterial and venous vascular networks. These vascular networks are arranged in parallel and connect at the level of the capillaries (Fig. 2.1). The heart is composed of two atria, which are low-pressure capacitance chambers that function to store blood during ventricular contraction (systole) and then fill the ventricles with blood during ventricular relaxation (diastole). The two ventricles are high-pressure chambers responsible for pumping blood through the lungs (right ventricle) and to the peripheral tissues (left ventricle). The left ventricle is thicker than the right, in order to generate the higher systemic pressures required for perfusion.

There are four cardiac valves that facilitate unidirectional blood flow through the heart. Each of the four valves is surrounded by a fibrous ring, or annulus, that forms part of the structural support of the heart. Atrioventricular (AV) valves separate the atria and ventricles. The mitral valve is a bileaflet valve that separates the left atrium and left ventricle. The tricuspid valve is a trileaflet valve that separates the right atrium and right ventricle. Thin, fibrous connective tissue (chordae tendineae) attaches the ventricular aspects of these valves to the papillary muscles of their respective ventricles for proper opening of the valves. Additional valves include the aortic valve that separates the left ventricle from the aorta, and the pulmonic valve that separates the right ventricle from the pulmonary artery.

A thin, double-layered membrane called the pericardium surrounds the heart. The inner, or visceral, layer adheres to the outer surface of the heart, also known as the epicardium. The outer layer is the parietal pericardium, which attaches to the sternum, vertebral column, and diaphragm to stabilize the heart in the chest. Between these two membranes is a pericardial space filled with a small amount of fluid (<50 mL). This fluid serves to lubricate contact surfaces and limit direct tissue-surface contact during myocardial contraction. A normal pericardium exerts minimal external pressure on the heart, thereby facilitating normal movement of the interventricular septum during the cardiac cycle. Too much fluid in this space (i.e., pericardial effusion) can cause impaired ventricular filling and abnormal septal movement. (Please refer to Chapter 68, "Pericardial Diseases," in ❖ *Goldman-Cecil Medicine*, 26th Edition).

CIRCULATORY PATHWAY

The purpose of the circulatory system is to bring deoxygenated blood, carbon dioxide, and other waste products from the tissues to the lungs for disposal and reoxygenation (see Fig. 2.1A). Deoxygenated blood drains from peripheral tissues through venules and veins, eventually entering the right atrium through the superior and inferior venae cavae during ventricular systole. Venous drainage from the heart enters the right atrium through the coronary sinus. During ventricular diastole, the blood in the right atrium flows across the tricuspid valve and into the right ventricle. Blood in the right ventricle is ejected across the pulmonic valve and into the main pulmonary artery, which bifurcates into the left and right pulmonary arteries and perfuses the lungs. After multiple bifurcations, blood reaches the pulmonary capillaries, where carbon dioxide is exchanged for oxygen across the alveolar-capillary membrane. Oxygenated blood then enters the left atrium from the lungs via the four pulmonary veins. Blood flows across the open mitral valve and into the left ventricle during diastole and is ejected across the aortic valve and into the aorta during systole. The blood reaches various organs, where oxygen and nutrients are exchanged for carbon dioxide and metabolic wastes, and the cycle begins again.

The heart receives its blood supply through the left and right coronary arteries, which originate in outpouchings of the aortic root called the *sinuses of Valsalva*. The left main coronary artery is a short vessel that bifurcates into the left anterior descending (LAD) and the left circumflex (LCx) coronary arteries. The LAD supplies blood to the anterior and anterolateral left ventricle through diagonal branches and to the anterior interventricular septum through septal perforator branches. The LAD travels anteriorly in the anterior interventricular groove and terminates at the cardiac apex. The LCx traverses posteriorly in the left AV groove (between left atrium and left ventricle) to perfuse the lateral aspect of the left ventricle (through obtuse marginal branches) and the left atrium. The right coronary artery (RCA) courses down the right AV groove to the *crux* of the heart, the point at which the left and right AV grooves and the inferior interventricular groove meet. The RCA gives off branches to the right atrium and acute marginal branches to the right ventricle.

The blood supply to the diaphragmatic and posterior aspects of the left ventricle varies. In 85% of individuals, the RCA bifurcates at the crux to form the posterior descending coronary artery (PDA), which travels in the inferior interventricular groove to supply the inferior left ventricle and the inferior third of the interventricular septum, and the posterior left ventricular (PLV) branches. This course is termed a *right-dominant circulation*. In 10% of individuals, the RCA terminates before reaching the crux, and the LCx supplies the PLV and PDA. This course is termed a *left-dominant circulation*. In the remaining individuals, the RCA gives rise to the PDA and the LCx gives rise to the PLV in a *co-dominant circulation*.

CONDUCTION SYSTEM

The sinoatrial (SA) node is a collection of specialized pacemaker cells, 1 to 2 cm long, located in the right atrium between the superior vena cava and the right atrial appendage (see Fig. 2.1B). The SA node is supplied by the SA nodal artery, which is a branch of the RCA in about 60% of the population and a branch of the LCx in about 40%. An

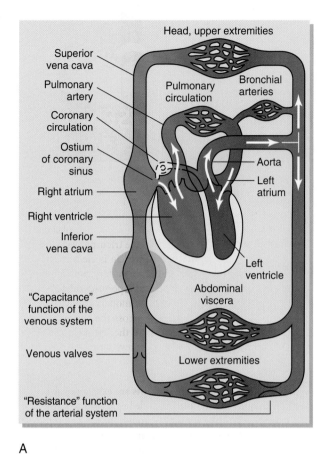

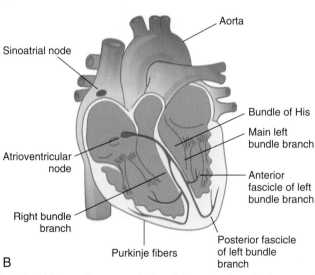

Fig. 2.1 (A) Schematic representation of the systemic and pulmonary circulatory systems. The venous system contains the greatest amount of blood at any one time and is highly distensible, accommodating a wide range of blood volumes (high capacitance). The arterial system is composed of the aorta, arteries, and arterioles. Arterioles are small muscular arteries that regulate blood pressure by changing tone (resistance). (B) A schematic representation of the cardiac conduction system.

electrical impulse originates in the SA and is conducted to the AV node by internodal tracts within the atria.

The AV node is a critical electrical interface between the atria and ventricles, because it facilitates electromechanical coupling. The AV node is located at the inferior aspect of the right atrium, between the coronary sinus and the septal leaflet of the tricuspid valve. The

AV node is supplied by the AV nodal artery, which is a branch of the RCA in about 90% of the population and a branch of the LCx in 10%. Electrical impulse conduction slows through the AV node and continues to the ventricles by means of the His-Purkinje system. The increased impulse time through the AV node allows for adequate ventricular filling.

The bundle of His extends from the AV node down the membranous interventricular septum to the muscular septum, where it divides into the left and right bundle branches, finally terminating in Purkinje cells, which are specialized cells that facilitate the rapid propagation of electrical impulses. The Purkinje cells directly stimulate myocytes to contract. The right bundle and the left bundle are supplied by septal perforator branches from the LAD. The distal and posterior portion of the left bundle has an additional blood supply from the AV nodal artery (PDA origin); for that reason, it is more resistant to ischemia. Conduction can be impaired at any point, from ischemia, medications (e.g., β-blockers, calcium channel blockers), infection, or congenital abnormalities. (Please refer to Chapter 55, "Principles of Electrophysiology," in *Goldman-Cecil Medicine*, 26th Edition.)

NEURAL INNERVATION

The autonomic nervous system is an integral component in the regulation of cardiac function. In general, sympathetic stimulation increases the heart rate (HR) (chronotropy) and the force of myocardial contraction (inotropy). Sympathetic stimulation commences in preganglionic neurons located within the superior five or six thoracic segments of the spinal cord. They synapse with second-order neurons in the cervical sympathetic ganglia and then propagate the signal through cardiac nerves that innervate the SA node, AV node, epicardial vessels, and myocardium. The parasympathetic system produces an opposite physiologic effect by decreasing HR and contractility. Its neural supply originates in preganglionic neurons within the dorsal motor nucleus of the medulla oblongata, which reach the heart through the vagus nerve. These efferent neural fibers synapse with second-order neurons located in ganglia within the heart that terminate in the SA node, AV node, epicardial vessels, and myocardium to decrease HR and contractility. Conversely, afferent vagal fibers from the inferior and posterior aspects of the ventricles, the aortic arch, and the carotid sinus conduct sensory information back to the medulla, which mediates important cardiac reflexes.

MYOCARDIAL STRUCTURE

The proper cellular organization of cardiac tissue (myocardium) is critical for the generation of efficient myocardial contraction. Disruptions in this structure and organization lead to cardiac dyssynchrony and arrhythmias, which cause significant morbidity and mortality. Atrial and ventricular myocytes are specialized, branching muscle cells that are connected end to end by intercalated disks. These disks aid in the transmission of mechanical tension between cells. The myocyte plasma membrane, or sarcolemma, facilitates excitation and contraction through small transverse tubules (T tubules). Subcellular features specific for myocytes include increased mitochondria number for production of adenosine triphosphate (ATP); an extensive network of intracellular tubules, called the *sarcoplasmic reticulum*, for calcium storage; and *sarcomeres*, which are myofibrils comprised of repeating units of overlapping thin actin filaments and thick myosin filaments and their regulatory proteins troponin and tropomyosin. Specialized myocardial cells form the cardiac conduction system (described earlier) and are responsible for the generation of an electrical impulse and

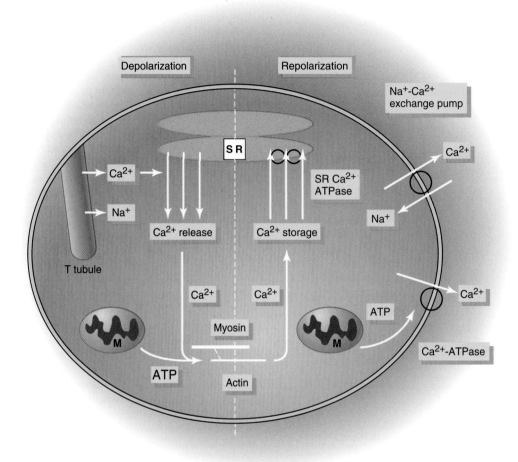

Fig. 2.2 Calcium dependence of myocardial contraction. (1) Electrical depolarization of the myocyte results in an influx of Ca^{2+} ions into the cell through channels in the T tubules. (2) This initial phase of calcium entry stimulates the release of large amounts of Ca^{2+} from the sarcoplasmic reticulum (SR). (3) The Ca^{2+} then binds to the troponin-tropomyosin complex on the actin filaments, resulting in a conformational change that facilitates the binding interaction between actin and myosin. In the presence of adenosine triphosphate (ATP), the actin-myosin association is cyclically dissociated as the thick and thin filaments slide past each other, resulting in contraction. (4) During repolarization, the Ca^{2+} is actively pumped out of the cytosol and sequestered in the SR. *ATPase*, Adenosine triphosphatase; *M*, mitochondrion.

organized propagation of that impulse to cardiac myocytes, which, in turn, respond by mechanical contraction.

MUSCLE PHYSIOLOGY AND CONTRACTION

Calcium-induced calcium release is the primary mechanism for myocyte contraction. When a depolarizing stimulus reaches the myocyte, it enters special invaginations within the sarcolemma called T tubules. These specialized channels open in response to depolarization, permitting calcium flux into the cell (Fig. 2.2). The sarcoplasmic reticulum closely proximates the T tubules, and the initial calcium current triggers the release of large amounts of calcium from the sarcoplasmic reticulum into the cell cytosol. Calcium then binds to the calcium-binding regulatory subunit, troponin C, on the actin filaments of the sarcomere, resulting in a conformational change in the troponin-tropomyosin complex. The myosin binding site on actin is now exposed, to facilitate binding of actin-myosin cross-bridges, which are necessary for cellular contraction. The energy for myocyte contraction

is derived from ATP. During contraction, ATP promotes dissociation of myosin from actin, thereby permitting the sliding of thick filaments past thin filaments as the sarcomere shortens.

The force of myocyte contraction is regulated by the amount of free calcium released into the cell by the sarcoplasmic reticulum. More calcium allows for more frequent actin-myosin interactions, producing a stronger contraction. On repolarization of the sarcolemmal membrane, intracellular calcium is rapidly and actively resequestered into the sarcoplasmic reticulum, where it is stored by various proteins, including calsequestrin, until the next wave of depolarization occurs. Calcium is also extruded from the cytosol by various calcium pumps in the sarcolemma. The active removal of intracellular calcium by ATP ion pumps facilitates ventricular relaxation, which is necessary for proper ventricular filling during diastole.

Circulatory Physiology and the Cardiac Cycle

The term *cardiac cycle* describes the pressure changes within each cardiac chamber over time (Fig. 2.3). This cycle is divided into *systole*,

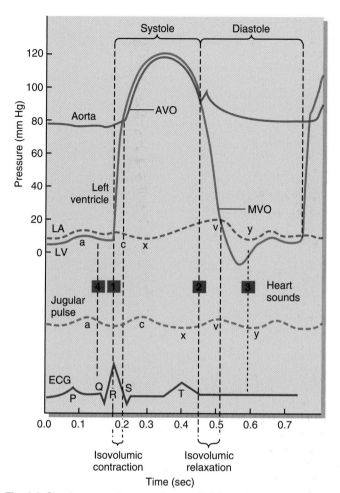

Fig. 2.3 Simultaneous electrocardiogram (ECG) and pressure tracings obtained from the left atrium (LA), left ventricle (LV), and aorta and the jugular venous pressure during the cardiac cycle. (For simplification, pressures on the right side of the heart have been omitted. Normal right atrial (RA) pressure closely parallels that of the LA, and right ventricular and pulmonary artery pressures are timed closely with their corresponding left-sided counterparts; they are reduced only in magnitude. Normally, closure of the mitral and aortic valves precedes closure of the tricuspid and pulmonic valves, whereas valve opening reverses this order. The jugular venous pulse lags behind the RA pulse.) During the course of one cardiac cycle, the electrical (ECG) events initiate and therefore precede the mechanical (pressure) events, and the latter precede the auscultatory events (heart sounds) that they themselves produce *(red boxes)*. Shortly after the P wave, the atria contract to produce the *a* wave. The QRS complex initiates ventricular systole, followed shortly by LV contraction and the rapid buildup of LV pressure. Almost immediately, LV pressure exceeds LA pressure, closing the mitral valve and producing the first heart sound. After a brief period of isovolumic contraction, LV pressure exceeds aortic pressure and the aortic valve opens (AVO). When the ventricular pressure once again falls to less than the aortic pressure, the aortic valve closes to produce the second heart sound and terminate ventricular ejection. The LV pressure decreases during the period of isovolumic relaxation until it drops below LA pressure and the mitral valve opens (MVO). See text for further details.

the period of ventricular contraction, and *diastole*, the period of ventricular relaxation. Each cardiac valve opens and closes in response to pressure gradients generated during these periods. At the onset of systole, ventricular pressures exceed atrial pressures, so the AV valves passively close. As myocytes contract, the intraventricular pressures rise initially, without a change in ventricular volume (isovolumic

contraction), until they exceed the pressures in the aorta and pulmonary artery. At this point, the semilunar valves open, and ventricular ejection of blood occurs. When intracellular calcium levels fall, ventricular relaxation begins; arterial pressures exceed intraventricular pressures, so the semilunar valves close. Ventricular relaxation initially does not change ventricular volume (isovolumic relaxation). At the point at which intraventricular pressures fall below atrial pressures, the AV valves open. This begins the rapid and passive ventricular filling phase of diastole, during which blood in the atria empties into the ventricles. At the end of diastole, active atrial contraction augments ventricular filling. When the myocardium exhibits increased stiffness due to age, hypertension, diabetes, or heart failure, the early passive phase of ventricular filling is decreased. To compensate for the reduction in passive ventricular filling, there is reliance on atrial contraction to sufficiently fill the ventricle during diastole. A pathologic consequence of atrial fibrillation, a disease in which the atrium does not contract, is that patients often have worse symptoms because this additional ventricular filling is lost.

Pressure tracings obtained from the periphery complement the hemodynamic changes exhibited in the heart. In the absence of valvular disease, there is no impediment to blood flow moving from the ventricles to the arterial beds, so the systolic arterial pressure rises sharply to a peak. During diastole, no further blood volume is ejected into the aorta, so the arterial pressure gradually falls as blood flows to the distal tissue beds and elastic recoil of the arteries occurs.

Atrial pressure can be directly measured in the right atrium, but the left atrial pressure is indirectly measured by occluding a small pulmonary artery branch and measuring the pressure distally (the pulmonary capillary *wedge* pressure). An atrial pressure tracing is shown in Fig. 2.3. It is composed of several waves. The *a wave* represents atrial contraction. As the atria subsequently relax, the atrial pressure falls, and the *x descent* is seen on the pressure tracing. The *x* descent is interrupted by a small *c wave*, generated as the AV valve bulges toward the atrium during ventricular systole. As the atria fill from venous return, the *v wave* is seen, after which the *y descent* appears as the AV valves open and blood from the atria empties into the ventricles. The normal ranges of pressures in the various cardiac chambers are shown in Table 2.1.

Cardiac Performance

The amount of blood ejected by the heart each minute is referred to as the cardiac output (CO). It is the product of the stroke volume (SV), which is the amount of blood ejected with each ventricular contraction, and the HR:

$$CO = SV \times HR$$

The cardiac index is a way of normalizing the CO to body size. It is the CO divided by the body surface area and is measured in L/min/m². The normal CO is 4 to 6 L/min at rest and can increase fourfold to sixfold during strenuous exercise.

The main determinants of SV are preload, afterload, and contractility (Table 2.2). *Preload* is the volume of blood in the ventricle at the end of diastole; it is primarily a reflection of venous return. Venous return is determined by the plasma volume and the venous compliance. Clinically, intravenous fluids increase preload, whereas diuretics or venodilators such as nitroglycerin decrease preload. When the preload is increased, the ventricle stretches, and the ensuing ventricular contraction becomes more rapid and forceful, because the increased sarcomere length facilitates actin and myosin cross-bridge kinetics by means of an increased sensitivity of troponin C to calcium. This phenomenon is known as the Frank-Starling relationship. Ventricular filling pressure (ventricular end-diastolic pressure, atrial pressure, or

TABLE 2.1 Normal Values for Common Hemodynamic Parameters	
Heart rate	60-100 beats/min
Pressures (mm Hg)	
Central venous	≤9
Right atrial	≤9
Right ventricular	
Systolic	15-30
End-diastolic	≤9
Pulmonary arterial	
Systolic	15-30
Diastolic	3-12
Pulmonary capillary wedge	≤12
Left atrial	≤12
Left ventricular	
Systolic	100-140
End-diastolic	3-12
Aortic	
Systolic	100-140
Diastolic	60-90
Resistance	
Systemic vascular resistance	800-1500 dynes-sec/cm^{-5}
Pulmonary vascular resistance	30-120 dynes-sec/cm^{-5}
Cardiac output	4-6 L/min
Cardiac index	2.5-4 L/min

TABLE 2.2   Factors Affecting Cardiac Performance
Preload (Left Ventricular Diastolic Volume)
Total blood volume
Venous (sympathetic) tone
Body position
Intrathoracic and intrapericardial pressures
Atrial contraction
Pumping action of skeletal muscle
Afterload (Impedance Against Which the Left Ventricle Must Eject Blood)
Peripheral vascular resistance
Left ventricular volume (preload, wall tension)
Physical characteristics of the arterial tree (elasticity of vessels or presence of outflow obstruction)
Contractility (Cardiac Performance Independent of Preload or Afterload)
Sympathetic nerve impulses
Increased contractility
Circulating catecholamines
Digitalis, calcium, other inotropic agents
Increased heart rate or post-extrasystolic augmentation
Anoxia, acidosis
Decreased contractility
Pharmacologic depression
Loss of myocardium
Intrinsic depression
Heart Rate
Autonomic nervous system
Temperature, metabolic rate
Medications, drugs

pulmonary capillary wedge pressure) is frequently used as a surrogate measure of preload.

Afterload is the force against which the ventricles must contract to eject blood. The main determinants of afterload are the arterial pressure and the dimensions of the left ventricle. As the arterial blood pressure increases, the amount of blood that can be ejected into the aorta decreases. Wall stress, a significant and often overlooked determinant of afterload, is directly proportional to the size of the ventricular cavity and inversely proportional to the ventricular wall thickness (Laplace's law). Diuretics reduce the increased wall stress associated with pathologic dilatation in cardiomyopathy by decreasing left ventricular volume and size. In addition, ventricular wall hypertrophy is a compensatory mechanism to reduce afterload caused by systemic hypertension. Drugs that treat hypertension, such as angiotensin-converting enzyme (ACE) inhibitors and hydralazine, reduce blood pressure (BP) and thereby reduce afterload.

Contractility, or inotropy, represents the force of ventricular contraction in the presence of constant preload and afterload. Inotropy is regulated at a cellular level through stimulation of catecholaminergic (epinephrine, norepinephrine, and dopamine) receptors, intracellular signaling cascades (phosphodiesterase inhibitors), and intracellular calcium levels (affected by levosimendan and, indirectly, by digoxin). Many antihypertensive medications (e.g., β-blockers, calcium channel antagonists) interfere with adrenergic receptor activation or intracellular calcium levels, which can decrease the strength of ventricular contractions. (Please refer to Chapter 47, "Cardiac and Circulatory ❖ Function," in *Goldman-Cecil Medicine*, 26th Edition.)

Physiology of the Coronary Circulation

The normally functioning heart maintains equilibrium between the amount of oxygen delivered to myocytes and the amount of oxygen consumed by them (myocardial oxygen consumption, or Mvo$_2$). If a myocyte works harder because it is contracting with increased frequency (HR), with increased intensity (contractility), or against an increased load (wall stress), then it will use more oxygen and its Mvo$_2$ will increase. In order to meet this increase in demand for more oxygen, the heart will have to either increase blood flow or increase its efficiency in extracting oxygen. The heart is unique in that its oxygen extraction is almost maximal at resting conditions. Therefore, increasing blood flow is the only reasonable means of increasing oxygen supply.

Microvascular blood flow in the coronary circulation is impaired during systole because the intramyocardial blood vessels are compressed by contracting myocardium. Therefore, most coronary flow occurs during diastole. Accordingly, the diastolic pressure is the major pressure driving flow within the coronary circulation. Systolic pressure impedes intramyocardial arterial blood flow but augments venous flow. On a clinical note, tachycardia is particularly detrimental because coronary flow is reduced when the diastolic filling time is abbreviated, and the Mvo$_2$ increases with increasing HR. In order to sustain constant perfusion to the myocardium, coronary blood flow is maintained constant over a wide range of pressures in a process called autoregulation.

In response to a change in Mvo$_2$, the coronary arteries dilate or constrict, which changes the vascular resistance and thereby appropriately changes flow. This regulation of arterial resistance occurs at the arterioles and is mediated by several factors. Adenosine, a metabolite of ATP, is released during contraction and acts as a potent vasodilator.

Other consequences of myocardial metabolism, such as decreased oxygen tension, increased carbon dioxide, hydrogen peroxide, acidosis, and hyperkalemia, also mediate coronary vasodilation. The endothelium produces several potent vasodilators, including nitric oxide and prostacyclin. Nitric oxide is released by the endothelium in response to acetylcholine, thrombin, adenosine diphosphate (ADP), serotonin, bradykinin, platelet aggregation, and an increase in shear stress (called *flow-dependent vasodilation*). Finally, the coronary arteries are innervated by the autonomic nervous system, and activation of sympathetic neurons mediates vasoconstriction or vasodilation through α- or β-receptors, respectively. Parasympathetic neurons from the vagus nerve secrete acetylcholine, which mediates vasodilation. Vasoconstricting factors, notably endothelin, are produced by the endothelium and may be important in conditions such as coronary vasospasm. (Please refer to Chapter 47, "Cardiac and Circulatory Function," in *Goldman-Cecil Medicine*, 26th Edition.)

Physiology of the Systemic Circulation

The normal cardiovascular system delivers appropriate blood flow to each organ of the body under a wide range of conditions. This regulation is achieved by maintaining BP through adjustments in cardiac output and tissue blood flow resistance by neural and humoral factors.

Poiseuille's law generally describes the relationship between pressure and flow in a vessel. Fluid flow (F) through a tube is proportional (proportionality constant = K) to the pressure (P) difference between the ends of the tube:

$$F = K \times \Delta P$$

K is equivalent to the inverse of resistance to flow (R); that is, K = 1/R. Resistance to flow is determined by the properties of both the fluid and the tube. In the case of a steady, streamlined flow of fluid through a rigid tube, Poiseuille found that these factors determine resistance:

$$R = 8\eta L \,/\, \pi r^4$$

Where r is the radius of the tube, L is its length, and η is the viscosity of the fluid. Notice that changes in radius have greater influence than changes in length, because resistance is inversely proportional to the fourth power of the radius. Poiseuille's law incorporates the factors influencing flow, so that:

$$F = \Delta P/R = \Delta P \pi r^4 / 8\eta L$$

Therefore, the most important determinants of blood flow in the cardiovascular system are ΔP and r^4. Small changes in arterial radius can cause large changes in flow to a tissue or organ. Practically, systemic vascular resistance (SVR) is the total resistance to flow caused by changes in the radius of resistance vessels (small arteries and arterioles) of the systemic circulation. The SVR can be calculated as the pressure drop across the peripheral capillary beds (mean arterial pressure − right atrial pressure) divided by the blood flow across the beds (i.e., SVR = BP/CO). It is normally in the range of 800 to 1500 dynes-sec/cm^{-5}.

The autonomic nervous system alters systemic vascular tone through sympathetic and parasympathetic innervation as well as metabolic factors (local oxygen tension, carbon dioxide levels, reactive oxygen species, pH) and endothelium-derived signaling molecules (NO, endothelin). Neural regulation of BP occurs by means of constitutive and reflex changes in autonomic efferent outflow to modulate cardiac chronotropy, inotropy, and vascular resistance.

The baroreflex loop is the primary mechanism by which BP is neurally modulated. Baroreceptors are stretch-sensitive nerve endings that are distributed throughout various regions of the cardiovascular system. Those located in the carotid artery (e.g., carotid sinus) and aorta are sometimes referred to as *high-pressure baroreceptors* and those in the cardiopulmonary areas as *low-pressure baroreceptors*. After afferent impulses are transmitted to the central nervous system, the signals are integrated, and the efferent arm of the reflex projects neural signals systemically through the sympathetic and parasympathetic branches of the autonomic nervous system. In general, an increase in systemic BP increases the firing rate of the baroreceptors. Efferent sympathetic outflow is inhibited (reducing vascular tone, chronotropy, and inotropy), and parasympathetic outflow is increased (reducing cardiac chronotropy). The opposite occurs when BP decreases. (Please refer to Chapter 47, "Cardiac and Circulatory Function," in *Goldman-Cecil Medicine*, 26th Edition.)

Physiology of the Pulmonary Circulation

Like the systemic circulation, the pulmonary circulation consists of a branching network of progressively smaller arteries, arterioles, capillaries, and veins. The pulmonary capillaries are separated from the alveoli by a thin alveolar-capillary membrane through which gas exchange occurs. The partial pressure of oxygen (P_{O_2}) is the main regulator of pulmonary blood to optimize blood flow toward well-ventilated lung segments and away from poorly ventilated segments.

SUGGESTED READINGS

Berne RM, Levy MN: Physiology: part IV. The cardiovascular system, ed 7, St. Louis, 2017, Elsevier.
Guyton AC, Hall JE: Textbook of medical physiology, ed 13, St. Louis, 2015, Elsevier.

3

Evaluation of the Patient With Cardiovascular Disease

James Kleczka, Noura M. Dabbouseh

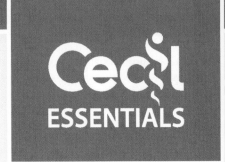

DEFINITION AND EPIDEMIOLOGY

Cardiovascular disease is a major cause of morbidity and mortality around the world, and its spectrum is wide-reaching. Included in this population of patients are people with coronary artery disease (CAD), congestive heart failure, stroke, hypertension, peripheral arterial disease, atrial fibrillation and other arrhythmias, valvular disease, and congenital heart disease. The impact of cardiovascular disease is unmistakable: It is the leading cause of death in both males and females in the United States, with reports estimating that heart disease accounts for between one in three and one in four deaths. It accounted for more inpatient hospital days in the years of 1990-2009 than other disorders such as chronic lung disease and cancer. The high number of inpatient days associated with cardiovascular disease led to a total economic cost of more than $297 billion in the year 2008 alone. In 2011, an estimated $316.6 billion in health care costs and lost productivity was attributable to heart disease and stroke.

Given these facts, the proper evaluation of a patient with cardiovascular disease is imperative in order to potentially decrease an individual's morbidity and mortality and potentially impact health care expenditures. An understanding of the basics of the pathophysiology of heart disease as well as a thorough history and detailed physical examination are required to accurately assess and manage patients with cardiovascular disease.

PATHOLOGY

The term *cardiovascular disease* encompasses a wide array of patient problems. The heart's circulation, myocardium, rhythm, valves, and pericardial structures may be affected, as can the arterial or venous vascular systems. *Coronary artery disease (CAD)*, discussed in depth in Chapter 8, is a leading cause of morbidity and mortality. While many patients do have silent CAD or asymptomatic coronary atherosclerosis, this still impacts patient morbidity. At presentation, patients with symptomatic CAD may have stable angina or an acute coronary syndrome, further stratified into unstable angina (UA), non–ST segment elevation myocardial infarction (NSTEMI), or ST segment elevation myocardial infarction (STEMI). The initial presentation for some patients with CAD is sudden cardiac death, the result of arrhythmia often caused by atherosclerosis of the coronary vasculature.

Congestive heart failure is the end result of many cardiac disorders and has been historically classified as systolic or diastolic in etiology. More recently, the terms heart failure with reduced ejection fraction (HFrEF) and heart failure with preserved ejection fraction (HFpEF), which is often due to diastolic dysfunction, have gained widespread acceptance. In patients with ventricular enlargement or systolic dysfunction, the term cardiomyopathy is appropriate whether or not a patient has clinically demonstrated signs of heart failure. Various forms of cardiomyopathy may lead to systolic dysfunction and a decline in ejection fraction. Without proper management, this will inevitably lead to alterations in hemodynamics that result in development of pulmonary vascular congestion, edema, and a decline in functional capacity, all symptoms of clinical heart failure. Diastolic dysfunction can be present with systolic dysfunction and is often the result of uncontrolled hypertension or infiltrative disorders such as hemochromatosis or amyloidosis. Various forms of heart failure are further discussed in Chapter 5.

Stroke is caused by cerebral hypoperfusion, which can result from such problems as carotid disease, thromboembolism, or emboli of infectious origin. A more detailed discussion can be found in Chapter 118.

Peripheral arterial disease (PAD), addressed in Chapter 12, includes such entities as aneurysms of the ascending, descending, and abdominal aorta and its branches; aortic or peripheral arterial dissection; carotid disease; and atherosclerosis of branch vessels of the aorta and vessels in the limbs. PAD is often present in patients with CAD.

Atrial fibrillation and *hypertension* (see Chapter 9) are not uncommon and increase in prevalence with age. Although they are not typically the primary cause of mortality, these problems often predispose to other causes of cardiovascular disease mortality, such as stroke and heart failure. Arrhythmias other than atrial fibrillation are also common and can lead to significant morbidity and mortality.

Valvular heart disease may lead to cardiomyopathy and is found in all age groups.

Congenital heart disease includes a wide variety of disorders, ranging from valve abnormalities and coronary anomalies to cardiomyopathy and other structural abnormalities including shunts and malformations of the cardiac chambers. With advances in surgical techniques and medical therapy, life expectancy has improved significantly for patients with congenital heart disease. Congenital heart disease is discussed further in Chapter 6.

CLINICAL PRESENTATION

Technologic advancements have allowed for specialized testing to assist in the diagnosis of cardiovascular diseases. We now rely on such tests as angiography, ultrasound scanning, and advanced imaging modalities such as high-resolution computed tomography and magnetic resonance imaging to determine how to manage an individual case. However, these techniques should be used not as a primary method of assessment but rather to supplement the findings from a thorough history and physical examination. Despite the availability of rather costly imaging techniques and laboratory tests, a relatively inexpensive but detailed history and physical examination is a clinician's strongest tool in helping to establish a diagnosis.

TABLE 3.1 Cardiovascular Causes of Chest Pain

Condition	Location	Quality	Duration	Aggravating or Alleviating Factors	Associated Symptoms or Signs
Angina	Retrosternal region: radiates to or occasionally isolated to neck, jaw, shoulders, arms (usually left), or epigastrium	Pressure, squeezing, tightness, heaviness, burning, indigestion	<2-10 min	Precipitated by exertion, cold weather, or emotional stress; relieved by rest or nitroglycerin; variant (Prinzmetal) angina may be unrelated to exertion, often early in the morning	Dyspnea; S_3, S_4, or murmur of papillary dysfunction during pain
Myocardial infarction	Same as angina	Same as angina, although more severe	Variable; usually >30 min	Unrelieved by rest or nitroglycerin	Dyspnea, nausea, vomiting, weakness, diaphoresis
Pericarditis	Left of the sternum; may radiate to neck or left shoulder, often more localized than pain of myocardial ischemia	Sharp, stabbing, knifelike	Lasts many hours to days; may wax and wane	Aggravated by deep breathing, rotating chest, or supine position; relieved by sitting up and leaning forward	Pericardial friction rub
Aortic dissection	Anterior chest; may radiate to back, interscapular region	Excruciating, tearing, knifelike	Sudden onset, unrelenting	Usually occurs in setting of hypertension or predisposition, such as Marfan syndrome	Murmur of aortic insufficiency; pulse or blood pressure asymmetry; neurologic deficit

A patient who is given the opportunity to outline his or her symptoms in his or her own words can help lead a clinician toward the right diagnosis. For example, many patients who deny chest pain when asked specifically about this symptom will go on to describe the symptom of chest pressure, which patients often feel is distinct from "pain." Gathering further historical details such as provoking factors (e.g., activity, extreme emotional stress, or rest or unprovoked symptoms), location, quality, intensity, and radiation of the symptom is imperative when taking a thorough history. One should delve into aggravating or alleviating factors and whether there are other symptoms that accompany the primary symptom. It is also important to note the pattern of the symptom in terms of stability or progression in intensity or frequency over time. An assessment of functional status should always be a part of the history in a patient with cardiovascular disease; a recent decline in exercise tolerance can help determine severity of disease.

A detailed past medical history and review of systems are necessary in order to understand if the cardiovascular condition is isolated or part of a syndrome. For example, a patient may have arrhythmias in the setting of hyperthyroidism. Rheumatologic disorders often affect the heart. And cancer can increase the risk of thromboembolism, of pericardial effusion and, with some therapies, cardiomyopathy. A comprehensive list of medications must be reviewed, and a social history must be taken detailing alcohol use, smoking, and occupational history. Patients should also be questioned regarding major risk factors such as hypertension, hyperlipidemia, and diabetes mellitus. A thorough family history is needed, not only to identify such entities as early-onset CAD but also to assess for other potentially inherited disorders, such as familial cardiomyopathy or arrhythmic disorders (e.g., long-QT syndrome).

Chest Pain

Chest pain is one of the cardinal symptoms of cardiovascular disease, but it may also be present in many noncardiovascular diseases (Tables 3.1 and 3.2). Chest pain may be caused by cardiac ischemia but also may be related to aortic pathology such as dissection, pulmonary disease such as pneumonia, gastrointestinal pathology such as gastroesophageal reflux, or musculoskeletal pain related to chest wall trauma. Issues with organs in the abdominal cavity such as the gallbladder or pancreas can also cause chest pain. It is therefore very important to characterize the pain in terms of location, quality, quantity, duration, radiation, aggravating and alleviating factors, and associated symptoms. These details will help determine the origin of the pain.

Myocardial ischemia due to obstructive CAD often leads to typical angina pectoris. Angina is often described as tightness, pressure, burning, or squeezing discomfort that patients may not identify as true pain. Patients frequently describe angina as a sensation of "bricks on the center of the chest" or an "elephant standing on the chest." Angina is more common in the morning, and the intensity may be affected by heat or cold, emotional stress, or eating. This discomfort is typically located in the substernal region or left side of the chest. Anginal pain may radiate to other parts of the body, such as the left shoulder and arm (particularly the ulnar aspect), the neck, the jaw, or the epigastrium. Pain that radiates to the back may raise suspicion for aortic dissection. Anginal chest pain is usually brought on with exertion, in particular with more intense activity or walking up inclines, in extremes of weather, or after large meals. It is typically brief in duration, lasting 2 to 10 minutes, and frequently resolves with rest or administration of nitroglycerine within 1 to 5 minutes. Associated symptoms often include nausea, diaphoresis, dyspnea, palpitations, and dizziness. Patients typically report a stable pattern of angina that is relatively predictable and reproducible with a given amount of exertion. When this pain begins to increase in frequency and severity or occurs with lesser amounts of exertion or at rest, one must then consider unstable angina. Anginal pain that occurs at rest with increased intensity and lasts longer than 30 minutes may represent acute myocardial infarction (MI). Some patients endorse a feeling of doom when suffering an MI. Angina-like pain at rest may also occur with coronary vasospasm and noncardiac chest pain.

There are several other potential causes of chest pain that may be confused with angina pectoris (see Table 3.2). Pain associated

TABLE 3.2 Noncardiac Causes of Chest Pain

Condition	Location	Quality	Duration	Aggravating or Alleviating Factors	Associated Symptoms or Signs
Pulmonary embolism (chest pain often not present)	Substernal or over region of pulmonary infarction	Pleuritic (with pulmonary infarction) or angina-like	Sudden onset (minutes to hours)	Aggravated by deep breathing	Dyspnea, tachypnea, tachycardia; hypotension, signs of acute right ventricular heart failure, and pulmonary hypertension with large emboli; pleural rub; hemoptysis with pulmonary infarction
Pulmonary hypertension	Substernal	Pressure; oppressive	—	Aggravated by effort	Pain usually associated with dyspnea; signs of pulmonary hypertension
Pneumonia with pleurisy	Located over involved area	Pleuritic	—	Aggravated by breathing	Dyspnea, cough, fever, bronchial breath sounds, rhonchi, egophony, dullness to percussion, occasional pleural rub
Spontaneous pneumothorax	Unilateral	Sharp, well localized	Sudden onset; lasts many hours	Aggravated by breathing	Dyspnea; hyperresonance and decreased breath and voice sounds over involved lung
Musculoskeletal disorders	Variable	Aching, well localized	Variable	Aggravated by movement; history of exertion or injury	Tender to palpation or with light pressure
Herpes zoster	Dermatomal distribution	Sharp, burning	Prolonged	None	Vesicular rash appears in area of discomfort
Esophageal reflux	Substernal or epigastric; may radiate to neck	Burning, visceral discomfort	10-60 min	Aggravated by large meal, postprandial recumbency; relief with antacid	Water brash
Peptic ulcer	Epigastric, substernal	Visceral burning, aching	Prolonged	Relief with food, antacid	—
Gallbladder disease	Right upper quadrant; epigastric	Visceral	Prolonged	Spontaneous or after meals	Right upper quadrant tenderness may be present
Anxiety states	Often localized over precordium	Variable; location often moves from place to place	Varies; often fleeting	Situational	Sighing respirations; often chest wall tenderness

with acute pericarditis is typically sharp, is located to the left of the sternum, and radiates to the neck, shoulders, and back. This may be rather severe pain that is present at rest and can last for hours. It typically improves with sitting up and forward and worsens with inspiration. Oftentimes history of causative viral prodrome can be elicited.

Acute aortic dissection usually causes sudden onset of severe tearing chest pain that radiates to the back between the scapulae or to the lumbar region. Typically, there is a history of hypertension, and pulses may be asymmetric between the extremities. A murmur of aortic regurgitation may also be heard. Pain associated with pulmonary embolism is also acute in onset and is usually accompanied by shortness of breath. This pain is typically pleuritic, worsening with inspiration.

Dyspnea

Dyspnea is another hallmark symptom of cardiovascular disease, but it is also a primary symptom of pulmonary disease. It is defined as an uncomfortable heightened awareness of breathing. This can be an entirely normal sensation in individuals performing moderate to extreme exertion, depending on their level of conditioning. When it occurs at rest or with minimal exertion, dyspnea is considered abnormal. Dyspnea may accompany a large number of noncardiac conditions such as anemia due to a lack of oxygen-carrying capacity,

pulmonary disorders such as obstructive or restrictive lung disease and asthma, obesity due to an increased work of breathing and restricted filling of the lungs, and deconditioning. In the cardiovascular patient, dyspnea may be caused by ventricular dysfunction, either systolic or diastolic; CAD and resultant ischemia; a large pericardial effusion causing impaired filling and resulting depressed cardiac output (cardiac tamponade); or valvular heart disease that, when severe, can lead to a drop in cardiac output. In cases of left ventricular dysfunction and valvular disease, the mechanism of dyspnea often involves increased intracardiac pressures that lead to pulmonary vascular congestion. Fluid then leaks into the alveolar space, impairing gas exchange and causing dyspnea.

Breathing difficulties can also be secondary to a low-output state without pulmonary vascular congestion. Patients often notice dyspnea with exertion, but it can also occur at rest in patients with severe cardiac disease. Shortness of breath at rest is also a symptom in patients with pulmonary edema, large pleural effusions, anxiety, or pulmonary embolism. A patient with left ventricular systolic or diastolic failure may describe the acute onset of breathing difficulty when sleeping. This problem, called paroxysmal nocturnal dyspnea (PND), is caused by pulmonary edema that is redistributed in a prone position; it is usually secondary to left ventricular failure. These patients often notice the acute onset of dyspnea followed by coughing roughly 2 to 4 hours after going to sleep. This can be a very uncomfortable feeling, and it leads the patient to sit up immediately or get out of bed. Symptoms typically resolve over 15 to 30 minutes. Patients with left ventricular failure also often complain of orthopnea, which is dyspnea that occurs when one assumes a prone position. This is relieved by sleeping on multiple pillows or remaining seated to sleep. In severe cases of dyspnea due to heart failure, patients may have an immediate feeling of shortness of breath when attempting a supine position.

Patients with sudden onset of dyspnea may be experiencing flash pulmonary edema, which is very rapid and acute accumulation of fluid in the lungs. This can be associated with severe CAD and may also be a cause of dyspnea in patients with coarctation of the aorta and renal artery stenosis. Sudden dyspnea is associated with pulmonary embolism, and this symptom is typically accompanied by pleuritic chest pain and possibly hemoptysis in such patients. Pneumothorax can cause dyspnea accompanied by acute chest pain. Dyspnea due to lung disease is present with exertion, although in severe cases it may be present at rest. This is often accompanied by hypoxia and is relieved by pulmonary bronchodilators or steroids or both. Dyspnea may also be an "angina equivalent." Not all patients with CAD develop typical anginal chest pain. Dyspnea that comes on with exertion or emotional stress, is relieved with rest, and is relatively brief in duration might be a manifestation of significant CAD. This type of dyspnea is also usually improved with the administration of nitroglycerine.

Palpitation

Palpitation is another symptom commonly seen in the cardiovascular patient. This is the subjective sensation of rapid or forceful beating of the heart. Patients are often able to describe in detail the sensation they feel, such as jumping, skipping, racing, fluttering, or an irregularity in the heartbeat. It is important to ask the patient about the onset of the palpitations because they may begin abruptly at rest, only with exertion, with emotional stress, or with ingestion of certain foods such as chocolate. One should also inquire about associated symptoms such as chest pain, dyspnea, dizziness, and syncope. It is important to note other medical issues, such as thyroid disease, and bleeding, which can lead to anemia, because these conditions may be associated with arrhythmias. A social history focusing on drug use and intake of alcohol, caffeine, or medications is important because use of many substances can lead to certain rhythm disturbances. Certain over-the-counter medicines contain pseudoephedrine, which can cause increased heart rate and palpitations. The family history is also important, because there are many inherited disorders (e.g., long-QT syndromes) that might lead to significant arrhythmias.

Potential etiologies of palpitations include premature atrial or ventricular beats, which are typically described as isolated skips and can be uncomfortable. Supraventricular tachycardias such as atrial flutter, AV nodal reentrant tachycardia, and paroxysmal atrial tachycardia often start and stop abruptly and can be rapid. Atrial fibrillation is an irregular heart rhythm originating from the atria. It can lead to rapid heart rates, which can be symptomatic. Even slowly conducted atrial fibrillation can be symptomatic for some patients. Ventricular arrhythmias are more often associated with severe dizziness or syncope. Gradual onset of tachycardia with a gradual decline in HR is more indicative of sinus tachycardia or anxiety.

Syncope

Syncope may be caused by a variety of cardiovascular diseases. It is the transient loss of consciousness due to inadequate cerebral blood flow. In the patient presenting with syncope as a primary complaint, one must try to differentiate true cardiac causes from neurologic issues such as seizure and metabolic causes such as hypoglycemia. Determination of the timing of the syncopal event and associated symptoms is very

helpful in determining the etiology. True cardiac syncope is typically very sudden, with no prodromal symptoms. It is typically caused by an abrupt drop in cardiac output that may be due to tachyarrhythmias such as ventricular tachycardia or fibrillation, bradyarrhythmias, such as complete heart block, severe valvular heart disease such as aortic or mitral stenosis, or obstruction of flow due to left ventricular outflow tract (LVOT) obstruction. It can also be caused by cardiac tamponade as well as by hemodynamically significant pulmonary embolism. True cardiac syncope often has no accompanying aura, though palpitations can be experienced in patients with tachyarrhythmia, or with pulmonary embolism or tamponade (due to frequently higher heart rates in these scenarios). In situations such as aortic stenosis or LVOT obstruction, syncope typically occurs with exertion. Patients may regain consciousness rather quickly with true cardiac syncope. It should be noted that some syncope is associated with a generalized shaking (i.e., convulsive syncope), which can mimic epileptic activity. Convulsive activity should not cause the clinician to rule out a cardiac etiology for syncope.

Neurocardiogenic syncope involves an abnormal reflexive response to a change in position. When one rises from a prone or seated position to a standing position, the peripheral vasculature usually constricts, and the HR increases, to maintain cerebral perfusion. With neurocardiogenic syncope, the peripheral vasculature abnormally dilates, the HR slows or doesn't increase normally, or both. This leads to a reduction in cerebral perfusion and syncope. A similar mechanism is responsible for carotid sinus syncope and syncope associated with micturition and cough. The patient usually describes a gradual onset of symptoms such as flushing, dizziness, diaphoresis, and nausea before losing consciousness, which lasts seconds. When these patients wake, they are often pale and have a lower HR.

In the patient with syncope due to seizures, a prodromal aura is typically present before loss of consciousness occurs. Patients regain consciousness much more slowly and at times are incontinent, complain of headache and fatigue, and have a "postictal" confusional state. Syncope due to stroke is rare, because there must be significant bilateral carotid disease or disease of the vertebrobasilar system causing brainstem ischemia. Neurologic deficits accompany the physical examination findings in these patients.

The history is very important in determining the cause of a syncopal episode. This was previously studied by Calkins and colleagues, who found that men older than 54 years of age who had no prodromal symptoms were more likely to have an arrhythmic cause of their episodes. However, those with prodromal symptoms such as nausea, diaphoresis, dizziness, and visual disturbances before passing out were more likely to have neurocardiogenic syncope. Many inherited disorders such as long-QT syndrome and other arrhythmias, hypertrophic cardiomyopathy with LVOT obstruction, and familial dilated cardiomyopathy lead to states conducive to syncope. For this reason, detailed family history is necessary.

Edema

Edema often accompanies cardiovascular disease but may be a manifestation of liver disease (cirrhosis), renal disease (nephrotic syndrome), thyroid disease (myxedema) or local issues such as chronic venous insufficiency or thrombophlebitis. Edema related to cardiac disease is caused by increased venous pressures that alter the balance between hydrostatic and oncotic forces. This leads to extravasation of fluid into the extravascular space. These patients, therefore, are intravascularly "volume up," which has implications for therapeutic approaches. Peripheral edema is common with right-sided heart failure, whereas the same process in left-sided heart failure leads to pulmonary edema. Left- and right-sided heart failure often coexist.

Edema due to a cardiac etiology is typically bilateral and begins distally with progression in a proximal fashion. The feet and ankles are affected first, followed by the lower legs, thighs, and, ultimately, the abdomen, sometimes accompanied by ascites. If edema is visible, it is usually preceded by a weight gain of at least 5 to 10 pounds. Edema with heart disease is typically pitting, leaving an indentation in the skin after pressure is applied to the area. The edema is usually worse in the evening, and patients often describe an inability to fit into their shoes. There may also be a feeling of abdominal fullness, depressed appetite, and difficulty fitting into other clothing, such as pants, normally. While these patients are lying prone, the edema can shift to the sacral region after several hours, only to accumulate again the next day when they are on their feet again (dependent edema).

Total body edema, or anasarca, may be caused by heart failure but is also seen in nephrotic syndrome, cirrhosis, and severe hypothyroidism. Unilateral edema is more likely associated with a localized issue such as deep venous thrombosis or thrombophlebitis. Other parts of the history may shed light on the etiology of edema. Patients who report PND and orthopnea are likely to have a cardiac etiology, and in fact, PND is the most specific historical finding in heart failure. If there is a history of alcohol abuse and jaundice is present, liver disease should be a considered cause. Edema of the eyes and face in addition to lower-extremity edema is more likely related to nephrotic syndrome, though this may also occur in heart failure. Edema associated with discoloration or ulcers of the lower extremities is often seen with chronic venous insufficiency. In a patient with insidious onset of edema progressing to anasarca and ascites, one must consider a diagnosis of chronic constrictive pericarditis.

Cyanosis

Cyanosis is defined as an abnormal bluish discoloration of the skin resulting from an increase in the level of reduced hemoglobin or abnormal hemoglobin in the blood. When present, it typically represents an oxygen saturation of less than 85% (normal, >90%). There are several types of cyanosis. Central cyanosis often manifests in discoloration of the lips or trunk and usually represents low oxygen saturations due to right-to-left shunting of blood. This can occur with structural cardiac abnormalities such as large atrial or ventricular septal defects, but it also happens with impaired pulmonary function, as in severe chronic obstructive lung disease. Peripheral cyanosis is typically secondary to vasoconstriction in the setting of low cardiac output. This can also occur with exposure to cold and can represent local arterial or venous thrombosis. When localized to the hands, peripheral cyanosis suggests Raynaud's phenomenon. Cyanosis in childhood often indicates congenital heart disease with right-to-left shunting of blood, causing lower oxygen content in systemically circulated blood.

Other

There are other, nonspecific symptoms that may indicate cardiovascular disease. Although fatigue is present with myriad medical conditions, it is common in patients with cardiac disease and can be a manifestation of coronary disease, volume overload, low cardiac output, hypotension, or hypertension. Iatrogenic causes of fatigue in cardiac patients include aggressive medical treatment of hypertension and overdiuresis in patients with heart failure. Fatigue may also be a direct result of medical therapy for cardiac disease itself, such as with β-blocking agents.

Although cough is commonly associated with pulmonary disease, it may also indicate high intracardiac pressures which can lead to pulmonary edema. Cough may be present in patients with heart failure or significant left-sided valve disease. A patient with congestive heart failure may describe a cough productive of frothy pink sputum, as opposed to frank bloody or blood-tinged sputum, which is more typically seen with primary lung pathology. Nausea and emesis can accompany acute myocardial infarction and are often the only symptoms of MI. These "abdominal" symptoms may also be a reflection of heart failure leading to hepatic or intestinal congestion due to high right heart pressures. Anorexia, abdominal fullness, and cachexia may occur with end-stage heart failure, and the term "cardiac cachexia" has been coined to describe this syndrome. Nocturia is also a symptom described with heart failure; renal perfusion improves when the patient lies in a prone position, leading to an increase in urine output. Hoarseness of voice can occur due to compression of the recurrent laryngeal nerve. This may happen with enlarged pulmonary arteries, enlarged left atrium, or aortic aneurysm (Ortner's syndrome).

Despite the myriad symptoms of cardiovascular disease described here, many patients with significant cardiac disease are asymptomatic. Patients with CAD may have periods of asymptomatic ischemia that can be documented on ambulatory electrocardiographic monitoring. Up to one third of patients who have suffered a myocardial infarction are unaware that they had an event. This is more common in diabetics and in older patients. A patient may have severely depressed ventricular function for some time before presenting with symptoms. In addition, patients with atrial fibrillation can be entirely asymptomatic, with this rhythm discovered only after a physical examination or electrocardiogram is performed.

It is also important to note that cardiovascular disease is a leading cause of morbidity and mortality in women, but women have not classically been included in large longitudinal or epidemiologic studies of cardiac disease. Thus, much of our knowledge has been gathered from the study of men, and women may have atypical symptoms and presentations for cardiovascular disease. A high clinical suspicion for cardiovascular disease, the leading cause of death in both men and women, is imperative during evaluation, especially of the patient with cardiovascular disease risk factors.

At times, patients do not report having symptoms related to usual activities of daily living, yet symptoms are present when functional testing is performed. Therefore, assessing functional capacity is a very important part of the history in a patient with known or suspected cardiovascular disease. The ability or inability to perform various activities plays a substantial role in determining the extent of disability and in assessing response to therapy and overall prognosis, and it can influence decisions regarding the timing and type of therapy or intervention. The New York Heart Association Functional Classification is a commonly used method to assess functional status based on "ordinary activity" (Table 3.3). Patients are classified in one of four functional classes. Functional class I includes patients with known cardiac disease who have no limitations with ordinary activity. Functional classes II and III describe patients who have symptoms with less and less activity, whereas patients in functional class IV have symptoms at rest. The Canadian Cardiovascular Society has provided a similar classification of functional status specifically for patients with angina pectoris. These tools are very useful in classifying a patient's symptoms at a given time, allowing comparison at a future point and determination as to whether the symptoms are stable or progressive.

DIAGNOSIS AND PHYSICAL EXAMINATION

General

Like the detailed history, the physical examination is also vital when assessing a patient with cardiovascular disease. This consists of more than simple cardiac auscultation. Many diseases of the cardiovascular system can affect and be affected by other organ systems. Therefore, a detailed general physical examination is essential. The general

TABLE 3.3 Classification of Functional Status[a]

Class I	Uncompromised	Ordinary activity does not cause symptoms; symptoms occur only with strenuous or prolonged activity.
Class II	Slightly compromised	Ordinary physical activity results in symptoms; no symptoms at rest.
Class III	Moderately compromised	Less than ordinary activity results in symptoms; no symptoms at rest.
Class IV	Severely compromised	Any activity results in symptoms; symptoms may be present at rest.

[a]*Symptoms* refers to undue fatigue, dyspnea, palpitations, or angina in the New York Heart Association classification and refers specifically to angina in the Canadian Cardiovascular Society classification.

appearance of a patient is helpful: Examination of skin color, breathing pattern, presence of pain, and overall nutritional status can provide clues regarding the diagnosis. Examination of the head may reveal evidence of hypothyroidism, such as hair loss and periorbital edema, and examination of the eyes may reveal exophthalmos associated with hyperthyroidism. Both conditions can affect the heart. Retinal examination may reveal macular edema or flame hemorrhages that can be associated with uncontrolled hypertension. Findings such as clubbing or edema when examining the extremities, and jaundice or cyanosis when evaluating the skin, may provide clues to undiagnosed cardiovascular disease.

Examination of the Jugular Venous Pulsations

Examination of the neck veins can provide a great deal of insight into right heart hemodynamics. The right internal jugular vein should be used, because the relatively straight course of the right innominate and jugular veins allows for a more accurate reflection of the true right atrial pressure. The longer and more winding course of the left-sided veins does not allow for as accurate a transmission of hemodynamics. For examination of the right internal jugular vein, the patient should be placed at a 45-degree angle—higher in patients with suspected elevated venous pressures and lower in those with lower venous pressures. The head should be turned slightly leftward, and a light shined at an angle over the neck can help the exam. Although the internal jugular vein itself is not visible, the pulsations from that vessel are transmitted to the skin and can be seen in most cases. The carotid artery lies in close proximity to the jugular vein, and its pulsations can sometimes be seen as well. Therefore, one must be certain one is observing the correct vessel.

Several techniques can help the clinician differentiate carotid and venous pulsations. A normal carotid pulsation pattern usually appears as a smooth and rapid upstroke, whereas a venous pulsation tends to have three "waves," the *a* wave of atrial contract, the *c* wave of the tricuspid valve closure, and the *v* wave of ventricular contraction. Variations in the appearance of these waves can help the clinician diagnose arrhythmia, constriction and tamponade, valvular heart disease, and heart failure. These are further discussed in the following text. The carotid and venous pulsations can further be distinguished by response to attempted compression of the pulsations or vessel. An arterial pulse will not be obliterated by this maneuver, whereas a venous pulse likely will become diminished or absent with compression. The arterial pulsations will not change with changes

in positioning, whereas venous pulsations, as they are essentially reflections of a column of fluid draining into the right heart, will appear higher in the neck/head when a patient is more supine and lower when a patient is more upright. Finally, compression of the abdomen will cause an elevation or increase in prominence of the appearance of a venous wave and will not affect an arterial waveform in the neck.

Both the level of venous pressure and the morphology of the venous waveforms should be noted. Once the pulsations have been located, the vertical distance from the sternal angle (angle of Louis) to the top of the pulsations is determined. Because the right atrium lies about 5 cm vertically below the sternal angle, this number is added to the previous measurement to arrive at an estimated right atrial pressure in centimeters of water. The right atrial pressure is normally 5 to 9 cm H_2O. It can be higher in patients with decompensated heart failure, disorders of the tricuspid valve (regurgitation or stenosis), restrictive cardiomyopathy, or constrictive pericarditis.

With inspiration, negative intrathoracic pressure develops, venous blood drains into the thorax, and venous pressure in the normal patient falls; the opposite occurs during expiration. In a patient with conditions such as decompensated heart failure, constrictive pericarditis, or restrictive cardiomyopathy, this pattern is reversed (Kussmaul sign), and the venous pressure increases with inspiration. When the neck veins are examined, firm pressure should be applied for 10 to 30 seconds to the right upper quadrant over the liver. In a normal patient, this will cause the venous pressure to increase briefly and then return to normal. In the patient with conditions such as heart failure, constrictive pericarditis, or substantial tricuspid regurgitation, the neck veins will reveal a sustained increase in pressure due to passive congestion of the liver. This finding is called hepatojugular reflux.

The normal waveforms of the jugular venous pulse are depicted in Fig 3.1A. The *a* wave results from atrial contraction. The *x* descent results from atrial relaxation after contraction and the pulling of the floor of the right atrium downward with right ventricular contraction. The *c* wave interrupts the *x* descent and is generated by bulging of the cusps of the tricuspid valve into the right atrium during ventricular systole. This occurs at the same time as the carotid pulse. Atrial pressure then increases as a result of venous return with the tricuspid valve closed during ventricular systole; this generates the *v* wave, which is typically smaller than the *a* wave. The *y* descent follows as the tricuspid valve opens and blood flows from the right atrium to the right ventricle during diastole.

Understanding of the normal jugular venous waveforms is paramount, as these waveforms can be altered in different disease states. Abnormalities of these waveforms reflect underlying structural, functional, and electrical abnormalities of the heart (see Fig. 3.1B to G). Elevation of the right atrial pressure leading to jugular venous distention can be found in heart failure (both systolic and diastolic), hypervolemia, superior vena cava syndrome, and valvular disease. The *a* wave is exaggerated in any condition in which a greater resistance to right atrial emptying occurs. Such conditions include pulmonary hypertension, tricuspid stenosis, and right ventricular hypertrophy or failure. *Cannon a waves* occur when the atrium contracts against a closed tricuspid valve, which can occur with complete heart block or any other situation involving AV dissociation. The *a* wave is absent during atrial fibrillation. With significant tricuspid regurgitation, the *v* wave becomes very prominent and may merge with the *c* wave, diminishing or eliminating the *x* descent. With tricuspid stenosis, there is impaired emptying of the right atrium, which leads to an attenuated *y* descent. In pericardial constriction and restrictive

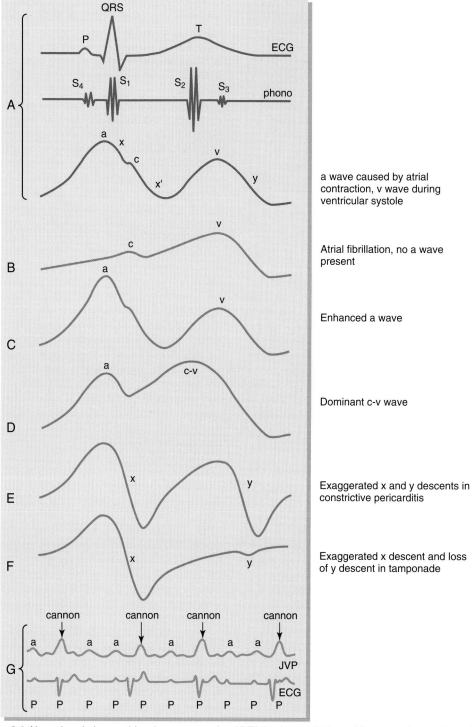

Fig. 3.1 Normal and abnormal jugular venous pulse (JVP) tracings. (A) Normal jugular pulse tracing with simultaneous electrocardiogram (ECG) and phonocardiogram. (B) Loss of the *a* wave in atrial fibrillation. (C) Large *a* wave in tricuspid stenosis. (D) Large *c-v* wave in tricuspid regurgitation. (E) Prominent *x* and *y* descents in constrictive pericarditis. (F) Prominent *x* descent and diminutive *y* descent in pericardial tamponade. (G) JVP tracing and simultaneous ECG during complete heart block demonstrates cannon *a* waves occurring when the atrium contracts against a closed tricuspid valve during ventricular systole. *P*, P waves correlating with atrial contraction; S_1 to S_4, heart sounds.

cardiomyopathy, the *y* descent occurs rapidly and deeply, and the *x* descent may also become more prominent, leading to a waveform with a w-shaped appearance. With pericardial tamponade, the *x* descent becomes very prominent while the *y* descent is diminished or absent.

Examination of Arterial Pressure and Pulse

Arterial blood pressure is measured noninvasively with the use of a sphygmomanometer. Before the blood pressure is taken, the patient ideally should be relaxed, allowed to rest for 5 to 10 minutes in a quiet room, and seated or lying comfortably. The cuff is typically applied

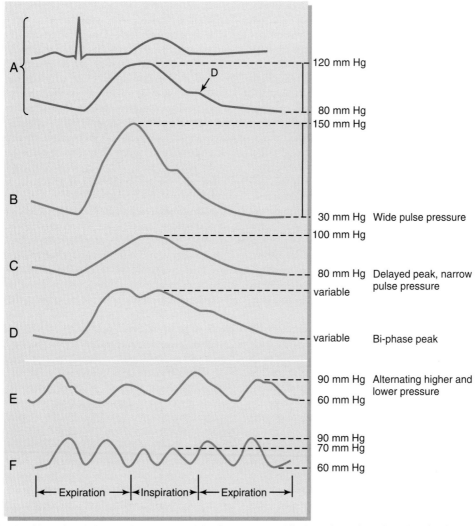

Fig. 3.2 Normal and abnormal carotid arterial pulse contours. (A) Normal arterial pulse with simultaneous electrocardiogram (ECG). The dicrotic wave *(D)* occurs just after aortic valve closure. (B) Wide pulse pressure in aortic insufficiency. (C) Pulsus parvus et tardus (small amplitude with a slow upstroke) associated with aortic stenosis. (D) Bisferiens pulse with two systolic peaks, typical of hypertrophic obstructive cardiomyopathy or aortic insufficiency, especially if concomitant aortic stenosis is present. (E) Pulsus alternans, characteristic of severe left ventricular failure. (F) Paradoxic pulse (systolic pressure decrease >10 mm Hg with inspiration), most characteristic of cardiac tamponade.

to the upper arm, approximately 1 inch above the antecubital fossa. A stethoscope is then used to auscultate under the lower edge of the cuff. The cuff is rapidly inflated to approximately 30 mm Hg above the anticipated systolic pressure and then slowly deflated (at approximately 3 mm Hg/sec) while the examiner listens for the sounds produced by blood entering the previously occluded artery. These sounds are the Korotkoff sounds. The first sound is typically a very clear tapping sound that, when heard, represents the systolic pressure. As the cuff continues to deflate, the sounds will disappear; this point represents the diastolic pressure.

In normal situations, the pressure in both arms is relatively equal. If the pressure is measured in the lower extremities rather than the arms, the systolic pressure is typically 10 to 20 mm Hg higher. If the pressures in the arms are asymmetric, this may suggest atherosclerotic disease involving the aorta, aortic dissection, or obstruction of flow in the subclavian or innominate arteries. The pressure in the lower extremities can be lower than arm pressures in the setting of abdominal aortic, iliac, or femoral disease. Coarctation of the aorta

can also lead to discrepant pressures between the upper and lower extremities. Leg pressure that is more than 20 mm Hg higher than the arm pressure can be found in the patient with significant aortic regurgitation, a finding called Hill's sign. A common mistake in taking the arterial blood pressure involves using a cuff of incorrect size. Use of a small cuff on a large extremity leads to overestimation of pressure. Similarly, use of a large cuff on a smaller extremity underestimates the pressure.

Examination of the arterial pulse in a cardiovascular patient should include palpation of the carotid, radial, brachial, femoral, popliteal, posterior tibial, and dorsalis pedis pulses bilaterally. The carotid pulse most accurately reflects the central aortic pulse. One should note the rhythm, strength, contour, and symmetry of the pulses. A normal arterial pulse (Fig. 3.2A) rises rapidly to a peak in early systole, plateaus, and then falls. The descending limb of the pulse is interrupted by the incisura or dicrotic notch, which is a sharp deflection downward due to closure of the aortic valve. As the pulse moves toward the periphery, the systolic peak is higher and the dicrotic notch is later and less noticeable.

The normal pattern of the arterial pulse can be altered by a variety of cardiovascular diseases (see Fig. 3.2B to F). The amplitude of the pulse increases in conditions such as anemia, pregnancy, thyrotoxicosis, and other states with high cardiac output. Aortic insufficiency, with its resultant increase in pulse pressure (difference between systolic and diastolic pressure), leads to a bounding carotid pulse often referred to as a Corrigan pulse or a water-hammer pulse. The amplitude of the pulse is diminished in low-output states such as heart failure, hypovolemia, and mitral stenosis. Tachycardia, with shorter diastolic filling times, also lowers the pulse amplitude. Aortic stenosis, when significant, leads to a delayed systolic peak and diminished carotid pulse, referred to as *pulsus parvus et tardus*. A bisferiens pulse is most perceptible on palpation of the carotid artery. It is characterized by two systolic peaks and can be found in patients with pure aortic regurgitation. The first peak is the percussion wave, which results from the rapid ejection of a large volume of blood early in systole. The second peak is the tidal wave, which is a reflected wave from the periphery. A bisferiens pulse may also be found in those with hypertrophic cardiomyopathy, in which the initial rapid upstroke of the pulse is interrupted by LVOT obstruction. The reflected wave produces the second impulse. Pulsus alternans is beat-to-beat variation in the pulse and can be found in patients with severe left ventricular systolic dysfunction.

Pulsus paradoxus is an exaggeration of the normal inspiratory fall in systolic pressure. With inspiration, negative intrathoracic pressure is transmitted to the aorta, and systolic pressure typically drops by as much as 10 mm Hg. In pulsus paradoxus, this drop is greater than 10 mm Hg and can be palpable when marked (>20 mm Hg). It is characteristic in cardiac tamponade but can also be seen in constrictive pericarditis, pulmonary embolism, hypovolemic shock, pregnancy, and severe chronic obstructive lung disease.

Because peripheral vascular disease often accompanies CAD, a detailed examination of the peripheral pulses is a crucial part of the physical exam of a patient with known or suspected ischemic heart disease. In addition to the carotid, brachial, radial, femoral, popliteal, dorsalis pedis, and posterior tibial pulses, the abdominal aorta should be palpated. When the abdominal aorta is palpable below the umbilicus, the presence of an abdominal aortic aneurysm is suggested. Impaired blood flow to the lower extremities can cause claudication, a cramping pain located in the buttocks, thigh, calf, or foot, depending on the location of disease. With significant stenosis in the peripheral vasculature, the distal pulses may be significantly reduced or absent. Blood flow in a stenotic artery may be turbulent, creating an audible bruit. With normal aging, the peripheral arteries become less compliant and this change may obscure abnormal findings.

Examination of the Precordium

A complete cardiovascular examination should always include careful inspection and palpation of the chest. Abnormalities of the chest wall including skin findings should be observed. The presence of pectus excavatum is associated with Marfan syndrome and mitral valve prolapse. Pectus carinatum can also be found in patients with Marfan syndrome. Kyphoscoliosis can lead to right-sided heart failure and secondary pulmonary hypertension. One should also assess for visible pulsations, in particular in the regions of the aorta (second right intercostal space and suprasternal notch), pulmonary artery (third left intercostal space), right ventricle (left parasternal region), and left ventricle (fourth to fifth intercostal space at the left midclavicular line). Prominent pulsations in these areas suggest enlargement of these vessels or chambers. Retraction of the left parasternal area can be observed in patients with severe left ventricular hypertrophy, whereas systolic retraction at the apex or in the left axilla (Broadbent sign) is more characteristic of constrictive pericarditis.

Palpation of the precordium is best performed when the patient, with chest exposed, is positioned supine or in a left lateral position with the examiner located on the right side of the patient. The examiner should then place the right hand over the lower left chest wall with fingertips over the region of the cardiac apex and the palm over the region of the right ventricle. The right ventricle itself is typically best palpated in the subxiphoid region with the tip of the index finger. In those patients who have chronic obstructive lung disease, are obese, or are very muscular, the normal cardiac pulsations may not be palpable. In addition, chest wall deformities may make pulsations difficult or impossible to palpate. The normal apical cardiac impulse is a brief and discrete (1 cm in diameter) pulsation located in the fourth to fifth intercostal space along the left midclavicular line. In a patient with a normal heart, this represents the point of maximal impulse (PMI). If the heart cannot be palpated with the patient supine, a left lateral position should be tried. If the left ventricle is enlarged for any reason, the PMI will typically be displaced laterally. With volume overload states such as aortic insufficiency, the left ventricle dilates, resulting in a brisk apical impulse that is increased in amplitude. With pressure overload, as in long-standing hypertension and aortic stenosis, ventricular enlargement is a result of hypertrophy, and the apical impulse is sustained. Often, it is accompanied by a palpable S_4 gallop. Patients with hypertrophic cardiomyopathy can have double or triple apical impulses. Those with apical aneurysm may have an apical impulse that is larger and dyskinetic.

The right ventricle is usually not palpable. However, in those with right ventricular dilation or hypertrophy, which can be related to severe lung disease, pulmonary hypertension, or congenital heart disease, an impulse may be palpated in the left parasternal region. In some cases of severe emphysema, when the distance between the chest wall and right ventricle is increased, the right ventricle is better palpated in the subxiphoid region. With severe pulmonary hypertension, the pulmonary artery may produce a palpable impulse in the second to third intercostal space to the left of the sternum. This may be accompanied by a palpable right ventricle or a palpable pulmonic component of the second heart sound (S_2). An aneurysm of the ascending aorta or arch may result in a palpable pulsation in the suprasternal notch. Thrills are vibratory sensations best palpated with the fingertips; they are manifestations of harsh murmurs caused by such problems as aortic stenosis, hypertrophic cardiomyopathy, and septal defects.

Auscultation
Techniques

Auscultation of the heart is accomplished by use of a stethoscope with dual chest pieces. The diaphragm is ideal for high-frequency sounds, whereas the bell aids in auscultation of low-frequency sounds. When one is listening for low-frequency tones, the bell should be placed gently on the skin with minimal pressure applied. If the bell is applied more firmly, the skin will stretch and higher-frequency sounds will be heard (as when using the diaphragm). Auscultation should ideally be performed in a quiet setting with the patient's chest exposed and the examiner best positioned to the right of the patient. Four major areas of auscultation are evaluated, starting at the apex and moving toward the base of the heart. The mitral valve is best heard at the apex or location of the PMI. Tricuspid valve events are appreciated in or around the left fourth intercostal space adjacent to the sternum. The pulmonary valve is best evaluated in the second left intercostal space. The aortic valve is assessed in the second right intercostal space. These areas should be evaluated from apex to base using the diaphragm and then evaluated again with the bell. Auscultation of the back, the axillae, the right side of the chest, and the supraclavicular areas should also be done. Having the patient perform maneuvers such as leaning forward, exhaling, standing, squatting, and performing a Valsalva maneuver may help to accentuate certain heart sounds (Table 3.4).

Normal Heart Sounds

All heart sounds should be described according to their quality, intensity, and frequency. There are two primary heart sounds heard during auscultation: S_1 and S_2. These are high-frequency sounds caused by closure of the valves. S_1 occurs with the onset of ventricular systole and is caused by closure of the mitral and tricuspid valves. S_2 is caused by closure of the aortic and pulmonic valves and marks the beginning of ventricular diastole. All other heart sounds are timed based on these two sounds.

S_1 has two components, the first of which (M_1) is usually louder, heard best at the apex, and caused by closure of the mitral valve. The second component (T_1), which is softer and thought to be related to closure of the tricuspid valve, is heard best at the lower left sternal border. Although there can be two components, S_1 is typically heard as a single sound. S_2 also has two components, which typically can be easily distinguished. A_2, the component caused by closure of the aortic valve, is usually louder and heard earlier and is best heard at the right upper sternal border. P_2, caused by closure of the pulmonic valve, is recognized best over the left second intercostal space. With expiration, a normal S_2 is perceived as a single sound. With inspiration, however, venous return to the right heart is augmented, and the increased capacitance of the pulmonary vascular bed results in a delay in pulmonic valve closure. A slight decline in pulmonary venous return to the left ventricle leads to earlier aortic valve closure. Therefore, physiologic splitting of S_2, with A_2 preceding P_2 during inspiration, is a normal finding.

Additional heart sounds can at times be heard in normal individuals. A third heart sound can sometimes be heard in healthy children and young adults. This is referred to as a physiologic S_3, which is rarely heard after the age of 40 years in a normal individual. A fourth heart sound is caused by forceful atrial contraction into a noncompliant ventricle; it is rarely audible in normal young patients but is relatively common in older individuals.

Murmurs are auditory vibrations generated by high flow across a normal valve or normal flow across an abnormal valve or structure. Murmurs that occur early in systole and are soft and brief in duration are not typically pathologic and are termed *innocent murmurs*. These usually are caused by flow across normal left ventricular or right ventricular outflow tracts and are found in children and young adults. Some systolic murmurs may be associated with high-flow states such as fever, anemia, thyroid disease, and pregnancy and are not innocent, although they are not typically associated with structural heart disease. They are called *physiologic murmurs* because of their association with altered physiologic states. All diastolic murmurs are pathologic.

Abnormal Heart Sounds

Abnormalities in S_1 and S_2 are related to either intensity (Table 3.5) or respiratory splitting (Table 3.6). S_1 is accentuated with tachycardia and with short PR intervals, whereas it is softer in the setting of a long PR interval. S_1 varies in intensity if the relationship between atrial and ventricular systole varies. In those patients with atrial fibrillation, atrial filling and emptying is not consistent because of the variable HR leading to beat-to-beat changes in the intensity of S_1. This also can occur with heart block or AV dissociation. In early mitral stenosis, S_1 is often accentuated, but with severe stenosis, there is decreased leaflet excursion and S_1 is diminished in intensity or altogether absent (Figs. 3.3 and 3.4). As previously mentioned, splitting of S_1 is not frequently heard. However, it is more apparent in conditions that delay closure of the tricuspid valve, including right bundle branch block and Ebstein's anomaly (Audio Clip 3.1, Ebstein Abnormalities).

TABLE 3.4 Effects of Physiologic Maneuvers on Auscultatory Events

Maneuver	Major Physiologic Effects	Useful Auscultatory Changes
Respiration	↑ Venous return with inspiration	↑ Right heart murmurs and gallops with inspiration; splitting of S_2 (see Fig. 3.3)
Valsalva (initial ↑ BP, phase I; followed by ↓ BP, phase II)	↓ BP, ↓ venous return, ↓ LV size (phase II)	↑ HCM ↓ AS, MR MVP click earlier in systole; murmur prolongs
Standing	↓ Venous return ↓ LV size	↑ HCM ↓ AS, MR MVP click earlier in systole; murmur prolongs
Squatting	↑ Venous return ↑ Systemic vascular resistance ↑ LV size	↑ AS, MR, AI ↓ HCM MVP click delayed; murmur shortens
Isometric exercise (e.g., handgrip)	↑ Arterial pressure ↑ Cardiac output	↑ Gallops ↑ MR, AI, MS ↓ AS, HCM
Post PVC or prolonged R-R interval	↑ Ventricular filling ↑ Contractility	↑ AS Little change in MR
Amyl nitrate	↓ Arterial pressure ↑ Cardiac output ↓ LV size	↑ HCM, AS, MS ↓ AI, MR, Austin Flint murmur MVP click earlier in systole; murmur prolongs
Phenylephrine	↑ Arterial pressure ↑ Cardiac output ↓ LV size	↑ MR, AI ↓ AS, HCM MVP click delayed; murmur shortens

↑, Increased intensity; ↓, decreased intensity; *AI*, aortic insufficiency; *AS*, aortic stenosis; *BP*, blood pressure; *HCM*, hypertrophic cardiomyopathy; *LV*, left ventricle; *MR*, mitral regurgitation; *MS*, mitral stenosis; *MVP*, mitral valve prolapse; *PVC*, premature ventricular contraction; *R-R*, interval between the R waves on an electrocardiogram.

TABLE 3.5 Abnormal Intensity of Heart Sounds

	S_1	A_2	P_2
Loud	Short PR interval Mitral stenosis with pliable valve	Systemic hypertension Aortic dilation Coarctation of the aorta	Pulmonary hypertension Thin chest wall
Soft	Long PR interval Mitral regurgitation Poor left ventricular function Mitral stenosis with rigid valve Thick chest wall	Calcific aortic stenosis Aortic regurgitation	Valvular or subvalvular pulmonic stenosis
Varying	Atrial fibrillation Heart block	—	—

A_2, Component of second heart sound caused by closure of aortic valve; P_2, component of second heart sound caused by closure of pulmonic valve; S_1, first heart sound.

S_2 can be accentuated in the presence of hypertension, when the aortic component will be louder, or in pulmonary hypertension, when the pulmonic component will be enhanced. In the setting of severe aortic or pulmonic stenosis, leaflet excursion of the respective valves is reduced and the intensity of S_2 is significantly diminished. It may become absent altogether if the accompanying murmur obscures what remains of S_2.

There are several patterns of abnormal splitting of S_2. S_2 can remain single throughout respiration if either A_2 or P_2 is not present or if they occur simultaneously. A_2 can be absent, as previously mentioned, with severe aortic stenosis. P_2 can be absent with a number of congenital abnormalities of the pulmonic valve. Splitting may be persistent throughout the respiratory cycle if A_2 occurs early or if P_2 is delayed, as in the presence of right bundle branch block. In that case, splitting is always present but the interval between A_2 and P_2 varies somewhat. In fixed splitting, the interval between A_2 and P_2 is consistently wide and unaffected by respiration. This finding is observed in the presence of an ostium secundum atrial septal defect or right ventricular failure. Paradoxical splitting of S_2 occurs when P_2 precedes A_2. This leads to splitting with expiration and a single S_2 with inspiration. It is commonly found in situations of delayed electrical activation of the left ventricle, as in patients with left bundle branch block or right ventricular pacing. It can also be seen with prolonged mechanical contraction of the left ventricle, as in patients with aortic stenosis or hypertrophic cardiomyopathy.

The third heart sound, S_3, is a low-pitched sound heard best at the apex in mid diastole. Because it is low pitched, it is best recognized with use of the bell on the stethoscope. As stated previously, S_3 can be physiologic in children but is pathologic in older individuals and often associated with underlying cardiac disease. An S_3 occurs during the rapid filling phase of diastole and is thought to indicate a sudden limitation of the expansion of the left ventricle. This can be seen in cases of volume overload or tachycardia. Maneuvers that increase venous return accentuate an S_3, whereas those that reduce venous return diminish the intensity. The fourth heart sound, S_4, is also a low-frequency sound, but in contrast to S_3, it is heard in late diastole, just before S_1. The S_4 gallop occurs as a result of active ejection of blood into a noncompliant left ventricle. Therefore, when atrial contraction is absent, such as in atrial fibrillation, an S_4 cannot be heard. This heart sound is also best recognized with the use of a bell at the apex. It can be heard in patients with left ventricular hypertrophy, acute myocardial infarction,

or hyperdynamic left ventricle. At times, an S_3 and an S_4 can be heard in the same patient. In tachycardic states, the two sounds can fuse in mid diastole to form a summation gallop.

S_3 and S_4 gallops are heard in mid diastole and late diastole, respectively. There are other abnormal sounds that can be heard during systole and early diastole. *Ejection sounds* are typically heard in early systole and involve the aortic and pulmonic valves. These are high-frequency sounds that can be heard with a diaphragm shortly after S_1.

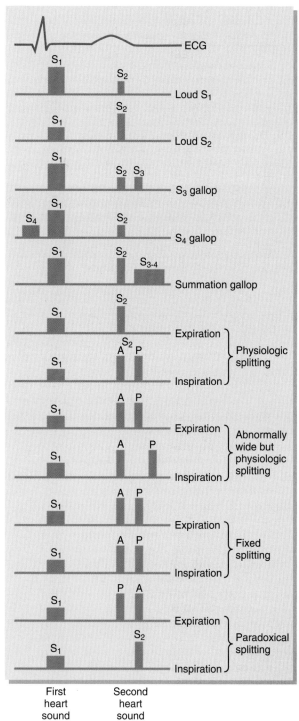

Fig. 3.3 Abnormal heart sounds can be related to abnormal intensity, abnormal presence of a gallop rhythm, or abnormal splitting of the second heart sound (S_2) with respiration. A_2, Component of S_2 caused by closure of aortic valve; *ECG*, electrocardiogram; P_2, component of S_2 caused by closure of pulmonic valve.

TABLE 3.6	Abnormal Splitting of S_2		
Single S_2	Widely Split S_2 With Normal Respiratory Variation	Fixed Split S_2	Paradoxically Split S_2
Pulmonic stenosis	Right bundle branch block	Atrial septal defect	Left bundle branch block
Systemic hypertension	Left ventricular pacing	Severe right ventricular dysfunction	Right ventricular pacing
Coronary artery disease	Pulmonic stenosis		Angina, myocardial infarction
	Pulmonary embolism		
Any condition that can lead to paradoxical splitting of S_2	Idiopathic dilation of the pulmonary artery		Aortic stenosis
	Mitral regurgitation		Hypertrophic cardiomyopathy
	Ventricular septal defect		Aortic regurgitation

S_2, Second heart sound.

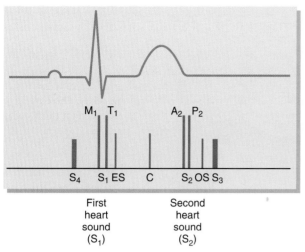

Fig. 3.4 The relationship of extra heart sounds to the normal first (S_1) and second (S_2) heart sounds. S_1 is composed of the mitral (M_1) and tricuspid (T_1) closing sounds, although it is frequently perceived as a single sound. S_2 is composed of the aortic (A_2) and pulmonic (P_2) closing sounds, which are usually easily distinguished. A fourth heart sound (S_4) is soft and low pitched and precedes S_1. A pulmonic or aortic ejection sound (ES) occurs shortly after S_1. The systolic click (C) of mitral valve prolapse may be heard in mid systole or late systole. The opening snap (OS) of mitral stenosis is high pitched and occurs shortly after S_2. A tumor plop or pericardial knock occurs at the same time and can be confused with an OS or an S_3, which is lower in pitch and occurs slightly later.

In figure labels: M₁ T₁, A₂ P₂, First heart sound (S_1), Second heart sound (S_2), S_4, S_1 ES, C, S_2 OS S_3

TABLE 3.7	Grading System for Intensity of Murmurs	
Grade	**Description**
1	Barely audible murmur
2	Murmur of medium intensity
3	Loud murmur, no thrill
4	Loud murmur with thrill
5	Very loud murmur; stethoscope must be on the chest to hear it; may be heard posteriorly
6	Murmur audible with stethoscope off the chest

These sounds are longer than individual heart sounds and should be described on the basis of their location, frequency, intensity, quality, duration, shape, and timing in the cardiac cycle. The intensity of a given murmur is typically graded on a scale of 1 to 6 (Table 3.7). Murmurs of grade 4 or higher are associated with palpable thrills. The intensity or loudness of a murmur does not necessarily correlate with the severity of disease. For example, a murmur can be quite harsh when it is associated with a moderate degree of aortic stenosis. If stenosis is critical, however, the flow across the valve is diminished and the murmur becomes rather quiet. In the presence of a large atrial septal defect, flow is almost silent, whereas flow through a small ventricular septal defect is typically associated with a loud murmur.

The frequency of a murmur can be high or low; higher-frequency murmurs are more correlated with high velocity of flow at the site of turbulence. It is also important to notice the configuration or shape of a murmur, such as crescendo, crescendo-decrescendo, decrescendo, or plateau (Fig. 3.5). The quality of a murmur (e.g., harsh, blowing, rumbling) and the pattern of radiation are also helpful in diagnosis. Physical maneuvers can sometimes help clarify the nature of a particular murmur (see Table 3.4).

Murmurs can be divided into three different categories (Table 3.8). Systolic murmurs begin with or after S_1 and end with or before S_2. Diastolic murmurs begin with or after S_2 and end with or before S_1. Continuous murmurs begin in systole and continue through diastole. Murmurs can result from abnormalities on the left or right side of the heart or in the great vessels. Right-sided murmurs become louder with inspiration because of increased venous return. This can help differentiate them from left-sided murmurs, which are unaffected by respiration.

Systolic murmurs should be further differentiated based on timing (i.e., early systolic, midsystolic, late systolic, and holosystolic murmurs). Early systolic murmurs begin with S_1, are decrescendo, and end typically before mid systole. Ventricular septal defects and acute mitral regurgitation may lead to early systolic murmurs. Midsystolic murmurs begin after S_1 and end before S_2, often in a crescendo-decrescendo shape. They are typically caused by obstruction to left ventricular outflow, accelerated flow through the aortic or pulmonic valve, or enlargement of the aortic root or pulmonary trunk. Aortic stenosis, when less than severe in degree, causes a midsystolic murmur that may be harsh and may radiate to the carotids. Pulmonic stenosis leads to a similar murmur that does not radiate to the carotid arteries but may change with inspiration. The murmur of hypertrophic cardiomyopathy may be mistaken for aortic stenosis; however, it does not radiate to the carotids and becomes exaggerated with diminished venous return. Innocent or benign murmurs may also occur as a result of aortic valve sclerosis, vibrations of a left ventricular false tendon, or vibration of normal pulmonary leaflets. They are generally less

Ejection sounds are caused by the opening of abnormal valves to their full extent, such as with a bicuspid aortic valve or congenital pulmonic stenosis. They are frequently followed by a typical ejection murmur of aortic or pulmonic stenosis. Ejection sounds can also be heard with systemic or pulmonary hypertension, in which case the exact mechanism is not clear.

Midsystolic to late systolic sounds are called *ejection clicks*. They are most commonly associated with mitral valve prolapse. They are also high pitched and easily auscultated with the diaphragm. The click occurs because of maximal displacement of the prolapsed mitral leaflet into the left atrium and resultant tensing of chordae and redundant leaflets (Audio Clip 3.2, Mitral Valve Prolapse). The click is usually followed by a typical murmur of mitral regurgitation. Any maneuver that decreases venous return will cause the click to occur earlier in systole, whereas increasing ventricular volume will delay the click (see Table 3.4).

The opening of abnormal mitral or tricuspid valves can be heard in early diastole. This *opening snap* is most frequently associated with rheumatic mitral stenosis. It is heard if the valve leaflets remain pliable and is generated when the leaflets abruptly dome during diastole. The frequency, intensity, and timing of the click have diagnostic significance. For example, the shorter the interval between S_2 and the opening snap, the more severe the degree of mitral stenosis, because this is a reflection of higher left atrial pressure. The *pericardial knock* of constrictive pericarditis and *tumor plop* generated by an atrial myxoma also occur in early diastole and may be confused with an opening snap. They can typically be differentiated from an S_3 gallop because they are higher-frequency sounds.

Murmurs

Murmurs are a series of auditory vibrations generated by either abnormal blood flow across a normal cardiac structure or normal flow across an abnormal cardiac structure, both of which result in turbulent flow.

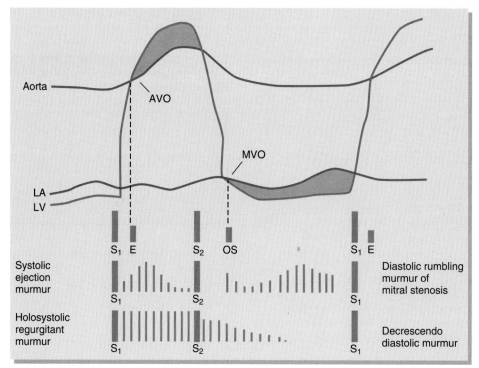

Fig. 3.5 Abnormal sounds and murmurs associated with valvular dysfunction displayed simultaneously with left atrial (LA), left ventricular (LV), and aortic pressure tracings. The *shaded areas* represent pressure gradients across the aortic valve during systole or across mitral valve during diastole; they are characteristic of aortic stenosis and mitral stenosis, respectively. *AVO,* Aortic valve opening; *E,* ejection click of the aortic valve; *MVO,* mitral valve opening; *OS,* opening snap of the mitral valve; S_1, first heart sound; S_2, second heart sound.

TABLE 3.8 Classification of Heart Murmurs

Class	Description	Characteristic Lesions
Systolic		
Ejection	Begins in early systole; may extend to mid or late systole	Valvular, supravalvular, and subvalvular aortic stenoses
	Crescendo-decrescendo pattern	Hypertrophic cardiomyopathy
	Often harsh in quality	Pulmonic stenosis
	Begins after S_1 and ends before S_2	Aortic or pulmonary artery dilation
		Malformed but nonobstructive aortic valve
		↑ Transvalvular flow (e.g., aortic regurgitation, hyperkinetic states, atrial septal defect, physiologic flow murmur)
Holosystolic	Extends throughout systole[a]	Mitral regurgitation
	Relatively uniform in intensity	Tricuspid regurgitation
		Ventricular septal defect
Late	Variable onset and duration, often preceded by a nonejection click	Mitral valve prolapse
Diastolic		
Early	Begins with A_2 or P_2	Aortic regurgitation
	Decrescendo pattern with variable duration	Pulmonic regurgitation
	Often high pitched, blowing	
Mid	Begins after S_2, often after an opening snap	Mitral stenosis
	Low-pitched *rumble* heard best with bell of stethoscope	Tricuspid stenosis
	Louder with exercise and left lateral position	↑ Flow across atrioventricular valves (e.g., mitral regurgitation, tricuspid regurgitation, atrial septal defect)
	Loudest in early diastole	
Late	Presystolic accentuation of mid-diastolic murmur	Mitral stenosis
		Tricuspid stenosis
Continuous		
	Systolic and diastolic components	Patent ductus arteriosus
	"Machinery murmurs"	Coronary atrioventricular fistula
		Ruptured sinus of Valsalva aneurysm into right atrium or ventricle
		Mammary soufflé
		Venous hum

A_2, Component of S_2 caused by closure of aortic valve; P_2, component of S_2 caused by closure of pulmonic valve; S_1, first heart sound; S_2, second heart sound.
[a]Encompasses both S_1 and S_2.

harsh and shorter in duration. High-flow states such as those found in patients with fever, during pregnancy, or with anemia may also lead to midsystolic "flow" murmurs.

Holosystolic murmurs begin with S_1 and end with S_2; the classic examples are the murmurs associated with mitral regurgitation and tricuspid regurgitation. They may also occur with ventricular septal defects and patent ductus arteriosus. Late systolic murmurs begin in mid to late systole and end with S_2. They can be characteristic of more severe aortic stenosis and are also typical of murmurs associated with mitral valve prolapse.

Diastolic murmurs are also classified by timing (i.e., early diastolic, mid diastolic, and late diastolic). Early diastolic murmurs begin with S_2 and can result from aortic or pulmonic regurgitation; they are usually decrescendo in shape. Shorter and quieter murmurs typically represent an acute process or mild regurgitation, whereas longer-lasting and louder murmurs are likely due to more severe regurgitation. Mid-diastolic murmurs begin after S_2 and are usually caused by mitral or tricuspid stenosis. They are low pitched and are often referred to as *diastolic rumbles*. Because they are of low frequency, they are better auscultated with the bell of the stethoscope. Similar murmurs can be heard with obstructing atrial myxomas. Severe chronic aortic insufficiency can lead to premature closure of the mitral valve, causing a mid-diastolic rumble called an Austin-Flint murmur. Late diastolic murmurs occur immediately before S_1 and reflect presystolic accentuation of the mid-diastolic murmurs resulting from augmented mitral or tricuspid flow after atrial contraction.

Continuous murmurs begin with S_1 and last though part or all of diastole. They are generated by continuous flow from a vessel or chamber with high pressure into a vessel or chamber with lower pressure. They are referred to as *machinery murmurs* and are caused by aortopulmonary connections such as a patent ductus arteriosus, AV malformations, or disturbances of flow in arteries or veins.

Other Cardiac Sounds

Pericardial rubs occur in the setting of pericarditis and are coarse, scratching sounds similar to rubbing leather. They are typically heard best at the left sternal border with the patient leaning forward and holding the breath at end-expiration. A classic pericardial rub has three components: atrial systole, ventricular systole, and ventricular diastole. One might also hear a pleural rub caused by localized irritation of surrounding pleura. Continuous venous murmurs, or *venous hums*, are almost always present in children. They can be heard in adults during pregnancy, in the setting of anemia, or with thyrotoxicosis. They are heard best at the base of the neck with the patient's head turned to the opposite direction.

Prosthetic Heart Sounds

Prosthetic heart valves produce characteristic findings on auscultation. Bioprosthetic valves produce sounds that are similar to those of native heart valves, but they are typically smaller than the valves that they replace and therefore have an associated murmur. Mechanical valves have crisp, high-pitched sounds related to valve opening and closure. In most modern valves such as the St. Jude valve, which is a bileaflet mechanical valve, the closure sound is louder than the opening sound.

An ejection murmur is common. If there is a change in murmur or in the intensity of the mechanical valve closure sound, dysfunction of the valve should be suspected.

For a deeper discussion of this topic, please see Chapter 45, ❖ "Approach to the Patient with Possible Cardiovascular Disease," in *Goldman-Cecil Medicine*, 26th Edition.

SUGGESTED READINGS

Agency for Healthcare Research and Quality, U.S. Department of Health and Human Services: Total expenses and percent distribution for selected conditions by type of service: United States, 2008. Medical Expenditure Panel Survey: Household Component Summary Tables. Available at: http://www.meps.ahrq.gov/mepsweb/data_stats/quick_tables_search.jsp?component=1&subcomponent=0. Accessed August 5, 2014.

Calkins H, Shyr Y, Frumin H, et al: The value of the clinical history in the differentiation of syncope due to ventricular tachycardia, atrioventricular block, and neurocardiogenic syncope, Am J Med 98:365–373, 1995.

Go AS: The epidemiology of atrial fibrillation in elderly persons: the tip of the iceberg, Am J Geriatr Cardiol 14:56–61, 2005.

Goldman L, Ausiello D: Cecil Medicine: part VIII. Cardiovascular disease, Philadelphia, 2012, Saunders.

Heart Disease Fact Sheet. CDC Division for Heart Disease and Stroke Prevention. https://www.cdc.gov/dhdsp/data_statistics/fact_sheets/fs_heart_disease.htm.

Hirsch AT, Criqui MH, Treat-Jacobson D, et al: Peripheral arterial disease: detection, awareness, and treatment in primary care, JAMA 286:1317–1324, 2001.

Hoffman JI, Kaplan S, Liberthson RR: Prevalence of congenital heart disease, Am Heart J 147:425–439, 2004.

National Heart, Lung and Blood Institute, National Institutes of Health. Unpublished tabulations of National Vital Statistics System mortality data. 2008. Available at: http://www.cdc.gov/nchs/nvss/mortality_public_use_data.htm. Accessed August 5, 2014.

National Heart, Lung and Blood Institute, National Institutes of Health, Unpublished tabulations of National Hospital Discharge Survey, 2009. Available at http://www.cdc.gov/nchs/nhds/nhds_questionnaires.htm. Accessed August 5, 2014.

National Heart, Lung and Blood Institute. Unpublished tabulations of National Health Interview Survey, 1965-2010. Available at: http://www.cdc.gov/nchs/nhis/nhis_questionnaires.htm. Accessed August 5, 2014.

National Heart, Lung and Blood Institute, National Institutes of Health. Morbidity and mortality: 2012 Chart book on cardiovascular, lung, and blood diseases. Available at https://www.nhlbi.nih.gov/research/reports/2012-mortality-chart-book.htm. Accessed September 26, 2014.

National Vital Statistics System, Centers for Disease Control and Prevention: Mortality tables. Available at http://www.cdc.gov/nchs/nvss/mortality_tables.htm. Accessed August 5, 2014.

Pickering TG, Hall JE, Appel LJ, et al: Recommendations for blood pressure measurement in humans and experimental animals: part 1. Blood pressure measurement in humans: a statement for professionals from the Subcommittee of Professional and Public Education of the American Heart Association Council on High Blood Pressure Research, Circulation 111:697–716, 2005.

4

Diagnostic Tests and Procedures in the Patient With Cardiovascular Disease

Esseim Sharma, Alan R. Morrison

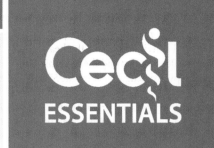

ELECTROCARDIOGRAPHY

The electrocardiogram (ECG) is one of the most basic yet powerful diagnostic tools in cardiovascular medicine. It is critical in the investigation of cardiac arrhythmias, myocardial infarction, and pericardial disease, and may provide additional insight into a variety of other cardiac and noncardiac conditions.

The ECG is a simple and noninvasive procedure that makes use of electrodes placed on the skin of the chest at specific locations in order to measure the electrical activity of the heart. The output is a scroll of wave forms represented as a temporal sequence of deflections on the ECG (Fig. 4.1). The horizontal axis of the graph paper represents time, and at a standard paper speed of 25 mm/second, which is also known as the sweep speed, each small box (1 mm) represents 0.04 seconds, and each large box (5 mm) represents 0.20 seconds. The vertical axis represents voltage or amplitude (1 mm = 0.1 mV). Because the standard ECG demonstrates a 10-second window of time, the heart rate can be calculated by simply counting the number of QRS complexes and multiplying by 6. Alternatively, the heart rate can be estimated by dividing the number of large boxes between complexes (i.e., R-R interval) into 300.

Lead Positioning

The standard ECG consists of 12 leads: six limb leads (I, II, III, aVR, aVL, and aVF) and six chest or precordial leads (V_1 to V_6) (Fig. 4.2). The limb leads view the electrical activity of the heart in the vertical plane, while the precordial leads view the horizontal plane. The electrical activity recorded in each lead represents the direction and magnitude (i.e., vector) of the electrical force as seen from that lead position. Electrical activity directed toward a particular lead is represented as an upward (positive) deflection, and electrical activity directed away from a particular lead is represented as a downward (negative) deflection. Accurate lead placement is essential to reliable interpretation of the ECG.

The limb leads consist of bipolar leads (I, II, and III) and unipolar or augmented leads (leads aVR, aVL, and aVF). The bipolar leads represent electrical forces between the two leads, while augmented leads represent the electrical forces towards the lead. Lead I measures electrical activity between the right and left arms (left arm positive), lead II between the right arm and left leg (left leg positive), and lead III between the left arm and left leg (left leg positive). A vector perpendicular to the limb leads would be isoelectric. In aVR, aVL, and aVF, the vector is positive if electrical forces are directed toward the right arm for aVR, left arm for aVL, and left leg for aVF. Taken together, the six limb leads form a frontal plane of 30-degree arc intervals (Fig. 4.3).

The six standard precordial leads (V_1 to V_6) are attached to the anterior chest wall and are also unipolar leads. Lead placement should be as follows: V_1: fourth intercostal space, right sternal border; V_2: fourth intercostal space, left sternal border; V_3: midway between V_2 and V_4; V_4: fifth intercostal space, left midclavicular line; V_5: level with V_4, left anterior axillary line; V_6: level with V_4, left midaxillary line.

Nonstandard lead configurations can be used in specific clinical scenarios. In patients where there is concern for right ventricular infarction, standard V_1 and V_2 leads are switched, and V_{3R} to V_{6R} are placed at locations on the right chest wall in a mirror image of the standard left-sided chest leads. Posterior leads may be used to increase the sensitivity for diagnosing lateral and posterior wall infarction or ischemia—areas that are often deemed to be *electrically silent* on traditional 12-lead ECGs. To do this, six additional leads are placed in the fifth intercostal space continuing posteriorly from the position of V_6. Shifting the right precordial leads (V_1-V_3) superiorly to the second intercostal space can be used to unmask Brugada syndrome.

Electrocardiographic Intervals

In the normal heart, the electrical impulse originates in the sinoatrial (SA) node, located superiorly in the right atrium, and is conducted through the atria. Given that depolarization of the SA node is too weak to be detected on the surface ECG, the first, low-amplitude deflection on the surface ECG represents a summation atrial vector and is called the *P wave*. The P wave has an electrical axis that moves in sum toward the AV node, generally downward and to the left. The interval between the onset of the P wave and the next rapid deflection (QRS complex) is known as the *PR interval*. It primarily represents the time taken for the impulse to travel through the atrioventricular (AV) node. The normal PR segment ranges from 0.12 to 0.20 seconds. A PR interval greater than 0.20 seconds defines first-degree AV nodal block.

After the wave of depolarization has moved through the AV node, the ventricular myocardium is depolarized in a sequence of four phases. The interventricular septum depolarizes from left to right. This phase is followed by depolarization of the right ventricle and inferior wall of the left ventricle, then the apex and central portions of the left ventricle, and finally the base and the posterior wall of the left ventricle. Ventricular depolarization results in a high-amplitude complex on the surface ECG known as the *QRS complex*. The first downward deflection of this complex is the Q wave, the first upward deflection is the R wave, and the subsequent downward deflection is the S wave. In some individuals, a second upward deflection may occur after the S wave, and it is called *R prime* (R'). Normal duration of the QRS complex is less than 0.10 second. Complexes longer than 0.12 seconds in duration are usually secondary to some form of interventricular conduction delay, including right or left bundle branch block.

The isoelectric segment after the QRS complex is the ST segment, which represents a brief period during which relatively little electrical activity occurs in the heart. The junction between the end of the QRS complex and the beginning of the ST segment is the J point. The upward deflection after the ST segment is the T wave, which represents ventricular repolarization. The QT interval, which reflects the duration and transmural gradient of ventricular depolarization and repolarization, is measured from the onset of the QRS complex to the end of the T wave. The observed QT (QT_{ob}) interval varies with heart rate, but for rates between 60 and 100 beats/minute, the normal QT interval ranges from 0.35 to 0.44 seconds. For heart rates outside this range, the QT interval can be corrected (QT_c) using the following formula (with R-R interval in seconds):

$$QTc = \frac{QTob}{\sqrt{R - R\ interval}}$$

Importantly, patients with interventricular conduction delay due to the presence of bundle branch blocks or pacing will have prolonged QT intervals due to the dispersion of ventricular repolarization, which is not necessarily pathologic. Adjustment of the QT interval in these cases remains controversial.

The TP segment is the isoelectric interval that follows the end of the T wave and lasts till the beginning of the P wave. Because it represents an electrically silent portion of the ECG, the TP segment can be used to measure excursions of other segments, such as the ST or PR segments, to determine the presence of elevation or depression. In some individuals, the T wave may be closely followed by a U wave (0.5 mm deflection, not shown in Fig. 4.1), which can be seen for a variety of reasons, including hypokalemia and central nervous system abnormalities.

Axis

The cardiac axis refers to the overall direction of myocardial depolarization measured in the vertical plane and provides clinically useful information. Though the axis can be calculated for any of the ECG segments mentioned above, the mean QRS axis is the most clinically useful.

Fig. 4.3 illustrates the axial reference system, a reconstruction of the Einthoven triangle, and the polarity of each of the six limb leads of the standard ECG. The normal QRS axis ranges from −30 to +90 degrees. An axis more negative than −30 defines left axis deviation, and an axis greater than +90 defines right axis deviation. Extreme axis deviation is present when the mean QRS axis is between −90 and +180 degrees. A positive QRS complex in leads I and aVF suggests a normal QRS axis between 0 and 90 degrees.

While the precordial leads are not useful in determining cardiac axis, they are helpful in determining the direction of cardiac activation in the horizontal plane. Normally, a small R wave occurs in lead V_1, reflecting septal depolarization, along with a deep S wave, reflecting predominantly left ventricular activation. From V_1 to V_6, the R wave becomes larger (and the S wave smaller) because the predominant forces directed at these leads originate from the left ventricle. The transition from a predominant S wave to a predominant R wave usually occurs between leads V_3 and V_4. A delay in this transition is termed "poor R wave progression" and can be seen in patients with prior anterior myocardial infarctions, among other conditions. In patients with ventricular arrhythmias, the pattern of S and R waves in the precordial leads is essential in localizing the foci of the arrhythmia.

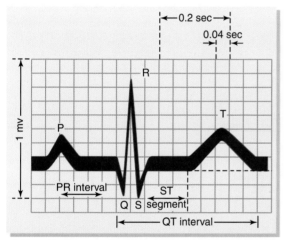

Fig. 4.1 Normal electrocardiographic complex with labeling of waves and intervals.

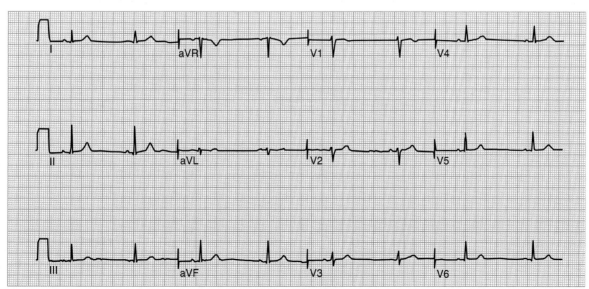

Fig. 4.2 Normal 12-lead electrocardiogram.

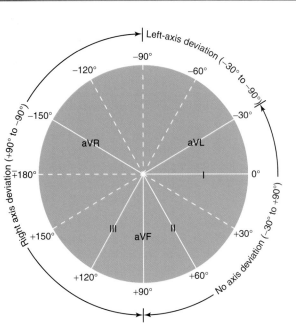

Fig. 4.3 Hexaxial reference figure for frontal plane axis determination, indicating values for abnormal left and right QRS axis deviations.

ABNORMAL ELECTROCARDIOGRAPHIC PATTERNS

Chamber Abnormalities and Ventricular Hypertrophy

Because of the downward and leftward vector direction, the P wave is normally upright in leads I, II, and aVF, inverted in aVR, and biphasic in V_1. Left atrial abnormality (i.e., enlargement, hypertrophy, or increased wall stress) is characterized by a wide P wave in lead II (0.12 second) and a deeply inverted terminal component in lead V_1 (able to contain one small box or 1 mm²). Right atrial abnormality is identified when the P waves in the limb leads are tall and peaked and at least 2.5 mm high and (able to contain two stacked small boxes).

Left ventricular hypertrophy may result in increased QRS voltage, slight widening of the QRS complex, late intrinsicoid deflection, left axis deviation, and abnormalities of the ST-T segments (Fig. 4.4A). Multiple criteria with various degrees of sensitivity and specificity for detecting left ventricular hypertrophy are available. The most frequently used criteria are given in Table 4.1.

Right ventricular hypertrophy is characterized by tall R waves in leads V_1 through V_3; deep S waves in leads I, aVL, V_5, and V_6; and right axis deviation (see Fig. 4.4B). The R wave is greater than 7 mm and the R-S ratio is greater than 1 in lead V_1. Other causes of a tall R-wave in V_1 must be excluded, including posterior wall myocardial infarction,

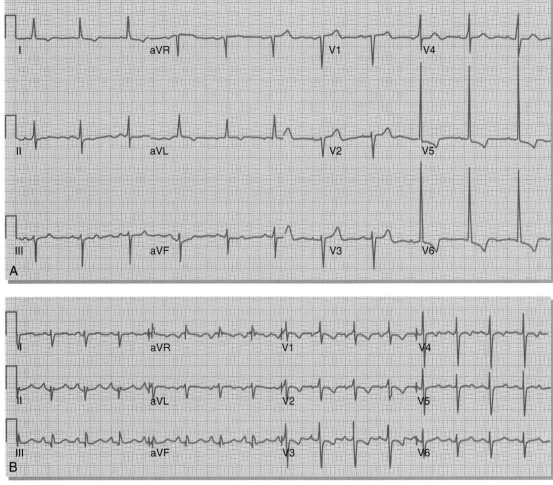

Fig. 4.4 (A) Left ventricular hypertrophy as seen on an electrocardiographic recording. Characteristic findings include increased QRS voltage in precordial leads (i.e., deep S in lead V_2 and tall R in lead V_5) and downsloping ST depression and T-wave inversion in lateral precordial leads (i.e., strain pattern) and leftward axis. (B) Right ventricular hypertrophy with tall R wave in right precordial leads, downsloping ST depression in precordial leads (i.e., RV strain), right axis deviation, and evidence of right atrial enlargement.

TABLE 4.1 Electrocardiographic Manifestations of Atrial Abnormalities and Ventricular Hypertrophy

Left Atrial Abnormality
P-wave duration ≥0.12 second
Notched, slurred P wave in leads I and II
Biphasic P wave in lead V_1 with a wide, deep, negative terminal component

Right Atrial Abnormality
P-wave duration ≤0.11 second
Tall, peaked P waves of ≥2.5 mm in leads II, III, and aVF

Left Ventricular Hypertrophy
Voltage criteria
R wave in lead aVL ≥12 mm
R wave in lead I ≥15 mm
S wave in lead V_1 or V_2 + R wave in lead V_5 or V_6 ≥35 mm
Depressed ST segments with inverted T waves in the lateral leads
Left axis deviation
QRS duration ≥0.09 second
Left atrial enlargement

Right Ventricular Hypertrophy
Tall R waves over right precordium (R-to-S ratio in lead V_1 >1.0)
Right axis deviation
Depressed ST segments with inverted T waves in leads V_1 to V_3
Normal QRS duration (if no right bundle branch block)
Right atrial enlargement

TABLE 4.2 Electrocardiographic Manifestations of Fascicular and Bundle Branch Blocks

Left Anterior Fascicular Block
QRS duration ≤0.1 second
Left axis deviation (more negative than −45 degrees)
rS pattern in leads II, III, and aVF
qR pattern in leads I and aVL

Right Posterior Fascicular Block
QRS duration ≤0.1 second
Right axis deviation (+90 degrees or greater)
qR pattern in leads II, III, and aVF
rS pattern in leads I and aVL
Exclusion of other causes of right axis deviation (e.g., chronic obstructive pulmonary disease, right ventricular hypertrophy)

Left Bundle Branch Block
QRS duration ≥0.12 second
Broad, slurred, or notched R waves in lateral leads (I, aVL, V_5, and V_6)
QS or rS pattern in anterior precordium leads (V_1 and V_2)
ST-T-wave vectors opposite to terminal QRS vectors

Right Bundle Branch Block
QRS duration ≥0.12 second
Large R′ wave in lead V_1 (rsR′)
Deep terminal S wave in lead V_6
Normal septal Q waves
Inverted T waves in leads V_1 and V_2

Wolff-Parkinson-White, right bundle branch block, muscular dystrophy, dextrocardia, and lead misplacement.

Interventricular Conduction Delays

The ventricular conduction system consists of two main branches, the right and left bundles. The left bundle further divides into the anterior and posterior fascicles. Conduction block can occur in either of the major branches or in the fascicles (Table 4.2).

Fascicular block results in a change in the sequence of ventricular activation but does not substantially prolong overall conduction time. Left anterior fascicular block abnormality is identified when extreme left axis deviation occurs (i.e., more negative than −45 degrees), when the R wave is greater than the Q wave in leads I and aVL, and when the S wave is greater than the R wave in leads II, III, and aVF. Left posterior fascicular block is relatively uncommon but is associated with right axis deviation (>90 degrees); small Q waves in leads II, III, and aVF; and small R waves in leads I and aVL. Fascicular blocks can be seen in conjunction with right bundle branch block (RBBB), and left or right axis deviations can indicate concurrent left anterior or posterior fascicular blocks, respectively.

Complete bundle branch blocks cause QRS prolongation greater than 120 milliseconds. A left bundle branch block (LBBB) can be indicative of underlying coronary or myocardial disease—most commonly fibrosis due to ischemic injury or hypertrophy. In LBBB, depolarization proceeds down the right bundle, across the interventricular septum from right to left, and then to the left ventricle. Characteristic electrocardiographic findings include a wide QRS complex; a broad R wave in leads I, aVL, V_5, and V_6; a deep QS wave in leads V_1 and V_2; and ST depression and T-wave inversion opposite the terminal deflection of the QRS (Fig. 4.5A). Given the abnormal sequence of ventricular activation and repolarization with LBBB, many ECG abnormalities, such as Q-wave myocardial infarction (MI) and left ventricular hypertrophy, are difficult to evaluate. Sgarbossa's criteria can help to identify the presence of MI in the setting of LBBB, though its sensitivity is limited. A new LBBB may be a sign of an acute myocardial infarction in the correct clinical setting (Fig. 4.6B).

With RBBB, the interventricular septum depolarizes normally from left to right, as this depolarization depends on the left bundle. Thus, the initial QRS deflection remains unchanged, and thus it is important to note that ECG abnormalities such as Q-wave MI can still be interpreted. After septal activation, the left ventricle depolarizes, followed by the right ventricle. The ECG is characterized by a wide QRS complex; a large R′ wave in lead V_1 (R-S-R′); and deep S waves in leads I, aVL, and V_6, representing delayed right ventricular activation (see Fig. 4.5B). Ventricular repolarization is still abnormal, and secondary ST and T wave changes will be present just as in LBBB. Although RBBB may be associated with underlying cardiac disease, it is quite common and may often reflect the fibrosis of aging.

Myocardial Ischemia and Infarction

Myocardial ischemia and myocardial infarction (MI) may be associated with abnormalities of the ST segment, T wave, and QRS complex. Myocardial ischemia primarily affects repolarization of the myocardium and is often associated with horizontal or downsloping ST-segment depression and T-wave inversion. These changes may be transient, such as during an anginal episode or an exercise-related stress, or they may be long-lasting in the setting of progressive angina or MI. T-wave inversion without ST-segment depression can be a nonspecific finding and must be correlated with the clinical findings

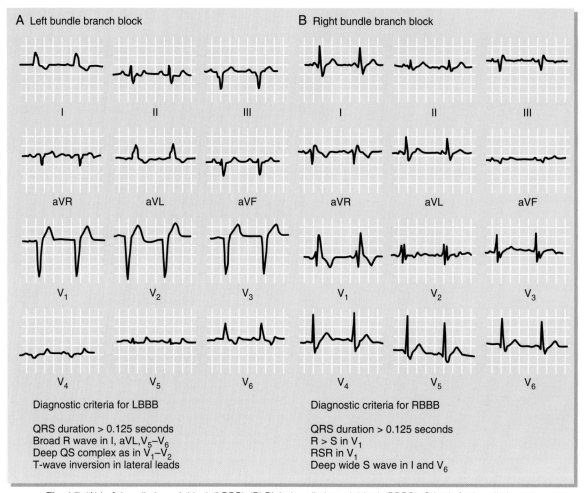

A Left bundle branch block

I   II   III

aVR   aVL   aVF

V₁   V₂   V₃

V₄   V₅   V₆

Diagnostic criteria for LBBB

QRS duration > 0.125 seconds
Broad R wave in I, aVL,V₅–V₆
Deep QS complex as in V₁–V₂
T-wave inversion in lateral leads

B Right bundle branch block

I   II   III

aVR   aVL   aVF

V₁   V₂   V₃

V₄   V₅   V₆

Diagnostic criteria for RBBB

QRS duration > 0.125 seconds
R > S in V₁
RSR in V₁
Deep wide S wave in I and V₆

Fig. 4.5 (A) Left bundle branch block (LBBB). (B) Right bundle branch block (RBBB). Criteria for bundle branch blocks are summarized in Table 4.2.

to invoke ischemia or injury. Diffuse T-wave inversions across the precordial leads are often seen in patients with acute cerebral disease, such as stroke or seizures.

ST-segment elevation of 2 mm or more in two or more contiguous leads suggests more extensive myocardial injury, and in the right clinical presentation, is often considered to be an acute MI until proven otherwise (Fig. 4.6A). Vasospastic or Prinzmetal angina may be associated with reversible ST-segment elevation without MI. ST-segment elevation may occur in other settings not related to acute ischemia or infarction. Persistent, localized ST-segment elevation in the same leads as pathologic Q waves is consistent with a ventricular aneurysm. Acute pericarditis is also associated with diffuse ST-segment elevation across multiple contiguous and noncontiguous leads but is also associated with PR depression relative to the TP interval. Diffuse J-point elevation in association with upward-coving ST segments is a normal variant common among young men and is often referred to as *early repolarization.*

A pathologic Q wave is one of the criteria used to diagnose MI. Infarcted myocardium is impaired at conducting normal electrical activity, and electrical forces are directed away from the surface electrode overlying the infarcted region, producing a Q wave on the surface ECG. A thorough understanding of contiguous leads allows for identification of each region of the myocardium relative to the surface lead, enabling the examiner to localize the area of infarction (Table

4.3). Pathologic Q waves are defined as follows: any Q wave 20 ms or greater or QS complex in leads V₂ to V₃, or a Q wave 30 ms or greater and 0.1 mV deep or greater or QS complex in leads I, II, aVL, aVF or V₄ to V₆ in any 2 leads of a contiguous lead grouping (I, aVL, V₆; V₄ to V₆; II, III, and aVF). Not all MIs result in the permanent formation of Q waves. Small R waves can return many weeks to months after an MI. Abnormal Q waves, or *pseudoinfarction* pattern, may be associated with nonischemic cardiac disease, such as ventricular preexcitation, cardiac amyloidosis, sarcoidosis, idiopathic or hypertrophic cardiomyopathy, myocarditis, and chronic lung disease.

Abnormalities of the ST Segment and T Wave

A number of drugs and metabolic abnormalities may affect the ST segment and T wave (Fig. 4.7). Hypokalemia may result in prominent U waves in the precordial leads along with prolongation of the QT interval. Hyperkalemia may result in tall, peaked T waves. Hypocalcemia typically lengthens the QT interval, whereas hypercalcemia shortens it. A commonly used cardiac medication, digoxin, often results in diffuse, scooped ST-segment depression. Cardiac pacing, LBBB, and RBBB affect ventricular repolarization and alter the ST segment and T-wave. Minor or *nonspecific* ST-segment and T-wave abnormalities may occur in many patients and have no definable cause. In these instances, the physician must determine the significance of the abnormalities based on clinical findings.

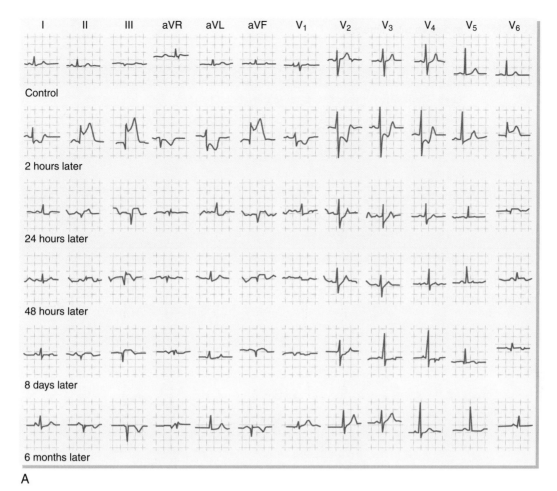

Control

2 hours later

24 hours later

48 hours later

8 days later

6 months later

A

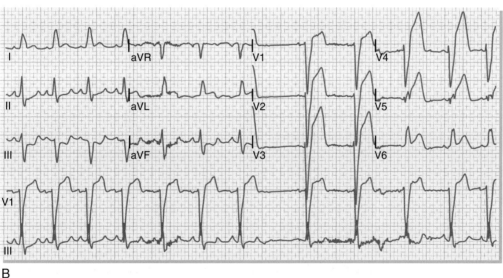

B

Fig. 4.6 (A) Evolutionary changes in a posteroinferior myocardial infarction (MI). Control tracing is normal. The tracing recorded 2 hours after onset of chest pain demonstrated development of early Q waves, marked ST-segment elevation, and hyperacute T waves in leads II, III, and aVF. A larger R wave, ST-segment depression, and negative T waves have developed in leads V_1 and V_2. These early changes indicate acute posteroinferior MI. The 24-hour tracing demonstrates further evolutionary changes. In leads II, III, and aVF, the Q wave is larger, the ST segments have almost returned to baseline, and the T wave has begun to invert. In leads V_1 to V_2, the duration of the R wave exceeds 0.04 seconds, the ST segment is depressed, and the T wave is upright. (In this example, electrocardiographic changes of true posterior involvement extend past lead V_2; ordinarily, only leads V_1 and V_2 may be involved.) Only minor further changes occur through the 8-day tracing. Six months later, the electrocardiographic pattern shows large Q waves, isoelectric ST segments, and inverted T waves in leads II, III, and aVF and shows large R waves, isoelectric ST segment, and upright T waves in leads V_1 and V_2, indicative of an old posteroinferior MI. (B) Electrocardiogram from a patient with an underlying left bundle branch block (LBBB) who experienced an acute anterior MI. Characteristic ST segment elevation and hyperacute T waves are seen in leads V_1 through V_6 and leads I and aVL despite the presence of the LBBB. This is not always the case, and a patient with typical symptoms, an LBBB, and no definite ischemic ST-segment elevations should be treated as if the individual is having a myocardial infarction or acute coronary syndrome.

TABLE 4.3	Electrocardiographic Localization of Myocardial Infarction	
Infarct Location	**Leads Depicting Primary Electrocardiographic Changes**	**Likely Vessel Involved[a]**
Inferior	II, III, aVF	RCA
Septal	V_1, V_2	LAD
Anterior	V_3, V_4	LAD
Anteroseptal	V_1 to V_4	LAD
Extensive anterior	I, aVL, V_1 to V_6	LAD
Lateral	I, aVL, V_5 to V_6	CIRC
High lateral	I, aVL	CIRC
Posterior[b]	Prominent R in V_1	RCA or CIRC
Right ventricular[c]	ST elevation in V_1; more specifically, V_4R in setting of inferior infarction	RCA

CIRC, Circumflex artery; *LAD*, left anterior descending coronary artery; *RCA*, right coronary artery.
[a]This is a generalization; variations occur.
[b]Usually in association with inferior or lateral infarction.
[c]Usually in association with inferior infarction.

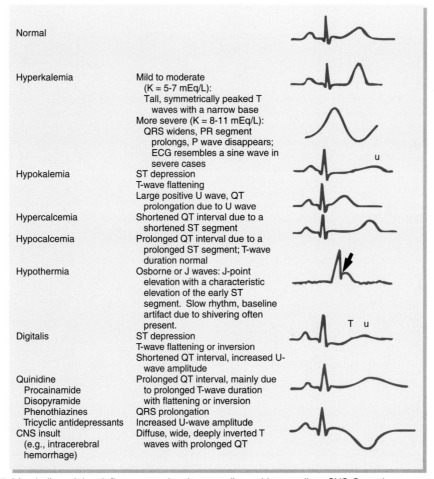

Normal	
Hyperkalemia	Mild to moderate (K = 5-7 mEq/L): Tall, symmetrically peaked T waves with a narrow base
	More severe (K = 8-11 mEq/L): QRS widens, PR segment prolongs, P wave disappears; ECG resembles a sine wave in severe cases
Hypokalemia	ST depression
	T-wave flattening
	Large positive U wave, QT prolongation due to U wave
Hypercalcemia	Shortened QT interval due to a shortened ST segment
Hypocalcemia	Prolonged QT interval due to a prolonged ST segment; T-wave duration normal
Hypothermia	Osborne or J waves: J-point elevation with a characteristic elevation of the early ST segment. Slow rhythm, baseline artifact due to shivering often present.
Digitalis	ST depression
	T-wave flattening or inversion
	Shortened QT interval, increased U-wave amplitude
Quinidine Procainamide Disopyramide	Prolonged QT interval, mainly due to prolonged T-wave duration with flattening or inversion
Phenothiazines	QRS prolongation
Tricyclic antidepressants	Increased U-wave amplitude
CNS insult (e.g., intracerebral hemorrhage)	Diffuse, wide, deeply inverted T waves with prolonged QT

Fig. 4.7 Metabolic and drug influences on the electrocardiographic recording. *CNS*, Central nervous system; *ECG*, electrocardiogram.

AMBULATORY ELECTROCARDIOGRAPHIC RECORDING

Ambulatory ECG monitoring allows clinicians to monitor and capture the presence and frequency of cardiac arrhythmias over a specified period of time. Multiple types of ambulatory recording modalities are available, and the decision to use one or the other largely depends on the duration of surveillance required. Determination of the surveillance duration is influenced by many factors, including the frequency of symptoms (daily, weekly, monthly, or longer), reason for the study (i.e., quantifying arrhythmia burden vs. catching an arrhythmic event), and severity of symptoms (lightheadedness vs. stroke).

A Holter monitor collects ECG data from two or three surface leads on a recorder that the patient wears under their clothing, typically for 24 to 72 hours. The device stores all data over this period of time. Patients are asked to write their symptoms in a diary, so that symptoms can be correlated with the rhythm at that time. From these recordings, algorithms analyze and identify abnormal strips for clinician review. Holter monitors are most useful for patients with frequent, daily symptoms, or for quantifying arrhythmic burden such as frequent premature ventricular contractions. Electrocardiographic devices are more recent innovations that also provide continuous ECG recordings through small ECG sensors placed on the chest, usually over a period of two weeks, and can be used instead of Holter monitors.

For patients with more infrequent symptoms, an event recorder can be used to record data for up to a month. Like Holter monitors, surface leads are placed on the chest and connected to a recording device. Unlike Holter monitors, the device only maintains data for 30 to 60 second loops, after which it is erased. Data are only saved when algorithms identify ECG abnormalities, or when patients press a button indicating the presence of symptoms. Therefore, patients must be able to trigger the device. These data are usually uploaded to a monitoring center, where patients can be called for further questioning or counseling.

Implantable loop recorders (ILRs) are small recording devices that are implanted subcutaneously in the left parasternal chest wall. They can record symptoms for up to two years. Like event recorders, data are maintained on a loop, though for a much greater period of time (about thirty minutes). Data are stored either automatically or through a small magnetic activator that patients pass over the device. A device programmer is then used to extract the data in the office. ILRs are especially useful in patients with rare but serious symptoms, or when quantifying arrhythmic burden, such as atrial fibrillation, may be critical to informing the treatment plan.

In addition to clinician prescribed monitoring devices, there has been a recent surge in the use of personal wearable devices such as smartwatches that have the capacity to record and store single lead ECG tracings. Some of these devices may even alert patients to the presence of abnormal heart rhythms. Though the diagnostic utility of these devices is unclear at this time, clinicians are likely to encounter them at an increasing rate in practice, and abnormalities seen on these devices may be used to prompt further investigation.

CHEST RADIOGRAPHY

Chest radiography is one of the most ubiquitous and commonly performed diagnostic tests in the world. It is an integral part of the initial evaluation and work-up for patients presenting with a number of cardiovascular-related complaints, particularly chest pain, shortness of breath, and postprocedural complaints involving cardiac devices. Regardless of the clinical indication, chest radiography provides useful information regarding cardiac structures that may provide additional insight into a patient's condition.

Routinely, chest radiography is performed in the posteroanterior and lateral projections (Fig. 4.8). In the posteroanterior view, cardiac enlargement may be identified when the transverse diameter of the cardiac silhouette is greater than one half of the transverse diameter of the thorax. The heart may appear falsely enlarged when it is displaced horizontally, such as with poor inflation of the lungs or when the image is taken in an anteroposterior projection, which magnifies the heart shadow. The differential diagnosis for cardiac silhouette enlargement

on chest radiography includes cardiomegaly, pericardial effusion, prominent epicardial fat pad, or an anterior mediastinal mass.

Left atrial enlargement is suggested when the left-sided heart border is straightened or bulges toward the left. Right atrial enlargement may be confirmed when the right-sided heart border bulges toward the right. Left ventricular enlargement results in downward and lateral displacement of the apex. A rounding of the displaced apex suggests ventricular hypertrophy. Right ventricular enlargement is best assessed on the lateral view and may be diagnosed when the right ventricular border occupies more than one third of the retrosternal space between the diaphragm and thoracic apex.

The aortic arch and thoracic aorta may become dilated and tortuous in patients with severe atherosclerosis, long-standing hypertension, and aortic dissection. A widened mediastinum, which is defined as a width of greater than 8.0 centimeters at the level of the aortic knob, can be seen in acute aortic dissection, although it is not very sensitive or specific for acute dissection.

Pulmonary venous congestion due to elevated left ventricular end-diastolic pressure results in redistribution of blood flow in the lungs and prominence of the apical vessels, which can be seen on chest radiography. Transudation of fluid into the interstitial space may result in fluid in the fissures and along the horizontal periphery of the lower lung fields (i.e., Kerley B lines). As venous pressures further increase, fluid collects in the alveolar space, which early on collects preferentially in the inner two thirds of the lung fields, resulting in a characteristic butterfly appearance.

Chest radiography is also used to evaluate device and lead positioning after implantation of defibrillators or pacemakers. The posteroanterior view helps to evaluate for device and lead integrity as well as potential device placement complications such as pneumothorax. A lateral view is necessary to evaluate ventricular lead positioning. In the lateral view, a right ventricular lead will course anteriorly, while a left ventricular lead will course posteriorly. The shape of the pulse generator can help in determining the device manufacturer, which is necessary to know for device interrogation.

ECHOCARDIOGRAPHY

Echocardiography is a widely used, noninvasive technique in which sound waves are used to image cardiac structures and evaluate blood flow. Transthoracic echocardiography is safe, simple, fast, and relatively inexpensive. It can provide a wealth of information on a patient's cardiovascular status, including ventricular function, valvular function, chamber size, possible coronary artery disease, pericardial disease, congenital heart disease, aortopathy, cardioembolic sources, volume status, and hemodynamics, among many other things.

A piezoelectric crystal housed in a transducer placed on the patient's chest wall produces ultrasound waves. As the sound waves encounter structures with different acoustic properties, some of the ultrasound waves are reflected to the transducer and recorded. Steering the ultrasound beam across a 90-degree arc multiple times per second creates two-dimensional imaging (Fig. 4.9). The development of three-dimensional echocardiographic imaging techniques allows for greater accuracy in measurements of chamber volumes and mass, as well as the assessment of geometrically complex anatomy and valvular lesions. Video 4.1 shows a three-dimensional image.

Doppler echocardiography allows assessment of the direction and velocity of blood flow in the heart and great vessels. When ultrasound waves encounter moving red blood cells, the energy reflected to the transducer is altered. The magnitude of this change (i.e., Doppler shift) is represented as velocity on the echocardiographic display and can be used to determine whether the blood flow is normal or abnormal

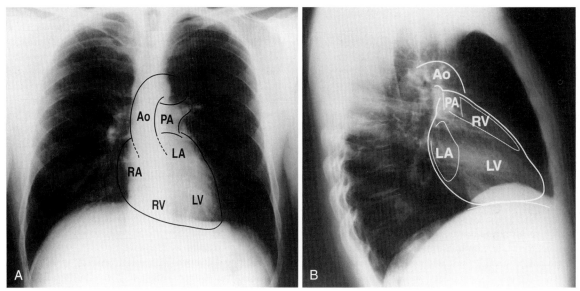

Fig. 4.8 Schematic illustration of the parts of the heart, outlines of which can be identified on a routine chest radiograph. (A) Posteroanterior chest radiograph. (B) Lateral chest radiograph. *Ao*, Aorta; *LA*, left atrium; *LV*, left ventricle; *PA*, pulmonary artery; *RA*, right atrium; *RV*, right ventricle.

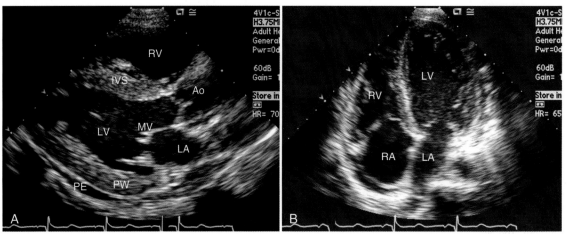

Fig. 4.9 Portions of standard two-dimensional echocardiograms show the major cardiac structures in a parasternal long-axis view (A) and apical four-chamber view (B). Video 4.3 shows a moving image of a two-dimensional echocardiogram. *Ao*, Aorta; *IVS*, interventricular septum; *LA*, left atrium; *LV*, left ventricle; *MV*, mitral valve; *PE*, pericardial effusion; *PW*, posterior left ventricular wall; *RV*, right ventricle. (Image courtesy Sheldon E. Litwin, MD, Division of Cardiology, University of Utah, Salt Lake City, Utah.)

(Fig. 4.10). The velocity of a particular jet of blood can be converted to pressure, allowing assessment of pressure gradients across valves or between chambers. Color Doppler imaging allows visualization of blood flow through the heart by assigning a color to the red blood cells based on their velocity and direction (Fig. 4.11, Video 4.2). By convention, blood moving away from the transducer is represented in shades of blue, and blood moving toward the transducer is represented in red. Color Doppler imaging is particularly useful in identifying valvular insufficiency and abnormal shunt flow between chambers. The use of Doppler techniques to record myocardial velocities or strain rates can aid in the assessment of myocardial function and hemodynamics.

Ultrasound contrast agents composed of microbubbles can be used in patients who have poorly visualized cardiac structures, such as obese patients or those with chronic lung disease. Ultrasound contrast opacifies the endocardial cavity and aids in assessment of cardiac function (Fig. 4.12). Video 4.3 shows a dynamic contrast echocardiographic image. These contrast agents are also necessary in the assessment of potential left ventricular thrombus. Agitated saline, commonly referred to as "bubbles," can be used to assess for intracardiac shunts.

Transesophageal echocardiography (TEE) allows two-dimensional and Doppler imaging of the heart through the esophagus by having the patient swallow a gastroscope mounted with an ultrasound crystal in its tip. Given the proximity of the esophagus to the heart, high-resolution images can be obtained, especially of the left atrium, mitral valve apparatus, and aorta. TEE is particularly useful in diagnosing left atrial appendage thrombi, aortic dissection, endocarditis, prosthetic valve dysfunction, and left atrial masses (Fig. 4.13, Video 4.4). TEE has been used for decades intraoperatively during cardiac surgery, and it is now being used with increasing frequency to guide percutaneous cardiac procedures such as transcatheter aortic valve replacement, transcatheter mitral valve repair, and left atrial appendage occlusion.

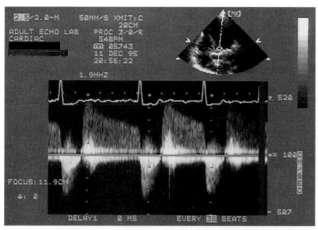

Fig. 4.10 Doppler tracing in a patient with aortic stenosis and regurgitation. The velocity of systolic flow is related to the severity of obstruction.

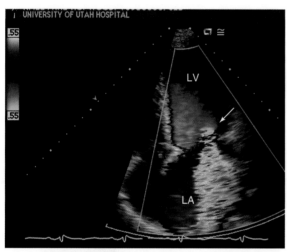

Fig. 4.11 Color Doppler recording demonstrates severe mitral regurgitation. The regurgitant jet seen in the left atrium is represented in *blue* because blood flow is directed away from the transducer. The *yellow* components are the mosaic pattern traditionally assigned to turbulent or high-velocity flow. The *arrow* points to the hemisphere of blood accelerating proximal to the regurgitant orifice (i.e., proximal isovelocity surface area [PISA]). The size of the PISA can be used to help grade the severity of regurgitation. Video 4.2 shows a dynamic echocardiographic image in a patient with mitral regurgitation. *LA,* Left atrium; *LV,* left ventricle. (Image courtesy Sheldon E. Litwin, MD, Division of Cardiology, University of Utah, Salt Lake City, Utah.)

NUCLEAR CARDIOLOGY

The traditional radiotracer approach to assess ventricular function is equilibrium radionuclide angiocardiography (ERNA), which uses technetium-99m-labeled red blood cells. Serial ERNA can be performed at rest and during various levels of exercise of pharmacologic perturbations to evaluate ventricular function and reserve. ERNA has high reproducibility because there are no geometric assumptions and there is much less operator dependence in the image acquisition. Diastolic parameters can be readily assessed from the ventricular volume curve, which may be very helpful in the assessment of diastolic dysfunction.

In radionuclide imaging of the heart, patients are injected with a radioactive tracer, which distributes throughout the myocardium in proportion to blood flow. Highly specialized cameras then capture the distribution of the radioactive tracer, which allows for quantification of left ventricular size, systolic function, and myocardial perfusion, depending on the tracer used. The two main types of myocardial imaging used in cardiology, often in stress testing, are single-photon emission tomography (SPECT) and positron emission tomography (PET).

In SPECT imaging, images of the heart are obtained for qualitative and quantitative analyses at rest and after stress (i.e., exercise or pharmacologic vasodilation). Radionuclide tracers are injected prior to rest images and just prior to the completion of stress. The most frequently used radionuclide in SPECT imaging is technetium-99m sestamibi. In the normal heart, the radioisotope is equally distributed throughout the myocardium at rest and stress. In patients with ischemia, a localized area of decreased radiotracer uptake occurs after stress but may partially or completely reverse during rest. A persistent defect at peak exercise and rest (i.e., fixed defect) is consistent with MI or scarring.

The use of new approaches such as combined low-level exercise and vasodilators, prone imaging, attenuation correction, and computerized data analysis has improved the quality and reproducibility of the data from these studies. New camera technologies, including those with solid state detector arrays, have demonstrated improved image resolution and allow for reduced radiation exposure. Myocardial perfusion imaging may also be combined with ECG-gated image acquisition (gated SPECT) to allow simultaneous assessment of ventricular function and perfusion. Using this technique, regional wall motion can be evaluated to help assess potential perfusion defects (Video 4.5).

PET has been widely used in oncology for many years but has become increasingly popular in cardiology (Video 4.5). The commonly used tracers in cardiac PET imaging include rubidium-82 and fluorine-18 fluorodeoxyglucose (FDG). When compared to SPECT, PET has several technical advantages, including higher spatial and temporal resolution, less radiation exposure, and the ability to quantify absolute rather than relative coronary blood flow. These advantages mean that PET is more sensitive and specific compared to SPECT in diagnosing coronary disease, especially in the presence of multivessel disease. Additionally, because PET gives an absolute rather than relative quantification of coronary blood flow, it can be used to assess abnormal microvascular coronary circulation. Despite these clinical advantages of PET over SPECT, the lack of availability of PET cameras and radiotracers, as well as high costs and reimbursement issues, limits the widespread adoption of PET.

In patients with suspected cardiac sarcoidosis, FDG-PET is the imaging modality of choice for diagnosis. FDG-PET can also be used to detect myocardial viability by the use of perfusion and metabolic tracers. In patients with left ventricular dysfunction, metabolic activity in a region of myocardium supplied by a severely stenotic coronary artery suggests viable tissue that may regain more normal function after revascularization (Fig. 4.14).

CARDIAC MAGNETIC RESONANCE IMAGING

Cardiac magnetic resonance imaging (cMRI) is a noninvasive method that is increasingly used for studying the heart and vasculature and has, in fact, become the gold standard for measuring myocardial function, volumes, and scarring. cMRI offers high-resolution dynamic and static images of the heart that can be obtained in any plane, allowing quantification of left ventricular and valvular function. High-quality images can be obtained in a larger proportion of subjects than is typically possible with echocardiography. Obesity, claustrophobia, inability to perform multiple breath-holds of 10 to 20 seconds, and arrhythmias are causes of reduced image quality.

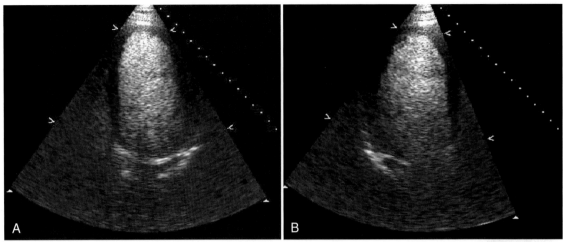

Fig. 4.12 Echocardiogram enhanced with intravenous ultrasound contrast agent: apical four-chamber view (A) and apical long-axis view (B). Highly echo-reflectant microbubbles make the left ventricular cavity appear white, whereas the myocardium appears dark. Video 4.3 shows a dynamic image of echocardiographic contrast. (Image courtesy Sheldon E. Litwin, MD, Division of Cardiology, University of Utah, Salt Lake City, Utah.)

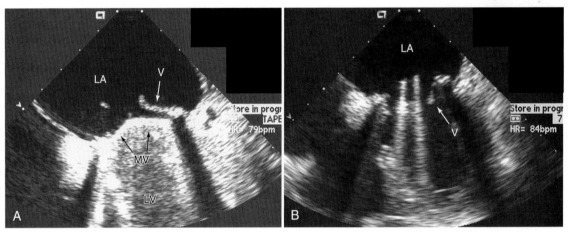

Fig. 4.13 Transesophageal echocardiogram demonstrates a vegetation *(arrow)* adherent to the ring of a bileaflet, tilting-disk mitral valve prostheses. (A) In systole, the leaflets are closed with the vegetation seen in the left atrium. (B) In diastole, the leaflets are open, with the vegetation prolapsing into the left ventricle. Transesophageal echocardiography is the diagnostic test of choice for assessing prosthetic mitral valves because the esophageal window allows unimpeded views of the atrial surface of the valve. Video 4.4 shows a dynamic transesophageal echocardiographic image. *LA,* Left atrium; *LV,* left ventricle; *MV,* prosthetic mitral valve disks; *V,* vegetation. (Courtesy Sheldon E. Litwin, MD, Division of Cardiology, University of Utah, Salt Lake City, Utah.)

cMRI also offers significant advantages over other imaging techniques for the characterization of tissues (e.g., muscle, fat, scar). cMRI is useful in the evaluation of ischemic heart disease because stress-rest myocardial perfusion (Fig. 4.15A) and areas of prior infarction (see Fig. 4.15B to D) can be visualized with excellent spatial resolution. Delayed or late gadolinium enhancement (LGE) in the myocardium is characteristic of scar or permanently damaged tissue (Video 4.6). The greater the transmural extent of LGE is in a given segment, the lower the likelihood of improved function in that segment after revascularization. Because of the better spatial resolution, LGE can identify localized or subendocardial scars that are not detectable with nuclear imaging techniques.

MRI is excellent for evaluating a variety of cardiomyopathies (Fig. 4.16). In addition to morphology and function, characteristic patterns of LGE have been reported in myocarditis, cardiac amyloidosis, sarcoidosis, and hypertrophic cardiomyopathy (HCM). In patients with

HCM, specific patterns on MRI can help identify those patients at highest risk of sudden cardiac death who would require defibrillators. Similarly, MRI has also been used to help assess right ventricular morphology and function in patients with suspected arrhythmogenic right ventricular cardiomyopathy. The role of MRI in all aspects of cardiac imaging continues to grow.

STRESS TESTING

Stress testing is an important noninvasive tool for evaluating patients with known or suggested coronary artery disease (CAD). During exercise, the increased demand for oxygen by the working skeletal muscles is met by increases in heart rate and cardiac output. In patients with significant CAD, the increase in myocardial oxygen demand cannot be met by a proportional increase in coronary blood flow, and myocardial ischemia may produce chest pain and characteristic ECG

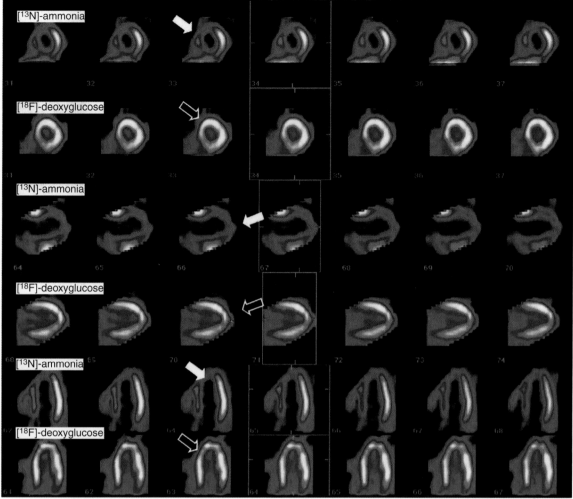

Fig. 4.14 Resting myocardial perfusion (obtained with [^{13}N]-ammonia) and metabolism (obtained with [^{18}F]-deoxyglucose) is seen in positron emission tomography images of a patient with ischemic cardiomyopathy. The study demonstrates a perfusion-metabolic mismatch (reflecting hibernating myocardium) in which large areas of hypoperfused *(solid arrows)* but metabolically viable *(open arrows)* myocardium involve the anterior, septal, and inferior walls and the left ventricular apex. Video 4.5 shows a dynamic image obtained with cardiac single-photon emission computed tomography imaging. (Courtesy Marcelo F. Di Carli, MD, Brigham and Women's Hospital, Boston, Mass.)

abnormalities. Combined with the hemodynamic response to exercise, these changes can give useful diagnostic and prognostic information for the patient with cardiac abnormalities. The most common indications for stress testing include establishing a diagnosis of CAD in patients with chest pain, assessing prognosis and functional capacity of patients with chronic stable angina or after an MI, evaluating exercise-induced arrhythmias, and assessing for ischemia after a revascularization procedure. Contraindications to stress testing include acute coronary syndromes, poorly controlled hypertension (blood pressure >220/110 mm Hg), severe aortic stenosis (valve area <1.0 cm^2), and decompensated congestive heart failure.

When to Stress Symptomatic Patients

Stress testing is most often used to evaluate symptoms concerning for flow-limiting coronary artery disease and make the diagnosis of CAD. The diagnostic accuracy of the stress test depends on several factors, including the pretest probability of CAD in a given patient, the sensitivity and specificity of the test results in that patient population, the adequacy of stress, and the criteria used to define a positive test. Stress testing, when used to diagnose CAD, is one of the most useful and cost-effective tests in symptomatic patients who have an intermediate pretest probability of CAD, which is defined as a 10% to 90% risk. This is because in patients with a low pretest probability, a positive test does not significantly increase the post-test probability of CAD, and in patients with a high pretest probability, a negative test does not significantly decrease the post-test probability of CAD. The pretest probability of CAD can be calculated through a variety of scores but is most commonly done based on a patient's description of angina (Table 4.4).

Angina has three important components:
1. Substernal chest pain or discomfort
2. The pain or discomfort is provoked by exertion or emotional stress
3. The pain or discomfort is relieved by rest and/or nitroglycerin.

Patients with all three components are said to have *typical angina*. Those with any two of the three components have *atypical angina*, and patients with *nonanginal* chest pain have only one or none of these components.

Other factors that are not solely based on the description of chest discomfort may be present that would increase a patient's pretest

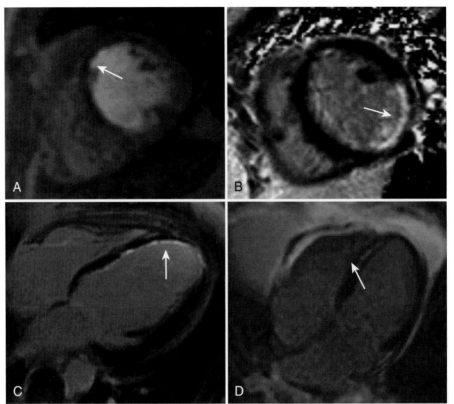

Fig. 4.15 Use of cardiac magnetic resonance imaging in the evaluation of chest pain or ischemic heart disease. (A) First-pass perfusion study during vasodilator stress shows a large septal perfusion defect *(arrow)*. The hypoperfused area appears dark compared with the myocardium with normal perfusion. (B) Example of delayed enhancement imaging of an almost transmural infarction of the mid-inferolateral wall, including the posterior papillary muscle. Infarcted myocardium appears *white*, whereas normal myocardium is *black (arrow)*. (C) Nontransmural (subendocardial) infarction of the septum and apex *(arrow)*. (D) Patient with acute myocarditis mimicking an acute coronary syndrome. Midmyocardial, rather than subendocardial, delayed enhancement is characteristic of myocarditis *(arrow)*.

probability of CAD. These include baseline ECG abnormalities suggestive of CAD and multiple CAD risk factors, such as diabetes, smoking, hypertension, dyslipidemia, or family history of premature CAD. These should be taken into consideration on an individual basis and may require an upward revision of pretest probability.

Stress Modalities

There are two essential components to any stress test: the type of stress and the imaging modality. Stress can either be exercise-induced or pharmacologic. Exercise level is deemed adequate if the patient achieves 85% of his or her maximal predicted heart rate. Submaximal stress tests can still be interpreted but may be limited in the ability to rule out disease due to decreased sensitivity. Indications for terminating a stress test include fatigue, severe hypertension (>220 mm Hg systolic), worsening angina during exercise, developing marked or widespread ischemic ECG changes, significant arrhythmias, or hypotension.

For patients who are able to exercise, the most commonly used exercise protocols are the Bruce and modified Bruce protocols. These protocols require a patient to walk on a treadmill as the speed and incline of the belt increases with each advancing stage. Any patient who can exercise should do so, as duration of exercise and provoked symptoms provide valuable clinical and prognostic information for the physician. The modified Bruce or similar protocols are ideal for older, overweight, unstable, or debilitated patients. Additionally, in patients

unable to exercise on a treadmill, bicycle or arm ergometer testing may also be used. In patients who cannot exercise or in those where exercise will interfere with image acquisition, pharmacologic agents may be used.

The most commonly used pharmacologic stress agents are dobutamine, adenosine, and regadenoson, an adenosine derivative and selective adenosine A2A receptor agonist. Dobutamine is a synthetic sympathomimetic that stimulates alpha-1, beta-1, and beta-2 receptors, increasing inotropy and chronotropy, thereby increasing myocardial oxygen demand. It should be used cautiously in patients with a history of atrial or ventricular arrhythmias as it can exacerbate both. Regadenoson is an adenosine receptor agonist that induces coronary vasodilation and is more commonly used in radionuclide myocardial perfusion imaging. Its use is contraindicated in patients with asthma or COPD and active wheezing as well as patients with significant bradyarrhythmias without a pacemaker. It should be used with caution in patients with a history of seizures as it can lower the seizure threshold.

STRESS IMAGING

Exercise or pharmacologic stress testing must be combined with imaging modalities to assess for characteristic changes seen in flow-limiting coronary artery disease. The most basic form of imaging is an ECG, which can be combined with adjunctive echocardiography or radionuclide imaging to increase the diagnostic accuracy of the testing.

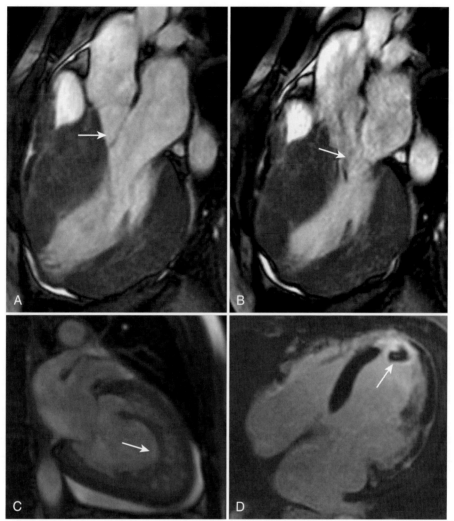

Fig. 4.16 Cardiac magnetic resonance imaging (MRI) is used in the evaluation of cardiomyopathies. (A) Severe left ventricular hypertrophy in a patient with hypertrophic cardiomyopathy. Diastolic frame shows open mitral valve *(arrow)*. (B) Systolic frame shows systolic anterior motion of the mitral valve with flow disturbance in the left ventricular outflow tract *(arrow)*. (C) Patient has left ventricular noncompaction as evidenced by deep trabeculations in the left ventricular apex *(arrow)*. (D) Patient with ischemic cardiomyopathy has transmural apical infarction and adjacent mural thrombus *(arrow)*. Video 4.6 shows a dynamic cardiac MRI image. (Images courtesy Sheldon E. Litwin, MD, Division of Cardiology, University of Utah, Salt Lake City, Utah.)

TABLE 4.4   Diamond and Forrester Pretest Probability of Coronary Artery Disease by Age, Sex, and Symptoms

Age (Years)	Sex	Typical/Definite Angina Pectoris	Atypical/Probable Angina Pectoris	Nonanginal Chest Pain
≤39	Men	Intermediate	Intermediate	Low
	Women	Intermediate	Very low	Very low
40-49	Men	High	Intermediate	Intermediate
	Women	Intermediate	Low	Very low
50-59	Men	High	Intermediate	Intermediate
	Women	Intermediate	Intermediate	Low
≥60	Men	High	Intermediate	Intermediate
	Women	High	Intermediate	Intermediate

High: >90% pretest probability. Intermediate: between 10% and 90% pretest probability. Low: between 5% and 10% pretest probability. Very low: <5% pretest probability.

From Wolk MJ, Bailey SR, Doherty JU, et al: ACCF/AHA/ASE/ASNC/HFSA/HRS/SCAI/SCCT/SCMR/STS 2013 Multimodality Appropriate Use Criteria for the Detection and Risk Assessment of Stable Ischemic Heart Disease. Journal of the American College of Cardiology 63:380-406, 2014.

Stress Electrocardiography

The normal physiologic response to exercise is an increase in heart rate and systolic and diastolic blood pressures. The ECG maintains normal T-wave polarity, and the ST segment remains unchanged or, if depressed, has a rapid upstroke back to baseline. An ischemic ECG response to exercise is defined as 1.5 mm of upsloping ST-segment depression measured 0.08 second past the J point, at least 1 mm of horizontal ST depression, or 1 mm of downsloping ST-segment depression measured at the J point. Given the large amount of artifact on the ECG that may occur with exercise, these changes must be seen in at least three consecutive depolarizations. Other findings that suggest more extensive CAD include early onset of ST depression (6 minutes); marked, downsloping ST depression (>2 mm), especially if present in more than five leads; ST changes persisting into recovery for more than 5 minutes; and failure to increase systolic blood pressure to 120 mm Hg or more or a sustained decrease of 10 mm Hg or more below baseline.

The ECG is not diagnostically useful in the setting of left ventricular hypertrophy, LBBB, Wolff-Parkinson-White syndrome, or chronic digoxin therapy. In these instances, further imaging modalities such as echocardiography, nuclear imaging, or positron-emission tomography (PET) are needed to help diagnose ischemia.

Stress Echocardiography

Two-dimensional echocardiography and Doppler echocardiography are often used in conjunction with exercise or pharmacologic stress testing. The pharmacologic agent typically used is dobutamine. A baseline echocardiogram is performed at rest and during stress. Changes in wall motion are indicative of ischemia and coronary artery disease. In areas of the left ventricle that have wall motion abnormalities at rest, improvement of these wall motion abnormalities with exercise or low-dose dobutamine is indicative of viability.

Relative to myocardial perfusion imaging, the sensitivity of stress echocardiography is slightly lower whereas the specificity is slightly higher. A poor baseline echocardiogram due to limited acoustic windows will limit stress test results. The estimated cost-effectiveness of stress echocardiography is significantly better than nuclear perfusion imaging because of the overall lower cost.

Myocardial Perfusion Imaging (See Also Nuclear Cardiology Section)

Stress testing, using myocardial perfusion imaging with SPECT to compare relative coronary blood flow at stress and at rest, helps to identify areas of perfusion mismatch, indicative of ischemia. Like with other stress modalities, exercise or pharmacologic stress can be used. Commonly used pharmacologic agents include dipyridamole, adenosine, and regadenoson, which are all coronary vasodilators. It is important to note that patients with LBBB have to undergo pharmacologic stress when receiving myocardial perfusion imaging, even if they are able to exercise, as the abnormal septal motion caused by the LBBB can lead to a false perfusion defect during exercise.

Stress Cardiac Magnetic Resonance Imaging

Though either exercise or pharmacologic stress may be combined with cMRI, the contemporary use of stress cMRI usually refers to stress perfusion cMRI with gadolinium contrast that is performed with regadenoson. This technique allows for evaluation of wall motion, perfusion, scar, viability, and microvascular dysfunction, as well as chamber quantification and function, allowing for a comprehensive evaluation of the myocardium and myocardial function. Changes in late gadolinium enhancement between rest and stress has performance characteristics for diagnosing CAD that are at least as good and likely superior to those of conventional stress tests using nuclear myocardial perfusion imaging or echocardiography, and on par with PET imaging.

COMPUTED TOMOGRAPHY OF THE HEART

Newer applications of computed tomography (CT) have greatly advanced our ability to diagnose cardiovascular disease noninvasively. The development of fast gantry rotation speeds and the addition of multiple rows of detectors (i.e., multidetector CT) have allowed unprecedented visualization of the great vessels, heart, and coronary arteries with images acquired during a single breath-hold lasting 10 to 15 seconds. CT is used to diagnose aortic aneurysm, acute aortic dissection, and pulmonary embolism, and it is useful for defining congenital abnormalities and detecting pericardial thickening or calcification associated with constrictive pericarditis. ECG-gated dynamic CT images have been used to quantify ventricular size, function, and regional wall motion (Video 4.7), and in contrast to echocardiography, CT is not limited by lung disease or chest wall deformity. However, obesity and implanted prosthetic materials (i.e., mechanical valves or pacing wires) may affect image quality.

The greatest excitement and controversy about cardiac CT relates to the evaluation of coronary atherosclerosis. Electron beam and multidetector CT scans can be used to quickly and reliably visualize and quantitate the extent of coronary artery calcification (Fig. 4.17). The presence of coronary calcium is pathognomonic of atherosclerosis, and the extent of coronary calcium (usually reported as an Agatston score) is a powerful marker of future cardiovascular events. The coronary calcium score adds substantial, independent improvement in risk prediction to the commonly employed clinical risk scores (e.g., Framingham risk score). Moreover, the calcium score is a good marker of the overall atherosclerotic burden. Indications for coronary calcium scoring continue to grow, especially in refining risk predictions in asymptomatic patients at intermediate risk for arteriosclerotic cardiovascular disease.

Contrast-enhanced coronary computed tomography angiography (CCTA) has improved dramatically in recent years. CCTA has a sensitivity of more than 95% in diagnosing significant coronary artery obstruction. Unlike myocardial perfusion imaging, CCTA is an anatomic test, and thus does not give information on perfusion or blood flow across a lesion. Thus, in patients with known coronary disease, CCTA cannot easily differentiate between ischemic and nonischemic chest pain. New technology is being developed to noninvasively determine the hemodynamic significance of a lesion through CCTA, similar to fractional flow reserve in coronary catheterization, though this technology still needs to be rigorously tested and standardized. Evaluation of coronary arteries with CCTA can be significantly limited in patients with extensive coronary calcifications, cardiac devices, or prior stents due to technical limitations.

Concerns that limit the widespread use of cardiac CT most frequently cite the risks of radiation and contrast exposure and the lack of prospective studies showing improvement in outcome with this testing modality. In early studies, the calculated radiation exposure of CCTA was about double that of a diagnostic invasive coronary angiogram, although with prospective ECG-gating, most studies are now equal to or less than a diagnostic angiogram. Contrast use is often higher in a CCTA than in a diagnostic invasive coronary angiogram. The role of CCTA in routine clinical practice continues to evolve.

CARDIAC CATHETERIZATION

Cardiac catheterization is an invasive technique in which fluid-filled catheters are introduced percutaneously into the arterial and/or venous circulation. This method allows direct measurement of intracardiac

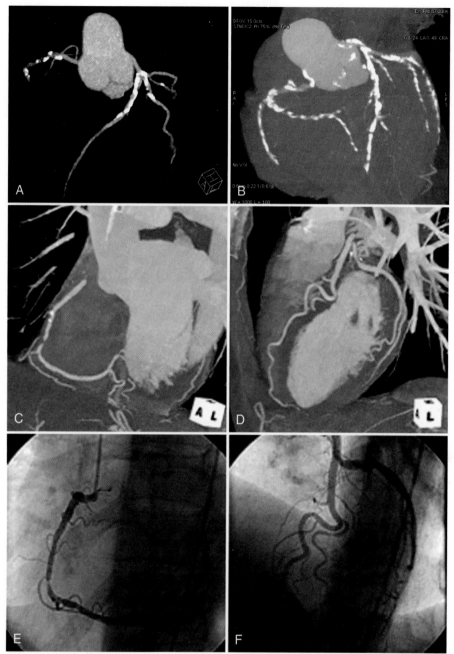

Fig. 4.17 Computed tomography coronary angiography compared with conventional radiographic contrast angiography. (A and B) Volume-rendering technique demonstrates stenosis of the right coronary artery and normal left coronary artery. (C and D) Maximal intensity projection of the same arteries demonstrates severe noncalcified plaque in the right coronary artery with superficial calcified plaque. (E and F) Invasive angiography of the same arteries. (From Raff GL, Gallagher MJ, O'Neill WW, et al: Diagnostic accuracy of noninvasive coronary angiography using 64-slice spiral computed tomography, J Am Coll Cardiol 46:552-557, 2005.)

pressures and oxygen saturation and, with the injection of a contrast agent, visualization of the coronary arteries, cardiac chambers, and great vessels. Cardiac catheterization is indicated when a clinically suggested cardiac abnormality requires confirmation and its anatomic and physiologic importance needs to be quantified. Coronary angiography for the diagnosis of CAD is the most common indication for this test.

Compared with catheterization, noninvasive testing with echocardiography is safer, often cheaper, and equally effective in the evaluation of most valvular and hemodynamic conditions. Most often, catheterization precedes some type of beneficial intervention, such as

coronary artery angioplasty, coronary bypass surgery, or valvular surgery. Although cardiac catheterization is usually safe (0.1% to 0.2% overall mortality rate), procedure-related complications such as vascular injury, renal failure, stroke, and MI can occur.

Left Heart Catheterization and Coronary Angiography

Left heart catheterization and coronary angiography first requires the introduction of wires and fluid-filled catheters into the arterial system of the body. In the past, femoral arterial access was the default route, but now, radial arterial access has become increasingly more common.

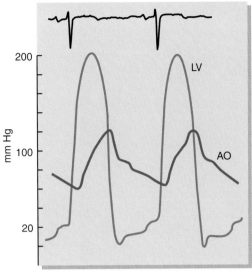

Fig. 4.18 Electrocardiographic tracing and left ventricular (LV) and aortic (AO) pressure curves in a patient with aortic stenosis. A pressure gradient occurs across the aortic valve during systole.

It has replaced femoral arterial access as the default access site in most centers. Radial arterial access is associated with less bleeding, fewer vascular complications, and increased patient comfort and early mobility after the procedure when compared with femoral arterial access. However, it is also associated with higher radiation exposure and increased procedural time.

After access is obtained, wires and fluid-filled catheters are advanced to the aortic root and through the aortic valve into the left ventricle under fluoroscopic guidance. Here, left ventricular size, wall motion, and ejection fraction can be accurately assessed by injecting contrast into the left ventricle (i.e., left ventriculography). Aortic and mitral valve insufficiency can be qualitatively assessed during angiography by observing the reflux of contrast medium into the left ventricle and left atrium, respectively. Left ventricular pressures can be directly measured and recorded, and the catheter can slowly be pulled back across the left ventricular outflow tract (LVOT) and aortic valve to directly assess for any pressure differential that would be consistent with aortic stenosis or LVOT obstruction (Fig. 4.18).

The coronary anatomy can be defined by injecting contrast medium into the coronary tree. Atherosclerotic lesions appear as narrowing of the internal diameter (lumen) of the vessel. A hemodynamically important stenosis is defined as 70% or more narrowing of the luminal diameter. However, the hemodynamic significance of a lesion can be underestimated by coronary angiography, particularly when the atherosclerotic plaque is eccentric or elongated. Intravascular ultrasound, optical coherence tomography, or miniaturized pressure sensors can be used during invasive procedures to help evaluate the severity or estimate the physiologic significance of intermediate lesions.

Right Heart Catheterization

Right heart catheterization is a useful invasive technique that can be performed at bedside or with fluoroscopic guidance. The pulmonary artery (Swan-Ganz) catheter, which is a balloon-tipped catheter used for right heart catheterization, can be left in a patient for a prolonged period of time in a critical care setting to provide continuous information on cardiovascular hemodynamics and filling pressures. Right heart catheterization can be helpful when used in appropriate situations, such as when differentiating noncardiogenic from cardiogenic

pulmonary edema, managing mixed shock, managing cardiogenic shock, and classifying and treating pulmonary hypertension.

Right heart catheterization is performed by first accessing the venous system. Common sites of entry for right heart catheterization include the internal jugular vein (usually the right), the right brachial vein, or the femoral veins. The procedure can be performed at the bedside or under fluoroscopic guidance with a balloon-tipped (Swan-Ganz) catheter. The catheter is advanced from the vein to the right atrium, right ventricle, and pulmonary artery, where pressures are measured and recorded. The catheter can then be advanced further until it *wedges* in the distal pulmonary artery. The transmitted pressure measured in this location originates from the pulmonary venous system and is known as the *pulmonary capillary wedge pressure*. In the absence of pulmonary venous disease, the pulmonary capillary wedge pressure reflects left atrial pressure, and if no significant mitral valve pathologic condition exists, it reflects left ventricular diastolic pressure. A more direct method of obtaining left ventricular filling pressures is through left heart catheterization, as described in the previous section. With these two methods of obtaining intracardiac pressures, each chamber of the heart can be directly assessed and the gradients across any of the valves determined (Fig. 4.19).

Cardiac output can be determined by one of two widely accepted methods: the Fick oxygen method and the indicator dilution technique. The basis of the Fick method is that total uptake or release of a substance by an organ is equal to the product of blood flow to that organ and the concentration difference of that substance between the arterial and venous circulation of that organ. If this method is applied to the lungs, the substance released into the blood is oxygen; if no intrapulmonary shunts exist, pulmonary blood flow is equal to systemic blood flow or cardiac output. The cardiac output can be determined by the following equation:

$$\text{Cardiac output} = \frac{\text{Oxygen consumption}}{\text{(Arterial oxygen content} - \text{Venous oxygen content)}}$$

Oxygen consumption is measured in milliliters per minute by collecting the patient's expired air over a known period while simultaneously measuring oxygen saturation in a sample of arterial and mixed venous blood (i.e., arterial and venous oxygen content, respectively, measured in milliliters per liter). The cardiac output is expressed in liters per minute and then corrected for body surface area (i.e., cardiac index). The normal range of cardiac index is 2.6 to 4.2 L/min/m^2. Cardiac output can also be determined by the indicator dilution technique, which most commonly uses cold saline as the indicator. With this method, cold saline is injected into the blood, and the resulting temperature change *downstream* is monitored. This action generates a curve in which temperature change is plotted over time, and the area under the curve represents cardiac output.

Detection and localization of intracardiac shunts can be performed by sequential measurement of oxygen saturation in the venous system, right side of the heart, and two main pulmonary arteries. In patients with left-to-right shunt flow, an increase in oxygen *step-up* (i.e., saturation increase from one chamber to the successive chamber) occurs as arterial blood mixes with venous blood. By using the Fick method for calculating blood flow in the pulmonary and systemic systems, the shunt ratio can be calculated. Noninvasive approaches have largely supplanted catheterization laboratory assessment of shunts.

In the past, the Swan-Ganz catheter was routinely used in most patients with shock; however, randomized trials have since been published suggesting no improvement in outcomes in critically ill patients in whom pulmonary artery catheterization was performed.

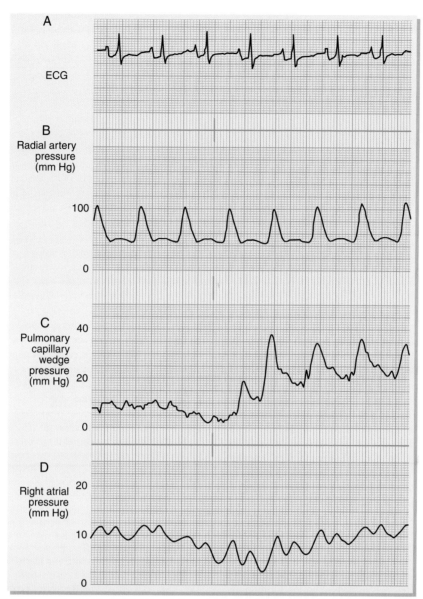

A ECG

B Radial artery pressure (mm Hg)

C Pulmonary capillary wedge pressure (mm Hg)

D Right atrial pressure (mm Hg)

Fig. 4.19 Electrocardiographic (ECG) (A) and Swan-Ganz flotation catheter (C) recordings are shown. The recordings of a catheter in the radial artery and Swan-Ganz floating catheter in the right atrium are shown in B and D, respectively. The left portion of tracing C was obtained with the balloon inflated, yielding the pulmonary arterial wedge pressure. The right portion of tracing C was recorded with the balloon deflated, depicting the pulmonary arterial pressure. In this patient, the pulmonary arterial wedge pressure (i.e., left ventricular filling pressure) is normal, and the pulmonary artery pressure is elevated because of lung disease.

Certainly, improvements in noninvasive imaging techniques have made the Swan-Ganz catheter much less important in diagnosing cardiac conditions such as cardiac tamponade, constrictive pericarditis, right ventricular infarction, and ventricular septal defect. This led to a decline in the routine use of Swan-Ganz catheters in intensive care units. However, the use of these catheters has resurged, likely due to the increased use of advanced heart failure therapies and mechanical support, where continuous hemodynamic monitoring is essential for optimal therapy titration (Table 4.5).

ENDOMYOCARDIAL BIOPSY

Biopsy of the right ventricular endomyocardium can be performed. With this technique, a bioptome is introduced into the venous system through the right internal jugular vein and guided into the right ventricle by fluoroscopy. Small samples of the endocardium are taken for histologic evaluation. The primary indication for endomyocardial biopsy is the diagnosis of rejection after cardiac transplantation and documentation of cardiac amyloidosis; however, endomyocardial biopsy may have some use in diagnosing specific etiologic agents responsible for myocarditis.

NONINVASIVE VASCULAR TESTING

Assessment for the presence and severity of peripheral vascular disease is an important component of the cardiovascular evaluation. Comparison of the systolic blood pressure in the upper and lower extremities is one of the simplest tests to detect hemodynamically important arterial disease. Normally, the systolic pressure in the thigh is similar to that in the brachial artery. An ankle-to-brachial pressure

TABLE 4.5   Differential Diagnosis Using a Bedside Balloon Flow-Directed (Swan-Ganz) Catheter

Disease State	Thermodilution Cardiac Output	PCW Pressure	RA Pressure	Comments
Cardiogenic shock	↓	↑	nl or ↓	↑ Systemic vascular resistance
Septic shock (early)	↑	↓	↓	↑ Systemic vascular resistance; myocardial dysfunction can occur late
Volume overload	nl or ↑	↑	↑	
Volume depletion	↓	↓	↓	
Noncardiac pulmonary edema	nl	nl	nl	
Pulmonary heart disease	nl or ↑	nl	↑	↑ PA pressure
RV infarction	↓	↓ or nl	↑	
Pericardial tamponade	↓	nl or ↑	↑	Equalization of diastolic RA, RV, PA, and PCW pressure
Papillary muscle rupture	↓	↑	nl or ↑	Large v waves in PCW tracing
Ventricular septal rupture	↑	↑	nl or ↑	Artifact caused by RA → PA sampling higher in PA than RA; may have large v waves in PCW tracing

nl, Normal; *PA,* pulmonary artery; *PCW,* pulmonary capillary wedge; *RA,* right atrium; *RV,* right ventricle; ↑, increased; ↓, decreased.

ratio (i.e., ankle-brachial index) of less than or equal to 0.9 is abnormal. Patients with claudication usually have an index ranging from 0.5 to 0.8, and patients with rest pain have an index less than 0.5. In some patients, measuring the ankle-brachial index after treadmill exercise may help to determine the importance of borderline lesions. During normal exercise, blood flow increases to the upper and lower extremities with corresponding decreases in peripheral vascular resistance, whereas the overall ankle-brachial index remains unchanged. In the presence of a hemodynamically significant lesion, the reduced flow across the lesions causes a consequent pressure decrease, and as a result, the ankle-brachial index decreases in proportion to the severity of the stenosis. Some patients, especially those with diabetes or chronic kidney disease, may have falsely elevated ankle-brachial indices due to vascular stiffness (>1.3). In these patients, a toe-brachial index can be measured. In general, a toe-brachial index less than 0.6 indicates abnormal perfusion in the foot, though the site of the occlusive disease would have to be identified with further studies.

After significant vascular disease in the extremities has been identified, plethysmography can be used to determine the location and severity of the disease. With this method, a pneumatic cuff is positioned on the leg or thigh, and when inflated, temporarily obstructs venous return. Volume changes in the limb segment below the cuff are converted to a pressure waveform, which can be analyzed. The degree of amplitude reduction in the pressure waveform corresponds to the severity of arterial disease at that level.

Doppler ultrasound uses reflected sound waves to identify and localize stenotic lesions in the peripheral arteries. This test is particularly useful for patients with severely calcified arteries, for whom pneumatic compression is not possible and ankle-brachial indices are inaccurate. In combination with real-time imaging (i.e., duplex imaging), this technique is useful in assessing specific arterial segments and bypass grafts for stenotic or occlusive lesions.

Magnetic resonance angiography and CTA allow high-quality and comprehensive imaging of the entire peripheral arterial circulation in a single study. The three-dimensional nature of these studies and the ability to perform extensive postprocessing views, including cross-sectional views, of all vessels, even those that are very tortuous, are attractive features of these modalities.

SUGGESTED READINGS

Fihn SD, Blakenship JC, Alexander KP, et al: 2014 ACC/AHA/AATS/PCNA/ SCAI/STS Focused update of the guideline for the diagnosis and management of patients with stable ischemic heart disease, Circulation 130:1749-1767, 2014.

Kligfield P, Gettes LS, Bailey JJ, et al: Recommendations for the standardization and interpretation of the electrocardiogram: part I: the electrocardiogram and its technology a scientific statement from the American Heart Association Electrocardiography and Arrhythmias Committee, Council on Clinical Cardiology; the American College of Cardiology Foundation; and the Heart Rhythm Society endorsed by the International Society for Computerized Electrocardiology, J Am Coll Cardiol 49:1109-1127, 2007.

Otto CM: Textbook of clinical echocardiography, ed 6, Chapter 2, Normal anatomy and flow patterns on transthoracic echocardiography, Philadelphia, Elsevier, pp. 33-65, 578p.

Rybicki FJ, Udelson JE, Peacock, WF, et al: 2015 ACR/ACC/AHA/AATS/ACEP/ ASNC/NASCI/SAEM/SCCT/SCMR/SCPC/SNMMI/STR/STS Appropriate utilization of cardiovascular imaging in emergency department patients with chest pain: a joint document of the American College of Radiology Appropriateness Criteria Committee and the American College of Cardiology Appropriate Use Criteria Task Force, J Am Coll Cardiol 13:e1-e29, 2016.

St. John Sutton M, Morrison AR, Sinusas AJ, Ferrari VA: Heart failure: a companion to braunwald's heart disease, ed 4, Mann DL, Felker GM, editors: Philadelphia, Elsevier Inc, 2019, Chapter 32, Cardiac imaging in heart failure, p.418-448. 739p.

Wolk MJ, Bailey SR, Doherty JU, et al: ACCF/AHA/ASE/ASNC/HFSA/HRS/ SCAI/SCCT/SCMR/STS 2013 Multimodality appropriate use criteria for the detection and risk assessment of stable ischemic heart disease, J Am Coll Cardiol 63:380-406, 2014.

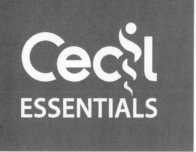

Heart Failure and Cardiomyopathy

Daniel J. Levine, Hyeon-Ju Ryoo Ali, Rayan Yousefzai

DEFINITION AND CLASSIFICATION

Heart failure (HF) is a clinical syndrome defined by inability of the heart to maintain output under normal filling pressures and/or impairment in relaxation of ventricles causing an increase in filling pressures. Patients experience fatigue and exercise intolerance if cardiac output is low and dyspnea and peripheral edema if the ventricular filling pressure is elevated. There are numerous ways to classify HF—by the type of cardiac impairment, causes of cardiomyopathy, patient's symptoms, or hemodynamic profiles.

Ejection Fraction

Most patients with HF have disorders in both systolic and diastolic function. However, ejection fraction (EF) is an important distinguishing characteristic in most clinical trials and, therefore, in guidelines for therapy. By imaging, cardiac function can be categorized as reduced EF (<40%) or preserved EF (≥50%). Patients with midrange EF (40% to 50%) are treated similarly to patients with reduced EF. HF with reduced EF (HFrEF) is associated with significant morbidity and mortality, especially in the elderly and those with severely low EF (<30%). HF with preserved EF (HFpEF) is less well studied with fewer effective targeted therapies. Increasing awareness of HFpEF has led to recognition of its prevalence with associated morbidity and mortality and the need for more research into optimal management.

Causes

Table 5.1 lists the common causes of cardiomyopathy leading to HF. Ischemic cardiomyopathy is the most common cause of HF and is estimated to account for about 60% of all HF admissions in the United States. This serves as a basis for clinical practice. Patients who present with new cardiomyopathy may undergo cardiac catheterization to exclude underlying coronary artery disease (CAD). Common causes of nonischemic cardiomyopathy include hypertension, chemotherapy, substance use, familial cardiomyopathy, and systemic disorders affecting the heart, such as amyloidosis and hemochromatosis. Worldwide, infections are a common cause of nonischemic cardiomyopathy including Chagas disease (endemic in South America), tuberculosis, and HIV.

Additional nonmyocardial processes that lead to HF include primary pericardial disorders. Pericardial tamponade limits the compliance of the heart, resulting in elevated filling pressures. Other causes include radiation-induced pericarditis, viral pericarditis, postsurgical pericardial thickening, and idiopathic fibrosis of the pericardium.

Valvular pathology including regurgitant and stenotic lesions can also lead to signs and symptoms of HF. Undetected, they can lead to morphologic changes in ventricular size and function. Most studies of HF exclude patients with uncorrected valvular diseases. Diagnosis and treatment of valvular heart disease is reviewed separately (see Chapter 7, "Valvular Heart Disease").

Types of Cardiomyopathy

Historically, cardiomyopathy has been classified morphologically as "dilated," "hypertrophic," and "restrictive." Dilated cardiomyopathy commonly leads to impairment in systolic function, or HFrEF. Common causes of dilated cardiomyopathy include myocardial infarction or infectious myocarditis.

Ventricular hypertrophy causes impairment in relaxation of ventricles, elevated filling pressures, and HFpEF. The most common cause of hypertrophy of ventricles is long-standing hypertension. Older women are at higher risk, as well as patients with diabetes, atrial fibrillation, obesity, hyperlipidemia, and CAD. Hypertrophic cardiomyopathy (HCM) is a genetic disorder in which a mutation in the sarcomeric proteins leads to thickening of ventricles and impaired filling. Patients with known family history of HCM should be tested by genetic analysis; current tests achieve a diagnostic yield of 30% to 60%. More than 130 genes associated with cardiomyopathy and arrhythmias have been identified. Genetic testing should be performed in centers with experienced geneticists and genetic counselors.

Restrictive cardiomyopathy also impairs ventricular relaxation and leads to HFpEF. This type of cardiomyopathy can be due to fibrosis as in radiation heart disease, or deposition of insoluble proteins as in amyloidosis. Restrictive cardiomyopathy is much less common than the other two types.

High-output HF is an under-recognized entity. It is characterized by an increased cardiac output that still fails to meet the metabolic and perfusion demands. Possible causes include obesity, anemia, hyperthyroidism, vitamin B1 deficiency, arteriovenous shunts and liver disease.

Functional Impairment

HF is a clinical syndrome with management strategies targeted to patients' symptoms and function status. Thus, it is paramount to have a unified language to stratify patients' degree of symptoms. Table 5.2 displays two classification methods: the "stages" as defined by the American College of Cardiology Foundation and the American Heart Association (ACCF/AHA) and the "classes" as defined by the New York Heart Association (NYHA).

ACCF/AHA Stages of HF

Patients in ACCF/AHA stage A have risk factors—such as hypertension, diabetes, metabolic syndrome, history of cardiac toxins, and family history of cardiomyopathy—without the diagnosis of CAD or cardiac remodeling. In stage B, patients may have prior history of MI or evidence of cardiomyopathy, but do not have symptoms. Stage C

TABLE 5.1 Causes of Cardiomyopathy

Myocardial infarction
Infection
  HIV
  Lyme
  Chagas
  Viral myocarditis
  Tuberculosis
Iatrogenic
  Chemotherapy: bleomycin, doxorubicin (Adriamycin)
  Antiretroviral medications
  Radiation
  Phenothiazines
  Chloroquine
  Clozapine
Toxins
  Alcohol
  Cocaine
  Methamphetamines
  Cobalt, lead, lithium, mercury, carbon monoxide, beryllium
Endocrine and metabolic
  Thyroid dysfunction
  Thiamine deficiency
  Pellagra
  Hypophosphatemia, hypocalcemia, uremia
Inflammatory
  Systemic lupus erythematosus
  Scleroderma
  Rheumatoid arthritis
  Giant cell arteritis
  Kawasaki disease
Infiltrative cardiomyopathy
  Amyloidosis
  Sarcoidosis
  Hemochromatosis
Other structural
  Valvular disease: progressive stenosis or regurgitation, acute chordae
    tendineae rupture, thrombosis of replaced valve
  Infective endocarditis
  Takotsubo cardiomyopathy
  Idiopathic dilated cardiomyopathy
  Idiopathic restrictive cardiomyopathy
  Peripartum cardiomyopathy
  Arrhythmogenic right ventricular dysplasia
Congenital heart disease
  Fabry disease
  Danon disease
  Friedreich's ataxia
  Myotonic dystrophy
  Duchenne-Becker muscular dystrophy
Rhythm
  Tachy-mediated cardiomyopathy
  Pacing-mediated cardiomyopathy

asymptomatic with ordinary activity and may also fall under stage B. Patients in class II have *some* limitation at *moderate* levels of physical activity while patients in class III have *any* limitations at *mild* levels of activity. Patients with symptoms at rest are categorized as class IV.

Hemodynamic Profiles

The impact of HF on circulatory physiology can be broadly categorized into four groups based on the degree of impairment of cardiac output and elevation of filling pressures (Fig. 5.1). Reduced cardiac output (cardiac index, CI ≤ 2.2 L/min/m^2) leads to impairment in end-organ perfusion. Patients may complain of fatigue, dizziness, or diminished urine output. On physical exam, extremities are cool due to low cardiac output and the compensatory vasoconstriction of the capillary beds to maintain perfusion. This finding helps identify the "cold" patients in the low-output state.

Elevated filling pressures can cause hydrostatic pressure to increase beyond the oncotic pressure, leading to extravasation of fluid into the interstitial space. Fluid may be retained in the lungs causing dyspnea, in the gut causing loss of appetite or nausea, and in the extremities causing peripheral edema.

Most patients who present in acute HF exacerbation are "warm and wet." Despite elevated filling pressures and congestion, they are still adequately perfused and can be treated with diuresis without hemodynamic support. "Cold and wet" patients are further decompensated. They require inotropic support to maintain adequate blood pressures and to perfuse the kidneys and permit effective diuresis. Some patients, despite diuresis, may remain in a poor perfusion state due to underlying cardiac disease. These patients are "cold and dry" and may require advanced therapies that will be described later.

PATHOPHYSIOLOGY

Frank-Starling Law

Under normal conditions, an increase in preload, or left ventricular end-diastolic pressure (LVEDP), increases stroke volume, as described by the Frank-Starling law (Fig. 5.2). In HF, the low cardiac output triggers an adaptive neurohormonal response that is designed to increase preload and stroke volume. However, due to the depressed myocardial contractility, the same increase in preload does not lead to increase in stroke volume or cardiac output. The consequence is dysregulation of an adaptive mechanism that leads to excessive filling pressures and fluid retention. Treatment consists of augmenting stroke volume by reducing afterload and increasing myocardial contractility with an inotrope. Diuresis can also reduce LVEDP, filling pressures, and congestive symptoms. Treatment of decompensated HF is discussed further in the section titled "Diagnosis and Management of Acute Decompensation."

Adaptive Neurohormonal Response

Our understanding of HF has changed over the years. It is no longer sufficient to consider morphologic characteristics or hemodynamic profiles of this clinical syndrome. HF is a clinical syndrome marked by sympathetic activation and neurohormonal dysregulation. The neurohormonal dysregulation and adaptive response are important targets for HF management strategies.

In response to low cardiac output, the sympathetic nervous system is triggered, releasing epinephrine and norepinephrine. The adrenalins increase heart rate and cause ventricular relaxation. They also trigger the G-coupled receptor pathways, increasing cyclic adenosine monophosphate (cAMP) production. Increased cAMP concentration leads to calcium influx and augments myocardial contractility.

In the kidneys, the juxtaglomerular cells in afferent arterioles sense decreased blood flow and in turn release renin. The consequent activation of the renin-angiotensin-aldosterone system (RAAS) is a cascade

constitutes clinical signs and symptoms of HF, while stage D encompasses patients whose HF is refractory to appropriate therapy.

NYHA Functional Classification of HF

The NYHA classification characterizes functional impairment of patients in symptomatic HF (ACCF/AHA stages C and D). Class I patients are

TABLE 5.2 ACCF/AHA Stages and NYHA Functional Classification of HF

ACCF/AHA Stages		NYHA Functional Classification	
A	Risk factors for HF without cardiomyopathy or HF symptoms	None	
B	Cardiomyopathy without HF symptoms	I	No HF symptoms
C	Cardiomyopathy with HF symptoms	I	No HF symptoms
		II	Some HF symptoms with moderate activity
		III	Any HF symptoms with mild activity
		IV	HF symptoms at rest
D	HF refractory to medical therapy	IV	HF symptoms at rest

ACCF, American College of Cardiology Foundation; *AHA,* American Heart Association; *HF,* heart failure; *NYHA,* New York Heart Association.
Data from Yancy CW, Jessup M, Bozkurt B, et al: 2013 ACCF/AHA guidelines for the management of heart failure: a report of the American College of Cardiology Foundation/American Heart Association Task Force on Practice Guidelines, *J Am Coll Cardiol* 62:e147-e239, 2013.

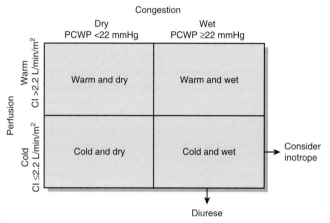

Fig. 5.1 Assessment of hemodynamic profiles in patients with heart failure. *CI,* Cardiac index; *PCWP,* pulmonary capillary wedge pressure. (Modified from Thibodeau JT, Drazner MH. The role of the clinical examination in patients with heart failure. JACC Hear Fail. 2019;6(7):544-551. https://doi.org/10.1016/j.jchf.2018.04.005.)

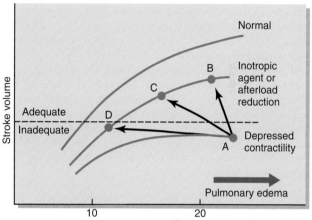

Fig. 5.2 Frank-Starling curve. Pulmonary edema occurs when the left ventricular end-diastolic pressure (LVEDP) is elevated such that hydrostatic pressures in pulmonary vasculature exceed oncotic pressures. For most patients, this threshold is approximately LVEDP = 20 mm Hg. Diuresis or venodilation reduces the filling pressures and can shift patients along the same curve correlating with lower LVEDP. Inotropic agents or afterload reduction can improve the cardiac output and improve stroke volume, shifting the pressure-volume curve upwards and to the left, moving patients from point A to point B. Adding diuresis or venodilation can shift patients from point A to point C. Excessive diuresis or venodilation shifting from point A to point D may cause excessive decline in LVEDP. While these patients may be at lower risk of pulmonary edema, their stroke volume may be impaired and result in inadequate cardiac output.

of enzyme activity that promotes end-organ perfusion by vasoconstriction, fluid retention at the level of the kidneys, and increased fluid intake by stimulating thirst.

Over time, these mechanisms become dysregulated. The adrenalins augment chronotropy and inotropy, which increase wall stress and myocardial oxygen consumption. Angiotensin II causes vasoconstriction that places the myocardium under higher afterload. Initially, cardiac muscles become hypertrophied to compensate for the workload; however, ventricles eventually dilate and lose contractility. Aldosterone also exacerbates ventricular remodeling, leading to progressive decline in cardiac function and loss of myocytes with subsequent fibrosis in a process known as apoptosis.

Atrial natriuretic peptide and brain natriuretic peptide (BNP) are counterregulatory hormones that are released in response to myocardial stress. They promote natriuresis and arterial vasodilation. Neprilysin degrades BNP and thereby inhibits the counterregulatory mechanism and inhibits natriuresis. This pathway is the target of novel drug therapies described in the section titled "Guideline-directed Medical Therapy."

DIAGNOSIS AND MANAGEMENT OF ACUTE DECOMPENSATION

Patients with HF frequently experience acute decompensation. Careful history and exam, as well as laboratory and imaging findings can help distinguish HF from other causes of dyspnea, such as chronic obstructive pulmonary disease (COPD) exacerbation or pneumonia.

History
Symptoms
HF is a clinical diagnosis. Thus, presenting symptoms, exam findings, and patients' response to HF treatments help establish the diagnosis.

Most patients with HF exacerbation present with dyspnea. Patients may also experience orthopnea (shortness of breath while lying flat) or paroxysmal nocturnal dyspnea or PND (waking up with shortness of breath) due to redistribution of fluid from the periphery to the lungs. Orthopnea and PND are specific for HF (specificity = 74% to 77% for orthopnea and 80% to 84% for PND) and can help discriminate among different etiologies for dyspnea.

Elevation of venous pressures (preload to the right ventricle) cause symptoms of systemic venous congestion. Patients may complain of decreased appetite, nausea, and abdominal fullness from intestinal edema of the gut. Transudation of fluid into the abdominal compartment may cause ascites and increased abdominal girth. Many patients complain of leg swelling or inability to fit into their shoes. Asking patients about sudden weight gain (e.g., 2-3 lb in a few days or 5 lb in a week) can also help assess the degree of fluid accumulation and identify targets for therapy.

Patients with inadequate cardiac output due to HF experience fatigue, exercise intolerance, or presyncope. Reduced end-organ perfusion can lead to altered mental status and diminished urine output. These symptoms are important clues to the hemodynamic profile of the patient and are critical for determining their need for inotropic support.

Precipitating Factors for Acute HF Exacerbation

Acute HF exacerbation may result from a new-onset primary cardiac dysfunction or decompensation of known chronic HF due to noncardiac causes. Cardiac dysfunction causes of acute HF exacerbation include acute myocardial infarction, other primary nonischemic cardiomyopathy, conduction disorders, valvular pathology, or pericardial issues (see Table 5.1 for a comprehensive list).

The most common noncardiac causes of heart failure exacerbation are diet indiscretion (increased salt intake or alcohol consumption) and medication noncompliance. Other common causes include infections (e.g., viral upper respiratory tract infection) or acute blood loss anemia. High blood pressure can also increase afterload acutely, increase filling pressures, and cause reduced cardiac output and/or worsening congestion.

Additional Information for New-Onset Cardiomyopathy

Once heart failure exacerbation diagnosis is established, additional history elements can help determine cause of cardiomyopathy. Questions should be focused on symptoms and risk factors of coronary artery disease, given that myocardial infarction is the most common cause of cardiomyopathy in the United States. Other helpful information includes past medical history including valvular disease, arrhythmias, autoimmune diseases, congenital heart disease, cancer, radiation, or cardiotoxic therapy, such as anthracycline derivatives. Social history should include duration and quantity of alcohol intake and cocaine use. Symptoms suggestive of other systemic disorders affecting the heart, such as neuropathy in amyloidosis, may be helpful and relevant for treatment options. Family history may be important in cases such as early-onset coronary artery disease, autoimmune disorders, congenital heart disease, and familial cardiomyopathies.

Exam Findings

Exam findings should be focused on signs of elevated filling pressures and reduced cardiac output to establish the diagnosis of heart failure. Other exam maneuvers not reviewed here include those relevant to myocardial ischemia, valvular disease, and arrhythmias that are reviewed in Chapters 7, 8, and 9.

Edema, JVD, and HJR

Elevated filling pressures in the heart are detected by several physical exam cues. Pulmonary auscultation may demonstrate rales, rhonchi, or even wheezing. Edema may be found in the lower extremities, but also in the abdomen in the form of ascites.

Jugular venous distension (JVD) is assessed with the patient situated at 30 to 45 degrees and breathing quietly. The vertical distance between the sternal notch and top of the JVD meniscus is the jugular venous height to which 5 cm should be added for true central venous pressure (normal range = 5-9 cm H_2O). Hepatojugular reflux (HJR) is

elevation of filling pressures by more than 3 cm H_2O while compressing the right upper quadrant for at least 10 seconds. Valvular disease, specifically tricuspid regurgitation, may falsely elevate the JVD meniscus and make these exam findings less reliable.

Cardiac Examination: S_3 and S_4

The point of maximal impulse (PMI) may be displaced (below the fifth intercostal space and lateral to the midclavicular line) suggestive of cardiomegaly. On auscultation of the heart, a third heart sound (S_3) may be heard in early diastole. The sound is the result of blood passively traveling from the atrium into an already filled ventricle. This is typically associated with left ventricular systolic dysfunction and incomplete ejection of blood during systole. S_4 is heard in late diastole and results from the atrial kick pushing the remaining fluid into a stiffened ventricle. S_4 suggests diastolic dysfunction.

Bendopnea

Bendopnea is a recently described simple stress maneuver that can be used if the aforementioned exams are not helpful in discriminating among the many causes of dyspnea. Patients are asked to bend forward while sitting in a chair for 30 seconds, which increases filling pressures. Patients may develop dyspnea or "bendopnea," particularly if they have a low cardiac index. This maneuver has been associated with increased 6-month mortality, composite end point of death, heart failure–related admission, and need for advanced therapies.

Square Wave Response

Another stress maneuver to assess the left ventricular filling pressure is the square wave response. This is particularly useful when the JVD and HJR are limited due to body habitus or tricuspid regurgitation. The blood pressure cuff is inflated to the point of hearing the first Korotkoff sound. Then the patient is asked to Valsalva (i.e., bear down) in order to reduce the preload and decrease pulmonary venous return to the left ventricle. In normal patients, the Korotkoff sound disappears due to a drop in blood pressure. In patients with pulmonary congestion, the pulmonary intravascular volume maintains forward flow during Valsalva, and the Korotkoff sound remains the same. The persistence of Korotkoff sound, therefore, is a positive test and is suggestive of elevated left ventricular pressures and pulmonary congestion.

Laboratory Data and Imaging

Patients who have symptoms and signs concerning for acute heart failure exacerbation should all receive an electrocardiogram (ECG) and a chest radiograph. An ECG may show evidence of new ischemia or old infarct suggesting MI as the potential cause for cardiomyopathy. A chest radiograph may demonstrate signs of pulmonary edema, such as Kerley B lines and pleural effusions (Fig. 5.3). The BNP is often elevated, although it is neither sensitive nor specific. In fact, BNP is most useful for its negative predictive value. A low BNP (or NT-pro-BNP) can exclude HF in patients with combined cardiopulmonary disease who present acutely with dyspnea. The troponin may be elevated in acute myocardial infarction or demand ischemia. Laboratory testing should include a basic metabolic panel to establish baseline electrolytes and kidney function. The liver function test results help assess the degree of congestion and cardiohepatic syndrome. The complete blood count can give clues to the etiology, such as leukocytosis in the setting of acute infection or anemia.

All patients with new-onset heart failure should have an echocardiogram. It may reveal wall motion abnormalities consistent with CAD, valvular stenosis or regurgitation, or pericardial effusion. Ventricular wall thickness and chamber sizes can also be assessed. Thickened ventricles may raise concerns for genetic hypertrophic cardiomyopathy,

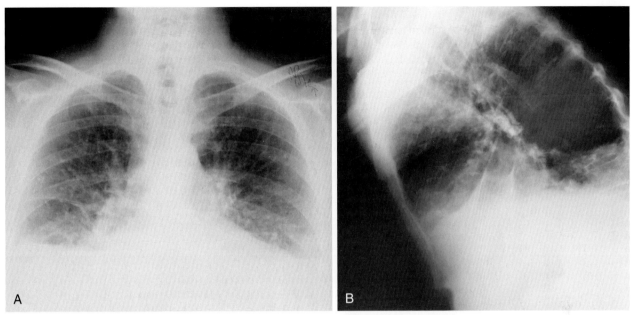

Fig. 5.3 (A) Posteroanterior chest radiograph demonstrating pulmonary edema. Notice the increased interstitial markings, more prominent in central zones, and Kerley B lines, which are horizontal markings at the lung periphery. There is also a prominent horizontal line in left lung, suggestive of fluid layering in the major fissure. Both costovertebral angles are obscured, suggesting bilateral pulmonary effusion. (B) Lateral chest radiograph demonstrating pulmonary edema. Fluid is layering in the lower lung zones suggestive of pulmonary effusion.

long-standing hypertension hypertrophic heart, or infiltrative disease such as amyloidosis (Fig. 5.4). Newer techniques including strain imaging can be used to evaluate for infiltrative disease as well as early changes due to toxic chemotherapeutic agents.

Additional Testing to Determine Etiology

Appropriate patients with symptoms, signs, ECG, and/or troponin results concerning for myocardial infarction causing heart failure exacerbation should undergo coronary angiography and revascularization. Some patients presenting with new heart failure diagnosis have a history of coronary artery disease but do not have typical anginal symptoms. For these patients, the Surgical Treatment for Ischemic Heart Failure (STITCH) trials demonstrated that myocardial viability assessment with nuclear stress testing does not, in fact, improve mortality. However, the ACCF/AHA 2013 guidelines make weak recommendations to obtain noninvasive imaging such as nuclear stress test or stress echocardiogram prior to proceeding with revascularization. Evidence of ischemia and significant myocardial viability may be one of the factors to be considered for catheterization.

If the above work-up is negative, additional testing for nonischemic cardiomyopathy can be pursued. A cardiac MRI can reveal specific patterns of enhancement that are indicative of infiltrative disorders (e.g., cardiac amyloidosis and sarcoidosis). Additional laboratory testing may include thyroid function test, human immunodeficiency virus (HIV) test, iron studies, and hepatitis C virus antibodies.

Prompt recognition and work-up for cardiac amyloidosis has become more important as novel therapies have become available that are important to initiate early in the disease progression. Features concerning for amyloidosis include low voltage on ECG, left ventricular hypertrophy, and evidence of other organ manifestation such as gastrointestinal symptoms (diarrhea, nausea), neuropathy, and chronic kidney disease. Laboratory testing should include levels of serum and urine protein electrophoresis (SPEP and UPEP) along with serum and/or urine immunofixation. Imaging techniques include echocardiography, specifically strain imaging that tends to spare the apex, and nuclear imaging called pyrophosphate (PYP) scan. The latter is sensitive and specific for transthyretin, or wild-type amyloidosis. Definitive diagnosis is achieved with direct visualization of the amyloid deposits in tissue samples. Biopsy can be done on the abdominal fat pad, cardiac muscle, rectal mucosa, salivary gland, and liver.

Right heart catheterization is another diagnostic tool for assessment of acute HF exacerbation. The routine use of pulmonary artery catheters (PACs) for patients with HF exacerbation has not been shown to improve mortality, length of stay, or rehospitalization rates (the Evaluation Study of Congestive Heart Failure and Pulmonary Artery Catheterization Effectiveness, ESCAPE). The ACCF/AHA 2013 guidelines still recommend use of PACs with patients who do not respond to standard therapies and when there is a degree of uncertainty regarding the patient's volume status despite routine clinical assessment. Right heart catheterization is also used to estimate cardiac output, assess candidacy for advanced therapy, and perform cardiac biopsy.

Acute Management
Diuresis

The mainstay treatment for acute HF exacerbation is intravenous (IV) loop diuretics. Intravenous administration of diuretics should be equal to or exceed the dose of home oral medications. Oral diuretics may be less effective in this setting due to bowel edema which can impair absorption via the gut. Diuresis should be targeted toward symptom management, improvement in vital signs, resolution of acute kidney injury (AKI), change in weight, and net output of urine. Some patients with prolonged diuretic use can develop resistance to loop diuretics. These patients may benefit from thiazide administration to block fluid reabsorption in the distal convoluted tubules. Patients who do not respond to maximal diuretic regimen can be considered for ultrafiltration.

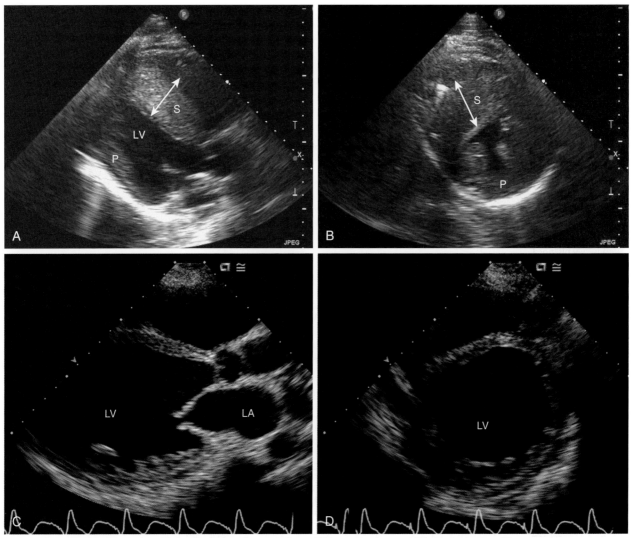

Fig. 5.4 Examples of hypertrophic cardiomyopathy on (A) long axis view and (B) short axis view. The posterior wall "P" and interventricular septum, "S" are markedly thickened. Examples of dilated cardiomyopathy on (C) long axis view and (D) short axis view. The left ventricular cavity "LV" and left atrium "LA" are enlarged.

Afterload Reduction

Patients may be hypertensive in the setting of HF exacerbation. Acutely lowering the blood pressure can quickly reduce the afterload, lower ventricular filling pressures, and reduce the degree of pulmonary vascular congestion. Patients in respiratory distress may experience prompt relief of their symptoms with afterload reduction. Intravenous therapy options for acute afterload reduction include nitroglycerin, nitroprusside, and nesiritide.

Cardiogenic Shock Management

Some patients in acute HF exacerbation present in "cold" hemodynamic profiles and have significantly reduced cardiac output. These patients may require inotropic support for end-organ perfusion. The use of inotropes can improve perfusion of kidneys and patients' response to diuresis. More information regarding the different types of inotropes and their use is detailed in the section titled "Inotropic Support."

Guideline-Directed Medical Therapy

In the current age, the goal in heart failure therapy is to not only control symptoms and slow progression of disease, but also to recover some cardiac function. New pharmacotherapies have become available that not only improve functional status but lower mortality and reduce hospitalizations. Thus, it is imperative to understand and follow guideline-directed medical therapy (GDMT) for all patients with HF (Fig. 5.5).

All patients with HF should be advised to make lifestyle modifications to reduce the risk of development or progression or cardiac disease. Blood pressure control, weight loss, and management of diabetes can significantly reduce the risk of CAD and ventricular remodeling. Patients with any stage of heart failure, regardless of whether they have symptoms, should be treated with ACE inhibitors or aldosterone receptor II blockers (ARBs), as well as statins if there is evidence of coronary artery disease or the atherosclerotic cardiovascular disease (ASCVD) risk score is greater than 7.5%.

For patients with HFrEF stage C (i.e., patients with any symptoms), several medications have been shown to reduce mortality and improve quality of life. All patients should be treated with specific β-blockers known to improve mortality in HFrEF patients, as well as a medication for afterload reduction (ACE inhibitors, ARBs, or angiotensin receptor blocker–neprilysin inhibitors, i.e., ARNIs). The other therapies described in the following sections have been proven effective for only certain subpopulations.

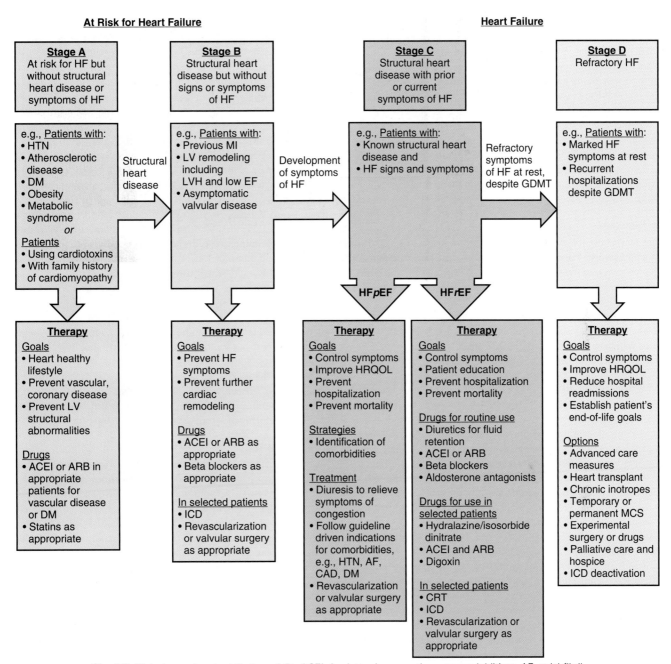

Fig. 5.5 Clinical overview by HF stage A-D. *ACEI*, Angiotensin-converting enzyme inhibitor; *AF*, atrial fibrillation; *ARB*, angiotensin receptor blocker; *CAD*, coronary artery disease; *CRT*, cardiac resynchronization therapy; *DM*, diabetes mellitus; *EF*, ejection fraction; *GDMT*, guideline-directed medical therapy; *HF*, heart failure; *HRQOL*, health-related quality of life; *HTN*, hypertension; *ICD*, implantable cardiac defibrillator; *LV*, left ventricular; *LVH*, left ventricular hypertrophy; *MCS*, mechanical circulatory support. (Adapted from ACCF/AHA 2013 Guidelines.)

ACE Inhibitor, ARB, and ARNI

All patients with stage C HFrEF, regardless of symptom burden, should be on an ACE inhibitor, an ARB, or an ARNI. By inhibiting RAAS, ACE inhibitors and ARBs reduce afterload and inhibit fibrosis. Multiple trials from the 1980s to the early 2000s including CONSENSUS, SOLVD, Val-HeFT, and CHARM demonstrated an improvement in mortality (by 16% to 40%) and reduced hospitalizations for HF exacerbations in patients treated with ACE inhibitors or ARBs.

The ARNI is a novel medication that combines the ARB, valsartan, with a neprilysin inhibitor called sacubitril. Neprilysin is an endopeptidase that breaks down vasoactive peptides such as BNP and bradykinin. By inhibiting neprilysin, the sacubitril promotes the action of the BNP, which increases diuresis. In the PARADIGM randomized controlled trial (RCT) ARNIs were found to be superior to ACE inhibitors (number needed to treat, NNT = 21 for composite end point of HF admissions or mortality). The PIONEER study also demonstrated ARNIs could be safely started during hospitalization and readmission due to HF exacerbations. The 2017 American College of Cardiology and American Heart Association (ACC/AHA) updates to the guidelines recommend patients on ACE inhibitors or ARBs should be switched to ARNIs. Patients on ACE inhibitors should have a wash-out period of 36 hours after ACE inhibitors are discontinued to avoid angioedema secondary to bradykinin accumulation.

The therapeutic potential of ACE inhibitors and ARBs for the HFpEF patient population has been investigated by several RCTs, including PEP-CHF, CHARM-preserved, and I-PRESERVE. These studies unfortunately showed ACE inhibitors and ARBs do not significantly reduce cardiovascular mortality or heart failure exacerbations in this patient group. The Prospective Comparison of ARNI with ARB Global Outcomes in HFpEF (PARAGON-HF) also demonstrated no significant risk reduction of mortality or HF-related hospitalizations for ARNIs. Guidelines currently do not recommend initiation of ACE inhibitors, ARBs, or ARNIs for HFpEF patients.

Beta-Blockers

The three types of β-blockers found to be effective in Stage C HFrEF are bisoprolol, carvedilol, and metoprolol succinate. β-Blockers inhibit the sympathetic nervous system, reduce myocardial work, improve endothelial integrity, and ultimately reduce ventricular remodeling. Numerous studies—MERIT-HF, CAPRICORN, COPERNICUS, COMET, and CIBIS-II—have demonstrated a significant reduction in mortality (31% to 40%) and the composite end point of mortality and heart failure exacerbation admissions. The trials on HFpEF patients are small and inadequately powered, but many show a trend toward improving mortality.

Aldosterone Antagonist

Patients with stage C HFrEF, NYHA class II-IV already on β-blockers and afterload reduction with an ACE inhibitor, ARB, or ARNI should be started on aldosterone receptor antagonists assuming creatinine clearance greater than 30 and normal potassium levels. The direct inhibition of aldosterone further reduces ventricular fibrosis and remodeling. The RALES trial showed a 30% reduction in all-cause mortality, sudden cardiac death, and HF hospitalizations for patients with NYHA class II-IV symptoms. EMPHASIS-HF also showed a 37% reduction in the composite end point of death and HF readmissions.

Patients with HFpEF may also benefit from aldosterone receptor antagonists. The Treatment of Preserved Cardiac Function Heart Failure with an Aldosterone Antagonist (TOPCAT) was an international, placebo-controlled, randomized study for patients with EF 45% or greater. The study showed a small effect size of spironolactone reducing HF hospitalizations (12.0% vs. 14.2%). However, subsequent analyses showed a significant regional variation, suggesting that North American participants may have been more compliant with the medications and likely may have derived greater benefit.

Ivabradine

Patients with symptomatic HFrEF (stage C, NYHA class II-IV) with high resting heart rate (≥70 beats per minute) despite treatment with a high dose of β-blocker may benefit from the addition of ivabradine. Ivabradine works by inhibiting I_f—the "funny channel"—at the sinus node. The SHIFT trial demonstrated that patients in NYHA II-IV class with EF 35% or less already on GDMT treated with ivabradine experienced a 5% absolute risk reduction in heart failure exacerbations and 2% absolute reduction in cardiovascular mortality.

Hydralazine and Nitrates

Vasodilators such as hydralazine and nitrates reduce afterload, myocardial work, and in theory, reduce ventricular remodeling. Their efficacy, however, has only been shown among African Americans with HFrEF stage C and NYHA III-IV symptoms already on GDMT. For patients with HFpEF, nitrates have been shown to improve exercise tolerance but do not improve mortality (NEAT-HFpEF, 2015). The

ACC/AHA 2017 updates to the guidelines do not yet recommend vasodilators for HFpEF patients.

Digoxin

Digoxin increases myocardial contractility by inhibiting sodium-potassium exchange, which increases intracellular calcium. Digoxin is associated with a decrease in HF hospitalizations, improvement in quality of life, and increase in exercise tolerance. The DIG trials, however, showed no impact on mortality. Digoxin also has an unfavorable side effect profile. It can cause arrhythmias (ectopic, re-entrant cardiac rhythms, and heart block), GI side effects (nausea, anorexia), and neurologic side effects (visual effects, disorientation, confusion). Patients who are elderly and have low body mass index or renal dysfunction are at higher risk. Many medications can increase the digoxin level and increase the risk of toxicity (clarithromycin, erythromycin, itraconazole, amiodarone, dronedarone, cyclosporine, propafenone, verapamil, and quinidine). Given these risks and benefits, patients with stage C HFrEF could benefit from digoxin.

Diuretics

For patients with chronic heart failure, diuretics are used to maintain euvolemia and target symptom management. Loop diuretics are most commonly used, but some patients develop resistance over time. Distal convoluted tubules become hypertrophied and water becomes reabsorbed past the loop of Henle, reversing the effect of loop diuretics. Small doses of thiazide and metolazone, which impact the distal nephrons, can significantly increase diuresis. Their use requires close and careful monitoring of serum electrolytes and renal function.

Device Therapy

Cardiomyopathy confers an increased risk of ventricular arrhythmias and sudden cardiac death (SCD). Patients with low EF of 35% or less and NYHA class II-III symptoms should receive an implantable cardiac defibrillator (ICD) for primary prevention (Fig. 5.6). Numerous trials—SCD-HeFT, CARE-HF, MADIT-CRT, and REVERSE—have demonstrated reduction in SCDs that outweigh the risk of device-related complications for HFrEF patients.

Patients with ischemic cardiomyopathy are at higher risk for SCDs due to the scar tissue that can be a nidus for ventricular arrhythmias. Thus, patients with ischemic cardiomyopathy (EF ≤30%) should also receive an ICD even if they do not have symptoms (NYHA class I). The evidence behind device therapy for HFpEF patients, however, is less clear. The DANISH trials demonstrated 3% mortality benefit but 1.5% device-related complications.

Device therapy in the form of cardiac resynchronization therapy (CRT), also termed "biventricular pacing," has also been shown to improve functional capacity, reduce HF rehospitalizations, and improve all-cause mortality. Patients derive their benefit from improved contractility and increased forward flow due to ventricular synchrony. Additional benefits include improvement in blood pressure, making it possible to intensify therapy with ACE inhibitors, ARBs, and ARNIs. Patients with HFrEF and a widened QRS of 150 ms or greater with a left bundle branch block pattern should be considered for CRT implantation.

Management of Atrial Fibrillation

HF patients with atrial fibrillation (AF) are at higher risk of stroke, HF exacerbations, and mortality. The AFFIRM trial demonstrated similar outcomes between rate and rhythm control strategies; however, patients with HFrEF were underrepresented. Theoretically, restoring sinus rhythm allows preservation of the atrial kick and improvement in A-V synchrony, which could reduce filling pressures and improve cardiac output. Recently, CASTLE-AF demonstrated that patients with HFrEF

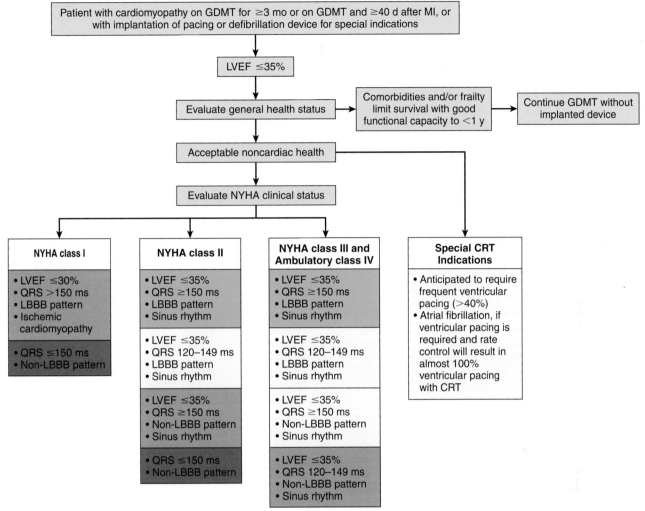

Fig. 5.6 Recommendations for implanted cardiac defibrillator (ICDs) and cardiac resynchronization therapy (CRT) depend on the ejection fraction (EF) and New York Heart Association (NYHA) functional class. *Green* indicates class I recommendations (evidence or agreement that treatment is useful and effective), *yellow* indicates class IIa recommendations (weight of evidence or opinion in favor of treatment), *orange* indicates IIb recommendations (usefulness/efficacy is less well established), and *red* indicates class III recommendations (evidence or general agreement that treatment is not useful/effect and in some cases may be harmful). *GDMT,* Guideline-directed medical therapy; *LBBB,* left bundle branch block; *MI,* myocardial infarction. (Adapted from ACCF/AHA 2013 guidelines.)

NYHA class II-IV experienced significant reduction in death (11.6%) and heart failure exacerbation (15.2%) after catheter ablation to restore sinus rhythm. Although not yet reflected in the guidelines, patients with HFrEF who are symptomatic should be considered for AF ablation.

Invasive Hemodynamic Monitoring of Ambulatory Patients

For patients with recurrent heart failure exacerbations, ambulatory monitoring devices can allow for early detection of increase in filling pressures and timely interventions. CardioMEMS is an implantable device placed in the pulmonary artery that communicates real-time hemodynamics measurements remotely to trained health care professionals. Multiple RCTs have demonstrated their effectiveness. In COMPASS-HF patients with NYHA class III monitored with CardioMEMS experienced a 36% reduction of HF hospitalizations. Similarly, CHAMPION-HF demonstrated CardioMEMS could achieve up to 37% relative risk reduction in HF exacerbations in the first 17 months. Device-related or systems-related complications were found to be exceedingly rare (freedom from complications estimated to be 98.6%). Currently, the device is FDA-approved for patients with heart failure with NYHA class III symptoms

who have been hospitalized in the past year. The GUIDE-HF trial is an ongoing investigation to determine the impact of CardioMEMS in the NYHA class II and IV patient population and patients with elevated BNP. Many ICDs now have the capacity to monitor physiologic parameters including heart rate variability and intrathoracic impedance, which may be helpful for patient assessment and management.

Advanced Therapy

Patients with HFrEF stage D, who are refractory to medical therapy, are challenging to manage. Appropriate patients with stage D symptoms despite optimal medical therapy should be referred to centers that provide advanced circulatory support. Recent advances in mechanical support technology have made possible implantation of durable pumps as destination therapy in patients ineligible for other therapy.

INTERMACS Profiles

Patients in HFrEF stage D can be further characterized with profiles developed by the Interagency Registry of Mechanically Assisted Circulatory Support (INTERMACS). The INTERMACS profiles

TABLE 5.3 INTERMACS Profiles

INTERMACS Profile	Description	Urgency of Interventions
1: Cardiogenic shock	"Crash and burn": critical cardiogenic shock despite increasing doses of inotropes confirmed with rising lactate or acidosis	Within hours
2: Progressive decline	"Sliding on inotropes": end-organ hypoperfusion evidenced by worsening renal failure and inability to maintain euvolemia despite inotropic support	Within days
3: Stable but inotrope dependent	"Dependent stability": adequate end-organ perfusion and symptom control while on inotropic support or temporary circulatory support device, but unable to wean from inotropes	Within weeks to months
4: Resting symptoms	Symptoms of congestion occur at rest	Within weeks to months
5: Exertion intolerant	"Housebound": comfortable at rest and basic activities of daily living but any other activity causes limiting symptoms	Depends upon nutrition, organ function, activity
6: Exertion limited	"Walking wounded": fatigues after a few minutes of activity. Could confirm cardiac impairment with hemodynamic measures or cardiopulmonary stress test	Depends upon nutrition, organ function, activity
7: Advanced NYHA III	Mild physical exertion is tolerable, but moderate activity causes symptoms	Not yet indicated

INTERMACS, Interagency Registry of Mechanically Assisted Circulatory Support; *NYHA,* New York Heart Association.
Data from Stevenson LW, Pagani FD, Young JB, et al. INTERMACS profiles of advanced heart failure: the current picture. *J Heart Lung Transplant.* 2009;28(6):535-541.

describe the range of symptoms from advanced NYHA class III (profile 7) to critical cardiogenic shock (profile 1) and can help assess the urgency to evaluate for mechanical circulatory support or transplants (Table 5.3). Patients in INTERMACS profiles 5 through 7 can be monitored without immediate plan for advanced heart failure therapy. Patients with resting symptoms (profile 4) or receiving inotropic support (profile 3) may need circulatory support sooner. Patients who are "sliding on inotropes" (profile 2)—demonstrating poor end-organ perfusion despite inotropic support—should be considered for immediate support within days and potentially transferred to a left ventricular assist device (LVAD) and transplant center. Patients in critical cardiogenic shock (profile 1) take precedence in mechanical circulatory support or heart transplant, which may be needed within hours.

Inotropic Support

Patients who have persistent symptoms despite GDMT and volume optimization, found to have elevated filling pressures and/or low cardiac output, may be appropriate candidates for ambulatory inotropic support. Ambulatory inotropes can be used for either bridge to durable mechanical support or palliation of symptoms. The current evidence suggests that ambulatory inotropes compared to GDMT do not improve mortality but may improve heart failure symptoms (improvement in NYHA class by 0.6 more than GDMT).

Inotropes commonly used include milrinone and dobutamine. Milrinone inhibits phosphodiesterase and thereby causes vasodilation. Hemodynamics improve due to reduction in afterload, decrease in pulmonary vascular resistance, and increase in cardiac contractility. Dobutamine is a sympathomimetic agent; it is an agonist for α-1, β-1, and β-2 receptor. This leads to an increase in myocardial contractility and stroke volume as well as decrease in total peripheral resistance, or afterload. Adverse effects include arrhythmias and significant hypotension due to vasodilation. If patients are hypotensive, norepinephrine (α-1 and β-1 receptor agonists) and dopamine (β-1 receptor agonist at medium doses and α-adrenergic receptor agonists at high doses) are preferred agents because they can vasoconstrict and increase blood pressure in addition to increasing myocardial contractility.

Mechanical Circulatory Support

In the setting of acute cardiogenic shock, several options are available for short-term mechanical support.

The intra-aortic balloon pump (IABP) is a counterpulsation pump placed in the aorta and synchronized to native cardiac beats. It reduces the afterload by deflating during systole and improves coronary perfusion pressure by inflating during diastole. The IABP-SHOCK II trials demonstrated no difference in 30-day mortality between patients treated with inotropes alone and those with IABP. Compared to other short-term mechanical supports, IABP provides only a small augmentation in cardiac output (500-600 mL/min/m²). Potential complications include limb ischemia, thrombosis, and vascular complications.

The Impella ventricular support system is an axial-flow pump that pulls blood from the left ventricle through an inlet area near the tip and expels blood from the catheter into the ascending aorta. There are different sizes of Impella including 2.5 or CP, which are designed for percutaneous peripheral insertion, as well as Impella 5.0 or LD, which are designed for surgical insertion. Depending on the type of Impella, it can provide 2.5 to 5 L/min/m² of augmentation. The ISAR-SHOCK and IMPRESS trials, however, have demonstrated no improvement in mortality. In addition to limb ischemia and vascular complications, the rotor in the pump can lyse red blood cells, causing significant hemolytic anemia.

Venous arterial extracorporeal membrane oxygenation (VA-ECMO) is a heart-lung bypass via venous and arterial cannulas that pump the blood from the body through an external oxygenator. Venous blood is drained from the right atrium and returned to the distal arterial system providing near complete temporary circulation support.

In addition to concerns of limb ischemia, hemolysis, and vascular injury due to the cannulas, the north-south syndrome is a feared complication. In this syndrome, only the lower body receives oxygenated blood through the arterial cannula, and the "north"—or the brain and upper body—receives perfusion with the deoxygenated blood. This may occur due to the position of the cannulas or the recovery of native heart function. VA-ECMO is considered as a last resort and is available at only select centers with the surgeons and infrastructure capabilities.

The advancement in durable mechanical circulatory support devices has now made it possible for HF patients in cardiogenic shock to be discharged and managed in ambulatory settings. Since the first heart lung machine in 1953, the durable circulatory supports have undergone significant transformation to reduce their size, noise, and device-related complications (Table 5.4). In order to reduce pump thrombosis, devices have evolved from axial-flow to centrifugal-flow.

TABLE 5.4 Parameters of Left Ventricular Assist Device

	HeartMate II	HeartMate III	HVAD
Flow configuration	Axial	Centrifugal	Centrifugal
Impeller bearings	Mechanical	Magnetic levitation	Hybrid
Weight	250 grams	220 grams	160 grams
Variation in speed	No	Yes	No
Implantation site	Chest and abdomen	Pericardial	Pericardial

In the latter configuration, impellers are perpendicular to the flow of the blood to reduce the risk of clot formation. Although older devices required mechanical bearings for the pumps, the latest designs employ magnetic levitation, further reducing thrombotic risks and improving durability. The newest FDA-approved device, HeartMate III, combines continuous flow with frequent variation in the speed, which can further reduce hemostasis and clot formation.

The prospective, multicenter RCT with the HeartMate III demonstrated up to 78% stroke-free 2-year survival rate. With these superior outcomes for the latest LVADs, advanced heart failure patients who are otherwise not candidates for heart transplants can now receive durable circulatory support as destination therapy. In fact, LVADs are now FDA-approved for patients with INTERMACS profiles 1 through 6. Patients who demonstrate signs of cardiorenal syndrome, intolerance to GDMT due to hypotension, and are persistently in NYHA functional classes III to IV despite GDMT should be referred to an advanced heart failure specialist for further evaluation.

Heart Transplant

Heart transplant remains an option for select patients with refractory HF. In recent years, the list of candidates for heart transplantation continues to grow without concurrent increase in available heart donors. Due to the scarcity of organs and high waitlist mortality, particularly in certain geographic areas, the United Network for Organ Sharing (UNOS) released a new set of allocation criteria in order to prioritize the sickest patients (Fig. 5.7). Those in status 1 or 2 will have access to organs that become available in a larger geographic area of up to 500 miles from the donor site.

Patients' survival after heart transplantation has improved but gains are mostly limited to the first year, with 1-year survival estimated to be 85%. The median survival is estimated to be 11 years; those who survive the first year have a longer median survival of 13 years. Survival may be improved by preoperative care including LVAD implantation as bridge to transplant, reducing allograft ischemic time intraoperatively, and optimization of postoperative immunosuppressants and cardiac rehabilitation. Patients are on multiple immunosuppressants, which places them at increased risk of developing opportunistic infections and malignancy. Inadequate immunosuppression can increase the risk of graft failure. These patients undergo close surveillance for the first year and continued monitoring for the rest of their lives.

Palliative Care

Despite advances in HF treatment and prevention, rates of hospitalization for acute decompensation, 30-day readmission, and mortality rates remain high. Only 50% of patients survive after 5 years and 29% die within the first year. Indicators of poor prognosis include functional status, low EF, pulmonary vascular and right ventricular remodeling due to left ventricular failure, cardiorenal and hepatic syndromes, and presence of arrhythmias.

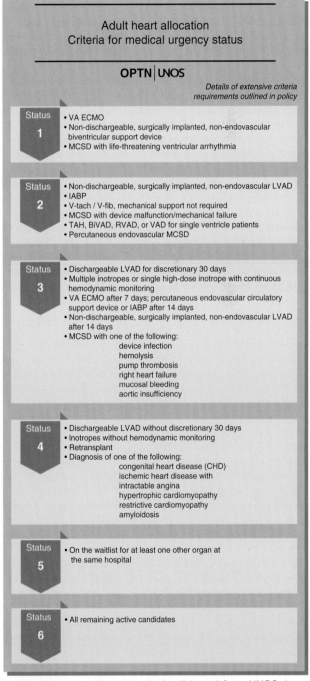

Fig. 5.7 Adult heart allocation criteria. (Adapted from UNOS, https://optn.transplant.hrsa.gov/learn/professional-education/adult-heart-allocation/.)

Toward the end of life, patients with HF have significant symptom burden that leads to loss of function and independence. Palliative care provides an interdisciplinary approach to meet the physical and emotional needs of the patient. Patients experience significant improvement in symptom burden, rates of anxiety and depression, as well as reduced hospitalization readmission rates. Palliative care can also assist with end-of-life transition and introduction of hospice care to patients and their families. Palliative care is a class I recommendation for stage D HFrEF patients. The optimization of HF symptom management and increasing access to palliative care are critical for improving care for advanced HF patients.

FUTURE DIRECTIONS

Prevention is still the key to success in treating HF. Treating hypertension and diabetes remain major public health objectives. Recent advances in pharmacologic and device therapies have improved HF-associated mortality and morbidity. Replacement of ACE inhibitors and ARBs with ARNIs has been shown to reduce mortality. CardioMEMs reduce 30-day readmission rates by more than 50%. Patients with advanced HF who are poor candidates for heart transplants can now receive LVADs as destination therapy. In addition, there is promising research and development in diagnosis and treatment of previously underrecognized conditions, such as HFpEF and amyloidosis.

However, access to care remains challenging in the modern health care environment. Currently, costs of novel therapies like ARNIs, cardioMEMs, and LVADs can be prohibitive. There is still limited access to palliative care services for advanced HF patients, even though this "low tech" intervention improves symptom management and reduces costs due to excessive acute care service utilization. Collaboration among health care providers, patient advocates, and policymakers can lead to improvement not only in survival and quality of life but reducing the financial burden to the society and the individual.

SUGGESTED READINGS

Abrahao Hajjar L, Teboul J-L: Mechanical Circulatory Support Devices for Cardiogenic Shock: State of the Art, 1–150, 2019, https://doi.org/10.1186/s13054-019-2368-y.

Gersh BJ, Maron BJ, Bonow RO, et al: 2011 ACCF/AHA Guideline for the diagnosis and treatment of hypertrophic cardiomyopathy: a report of the American College of Cardiology Foundation/American Heart Association Task Force on Practice guidelines developed in collaboration with the American Association for Thoracic Surgery, American Society of Echocardiography, American Society of Nuclear Cardiology, Heart Failure Society of America, J Am Coll Cardiol 58(25):e212–e260, 2011, https://doi.org/10.1016/j.jacc.2011.06.011.

Hershberger RE, Givertz MM, Ho CY, et al: Genetic evaluation of cardiomyopathy—a Heart Failure Society of America Practice Guideline, J Card Fail 24(5):281–302, 2018, https://doi.org/10.1016/j.cardfail.2018.03.004.

Kavalieratos D, Gelfman LP, Tycon LE, et al: Palliative care in heart failure: rationale, evidence, and future priorities, J Am Coll Cardiol 70(15):1919–1930, 2017, https://doi.org/10.1016/j.jacc.2017.08.036.

Martin N, Manoharan K, Thomas J, Davies C, Lumbers RT: Beta-blockers and inhibitors of the renin-angiotensin aldosterone system for chronic heart failure with preserved ejection fraction, Cochrane Database Syst Rev 2018(6), 2018, https://doi.org/10.1002/14651858.CD012721.pub2.

Thibodeau JT, Drazner MH: The role of the clinical examination in patients with heart failure, JACC Hear Fail 6(7):544–551, 2019, https://doi.org/10.1016/j.jchf.2018.04.005.

Yancy CW, Jessup M, Bozkurt B, et al: 2013 ACCF/AHA Guideline for the management of heart failure: a report of the American College of Cardiology Foundation/American Heart Association Task Force on practice guidelines, Circulation 128(16):e240–e327, 2013, https://doi.org/10.1161/CIR.0b013e31829e8776.

Yancy CW, Jessup M, Bozkurt B, et al: 2017 ACC/AHA/HFSA focused update of the 2013 ACCF/AHA guideline for the management of heart failure: a report of the American College of Cardiology/American Heart Association Task Force on Clinical Practice Guidelines and the Heart Failure Society of America, Circulation 136:e137–e161, 2017, https://doi.org/10.1161/CIR.0000000000000509.

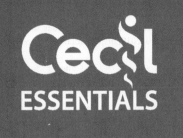

6

Congenital Heart Disease

Scott Cohen, Michael G. Earing

INTRODUCTION

Congenital heart defects are the most common group of birth defects, occurring in approximately 9 of 1000 live births. Without treatment, most patients die in infancy or childhood, with only 5% to 15% surviving into adulthood. Advancements in surgical and medical practices have resulted in survival of approximately 90% of these children to adulthood. Estimates suggest that more adults than children are living with congenital heart disease in the United States and that there is a 5% increase in the size of the adult congenital heart disease population every year.

Most adults living with congenital heart disease have had interventions performed (Table 6.1). Although most children who undergo surgical intervention survive to adulthood, total correction usually is not the rule. Adult patients with congenital heart disease are surviving longer than ever before, and it is becoming apparent that even the simplest lesions can be associated with long-term cardiac complications (i.e., arrhythmias and conduction abnormalities, ventricular dysfunction, residual shunts, valvular lesions, hypertension, and aneurysms) and noncardiac complications (i.e., renal dysfunction, restrictive lung disease, neurocognitive deficits, anxiety, depression, and liver dysfunction). Most adults with congenital heart disease need lifelong follow-up.

ACYANOTIC HEART DISEASE

Atrial Septal Defects

Definition and Epidemiology

Atrial septal defects (ASDs) are communications between the atria that allow shunting of blood from one atrium to the other. They are among the most common congenital anomalies seen in adolescents and young adults, occurring in 1 of 1500 live births and constituting 6% to 10% of all congenital heart defects.

There are four main types of ASDs. Ostium secundum defects are the most common, accounting for 75% of all ASDs. This defect occurs in the region of the fossa ovalis and results from excessive absorption of the septum primum or insufficient development of the septum secundum, or both.

Ostium primum defects represent about 20% of all ASDs and represent a form of atrioventricular septal defect (i.e., partial or incomplete atrioventricular canal). These defects are located in the inferior aspect of the atrial septum adjacent to the mitral and tricuspid valves. The defects result from lack of closure of the ostium primum by the endocardial cushions, which are embryologic swellings in the heart that form the primum atrial septum, the inlet portion of the ventricular septum, and parts of the mitral and tricuspid valve. The lesions often are associated with clefts in the mitral and tricuspid valves.

Sinus venosus ASDs represent 5% of all ASDs and are located at the entry of the superior vena cava or inferior vena cava into the right atrium. Frequently, there is associated partial anomalous drainage of the right upper pulmonary vein with the superior sinus venosus defect. This type of defect results from resorption of the wall between the vena cava and pulmonary veins.

An unroofed coronary sinus is a rare form of ASD, representing less than 1% of all ASDs. The coronary sinus is in apposition to the posterior aspect of the left atrium, but the orifice is in the right atrium. When a defect exists in the roof of the coronary sinus, a communication between the left atrium and right atrium exists, allowing shunting.

Pathology

All four types of ASDs allow oxygenated blood to pass from the left atrium into the right atrium, resulting in volume overload of the right atrium and right ventricle (Fig. 6.1). The degree of shunting is determined by the size of the ASD and the compliance of the left and right cardiac chambers. Comorbidities that increase left-sided filling pressures (i.e., left ventricular [LV] diastolic dysfunction, myocardial infarction, and mitral stenosis) may result in an increased left-to-right shunt. Over time, significant left-to-right shunting can cause enlargement of the right atrium and right ventricle, eventually leading to right ventricular (RV) systolic dysfunction and failure. Pulmonary hypertension may occur in approximately 26% of patients with a secundum ASD. However, significant elevation in pulmonary vascular resistance is rare.

Clinical Presentation

Although most individuals with an ASD are diagnosed during childhood after a murmur is noticed, a few patients have symptoms for the first time as adults. Most patients are asymptomatic during the first and second decades of life. In the third decade, increasing numbers of patients develop exercise intolerance, palpitations due to atrial arrhythmias, and cardiac enlargement on the chest radiograph. In patients with ASDs, the RV impulse at the left lower sternal border often has increased force compared with normal. On auscultation, the second heart sound typically is widely split and fixed (i.e., does not vary with inspiration).

All patients have a systolic ejection murmur, which is best heard at the left upper sternal border and is related to increased flow across a usually normal pulmonary valve. When there is a large left-to-right shunt, a mid-diastolic murmur can be heard at the left lower sternal border; it is related to increased flow across a normal tricuspid valve. When a mid-diastolic murmur is identified, the degree of left-to-right shunt is considered to be 1.5 times normal. In the setting of a primum

TABLE 6.1 Most Common Congenital Heart Defects Surviving to Adulthood Without Surgery or Interventional Catheterization

Mild pulmonary valve stenosis

Bicuspid aortic valve

Small to moderate size atrial septal defect

Small ventricular septal defect

Small patent ductus arteriosus

Mitral valve prolapse

Partial atrioventricular canal (ostium primum atrial septal defect and cleft mitral valve)

Marfan syndrome

Ebstein's anomaly

Congenitally corrected transposition (atrioventricular and ventriculoarterial discordance)

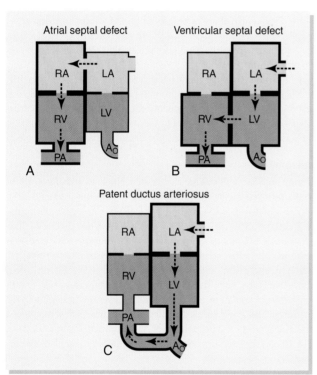

Fig. 6.1 The diagram shows three types of shunt lesions that commonly survive until adulthood and their effects on chamber size. (A) Uncomplicated atrial septal defect with left-to-right shunt flow across the interatrial septum, resulting in dilation of the right atrium (RA), right ventricle (RV), and pulmonary artery (PA). (B) Uncomplicated ventricular septal defect, resulting in dilation of the RV, left atrium (LA), and left ventricle (LV). (C) Uncomplicated patent ductus arteriosus, resulting in dilation of the LA, LV, and PA. *Ao,* Aorta. (From Liberthson RR, Walkdman H: Congenital heart disease in the adult. In Kloner RA, editor: Guide to cardiology, ed 3, Greenwich, Conn., 1991, Le Jacq Communications, pp 24-27.)

ASD, an additional holosystolic murmur at the apex may be caused by a cleft in the anterior leaflet of the mitral valve, resulting in mitral regurgitation.

Diagnosis

On the electrocardiogram (ECG), the features of ASD depend on the size and type of defect. In the setting of a large ostium secundum, sinus

venosus, or unroofed coronary sinus defect, the ECG typically demonstrates evidence of right atrial (RA) enlargement, RV hypertrophy, and right axis deviation. In the setting of an ostium primum ASD, like other forms of atrioventricular defects, there is a superior axis. The chest radiograph is helpful for evaluating the degree of left-to-right shunting. With a small shunt, the radiograph will be normal. As the shunt increases in size, the heart size and pulmonary vascular markings also increase.

The diagnosis of an ASD and its location are confirmed by transthoracic echocardiography in most cases. A sinus venosus ASD is the exception. In this setting, transesophageal echocardiography may be necessary. Cardiac catheterization is rarely performed to diagnose an ASD. CT scan or cardiac MRI may be useful in defining the pulmonary venous anatomy especially in defects associated with anomalous pulmonary veins.

Treatment

The treatment of ASDs involves surgical or transcatheter device closure and is indicated in the setting of impaired functional capacity, right atrial and/or right ventricular enlargement or a Qp:Qs (pulmonary to systemic blood flow) ratio of 1.5:1 or greater. Individuals with an ASD and a PA systolic pressure greater than two-thirds of systemic, pulmonary vascular resistance greater than two-thirds of systemic, and/or a net right to left shunt should not undergo ASD closure. However, individuals with significantly elevated PA systolic pressure or pulmonary vascular resistance can be assessed for reversibility during a hemodynamic catheterization (usually with nitric oxide) and if found to have reversible pulmonary vascular disease they can be considered for repair. Those that are not reversible can be placed on pulmonary hypertension targeted therapy and undergo a hemodynamic reassessment after 6 months. A reduction in pulmonary vascular resistance of greater than 20% is associated with a favorable prognosis after ASD closure, and closure with a pulmonary vascular resistance of 6.5 Wood units or less has been associated with improved RV function. For a secundum ASD, surgical closure and transcatheter device closure are accepted treatment options. Device closure is the most commonly used technique for closure of secundum defects. This technique, however, requires an adequate rim of septal tissue around the entire defect to allow for device stabilization. For ostium primum, sinus venosus, and unroofed coronary sinus forms of ASDs, surgical closure remains the only option.

Prognosis

Most patients who have undergone early closure of a defect have excellent long-term survival rates with low morbidity rates if repair is undertaken before 25 years of age. Older age at repair is associated with decreased late survival rates and an associated increased risk of atrial arrhythmias, thromboembolic events, and pulmonary hypertension. After the age of 40 years for patients with unrepaired ASDs, the mortality rate increases by 6% per year, and more than 20% of patients develop atrial fibrillation. By 60 years of age, the number of patients with atrial fibrillation increases to more than 60%. In asymptomatic patients, it is reasonable to close a hemodynamically significant ASD in the absence of significant pulmonary hypertension; however, comorbidities (especially in older adults) may impact the benefit of ASD closure on improving symptoms and functional capacity. Long-term rates of late complications and survival after transcatheter device closure remain unknown.

Ventricular Septal Defects
Definition and Epidemiology

Ventricular septal defects (VSDs) occur in 1.5 to 3.5 of 1000 live births. They constitute 20% of congenital heart defects.

There are four types of VSD: perimembranous, muscular, supracristal, and inlet. Perimembranous VSDs are the most common, comprising 70% of all VSDs. The membranous septum is relatively small and sits directly under the aortic valve. Perimembranous VSDs involve the membranous septum and typically extend into the muscular tissue adjacent to the membranous septum. If not large, these defects may close spontaneously by tissue from the septal leaflet of the tricuspid valve.

Muscular VSDs are the second most common VSD and account for 5% to 20% of all VSDs. Multiple muscular VSDs commonly are found at the time of diagnosis. Muscular VSDs have the highest rate of spontaneous closure.

Supracristal VSDs represent 5% to 8% of all VSDs. These defects are located superior to the crista supraventricularis (i.e., within the RV outflow tract directly below the right cusp of the aortic valve). These defects are associated with prolapse of the right aortic cusp, which can lead to progressive aortic regurgitation. In some cases, the prolapsed right aortic cusp may restrict the defect, but rarely do they spontaneously close.

Inlet VSDs are located in the posterior ventricular septum, just inferior to the tricuspid and mitral valve. They account for 5% to 8% of all VSDs and never close spontaneously.

Pathology

Shunting through a VSD is typically left to right and can cause overcirculation of the pulmonary vasculature and increased pulmonary venous return, resulting in left-sided chamber enlargement (see Fig. 6.1). The degree of shunting depends on the size of the defect and the pulmonary vascular resistance. Small defects (i.e., restrictive defects) typically have a small degree of shunting and normal pulmonary artery pressure. Moderate-sized defects have enough left-to-right shunting to cause mildly elevated pulmonary artery pressures and some left-sided chamber enlargement. Large defects (i.e., nonrestrictive defects) allow LV systolic pressures to be transmitted to the pulmonary circulation. This can cause irreversible obstructive pulmonary vascular disease early in childhood. Eventually, if the pulmonary vascular resistance exceeds the systemic vascular resistance, the shunt may reverse to right to left (i.e., Eisenmenger's physiology).

Clinical Presentation

The physical findings for a patient with a VSD depend on the size of the VSD, magnitude of the shunt, and the level of pulmonary artery hypertension. For patients with a small VSD, the apical impulses of the right ventricle and left ventricle typically have normal intensity on palpation, but there may be a palpable thrill. The first and second heart sounds typically are normal, and in most cases, there is a holosystolic murmur of moderate intensity at the left lower sternal border.

Patients with Eisenmenger's syndrome have cyanosis and secondary erythrocytosis. The RV impulse usually is increased at the left lower sternal border, and the pulmonary component of the second heart sound may be palpable. Typically, no systolic murmur is detected, but a diastolic murmur is often heard at the left upper sternal border due to a severely dilated main pulmonary artery and resultant pulmonary regurgitation.

Diagnosis

The ECG should be normal for patients with small VSDs. For those with Eisenmenger's syndrome, the ECG usually demonstrates RV hypertrophy with right axis deviation. Patients with a small VSD have a normal chest radiograph. Patients with Eisenmenger's syndrome may have mild cardiac enlargement with enlarged proximal pulmonary arteries and peripheral pruning with oligemic lung fields. Echocardiography

allows confirmation of the diagnosis, localization of defect, identification of long-term complications, and estimation of pulmonary artery pressure. Cardiac catheterization allows direct measurement of the degree of left-to-right shunting, pulmonary artery pressure, and pulmonary vascular reactivity.

Treatment

Because the majority of adult patients with an isolated VSD have no significant hemodynamic abnormalities, closure of the VSD is typically not needed. Closure of a VSD is indicated if there is evidence of left ventricular volume overload and a hemodynamically significant shunt (Qp:Qs >1.5). Small VSDs that are asymptomatic should be followed conservatively. Because of the long-term risks, they need intermittent follow-up for life to monitor for the development of late complications. The exceptions to this rule are those with small supracristal or perimembranous VSDs with associated prolapse of the aortic cusp into the defect that results in progressive aortic regurgitation. These patients should be considered for surgical repair at the time of diagnosis to prevent progressive aortic valve damage.

Prognosis

Although isolated VSDs are common forms of congenital heart disease, the diagnosis of a VSD in an adult is rare. Most patients with a hemodynamically significant VSD have undergone repair in childhood or died earlier in life. As a result, the spectrum of isolated VSDs in adults is limited to those with small restrictive defects, those with Eisenmenger's syndrome, and those who had their defects closed in childhood.

For patients with small restrictive VSDs, long-term survival is excellent, with an estimated 25-year survival rate of 96%. The rate of long-term morbidity for patients with a restrictive VSD also appears to be low. However, the clinical course is not completely benign. Reported long-term complications include endocarditis, progressive aortic regurgitation due to prolapse of aortic valve into the defect (i.e., highest risk for the supracristal type but can occur with a perimembranous defect), and the development of right and left outflow tract obstruction from a double-chamber right ventricle or a subaortic membrane.

For patients who develop Eisenmenger's syndrome, survival into the third decade is common. However, with increasing age, the long-term complications of right heart failure, paradoxical emboli, and erythrocytosis usually result in a progressive drop in survival, with an average age of death of 37 years. Adults with previous VSD closure and without pulmonary hypertension or residual defects have a normal life expectancy.

Complete Atrioventricular Septal Defects
Definition and Epidemiology

Complete atrioventricular septal defects (AVSDs) consist of several cardiac malformations that result from abnormal development of the endocardial cushions. AVSDs account for 4% to 5% of congenital heart defects. Down syndrome is a common association; 40% of Down syndrome patients have congenital heart disease, and 40% of these have some form of AVSD.

AVSDs are categorized as partial (or incomplete) or complete. Both forms share common structural abnormalities—ostium primum ASD, inlet VSD, and cleft anterior mitral and septal tricuspid leaflet—in various combinations.

Pathology

A combination of the previously described defects results in interatrial and interventricular shunts, LV-to-RA shunt, and atrioventricular regurgitation. Because these defects include deficiency of the inlet portion of the ventricular septum, the LV outflow tract is lengthened and may be narrowed, producing the characteristic goose-neck deformity.

The natural history for patients with complete AVSD is characterized by the early development of pulmonary vascular disease, leading to irreversible damage that often occurs by 1 year of age, particularly for patients with Down syndrome. Surgery needs to be undertaken early if it is to be successful. Patients who are diagnosed in adulthood can be categorized in two groups: those with Eisenmenger's syndrome and those who had their defects closed in childhood.

Clinical Presentation

On physical examination, most previously repaired patients are cardiovascularly normal. However, patients with significant left atrioventricular (AV) valve regurgitation have a grade 3 or 4 (of 6) holosystolic regurgitant murmur at the apex. For the rare patient with subaortic stenosis, a grade 2 or 3 systolic murmur can be detected at the left midsternal border and radiating to the neck. The physical examination findings for patients with Eisenmenger's syndrome are similar to those for patients with unoperated VSDs.

Diagnosis

On the ECG, first-degree heart block is a common finding for patients with AVSD. All patients have a superior, leftward QRS axis. For those with Eisenmenger's syndrome, the chest radiograph demonstrates cardiomegaly, large proximal pulmonary arteries, and small peripheral pulmonary arteries (i.e., peripheral pruning). Patients who underwent previous repair and have significant systemic left AV valve regurgitation have cardiomegaly with increased vascular markings.

Treatment

Patients who underwent previous repair with significant left AV valve regurgitation causing symptoms, atrial arrhythmias, or deterioration in ventricular function should undergo elective repair or replacement. Previously repaired patients who develop significant subaortic stenosis (i.e., peak cardiac catheterization or echo gradient of ≥50 mm Hg or less in the presence of heart failure or moderate to severe mitral regurgitation) should undergo surgical repair.

Prognosis

Overall, for patients who underwent early repair before the development of pulmonary vascular disease, the long-term prognosis is good. The most common long-term complication is left AV valve regurgitation, with approximately 5% to 10% of patients requiring surgical revision for left AV valve repair or replacement during follow-up. The second most common long-term complication for this group is subaortic stenosis, occurring in up to 5% of patients after repair. Other long-term complications include residual atrial- or ventricular-level shunts, complete heart block, atrial and ventricular arrhythmias, and endocarditis.

Patients with Eisenmenger's syndrome are symptomatic with exertional dyspnea, fatigue, palpitations, edema, and syncope. Survival is similar to that for other forms of Eisenmenger's syndrome, with a mean age at death of 37 years. In retrospective studies, strong predictors for death included syncope, age at presentation of symptoms, poor functional class, low oxygen saturation (≤85%), increased serum creatinine and serum uric acid concentrations, and Down syndrome.

Coarctation of the Aorta
Definition

Coarctation of the aorta is an abnormal narrowing of the aortic lumen. It constitutes 5% of congenital heart defects. Coarctation of the aorta may occur anywhere along the descending aorta, even below the diaphragm, but in more than 95% of cases, the narrowing is just below the takeoff of the left subclavian artery. In 50% to 85% of cases, there is an associated bicuspid aortic valve. Other associated lesions include VSDs, subaortic stenosis, and mitral valve stenosis.

Pathology

Coarctation of the aorta is an aortopathy of the entire aorta rather than a localized abnormality. In the young, significant coarctation can decrease blood flow to the kidneys, gut, and lower extremities, resulting in severe acidosis and shock requiring immediate treatment. Unrepaired coarctation of the aorta can be seen in adults, but it is rare. Affected individuals develop extensive arterial collateralization to maintain distal perfusion. Most patients seen in adulthood are patients who have had previous coarctation of the aorta repair using a variety of different techniques.

Even after successful repair to relieve the obstruction, multiple studies have demonstrated that patients have persistent abnormalities in the media of the aorta proximal and distal to the coarctation repair site. The stiff aortic wall is characterized by decreased distensibility and endothelial and vascular dysfunction. These can result in resting and exercise-induced hypertension, increased carotid intimal thickness, and abnormal peripheral arterial responses to augmented blood flow and nitroglycerin.

Clinical Presentation

The clinical presentation of coarctation of the aorta depends on the severity of obstruction and the associated anomalies. Unrepaired coarctation of the aorta typically manifests with symptoms before adulthood. Symptoms include headaches related to hypertension, leg fatigue or cramps, exercise intolerance, and systemic hypertension. Untreated patients surviving to adulthood typically have only mild coarctation of the aorta.

Cardinal clinical features in the setting of a significant coarctation of the aorta include upper body hypertension, weak and delayed femoral pulses, and a blood pressure gradient between the right arm and right leg determined by blood pressure cuff. On auscultation, the aortic valve closure sound is usually loud; in the setting of a bicuspid aortic valve, an ejection click, often with a crescendo-decrescendo systolic murmur, is heard at the right upper sternal border. Often, a continuous systolic murmur is heard over the left scapula. It is related to continuous flow across the coarctation of the aorta.

Diagnosis

Patients with significant coarctation of the aorta typically show various degrees of left atrial (LA) and LV enlargement on an ECG. The chest radiograph typically demonstrates normal heart size with dilation of the ascending aorta and kinking or double contouring in the region of the descending aorta in the area of the coarctation, producing the characteristic figure-3 sign.

Most adult patients have rib notching. It is caused by the dilated intercostal collateral arteries eroding the undersurface of the ribs. Echocardiography is used to identify site, structure, and degree of stenosis or restenosis. Echocardiography is valuable for identifying other lesions, LV systolic function, and degree of LV hypertrophy.

Magnetic resonance imaging (MRI) and CT angiography are quite good for imaging the coarctation, defining the arch vessel anatomy, and identifying collaterals. Cardiac catheterization remains the gold standard for determining the anatomy and absolute degree of stenosis.

Treatment

Patients with hypertension and a significant native or residual coarctation of the aorta (i.e., upper extremity/lower extremity resting peak to peak gradient >20 mm Hg or mean Doppler systolic gradient >20 mm Hg, upper extremity/lower extremity gradient >10 mm Hg or mean

Doppler gradient >10 mm Hg plus either decreased LV systolic function of aortic regurgitation, upper extremity/lower extremity gradient >10 mm Hg or mean Doppler gradient >10 mm Hg with collateral flow) should be considered for surgical repair or catheter intervention with balloon angioplasty with or without stent placement. Surgical repair in the adult patient is technically difficult and is associated with high rates of morbidity. As a result, catheter-based intervention has become the preferred method in most experienced congenital heart disease centers, and balloon angioplasty for a native or recurrent coarctation of the aorta should be considered if stent placement or surgery is not an option.

Prognosis

After surgical repair, long-term survival is good but directly correlates with the age at repair. Those repaired after 14 years of age have a lower 20-year survival rate than those repaired earlier (79% vs. 91%). Long-term outcome data for catheter-based treatment is limited, but studies suggest that stented patients have lower acute and long-term complications at 60 months (25% for surgery vs. 12.5% for stents). Irrespective of the type of repair, the most common long-term complication is persistent or new systemic hypertension at rest or during exercise. Other long-term complications include aneurysms of the ascending or descending aorta (especially after Dacron patch repair), recoarctation at the site of previous repair, coronary artery disease, aortic stenosis or regurgitation (in the setting of a bicuspid aortic valve), and endarteritis. Intracranial aneurysms are seen in approximately 10% of patients with a coarctation, and increasing age and hypertension have been identified as risk factors.

Patent Ductus Arteriosus
Definition and Epidemiology

Patent ductus arteriosus (PDA) represents 9% to 12% of congenital heart defects. It is patent in the fetus but normally closes within several days of birth. However, it remains open in about 1 of 2500 to 5000 births. In infants born prematurely, the incidence is even higher, occurring in 8 of 1000 live births. The incidence of PDA is 30 times greater for babies born at high altitudes than for those born at sea level.

Pathology

A PDA allows transit of blood from the aorta into the pulmonary artery and recirculation through the pulmonary vasculature and the left side of the heart. This can result in left-sided chamber enlargement (see Fig. 6.1). As with VSDs, the size of the defect is the primary determinant of the clinical course in the adult patient. PDAs can be clinically categorized as silent PDAs; small, hemodynamically insignificant PDAs; moderate-size PDAs; large PDAs; and previously repaired PDAs.

Clinical Presentation

A silent PDA is a tiny defect that cannot be heard by auscultation and is detected only by other nonclinical means such as echocardiography. Life expectancy is always normal for this population, and the risk of endocarditis is extremely low.

Patients with a small PDA have an audible, long-ejection or continuous murmur that is heard best at the left upper sternal border and radiating to the back. They have normal peripheral pulses. Because there is negligible left-to-right shunting, these patients have normal LA and LV sizes and normal pulmonary artery pressure. Like those with silent PDAs, these patients are asymptomatic and have a normal life expectancy. However, they do have a higher risk of endocarditis.

Patients with moderate-size PDAs may be diagnosed during adulthood. These patients often have wide, bouncy peripheral pulses and an audible, continuous murmur. They have significant volume overload and develop some degree of LA and LV enlargement and some degree of pulmonary hypertension. These patients are symptomatic with dyspnea, palpitations, and heart failure. Patients with large PDAs typically have signs of severe pulmonary hypertension and Eisenmenger's syndrome. By adulthood, the continuous murmur is typically absent, and there is differential cyanosis (i.e., lower extremity saturations are lower than the right arm saturation).

Diagnosis

Patients with silent and small PDAs appear normal by echocardiography and chest radiography. Calcifications may be seen on the postero-anterior and lateral films of an older patient with a PDA. In patients with significant left-to-right shunting, there typically is dilation of the central pulmonary arteries with increased pulmonary vascular markings. On an ECG, broad P waves and tall QRS complexes suggest LA and LV volume overload. A tall R wave in lead V_1 with a right axis deviation suggests significant pulmonary hypertension. Measurement of oxygen saturation should be performed in feet and both hands in adults with moderate or large PDAs to assess for the presence of right to left shunting. Echocardiography is important to estimate the size of the defect, degree of LA or LV enlargement, and degree of pulmonary artery hypertension.

Treatment

PDA closure is recommended if there is left atrial or left ventricular enlargement present that is attributable to a PDA with left-to-right shunting. Patients with a PDA and severe, irreversible pulmonary hypertension should not have their PDA closed. Catheter device closure is the preferred method in most centers. Surgical closure is reserved for patients with PDAs too large for device closure and for distorted anatomy such as a large ductal aneurysm. Because patients with clinical evidence of a PDA are at increased risk for endocarditis and the low risk of catheter-based device closure, a small audible PDA should be considered for device closure.

Prognosis

Patients with a large PDA who have developed Eisenmenger's syndrome have a prognosis similar to that of other patients with Eisenmenger's syndrome. Patients who underwent PDA repair before the development of pulmonary hypertension have a normal life expectancy without restrictions.

Pulmonary Valve Stenosis
Definition and Epidemiology

Pulmonary valve stenosis occurs in approximately 4 of 1000 live births and constitutes 5% to 8% of congenital cardiac defects. It is one of the most common adult forms of unoperated congenital heart disease. It can occur in isolation or with other congenital heart defects, such as an ASD.

Pathology

In congenital pulmonary valve stenosis, the pulmonary valve leaflets are often fused or thickened, which obstructs blood flow out of the right ventricle. The obstruction elevates RV pressure, and compensatory RV hypertrophy develops. Pulmonary stenosis is often tolerated better than aortic stenosis. Over time, RV dilation and dysfunction may occur.

Clinical Presentation

Most patients with pulmonary valve stenosis are asymptomatic and have a cardiac murmur at presentation. Most unoperated adults with severe stenosis have jugular venous distention, and on palpation, an RV lift at the left lower sternal border and a thrill at the left upper sternal border can be identified. On auscultation, the second heart sound is widely split, and a systolic ejection click may or may not be heard, depending on the mobility of the pulmonary valve leaflets. In most cases, there is a harsh, crescendo-decrescendo systolic ejection murmur, which is heard best at the left upper sternal border; it radiates to the back and varies with inspiration.

Diagnosis

With moderate to severe pulmonary valve stenosis, the ECG demonstrates right axis deviation, RV hypertrophy, and RA enlargement. The ECG is usually normal for patients with mild pulmonary valve stenosis. On the chest radiograph, a prominent main pulmonary artery caused by poststenotic dilatation is a common finding regardless of the degree of stenosis. In patients with severe pulmonary valve stenosis, cardiomegaly due to RA and RV enlargement is often seen.

Echocardiography is the diagnostic method of choice. It allows visualization of the valve anatomy and degree of stenosis and enables estimation of the valve gradient.

Treatment

Survival into adult life and the need for intervention directly correlate with the degree of obstruction. In the Second Natural History Study of Congenital Heart Disease, patients with trivial stenosis (i.e., peak gradient ≤25 mm Hg) who were followed for 25 years remained asymptomatic and had no significant progression of obstruction over time. For those with moderate pulmonary valve stenosis (i.e., peak gradient between 25 and 49 mm Hg), there was an approximately 20% chance of requiring intervention by 25 years of age. Most patients with severe stenosis (i.e., peak gradient of ≥50 mm Hg) require intervention (i.e., surgery or balloon valvuloplasty) by age 25 years. Patients with moderate to severe pulmonary stenosis may be considered for intervention even in the absence of symptoms.

Since 1985, percutaneous balloon valvuloplasty has been the accepted treatment for patients of all ages. Before 1985, surgical valvotomy had been the gold standard. Today, adults with moderate or severe valvular pulmonary stenosis and otherwise unexplained symptoms of heart failure, cyanosis from interatrial right to left shunting, or exercise are recommended to undergo balloon valvuloplasty if feasible; otherwise surgical valvotomy is recommended (if the valve is extremely dysplastic or calcified).

Prognosis

After surgical valvotomy for isolated pulmonary stenosis, long-term survival is excellent. However, with longer follow-up the incidence of late complications and the need for reintervention do increase. The most common indication for reintervention is pulmonary valve replacement for severe pulmonary regurgitation. Other long-term complications include recurrent atrial arrhythmias, endocarditis, and residual subpulmonary obstruction.

Aortic Valve Stenosis
Definition and Epidemiology

Aortic valve stenosis is a common abnormality in adults with congenital heart disease. It is usually caused by a bicuspid aortic valve, which occurs in 1% to 2% of adults and is three times more common in males. It typically is an isolated lesion but can be associated with a dilated ascending aorta and other defects such as coarctation of the aorta or VSD.

Pathology

Aortic valve stenosis results in pressure overload of the left ventricle, which increases wall stress and causes compensatory LV hypertrophy. Diastolic dysfunction and oxygen delivery-demand mismatch ensues. The patient may remain well compensated and asymptomatic for many years, but compensatory mechanisms eventually begin to fail and LV dysfunction can develop. Patients with a bicuspid aortic valve have abnormal structure of the aortic wall that often leads to ascending aortic dilation.

Clinical Presentation

Most patients with aortic valve stenosis are asymptomatic and are diagnosed after a murmur is detected. The severity of obstruction at the time of diagnosis correlates with the pattern of progression. Symptoms are rare until patients have severe aortic valve stenosis (i.e., mean gradient by echocardiography of ≥40 mm Hg). Symptoms include chest pain, exertional dyspnea, near-syncope, and syncope. With any of these symptoms, the risk of sudden cardiac death is very high, and surgical intervention is mandated.

Patients with moderate to severe stenosis typically have decreased peripheral pulses, an increased apical impulse, and a palpable thrill at the base of the heart. On auscultation, these patients have an ejection click followed by a crescendo-decrescendo systolic murmur, which is heard best at the left midsternal border and radiating to the right upper sternal border and the neck. Correlation between the degree of stenosis and the intensity of the murmur is not good. However, it is rare for a murmur of 2/6 or less to be associated with severe stenosis. Some patients with aortic stenosis also have aortic regurgitation, in which case a decrescendo diastolic murmur at the left midsternal border that radiates to the apex is detected at presentation.

Diagnosis

Many patients with significant aortic stenosis have LV hypertrophy identified on the ECG. However, the correlation between the severity of stenosis and the finding of LV hypertrophy on the ECG is unreliable. On chest radiography, most patients with severe aortic stenosis have a normal heart size unless there is concurrent aortic regurgitation. Post-stenotic dilation of the ascending aorta is common irrespective of degree of stenosis, and ascending aorta dilation is a common finding. It appears on the chest radiograph as a widened mediastinum.

Echocardiography is the gold standard for evaluation of the severity of aortic valve stenosis and the anatomic morphology of the aortic valve. Cardiac catheterization is primarily indicated to evaluate coronary artery disease before surgical intervention, because approximately one-half of adults with symptomatic aortic valve stenosis have concurrent coronary artery disease.

Treatment

Patients with severe aortic stenosis and symptoms or asymptomatic patients with severe aortic valve stenosis and reduced LV systolic function (<50%) should be considered for intervention. Treatment involves manipulating the valve to reduce stenosis. This can be accomplished by transvenous balloon dilation of the valve, open surgical valvotomy, or surgical or catheter-based valve replacement. In absence of significant aortic regurgitation, most centers favor balloon dilation or surgical valvotomy for children who have pliable valves with fusion of the commissures. In adults, aortic valve replacement is the treatment of choice. Aortic valve replacement may be done with a mechanical valve, bioprosthetic valve, or the Ross procedure (placing the pulmonary autograft in the aortic position and putting a new valve in the pulmonary position). The ascending aorta may be replaced if it is 5.5 cm (5.0 cm in the setting of high-risk features, such as growth >0.5 cm/year or family history of dissection) or 4.5 cm at the time of an aortic valve replacement.

Prognosis

The natural history of aortic valve stenosis in adults varies but is characterized by progressive stenosis over time. By 45 years of age, approximately 50% of bicuspid aortic valves have some degree of stenosis. Most patients requiring surgical valvotomy to relieve the stenosis before adulthood do well. However, by the 25-year follow-up, up to 40% of patients required a second operation for residual stenosis or regurgitation.

CYANOTIC HEART DISEASE

Tetralogy of Fallot

Definition and Epidemiology

Tetralogy of Fallot (TOF) is the most common cyanotic heart disease seen in adulthood, and it represents 10% of congenital heart defects. It consists of a large VSD, pulmonary stenosis (which may be valvular, subvalvular, and or supravalvular), an aorta that overrides the VSD, and RV hypertrophy.

Pathology

Newborns with TOF are cyanotic because of the right-to-left shunt through the VSD and decreased pulmonary blood flow. The amount of pulmonary blood flow depends on the severity of the obstruction through the RV outflow tract. By the time TOF patients reach adulthood, most have had complete repair or palliative surgery.

Many adults with repaired TOF have had a transannular patch (i.e., synthetic patch across the pulmonary annulus) placed to relieve the RV outflow tract obstruction. This patch causes obligatory free pulmonary regurgitation. Free pulmonary regurgitation can be well tolerated by the right ventricle for many years, but usually in the third or fourth decades, the right ventricle begins to dilate, and it may become dysfunctional. Significant RV dilation and dysfunction can lead to LV dysfunction, significant tricuspid regurgitation, and atrial or ventricular arrhythmias. Almost 29% of adults with repaired TOF also have a dilated ascending aorta due to increased blood flow through the aorta before repair.

Clinical Presentation

Patients with repaired TOF typically have normal oxygen saturation levels. On palpation, there often is an RV lift at the left lower sternal border. On auscultation, there typically is a widely split second heart sound with a to-and-fro murmur in the pulmonary area due to significant pulmonary regurgitation or, less commonly, aortic regurgitation. A holosystolic murmur due to tricuspid regurgitation may be heard at the left lower sternal border. Symptoms in the adult with repaired TOF may include exertional dyspnea, palpitations, syncope, and sudden cardiac death.

Diagnosis

The ECG almost universally reveals a right bundle branch block pattern in patients who underwent repair of TOF. The QRS duration from the standard surface ECG correlates with the degree of RV dilation and dysfunction. A maximum QRS duration of 180 milliseconds or more is a highly sensitive and relatively specific marker for sustained ventricular tachycardia and sudden cardiac death. Patients with significant pulmonary regurgitation often have cardiomegaly with dilated central pulmonary arteries identified on the chest radiograph. A right aortic arch occurs in 25% of cases, and it can be detected by close observation of the chest radiograph. An echocardiogram is useful for evaluating the RV outflow tract (e.g., pulmonary regurgitation, residual stenosis), biventricular size and function, tricuspid valve function, and ascending aortic size. MRI is the gold standard for assessing RV size and function

(Fig. 6.2). It can also give an accurate assessment of the degree of pulmonary insufficiency and branch pulmonary artery anatomy.

Treatment

Treatment for TOF is surgical repair. Repair is typically performed between 3 to 12 months of age and consists of patch closure of the VSD and relief of the pulmonary outflow tract obstruction by patch augmentation of the RV outflow tract or pulmonary valve annulus, or both. Reintervention is necessary in approximately 10% of adults with repaired TOF after 20 years of follow-up. With longer follow-up, the incidence of reintervention continues to increase. The most common indication for reintervention is pulmonary valve replacement in patients with moderate or greater pulmonary valve regurgitation and symptoms. Pulmonary valve replacement is also reasonable for preservation of ventricular size and function in asymptomatic patients with repaired tetralogy of Fallot and ventricular enlargement or dysfunction and moderate or greater pulmonary regurgitation. Pulmonary valve replacement can be performed surgically, or in some patients, percutaneously. Patients with repaired tetralogy of Fallot may be considered for an ICD for primary prevention if multiple risk factors for sudden death are present, including LV systolic or diastolic dysfunction, nonsustained ventricular tachycardia, QRS greater than 180 ms, extensive right ventricular scarring or inducible sustained ventricular tachycardia at an electrophysiologic study.

Prognosis

In the developed world, the unoperated adult with TOF has become a rarity because most patients undergo palliation (i.e., stenting) or repair in childhood. Survival of the unoperated patient to the seventh decade has been described but is rare. Only 11% of unrepaired patients are alive at 20 years of age and only 3% at 40 years.

Late survival after repair of TOF is excellent. Survival rates at 32 and 35 years are 86% and 85%, respectively, compared with 95% for age- and sex-matched controls. Importantly, most patients live an unrestricted life. However, many patients over time develop late symptoms related to numerous, long-term complications after TOF repair. Late complications include endocarditis, aortic regurgitation with or without aortic root dilation (typically due to damage of the aortic valve during VSD closure or to an intrinsic aortic root abnormality), LV dysfunction (from inadequate myocardial protection during previous repair or chronic LV volume overload due to long-standing palliative arterial shunts), residual pulmonary obstruction, residual pulmonary valve regurgitation, RV dysfunction (due to pulmonary regurgitation or pulmonary stenosis), atrial arrhythmias (typically atrial flutter), ventricular arrhythmias, and heart block.

Transposition of the Great Arteries

Definition and Epidemiology

Transposition of the great arteries (TGA) represents 3.8% of all congenital heart disease. In complete TGA, the aorta arises from the right ventricle and the pulmonary artery from the left ventricle. As a result, the systemic venous flow (i.e., blood with low oxygen content) is returned to the right ventricle and is then pumped to the body through the aorta without passing through the lungs for gas exchange. The pulmonary venous flow (i.e., oxygenated blood) returning to the left ventricle is then pumped back to the lungs. As a result, the systemic and pulmonary circulations run in parallel. Oxygenation and survival depend on mixing between the systemic and pulmonary circulations at the atrial, ventricular, or PDA level. In 50% of cases, there are other anomalies: VSD (30%), pulmonary stenosis (5% to 10%), aortic stenosis, and coarctation of the aorta (≤5%).

The first definitive operations for TGA (i.e., atrial switch procedures) were described by Senning in 1959 and Mustard in 1964. In these procedures, the systemic and pulmonary venous returns are

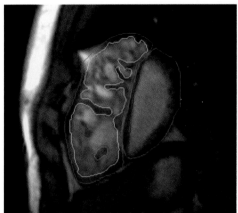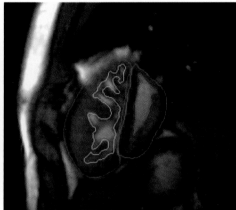

Fig. 6.2 Short axis magnetic resonance images of the right and left ventricles with epicardial and endocardial tracings of both ventricular cavities. There are a predefined number of slices through the heart with a constant thickness. The volumes of the left and right ventricles in each slice are calculated and summed together in end diastole and end systole to determine the total right and left ventricular volumes (i.e., Simpson's method).

rerouted in the atrium by constructing baffles. The systemic venous return from the superior and inferior vena cavae is directed through the mitral valve and into the left ventricle, which is connected to the pulmonary artery. The pulmonary venous return is then directed through the tricuspid valve into the right ventricle, which is connected to the aorta. These procedures leave the left ventricle as the pulmonary ventricle and the right ventricle as the systemic ventricle.

Over the past 20 years, the arterial switch procedure has gained popularity. During the procedure, the great arteries are transected and reanastomosed to the correct ventricle (i.e., left ventricle to the aorta and right ventricle to the pulmonary artery) along with coronary artery transfer. Operative survival after the arterial switch procedure is very good, with a surgical mortality rate of 2% to 5%.

Pathology

Most infants who do not have surgical intervention die in the first few months of life. For adults born with complete TGA who have had an atrial switch procedure, the right ventricle continues to be the systemic ventricle, and the left ventricle is the subpulmonic ventricle. Long-term follow-up series have demonstrated that the right ventricle can function as the systemic ventricle for 30 to 40 years, but with longer follow-up, systemic ventricular dysfunction continues to increase. At the 35-year follow-up, approximately 61% of patients have developed moderate or severe RV dysfunction.

Another common postoperative problem is the tricuspid valve. After the atrial switch procedure, the tricuspid valve remains the systemic atrioventricular valve and must tolerate systemic pressures. Due to changes in RV morphology and abnormal chordal attachments, the tricuspid valve is prone to become dysfunctional and develop significant regurgitation.

Significant coronary lesions, such as occlusions or stenoses, occur in 6.8% of patients who have had the arterial switch procedure. These lesions are likely related to suture lines or kinking at the time of reimplantation of the coronary arteries into the neo-aorta. Systemic LV function is usually normal. LV dysfunction is associated with coronary anomalies.

Clinical Presentation

In the repaired adult with an atrial switch procedure, the physical examination may reveal a murmur consistent with tricuspid valve insufficiency and a prominent second heart sound due to the anterior position of the aorta. Patients who have had an atrial switch procedure tend to have worsening functional status as the length of follow-up increases. They often have resting sinus bradycardia or a junctional rhythm. Palpitations due to atrial arrhythmias are common, occurring in up to 48% of patients 23 years after the atrial switch procedure.

In those who undergo the arterial switch procedure, the physical examination may reveal a murmur of neo-aortic or neo-pulmonic regurgitation. These patients usually have normal function status, but because of denervation of the heart, myocardial ischemia may manifest as atypical chest discomfort.

Diagnosis

After the atrial switch procedure, the ECG may show a loss of sinus rhythm with evidence of RV hypertrophy. Ambulatory monitors are important to monitor for bradyarrhythmias, sinus node dysfunction, and atrial arrhythmias. Chest radiographs may show an enlarged cardiac silhouette in those with a dilated systemic right ventricle. An echocardiogram can demonstrate qualitative systemic RV size and function and the degree of tricuspid regurgitation. MRI is often used to accurately quantify systemic RV size and function, tricuspid valve function, and atrial baffle anatomy.

After the arterial switch, echocardiography is used to assess pulmonary artery and branch pulmonary artery stenosis, neo-aortic and neo-pulmonic valve regurgitation, and ventricular function. MRI or computed tomography may be used to assess the anatomy of the branch pulmonary arteries. An exercise stress test is often used to evaluate myocardial ischemia.

Treatment

Treatment options are limited for adults with complete TGA repaired by atrial switch who have failing systemic right ventricles or significant tricuspid regurgitation, and evidence of significant benefit is lacking. However, potential treatments include medical therapy, revision of atrial baffles, pulmonary artery banding, resynchronization therapy, ventricular assist devices, and possible transplantation. Medical therapy, including consideration of anticoagulation, in patients with atrial tachyarrhythmias is recommended.

After the arterial switch procedure, catheter-based or surgical reintervention for pulmonary artery stenosis may be required in 5% to 25% of patients. Coronary artery revascularization is rarely required (0.46% of patients), as is neo-aortic valve repair or replacement (1.1%

of patients). Guideline-directed recommendations for aortic valve replacement are reasonable to follow for patients with d-TGA and severe neo-aortic valve regurgitation.

Prognosis

Long-term follow-up studies after the atrial switch procedure show a small but ongoing attrition rate, with numerous intermediate- and long-term complications. Long-term complications include systemic RV dysfunction and tricuspid valve regurgitation, loss of sinus rhythm with the development of atrial arrhythmias (50% incidence by age 25), endocarditis, baffle leaks, baffle obstruction, and sinus node dysfunction requiring pacemaker placement. Intermediate-term complications related to the arterial switch procedure include coronary artery compromise, pulmonary outflow tract obstruction (at the supravalvular level or takeoff of the peripheral pulmonary arteries), neo-aortic valve regurgitation, endocarditis, and neo-aorta dilation.

As a result of the long-term complications associated with the atrial switch procedure, the arterial switch operation has been the procedure of choice since 1985. Long-term data on the survival after the arterial switch operation do not exist, but intermediate-term results are promising: 88% at 10 and 15 years.

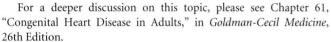 For a deeper discussion on this topic, please see Chapter 61, "Congenital Heart Disease in Adults," in *Goldman-Cecil Medicine*, 26th Edition.

SUGGESTED READINGS

Bradley EA, Ammash N, Martinez SC: "Treat to close": Non-repairable ASD-PAH in the adult, Int J Card 291:127–133, 2019.

Campbell M: Natural history of atrial septal defect, Br Heart J 32:820–826, 1970.

Cohen M, Fuster V, Steele PM, et al: Coarctation of the aorta. Long-term follow-up and prediction of outcome after surgical correction, Circulation 80:840–845, 1989.

Cohen SB, Ginde S, Bartz PJ, et al: Extracardiac complications in adults with congenital heart disease, Congenit Heart Dis 8:370–380, 2013.

Co-Vu JG, Ginde S, Bartz PJ, et al: Long-term outcomes of the neoaorta after arterial switch operation for transposition of the great arteries, Ann Thorac Surg 95:1654–1659, 2013.

Cramer JW, Ginde S, Bartz PJ, et al: Aortic aneurysms remain a significant source of morbidity and mortality after use of Dacron patch aortoplasty to repair coarctation of the aorta: results from a single center, Pediatr Cardiol 34:296–301, 2013.

Crumb SR, Dearani JA, Fuller S, et al: 2018 AHA/ACC guideline for the management of adults with congenital heart disease, J Am Coll Cardiol 1–175.

Earing MG, Connolly HM, Dearani JA, et al: Long-term follow-up of patients after surgical treatment for isolated pulmonary valve stenosis, Mayo Clin Proc 80:871–876, 2005.

Earing MG, Webb GD: Congenital heart disease and pregnancy: maternal and fetal risks, Clin Perinatol 32:913–919, 2005.

Gatzoulis MA, Freeman MA, Siu SC, et al: Atrial arrhythmia after surgical closure of atrial septal defects in adults, N Engl J Med 340:839–846, 1999.

Gunther T, Mazzitelli D, Haehnel CJ, et al: Long-term results after repair of complete atrioventricular septal defects: analysis of risk factors, Ann Thorac Surg 65:754–759, 1998, discussion 759-760.

Hickey EJ, Gruschen V, Bradely TJ, et al: Late risk of outcomes for adults with repaired tetralogy of Fallot from an inception cohort spanning four decades, Eur J Cardiothorac Surg 35:156–164, 2009.

Khairy P, Van Hare GF, Balaji S: PACES/HRS expert consensus statement on the recognition and management of arrhythmias in adult congenital heart disease, Can J Cardiol e1–e63, 2014.

Losay J, Touchot A, Serraf A, et al: Late outcome after arterial switch operation for transposition of the great arteries, Circulation 104(Suppl 1):I121–I1126, 2001.

Perloff JK, Warnes CA: Challenges posed by adults with repaired congenital heart disease, Circulation 103:2637–2643, 2001.

Soto B, Becker AE, Moulaert AJ, et al.: Classification of ventricular septal defects, Br Heart J 43:332–343, 1980.

Stout KK, Daniels CJ, Aboulhosn JA, et al.: Transposition of the great arteries, Circulation 114:2699–2709, 2006.

7

Valvular Heart Disease

Christopher Song

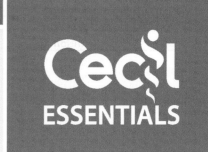

INTRODUCTION

In developing countries, rheumatic heart disease (RHD) remains a common cause of valvular heart disease (VHD). In industrialized countries, the burden of rheumatic disease has significantly decreased, and the most common etiology is degenerative disease. The prevalence of VHD in the US adult population is 2.5%. Prevalence increases with age to as high as 13.3% in those 75 years and older. Moderate or severe VHD is associated with excess mortality. Therefore, with an aging population, valvular heart disease is and will continue to be a major public health problem.

The "2014 AHA/ACC Guideline for the Management of Patients with Valvular Heart Disease" provides a classification of the progression of VHD with 4 stages, A through D (Table 7.1). Timing of intervention for most VHD is guided by the onset of symptoms, severity of VHD, and evidence of adverse cardiac remodeling. Therefore, a thorough history and physical examination along with a comprehensive transthoracic echocardiogram (TTE) are essential in the evaluation of patients with known or suspected VHD. Other cardiac testing modalities can help to determine the severity of VHD and the presence of symptoms. Once intervention is contemplated, each individual patient's surgical risk should be assessed. If surgical risk is high or prohibitive, transcatheter approaches may be an option.

AORTIC STENOSIS

Definition and Etiology

Valvular aortic stenosis (AS) is defined by restriction in leaflet motion resulting in left ventricular (LV) outflow obstruction. Less common causes of LV outflow obstruction include lesions at the supravalvular or subvalvular level. There are three primary etiologies of valvular AS: congenital, rheumatic, and calcific disease.

The etiology often dictates age at presentation. Patients with congenital aortic stenosis and unicuspid aortic valves usually present before the age of 30. Those with a bicuspid aortic valve or rheumatic valve disease typically present between the age of 40 and 60. Patients with calcific trileaflet valve typically present after age 70. However, patients with Paget disease or end-stage renal disease may present at a younger age.

Pathophysiology

The initiation phase of calcific aortic valve disease is similar to atherosclerosis. The process is thought to begin with mechanical stress and endothelial damage leading to inflammation and lipid deposition. The propagation phase is dominated by calcification leading to progressive restriction of the valve leaflets and eventual LV outflow obstruction.

In bicuspid aortic valves there is an associated increase in mechanical stress which leads to accelerated calcification of the valve leaflets. Bicuspid aortic valve occurs in about 1% of the population and it is twice as common in males as in females. Patients with a bicuspid aortic valve often have an associated aortopathy such as coarctation or aortic aneurysm.

Once AS becomes hemodynamically significant, it leads to resistance in LV ejection and an increase in LV systolic pressure and wall stress. In order to maintain normal wall stress, wall thickness increases resulting in concentric hypertrophy. The left ventricle can remain in this compensated state for a prolonged period. However, as valvular stenosis and hypertrophy progress, LV end-diastolic pressure increases and, eventually, LV dilation and systolic dysfunction ensue.

Natural History and Clinical Presentation

Patients with AS are usually asymptomatic for a prolonged period. Symptom onset occurs when valve obstruction is severe and usually prior to the onset of LV systolic dysfunction. In fact, LV chamber size and systolic function can remain normal until the AS is end-stage. The onset of symptoms in AS indicates a significant increase in mortality risk. This was first described by Ross and Braunwald in their seminal paper in 1968. They also found that specific symptoms were associated with different survival rates. The average survival of patients with symptoms of angina, syncope, and heart failure was 5, 3, and 2 years, respectively (Fig. 7.1).

These "classic" symptoms are now thought to be symptoms of end-stage disease. With the advent of echocardiography and close follow-up of patients, the most common presenting symptoms are dyspnea on exertion or decreased exercise tolerance, exertional dizziness, and exertional angina. Given the nonspecific nature of these symptoms along with the prognostic and therapeutic implications of diagnosing a patient with severe symptomatic AS, one must be thorough in screening patients for these symptoms but also be cautious in attributing these symptoms to AS.

Physical Examination

The physical examination is useful in the initial detection of AS and correlates with severity (Table 7.2). However, no physical examination findings can reliably exclude severe AS.

When palpating the carotid artery, a delayed, low amplitude pulse may be appreciated (*pulsus parvus et tardus*). With precordial palpation, a heaving and sustained apical impulse may be noted due to LV hypertrophy or systolic dysfunction. A fourth heart sound (S_4) can be palpable in the setting of a noncompliant left ventricle. In addition, a

TABLE 7.1   Stages of Progression of VHD

Stage	Definition	Description
A	At risk	Patients with risk factors for development of VHD
B	Progressive	Patients with progressive VHD (mild-moderate severity and asymptomatic)
C	Asymptomatic severe	Asymptomatic patients who have the criteria for severe VHD:
		C1: asymptomatic patients with severe VHD in whom the left and right ventricle remain compensated
		C2: asymptomatic patients with severe VHD with decompensation of the left or right ventricle
D	Symptomatic severe	Patients who have developed symptoms as a result of VHD

Data from Nishimura R, Otto C, Bonow RO, et al: 2014 AHA/ACC guideline for the management of patients with valvular heart disease. J Am Coll Cardiol 2014;63:e57-e185.

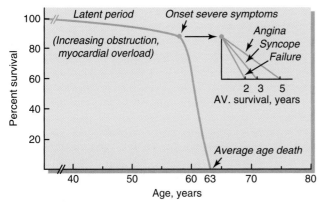

Fig. 7.1 Natural history of severe aortic stenosis without surgery once symptoms develop. (Data from Ross J Jr, Braunwald E: Aortic stenosis, Circulation 38:61, 1968.)

precordial thrill may be appreciated due to turbulent blood flow across a stenotic aortic valve.

The findings on cardiac auscultation are reflective of reduced mobility and delayed closure of the aortic valve leaflets and resistance to flow. The aortic component (A_2) of the second heart sound (S_2) becomes delayed to occur simultaneously with the pulmonic component (P_2) forming a single S_2. In severe AS, A_2 may become inaudible or paradoxical S_2 can be observed. An aortic ejection click can be heard in mild to moderate AS, when the leaflets are stiff but still mobile. The classic murmur AS is described as a harsh crescendo-decrescendo systolic murmur that is best heard at the right upper sternal border that radiates to the carotid arteries. The murmur begins after the first heart sound (S_1) and ends before S_2. Like the carotid pulse, the timing of the murmur correlates with severity of AS. An early peaking murmur is indicative of mild or moderate AS whereas a late peaking murmur is typically a sign of severe AS. The murmur may also radiate to the apex where a distinct musical quality can be appreciated. This is known as Gallavardin's phenomenon and often mistaken as the presence of concomitant mitral regurgitation (MR).

Diagnosis

An electrocardiogram (ECG) and chest radiograph are commonly obtained and can have nonspecific findings such as LV hypertrophy or cardiomegaly, respectively. The primary tool for diagnosing AS is echocardiography. TTE can accurately assess the aortic valve structure, the severity of AS, and the effects of AS on the cardiac chambers. Doppler imaging can be used to estimate the gradients across a stenotic aortic valve and calculate an aortic valve area. Criteria for mild, moderate, and severe AS are well established (Table 7.3).

In most cases the severity of AS by TTE correlates with the clinical evaluation. If there is a discrepancy, further testing can be considered.

An exercise treadmill study can be done to objectively assess functional capacity. A cardiac catheterization with hemodynamic measurements provides an alternative assessment of the severity of AS. Computed tomography can quantify aortic valve calcium, which has been shown to correlate with AS severity by TTE and with clinical outcomes.

In patients with LV systolic dysfunction, it may be unclear if a patient has true severe AS or pseudosevere AS. A low-dose dobutamine stress echocardiogram can help to differentiate between the two. In true severe AS the valve area is fixed, regardless of dobutamine. In pseudosevere AS the aortic valve opening is limited by the low LV outflow and the valve area will increase with dobutamine. This test can also provide information about the contractile reserve of the left ventricle, which has prognostic implications when considering valve replacement.

Treatment

The management of asymptomatic AS involves close monitoring, early detection of symptoms, and treatment of cardiovascular risk factors and comorbidities such as hypertension, hyperlipidemia, and coronary artery disease. No treatments have been shown to prevent the progression of AS.

Once a patient develops severe symptomatic AS, medical therapy has limited benefit and aortic valve replacement (AVR) is recommended. Medical therapy should focus on preventing and optimizing concomitant cardiovascular conditions and treating symptoms. Nonetheless, AVR has been shown to improve symptoms and survival and it is the only effective treatment in severe symptomatic AS. Those with severe asymptomatic AS may also meet indications for AVR if they have concurrent LV systolic dysfunction, very severe AS, rapidly progressing AS, or if they are undergoing another cardiac surgery.

There are two broad approaches to AVR: surgical and transcatheter. For decades, surgical AVR was the mainstay of therapy for severe AS. With surgical AVR, either a mechanical or bioprosthetic valve can be considered. With favorable flow characteristics, mechanical valves can last for the patient's lifetime (Fig. 7.2). However, these valves require anticoagulation with warfarin. While bioprosthetic valves, made from bovine or porcine material, do not require anticoagulation, they are less durable and typically require re-replacement after 10 to 20 years (Fig. 7.3).

Rather than an open procedure requiring sternotomy, transcatheter aortic valve implantation (TAVI) most commonly involves accessing the femoral artery and using a catheter to deliver a bioprosthetic valve into position by expanding a balloon and effectively crushing the native aortic valve against the aortic wall (Fig. 7.4). Less common approaches include transapical, transaortic, and subclavian. The role of TAVI was initially established in patients with severe symptomatic AS and prohibitive surgical risk. TAVI led to significant mortality benefit

TABLE 7.2   AS Exam Findings by Severity

Exam Finding	Mild	Moderate	Severe
Carotid pulse	Normal	Slow rising	Parvus et tardus
Apical impulse	Normal	Heaving	Heaving and sustained
S_4 gallop	Absent	May be present	Present
Systolic ejection click	Present	May be present	Absent
Systolic murmur peak	Early systole	Mid systole	Mid or late systole
S_2	Normal	Normal or single	Single or paradoxical

TABLE 7.3   Measures of AS Severity on Echocardiography

Indicator	Normal	Mild	Moderate	Severe
Aortic valve area (cm^2)	>2.0	1.5-2.0	1.0-1.5	<1.0
Mean gradient (mm Hg)		<25	25-40	>40
Peak jet velocity (m/s)	<2.0	2-3	3-4	>4

Data from Baumgartner H, Hung J, Bermego J, et al: Echocardiographic assessment of valve stenosis: EAE/ASE recommendations for clinical practice. J Am Soc Echocardiogr 2009;22:1-22.

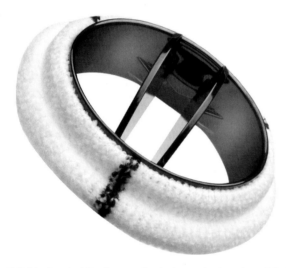

Fig. 7.2 Medtronic bileaflet mechanical prosthetic valve. (Modified from Medtronic, Inc.)

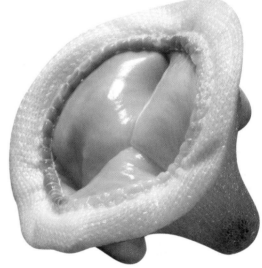

Fig. 7.3 Medtronic Hancock II bioprosthetic valve. (Modified from Medtronic, Inc.)

in this patient population when compared to standard therapy. Since the landmark trial in 2010, TAVI has emerged as an effective therapy for severe symptomatic AS in patients across the entire spectrum of surgical risk, from extreme risk to low risk.

Patients being considered for AVR should undergo a thorough individualized evaluation by a multidisciplinary heart valve team. The patient's life expectancy, surgical risk, comorbidities, frailty, anatomy, quality of life, values, and preferences should all be considered before making an informed shared decision on treatment strategy.

MITRAL STENOSIS

Definition and Etiology

Mitral stenosis (MS) is defined by the restriction of blood flow from the left atrium (LA) to the left ventricle during diastole. RHD is by far the most common cause of MS. In developed nations, rheumatic MS has become less common with the decreasing incidence of rheumatic fever. However, in developing nations, RHD remains a significant

public health problem. Less common causes of MS include mitral annular calcification, radiation exposure, congenital, or mechanical obstruction from an atrial myxoma, vegetation, or thrombus.

Pathophysiology

Rheumatic fever is the result of an abnormal immune response usually occurring after 10 days to 3 weeks after untreated group A streptococcal pharyngitis. It typically affects children between the ages of 6 and 15 years. The diagnosis can be made based on clinical manifestations and the revised Jones criteria (Table 7.4).

In RHD, there is inflammatory process thought to be due to cross-reactivity between streptococcal antigen and valve tissue. This along with chronic turbulent flow through a deformed valve results in thickening and calcification of the mitral leaflets, thickening and shortening of the chordae tendineae, and fusion of the leaflet commissures (Fig. 7.5). This ultimately leads to a reduced orifice through which blood can flow from the LA to the left ventricle during diastole.

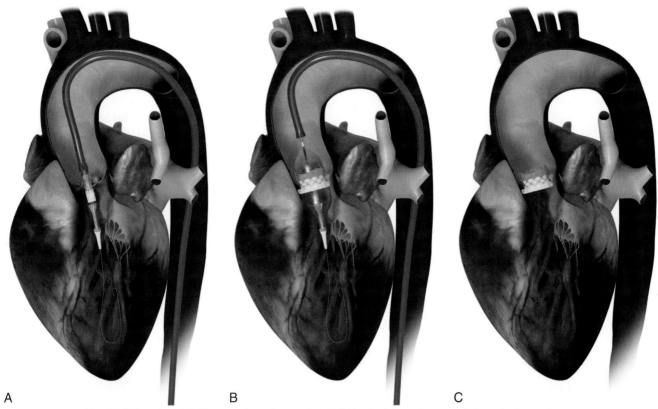

Fig. 7.4 Edwards SAPIEN transcatheter heart valve. (A) Valve is delivered retrograde from the femoral artery and positioned at the level of the aortic annulus. (B) Balloon inflated, deploying the valve. (C) Deployed valve. (From Cardiology Secrets, 5th ed, Elsevier, 2018.)

TABLE 7.4 Revised Jones Criteria[a]

Major Criteria	Minor Criteria
Carditis (pleuritic chest pain, friction rub, heart failure)	Fever
Polyarthritis	Arthralgia
Chorea	Previous rheumatic fever or known rheumatic heart disease
Erythema marginatum	
Subcutaneous nodules	

[a]Rheumatic fever is diagnosed based on the presence of two major criteria or one major and two minor criteria after a recent documented group A streptococcal infection.

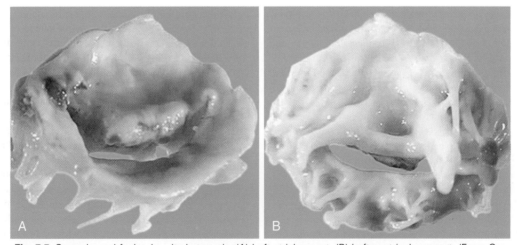

Fig. 7.5 Commissural fusion in mitral stenosis. (A) Left atrial aspect. (B) Left ventricular aspect. (From Cardiovascular Pathology, Fourth Ed, Elsevier, 2016.)

The hemodynamic consequences of MS primarily affect the pulmonary capillary bed, pulmonary artery, and right ventricle. In pure MS, the left ventricle remains unaffected. With resistance to left atrial emptying during diastole, left atrial pressure (LAP) increases. This pressure is reflected back to the capillary bed and pulmonary artery, which can result in pulmonary edema and pulmonary hypertension. This can lead to pressure overload of the right ventricle with subsequent right ventricle hypertrophy (RVH), tricuspid regurgitation (TR), and eventual right ventricular (RV) failure.

Natural History and Clinical Presentation

In developed countries, rheumatic MS is usually a slow progressive disease with a prolonged asymptomatic period of up to several decades. In developing countries, the disease course can be more rapid with symptoms in young adults and children. Symptom onset occurs once the mitral valve area is less than 1.5 cm^2. Once symptom onset occurs, the prognosis becomes worse. Mortality has been linked to New York Heart Association (NYHA) functional class. The presence of atrial fibrillation (AF) and pulmonary hypertension has also been established as a poor prognostic indicator.

Patients often present with dyspnea on exertion and decreased exercise tolerance. This is a consequence of elevated LAP and pulmonary pressures. Additionally, with exertion, an increase in heart rate leads to a decrease in diastolic filling time and increase in the diastolic gradient across the mitral valve.

Elevated LAP leads to left atrial dilation and AF. This can often precipitate or exacerbate the symptoms of MS in two possible ways. First, in AF, there is the loss of atrial contraction which further impedes diastolic flow across a stenotic mitral valve. Second, AF often leads to high heart rates and decreases diastolic filling time. Also, with AF associated with MS, there is an increased thromboembolic risk. If the LA becomes severely dilated, it can compress the recurrent laryngeal nerve and cause hoarseness (Ortner syndrome) or coughing.

Increases in pulmonary pressures and vascular congestion can lead to hemoptysis. As pulmonary hypertension progresses, it affects the right heart and right-sided filling pressures, ultimately leading to symptoms of right heart failure such as ascites and peripheral edema.

Symptoms can be provoked with any state causing an increase in cardiac output or heart rate such as exertion, stress, illness, infection, or arrhythmia. Symptoms may be unmasked in previously asymptomatic women with MS who become pregnant given the increase in heart rate and cardiac output associated with pregnancy.

Physical Examination

Several components of the physical examination need to be carefully assessed when evaluating patients with MS. The patient should be examined in a quiet room and positioned in the left lateral decubitus position because certain characteristic findings of MS may be difficult to appreciate.

S_1 is loud early on in the disease as elevated LAP leads to increased excursion of the mitral leaflets. However, as the disease progresses and the leaflets become calcified and rigid, S_1 diminishes. The S_2 is initially normal but P_2 can increase in intensity as pulmonary pressures rise. Eventually a single S_2 can result. S_3 is typically not heard but S_4 can be heard due to right ventricular hypertrophy (RVH).

A diastolic opening snap (OS) can be heard due to the initial rapid opening of the mitral leaflets followed by an abrupt halt due to fusion of the leaflet tips. The interval between S_2 and OS varies inversely with the severity of MS. The earlier in diastole the OS occurs, the more severe the MS as this is reflective of higher LAP.

The murmur appreciated in MS is a low-pitched diastolic rumble best heard at the apex and at end expiration using the bell of the stethoscope. In mild MS, the murmur may be heard only in late diastole. As MS progresses the murmur may be heard throughout diastole, and if the MS is very severe the murmur may be very soft or absent due to slow flow across the mitral valve.

Patients with symptomatic MS may have signs of heart failure such as rales, jugular venous distension, hepatomegaly, and peripheral edema. If there is significant pulmonary hypertension, a parasternal lift or RV heave may be appreciable.

Diagnosis

ECG and chest radiograph can have nonspecific findings. ECG can show left atrial enlargement, AF, or RVH. Chest radiograph may demonstrate pulmonary vascular congestion, RV dilation, pulmonary artery dilation, or left atrial enlargement ("double density" sign).

TTE is the diagnostic test for MS. TTE is also used to evaluate the severity of MS, assess the effects of the MS on the cardiac chambers and pulmonary pressures, assess for concomitant valvular disease, and assess for suitability of valve anatomy for percutaneous mitral balloon valvotomy (PMBV). On TTE, the mitral leaflets appear thickened and deformed. In rheumatic MS, leaflet motion during diastole is restricted and results in a characteristic "hockey stick" appearance. Doppler interrogation can provide an estimation of mitral valve area and pulmonary artery pressure. The TTE can also assess for the other findings associated with MS such as left atrial dilation, RVH or RV dilation, and TR. With the findings on TTE and the patient's symptoms, MS severity can be staged (Table 7.5).

When there is a discrepancy between the TTE findings and clinical findings, exercise stress echocardiography can be performed to evaluate the mitral valve gradients and pulmonary pressures during exercise. Alternatively, cardiac catheterization can be considered to obtain direct measurements of the cardiac chambers and mitral gradients.

Treatment

There is a limited role for medical therapy in the treatment of MS. If patients have symptoms of heart failure, diuretics can be used to alleviate symptoms. Slowing the heart rate with β-blockers or calcium-channel blockers will increase diastolic filling time and decrease mitral gradients. Rate control is particularly important in AF. Anticoagulation with a vitamin K antagonist is recommended in patients with MS and AF, prior embolic event, or left atrial thrombus. Direct oral anticoagulants have not been approved for this indication.

The decision to proceed with an intervention of the mitral valve depends on the severity of MS and the presence of symptoms, AF, and pulmonary hypertension. Valve morphology, presence of concomitant MR, presence of left atrial thrombus, and the patient's surgical risk will guide whether the patient undergoes a surgical mitral valve replacement or PMBV. Contraindications for PMBV include the presence of left atrial thrombus and more than moderate MR. TTE can be used to assess the suitability for PMBV by assessing the mobility, thickening, and calcification of the mitral leaflets and the degree of subvalvular thickening. Refer to Table 7.6 for a summary of the recommendations for mitral valve intervention described in the 2014 AHA/ACC valve guidelines.

PULMONIC STENOSIS

Definition and Etiology

Pulmonic stenosis (PS) is defined by a restriction in leaflet motion resulting in RV outflow obstruction and a pressure gradient between the right ventricle and main pulmonary artery. The etiology of PS is almost always congenital and usually occurs as an isolated lesion. However, it can also be associated with other congenital conditions such as tetralogy of Fallot, congenital rubella syndrome, and Noonan syndrome.

TABLE 7.5 Stages of MS

Stage	Definition	Valve Anatomy	Hemodynamic Consequences	Symptoms
A	At risk of MS	Doming of mitral leaflets during diastole	None	None
B	Progressive MS	Rheumatic valve changes with commissural fusion and diastolic doming of the mitral leaflets MVA >1.5 cm^2	Mild to moderate LA enlargement Normal pulmonary pressure at rest	None
C	Asymptomatic severe MS	Rheumatic valve changes with commissural fusion and diastolic doming of the mitral leaflets MVA ≤1.5 cm^2 (MVA <1.0 cm^2 with very severe MS)	Severe LA enlargement Elevated pulmonary artery pressure	None
D	Symptomatic severe MS	See Stage C	See Stage C	Decreased exercise tolerance Exertional dyspnea

Modified from Nishimura R, Otto C, Bonow RO, et al: 2014 AHA/ACC guideline for the management of patients with valvular heart disease. J Am Coll Cardiol 2014;63:e57-e185.

TABLE 7.6 Summary of Recommendations for Mitral Valve Intervention in MS

Recommendation	Class of Recommendation
PMBV is recommended for symptomatic patients with severe MS (MVA ≤1.5 cm^2, stage D) and favorable valve morphology in the absence of contraindications	I
MVR is indicated in severely symptomatic patients (NYHA class III/IV) with severe MS (MVA ≤1.5 cm^2, stage D) who are not high risk for surgery and who are not candidates for or failed previous PMBV	I
Concomitant MVR is indicated for patients with severe MS (MVA ≤1.5 cm^2, stage C or D) undergoing other cardiac surgery	I
PMBV is reasonable for asymptomatic patients with very severe MS (MVA ≤1.0 cm^2, stage C) and favorable valve morphology in the absence of contraindications	IIa
MVR is reasonable for severely symptomatic patients (NYHA class III/IV) with severe MS (MVA ≤1.5 cm^2, stage D), provided there are other operative indications	IIa
PMBV may be considered for asymptomatic patients with severe MS (MVA ≤1.5 cm^2, stage C) and favorable valve morphology who have new onset of AF in the absence of contraindications	IIb
PMBV may be considered for symptomatic patients with MVA >1.5 cm^2 if there is evidence of hemodynamically significant MS during exercise	IIb
PMBV may be considered for severely symptomatic patients (NYHA class III/IV) with severe MS (MVA ≤1.5 cm^2, stage D) who have suboptimal valve anatomy and are not candidates for surgery or at high risk for surgery	IIb
Concomitant MVR may be considered for patients with moderate MS (MVA 1.6 to 2.0 cm^2) undergoing other cardiac surgery	IIb
MVR and excision of the left atrial appendage may be considered for patients with severe MS (MVA ≤1.5 cm^2, stages C and D) who have had recurrent embolic events while receiving adequate anticoagulation	IIb

Modified from Nishimura R, Otto C, Bonow RO, et al: 2014 AHA/ACC guideline for the management of patients with valvular heart disease. J Am Coll Cardiol 2014;63:e57-e185.

Pathophysiology

In PS, the valve is typically trileaflet with thickening and fusion of the commissures resulting in restricted leaflet opening during systole. Post-stenotic dilation of the main pulmonary artery can occur due to eccentric flow through the stenotic valve. Over time, RVH can occur due to increased afterload.

Natural History and Clinical Presentation

Isolated PS is generally well tolerated and survival is comparable to the general population. Patients with mild PS are asymptomatic and may not be diagnosed with PS until adulthood. Moderate PS is usually identified in childhood and patients are usually symptomatic due to RV pressure overload. Decreasing right-sided cardiac output leads to symptoms of dyspnea on exertion and fatigue. In more advanced disease, patients can have RV failure and cyanosis.

Physical Examination

On physical examination, patients with PS can have a parasternal lift as a result of RVH. The jugular veins may demonstrate prominent a waves. The murmur of PS is a systolic ejection murmur best heard at the left upper sternal border radiating to the back with the duration correlating with severity. A late peaking murmur indicates more severe disease. A systolic ejection click may be heard in mild to moderate PS. S_2 can have wide splitting due to prolonged ejection time of the right ventricle. Fixed splitting of S_2 occurs in severe disease when the RV output becomes fixed.

Diagnosis

TTE can be used to diagnose PS, assess the severity of PS, and evaluate the right ventricle. Using Doppler measurements, the gradients across a stenotic pulmonic valve can be estimated. If TTE is inconclusive or for patients with complex anatomy, cardiac magnetic resonance imaging (CMR) can be considered as an alternative imaging modality to assess the severity of valve disease and quantitatively measure RV size and function.

Treatment

Intervention is guided by the valve anatomy, gradients measured on TTE, and the presence of symptoms. Percutaneous balloon valvotomy is recommended in asymptomatic patients with a peak gradient of greater than 60 mm Hg or a mean gradient of 40 mm Hg, or in symptomatic patients with a peak gradient of 50 mm Hg or a mean gradient of 30 mm Hg. A surgical approach is usually recommended for dysplastic valves, in the presence of severe pulmonic regurgitation, or if there is another indication for surgery.

TRICUSPID STENOSIS

Definition and Etiology

In tricuspid stenosis (TS), there is restriction of blood flow between the right atrium and right ventricle. The etiology of TS is most commonly rheumatic and is generally associated with MS. Isolated TS is rare but can be seen in congenital tricuspid valve atresia, right heart tumors, carcinoid syndrome, and endocarditis.

Pathophysiology

TS causes flow obstruction at the level of the tricuspid valve resulting in a diastolic pressure gradient between the right atrium and right ventricle. This leads to elevated right atrial pressure (RAP) and systemic venous congestion. With exertion or tachycardia, diastolic filling time decreases and the diastolic pressure gradient increases. With inspiration, the decrease in intrathoracic pressure results in increased venous return which also increases the pressure gradient across the tricuspid valve. Conversely, expiration leads to a decrease in the pressure gradient.

Natural History and Clinical Presentation

The natural history of patients with TS is variable. Most patients with rheumatic TS have concomitant significant aortic and/or mitral valve disease. Tricuspid valve atresia is managed with multiple surgeries starting in the neonatal period into early childhood.

Patients present with signs and symptoms of systemic venous congestion including ascites, peripheral edema, and hepatomegaly. Patients may report a fluttering sensation in the neck from prominent *a* waves.

Physical Examination

With an increase in RAP there is jugular venous distension. A prominent *a* wave can often be appreciated. A rise in jugular venous pressure with inspiration (Kussmaul sign) may also be seen. Other signs of systemic venous congestion can be present including hepatomegaly, ascites, peripheral edema, and anasarca. The murmur of TS is described as a low-frequency, diastolic murmur best heard at the left lower sternal border. There may also be an opening snap. These sounds are difficult to distinguish from the murmur and opening snap of MS. However, with right-sided murmurs, the intensity of the TS murmur should increase with inspiration (Carvallo sign).

Diagnosis

TS can be diagnosed using TTE. In rheumatic TS, as seen in MS, the leaflets are restricted, thickened, and calcified. TTE is also used to assess for concomitant valve disease and to estimate the right atrial size and pressure. Using Doppler, the diastolic pressure gradients can be measured across the tricuspid valve and the tricuspid valve area can be estimated. A valve area of 1.0 cm^2 or less is considered to be severe TS.

Treatment

There are limited data to guide treatment in TS. Options include medical therapy such as diuretics to help with systemic venous congestion, surgical intervention, or percutaneous balloon valvotomy. The decision for surgical versus percutaneous approach should be individualized and based on valve anatomy, surgical risk, and operator experience. A surgical approach is typically reserved for symptomatic patients with severe TS or asymptomatic patients with severe TS requiring cardiac surgery for another indication.

AORTIC REGURGITATION

Definition and Etiology

Aortic regurgitation (AR) is the result of inadequate coaptation of the aortic valve leaflets during diastole leading to regurgitant flow of blood from the aorta to the left ventricle. The ability of the left ventricle to accommodate this additional volume is dependent on the chronicity of the disease. Therefore, acute severe AR and chronic AR should be considered as separate disease processes.

The two most common causes of acute severe AR in a native aortic valve are endocarditis and aortic dissection. Endocarditis can lead to leaflet destruction, leaflet perforation, or perivalvular abscess that can rupture into the left ventricle. Aortic dissection can result in AR by dilation of the sinuses, involvement of the commissures or leaflets, or prolapse of the dissection flap across the aortic valve.

In developing countries, chronic AR is usually due to rheumatic heart disease. In developed countries, aortic root dilation, calcific degeneration, and bicuspid aortic valve are the most common causes. However, many other disease processes can affect the aortic valve or the ascending aorta and lead to chronic AR (Table 7.7).

Pathophysiology

In acute severe AR, a large regurgitant volume enters an unprepared left ventricle which results in a decrease in effective stroke volume and rapid increase in LV end-diastolic pressure with subsequent pulmonary edema, cardiogenic shock, and possible hemodynamic collapse.

In chronic AR, the left ventricle is able to make compensatory changes to maintain cardiac output. The regurgitant flow from the aorta into the left ventricle results in an increase in LV end-diastolic volume and wall stress. In response, there is eccentric hypertrophy, chamber dilation, and an increase in ventricular compliance. Therefore, LV end-diastolic pressure can remain normal despite a significant increase in LV volume. In addition, these compensatory changes can lead to an increase in total stroke volume, which results in an elevation in systolic pressure. During diastole, there is rapid equalization of pressures between the aorta and left ventricle resulting in a low diastolic pressure. This accounts for the wide pulse pressure and several of the characteristic physical examination findings seen in chronic AR.

Natural History and Clinical Presentation

Patients with acute severe AR often present with pulmonary edema and cardiogenic shock. Other presenting symptoms will depend on the etiology, which is usually aortic dissection or endocarditis.

In contrast, there is a prolonged asymptomatic period in chronic AR. Even with severe AR, exercise tolerance can be preserved as an increase in heart rate during exercise leads to shorter diastolic filling times, and thus less AR. However, with progressive LV dilation,

TABLE 7.7 Causes of Chronic Aortic Regurgitation

Mechanism	Etiology
Congenital/leaflet abnormalities	Bicuspid, unicuspid, or quadricuspid aortic valve
	Ventricular septal defect
Acquired leaflet abnormalities	Senile calcification
	Infective endocarditis
	Rheumatic disease
	Radiation-induced valvulopathy
	Toxin-induced valvulopathy: anorectic drugs, 5-hydroxytryptamine
Congenital/genetic aortic root abnormalities	Annuloaortic ectasia
	Connective tissue disease: Loeys Dietz, Ehlers-Danlos, Marfan syndrome, osteogenesis imperfecta
Acquired aortic root abnormalities	Idiopathic aortic root dilation
	Systemic hypertension
	Autoimmune disease: systemic lupus erythematosus, ankylosing spondylitis, reactive arthritis
	Aortitis: syphilis, Takayasu arteritis
	Aortic dissection
	Trauma

Modified from: Zoghbi W, Adams D, et al: Recommendations for noninvasive evaluation of native valvular regurgitation. JASE 2017;30:303-371.

patients can develop LV systolic dysfunction and symptoms of heart failure.

Physical Examination

Patients with acute severe AR will have physical examination findings consistent with cardiogenic shock and pulmonary edema such as hypotension, pallor, peripheral vasoconstriction, and rales. Wide pulse pressures and the characteristic findings seen in chronic AR are typically not appreciated.

With regards to the heart sounds in acute severe AR, A_2 may be diminished, P_2 is more prominent due to pulmonary hypertension, and S_3 can be heard. The murmurs heard in acute AR include an early, low-pitched, diastolic murmur and a soft systolic murmur due to increased flow across the aortic valve. The presence of both results in a characteristic "to-and-fro" murmur. However, depending on the diastolic gradient between the aorta and left ventricle, these murmurs may be inaudible.

The wide pulse pressure seen in chronic AR can lead to several physical findings (Table 7.8). The murmur of chronic AR is a blowing early diastolic murmur best heard at the left upper sternal border with the patient sitting up, leaning forward, and at end-expiration. As AR progresses, this murmur can become holodiastolic and harsher in quality. In very severe AR, the murmur can become soft or even absent.

An Austin-Flint murmur, a mid to late diastolic rumble best heard at the apex in severe AR and due to vibration of the anterior mitral leaflet as it is struck by the jet of AR, may also be appreciated. Additionally, a short midsystolic ejection murmur radiating to the neck can be heard as a result of increased stroke volume.

Diagnosis

In both acute and chronic AR, echocardiography can evaluate the presence, severity, and mechanism of AR, the effect of AR on the other cardiac chambers, and the presence of concomitant valve disease. In the case of acute severe AR with suspected aortic dissection or endocarditis, a transesophageal echocardiogram (TEE) should be considered over TTE given its superior sensitivity and specificity for these diagnoses. Computed tomography (CT) imaging has similar sensitivity and specificity for diagnosing aortic dissection. However, TEE also allows for concomitant evaluation of the aortic valve structure, AR, and the other cardiac structures.

In the assessment of chronic AR, when the TTE results are inconclusive or discrepant from clinical findings, alternative imaging modalities can be considered. TEE generally provides superior image quality compared to TTE. CMR can accurately quantify the severity of AR as well as chamber sizes and LV systolic function. Aortography and cardiac catheterization may also be considered to evaluate AR, aortic root, and left-sided filling pressures. However, their role has diminished because of the availability and accuracy of noninvasive imaging.

Treatment

In acute severe AR, emergent or urgent surgical intervention is usually indicated in the setting of aortic dissection or infective endocarditis. Prior to surgery, the mainstay of medical therapy is afterload reduction. This can be achieved with intravenous nitroprusside. Diuretics and ionotropic agents may be helpful in the setting of cardiogenic shock and pulmonary edema. Beta-blockers, while helpful for aortic dissection, can lead to further hemodynamic deterioration as the increase in diastolic filling time leads to more AR. Vasopressors and intra-aortic balloon pumps are contraindicated in this setting.

With chronic AR, there is a limited role for medical therapy. Vasodilators such as hydralazine, angiotensin-converting enzyme (ACE) inhibitors, and calcium-channel blockers can be used in patients who are asymptomatic and hypertensive. There is conflicting evidence for their use to delay surgery. AVR is recommended once a patient has severe symptomatic AR or severe asymptomatic AR with a LV systolic dysfunction (left ventricular ejection fraction (LVEF) of less than 50%) or chamber dilation (LV end systolic diameter (LVESD) of greater than 50 mm or LV end diastolic diameter (LVEDD) of greater than 65 mm). AVR is also indicated in patients with severe asymptomatic AR if there is another indication for cardiac surgery.

The options for mechanical and biologic prostheses are similar to those for surgical AVR for AS. However, a percutaneous approach is not available.

MITRAL REGURGITATION

Definition and Etiology

Mitral regurgitation (MR) is defined by the inadequate coaptation of the mitral leaflets during systole resulting in regurgitant flow from the left ventricle to the left atrium. Similar to AR, MR leads to LV volume overload

TABLE 7.8   Signs of Chronic Aortic Regurgitation

Name	Description
Corrigan pulse	Rapid upstroke and collapse of pulses; "water hammer pulses"
Musset sign	Head bob with each heartbeat
Traube sign	Systolic and diastolic sounds heard over femoral arteries; "pistol shot pulse"
Duroziez sign	Systolic and diastolic bruit heard with compression of femoral artery
Quincke pulses	Capillary pulsations
Mueller sign	Pulsation of uvula
Becker sign	Pulsation of retinal arteries and pupils
Hills sign	Popliteal systolic cuff pressure exceed brachial pressure by >20 mm Hg
Mayne sign	>15 mm Hg decrease in diastolic blood pressure with arm elevation
Rosenbach sign	Pulsations of liver
Gerhard sign	Pulsations of spleen

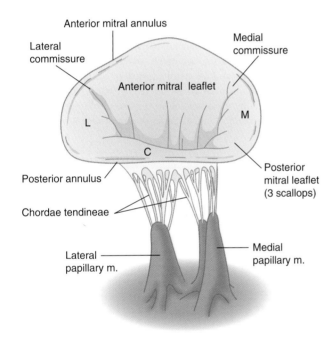

Fig. 7.6 Mitral apparatus. (From Otto C: Textbook of Clinical Echocardiography, 6th ed., Elsevier, 2018.)

and the ability of the left ventricle to compensate for this additional volume is dependent upon chronicity. Therefore, like AR, acute severe MR and chronic MR should be considered as two distinct disease processes.

The mitral apparatus consists of the left atrial wall, mitral annulus, anterior and posterior leaflets, chordae tendineae, papillary muscles, and the LV myocardium underlying the papillary muscles (Fig. 7.6). Disturbance to any component of the mitral apparatus can result in MR.

Acute MR can be caused by ischemic and nonischemic etiologies. Papillary muscle rupture or displacement can be seen in the setting of an acute myocardial infarction or ischemia. Nonischemic causes include infective endocarditis, ruptured chordae tendineae, trauma, RHD, and dynamic LV outflow obstruction.

Given the complexity of the mitral apparatus, it is useful to categorize the causes of MR as primary or secondary (Table 7.9). Primary MR is due to an intrinsic abnormality of the mitral leaflets. Secondary MR is a result of distortion of the mitral annulus in the setting of ventricular remodeling. Distinguishing between primary and secondary MR is important because the management and outcomes differ. Alternatively, MR can be classified based on leaflet motion using the Carpentier classification (Fig. 7.7).

Pathophysiology

The pathophysiology of MR and the differences in the pathophysiology between acute and chronic MR are illustrated in Fig. 7.8. In acute severe MR, there is a sudden increase in preload and decrease in afterload. This leads to an increase in the total stroke volume (TSV) and LVEF. However, the forward stroke volume (FSV) decreases resulting in reduced cardiac output. Simultaneously, there is an acute rise in LAP causing pulmonary edema. This ultimately leads to cardiogenic shock.

In chronic compensated MR, the progressive rise in LV preload leads to increased wall stress. In response, there is eccentric hypertrophy of the left ventricle and an increase in the LV end diastolic volume. This not only increases LVEF and TSV, but it also allows for the maintenance of a normal FSV. However, as MR progresses, LV systolic dysfunction and dilation occur. In this setting, LVEF, TSV, and FSV all decrease, resulting in chronic decompensated MR.

In chronic MR, the compliant left atrium is able to accommodate a large regurgitant volume from the left ventricle. However, this eventually results in left atrial dilation and pulmonary hypertension.

Natural History and Clinical Presentation

Patients with acute severe MR are acutely ill and often in cardiogenic shock. Along with hemodynamic instability, patients may have symptoms related to the etiology of MR. For example, in the setting of an acute myocardial infarction with papillary muscle rupture, a patient may present with chest pain along with ischemic ECG changes and elevated cardiac enzymes. Patients with infective endocarditis may have fevers, positive blood cultures, vascular phenomena, immunologic phenomena, or a predisposing condition such as intravenous drug use.

With chronic MR, the natural history and clinical presentation are quite different because the left ventricle has time to remodel and compensate via the mechanisms noted above. Often times, patients have a prolonged asymptomatic phase. Over time, as the left-sided filling pressures increase, patients may develop fatigue or decreased exercise tolerance. Eventually, patients can have signs and symptoms of congestive heart failure (CHF) such as dyspnea on exertion, orthopnea, paroxysmal nocturnal dyspnea, and/or peripheral edema. With left atrial dilation, patients may develop AF.

Physical Examination

Patients with acute severe MR are often in pulmonary edema and cardiogenic shock. Physical examination may be remarkable for pallor, cool extremities due to peripheral vasoconstriction, rales, jugular venous distension, and diminished peripheral pulses. The murmur of acute severe MR is usually soft, low-pitched, decrescendo, and early systolic. However, in about half of the patients, no murmur may be appreciated due to the low-pressure gradient between the left ventricle and the left atrium. Therefore, the absence of a systolic murmur does not necessarily rule out acute severe MR.

In chronic MR, S_1 is diminished due to inadequate coaptation of the mitral leaflets. S_2 is widely split with a reduced forward stroke volume leading to an early A_2 and pulmonary hypertension delaying P_2. An S_3 can also be appreciated with the increased diastolic flow across the mitral valve into a left ventricle. The murmur of chronic MR is

TABLE 7.9 Mechanisms of Mitral Regurgitation

	Valvular Abnormality
Primary Mitral Regurgitation	
Degenerative	Mitral valve prolapse, thickening/calcification
Rheumatic	Leaflet thickening/restriction
Infectious endocarditis	Vegetations, tissue destruction, leaflet perforation
Systemic inflammatory conditions	Libman-Sacks lesions
Malignancy associated	Marantic endocarditis
Genetic connective tissue disorders (Marfan syndrome, Ehlers-Danlos syndrome)	Elongated, redundant leaflet tissue
Irradiation	Diffuse leaflet thickening/calcification
Drug-induced (anorexigen, ergotamine)	Diffuse leaflet thickening
Congenital	Cleft/parachute mitral valve
Secondary Mitral Regurgitation	
	Ventricular distortion of mitral apparatus (coronary artery disease, cardiomyopathy)
	Mitral annular dilation (usually with atrial fibrillation)

Modified from Otto C: Practice of Clinical Echocardiography, Fifth Edition. Philadelphia, Elsevier, 2017.

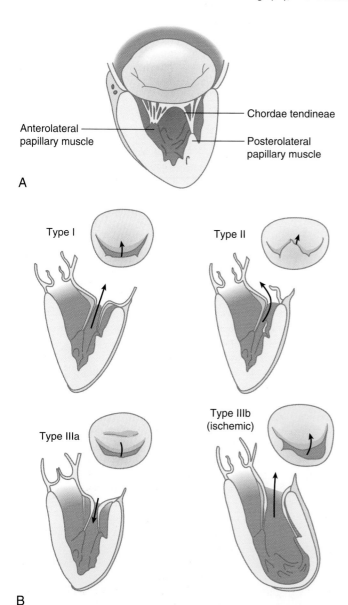

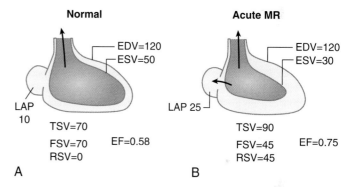

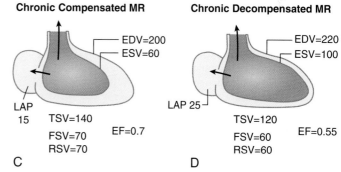

Fig. 7.8 Pathophysiology of mitral regurgitation. (From Otto C: Textbook of Clinical Echocardiography, 5th ed., Elsevier, 2013.)

Fig. 7.7 (A) Mitral apparatus. (B) Carpentier classification of mitral regurgitation. (From Interventional Cardiology Clinics, Volume 5, Issue 1, 2016.)

most commonly a blowing, high-pitched, holosystolic murmur best heard at the apex. Depending on the direction of the MR jet, the murmur may radiate toward the axilla or the neck. In MR due to mitral valve prolapse, a midsystolic click can be heard followed by a mid or late systolic murmur.

Diagnosis

An electrocardiogram (ECG) and chest radiograph may have nonspecific findings such as left atrial enlargement or cardiomegaly, respectively. Pulmonary edema can be seen on chest radiograph in the setting of CHF. However, the diagnosis of MR is ultimately made by TTE, which can assess for the presence and severity of MR, the effect of MR on the other cardiac chambers, the presence of concomitant valve disease, and possibly the etiology of MR. If TTE is inadequate, there are other imaging modalities that are useful. CMR can be used to accurately quantify the chamber sizes, LVEF, and the severity of MR. TEE can provide superior image quality to TTE, including three-dimensional imaging, and help to clarify the severity and anatomic mechanism of MR. In the case of acute severe MR, if the level of suspicion is high and the TTE does not show significant MR, a TEE can be performed. Alternatively, a right heart catheterization can be considered. In the presence of significant MR, the pulmonary capillary wedge waveform would have prominent *v* waves from the regurgitant flow from the left atrium. Finally, in patients who have symptoms that are out of proportion to the severity of MR, exercise echocardiography can be considered to assess for changes in MR and pulmonary artery pressure with exercise.

Treatment

In acute severe MR, emergent or urgent surgical intervention is usually indicated. Until surgery can be performed, afterload reduction is essential. This is achieved with an intra-aortic balloon pump which not only reduces afterload but also improves cardiac output and coronary blood flow. Nitroprusside can also be given to reduce afterload and ionotropic agents can be given for hemodynamic support. In the absence of hypotension, diuretics can be given to treat pulmonary edema.

There is no clear role for medical therapy in treating the primary process of chronic MR. The use of vasodilators in normotensive patients with normal LV systolic function is not recommended. Hypertensive patients can be treated with standard antihypertensive therapy which may limit worsening of MR. Patients with LV systolic dysfunction can be given guideline-directed medical therapy (ACE inhibitors/angiotensin-receptor blockers/angiotensin receptor–neprilysin inhibitor, β-blocker, aldosterone antagonist, and diuretics).

The indication for mitral valve intervention depends on several factors. If a patient has severe symptomatic MR, mitral valve surgery is recommended. If a patient has severe asymptomatic MR and LVEF between 30% and 60%, LVESD 40 mm or greater, or if there is a progressive decrease in LVEF or increase in LVESD, then mitral valve surgery is also recommended. Also, in patients with severe asymptomatic MR with new onset AF or pulmonary hypertension, mitral valve repair can be considered if the likelihood of successful repair is greater than 95% and the expected mortality is less than 1%. In general, there is a higher chance of successful repair in primary MR involving the posterior leaflet. Mitral valve repair is preferred over mitral valve replacement, when possible.

For patients with prohibitive surgical risk, transcatheter mitral valve repair (TMVR) can be considered (Figs. 7.9 and 7.10). Patients with prohibitive surgical risk, at least moderate to severe primary MR with NYHA class III or IV symptoms despite optimal medical therapy, favorable anatomy, and reasonable life expectancy (≥2 years), should be referred to a heart valve team for evaluation for TMVR. Trials assessing the benefit of TMVR in secondary MR have yielded conflicting results. Nonetheless, TMVR has been approved for moderate to severe or severe secondary MR.

PULMONIC REGURGITATION

Definition and Etiology

Pulmonic regurgitation (PR) is a result of inadequate coaptation of the pulmonic leaflets resulting in diastolic flow from the pulmonary artery to the right ventricle. Physiologic to mild PR is common in normal adults. Primary PR is due to an abnormality of the valve leaflets. Causes of primary PR include iatrogenic, endocarditis, RHD, carcinoid syndrome, and congenital. Secondary PR occurs in the setting of normal valve leaflets and can be seen in patients with pulmonary artery dilation or severe pulmonary arterial hypertension. Severe PR is most

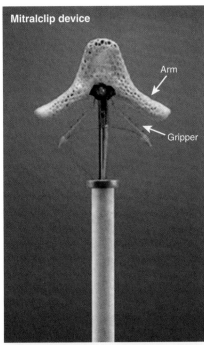

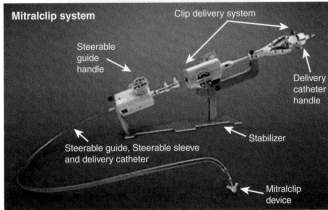

Fig. 7.9 Mitralclip delivery system. (Modified from Abbott Vascular.)

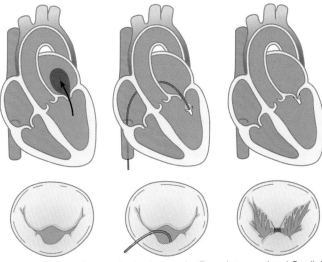

Fig. 7.10 Transcatheter mitral valve repair. (From Interventional Cardiology Clinics, Volume 5, Issue 1, 2016.)

commonly seen in patients with of tetralogy of Fallot who underwent surgical valvotomy or balloon valvuloplasty.

Pathophysiology

Regurgitant diastolic flow from the main pulmonary artery to the right ventricle leads to RV volume overload. Eventually, patients may develop RV dilation, RV dysfunction, and TR.

Natural History and Clinical Presentation

Patients with PR typically have a prolonged asymptomatic phase. As RV systolic function declines, cardiac output decreases and patients can develop fatigue or decreasing exercise tolerance. With RV dilation, TR and elevated right-sided filling pressure may develop along with signs and symptoms of right-sided heart failure such as ascites, peripheral edema, and hepatosplenomegaly.

Physical Examination

The murmur of PR is an early diastolic murmur best heard over the left upper sternal border that increases in intensity with inspiration. A systolic ejection murmur may also be heard with more significant amounts of PR due to increased RV flow. With concomitant pulmonary hypertension, a high frequency, blowing, diastolic murmur (Graham-Steell murmur) may be present. On examination of the neck veins, a prominent *a* wave can be seen in pulmonary hypertension and a prominent *v* wave in TR.

Diagnosis

ECG may have nonspecific findings such as RVH or arrhythmias. A right bundle branch block with intraventricular conduction delay can be observed in patients with a history of tetralogy of Fallot repair and severe PR. RV dilation may be seen on chest radiograph.

TTE can confirm the diagnosis of PR and also evaluates the severity, etiology, and, hemodynamic effects of PR, as well as concomitant valvular disease or pulmonary hypertension. CMR can also provide a quantitative assessment of PR and RV size and function.

Treatment

Medical therapy of secondary PR should target the underlying cause. Patients with right-sided heart failure can be given diuretics. However, surgical intervention is recommended for severe symptomatic PR. Surgery can also be considered for patients with severe asymptomatic PR with RV dilation or dysfunction, symptomatic arrhythmias, or progressive TR. In general, patients with native PR undergo surgical valve replacement. Due to the risk of prosthesis regurgitation and device embolization, a percutaneous approach is rarely recommended for native PR. Alternatively, for those with prosthetic PR, percutaneous valve replacement is an option.

TRICUSPID REGURGITATION

Definition and Etiology

TR is defined by the inadequate coaptation of the tricuspid leaflets during systole resulting in regurgitant flow from the right ventricle to the right atrium. Physiologic TR is present in about 70% of healthy adults.

Primary TR, a result of an abnormality of the valve structure, is rare. Possible causes include iatrogenic direct valve injury, chest wall trauma or deceleration injury, endocarditis, RHD, carcinoid syndrome, ischemic heart disease (causing papillary muscle dysfunction), myxomatous degeneration, Marfan syndrome, or drug-induced (fenfluramine, phentermine). The most common congenital heart disease affecting the tricuspid valve is Ebstein's anomaly.

Secondary TR occurs in the setting of normal valve anatomy and is much more common. TR is most often a result of RV dilation, annular dilation, or leaflet tethering. This can occur in any condition with increased right-sided filling pressures or pulmonary hypertension such as left-sided heart failure, mitral valve disease, stenosis of the pulmonic valve or pulmonary artery, primary pulmonary disease, left-to-right shunting, and Eisenmenger syndrome.

Pathophysiology

With regurgitant systolic flow into the right atrium, there is a progressive increase in RAP and RV volume. This leads to signs and symptoms of right-sided heart failure and low cardiac output due to RV systolic dysfunction.

Natural History and Clinical Presentation

Since the right atrium is a compliant chamber, it is able to accommodate the regurgitant volume when TR is mild or moderate. Therefore, patients are usually asymptomatic. Once severe, patients may have symptoms of venous congestion and right-sided heart failure such as hepatosplenomegaly, ascites, and peripheral edema. Patients with significant pulmonary hypertension may have signs of reduced cardiac output such as fatigue and dyspnea on exertion.

Physical Examination

TR leads to elevated RAP. This is demonstrated on physical examination by distended jugular veins. A prominent *c-v* wave due to the regurgitant flow may be observed. Kussmaul sign, a paradoxical rise in jugular venous pressure with inspiration, can be seen in the setting of RV dysfunction. With right-sided heart failure, peripheral edema, ascites, anasarca, and painful hepatosplenomegaly may be present.

On cardiac exam, wide splitting of S_2 and a loud P_2 can be heard with pulmonary hypertension. S_3 or S_4 may also be present in the setting of RV dilation or hypertrophy. The murmur of TR is holosystolic and best heard at the mid left sternal border. The intensity of the murmur will increase with maneuvers that increase venous return such as inspiration, leg raise, and hepatic compression. An RV heave may be appreciated on palpation in the setting of RV dilation.

Diagnosis

TR is diagnosed by TTE. Echocardiography can help to determine the severity and etiology of TR and RV size and function. In addition, Doppler can be used to estimate the pulmonary artery systolic pressure. If the TTE is inconclusive, CMR can quantify TR, RV size, and RV function. Right heart catheterization can provide direct measurements of right-sided pressures, pulmonary pressures, and pulmonary vascular resistance.

Treatment

Medical therapy for severe TR and right-sided heart failure consists of diuretics to treat volume overload. If possible, the primary disease process should be treated such as in ischemic heart disease, left-sided heart failure, mitral valve disease, and pulmonary arterial hypertension.

Isolated tricuspid valve surgery is only recommended in patients with severe symptomatic primary TR or severe asymptomatic TR with progressive RV dysfunction. If a patient is undergoing left-sided valve surgery, tricuspid valve surgery is recommended for those with concomitant severe TR or at least mild functional TR with tricuspid annular dilation or right-sided heart failure.

SUGGESTED READINGS

Mack M, Leon M, et al: Transcatheter aortic-valve replacement with a balloon-expandable valve in low risk patients, NEJM 380:1695–1705, 2019.

Nishimura R, Otto C, Bonow RO, et al.: 2014 AHA/ACC Guideline for the management of patients with valvular heart disease, J Am Coll Cardiol 63:e57–e185, 2014.

Nishimura R, Otto C, Bonow RO, et al.: 2017 AHA/ACC focused update of the 2014 AHA/ACC Guideline for the management of patients with valvular heart disease, J Am Coll Cardiol 70:252–289, 2017.

Nkomo V, Gardin J, et al.: Burden of valvular heart diseases: a population-based study, Lancet 368:1005–1011, 2006.

Obadia J, Messika-Zeitoun D, et al.: Percutaneous repair or medical treatment for secondary mitral regurgitation, NEJM 379:2297–2306, 2018.

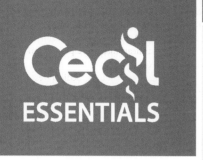

8

Coronary Heart Disease

David E. Lewandowski, Michael P. Cinquegrani

DEFINITION AND EPIDEMIOLOGY

The term *coronary heart disease* (CHD) describes a number of cardiac conditions that result from the presence of atherosclerotic lesions in the coronary arteries. The development of atherosclerotic plaque within the coronary arteries can result in obstruction to blood flow, producing ischemia, which can be acute or chronic in nature. Atherosclerosis is a disease process that starts at a young age and can be present for years in an asymptomatic form until the degree of vessel obstruction leads to ischemic symptoms. Obstructive atherosclerotic lesions can cause chronic symptoms of exercise- or stress-related angina; or, in the case of plaque rupture and acute thrombosis, sudden death, unstable angina, or myocardial infarction (MI) may ensue.

In the United States, more than 18 million people experience some form of CHD. Approximately 10 million suffer from symptoms of angina, and at least 360,000 deaths occur each year from acute MI or CHD-related sudden death. Despite progress in therapy and overall reductions in CHD-related mortality, CHD remains the number one cause of death in both men and women, accounting for 27% of deaths in women (more than deaths due to cancer). The incidence of CHD increases with age for both men and women. There are at least 1.3 million MIs per year in the United States and many more cases of unstable angina. CHD frequently results in lifestyle-limiting symptoms due to angina or impairment of left ventricular (LV) function. The cost of care related directly to CHD and indirectly to lost productivity from CHD is in the range of $156 billion per year. CHD remains a major life-threatening disease process associated with significant economic impact.

RISK FACTORS FOR ATHEROSCLEROSIS

There are a number of well-known risk factors for coronary artery disease (CAD), some of which are modifiable (Table 8.1). Although women ultimately also carry a significant atherosclerotic burden, men develop CAD at younger ages, and the prevalence of the disease also increases as men age. Another potent risk factor for the development of CAD is a family history of premature CAD. This speaks to a non-modifiable, genetically based risk. Commonly, multiple family members develop symptomatic CAD before the age of 55 years (65 years for women). Risks are additive, making it very important to appreciate the modifiable risk factors such as hyperlipidemia, hypertension, diabetes mellitus, metabolic syndrome, cigarette smoking, obesity, sedentary lifestyle, and heavy alcohol intake. Patients are risk-stratified for the likelihood of developing clinically significant coronary artery disease through the ASCVD (atherosclerotic cardiovascular disease)

score. Taking into account multiple patient-specific factors, the score estimates the patient's 10-year probability of experiencing an adverse event such as nonfatal MI, cardiovascular death, or stroke. The score can help guide blood pressure goals, the need for statin therapy, and other key preventative measures against CAD.

Metabolic syndrome deserves particular attention given that up to 25% of the adult US population may satisfy the definition of the disorder as laid out by the National Cholesterol Education Program Adult Treatment Panel. The definition of metabolic syndrome requires the presence of at least three of the following five criteria: waist circumference greater than 102 cm in men or 88 cm in women, triglyceride level 150 mg/dL or higher, high-density lipoprotein (HDL) cholesterol level lower than 40 mg/dL in men or 50 mg/dL in women, blood pressure 130/85 mm Hg or higher, and fasting serum glucose level 110 mg/dL or higher. The features of metabolic syndrome are largely modifiable risk factors for CAD.

Hyperlipidemia, in particular elevated levels of low-density lipoprotein (LDL) cholesterol, plays a pivotal role in the development and evolution of atherosclerosis. HDL-cholesterol is believed to be protective, likely due to its role in transporting cholesterol from the vessel wall to the liver for degradation. Increased levels of HDL are inversely proportional to the risk of CAD-related problems. The interplay among circulating lipids is complex. Elevated levels of triglycerides are a risk factor for CAD and are frequently associated with reduced levels of protective HDL. Hyperlipidemia is highly modifiable, and clinical trials have shown that drug treatment directed at lowering LDL-cholesterol significantly reduces the risk of CAD-related complications or death.

As with hyperlipidemia, hypertension contributes to the risk of CAD-related complications. Hypertension, probably through sheer stress, causes vessel injury that supports the development of atherosclerotic plaque. Increasing severity of hypertension is associated with greater risk of CAD. Control of hypertension is associated with a reduced risk of CAD. Recent guidelines advise more aggressive blood pressure goals for patients at high risk for coronary artery disease. Antihypertensive medications are advised for patients with a blood pressure greater than 130/80 and diabetes, chronic kidney disease, or an ASCVD 10-year risk of greater than 10%.

Diabetes mellitus is a prominent risk factor for CAD, and the disease is becoming epidemic. Diabetes mellitus typically is associated with other risk factors, such as elevated triglycerides, reduced HDL, and hypertension, which accounts for the enhanced risk of CAD-related problems in diabetic patients. It is not clear that control of hyperglycemia in diabetic patients translates into a reduced risk of CAD, but the presence of diabetes mellitus drives the need to ensure good treatment

TABLE 8.1   Risk Factors and Markers for Coronary Artery Disease

Nonmodifiable Risk Factors

Age

Male sex

Family history of premature coronary artery disease

Modifiable Independent Risk Factors

Hyperlipidemia

Hypertension

Diabetes mellitus

Metabolic syndrome

Cigarette smoking

Obesity

Sedentary lifestyle

Heavy alcohol intake

Markers

Elevated lipoprotein(a)

Hyperhomocysteinemia

Elevated high-sensitivity C-reactive protein (hsCRP)

Coronary arterial calcification detected by EBCT or MDCT

EBCT, Electron beam computed tomography; *MDCT,* multidetector computed tomography.

of other modifiable risk factors. Although metformin remains the first-line agent for glycemic control, the new sodium-glucose cotransporter-2 (SGLT-2) inhibitors and the glucagon-like peptide-1 (GLP-1) receptor agonists have shown improvements in ASCVD outcomes in patients with diabetes and established CAD.

Chronic kidney disease (CKD) is increasingly being recognized as a unique risk factor in the development of CAD. Although not recognized as a CAD risk equivalent to diabetes, patients with CKD, particularly end-stage renal disease (ESRD) on dialysis, have dramatically elevated risks of CAD compared to the general population. In addition, outcomes of acute coronary syndrome (ACS) in CKD patients are worse compared to the general population.

Cigarette smoking has long been known as a significant risk factor for both CAD and lung cancer. Cigarette smoking is associated with increased platelet reactivity and increased risk of thrombosis, as well as lipid abnormalities. This addictive habit is modifiable, and smoking cessation can lead to a decrease in CAD event rates by 50% in the first 2 years of cessation.

Similar to diabetes mellitus, obesity (body mass index >30 kg/m^2) is associated with risk factors such as hypertension, hyperlipidemia, and glucose intolerance. Although multiple risk factors are frequently present in obese people, obesity itself carries some independent risk for CAD. The location and type of adipose tissue appear to influence CAD risk, with abdominal obesity posing a greater risk for CAD in men and women.

Numerous clinical studies have shown the benefit of regular aerobic exercise in decreasing the risk for CAD-related problems, both in the people without known CAD and in those with the disease. Sedentary lifestyles carry an increased risk that is modifiable through exercise.

Another common attribute of life, alcohol consumption, can influence the risk of CAD in both directions. One to two ounces of alcohol per day may reduce the risk for CAD-related events, but more than 2 ounces of alcohol per day is associated with an increased risk of events. Lower levels of alcohol consumption can increase HDL levels, although it is not clear that this is the mechanism of benefit. In contrast, excessive alcohol consumption is associated with hypertension, a definite risk for CAD, although other effects of high-dose alcohol may also be at play.

Additional factors that may have some role in adding CAD risk include lipoprotein(a) and homocysteine. Lipoprotein(a) is structurally similar to plasminogen and may interfere with the activity of plasmin, thus contributing to a prothrombotic state. Hyperhomocysteinemia has been associated with increased vascular risks, including coronary, cerebral, and peripheral vascular disease. It is not clear that a causal link exists, and the use of folic acid supplementation to lower homocysteine levels has not been shown to reduce the risk of MI or stroke.

C-reactive protein (CRP) is a marker of systemic inflammation, and it indicates an increased risk for coronary plaque rupture. High-sensitivity assays for CRP (hsCRP) have measured elevated levels that correlate with risk for MI, stroke, peripheral vascular disease, and sudden cardiac death. Another marker for the presence of CAD is coronary calcification. The process of atherosclerosis is often associated with deposition of calcium within the plaque.

Coronary artery calcification can be detected by fluoroscopy during cardiac catheterization as well as by computed tomography (CT) scanning using multidetector computed tomography (MDCT). CT technology allows for a quantitative measure of coronary calcium deposits that correlates with the probability of having significant obstructive lesions. Advantages to this method include low cost and relatively low radiation exposure. This technology can be used in conjunction with ASCVD score stratification to identify patients at elevated risk for MI. Patients in whom coronary calcification is identified should be approached with aggressive risk-factor modification.

Historically, low-dose aspirin therapy (75-162 mg daily) has been recommended for patients deemed "high-risk" for CAD for the prevention of CAD-related adverse events. More recently, several trials looking at aspirin use for patients without CAD (primary prevention) failed to find a mortality benefit. Furthermore, in patients over age 70 there was a significantly increased risk of bleeding associated with aspirin use that outweighed any small reduction in ASCVD events. Given these findings, the use of aspirin for patients without established CAD is no longer routinely recommended. Aspirin use in patients with established CAD (secondary prevention) is still highly recommended.

PATHOLOGY

The process of atherosclerosis is known to begin at a young age. Autopsies of teenagers frequently demonstrate the presence of atherosclerotic changes in coronary arteries. Atherosclerosis is a process linked to the subintimal accumulation of small lipoprotein particles that are rich in LDL. Subintimal deposits of LDL are oxidized, setting off a cascade of events that culminate in not only the development of atherosclerotic plaque but also vascular inflammation. Vascular inflammation drives progression of atherosclerosis as well as the potential rupture of plaque leading to vessel occlusion. The process of lipoprotein uptake by the vessel wall is enhanced by vascular endothelial injury, which may be triggered by hypercholesterolemia, the toxic effects of cigarette smoking, sheer stresses associated with hypertension, or vascular effects of diabetes mellitus.

Oxidized LDL aggregates trigger the expression of endothelial cell surface adhesion molecules, including vascular adhesion molecule-1, intracellular adhesion molecule-1, and selectins, which results in the binding of circulating macrophages to the endothelium. In response to cytokines and chemokines released by endothelial and smooth muscle cells, macrophages migrate into the subintimal region, where they ingest oxidized LDL aggregates. These LDL-laden macrophages are also called foam cells (based on the microscopic appearance), and the accumulation of foam cells represents the development of atherosclerosis.

Foam cells break down, releasing pro-inflammatory substances that promote ongoing accumulation of both macrophages and T lymphocytes. This process potentiates the development of atherosclerotic plaque. Growth factors are also released that promote smooth muscle cell and fibroblast proliferation. The net result is the development of a fibrous cap, which covers a lipid-rich core.

Important contributors to the pathologic evolution of atherosclerotic plaque include impaired endothelial synthesis of nitric oxide and prostacyclin, both of which play major roles in vascular homeostasis. The loss of these vasodilators leads to abnormal regulation of vascular tone and also plays a role in evolving a local prothrombotic state. Platelets adhere to areas of vascular injury and are not only prothrombotic but also release growth factors that help drive the aforementioned proliferation of smooth muscle cells and fibroblasts. A key structural constituent of the fibrous cap is collagen, and its synthesis by fibroblasts is inhibited by cytokines elaborated by accumulating T lymphocytes. Foam cell degradation also releases matrix metalloproteinases that break down collagen, leading to weakening of the fibrous core and making it prone to rupture. T lymphocytes tend to accumulate at the border of plaque, which is the frequent site of plaque rupture.

As the fibrous cap thins through collagen degradation and eventually ruptures, blood is exposed to the thrombogenic triggers of collagen and lipid. In this setting, platelets are activated and begin to aggregate at the site of rupture. Platelets release vasoconstrictor substances thromboxane and serotonin, but more importantly, they serve as the trigger for thrombin formation, which leads to local thrombosis. Thrombin accumulation along with ongoing platelet activation can lead to rapid accumulation of thrombus in the vessel lumen. The combination of platelet-mediated thrombus accumulation and vasoconstriction can significantly limit blood flow, leading to myocardial ischemia. The degree of ischemia and its duration can culminate in MI. Complete vessel occlusion by thrombus leads to the greatest degree of myocardial ischemia and infarction, typically resulting in an ST elevation myocardial infarction (STEMI). Incomplete vessel occlusion limits blood flow enough to cause symptomatic myocardial ischemia and lesser degrees of MI, resulting in the syndromes of unstable angina or non–ST segment elevation myocardial infarction (NSTEMI).

MI is the most profound consequence of atherosclerotic plaque pathology, but significant disability can also develop when atherosclerotic plaques expand in size, leading to obstruction of blood flow and resultant myocardial ischemia. Plaque growth, driven by smooth muscle cell proliferation, initially causes the vessel to expand toward the adventitia (Glagov remodeling). Once a limit of lateral expansion is reached, the enlarging plaque encroaches on the vessel lumen. Typically, when the diameter of the lumen is decreased by at least 70%, myocardial ischemia and symptoms of angina can develop under conditions of increasing demand for blood flow. In the case of exercise, increases in heart rate and blood pressure lead to increasing myocardial oxygen demand; when flow-limiting atherosclerotic lesions are present, oxygen demand may not be met by supply and myocardial ischemia ensues. The greater the degree of vessel obstruction, the more likely it is that myocardial ischemia and angina will occur at low workloads, even to the point of angina at rest. Fig. 8.1 shows an angiogram demonstrating a coronary artery obstruction before and after angioplasty. Other forms of stress, such as emotional stress or cold exposure, can also cause symptoms of angina in patients with significant obstructive plaque through mechanisms such as hypertension (increased myocardial oxygen demand) or sympathetically mediated vasoconstriction and tachycardia.

CLINICAL PRESENTATIONS OF CORONARY ARTERY DISEASE

The clinical syndromes that patients experience due to the presence of CAD principally relate to the occurrence of myocardial ischemia. Myocardial ischemia develops when there is a mismatch of oxygen delivery and oxygen demand. Given that extraction of oxygen by the myocardium is very high, any increase in oxygen demand must be met with an increase in coronary blood flow. Oxygen demand is directly related to increases in heart rate, myocardial contractility, and wall stress (which are related to blood pressure and cardiac dimensions). There is a reflex increase in myocardial oxygen demand driven by these factors as the heart is required to deliver more systemic blood flow in the face of various stresses, the most common of which is increased exertion. Coronary blood flow also depends on the vascular tone of arterioles that are under the control of vasodilators derived from normal functioning endothelium and autonomic tone.

Coronary blood flow increases to meet an increase in myocardial oxygen demand through endothelium-mediated vasodilation. In the face of atherosclerosis, endothelial dysfunction may develop, resulting in reduced endothelium-mediated vasodilation. Endothelial dysfunction coupled with a flow-limiting stenosis sets the stage for the development of myocardial ischemia. The coronary vessel distal to a flow-limiting stenosis tends to be maximally dilated. As myocardial oxygen demand increases, the myocardium distal to a flow-limiting stenosis is no longer able to augment flow by additional dilation. An overall limitation in the ability to increase coronary blood flow due to flow-limiting stenosis and endothelial dysfunction results in supply/demand mismatch and myocardial ischemia.

The major clinical manifestation of myocardial ischemia is chest discomfort (angina pectoris), which is usually described as a pressure or sensation of midsternal tightness. It may be quite pronounced in intensity or relatively subtle. Myocardial ischemia produces not only the sensation of angina pectoris but also a number of derangements in myocyte function. As in any tissue, inadequate oxygen delivery leads to a transition to anaerobic glycolysis, increased lactate production causing cellular acidosis, and abnormal calcium homeostasis. The net consequences of these cellular abnormalities include reductions in myocardial contractility and relaxation. Decreased myocardial contractility results in systolic wall motion abnormalities in the area of ischemia, and the abnormality of relaxation causes reduced ventricular compliance. These changes cause an increase in LV filling pressures above the normal range. The cellular abnormalities related to myocardial ischemia also translate into changes in cellular electrical activity that appear as abnormalities in the electrocardiogram (ECG). Myocardial ischemia may result in either ST depression or ST elevation, depending on the duration, severity, and location of the ischemia. The cellular, mechanical, and electrical abnormalities caused by ischemia typically precede the patient's perception of angina.

Myocardial dysfunction due to ischemia may recover quickly to normal if the duration of ischemia is brief. Prolonged myocardial ischemia can lead to conditions of myocardial stunning or myocardial hibernation. In the case of stunning, the mechanical dysfunction induced by prolonged ischemia persists for hours or days until function returns to normal. In the face of chronic ischemia, myocyte viability may be maintained, but because of ischemia, mechanical dysfunction persists; in this condition, known as hibernation, restoration of blood flow can result in recovery of myocardial function.

The heart's conduction system is less prone to ischemic injury, but ischemia can lead to impaired conduction. Ischemic disruption of myocyte electrical homeostasis also sets the stage for potentially life-threatening arrhythmias.

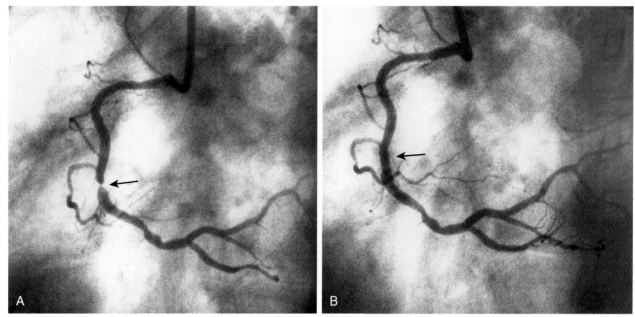

Fig. 8.1 Angiograms of the right coronary artery. (A) Discrete stenosis is observed in the middle segment of the artery *(arrow)*. (B) The same artery is shown after successful balloon angioplasty of the stenosis and placement of an intracoronary stent *(arrow)*.

Angina Pectoris and Stable Ischemic Heart Disease

Definition

Angina pectoris is a clinical manifestation of obstructive CAD, which in turn is usually the result of atherosclerotic plaque formation over a number of years. The term *angina pectoris* refers to the symptom of chest discomfort that may be described by the patient as a sensation of chest tightness or burning. Of the 18,000,000 adults in the United States with heart disease, as many as 9,400,00 have angina pectoris. It is estimated that 785,000 people experience a new ischemic episode annually, and recurrent events occur in at least 470,000 Americans each year.

Pathology

As a symptom, angina pectoris is experienced when myocardial ischemia develops. Myocardial ischemia and angina pectoris may occur in the face of obstructive atherosclerotic plaque that limits blood flow in the face of increased demand such as exertion or emotional excitement. Myocardial oxygen demand is directly related to increases in heart rate and blood pressure; these variables, in turn, can be manipulated with medical therapy to reduce the demand. Restricted oxygen supply, in the form of reduced blood flow, can also induce myocardial ischemia. Blood flow reduction is a prominent feature of acute presentations of CAD such as NSTEMI and STEMI, but atherosclerosis-mediated coronary vasoconstriction, or coronary vasospasm, is also a potential cause of flow limitation leading to myocardial ischemia. Another example of supply limitation is anemia, whereby reduced oxygen-carrying capacity coupled with obstructive lesions leads to myocardial ischemia and symptoms of angina pectoris. The term *stable* angina pectoris refers to myocardial ischemia caused by either plaque-mediated flow limitation in the face of excess demand or supply limitation due to coronary vasospasm.

Clinical Presentation

Angina pectoris may manifest in either stable or unstable patterns (Table 8.2), but the symptom expression is similar. Typically, patients complain of retrosternal discomfort that they may describe as pressure,

tightness, or heaviness. The symptom can be subtle in its presentation, and inquiry as to the presence of "chest pain" may lead to a negative response in a patient experiencing angina pectoris. When taking a history aimed at discerning angina pectoris, one needs to seek answers to these more nuanced descriptions of symptoms. In addition to chest discomfort, patients may have associated discomfort in the arm, throat, back, or jaw. They also may experience dyspnea, diaphoresis, or nausea associated with angina pectoris.

There is a good deal of variability in the expression of symptoms related to myocardial ischemia, although each person tends to have a unique signature of symptoms. Some have no chest discomfort but only radiated arm, throat, or back symptoms; dyspnea; or abdominal discomfort. Myocardial ischemia can also manifest in a "silent" form, particularly in the elderly and in patients with long-standing diabetes mellitus. The duration of angina pectoris varies, probably depending on the magnitude of the underlying myocardial ischemia. Exertion-related angina pectoris, the hallmark of stable obstructive CAD, typically resolves with rest or with decreased intensity of exercise. In stable angina pectoris, the duration of events is usually in the range of 1 to 3 minutes. Prolonged symptoms in the 20- to 30-minute range are indicative of a more serious problem such as NSTEMI or STEMI.

The physical examination of patients with CAD is typically normal. However, if the patient is physically examined during an episode of myocardial ischemia, either at rest or after exertion, significant changes may be present. As with any form of discomfort, there may be a reflex increase in heart rate and blood pressure. Elevated heart rate and blood pressure may act to sustain the duration of angina by increasing myocardial oxygen demand in the face of supply-limiting coronary stenosis. Acute mitral regurgitation can develop if the distribution of myocardial ischemia includes a papillary muscle, the supporting structure of the mitral valve. The physical examination in such cases would demonstrate a new systolic murmur consistent with mitral regurgitation. If severe enough in degree, this mitral regurgitation will cause decreased LV compliance and, consequently, an acute elevation in left atrial and pulmonary vein pressure leading to pulmonary congestion. In this setting, the patient will have not only

TABLE 8.2 Angina Pectoris

Type	Pattern	ECG	Abnormality	Medical Therapy
Stable	Stable pattern, induced by physical exertion, exposure to cold, eating, emotional stress	Baseline often normal or non-specific ST-T changes	≥70% Luminal narrowing of one or more coronary arteries from atherosclerosis	Aspirin Sublingual nitroglycerin
	Lasts 5-10 min Relieved by rest or nitroglycerin	Signs of previous MI ST-segment depression during angina		Anti-ischemic medications Statin
Unstable	Increase in anginal frequency, severity, or duration Angina of new onset or now occurring at low level of activity or at rest May be less responsive to sublingual nitroglycerin	Same as stable angina, although changes during discomfort may be more pronounced Occasional ST-segment elevation during discomfort	Plaque rupture with platelet and fibrin thrombus, causing worsening coronary obstruction	Aspirin and clopidogrel Anti-ischemic medications Heparin or LMWH Glycoprotein IIb/IIIa inhibitors
Prinzmetal or variant angina	Angina without provocation, typically occurring at rest	Transient ST-segment elevation during pain Often with associated AV block or ventricular arrhythmias	Coronary artery spasm	Calcium-channel blockers Nitrates

AV, Atrioventricular; *ECG*, electrocardiography; *LMWH*, low-molecular-weight heparin; *MI*, myocardial infarction.

the symptom of angina pectoris but also the symptom of dyspnea and the physical finding of rales. Ischemia-induced increases in LV filling pressure due to diminished compliance also can occur independently of ischemia-induced mitral regurgitation. Decreased LV compliance can produce the abnormal heart sound S_4; in the case of severe diffuse myocardial ischemia causing LV systolic dysfunction, an S_3 may also be perceived. Resolution of myocardial ischemia results in not only a cessation of angina pectoris but also a return to the patient's baseline physical examination status.

Diagnosis and Differential Diagnosis

Three basic forms of testing have played major roles in assessing patients with chest discomfort possibly due to CAD. All of these tests capitalize on the effect of myocardial ischemia on various aspects of cardiac physiology. First, myocardial ischemia induced by exercise or by spontaneous coronary occlusion results in subendocardial ischemia, which appears on an ECG as diffuse ST depression (Fig. 8.2). Once ischemia resolves, the ECG returns to normal. Second, myocardial ischemia typically affects a segment of heart muscle, and that territory develops a wall motion abnormality that can be detected by either echocardiography or nuclear scintigraphy. Third, the basis for myocardial ischemia is a decrease in coronary and myocardial blood flow. This abnormality can be detected by assessing the distribution of radioactive tracers such as thallium 201 or technetium sestamibi using specialized detectors for imaging myocardial perfusion. All stress test techniques used in diagnosing patients with possible CAD rely on these means of detecting the impact of myocardial ischemia on cardiac electrical activity, mechanical function, or myocardial perfusion.

Stress testing in its various forms frequently plays a pivotal role in the assessment of patients with possible CAD. In using stress testing, it is important to understand the significance of pretest probability of CAD in interpreting the results of any stress test method. For a patient with a high pretest probability of CAD, a positive test is highly predictive of underlying CAD, and a negative test carries the weight of being falsely negative. The opposite is true in a patient with a low pretest probability of CAD: A negative test is associated with a high negative predicative value for the presence of CAD, but a positive test is likely to be falsely positive.

Stress testing is useful not only as a diagnostic tool but also in the long-term management of established CAD. Exercise stress testing, through its ability to quantify exercise capacity, can monitor the effectiveness of medical therapy directed at reducing myocardial ischemia. The findings of an exercise stress test also have predictive value in that patients with ischemia induced at low workloads are more likely to have extensive multivessel disease, whereas those who achieve high workloads are less prone to ischemic complications of CAD. A higher risk for poor outcomes related to CAD is implied by (1) ECG changes of ST depression early during exercise and persisting late into recovery; (2) exercise-induced reduction in systolic blood pressure; and (3) poor exercise tolerance (<6 minutes on the Bruce stress test protocol).

Patients with a normal resting ECG can reliably be assessed by standard exercise stress testing with ECG monitoring (Fig. 8.3). The specificity of ST changes with exertion is significantly reduced in the face of baseline ECG abnormalities related to LV hypertrophy, left bundle branch block (LBBB), preexcitation, or use of digoxin. Various imaging techniques (echocardiography, nuclear scintigraphy, magnetic resonance imaging) have been developed to overcome the impact of baseline ECG abnormalities on the validity of stress testing. Because women also have lower specificity for ECG changes during exercise testing than men, an imaging technique is frequently used in the assessment of women. Overall, the addition of an imaging technique to stress testing significantly improves the sensitivity, specificity, and predictive value of the stress test but also greatly increases its cost.

Radionuclide stress testing is a common form of imaging-based stress test. Near peak exertion, a radionuclide tracer (thallium-201, technetium-99, or tetrofosmin) is administered intravenously. The tracer is distributed to the myocardium in a quantity directly proportional to blood flow. This type of image testing relies on a disparity of tracer uptake to detect an area of ischemia. Thallium-201 redistributes over 4 hours to viable myocardium, allowing for comparison of stress-induced ischemia to a baseline state. The other tracers do not share this redistribution feature, and tests using technetium-99 or tetrofosmin require both "rest" and "stress" injections of tracer to differentiate ischemic myocardium. Patients with normal perfusion studies have a low risk of coronary events (<1%/year). The presence of a positive perfusion study confers a risk of about 7%/year for coronary events, with the risk increasing relative to the extent of perfusion abnormality.

An alternative means of imaging for exercise testing is the use of echocardiography to detect ischemia-induced wall motion abnormalities. This form of testing is increasingly favored because there is no

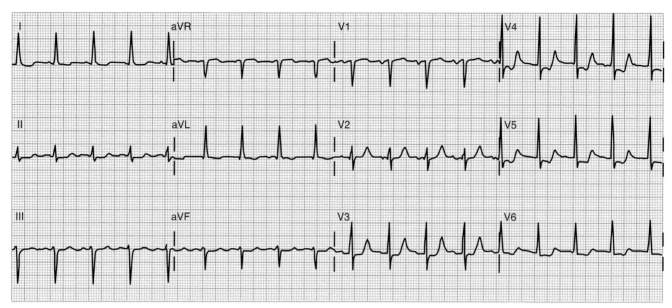

A

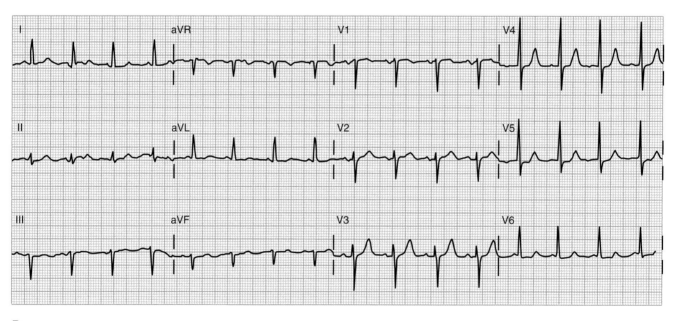

B

Fig. 8.2 Electrocardiogram obtained during angina (A) and after the administration of sublingual nitroglycerin and subsequent resolution of angina (B). During angina, transient ST-segment depression and T wave abnormalities are present.

radiation associated with its use, whereas radionuclide tracers expose the patient to a significant dose of radiation. Stress echocardiography carries with it the same enhancement in sensitivity, specificity, and predictive value as radionuclide imaging. An additional benefit of echocardiography imaging is more discrete anatomic data on valve function. If it is coupled with Doppler flow imaging, information regarding exercise-induced mitral regurgitation can be obtained.

Another means of assessing for exercise-induced wall motion abnormalities is the use of radionuclide ventriculography or multigated acquisition scanning (MUGA). This technique is usually included as part of the interpretation of an exercise stress radionuclide study. This imaging technique does not provide the anatomic detail associated with echocardiography, and it has the negative feature of significant radiation exposure.

An additional imaging technique for stress testing is the use of magnetic resonance imaging. Radiation is not a concern, and cardiac structural imaging can match echocardiography (or exceed it in patients with poor images on echocardiography). The technique is not as easy to execute as echocardiography and is not as frequently utilized.

Not all patients who require noninvasive testing for CAD are able to exercise to a degree sufficient to induce ischemia, and for some patients exercise testing is not an option at all. For these patients,

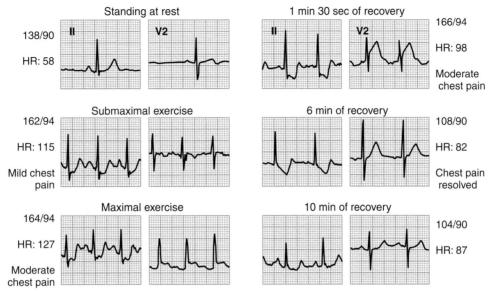

Standing at rest
138/90
HR: 58
II   V2

1 min 30 sec of recovery
166/94
HR: 98
II   V2
Moderate chest pain

Submaximal exercise
162/94
HR: 115
Mild chest pain

6 min of recovery
108/90
HR: 82
Chest pain resolved

Maximal exercise
164/94
HR: 127
Moderate chest pain

10 min of recovery
104/90
HR: 87

Fig. 8.3 Treadmill exercise test demonstrates a markedly ischemic electrocardiogram (ECG) response. The resting ECG is normal. The test was stopped when the patient developed angina at a relatively low workload, accompanied by ST-segment depression in lead II and ST-segment elevation in lead V_2. These changes worsened early in recovery and resolved after administration of sublingual nitroglycerin. Only leads II and V_2 are shown; however, ischemic changes were seen in 10 of the 12 recorded leads. Severe atherosclerotic disease of all three coronary arteries was documented at subsequent cardiac catheterization.

pharmacologic stress testing has evolved as a viable alternative to exercise testing. The prognostic benefit of exercise workload is not available from this form of testing, but information regarding the presence of ischemia-inducing atherosclerosis is obtainable. One common form of pharmacologic testing relies on inducing coronary vasodilation (as with dipyridamole, adenosine, or regadenoson), which produces a disparity of myocardial blood flow based on the presence of coronary stenosis. Radionuclide administered during the infusion of the coronary vasodilator allows for detection of myocardial ischemia similar to that observed with exercise testing. An alternative pharmacologic approach uses the inotropic and chronotropic effects of dobutamine to increase myocardial oxygen demand and induce segmental ischemia. Echocardiography is commonly used to detect dobutamine-induced wall motion abnormalities with this approach, although radionuclide or magnetic resonance imaging could also be used.

All of the stress testing techniques discussed here are able to assess for the presence of inducible myocardial ischemia associated with CAD. The presence of CAD can also be determined by assessment of coronary calcification using either EBCT or the now more common MDCT. Coronary calcification is present only because of underlying CAD. Although detecting its presence does not directly indicate the presence of obstructive CAD as would an abnormal imaging stress test, studies have shown a direct correlation between the amount of coronary calcification and the probability that a 70% stenosis is present.

Multidetector computed tomography (MDCT) scanners can reliably perform coronary angiography with the use of intravenous contrast agents and specifically timed imaging protocols. This can provide insight into coronary anatomy that stress testing cannot. When this technique is coupled with newer techniques such as CT fractional flow reserve (FFR), it can provide a functional assessment as well. The PLATFORM trial demonstrated that in patients with stable chest pain, CTA + FFR guiding the need for invasive coronary angiography (ICA) resulted in similar outcomes but with lower costs compared to standard of care. A negative study carries a high negative predictive value for the occurrence of coronary events and thus is useful in patients with low-intermediate pretest probability for coronary artery disease. MDCT is also valuable in defining coronary anomalies.

Invasive coronary angiography (ICA) has been considered the "gold standard" for detecting the extent and severity of underlying CAD. This approach carries a small risk of MI, stroke, or death, so it must not be taken lightly. In the case of patients with positive stress tests, particularly those with high-risk features, coronary angiography adds more discrete information regarding the underlying disease and guides the potential use of revascularization techniques (i.e., percutaneous coronary intervention or coronary artery bypass surgery) versus medical therapy to treat CAD (Table 8.3). Additional tools, such as pressure wires used to perform FFR, add to the diagnostic power of invasive catheterization by allowing one to discriminate between physiologically significant lesions and those not likely to cause ischemia. Revascularization is not indicated for lesions that do not cause ischemia.

The physician must also be cognizant of the fact that not all chest discomfort is related to CAD. Other causes of chest discomfort include esophageal disease (esophageal reflux may mimic typical angina pectoris), chest wall–related pain, pulmonary embolism, pneumonia, and trauma. The clinical presentation of the patient usually points in one direction or another, but patients with chest discomfort commonly undergo an evaluation for CAD, typically with the use of stress testing. Once CAD is reliably ruled out, the physician needs to consider alternative causes of the symptom. In the acute setting of severe chest discomfort, particularly in a hemodynamically unstable patient, the differential diagnosis includes acute MI, pulmonary embolism, and aortic dissection. Prompt and accurate diagnostic evaluation, commonly with the use of invasive or CT angiography, can be lifesaving in this situation.

Treatment

Medical management of stable angina. The treatment of CAD and angina pectoris is multifaceted. The presence of CAD with or without angina requires the physician to recommend risk factor modification, frequently associated with lifestyle changes. For angina pectoris, pharmacologic therapy is typically used to control symptoms, allowing for maintenance of reasonable exercise tolerance. Revascularization is commonly used to control symptoms to a degree better than what can be achieved with medications alone, but only a small group of patients with CAD benefit from revascularization in terms of increased longevity.

Other medical conditions can lower the threshold for angina, causing worsening symptoms and affecting quality of life. Anemia is a common medical problem that, when addressed, can significantly reduce the frequency of angina pectoris. Hyperthyroidism, with its increased metabolic demand and tachycardia, can increase the frequency of angina pectoris. Uncompensated congestive heart failure lowers the anginal threshold through the effects of LV dilation and filling pressure elevation on myocardial oxygen demand. Chronic obstructive pulmonary disease (COPD) and obstructive sleep apnea leading to hypoxemia can trigger angina pectoris. The use of illicit substances such as cocaine can also lead to angina through increased metabolic demand as well as coronary vasospasm.

Attention to the major modifiable risk factors for CAD is a cornerstone of therapy. Poorly controlled diabetes mellitus, hypertension, hyperlipidemia, and ongoing smoking all drive the progression of CAD and increase the risk for catastrophic events such as MI or sudden death. The wealth of clinical research on preventing death and disability from CAD has led to the development of evidence-based guidelines that form the basis of contemporary therapy for CAD (Table 8.4). Complete smoking cessation is a must for patients with CAD regardless of the presence of symptoms. Control of hypertension is also important. The use of statin medications to reduce LDL cholesterol has revolutionized the therapy for CAD and remains the cornerstone of lipid therapy. Statins have been shown to reduce the risk of MI in patients with proven CAD (goal LDL <70 mg/dL) and in those at significant risk (goal to lower LDL levels by >30% in intermediate risk patients and >50% in high-risk patients). If LDL levels do not reach the goal with statin monotherapy, ezetimibe can be utilized as an adjunctive agent. A new class of drug, PCSK-9 inhibitors (alirocumab and evolocumab), can have a dramatic impact on a patient's lipid profile but are somewhat cost-prohibitive. These are considered for secondary prevention in patients who have refractory hyperlipidemia to statin therapy as well as patients with familial hyperlipidemia syndromes who are at extreme risk for developing clinical ASCVD. There is also interest in low HDL levels, which appear to confer increased risk for coronary events. Exercise increases HDL levels and may confer protective effects through other mechanisms. Pharmacologic strategies to elevate HDL including niacin have not been proven to be beneficial.

Antiplatelet therapy is known to reduce the risk of MI in those who have known CAD. Patients should be instructed to take aspirin, 75 to 162 mg/day (clopidogrel 75 mg/day may be used in those who are aspirin intolerant or allergic). Angiotensin-converting enzyme (ACE) inhibitors reduce the risk of recurrent MI and are also beneficial for patients with diabetes mellitus or reduced LV function. Angiotensin receptor blockers (ARBs) can be substituted in those who experience significant side effects from ACE inhibitors.

Regular aerobic exercise can benefit patients with CAD by reducing their risk for complications related to the disease. Aerobic exercise also increases exercise tolerance and may reduce the frequency of exercise-related angina pectoris. Positive benefits also accrue from weight loss related to exercise and improved blood pressure control. In sedentary individuals, isometric activities such as snow shoveling can trigger MI and should be avoided. There may be some benefits to judicious weight training in patients with CAD.

TABLE 8.3 Indications for Coronary Angiography in Patients With Stable Angina Pectoris

Unacceptable angina despite medical therapy (for consideration of revascularization)

Noninvasive testing results with high-risk features

Angina or risk factors for coronary artery disease in the setting of depressed left ventricular systolic function

For diagnostic purposes, in the individual in whom the results of noninvasive testing are unclear

TABLE 8.4 Goals of Risk Factor Modification

Risk Factor	Goal
Dyslipidemia	
Elevated LDL-cholesterol level	
Patients with CAD or CAD equivalent[a]	LDL <70 mg/dL
Without CAD, ≥2 risk factors[b]	LDL <130 mg/dL (or <100 mg/dL[c])
Without CAD, 0-1 risk factors[c]	LDL <160 mg/dL
Elevated TG	TG <200 mg/dL
Reduced HDL-cholesterol level	HDL >40 mg/dL
Hypertension	Systolic blood pressure <140 mm Hg
	Diastolic blood pressure <90 mm Hg
Smoking	Complete cessation
Obesity	<120% of ideal body weight for height
Sedentary lifestyle	30-60 min moderately intense activity (e.g., walking, jogging, cycling, rowing) five times per week

CAD, Coronary artery disease; CRP, C-reactive protein; HDL, high-density lipoprotein; hsCRP, high-sensitivity C-reactive protein; LDL, low-density lipoprotein; TG, triglycerides.

[a]CAD equivalents include diabetes mellitus, noncoronary atherosclerotic vascular disease, or >20% 10-year risk for a cardiovascular event as predicted by the Framingham risk score.

[b]Risk factors include cigarette smoking, blood pressure ≥140/90 mm Hg or taking antihypertensive medication, HDL-cholesterol level <40 mg/dL, family history of premature coronary atherosclerosis (male, <45 yr; female, <55 yr).

[c]Target of 100 mg/dL should be strongly considered for men ≥60 yr and for individuals with a high burden of subclinical atherosclerosis (coronary calcification >75th percentile for age and sex), hsCRP >3 mg/dL, or metabolic syndrome.

TABLE 8.5 Medications for Angina Pectoris

Drug Class	Examples	Antianginal Effect	Physiologic Side Effects	Comments
Nitroglycerin	Sublingual Topical Intravenous Oral	Decreased preload and afterload Coronary vasodilation Increased collateral blood flow	Headache Flushing Orthostasis	Tolerance develops with continuous use
β-Adrenergic blocking agents	Metoprolol Atenolol Propranolol Nadolol	Decreased heart rate Decreased blood pressure Decreased contractility	Bradycardia Hypotension Bronchospasm Depression	May worsen heart failure and AV conduction block; avoid in vasospastic angina
Calcium-channel blocking agents (non-dihydropyridine)	Phenylalkylamine (verapamil) Benzothiazepine (diltiazem)	Decreased heart rate Decreased blood pressure Decreased contractility Coronary vasodilation	Bradycardia Hypotension Constipation with verapamil	May worsen heart failure and AV conduction
Calcium-channel blocking agents	Dihydropyridine (nifedipine, amlodipine)	Decreased blood pressure Coronary vasodilation	Hypotension, reflex tachycardia Peripheral edema	Short-acting nifedipine is associated with increased risk for cardiovascular events.
Late sodium current blocking agents	Ranolazine	Inhibits cardiac late I_{Na} Prevents calcium overload	Dizziness Headache Constipation Nausea	No effects on blood pressure or heart rate Modest QTc prolongation

AV, Atrioventricular; I_{Na}, sodium current.

In addition to antiplatelet therapy, the commonly employed medications to control angina pectoris include β-blockers, nitrates, and calcium-channel blockers. These agents work by correcting supply/demand blood flow mismatch that is the cause of myocardial ischemia and angina pectoris (Table 8.5). Interestingly, these drugs principally control symptoms in chronic stable angina pectoris, but they do not reduce mortality risk as therapy with aspirin or statins does.

Nitrates in various forms have a long history of use in patients with symptomatic CAD and can be very effective in controlling exertion-related angina. Nitrates work by venodilating large-capacitance veins and thus shifting blood out of the heart, reducing preload and myocardial oxygen demand. Nitrates are also potent coronary vasodilators and can reverse coronary spasm, allowing for improved perfusion. Short-duration but quick-acting sublingual nitroglycerin has been a mainstay both for treatment of an anginal episode and for prophylaxis against angina in situations where it is likely to occur. Patients who respond well to nitrates are frequently treated with long-acting oral or topical preparations. Both methods can effectively prevent angina pectoris, but continued use can induce tolerance. There is a recognized need for patients to have a nitrate-free period of about 8 hours every day to prevent tolerance. This usually involves cessation of use during sleep. Intravenous nitroglycerin administered by continuous drip is reserved for patients with unstable angina or acute MI.

β-Blocker therapy is very effective at reducing the likelihood of exertion-related angina. β-Blockers bind to cell surface β-receptors and by so doing reduce heart rate, contractility, and blood pressure, all of which tip the balance in favor of reduced oxygen demand and less angina. The use of β-blockers can be limited by the degree of bradycardia they induce or by baseline atrioventricular (AV) conduction abnormalities. In patients with higher degrees of AV block, β-blockers can induce complete heart block. These drugs also vary in their β-receptor selectivity. Blockade of β2-adrenergic receptors can lead to bronchospasm and vasoconstriction. Even selective β1-adrenergic antagonists such as atenolol and metoprolol have some β2 activity at higher doses. Intolerance of β-blockers can limit their use in patients with significant COPD or peripheral vascular disease. β-Blockers may also add to glucose intolerance and may affect lipids by increasing triglycerides or reducing HDL. In general, these effects do not preclude their use if they prove effective in controlling angina pectoris.

Calcium-channel blocking drugs can decrease myocardial oxygen demand by causing arterial vasodilation, bradycardia, and decreased contractility. The magnitude of these effects varies according to the class of agent used. Dihydropyridines such as nifedipine and amlodipine cause arterial vasodilation leading to a blood pressure–lowering effect. In the dose ranges administered, they have no significant effect on contractility or heart rate. In contrast, verapamil, a phenylalkylamine, has significant effects on heart rate, AV conduction, and contractility. Benzothiazepine agents such as diltiazem manifest less vasodilation than dihydropyridines and less effect on contractility than phenylalkylamine drugs. The net effect of calcium-channel blocking drugs is reduced myocardial oxygen demand resulting in less angina pectoris. Diltiazem should be used with caution in patients who are also taking a β-blocker, because severe bradycardia or heart block can occur. Verapamil should not be co-administered with a β-blocker.

A newer class of antianginal drug is represented by ranolazine. This drug is a selective inhibitor of late sodium current and reduces sodium-induced calcium overload in myocytes. Although it has no effect on heart rate or blood pressure, ranolazine demonstrates antianginal properties. It is typically used when other medical therapy is insufficient in controlling angina.

Revascularization therapy for chronic stable angina pectoris. Revascularization therapy is an option to be considered when medical therapy is not sufficiently controlling symptoms leading to impaired lifestyle. It is also frequently pursued in the face of high-risk situations such as unstable angina, STEMI, heart failure complicated by angina, arrhythmias associated with angina, or the presence of large areas of myocardial ischemia documented by noninvasive imaging. The two types of revascularization procedures are coronary bypass grafting (CABG) and percutaneous coronary intervention (PCI).

Percutaneous transluminal coronary angioplasty was the initial mode of catheter-based revascularization introduced in the late 1970s (see video, Angioplasty, http://www.heartsite.com/html/ptca.html). In this technique, a guidewire is placed through a stenotic segment of artery, after which a balloon-tipped catheter is threaded over the wire to the area of stenosis and then inflated. Angioplasty of this form enlarges the vessel lumen in an irregular geometry through disruption of the plaque and injury to the vessel intima. Plain old balloon angioplasty (POBA), as the procedure later became known, was effective at improving myocardial perfusion and reducing exercise-related angina. However, because of plaque disruption, there was a 2% to 5% risk of abrupt vessel closure frequently leading to MI. In addition, there was a high incidence of injury-mediated restenosis (up to 50%) during the first 3 to 6 months after the procedure. The process of restenosis involved intimal hyperplasia and remodeling, yielding a recurrent stenosis sometimes more severe in nature than the original lesion.

The innovation of coronary stents pioneered through the 1980s and clinically available in the early 1990s represented a significant advance in PCI (see video, Intracoronary Stenting, http://www.heartsite.com/html/stent.html). Coronary stents are expandable metallic mesh tubes that are mounted on an angioplasty balloon, allowing delivery to an area of stenosis, where balloon inflation expands the stent into the vessel wall. The stent becomes permanently embedded in the vessel wall and scaffolds the artery to keep it open. This procedure not only reduces the risk of abrupt vessel occlusion to 1% or less, but it is also associated with a significant reduction in restenosis risk (20% to 25%, compared with 50% for POBA). The benefit of stenting for a patient is clear in terms of less risk of procedure-related acute MI and less need for repeat procedures. Vessels smaller than 2 mm in diameter are not good targets for stenting, because the smallest-diameter stent is 2 mm. Stents do have a risk of thrombosis, necessitating lifelong aspirin therapy and the use of clopidogrel for 4 weeks to 1 year after the procedure (there may be some advantage to longer-duration clopidogrel for 1 year).

Despite the reduction achieved with coronary stents, there was still a significant risk of restenosis, leading investigators to search for a means to lower that risk. Drug-eluting stents (DES) were found to significantly reduce the risk of restenosis compared to bare metal stents. The first DES, released for use in 2003, was coated with either sirolimus or paclitaxel, both of which inhibited the hyperplastic response in the vessel wall triggered by PCI. The current generations of DES are coated with either zotarolimus or everolimus, both very effective at reducing restenosis. The predicted restenosis rate for current-generation DES is in the range of 5% to 10%. Vessel diameter affects restenosis risk, with larger-diameter vessels demonstrating less restenosis. The benefit of inhibiting tissue overgrowth within the stent is also associated with delayed endothelialization of the stent, which increases the risk of stent thrombosis for a longer time than with bare metal stents. For this reason P2Y12 inhibitors, in conjunction with aspirin, are prescribed to patients with stents to prevent stent thrombosis. If a situation arises in which the P2Y12 inhibitor must be discontinued the minimum time post-stent implantation at which it can safely be held depends on the type of stent implanted: 1 month for a bare metal stent (BMS) and 3 to 6 months for a drug-eluting stent. The decision regarding whether to implant a DES or a BMS is based on patient characteristics such as risk of bleeding or need for urgent surgical procedure. However, the use of BMS has declined over recent years as the safety and effectiveness of newer generation DES has been demonstrated. Aspirin should be continued indefinitely, to minimize the risk of late stent thrombosis.

A host of other devices to treat stenotic coronary arteries have come and gone over time. In this era, rotational atherectomy plays a role in treating calcified lesions in about 5% of patients. Routine use of catheter-based aspiration of thrombus led to an increased incidence of stroke and thus is no longer recommended on a routine basis. Intravascular ultrasound is an important imaging adjunct that can be helpful in interrogating lesions or defining the end result of stent placement.

CABG emerged in the 1970s as an effective means of coronary revascularization for the control of angina. Bypass grafts take the form of saphenous vein from the leg, free radial artery segments, or intact left or right internal mammary artery grafts. The vein or radial artery grafts are placed on the ascending aorta and then anastomosed to the coronary vessels distal to the site of obstruction. In contrast, left or right internal mammary arteries are left intact at their origins and anastomosed distal to the obstruction. The left internal mammary artery is typically placed onto the left anterior descending coronary artery. This is the most important vessel to graft because of its size and distribution, and the left internal mammary artery is ideal given an expected patency rate of 90% at 10 years. Saphenous vein grafts degenerate over time, leading to episodes of symptomatic abrupt occlusion and a 50% patency rate at 10 years. Free radial artery grafts perform better than vein grafts but less well than intact mammary artery grafts. CABG is a major cardiac surgical procedure, but in skilled hands the mortality rate is expected to be 1% to 2%, with a similar risk of stroke. Periprocedural MI rates are in the range of 5% to 10%. There has been controversy over whether the use of the heart-lung machine to support CABG causes more problems for patients than "beating heart" surgery does. Recent studies suggest there is no long-term difference in outcomes, such as death, MI, or stroke, for patients undergoing CABG, either on- or off-pump.

Most CABG procedures are performed for symptom control and are not likely to enhance longevity. The categories of patients likely to have life prolonged by CABG include those with a left main coronary artery more than 50% narrowed, those with severe three-vessel obstructive disease associated with a decrease in ejection fraction (EF, 35% to 50%), and those with two- or three-artery disease whose proximal left anterior descending artery is severely stenosed.

Clinical trials comparing CABG and PCI have consistently shown that patients undergoing CABG require fewer repeat procedures during the first 2 years after surgery. In the first 2 years, it is more likely that patients with PCI will experience symptomatic restenosis than that patients with CABG will have graft failure. Over time, this advantage is lost as vein grafts begin to fail 5 to 10 years after surgery. However, there is evidence that a survival advantage exists for diabetic patients with multivessel CAD who undergo CABG as opposed to PCI. A recent study also demonstrated long-term survival benefit for CABG over PCI in the face of multivessel CAD. Some of the survival advantages in favor of CABG may be linked to the use of the left internal mammary artery as a graft.

Despite the use of either revascularization technique, patients remain prone to progressive atherosclerotic disease with the potential to form plaque at previously unaffected sites. This necessitates aggressive long-term medical therapy and risk factor modification to achieve the lowest possible risk of symptomatic progression or MI. Retreatment with CABG is possible but is fraught with higher risk, and the outcome of repeat stenting for in-stent restenosis is never as good as for de novo lesions.

In a small group of patients, PCI and/or CABG fails and the patient has refractory angina. Once medical therapy has been maximized, few truly effective options remain. Transmyocardial laser revascularization in areas of ischemia has been used to reduce symptoms, but this technique is now of uncertain value. External counterpulsation is a technique whereby blood pressure cuffs are placed on each leg, inflated during diastole and deflated during systole. Patients typically have a 1-hour session that may be repeated 35 times. Angina relief has been reported with this procedure and may reflect some beneficial effect on endothelial function. Spinal cord stimulation using electrodes placed in the C7-T1 dorsal epidural space can reduce anginal symptoms in the short term, although the long-term role needs definition.

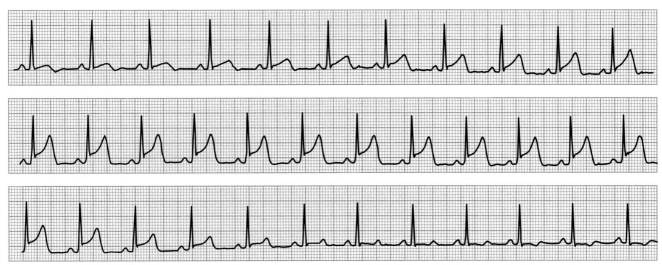

Fig. 8.4 Continuous electrocardiogram recording in a patient with Prinzmetal (variant) angina. The spontaneous onset of chest discomfort began during the top strip, accompanied by transient ST-segment elevation. By the bottom strip, several minutes later, both discomfort and ST-segment elevation had resolved.

Other Anginal Syndromes

Variant angina. Whereas typical angina pectoris is usually triggered by physical or emotional stress, some patients experience a syndrome termed variant angina. Variant angina was first described in 1959 by Prinzmetal and colleagues, who observed patients with chest discomfort at rest, not triggered by physical or emotional stress, and associated with ST-segment elevation (Fig. 8.4). Episodes of AV block and ventricular ectopy were observed, but MI was not a common feature. These patients typically did not have the common CAD risk factors other than smoking. Coronary angiography demonstrated these patients to be experiencing transient coronary vasospasm. The vasospasm tended to occur in an area of atherosclerotic plaque, but some patients had spasm in angiographically normal segments of coronary artery.

In the course of investigating the pathophysiology of variant angina, a number of provocative tests were developed to induce coronary spasm in susceptible individuals. Intracoronary ergonovine or acetylcholine can induce spasm in patients with variant angina, probably as a result of underlying endothelial dysfunction. Other spasm-inducing provocations include the cold pressor test (placing a hand in an ice bath), the induction of alkalosis (hyperventilation or intravenous bicarbonate), and histamine infusion. Provocative testing to induce coronary vasospasm has fallen out of favor in the routine assessment of patients with angina.

Coronary vasospasm usually resolves promptly with the administration of nitroglycerin (sublingual, intravenous, or intra-arterial). The combination of oral nitrates and calcium-channel blockers is often used to prevent spasm. β-Blockers may aggravate coronary spasm by inhibiting the action of vasodilating β2-receptors, allowing for unopposed α-receptor induced vasoconstriction. Rare patients do not respond to vasodilator medical therapy and may benefit from coronary stent placement in spasm-prone atherosclerotic lesions.

Microvascular angina with normal coronary arteries. Angina can occur in some patients in the face of normal-appearing coronary arteries and no provocable spasm. Decreased endothelium-dependent vasodilation may be the underlying pathophysiology of microvascular angina. Patients with this condition may demonstrate an increase in coronary resistance and an inability to increase coronary blood flow sufficiently when challenged by increases in myocardial oxygen demand. Women are more likely to be affected with microvascular angina, and the symptoms not uncommonly occur at rest or with emotional stress. Exercise can also trigger angina.

A host of diagnostic tests can detect the presence of ischemia in patients with microvascular angina. In the case of stress testing, ST changes of ischemia can be detected as well as nuclear perfusion defects and transient wall motion abnormalities on echocardiography. More sophisticated invasive testing may demonstrate the presence of stress-induced metabolic abnormalities characteristic of ischemia and endothelial dysfunction.

Exercise-related ischemic symptoms may respond to β-blocker therapy. Microvascular angina also tends to respond well to nitrates, both short-acting sublingual nitroglycerin and long-acting oral nitrates. Calcium-channel antagonists are sometimes used together with nitrates to control angina related to microvascular ischemia.

Silent myocardial ischemia. Not all episodes of myocardial ischemia are associated with angina. Some patients may only experience episodes of silent myocardial ischemia as evidenced by transient ST depression with ECG monitoring. Such patients can also have silent MI. It is also possible, and probably not uncommon, for patients to have both silent myocardial ischemia episodes and typical angina; this is termed mixed angina. Episodes of silent myocardial ischemia can be observed in all settings of CAD: chronic stable angina, unstable angina, and coronary vasospasm. Silent ischemia is more common in diabetic patients. Medical therapy directed at controlling symptomatic angina also reduces the number of episodes of silent ischemia.

Prognosis

Contemporary therapies for stable ischemic heart disease have significantly reduced the risks of cardiac events and mortality. The annual rate of major ischemic events such as MI is in the range of 1% to 2%, and the yearly mortality rate is 1% to 3%. CAD is frequently associated with systemic vascular disease, making these patients prone to a host of other events. Patients with stable ischemic heart disease have a yearly combined outcome risk for cardiovascular death, MI, or stroke in the range of 4.5%.

Despite advances in medical and revascularization therapies, up to 30% of patients face some limiting symptoms of recurrent angina.

Revascularization does not abolish the need for ongoing antianginal medical therapy in 80% of patients.

Patients with stable ischemic heart disease should first be treated with medical therapy appropriate to reduce the risk of ischemic events (aspirin, statins) and to control symptoms of angina (nitrates, β-blockers, calcium-channel antagonists). Revascularization therapy with either PCI or CABG is an option for patients who continue to have lifestyle-limiting symptoms despite the use of medical therapy and risk factor modification. The goal of all therapies for patients with stable ischemic heart disease should be individualized, taking advantage of information from controlled trials and directed at improving overall lifestyle and reducing the risk of death and disability due to progressive CAD or systemic vascular disease.

Acute Coronary Syndrome: Unstable Angina and NSTEMI

Definition

Asymptomatic CAD or chronic stable angina may undergo transition to a more aggressive stage of disease called acute coronary syndrome (ACS). ACS comprises a spectrum of clinical presentations, ranging from unstable angina to NSTEMI or STEMI. Unstable angina represents the new onset of angina at rest or on exertion, or an increase in frequency of previously stable anginal symptoms, particularly at rest. ACS manifesting as MI, either NSTEMI or STEMI, is differentiated from unstable angina on the basis of prolonged symptoms, characteristic ECG changes, and the presence of biomarkers in blood. Unstable angina may be a harbinger of either NSTEMI or STEMI, and the diagnosis of unstable angina identifies a patient who requires careful assessment and treatment.

Epidemiology

The occurrence of ACS represents a significant clinical event in up to 1.3 million Americans annually. One third of those categorized as having ACS are diagnosed with NSTEMI. More than half of patients with NSTEMI are 65 years of age or older, and approximately one half are women. NSTEMI is more common in patients with diabetes, peripheral vascular disease, or chronic inflammatory disease (e.g., rheumatoid arthritis).

Primary ACS is the most common form of the disease and reflects underlying plaque rupture leading to intracoronary thrombus formation and limitation of blood flow. This is in contrast to demand ischemia that reflects imbalances in myocardial oxygen supply and demand leading to myocardial ischemia. Examples of decreased oxygen supply include profound anemia, systemic hypotension, and hypoxemia. Increased demand occurs in the face of severe systemic hypertension, fever, tachycardia, and thyrotoxicosis. Demand ischemia not uncommonly unmasks previously asymptomatic obstructive CAD, but it may also occur in the absence of CAD. Treatment of demand ischemia is directed at correcting the underlying medical condition.

Pathology

Most patients who experience NSTEMI do so as a result of plaque rupture with subsequent thrombosis causing subtotal occlusion of the coronary artery. The limitation of coronary blood flow in this situation leads to subendocardial ischemia in the distribution of the affected coronary artery. The same pathology underlies STEMI, although in that case complete vessel occlusion occurs, leading to more extensive MI. It is possible for patients with obstructive CAD to develop collateral support of the affected artery, and in that case plaque rupture with complete vessel occlusion may lead to NSTEMI as opposed to STEMI.

A smaller percentage of patients have ACS due to coronary vasospasm, which, if severe and prolonged, can lead to myocardial necrosis. Vasospasm may occur in regions of endothelial dysfunction induced by atherosclerotic plaque, or it may be triggered by exogenous vasoconstrictors such as cocaine ingestion, the use of serotonin agonists (for migraine therapy), or chemotherapeutic agents (e.g., 5-fluorouracil). A less common cause of ACS is coronary vasculitis.

An alternative coronary artery pathology that can lead to MI is spontaneous coronary artery dissection (SCAD). Less is known about the underlying pathology of SCAD in contrast with MI due to plaque rupture, but its recognition is critical to appropriate treatment. SCAD has a predilection for a younger patient population with a strong bias toward females and is associated in particular with pregnancy and in patients with fibromuscular dysplasia. Rapid diagnosis can be challenging given that the patient population is one with few risk factors for CAD, and so a high index of suspicious is critical. Treatment differs from traditional MI in that a conservative approach is more often taken owing to increased complexity of percutaneous coronary intervention (PCI) on coronary dissection. Medical therapy for SCAD is similar to plaque rupture MI.

Atherosclerotic plaques rich in LDL are prone to develop inflammation, which in turn degrades the collagen-rich fibrous cap, leading to rupture and thrombosis as described previously. Systemic inflammatory conditions may also play a role in plaque rupture in some patients. It is possible to have multiple sites of plaque ulceration or rupture.

Plaque rupture leads to platelet adherence and subsequent activation at the site of rupture. As platelets aggregate, the thrombosis cascade is triggered, leading to progressive accumulation of intravascular thrombus. The severity of myocardial ischemia and MI depends on the degree to which thrombus occludes the vessel. It is also possible for ACS to occur as a result of embolization of platelet aggregates or thrombus.

Clinical Presentation

ACS may manifest as a first symptom of angina pectoris in a previously asymptomatic patient. Alternatively, patients with preexisting angina pectoris experience more frequent angina, angina at lower levels of exertion, or angina at rest. Patients who have developed ACS commonly experience their typical symptom of angina in terms of location and radiation but with increased intensity and duration. Patients with subtotal or total occlusion of a coronary artery may be much less responsive or completely unresponsive to the effects of nitroglycerin.

Physical examination during myocardial ischemia may reveal a patient who is clearly anxious and uncomfortable and who may also be experiencing dyspnea, nausea, or vomiting. Sinus tachycardia and hypertension is a common response to the discomfort of ACS, but in some instances sinus bradycardia and varying degrees of heart block may be observed. Bradyarrhythmias may also be associated with hypotension. Auscultation may reveal the presence of an S_4, reflecting diminished LV compliance, or an S_3 if there is extensive LV dysfunction. In the case of ischemia-induced papillary muscle dysfunction, the systolic murmur of mitral regurgitation can be heard. Patients with large areas of ischemic myocardium develop elevated LV filling pressures leading to pulmonary congestion, dyspnea, and the physical finding of rales on lung auscultation.

Diagnosis

Patients presenting with ACS require urgent care directed at rapid diagnosis and treatment. The ECG is critically important in early diagnosis of presumed ACS. The finding of ST elevation in multiple leads (Fig. 8.5) is diagnostic of STEMI and portends a more extensive MI

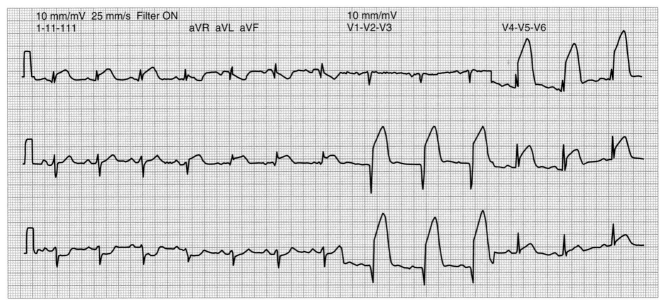

Fig. 8.5 Acute anterolateral myocardial infarction. Leads I, aVL, and V$_2$ to V$_6$ demonstrate ST-segment elevation. Reciprocal ST-segment depression is seen in leads II, III, and aVF. Deep Q waves have developed in leads V$_2$ and V$_3$.

and the need for prompt revascularization. The distribution of ST elevation reflects the region of myocardium affected by thrombotic coronary occlusion. For example, ST elevation in leads II, III, and aVF reflects an inferior MI due to occlusion of the right coronary artery (or circumflex coronary artery in some cases). ST elevation in leads V$_2$ through V$_6$ (see Fig. 8.5) reflects an anterior MI caused by obstruction of the left anterior descending coronary artery.

Unstable angina or NSTEMI is caused by subtotal vessel occlusion by thrombus leading to reduced coronary blood flow. This results in subendocardial ischemia and the characteristic ECG changes of ST depression (Fig. 8.6). It is important to recognize that up to half of patients with acute MI do not have significant ECG abnormalities on the initial study. Sequential ECGs are frequently required to establish a diagnosis. If there is a high index of suspicion for MI and ECGs are persistently nondiagnostic, the use of leads extending to the patient's back (V$_7$ to V$_9$) may demonstrate ST changes related to posterior LV ischemia (usually a circumflex coronary artery occlusion). Echocardiography showing regional wall motion abnormalities can also help to establish the diagnosis of acute MI.

Serum biomarkers also play an important role in the diagnosis of acute MI. Myocardial necrosis leads to the release of biomarkers that can be measured in serial fashion to document the occurrence of MI. The presence of specific biomarkers is definitive evidence of MI, and they are particularly helpful to provide prognostic significance when symptoms are mild and ECG changes are minimal. Common biomarkers include creatine kinase (CK), troponin I, troponin T, lactate dehydrogenase (LDH), and aspartate aminotransferase (AST). Sequential measurement of biomarkers demonstrates their various time courses for abnormal elevation after an acute MI (Fig. 8.7). This information can be helpful in retrospectively timing the occurrence of an event. In contemporary practice, troponin has become the most frequently measured biomarker. LDH, CK, and AST are no longer routinely measured for the diagnosis of MI. Some centers are adopting the "high-sensitivity troponin," which can detect more subtle degrees of myocardial injury than its predecessors. In principle this allows for more rapid triaging of patients presenting with chest pain while maintaining high sensitivity as the test will pick up on troponin release very early in the course of ACS.

Troponins I and T are the most sensitive and most specific markers of myocardial necrosis, and as a consequence, they have become the standard in the biochemical diagnosis of acute MI. The myocardial-specific isozyme CK-MB may be in the normal range while concomitant measurement of troponin I or T reveals the presence of myocardial necrosis. Troponins I and T begin to rise within 4 hours of myocardial necrosis and remain elevated for 7 to 10 days after the MI event. Confounding elevations of troponin T occur in patients with renal failure and congestive heart failure not related to ACS. Troponin release also occurs in the case of demand ischemia not related to coronary thrombosis. This requires careful attention to the entire clinical presentation in discerning the likelihood of underlying ACS due to coronary thrombosis.

In the absence of clear evidence of NSTEMI (i.e., normal examination, ECG findings, and biomarkers), patients who present with the diagnosis of unstable angina should undergo stress testing. A negative exercise stress test is very helpful for distinguishing those patients who require more aggressive diagnostic testing (e.g., catheterization) from those who can be monitored as outpatients. Some centers have embraced the use of CT coronary angiography in the assessment of low-risk patients. This technique has a high negative predictive value for ACS by demonstrating the absence of obstructive CAD.

Echocardiography can be helpful in patients with equivocal ECG findings for ischemia and normal biomarkers. The presence of regional wall motion abnormalities, particularly if they correlate with the distribution of ECG abnormalities, raises the risk for underlying CAD as a cause of symptoms. The echocardiogram may also show evidence of other abnormalities as causes of chest discomfort, such as pericarditis, pulmonary embolism, or aortic dissection.

Patients with a high risk for future coronary events should be directed toward coronary angiography. In the absence of contraindications, coronary angiography is indicated for patients with clear evidence of NSTEMI based on clinical presentation of symptoms, ECG changes, and positive biomarkers. Patients undergoing evaluation for unstable angina who have significant stress test abnormalities are also candidates for coronary angiography. Some patients who have ambiguous stress test findings or ongoing symptoms in the absence of other

Boston University Hospital

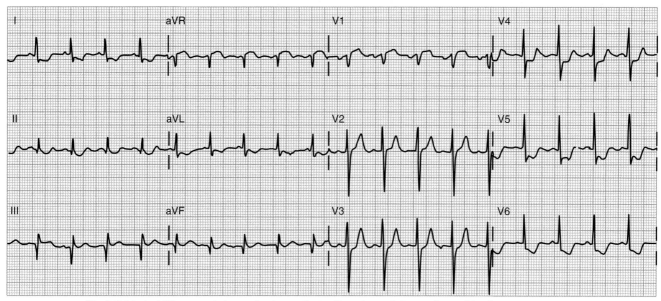

Fig. 8.6 Marked ST-segment depression in a patient with prolonged chest pain resulting from an acute non–ST segment elevation myocardial infarction. Between 1 and 3 mm of ST-segment depression is seen in leads I, aVL, and V_4 to V_6. The patient was known to have had a previous inferior myocardial infarction.

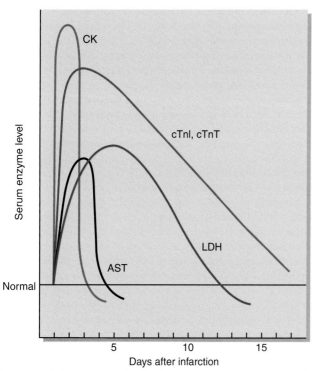

Fig. 8.7 Typical time course for the detection of enzymes released after myocardial infarction. *AST,* Serum aspartate aminotransferase; *CK,* creatine kinase; *cTnI,* cardiac troponin I; *cTnT,* cardiac troponin T; *LDH,* lactate dehydrogenase.

findings of NSTEMI require coronary angiography to resolve the issue as to whether underlying CAD is present.

Up to 15% of patients undergoing coronary angiography for NSTEMI have no significant obstructive CAD. In a number of patients, there will be a clear "culprit" lesion showing the earmarks of plaque rupture with ulceration, associated thrombus, or reduced coronary flow. Lesions that may have played a role in symptoms, ECG findings, or biomarker release that are not clearly stenotic may be assessed for physiologic significance with the use of a fractional flow reserve (FFR) study using a pressure wire device.

Patients who have new-onset chest pain require careful monitoring in an appropriate care setting that allows for rhythm monitoring as well as repeat evaluations of ECG findings and biomarker measurements. Risk assessment is aided by the use of risk scores calculated with either the Thrombolysis in Myocardial Infarction (TIMI) or the Global Registry of Acute Coronary Events (GRACE) algorithms (see Chapter 63, "Acute Coronary Syndrome: Unstable Angina and Non-ST Elevation Myocardial Infarction," in *Goldman-Cecil Medicine*, 26th Edition). The overall assessment in cases of new symptoms of ❖ chest discomfort aims to triage patients based on risk for coronary events. Low-risk patients can be spared aggressive anticoagulation protocols and coronary angiography, whereas high-risk patients are likely to benefit from these approaches. The use of appropriate therapies in high-risk patients (medical therapy or revascularization or both) leads to a 20% to 40% decrease in recurrent ischemic events and a 10% reduction in mortality.

Differential Diagnosis

The initial assessment of patients with possible ACS should include consideration of other potentially life-threatening conditions such as pulmonary embolism and aortic dissection. These considerations are particularly important if the patient's presentation does not entirely fit that of ACS. Pulmonary embolism can be associated with ECG changes and troponin elevation, and such findings lead to early use of coronary angiography. If there is no CAD-related explanation of the patient's presentation, prompt investigation for pulmonary embolism is warranted. If the patient has findings suggestive of aortic dissection, that diagnosis should be aggressively pursued with appropriate imaging techniques, given the high risk of mortality associated with that disease. Valvular heart diseases such as aortic stenosis or regurgitation and hypertrophic cardiomyopathy can manifest with symptoms and ECG findings suggestive of ACS. Physical examination should aid in consideration of these conditions. Pericarditis and myopericarditis can also present diagnostic dilemmas related to chest pain, ECG abnormalities (ST and T wave changes mimicking ischemia), and positive biomarkers. Stress cardiomyopathy (takotsubo syndrome) also manifests with chest pain, T wave inversion, and positive biomarkers. Patients with this diagnosis frequently undergo urgent catheterization to assess for CAD. The absence of a culprit lesion and findings of characteristic wall motion abnormalities establish the diagnosis.

Treatment

Patients with chest pain suggestive of ACS need urgent evaluation for evidence of ischemia (serial ECGs) and myocardial necrosis (serial biomarkers). Serial biomarker measurements, in the current era usually troponin, establish the diagnosis of MI. Continuous ECG monitoring is important given the risk of ischemia-mediated arrhythmias, and serial ECGs establish a pattern of ST changes consistent with ischemia. Patients are also placed on activity limitations up to and including bedrest for patients with particularly difficult to control angina. Supplemental oxygen is provided to patients who are hypoxemic, but routine administration of supplemental oxygen to patients with ACS has not been shown to provide any benefit. Those with a high index of suspicion for ACS require hospital admission for observation and appropriate diagnostic testing. Chest pain lends itself well to diagnosis and treatment algorithms that guide the clinician through decision trees based on expert opinion and evidence-based medicine (see Chapter 63, "Acute Coronary Syndrome: Unstable Angina and Non-ST Elevation Myocardial Infarction," in *Goldman-Cecil Medicine*, 26th Edition). STEMI is typically diagnosed at the time of initial presentation. Those without evidence of ST elevation can be risk stratified, as discussed earlier, using the guidance of recurrent symptoms, ECG changes, or abnormal biomarker levels. Treatment of patients who are categorized as having unstable angina or NSTEMI is directed by their allocation to either low- or high-risk status.

Once recognized as having ACS, patients require antiplatelet therapy because plaque rupture and thrombosis is a frequent underlying pathology, and antiplatelet therapy significantly reduces mortality risk in patients with NSTEMI. Patients should be given aspirin (75 to 162 mg per day) and a P2Y12 inhibitor (either clopidogrel or ticagrelor). Given prasugrel and ticagrelor's increased strength and rapidity of platelet inhibition compared to clopidogrel they are favored in the ACS setting. Note that prasugrel is reserved for patients undergoing PCI and is contraindicated in patients with a history of stroke or transient ischemic attack.

The use of these more potent antiplatelet agents must be weighed against an increased risk of bleeding that accompanies this effect. The aspirin/P2Y12 inhibitor combination is indicated as ongoing therapy in the year following diagnosis of NSTEMI.

Symptoms of chest discomfort can be treated with nitrates (sublingual, topical, or intravenous drip) and β-blockers. The latter therapy slows heart rate and reduces blood pressure, effects that translate into reduced myocardial oxygen demand in the face of limited supply. It is important not to give nitrates to patients who have taken phosphodiesterase-5 inhibitors (sildenafil, tadalafil, or vardenafil) within the previous 24 to 48 hours. Attention to this detail minimizes the risk for nitrate-induced hypotension. Calcium-channel antagonists may be used in lieu of β-blockers, particularly if there is a need for blood pressure control, but they should be avoided in patients with reduced EF or overt heart failure. The dihydropyridine calcium-channel blocker nifedipine can be effective in controlling blood pressure and promoting coronary vasodilation, but it should be given in conjunction with a β-blocker because of the potential for the drug to induce reflex tachycardia and thereby increase myocardial oxygen demand.

Glycoprotein IIb/IIIa inhibitors block platelet aggregation and can reduce ischemic events in patients undergoing PCI as treatment for NSTEMI. These drugs are usually reserved for high-risk patients at the time of PCI. They require intravenous administration and are given for 12 to 24 hours after PCI. The use of this class of drugs for PCI has decreased in light of data suggesting advantages of bivalirudin, a direct thrombin inhibitor, over the glycoprotein IIb/IIIa inhibitors.

Heparin, given in its unfractionated form or as a low-molecular-weight (LMW) preparation, has been shown to reduce the risk of ischemic complications in patients with NSTEMI. Heparin acts by activating antithrombin and thereby inhibiting the formation and activity of thrombin. The anti-ischemic effect of heparin is additive to that of aspirin. Unfractionated heparin is given by continuous intravenous drip for up to 48 hours. It is usually not continued after revascularization. Heparin may be associated with mild thrombocytopenia, and 1% to 5% of patients experience profound antibody-mediated thrombocytopenia. These patients usually have been exposed to heparin in the past, and a known diagnosis of heparin-induced thrombocytopenia necessitates the use of alternative antithrombin therapy.

LMW heparins are fragments of unfractionated heparin that are more predictable in their antithrombin activity and are associated with reduced risks for thrombocytopenia and bleeding complications. The drug should be avoided in patients who have a history of heparin-induced thrombocytopenia. Clinical studies of patients with NSTEMI have shown superiority of LMW heparin over unfractionated heparin in reducing the end point of death or MI during hospitalization. LMW heparin, either enoxaparin or dalteparin, is administered subcutaneously for up to 8 days after hospitalization. As with unfractionated heparin, LMW heparin is not continued after revascularization. Dosing of LMW heparin is based on renal function status, age, and weight. LMW heparin has a long duration of action and cannot be reversed with protamine. Unfractionated heparin has a shorter duration of action and is reversible with protamine, making unfractionated heparin the preferred anticoagulant for patients who may require CABG.

Fondaparinux is a selective factor Xa inhibitor that does not induce thrombocytopenia. It can reduce ischemic events in patients with NSTEMI and is associated with a lower risk of bleeding than is seen with enoxaparin. There is an increased risk of catheter-related thrombosis in patients treated with fondaparinux who are undergoing coronary angiography. This drug is reserved for cases that will be managed noninvasively and where there is a higher risk for heparin-related bleeding.

Bivalirudin, a direct thrombin inhibitor, is an alternative to heparin for patients who are undergoing PCI. It is as effective as the combination of heparin and glycoprotein IIb/IIIa inhibitor in reducing the risk of ischemic complications related to PCI, and it is associated with a reduced risk of postprocedure bleeding. Bivalirudin is used preferentially in patients with a history of heparin-induced thrombocytopenia.

Statin therapy is also indicated in patients with NSTEMI at presentation. Statins act to stabilize plaque and improve endothelial function. These drugs should be initiated at the time of admission to the hospital and continued after discharge. There is evidence that high-dose atorvastatin (80 mg/day) given to patients with NSTEMI reduces the risk of subsequent ischemic events.

Risk stratification is important in appropriately evaluating patients with ACS. Low-risk patients (age <75 years, normal troponin levels, 0 to 2 TIMI risk factors) should be evaluated with noninvasive testing, either exercise or pharmacologic stress testing before hospital discharge. Those whose tests are positive for ischemia should be considered for predischarge coronary angiography. This approach leads to selective use of invasive testing and subsequent revascularization. Patients with high-risk ACS profiles (age >75 years, elevated troponin levels, ≥3 TIMI risk factors) are candidates for coronary angiography and, when appropriate, revascularization. The high-risk ACS patient group will have fewer subsequent ischemic events when approached in this way. Risk stratification occurs early after admission for possible ACS. An early invasive strategy (coronary angiography within 24 hours of admission) for high-risk patients has been shown to reduce the combined end point of death, MI, or stroke compared with a delayed invasive approach. The occurrence of acute heart failure, hypotension, or ventricular arrhythmias in the face of ACS prompts urgent coronary angiography to identify patients with high-risk coronary anatomy that requires urgent revascularization (see video, Cardiac Cath, http://www.heartsite.com/html/cardiac_cath.html).

Invasive coronary angiography always carries with it a risk of bleeding complications that is no doubt enhanced by the concomitant use of potent antiplatelet and antithrombin therapies. Those at increased risk for bleeding complications include patients with female gender, low body weight, diabetes mellitus, renal insufficiency, low hematocrit, and hypertension. The risks of bleeding as well as vascular complications are lower via radial artery catheterization compared to a femoral artery approach at the cost of some increased difficulty in catheter manipulation. Utilization of a radial approach is becoming more commonplace and has become the preferred method of access for a large number of interventional cardiologists.

Prognosis

The extent and magnitude of ST depression noted on ECG in patients with NSTEMI predicts mortality risk. Patients who exhibit 2 mm or more of ST depression in multiple leads have a 10-fold increased mortality rate at 1 year. The degree of elevation in troponin also identifies patients with an increased risk of mortality during the following year. It has also been observed that the combined measurement of troponin, hsCRP, and B-type natriuretic peptide (BNP) predicts an increased mortality risk better than any individual biomarker.

Contemporary practice significantly reduced the risk of mortality for patients with ACS at presentation. Risk stratification with appropriate revascularization and use of antiplatelet therapy, statins, and overall coronary risk factor reduction also contribute to this decrease in mortality risk. Whereas the immediate mortality risk for patients with NSTEMI is lower than for patients with STEMI (5% vs. 7%), those with NSTEMI are more prone to subsequent recurrent coronary events. The cumulative mortality rate for STEMI and NSTEMI is similar at 6 months after presentation (12% vs.13%). NSTEMI identifies a patient group with significant long-term mortality risk who require aggressive attention to modifiable coronary risk factors.

Acute STEMI and Complications of Myocardial Infarction
Definition and Epidemiology

Sustained myocardial ischemia, regardless of its cause, can result in myocardial necrosis, which underlies the clinical syndrome of MI. MI represents a spectrum of myocardial necrosis, from relatively small amounts of muscle in the case of demand ischemia, to more extensive subendocardial MI that characterizes NSTEMI, to typically large transmural MIs commonly manifesting as STEMI. The current accepted definition of acute MI accounts for clinical setting and mechanism. STEMI represents the range of large MIs that are almost always caused by total occlusion of an epicardial coronary artery resulting in extensive transmural myonecrosis (Fig. 8.8). In contrast, NSTEMI reflects subtotal coronary occlusion leading to subendocardial myonecrosis. Whereas both NSTEMI and STEMI are life-threatening, their different underlying mechanisms mandate different therapeutic strategies and affect the urgency with which they are applied.

One half of all deaths in the United States and developed countries are related to cardiovascular disease. In the United States, there are over one million nonfatal or fatal MIs each year. CAD plays a role in 360,000 deaths each year, and 110,000 deaths are caused by acute MI. One half of patients with acute MI at presentation die within 1 hour of onset, before therapy can be instituted. Of the 5 million patients who come to emergency rooms with chest pain, 1.3 million are admitted to hospital with ACS. In this group of patients, the presence of ST elevation on ECG or an LBBB indicates the diagnosis of STEMI and the need for prompt intervention to open an occluded coronary artery. STEMI accounts for 30% of all MIs, but this mechanism of MI is associated with the highest immediate mortality risk, prompting the need for urgent therapeutic intervention.

Pathology
Lipid-rich coronary plaques are subject to inflammation incited by the response to oxidation of LDL-cholesterol within the plaque. A sequence of inflammatory events leads to macrophage accumulation and the elaboration of metalloproteinases that degrade collagen in the fibrous cap of the plaque. Thinning of the fibrous cap makes the plaque vulnerable to rupture and exposure of blood to thrombogenic stimuli, resulting in platelet aggregation and activation, thrombin generation, and the evolution of fibrin-based thrombus. If the occlusion is total, transmural myocardial ischemia and necrosis ensue and the ECG demonstrates ST elevation. In contrast, partially occlusive thrombus can result in unstable angina or NSTEMI (subendocardial MI). The presence of coronary collaterals can limit the extent of ischemia and necrosis in either scenario. Both STEMI and NSTEMI can set the stage for arrhythmias and LV dysfunction. Whereas coronary thrombosis is the cause of most MIs, there are patients who develop MI related to coronary embolization, coronary vasospasm, vasculitis, coronary anomalies, dissection of the aorta or a coronary artery, or trauma.

One key feature of the pathology of MI is its time-dependent nature. Experimental and clinical studies have documented that coronary occlusion leads to ischemia and myonecrosis in a wavefront manner, from endocardium to epicardium. Restoration of flow to the vessel within 6 hours after occlusion is associated with limitation of infarct size and a favorable effect on mortality risk. The principle of time dependency of MI drives the need to aggressively reperfuse occluded coronary arteries, and this is the cornerstone of contemporary therapy for STEMI.

Clinical Presentation
Patients with acute MI usually have a combination of chest discomfort, ECG changes (ST elevation in contiguous leads or LBBB), and elevation in biomarkers such as CK-MB and troponin. The high sensitivity and high specificity of troponin have made it the preferred biomarker in the diagnosis of MI. The chest discomfort associated with MI is similar to angina pectoris but more severe in nature. It is usually described as substernal pressure, tightness, or fullness. Patients may have symptoms of discomfort that radiate to the neck, jaw, one or both arms, or the back. Not uncommonly, patients with symptoms of acute MI also experience nausea, vomiting, diaphoresis, apprehension, dyspnea, or weakness. In contrast to angina pectoris associated with stable CAD, acute MI symptoms last longer than 20 to 30 minutes (up to hours).

Occasionally, patients only have symptoms in the non-chest areas usually associated with radiation. Up to 20% of patients, particularly the elderly and diabetics, do not have typical chest discomfort at presentation. The index of suspicion for acute MI should be high in these groups if the patient exhibits profound weakness, acute dyspnea or pulmonary edema, nausea, vomiting, ventricular arrhythmias, or hypotension. The differential diagnosis for patients with chest

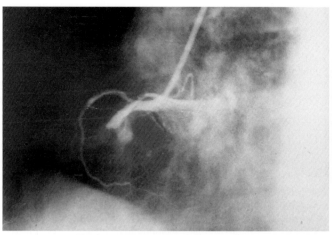 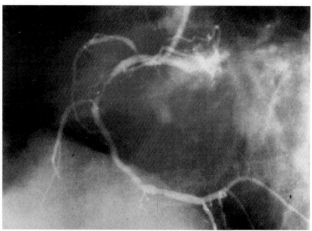

Fig. 8.8 Right coronary artery angiogram in a patient with acute inferior myocardial infarction. The left panel demonstrates total occlusion of the right coronary artery. The right panel depicts restoration of flow 90 minutes after the intravenous administration of tissue-type plasminogen activator.

discomfort suspicious for acute MI includes aortic dissection, pulmonary embolism, chest wall pain, esophageal reflux, acute pericarditis, pleuritis, and panic attacks. Given the life-threatening nature of aortic dissection and pulmonary embolism, these diagnoses should always be paramount, along with acute MI, in patients presenting with chest discomfort.

Physical examination. A comprehensive examination should be undertaken if acute MI is suspected. Attention must be paid to vital signs, because patients may be either hypertensive or hypotensive during the course of an MI. In some cases, such as inferior MI, profound bradycardia may be present. Auscultation of the heart may reveal an S_4. In the case of a large MI, the patient may have symptoms and signs of heart failure such as dyspnea, rales, elevated central venous pressure, and an S_3. Severe heart failure may lead to cardiogenic shock with hypotension and vasoconstriction causing the extremities to be cool to touch. Patients with acute MI are also subject to mechanical problems such as mitral regurgitation due to papillary muscle dysfunction.

Electrocardiogram. The ECG is an important tool in the diagnosis of acute MI. ST elevation of 1 mm or greater in contiguous leads is seen in most patients with acute MI. The initial ECG may be nondiagnostic, so it is important to obtain serial tracings no more than 20 minutes apart to detect the evolutionary changes characteristic of STEMI. The first stage of ECG presentation is ST elevation that subtends the region of the heart affected by transmural ischemia. ST depression may be present in opposing leads, and these are termed reciprocal changes (see Chapter 64, "ST Elevation Acute Myocardial Infarction and Complications of Myocardial Infarction," in *Goldman-Cecil Medicine*, 26th Edition). The presence of reciprocal changes may indicate a larger and more threatening MI. As the MI progresses, ST elevation gives way to T wave inversion. Varying degrees of resolution of ST and T wave changes occur over time, but patients with transmural MI develop pathologic Q waves in the leads subtending the infarcted muscle. Other causes of ST elevation include pericarditis and a chronic repolarization finding of "early repolarization." The presence of either cause of ST elevation can confound the early ECG diagnosis of acute MI.

Approximately 30% of acute MIs originate from the circumflex coronary artery on the posterior wall of the heart. This type of MI appears on the ECG as precordial ST depression. The presence of precordial ST depression should raise suspicion of the presence of "true posterior MI," and additional leads placed through the axilla to the back may reveal the presence of posterior ST elevation. Echocardiography

demonstrating posterior hypokinesis is also useful in discriminating true posterior MI. Acute inferior MI due to occlusion of the right coronary artery can also be associated with right ventricular infarction if the right coronary artery's acute marginal branch is compromised. Right ventricular infarction can lead to some challenging management issues, and its diagnosis is aided by the use of right precordial leads to detect ST elevation.

LBBB or ventricular pacing can mask ST elevation due to acute MI. Patients with clinical features of acute MI who have an LBBB (particularly a new LBBB) should be presumed to have STEMI and treated appropriately. Right bundle branch block (RBBB) does not mask the ST elevation of STEMI.

Differential Diagnosis

The diagnosis of STEMI is usually straightforward based on symptoms and ECG findings, but a number of conditions can mimic the ST elevation of STEMI and confound the diagnosis. The ECG changes of early repolarization, takotsubo syndrome, acute myocarditis, or pericarditis can be difficult or impossible to distinguish from those of STEMI. In the face of ST elevation and chest discomfort, it may be necessary to perform coronary angiography in patients who ultimately are diagnosed with a condition other than STEMI so as to not miss this critical diagnosis.

Diagnostic testing. Cardiac troponins (cTnI and cTnT) are sarcomere proteins that, when measured in blood, are specific for myocardial injury. The troponin level becomes elevated 2 to 4 hours after the onset of injury, and the abnormal elevation can persist for up to 2 weeks after the event. The CK-MB isomer is not as specific for heart injury as troponin, but it can still be useful in documenting the presence of MI. CK-MB is found elevated within 4 hours after an acute MI, but it clears more rapidly than troponin. In the case of persistently elevated troponin, a measurable increase in CK-MB may herald another episode of myocardial necrosis. Chronic renal insufficiency is associated with false-positive elevations of troponin T, more so than troponin I. In addition to biomarkers of myocardial injury, other laboratory studies obtained in patients with acute MI include a complete blood count, blood chemistries, lipid panel, prothrombin time (PT), and partial thromboplastin time (PTT). Leukocytosis is a common finding in acute MI, reflecting the inflammatory nature of myocardial necrosis.

At the time of admission, chest radiographs are obtained to assess for the presence of pulmonary edema or mediastinal widening suspicious for dissection. Echocardiography is important in delineating the extent of MI and assessing EF. In cases of diagnostic ambiguity, early use of echocardiography can demonstrate the presence of regional wall motion abnormalities consistent with acute MI. Echocardiography with color Doppler is also helpful in diagnosing complications of acute MI such as infarct-related mitral regurgitation or ventricular septal defect (VSD), pericardial effusion, or evidence of pseudoaneurysm as a result of myocardial rupture. Follow-up echocardiography in the months after acute MI can also reveal recovery of LV function. Radionuclide tracer studies are not useful in diagnosing acute MI. CT, cardiac MRI, and transesophageal echocardiography are all useful in diagnosing aortic dissection when there is an increased index of suspicion. Cardiac MRI can also distinguish myopericarditis.

Treatment

Acute STEMI is caused by occlusion of the epicardial coronary artery by thrombus after rupture of a vulnerable plaque. The process of myocardial necrosis is time dependent, so diagnosis and treatment of STEMI to preserve myocardium must occur as quickly as possible. More than half of deaths occur within 1 hour after onset of symptoms, before the patient can be reached for emergency care. Patients often delay seeking care for symptoms of acute MI despite efforts to alert the public to the risk of ignoring symptoms of chest discomfort. Emergency medical personnel who respond to patients with possible MI begin to institute initial therapy in the field. Patients are monitored with ECG for rhythm disturbances such as ventricular tachycardia (VT) or ventricular fibrillation (VF) that require prompt cardioversion or defibrillation. Oxygen is administered via nasal cannula, and intravenous access is established. Aspirin (162 to 325 mg) is administered to the patient, and sublingual nitroglycerin may also be given in an attempt to relieve chest discomfort. Some emergency response systems perform 12-lead ECGs and telemeter the results to the emergency department, allowing for early diagnosis of STEMI and early decision making regarding revascularization strategies.

Once the patient arrives in the emergency department, an ECG, if not already available, will be performed within 5 minutes. If the ECG is nondiagnostic, a second study is obtained no more than 20 minutes after presentation. A diagnosis of STEMI triggers decision making regarding reperfusion strategies that are used by the particular institution (see Chapter 64, "ST Elevation Acute Myocardial Infarction and Complications of Myocardial Infarction," in *Goldman-Cecil Medicine*, 26th Edition). Hospitals that are capable of performing emergency cardiac catheterization for the purpose of reperfusion therapy have an established rapid response system to activate the catheterization laboratory for this urgent therapy. There is evidence that primary PCI therapy for STEMI is superior to fibrinolytic therapy, but its use depends on the timely availability of a well-trained catheterization team. The quality of primary PCI is signified by a so-called door-to-balloon time of less than 90 minutes. Likewise, the standard for fibrinolytic therapy is a door-to-needle time of less than 30 minutes. Regardless of the means of reperfusion, it is important for the hospital treating patients with STEMI to have a structured protocol for timely diagnosis, decision making, and initiation of therapy.

In addition to aspirin, the patient should be given a loading dose of a P2Y12 inhibitor (ticagrelor 180 mg, clopidogrel 600 mg or prasugrel 60 mg), assuming he or she will be treated with primary PCI. Unfractionated heparin in a dose of 60 IU/kg should be administered (no more than 4000 IU bolus) with a drip rate of 12 IU/kg/hour (maximum dose, 1000 IU/hour). LMW heparin may also be used (enoxaparin 30 mg IV bolus with 1 mg/kg subcutaneously every 12 hours for patients younger than 75 years of age who have normal renal function). Other agents such as glycoprotein IIb/IIIa inhibitors or bivalirudin

are administered depending on the protocols of the catheterization laboratory.

Patients are commonly given sublingual nitroglycerin 0.4 mg (repeat every 5 minutes for no more than three total doses), which often helps to diminish chest discomfort. Intravenous nitroglycerin may be helpful for control of both persistent pain and hypertension if present. Intravenous morphine (2 to 4 mg, repeated every 5 to 15 minutes as needed) is also frequently used for pain control. Although there has been no consensus statement on the use of morphine in ACS, recently there have been several studies that have suggested an increased risk of in-hospital mortality associated with its use presumed secondary to reduced antiplatelet activity of P2Y12 inhibitors. Intravenous β-blockers such as metoprolol (5-mg bolus every 10 minutes for a total dose of 15 mg) are indicated in the treatment of STEMI but should be avoided in the face of heart failure, severe COPD, hypotension, or bradycardia. β-Blockers (metoprolol, propranolol, atenolol, timolol, and carvedilol) have been shown to significantly reduce the risk of future MI and cardiovascular mortality. Statin therapy, as mentioned for NSTEMI, is recommended for all patients with STEMI as a presenting symptom regardless of their history of hypercholesterolemia. Other adjunctive measures include bedrest for the first 12 hours, ongoing oxygen by nasal cannula with pulse oximeter monitoring, continuous rhythm monitoring, anxiolytic agents as needed, and stool softeners. Atropine is kept in reserve for the treatment of hemodynamically significant bradycardia, which may occur with inferior MI.

ACE-inhibitor therapy also plays an important role in the long-term survival of patients after STEMI. ACE-inhibitor therapy has been shown to reduce the incidence of heart failure, recurrent MI, and long-term mortality after STEMI. ACE inhibitors commonly used for this purpose include lisinopril, captopril, enalapril, and ramipril. The decision to initiate ACE-inhibitor therapy is directed by the patient's tolerance. Care is warranted early after STEMI, because the patient may be prone to hypotension related to ACE-inhibitor therapy. A low dose should be administered first, with gradual upward titration.

Aldosterone receptor blockade with eplerenone (25 to 50 mg/day) reduces cardiovascular mortality after MI in patients with heart failure and a reduced EF of less than 40% or diabetes. Spironolactone also reduces mortality in patients with heart failure and a history of remote MI.

Reperfusion therapy. Timely reperfusion therapy, either thrombolytic therapy or primary PCI, is critical to limiting the extent of MI and reducing the risks of future morbidity and mortality. Primary PCI has been shown to have advantages over thrombolytic therapy, with higher immediate and long-term vessel patency. Primary PCI depends on the availability of cardiac catheterization facilities and staff to conduct the reperfusion procedure quickly (see earlier discussion). If the patient has not had access to a catheterization facility for longer than 2 hours after presentation, thrombolytic therapy is a reasonable alternative.

In the randomized, placebo-controlled Gruppo Italiano per lo Studio della Streptochinasi nell'Infarto (GISSI) study, thrombolytic therapy with intravenous streptokinase was shown to reduce the risk of mortality in patients with STEMI if it was administered early after presentation. The time-dependent nature of therapy was also demonstrated, in that patients treated more than 12 hours after the onset of symptoms had no measurable benefit from thrombolysis. The next generation of thrombolytic agents, recombinant tissue-type plasminogen activators (rt-PA), improved on mortality reduction when compared with streptokinase (30-day mortality rate, 7.3% with streptokinase vs. 6.3% with rt-PA). The advantage of rt-PA appeared to be related to enhanced vessel patency at 90 minutes after administration (80% with rt-PA vs. 53% to 60% with streptokinase). Subsequent forms of rt-PA, although easier to administer, did not further reduce mortality. The major attribute of thrombolytic therapy is its ease of administration, but there is a significant risk (0.5% to 1%) of catastrophic bleeding complications in the form of intracerebral hemorrhage. Age older than 75 years, female gender, hypertension, and concomitant use of heparin increase the risk of this complication. In the case of failed thrombolytic therapy, rescue PCI may be pursued.

Primary PCI has been shown to be superior to thrombolytic therapy based on lower overall mortality rates and reduced risk of recurrent nonfatal MI. It is also associated with higher vessel patency rates and a low risk of intracranial hemorrhage. Primary PCI is frequently performed by mechanical aspiration of thrombus and placement of a coronary stent. Balloon angioplasty may or may not be needed during this procedure. Patients should receive preprocedure P2Y12 inhibitor (ticagrelor 180 mg, clopidogrel 600 mg or prasugrel 60 mg). For patients who are not able to take oral medications, whose platelet inhibition may not be at therapeutic levels at the time of stent placement, or who are at high risk for life-threatening bleeding requiring cessation of antiplatelet therapy, cangrelor (an intravenous P2Y12 inhibitor given at 30 mcg/kg bolus followed by infusion of 4 mcg/kg/minute) may be considered given its rapid onset and offset of platelet inhibition.

Bivalirudin was shown in a clinical trial of primary PCI to be superior to both heparin- and glycoprotein IIb/IIIa–based anticoagulation with lower post-MI mortality and fewer bleeding complications. Centers that are dedicated to primary PCI as the preferred therapy are likely to have the best outcomes when operators are sufficiently skilled and the institution cares for this patient population on a regular basis. Primary PCI is the best option for patients in cardiogenic shock (within 18 hours after onset of shock), for patients with prior CABG (graft occlusion is not amenable to thrombolysis), and for patients older than 70 years of age (conferring a reduced risk of intracerebral hemorrhage compared with thrombolysis).

Complications of Myocardial Infarction
Recurrent Chest Pain

MI is associated with a number of possible problems related to the extent of injury (Table 8.6). Patients can experience post-infarction angina that may reflect re-occlusion of the infarct related vessel. This can occur either in patients who underwent primary PCI with stent placement (stent thrombosis) or thrombolysis. Post-infarction angina usually requires cardiac catheterization for appropriate diagnosis and treatment. Patients with transmural MI are also subject to pericarditis 2 to 4 days after the event. This diagnosis is usually established by the symptom nature and pattern (worse with inspiration or supine position, improved with sitting), which is different from their initial presentation with acute MI. A less common event is the development of pericarditis due to Dressler syndrome up to 10 weeks after acute MI. This is likely an immune-mediated phenomenon. Pericarditis is treated with aspirin or nonsteroidal anti-inflammatory drugs.

Arrhythmias

The highest risk of life-threatening arrhythmias is during the first 24 to 48 hours after the onset of acute MI. Ischemic myocardium is susceptible to arrhythmia generation, probably based on micro-reentry associated with ischemic myocardium. The significant mortality risk in the early hours of acute MI is largely attributed to arrhythmias such as VF or VT. The risk of VF is about 3% to 5% in the early hours of MI and diminishes over 24 to 48 hours. One of the benefits of rhythm monitoring during the first 48 hours after presentation is prompt recognition and treatment of life-threatening ventricular arrhythmias.

TABLE 8.6	Complications of Acute Myocardial Infarction

Functional
Left ventricular failure
Right ventricular failure
Cardiogenic shock

Mechanical
Free-wall rupture
Ventricular septal defect
Papillary muscle rupture with acute mitral regurgitation

Electrical
Bradyarrhythmias (first-, second-, and third-degree atrioventricular blocks)
Tachyarrhythmias (supraventricular, ventricular)
Conduction abnormalities (bundle branch and fascicular blocks)

Accelerated idioventricular rhythm occurs early in the course of MI and may be associated with reperfusion. This arrhythmia is well tolerated and does not require specific therapy.

Ventricular arrhythmias occurring late (>48 hours) after acute MI usually are associated with large underlying MIs and heart failure. Late episodes of VF or VT portend a poor prognosis. Immediate therapy for VF is electrical defibrillation. VT that causes hemodynamic embarrassment is treated with synchronized electrical cardioversion. β-Blocker therapy may help to suppress arrhythmias in patients who are prone to them, as may the use of amiodarone. Correction of residual ischemia may also play a role in controlling VF or VT events. Patients with late VF or hemodynamically significant VT are candidates for an implantable cardioverter defibrillator device (ICD). An ICD can also improve survival in asymptomatic patients with a persistently reduced EF less than 30% at 40 days after their acute MI. ICD therapy is also indicated if the EF is less than 35% at 40 days after MI in a patient with symptomatic heart failure.

Atrial fibrillation (AF) occurs in 10% to 15% of patients after MI. Those more prone to AF include patients with older age, large MI, hypokalemia, hypomagnesemia, hypoxia, or increased sympathetic activity. Rate control with β-blockers (e.g., metoprolol), digoxin, calcium-channel blockers (e.g., diltiazem) or some combination of these agents is warranted, as is the use of intravenous heparin to reduce the risk of systemic embolization. Cardioversion is warranted in the face of rapid rates that cause ischemia, heart failure, or hypotension. Amiodarone is sometimes used to help maintain sinus rhythm for the first few months after MI-related AF.

Sinus bradycardia or AV block due to increased vagal tone is common in cases of inferior MI (30% to 40%). Reperfusion of the right coronary artery may be associated with significant bradycardia (Bezold-Jarisch reflex). Atropine (0.5 to 1.5 mg IV) can resolve severe inferior MI–related bradycardia. In contrast, heart block and wide-complex escape rhythms associated with anterior MI suggest an infra–AV node block. This may be worsened by the use of atropine.

Advanced degrees of heart block may require the placement of a permanent pacemaker. Intermittent second-degree or third-degree AV block associated with bundle branch block or symptomatic AV block are indications for a permanent pacemaker. Type I AV block (Wenckebach) is usually not persistent and rarely causes symptoms that warrant a permanent pacemaker.

Heart Failure and Low-Output States

MI involving 20% to 25% of the left ventricle can result in significant heart failure manifesting with dyspnea due to pulmonary congestion and findings of LV dysfunction such as an S_3 or S_4. Cardiogenic shock is associated with loss of 40% of the myocardium. This condition carries a very high risk of mortality. In the era of widespread use of reperfusion therapy, the incidence of post-MI heart failure or cardiogenic shock has declined. Early use of reperfusion therapies limits infarct size and the risk of complications related to heart failure. When acute heart failure occurs with MI, therapeutic interventions including oxygen, intravenous morphine, and diuretics can help stabilize the patient. Nitroglycerin can also help by reducing the elevated preload. Long-term therapy for heart failure related to reduced EF after acute MI includes the use of ACE inhibitors (or ARBs), appropriate β-blockers, aldosterone receptor antagonists such as eplerenone or spironolactone, and diuretics as needed.

The acutely infarcted ventricle requires an increased filling pressure and volume to optimize its performance. Patients with acute MI may become relatively fluid depleted due to nausea, vomiting, or decreased fluid intake, leading to reduced LV volume and a fall in cardiac output. This can translate into hypotension that is best treated by judicious administration of fluids.

Acute inferior MI is usually associated with a low mortality risk once the early arrhythmia-prone hours have passed. Occlusion of the right coronary artery and a significant acute marginal branch can lead to right ventricular infarction. Approximately 10% to 15% of patients with inferior MI have associated right ventricular infarction. This condition produces a significant increase in mortality risk (in-hospital mortality, 25% to 30% vs. <6%). Hallmarks of right ventricular infarction include elevated jugular venous pressure with Kussmaul sign and hypotension. Right ventricular function frequently recovers, but it may be necessary to administer sufficient volume to maintain right heart output. Short-term inotropic support with dobutamine is sometimes needed, and venodilators and diuretics should be avoided. High-degree AV block, usually transient with inferior MI, may worsen hemodynamics and necessitate temporary AV sequential pacing. AF may not be tolerated and may require cardioversion.

Cardiogenic Shock

Cardiogenic shock is a clinical syndrome associated with extensive loss of myocardium, which leads to a reduced cardiac index (<1.8 L/min/m^2) in the face of elevated LV filling pressures (pulmonary capillary wedge pressure >18 mm Hg), resulting in systemic hypotension and reduced organ perfusion. This shock state is associated with mortality rates in the range of 70% to 80%. Aggressive diagnosis with hemodynamic monitoring and appropriate support with an inotropic agent and invasive mechanical support as indicated can help to stabilize the patient. Mechanical circulatory support includes the intra-aortic balloon pump (IABP), Impella ventricular assist device (VAD), and extracorporeal membrane oxygenation (ECMO). One benefit of the IABP is that it can quickly be placed in the cath lab to both augment cardiac output as well as diastolic filling of the coronary arteries. IABP therapy is at best temporizing, and the patient's survival depends on the presence of reversible factors such as ischemia that respond to revascularization or correction of a mechanical complication of MI (e.g., mitral regurgitation or VSD). IABP therapy cannot be used in the face of significant aortic insufficiency and may not be feasible in the presence of significant peripheral vascular disease. Despite the hemodynamic support it provides, the IABP has never been proven in a randomized trial to improve mortality, and thus its use is based on clinician decision making rather than routine use. Some centers now are opting for more advanced levels of support in particularly ill patients including the Impella or ECMO as a bridge to recovery or long-term VAD/transplant.

In patients with cardiogenic shock secondary to acute MI it is key to reestablish perfusion to affected areas of the heart as able. More recent theories have suggested that rather than the "door to balloon time" emphasized in STEMI, the emphasis in patients in shock should be to achieve early improvement in perfusion with mechanical support as needed and then address revascularization. If multivessel disease is discovered in a patient in shock, the culprit lesion should be addressed, and other high-grade diseases can be addressed at a later time.

Mechanical Complications

Mechanical complications of acute MI include mitral regurgitation (due to ischemic papillary muscle dysfunction or rupture), VSD, free wall rupture, and LV aneurysm formation. These problems usually occur during the first week after MI, and they account for as much as 15% of MI-related mortality. A new murmur, sudden onset of heart failure, or hemodynamic collapse should also raise suspicion of a mechanical complication of MI. Patients who either were not reperfused or were reperfused late after onset of MI are most at risk for these problems. Echocardiography usually identifies the mechanical problem, and hemodynamic assessment with right heart catheterization can aid the diagnosis. Surgical correction of the defect is usually required.

Papillary muscle rupture or dysfunction leading to acute severe mitral regurgitation results in severe heart failure and up to 75% mortality within 24 hours after onset. Afterload reduction with intravenous nitroprusside and the use of IABP can help to stabilize the patient, but surgical valve repair or replacement will be needed to provide some chance of survival. Surgery is associated with a 25% to 50% mortality risk, but that still is better than the risk with medical or IABP therapy only.

Elderly patients, particularly those with hypertension, are more prone to MI-related VSD. Thrombolytic therapy may also place patients at risk for this complication. Acute VSD with resultant left-to-right shunting can produce severe hemodynamic instability. As with acute mitral regurgitation, afterload reduction and IABP may help to stabilize the patient, but ultimately surgical repair will be required. Moderate to large VSDs are not well tolerated and are associated with significant mortality risk. VSDs related to anterior MI may offer a better opportunity for surgical repair than those resulting from inferior MI. Some patients have been helped by the use of percutaneous closure devices, which can afford an opportunity to delay surgery until there is better tissue healing in the infarct area.

LV free wall rupture is similar to VSD in terms of risk for occurrence and underlying myocardial pathology. Free wall rupture is usually associated with sudden death due to cardiac tamponade. On occasion, a pseudoaneurysm forms and the patient can be treated surgically.

Thromboembolic Complications

In earlier years, thromboembolism in the form of either cardioembolic stroke or pulmonary embolism contributed to 25% of post-MI in-hospital mortality, and clinical events were diagnosed in 10% of patients. The risk of thromboembolism is linked to the presence of LV mural clot, which is more likely to be found in anterior MI with associated apical akinesis and deep venous thrombosis due to prolonged bedrest. Contemporary methods of care for acute MI have greatly reduced the risk of post-MI thromboembolism.

Reperfusion therapy, when applied in a timely fashion, results in less extensive MI and less impairment of LV function. Patients with anterior MI treated with reperfusion therapy are less likely to have extensive apical akinesis, which is the breeding ground for mural thrombus. It is advised that patients treated for acute MI have an echocardiogram to assess for overall LV function; in the case of anterior MI, the presence of apical mural thrombus can be detected by echocardiography.

If LV mural thrombus is present, the patient should receive therapeutic anticoagulation with unfractionated or LMW heparin while oral anticoagulation with warfarin is initiated. Warfarin therapy should be continued for 6 months after MI when LV apical mural thrombus is detected. Early ambulation after MI, along with the use of compression stockings and subcutaneous heparin prophylaxis (unfractionated or LMW) for deep venous thrombosis, has greatly diminished the threat of pulmonary embolism.

PROGNOSIS

Risk Stratification After Myocardial Infarction

Key to understanding an individual patient's risk for future coronary events or mortality related to MI is a thorough assessment of drivers for those risks: status of LV function and its impact on clinical functional status, residual myocardial ischemia, and spontaneous or exercise-induced arrhythmias. Appropriate predischarge assessments provide a comprehensive picture of the patient's risk status and prognosis.

Electrocardiographic Monitoring

Patients are routinely monitored by telemetry systems that capture arrhythmic events in the first 48 hours after MI. Late ventricular arrhythmias such as VF or sustained VT identify patients who are likely to benefit from ICD therapy. This is particularly true if EF is reduced to less than 40%. ICD implantation is also indicated for patients with persistently reduced EF (<30%).

Cardiac Catheterization and Noninvasive Testing

Predischarge risk stratification may involve cardiac catheterization, submaximal predischarge exercise stress testing (on days 4 to 6), or maximal exercise stress testing after discharge (at 2 to 6 weeks). The presence or absence of high-risk coronary anatomy is demonstrated for patients who have undergone primary PCI at the time of presentation. Many patients who have been treated with thrombolytic therapy undergo coronary angiography before discharge to determine the extent and severity of underlying CAD as well as the status of the culprit lesion. If coronary angiography is not performed, predischarge submaximal exercise testing (up to 70% of maximal predicted heart rate) is done to identify those who are at increased risk for postdischarge coronary ischemic events. Patients who undergo submaximal exercise stress testing in lieu of coronary angiography frequently have a follow-up maximal exercise stress test within 2 to 6 weeks after discharge. During stress testing, positive results that suggest the need for coronary angiography include exercise-induced angina, ST changes of ischemia (ST depression), exercise-induced hypotension, exercise-induced ventricular arrhythmias, and low functional capacity. The sensitivity and specificity of stress testing after MI is enhanced by the use of imaging modalities such as stress echocardiography or nuclear perfusion imaging. All patients should have their EF assessed, typically by echocardiography, before discharge.

Secondary Prevention, Patient Education, and Rehabilitation

The goal of secondary prevention is to reduce the risk of recurrent MI and cardiovascular mortality. Risk factor modification is key to the secondary prevention strategy. All patients should have their lipid status assessed at the time of admission, but statin therapy is warranted in patients with acute MI at presentation. The target LDL level is less than 100 mg/dL, preferably closer to 70 mg/dL. Smoking cessation is of critical importance because it can reduce the risk of reinfarction, and ongoing smoking can double the risk of recurrent MI or mortality in the first year after MI. Structured smoking cessation programs and the use of pharmacologic aids (e.g., nicotine patches or gum, bupropion, varenicline) can increase the success of smoking cessation efforts.

Antiplatelet therapy with aspirin (75 to 162 mg/day) is given indefinitely to all patients after MI. Regardless of whether primary PCI has been performed, patients will benefit from the additional use of a P2Y12 inhibitor for the first year after MI. Those patients who have received a stent during primary PCI should continue clopidogrel 75 mg/day, ticagrelor 90 mg twice daily, or prasugrel 10 mg/day for one year. There are some data suggesting that if the patient is tolerating dual-antiplatelet therapy (DAPT) well and has a low bleeding risk, there may be additional benefit to continuing DAPT even for up to three years.

The use of anticoagulation is indicated for patients with systemic or pulmonary thromboembolism, as well as persistent or paroxysmal AF, guided by their CHADS-2 score (congestive heart failure, hypertension, age ≥75 years, diabetes mellitus, and stroke). Patients who are at high risk for thromboembolism after acute MI, such as those with low EF related to anterior MI, can also be considered for prophylactic anticoagulation; however, there is no strong randomized data for this indication.

The high prevalence of patients who have both AF and the need for stent placement creates a conundrum involving the need for both anticoagulation and antiplatelet agents leading to a significantly increased risk of bleeding. Warfarin (target international normalized ratio [INR], 2.0 to 3.0) has been the historical choice for anticoagulation. Its use in conjunction with patients having undergone stenting was evaluated in several clinical trials that suggested that therapy with warfarin and clopidogrel had similar outcomes for ischemic or embolic events compared to "triple therapy" (warfarin, clopidogrel, and aspirin) but afforded a lower risk of bleeding. Since then, newer anticoagulant medications have been developed for nonvalvular AF that have merited their own series of trials, including the thrombin inhibitor dabigatran and the direct factor Xa inhibitors apixaban, edoxaban, and rivaroxaban. These drugs were also demonstrated to be effective when paired with clopidogrel with a lower bleeding risk compared to triple therapy. None of the trials referenced above utilized any other P2Y12 inhibitors aside from clopidogrel. Ultimately the decision regarding antithrombotic therapy length and composition will be provider dependent but should be based upon an assessment of the patient's bleeding and ischemic risk.

Acute anterior MI that has resulted in significant injury to the ventricle with an EF of less than 40% places the patient at risk for future negative remodeling of the left ventricle and potential heart failure. ACE-inhibitor therapy has been shown to reduce the risk of negative remodeling and the occurrence of heart failure in such patients. This group of patients also experiences a reduction in future recurrent MI risk with the use of ACE-inhibitor therapy. This observation does not appear to carry over to patients with stable CAD. ACE-inhibitor therapy (captopril, ramipril, lisinopril) is indicated for all patients after MI. The use of ARBs (e.g., valsartan, losartan) is reasonable for patients who are intolerant of ACE-inhibitor therapy. The aldosterone receptor antagonist eplerenone (25 mg/day, titrated to 50 mg/day) is indicated as additive therapy to ACE or ARB in MI patients who have reduced EF (<40%) or diabetes. Careful monitoring of serum potassium is required after initiation of eplerenone together with ACE or ARB.

β-Blocker therapy reduces mortality risk in patients who have reduced EF post-MI. This therapy should be avoided in patients with uncompensated heart failure early after MI or the presence of other contraindications. Metoprolol succinate (25 mg/day titrated up to 200 mg/day) or carvedilol (3.125-6.25 mg titrated to 25 mg twice each day) should be initiated at low doses and titrated upward as tolerated. The role of β-blockers in patients with no residual myocardial ischemia, arrhythmias, or normal EF is not clear.

Nitrates, either short-acting sublingual nitroglycerin or long-acting versions, may be useful in the treatment of stable angina. Calcium-channel blocking drugs should be avoided in patients with reduced EF (<40%). In patients with normal EF, either diltiazem or verapamil may useful as a substitute in patients who are intolerant of β-blockers when either antianginal therapy or rate control for AF is needed. The dihydropyridine, amlodipine, may be a useful adjunct for control of hypertension or treatment of angina. It should be used with caution in the face of reduced EF.

After acute MI, women should refrain from initiating hormone therapy with estrogen or estrogen/progesterone preparations; these agents do not decrease the risk of recurrent MI but do increase the risk of thromboembolic events. The ongoing use of hormone therapy in women already receiving treatment should be individualized, with a bias toward discontinuing therapy. Diabetic patients need attention to their degree of glycemic control, with a target of hemoglobin A_{1c} less than 7%. Vitamin supplements have no clear role in therapy for MI patients. Fish oil supplements do not appear to benefit patients who have experienced acute MI.

Patient Education and Cardiac Rehabilitation

It is important to begin the education of patients early after acute MI so that they understand the value of their various prescribed medical therapies and the need for risk factor modification. Cardiac rehabilitation programs are very useful in the ongoing education of patients; they reinforce positive lifestyle changes and provide exercise training in the post-MI period. Such programs not only educate patients but also help them to regain confidence in their ability to perform the tasks of daily living and other activities they enjoy. Early follow-up with the physician after discharge is also important to ensure clinical stability and tolerance of medical therapy and to monitor the progress of lifestyle changes.

SUGGESTED READINGS

Amsterdam EA, Wenger NK, Brindis RG, et al: 2014 AHA/ACC Guideline for the Management of Patients with Non–ST-Elevation Acute Coronary Syndromes, J Am Coll Cardiol 64(24):e139–e228, 2014.

Arnett DK, Blumenthal RS, Albert MA, et al.: 2019 ACC/AHA Guideline on the primary prevention of cardiovascular disease: A Report of the American College of Cardiology/American Heart Association Task Force on Clinical Practice Guidelines, Circulation 140:e596–e646, 2019.

Fihn SD, Gardin JM, Abrams J, et al.: 2012 ACCF/AHA/ACP/AATS/PCNA/SCAI/STS Guideline for the diagnosis and management of patients with stable ischemic heart disease: a report of the American College of Cardiology Foundation/American Heart Association Task Force on Practice Guidelines, and the American College of Physicians, American Association for Thoracic Surgery, Preventive Cardiovascular Nurses Association, Society for Cardiovascular Angiography And Interventions, and Society of Thoracic Surgeons, J Am Coll Cardiol 60:e44–e164, 2012.

Hillis LD, Smith PK, Anderson JL, et al.: 2011 ACCF/AHA Guideline for coronary artery bypass graft surgery: A report of the American College of Cardiology Foundation/American Heart Association Task Force on Practice Guidelines. Developed in collaboration with the American Association for Thoracic Surgery, Society of Cardiovascular Anesthesiologists, and Society of Thoracic Surgeons, J Am Coll Cardiol 58:e123–e210, 2011.

Levine GN, Bates ER, Bittl JA, et al.: 2016 ACC/AHA Guideline focused update on duration of dual antiplatelet therapy in patients with coronary artery disease, J Am Coll Cardiol 68(10):1082–1115, 2016.

Levine GN, Bates ER, Blankenship JC, et al.: 2011 ACCF/AHA/SCAI guideline for percutaneous coronary intervention: a report of the American College of Cardiology Foundation/American Heart Association Task Force on Practice Guidelines and the Society for Cardiovascular Angiography and Interventions, J Am Coll Cardiol 58:e44–e122, 2011.

Levine GN, Bates ER, Blankenship JC, et al.: 2015 ACC/AHA/SCAI focused update on primary percutaneous coronary intervention for patients with ST-elevation myocardial infarction, J Am Coll Cardiol 67(10):1235–1250, 2016.

O'Gara PT, Kushner FG, Ascheim DD, et al.: 2013 ACCF/AHA Guideline for the management of ST-elevation myocardial infarction: a report of the American College of Cardiology Foundation/American Heart Association Task Force on Practice Guidelines, J Am Coll Cardiol 61(4):e78–e140, 2013.

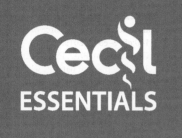

9

Cardiac Arrhythmias

Marcie G. Berger, Jason C. Rubenstein, James A. Roth

BASIC CELLULAR ELECTROPHYSIOLOGY

Cardiac myocytes actively maintain a negative resting membrane potential (E_m) through the differential distribution of ions between intracellular and extracellular compartments, which is an energy-dependent process that relies on ion channels, pumps, and exchangers. Transmembrane differences in voltage and ionic concentration create electrical and chemical forces that drive charged ions in and out of cells.

The resting E_m of cardiac myocytes is controlled by potassium ions (K^+). Active K^+ transport by the sodium-potassium adenosine triphosphatase pump (Na^+, K^+-ATPase) produces a transmembrane ionic gradient, with the intracellular concentration of K^+ exceeding the extracellular concentration. This favors the net efflux of K^+ from cells, down the chemical concentration gradient, yielding a resting negative charge within the cardiac myocytes. K^+ continues to flow from the intracellular to the extracellular compartment until the negative intracellular charge counterbalances the transmembrane K^+ concentration gradient at a potential called the *equilibrium potential* for K^+. This potential, at which the net K^+ current is zero, is close to the resting E_m of nonpacemaker cardiac myocytes. Pacemaker cells (i.e., sinoatrial and atrioventricular [AV] nodal cells) are characterized by a resting E_m of −50 to −60 mV. The resting E_m of atrial and ventricular myocytes is typically −80 to −90 mV.

The depolarization of a cardiac myocyte to threshold potential triggers a sequence of ionic movements resulting in a cardiac action potential (Fig. 9.1). The action potential is divided into five phases. Phase 0 is the rapid depolarization of nonpacemaker myocytes resulting from rapid sodium ion (Na^+) entry through fast Na^+ channels. These channels have three conformational states: closed (resting state), open (conducting Na^+ current), and inactivated, from which recovery is voltage dependent. Phase 1 is early, rapid, partial repolarization of the cell mediated by K^+ efflux. During phase 2, the plateau phase, there is a small net current flow, with inward calcium ion (Ca^{2+}) flow balanced by outward K^+ flow.

During phase 3, repolarization is mediated by an increase in K^+ efflux and a decline in Ca^{2+} influx. The dominant repolarizing current is I_{Kr}, the rapidly activating delayed rectifier K^+ current, a channel encoded by the *KCNE2* gene (also called *HERG*). The I_{Ks} current, or slowly activating delayed rectifier K^+ current, also contributes to repolarization. Phase 3 determines to a large degree the cellular refractory period. Importantly, I_{Kr} is inhibited by a large number of drugs that prolong the action potential duration.

Phase 4 is particularly significant in cardiac pacemaker cells because slow depolarization occurs from the resting membrane potential to the threshold potential. The resting E_m, rate of spontaneous phase 4 depolarization, and rate of phase 0 depolarization differentiate slow-response from fast-response cardiac myocytes. Slow-response cells, located in the sinoatrial node and AV node, normally display automaticity or spontaneous depolarization during phase 4. Resting E_m in slow-response cells is less negative, and Ca^{2+} current mediates phase 0 depolarization. Conduction in these pacemaker cells is slow, and recovery from inactivation is time dependent. The fast-response cells found in atrial myocytes, ventricular myocytes, and the His-Purkinje system display slow phase 4 depolarization and do not typically display automaticity. Their resting E_m is more negative, and the fast Na^+ current drives rapid phase 0 depolarization and rapid conduction. Recovery from inactivation in these cells is voltage dependent.

The sinus node typically displays the fastest phase 4 depolarization. Other cardiac tissues have the capacity to depolarize spontaneously, and subsidiary pacemakers may take over when sinus rates slow and under conditions of increased automaticity. Typically, the AV node, located above the AV ring, serves as the heart's secondary pacemaker, with a spontaneous rate of depolarization of 40 to 50 beats per minute. Automaticity of cardiac myocytes is increased when the slope of phase 4 depolarization increases, with a shift of threshold potentials to more negative values, or in the presence of more positive maximal diastolic potentials.

The sinus node is the primary intrinsic pacemaker, and spontaneous depolarization leads to action potential generation, with normal resting rates of 60 to 100 beats per minute. Depolarization then spreads through the atria to the AV node, where conduction slows, introducing a delay between atrial and ventricular activation, and then to the His-Purkinje system fibers, which originate at the AV node with the bundle of His and split to form the left bundle branch and the right bundle branch, rapidly conducting depolarization to the ventricular myocardium. Cardiac myocytes are joined by electrical synapses called *gap junctions*, which permit the flow of intracellular current from cell to cell.

Classification of Arrhythmias

Mechanistically, cardiac arrhythmias can be broadly divided into disorders of action potential formation and disorders of impulse conduction. Clinically, arrhythmias are classified as bradycardias and tachycardias, with further categorization according to arrhythmia origin. This information is used to guide evaluation and management strategies.

Electrophysiologic Mechanisms of Arrhythmias

Automaticity is a normal function of pacemaker cells, occurring during phase 4 depolarization. *Enhanced automaticity* occurs when pacemaker cells depolarize at a faster rate due to an increased slope of phase 4 depolarization, a shift of threshold potential to a more negative value,

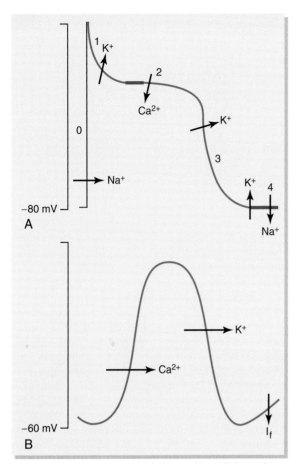

Fig. 9.1 Electrophysiologic basis of the cardiac cellular action potential. (A) Fast-response cells found in working myocardium and the specialized infranodal conduction system maintain a strongly negative resting membrane potential and a brisk phase 0 upstroke mediated by rapid sodium influx at the start of the action potential. (B) In contrast, slow-response cells found in the sinus node and atrioventricular nodal tissue exhibit less-negative resting membrane potentials, slower calcium-channel–dependent action potential upstrokes, and phase 4 depolarization.

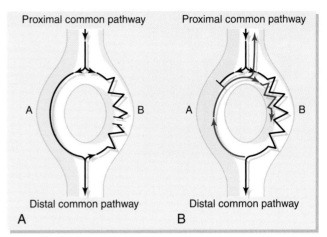

Fig. 9.2 Mechanism of reentry. Reentry requires two distinct pathways with different refractoriness and a region of slowed conduction. One pathway *(A)* has normal rapid conduction but a long refractory period. The second pathway *(B)* has slowed conduction but a relatively shorter refractory period. To initiate reentry, conduction must fail down one pathway in the antegrade direction but then permit later retrograde reactivation of this pathway. This is referred to as a *unidirectional block.* A fixed or functional obstacle must maintain separation of the two pathways. Although drawn schematically as a circular loop, the anatomy of circuits is often complex and circuitous and is different in different arrhythmia mechanisms. (A) In normal rhythm, the circuit is activated in an antegrade direction down both pathways. However, because of slowed conduction in the *B* limb, distal activation is mediated by the faster *A* pathway, which arrives first and may activate the slowly conducting pathway in a retrograde direction. This retrograde conduction is electrocardiographically concealed (invisible), collides with the antegrade wave front, and is extinguished, and no tachycardia results. (B) Reentry is usually initiated by a premature beat originating independently of the circuit. The premature beat fails to propagate down the rapidly conducting *A* limb due to differential refractoriness of the two limbs, but it is able to propagate down the slowly conducting *B* pathway, where it may encounter substantial delay due to increased conduction time with prematurity (i.e., decremental conduction), allowing recovery of the previously blocked rapidly conducting *A* limb. This permits the rapidly conducting *A* limb to act as a return path and for ultimate reentrant reactivation of the slowly conducting *B* pathway, initiating sustained reentrant tachycardia in the circuit.

or a shift of the maximal diastolic potential to a more positive value. These changes may occur with sympathetic stimulation. Enhanced automaticity may be normal (e.g., appropriate sinus tachycardia) or abnormal (e.g., inappropriate sinus tachycardia). Spontaneous depolarization occurring in nonpacemaker cardiac myocytes is called *abnormal automaticity.* Conditions such as ischemia, electrolyte abnormalities, and sympathetic stimulation may produce abnormal automaticity. Premature atrial and ventricular depolarizations, atrial tachycardia, and ventricular tachycardia (VT) may result.

Triggered activity occurs when secondary cardiac depolarizations are initiated by prior depolarizations. If these secondary depolarizations reach threshold potential, they may generate action potentials during or immediately after phase 3 of the action potential. *Early afterdepolarizations* (EADs) are observed when triggered depolarization occurs during phase 3 of the action potential. Inciters of EADs include QT-prolonging drugs, hypokalemia, and bradycardia. Patients with congenital long QT syndrome (LQTS) are prone to develop EADS, resulting in *torsades de pointes* (TdP).

When triggered activity occurs during phase 4, *delayed afterdepolarizations* (DADs) result. DADs are exaggerated at rapid heart rates and observed with digoxin toxicity and high-level catecholamine

states, conditions that are associated with intracellular calcium overload. DADs are thought to be the chief arrhythmic mechanism underlying catecholaminergic polymorphic VT (CPVT).

Reentry is the dominant mechanism underlying clinical tachyarrhythmias. Reentry describes the reexcitation of a localized region of cardiac tissue by the same impulse, requiring bifurcating conduction pathways with different velocities and refractory periods. To permit reentry, unidirectional block in one pathway and slowed conduction in the other are required. Reentry is further categorized as anatomic, circling around a fixed anatomic obstacle, or functional, in which the unexcitable center of a reentrant circuit is not fixed but functionally refractory. Fig. 9.2 illustrates reentry as an arrhythmic mechanism. The two pathways join proximally and distally. Pathway *A* conducts rapidly but has a long refractory period. Pathway *B* is slowly conducting but has a shorter refractory period. A normally timed impulse enters the two pathways through the proximal common pathway, conducting rapidly down *A* and slowly down *B*. As the impulse from pathway *A* reaches the distal common pathway, while continuing distally, it may also turn around to activate *B* retrogradely. This impulse collides with the slowly conducting antegrade impulse in pathway *B*, extinguishing the impulse. However, a sufficiently premature stimulus

TABLE 9.1 Singh–Vaughan Williams Classification of Antiarrhythmic Drugs

Class	Physiologic Effect[a]	Examples
I	Blocks sodium channels; predominantly reduces the maximum velocity of the upstroke of the action potential (phase 0)	
IA	Intermediate-potency blockade	Quinidine, procainamide, disopyramide
IB	Least-potent blockade	Lidocaine, tocainide, mexiletine, phenytoin
IC	Most-potent blockade	Flecainide, propafenone, moricizine
II	β-Adrenergic receptor blockade	Propranolol, metoprolol, atenolol
III	Potassium-channel blockade: predominantly prolongs action potential duration	Amiodarone, sotalol, bretylium, ibutilide, dofetilide, dronedarone
IV	Calcium-channel blockade	Verapamil, diltiazem

[a]Several agents have physiologic effects characteristic of more than one class.

may enter the proximal common pathway, finding pathway *A* with its long refractory period unexcitable, traveling slowly down pathway *B*, and finally reaching the distal common pathway. Due to the slow conduction velocity in pathway *B*, pathway *A* may no longer be refractory, and the impulse may successfully travel retrograde up pathway *A*, potentially repeatedly activating the circuit. Reentry is the most common mechanism producing supraventricular tachycardia (SVT) and VT.

❖ For a deeper discussion on this topic, please see Chapter 55, "Principles of Electrophysiology," in *Goldman-Cecil Medicine*, 26th Edition.

GENERAL APPROACH TO MANAGEMENT

Diagnostic Procedures

Electrocardiography

The baseline 12-lead electrocardiogram (ECG) is essential for the initial evaluation of patients with arrhythmic symptoms. The baseline ECG may indicate underlying structural heart disease, with Q waves or fractionated QRS complexes suggesting prior myocardial infarction (MI). Slow sinus rates or AV conduction abnormalities may point to susceptibility to symptomatic bradycardia. Delta waves confirm an accessory pathway and direct the evaluation of arrhythmic symptoms toward the diagnosis of Wolff-Parkinson-White (WPW) syndrome while localizing the accessory pathway.

Evidence for hereditary cardiomyopathies and cardiac ion channel disorders that predispose to sudden death may be detected on a baseline ECG. Patients with arrhythmogenic right ventricular (RV) dysplasia may have epsilon waves and inverted T waves in the right precordial leads. QT interval prolongation or shortening may indicate congenital or acquired long QT or short QT syndrome, respectively. Brugada syndrome can be diagnosed based on coved ST-segment elevation in leads V_1 and V_2.

A 12-lead ECG obtained during arrhythmic symptoms can establish the cause of a patient's symptoms. The specific mechanism underlying bradycardia and tachycardia can often be inferred from the ECG. Documentation of QRS morphology during VT or accessory pathway–mediated tachycardia on a 12-lead ECG aids in localizing the site of origin and guiding catheter ablation.

Ambulatory Monitoring

Although a 12-lead ECG obtained during arrhythmic symptoms is ideal, it is difficult to obtain in practice because of the transient and intermittent nature of these symptoms. Ambulatory recording devices permit electrocardiographic monitoring over longer periods to establish symptom-rhythm correlations.

Three types of monitoring devices are available. *Holter monitors* typically provide continuous electrogram storage for 24 to 48 hours.

Holter monitoring is helpful for patients with frequent symptoms. The comprehensive rhythm record obtained during this sampling period provides useful information about heart rate variability, rate control with atrial fibrillation (AF), AF burden, asymptomatic arrhythmias, and the frequency of ventricular ectopy.

External event monitors or loop recorders, which can be worn for 30 days, store electrograms when triggered by patients for symptoms. Additionally, loop monitors employ algorithms to automatically detect tachycardia, bradycardia, and atrial fibrillation. Episode storage varies from seconds to minutes. After events are recorded, patients transmit the data by telephone. External loop recorders are intended to identify cardiac rhythm disturbances underlying infrequent symptoms.

For patients with arrhythmia symptoms occurring less than once per month, *implantable loop recorders* may be useful. These small devices implanted in a subcutaneous pocket in the left chest record patient-triggered and auto-triggered ECGs based on heart rate and AF detection criteria. With a 3-year anticipated battery longevity, implantable loop recorders are valuable in establishing the cause of recurrent infrequent syncope and arrhythmic symptoms. Implantable loop recorders, with a reported 98% sensitivity for AF detection, are useful both for AF management and AF surveillance in the setting of cryptogenic stroke, resulting in higher utilization of appropriate oral anticoagulation following stroke.

Electrophysiologic Testing

To perform electrophysiologic studies, temporary transvenous pacing catheters are positioned in multiple locations in the heart, permitting pacing and recording of intracardiac electrograms. Catheters are typically placed in the right atrium, the right ventricle, close to the bundle of His, and in the coronary sinus for left atrial recording and pacing. Electrophysiologic studies can define the mechanism of tachyarrhythmias and guide therapy. In patients with prior MI, induction of VT may assist in determining patient susceptibility to life-threatening arrhythmias and inform decisions regarding defibrillator implantation. Electrophysiologic testing also can evaluate sinus node function and AV conduction.

Pharmacologic Therapy

Antiarrhythmic drugs are traditionally divided according to the Singh–Vaughan Williams classification, which categorizes agents based on their primary physiologic effect (Table 9.1). When this classification system was first proposed, knowledge of electrophysiologic mechanisms was limited. Although the simplicity of categorizing antiarrhythmic drugs according to Singh–Vaughan Williams classes I through IV is appealing, the system has many limitations. A hybrid classification system, class I and III agents block ion channels, and class II and IV drugs block receptors. Some drugs cross classes and have several

TABLE 9.2   Selected Characteristics of Antiarrhythmic Drugs

Drug	Effect on Surface ECG	Effect on LV Function	Important Drug Interactions	Effect on Pacing and Defibrillation Thresholds	Major Route of Elimination
Quinidine	Prolongs QRS and QT	Negative inotrope	Increases digoxin level and warfarin effect Cimetidine increases quinidine level Phenobarbital, phenytoin, and rifampin decrease quinidine level	Increases PT and DT at high doses	Liver (CYP3A4) and kidney
Procainamide	Prolongs PR, QRS, and QT	Negative inotrope	Cimetidine, alcohol, and amiodarone increase procainamide level	Increases PT at high doses	Liver and kidney
Disopyramide	Prolongs QRS and QT	Negative inotrope	Phenobarbital, phenytoin, and rifampin decrease disopyramide level	Increases PT at high doses	Liver (CYP3A4) and kidney
Lidocaine	Shortens QT	None	Propranolol, metoprolol, and cimetidine increase lidocaine level	Increases DT	Liver (CYP2D6)
Mexiletine	Shortens QT	None	Increases theophylline level Phenobarbital, phenytoin, and rifampin decrease mexiletine level	Various effects	Liver (CYP2D6)
Flecainide	Prolongs PR and QRS	Negative inotrope	Increases digoxin level	Increases PT; variable effect on DT	Liver (CYP2D6) and kidney
Propafenone	Prolongs PR and QRS	Negative inotrope	Increases digoxin, theophylline, and cyclosporine levels; increases warfarin effect Phenobarbital, phenytoin, and rifampin decrease propafenone level Cimetidine and quinidine increase propafenone level	Increases PT; variable effect on DT	Liver (CYP2D6)
Dronedarone	Prolongs PR and QT; slows sinus rate	Negative inotrope	CYP3A4 inhibitors (ketoconazole, clarithromycin, calcium-channel blockers) increase dronedarone levels; additive effect with drugs that prolong QT (macrolides, class I and III antiarrhythmics) increasing risk of TdP; increases dabigatran levels	Little effect	Liver (CYP3A4)
Amiodarone	Prolongs PR and QT; slows sinus rate	None	Increases digoxin and cyclosporine levels; increases warfarin effect	Increases DT	Liver (CYP3A4)
Sotalol	Prolongs PR and QT; slows sinus rate	Negative inotrope	Additive effects with other β-blockers	Decreases DT	Kidney
Ibutilide	Prolongs PR and QT	None	Additive effect on QT prolongation with class IA and other class III antiarrhythmic agents	Decreases DT	Liver
Dofetilide	Prolongs QT	None	Verapamil, diltiazem, Cimetidine, and ketoconazole increase dofetilide level	Decreases DT	Liver and kidney

DT, Defibrillation threshold; *ECG*, electrocardiogram; *LV*, left ventricle; *PT*, pacing threshold; *TdP*, torsades de pointes.

mechanisms of action. There are drugs with antiarrhythmic action that are excluded from the classification, such as digitalis and adenosine. The system categorizes drugs based on their in vitro electrophysiologic effects in normal cardiac tissues.

Available antiarrhythmic drugs have limited efficacy and carry the risk of adverse events, including proarrhythmic potential. Knowledge of drug metabolism, interactions, electrophysiologic effects, and side effects is essential. Certain antiarrhythmics may suppress left ventricular systolic function and may impact pacing and defibrillation thresholds. Excepting β-blockers, none of the antiarrhythmics has been demonstrated to reduce mortality rates. In fact, the use of antiarrhythmic agents may confer an increased risk of cardiovascular mortality, particularly in heart failure patients. Tables 9.2 and 9.3 summarize major characteristics and side effects of commonly used antiarrhythmic drugs.

Class I Antiarrhythmic Agents

Class I antiarrhythmic drugs include sodium-channel blockers that bind fast sodium channels in their open and inactivated states and dissociate from sodium channels during their resting state. Blocking voltage-gated fast sodium channels slows phase 0 depolarization and conduction velocity. Class I agents demonstrate use-dependent blockade, and their effect is potentiated at faster heart rates. The drug dissociation rate from sodium channels during phase 4 of the action potential determines the degree to which these agents depress cardiac conduction velocity.

Class IA agents have a slow rate of drug dissociation from sodium channels, conferring moderate potency. In addition to blocking voltage-gated fast sodium channels, class IA drugs block delayed rectifier potassium channels. Slowing of conduction velocity and action potential prolongation are observed. All are antimuscarinic, especially

TABLE 9.3 Common Side Effects of Select Antiarrhythmic Drugs

Drug	Major Side Effects
Quinidine	Nausea, diarrhea, abdominal cramping
	Cinchonism: decreased hearing, tinnitus, blurred vision, delirium
	Rash, thrombocytopenia, hemolytic anemia
	Hypotension, torsades de pointes (quinidine syncope)
Procainamide	Drug-induced lupus syndrome
	Nausea, vomiting
	Rash, fever, hypotension, psychosis, agranulocytosis
	Torsades de pointes
Disopyramide	Anticholinergic: dry mouth, blurred vision, constipation, urinary retention, closed angle glaucoma
	Hypotension, worsening heart failure
Lidocaine	CNS: dizziness, perioral numbness, paresthesias, altered consciousness, coma, seizures
Mexiletine	Nausea, vomiting
	CNS: dizziness, tremor, paresthesias, ataxia, confusion
Flecainide	CNS: blurred vision, headache, ataxia, tremor
	Congestive heart failure, ventricular proarrhythmia
Propafenone	Nausea, vomiting, constipation, metallic taste to food
	Dizziness, headache, exacerbation of asthma, ventricular proarrhythmia
β-Blockers	Bronchospasm, bradycardia, fatigue, depression, impotence
	Congestive heart failure
Calcium-channel blockers	Congestive heart failure, bradycardia, heart block, constipation
Amiodarone	Agranulocytosis, pulmonary fibrosis, hepatopathy, hyperthyroidism or hypothyroidism, corneal microdeposits, bluish discoloration of the skin, nausea, constipation, bradycardia, tremor, ataxia
Sotalol	Same as β-blockers, torsades de pointes
Dronedarone	Diarrhea, QT prolongation and torsades de pointes, death, bradycardia, congestive heart failure, hepatocellular injury, interstitial lung disease
Ibutilide	Torsades de pointes
Dofetilide	Torsades de pointes, headache, dizziness, diarrhea

CNS, Central nervous system.

disopyramide. Clinical applications include SVT, AF, atrial flutter, and VT. In the setting of atrial flutter and AF, class IA drugs are vagolytic. They may improve AV nodal conduction and should be used in conjunction with a β-blocker or calcium-channel blocker to avoid uncontrolled ventricular response rates. Quinidine is infrequently used due to its side effect profile, including diarrhea, thrombocytopenia, and QT prolongation, triggering polymorphic VT. Clinical studies highlight the proarrhythmic risk and increased mortality associated with quinidine therapy. Procainamide, available as an intravenous formulation, has an active metabolite *N*-acetylprocainamide (NAPA) and may induce a reversible lupus-like syndrome. Disopyramide, with its potent negative inotropic and antimuscarinic activity, has been used to treat vagally mediated AF.

Class IB agents rapidly dissociate from sodium channels during phase 4, providing weak sodium-channel blockade. Their therapeutic role is restricted to ventricular arrhythmias due to a lack of effect on the sinoatrial node, AV node, and atrial tissue. Lidocaine, which is available parentally, undergoes extensive first-pass hepatic inactivation. Lidocaine is more effective in relatively depolarized ventricular tissue due to preferential affinity for inactivated sodium channels; the drug is more potent in ischemic tissue. Mexiletine, which is available orally, has slower hepatic metabolism and a longer half-life than lidocaine.

Class IC drugs are potent fast sodium-channel blockers with little effect on K^+ current. These agents have a role in the therapy of SVTs and VTs. Their use is relegated to patients without coronary disease or significant structural heart disease. The Cardiac Arrhythmia Suppression Trial proved that the use of flecainide and moricizine to suppress ventricular arrhythmias after MI increased mortality rates. These agents may convert AF to atrial flutter and slow atrial conduction sufficiently to permit 1:1 AV conduction during atrial flutter, necessitating the simultaneous use of AV nodal–blocking therapies in patients with atrial arrhythmias. Flecainide is associated with bronchospasm, leukopenia, thrombocytopenia, and neurologic side effects. Flecainide, which inhibits Ca^{2+} release from the sarcoplasmic reticulum cardiac ryanodine receptor, may be useful in the therapy for CPVT. Propafenone has β-blocking effects and can cause agranulocytosis, anemia, and thrombocytopenia.

Class II and IV Antiarrhythmic Agents

β-Adrenoceptor antagonists, the class II agents, inhibit sympathetic activation of cardiac automaticity and conduction, resulting in slowing of the heart rate, decreased AV node conduction velocity, and prolongation of the AV node refractory period. Side effects include bradycardia, hypotension, exacerbation of reactive airway disease, fatigue, worsening symptoms of peripheral vascular disease, and depression. β-Blockers have different half-lives, lipid solubilities, elimination routes, and specificities for β_1 and β_2 receptors.

Class IV agents include the nondihydropyridine calcium-channel blockers. Blockade of voltage-gated L-type calcium channels decreases AV nodal conduction velocity, increases AV nodal refractory period, slows sinus node automaticity, and decreases myocardial contractility. Calcium-channel blockers may cause hypotension, bradycardia, and heart failure. Clinical applications for these agents include rate control for atrial tachyarrhythmias, termination and suppression of SVT, and normal heart VT. In the setting of atrial arrhythmias with underlying WPW, they can potentiate accessory pathway conduction and should be avoided.

Class III Antiarrhythmic Agents

Class III antiarrhythmic agents are a heterogeneous group of drugs that block the potassium delayed rectifier currents responsible for phase 3 cardiac repolarization, prolonging the cardiac action potential duration and refractory period. These agents demonstrate reverse-use dependence, with more potent potassium-channel blockade at slower heart rates. Prolonging the action potential duration can be therapeutic or proarrhythmic (e.g., TdP). This class represents the dominant category of antiarrhythmic agents in use.

Amiodarone is an iodinated compound available orally and parentally. With oral administration, it is slowly absorbed. Because it concentrates in fat tissues, amiodarone has a large volume of distribution. This characteristic prolongs the time to reach steady-state levels and produces a long elimination half-life, approximately 35 to 100 days. Amiodarone's pharmacology is complex, with class I through IV activity, although its primary therapeutic mechanism is prolongation of the action potential duration. It is effective in treating SVTs and VTs. It is hepatically metabolized and proven safe to use in the setting of congestive heart failure. Amiodarone is commonly used to treat atrial and ventricular arrhythmias in patients with structural heart disease and renal failure. Amiodarone is the only antiarrhythmic agent to demonstrate improved survival to hospital admission after cardiac arrest. This finding led to amiodarone prioritization within the ACLS pulseless

VT/VF algorithm. Widespread chronic use of amiodarone has been limited by significant side effects necessitating drug discontinuation in up to 20% of patients. Serious adverse effects include potentially irreversible pulmonary fibrosis, optic neuropathy producing visual impairment, hyperthyroidism, and severe hepatic toxicity. Less serious adverse effects include hypothyroidism, neurologic toxicity, sun sensitivity, QT prolongation, and bradycardia.

Sotalol blocks β-adrenoreceptors and delayed rectifier K^+ channels, decreasing sinoatrial node automaticity, slowing AV conduction velocity, and prolonging repolarization. It effectively treats a large number of ventricular and supraventricular arrhythmias.

Dofetilide, a selective class III agent used primarily to treat atrial arrhythmias, blocks delayed rectifier K^+ channels to prolong action potential duration and QT intervals. The risk of TdP is about 1% among patients without structural heart disease but as high as 4.8% among patients with congestive heart failure.

Ibutilide, an intravenous class III agent, is used for the acute termination of recent-onset AF and atrial flutter. The risk of polymorphic VT with administration of ibutilide is 8.3%.

Dronedarone is an orally available class III drug demonstrated to reduce the risk of first hospitalization due to cardiovascular events or death from any cause for patients in sinus rhythm with a history of paroxysmal or persistent AF. Dronedarone may not be used in the setting of permanent AF or in patients with New York Heart Association (NYHA) class IV heart failure or symptomatic heart failure with recent decompensation because the drug increases the risk of cardiovascular death in these populations. Other major side effects of dronedarone are severe hepatotoxicity, interstitial lung disease, bradycardia, and QT prolongation.

Other Antiarrhythmic Agents

The Singh–Vaughan Williams classification scheme does not describe several agents commonly used in cardiac arrhythmia management. *Adenosine* is a parenteral agent with an elimination half-life of 1 to 6 seconds. The drug binds to A1 receptors to activate K^+ channels, decreasing the action potential duration and hyperpolarizing membrane potentials in the atria, sinoatrial node, and AV node. Indirectly, adenosine blocks catecholamine-stimulated adenylate cyclase activation, decreasing cAMP and consequently decreasing Ca^{2+} influx. Used clinically for its ability to produce transient AV block, adenosine can terminate SVT when the AV node contributes to the reentrant circuit. By slowing atrial-ventricular conduction, adenosine can also establish the presence of underlying atrial tachycardia or atrial flutter when the arrhythmia mechanism is unclear.

Digoxin inhibits Na^+, K^+-ATPase, increasing intracellular Na^+ concentrations and stimulating the Na^+-Ca^{2+} exchanger to increase intracellular Ca^{2+}, accounting for its positive inotropic effect. Digoxin also acts through the autonomic nervous system to enhance vagal tone, slowing sinus rates, shortening the atrial refractory period, and prolonging AV conduction. Digoxin is therefore used for rate control in patients with atrial arrhythmias. Renally excreted, digoxin has a narrow therapeutic range. Digoxin toxicity may lead to high-grade AV block, tachyarrhythmias, blurred vision, nausea, dizziness, and severe hyperkalemia.

Cardioversion and Defibrillation

Direct current cardioversion and defibrillation represent the cornerstone of acute therapy for unstable tachyarrhythmias and play an important role in the termination of medication-refractory stable tachyarrhythmias. Organized VTs and SVTs may be terminated by synchronized cardioversion—shock delivery synchronized to the QRS complex—to restore normal rhythm. Synchronization is critical to avoid induction of VF by delivering energy during the relative refractory period of the cardiac cycle. Defibrillation entails the asynchronous delivery of electrical current to depolarize a critical mass of myocardium and terminate VF. Successful defibrillation is time dependent, with the likelihood of success declining by approximately 10% per minute from the onset of VF.

Defibrillation may be delivered internally through an implantable cardioverter-defibrillator (ICD) or externally through an automatic external defibrillator (AED). Current-generation AEDs use biphasic waveforms, achieving greater first-shock efficacy compared with older devices delivering monophasic waveforms. ICDs, implanted in patients for primary and secondary prevention of sudden cardiac death (SCD), deliver defibrillation shocks directly to the endocardium through an RV lead. With direct delivery of energy, relatively lower energy levels (<40 J) are typically effective.

Ablation

Catheter ablation plays an important role in the therapy of a broad range of arrhythmias, such as SVT, atrial arrhythmias, and VT. The ascendance of catheter ablation derives in part from the poor efficacy and side effect profiles of available antiarrhythmic drugs. Radiofrequency ablation (i.e., applying radiofrequency-range energy) and cryoablation (i.e., administering freezing temperatures, to produce localized cellular and tissue injury) are commonly used.

Focal and reentrant arrhythmias are defined and localized, permitting targeted delivery of ablation energy to eliminate the tachyarrhythmia. Ablation is associated with varied success and complication rates, depending on the mechanism and location of the arrhythmogenic focus. Cure rates for typical tricuspid-caval isthmus–dependent atrial flutter, AV nodal reentry tachycardia (AVNRT), and accessory pathway–mediated tachycardias exceed 95%, with low complication rates of about 2%. Although an important therapeutic option in the treatment of AF and VT, success rates are lower and procedural risks are higher.

For a deeper discussion on this topic, please see Chapter 56, ❖ "Approach to the Patient with Suspected Arrhythmia," in *Goldman-Cecil Medicine,* 26th Edition.

BRADYCARDIA

Bradycardia, defined as a heart rate of less than 60 beats per minute, may occur as a consequence of physiologic adaptations or pathology. Bradycardia always results from failure of sinus node function or AV conduction disturbances, or both processes. Clinically significant bradycardia or pauses may result from autonomic disturbances, drugs, chronic intrinsic conduction system disease, or acute cardiac damage as occurs with endocarditis or infarction.

Normal Conduction System: Anatomy and Physiology

Because of the normal gradient of intrinsic automaticity, heart rate usually is determined by intrinsic automaticity of the sinus node. The sinus node is a complex of cells that extends from the superior vena cava and along the upper right atrial free wall in the sulcus terminalis. Blood supply is derived from the sinus node artery, which arises from the right coronary in 66% or left coronary in 34% of patients.

Activation proceeds through the right atrium to the AV node, which is located in the low interatrial septum adjacent to the tricuspid annulus. The AV node is a complex structure with at least three preferential atrial insertions. The anterior atrial insertion has a short conduction time and usually determines the normal AV conduction time in sinus rhythm. The posterior right and left atrial insertions have long conduction times. Because they do not normally mediate

AV conduction in humans, they are functionally vestigial. However, the posterior slowly conducting insertions become important in mediating paroxysmal supraventricular tachycardia (PSVT). The AV node derives its blood supply from the AV nodal artery, which is supplied by the right coronary artery in 73% or the left coronary artery in 27% of patients.

After entry into the AV node, conduction proceeds to the His bundle through the fibrous annulus and along the membranous septum before splitting into a leftward Purkinje branch, the left bundle, which ramifies over the left ventricular endocardium, and a rightward branch, the right bundle, which similarly ramifies over the RV endocardium. The leftward branch may be damaged proximally, resulting in full left bundle branch block, or damaged more distally in its anterior or posterior divisions, resulting in fascicular hemiblock patterns.

Normal Autonomic Regulation of Heart Rate

Normal heart rate is a consequence of tonic and phasic autonomic modulation of intrinsic sinus node automaticity. The intrinsic heart rate in the absence of autonomic modulation ranges from 85 to 110 beats per minute and is somewhat faster than normal resting heart rates. That the normal heart rate is slower than the intrinsic rate is a consequence of the dominance of parasympathetic tone over adrenergic tone in the resting state.

Based on a review of Holter recordings in a normal population, the normal resting heart rate is 46 to 93 beats per minute in men and 51 to 95 beats per minute in women. It has been proposed that 50 to 90 is a clinically more accurate working definition of normal heart rate for adults than the traditional 60 to 100 beats per minute commonly used by consensus. However, heart rates well below these estimates may be seen in normal people, especially during hours of sleep. For these reasons, defining a cutoff value for pathologic bradycardia in the absence of symptoms is problematic for an otherwise healthy patient.

The maximal stress-induced heart rate (HR_{max}) is related to maximal sympathetic stimulation, accompanied by withdrawal of parasympathetic tone. This is commonly estimated as $HR_{max} = (220 - age)$.

Sinus Node Dysfunction

Sick sinus syndrome, also called *sinus node dysfunction,* is a common clinical syndrome that increases in prevalence with age. The estimated prevalence is 1 case per 600 patients older than 65 years of age, and it accounts for about one half of all pacemaker implantations. Sinus node dysfunction is a consequence of two distinct processes: failure of intrinsic automaticity and failure of propagation of sinus node impulses to the surrounding atrial tissue, also referred to a *sinus node exit block.*

Sinus node dysfunction manifests clinically as one of several patterns: persistent or episodic sinus bradycardia, inability to appropriately augment rate with exercise (i.e., chronotropic incompetence), sinus pauses, or commonly a combination of these patterns. The sinus node is at the top of a cascade of automaticity and is normally backed up by a competent AV junctional escape mechanism. Severe bradycardia and associated symptoms due to sinus node dysfunction always imply sinus node dysfunction and simultaneous failure of normal subsidiary escape mechanisms. In the setting of a competent escape mechanism, even severe sinus node dysfunction may be completely asymptomatic, clinically well tolerated, and require no specific therapy.

Resting Sinus Bradycardia

Sinus bradycardia is frequently observed during routine clinical practice. Modest sinus bradycardia in the high 40s in men and 50s in women is normal and called *bradycardia* only because of the conventional choice of 60 beats per minute as the lower limit of normal rates.

Because there is no set rate at which sinus bradycardia can be labeled as pathologic, pathologic sinus node dysfunction is best defined as significant bradycardia associated with symptoms plausibly attributable to bradycardia.

Modest persistent bradycardia is often asymptomatic. When symptoms occur, they are commonly nonspecific, such as fatigue, listlessness, or dyspnea, making the attribution of symptoms to resting bradycardia difficult. Sinus bradycardia may also exacerbate congestive heart failure and limit effective use of β-blocker therapy, a cornerstone of therapy for heart failure, coronary disease, and tachyarrhythmias. When inappropriate sinus bradycardia is persistent, especially when severe, plausible symptoms are present, and alternative causes of symptoms have been excluded, pacemaker implantation is reasonable. Asymptomatic sinus bradycardia should rarely be treated with pacing unless a need for medical therapy is expected to further exacerbate bradycardia.

Chronotropic Incompetence

Cardiac output during exercise is increased by augmentation in stroke volume and an increase in heart rate. If heart rate rise with exercise is inadequate, exertional symptoms such as fatigue or dyspnea may ensue. As in the case of resting sinus bradycardia, unless severe, attribution of symptoms to chronotropic incompetence is difficult. Various criteria for this condition have been proposed that rely on the inability to achieve a set fraction of age-predicted heart rate or heart rate reserve. As for resting sinus bradycardia, the decision to implant a pacemaker for chronotropic incompetence is a matter of judgment more than criteria.

Sinus Pauses or Arrest

An abrupt failure of sinus node automaticity or failure of propagation from the sinus node to the atrium can result in a pause in atrial activity. P waves are absent, and if of adequate duration and not accompanied by a competent subsidiary escape mechanism, it can result in abrupt symptoms of lightheadedness, presyncope or true syncope. Sinus pauses of less than 3 seconds are commonly seen for normal subjects, who are rarely symptomatic. Sinus pauses exceeding 3 seconds and not occurring during sleep are often pathologic and may result in symptoms. Sinus pauses associated with simultaneous symptoms and documentation of pauses lasting 3 seconds or longer in patients with a history of symptoms plausibly related to bradycardia are indications for pacemaker therapy.

Sinoatrial Exit Block

Sinus node dysfunction is often accompanied by significant atrial fibrosis, which may lead to a block in the tissues surrounding the sinus node complex and impede propagation to the atrial tissue. Bradycardia due to sinus node dysfunction may result, not from a failure of automaticity, but from failure of propagation from the sinus node complex to the atrium. Because sinus node activity is not directly apparent from the surface ECG, the diagnosis is made indirectly by the observation of abrupt halving in the sinus P-wave rate, followed by an abrupt return to the baseline sinus rate (Fig. 9.3C and D). Although other patterns may be observed, 2:1 exit block is the most common. Therapy for sinoatrial exit block is identical to that for intermittent sinus bradycardia (discussed earlier).

Bradycardia-Tachycardia Syndrome as a Consequence of Sinus Node Dysfunction

Bradycardia-tachycardia ("brady-tachy") syndrome refers to a clinically significant tachyarrhythmia sometimes accompanied by clinically significant bradycardia. The term may be confusing because the mechanism of tachycardia is often unrelated to the mechanism of bradycardia.

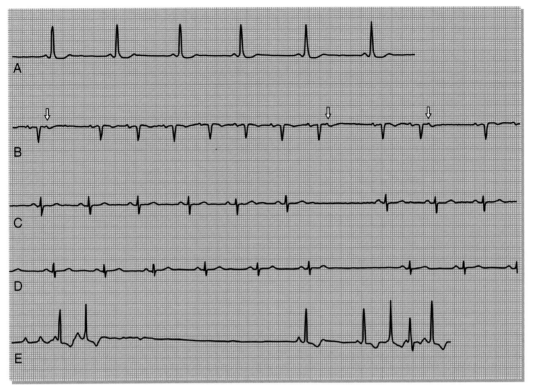

Fig. 9.3 Sinus node dysfunction. (A) Sinus bradycardia in a patient receiving metoprolol. This bradycardia results from diminished normal automaticity of the sinus node. (B) Pauses related to blocked premature atrial contractions (PACs). Blocked PACs are a common cause for apparent sinus pauses because the PAC may be early enough to be concealed by the T wave of the preceding beat *(arrows)*. The pauses are not a sign of sinus node dysfunction but rather a physiologic response to an early coupled PAC. (C) The sinus pause is an abnormal finding that suggests sinus node disease. The pause is exactly two sinus cycles and may represent sinoatrial exit block. (D) Sinoatrial Wenckebach type exit block. As is the case with the RR interval preceding atrioventricular nodal Wenckebach, progressive shortening of the PP interval preceding a doubling in sinus cycle length likely represents Wenckebach exit block from the sinus node tissue to the atrium. (E) Bradycardia-tachycardia syndrome due to sinus node dysfunction. An episode of rapidly conducted atrial fibrillation or flutter terminates and is followed for a protracted period of sinus arrest before recovery of sinus rhythm and ultimate relapse of rapidly conducted atrial fibrillation. These pauses may result in syncope or near-syncope.

This syndrome most commonly manifests as intermittent pathologic atrial arrhythmias, often intermittent AF with concomitant sinus node dysfunction resulting in long pauses or symptomatic sinus bradycardia when the patient is in sinus rhythm. A typical manifestation of this syndrome is a prolonged period of asystole after termination of AF (see Fig. 9.3E) due to slow recovery of sinus node automaticity with resultant presyncope or syncope.

The combination of two seemingly independent processes is in part a consequence of the high prevalence of AF and sinus node dysfunction in the elderly and the need to use potent drugs to decrease ventricular response during AF with resultant unintended secondary sinus node dysfunction between periods of atrial arrhythmias. This type of bradycardia-tachycardia syndrome represents an important form of clinical sinus node dysfunction and is a common indication for pacemaker implantation.

Sinus node dysfunction causing bradycardia-tachycardia should be distinguished from a common, unrelated form of bradycardia-tachycardia syndrome, which is characterized by chronic rather than intermittent AF with periods of rapid and slow ventricular responses. This condition is often incorrectly referred to as *sick sinus syndrome*. However, in this syndrome, the atrium is chronically fibrillating, and the sinus node therefore has no influence on heart rate. Bradycardia or protracted pauses in the setting of chronic AF is a consequence of impaired AV conduction and is unrelated to sinus node dysfunction.

Atrioventricular Conduction Disturbances

AV conduction disturbances include disorders in which the normal physiologic AV relationship is not maintained due to pathologic delay in AV conduction or to intermittent or complete loss of AV conduction. The PR interval includes three distinct phases of AV conduction. Although the individual components of AV conduction can be readily recorded by a His bundle catheter in an electrophysiology laboratory, the salient features of AV conduction disturbances can usually be elucidated by careful interpretation of the surface ECG without resorting to invasive recording techniques.

The right atrial conduction time from the area of the sinus node where the P wave begins to the region of the AV node occupies a short first portion of the PR interval and usually lasts no more than 30 milliseconds. Because the atrial conduction time is short and does not change much over time in a given patient, it can conveniently be ignored when assessing AV conduction. The second portion of the PR interval is the propagation time through the AV node, which is normally 50 to 120 milliseconds. The last component of the PR interval is the time for propagation through the His bundle and bundle branches, which is typically 30 to 55 milliseconds. Although this last portion, constituting His-Purkinje conduction, is short, it is the major prognostic component of AV conduction and therefore clinically important. Because the last portion of the PR interval is the time from the onset

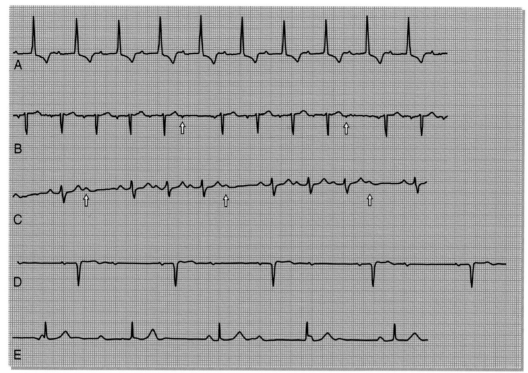

Fig. 9.4 Heart block. (A) First-degree atrioventricular (AV) block is associated with 1:1 conduction but a pro-longed PR interval more than 200 milliseconds. (B) Mobitz type I (Wenckebach) second-degree AV block. Notice the progressive PR prolongation preceding the blocked P wave *(arrows)* followed by recovery of conduction with a shorter PR interval before repetition of the same pattern. (C) Mobitz type II second-degree AV block. Notice that the PR interval does not prolong in the beat preceding the blocked P wave *(arrows)*. (D) A 2:1 second-degree AV block. Notice that every other P wave fails to conduct. Because there are never two consecutively conducted P waves to assess for the presence or absence of progressive prolongation, this type of block is neither Mobitz I nor Mobitz II. (E) Complete heart block with a junctional escape rhythm. Notice that the atrial rate is faster than the ventricular rate and that there is AV dissociation. The narrow QRS escape rhythm implies a level of block high in the conduction system near the AV node.

of His bundle to the time of ventricular activation, it is commonly referred to as the HV interval. Although the HV interval cannot be measured directly from the surface ECG, a block in the His-Purkinje system can be inferred from the characteristic features that can be gleaned from review of the surface ECG.

First-Degree Atrioventricular Block

First-degree AV block is defined as a PR interval exceeding 0.2 seconds (200 milliseconds) in the setting of otherwise preserved AV conduction (Fig. 9.4A). First-degree block implies a conduction delay in one of the components of AV conduction, usually at the level of the AV node or His-Purkinje system (i.e., infranodal conduction system). First-degree AV block is usually asymptomatic, but it is a sign of AV conduction system disease and may be a diagnostic clue to the mechanism of intermittent electrocardiographically undocumented symptoms in a patient with unexplained syncope.

Second-Degree Atrioventricular Block

Second-degree AV block is defined as intermittent failure of AV conduction with interspersed periods of intact AV conduction. Second-degree AV block, like sinus bradycardia and pauses, may be seen normally during hours of sleep as well as in athletes with high parasympathetic tone. Alone, it is not an indication of AV conduction system disease.

Second-degree block may be asymptomatic, may be associated with mild symptoms such as palpitations, or if resulting in protracted

pauses or persistent bradycardia, may result in hemodynamic symptoms, including lightheadedness, syncope, and fatigue. Second-degree AV block at the level of the AV node is usually indolent and gradually progressive. Because of stable junctional escape mechanisms associated with progression to complete heart block at the level of the AV node, second-degree AV block at this level tends to have a benign prognosis and, in the absence of symptoms, can be followed safely without intervention.

Second-degree block in the infranodal conduction system, which is composed of the His bundle and bundle branches, can be malignant with a tendency to progress abruptly and unpredictably to higher degrees of AV block accompanied by unstable or absent subsidiary escape mechanisms. After a patient becomes symptomatic, the infranodal block may progress to complete heart block and, in some cases, to sudden death. Despite its malignant nature, SCD is rarely attributable to complete heart block, suggesting that most patients have symptoms permitting intervention before progression to sudden death.

Because of the profound difference in natural history of second-degree AV block at the AV node and that at an infranodal level, the major clinical task in evaluating patients with second-degree AV block is to establish the probable level of the block. The surface ECG and pattern of block are quite useful.

Mobitz type I second-degree atrioventricular block. Also referred to a Wenckebach block, *Mobitz type I second-degree AV block* is a progressive prolongation in the PR interval before development of AV block, usually for one cycle followed by recovery of conduction with a return to the baseline PR interval (see Fig. 9.4B). Because the degree of prolongation of the PR interval is less with each successive beat before the block, the RR intervals can paradoxically shorten in the final beats before the block.

Mobitz I AV block typically is associated with block at the level of the AV node. However, this pattern is rarely seen with advanced infranodal disease in the His bundle and bundle branches. Because Mobitz type I AV block usually occurs at the level of the AV node, infranodal conduction is commonly normal and associated with a narrow conducted QRS complex. In ambiguous cases, other clues may be helpful. Because AV node function is improved with exercise, Mobitz I block tends to normalize with activity and return at rest. Second-degree block at the level of the AV node is improved with atropine and exacerbated by carotid sinus massage. If associated with periods of complete heart block, a block at the level of the AV node is associated with a junctional escape with a QRS morphology similar to that in conducted sinus rhythm. In contrast, the observation of a wide complex escape that is different from the conducted QRS points to infranodal causes of block in the His-Purkinje system. The block may be malignant (discussed later) and require expeditious use of ventricular pacing to prevent catastrophic bradycardia.

Mobitz type II second-degree atrioventricular block. Mobitz *type II second-degree AV block* is intermittent failure of AV conduction during stable atrial rates without antecedent PR prolongation and followed by recovery of AV conduction (see Fig. 9.4C). Mobitz II AV block is believed to always be a sign of block in the infranodal tissues, including the His bundle and bundle branches. Whereas infranodal block may rarely display Mobitz I (Wenckebach) periodicity, AV block at the level of the AV node does not result in true Mobitz II AV block periodicity.

The finding of Mobitz II AV block is always reason for concern. Although it may result from block in the His bundle or subsidiary bundle branches, block within the His bundle accompanied by a narrow QRS complex is uncommon. In practice, Mobitz II AV block is usually preceded by the development of fixed bundle branch block. It has been believed that such bundle branch block patterns implied disease of the bundle branches themselves as they ramify within the ventricles. However, in many cases of left bundle branch block, the disease process may actually be within the His bundle affecting fibers that will ultimately extend to the left bundle branch. Regardless of the exact anatomic level of clinical bundle branch block, it remains a good clinical rule that most patients exhibiting Mobitz II AV block will also exhibit a full bundle branch block pattern during periods of conduction between episodes of second-degree AV block.

In ambiguous cases, other clues may be helpful. Because infranodal function improves relatively little with exercise, infranodal block tends to worsen with the increasing heart rates associated with exercise or stress. Atropine is not helpful for infranodal block, and because it may accelerate sinus rates, it may cause a patient to progress to higher degrees of AV block with a consequent decrease in the conducted ventricular rate. Exogenous catecholamines such as isoproterenol infusion may be helpful acutely but should not be relied on. Because of its malignant potential, hemodynamically significant Mobitz II AV block should be addressed with early temporary or permanent pacing.

2:1 and High-Grade Atrioventricular Blocks

2:1 AV block is a failure of conduction of every other P wave (see Fig. 9.4D). This pattern is most commonly seen with an infranodal block in the His bundle or bundle branches. However, 2:1 AV block may also be observed in advanced AV nodal disease. It can be distinguished from the more common infranodal form of 2:1 block by the typical Mobitz

I periodicity accompanied by a usually narrow QRS complex at other times in the same patient. Because two consecutive conducted P waves are not available to assess the Mobitz pattern, a 2:1 AV block is neither truly Mobitz I nor Mobitz II, although it is common in clinical practice to describe 2:1 block as Mobitz II.

High-grade AV block is second-degree AV block with conduction failure of two or more consecutive P waves. High-grade AV block is neither Mobitz I nor Mobitz II. Although Mobitz periodicity cannot be assigned, like other forms of second-degree AV blocks, the level of block must be established to assess prognosis and guide therapy. In this case, the ancillary clues described for Mobitz blocks remain useful.

Third-Degree Atrioventricular Block

Third-degree AV block or equivalently complete heart block is a complete failure of AV conduction. In the setting of underlying sinus rhythm, this is an atrial rate faster than the ventricular rate associated with AV dissociation (see Fig. 9.4E). However, when the underlying rhythm is AF, the definition of complete heart block cannot rely on the demonstration of AV dissociation. Because conducted AF always results in an *irregular* ventricular response, the finding of a *regular and slow* ventricular response during AF implies an associated complete heart block.

As is the case for second-degree AV block, the level of the third-degree block determines the clinical behavior and prognosis of complete heart block. Complete heart block at the level of the AV node is associated with a generally stable junctional escape with rates between 40 and 50 beats per minute and usually with a narrow QRS complex. If the patient had a bundle branch block before the development of complete heart block, a block at the level of the AV node is associated with a wide QRS escape, identical to the conducted QRS before the development of a block.

Complete heart block at an infranodal level is associated with a wide and slow ventricular escape rhythm, which often is slower than 40 beats per minute with a QRS different from the antecedent conducted morphology. Unfortunately, infranodal escape rhythms may be absent entirely, leading to asystole and loss of consciousness. When infranodal complete heart block is suspected, regardless of tolerance of the ventricular escape rhythm, prompt institution of temporary or permanent ventricular pacing is appropriate.

TACHYCARDIAS

Overview and Classification

Tachyarrhythmias are categorized as supraventricular and ventricular arrhythmias. SVT relies mechanistically on the atrium, the AV node, or both. During SVT, normal depolarization of the ventricles by the His-Purkinje system typically produces a narrow complex tachycardia. SVT can manifest as a wide-complex tachycardia in the setting of aberrancy with left bundle branch block or right bundle branch block conduction, or antegrade conduction down an accessory pathway, producing an abnormal sequence of ventricular activation. Ventricular tachyarrhythmias do not depend on the atrium or AV node; they originate in the ventricles, generating a wide-complex tachycardia.

Supraventricular Tachycardias

SVTs can be categorized as paroxysmal supraventricular tachycardia (PSVT), focal atrial tachycardia, atrial flutter, and AF. This classification scheme, which addresses the underlying arrhythmic mechanism, clinical presentation, and prognosis, guides evaluation and therapy.

PSVT typically manifests in young patients without structural heart disease. The PSVT syndrome is characterized by recurrent tachypalpitations with abrupt onset and offset. Focal atrial tachycardia is more often observed in patients with underlying atrial enlargement and valvular heart disease. AF and atrial flutter are associated with advancing age, hypertension, structural heart disease, diabetes, obstructive sleep apnea, and pulmonary disease. Unlike PSVT, AF carries an increased risk of stroke, heart failure, and death.

Paroxysmal Supraventricular Tachycardia

The incidence of PSVT is 35 cases per 100,000 person-years, with a prevalence of 2.25 per 1000 person-years. Patients report recurrent tachypalpitations. Associated symptoms may include shortness of breath, lightheadedness, chest pain, and syncope. Anginal chest pain and ischemic ST-segment depression are common and related to increased myocardial oxygen demand coupled with the loss of normal diastolic coronary perfusion time. These findings do not necessarily indicate underlying coronary artery disease and typically resolve with tachycardia termination.

PSVT typically occurs independent of structural heart disease and may manifest at any point from infancy to advanced age. PSVT relies on reentry, which is localized in the AV node in approximately 60% of cases and uses a concealed or manifest accessory pathway in 40%. Unless a delta wave indicative of WPW is identified, the underlying mechanism of PSVT may not be apparent on initial clinical presentation.

An ECG obtained during PSVT can provide useful clues to establish the diagnosis and guide management. The AV relationship should be assessed during tachycardia. By ascertaining the relationship of the P wave to the preceding QRS complex, it is possible to classify PSVT as a short RP tachycardia or a long RP tachycardia. Short RP tachycardias demonstrate a short RP pattern with P waves embedded within or occurring closely after the preceding QRS complex. Short RP tachycardias occur with reentrant SVT when the retrograde VA conduction time is shorter than the antegrade AV conduction time. This pattern is observed in the two most common forms of PSVT: typical AV nodal reentry tachycardia and reciprocating AV tachycardia related to an accessory pathway.

Long RP tachycardias are characterized by an RP interval that is longer than the next PR interval during tachycardia. This pattern occurs when the retrograde VA conduction time in reentrant arrhythmias is long due to a slowly conducting retrograde pathway during tachycardia. Atypical AV node reentry, in which retrograde conduction occurs over the slow AV nodal pathway, is the most common example of a long RP reentrant tachycardia.

Atrioventricular nodal reentry tachycardia. AVNRT is the most common form of PSVT. The arrhythmic mechanism depends on two distinct pathways in the AV node: a slowly conducting pathway with a short effective refractory period (i.e., slow pathway) and a rapidly conducting pathway with a longer refractory period (i.e., fast pathway). The fast pathway is located anteriorly near the bundle of His, and the slow pathway posteriorly near the coronary sinus ostium. Although dual pathways are a common feature of the AV node, patients with clinical tachycardia have more robust slow pathway conduction.

Tachycardia is most commonly triggered by a premature atrial contraction that blocks in the fast pathway due to its prolonged refractory period and conducts slowly antegrade down the slow pathway, producing a long PR interval on the ECG. On reaching the distal common pathway where the fast and slow AV nodal inputs meet, if the fast pathway is no longer refractory, the impulse may penetrate the fast pathway in a retrograde direction and rapidly activate the atrium, producing a short RP interval and reinitiating reentry down the slow pathway and up the fast pathway. In typical slow-fast AVNRT, the RP interval is so short that the P wave is often buried in the preceding QRS complex (Fig. 9.5A).

Atypical fast-slow AVNRT may occur with antegrade conduction over the fast pathway and retrograde conduction over the slow pathway. This form of AVNRT is uncommon and produces a long RP pattern on the ECG with characteristically deeply inverted retrograde P waves in leads II, III, and aVF.

Vagal maneuvers cause temporary AV nodal blockade and may terminate sustained AVNRT. Alternatively, intravenous adenosine is a highly effective acute therapy. The need for chronic or definitive therapy is determined by symptoms, arrhythmia frequency, and patient preference. Catheter ablation of the slow pathway at the posterior AV node is highly successful, eliminating AVNRT with a greater than 95% success rate and a low risk of complications. Drug therapy with β-blockers and calcium-channel blockers directed at the AV node may be helpful for chronic suppression. Occasionally, class IC and III antiarrhythmics may be required. AVNRT should be easily distinguished from automatic junctional tachycardia, with a narrow complex and rapid, irregular rhythm typically demonstrating AV dissociation (see Fig. 9.5B).

Reciprocating atrioventricular tachycardia and preexcitation syndromes. Congenital anomalous extranodal AV muscle fibers or accessory pathways may arise as a consequence of incomplete development of the AV annulus. These pathways are usually observed in patients with otherwise anatomically normal hearts, although right-sided accessory pathways are infrequently associated with Ebstein's anomaly and left-sided accessory pathways with hypertrophic cardiomyopathy.

Accessory pathways, or bypass tracts, may conduct antegrade, retrograde, or bidirectionally. They typically fail to demonstrate decremental conduction or the slowed conduction with increasingly frequent stimulation that characterizes the AV node. Accessory pathways capable of antegrade conduction produce early activation of the ventricle in sinus rhythm because conduction over the accessory pathway surpasses conduction over the AV node. The relatively rapid AV conduction produces a shortened PR interval, and eccentric ventricular activation over the pathway slurs the QRS onset, resulting in a delta wave (see Fig. 9.5C). If the accessory pathway is capable only of retrograde conduction, the baseline ECG in sinus rhythm does not show evidence of an accessory pathway, and the extranodal AV connection is called *concealed*.

Short PR intervals during sinus rhythm are also observed in patients with Lown-Ganong-Levine syndrome. These patients have a normal-appearing QRS complex without a delta wave because ventricular activation occurs through the His-Purkinje system (see Fig. 9.5D).

Whether accessory pathways are concealed or manifest, the most common associated arrhythmia is *orthodromic AV reentrant tachycardia* (AVRT). Tachycardia is mediated by antegrade conduction down the AV node to the ventricle and subsequent retrograde conduction up the accessory pathway to activate the atrium, then antegrade again down the AV node. Because the ventricles are activated during tachycardia exclusively over the AV node, the resulting tachycardia is typically a narrow complex unless aberrancy occurs (see Fig. 9.5E). A short RP pattern is observed on the ECG, although the RP is slightly longer than commonly observed in a typical AVNRT. Because the atria and ventricles constitute portions of the reentrant circuit, tachycardia depends on 1:1 AV conduction.

Less frequently, *antidromic AV reentrant tachycardia* is seen in patients with accessory pathways capable of antegrade conduction. The accessory pathway provides the antegrade limb of the reentrant circuit, and the AV node serves as the retrograde pathway, resulting in a wide QRS tachycardia due to complete preexcitation of the ventricles, or activation of the ventricles entirely over the accessory pathway.

Special considerations for patients with supraventricular tachycardia and delta waves in sinus rhythm. Asymptomatic patients may have delta waves on the ECG, which is called a *WPW pattern*. Prevalence

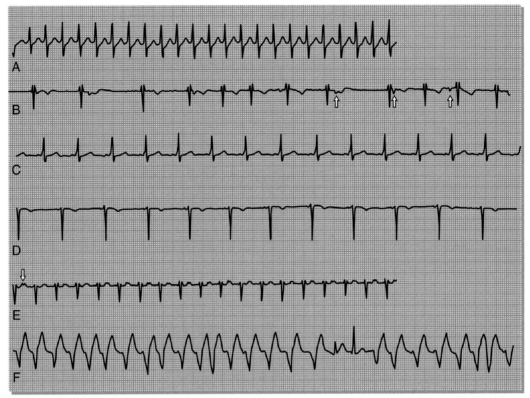

Fig. 9.5 Atrioventricular (AV) nodal (junctional) rhythm disturbances. (A) Supraventricular tachycardia. The lack of visible P waves during tachycardia suggests that they are concealed within the QRS complex, a pattern indicative of underlying AV nodal reentrant tachycardia. (B) Automatic junctional tachycardia. Notice the AV dissociation during tachycardia. The P waves *(arrows)* are dissociated from the QRS complexes. (C) Sinus rhythm with a short PR interval due to the presence of delta waves in a patient with Wolff-Parkinson-White (WPW) syndrome. The slurred QRS upstroke of the delta wave results from early activation of the ventricle by the extranodal bypass tract, followed by fusion with rapid conduction down the normal conduction system and resulting in narrowing of the terminal QRS. (D) Sinus rhythm with a short PR interval but no delta waves. Despite the short PR, the P wave is normally vectored, excluding a junctional rhythm that appears similar but with an inverted P wave. A short PR interval in sinus rhythm without delta waves is caused by an abnormally rapid AV nodal conduction and is described as a Lown-Ganong-Levine pattern. (E) Supraventricular tachycardia. Unlike tracing A, there is a clear P wave *(arrow)* inscribed immediately after each QRS in the ST segment. This pattern is seen most commonly with orthodromic AV reciprocating tachycardia in a patient with WPW syndrome. The early P wave in WPW is caused by retrograde conduction up the accessory pathway after ventricular activation during tachycardia. (F) Preexcited atrial fibrillation (AF) in a patient with WPW syndrome. Notice the rapid and irregular ventricular response with widening of the QRS due to preexcitation. This pattern results from rapid conduction of the AF down the accessory pathway, bypassing the normal conduction system. As in this arrhythmia, occasional conduction down the AV node may occur during ongoing tachycardia, resulting in periods with a narrow QRS complex.

of the WPW pattern in the general population is approximately 1 case per 1000 people. Accessory pathways may be poorly conducting and less likely to promote tachycardia, accounting for the absence of symptoms. These patients have a favorable prognosis, particularly if spontaneous and abrupt cessation of ECG preexcitation (delta wave) occurs with exercise or during ambulatory monitoring. In many cases, no specific therapy is required for asymptomatic patients.

Asymptomatic young patients participating in high-risk activities with WPW pattern may be subjected to invasive electrophysiologic testing for risk stratification. Patients with delta waves demonstrating clinical SVT or suggestive arrhythmic symptoms are said to have WPW syndrome, and invasive electrophysiologic testing is ordinarily recommended in these patients. Invasive testing helps to stratify the risk of sudden cardiac death.

Curative ablation is highly effective, with a success rate of 95%, and poses a low risk of procedural complications. Chronic therapy with

antiarrhythmic drugs that prolong the accessory pathway refractory period (i.e., class IA, IC, or III agents) may be effective, but the potential for adverse drug effects has made accessory pathway ablation the treatment of choice for symptomatic and high-risk patients.

The use of agents that slow AV nodal conduction in patients with WPW syndrome warrants special mention. Digoxin, β-blockers, and calcium-channel blockers should not be used in patients with WPW because they slow conduction through the AV node, resulting in preferential excitation of the ventricles over the accessory pathway. In the setting of AF or atrial flutter, this may cause rapid ventricular rates and hemodynamic instability.

Wolff-Parkinson-White syndrome and atrial fibrillation. WPW syndrome is associated with a 0.25% per year risk of sudden cardiac death (SCD), which is related to the development of AF with rapid antegrade conduction over the accessory pathway producing VF. This risk is greatest for patients demonstrating very short preexcited RR

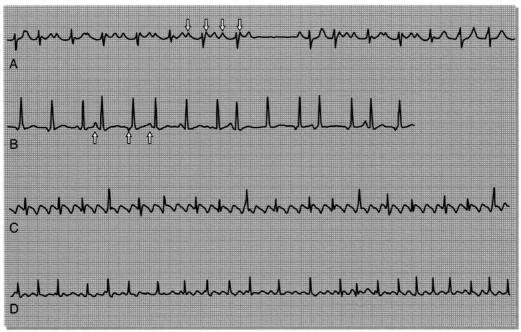

Fig. 9.6 Atrial arrhythmias. (A) Runs of focal atrial tachycardia with variable atrioventricular (AV) block. The tachycardia occurs in salvos with interspersed periods of sinus rhythm. The P waves *(arrows)* during tachycardia appear uniform although their cycle length varies, resulting in variable patterns of AV conduction and an irregular ventricular rate. (B) Multifocal atrial tachycardia. Notice the incessant atrial premature beats *(arrows)* with at least three distinct morphologies. Because of the irregularly irregular response, this arrhythmia can be easily misdiagnosed as atrial fibrillation (which lacks discrete P waves) if the tracing is not carefully reviewed. (C) Atrial flutter with rapid, variable conduction. Notice the continuous sawtooth atrial activity. Although commonly manifesting with stable 2:1 block and a regular response, the block varies in this patient, progressing through periods of 2:1 and 3:1 ratios and resulting in an irregular ventricular response. (D) Atrial fibrillation with a rapid ventricular response. Notice the wavering baseline without distinct P waves and an irregularly irregular response.

intervals during AF. For some WPW patients, SCD may be the initial presentation. Successful catheter ablation of the accessory pathway eliminates this possibility.

Patients with WPW and rapidly conducted AF have the characteristic electrocardiographic findings of a rapid, irregularly irregular, wide QRS rhythm with various degrees of QRS widening or preexcitation from beat to beat (see Fig. 9.5F). During AF in the setting of underlying WPW, activation of the ventricle over the AV node produces concealed retrograde activation of the accessory pathway, prolonging the refractory period of the pathway and moderating the rate of antegrade accessory pathway conduction.

Treating patients with AV nodal–blocking therapy decreases concealed retrograde activation of the pathway, facilitating antegrade accessory pathway conduction and potentiating hemodynamic instability. Appropriate acute therapy includes drugs that prolong the accessory pathway refractory period, such as intravenous procainamide, ibutilide, or amiodarone. In the event of hemodynamic instability, electrical cardioversion is preferred.

Role of catheter ablation in Wolff-Parkinson-White syndrome. Catheter ablation is highly effective for treating WPW, with success rates of approximately 95% and recurrence rates of only 5%. Procedural complications are uncommon, with major complications occurring in 2% to 4% of cases and deaths related to ablation occurring in 0.1%.

Although antiarrhythmic drug therapy may control symptoms, the expense and risks of pharmacologic therapy along with the safety and efficacy of ablation have made radiofrequency ablation the first-line therapy for symptomatic WPW. Because older patients with asymptomatic WPW patterns have a favorable prognosis, they should not routinely be subjected to ablation.

Atrial Arrhythmias
Overview and Classification
Atrial arrhythmias depend entirely on the atria but are mechanistically independent of AV conduction. As a consequence, intra-atrial arrhythmias persist despite the development of spontaneous or pharmacologically induced AV block. Tachycardias originating in the atria may be organized and repetitive, resulting from automaticity or intra-atrial reentry, or may be chaotic and disorganized, as is the case in AF. Therapy is directed at moderating the ventricular response during episodes of tachycardia or suppressing the underlying atrial arrhythmia.

Focal arrhythmias originate from a point source in one of the atria, and circumferential spread encompasses the remainder of the atrium. These arrhythmias display distinct P waves separated by a clear isoelectric segment. Focal arrhythmias commonly have an automatic mechanism, but in some cases, they may result from micro-reentry involving an anatomically small portion of the atrium (e.g., around a single pulmonary vein), followed by radial spread to the rest of the atrium. Although most commonly a single abnormal focus may be active, in the setting of severe physiologic stress, multiple foci may be active simultaneously, leading to a chaotic electrocardiographic appearance with multiple distinct P waves, referred to as *multifocal atrial tachycardia* (MAT) (Fig. 9.6B). Automatic arrhythmias tend to be episodic and nonsustained, sometimes recurring incessantly. Cycle length often varies within a run, between runs, and with changes in autonomic tone.

Macro-reentrant atrial arrhythmias are a consequence of stable reentrant circuits, which encompass large portions of the atria. All such circuits require a central obstacle and a region of slowed atrial conduction related to atrial dilation or fibrosis. The most common of these arrhythmias is *typical atrial flutter,* which is mediated by right atrial reentry around normal anatomic obstacles. In addition to typical flutter, reentry may occur around acquired obstacles, most commonly scars resulting from prior cardiac surgery or ablation involving the atria. Reentrant arrhythmias tend to manifest clinically as paroxysmal sustained or persistent arrhythmias. Although they may be self-terminating and episodic, individual episodes tend to be protracted.

The final mechanism of atrial arrhythmia is AF. This arrhythmia involves components of focal automatic mechanisms and reentry. The major advances made in the understanding and management of this common arrhythmia are reviewed in the following sections.

Focal Atrial Tachycardia

Focal atrial tachycardia also is referred to as ectopic atrial tachycardia and automatic atrial tachycardia. These terms describe a characteristic clinical pattern that usually manifests as runs of unifocal PACs lasting for seconds or minutes, usually followed by spontaneous termination and subsequent spontaneous reinitiation of additional salvos of tachycardia (see Fig. 9.6A). This arrhythmia less commonly manifests as a paroxysmal sustained tachycardia. When mapped in the electrophysiologic laboratory, these arrhythmias have a focal origin, and although they are sometimes triggered by rapid pacing, suggesting triggered activity, they appear to be automatic rather than a reentrant mechanism.

The electrocardiographic features are characteristic and usually permit accurate diagnosis. Because the arrhythmia is focal and automatic, the morphology of the first PAC of the run is identical to the subsequent PACs. Cycle length tends to vary between and within runs, and tachycardia is unaffected by intermittent AV block, which may occur during the runs. The same focus often fires erratically between runs, resulting in frequent atrial ectopy that is morphologically similar to the P wave observed during the runs.

The arrhythmia appears to be caused by intracellular calcium overload and resultant triggered activity related to delayed afterdepolarizations, making it responsive to calcium-channel blockers and β-blockers. The paroxysmal sustained form of this arrhythmia is also adenosine responsive, giving the false impression of dependence on AV conduction. The use of digoxin may exacerbate triggered causes of atrial tachycardia. Class IC agents, such as flecainide and propafenone, may be useful in patients without structural heart disease or coronary artery disease. Amiodarone can also be used in these patients for rhythm control. The arrhythmia is readily amenable to catheter ablation if ectopy occurs frequently enough to permit mapping.

Typical Atrial Flutter

Atrial flutter is a persistent atrial arrhythmia with an atrial rate of at least 250 beats per minute (see Fig. 9.6C). Because the normal AV node cannot conduct 1:1 at these rates, this arrhythmia characteristically manifests with 2:1 conduction and a ventricular response of about 140 to 150 beats per minute. During 2:1 conduction, the difficulty in perceiving flutter waves may lead to diagnostic confusion. Typical atrial flutter is the most common form of this arrhythmia, and it is mediated by macro-reentry restricted to the right atrium. The central obstacles in this circuit consist of normal anatomic structures, accounting for its stereotyped pattern.

Typical atrial flutter is mediated by counterclockwise reentry around the tricuspid valve as viewed from the ventricle. The valve prevents anterior collapse of the circuit, and posteriorly a long ridge in

the atrial wall (i.e., crista terminalis) forms a functional line of block, preventing the circuit from collapsing posteriorly. Because the normal obstacles already exist, flutter development results from the abnormally slowed conduction related to atrial enlargement, fibrosis, or edema, which sometimes is combined with shortened atrial refractory periods due to catecholamine stress. Typical counterclockwise atrial flutter demonstrates a deeply negative F wave in leads II, III, and aVF; a sharply positive F wave in V_1; and a negative F wave in V_6.

A less common reversed form of this arrhythmia is caused by clockwise reentry around the tricuspid valve. It demonstrates an ECG exactly opposite to the counterclockwise form, with a strongly positive F wave in leads II, III, and aVF; a sharply negative F wave in V_1; and a positive F wave in V_6. In both cases, the F waves are often difficult to perceive because of 2:1 conduction. If the unusual F-wave vector is not recognized, the ECG may be misinterpreted as sinus tachycardia. Clues to identification of atrial flutter are persistent, unexplained heart rates of about 150 beats per minute with a variation of only a few beats per minute over time and the finding of a negative P wave in the inferior leads, which is expected to be positive in sinus rhythm.

The most fruitful method of diagnosis is the provocation of transient AV block with carotid sinus massage or adenosine infusion. This transiently exposes the underlying flutter waves but does not terminate the arrhythmia.

Although acute therapy involves rate control or cardioversion if drugs are poorly tolerated, long-term rate control for this arrhythmia is difficult. Drug doses that result in acceptable block at rest often fail to control exercise rates, and doses that result in exercise rate control often provoke bradycardia at rest. Early restoration of sinus rhythm is preferred for this arrhythmia.

Atrial flutter is a common transient arrhythmia in acute care hospital settings. The right atrial wall is thin, and pericarditis resulting from cardiac or thoracic surgery results in atrial edema and inflammation that may permit adequate slowing and promote transient atrial flutter. Acute pulmonary decompensation may result in right heart failure and may promote transient atrial flutter. In all of these settings, endogenous or pharmacologic catecholamine stimulation exacerbates the arrhythmia. Transient therapy for up to a month is appropriate in these settings.

When atrial flutter occurs in the absence of an acute precipitant, long-term therapy is required. Given the difficulty of achieving rate control in atrial flutter and the need for antiarrhythmic agents with associated potential morbidity to maintain sinus rhythm, catheter ablation has become the primary means of treating this arrhythmia. Antiarrhythmic therapy for atrial flutter is similar to that for AF (discussed later). Antiarrhythmic drug therapy should be reserved for temporary treatment of likely transient flutter or for patients who are not suitable candidates for invasive management. Catheter ablation of typical atrial flutter is a low-risk procedure with a long-term success rate exceeding 90% in experienced centers.

Atypical Atrial Flutter and Macro-Reentrant Atrial Tachycardia

In addition to the typical atrial flutter circulating around normal anatomic obstacles, atrial disease with associated fibrosis or, more commonly, atrial scars created at the time of prior catheter or surgical ablation or cardiac surgery for valvular or congenital heart disease may create alternative substrates for intra-atrial reentry. Common to these arrhythmias is a significant region of scar with a channel of surviving myocardium bridging the scar or between the scar and a normal anatomic obstacle. Within the channel, conduction is slow and electrocardiographically silent, resulting in an isoelectric PP interval. Because the circuit is different from that of typical atrial flutter, the P-wave morphology is atypical.

When the rate is 250 beats per minute or greater, the arrhythmia is arbitrarily classified as atypical atrial flutter, and when the rate is less than 250 beats per minute, it is arbitrarily classified as atrial tachycardia. Like typical atrial flutter, these arrhythmias are paroxysmal sustained or persistent arrhythmias, and when manifesting with 2:1 conduction, they may be misdiagnosed as sinus tachycardia if the abnormal P-wave vector and fixed heart rate over time are not recognized. Therapy and prognosis are otherwise similar to those for typical atrial flutter.

Atrial Fibrillation
Overview and Classification
AF is a chaotic atrial rhythm related to continuous and variable activation of the atria. There are no distinct P waves or periods of atrial quiescence. It is characterized electrocardiographically by a wavering baseline associated with an irregular ventricular response (see Fig. 9.6D).

AF is the most common clinically significant arrhythmia. It affects 2.2 million people in the United States. Its prevalence is between 0.4% and 1% in the general population, and it increases with age, reaching 8% in those older than 80 years. Patients with AF have a higher risk of stroke, heart failure, and mortality. However, the role of AF as an independent determinant of mortality is uncertain because it commonly coexists with other important conditions. Patients with lone AF do not have an increased mortality rate, and carefully designed trials exploring the benefit of maintenance of sinus rhythm over rate control show, in most populations, no survival benefit for sinus rhythm. One exception may be in patients with systolic heart failure in addition to AF where ablation of AF may have a survival advantage. The recently completed CASTLE-AF (Catheter Ablation vs. Standard Conventional Treatment in Patients with LV Dysfunction and AF) showed a significant reduction in mortality with catheter ablation of AF in this select population. AF is often classified by its clinical presentation and pattern. When AF is first detected, it is called *new onset*, and its ultimate pattern is initially undetermined. When AF relapses during follow-up, it is called *recurrent* and classified by its clinical pattern. If AF terminates spontaneously, it is called *paroxysmal* AF. Although episodes lasting up to 7 days are defined as paroxysmal, most episodes of paroxysmal AF terminate within the first 24 hours and many terminate within minutes or hours of onset. When AF lasts longer than 7 days, it is designated as *persistent*. AF that persists for a long interval, typically more than a year, without return of an interim period of sinus rhythm (spontaneously or as a result of medical intervention such as cardioversion) is termed long-standing persistent AF. Finally, when a clinical decision is made to no longer try to maintain sinus rhythm, the term *permanent* AF is used.

Mechanisms of Atrial Fibrillation
Because of its chaotic nature, it has been difficult to study AF, and its mechanisms remain incompletely understood. The initiation of spontaneous AF is a consequence of rapid electrical firing from preferential focal sites of origin. The most common site of focal origin is from left atrial muscle sleeves extending along the outer surface of the pulmonary veins. When firing does not originate from a pulmonary vein, it is commonly from the left atrial tissue immediately adjacent to one of the veins or occasionally from one of the other thoracic veins such as the ostium of the superior vena cava or the ostium of the coronary sinus. Atrial rates recorded in and around the pulmonary veins are significantly higher than at other atrial sites, suggesting that activity in the region of the veins is important in perpetuating AF after initiation.

These insights have produced highly effective techniques for the cure of AF. Ablation techniques designed to isolate these trigger sites from the atrium have success rates of 70% to 80% for the cure of

paroxysmal AF and somewhat lower rates for the cure of persistent AF. Ablation restricted to the region of the pulmonary veins and adjacent left atrium is curative in most patients with AF, implying that most cases of AF are arrhythmias entirely contained within and maintained by the left atrium and connecting veins. In the same way that typical atrial flutter is the characteristic arrhythmia of the right atrium, AF is the characteristic arrhythmia of the left atrium.

Anticoagulation and Atrial Fibrillation
During AF (and to some extent, atrial flutter), the atria have incomplete and ineffective contractions. Blood stasis occurs and may result in the formation of intracardiac thrombus, which may lead to thromboembolism and stroke. The overall risk of stroke in patients with AF is 5% per year. Certain risk factors may adjust this risk, including age, gender, rheumatic heart disease, prior stroke, left ventricular dysfunction, vascular disease, hypertrophic cardiomyopathy, left atrial enlargement, hypertension, and diabetes.

Scoring systems have been developed to estimate a patient's AF-related stroke risk based on his or her constellation of risk factors. Formerly, the most used system was the $CHADS_2$ score (*c*ardiac failure, *h*ypertension, *a*ge $\geq$75 years, *d*iabetes mellitus, and prior *s*troke). This system has been well validated in assessing the stroke risk of patients with AF. It assigns a single point for age of 75 years or older, diabetes, history of heart failure, and hypertension. It assigns two points for a history of stroke or transient ischemic attack. A score of 0 correlates with a relatively low risk of stroke at 1.9% per year, a score of 1 has a stroke risk of 2.8% per year, a score of 2 has a risk of 4.0% per year, and a score of 3 or higher has a stroke risk of more than 5.9% per year.

The $CHADS_2$ underwent further refinement to increase the granularity of stroke risk stratification with the creation of the CHA_2DS_2-VASc (*v*ascular disease, *a*ge, and *s*ex) scoring system, currently the primary score for thromboembolic risk stratification. In this system, congestive heart failure, hypertension, diabetes mellitus, vascular disease, age between 65 and 74 years, and female gender are assigned 1 point, and age of 75 years or older and prior stroke are assigned 2 points. A CHA_2DS_2-VASc score of 0 was associated with a 0% stroke rate, a score of 1 with a 0.6% per year risk, a score of 2 with a 1.6% risk, and a score of 3 with a risk of 3.9%. This system may be most useful for identifying truly low-risk patients.

After a patient's individualized stroke risk is determined, it can be balanced against the risk of anticoagulation to determine what would be appropriate for stroke prevention. A useful tool for estimating bleeding risk due to oral anticoagulation is the HAS-BLED (*h*ypertension, *a*bnormal renal/liver function, *s*troke, *b*leeding history or predisposition, *l*abile international normalized ratio, *e*lderly, *d*rugs/alcohol) score. Patients with a HAS-BLED score of 0 had a risk of 0.59 severe bleeds per 100 patient-years, those with a score of 1 had a risk of 1.51, those with a score of 2 had a risk of 3.20, and those with a score of 3 had a risk of 19.51.

In patients with an acceptable bleeding risk, and with a CHA_2DS_2-VASc score of 2 or greater in men or 3 or greater in women, the 2019 AHA guidelines recommend oral anticoagulation to help prevent embolic stroke. Recommended agents include warfarin, dabigatran, rivaroxaban, apixaban or edoxaban. For patients with low CHA_2DS_2-VASc scores, aspirin is no longer recommended. Oral anticoagulants might be reasonable for intermediate CHA_2DS_2-VASc scores (1 in men and 2 for women), but this has less evidence.

Warfarin is the longest-studied antithrombotic used for reducing the rate of AF-related stroke and reduces the risk by 50%. Warfarin can be difficult to administer; the level of blood-thinning effect must be constantly monitored with international normalized ratio (INR) blood testing. An INR less than 2.0 is associated with higher rates of ischemic stroke; a level greater than 3.0 is associated with increased intracranial bleeding. On average, a therapeutic INR (between 2.0 and 3.0) is maintained in only two thirds of cases, and there are many drug and dietary interactions with warfarin.

Several newer oral anticoagulants (NOACs) have effectiveness and bleeding risk rates similar to warfarin, but they do not require drug level monitoring. They include dabigatran, rivaroxaban, apixaban, and edoxaban. These drugs have been studied in large patient groups and found to be noninferior to warfarin, and some may be superior in certain aspects. NOACs are preferred in eligible patients over warfarin except in cases of moderate-to-severe mitral stenosis or the presence of a mechanical heart valve.

Percutaneous occlusion of the left atrial appendage with the Watchman device has been compared to Coumadin in patients with nonvalvular atrial fibrillation and found generally to offer similar protection against stroke. Oral anticoagulation remains the preferred therapy for stroke prevention in most patients; however, in those who are poor candidates for long-term anticoagulation (because of the propensity for bleeding or poor drug tolerance or adherence), the Watchman device provides an alternative.

The highest risk of stroke related to AF occurs at time of conversion to sinus rhythm achieved spontaneously or by chemical or electrical cardioversion. If thrombus has formed within the left atrium or left atrial appendage, it may not leave the atria during AF due to ineffective atrial mechanics. However, after sinus rhythm is restored, the improved atrial function may eject the thrombus and cause embolic stroke or other systemic embolic sequelae. Even with restoration of electrical atrial systole, the recovery of normal atrial mechanics may be delayed several days to weeks (i.e., atrial stunning). To reduce the risk of pericardioversion stroke, it is important to reduce the risk of preexisting thrombus and to prevent formation in the time period immediately after cardioversion.

The risk of preexisting thrombus can be reduced by 3 weeks of oral anticoagulation or Doppler transesophageal echocardiography (TEE) before cardioversion. These steps are recommended for any patient who has been in AF for an unknown period or has been documented to be in AF more than 48 hours. Although thrombi have been identified in patients with AF for shorter periods, current clinical practice presumes that most thrombus formation requires at least 48 hours. Thrombus related to AF occurs most commonly in the left atrial appendage, which cannot be well visualized by transthoracic echocardiography; TEE is often recommended before cardioversion for optimal imaging of the left atrial appendage. After cardioversion, at least 4 weeks of oral anticoagulation is recommended for everyone, with the exception of low CHA_2DS_2-VASc score patients (0 in men or 1 in women) who had AF less than 48 hours prior to the cardioversion, in whom postconversion anticoagulation may be omitted.

Acute Management of Atrial Fibrillation: Rate Control

The acute management of AF centers on the control of the ventricular response, timely restoration of sinus rhythm, and identification of potentially reversible factors that might have precipitated the arrhythmia. AF with rapid ventricular response results in acute deterioration in stroke volume and cardiac output and an increase in myocardial oxygen demand with the potential for coronary ischemia. Patients who are symptomatic must be controlled promptly. When pursuing rate control for acute AF of recent onset, the fastest way to achieve rate control is the restoration of sinus rhythm. If rate control in ongoing rapidly conducted AF proves difficult or is not well tolerated, cardioversion should be undertaken early.

For the acute control of rapidly conducted AF, intravenous administration of a β-blocker (i.e., esmolol, metoprolol, or propranolol) or a nondihydropyridine calcium-channel blocker (i.e., diltiazem or verapamil) is preferred. In the setting of decompensated heart failure, the use of a calcium-channel blocker may exacerbate heart failure and should be avoided. In this setting, digoxin is a useful agent for resting rate control. Digoxin is also a useful second-line drug in addition to a calcium-channel or β-blocker for resting rate control. If this therapy is ineffective or not tolerated, intravenous amiodarone is a useful rate control agent, especially in the setting of congestive heart failure, and it may facilitate restoration of sinus rhythm.

Long-term targets for rate control of permanent AF have been a matter of debate. The Rate Control Efficacy in Permanent Atrial Fibrillation II (RACE II) study showed no advantage to strict rate control. Targeting a resting rate of less than 80 beats per minute showed no advantage over a target of less than 110 and was much harder to achieve. For long-term management, the results suggest that achieving a resting heart rate of less than 110 beats per minute may be sufficient and safe.

Acute Management of Atrial Fibrillation: Restoration of Sinus Rhythm

When sinus rhythm is restored in the first 48 hours of acute AF, the thromboembolic risk is low, and anticoagulation is not required. New-onset AF should be managed with a plan to restore sinus rhythm during this period if possible. At least one half of new-onset AF episodes terminate spontaneously in the first 24 to 48 hours.

Pharmacologic conversion of atrial fibrillation. Pharmacologic conversion of AF can be undertaken when restoration of sinus rhythm is not urgent. Several antiarrhythmic drugs have been effective in increasing the rate of early conversion of AF. Pharmacologic conversion usually is more successful with AF of recent onset than with chronic AF.

Oral agents with efficacy in the early conversion of AF include flecainide, propafenone, and dofetilide. Oral amiodarone and sotalol have been associated with a 27% and 24% conversion rate, respectively, occurring after 28 days of therapy. However, due to low early conversion rates, these oral drugs are not recommended for conversion. Intravenous agents with efficacy for early conversion include ibutilide and amiodarone. Ibutilide is limited by a relatively high 4% rate of drug-induced QT prolongation and TdP VT. This risk is even higher in the setting of LV dysfunction, electrolyte disturbances, or heart failure. Ibutilide should be reserved for the pharmacologic conversion of stable patients with a baseline normal QT interval. In contrast, intravenous amiodarone is well tolerated by unstable patients and is the preferred pharmacologic agent for conversion in the critically ill.

Electrical cardioversion of atrial fibrillation. Electrical cardioversion should be performed urgently in the case of severe compromise related to acute AF, including angina, heart failure, hypotension, and shock. Cardioversion should also be attempted at least once electively in most cases of new-onset AF regardless of tolerance. When performing electrical cardioversion, an anterior-posterior patch or paddle position is more effective than the conventional anterior-to-lateral patch or paddle position used for ventricular defibrillation. Although low-output discharges may be effective in some patients, a strategy of starting at higher outputs decreases the number of shocks required and the average cumulative energy delivered. An initial shock energy of 200 J is recommended. After a failed initial shock, full output should be used for the next attempt.

Long-Term Maintenance of Sinus Rhythm

Antiarrhythmic therapy. Despite the association of AF with an increase in stroke-related and all-cause mortality, no study has established a benefit for pharmacologic maintenance of sinus rhythm in terms of stroke risk or survival. This may be because AF is merely a marker and not a mechanism of mortality. It may also be a consequence of the relative inefficacy of pharmacologic therapy in the maintenance of sinus rhythm and the difficulty of establishing whether patients thought to be in sinus rhythm are consistently in sinus rhythm at follow-up.

The largest and best designed trial addressing this issue was the Atrial Fibrillation Follow-up Investigation of Rhythm Management (AFFIRM) trial. The study included 4060 patients randomly assigned to rhythm control with antiarrhythmic drugs, most commonly amiodarone, or to rate control without attempts to maintain sinus rhythm. AFFIRM demonstrated no advantage in stroke or mortality rates using a strategy of sinus rhythm maintenance compared with rate control. Either strategy can be offered to patients with an expectation of similar outcomes with regard to hard end points. The decision to pursue sinus rhythm usually is determined by the management of symptoms that may be better addressed by maintaining sinus rhythm in selected patients.

In the absence of antiarrhythmic drugs, more than 80% of patients relapse during the first year after cardioversion of AF. Antiarrhythmic drugs remain the primary strategy for maintaining sinus rhythm after cardioversion and for preventing symptomatic episodes in patients with paroxysmal AF. However, antiarrhythmic therapy has many limitations, and alternative ablative therapies may over time overtake antiarrhythmic therapy in the management of AF.

All antiarrhythmic drugs have the potential for proarrhythmia, the unintended precipitation of a new arrhythmic problem caused by the drug. Adverse rhythm effects of drugs may include sinus node dysfunction, heart block, promotion of drug-slowed atrial flutter permitting rapid 1:1 conduction, and promotion of potentially lethal ventricular arrhythmias. Class I drugs such as flecainide, propafenone, and disopyramide may result in significant direct myocardial depression and consequent exacerbation of heart failure. The array of potential adverse effects of antiarrhythmic drugs is beyond the scope of this chapter, but certain essential concepts are important to recognize.

Class I drugs such as flecainide and propafenone, which work by slowing conduction, have a high risk of ventricular proarrhythmia and potential for sudden death in the setting of heart failure, LV dysfunction, and coronary artery disease. Use of these drugs is restricted to patients with preserved cardiac function and no evidence of obstructive coronary artery disease. However, in this selected group of patients with normal hearts, these drugs are exceedingly safe, well tolerated, and often effective.

Class III drugs, which prolong repolarization and refractoriness, include sotalol, dofetilide, dronedarone, and amiodarone. They are safe for patients with coronary artery disease, and in the case of dofetilide and amiodarone, they are safe for those with congestive heart failure. However, sotalol and dofetilide may provoke TdP, even in patients with normal cardiac function, and they must be used with caution. Amiodarone has greater long-term efficacy than other drugs and a lower risk of proarrhythmia, but long-term somatic toxicity consisting of thyroid dysfunction, pulmonary, and occasional hepatotoxicity limits the use of this drug in older patients or those with limited expected longevity or an inability to safely tolerate alternative agents due to advanced cardiac disease or proarrhythmia. Amiodarone is highly effective for the short-term, acute management of arrhythmias in critically ill patients when the potential risk of long-term toxicity is not an issue.

Dronedarone was derived by modification of the amiodarone molecule. Like amiodarone, the drug has a low risk of proarrhythmia and TdP VT. Unlike amiodarone, the drug does not cause thyroid toxicity. In common use, hepatotoxicity is also uncommon with dronedarone. However, rare cases of hepatic failure have been associated

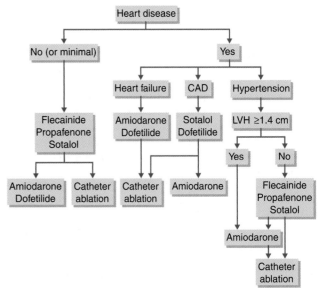

Fig. 9.7 A strategy for the selection of therapy to maintain sinus rhythm in patients with recurrent atrial fibrillation. Patients are stratified by the presence or absence of structural heart disease, and drugs expected to have the greatest efficacy and lowest therapeutic risk in each group are selected. Catheter ablation becomes a therapeutic option after failure of at least one antiarrhythmic drug. The class IC drugs flecainide and propafenone are not advised for patients with heart failure or coronary artery disease (CAD). Amiodarone is an acceptable first-line drug for those with heart failure and severe left ventricular hypertrophy. Because of its potential for somatic toxicity, amiodarone is otherwise reserved as a second-line agent that is used as an alternative to catheter ablation.

with dronedarone use. Dronedarone has increased mortality rates for patients with recently decompensated heart failure and when used as a simple rate control agent in patients with permanent AF. It is contraindicated in these settings.

In addition to being useful agents for the prevention of AF, sotalol, dronedarone, and amiodarone provide substantial rate control during relapses of AF. However, rate control with other antiarrhythmic agents may not be adequate to prevent rapid conduction with relapse, and class I drugs such as flecainide may accelerate response at the time of relapse. Antiarrhythmic drugs other than sotalol, dronedarone, or amiodarone should therefore be combined with a rate control agent such as a β-blocker or nondihydropyridine calcium-channel blocker during long-term therapy. Fig. 9.7 is a proposed strategy for antiarrhythmic drug selection for the long-term maintenance of sinus rhythm in patients with AF.

Surgical ablation of atrial fibrillation. The surgical treatment of AF was pioneered by Cox with the development of the atrial maze procedure. The procedure was predicated on the concept that AF was maintained by multiple interacting wave fronts of activity. By surgically dividing the atria into narrow channels, most with connection back to the sinus node, it was thought that AF could be abolished while preserving physiologic activation and contraction of the atrium. The circuitous path left for atrial activation and the multiple barriers created in the atrium intended to prevent AF gave rise to the term *maze procedure* to describe the technique. The initial procedure was thought to be highly successful but was associated with significant surgical risks and problems with sinus node dysfunction. Because of the surgical complexity of making and then closing multiple incisions in the atria and the complications associated with the procedure, the initial cut-and-sew maze procedure has fallen out of clinical use.

Although the original maze procedure is no longer used, many techniques have been developed to simplify the operation by substituting linear thermal ablation (by heating or cooling tissue) to create lines of conduction block in the atria without the need for extensive atrial dissection and reconstruction. Surgical ablation is commonly applied in patients with a history of AF who are undergoing concomitant heart operations for other indications such as valvular or coronary disease. Less frequently, surgical ablation has been applied as a stand-alone procedure for the sole management of AF. In that setting, various minimally invasive techniques have been developed. However, the techniques used vary widely from one center to another and long-term reporting of outcomes is inconsistent. In a large series that included 282 patients undergoing an open bi-atrial ablation procedure, 78% were in sinus rhythm without antiarrhythmic therapy at the 1-year follow-up evaluation.

Another important potential benefit of surgical ablation for AF is that it provides an opportunity to eliminate the left atrial appendage as a potential site of thrombus formation and source of thromboembolism. This can be accomplished by complete amputation of the appendage with oversewing of the appendage or clamping off the opening to the appendage with special devices designed for this purpose. This may be especially important in patients with absolute or relative contraindications to anticoagulation.

Catheter ablation of atrial fibrillation. Catheter ablation has become a common procedure for the management of AF after failure of initial attempts at medical therapy. Initial attempts to cure AF using catheter techniques were based on attempts in the early 1990s to emulate the linear lesion set of the Cox maze procedure with multiple endocardial lesions. High complication rates and limited efficacy led to abandonment of this approach.

In 1998, Haissaguerre reported the important role of rapid activity originating in the musculature of the pulmonary veins in initiation of paroxysmal AF. This led to the development of procedures designed to target the pulmonary veins and eventuated in the technique of electrical pulmonary vein isolation (PVI), which is currently the primary ablative approach to treatment of paroxysmal AF by catheter techniques. This technique has had acceptably high success rates (≈70%) at multiple centers for the treatment of paroxysmal AF without antiarrhythmic therapy.

Despite the high success rate of catheter PVI ablation for the treatment of paroxysmal AF, this technique has not proved reliably effective in the management of more persistent forms of AF, especially long-standing persistent AF. This likely reflects the importance of factors other than pulmonary vein activity in the initiation and maintenance of persistent AF that are not addressed by PVI ablation. Multiple ablative techniques are currently used in an attempt to increase the success rates for patients with persistent AF. They have included addition of linear lesions to block reentrant wave fronts, ablation of regions of unusually rapid atrial activity during ongoing AF, and interruption of stable rotors of atrial activity identified during multisite mapping of AF. Although these techniques have improved success rates in limited series, it is uncertain which, if any, of these methods represents the optimal approach to the ablation of long-standing persistent AF.

In summary, catheter ablation is the preferred secondary strategy for treatment of symptomatic AF after initial attempts at medical therapy have failed. Simple pulmonary vein isolation has a high success rate for the management of patients with paroxysmal AF. Success rates for all ablative techniques are lower for persistent AF, especially for long-term AF. As in the case of surgical ablation, multiple techniques are used at various centers, and the different strategies for follow-up and definitions of response have made it difficult to ascertain the relative efficacy of the various approaches in common use.

Catheter ablation of the atrioventricular node. Although less commonly used today than in the past, the older technique of catheter ablation of the AV node resulting in complete heart block followed by placement of a ventricular pacemaker to maintain physiologic heart rates remains an option for patients when rate control cannot be achieved medically. This technique continues to have an important role in the management of patients who are too infirm to safely undergo AF ablation or in patients for whom ablative techniques have failed to control the arrhythmia.

For a deeper discussion on this topic, please see Chapter 58, "Supraventricular Cardiac Arrhythmias," in *Goldman-Cecil Medicine*, 26th Edition.

SYNCOPE

Syncope is a sudden loss of consciousness that is transient. Syncope has cardiac causes (e.g., low cerebral blood pressure) and noncardiac causes. Common causes and categories of syncope are outlined in Table 9.4. Cerebrovascular disease or stroke uncommonly manifests as syncope unless a large cerebral territory is involved. Syncope is a common reason for emergency room or hospital admission.

The diagnostic approach to a patient with syncope is given in Fig. 9.8. Most causes can be identified by the medical history and physical examination alone. Conditions surrounding the syncopal episode often suggest a cause. For example, vasovagal episodes often occur during stress, pain, straining, coughing, or urination. Exercise-induced syncope may indicate obstructive coronary disease, channelopathies such as long QT or CPVT, obstructive cardiomyopathy, aortic stenosis, or arrhythmia. A history of palpitations or syncope with no warning may be related to cardiac arrhythmias. Very long episodes of syncope (>5 minutes) suggest noncardiac causes. A recent change in medications or dizziness with position changes suggests orthostatic hypotension. Witnessed limb movements or posturing is not specific for neurologic causes and can result from any type of cerebral hypoperfusion, even from cardiac causes.

Beyond the history, physical examination, and routine ECG, further testing has little diagnostic utility. Holter or loop recorders may be useful. Implantable loop recorders may have utility in cases of recurrent, infrequent syncope. Electrophysiologic testing may be useful in some patients with other abnormalities suggesting an arrhythmic cause.

Despite thorough evaluations, more than 30% of patients with syncope have no identifiable cause. Cardiac causes of syncope have the highest morbidity and mortality rates. Because patients with unknown causes of syncope have long-term outcomes similar to those with noncardiac syncope, the major goal of an evaluation is to identify cardiac causes of syncope.

VENTRICULAR ARRHYTHMIAS AND SUDDEN CARDIAC DEATH

Ventricular ectopy is defined as cardiac beats that originate from within the right or left ventricular muscle or conduction system. Premature ventricular contractions (PVCs) can occur singly or as ventricular couplets or triplets. VT is four or more consecutive beats that originate from the ventricle at a rate of at least 100 beats per minute. VT is classified as *sustained* if it lasts longer than 30 seconds or requires termination due to hemodynamic instability; otherwise, it is classified as *nonsustained* VT (NSVT).

Ventricular ectopy also may be classified based on maintenance of a similar electrocardiographic morphology. The beats of monomorphic VT (MMVT) appear to be identical and usually originate from

TABLE 9.4 Causes of Syncope

Cause	Features
Peripheral Vascular or Circulatory	
Vasovagal syncope (neurally mediated)	Prodrome of pallor, yawning, nausea, diaphoresis; precipitated by stress or pain; occurs when patient is upright, aborted by recumbency; fall in blood pressure with or without a decrease in heart rate
Micturition syncope	Syncope with urination (probably vagal)
Post-tussive syncope	Syncope after paroxysm of coughing
Hypersensitive carotid sinus syndrome	Vasodepressor and/or cardioinhibitory responses with light carotid sinus massage
Drugs	Orthostasis; occurs with antihypertensive drugs, tricyclic antidepressants, phenothiazines
Volume depletion	Orthostasis; occurs with hemorrhage, excessive vomiting or diarrhea, Addison's disease
Autonomic dysfunction	Orthostasis; occurs in diabetes, alcoholism, Parkinson's disease, deconditioning after a prolonged illness
Central Nervous System	
Cerebrovascular	Transient ischemic attacks and strokes are unusual causes of syncope; associated neurologic abnormalities are usually identified
Seizures	Warning aura sometimes present, jerking of extremities, tongue biting, urinary incontinence, postictal confusion
Metabolic	
Hypoglycemia	Confusion, tachycardia, jitteriness before syncope; patient may be taking insulin
Cardiac	
Obstructive	Syncope is often exertional; physical findings consistent with aortic stenosis, hypertrophic obstructive cardiomyopathy, cardiac tamponade, atrial myxoma, prosthetic valve malfunction, Eisenmenger's syndrome, tetralogy of Fallot, primary pulmonary hypertension, pulmonic stenosis, massive pulmonary embolism
Arrhythmias	Syncope may be sudden and occurs in any position; episodes of dizziness or palpitations; may be history of heart disease; bradyarrhythmias or tachyarrhythmias may be responsible—check for hypersensitive carotid sinus

the same area of the heart. *Ventricular flutter* is a term that may be used to describe MMVT with rates of more than 300 beats per minute. Polymorphic VT (PMVT) has a more variable appearance on the ECG than MMVT. TdP is a special form of PMVT that has a repetitive, undulating periodicity and usually implies a long-QT triggered mechanism. VF is the most chaotic form of ventricular ectopy. It is associated with no meaningful cardiac output and usually leads to death unless rapidly treated. The other forms of VT may eventually degrade into VF.

Determining whether a patient has a rhythm of ventricular origin usually is done by 12-lead surface ECG. Ventricular ectopy typically has a wide QRS morphology (Fig. 9.9). Not all wide QRS morphologies are ventricular in origin, and there are criteria for determining whether a wide-complex tachycardia is supraventricular or ventricular. SVT may appear as a wide-complex tachycardia if it conducts to the ventricle with aberrancy (e.g., bundle branch block) or through an accessory pathway (e.g., WPW syndrome). Features that may help distinguish between SVT and VT include AV dissociation with capture beats and fusion beats and the QRS morphology and duration (Table 9.5). The Brugada algorithm is commonly used for determining the site of origin of wide-complex tachycardia. The tachycardia has a ventricular origin in more than 90% of patients with a history of ischemic heart disease.

VT may occur by the same mechanisms as other tachycardias, such as reentry, enhanced automaticity, or triggered activity. VT often occurs as a reentrant tachycardia around an area of prior MI scar in the left ventricle. VT in the chronic phase of ischemic heart disease is mediated by reentry through channels or sheets of surviving myocardium, especially in the partially spared border zone of a region of scar resulting from a prior MI. In these channels, conduction is abnormally slow due to poor coupling between sparse surviving myocytes. Susceptibility to sustained VT increases with worsening left ventricular dysfunction, likely due to the greater extent of ventricular scar.

VT can occur in the absence of ischemic heart disease in the form of idiopathic VT, nonischemic cardiomyopathies, hypertrophic cardiomyopathies, arrhythmogenic RV dysplasia, bundle branch reentry, cardiac ion channel disorders, or electrolyte disturbances. The right ventricular outflow tract (RVOT) is the most common origin of idiopathic VT, which is likely caused by triggered activity. This form of VT (or PVCs) is usually sensitive to catecholamines and may terminate with adenosine (i.e., adenosine-sensitive VT). Another common form of idiopathic VT originates from the left ventricular conduction system (i.e., fascicular VT) and may be verapamil sensitive. Idiopathic VTs are common targets for successful catheter ablation.

Nonsustained VT usually does not require specific therapy unless the patient is symptomatic. The Cardiac Arrhythmia Suppression Trial treated PVCs and NSVT after the acute phase of MI with class I antiarrhythmic drugs, and the trial demonstrated increased mortality rates when the arrhythmias were treated. If VT is attributed to reversible causes such as electrolyte disturbances or acute ischemia, the underlying mechanism should be treated. VT not due to reversible causes may be treated with β-blockers, antiarrhythmic drug therapy (e.g., amiodarone), or catheter ablation. If urgent treatment is required due to hemodynamic instability, direct current cardioversion is performed. It should be synchronized to the QRS complex if a regular morphology exists; otherwise, it should be nonsynchronized. Performing direct current cardioversion during the refractory period (T wave) of MMVT may degrade the rhythm to VF. An ICD often is used in patients who survive VT or VF to quickly treat recurrent episodes. Endocardial and epicardial catheter ablation has become an effective treatment for VT.

Prevention of Sudden Cardiac Death

SCD is defined as death within 1 hour of the onset of symptoms. It may result from a variety of cardiac or noncardiac conditions (Table 9.6). SCD is one of the most common causes of death, with 400,000 events occurring annually in the United States. The most common cause of SCD is VT

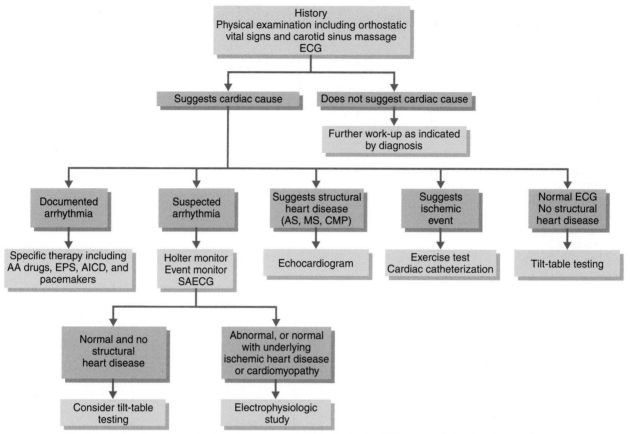

Fig. 9.8 Approach to the evaluation of syncope. *AA,* Antiarrhythmic; *AICD,* automatic implantable cardioverter-defibrillator; *AS,* aortic stenosis; *CMP,* cardiomyopathy; *ECG,* electrocardiogram; *EPS,* electrophysiologic study; *MS,* mitral stenosis; *SAECG,* signal-averaged ECG.

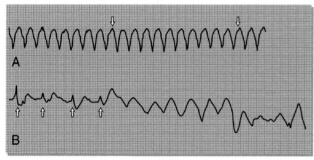

Fig. 9.9 Ventricular arrhythmias. (A) Monomorphic ventricular tachycardia (VT). Notice the wide QRS with a stable appearance with each beat. Detecting P waves during VT is difficult due to the overlying ventricular activity, but it is visible at several points on this tracing, some of which are marked by *arrows.* The AV dissociation is diagnostic of VT and excludes supraventricular tachycardia. (B) An initially organized agonal (preterminal) rhythm *(arrows)* degenerates into coarse ventricular fibrillation. Notice the irregular baseline and the absence of organized QRS complexes. During ventricular fibrillation, there is no forward cardiac output, and cardiac arrest immediately ensues.

TABLE 9.5   Differentiation of Ventricular Tachycardia From Supraventricular Tachycardia With Aberrancy

Helpful Features	Implications
Positive QRS concordance	Diagnostic of VT
AV dissociation, capture beats, or fusion beats	Diagnostic of VT
Atypical RBBB (monophasic R, QR, RS, or triphasic QRS in V$_1$; R:S ratio <1, QS or QR, monophasic R in V$_6$)	Suggests VT
Atypical LBBB (R >30 min or R to S [nadir or notch] >60 min in V$_1$ or V$_2$; R:S ratio <1, QS or QR in V$_6$)	Suggests VT
Shift of axis from baseline	Suggests VT
History of CAD	Suggests VT
QRS during tachycardia identical to QRS during sinus rhythm	Suggests SVT
Termination with adenosine	Suggests SVT

AV, Atrioventricular; *CAD,* coronary artery disease; *LBBB,* left bundle branch block; *RBBB,* right bundle branch block; *SVT,* supraventricular tachycardia; *VT,* ventricular tachycardia.

or VF. Cardiac conditions that increase the risk of SCD include LQTS, hypertrophic cardiomyopathy, Brugada syndrome, arrhythmogenic RV dysplasia, and nonischemic or ischemic cardiomyopathy. The most common cardiac condition that may lead to SCD is acute or distant MI.

The successful treatment of SCD due to VF usually requires rapid access to cardioversion; if treatment is delayed by more than 5 to 10 minutes, permanent brain injury is common. AEDs can reduce the time to defibrillation and improve survival when placed in public areas, although they have been less effective when installed in private residences, even for patients at risk for SCD.

ICDs used in the treatment of SCD have improved mortality rates. Patients who are at high risk for SCD are often offered an ICD to enable rapid defibrillation before the onset of anoxic brain injury. If a patient survives the first episode of SCD due to documented or presumed VT

TABLE 9.6 Causes of Sudden Cardiac Death

Noncardiac Causes
Central nervous system hemorrhage
Massive pulmonary embolus
Drug overdose
Hypoxia secondary to lung disease
Aortic dissection or rupture

Cardiac Causes
Ventricular fibrillation
Myocardial ischemia or injury
Long QT syndrome
Short QT syndrome
Brugada syndrome
Arrhythmogenic right ventricular dysplasia
Ventricular tachycardia
Bradyarrhythmias, sick sinus syndrome
Aortic stenosis
Tetralogy of Fallot
Pericardial tamponade
Cardiac tumors
Complications of infective endocarditis
Hypertrophic cardiomyopathy (arrhythmia or obstruction)
Myocardial ischemia
Atherosclerosis
Prinzmetal angina
Kawasaki arteritis

TABLE 9.7 Predictors of Sudden Cardiac Death After Myocardial Infarction

Decreased left ventricular ejection fraction
Residual ischemia
Delayed enhancement on cardiac MRI
Late potentials on signal-averaged electrocardiography
Decreased heart rate variability
Prolonged QT on ECG
Induction of sustained MMVT with programmed electrical stimulation
Complex ventricular ectopy (e.g., NSVT) on ambulatory monitoring

ECG, Electrocardiogram; *MMVT,* monomorphic ventricular tachycardia; *MRI,* magnetic resonance imaging; *NSVT,* nonsustained ventricular tachycardia.

or VF from nonreversible or unknown causes, he or she is offered an ICD. ICDs are extremely successful in the detection and treatment of VT or VF. They do not always prevent loss of consciousness because it takes 15 to 20 seconds to treat the arrhythmia, and low cardiac output may cause syncope before restoration of normal rhythm, especially if several cardioversions are required.

The earliest ICD trials examined their use in the secondary prevention of SCD (i.e., treating patients who had already survived an episode of cardiac arrest). The largest study was the Antiarrhythmics Versus Implantable Defibrillators (AVID) trial, which randomized patients with a history of poorly tolerated sustained VT or cardiac arrest to empirical amiodarone or ICD implantation. In this trial and several others, ICD therapy was associated with a lower risk of arrhythmic and all-cause death compared with antiarrhythmic therapy.

Several trials have examined the use of ICDs for the primary prevention of SCDs (i.e., treating patients who are at risk for SCD). The first was the Multicenter Automatic Defibrillator Implantation Trial (MADIT), which enrolled patients with a prior MI and an ejection fraction of 35% or less who had frequent ventricular ectopy and inducible VT at electrophysiologic testing. The study demonstrated a substantial mortality reduction with ICD therapy. MADIT-II enrolled patients with a prior MI and an ejection fraction of 30% or less in the chronic phase, without requiring invasive testing. A significant mortality benefit was associated with ICD therapy.

The Sudden Cardiac Death in Heart Failure trial enrolled a broader population consisting of patients with ischemic and nonischemic cardiomyopathy, symptomatic heart failure, and an ejection fraction of 35% or less. A survival benefit was found for patients treated with an ICD compared with conventional therapy or empirical amiodarone therapy. The degree of benefit was similar for patients with ischemic or nonischemic cardiomyopathy, suggesting that primary prevention with ICDs for patients with prior MI or nonischemic cardiomyopathy and heart failure was appropriate.

The risk of SCD after MI is highest in the few months after the index event. However, ICDs have not been effective when implanted immediately after MI or revascularization procedures. The reason for this is unclear; it may reflect the large percentage of patients who have improved cardiac function early on, which decreases the risk of SCD and therefore the benefit of an ICD. Alternatively, the mechanism for SCD in the early period after an MI or revascularization procedure may be recurrent ischemia rather than reentrant tachycardia and therefore less amenable to ICD therapy. The Defibrillator in Acute Myocardial Infarction Trial (DINAMIT) randomized 675 patients with low ejection fractions immediately after MI to ICD or medical therapy; no difference in mortality rates was seen. The current recommendations are to avoid primary prevention with ICDs within 40 days of an MI or 3 months of revascularization.

A significant challenge in modern medicine is identifying patients who have an elevated risk of SCD to allow effective use of primary prevention interventions such as ICDs. Some known predictors of SCD after MI are shown in Table 9.7, but many are not specific or sensitive enough for practical use. Reduced ejection fraction has been the most successful noninvasive measure that can predict increased risk of SCD. An electrophysiologic study is a minimally invasive catheter procedure that with electrical stimulation can help to identify patients who are prone to VT. Electrophysiologic studies are most sensitive in patients with prior MI, but they may be less useful in other cardiac conditions. Cardiac magnetic resonance imaging (MRI), which can directly image cardiac function and cardiac scar or fibrosis, is showing great promise as a more sensitive and specific, noninvasive risk predictor of SCD.

Ventricular Tachycardia and Ventricular Fibrillation Without Evident Heart Disease

Ventricular arrhythmias occurring in the absence of structural heart disease usually carry a benign prognosis but can be associated with SCD in patients with genetic arrhythmic syndromes predisposing to life-threatening polymorphic VT. Genetic screening for these syndromes is important to identify at-risk family members.

Idiopathic Ventricular Tachycardia

Idiopathic VT most commonly originates from the outflow tracts, with approximately 80% localized to the RVOT and the remainder originating in the left ventricular outflow tract (LVOT), the aortic sinuses of Valsalva, and the region of the aortomitral continuity. Idiopathic RVOT VT manifests with the characteristic electrocardiographic findings of left bundle branch block and inferior axis VT QRS morphology. Triggered activity is the mechanism underlying outflow tract tachycardias. This calcium-dependent mechanism explains why an outflow tract VT often terminates with adenosine, β-blockers, and calcium-channel blockers.

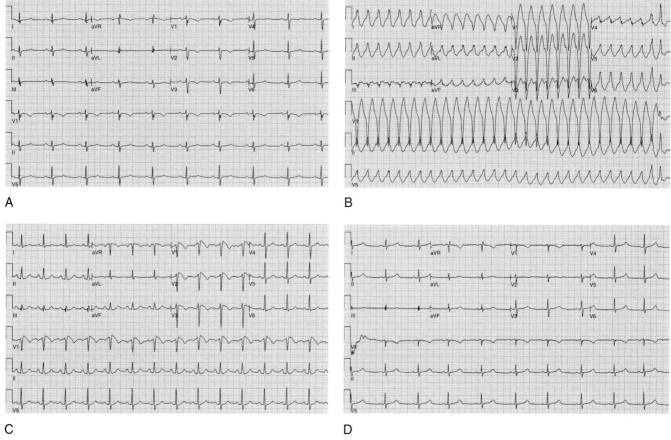

Fig. 9.10 Characteristic electrocardiograms associated with genetic disorders predisposing to SCD. (A) ARVC ECG demonstrating inverted T waves V_1-V_3 during sinus rhythm. (B) Monomorphic ventricular tachycardia with left bundle branch block morphology characteristic of ARVC. (C) Type I Brugada ECG pattern with coving ST elevation and T inversion in V_1-V_2. (D) ECG from patient with hereditary LQT1, with mutation KCNQ1.

Patients in their third or fourth decade typically have palpitations, shortness of breath, and lightheadedness at presentation. Reports of cardiac arrest are rare, and treatment is directed at controlling symptoms. β-Blockers and calcium-channel blockers are often used initially, although some patients require catheter ablation or antiarrhythmic drug therapy. A subset of asymptomatic patients may develop tachycardia-mediated cardiomyopathy due to frequent ventricular ectopy. The PVC burden posing the greatest risk for producing left ventricular dysfunction is likely more than 10,000 PVCs daily. Fortunately, PVC suppression with catheter ablation usually improves ventricular function.

Arrhythmogenic Right Ventricular Cardiomyopathy or Dysplasia

Arrhythmogenic right ventricular cardiomyopathy (ARVC) is an inherited cardiomyopathy with typically autosomal dominant transmission. It is associated with mutations affecting desmosomes, which are molecular complexes of cell adhesion proteins that bind cardiac myocytes. Although morphologic changes in the RV free wall predominate, biventricular or primary left ventricular variants occur. Due to myocyte death, large portions of the right ventricle are replaced with adipose tissue, leading to wall motion abnormalities, cardiac dysfunction, and aneurysm formation. Structural changes spread from the epicardium to the endocardium. RV imaging classically demonstrates RV enlargement with focal wall motion abnormalities and RV hypokinesis. The RV free wall is not well imaged by routine cardiac echocardiography, and MRI has become the gold standard for the diagnosis of ARVC.

ARVC patients develop ventricular arrhythmias with associated symptoms, including palpitations, lightheadedness, syncope, and SCD. Given the typical RV origin of arrhythmias in ARVC, the ventricular arrhythmias have a left bundle branch morphology (Fig. 9.10B). The surface ECG during sinus rhythm may demonstrate inverted T waves in the V_1 to V_3 leads or epsilon waves, which are low-amplitude deflections at the end of the QRS complex in the right precordial leads resulting from slowed RV conduction (Fig. 9.10A).

Distinguishing ARVC from idiopathic RVOT VT is essential because of the different prognostic and therapeutic implications of the two diagnoses. The diagnosis of ARVC is established by the ARVC Task Force Criteria. Risk factors for SCD of ARVC patients include prior aborted episodes of SCD, syncope, young age, LV dysfunction, and markedly diminished RV function.

Patients with documented ARVC typically receive ICDs. Adjunctive therapy with antiarrhythmic drugs or ablation, particularly strategies incorporating combined epicardial and endocardial ablation, may be useful in treating symptomatic VT.

Congenital Long QT Syndrome

Congenital LQTS is a genetic disorder characterized by abnormal cardiac repolarization producing QT prolongation on the ECG (corrected QT [QTc] >440 milliseconds in men and >460 milliseconds in women) (Fig. 9.10D). It is a leading cause of SCD in the young.

Mutations in 16 genes that participate in cardiac repolarization have been identified in patients with LQTS. Mutations of *KCNQ1* (encodes the α-subunit of the I_{Ks} potassium channel) produce LQT1; mutations of *KCNH2* (encodes the α-subunit of the I_{Kr} potassium channel) produce LQT2; and mutations of *SCN5A* (encodes the α-subunit of the cardiac sodium channel) cause LQT3. Together, they account for 75% of cases of congenital LQTS.

Decreased outward potassium currents or increased inward sodium currents prolong action potential duration, predisposing to early afterdepolarizations and TdP, a specific type of polymorphic VT. Symptoms typically begin during adolescence and include syncope, seizures, and SCD. The arrhythmia triggers in LQTS are gene specific. Patients with LQT1 are at risk during high adrenergic states, such as exercise; arrhythmias in LQT2 are triggered by sudden noises such as alarms; and LQT3 patients are more likely to experience arrhythmias during sleep. The autosomal dominant Romano-Ward variant has a prevalence of 1 case in 2000 live births.

Chronic treatment is directed at prevention of SCD. Initial therapy includes avoidance of QT-prolonging agents and initiation of β-blockers in symptomatic patients and asymptomatic patients with significant QT prolongation. ICDs are recommended after resuscitation from a cardiac arrest and for recurrent syncope despite β-blockade. The acute treatment of TdP is different from that of other forms of VT because many antiarrhythmic agents prolong the QT interval and should therefore be avoided.

Brugada Syndrome

The Brugada syndrome is a genetic disorder predisposing to polymorphic VT and SCD. The ECG characteristically displays coving ST elevation in the right precordial leads, V_1 to V_3, and a right bundle branch block pattern (Fig. 9.10C). These electrocardiographic abnormalities may be dynamic, and they are characteristically exacerbated by fever and therapy that blocks sodium channels.

The syndrome is linked to mutations in *SCN5A*, which encodes the cardiac sodium channel. Mutations result in a reduction in the sodium current. The mode of transmission is autosomal dominant. Patients typically have syncope or cardiac arrest, often occurring during sleep.

Although quinidine, by virtue of its ability to block transient outward potassium current (I_{to}), may have a therapeutic role, there are no established medical therapies to prevent VT in Brugada syndrome. Intravenous β-adrenergic stimulation with isoproterenol or a similar agent, by virtue of its ability to augment the sodium current, is potentially useful in the acute management of recurrent VT or VF in Brugada syndrome. Paradoxically, because of a protective effect of catecholamine stimulation, β-blockers are potentially harmful in patients with Brugada syndrome and should be avoided.

ICDs represent the only proven therapy for prevention of cardiac arrest. ICD therapy is recommended for secondary prevention of SCD. For high-risk patients with a spontaneous Brugada electrocardiographic pattern and syncope, primary prevention with an ICD is indicated.

Catecholaminergic Polymorphic Ventricular Tachycardia

CPVT is a genetic disorder that alters myocardial calcium handling, resulting in exercise-induced polymorphic or bidirectional VT. Exercise-triggered syncope or SCD during childhood is the common presenting symptom. About 50% to 60% of patients have an inherited or sporadic autosomal dominant mutation affecting the cardiac ryanodine receptor gene (*RYR2*), producing abnormal calcium-induced calcium release from the sarcoplasmic reticulum and intracellular calcium overload.

β-Blockers along with exercise restriction represent the primary therapy, although arrhythmia breakthrough is common. ICD therapy may be used for secondary prevention, although ICD shocks can produce catecholamine surges that may exacerbate the underlying arrhythmia. Left cardiac sympathetic denervation is useful in selected cases.

Acquired Long QT Syndrome

Environmental factors may prolong cardiac repolarization and produce QTc prolongation, leading to the development of early afterdepolarizations and TdP. Patients with acquired LQTS may have background genetics predisposing them to develop excessive QTc prolongation and polymorphic VT in response to electrolyte abnormalities (i.e., hypokalemia, hypomagnesemia, and hypocalcemia), bradycardia, and the use of QT-prolonging medications. Most QTc-prolonging drugs block the rapid component of the delayed rectifier potassium channel (I_{Kr}) encoded by the *KCNE2* gene. Drugs known to prolong the QTc interval are updated on an Internet registry. Therapy for acquired LQTS requires reversal of inciting physiologic factors and discontinuation of offending medications.

Genetic Testing for Channelopathies

Commercial laboratories offer genetic testing for congenital LQTS, Brugada syndrome, and CPVT. The yields of genetic testing vary from 25% for Brugada syndrome up to 80% for congenital LQTS. The limited sensitivity of current assays and the common finding of genetic variants of unknown significance represent ongoing challenges. Despite these considerations, cascade screening or screening of family members for a disease-causing mutation once characterized in a proband has been effectively used to identify mutation carriers.

Mutation-positive family members may benefit from prophylactic therapy. Reassurance for mutation-negative individuals is also valuable. Before ordering genetic testing, patients should be thoroughly informed of the risks, benefits, and limitations of testing. Genetic counselors ideally play an important advisory role.

For a deeper discussion on this topic, please see Chapter 59, ❖ "Ventricular Arrhythmias," in *Goldman-Cecil Medicine*, 26th Edition.

SUMMARY

Cardiac arrhythmias are caused by disorders of action potential formation or propagation and are broadly categorized as abnormally slow rhythms (i.e., bradycardias) or abnormally rapid rhythms (i.e., tachycardias). The cardiac cellular action potential is composed of five phases determined by the activity of multiple ion channels, including the rapid sodium channel, several potassium channels, and a calcium current. Disruptions of these currents may lead to abnormal automaticity and triggered activity, which may mediate pathologic tachyarrhythmias. Reentry is the dominant mechanism of clinically significant tachyarrhythmias and requires a functional or fixed obstacle to propagation, an area of slowed conduction, and differential refractoriness for initiation and perpetuation of the arrhythmia.

Antiarrhythmic drugs are commonly divided into four broad groups using the Singh–Vaughan Williams classification. Despite its clinical utility, many antiarrhythmic drugs have multiple effects and do not fit neatly into this framework. Some, such as adenosine and digoxin, fall completely outside of it. Class I drugs slow membrane conduction by blockade of the sodium channel. Class II drugs, or β-blockers, function by blockade of the cardiac β-receptor. Class III drugs prolong repolarization and the QT interval. Class IV drugs block the slow calcium channel and are primarily active in slow-response myocytes such as the sinus and AV node.

All bradycardia is a consequence of impairment of sinus node function or AV conduction, or both. Sinus and AV nodal function is strongly influenced by autonomic tone. Parasympathetic tone dominates at rest, and significant bradycardia and second-degree

AV block may be observed in normal patients due to increased parasympathetic tone, especially during sleep or athletic training. Clinical sinus node dysfunction manifests as one of several syndromes, including sinus bradycardia, chronotropic incompetence, exit block, and bradycardia-tachycardia syndrome due to sinus pauses and bradycardia when concomitant atrial arrhythmias terminate to sinus rhythm.

AV conduction disturbances may occur at the AV nodal level or infranodal level. A block at the level of the AV node tends to be indolent, characterized by gradual progression and competent subsidiary escapes that usually protect the patient from catastrophic bradycardia. This permits asymptomatic patients to be followed clinically for the development of symptoms before intervention. In contrast, second- or third-degree infranodal block at the His bundle, or more commonly at the level of the bundle branches, is potentially malignant and is often not accompanied by stable escape mechanisms. If not managed appropriately, it can cause sudden death. Clues to an infranodal level of block are Mobitz II periodicity, associated bundle branch block, worsening heart block with tachycardia or exercise, and a wide QRS escape rhythm different from the conducted QRS in the setting of a high-degree or third-degree AV block.

Tachycardias are broadly categorized as SVTs, which depend on the atrium and AV conduction system, and ventricular arrhythmias, which depend on the ventricular myocardium. Supraventricular arrhythmias are further categorized as PSVTs, which depend on AV nodal conduction, and intra-atrial arrhythmias, which depend only on atrial tissue and not on AV conduction. The PSVTs include AVNRT and AV reciprocating tachycardia related to WPW syndrome. Intra-atrial arrhythmias include organized atrial arrhythmias, such as focal atrial tachycardia, atrial flutter, macro-reentrant atrial tachycardia, and AF, a common disorganized atrial arrhythmia. Recurrent atrial flutter and AF carry a risk of thromboembolism and, based on risk stratification, should be treated with antithrombotic therapy when appropriate. Catheter ablation has an important role in the management of all supraventricular arrhythmias but remains a second-line strategy for AF, for which success rates are lower and complication rates are higher than for other supraventricular arrhythmias.

Ventricular arrhythmias include isolated ventricular premature beats; short, nonsustained runs of tachycardia; and sustained ventricular arrhythmias. Sustained VT lasts more than 30 seconds or requires intervention before then. It is classified as monomorphic if beats all share a single electrocardiographic morphology, polymorphic if the electrocardiographic morphology is variable, TdP when the morphology is variable and the arrhythmia is associated with pathologic QT prolongation, and VF when the surface ECG continuously varies without distinct QRS complexes. VT is poorly tolerated and is the major cause of cardiac arrest. Although commonly seen in the setting of ischemic heart disease, idiopathic VT may be seen in the absence of structural heart disease.

Antiarrhythmic drugs have not been effective in reducing the risk of SCD after MI. In contrast, ICDs have been shown to improve mortality rates for patients with impaired LV function after an MI and patients with heart failure and impaired LV function with or without coronary disease.

In addition to advanced structural heart disease as a cause for VT, several syndromes may result in VT in the absence of evident structural heart disease. They include the syndrome of idiopathic VT, ARVC, arrhythmogenic RV dysplasia, congenital LQTS, Brugada syndrome, and CPVT. Several of these conditions are familial, and genetic testing and family screening have important roles in their management.

SUGGESTED READINGS

Al-Khatib SM, Stevenson WG, Ackerman MJ, et al.: 2017 AHA/ACC/HRS guideline for management of patients with ventricular arrhythmias and the prevention of sudden cardiac death, *Circulation* 138:e272–e391, 2018.

Calkins H, Hindricks G, Cappato R, et al.: 2017 HRS/EHRA/ECAS/APHRS/ SOLAECE expert consensus statement on catheter and surgical ablation of atrial fibrillation, *Heart Rhythm* 14:e275–e444, 2017.

January CT, Wann LS, Calkins H, et al. AHA/ACC/HRS Focused Update of the 2014 AHA/ACC/HRS Guideline for the Management of Patients With Atrial Fibrillation. A Report of the American College of Cardiology/American Heart Association Task Force on Clinical Practice Guidelines and the Heart Rhythm Society 2019:25873.

Priori SG, Wilde AA, Horie M, et al.: Executive summary: HRS/EHRA/APHRS expert consensus statement on the diagnosis and management of patients with inherited primary arrhythmia syndromes, *Heart Rhythm* 10:e85–e108, 2013.

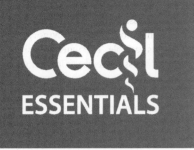

10

Pericardial and Myocardial Disease

Jennifer L. Strande

PERICARDIAL DISEASE

The pericardium is a thin, fibrous sac that envelops the heart and consists of two layers: visceral and parietal. The space between these two layers contains a small amount of fluid (15 to 50 mL), which is a plasma ultrafiltrate. The pericardium has mechanical, immunologic, and anatomic barrier functions.

Due to a paucity of randomized trial data and absence of practice guideline statements, the recommendations for assessment and treatment of pericardial disorders in this chapter are largely based on expert opinion and professional consensus.

Acute Pericarditis
Definition and Epidemiology
Acute pericarditis or inflammation of the pericardium has several causes. The exact incidence of acute pericarditis is unknown because a subclinical course is common.

Pathology
About 85% of cases are from idiopathic or viral causes. Less commonly, infection (other than viral), uremia, trauma, metabolic disorders, autoimmune disorders, and neoplastic involvement can also cause pericarditis. Causes of acute pericarditis are listed in Table 10.1.

Clinical Presentation
The classic manifestation of acute pericarditis is severe and sharp chest pain, which is often aggravated by a supine position, inspiration, and cough and relieved by sitting up and leaning forward. The pain is usually substernal and left precordial, and may radiate to the neck, shoulder, and scapular ridge, mimicking that of myocardial ischemia. Chest discomfort may be mild or absent in patients with connective tissue disorders, uremia, or neoplastic involvement. Patients may also have symptoms of low-grade fever, malaise, dyspnea, and less frequently, hiccups (i.e., phrenic nerve irritation).

In the absence of significant pericardial effusion, results of the inspection and palpation of the precordium are normal. A high-pitched, rasping pericardial friction rub is heard on cardiac auscultation in most patients with acute pericarditis. It may have three components corresponding to atrial contraction, ventricular systole, and early diastole, and it is best appreciated at end expiration with the patient leaning forward. It can be intermittent, and serial auscultation is recommended.

Diagnosis
The electrocardiographic (ECG) changes of acute pericarditis typically evolve over days to weeks. The early stage findings are characterized by diffuse ST segment elevation (i.e., concave upward) with upright T waves and PR depression. PR depression occasionally precedes the ST segment elevation. Resolution of the ST elevations is followed by diffuse T wave inversion. These ECG changes are not always seen and serial tracings should be obtained.

The laboratory findings of acute idiopathic pericarditis are not specific and consist of mild elevation of the white blood cell count, sedimentation rate, and C-reactive protein level. If indicated, specific testing for tuberculosis, human immunodeficiency virus (HIV), thyroid disease, or autoimmune disorders is recommended. However, routine performance of viral serologic testing has limited utility. Elevation of serum cardiac biomarkers (e.g., creatine kinase, troponin) reflects involvement of the adjacent myocardium. In uncomplicated acute pericarditis, the chest radiograph and echocardiographic findings are normal. Although not essential for the diagnosis of pericarditis, echocardiography is the diagnostic imaging modality of choice for the detection and determination of the hemodynamic significance of a pericardial effusion.

Treatment
Patients with uncomplicated idiopathic or viral pericarditis can be managed as outpatients. For patients with fever, large pericardial effusions, or elevated levels of cardiac biomarkers and for those with possible secondary causes or immunocompromised status, hospitalization for further investigation and treatment should be considered. Treatment consisting of high-dose nonsteroidal anti-inflammatory drugs (NSAIDs) is usually effective. Colchicine with NSAIDs or as monotherapy provides prompt resolution of symptoms and decreases the recurrence rate. The use of glucocorticoids results in rapid symptomatic improvement. However, glucocorticoids are associated with higher rates of symptomatic recurrence.

Prognosis
Most patients with idiopathic or viral pericarditis have an uneventful clinical course with complete recovery. Possible complications include recurrent pericarditis, cardiac tamponade, and constrictive pericarditis.

Pericardial Effusion and Cardiac Tamponade
Definition and Epidemiology
Pericardial effusion, an abnormal collection of fluid in the pericardial space, is a relatively common and incidental echocardiographic finding that is encountered in approximately 10% of studies. Cardiac tamponade occurs when fluid accumulation results in increased intrapericardial pressure, leading to cardiac compression, impaired ventricular filling, and reduced cardiac output. Accumulation of pericardial fluid can be caused by virtually any type of acute pericarditis. Pericardial effusions due to bacterial pericarditis (including tuberculosis), neoplastic involvement, uremic pericarditis, and trauma have a high incidence of progression to tamponade.

TABLE 10.1   Causes of Pericarditis

Idiopathic
Infectious
  Viral (echovirus, coxsackievirus, adenovirus, cytomegalovirus, hepatitis B virus, Epstein-Barr virus, human immunodeficiency virus)
  Bacterial (*Staphylococcus, Streptococcus,* and *Mycoplasma* species; *Borrelia burgdorferi, Haemophilus influenzae, Neisseria meningitidis*)
  Mycobacterial *(Mycobacterium tuberculosis, Mycobacterium avium-intracellulare)*
  Fungal (*Histoplasma* and *Coccidioides* species)
  Protozoal
Immune or inflammatory
  Connective tissue disease (systemic lupus erythematosus, rheumatoid arthritis, scleroderma)
  Arteritis (polyarteritis nodosa, temporal arteritis)
  Late after myocardial infarction (Dressler syndrome), late postcardiotomy or thoracotomy
Drug induced
  Procainamide, hydralazine, isoniazid, cyclosporine
Trauma or damage to adjacent structures
  Penetrating trauma
  Acute myocardial infarction, cardiac surgery, coronary angioplasty, implantable defibrillators, pacemakers
  Pneumonia
Neoplastic disease
  Primary: mesothelioma, fibrosarcoma, lipoma
  Secondary (metastatic or direct extension): breast, lung, thyroid carcinoma, lymphoma, leukemia, melanoma
Radiation induced
Miscellaneous
  Uremia
  Hypothyroidism
  Gout

Pathology

The hemodynamic consequences of a pericardial effusion depend on the rate of accumulation. The normal pericardium has relatively limited reserve volume. The mechanical properties of the parietal pericardium are such that when stretched, it becomes rapidly inelastic and resistant to further expansion. As a result, rapidly accumulating effusions may result in significant hemodynamic compromise with only 100 to 200 mL of fluid. Conversely, when the accumulation of fluid is slow, the pericardium undergoes adaptive changes and can accommodate large (>1500 mL) effusions without the development of tamponade.

Clinical Presentation

The clinical manifestations of a pericardial effusion depend on the size and rate of fluid accumulation and may range from dyspnea, chest discomfort, and orthopnea to circulatory collapse, pulseless electrical activity, and death. Compression of adjacent structures such as the phrenic nerve and the recurrent laryngeal nerve can result in cough or hiccups and hoarseness, respectively. Compression of the esophagus may cause dysphasia.

A normal cardiac examination is not uncommon in patients with small effusions. With larger effusions, the apical impulse can be decreased or absent, and the cardiac sound may be muffled. In patients with acute pericarditis, disappearance of the pericardial friction rub may indicate development of an effusion. Compression of the left lung base can result in dullness to percussion, egophony, and bronchial breath sounds under the left scapula (i.e., Ewart sign).

Patients with tamponade usually appear to be in distress with tachypnea and tachycardia. The classic physical findings include hypotension, jugular venous distention with an absent *y* descent, and muffled or absent heart sounds. Pulsus paradoxus, a characteristic physical finding, is defined as a greater than 10 mm Hg of inspiratory decline of the systolic blood pressure. This results from the inspiratory decrease of the left ventricular stroke volume and systemic blood pressure. Under normal conditions, the intrathoracic pressure decreases during inspiration, resulting in enhanced right ventricular filling and enlargement. In cases of cardiac tamponade, the total heart volume is fixed, and the right ventricular expansion displaces the interventricular septum toward the left ventricle, with consequent reduction of the left ventricular stroke volume and systemic hypotension. Pulsus paradoxus is not pathognomonic of cardiac tamponade and can be detected in severe chronic obstructive airway disease, pulmonary embolism, bronchial asthma, constrictive pericarditis, and hypovolemic shock.

Diagnosis

The ECG findings of moderate to large pericardial effusions include low-voltage QRS complexes and occasionally electrical (QRS) alternans caused by the heart's swinging motion within the fluid-filled pericardium. The chest radiograph demonstrates an enlarged cardiac silhouette. Transthoracic echocardiography, the imaging modality of choice, provides information regarding the size, location (circumferential vs. loculated), and most importantly, the hemodynamic consequences of the pericardial effusion suggesting tamponade.

The two-dimensional findings of tamponade include right atrial and right ventricular collapse, distention of the inferior vena cava, and evidence of increased ventricular interdependence (Fig. 10.1). Doppler quantification of the mitral and tricuspid inflow velocity respiratory variation is more sensitive than two-dimensional echocardiography for determining the hemodynamic significance of pericardial effusions. Right heart catheterization demonstrates decreased cardiac output, elevated right atrial pressure with diminished or absent *y* descent, and equalization of the cardiac filling pressures (i.e., right atrial, pulmonary wedge, and diastolic pulmonary artery pressures).

Computed tomography (CT) and magnetic resonance imaging (MRI) can accurately identify pericardial effusions and may be used along with echocardiography to assess for loculated effusions, pericardial thickening, and extracardiac structures. A diagnostic pericardiocentesis should be performed for evaluating for bacterial, tuberculous, or malignant causes.

Treatment

Routine drainage of pericardial effusions is unnecessary in the absence of hemodynamic compromise. Cardiac tamponade is a life-threatening emergency requiring urgent drainage of the pericardial effusion. Fluid resuscitation should be initiated to increase preload and filling of the cardiac chambers. Inotropic and vasopressor support has limited utility. Surgical drainage is appropriate and therapeutic for loculated, purulent, and tuberculous effusions and for tissue biopsy.

Fluid should be analyzed for pH, cell count, glucose, protein, cholesterol, triglycerides, and acid-fast bacilli by Gram stain, culture, cytology, and laboratory tests. For patients with chronic, recurring effusions, the surgical creation of a pleuropericardial window provides a long-term solution.

Prognosis

The underlying cause of the pericardial effusion and the availability of effective treatment determine the prognosis.

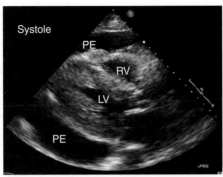
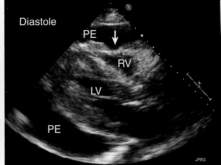

Fig. 10.1 Parasternal long axis echocardiographic views of the right ventricle in systole and diastole show right ventricular diastolic collapse *(arrow)* in a patient with a large, circumferential pericardial effusion. *LV,* Left ventricle; *PE,* pericardial effusion; *RV,* right ventricle.

Constrictive Pericarditis

Definition and Epidemiology

Pericardial constriction is caused by pericardial inflammation and is a condition characterized by a rigid, scarred pericardium that limits diastolic filling of the ventricles, resulting in increased intracardiac pressures. The most common causes are infection, prior cardiac surgery, trauma, and irradiation. Less common causes include connective tissue disorders, uremia, and neoplastic involvement of the pericardium. In developing countries, tuberculous pericarditis is a more common cause of pericardial constriction. Often a specific cause cannot be determined.

Pathology

Constriction is the end result of pericardial inflammation with scarring, fibrosis, calcification, and adhesion of the parietal and visceral layers of the pericardium. Although pericardial thickening is a usual pathologic finding, its absence does not exclude constriction.

Clinical Presentation

In the early stages, symptoms consist of dyspnea, fatigue, decreased exercise tolerance, and lower extremity edema. As the disease progresses, early signs and symptoms may be accompanied by ascites, anasarca, cachexia, and muscle wasting.

Physical examination reveals jugular venous distention with prominent *x* and *y* descents and an increase (or failure to decrease) of central venous pressure with inspiration (i.e., Kussmaul sign). The arterial blood pressure is usually normal, and pulsus paradoxus is absent in most patients. Ascites and hepatomegaly can be prominent with advanced disease. On cardiovascular examination, the apical impulse may be decreased, and the cardiac sounds muffled. An early diastolic sound (i.e., pericardial knock) corresponding to the abrupt cessation of early ventricular diastolic filling is pathognomonic of pericardial constriction, but it is not always detected.

Diagnosis

The diagnosis of pericardial constriction may be challenging and frequently requires the use of multiple imaging modalities. The electrocardiogram may display low QRS voltage, left atrial enlargement, and nonspecific T-wave changes. Atrial fibrillation occurs in one third of cases. The chest radiograph may reveal pleural effusions and pericardial calcification, which are best appreciated in the lateral projection.

Transthoracic echocardiography shows dilation of the inferior vena cava, abnormal interventricular septal motion, and pericardial thickening. Doppler echocardiography demonstrates abnormal respirophasic variations of the pulmonary and hepatic venous flow and mitral valve inflow. CT and MRI can accurately measure pericardial thickness.

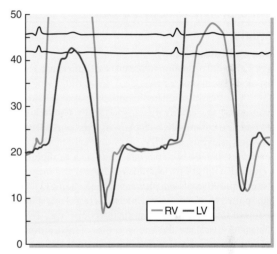

Fig. 10.2 Pressure recordings from a patient with constrictive pericarditis. Simultaneous right ventricular and left ventricular pressure tracings show equalization of diastolic pressure and dip-and-plateau morphology. *LV,* Left ventricle; *RV,* right ventricle.

Cardiac catheterization is essential in the diagnosis of pericardial constriction and differentiation from restrictive cardiomyopathy (RCM). The right atrial pressure tracing shows prominent *x* and *y* descents with equalization of the end-diastolic atrial and ventricular pressures. The ventricular pressure tracings show a rapid early diastolic filling of the ventricles, with abrupt cessation in middle and end diastole due to the finite volume of the rigid pericardium (i.e., dip-and-plateau morphology or the square root sign) (Fig. 10.2). Enhanced ventricular interdependence demonstrated by simultaneous measurement of right and left ventricular pressures during respiration is a more specific finding of pericardial constriction.

Treatment

Medical therapy with sodium restriction and diuretics is of limited efficacy and is only appropriate in patients who are not surgical candidates due to comorbidities. Pericardiectomy is the only definitive treatment for constrictive pericarditis.

Prognosis

Pericardiectomy is associated with substantial operative risk that depends on the extent of cardiac involvement and existence of comorbid conditions. Successful pericardial resection leads to resolution of the symptoms of constriction over a period of weeks to months. For patients who are not surgical candidates, the prognosis is poor.

Effusive Constrictive Pericarditis

Effusive constrictive pericarditis is characterized by a pericardial effusion and a noncompliant or fibrotic parietal and visceral pericardium. Although it may result from any type of pericardial inflammation, it is usually seen after cardiac surgery or radiation injury. It likely represents a transition stage between acute pericarditis with effusion and pericardial constriction. It shares the clinical and hemodynamic features of both conditions.

Typically, drainage of the effusion does not result in resolution of symptoms, and the central venous and right atrial pressures remain elevated. In the early stage of the disease, patients may respond to prolonged treatment with NSAIDs. However, visceral and parietal pericardiectomy is often required. For a deeper discussion of this topic, please see Chapter 68, "Pericardial Diseases," in *Goldman-Cecil Medicine*, 26th Edition.

DISEASES OF THE MYOCARDIUM

Myocarditis
Definition and Epidemiology

Myocarditis is an inflammation of the myocardium caused by a variety of toxins, medications, and viruses. Viral myocarditis, which accounts for about 20% of cases of dilated cardiomyopathy (DCM), is commonly caused by the enteroviruses, specifically Coxsackie group B serotypes and, less commonly, adenoviruses, parvovirus B19, hepatitis C virus, cytomegalovirus, and HIV.

Other causes include bacterial infections such as diphtheria, brucellosis, clostridial infections, legionnaires disease, and meningococcal, streptococcal, and *Mycoplasma pneumoniae* infections. Q fever, Rocky Mountain spotted fever, spirochetal infections (e.g., leptospirosis, Lyme disease), fungal infections, and parasitic infections (e.g., *Trypanosoma cruzi* [Chagas' disease]) are also known causes of myocarditis.

Pathology

The pathogenesis of viral myocarditis is thought to begin with direct viral invasion of the myocardium and subsequent immunologic activation. Normal cellular and antibody-mediated immune responses lead to viral clearing and myocardial healing. However, a few patients go on to develop DCM and heart failure due to an abnormal immune response that furthers myocardial damage. The exact mechanisms are unknown, but they involve cytokines, autoantibodies, and possibly other processes associated with persistent, low-level viral replication in myocytes, leading to myocyte atrophy, myocyte apoptosis, and adverse remodeling of the ventricles. In nonviral infections, the damage is attributed to the bacterial toxins or abnormal immune responses, and in parasitic infections, it is largely immune mediated.

Multiple chemicals and drugs can lead to myocardial inflammation by direct effect or as part of a hypersensitivity reaction. Some of the common causes include cocaine, chemotherapeutics (e.g., daunorubicin, doxorubicin), and antibiotics.

Giant cell myocarditis is a rare disorder of uncertain origin, but it can be rapidly fatal. It is usually associated with ventricular arrhythmias and progressive, severe heart failure. Multinucleated giant cells seen on myocardial biopsy are pathognomonic.

Clinical Presentation

The clinical manifestations range from asymptomatic ECG abnormalities to cardiogenic shock. Patients report heart failure symptoms, including exercise intolerance, shortness of breath, fluid retention, and persistent fatigue. In the setting of viral myocarditis, they often report a viral prodrome, including fever, myalgia, fatigue, respiratory symptoms, or gastroenteritis that precedes the heart failure symptoms.

Patients are often tachycardic and hypotensive. They may have an elevated jugular venous pressure, S_3 gallop, crackles, and peripheral edema. Myocarditis can masquerade as an acute coronary syndrome.

Diagnosis

Testing is performed to determine a possible infectious cause. Rising viral titers are often seen in cases of viral myocarditis. Serum cardiac enzymes (e.g., troponin, creatine kinase) are measured when myocarditis is suspected. Sinus tachycardia and nonspecific ST- and T-wave abnormalities are common ECG findings. When the pericardium is also involved by the inflammatory process, diffuse ST-segment elevations typical for acute pericarditis are also seen. Ventricular ectopy is common, and atrioventricular conduction defects are seen in myocarditis associated with Lyme disease.

Echocardiography is recommended in the initial diagnostic evaluation to identify ventricular remodeling, including increasing chamber size and ventricular systolic dysfunction. Cardiac MRI is a promising technique to detect myocardial inflammation and injury based on small, observational clinical studies.

Transvenous endomyocardial biopsy should be performed only when there is rapid deterioration of the clinical condition. Histopathologic abnormalities such as infiltrating white cells (i.e., macrophages, lymphocytes, and eosinophils), evidence of myocardial damage, and interstitial fibrosis help to establish acute myocarditis, but the determination is subject to significant intraobserver and interobserver variability. Often the biopsy does not provide a conclusive diagnosis. The endomyocardial biopsy is helpful in diagnosing giant cell myocarditis (i.e., multinucleated giant cells are seen) or hypersensitivity myocarditis (i.e., eosinophilic infiltrate is seen). Polymerase chain reaction testing can detect specific viral genomes in the myocardium.

Treatment

Supportive care is the mainstay of treatment. A few patients with fulminant or acute myocarditis require an intensive level of hemodynamic support and aggressive pharmacologic intervention similar to that for patients with advanced heart failure.

After initial hemodynamic stabilization, treatment should follow current American College of Cardiology and American Heart Association (ACC/AHA) recommendations for the management of left ventricular systolic dysfunction. Treatment includes β-adrenergic blockers, angiotensin-converting enzyme inhibitors, aldosterone receptor blockers, and diuretics.

No evidence-based guided therapy for viral myocarditis has been established. Clinical trials of various forms of antiviral or immunosuppressive therapy (e.g., prednisone, cyclosporine, azathioprine, intravenous immunoglobulin, interferon immunoadsorption) have not resulted in conclusive evidence of benefit. Treatment of nonviral myocarditis is aimed at eradication of the specific infectious agent. For Chagas' disease, treatment with antiprotozoal therapy, if initiated early in the course of infection, may be beneficial.

Hypersensitivity myocarditis and myocarditis associated with toxins respond to withdrawal of the offending agent. Immunosuppressive therapy has been effective in giant cell myocarditis.

Prognosis

The diverse clinical presentations and causes of myocarditis have limited the understanding of its natural history. It is thought that one third of the patients fully recover, one third of the patients have some sequelae in the form of left ventricular systolic dysfunction but are stable on medical therapy, and one third of patients progress to advanced heart failure. Patients who progress to chronic DCM have 5-year survival rates of less than 50%.

TABLE 10.2   Cardiomyopathies

Disorder	Description and Cause
Dilated cardiomyopathy	Dilation and impaired systolic function of the left or both ventricles
Familial (genetic)	Known or unknown genetic mutations
Nonfamilial	Viral myocarditis, nonviral infective myocarditis, idiopathic (immune) myocarditis
	Toxins (drugs, alcohol)
	Pregnancy (peripartum cardiomyopathy)
	Nutritional (thiamine deficiency [beriberi], vitamin C deficiency [scurvy], selenium deficiency)
	Endocrine (diabetes mellitus, hyperthyroidism, hypothyroidism, hyperparathyroidism, pheochromocytoma, acromegaly)
	Autoimmune (rheumatoid arthritis, systemic lupus erythematosus, dermatomyositis)
	Tachycardia induced
Hypertrophic cardiomyopathy	Left and/or right ventricular hypertrophy, often asymmetrical (usually more prominent hypertrophy of the interventricular septum)
Familial (genetic)	Mutations of sarcoplasmic proteins (several hundred described)
	Metabolic storage diseases of the myocyte
Restrictive cardiomyopathy	Restrictive filling of the ventricles; ventricles are usually small, atria are markedly enlarged
Familial (genetic)	Mutations of sarcomeric proteins
	Familial amyloidosis (transthyretin, apolipoprotein)
	Hemochromatosis
	Desminopathy, pseudoxanthoma elasticum, glycogen storage diseases
	Unknown genetic mutations
Nonfamilial	Amyloidosis, sarcoidosis, carcinoid, scleroderma
	Endomyocardial fibrosis (hypereosinophilic syndrome, idiopathic, chromosomal defect, drugs)
	Radiation, metastatic cancer, anthracycline toxicity
Arrhythmogenic right ventricular	Progressive fibrofatty replacement of the right and, to a lesser degree, left ventricular cardiomyopathy
Familial	Unknown gene mutation
	Mutations of intercalated disk protein, cardiac ryanodine receptor, transforming growth factor-β3
Unclassified Cardiomyopathies	
Takotsubo (stress-induced) cardiomyopathy	Transient dilation and dysfunction of the distal parts of the left ventricle (apical ballooning) in the setting of a stressful situation; usually resolves within weeks
Left ventricular noncompaction	Characterized by prominent left ventricular trabeculae and deep intertrabecular recesses; familial in most cases, caused by arrest in the normal embryogenesis of the heart; apex and periapical regions of the left ventricle most affected; some patients remain asymptomatic, but others develop left ventricular dilation and systolic dysfunction
Cardiomyopathies associated with muscular dystrophies and neuromuscular disorders	Duchenne-Becker muscular dystrophy, Emery-Dreifuss muscular dystrophy, myotonic dystrophy, Friedreich's ataxia, neurofibromatosis, tuberous sclerosis
Ion channelopathies	Disorders caused by mutations in genes encoding ionic channel proteins; not considered cardiomyopathies because they are not associated with typical structural changes of the heart but rather manifest with electrical dysfunction; some classifications include these disorders as cardiomyopathies: long QT syndrome, short QT syndrome, Brugada syndrome, catecholaminergic polymorphic ventricular tachycardia

Cardiomyopathies

Cardiomyopathies are a heterogeneous group of diseases in which the major structural abnormality is limited to the myocardium. The four main cardiomyopathic groups are dilated, hypertrophic, restrictive, and arrhythmogenic right ventricular cardiomyopathy. Atrophic cardiomyopathy is a newer recognized group. Familial (genetic) and nonfamilial (acquired) forms of the diseases have been described.

Dilated Cardiomyopathy

Definition and epidemiology. Cardiac enlargement and systolic dysfunction in DCM result from a wide spectrum of genetic, inflammatory, toxic, and metabolic causes (Table 10.2), although most cases are idiopathic. Abnormal loading conditions such as hypertension, valvular disease, or coronary artery disease can lead to similar structural and functional changes; these conditions are not considered to be part of the DCM group and are discussed elsewhere.

Most cases are thought to result from acute viral myocarditis, a process described earlier. Exposures to cardiac toxins such as chemotherapeutic agents, alcohol, cocaine, and radiation, along with deficiency of nutrients such as thiamine (causes beriberi), vitamin C (causes scurvy), carnitine, selenium, phosphate, and calcium, can cause DCM. Peripartum cardiomyopathy is a rare cause of DCM that can develop during the last month of pregnancy and up to 6 months after delivery. The pathogenesis of this peripartum cardiomyopathy is not completely understood, and it is a diagnosis of exclusion. Risk factors include older maternal age, being African American, and having multiple pregnancies. Prolonged periods of supraventricular or ventricular tachycardia can lead to idiopathic DCM (i.e., tachycardia-induced cardiomyopathy). The structural and functional changes usually reverse after the rapid heart rhythm is controlled.

Familial forms of DCM may be responsible for 20% to 30% of cases. Specific mutations involve genes that encode proteins of the sarcomere, cytoskeleton, nuclear membrane, and mitochondria; many mutations remain unknown. The mode of inheritance is typically autosomal dominant, but it can be an X-linked or mitochondrial pattern.

Pathology. Marked enlargement of all four cardiac chambers is typical of DCM, although the disease sometimes is limited to the left or right chambers. The dilation is out of proportion to the ventricular thickness. Histology reveals evidence of myocyte degeneration with irregular hypertrophy and atrophy of myofibers with often extensive interstitial and perivascular fibrosis.

Clinical presentation. DCM usually manifests with symptoms of heart failure such as fatigue, weakness, dyspnea, and edema. In some patients, the presenting episode is related to arrhythmia or an embolic event. On physical examination, signs of decreased cardiac output are often found, including cool extremities, narrow pulse pressure, and tachycardia. The cardiac examination reveals a laterally displaced apex. An S_3 gallop is common, along with murmurs of mitral and tricuspid regurgitation. Pulmonary edema manifests as auscultatory crackles over the lung fields, and breath sounds may be diminished if there are pleural effusions. In some patients, the clinical features of right ventricular heart failure may predominate, with jugular venous distention hepatomegaly, ascites, and peripheral edema.

Diagnosis. Standard diagnostic procedures include a chest radiograph, an electrocardiogram, serum markers, and echocardiography. The radiograph shows cardiomegaly, pulmonary venous congestion, and pleural effusions. The electrocardiogram may reveal enlargement of the heart chambers along with other nonspecific ST- and T-wave abnormalities. Serum B-type natriuretic peptide (BNP) levels are elevated.

Echocardiography provides a comprehensive evaluation of ventricular size and function and valvular function, and it can show a ventricular thrombus. Similar information can be obtained with MRI.

A complete work-up should rule out ischemic, valvular, and hypertensive heart disease as the cause of myocardial dysfunction, and it should include evaluation for potentially reversible causes of DCM (e.g., alcohol, nutritional deficiencies). Myocardial biopsy may be considered if the cause of DCM is in question. In patients with a strong family history, a referral for genetic testing should be considered.

Treatment. Potential reversible causes of DCM should be addressed (e.g., alcohol cessation, correction of nutritional deficiencies, removal of cardiotoxic agents). Treatment should follow current ACC/AHA recommendations for the management of left ventricular systolic dysfunction and include β-adrenergic blockers, angiotensin-converting enzyme inhibitors, aldosterone receptor blockers, and diuretics.

Patients with idiopathic DCM who have persistent, moderate to severe symptoms of heart failure and a QRS duration longer than 120 milliseconds may benefit from cardiac resynchronization therapy with a biventricular pacemaker. Survival of patients with a left ventricular ejection fraction less than 35% despite maximal medical management is improved with the use of implantable cardioverter-defibrillators (ICDs). Patients with limiting heart failure symptoms despite use of the previously described therapies may be considered for heart transplantation or support with a left ventricular assist device.

Prognosis. The prognosis of patients with DCM depends on the response to medical therapy. Some patients have a significant improvement in symptoms and cardiac function, but in others, the disease is progressive and associated with a high mortality rate.

Hypertrophic Cardiomyopathy

Definition and epidemiology. Hypertrophic cardiomyopathy (HCM) is a disease state characterized by left ventricular hypertrophy with nondilated ventricular chambers in the absence of an apparent cause for hypertrophy (e.g., hypertensive disease, aortic stenosis). This is a relatively common genetic disease (1 case in 500 people in the general population) with autosomal dominant inheritance, although spontaneous mutations have been described. More than 1400 mutations identified among at least eight genes encoding proteins of the cardiac sarcomere have been described, with mutations of the β-myosin heavy chain being the most common.

Pathology. The main pathophysiologic abnormalities seen in HCM are left ventricular outflow obstruction, diastolic dysfunction, mitral regurgitation, and arrhythmias. Obstruction of left ventricular outflow occurs in roughly one half of the patients. During systole, the hypertrophied septum bulges into the left ventricular outflow tract, creating a gradient between the lower part of the left ventricular cavity and the left ventricular outflow. This causes high-velocity turbulent flow through the narrowed path, which results in a suction force (i.e., Venturi effect) that pulls the anterior leaflet of the mitral valve into the outflow tract. This worsens the obstruction and causes mitral regurgitation. Diastolic dysfunction from impaired relaxation properties of the abnormal myocardium causes marked elevation of left ventricular filling and pulmonary venous pressures, pulmonary congestion, and limitation in cardiac output. Patients with HCM are also predisposed to supraventricular and ventricular arrhythmias.

Clinical presentation. HCM is a heterogeneous cardiac disease with a diverse course and clinical manifestations. Most patients probably do not suffer sequelae from this disease during their lifetimes. When the disease does result in complications, there are three relatively discrete but not mutually exclusive clinical manifestations: sudden cardiac death due to unpredictable ventricular tachyarrhythmia, most commonly in young asymptomatic patients (<35 years of age); heart failure characterized by exertional dyspnea (with or without chest pain) that may progress despite preserved systolic function and sinus rhythm; and atrial fibrillation that associates with various degrees of heart failure.

Heart failure symptoms result from the dynamic obstruction to left ventricular outflow and diastolic dysfunction. The most frequent symptom is dyspnea on exertion, followed by ischemic chest pain due to the increased oxygen demand by the hypertrophied ventricle and elevated wall tension that reduces blood flow to the subendocardium. Abnormalities of the structure of small myocardial arteries in HCM can contribute to myocardial ischemia. Presyncope or syncope can result from outflow tract obstruction and an inability to increase cardiac output during exertion or from arrhythmias that can be triggered by exertion. In some, sudden death caused by ventricular arrhythmia is the initial manifestation of the disease.

Physical examination findings include pulsus bisferiens, a brisk initial upstroke in pulse followed by a midsystolic dip corresponding to the development of left ventricular outflow tract obstruction, followed by another rise in late systole. Cardiac examination may reveal a forceful and sustained apical impulse, an audible S_4 gallop, and a harsh crescendo-decrescendo systolic murmur best heard along the left sternal border with radiation to the base of the heart.

Patients may also have an apical holosystolic murmur of mitral regurgitation. The intensity of the murmur of HCM varies with changing degrees of obstruction. This can be observed with physiologic or pharmacologic maneuvers that change preload (i.e., left ventricular filling) or contractility. The intensity of the murmur increases with a Valsalva maneuver, with assuming a standing position, and after administration of nitroglycerin or inotropic drugs. The intensity of the murmur decreases with squatting, volume loading, and administration of β-blockers.

Diagnosis. Clinical diagnosis is made most commonly with echocardiography and increasingly with cardiac MRI. The diagnosis is based on a maximal left ventricular wall thickness of 15 mm or more; a wall thickness of 13 to 14 mm is considered borderline. The diagnosis can be made in the setting of other compelling information (e.g., family history of HCM). Genetic testing is available to confirm the diagnosis and to screen family members.

Treatment. The ACC/AHA hypertrophic cardiomyopathy guideline recommends tailored therapy based on the individual patient. For

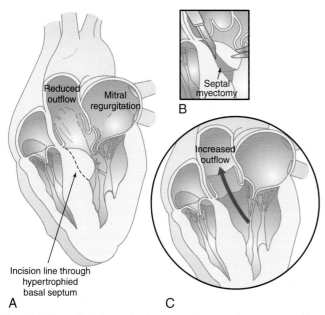

Fig. 10.3 (A to C) Schematic diagrams of a septal myectomy. (From Nishimura RA, Holmes DR Jr: Clinical practice: hypertrophic obstructive cardiomyopathy, N Engl J Med 350:1320-1327, 2004.)

asymptomatic patients, the usefulness of β-blockade and verapamil may be considered. For patients symptomatic with dyspnea or angina, β-blockers and verapamil are recommended. If patients remain symptomatic, it is reasonable to add disopyramide to a β-blocker or verapamil.

Nonpharmacologic therapies should be considered in patients with considerable symptoms despite medical management. Septal reduction therapy is recommended only for patients with severe drug-refractory symptoms and left ventricular outflow tract obstruction (Fig. 10.3). Use of ICD therapy for prevention of sudden death is guided by the perceived risk for ventricular arrhythmias in individual patients. Some of the characteristics that have been associated with this risk are prior cardiac arrest or sustained ventricular tachycardia; great (>30 mm) ventricular wall thickness; syncope, especially if exertional or recurrent; and a first-degree relative with sudden cardiac death. Certain genotypes appear to convey an increased risk of sudden cardiac death. Patients with HCM should be excluded from most competitive sports and should avoid strenuous exercise.

Prognosis. The clinical course of HCM varies. Sudden cardiac death is the leading cause of mortality. Heart failure symptoms may gradually progress and patients who are unresponsive to conventional therapy may require heart transplantation.

Restrictive Cardiomyopathies

Definition and epidemiology. RCM is an uncommon form of cardiomyopathy characterized by impaired ventricular filling of nondilated ventricles. RCM can be genetic or acquired. Causes include infiltrative disorders (e.g., amyloidosis, sarcoidosis, Gaucher's disease, Hurler's syndrome, fatty infiltration), storage diseases (e.g., hemochromatosis, Fabry's disease, glycogen storage disease), other disorders (e.g., hypereosinophilic syndrome, carcinoid heart disease), drugs (e.g., serotonin, methysergide, ergotamine), and cancer treatment (e.g., irradiation, chemotherapy).

Pathology. In the purest form of the disease, the atria are disproportionately dilated compared with the normal ventricular size, and the left ventricle has normal or near-normal systolic function

in the absence of hypertrophy. Histology is normally nondistinctive and can reveal normal findings or nonspecific degenerative changes, including myocyte hypertrophy, disarray, and degrees of interstitial fibrosis.

Clinical presentation. Patients often have symptoms and signs of pulmonary and systemic congestion. The most common symptoms include dyspnea, palpitations, fatigue, weakness, and exercise intolerance due to poor cardiac output. As central venous pressure continues to increase in advanced cases, there may be hepatosplenomegaly, ascites, and anasarca. The chest radiograph shows atrial enlargement, pulmonary venous congestion, and pleural effusions.

Diagnosis. The diagnosis of RCM should be considered for patients with predominantly right ventricular heart failure without evidence of cardiomegaly or systolic dysfunction. The correct diagnosis often is not made until months or years after symptom onset. Constrictive pericarditis can mimic RCM and establishing the correct diagnosis can be challenging. Distinctive features of the two disorders are described in Table 10.3.

Treatment. Treatment of RCM focuses on alleviating the symptoms of heart failure. Diuretics are used for decongestion, but intravascular depletion may compromise ventricular filling and lead to reduced cardiac output and hypotension. Supraventricular tachyarrhythmias are poorly tolerated. In patients with conduction system disease such as advanced atrioventricular block, a permanent pacemaker may be indicated. Specific therapies for underlying disorders include chemotherapy in amyloidosis, phlebotomy and iron chelation therapy in hemochromatosis, and steroids in sarcoidosis and endomyocardial fibrosis.

Prognosis. The course of RCM depends on the pathology, and treatment is often unsatisfactory. In the adult population, the prognosis usually is poor, with progressive deterioration and death due to low-output heart failure.

Arrhythmogenic Right Ventricular Cardiomyopathy

Definition and epidemiology. Arrhythmogenic right ventricular cardiomyopathy (ARVC) is an autosomal dominant disease characterized by specific myocardial pathology. The estimated prevalence of ARVC is about 1 case in 2000 to 5000 people, and it has a male predominance.

Pathology. The myocardium of the right ventricular free wall is progressively replaced by fibrous and adipose tissue. Right ventricular function is abnormal, with regional akinesis or dyskinesis or global right ventricular dilation and dysfunction.

Clinical presentation. The disease typically manifests in young adults as palpitations, dizziness or syncope, or sudden cardiac death. Symptoms of right ventricular failure are rare, despite evidence of right ventricular dysfunction on imaging studies.

Diagnosis. The clinical diagnosis of ARVC is suggested by integration of the information from the clinical presentation (e.g., arrhythmias), electrocardiogram, family history, and imaging studies. When available, histologic examination of the right ventricle confirms the diagnosis. The resting electrocardiogram may be normal, but common abnormalities include incomplete or complete right bundle branch block, the so-called epsilon waves that follow the QRS complex, and inverted T waves in the precordial leads. Right ventricular dilation and systolic dysfunction can be seen with echocardiography and MRI. The latter modality can also show myocardial fat.

Treatment. Treatment consists of ICD therapy to prevent sudden cardiac death, but the indications for implantation are not well defined. Antiarrhythmics and radiofrequency ablation of ventricular tachycardia are used in patients with frequent arrhythmias, but they have not been shown to reduce the risk of sudden cardiac death.

TABLE 10.3 Differentiation of Restrictive Cardiomyopathy From Constrictive Pericarditis

Type of Evaluation	Restrictive Cardiomyopathy	Constrictive Pericarditis
Physical examination	Kussmaul sign present	Kussmaul sign may be present
	Apical impulse may be prominent	Apical impulse usually not palpable
	Regurgitant murmurs are common	Pericardial knock may be present
Electrocardiography	Low QRS voltage (especially in amyloidosis)	Low QRS voltage
	Pseudoinfarction pattern	Repolarization abnormalities
	Bundle branch blocks	
	AV conduction disturbances	
	Atrial fibrillation	
Chest radiography		Calcification of the pericardium may be present
Echocardiography	Marked enlargement of the atria	Atria usually of normal size
	Increased wall thickness (especially in amyloidosis)	Normal wall thickness
		Pericardial thickening may be seen
Doppler echocardiography	Restrictive mitral inflow (dominant E wave with short deceleration time)	Restrictive mitral inflow (dominant E wave with short deceleration time)
	No significant variation (<10%) of transvalvular velocities with respiration	Increased velocity of RV filling and decreased velocity of LV filling with inspiration; opposite with expiration; variation in velocity exceeds 15%
	Reversal of forward flow in hepatic veins during inspiration	Reversal of forward flow in hepatic veins during expiration
Cardiac catheterization	Prominent atrial x and y descents (w sign)	Prominent atrial x and y descents (w sign)
	Dip-and-plateau appearance of ventricular diastolic pressure	Dip-and-plateau appearance of ventricular diastolic pressure
		Increase and equalization of diastolic pressures
	Diastolic pressures increased but not equalized; LV diastolic pressure higher than RV diastolic pressure	Discordance of RV and LV peak systolic pressures (with inspiration, RV systolic pressure increases and LV systolic pressure decreases)
Endomyocardial biopsy	May reveal specific cause of restrictive cardiomyopathy	No specific findings on endomyocardial biopsy
		Pericardial biopsy may reveal abnormality
Computed tomography, magnetic resonance imaging		Pericardial thickening

AV, Atrioventricular; *LV,* left ventricular; *RV,* right ventricular.

Patients with a probable or definite diagnosis of ARVC should be excluded from competitive sports.

Prognosis. The prognosis for these patients remains uncertain.

Unclassified Cardiomyopathies

Some cardiomyopathies that do not fit the current categories are described in Table 10.2.

❖ For a deeper discussion of this topic, please see Chapter 54, "Diseases of the Myocardium and Endocardium," in Goldman-Cecil Medicine, 26th Edition.

SUGGESTED READINGS

Elliott P, Andersson B, Arbustini E, et al: Classification of the cardiomyopathies: a position statement from the European Society of Cardiology Working Group on Myocardial and Pericardial Diseases, Eur Heart J 29:270–276, 2008.

Gersh BJ, Maron BJ, Bonow RO, et al: 2011 ACCF/AHA guideline for the diagnosis and treatment of hypertrophic cardiomyopathy: a report of the American College of Cardiology Foundation/American Heart Association Task Force on Practice Guidelines. Developed in collaboration with the American Association for Thoracic Surgery, American Society of Echocardiography, American Society of Nuclear Cardiology, Heart Failure Society of America, Heart Rhythm Society, Society for Cardiovascular Angiography and Interventions, and Society of Thoracic Surgeons, J Am Coll Cardiol 58:e212–e260, 2011.

Kindermann I, Barth C, Mahfoud F, et al: Update on myocarditis, J Am Coll Cardiol 59:779–792, 2012.

Maron BJ, Ackerman MJ, Nishimura RA, et al: Task Force 4: HCM and other cardiomyopathies, mitral valve prolapse, myocarditis, and Marfan syndrome, J Am Coll Cardiol 45:1340–1345, 2005.

Maron BJ, Towbin JA, Thiene G, et al: Contemporary definitions and classification of the cardiomyopathies: an American Heart Association scientific statement from the Council on Clinical Cardiology, Heart Failure and Transplantation Committee; Quality of Care and Outcomes Research and Functional Genomics and Translational Biology Interdisciplinary Working Groups; and Council on Epidemiology and Prevention, Circulation 113:1807–1816, 2006.

Yancy CW, Jessup M, Bozkurt B, et al: 2013 ACCF/AHA guideline for the management of heart failure: a report of the American College of Cardiology Foundation/American Heart Association Task Force on Practice Guidelines, Circulation 128:1810–1852, 2013.

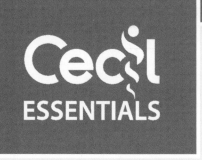

11

Other Cardiac Topics

Jinnette Dawn Abbott, Sena Kilic

CARDIAC DISEASE IN PREGNANCY

Pregnancy is associated with dramatic changes in the cardiovascular system that may result in significant hemodynamic stress to the patient with underlying heart disease. During a normal pregnancy, plasma volume increases an average of 50%, beginning in the first trimester and peaking between the 20th and 24th weeks of gestation. This change is accompanied by increases in stroke volume, heart rate, and, accordingly, cardiac output. In addition, a concomitant fall in systemic vascular resistance and mean arterial pressure occurs because of the effects of gestational hormones on the vasculature and the creation of a low-resistance circulation in the pregnant uterus and placenta. During labor, uterine contractions result in a transient increase of up to 500 mL of blood in the central circulation, resulting in further increases in stroke volume and cardiac output. After delivery, intravascular volume and cardiac output increase further as compression of the inferior vena cava by the gravid uterus is relieved and extravascular fluid is mobilized. The American Heart Association guidelines for the prevention of cardiovascular disease in women identified pregnancy complications as risk factors for cardiovascular disease in women. Hypertensive disorders of pregnancy and gestational diabetes mellitus are independently associated with increased 10-year cardiovascular risk.

Most women with cardiovascular disease can complete a pregnancy and delivery with proper follow-up. While cardiac disease may sometimes be manifested for the first time in pregnancy, the symptoms and signs that may mimic cardiac disease often accompany the usual hemodynamic changes of pregnancy, including fatigue, reduced exercise tolerance, lower-extremity edema, distention of the neck veins, S_3 gallop, and new systolic murmurs. Differentiating symptoms produced by cardiac disease from those attributable to a normal pregnancy can be difficult. Under such circumstances, echocardiography can be a safe and helpful noninvasive test to assess cardiac structure and function in the pregnant patient.

Certain cardiac conditions, including pulmonary hypertension, cardiomyopathy, valvular heart disease and connective tissue disorders including Marfan syndrome with a dilated aortic root, are associated with a high risk for cardiovascular complications and maternal death and require special consideration and counseling. The risk for cardiac complications during pregnancy depends on the maternal conditions as summarized in Table 11.1.

Specific Cardiac Conditions
Valvular Heart Disease

Due to the declining incidence of rheumatic heart disease in Western countries, valvular heart disease is infrequent in North America but remains prevalent in developing countries. Bicuspid aortic stenosis and mitral stenosis are the most common valvular diseases encountered during pregnancy. When aortic stenosis complicates pregnancy, it is usually secondary to a congenital bicuspid aortic valve whereas mitral stenosis is the most common rheumatic valvular disease encountered during pregnancy. These valvular conditions tend to worsen during pregnancy due to the increased cardiac output and tachycardia. Congestive heart failure may develop as the pregnancy progresses and may be worsened by the onset of atrial fibrillation. Careful echocardiographic assessment is recommended, and the cornerstone of therapy for the symptomatic patient is β-blockade. In patients with symptoms refractory to medical therapy aortic balloon valvuloplasty for aortic stenosis or mitral balloon valvotomy for mitral stenosis can be considered. Mitral and aortic regurgitation are usually well tolerated in pregnancy provided the regurgitation is no more than moderate in severity, the woman is symptom-free before pregnancy, and the left ventricular function is normal.

Prosthetic valves. When selecting a prosthetic valve for women of childbearing age, careful consideration has to be made with regards to the type of valve. Mechanical valves have greater longevity but routinely involve the use of warfarin, which is associated with a higher chance of fetal loss, placental hemorrhage, and prosthetic valve thrombosis. Tissue valves are less thrombogenic but tend to degenerate after an average of 10 years, necessitating a re-operation, which carries certain operative risks including mortality.

There is no universal consensus on the management of a pregnancy when the mother has a mechanical valve prosthesis. Prepregnancy counseling should include a detailed discussion of the risks to the patient. During pregnancy, increased platelet adhesiveness, increased concentration of clotting factors, and decreased fibrinolysis increase the risk of maternal valve thrombosis and thromboembolism. Unfractionated heparin, used subcutaneously or intravenously, is begun in the first trimester, as soon as pregnancy is diagnosed, to minimize fetal exposure to the teratogenic effects of warfarin. It is usually continued until week 13 or 14 of pregnancy, when fetal embryogenesis is complete, after which warfarin is resumed. Continuing heparin throughout pregnancy has been shown to increase valve thrombosis risk to 33%. Low-molecular-weight heparin is an alternative to unfractionated heparin but its use remains controversial with no large prospective studies or evidence base to support its use and therapeutic monitoring.

Marfan Syndrome

Pregnant women with Marfan syndrome are at increased risk for aortic dissection and rupture, especially during the third trimester and the first postpartum month. Pregnancy is contraindicated in women with an aortic root diameter greater than 40 mm. Periodic echocardiographic surveillance every 6 to 8 weeks is recommended to monitor the mother's aortic root size and treatment with β-adrenergic blockers is recommended. Vaginal delivery is safe in patients with Marfan syndrome with an aortic diameter less than 40 mm. To

TABLE 11.1 **Specific Maternal Cardiac Conditions and Risk for Cardiac Complications During Pregnancy**

Low Risk	Intermediate Risk	High Risk
Small left-to-right shunts	Large left-to-right shunt	New York Heart Association class III or IV symptoms
Repaired lesions without residual dysfunction	Unrepaired or palliated cyanotic congenital heart disease	Severe pulmonary hypertension
Mitral valve prolapse without regurgitation	Mechanical prosthetic valves	Marfan syndrome with aortic root dilation or major valvular disease
Bicuspid aortic valve without stenosis	Mitral or aortic valve stenosis	Severe aortic stenosis
Mild to moderate pulmonic stenosis	Severe pulmonic stenosis	History of peripartum cardiomyopathy with residual ventricular dysfunction
Valvular regurgitation with normal ventricular systolic function	Moderate to severe ventricular dysfunction	
	Unrepaired coarctation of the aorta	
	History of peripartum cardiomyopathy without residual ventricular dysfunction	

minimize pain and hemodynamic changes, epidural anesthesia and β-blockers or vasodilators should be used and forceps or vacuum use is recommended to shorten the second stage of labor. In patients with aortic diameter 40 mm or greater, delivery via elective C-section should be performed in a tertiary care center with cardiothoracic surgical expertise.

Congenital Heart Disease

Congenital heart disease is the predominant maternal cardiac disease in Western societies, and all patients with a history of congenital heart disease, whether or not they have had repair, should receive a detailed evaluation and appropriate counseling before conception. Patients with uncomplicated atrial or ventricular septal defects usually tolerate pregnancy without complications unless they have concomitant pulmonary hypertension or atrial fibrillation. In patients with pulmonary hypertension, pregnancy is contraindicated. The added volume load of pregnancy may potentially precipitate left ventricular failure in patients with large intracardiac shunts.

In women with coarctation of the aorta, symptoms may first present during pregnancy, typically as systemic hypertension. Therapeutic options such as antihypertensive therapy, percutaneous stenting of the coarctation, and surgical intervention are available and most women will have a successful pregnancy with proper care.

Women with uncorrected tetralogy of Fallot should undergo palliative or definitive repair before conception to improve maternal and fetal outcomes. Women with residual obstruction of the right ventricular outflow tract are at risk of worsening cyanosis and risk to both mother and fetus during pregnancy.

Heart Disease Arising During Pregnancy
Hypertension

Hypertension is the most common medical problem in pregnancy. It is defined as absolute blood pressure values greater than 140 mm Hg systolic or 90 mm Hg diastolic. The major forms of hypertension that may develop during pregnancy are essential or primary hypertension, gestational hypertension, preeclampsia superimposed on essential hypertension, and preeclampsia. Essential hypertension is defined as hypertension, without a secondary cause, present before pregnancy or that is diagnosed before week 20 of gestation. Gestational hypertension is new hypertension without proteinuria that occurs after the 20th week of gestation and resolves within 2 weeks after delivery.

The mainstay of treatment of hypertension in pregnancy is antihypertensive medications, which are usually effective in treating essential hypertension but not effective in preventing preeclampsia. Agents that have been safely used in pregnancy include hydralazine, α-methyldopa, clonidine, β-blockers, and labetalol. Diuretics should be used with caution because of the increased risk for placental hypoperfusion. When preeclampsia develops, typically characterized by hypertension and proteinuria, bedrest, salt restriction, and close monitoring are initiated and magnesium sulfate can be administered to prevent eclamptic seizures and prolong pregnancy to facilitate fetal maturity. Blood pressure usually normalizes rapidly with delivery.

Peripartum Cardiomyopathy

Peripartum cardiomyopathy (PCM) is a form of dilated cardiomyopathy that may begin during the last trimester of pregnancy or within 5 months of delivery in a previously healthy woman. The true incidence of the disease is unknown, but estimates conclude that 1 in every 2500 to 4000 pregnancies is affected in the United States. Although the cause of PCM is unknown, myocardial injury is thought to be immunologically mediated with inflammation playing a key role as evidenced by elevated serum markers of inflammation in many patients. Known risk factors include multiparity, black race, older maternal age and preeclampsia. Women usually exhibit symptoms and signs of congestive heart failure and cardiac imaging, usually with a transthoracic echocardiogram, establishes the diagnosis.

Management is similar to that for congestive heart failure (see Chapter 5) and usually includes the use of hydralazine, β-blockers, digoxin, and diuretics for symptom management and preload reduction. Diuretics may potentially reduce placental blood flow and must be used with caution. Angiotensin-converting enzyme inhibitors have been associated with increased fetal wastage in pregnant animals and aldosterone antagonists may have antiandrogenic effects on the fetus; therefore both classes of drugs should be avoided. Nitrates and inotropes may be necessary in severe cases and early fetal delivery may be necessary. Mechanical circulatory support may be necessary and cardiac transplantation may be considered in those cases refractory to mechanical circulatory support.

The outcome with PCM is variable. Left ventricular function normalizes in approximately 23% to 54% of women and death or progressive heart failure occurs in one third of affected women. The recurrence rate with subsequent pregnancies is 30%. In patients with full recovery of left ventricular function, mortality is negligible in subsequent pregnancies; however, women with a left ventricular ejection fraction less than 25% at diagnosis or persistent left ventricular dysfunction should be counseled against a subsequent pregnancy.

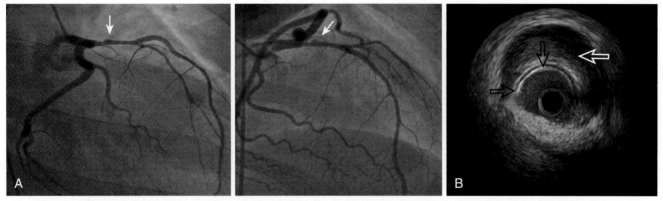

Fig. 11.1 Postpartum anterior wall myocardial infarction from spontaneous coronary dissection of the left anterior descending and diagonal arteries demonstrated by (A) left coronary angiography showing diffusely narrowed coronary lumen (proximal left anterior descending artery indicated by the *arrow*), and (B) intravascular ultrasound confirming hematoma in the medial-adventitial layer of the vessel. The imaging catheter is central in the lumen. *Black arrows* indicate the vessel media and the *white arrow* the hematoma. The intima of the vessel is thin and normal.

Spontaneous Coronary Artery Dissection

Spontaneous coronary artery dissection (SCAD) is defined as a separation of the arterial wall and subsequent coronary artery obstruction caused by the formation of an intramural hematoma that is not associated with atherosclerosis, trauma or iatrogenic injury (Fig. 11.1). While SCAD is the most common cause of pregnancy-associated myocardial infarction, pregnancy-associated SCAD represents a relatively small proportion of SCAD cases. The prevalence is 1.81 SCAD events per 100,000 pregnancies during pregnancy or in the postpartum period. SCAD has been reported as early as 5 weeks' gestation and up to a year or more postpartum, particularly in lactating women.

The cause of pregnancy-associated SCAD is not fully understood; however, hormonal changes of pregnancy are thought to alter the architecture of the arterial wall, weakening the wall and making it prone to rupture, intramural hematoma, and the subsequent development of clinical symptoms. Risk factors for pregnancy-associated SCAD include black race, chronic hypertension, lipid abnormalities, chronic depression, migraines, advanced maternal age, multiparty, and treatment for infertility.

Women with pregnancy-associated SCAD have poorer prognosis than women with SCAD not related to pregnancy. They have larger infarcts, more proximal artery dissections, and lower mean left ventricular ejection fraction immediately and at follow-up. Maternal complications of pregnancy-associated SCAD include cardiogenic shock, ventricular fibrillation, and mechanical circulatory support. In-hospital mortality has been reported to be as high as 4%.

CARDIAC TUMORS

Cardiac tumors are broadly divided into primary and secondary tumors. Primary cardiac tumors, defined as benign or malignant neoplasms that arise from any tissue of the heart, are extremely rare, with an autopsy incidence of 0.001% to 0.03%. Secondary, or metastatic, cardiac tumors are 30 times more common than primary tumors, with an autopsy incidence of 1.7% to 14%.

It is not uncommon for patients with cardiac tumors to initially have no symptoms or physical findings, but rather present with abnormalities on imaging. Alternatively, patients may present with a constellation of nonspecific symptoms or findings on physical examination.

The initial evaluation is typically imaging such as a two-dimensional transthoracic echocardiogram or magnetic resonance imaging (MRI). Once a mass is identified and described, additional imaging may be undertaken

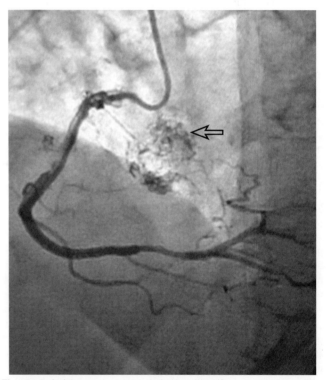

Fig. 11.2 Atrial myxoma vascularization identified on cardiac catheterization. Selective right coronary angiography demonstrates that the vascular supply to the tumor originates from atrial branches. The vascularized tumor is indicated by the *arrow*.

such as three-dimensional echocardiography with contrast, transesophageal echocardiography for anatomic information, MRI with gadolinium, coronary angiography to define coronary anatomy, position emission tomography (PET) for staging, and/or computed tomography (CT) to delineate other intrathoracic structures. When assessing a cardiac mass, the clinical context is critical to the diagnosis. The differential diagnosis of a cardiac mass is broad and includes tumors, thrombi, infection, and artifact.

Benign Primary Cardiac Tumors

Most primary cardiac tumors are benign, and myxoma is the most common primary tumor of the heart (Fig. 11.2). Most myxomas are

TABLE 11.2 Cardiac Trauma Categorized by Mechanism of Injury

Penetrating	Nonpenetrating (Blunt)
Stab wounds (e.g., knives, swords, ice picks)	Motor vehicle accident
Gunshot wounds (e.g., handguns, nail guns)	Vehicular-pedestrian accident
Shotgun wounds	Falls from height
Blast fragments	Crush (e.g., industrial accidents)
	Blast (e.g., explosives)

found in the left atrium. Less commonly, they may be found in the right atrium, right ventricle, and left ventricle in decreasing frequencies. While most myxomas occur sporadically, a familial pattern of myxomas can occur in an autosomal dominant manner. In a particular syndrome called the Carney complex, patients may present with cardiac myxomas, cutaneous myxomas, breast fibroadenomas, hyperpigmented nevi, hyperactive adrenal or testicular glands, and pituitary tumors. The Carney complex occurs in young individuals and should be considered in myxomas in atypical locations in the heart. Surgical removal is the only definitive treatment of cardiac myxomas. Myxomas tend to recur with rates varying from 5% to 14%; therefore, it is imperative that lifelong follow-up continue after surgical removal.

Less common benign tumors include rhabdomyomas, fibromas, lipomas, and papillary fibroelastomas. Rhabdomyomas are the most common cardiac tumors found in children and are usually located in the ventricle. They are often associated with a family history of tuberous sclerosis. Surgery can often be avoided unless the patient develops clinical evidence of arrhythmias and heart failure. Fibromas are composed of fibroblasts or collagen and typically occur in childhood. They are most often located on the interventricular septum and patients may present with chest pain, pericardial effusion, heart failure, arrhythmias, and sudden death. While both occur in the ventricle, the distinguishing feature of fibromas, in contrast to rhabdomyomas, is the presence of calcification. Lipomas are rare and occur most frequently in the left ventricle and the right atrium, although they can be found anywhere in the heart and the pericardium. They are frequently asymptomatic but can grow large enough to cause obstructive symptoms. Papillary fibroelastomas are pedunculate tumors with filiform attachments that typically arise from the aortic or mitral valve. They carry an elevated risk of embolic phenomena and, when situated on the aortic valve, can cause coronary ostial occlusion. Complete surgical resection is recommended because of the risk of systemic embolism. Recurrence rates are low and long-term anticoagulation is not recommended unless the patient has other indications.

Malignant Primary Cardiac Tumors

Malignant primary cardiac tumors commonly cause symptoms via three mechanisms: obstruction, embolization, and arrhythmia. Obstructive tumors can present with syncope, chest pain, dyspnea or heart failure. Pericardial invasion and tamponade are rarely the first manifestation of the disease. Primary cardiac sarcoma is the most common malignant primary cardiac tumor. Once diagnosed, treatment for cardiac sarcomas is primarily surgical with complete resection as the goal followed by adjacent chemotherapy. Cardiac sarcomas carry a very poor overall prognosis.

Secondary Cardiac Tumors

Cardiac metastases are common and can be found in up to 14% of patients dying with a known malignancy. Cardiac metastases can occur either by direct extension, by way of the bloodstream or lymphatics, or by intracavitary diffusion through the inferior vena cava (IVC). Metastases to the pericardium are most common, followed by epicardium, myocardium, and endocardium. Primary thoracic cancers, including breast and lung cancer, tend to invade the pericardium directly whereas abdominal and pelvic tumors reach the right atrium usually through the IVC. Renal cell carcinoma is the most common tumor to exhibit this tendency. In men and women, lung cancer is the most frequent cause of cardiac metastasis. In men, this is followed by esophageal cancer and lymphoma whereas in women it is followed by lymphoma and breast cancer.

The prognosis of metastatic cardiac tumors is poor, with 1-year mortality being 50%. Treatment therefore is primarily palliative and may include radiation therapy, chemotherapy, and surgical resection, if possible. Malignant pericardial effusion is typically managed with pericardiocentesis and may need a pericardiotomy to reduce subsequent reaccumulation of pericardial fluid.

TRAUMATIC HEART DISEASE

Traumatic heart disease can be categorized based on the mechanism of injury (Table 11.2).

Nonpenetrating Cardiac Trauma

Nonpenetrating or blunt cardiac trauma accounts for about 10% of all traumatic heart disease. Nonpenetrating cardiac trauma can manifest as a spectrum of pathology including septal rupture, free wall rupture, coronary artery thrombosis or dissection, rupture of the cordae tendinae or papillary muscle, pericarditis or cardiac tamponade, and arrhythmias. Commotio cordis is a type of nonpenetrating cardiac trauma that occurs more often in child athletes as a result of a projectile such as a ball striking the chest, resulting in ventricular fibrillation and sudden cardiac death.

Nonpenetrating cardiac trauma can present with clinically significant or clinically insignificant injury. Conduction disturbances are common and a screening 12-lead electrocardiogram (ECG) can be useful for initial evaluation. Sinus tachycardia is the most common ECG abnormality. Other possible findings on ECG include T-wave and ST-segment changes, bradycardia, first- and second-degree atrioventricular block, right bundle branch block, third-degree heart block, atrial fibrillation, premature ventricular complexes, ventricular tachycardia, and ventricular fibrillation. Elevated cardiac enzymes are not specific for blunt cardiac trauma and may be related to severity of noncardiac injury or underlying coronary disease. In one study, only 485 of patients with elevated troponin were clinically found to have significant blunt cardiac trauma. A negative troponin, however, had a negative predictive value of 93%. The major use of transthoracic echocardiography in the evaluation of nonpenetrating cardiac trauma is for the assessment of pericardial effusion, the presence of which is concerning for chamber rupture. Transesophageal echocardiography is a more sensitive test for the evaluation of more subtle features of blunt cardiac injury.

Most patients who present with suspected blunt cardiac injury can be managed with observation and monitoring. Patients in cardiogenic shock in whom structural injury is confirmed should be promptly referred to cardiothoracic surgery for surgical repair.

Penetrating Cardiac Trauma

Penetrating cardiac injury is the most common cause of significant cardiac injury, most often by firearms and knives. Due to their anterior location on the chest wall, the right and left ventricles are at the greatest risk for injury. Most penetrating cardiac injuries involve the myocardium, sparing additional structures, and are managed effectively with surgical intervention and rarely requiring reoperation for a residual defect.

Penetrating injury to the epigastrium and precordium should raise suspicion for penetrating cardiac injury. The clinical presentation

TABLE 11.3 Key Features of Available Left Ventricular Percutaneous Assist Devices

	IABP	Impella 2.5	Impella CP	Impella 5.0	TandemHeart	V-A ECMO
Mechanism	Aorta	LV → Aorta	LV → Aorta	LV → Aorta	LA → Aorta	RA → Aorta
Flow (L/min)	0.3-0.5	1.0-2.5	3.7-4.0	Max 5.0	2.5-5.0	3.0-7.0
Max implant time	—	7-10 days	7-10 days	2-3 weeks	2-3 weeks	3-4 weeks
Ability to oxygenate	No	No	No	No	No	Yes
Cardiac Power	↑	↑↑	↑↑	↑↑	↑↑	↑↑↑
Afterload	↓	↓	↓	↓	↑	↑↑↑
MAP	↑	↑↑	↑↑	↑↑	↑↑	↑↑
LVEDP	↓	↓	↓↓	↓↓	↓↓	↔
PCWP	↓	↓↓	↓↓	↓↓	↓↓	↔
LV preload	—	↓↓	↓↓	↓↓	↓↓	↓
Coronary perfusion	↑	↑	↑	↑	—	—

IABP, Intraaortic balloon pump; *LA*, left atrium; *LV*, left ventricle; *LVEDP*, left ventricular end-diastolic pressure; *MAP*, mean arterial pressure; *PCWP*, pulmonary capillary wedge pressure; *RA*, right atrium; *V-A ECMO*, veno-arterial extracorporeal membrane oxygenation.

could be varied from normal vital signs to circulatory collapse. This is because after a weapon injuring the myocardium and pericardium is withdrawn, blood filling the pericardium may not be able to escape. As pericardial fluid accumulates, ventricular filling is impaired and stroke volume decreases. In response to a decrease in stroke volume, there is a catecholamine surge resulting in tachycardia and increased right-sided filling pressures. As little as 60 mL to 100 mL of blood in the pericardial sac can result in clinical pericardial tamponade where the limits of distensibility are reached and there is bowing of the interventricular septum, further compromising left ventricular function, reducing cardiac output, and resulting in irreversible shock. The classic findings of Beck triad (muffled heart sounds, hypotension and distended neck veins) is rarely seen. Pulsus paradoxus (a fall in systolic blood pressure of 20 mm Hg or more during inspiration) and Kussmaul sign (increase in jugular venous distention on inspiration) may be present but not reliably predictive of pericardial tamponade. Narrowing of the pulse pressure, however, is a reproducible sign of tamponade. In the case of penetrating cardiac injury, definitive treatment involves surgical intervention.

PERCUTANEOUS MECHANICAL CIRCULATORY SUPPORT

Mechanical circulatory support (MCS) is a term that refers to mechanical pumps designed to assist or replace the function of the left ventricle, right ventricle or both ventricles of the heart. There are several MCS systems available including the intra-aortic balloon pump (IABP), extracorporeal membrane oxygenation (ECMO) or extracorporeal life support (ECLS), ventricular assist devices (VADs), and total artificial hearts (TAHs). Further details on the disease process and management of chronic heart failure are covered in Chapter 5. The following discussion will focus on temporary or percutaneous MCS as indicated in patients with cardiogenic shock refractory to medical therapy when the objective is rapid augmentation of cardiac output, reduction of ventricular filling pressures, and life support. Longer-term support, with VADs, TAHs, and cardiac transplantation are covered elsewhere. A comparison of the key features of the available percutaneous assist devices is summarized in Table 11.3.

Percutaneous Left Ventricular Assist Devices
Intra-Aortic Balloon Pump
The IABP remains the most commonly used form of circulatory support. A polyethylene helium-filled balloon is placed percutaneously through the femoral artery into the thoracic aorta, just distal to the left subclavian artery. Timing of balloon inflation and deflation is based on the ECG or the arterial waveform of the patient. The balloon inflates with the onset of diastole and deflates at the onset of left ventricular systole. Balloon inflation during diastole increases diastolic blood pressure, referred to as diastolic augmentation, allowing for maximal delivery of oxygenated blood to the coronary arteries. Deflation during systole decreases the afterload and myocardial oxygen consumption while modestly enhancing cardiac output. The IABP reduces myocardial oxygen demand but provides only modest ventricular unloading. Patients must have some left ventricular function and electrical stability for an IABP to be most effective because the device only results in an increase in cardiac output of 0.5 to 1.0 liter per minute.

The major contraindication for IABP is greater than mild aortic valve regurgitation because the diastolic inflation of the balloon may worsen the degree of regurgitation. Severe peripheral arterial disease or aortic disease increases the risk of vascular complication such as thromboembolism and lower extremity and visceral ischemia. Potential major complications include balloon leak, severe bleeding (e.g., retroperitoneal), thromboembolic events, major limb or visceral ischemia, vascular trauma, thrombocytopenia from platelet deposition in the IABP membrane, and infection.

Impella
The Impella (Abiomed, Danvers, Mass.) is a nonpulsatile axial flow Archimedes-screw pump that propels blood from the left ventricle into the proximal ascending aorta. Depending on the version used, these devices can deliver up to 5.0 L/min of maximal flow. Designed to be placed via the femoral artery, delivery can either be percutaneous (Impella 2.5 and CP) or via a surgical cutdown (Impella 5.0). At the tip of the catheter there is a flexible pigtail loop that stabilizes the device in the left ventricle. The main body of the device contains the pump inlet and outlet areas, motor housing, and pump pressure monitor. Unlike the IABP, the Impella does not require ECG or arterial pressure timing and therefore provides stability despite transient arrhythmias.

The hemodynamic effects of the Impella are to unload the left ventricle and increase forward flow, reducing myocardial oxygen consumption, improving mean arterial pressure, and reducing pulmonary capillary wedge pressure. Compared to the IABP, the Impella delivers a significant increase in cardiac output. Adequate right ventricular function is necessary to maintain left ventricular preload and hemodynamic support. In cases where there is significant biventricular failure or unstable ventricular arrhythmias, a concomitant right ventricular assist device may be necessary.

Contraindications to the use of the Impella are the presence of a mechanical aortic valve, left ventricular thrombus, severe aortic stenosis, moderate to severe aortic insufficiency, severe peripheral arterial disease, and the inability to tolerate systemic anticoagulation. Possible complications of Impella use include limb ischemia, vascular complications, hemolysis due to mechanical erythrocyte shearing, and bleeding requiring blood transfusion.

TandemHeart

The TandemHeart (TandemLife, Pittsburgh, Penn.) is a percutaneous centrifugal pump that provides up to 4 L/min of mechanical circulator support via a continuous-flow centrifugal pump. The TandemHeart is inserted through the femoral vein and advanced across the interatrial septum into the left atrium. Oxygenated blood is then withdrawn from the left atrium via a 21-Fr inflow cannula and reinjected into the lower abdominal aorta or iliac arteries via a 15-Fr to 17-Fr outflow cannula. The need for transseptal puncture is a limitation to the widespread use of this device. The potential complications of the TandemHeart include the need for blood transfusion, sepsis/systemic inflammatory response syndrome, bleeding around the cannula, gastrointestinal bleeding, coagulopathy, stroke, left atrial perforation, and device-related limb ischemia.

Right Ventricular Support

Acute right ventricular (RV) failure may occur in a number of clinical settings such as acute myocardial infarction, fulminant myocarditis, acute pulmonary embolism, pulmonary hypertension, postcardiotomy shock, postcardiac transplantation, and following LVAD implantation. The mainstay of therapy for RV failure is inotropic and pulmonary vasodilator support and volume status optimization. Vasopressors are often used to maintain coronary perfusion pressure and inhaled nitric oxide can be used to reduce RV afterload. When these measures are insufficient to augment RV systolic function, mechanical circulatory support may be required to unload the RV, ensure adequate LV preload, and optimize tissue perfusion.

There are both surgical and percutaneous options for RV mechanical circulatory support. The surgical right ventricular assist device (RVAD) was associated with worse outcomes when compared to patients with RV failure who did not need an RVAD. Unfavorable outcome data and the need for repeat sternotomy for both insertion and removal of the device has limited clinical utilization. There are two percutaneous devices currently available for RV support: (1) Impella RP (Abiomed, Danvers, Mass.), an axial catheter-based pump and (2) the Protek Duo (Cardiac Assist Inc., Pittsburgh, Penn.), a catheter with an extracorporeal centrifugal pump. The Impella RP provides RV unloading with up to 4 L/min of continuous flow from the inlet in the inferior vena cava through a cannula to the outlet in the pulmonary artery. The pump is inserted via a 23-Fr sheath in the femoral vein into the atrium and across the tricuspid and pulmonic valves into the main pulmonary artery. The Protek Duo is a dual-lumen cannula that is inserted percutaneously via the internal jugular vein. The inflow lumen is positioned in the right atrium and the outflow lumen is positioned in the main pulmonary artery. The extracorporeal pump allows flows up to 5 L/min and an oxygenator can also be introduced into the circuit to allow for oxygenation support.

Extracorporeal Membrane Oxygenation

ECMO provides cardiopulmonary support in patients whose heart and/or lungs no longer provide adequate physiologic support. ECMO can be either veno-venous (V-V ECMO) for isolated pulmonary failure only or veno-arterial (V-A ECMO) for pulmonary and cardiac failure. Cannulas are placed in the right side of the heart, from the vena cava, to drain blood into the ECMO circuit for oxygenation. Blood can then either be returned to the right side of the heart in V-V ECMO or to the arterial system (proximal or distal aorta) in V-A ECMO. The bypass circuit in ECMO is composed of a centrifugal, nonpulsatile pump for blood propulsion, and a membrane oxygenator for gas exchange. V-A ECMO requires anticoagulation while V-V ECMO does not. Complications relate to bleeding, thromboembolism, and mechanical complications such as hemolysis and arterial insufficiency.

V-V ECMO offers gas exchange and is useful for conditions resulting in severe impairment of gas exchange such as ARDS or pulmonary embolism. V-V ECMO does not provide hemodynamic support. Alternatively, V-A ECMO provides additional hemodynamic support with flows sometimes exceeding 6 L/min depending on the cannula French size and length and properties of the pump. V-A ECMO alone, however, does not reduce ventricular wall stress and the use of a concomitant MCS such as IABP or percutaneous VAD is usually needed to vent or unload the left ventricle.

NONCARDAIC SURGERY IN THE PATIENT WITH CARDIOVASCULAR DISEASE

Noncardiac surgery in patients with known cardiovascular disease may be associated with an increased risk for death or cardiac complications such as MI, congestive heart failure, and arrhythmias. To determine an individual patient's risk for a procedure, the consulting physician must have knowledge of the type and severity of the patient's cardiac disease, the comorbid risk factors, and the type and urgency of surgery. In general, the preoperative evaluation and management are the same as in the nonoperative setting; for patients who are at risk, additional noninvasive and invasive testing may be performed if the results would affect treatment or outcome.

Estimation of a patient's perioperative risk can be determined by a careful clinical evaluation, including a history, physical examination, ECG, and type of surgery. Risk models can then be applied to guide the clinician with regards to additional testing and treatment. The most widely used risk model was developed in a study of 4315 patients 50 years or older undergoing major noncardiac procedures in a tertiary care teaching hospital and has been validated over the past 15 years. The index includes six independent predictors of complications in a revised cardiac risk index (RCRI): high-risk type of surgery, history of cerebrovascular disease, preoperative treatment with insulin, history of ischemic heart disease, history of congestive heart failure, and preoperative serum creatinine concentration greater than 2.0 mg/dL. The evaluating clinician can risk stratify the patients into low, intermediate, or high cardiovascular risk on the basis of having zero, one to two, or three or more risk factors, respectively. Another risk model was developed from the American College of Surgeons 2007 National Surgical Quality Improvement Program database (NSQIP), which identified five predictors of perioperative myocardial infarction or cardiac arrest: type of surgery, dependent functional status, abnormal creatinine level, American Society of Anesthesiologists class, and increasing age.

Once the clinical evaluation is complete and the type of surgery is known, the need for additional testing and treatment can be determined. Very high-risk patients are defined as those with recent myocardial infarction (within 60 days), unstable angina, decompensated heart failure, and hemodynamically important valvular disease. These patients are at very high risk of preoperative myocardial infarction, heart failure, fatal arrhythmia, and cardiac death. All such patients should be optimally treated and referred to a cardiologist for evaluation.

If emergency surgery is contemplated, little in the way of cardiac assessment can be performed, and recommendations may be directed at perioperative medical management and surveillance. If surgery is not urgent, additional evaluation is based on the clinical assessments of the risk and type of surgery.

Disease-Specific Approaches
Ischemic Heart Disease

About 70% of MIs occur within the first 6 days after an operation, with the peak incidence between 24 and 72 hours. Multiple stresses associated with surgery such as volume shifts, anemia, and infection can increase the heart rate and blood pressure perioperatively and can provoke myocardial ischemia. Identification of known or symptomatic stable coronary artery disease or risk factors for coronary artery disease can guide further evaluation or changes in perioperative management.

Patients with stable angina represent a continuum from mild to severe. In mild cases, patients manifest angina only after strenuous exercise and do not have signs of left ventricular dysfunction. These patients can be stabilized with optimal medical therapy with aspirin, β-adrenergic blocking agents and statins. On the severe end of the continuum, patients with angina on mild exertion are at high risk for development of perioperative major cardiovascular events and warrant consideration of additional cardiovascular testing.

Coronary angiography and revascularization should be reserved for individuals in whom this treatment would otherwise result in significant improvement in symptoms or long-term survival. Current data do not support a clear benefit of preoperative coronary revascularization.

The preoperative management of patients with a history of recent coronary artery revascularization on antiplatelet therapy is challenging as clinicians balance the cardiac risks of discontinuing therapy with the bleeding risks of continuing antiplatelet agents. Several large observational studies have shown an increased risk of adverse cardiovascular events in patients undergoing noncardiac surgery, particularly within 6 weeks of receiving a coronary stent. While the risk extends to 12 months, it stabilizes without significant decrease in risk from 6 to 12 months. The American College of Cardiology (ACC) and American Heart Association (AHA) guidelines recommend the following algorithm for patients with a coronary stent. If surgery is elective and can be safely delayed, the optimal timing is 12 months after PCI. For those in whom surgery cannot be delayed and are within 30 days of bare metal or 6 months of a drug-eluting stent, dual-antiplatelet therapy with aspirin and P2Y$_{12}$ inhibitor should be continued. If the risk of bleeding is prohibitive, the P2Y$_{12}$ inhibitor is temporarily interrupted (for 5 to 7 days) and aspirin is continued throughout the perioperative period because typically aspirin provides benefits that outweigh the bleeding risk. Possible exceptions to this include intracranial procedures, transurethral prostatectomy, intraocular procedures, and operations with extremely high bleeding risk. In clinical practice, the decision is made with a multidisciplinary team approach considering a number of factors such as the risk of stent thrombosis if DAPT needs to be interrupted, the consequences of delaying the surgical procedure, the increased intra- and periprocedural bleeding risks, and possible consequences of such bleeding if DAPT is continued.

Heart Failure

Studies have shown that heart failure is associated with increased perioperative cardiac morbidity after noncardiac surgery. During the postoperative period, congestive heart failure most commonly occurs in the first 24 to 48 hours, when fluid administered during surgery is mobilized from the extravascular space. However, heart failure may also result from myocardial ischemia and new arrhythmias. Initial management includes identification and treatment of the underlying cause. In addition, intravenous diuretics usually provide rapid relief of pulmonary congestion. If heart failure is complicated by hypotension or poor urine output, insertion of a pulmonary artery catheter may be helpful to guide additional therapy.

Valvular Heart Disease

In regard to valvular heart disease the greatest risk for complications after noncardiac surgery is in those with aortic or mitral stenosis. Patients with symptomatic, severe aortic or mitral stenosis should be evaluated for valve replacement before high-risk noncardiac surgery. In patients with mild to moderate aortic or mitral stenosis, careful attention to volume status and heart rate control are necessary to optimize left ventricular filling and avoid pulmonary congestion. In patients with valve disease or prosthetic heart valves, prophylactic antibiotics are recommended if appropriate. Lifelong anticoagulation with an oral vitamin K antagonist (VKA) is recommended for all patients with mechanical prosthetic heart valves. In addition to the thrombogenic nature of the intravascular prosthetic material, mechanical valves create abnormal flow conditions and areas of high-shear stress, both of which can result in platelet activation leading to valve thrombosis and embolic events. The preoperative management of patients with mechanical heart valves in whom interruption of anticoagulation therapy is needed for diagnostic or surgical procedures should account for the type of procedure, risk factors, and type, location, and number of heart valve prostheses. The ACC/AHA guidelines recommend continuation of VKA anticoagulation with a therapeutic INR in patients undergoing minor procedures (such as dental extractions or cataract removal) where uncontrolled bleeding risk is low. The guidelines recommend bridging anticoagulation with either intravenous unfractionated heparin or subcutaneous low-molecular-weight heparin during the time interval when INR is subtherapeutic in patients who are undergoing invasive or surgical procedures with (1) mechanical aortic valves and any thromboembolic risk factor, (2) older-generation mechanical aortic valves, or (3) mechanical mitral valves.

Arrhythmias and Conduction Defects

Patients with symptomatic, high-grade conduction disturbances, such as third-degree atrioventricular (AV) block, have an increased perioperative risk for cardiac complications and should have a temporary pacemaker inserted before surgery. Patients with first-degree AV block, Mobitz type I AV block, or bifascicular block (right bundle branch block and left anterior fascicular block) do not require prophylactic pacemaker insertion.

Atrial arrhythmias such as atrial fibrillation are common after surgery and usually are not associated with significant complications if the ventricular rate is well controlled. Mounting evidence suggests that new-onset postoperative atrial fibrillation following noncardiac surgery carries a similar risk of thromboembolism as in patients with nonvalvular atrial fibrillation. Therefore, the long-term management of these patients should be similar with regards to anticoagulation.

Ventricular premature beats and nonsustained ventricular tachycardia are also common after noncardiac surgery and do not require specific therapy unless they are associated with myocardial ischemia or heart failure. In most instances, treatment of the underlying cause (e.g., hypoxia, metabolic abnormalities, ischemia, volume overload) results in significant improvement or resolution of the rhythm disturbance without specific antiarrhythmic therapy.

SUGGESTED READINGS

Brickner ME: Cardiovascular management in pregnancy: congenital heart disease, *Circulation* 130:273–282, 2014.

Butt JH, Olesen JB, Havers-Borgersen E, et al.: Risk of thromboembolism associated with atrial fibrillation following noncardiac surgery, *J Am Coll Cardiol* 72:2027–2036, 2018.

Douketis JD, Spyropoulos AC, Kaatz S, et al.: Perioperative bridging anticoagulation in patients with atrial fibrillation, *N Engl J Med* 373:823–833, 2015.

Hayes SN, Kim ESH, Saw J, et al.: Spontaneous coronary artery dissection: current state of the science: a scientific statement from the American Heart Association, *Circulation* 137:e523–e557, 2018.

Huis In't Veld MA, Craft CA, Hood RE: Blunt cardiac trauma review, *Cardiol Clin* 36:183–191, 2018.

Maleszewski J, Anavekar N, Moynihan T, et al.: Pathology, imaging, and treatment of cardiac tumours, *Nat Rev Cardiol* 14:536–549, 2017.

Nanna M, Stergiopoulos K: Pregnancy complicated by valvular heart disease: an update, *J Am Heart Assoc* 3:e000712, 2014.

Nishimura RA, Otto CM, Bonow RO, et al.: 2014 AHA/ACC guideline for the management of patients with valvular heart disease: executive summary: a report of the American College of Cardiology/American Heart Association Task Force on Practice Guidelines, *Circulation* 129:2440–2492, 2014.

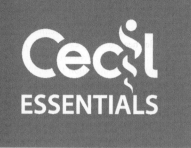

12

Vascular Diseases and Hypertension

Thomas Sperry, Wanpen Vongpatanasin

INTRODUCTION

Diseases of the systemic and pulmonary vasculature are among the most common clinical problems encountered in internal medicine. Yet these important diseases are not often given the emphasis they deserve; they fall between the cracks of traditional medical subspecialties. Early clinical recognition is important because effective therapy often can prevent or at least delay needless suffering and death. This chapter reviews the causes, clinical manifestations, diagnostic evaluations, and therapeutic approaches to the major forms of systemic and pulmonary vascular diseases, as well as arterial hypertension.

SYSTEMIC VASCULAR DISEASE

Peripheral Arterial Disease

Peripheral arterial disease (PAD) refers to atherosclerotic vascular disease of mainly the lower extremities. The prevalence increases with age, ranging from 2% to 6% for adults under the age of 60 years to 20% to 30% for those over age 70. As with coronary atherosclerosis, the major reversible risk factors are cigarette smoking, diabetes mellitus, hyperlipidemia, and hypertension. The diagnosis of PAD may at times be elusive, as only 30% to 50% of patients with PAD become symptomatic. PAD may present with symptoms of intermittent claudication, critical limb ischemia, or acute limb ischemia. Roughly 10% to 15% of patients present with the classic syndrome of intermittent claudication, which refers to ischemic muscle pain or weakness brought on by exertion and promptly relieved by rest. A larger proportion of PAD patients (50%) have more atypical leg symptoms different from classic claudication, which either may not limit an individual from walking or may not resolve within 10 minutes of rest. Claudication is also associated with a significant 10-year risk of morbidity and mortality. Approximately 10% to 20% of patients will develop worsening claudication or critical limb ischemia, 5% will require amputation, 10% to 20% will require revascularization, and up to 30% will die of a cardiovascular event (e.g., heart attack, stroke) as a result of concomitant coronary and/or cerebrovascular atherosclerosis. To minimize progression of PAD and avoid complications, risk factor modification is absolutely essential. This includes tight control of blood pressure (BP), plasma lipids, and blood glucose. Complete cessation of tobacco use is a must.

The diagnosis of PAD begins with a careful history and physical examination and is confirmed with noninvasive laboratory testing. Ischemic pain occurs in the leg muscles supplied by arterial segments that are distal to the site of stenosis. Calf claudication is the hallmark of femoral-popliteal disease, whereas discomfort in the thigh, hip, or buttock associated with impotence indicates aortoiliac disease (Leriche syndrome). Depending on the severity of the stenosis, the pain is experienced at a predictable walking distance and is promptly relieved by rest. Claudication must be differentiated from the pseudoclaudication of lumbar degenerative spinal canal stenosis. In the latter condition, walking can also aggravate leg pain, but it is not relieved simply by the cessation of exercise. Rather, assuming positions that minimize lumbar extension such as stooping forward or sitting alleviates the pain. The characteristic physical findings of PAD are absent or diminished pulses distal to the stenosis, bruits over the diseased artery, hair loss, thin shiny skin, and muscle atrophy. Severe ischemia causes pallor, cyanosis, decreased skin temperature, ulceration, and gangrene.

Noninvasive techniques are quite good in the diagnosis of PAD. The *ankle-brachial index* (ABI) is the ratio of the highest systolic BP measured from either the dorsalis pedis or posterior tibialis artery to the highest systolic BP obtained from the brachial artery of either arm using a Doppler stethoscope. The normal ABI range is 1.0 to 1.4. An ABI of 0.9 or less indicates PAD. This simple noninvasive test has a sensitivity and specificity of 68% to 84% and 84% to 99%, respectively, when compared to vascular imaging. In the occasional patient with a high likelihood of PAD but with borderline (between 0.9-1.0) or normal ABI, ABI obtained during exercise treadmill testing may prove useful in the diagnosis. In some patients with diabetes mellitus or renal failure, the media of the affected leg vessels become so heavily calcified that they resist compression except during very high levels of cuff inflation. The result is a falsely elevated ankle BP and an artificially normal or supernormal ABI of greater than 1.4 (Table 12.1). Measurement of toe BP to obtain toe-brachial index in that situation is recommended to verify presence of PAD. Patients with a toe-brachial index of less than or equal to 0.70 are considered to have hemodynamically significant PAD.

Duplex ultrasonography is an important adjunct to the ABI, with a similar sensitivity and specificity. This test is particularly useful to diagnose PAD in patients with noncompressible vessels from medial wall calcification. The Doppler velocity waveform remains abnormal, despite a spuriously normal or elevated ABI. Magnetic resonance (MR) angiography and computed tomographic (CT) angiography also

TABLE 12.1	Interpretation of Ankle-Brachial Index	
Ankle-Brachial Index	**Interpretation**
1.00-1.40	Normal
0.90-0.99	Borderline
0.70-0.89	Mild PAD
0.40-0.69	Moderate PAD
<0.40	Severe PAD
>1.40	Noncompressible vessels

PAD, Peripheral arterial disease.

permit excellent visualization of vascular stenosis and identification of runoff vessels. With these noninvasive imaging modalities, spatial resolution is comparable with that of traditional invasive angiography, which now is reserved for patients undergoing revascularization.

The medical management of PAD includes lifestyle and risk factor modification, as well as antiplatelet therapy. Smoking cessation reduces the risk of limb loss, myocardial infarction, and death. Lipid-lowering therapy with high-intensity statin therapy should be initiated and intensified to reduce the rate of vascular events regardless of cholesterol levels. In addition, PAD patients with LDL-C greater than 70 mg/dL despite maximally tolerated statin therapy should be considered for additional lipid-lowering therapy such as ezetimibe. Those with persistently elevated LDL-C despite statin and ezetimibe may then be considered for PCSK9 inhibition. Antihypertensive medication should be initiated and intensified until BP is less than 130/80 mm Hg. Choice of antihypertensive regimen should be based on corresponding comorbidities, but there is some evidence to support the use of ACE inhibitors or angiotensin-receptor blockers. β-Adrenergic blockers do not reduce walking capacity or worsen intermittent claudication in patients with PAD. Aspirin reduces the risk of myocardial infarction, death, and stroke. However, clopidogrel is an effective alternative treatment and is more effective than aspirin in reducing cardiovascular events. Newer antiplatelet agents, such as ticagrelor, have not been proven to be more effective than clopidogrel in reducing cardiovascular events or limb ischemia in patients with symptomatic PAD. More recently, the combination of low-dose factor Xa inhibitor rivaroxaban (2.5 mg twice daily) and low-dose aspirin of (≤100 mg) was shown to reduce the risk of cardiovascular events and limb amputation in PAD patients when compared to low-dose aspirin alone. While the overall bleeding risk is increased with the combination therapy, fatal bleeding is not. Therefore, this combination should be considered in PAD patients with high cardiovascular risk but low bleeding risk. Each patient also needs an exercise prescription as exercise training improves walking capacity and quality of life. This exercise training should be conducted in a medical facility or clinic at a minimal frequency of three times weekly for 12 weeks, preferably for 30 to 45 minutes per session. Cilostazol, a phosphodiesterase-3 inhibitor, is effective in improving claudication symptoms but is not effective in preventing cardiovascular events. Side effects of cilostazol include headache, diarrhea, dizziness, and palpitation. However, cilostazol must be avoided in patients with congestive heart failure because its use in such patients may increase mortality. Pentoxifylline should not be used in PAD as it is no more effective than placebo for intermittent claudication.

Revascularization (percutaneous or surgical) is indicated for patients with severe claudication that is resistant to medical therapy, limb-threatening ischemia, or ischemia-induced impotence (Fig. 12.1). A variety of devices are now available for aortoiliac, femoropopliteal, and infrapopliteal percutaneous interventions, including drug-coated balloons, cutting balloons, laser atherectomy, self-expanding stents, and drug-coated stents. However, efficacy of these newer devices has not been directly compared to each other or to surgical revascularization. In general, surgical revascularization is more suitable for longer areas of stenosis and remains the best option for some patients. The decision between surgery versus endovascular intervention also depends on a patient's life expectancy and other comorbid conditions. Overall, the selection of surgery versus percutaneous intervention as the initial mode of revascularization in patients with limb-threatening ischemia is complex and should be a decision made amongst an interdisciplinary team of physicians.

Acute limb ischemia (ALI) is a vascular emergency. Sudden occlusion of a peripheral artery is caused by either arterial embolism or thrombosis in situ. Arterial emboli usually originate in the cardiac chambers in the setting of preexisting cardiac disease such as myocardial infarction (e.g., left ventricular mural thrombus), congestive heart failure, or atrial arrhythmias (e.g., left atrial thrombus in a patient with atrial fibrillation). Thrombosis in situ usually occurs in arteries with a preexisting severe stenosis in the setting of long-standing PAD with or without previous vascular surgery. Patients with arterial embolism usually experience sudden onset of symptoms without a history of claudication, whereas those with thrombosis in situ typically have a history of claudication that has previously been stable and then suddenly assumes a crescendo pattern over a period of days. In either case, the physical examination reveals a cold, cyanotic (bluish) extremity with absent pulses distal to the site of arterial occlusion and diminished

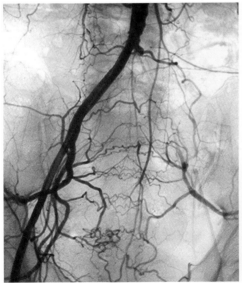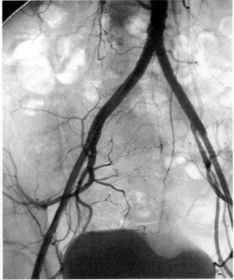

Fig. 12.1 Angiogram of the distal abdominal aorta and iliac arteries demonstrates an occluded left common iliac artery with extensive collateral circulation from the contralateral internal iliac artery *(left)*, which resolved after successful stent implantation *(right)*. (Courtesy of Bart Domatch, MD, Radiology Department, University of Texas Southwestern Medical Center, Dallas, Texas.)

motor and/or sensory function. A handheld Doppler device is used to assess signals at different arterial segments and confirms the diagnosis of acute vascular occlusion. Anticoagulation should be initiated immediately with intravenous heparin titrated to maintain the activated partial thromboplastin time equal to 2.0 to 2.5 times control. Catheter-directed infusion of thrombolytic therapy offers a similar success rate in salvaging the limbs as surgical revascularization (thromboembolectomy or bypass surgery). However, survival rate is higher with catheter-based therapy, likely related to the multiple comorbidities of patients with ALI. Patients with irreversible tissue necrosis, regardless of the cause, should be treated with emergent amputation rather than revascularization to reduce the risk of kidney failure (myoglobinuria), sepsis, and multiorgan failure.

Aortic Aneurysm

An aortic aneurysm is commonly defined as a dilation of all three layers of the vessel to more than 50% of the expected normal diameter. The two main types are thoracic aortic aneurysms (TAA), which occur above the diaphragm, and abdominal aortic aneurysms (AAA), which occur below the diaphragm. Abdominal aortic aneurysm is a common vascular disease in older adults, affecting 4% to 8% of men and 0.5% to 1.5% of women over the age of 65 years. Thoracic aortic aneurysm is much less prevalent (0.4% to 0.5%). Besides age, the major risk factors for abdominal aortic aneurysms are cigarette smoking, hypertension, and a family history of aortic aneurysms. Atherosclerosis is responsible for most cases of abdominal aortic aneurysm, while other causes such as genetic (Marfan syndrome, Ehlers-Danlos syndrome, Loeys-Dietz, Turner syndrome, or bicuspid aortic valve), vasculitis with connective tissue disease (Takayasu's arteritis, giant-cell arteritis), chronic infection (syphilitic aortitis), and trauma may cause thoracic or abdominal aortic aneurysms. Abdominal aortic aneurysms gradually grow in size over time at an average rate of 1 to 4 mm per year. The risk of rupture is low until the diameter reaches 5 cm, and then it increases exponentially. The risk of aortic rupture is 1% per year for aneurysms between 3.5 and 4.9 cm in diameter and 5% per year for aneurysms larger than 5 cm.

Most cases of aortic aneurysms are asymptomatic and detected incidentally during routine screening or imaging for other indications. However, some patients with AAA may develop vascular complications such as aneurysm expansion with compression of adjacent structures. Occasionally, mural thrombi form within the aneurysm and embolize, causing acute occlusion of distal arterial segments. Patients with iliac aneurysm may develop hydronephrosis or recurrent urinary tract infection from ureteral compression. Others develop neurologic symptoms from compression of sciatic or femoral nerves. The classic physical finding is a pulsatile nontender mass below the umbilicus (distal to the origin of the renal arteries). In thin patients, normal aortic pulsations are often palpable but above the umbilicus. Hypotension and acute abdominal pain should prompt consideration of aneurysm rupture, which requires emergent operative repair. Duplex ultrasonography is an accurate and reliable diagnostic tool for abdominal aortic and iliac aneurysms. Routine screening for AAA with ultrasonography is recommended for all men between the ages of 65 and 75 years who have ever smoked or men above the age of 60 with family history of AAA among first-degree relatives. Such screening has a proven mortality benefit. CT and MR angiography allow visualization of the thoracic and abdominal aorta, as well as the iliac arteries and its branches (Fig. 12.2).

Medical treatment for aortic aneurysm includes smoking cessation, tight BP control to less than 130/80 mm Hg, and intensive statin therapy. Although transforming growth factor-β has been implicated in the pathogenesis of aortic aneurysm in Marfan syndrome, which is mediated by angiotensin-II receptor activation, losartan was not shown to more effective than beta adrenergic receptor blockade in reducing the

rate of aortic root enlargement. β-Adrenergic blockade has not proven beneficial in patients with abdominal aortic aneurysm from other causes. Similarly, a randomized clinical trial failed to demonstrate superiority of angiotensin-converting enzyme inhibitors (ACEI) over calcium-channel blockers in preventing AAA expansion. However, small sample size and inclusion of patients with well-controlled hypertension may have limited the investigators' ability to detect a difference. Patients who develop symptoms from thoracic aneurysms of any size should undergo repair. For asymptomatic patients, presence of large aneurysms (diameter 5.5 cm or above) or rapid aneurysm expansion regardless of the size are also indications for aneurysm repair (Table 12.2). Open surgical repair remains the treatment of choice for thoracic aneurysms involving the aortic root, ascending aorta, or aortic arch. However, thoracic endovascular aortic repair (TEVAR) has now emerged as the procedure of choice for descending thoracic aneurysm given lower early morbidity and mortality compared to open surgical repair in several observational studies. Elective abdominal aortic aneurysm repair carries a perioperative mortality rate of 2% to 6%.

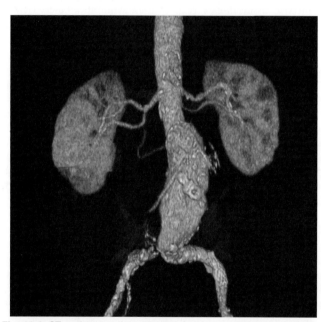

Fig. 12.2 CT angiogram of the distal abdominal aorta shows abdominal aortic aneurysm with the largest diameter of 6.2 cm and severe stenosis at the origin of the right common iliac artery. (Courtesy of Bart Domatch, MD, Radiology Department, University of Texas Southwestern Medical Center, Dallas, Texas.)

TABLE 12.2 Indications for Surgical Treatment of Arterial Aneurysms

Symptoms from expansion of aneurysm or compression of adjacent structure
Rupture of aneurysm
Rapid aortic aneurysm expansion of ≥1 cm per year
Asymptomatic with large size
   Thoracic aneurysm (ascending or descending aneurysm) with diameter >5.5 cm in adults
   For genetic cause of thoracic aneurysm (such as Marfan, Loeys-Dietz, Ehlers-Danlos, Turner syndrome, or bicuspid aortic valve), a lower diameter or aortic size may be considered (generally of at least 5 cm or >4.5 cm in the presence of family history of aortic dissection)
   Abdominal aorta >5.5 cm
   Iliac aneurysm >3 cm

Furthermore, a large randomized study failed to demonstrate any benefit of surgery in patients with aneurysms 4.0 to 5.4 cm in diameter. For these reasons, patients with small aortic aneurysms (4.0 to 5.4 cm in diameter) should be treated medically with close monitoring of aneurysm size with periodic imaging studies every 6 to 12 months (see Table 12.2).

Percutaneous endovascular aneurysm repair (EVAR) is an alternative method to open surgical repair for treatment of abdominal aortic aneurysm. EVAR offers lower perioperative death than surgical repair with equivalent long-term survival. However, EVAR should be reserved for patients with favorable anatomy who are able to return for follow-up visits and repeated imaging studies of the aneurysm sites to ensure that the stent graft is free from endovascular leaks or displacement.

Aortic Dissection

In aortic dissection, the intimal layer is torn from the aortic wall leading to the formation of a false lumen in parallel with the true lumen. Risk factors include hypertension, cocaine use, trauma, hereditary connective tissue disease (e.g., Marfan syndrome, Ehlers-Danlos syndrome), vasculitis (e.g., Takayasu's arteritis, giant-cell arteritis), Behçet's disease, bicuspid aortic valve, and aortic coarctation. Aortic dissection can be classified as types A and B (Stanford system). Type A dissection involves the ascending aorta, whereas type B dissection involves the distal aorta. The DeBakey system subdivides aortic dissection into three subtypes—types I, II, and III. Type 1 dissection involves the entire aorta, whereas type II involves only the ascending aorta and type III involves only the descending aorta. Aortic dissection involving the ascending aorta carries a high mortality rate of 1% to 2% per hour during the first 24 to 48 hours. Patients usually develop acute onset of severe chest or back pain. Abdominal pain, syncope, and stroke are common. Retrograde propagation of the dissection can cause pericardial tamponade or coronary artery dissection with acute myocardial infarction. Dissection involving the aortic valve causes acute severe aortic insufficiency with acute pulmonary edema. The dissection plane may propagate in an antegrade direction to compromise flow in the carotid and subclavian arteries, producing a stroke or acute upper limb ischemia. Patients with distal (type B) aortic dissection exhibit acute onset of back pain or chest pain often accompanied by lower extremity ischemia and ischemic neuropathy.

The physical findings include pulse deficits, neurologic deficits, or a diastolic murmur of aortic regurgitation. However, acute aortic regurgitation into an unprepared ventricle produces only a short, soft diastolic murmur that is often missed. The widened pulse pressure and associated physical findings of chronic aortic regurgitation are absent, and the clinical picture is that of an acutely ill patient with tachypnea, tachycardia, and a narrow pulse pressure. Hypotension, jugular venous distention, and pulsus paradoxus should prompt the diagnosis of pericardial tamponade. Transesophageal echocardiography, MR angiography, or CT angiography confirm the diagnosis by demonstrating an intimal flap that separates the true lumen from the false lumen (Fig. 12.3). Type A aortic dissection is uniformly fatal without emergent surgical repair. With surgery, mortality is reduced to 10% at 24 hours and 20% at 30 days. Patients with type B aortic dissection should be treated medically because 1-year survival is higher with medical therapy than it is with surgery (75% versus 50%). However, surgery is indicated if type B dissection compromises blood flow to the legs, kidneys, or other viscera. Tight control of BP is essential because aortic aneurysm was found to develop in 30% to 50% of patients with type B aortic dissection when studied over 4 years.

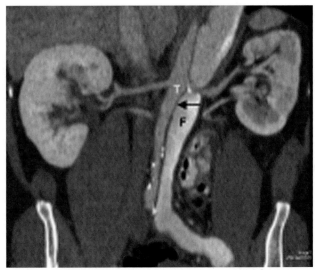

Fig. 12.3 CT angiogram of the aorta shows type B aortic dissection. The intimal flap *(arrow)* separates the true lumen *(T)* from the false lumen *(F)* and compromises blood flow to the right kidney causing renal atrophy and cortical thinning. (Courtesy of Bart Domatch, MD, Radiology Department, University of Texas Southwestern Medical Center, Dallas, Texas.)

Penetrating Aortic Ulcers and Intramural Hematoma

Penetrating aortic ulcers and intramural hematomas exhibit chest pain that is indistinguishable from that of aortic dissection. In contrast to aortic dissection, however, the pathologic condition is localized. No identifiable intimal flap and thus no branch vessel occlusion are produced. Disruption of the internal elastic lamina produces aortic ulcers that erode into the medial wall and protrude into the surrounding structures. Rupture of the vasa vasorum causes formation of localized hematoma underneath the adventitia with resultant asymmetric thickening of the aortic wall. Patients with either condition typically are older than those with aortic dissection, have a larger aortic size, and have a higher prevalence of abdominal aortic aneurysm. Aortic rupture is the major complication of both penetrating ulcers and intramural hematomas, particularly with those aneurysms located in the ascending aorta. The diagnosis is made with invasive angiography, CT angiography, or MR angiography (Fig. 12.4). Surgical intervention should be considered for ulcers and hematomas of the ascending aorta, deeply penetrating ulcers, or severely bulging hematomas, irrespective of their location. Ulcers and hematomas of the descending aortic may be managed successfully with β-adrenergic blockade and tight control of BP.

Other Arterial Diseases

Buerger's disease, or thromboangiitis obliterans is a nonatherosclerotic disease of the arteries, veins, and nerves of the arms and legs affecting mostly young men before the age of 45 years. The mechanism is unknown, but all patients have a history of heavy tobacco addiction. The presenting symptom is claudication of the feet, legs, hands, or arms. Multiple-limb involvement and superficial thrombophlebitis are common. The C-reactive protein and Westergren sedimentation rate typically are normal, and a search for serologic markers for connective tissue disease (e.g., antinuclear antibody or rheumatoid factor, antiphospholipid antibody) is negative. The diagnosis is based on the typical clinical presentation. If the presentation is atypical, then biopsy is needed to make the diagnosis. The histologic hallmark is inflammatory intramural thrombi within the arteries and veins with sparing of internal elastic lamina and other arterial wall structures. The most effective

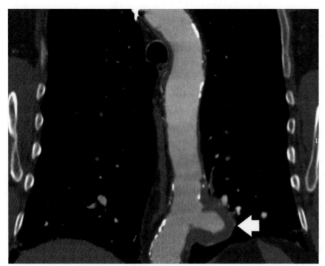

Fig. 12.4 CT angiogram of the descending thoracic aorta shows a large penetrating aortic ulcer above the diaphragm *(arrow)*. (Courtesy of Bart Domatch, MD, Radiology Department, University of Texas Southwestern Medical Center, Dallas, Texas.)

treatment for Buerger's disease is complete tobacco abstinence. The prostacyclin analog iloprost constitutes adjunctive therapy to reduce limb ischemia and improve wound healing.

Raynaud's phenomenon is a vasospastic disease of the small arteries of mainly the fingers and toes. Primary (idiopathic) Raynaud's phenomenon occurs in the absence of underlying disorders. Secondary Raynaud's phenomenon occurs in association with connective tissue diseases (e.g., scleroderma, polymyositis, rheumatoid arthritis, systemic lupus erythematosus), as well as with repeated mild physical trauma (e.g., use of jackhammers), certain drugs (e.g., antineoplastic chemotherapeutic agents, interferon, monamine-reuptake inhibitors such as tricyclic antidepressants, serotonin agonists), and Buerger's disease. Patients usually complain of recurrent episodes of digital ischemia, with a characteristic white-blue-red color sequence. Pallor is followed by cyanosis if ischemia is prolonged and then by erythema (reactive hyperemia) when the episode resolves. Episodes are precipitated by cold temperature or emotional stress. Physical examination can be entirely normal between attacks with normal radial, ulnar, and pedal pulses. Some patients may have digital ulcers or thickening of fat pad (sclerodactyly). Patients should be instructed to avoid cold temperatures and dress warmly. Calcium-channel blockers (CCBs) reduce the frequency and severity of vasospastic episodes.

Giant-cell arteritis is an immune-mediated vasculitis predominantly involving medium-sized and large arteries such as the subclavian artery, axillary artery, and aorta of the older adult with a strong male predominance. Approximately 40% of patients with giant-cell arteritis also have polymyalgia rheumatica, a syndrome characterized by severe stiffness and pain originating in the muscles of the shoulders and pelvic girdle. Patients may exhibit headache from temporal arteritis, jaw claudication from ischemia of the masseter muscles, or visual loss from involvement of the ophthalmic artery. Chest pain suggests the coexistence of aortic aneurysm or dissection. Physical findings include low-grade fever, scalp tenderness in the temporal area, pale and edematous fundi, or a diastolic murmur of aortic regurgitation. BP difference of more than 15 mm Hg between arms suggests subclavian artery stenosis. Laboratory findings include significantly elevated C-reactive protein and Westergren sedimentation rate plus anemia. The diagnosis is confirmed by histologic examination of the arterial tissue (frequently from temporal artery biopsy), showing infiltration

of lymphocytes and macrophages (i.e., giant cells) in all layers of the vascular wall. High-dose corticosteroids are highly effective and should be initiated immediately when the diagnosis is suspected to prevent potentially permanent blindness. To minimize complications from long-term corticosteroid administration, the steroid dose should be tapered to find the lowest dose needed to suppress symptoms, which often wane. Every attempt should be made to discontinue corticosteroids over time, and treatment with methotrexate or the interleukin-6 receptor antagonist tocilizumab may be used as steroid sparing agents.

Takayasu's arteritis is an idiopathic granulomatous vasculitis of the aorta, its main branches, and the pulmonary artery. This condition is particularly common in young women of Asian descent, but it also occurs in non-Asian women and men. The inflammatory process in the vascular wall can lead to stenosis and/or aneurysm formation. Hypertension, as a result of renal artery stenosis or aortic coarctation, is the most common manifestation and is present in as many as 80% of affected individuals. Because the vascular involvement is so widespread, patients may have symptoms and signs of coronary ischemia, congestive heart failure, stroke, vertebrobasilar insufficiency, or intermittent claudication. Physical findings include bruits over the subclavian arteries or aorta, as well as diminished brachial pulses and thus a low brachial artery BP. The diagnosis is based primarily on this clinical presentation. First-line treatment is with corticosteroids. Other immunosuppressive agents such as methotrexate or cyclophosphamide are often added to prevent disease progression and relapse, and newer biologics such as anti-TNF inhibitors (infliximab, etanercept) provide a viable alternative. Immunosuppressive therapy does not cause regression of preexisting vascular stenoses or aneurysms. For this reason, percutaneous or surgical revascularization is usually required.

Arteriovenous (AV) fistulas are abnormal vascular communications that shunt blood flow from the arterial system directly into the venous system, bypassing the capillary beds that normally ensure optimal tissue perfusion and nutrient exchange. AV fistulas may be congenital, as in AV malformation (AVM), or acquired. The main causes of acquired AV fistula are penetrating trauma (e.g., gunshot, knife wound) and surgically created shunts for hemodialysis access. Patients may exhibit a pulsatile mass, symptoms related to compression of an adjacent organ, or bleeding from spontaneous rupture of an AVM. Systolic and diastolic bruits or thrills may be detectable over the fistula or AVM. An AVM in skeletal muscle may lead to bone malformation or a pathologic fracture, whereas AVM in the brain may result in neurologic deficits or seizures. High-output heart failure is another complication from a large AVM or fistula. MR angiography, CT angiography, or conventional angiography confirms the diagnosis. Depending on the size and location of the AVM, treatment options include surgical resection, transcatheter embolization, or pulse laser irradiation. Patients with acquired AV fistulas from trauma usually need surgical closure.

PULMONARY VASCULAR DISEASE

Pulmonary hypertension is characterized by elevated mean pulmonary artery pressure (PAP) of greater than 20 mm Hg at rest. The many causes of pulmonary hypertension are summarized in Table 12.3.

Patients with pulmonary hypertension not only have an elevated pulmonary arterial pressure but also a low cardiac output, causing symptoms of exertional dyspnea, fatigue, and syncope. Pulmonary capillary wedge pressure is usually normal (≤15 mm Hg) except in patients with pulmonary hypertension due to impaired left ventricular systolic or diastolic function or left-sided valvular heart disease.

TABLE 12.3 Classification of Pulmonary Hypertension

Category 1: Pulmonary Arterial Hypertension (PAH)
Primary pulmonary hypertension (PPH) or idiopathic pulmonary hypertension (IPAH):
  Sporadic
  Familial
PPH associated with:
  Connective tissue disease
  Congenital heart disease
  Portal hypertension
  Human immunodeficiency viral infection
  Drugs and toxins: Anorexigens, cocaine, methamphetamine

Category 2: Pulmonary Venous Hypertension
Left ventricular heart failure
Left ventricular valvular heart disease

Category 3: Pulmonary Hypertension Associated With Chronic Respiratory Disease or Hypoxemia
Chronic obstructive pulmonary disease
Obstructive sleep apnea

Category 4: Pulmonary Hypertension Associated With Chronic Venous Thromboembolism
Left ventricular valvular heart disease

Category 5: Pulmonary Hypertension Due to Miscellaneous Disorders Directly Affecting the Pulmonary Vasculature
Sarcoidosis, histiocytosis X, compression of pulmonary vessels (adenopathy, tumor, fibrosing mediastinitis)

Pulmonary Arterial Hypertension

Pulmonary arterial hypertension (PAH) is caused by a combination of pulmonary vasoconstriction, endothelial cell and/or smooth muscle proliferation, intimal fibrosis, and thrombosis in the pulmonary capillaries and arterioles. PAH is either idiopathic (primary pulmonary hypertension [PPH]) or secondary to connective tissue disease, congenital heart disease, portal hypertension, or human immunodeficiency viral (HIV) infection, as well as anorexigenic drugs or toxins. Connective tissue diseases, particularly scleroderma, are the most common secondary causes of PAH.

Patients with mild PAH can be asymptomatic, but patients with more advanced disease complain of exertional dyspnea, chest pain, syncope, or presyncope. Orthopnea is an uncommon symptom associated with PAH and more commonly identified in patients with pulmonary hypertension from left-sided heart disease. Physical findings include a left parasternal lift, loud pulmonary component of the second heart sound, murmur of tricuspid or pulmonic regurgitation, hepatomegaly, peripheral edema, or ascites. Associated ECG abnormalities indicate right ventricular hypertrophy, right atrial enlargement, or right axis deviation. Echocardiography provides important information about the severity of the pulmonary hypertension (i.e., estimated pulmonary artery pressure, right ventricular dimensions and function) and its potential causes (e.g., left ventricular failure, valvular lesions, congenital heart disease with left-to-right shunts). Pulmonary function tests, ventilation-perfusion ($\dot{V}/\dot{Q}$) lung scans, polysomnography or overnight oximetry, autoantibody tests, HIV serology, and liver-function tests also should be performed to determine other potential causes. Right ventricular catheterization should be performed in all patients with suspected PAH. Under basal conditions in the catheterization laboratory, an elevated mean pulmonary artery pressure exceeding 20 mm Hg, a pulmonary capillary wedge pressure below 15 mm Hg, and a pulmonary vascular resistance exceeding 3 units confirm the diagnosis. Acute vasodilator drug challenge should be performed during right ventricular catheterization to guide appropriate treatment.

Without treatment, the prognosis of PAH is poor with a median survival of less than 3 years. Patients with high-risk features for clinical deterioration or death, including poor functional capacity, history of syncope, or right ventricular failure, should be treated with intravenous epoprostenol (a prostacyclin analog) because of its proven efficacy to improve exercise capacity and overall survival. Other prostacyclin analogs such as beraprost, treprostinil, and iloprost or prostacyclin-receptor agonists such as selexipag are also effective in reducing pulmonary artery pressure and improving exercise capacity. Other classes of medications approved for treatment of PAH include drugs that target the endothelin pathway and nitric oxide (NO) pathway. Currently available endothelin-receptor antagonists (ERAs) include bosentan, ambrisentan, macitentan. Drugs in the NO pathway include soluble guanyl cyclase stimulators (riociguat), and phosphodiesterase (PDE)5 inhibitors (sildenafil, tadalafil). Combination therapy of two to three drugs from different classes improves exercise capacity when compared to monotherapy and should be considered in patients with severe disease or those who fail to improve with monotherapy. Oral calcium-channel blockers (CCBs) are indicated only for the small subset of patients with mild-to-moderate symptoms who demonstrate significant reduction in pulmonary pressure with acute CCB challenge (decrease in mean PAP of at least 10 mm Hg to an absolute level of less than 40 mm Hg without a decrease in cardiac output). Supplemental home oxygen is indicated for all patients with hypoxemia. Travel to high elevations exacerbates hypoxia, and relocation to sea level improves symptoms. Oral anticoagulation should be considered for patients with PAH, particularly in those with a chronic indwelling central venous catheter for intravenous epoprostenol. Iron status should be monitored regularly to avoid iron deficiency anemia to prevent further deterioration in functional capacity. Diuretics should be prescribed for patients with peripheral edema or hepatic congestion. Lung transplantation is recommended only for patients in whom severe symptoms occur despite intensive medical therapy.

VENOUS THROMBOEMBOLIC DISEASE

Venous thromboembolism (VTE) encompasses both deep vein thrombosis (DVT) and pulmonary embolism (PE). Among the adult United States population, the overall combined annual incidence is as high as 2 new cases per 1000 persons. The incidence of VTE is higher in men than it is in women and higher in African Americans and white individuals than it is in Asians and Hispanics. Over 150 years ago, Dr. Rudolf Virchow recognized three predisposing factors: (1) endothelial damage, (2) venous stasis, and (3) hypercoagulation (Virchow's triad). Endothelial damage is common with surgery or trauma, venous stasis is common with prolonged bedrest or immobilization (leg cast), and hypercoagulation is more prevalent with cancer, oral estrogen use, and pregnancy. Trousseau syndrome consists of migratory thrombophlebitis with noninfectious vegetations on the heart valves (marantic endocarditis) typically in the setting of mucin-secreting adenocarcinoma. Dr. Trousseau, a pathologist, diagnosed his own pancreatic carcinoma on the basis of the association that now bears his name. Hypercoagulable states include hereditary diseases such as deficiencies in antithrombin III, protein C, or protein S; mutation in factor V gene (factor V Leiden) or factor II gene (prothrombin G20210A); as well as hyperhomocysteinemia. However, a thorough search for identifiable risk factors will come up negative in 25% to 50% of patients with VTE.

Deep Vein Thrombosis

Most DVT starts in the calf veins. Without treatment, 15% to 30% of these clots propagate to the proximal calf veins. The risk of a subsequent PE is much higher with proximal DVT than with clots confined to the distal calf vessels (40% to 50% versus 5% to 10%, respectively). Involvement of the upper extremities is much less common, but subclavian and/or axillary vein thrombosis also can lead to PE in as many as 30% of affected individuals. The same risk factors that cause lower extremity DVT also cause upper extremity DVT. In addition, other specific causes of upper extremity DVT include traumatic damage of the vessel intima from heavy exertion such as rowing, wrestling, or weight lifting (Paget-Schroetter syndrome), from extrinsic compression at the level of thoracic inlet (thoracic outlet obstruction), or from insertion of central venous catheters or pacemakers. Pain and/or swelling are the major complaints from patients with DVT; however, a large number of patients with DVT are asymptomatic, particularly if the DVT is restricted to the calf. Patients with upper-extremity DVT can develop the superior vena caval syndrome of facial swelling, blurred vision, and dyspnea. Thoracic outlet obstruction can compress the brachial plexus leading to unilateral arm pain associated with hand weakness. Physical examination frequently reveals tenderness, erythema, warmth, and swelling below the site of thrombosis. Pain with dorsiflexion of the foot (Homan's sign) may be present, but the low sensitivity and the low specificity limit its usefulness in the diagnosis of lower extremity DVT. A palpable tender cord, dilated superficial veins, and low-grade fever occur in some patients. Upper extremity DVT can cause brachial plexus tenderness in the supraclavicular fossa and atrophic hand muscles. For patients with probable thoracic outlet obstruction, several provocative tests should be performed. Adson test is positive if the radial pulses weaken during inspiration and during extension of the arm of the affected side while rotating the head to the same side. Wright test is positive if the radial pulses become weaker and painful symptoms are reproduced while abducting the shoulder of the affected side with the humerus externally rotated.

The laboratory diagnosis of DVT includes measurement of D-dimers, which are fibrin degradation products. D-dimer elevation is a highly sensitive indicator of DVT that can be performed rapidly in the emergency department. In a patient with low to intermediate probability, a negative D-dimer test effectively excludes the diagnosis of DVT. However, the test is not specific and can be elevated in many other conditions frequently encountered in hospitalized patients (e.g., inflammation, recent surgery, malignancy). Duplex ultrasonography can be used to demonstrate the presence of a blood clot and/or noncompressibility of the affected veins proximal to the site of occlusion. Duplex ultrasonography has greater sensitivity in detecting proximal DVT (90% to 100%) than distal DVT (40% to 90%) of the lower extremities. With upper extremity DVT, acoustic shadowing of the clavicle may obscure detection of thrombosis in subclavian vein segments. MR angiography is particularly helpful in making the diagnosis of upper extremity DVT and pelvic vein thrombosis. Contrast venography is the conventional gold standard test, but it is invasive and technically difficult in patients with edematous extremities. Therefore, invasive venography should be reserved for patients in whom the clinical suggestion is high, despite negative or inconclusive results from noninvasive imaging.

Patients with DVT should be treated initially with subcutaneous low-molecular-weight heparin (LMWH), or subcutaneous selective factor Xa inhibitor fondaparinux to prevent thrombus propagation and to maintain the patency of venous collaterals. Oral administration of factor Xa inhibitors, rivaroxaban or apixaban, may also be used in the initial monotherapy without pretreatment with heparin. In contrast, other direct anticoagulants such as dabigatran and edoxaban should be started only after an initial parenteral heparin or fondaparinux therapy for 3 to 5 days. Intravenous unfractionated heparin (UFH) should be given as a bolus, followed by continuous infusion to maintain an activated partial thromboplastin time of at least 1.5 times the control value. LMWH and fondaparinux has a longer half-life than UFH and can be given once or twice daily with similar efficacy. Oral anticoagulation should be initiated after the acute phase. In general, direct anticoagulants (DOACs) including dabigatran, rivaroxaban, apixaban, and edoxaban are preferred over warfarin because of lower risk of intracranial hemorrhage without compromising antithrombotic efficacy. If warfarin is chosen, it should be initiated without delay with an overlap period with LMWH, UFH, or fondaparinux therapy and titrated until the international normalized ratio (INR) reaches a value between 2 and 3. DOACs, however, have rapid onset of action and should be started at the discontinuation of UFH, LMWH, or fondaparinux without overlap period to avoid bleeding complication. After the acute phase, oral anticoagulants should be continued for 3 months in most patients. Lifelong anticoagulation should be considered in patients with unprovoked proximal DVT (either first episode or recurrent event) as well as patients with cancer-associated DVT with low to moderate bleeding risk. Furthermore, avoidance of frequent clinic visits to monitor INR during the initial period of warfarin titration is another major advantage of DOACs. When DVT is confined to the calf, the risk of PE is lower than proximal DVT. Therefore, anticoagulants should be started only in patients with severe symptoms or those with high-risk features for clot expansion, such as elevated D-dimer, large thrombus with greater than 5 cm in length, multiple vein involvement, history of thromboembolic events or active cancer, unprovoked DVT, or inpatient status. Oral anticoagulants should be continued for 3 months in most patients. In the absence of severe symptoms or risk factors for clot extension, patients with isolated distal DVT should be treated conservatively without anticoagulation with close monitoring via serial imaging of the deep veins for 2 weeks.

When upper extremity DVT occurs in the subclavian veins or axillary veins in patients who are severely symptomatic but otherwise healthy with low risk of bleeding, catheter-directed thrombolysis should be considered as it carries lower risk of bleeding than systemic thrombolytic therapy. The purpose of thrombolysis is to prevent or minimize the post-thrombotic syndrome, which includes chronic arm pain, swelling, hyperpigmentation, and ulceration from residual venous obstruction. In asymptomatic patients with occlusion in the more distal location, anticoagulation is preferred. If anticoagulation is stopped prematurely for any reason, aspirin should be considered in the absence of contraindication as it has been shown to reduce recurrent venous thromboembolism by 20% to 40% without increased risk of bleeding.

Catheter-based direct thrombolysis is effective in restoring venous patency and reducing post-thrombotic syndrome of venous congestion but increases risk of bleeding. Therefore, it should be considered for patients with iliofemoral DVT of recent onset who have low risk of bleeding. Vena cava filters are effective in reducing the incidence of PE, but they increase the risk of recurrent DVT. Consequently, IVC filters should be removed after 3 months. In patients treated with anticoagulation, addition of an IVC filter to anticoagulation offers no additional benefit in reducing recurrent venous thromboembolism compared to anticoagulation alone. Therefore, it should be considered only in patients in whom anticoagulation is contraindicated.

Pulmonary Embolism

PE occurs when a thrombus dislodges from the deep veins of the upper or lower extremities. Pulmonary vascular resistance and pulmonary arterial pressure increase from two mechanisms: (1) anatomic reduction in cross-sectional area of the pulmonary vascular bed and (2) functional hypoxia-induced pulmonary vasoconstriction. The pressure overload on the right ventricle can lead to dilation, hypokinesis, and tricuspid regurgitation. When severe, elevated right ventricular end-diastolic pressure can compress the right coronary artery, causing subendocardial ischemia. In acute PE, areas of lung tissue are ventilated but underperfused. This V̇/Q̇ mismatch and the resultant redistribution of pulmonary blood flow from the obstructed pulmonary artery to other lung regions with lower V̇/Q̇ ratios cause arterial hypoxemia. In patients with a patent foramen ovale, hypoxemia worsens when the sudden elevation in right atrial pressure causes right-to-left shunting across the foramen.

The classic symptoms of acute PE are the sudden onset of dyspnea and pleuritic chest pain. Additional symptoms include anginal chest pain from right ventricular ischemia, hemoptysis from pulmonary infarction, and syncope or presyncope from massive PE with acute right ventricular failure (cor pulmonale). The most common physical findings are tachypnea and tachycardia. Additional physical findings include a right ventricular lift, inspiratory crackles, a loud pulmonary component of the second sound, expiratory wheezing, and a pleural rub. Symptoms and signs of proximal DVT are present in 10% to 20% of patients. Arterial blood gas analysis often reveals hypoxemia, respiratory alkalosis, and a high alveolar-to-arterial oxygen tension gradient. However, normal arterial blood gases values do not exclude the diagnosis. The most common finding with ECG analysis is sinus tachycardia. Atrial fibrillation, premature atrial contraction, and supraventricular tachycardia are less common. Other ECG changes suggest acute right ventricular strain. These include the S1-Q3-T3 pattern, a new right bundle branch block or right-axis deviation, and P-wave pulmonale. However, these findings are present in only 30% of patients with even massive PE. Common but nonspecific abnormalities with chest radiographic studies include atelectasis, pleural effusion, and pulmonary infiltrates. Less common but more specific radiographic findings include Hampton's hump (i.e., wedge-shaped infiltrate in the peripheral lung field), which is indicative of pulmonary infarction and Westermark's sign (decreased vascularity). The plasma D-dimer test is elevated in most patients with PE as a result of activation of the endogenous fibrinolytic system, which is not sufficient to dissolve the clot. Commercially available D-dimer assays have a high sensitivity and negative predictive value but low specificity, particularly with increasing age. Therefore, it is important to use age-adjusted cut-off values (age × 10 μg/L) in patients older than 50 years old to improve specificity without compromising sensitivity of detection to above 97%. A normal age-adjusted D-dimer test effectively excludes the diagnosis of PE in patients in whom the clinical suggestion is low or intermediate. However, it should not be used to screen patients with high index of suspicion because of low negative predictive value. Elevated levels of cardiac troponin I and troponin T and other markers of myocardial injury can be found in patients with PE and are indicative of right ventricular dysfunction and a poor prognosis. Similarly, elevated natriuretic peptides, including B-type natriuretic peptide (BNP) and N-terminal pro-BNP have been shown to be predictive of adverse outcomes.

CT angiography is the imaging modality of choice in patients with suspected PE and high clinical probability because of its excellent visualization of the pulmonary artery (Fig. 12.5). The resolution of 1 mm

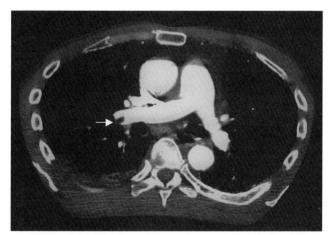

Fig. 12.5 Spiral chest CT angiogram shows a large thrombus in the right main pulmonary artery *(arrow)*. (Courtesy of Michael Landay, MD, Department of Radiology, University of Texas Southwestern Medical Center, Dallas, Texas.)

or less rivals that of conventional invasive angiography. The speed of the newer generation of scanners allows acquisition of all images within a single breath-hold, avoiding respiratory motion artifacts. The overall negative predictive value of multidetector CT angiography exceeds 99%. A negative CT excludes the diagnosis of PE and eliminates the need for further diagnostic testing. The CT scan also permits detection of other pathologic conditions involving the lung parenchyma, pleura, and mediastinal structures. Such pathologic findings may mimic PE and constitute alternative causes of chest pain and dyspnea. The requirement for intravenous injection of iodinated contrast material restricts applicability to those without a history of kidney disease or an allergic reaction to contrast dye. In such patients, V̇/Q̇ scan is a more suitable imaging modality. A completely normal V̇/Q̇ scan effectively excludes the diagnosis without further testing. However, less than 10% of V̇/Q̇ scans are interpreted as definitively normal. In patients in whom a moderate or high level of clinical probability of PE exists, a high-probability V̇/Q̇ scan has a diagnostic accuracy of 90% to 100%; however, a low or intermediate probability scan is no more helpful than a coin flip. Fig. 12.6 presents an algorithm for the work-up of PE based on current evidence. Echocardiography may directly detect thrombi in the right atrium, right ventricle, or pulmonary artery or indirectly demonstrate right ventricular dysfunction, signifying presence of hemodynamically significant emboli. Therefore, it is helpful in diagnosis of PE in patients with hypotension or shock. Invasive pulmonary angiography should be reserved for patients in whom noninvasive testing is inconclusive.

Once diagnosis of PE is made, clinical risk assessment should be made to guide treatment approach. Patients with low risk based on stable hemodynamic parameters without history of cardiovascular disease or excessive bleeding risk for anticoagulation treatment may be suitable for outpatient treatment or a brief inpatient observation. Similar to the treatment of DVT described previously, oral direct anticoagulants with or without initial parenteral therapy are preferred over warfarin because of lower risk of intracranial bleeding and increased ease of use associated with DOACs. PE patients with moderate to high risk features for cardiovascular decompensation (Table 12.4) should be admitted and monitored closely (PESI class III-V, or simplified PESI of at least 1). Aggressive parenteral therapy is preferred when patients have one or more features of high clinical risk. Thrombolytic therapy with recombinant tissue plasminogen activator (rt-PA) is indicated for patients with hypotension or shock. In patients with right

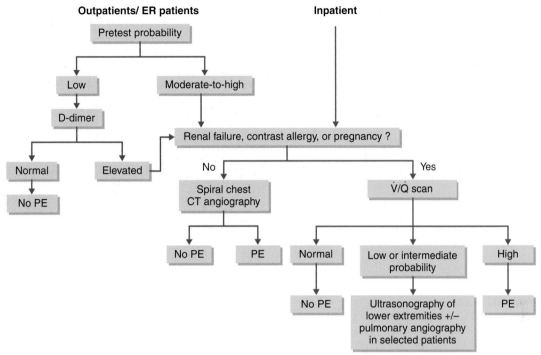

Fig. 12.6 Diagnostic algorithm for patients with suggested pulmonary embolism (PE).

TABLE 12.4 Pulmonary Embolism Severity Index (PESI)

Parameter	Original[a]	Simplified[a]
Age	Years	1 (for age >80 yrs)
Male sex	+10	—
Cancer	+30	1
Chronic heart failure	+10	1
Chronic pulmonary disease	+10	
HR at least 110 bpm	+20	1
SBP <100 mm Hg	+30	1
Respiratory rate >30 breaths per min	+20	—
Temperature <36° C	+20	—
Altered mental status	+60	—
Arterial oxyhemoglobin saturation <90%	+20	1

[a]Original: Total Score Class
≤65: I
66-85: II
86-105: III
106-125: IV
>125: V
Simplified:
0= low risk
≥1 = high risk

ventricular enlargement or dysfunction alone without hypotension (known as submassive PE), thrombolytic therapy reduces the risk of hemodynamic decompensation at the cost of increased risk of major hemorrhage and stroke. Thus, anticoagulation alone is preferred in most cases of submassive PE. After initial treatment with heparins or fondaparinux in high-risk patients, DOACs should be administered in a similar manner to treatment of DVT. If warfarin therapy is chosen instead of DOACs, parenteral anticoagulation should be administered until a therapeutic INR of 2 to 3 is reached. Surgical or percutaneous

removal of emboli should be considered in patients with massive PE who have contraindications for thrombolytic therapy.

The time necessary to continue anticoagulation after an acute PE or DVT episode depends on the presence or absence of reversible risk factors for recurrent VTE. Patients with a history of trauma or surgery generally have a low rate of recurrent VTE; therefore, warfarin can be discontinued after 3 months of administration. Patients with cancer and VTE should be treated initially with subcutaneous fixed-dose LMWH for 3 to 6 months because of its greater efficacy than warfarin in preventing recurrent thromboembolism in this setting. Preliminary studies indicated that DOACs are as effective as LMWH in preventing thromboembolic events though the bleeding risk is higher with DOACs. After this initial period, treatment with LMWH or DOACs should be continued indefinitely unless the cancer is cured. Patients with unprovoked PE with low risk of bleeding should be treated with oral anticoagulation for more than 3 months while those with high bleeding risk should be on treatment for at least 3 months. Beyond 3 months, aspirin is an alternative to long-term warfarin and should be considered for patients who have contraindication for anticoagulation or high bleeding risk.

Venous Thromboembolism Prophylaxis

Patients who are at high risk for VTE should receive pharmacologic prophylaxis. Subcutaneous LMWH is generally preferred over subcutaneous UFH because of a modest reduction in venous thromboembolism in high-risk patients. UFH is usually reserved for patients with creatinine clearance less than 30 mL/min). Patients at high risk include those who are hospitalized with acute medical illness—particularly congestive heart failure, acute respiratory illness, acute inflammatory diseases—those who are expected to be immobilized for 3 days or longer, or patients with previous VTE. Major surgery, either elective or emergent, is an important indication for VTE prophylaxis. Subcutaneous LMWH has a marginal advantage over UFH in preventing symptomatic DVT in patients undergoing general surgery, gynecologic surgery, or neurosurgery in some but not all studies. However, LMWH is more effective than UFH and adjusted dose warfarin (INR between 2-3) and is preferred for prevention of DVT in orthopedic surgery such as hip surgery or total knee replacement because of superior efficacy (level of evidence A). DOACs, such as dabigatran, rivaroxaban, and apixaban, have similar efficacy and safety when compared with LMWH in preventing VTE after knee surgery without increasing perioperative bleeding. Efficacy of DOACs in preventing VTE after hip surgery relative to LMWH has not been directly tested in the randomized trials. DVT prophylaxis should be continued for 10 to 14 days after knee surgery and 35 days after hip surgery. Patients undergoing major cancer surgery should receive continued prophylaxis after discharge up to 28 days. Mechanical prophylaxis with intermittent pneumatic compression has not been shown to confer additional benefit in preventing VTE in medical, surgical, and trauma ICU patients when used in combination with pharmacologic thromboprophylaxis versus pharmacologic thromboprophylaxis alone. However, it should be considered in patients with high risk of bleeding in whom anticoagulation is contraindicated.

ARTERIAL HYPERTENSION

Arterial hypertension is the leading cause of death in the world, affecting 103 million adults in the United States and 1.4 billion people worldwide. It is the most common cause for an outpatient visit to a physician and the most easily recognized treatable risk factor for stroke, myocardial infarction, heart failure, peripheral vascular disease, aortic dissection, atrial fibrillation, and end-stage kidney disease. Despite this knowledge and unequivocal scientific proof that treating hypertension with medication dramatically reduces its attendant morbidity and mortality, hypertension remains untreated or undertreated in the majority of affected individuals in all countries, including those with the most advanced systems of medical care. The 2017 American Heart Association/American College of Cardiology guideline has introduced the new threshold for diagnosis and treatment of hypertension to less than 130/80 mm Hg while most other countries in the world have continued the old thresholds of less than 140/90 mm Hg in their guidelines. Fewer than one in two Americans with hypertension have their blood pressure treated and controlled to below the new 130/80 mm Hg guideline. Globally, hypertension control rates among treated individuals have plateaued at the range below 70% since the mid-2000s (Fig 12.7). Thus, hypertension remains one of the world's great public health problems. The asymptomatic nature of the condition impedes early detection, which requires regular BP measurement. Because most cases of hypertension cannot be cured, BP control requires lifelong treatment with prescription medications, which can be costly. Effective hypertension management requires continuity of care by a regular and knowledgeable medical provider, as well as sustained active participation by an educated patient. This section reviews the most important principles in the early detection and effective treatment of hypertension.

Initial Evaluation for Hypertension

The initial evaluation for hypertension needs to accomplish three goals: (1) staging of BP, (2) assessing the patient's overall cardiovascular risk, and (3) detecting clues of secondary hypertension. The initial clinical data needed to accomplish these goals are obtained through a thorough history and physical examination, routine blood tests, a spot (preferably first morning) urine specimen, and a resting 12-lead ECG. Home BP monitoring is indicated in most patients to confirm the diagnosis of hypertension and to exclude white coat syndrome. In most cases, home BP or 24-hour ambulatory BP monitoring provides helpful additional data about the time-integral burden of BP on the cardiovascular system.

Goal 1: Accurate Assessment of Blood Pressure

Across populations, the risks of heart disease and stroke increase continuously and logarithmically with increasing levels of systolic and diastolic BPs at or above 115/75 mm Hg (Fig. 12.8). Thus, the dichotomous separation of *normal* from *high* BP is artificial. BP is currently staged as normal, elevated, or hypertension based on the average of two or more readings taken on at least two separate occasions. When a patient's average systolic and diastolic pressures fall into different stages, the higher stage applies (Table 12.5). *Elevated BP* is designated as BP in the 120 to 129 mm Hg systolic in the presence of diastolic BP below 80 mm Hg. Individuals with elevated BP are at higher risk for progression into hypertension and cardiovascular events.

BP normally varies dramatically throughout a 24-hour period. To minimize variability in readings, BP should be measured at least twice after 5 minutes of rest with the patient seated, the back supported, and the arm bare and at heart level. The most common mistake in measuring BP is using a standard-issue cuff that is too small for a large arm, producing spuriously elevated readings. Most overweight adults will require a large adult cuff. Tobacco and caffeine should be avoided for at least 30 minutes. To avoid underestimation of systolic pressure in older adults who may have an *auscultatory gap* as a result of arteriosclerosis, radial artery palpation should be performed to estimate systolic pressure; then the cuff should be inflated to a value 20 mm Hg higher than the level that obliterates the radial pulse and deflated at a rate of 3 to 5 mm Hg per second. BP should be measured in both arms and after 5 minutes of standing, the latter to exclude a significant postural fall in BP, particularly in older persons and in those with diabetes or other conditions (e.g., Parkinson's disease) that predispose the patient to autonomic insufficiency.

However, out-of-office readings either with home or ambulatory BP monitoring are required to accurately assess a person's typical BP. Because of the anxiety of going to the physician, BPs often are higher in the physician's office than when measured at home or during normal daily life outside the home. Self-monitoring of BP outside of the physician's office actively engages a patient in his or her own health care and provides a better estimate of a person's usual BP for medical decision making. BP should be measured in early morning and evening times. Three BP readings should be obtained during each measurement, separated by at least 1 minute. Because the first BP tends to be the highest, average BP should be used to assess home BP. Many electronic home monitors are available, but only a handful of models have been rigorously validated against mercury sphygmomanometry and can be recommended.

Ambulatory monitoring provides automated measurements of BP over a 24- or 48-hour period while patients are engaged in their usual activities, including sleep (Fig. 12.9). The *normal limits of 24-hour* ambulatory BP, which are corresponding to office BP of 130/80 mm Hg, are a mean daytime BP of less than 130/80 mm Hg, mean nighttime BP of 110/65 mm Hg, and a mean 24-hour BP of less than 125/75 mm Hg. To avoid undertreating hypertension, these lower treatment thresholds must be used when incorporating ambulatory monitoring in medical decision making. With self-monitoring of BP at home, an average value of less than 130/80 mm Hg should be considered the upper limit of normal.

Up to one third of patients with elevated office BPs have normal home or ambulatory BPs. If the 24-hour BP profile is completely normal and no target organ damage has occurred despite consistently elevated office readings, then the patient has *office only,* or *white coat,* hypertension, presumably the result of a transient adrenergic response to the measurement of BP in the physician's office (see Fig. 12.9). In other patients, office readings underestimate ambulatory BP,

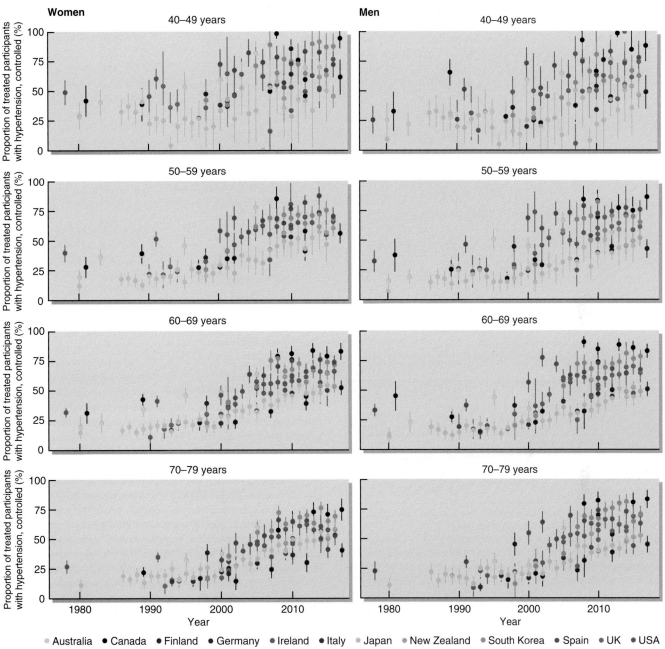

Women

Men

40–49 years

50–59 years

60–69 years

70–79 years

● Australia ● Canada ● Finland ● Germany ● Ireland ● Italy ● Japan ● New Zealand ● South Korea ● Spain ● UK ● USA

Fig. 12.7 Trends in hypertension control rates in 12 high-income countries. (NCD Risk Factor Collaboration [NCD-RisC], Lancet July 2019;10199:639-651.)

presumably because of sympathetic overactivity in daily life owing to job or home stress, tobacco use, or other adrenergic stimulation that dissipates when coming to the office (Fig. 12.10). Such documentation prevents underdiagnosing and undertreating this *masked hypertension,* which is also associated with high cardiovascular risks and identified in 10% of hypertensive patients in general, up to 40% of those with diabetes, and 70% of African American patients with hypertensive kidney disease.

Goal 2: Cardiovascular Risk Stratification

The great majority of patients with BPs in the prehypertensive or hypertensive range will have one or more additional modifiable risk factors for atherosclerosis (e.g., hypercholesterolemia, cigarette smoking, diabetes). The Pooled Cohort Equations (PCEs) is now recommended to estimate the 10-year risk of ASCVD

(atherosclerotic cardiovascular disease) among patients without history of cardiovascular disease in hypertensive patients. Patients with 10-year ASCVD risk of 10% or higher with BP of at least 130/80 mm Hg should be started on antihypertensive drug treatment without delay. In addition to ASCVD risk, presence of target organ involvement, such as left ventricular hypertrophy or proteinuria, which are not captured by PCEs but should be considered as a high-risk feature.

Goal 3: Identification of Secondary (Identifiable) Causes of Hypertension

A thorough search for secondary causes is not cost-effective in most patients with hypertension, but it becomes critically important in two circumstances: (1) when a compelling cause is found on the initial evaluation, or (2) when the hypertensive process is so severe that

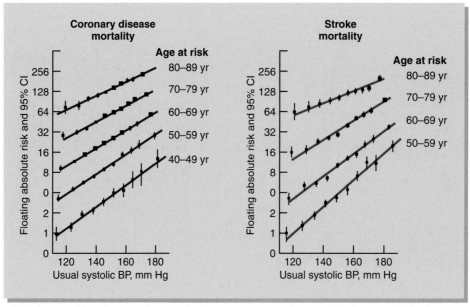

Fig. 12.8 Age-specific relevance of usual blood pressure to vascular mortality. Increased risk of myocardial infarction and stroke was observed with increasing levels of systolic BP beginning at the level of 115 mm Hg. (From Lewington S, et al. Age-specific relevance of usual blood pressure to vascular mortality: A meta-analysis of individual data for one million adults in 61 prospective studies. The Lancet 2002:360:1903-1913.)

TABLE 12.5   Staging of Office Blood Pressure[a]

Blood Pressure Category	Systolic Blood Pressure (mm Hg)	Diastolic Blood Pressure (mm Hg)
Normal	<120	and <80
Elevated	120-129	and <80
Stage 1 hypertension	130-139	or 80-89
Stage 2 hypertension	≥140	or ≥90

[a]Calculation of seated blood pressure is based on the mean of two or more readings on at least two separate occasions.
From Whelton PK, Carey RM, Aronow WS, et al. 2017 ACC/AHA/AAPA/ABC/ACPM/AGS/APhA/ASH/ASPC/NMA/PCNA guideline for the prevention, detection, evaluation, and management of high blood pressure in adults: a report of the American College of Cardiology/American Heart Association Task Force on Clinical Practice Guidelines. Circulation 2018. 138(17):e426-e483.

it either is refractory to intensive multiple-drug therapy or requires hospitalization. Table 12.6 summarizes the major causes of secondary hypertension that should be suggested on the basis of a good history, physical, and routine laboratory tests.

Renal Parenchymal Hypertension

Chronic kidney disease is the most common cause of secondary hypertension. Hypertension is present in more than 85% of patients with chronic kidney disease and is a major factor causing their increased cardiovascular morbidity and mortality. The mechanisms causing the hypertension include an expanded plasma volume and peripheral vasoconstriction, with the latter caused by both activation of vasoconstrictor pathways (renin-angiotensin and sympathetic nervous systems) and inhibition of vasodilator pathways (nitric oxide). Renal insufficiency should be considered when microalbuminuria of more than 30 mg/gram of creatinine is present or when the estimated glomerular filtration rate (eGFR) is below 60 mL/min/1.73 m^2.

Renovascular Hypertension

Unilateral or bilateral renal artery stenosis is present in less than 2% of patients with hypertension in a general medical practice but up to 30% in patients with medically refractory hypertension. The main causes of renal artery stenosis are atherosclerosis (85% of patients), typically in older adults with other clinical manifestations of systemic atherosclerosis and fibromuscular dysplasia (15% of patients), typically in women between the ages of 15 and 50 years. Unilateral renal artery stenosis leads to underperfusion of the juxtaglomerular cells, thereby producing renin-dependent hypertension even though the contralateral kidney is able to maintain normal blood volume. In contrast, bilateral renal artery stenosis (or unilateral stenosis with a solitary kidney) constitutes a potentially reversible cause of progressive renal failure and volume-dependent hypertension. The following clinical clues increase the suggestion of renovascular hypertension: any hospitalization for urgent or emergent hypertension; recurrent *flash* pulmonary edema; recent worsening of long-standing, previously well-controlled hypertension; severe hypertension in a young adult or in an adult after 50 years of age; precipitously and progressively worsening of renal function in response to angiotensin-converting enzyme (ACE) inhibition or angiotensin II-receptor blockade (ARB); unilateral small kidney by any radiographic study; extensive peripheral arteriosclerosis; or a flank bruit. The diagnosis is confirmed by noninvasive testing with MR or spiral computed tomographic (CT) angiography (Fig. 12.11). Renal artery angioplasty often cures fibromuscular dysplasia. Atherosclerotic renal artery stenosis should be treated with intensive medical management of atherosclerotic risk factors (hypertension, lipids, smoking cessation). Revascularization should be considered for the following indications: (1) medically refractory hypertension, (2) progressive renal failure on medical therapy, and (3) bilateral renal artery stenosis or stenosis of a solitary functioning kidney.

Primary Aldosteronism

The most common causes of primary aldosteronism are (1) a unilateral aldosterone-producing adenoma and (2) bilateral adrenal hyperplasia. Because aldosterone is the principal ligand for the mineralocorticoid

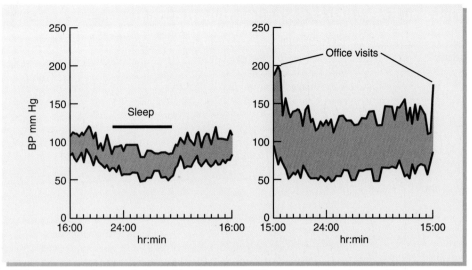

Fig. 12.9 Twenty-four hour ambulatory blood pressure (BP) monitor tracings in two different patients. (A) Optimal blood pressure (BP) in a healthy 37-year-old woman. The normal variability in BP, the nocturnal dip in BP during sleep, and the sharp increase in BP on awakening are noted. (B) Pronounced white coat effect in an 80-year-old woman referred for evaluation of medically refractory hypertension. Documentation of the white coat effect prevented overtreatment of the patient's isolated systolic hypertension.

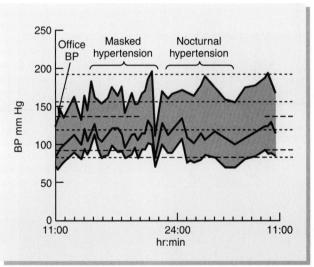

Fig. 12.10 Twenty-four hour ambulatory blood pressure (BP) monitor tracing shows both masked hypertension and nocturnal hypertension in a 55-year-old man with stage 3 chronic kidney disease. Treatment with three different antihypertensive medications in this patient produced an office BP of 125/75 mm Hg, which seems to be at goal. However, progressive hypertensive heart disease and deterioration of renal function suggested masked hypertension. Ambulatory monitoring revealed that the patient's treated BP was much higher out of the office, documenting both masked hypertension (ambulatory BP of 175/95 mm Hg) and sustained nocturnal hypertension (BP of 175/90 mm Hg). Additional medication was added. (Courtesy of Ronald G. Victor, MD, Hypertension Division, Department of Internal Medicine, University of Texas Southwestern Medical Center, Dallas, Texas.)

receptor in the distal nephron, excessive aldosterone production causes excessive renal Na^+-K^+ exchange, often resulting in hypokalemia. The diagnosis should always be suggested when hypertension is accompanied by either unprovoked hypokalemia (serum K^+ less than 3.5 mmol/L in the absence of diuretic therapy) or a tendency to develop excessive hypokalemia during diuretic therapy (serum K^+ less than 3.0

mmol/L). However, more than one third of patients do not have hypokalemia on initial presentation, and the diagnosis should be considered in any patient with refractory hypertension. The diagnosis is confirmed by the demonstration of nonsuppressible hyperaldosteronism during salt loading, followed by adrenal vein sampling to distinguish between a unilateral adenoma and bilateral hyperplasia. Laparoscopic adrenalectomy is the treatment of choice for unilateral aldosterone-producing adenoma, whereas pharmacologic mineralocorticoid-receptor blockade with eplerenone is the treatment for bilateral adrenal hyperplasia.

Mendelian Forms of Hypertension

Nine very rare forms of severe early-onset hypertension are inherited as Mendelian traits. In each case, the hypertension is mineralocorticoid-induced and involves excessive activation of the epithelial sodium channel (*ENaC*), the final common pathway for reabsorption of sodium from the distal nephron. The resultant salt-dependent hypertension can be caused by both gain-of-function mutations of *ENaC* (Liddle's syndrome) or the mineralocorticoid receptor (i.e., a rare form of pregnancy-induced hypertension) and by increased production or decreased clearance of mineralocorticoids. These include aldosterone (glucocorticoid-remediable aldosteronism), deoxycorticosterone (17-hydroxylase deficiency), and cortisol (syndrome of apparent mineralocorticoid excess). Mutations in the potassium channel subunit KCNJ5 and chloride channel CLCN2 have been linked to familial aldosteronism by increasing aldosterone release and or increasing proliferation of zona glomerulosa cells.

Pheochromocytoma and Paraganglioma

Pheochromocytomas are rare catecholamine-producing tumors of the adrenal chromaffin cells. Paragangliomas are even rarer extra-adrenal catecholamine-producing or nonfunctional tumors of sympathetic and parasympathetic ganglia. The diagnosis should be suggested when hypertension is accompanied by paroxysms of headaches, palpitations, pallor, or diaphoresis. However, the most common presentation of pheochromocytoma is an adrenal incidentaloma, an incidental adrenal mass discovered unexpectedly on abdominal imaging for another indication. In some patients,

TABLE 12.6 Guide to Evaluation of Secondary Hypertension

Probable Diagnosis	Clinical Clues	Diagnostic Testing
Renal parenchymal hypertension	Estimated GFR <60 mL/min/1.73 m² Urine albumin:creatinine >30 mg/g	Renal ultrasound
Renovascular disease	New elevation in serum creatinine, significant elevation in serum creatinine with initiation of ACEI or ARBs, refractory hypertension, flash pulmonary edema, abdominal bruit	MR or CT angiography, invasive angiogram
	Coarctation of the aorta pulses, arm BP >leg BP, chest bruits, rib notching on chest radiograph	Arm pulses >leg chest MR or CT, aortogram
Primary aldosteronism	Hypokalemia, refractory hypertension	Plasma renin and aldosterone, 24-hr urine potassium, 24-hr urine aldosterone and potassium after salt loading, adrenal CT scan, adrenal vein sampling
Cushing's syndrome	Truncal obesity, wide and blanching	24-hr urine cortisol, purple striae, muscle weakness, dexamethasone suppression test, adrenal CT scan
Pheochromocytoma	Spells of paroxysmal hypertension, palpitations, perspiration, pallor Pain in the head Diabetes	Plasma and 24-hr urine metanephrines and catecholamines, adrenal CT scan
Obstructive sleep apnea	Loud snoring, daytime somnolence, obesity, large neck	Sleep study

ACEI, Angiotensin-converting enzyme inhibitor; *ARBs,* angiotensin-receptor blockers; *BP,* blood pressure; *CT,* computed tomography; *GFR,* glomerular filtration rate; *MR,* magnetic resonance.

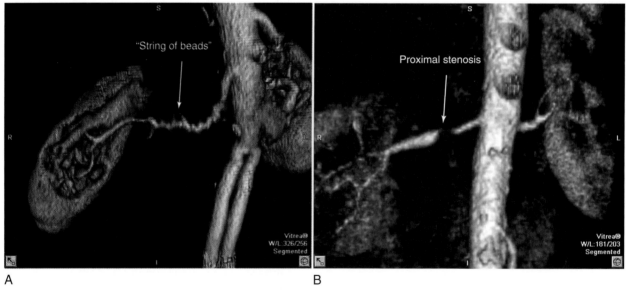

A   B

Fig. 12.11 Computed tomography (CT) angiogram with three-dimensional reconstruction. (A) Classic *string-of-beads* lesion of fibromuscular dysplasia. (B) Severe proximal atherosclerotic stenosis of the right renal artery. (Courtesy of Bart Domatch, MD, Radiology Department, University of Texas Southwestern Medical Center, Dallas, Texas.)

pheochromocytoma is misdiagnosed as panic disorder. A family history of early-onset hypertension may suggest pheochromocytoma as part of the multiple endocrine neoplasia syndromes or familial paraganglioma. If the diagnosis is missed, then outpouring of catecholamines from the tumor can cause an unsuspected hypertensive crisis during unrelated radiologic or surgical procedures; the perioperative mortality exceeds 80% in such patients.

Laboratory confirmation of pheochromocytoma is made by demonstrating elevated levels of plasma or urinary metanephrines; these are methylated derivatives of norepinephrine and epinephrine that are made in the adrenal medulla and continually leak out into the plasma even between blood pressure spikes. Pheochromocytomas are typically large adrenal tumors that can usually be localized by CT or MR imaging, although nuclear scanning with specific isotopes that localize to chromaffin tissue is occasionally needed to identify smaller tumors and paragangliomas.

Treatment of these tumors is surgical resection. Patients must receive adequate preoperative management with α-blockade followed by β-blockade and volume expansion to prevent the hemodynamic swings that can occur during surgical manipulation of the tumor. For unresectable tumors, chronic therapy with the α-adrenergic blocker phenoxybenzamine is usually effective.

TABLE 12.7 Oral Antihypertensive Agents

Drug	Dose Range, Total mg/day (Doses Per Day)	Drug	Dose Range, Total mg/day (Doses Per Day)
Diuretics		Ramipril	2.5-20 (1)
Thiazide Diuretics		Trandolapril	1-8 (1)
Hydrochlorothiazide (HCTZ)	6.25-50 (1)		
Chlorthalidone	12.5-25 (1)	**Angiotensin-Receptor Blockers**	
Indapamide	1.25-5 (1)	Azilsartan	40-80 mg (1)
Metolazone	2.5-5 (1)	Candesartan	8-32 (1)
		Eprosartan	400-800 (1-2)
Loop Diuretics		Irbesartan	150-300 (1)
Furosemide	20-160 (2)	Losartan	25-100 (2)
Torsemide	2.5-20 (1-2)	Olmesartan	5-40 (1)
Bumetanide	0.5-2 (2)	Telmisartan	20-80 (1)
Ethacrynic acid	25-100 (2)	Valsartan	80-320 (1-2)
Potassium-Sparing		**Direct Renin Inhibitor**	
Amiloride	5-20 (1)	Aliskiren	75-300 (1)
Triamterene	25-100 (1)		
Spironolactone	12.5-400 (1-2)	**α-Blockers**	
Eplerenone	25-100 (1-2)	Doxazosin	1-16 (1)
		Prazosin	1-40 (2-3)
β-Blockers		Terazosin	1-20 (1)
Acebutolol	200-800 (2)	Phenoxybenzamine	20-120 (2) for pheochromocytoma
Atenolol	25-100 (1)		
Betaxolol	5-20 (1)	**Central Sympatholytics**	
Bisoprolol	2.5-20 (1)	Clonidine	0.2-1.2 (2-3)
Carteolol	2.5-10 (1)	Clonidine patch	0.1-0.6 (weekly)
Metoprolol	50-450 (2)	Guanabenz	2-32 (2)
Metoprolol XL	50-200 (1-2)	Guanfacine	1-3 (1) (q hs)
Nadolol	20-320 (1)	Methyldopa	250-1000 (2)
Nebivolol	5-40 (1)	Reserpine	0.05-0.25 (1)
Penbutolol	10-80 (1)		
Pindolol	10-60 (2)	**Direct Vasodilators**	
Propranolol	40-180 (2)	Hydralazine	10-200 (2)
Propranolol LA	60-180 (1-2)	Minoxidil	2.5-100 (1)
Timolol	20-60 (2)		
		Fixed-Dose Combinations	
β/α-Blockers		Aliskiren/HCTZ	75-300/12.5-25 (1)
Labetalol	200-2400 (2)	Amiloride/HCTZ	5/50 (1)
Carvedilol	6.25-50 (2)	Amlodipine/benazepril	2.5-5/10-20 (1)
		Amlodipine/valsartan	5-10/160-320 (1)
Calcium-Channel Blockers		Amlodipine/olmesartan	5-10/20-40 (1)
Dihydropyridines		Atenolol/chlorthalidone	50-100/25 (1)
Amlodipine	2.5-10 (1)	Azilsartan/chlorthalidone	40-80/12.5-25 (1)
Felodipine	2.5-20 (1-2)	Benazepril/HCTZ	5-20/6.25-25 (1)
Isradipine CR	2.5-20 (2)	Bisoprolol/HCTZ	2.5-10/6.25 (1)
Nicardipine SR	30-120 (2)	Candesartan/HCTZ	16-32/12.5-25 (1)
Nifedipine XL	30-120 (1)	Enalapril/HCTZ	5-10/25 (1-2)
Nisoldipine	10-40 (12)	Eprosartan/HCTZ	600/12.5-25 (1)
		Fosinopril/HCTZ	10-20/12.5 (1)
Nondihydropyridines		Irbesartan/HCTZ	15-30/12.5-25 (1)
Diltiazem CD	120-540 (1)	Losartan/HCTZ	50-100/12.5-25 (1)
Verapamil HS	120-480 (1)	Olmesartan/amlodipine	20-40/5-10 (1)
		Olmesartan/HCTZ	20-40/12.5-25 (1)
Angiotensin-Converting Enzyme Inhibitors		Olmesartan/amlodipine/HCTZ	20-40/5-10/12.5-25 (1)
Benazepril	10-80 (12)	Spironolactone/HCTZ	25/25 (1/2-1)
Captopril	25-150 (2)	Telmisartan/HCTZ	40-80/12.5-25 (1)
Enalapril	2.5-40 (2)	Trandolapril/verapamil	2-4/180-240 (1)
Fosinopril	10-80 (1-2)	Triamterene/HCTZ	37.5/25 (1/2-1)
Lisinopril	5-80 (1-2)	Valsartan/HCTZ	80-160/12.5-25 (1)
Moexipril	7.5-30 (1)	Valsartan/amlodipine/HCTZ	80-160/5-10/12.5-25 (1)
Perindopril	4-16 (1)		
Quinapril	5-80 (1-2)		

Pheochromocytoma is a great masquerader and the large differential diagnosis includes causes of neurogenic hypertension such as sympathomimetic agents (cocaine, methamphetamine), baroreflex failure, and obstructive sleep apnea. A history of surgery and radiation therapy for head-and-neck tumors suggests the possibility of baroreceptor damage. Loud snoring, obesity, and somnolence suggest obstructive sleep apnea. Weight loss, continuous positive airway pressure, and corrective surgery improve BP control in some patients with sleep apnea.

Other causes of secondary hypertension include nonsteroidal anti-inflammatory drugs (NSAIDs), hypothyroidism, hyperthyroidism coarctation of the aorta, and immunosuppressive drugs, especially cyclosporine and tacrolimus.

TREATMENT OF HYPERTENSION

Prescription medication is the cornerstone of treating hypertension. Lifestyle modification should be used as an adjunct but not as an alternative to life-saving BP medication. Most dietary sodium (Na^+) comes from processed foods, and daily salt consumption should be reduced to less than 4 grams, which is equivalent to 1500 mg or 65 mmol of Na^+. The **Dietary Approach to Stop Hypertension** (DASH diet), which is rich in fresh fruits and vegetables (for high potassium content) and low-fat dairy products, has been shown to lower BP in feeding trials. Other lifestyle modifications that can lower BP include weight loss in overweight patients with hypertension, regular aerobic exercise, smoking cessation, and moderation in alcohol intake.

The list of antihypertensive drugs marketed for the treatment of hypertension in the United States is shown in Table 12.7. Major contraindications and side effects of these drugs are summarized in Table 12.8.

Patients With Uncomplicated Hypertension

The three first-line drug classes for uncomplicated hypertension are: (1) CCB, (2) ACEI or ARB, and (3) thiazide diuretic. The 2017 ACC/AHA high blood pressure guideline, recommended any one of these three drug classes as initial therapy for most patients with hypertension. It also recommended initiating therapy with two first-line drugs of different classes, either as separate agents or in a fixed-dose combination for individuals with BP more than 20/10 mm Hg above their target goal. β-Blockers are not recommended as first-line therapy unless patients have other compelling indications (such as heart failure or ischemic heart disease) because it is inferior to three first-line drug classes in preventing target organ damage and cardiovascular events. In contrast, the European Society of Hypertension endorses β-blocker as the first-line agent, arguing that the most effective drugs are those that the patient will tolerate and take. Long-term patient adherence is best with an ARB, intermediate with an ACEI or CCB, and worst with a thiazide. Initiation of single pill combination therapy is encouraged as it allows BP control to reach target goal faster and improves long-term adherence. The European Society of Hypertension advocates a treatment strategy that is based on the patient's age and ethnicity. It recommends upfront combination therapy of RAS blocker (either an ACE inhibitor or an ARB) with a CCB or diuretic except in frail older adults with mild hypertension, in whom a monotherapy is recommended.

A growing body of evidence from clinical trials emphasizes the overriding importance of lowering BP with combinations of drugs rather than belaboring the choice of a single, best agent to begin therapy. Primary hypertension is multifactorial, and typically several medications (at least two or more) with different mechanisms of action (see Table 12.7) are required simultaneously to reach BP goal. In most patients with hypertension, low-dose combination drug therapy is the only way to control BP adequately and to minimize side effects. With many classes of antihypertensive medication, the dose-response relationship for BP is rather flat. Most of the BP lowering occurs at the lower end of the dose range. However, many of the side effects are steeply dose-dependent, becoming problematic mainly at the high end of the clinical dose range. Thus, low-dose combinations achieve therapeutic synergy and minimize side effects. Fixed-dose combinations reduce pill burden and cost.

One highly effective well-tolerated combination is a CCB plus an ACEI or ARB. A large benefit of combination therapy with an ACEI plus a dihydropyridine CCB over the combination of an ACEI plus a thiazide diuretic is reducing cardiovascular events in high-risk patients. In contrast, the combination of ARB plus an ACEI or direct renin inhibitor ("dual renin-angiotensin system blockade") should be avoided because it results in deterioration of renal function and increases risk of hypotension without added cardiovascular benefit.

Kaiser-Permanente of Northern California, a large managed care organization, has increased the control of hypertension among its membership over the past decade from 44% to an astounding 80% by: increasing access with walk-in BP checks by medical assistants, registry rounds to identify and contact patients with elevated office BP, and institution of a system-wide simple medication treatment protocol that features once-daily combination therapy.

Along with antihypertensive medication, statin therapy should be strongly considered as an integral part of most antihypertensive regimens in patients with 10-year ASCVD risk of at least 7.5%.

Hypertension in African Americans

Hypertension disproportionately affects African Americans. The explanation is unknown, but the dominant importance of environmental factors is indicated by geographic variation in hypertension prevalence among African-origin and European-origin populations. Hypertension is rare among Africans living in Africa and is more prevalent in several European countries than it is in the United States. As monotherapy for hypertension, an ACEI (or ARB) generally yields a smaller decrease in BP in black African patients than it does in non-black patients and thus affords less protection against stroke. However, when an ACEI or ARB is used in combination with a CCB or a diuretic, antihypertensive efficacy is amplified and ethnic differences disappear. In addition, combination of CCB with an ACEI (or ARB) or a diuretic is superior to combination of ACEI and diuretics in lowering BP in this population. Nevertheless, an ACEI-based treatment should be considered in African American patients with hypertensive nephrosclerosis as it slows the deterioration in renal function.

Hypertensive Nephrosclerosis

Hypertension is the second most common cause of chronic kidney disease, accounting for over 25% of cases. Hypertensive nephrosclerosis is the result of persistently uncontrolled hypertension, causing chronic glomerular ischemia. Typically, proteinuria is mild (<0.5 g/24 hr). Nondiabetic chronic kidney disease is a compelling indication for ACEI-based or ARB-based antihypertensive therapy. ACEIs cause greater dilation of the efferent renal arterioles, thereby minimizing intraglomerular hypertension. In contrast, arterial vasodilators such as dihydropyridine CCBs, when used without an ACEI or ARB, preferentially dilate the afferent arteriole and impair renal autoregulation. Glomerular hypertension can result if systemic BP is not sufficiently lowered. The ACEI should be withdrawn only if the rise in serum creatinine exceeds 30% of the baseline value or the serum K increases to greater than 5.6 mmol/L.

TABLE 12.8 Major Contraindications and Side Effects of Antihypertensive Drugs

Drug Class	Major Contraindications	Side Effects
Diuretics		
Thiazides	Gout	Insulin resistance, new onset type 2 diabetes (especially in combination with β-blockers)
		Hypokalemia, hyponatremia
		Hypertriglyceridemia
		Hyperuricemia, precipitation of gout
		Erectile dysfunction (more than other drug classes)
		Potentiate nondepolarizing muscle relaxants
		Photosensitive dermatitis
Loop diuretics	Hepatic coma	Interstitial nephritis
		Hypokalemia
		Potentiate succinylcholine
		Potentiate aminoglycoside ototoxicity
Potassium-sparing diuretics	Serum K >5.5 mEq/L	Fatal hyperkalemia if used with salt substitutes, ACE inhibitors, ARBs, high-potassium foods, NSAIDs
	GFR <30 mg/mL/1.73 m^2	
β-Blockers	Heart block	Insulin resistance, new onset type 2 diabetes (especially in combination with thiazides)
	Asthma	Heart block, acute decompensated CHF
	Depression	Bronchospasm
	Cocaine and/or methamphetamine abuse	Depression, nightmares, fatigue
		Cold extremities, claudication (β2 effect)
		Stevens-Johnson syndrome
		Agranulocytosis
ACEIs	Pregnancy	Cough
	Bilateral renal artery stenosis	Hyperkalemia
	Hyperkalemia	Angioedema
		Leukopenia
		Fetal toxicity
		Cholestatic jaundice (rare fulminant hepatic necrosis if the drug is not discontinued)
ARBs	Pregnancy	Hyperkalemia
	Bilateral renal artery stenosis	Angioedema (very rare)
	Hyperkalemia	Fetal toxicity
Direct Renin Inhibitors	Pregnancy	Hyperkalemia
	Bilateral renal artery stenosis	Diarrhea
	Hyperkalemia	Fetal toxicity
Dihydropyridine CCBs	As monotherapy in chronic kidney disease with proteinuria	Headaches
		Flushing
		Ankle edema
		CHF
		Gingival hyperplasia
		Esophageal reflux
Nondihydropyridine CCBs	Heart block	Bradycardia, AV block (especially with verapamil)
	Systolic heart failure	Constipation (often severe with verapamil)
		Worsening of systolic function, CHF
		Gingival edema and/or hypertrophy
		Increase cyclosporine blood levels
		Esophageal reflux
α-Blockers	Monotherapy for hypertension	Orthostatic hypotension
	Orthostatic hypotension	Drug tolerance (in the absence of diuretic therapy)
	Systolic heart failure	Ankle edema
	Left ventricular dysfunction	CHF
		First-dose effect (acute hypotension)
		Potentiate hypotension with PDE5 inhibitors (e.g., sildenafil)
Central sympatholytics	Orthostatic hypotension	Depression, dry mouth, lethargy
		Erectile dysfunction (dose dependent)

Continued

TABLE 12.8	Major Contraindications and Side Effects of Antihypertensive Drugs—cont'd	
Drug Class	Major Contraindications	Side Effects
Direct vasodilators	Orthostatic hypotension	Rebound hypertension with clonidine withdrawal Coombs positive hemolytic anemia and elevated LFTs with α-methyldopa Reflex tachycardia Fluid retention Hirsutism, pericardial effusion with minoxidil Lupus with hydralazine

ACE, Angiotensin-converting enzyme; *ARBs,* angiotensin-receptor blockers; *AV,* arteriovenous; *CCBs,* calcium channel blockers; *CHF,* congestive heart failure; *GFR,* glomerular filtration rate; *LFTs,* liver function tests; *MI,* myocardial infarction; *NSAIDs,* nonsteroidal anti-inflammatory drugs; *PDE5,* phosphodiesterase type 5.

Hypertensive Patients With Diabetes

Compared with its 25% prevalence in the general adult population, hypertension is present in 75% of patients with diabetes and is a major factor contributing to excessive risk of myocardial infarction, stroke, heart failure, microvascular complications, and diabetic nephropathy progressing to end-stage renal disease. The Action to Control Cardiovascular Risk in Diabetes blood pressure trial (ACCORD BP) failed to show benefit of lowering systolic BP below 120 mm Hg in patients with type 2 diabetes mellitus in terms of reducing overall mortality or cardiovascular mortality. However, the risk of stroke was reduced by 60% in these patients. ACCORD trial also tested intensive versus standard glycemic targets (glycated hemoglobin <6% versus 7.0% to 7.9%). A more recent analysis has demonstrated benefit of intensive BP lowering in lowering cardiovascular events in diabetic patients in the standard glycemia arm but not in the intensive glycemic arm. Increased hypoglycemic events associated with intensive glycemic control may negate potential cardiovascular benefit of intensive BP lowering in this population. The Systolic Blood Pressure Intervention Trial (SPRINT), which was conducted in nondiabetic patients and has similar study design to the ACCORD trial, showed benefit of intensive BP lowering in patients with prediabetes. Consequently, the 2017 ACC/AHA guideline endorses a BP target of less than 130/80 mm Hg for diabetic patients. The 2019 American Diabetes Association endorses lower targets only in diabetic patients with 10-year ASCVD risk of greater than 15%. In general, an ACEI or ARB plus a CCB is an excellent combination to treat hypertension in patients with diabetes. Thiazide diuretics and standard β-blockers exacerbate glucose intolerance, whereas the vasodilating β-blockers such as carvedilol and nebivolol have neutral or possibly beneficial effects.

Hypertensive Patients With Coronary Artery Disease

To lower myocardial oxygen demands in patients with coronary disease, the antihypertensive regimen should reduce BP without causing reflex tachycardia. For this reason, a β-blocker is often prescribed in conjunction with a dihydropyridine CCB such as amlodipine. β-Blockers are indicated for patients with hypertension who have sustained a myocardial infarction and for most heart failure patients with reduced ejection fraction (HFrEF). In contrast, diuretics are recommended as the first therapy in heart failure patients with preserved ejection fraction (HFpEF) with evidence of volume overload. After euvolemia is achieved, ACEIs, ARBs, or spironolactone may be considered in patients with persistently elevated BP. In patients with stable coronary artery disease, a cardioprotective effect of ACE inhibition has also been demonstrated in patients with moderate cardiovascular risk profiles but not in those with lower risk profiles.

Isolated Systolic Hypertension in Older Adults

In developed countries, systolic pressure rises progressively with age; if individuals live long enough, then almost all (>90%) develop hypertension. Diastolic pressure rises until the age of 50 years and decreases thereafter, producing a progressive rise in pulse pressure (i.e., systolic pressure minus diastolic pressure) (Fig. 12.12).

Different hemodynamic faults underlie hypertension in younger and older persons. Patients who develop hypertension before 50 years of age typically have *combined systolic and diastolic hypertension*: systolic pressure greater than 140 mm Hg *and* diastolic pressure greater than 90 mm Hg. The main hemodynamic fault is vasoconstriction at the level of the resistance arterioles. In contrast, the majority of patients who develop hypertension after 50 years of age have *isolated systolic hypertension*: systolic pressure greater than 140 mm Hg but diastolic pressure less than 90 mm Hg (often less than 80 mm Hg). In isolated systolic hypertension, the primary hemodynamic fault is decreased distensibility of the aorta and other large conduit arteries (see Fig. 12.12). Collagen replaces elastin in the elastic lamina of the aorta, an age-dependent process that is accelerated by atherosclerosis and hypertension. The cardiovascular risk associated with isolated systolic hypertension is related to pulsatility, the repetitive pounding of the blood vessels with each cardiac cycle and a more rapid return of the arterial pulse wave from the periphery, both begetting more systolic hypertension. In the United States and Europe, the majority of uncontrolled hypertension occurs in older patients with isolated systolic hypertension. A BP of 160/60 mm Hg (pulse pressure of 100 mm Hg) carries twice the risk of fatal coronary heart disease as 140/110 mm Hg (pulse pressure of 30 mm Hg) (Fig. 12.13).

In older persons with isolated systolic hypertension, lowering systolic pressure from higher than 160 to lower than 150 mm Hg reduces the risks of stroke, myocardial infarction, and overall cardiovascular mortality; it also reduces heart failure admissions and slows the progression of dementia. Trial data do not yet exist in older persons to determine whether the treatment of isolated elevations in systolic pressure below 140 mm Hg is beneficial; however, in the absence of such data, treatment may be warranted to prevent progression of systolic hypertension if patients can tolerate treatment without side effects such as orthostatic hypotension.

The combination of a low-dose thiazide diuretic with a dihydropyridine CCB or with an ACEI reduces the risk of CV events in older patients with isolated systolic hypertension. According to the 2017 ACC/AHA high BP guideline, chlorthalidone is the preferred thiazide diuretic given its long half-life and more consistent reduction in cardiovascular events in clinical trials than other thiazide diuretics. To prevent orthostatic hypotension, medication should be titrated to standing BP and one low-dose medication should be started at a time.

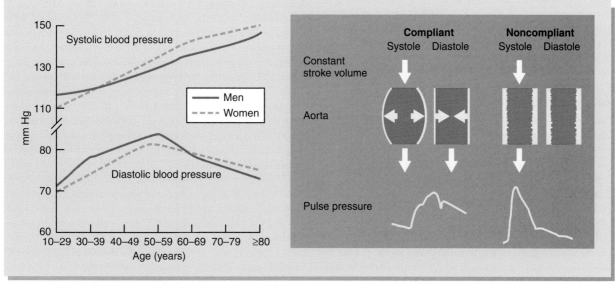

Fig. 12.12 Age-dependent changes in systolic and diastolic blood pressure (BP) in the United States *(left panel)*. Schematic diagram explains the relation between aortic compliance and pulse pressure *(right panel)*. *(Left panel,* From Burt V, Whelton P, Rocella EJ, et al: Prevalence of hypertension in the U.S. adult population: Results from the Third National Health and Nutrition Examination Survey, 1988–1991. Hypertension 25:305-313, 1995. *Right panel,* Courtesy of Dr. Stanley Franklin University of California at Irvine. Used with permission.)

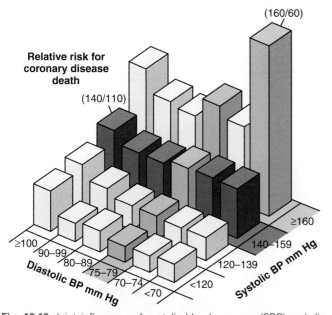

Fig. 12.13 Joint influences of systolic blood pressure (SBP) and diastolic BP on coronary heart disease (CHD) risk in the Multiple Risk Factor Intervention Trial. (Neaton JD, Wentworth D: Serum cholesterol, blood pressure, cigarette smoking, and death from coronary heart disease: Overall findings and differences by age for 316,099 white men. Arch Intern Med 152:56-64, 1992.)

Blood Pressure Lowering for Secondary Prevention of Stroke

Most neurologists do not recommend BP reduction during an acute stroke unless BP is extremely elevated (see section Acute Severe Hypertension). After the acute phase, BP should be lowered with a thiazide diuretic, adding an ACEI or additional drugs as needed to achieve BP lower than 140/90 mm Hg; whether BP should be lowered further remains unsettled. Lower BP target of less than 130/80 mm Hg for patients may be reasonable for patients with transient ischemic attack or lacuna infarct to prevent intracranial hemorrhage.

Blood Pressure Lowering for Prevention of Cognitive Impairment

Increasing number of studies have shown that high BP and other cardiovascular risk factors such as hyperlipidemia predisposes not only to increased cardiovascular damage but also brain injury and cognitive impairment in older adults, which is independent of stroke (i.e., what is good for the heart is good for the brain). The recent SPRINT MIND clinical trial showed that intensive lowering of systolic BP to below 120 mm Hg in adults with high cardiovascular risk but without history of stroke prevents development of cognitive impairment. There was no significant reduction in new cases of dementia but the trial was limited by short duration of follow-up. Additional studies are needed to clarify optimal BP target to prevent cognitive dysfunction in hypertensive adults.

Hypertensive Disorders of Women

Oral contraceptives cause a small increase in BP in most women but rarely cause a large increase into the hypertensive range. If hypertension develops, oral contraceptive therapy should be discontinued in favor of other methods of contraception. Oral estrogen replacement therapy seems to cause a small increase in BP. In contrast, transdermal estrogen (which bypasses first-pass hepatic metabolism) seems to avoid this side effect.

Hypertension, the most common nonobstetric complication of pregnancy, is present in 10% of all pregnancies. Of these women, one third are caused by chronic hypertension and two thirds are due to preeclampsia, which is defined as an increase in BP to 140/90 mm Hg or greater after the twentieth week of gestation accompanied by proteinuria (>300 mg/24 hr) and pathologic edema. This is sometimes accompanied by seizures (eclampsia) and the multisystem HELLP syndrome of hemolysis (H), elevated liver enzymes (EL), and low platelets (LP). Although the cause remains an enigma, preeclampsia is the most common cause of maternal mortality and perinatal mortality. Nifedipine and α-methyldopa are considered to be first-line drug therapy for preeclampsia and chronic hypertension in pregnancy. Labetalol is also effective in lowering BP but may result in intrauterine growth restriction.

Resistant Hypertension

Defined as persistence of usual BP above 140/90 mm Hg despite treatment with full doses of three or more different classes of medications in rational combination and including a diuretic, *resistant hypertension* is the most common reason for referral to a hypertension specialist. In practice, the majority of these patients have pseudoresistant hypertension due to: (1) *white coat aggravation,* a white coat reaction superimposed on chronic hypertension that is well-controlled with medication outside the physician's office; (2) an inadequate medical regimen; (3) nonadherence to medication, which is present in 30% to 60% of patients using direct measurement of drugs levels in the plasma or urine; and (4) ingestion of pressor substances. Common shortcomings of the medical regimen include under-treatment of hypertension with monotherapy and clonidine, a potent central sympatholytic that causes rebound hypertension between doses particularly with PRN dosing. Several common causes of pseudoresistant hypertension are related to the patient's behavior: medication nonadherence, recidivism with lifestyle modification (e.g., obesity, a high-salt diet, excessive alcohol intake), or habitual use of pressor substances such as sympathomimetics (e.g., tobacco, cocaine, methamphetamine, phenylephrine-containing cold or herbal remedies) or NSAIDs, with the latter causing renal sodium retention. Once these behavioral factors have been excluded, the search should begin for secondary hypertension.

The most common forms of secondary hypertension include obstructive sleep apnea, chronic kidney disease, and primary aldosteronism. Either a loop diuretic such a furosemide or a potent thiazide-type diuretic such as chlorthalidone may be required to control hypertension in patients with resistant hypertension and chronic kidney disease. The treatment of primary aldosteronism was discussed earlier. After excluding pseudoresistant hypertension and secondary hypertension, some patients have severe drug-resistant primary hypertension. Fourth- and fifth-line therapy includes a vasodilating β-blocker and spironolactone (even in the absence of primary aldosteronism). Percutaneous catheter-based renal denervation is proposed as a novel interventional approach to treat drug-resistant hypertension. Although the initial results raised enormous enthusiasm, subsequent randomized controlled trials have been disappointing as the magnitude of reduction in BP is modest (less than 10 mm Hg) when compared to the sham control arm. A number of studies that use other neuromodulation techniques, such as baroreflex activation, to reduce overall sympathetic tone beyond renal sympathetic activity alone, are being conducted to determine BP outcome in this population.

Acute Severe Hypertension

Of all the patients in the emergency department, 25% have an elevated BP. *Hypertensive emergencies* are acute, often severe elevations in BP that are accompanied by acute or rapidly progressive target organ dysfunction such as myocardial or cerebral ischemia or infarction, pulmonary edema, or renal failure. *Hypertensive urgencies* are severe elevations in BP without severe symptoms and without evidence of acute or progressive target organ dysfunction. Thus, the key distinction and approach to the patient depends on the state of the patient and the assessment of target organ damage, not simply the absolute level of BP. The full-blown clinical picture of a hypertensive emergency is a critically ill patient with a BP greater than 220/140 mm Hg,

headaches, confusion, blurred vision, nausea and vomiting, seizures, heart failure, oliguria, and grade III or IV hypertensive retinopathy (Fig. 12.14). Hypertensive emergencies require immediate admission in an intensive care unit (ICU) for intravenous therapy and continuous BP monitoring, whereas hypertensive urgencies can often be managed with oral medications and appropriate outpatient follow-up in 24 to 72 hours. The most common hypertensive cardiac emergencies include hypertension associated with acute aortic dissection, coronary artery bypass graft surgery, acute myocardial infarction, and unstable angina. Other hypertensive emergencies include those accompanying eclampsia, head trauma, severe body burns, postoperative bleeding from vascular suture lines, and epistaxis that cannot be controlled with anterior and posterior nasal packing. Neurologic hypertensive emergencies, which include acute ischemic stroke, hemorrhagic stroke, subarachnoid hemorrhage, and hypertensive encephalopathy, can be difficult to distinguish from one another. Hypertensive encephalopathy is characterized by severe hypertensive retinopathy (i.e., retinal hemorrhages and exudates, with or without papilledema) and a posterior leukoencephalopathy affecting mainly the white matter of the parieto-occipital regions as seen on cerebral MR imaging or CT scanning. A new focal neurologic deficit suggesting a stroke-in-evolution demands a much more conservative approach to correcting the elevated BP.

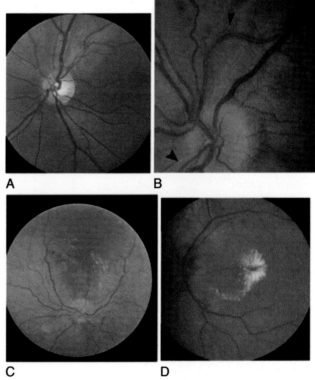

Fig. 12.14 Hypertensive retinopathy is traditionally divided into four grades. (A) Grade 1 shows very early and minor changes in a young patient; increased tortuosity of a retinal vessel and increased reflectiveness (silver wiring) of a retinal artery are seen at the 1-o'clock position in this view. Otherwise, the fundus is completely normal. (B) Grade 2 also shows increased tortuosity and silver wiring *(arrowheads)*. In addition, *nipping* of the venules at arteriovenous (AV) crossings is visualized *(arrow)*. (C) Grade 3 shows the same changes as grade 2 plus flame-shaped retinal hemorrhages and soft *cotton-wool* exudates. (D) In grade 4, swelling of the optic disc (papilledema) is observed, retinal edema is present, and hard exudates may collect around the fovea, producing a typical *macular star*. (From Forbes CD, Jackson WF: Color atlas and text of clinical medicine, 3rd ed. London, Mosby, 2003, with permission.)

In most other hypertensive emergencies, the goal of parenteral therapy is to achieve a controlled and gradual lowering of BP. The rapidity of BP reduction is highly dependent on clinical presentation. Patients with acute aortic dissection require rapid reduction to the 120/80 mm Hg range almost immediately to reduce shear stress and prevent further intimal tear in the aortic wall, which could be life-threatening. On the other hand, patients with acute ischemic stroke who are not candidates for intravenous thrombolysis or endovascular treatment should not be treated with antihypertensive agents unless BP is 220/120 mm Hg or higher. Following initial therapy, a more conservative BP reduction goal to no more than 15% during the first 24 hours after onset of stroke is recommended. In those who are candidates for thrombolysis, however, BP should be less than 185/110 mm Hg before administration of intravenous tissue plasminogen activator and should be maintained below 180/105 mm Hg for at least the first 24 hours after initiating drug therapy. The widely cited goal of BP lowering by 10% in the first hour and by an additional 15% over the next 3 to 12 hours is limited to patients who present with hypertensive encephalopathy or other presentations. Unnecessarily rapid correction of the elevated BP to completely normal values places the patient at high risk for worsening cerebral, cardiac, and renal ischemia. In chronic hypertension, cerebral autoregulation is reset to higher-than-normal BPs. This compensatory adjustment prevents tissue overperfusion (i.e., increased intracranial pressure) at very high BPs, but it also predisposes the patient to tissue underperfusion (i.e., cerebral ischemia) when an elevated BP is lowered too quickly.

Parenteral agents for the treatment of hypertensive emergency are summarized in Table 12.9. Sodium nitroprusside, a nitric oxide donor, is the most popular agent because it can be titrated rapidly to control BP. Intravenous nitroglycerin, another nitric oxide donor, is indicated mainly for hypertension in the setting of acute coronary syndrome or decompensated heart failure. Nicardipine is a parenteral dihydropyridine CCB that is particularly useful in the postoperative cardiac patient and patients with renal failure to avoid the thiocyanate toxicity with nitroprusside. Clevidipine is another intravenous CCB with shorter half-life than nicardipine of only 1 minute. Fenoldopam is a selective dopamine-1-receptor agonist that causes both systemic and renal vasodilation, as well as increased glomerular filtration, natriuresis, and diuresis. Intravenous labetalol is an effective treatment of a hypertensive crisis particularly in the setting of myocardial ischemia with preserved ventricular function.

Most patients in the emergency department with hypertensive urgencies are either nonadherent with their medical regimen or are being treated with an inadequate regimen. To expedite the necessary changes in medications, outpatient follow-up should be arranged within 72 hours. To manage the patient during the short-interim period, effective oral medication includes labetalol, clonidine, or captopril, which is a short-acting ACEI.

BPs greater than 160/110 mm Hg are a common incidental finding among patients in emergency departments and other acute care settings for urgent medical or surgical care of symptoms that are unrelated to BP (e.g., musculoskeletal pain, orthopedic injury). In these settings, the elevated BP is more often the first indication of chronic hypertension than a simple physiologic stress reaction, providing an important opportunity to initiate primary care referral for formal evaluation and treatment of chronic hypertension. Home and ambulatory BP monitoring are indicated to determine whether the patient's BP normalizes completely once the acute illness has resolved.

TABLE 12.9 Parenteral Agents for Management of Hypertensive Emergencies

Agent	Dose	Onset of Action	Precautions
Parenteral Vasodilators			
Sodium nitroprusside	0.25-10 mcg/kg/min IV infusion	Immediate	Thiocyanate toxicity with prolonged use
Nitroglycerin	5-100 mcg/min IV infusion	2-5 min	Headache, tachycardia, tolerance
Nicardipine	5-15 mg/hr IV infusion	1-5 min	Protracted hypotension after prolonged use
Clevidipine	1-21 mg/hr IV infusion	2-4 min	Tachycardia
Fenoldopam mesylate	0.01-0.3 mcg/kg/min IV infusion	1-5 min	Headache, tachycardia, increased intraocular pressure
Hydralazine	5-10 mg as IV bolus or 10-40 mg IM; repeat every 4-6 hrs	10 min IV 20 min IM	Unpredictable and excessive falls in tachycardia; angina exacerbation; blood pressure
Enalaprilat	0.625-1.25 mg every 6 hr IV bolus	15-60 min	Unpredictable and excessive falls in blood pressure; acute renal failure in patients with stenosis bilateral renal artery
Parenteral Adrenergic Inhibitors			
Labetalol	20-80 mg as slow IV injection every 10 min, or 0.5-2.0 mg/min IV as infusion	5-10 min	Bronchospasm, heart block, orthostatic hypotension
Metoprolol	5 mg IV every 10 min for three doses	5-10 min	Bronchospasm, heart block, heart failure, exacerbation of cocaine-induced myocardial ischemia
Esmolol	500 mcg/kg IV over 3 min; then 25-100 mg/kg/min as IV infusion	1-5 min	Bronchospasm, heart block, heart failure
Phentolamine	5-10 mg IV bolus every 5-15 min	1-2 min	Tachycardia, orthostatic hypotension

IM, Intramuscular; *IV,* intravenous.

PROGNOSIS

One of the most important prognostic factors in hypertension is ECG or echocardiographic LVH, with the latter already present in as many as 25% of patients with newly diagnosed hypertension. LVH predisposes the patient to heart failure, atrial fibrillation, and sudden cardiac death.

Because of their relatively short duration (typically <5 years), randomized controlled trials underestimate the lifetime protection against premature disability and death afforded by several decades of antihypertensive therapy in clinical practice. In the Framingham Heart Study, treating hypertension for 20 years in middle-aged adults reduced total cardiovascular mortality by 60%, which is considerably greater than the results of most randomized trials despite the less intense treatment guidelines when therapy was initiated in the 1950s through the 1970s.

PROSPECTS FOR THE FUTURE

- Further delineation of genetic causes of hypertension and application of this research to the treatment and prevention of hypertension, including development of pharmacologic and non-pharmacologic therapy that target the various signaling pathways in hypertension
- Determination of antihypertensive drug classes that are most effective in preventing dementia and cognitive decline
- Evaluation of the comparative efficacy and safety of DOACs against LMWH in preventing VTE in patients with active malignancy
- Further assessment of safety and efficacy of combination of direct anticoagulants and antiplatelet therapy in patients with atrial fibrillation, venous thromboembolism, and vascular disease

SUGGESTED READINGS

Arabi YM, Al-Hameed F, Burns KEA, et al: Adjunctive intermittent pneumatic compression for venous thromboprophylaxis, *N Engl J Med* 380:1305–1315, 2019.

Gerhard-Herman MD, Gornik HL, Barrett C, et al: 2016 AHA/ACC guideline on the management of patients with lower extremity peripheral artery disease: a report of the American College of Cardiology/American Heart Association Task Force on Clinical Practice Guidelines, Circulation 135:e726–e779, 2017.

Group SMIftSR, Williamson JD, Pajewski NM, et al: Effect of intensive vs standard blood pressure control on probable dementia: a randomized clinical trial, JAMA 321:553–561, 2019.

Kearon C, Akl EA, Ornelas J, et al: Antithrombotic therapy for VTE disease: chest guideline and expert panel report, Chest 149:315–352, 2016.

Konstantinides SV, Meyer G, Becattini C, et al: 2019 ESC Guidelines for the diagnosis and management of acute pulmonary embolism developed in collaboration with the European Respiratory Society (ERS): the Task Force for the diagnosis and management of acute pulmonary embolism of the European Society of Cardiology (ESC), Eur Respir J 54(3):1901647, 2019.

Ojji DB, Mayosi B, Francis V, et al.: Comparison of dual therapies for lowering blood pressure in black africans, N Engl J Med 380:2429–2439, 2019.

Simonneau G, Montani D, Celermajer DS, et al: Haemodynamic definitions and updated clinical classification of pulmonary hypertension, Eur Respir J 53, 2019.

Vongpatanasin W: Resistant hypertension: a review of diagnosis and management, JAMA 311(21):2216–2224, 2014.

Vongpatanasin W, Ayers C, Lodhi H, et al.: Diagnostic thresholds for blood pressure measured at home in the context of the 2017 hypertension guideline, Hypertension 72:1312–1319, 2018.

Whelton PK, Carey RM, Aronow WS, et al: 2017 ACC/AHA/AAPA/ABC/ACPM/AGS/APhA/ASH/ASPC/NMA/PCNA Guideline for the prevention, detection, evaluation, and management of high blood pressure in adults: Executive summary: A report of the American College of Cardiology/American Heart Association task force on clinical practice guidelines, Circulation 138:e426–e483, 2018.

Williams B, Mancia G, Spiering W, et al: 2018 ESC/ESH Guidelines for the management of arterial hypertension, Eur Heart J 39:3021–3104, 2018.

Pulmonary and Critical Care Medicine

13

Lung in Health and Disease

Sharon Rounds, Debasree Banerjee, Eric J. Gartman

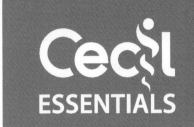

INTRODUCTION

The lung is part of the respiratory system and consists of conducting airways, blood vessels, and gas exchange units with alveolar gas spaces and capillaries (Fig. 13.1). The neural control of the respiratory system includes the brain cortex and medulla, the spinal cord, and peripheral nerves that innervate the skeletal muscles of respiration, airways, and vessels. The airways of the respiratory system include the upper airway—the nose, pharynx, and larynx—where inspired air is humidified and particulate matter is filtered. The intrathoracic airways continue down the trachea to the carina where the mainstem bronchi branch defining the right- and left-sided airways. Bronchi continue to branch into smaller airways (bronchioles) that eventually take on gas exchange capacity and end in alveolar sacs. Both pulmonary arteries and veins and lymphatics follow the branching patterns of the airways. The lung also has systemic circulation via the bronchial arteries. The bony structure of the chest wall protects the heart, lungs, and liver, and the lungs are maintained in an inflated state by mechanical coupling of the chest wall with the lungs. The skeletal muscles of respiration include the

diaphragm and the accessory muscles; the latter are important when disease causes diaphragm fatigue.

The lung is a complex organ with an extensive array of airways and vessels arranged to efficiently transfer the gases necessary for sustaining life. The organ has an immense capacity for gas exchange and can accommodate increased demand during exercise in healthy individuals. In lung disease, however, as exchange becomes compromised, the host's activities and function become increasingly compromised. The most dramatic consequence of acute and chronic abnormalities in lung function is systemic hypoxemia, which causes tissue hypoxia in multiple other organs.

In addition to gas exchange, the lungs have other functions, such as defense against inhaled infectious agents and environmental toxins. The entire cardiac output passes through the pulmonary circulation, which serves as a filter for blood-borne clots and infections. Additionally, the massive surface area of endothelial cells lining the pulmonary circulation has metabolic functions, such as conversion of angiotensin I to angiotensin II.

Lung disorders are common and range from well-known conditions such as asthma and chronic obstructive pulmonary disease (COPD) to rarely encountered disorders such as lymphangioleiomyomatosis. The chapters in Section III discuss the diagnosis, evaluation, and management of pulmonary disorders that develop in direct response to lung injury and those that develop indirectly through injuries to other organs. Section III also addresses critical illness such as acute lung injury, which is frequently managed by pulmonary or critical care specialists.

This chapter reviews the structural-functional relationships of the lung during development, the epidemiology of pulmonary disease, and the classification of pulmonary disorders.

LUNG DEVELOPMENT

The lung begins to develop during the first trimester of pregnancy through complex and overlapping processes that transform the embryonic lung bud into a functioning organ with an extensive airway network, two complete circulatory systems, and millions of alveoli responsible for the transfer of gases to and from the body. Lung development occurs in five consecutive stages: embryonic, pseudoglandular, canalicular or vascular, saccular, and alveolar postnatal (Table 13.1).

During the embryonic stage (between 21 days and 7 weeks' gestation), the rudimentary lung emerges from the foregut as a single epithelial bud surrounded by mesenchymal tissue. This stage is followed by the pseudoglandular stage (between 5 and 17 weeks' gestation), during which repeated extensive branching forms rudimentary airways, a process called *branching morphogenesis* (Fig. 13.2). Coinciding with airway formation, new bronchial arteries arise from the aorta.

The Respiratory System

Brain

Upper respiratory tract

Spinal cord

Airways

Peripheral nerves

Bony chest wall

Respiratory muscles

Alveoli

Capillaries

Fig. 13.1 The respiratory system includes neural structures that control breathing, the chest wall and skeletal muscles of breathing, the upper airway, and lung parenchyma.

TABLE 13.1   Stages of Lung Development

Stage	Period	Comments
Embryonic	3-7 wk	Embryonic lung bud emerges from the foregut.
Pseudoglandular	5-17 wk	Airway tree is formed through a process of extensive branching accompanied by growth.
Canalicular	17-24 wk	Angiogenesis and vasculogenesis form the developing vascular network.
Saccular	24-38 wk	Alveoli begin to form through thinning of the mesenchyme, apposition of vascular structures with the air spaces, and maturation.
Alveolar (postnatal)	36 wk-2 yr	Further alveoli development and maturation occurs.

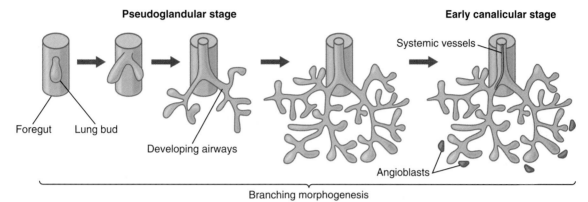

Fig. 13.2 Lung branching morphogenesis occurs during the pseudoglandular stage of lung development. It is the process by which the embryonic lung develops the primitive airway system through extensive branching.

The canalicular stage (between 17 and 24 weeks' gestation) is characterized by the formation of the acinus, differentiation of the acinar epithelium, and development of the distal pulmonary circulation. Through the processes of angiogenesis and vasculogenesis, capillary networks derived from endothelial cell precursors are formed, extend from and around the distal air spaces, and connect with the developing pulmonary arteries and veins. By the end of this stage, the thickness of the alveolar capillary membrane is similar to that in the adult.

During the saccular or prenatal alveolar stage (between 24 and 38 weeks' gestation), vascularized crests emerging from the parenchyma divide the terminal airway structures called *saccules*. Thinning of the interstitium continues, bringing capillaries from adjacent alveolar structures into close apposition and producing a double capillary network. Near birth, capillaries from opposing networks fuse to form a single network, and capillary volume increases with continuing lung growth and expansion.

During the alveolar postnatal stage (between 36 weeks' gestation and 2 years of age), alveolar development continues, and maturation occurs. The lung continues to grow through the first few years of childhood with the creation of more alveoli through septation of the air sacs. By age 2 years, the lung contains double arterial supplies and venous drainage systems, a complex airway system designed to generate progressive decreases in resistance to airflow as the air travels distally, and a vast alveolar network that efficiently transfers gases to and from the blood.

The processes that drive lung development are tightly controlled, but mishaps occur. Congenital lung disorders include cystic adenomatoid malformation of the lung, lung hypoplasia or agenesis, bullous changes in the lung parenchyma, and abnormalities in the vasculature, including aberrant connections between systemic vessels and lung compartments (e.g., lung sequestration) and congenital absence of one or both pulmonary arteries. In children without congenital abnormalities, lung disorders are uncommon, except for those caused by infection and accidents.

Congenital lung disorders are rare compared with the number of infants born annually with abnormal lung function as a result of prematurity. In premature infants, the type II pneumocytes of the lung are underdeveloped and produce insufficient quantities of surfactant, a surface-active substance produced by specific alveolar epithelial cells that helps to decrease surface tension and prevent alveolar collapse. This disorder is called neonatal *respiratory distress syndrome* (RDS). The treatment of neonatal RDS is administration of exogenous surfactant and corticosteroids to enhance lung maturation. To sustain life while allowing maturation, mechanical ventilation and oxygen supplementation are required but may promote the development of bronchopulmonary dysplasia (see Chapter 21 for further discussion).

PULMONARY DISEASE

Epidemiology

Diseases of the adult respiratory system are some of the most common clinical entities confronted by physicians. According to the Centers for Disease Control and Prevention data for 2017, chronic lower respiratory diseases, influenza or pneumonia, and cancer (including lung cancer) are among the top 10 causes of death due to medical illnesses in the United States.

COPD is a leading cause of both death and disability in the United States. At a time when the age-adjusted death rate for other common disorders such as coronary artery disease and stroke is decreasing, the death rate for COPD continues to increase. More than 16 million Americans are estimated to have COPD, but the number is expected to rise because COPD takes years to develop and the incidence of cigarette smoking (the most common etiologic factor for COPD) is staggering. In 2017, more than

34.3 million Americans were daily smokers and 16 million Americans had a smoking-related illness. The true disease burden of COPD is much greater than these numbers indicate.

Other pulmonary conditions are also common. Asthma affects 8% of adults and 9.5% of children in the United States. The prevalence, hospitalization rate, and mortality rate related to asthma continue to increase. In 2016, there were 257,000 hospital visits related to pneumonia and almost 50,000 deaths. Sleep-disordered breathing affects an estimated 7 to 18 million people in the United States, and 1.8 to 4 million of them have severe sleep apnea. Interstitial lung diseases are increasingly recognized, and their true incidence appears to have been underestimated. For example, idiopathic pulmonary fibrosis, the most common of the idiopathic interstitial pneumonias, affects 85,000 to 100,000 Americans annually.

These conditions affect males and females of all ages and races. However, a disproportionate increase in the incidence, morbidity, and mortality related to lung diseases exists for minority populations. This finding is true for COPD, asthma, certain interstitial lung disorders, and other diseases. Although these differences point to genetic differences among these populations, they also indicate differences in culture, socioeconomic status, exposure to pollutants (e.g., inner-city living), and access to health care.

Classification

Lung diseases are often classified on the basis of the affected anatomic areas of the lung (e.g., interstitial lung diseases, pleural diseases, airways diseases) and the physiologic abnormalities detected by pulmonary function testing (e.g., obstructive lung diseases, restrictive lung diseases). Classification schemes based exclusively on physiologic factors are inaccurate because distinctly different disorders with different causes, consequences, and responses to therapy have similar physiologic abnormalities (e.g., restriction from pulmonary fibrosis versus restriction from neuromuscular disease) (Fig. 13.3).

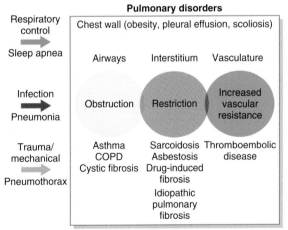

Pulmonary disorders

Fig. 13.3 Lung diseases are caused by abnormalities in the lung structure (e.g., airways, interstitium, vasculature) or in the chest wall or by external forces (e.g., infection). Disorders affecting the lung structure cause physiologic derangements (e.g., obstruction to airflow, restricted lung volumes, pulmonary hypertension, hypoxia). These derangements are not necessarily specific to any particular lung diseases, but there is extensive overlap among them, so that different disorders can have similar physiologic abnormalities. *COPD,* Chronic obstructive pulmonary disease.

The obstructive lung diseases have in common a limitation of airflow, called an *obstructive pattern,* as determined by pulmonary function testing. Obstructive lung diseases include COPD, asthma, and bronchiectasis.

The interstitial lung diseases are less common disorders and are more difficult to categorize because they include more than 120 distinct entities, some of which are inherited, but most of which are without an obvious cause. These disorders are characterized by a restrictive physiologic condition due to decreased lung compliance and small lung volumes, which is the reason they are often referred to as *restrictive lung disorders* (e.g., idiopathic pulmonary fibrosis). However, not all interstitial lung diseases exhibit a purely restrictive pattern on pulmonary function testing. They may have airflow limitation as a result of small airway involvement (e.g., sarcoidosis, cryptogenic organizing pneumonia).

In the pulmonary vascular diseases, involvement of the pulmonary vasculature causes increased pulmonary vascular resistance. These diseases range from disorders caused by obstruction to blood flow as a result of blood clots (e.g., pulmonary embolus) to disorders characterized by tissue remodeling and obliteration of blood vessels by vascular remodeling (e.g., pulmonary arterial hypertension).

Disorders of respiratory control include conditions in which extrapulmonary abnormalities cause respiratory system dysfunction and abnormal ventilation. Included are sleep disorders such as obstructive sleep apnea and neuromuscular system disorders such as myasthenia gravis and polymyositis, in which ventilatory abnormalities result from poor excursion of the respiratory muscles.

Disorders of the pleura, chest wall, and mediastinum are classified as such because they affect these structures. Infectious agents, commonly viruses and bacteria, cause infectious diseases of the lung. Neoplastic disorders of the lung include benign (e.g., hamartomas) and malignant (e.g., lung carcinoma) tumors, which can affect the lung parenchyma or its surrounding pleura (e.g., mesothelioma).

PROSPECTUS FOR THE FUTURE

Important questions about lung development remain. What are the primary stimuli for branching morphogenesis? How does gene regulation alter lung development? How is lung airway and blood vessel development coordinated? What are the environment-gene interactions that cause abnormal lung development and subsequent lung diseases? What impact does air pollution and climate change have on our lung health?

There are important fundamental questions about the epidemiology of lung diseases. For example, it is not clear whether or how childhood asthma and adult COPD are related. The role of fine particulate matter air pollution in the pathogenesis of lung diseases is unknown, and the causes and pathogenesis of many lung diseases, such as sarcoidosis, are unclear.

SUGGESTED READINGS

Schraufnagel DE, editor: Breathing in America: diseases, progress, and hope, New York, 2010, American Thoracic Society.

Whitsett JA, Haitchi HM, Maeda Y: Intersections between pulmonary development and disease, Am J Respir Crit Care Med 184:401–406, 2011.

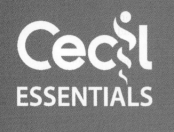

14

General Approach to Patients With Respiratory Disorders

Michael Raymond Goggins, Brian Casserly, Eric J. Gartman

INTRODUCTION

History taking is of paramount significance in the assessment of a patient who may have pulmonary disease. Patients with respiratory disorders often complain of one or more of the following symptoms: dyspnea, fatigue, exercise intolerance, wheeze, cough, sputum production, hemoptysis, and chest pain. Aside from the establishment of a trusting doctor-patient partnership, history taking gives the physician the opportunity to ask critical questions and clarify crucial details that may point towards a specific diagnosis.

Common symptoms of respiratory disease, such as chest pain and fever, frequently occur with diseases of other organ systems (Table 14.1). For example, chest pain is a cardinal symptom of cardiovascular disease. Fever, though it is commonly observed in pneumonia, may also be attributable to a wide array of hematologic and rheumatologic conditions. A thorough assessment of the past medical history, family history, social history, and occupational history combined with a focused physical examination and an understanding of the symptomatology are the pertinent aspects of a systemic approach to patients with respiratory disease. Applying a structured process guides the investigations necessary to determine the underlying respiratory pathology.

❖ For a deeper discussion on this topic, please see Chapter 77, "Approach to the Patient with Respiratory Disease," in *Goldman-Cecil Medicine*, 26th Edition.

CLINICAL PRESENTATION

Dyspnea (i.e., breathlessness) is perhaps the most common presentation of patients with respiratory conditions (Table 14.2). The time of onset (i.e., nocturnal), rate of onset (swift vs. gradual), exacerbating and alleviating factors (i.e., environmental triggers), frequency, and degree of functional impairment are fundamental components of the history. Determining the associated symptoms such as cough, hemoptysis, chest pain, wheeze, orthopnea, stridor, allergic rhinitis, sinusitis, and paroxysmal nocturnal dyspnea is also imperative in developing a differential diagnosis. For example, if dyspnea is of sudden onset and accompanied by chest pain then the list of differential diagnoses should include the following: pneumothorax, pulmonary embolism, myocardial infarction, and flash pulmonary edema. Conversely, long-standing dyspnea indicates that chronic conditions such as chronic obstructive pulmonary disease (COPD), interstitial lung disease, pulmonary arterial hypertension, and neuromuscular disorders are most likely.

The evolution of chronic dyspnea may be insidious, thus questions regarding variations in functional capacity over time are essential. Exertion may precipitate dyspnea or it may occur at rest. Intermittent exertional dyspnea suggests parenchymal lung disease or cardiovascular disease. Dyspnea that is seasonal or provoked by environmental exposure suggests diseases such as asthma and hypersensitivity pneumonitis.

Positional dyspnea can develop in patients with severe obstructive airway disease, diaphragmatic paralysis or neuromuscular weakness.

Orthopnea, dyspnea occurring in the supine position, may result from a reduction in vital capacity caused by abdominal contents applying pressure upon the diaphragm. Paroxysmal nocturnal dyspnea, a sudden onset of shortness of breath transpiring one to several hours after lying flat, is a commonly described symptom of decompensated congestive cardiac failure. This condition is a result of interstitial pulmonary edema secondary to increased venous return to the heart. Nocturnal dyspnea in the setting of asthma has also been frequently documented and is understood to be the consequence of decreased vital capacity in the supine position, decreased production of endogenous agents with bronchodilator functions, and increased exposure to allergens in bedclothes. Exercise-induced asthma causes dyspnea disproportionate to the level of exertion, with symptoms often being most distressing in the 15 to 30 minutes after cessation of exercise.

Wheeze, the continuous whistling noise of air passing through a narrowed tube, while often associated with asthma, may be the result of a variety of conditions. The presence of wheeze does not definitively establish asthma as the diagnosis, nor does the absence of wheeze exclude asthma as a diagnosis. Congestive heart failure, endobronchial obstruction, vocal cord abnormalities, and acute bronchitis are all causes of wheeze.

Cough is often a frustrating symptom because the underlying diagnosis may be surreptitious. The three most common sources of a chronic cough are postnasal drip, asthma, and gastroesophageal reflux disease. Cough may be mild and sporadic. However, it may also be forceful enough to provoke emesis or syncope. Cough may be dry or may generate sputum or blood (i.e., hemoptysis). The symptom may commence months after initiation of a drug (e.g., angiotensin-converting enzyme [ACE] inhibitors), resulting in a dry, hacking cough. *Bordetella pertussis* infection (i.e., whooping cough) and viral lower respiratory tract infections can produce a cough that may last longer than 3 months. Patients with asthma often have a cough, and occasionally it is their only symptom (cough-variant asthma). Nocturnal cough suggests asthma, heart failure, or gastroesophageal reflux disease.

Sputum expectoration occurring more than seldom is atypical and should be characterized with regard to volume, color, timing, frequency, diurnal variation, and presence or absence of blood. Chronic bronchitis is defined as a productive cough for more than 3 months in each of the past 3 years. Asthma patients often have a productive cough due to excess mucus production. Colored sputum may not always represent bacterial infection because the concentration of cellular debris—predominantly white cells in inflammatory processes—affects sputum color. Poorly controlled asthma and the finding of brown plugs or casts of the small bronchi in sputum may indicate allergic bronchopulmonary aspergillosis.

TABLE 14.1 Major Symptoms of Respiratory Disease

Cough
Sputum
Hemoptysis
Dyspnea (acute, progressive, or paroxysmal)
Wheeze
Chest pain
Fever
Hoarseness
Night sweats

TABLE 14.2 Causes of Dyspnea

Classification	Examples
Airways disease	Chronic obstructive pulmonary disease
	Asthma
	Laryngeal disorders
	Epiglottitis, bronchiolitis, and croup in children
	Tracheal stenosis or obstruction (foreign body or tumor)
	Tracheomalacia
	Bronchiectasis (immunodeficiency states, allergic bronchopulmonary aspergillosis, ciliary dyskinesia, cystic fibrosis)
Parenchymal lung disease	Pneumonia
	Interstitial lung diseases
	Obliterative bronchiolitis
	Pulmonary edema due to increased vascular permeability (acute respiratory distress syndrome)
	Infiltrative and metastatic malignancies
Pulmonary circulation disorders	Pulmonary thromboembolism
	Pulmonary arterial hypertension
	Pulmonary arteriovenous malformation
Chest wall and pleural disorders	Pneumothorax
	Pleural effusion or large-volume ascites
	Pleural tumor
	Fractured ribs, flail chest
	Chest wall deformities
	Neuromuscular diseases
	Bilateral diaphragmatic paresis
Cardiac disorders	Pulmonary edema due to left heart failure
	Myocardial infarction
	Pericardial effusion or constrictive pericarditis
	Intracardiac shunt
Hematologic disorders	Anemia
	Methemoglobinemia
	Carbon monoxide poisoning
	Acute chest syndrome (sickle cell disease)
Noncardiorespiratory disorders	Psychogenic diseases (hyperventilation)
	Midbrain lesion
Metabolic or endocrine disorders	Metabolic acidosis (diabetic ketoacidosis, sepsis, severe dehydration, inborn errors of metabolism)
	Hyperthyroidism
	Hypothyroidism
	Hyperammonemia
	Hypocalcemia (laryngospasm)
	Anaphylaxis
	Smoke inhalation
	Chemical agent exposures (phosgene, chlorine, cyanide)
	Drug overdose (salicylates)
Other causes	Biologic and chemical weapons (anthrax, tularemia, phosgene, nitrogen mustard, nerve agents, ricin)
	Submersion injury (near-drowning)

Hemoptysis is an alarming symptom. The volume of blood may be scant or considerable enough to cause asphyxiation or exsanguination. Bronchitis is the most common cause of hemoptysis in the United States, whereas pulmonary tuberculosis is the predominant cause worldwide. Hemoptysis is frequently small in volume and self-limited or resolves with treatment of the underlying process. Massive hemoptysis, variably defined as 250 to 500 mL of blood in 24 hours, is a rare medical emergency caused by the following: lung cancer, lung cavities containing mycetomas, cavitary tuberculosis, pulmonary hemorrhage syndromes, pulmonary arteriovenous malformations, and bronchiectasis. Clinicians should distinguish hemoptysis from epistaxis and hematemesis with comprehensive upper airway examination as many patients have difficulty identifying the source of the hemorrhage.

Chest pain attributable to a respiratory cause results from pleural disease, pulmonary vascular disease, or musculoskeletal pain precipitated by coughing as no pain receptors exist in the lung parenchyma. For example, lung cancer does not cause pain until it invades the pleura, chest wall, vertebral bodies, or mediastinal structures. Disease or inflammation of the pleura causes pleuritic chest pain characterized as a sharp or stabbing pain with deep inspiration. Pulmonary emboli, infection, pneumothorax, and collagen vascular disease often cause pleuritic chest pain. Pulmonary hypertension causing right ventricular strain and demand ischemia may produce dull anterior chest pain unrelated to respiration. Additional examples of noncardiac chest pain are esophageal disease, herpetic neuralgia, musculoskeletal pain, and trauma. Thoracic pain secondary to vertebral compression or rib fractures may be seen in elderly patients or those with a history of chronic systemic steroid use.

Adequate analgesic relief, including narcotic use, in patients with chest pain and respiratory disease is essential to prevent a reduction in vital capacity due to splinting of the chest in reaction to the pain. Musculoskeletal chest pain, which is often reproducible with movement or palpation over the affected area, should only be considered as a diagnosis once other causes have been excluded.

HISTORY

The examiner should always inquire about previous respiratory illness, including pneumonia, tuberculosis, or chronic bronchitis, and chest radiograph abnormalities that have been reported to the patient. Acquired immunodeficiency syndrome (AIDS) increases the risk of developing *Pneumocystis jirovecii* pneumonia and other respiratory infections, including tuberculosis. Immunosuppression from chronic steroid use may predispose to tuberculosis and other lung infections.

Many classes of drugs can be linked to lung toxicity. Examples include pulmonary embolism due to the oral contraceptive pill, interstitial lung disease from cytotoxic agents (e.g., methotrexate, cyclophosphamide, bleomycin), bronchospasm from β-adrenergic receptor blockers or nonsteroidal anti-inflammatory drugs, and cough from ACE inhibitors. Physicians should be conscious that illicit substances known to cause lung disease (e.g., cocaine, heroin) may not be mentioned by the patient.

An accurate history of tobacco use and other toxic and environmental exposures is vital for patients with respiratory symptoms. Tobacco smoke is the primary environmental toxin causing lung disease. It is the physician's obligation to ask about tobacco use and attempt to motivate patients to quit smoking. The risk of smoking-related lung disease is directly correlated to individual genetic susceptibility and the total pack-years history, while it is inversely related to the age at onset of smoking and, in the case of lung cancer, the interval since smoking cessation.

A history of exposure to other inhaled toxins, irritants, or allergens should be elicited. A thorough occupational history can uncover exposure to inorganic dust or fibers such as asbestos, silica, or coal dust. Organic dusts predispose to hypersensitivity pneumonitis and other interstitial lung diseases. Solvents and corrosive gases also induce pulmonary disease. The presence of house pets should be documented. Cats are the most allergenic for asthma while birds may cause hypersensitivity or fungal lung disease.

A travel history is pertinent in evaluating infectious causes of pulmonary disease. For example, histoplasmosis is endemic to the Ohio and Mississippi River valleys whereas coccidioidomycosis is observed in the desert Southwest. Travel to or immigration from developing countries heightens the risk of exposure to tuberculosis. A family history is crucial to establish the risk of genetic lung diseases such as cystic fibrosis and α_1-antitrypsin deficiency and predisposition to asthma, emphysema, or lung cancer.

PHYSICAL EXAMINATION

The physical examination should be comprehensive while also focusing on areas highlighted by the history. Observation and inspection when the patient's chest is bare are the initial steps in the physical examination of the patient with pulmonary disease. The physician should begin by assessing the patient's general appearance with particular attention given to the presence or absence of respiratory distress. This observation points toward the diagnosis and identifies the level of urgency.

Body habitus is relevant because morbid obesity in a patient with exercise intolerance and somnolence suggests a diagnosis of sleep-disordered breathing, whereas dyspnea in a thin, middle-aged individual with pursed lips may indicate emphysema. Race and sex are relevant as specific cohorts have a predisposition for certain conditions. For example, sarcoidosis is frequently encountered in African Americans in the Southeast, whereas lymphangioleiomyomatosis is a rare disorder that principally affects young women of childbearing age. Tachycardia and pulsus paradoxus are essential signs of severe asthma.

The physician should observe the effort required for breathing. Increased respiratory rate, accessory muscles use, pursed-lip breathing, and paradoxical abdominal movement indicate increased work of breathing. Paradoxical abdominal movement signifies diaphragm weakness and imminent respiratory failure. An inability to complete full sentences indicates severe airway obstruction or neuromuscular weakness. The potential presence of a cough should be discerned and the strength of the cough observed because it may signal respiratory muscle weakness or severe obstructive lung disease. The rib cage should expand symmetrically with inspiration. The shape of the thoracic cage should be considered. Increased anteroposterior diameter is appreciated in the setting of hyperinflation secondary to obstructive lung disease. Severe kyphoscoliosis, pectus excavatum, ankylosing spondylitis, and morbid obesity can produce restrictive ventilatory disease due to distortion and restriction of the thoracic cavity volume.

Hand examination may yield significant signs of respiratory pathology. Clubbing is often associated with respiratory disease. An uncommon association with clubbing is hypertrophic pulmonary osteoarthropathy (HPO) characterized by periosteal inflammation, swelling, and tenderness at the distal ends of long bones, the wrists, the ankles, the metacarpals and metatarsals. Rarely, HPO may occur without clubbing. The causes of HPO include pleural mesothelioma, pulmonary fibrosis, and chronic lung infections, such as lung abscess.

Finger staining (caused by tar because nicotine is colorless) is a sign of cigarette smoking. Dorsiflex of the wrists with the arms outstretched and fingers spread may result in a flapping tremor (i.e., asterixis) seen with severe carbon dioxide retention. Wasting and weakness are signs of cachexia due to malignancy or end-stage emphysema. Peripheral lung tumor compression and infiltration of a lower trunk of the brachial plexus produces wasting of the small muscles of the hand and finger abduction weakness.

Head and neck examination is critical. The eyes are inspected for Horner syndrome (i.e., constricted pupil, partial ptosis, and loss of sweating), which may result from an apical lung tumor compressing the sympathetic nerves in the neck. The voice is evaluated for hoarseness, which may indicate recurrent laryngeal nerve palsy associated with lung carcinoma (usually left-sided) or laryngeal carcinoma. However, the most common cause is laryngitis.

The nose is evaluated for nasal polyps (associated with asthma), engorged turbinates (various allergic conditions), and a deviated septum (nasal obstruction). Sinusitis is indicated by tenderness over the sinuses on palpation.

The tongue is examined for central cyanosis. The mouth may hold evidence of an upper respiratory tract infection (e.g., erythematous pharynx, tonsillar enlargement with or without a coating of pus). A damaged tooth or gingivitis may predispose to lung abscess or pneumonia. Superior vena cava obstruction can cause facial plethora or cyanosis. Obstructive sleep apnea patients may be obese and have a receding chin, a small pharynx, and a short, thick neck.

Chest palpation is performed by first palpating the accessory muscles (i.e., scalene and sternocleidomastoid) of respiration in the neck. Hypertrophy and contraction suggest increased respiratory effort. Tracheal palpation should demonstrate the trachea residing in the midline of the neck. Deviation is suggestive of lung collapse or a mass. Neck masses should be documented.

The physician should place both hands on the lower half of the patient's posterior thorax with thumbs touching and fingers spread; the hands should be kept in place while the patient takes several deep inspirations. The physician's thumbs should separate slightly and the hands should move symmetrically apart during the patient's inspiration. Causes of asymmetry include pain, chest wall abnormalities, consolidation, and tension pneumothorax.

Fremitus is a subtle vibration appreciated best with the edge of the hand against the patient's chest wall while the patient speaks. Increased fremitus occurs in areas with underlying lung consolidation, and decreased fremitus occurs over pleural effusions. Next, the patient's chest should be percussed and the diaphragm level should be determined bilaterally. The percussion note should be compared on each side starting at the apex and moving down, including the posterior, anterior, and lateral aspects. Pleural effusions, consolidation, masses, or elevated diaphragms can produce dullness to percussion and pneumothoraces or hyperinflation can cause hyperresonance.

Lung auscultation is utilized to gauge the quality of the breathing and to detect extra sounds not heard in normal lungs. Normal breath sounds have two qualities, vesicular and bronchial. Bronchial breath sounds are heard over the central airways and are louder and coarser than vesicular breath sounds, which are heard at the lung peripheries and bases. Bronchovesicular sounds are a combination of the two and are heard over medium-sized airways. Bronchial sounds have a longer inspiratory component, whereas vesicular sounds have an elongated expiratory component and are much softer. Bronchial breath sounds and bronchovesicular breath sounds at the lung peripheries are abnormal and may be due to underlying consolidation. In the setting of consolidation, increased vocal sound transmission, called *whispered pectoriloquy,* ensues; *egophony,* in which the spoken letter *e* sounds like an *a* over the area of consolidation, is heard and sometimes likened to the bleating of a goat.

Abnormal or extrapulmonary sounds are crackles, wheezes, and rubs. Crackles can be coarse rattles or fine, velcro-like sounds. Airway mucus or the opening of large- and medium-sized airways often causes coarse crackles. In bronchiectasis, alteration of crackles occurs with coughing. Fine inspiratory crackles, caused by the opening of collapsed alveoli, are most common at the bases and are often heard in pulmonary edema or interstitial fibrosis.

Wheeze is a higher-pitched sound suggestive of large airway obstruction when heard locally. Wheeze in the setting of asthma or congestive heart failure is lower in pitch and heard diffusely over all lung fields. Localized wheezing can be heard in conditions such as pulmonary embolism, bronchial obstruction by a tumor, and foreign-body aspiration.

A pleural rub is a sound generated by inflamed pleural surfaces rubbing together, often compared to the sound of pieces of leather rubbing against each other. Rubs, which are often transient and dependent upon the amount of fluid in the pleural space, can develop post large-volume thoracentesis, along with pleuritic chest pain.

A crunching sound timed with the cardiac cycle, called *Hamman crunch* or *Hamman sign*, is heard in patients with a pneumomediastinum. The complete absence of breath sounds on one side should cause one to consider pneumothorax, hydrothorax, or hemothorax; obstruction of a main stem bronchus; or surgical or congenital absence of the lung.

EVALUATION

A differential diagnosis should be established based on a comprehensive history and a thorough physical examination. The preliminary differential diagnosis determines the battery of tests requested, recognizing that these investigations may reveal disorders not considered in the initial assessment. The objective of this extended evaluation is twofold: to affirm a diagnosis or disregard other disorders and to assess the severity of the lung derangement.

Patients with a suggested lung disorder should undergo pulmonary function testing (see Chapter 15). Spirometry evaluates airflow and helps differentiate between the obstructive pattern characteristic of COPD, asthma, and related disorders and the restrictive pattern observed in fibrotic lung disease. Spirometry also illustrates the severity of the physiologic alteration.

Lung volume measurements are effective in assessing hyperinflation or confirming a restrictive process. Calculating the diffusing capacity of the lung for carbon monoxide (DLCO) elucidates alterations in gas-exchanging capability. The recording of oxygen saturation via pulse oximetry can be utilized to further assess gas exchange.

Information regarding oxygenation and acid-base status is obtained from arterial blood gas determination. A 6-minute walk test, which evaluates oxygenation during exertion, can demonstrate that patients require supplemental oxygen. Other, more specialized tests (e.g., bronchoprovocation, cardiopulmonary stress testing, polysomnography) may be necessary, depending on the context.

Imaging studies of the chest are beneficial in evaluating pulmonary structure. The chest radiograph displays the lung parenchyma and pleura, the cardiac silhouette, mediastinal structures, and body habitus. Examining old chest radiographic images is essential to assess for disease progression.

Computed tomography (CT) provides a more comprehensive assessment of the pulmonary and mediastinal structures and is essential in the evaluation of interstitial lung disease, lung masses, and other disorders. Together with ventilation-perfusion scanning and pulmonary angiography, CT is one of several resources used to evaluate the lung vasculature. Positron emission tomography is used to assess metabolic activity of lung masses and can indicate a diagnosis of malignancy.

Standard blood tests such as the blood counts and blood chemistry point to specific disorders or may provide information about the severity of a lung disorder (e.g., polycythemia in chronic hypoxemia, leukocytosis in lung infection). Some specialized tests should be reserved for specific diagnoses such as connective tissue disorders (e.g., rheumatoid factor, antinuclear antibodies) or hypersensitivity pneumonitis (hypersensitivity profile).

Together with the history and physical examination, these investigations are useful for narrowing a diagnosis to establish a specific management plan that can often be devised in a single visit. However, patients frequently require several follow-up visits in which the physician assesses disease progression, patient compliance, and response to treatment.

If noninvasive tests do not yield a diagnosis of the problem, more invasive tests may be necessary. Fiberoptic or rigid bronchoscopy allows direct visualization of the airways and acquisition of valuable clinical samples for examination. Transthoracic percutaneous needle aspiration or navigational bronchoscopy is useful in evaluating peripheral lung lesions. Ultimately, surgery may be required to obtain tissue through open or video-assisted thoracoscopically guided lung biopsy.

For a deeper discussion on this topic, please see Chapter 78, "Imaging in Pulmonary Disease," and Chapter 93, "Interventional and Surgical Approaches to Lung Disease," in *Goldman-Cecil Medicine*, 26th Edition.

PROSPECTUS FOR THE FUTURE

The predictive values of various facets of the history and physical examination need to be clarified. The role of quantitative CT analysis in the diagnosis and assessment of disability from lung diseases should be refined. The role of interventional pulmonary procedures must be ascertained for the diagnosis and treatment of lung diseases.

SUGGESTED READINGS

Davis JL, Murray JF: History and physical examination. In Mason RJ, Murray JF, Broaddus VC, et al, editors: Murray and Nadel's textbook of respiratory medicine, ed 6, Philadelphia, 2016, Elsevier.

Hollingsworth H: What's new in pulmonary and critical care medicine. https://www.uptodate.com/contents/whats-new-in-pulmonary-and-critical-care-medicine. Accessed August 5, 2019.

Ryder REJ, Mir MA, Freeman EA: An aid to the MRCP PACES, vol 1, ed 4, Chichester, 2012, Wiley-Blackwell Publishing.

Weiner DL: Causes of acute respiratory distress in children. Available at: https://www.uptodate.com/contents/causes-of-acute-respiratory-distress-in-children. Accessed August 5, 2019.

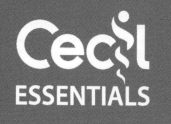

15

Evaluating Lung Structure and Function

Patrick Koo, F. Dennis McCool, Jigme Michael Sethi

INTRODUCTION

The satisfactory functioning of all organ systems depends on their capacity to consume oxygen and eliminate carbon dioxide. The primary function of the lung is to deliver oxygen to the pulmonary capillary blood and to excrete carbon dioxide. To accomplish this, the lung must generate a flux of air into and out of the alveoli (ventilation) while absorbing oxygen into the pulmonary blood and eliminating carbon dioxide from alveolar air (gas exchange). This is accomplished in a manner that attempts to optimize gas exchange (ventilation-perfusion matching). This remarkably efficient process allows the human to maintain optimal oxygenation and acid-base balance over a range of activities, from resting breathing to moderately strenuous activity. This chapter provides an overview of the anatomy and physiology that enable the respiratory system to perform its life-sustaining functions as well as a discussion of tests available to evaluate lung structure and function.

ANATOMY

Airway

Inspired air travels through the nose and nasopharynx, where it is warmed to body temperature, humidified, and filtered of airborne particles greater than 10 μm in diameter. Air then enters a complex system of dichotomously branching airways that form a tree occupying the thorax. The first 15 divisions, beginning with the trachea, the mainstem bronchi, segmental and subsegmental bronchi down to the terminal bronchioles, are simply a set of conducting tubes that do not participate in gas exchange. Together, they constitute the *conducting zone* of the lung, also known as the *anatomic dead space* (about 1 mL per pound of ideal body weight, or approximately 150 mL) (Fig. 15.1). Cartilaginous rings help to maintain the patency of these large airways. In the mainstem bronchi, the rings are circumferential, whereas in the trachea, the cartilaginous rings are U-shaped, with the posterior membrane of the trachea sharing a wall with the esophagus. The branching pattern of these first 15 divisions of the airways follows the principles of fractal geometry: The reduction of airway diameter and length between each generation is similar, by a factor of 0.79, serving to densely compact the airways into the available space of the thorax (Fig. 15.2A and B). This geometry reduces bronchial path length from the trachea to the periphery and minimizes both dead space volume and resistance to convective airflow.

The remaining eight generations of airways comprise the respiratory bronchioles and alveolar ducts lined with alveolar sacs. This area of the lung is referred to as the *respiratory zone*, and the terminal respiratory unit is called the acinus. Gas exchange commences in the

Airway subdivision		Order No.	Cross-sectional area (cm²)	Resistance (cm H₂O • L⁻¹ • sec)
Larynx		0		0.5
Trachea		0	2.5	0.5
Bronchi		1	2.0	0.5
		2		
Bronchioles			5.0	0.2
		16	1.8 x 10²	
Respiratory bronchioles		17		
		19	9.4 x 10²	
Alveolar ducts				
		22	5.8 x 10³	
Alveoli		23	5.6 x 10⁷	

Fig. 15.1 The subdivisions of the airways and their nomenclature. (Modified from Weibel ER: Morphometry of the human lung, Berlin, 1963, Springer.)

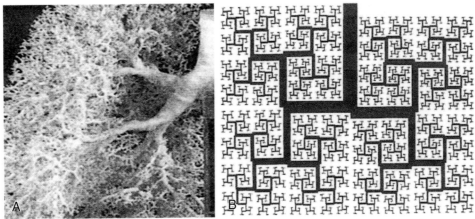

Fig. 15.2 (A) Cast of the right lung demonstrates branching of airways. (B) The branching airways can be modeled by use of the principles of fractal geometry, which allow for efficient filling of the thoracic space.

respiratory zone but primarily occurs in the alveoli. Inspired air moves down the conducting zone primarily by bulk convective flow, whereas the movement of oxygen in the respiratory zone is by diffusion.

In total, there are an average of 23 subdivisions of the airway from the trachea to the alveolar ducts. Although it might be suspected that resistance to convective flow would be highest in the small airways because of their small diameter, the opposite is the case. The enormous number of small airways together provide a huge net cross-sectional area for airflow. For example, the cross-sectional area of the trachea is 2.5 cm², compared with a total cross-sectional area of 300 cm² for all of the alveolar ducts combined. As a result, 80% of the resistance to airflow occurs in the first seven generations of bronchi, and the remaining "small" airways (diameters <2 mm) contribute only 20% of the resistance to airflow (Fig. 15.3). As the lung expands during inspiration, the net cross-sectional area of the alveolar ducts doubles, further reducing resistance to airflow.

Alveoli

The alveoli are the grapelike clusters of air sacs that interface with the pulmonary capillaries. There are about 300 million individual alveolar sacs, or 10,000 in each of the 30,000 acini. The alveoli are thin-walled structures with a total surface area of about 130 m². This is roughly half the size of a doubles tennis court. The surface of the alveoli is lined by two types of cells. The flat type I pneumocytes constitute 95% of the cells. Type II pneumocytes, which account for about 5% of the alveolar lining cells, secrete surfactant, a complex lipoprotein whose role in lowering surface tension in the alveolar space is critical to reducing the forces needed to expand the lung. Surfactant is also important in preventing alveolar collapse at low lung volumes and thereby promoting normal gas exchange. The capillaries run in the exceedingly thin septa that separate the alveoli and are therefore exposed to the air from surrounding alveoli. The epithelial lining of the alveoli, the endothelial lining of the capillaries, and the intervening fused basement membrane form the alveolar-capillary interface. Normally, this interface is less than 1 μm thick and does not significantly interfere with gas exchange.

Blood Vessels

The pulmonary artery arises from the right ventricle and branches until it terminates in a meshwork of capillaries that surround the alveoli. This creates a large surface area that facilitates gas exchange. Blood returns to the heart through pulmonary veins that course through the lungs, coalesce into four main pulmonary veins, and empty into the left atrium. The pulmonary circulation is a low-resistance circuit; pulmonary vascular resistance is about one tenth of the resistance in

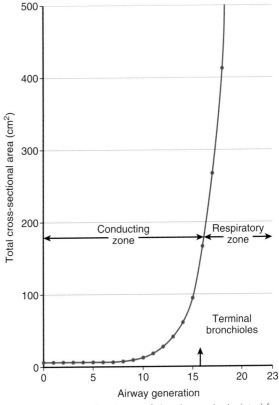

Fig. 15.3 Total cross-sectional area of the airways is depicted for several generations of airways. The total cross-sectional area increases dramatically in the respiratory zone. Consequently, the velocity of gas entering the respiratory zone decreases and resistance is low.

the systemic circulation. Pulmonary vessels can easily be recruited to accommodate increases in blood flow while maintaining low pressure and resistance. Accordingly, during exercise, any increase in cardiac output can be distributed through the lung without significantly increasing pulmonary arterial pressures.

A separate vascular system, the bronchial system, also supplies the lung. The bronchial arteries originate from the aorta and, in contrast to the pulmonary arteries, are under systemic pressure. These vessels provide nutrients to lung structures proximal to the alveoli. Two thirds of the bronchial circulation drains into the pulmonary veins and then empties into the left atrium. This blood, which has low oxygen content, mixes

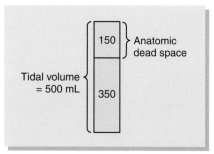

Fig. 15.4 Schematic diagram of the inspired volume of air that participates in gas exchange (V_A, 350 mL) and the volume of anatomic dead space (V_D, 150 mL), which together provide a tidal breath (V_T) of 500 mL.

with the freshly oxygenated blood from the pulmonary veins to lower the oxygen content of the blood that enters the systemic circulation.

PHYSIOLOGY

Ventilation

Ventilation refers to the bulk transport of air from the atmosphere to the alveolus. The product of tidal volume (V_T) and breathing frequency (f) represents the total volume of air delivered to the lung per minute (minute ventilation). However, not all air entering the lung is in contact with gas-exchanging units. The portion of V_T that fills the respiratory zone and alveoli and is available for gas exchange constitutes the alveolar volume (V_A), whereas the portion remaining in the conducting airways is the anatomic dead space volume (V_D) (Fig. 15.4). The ratio of V_D to V_T is called the *dead space ratio* (V_D/V_T). Normally, one third of a breath is dead space ($V_D/V_T = \frac{1}{3}$). The amount of fresh air reaching the alveoli is $V_T - V_D$. With large breaths, the dead space becomes a smaller fraction of the total tidal volume. Therefore, for a given V_T, slow, deep breathing results in greater V_A and improved gas exchange compared with rapid, shallow breathing.

The V_D/V_T ratio can be calculated by the Bohr method, as follows:

$$V_D/V_T = (Pa_{CO_2} - Pe_{CO_2})/Pa_{CO_2}$$

where Pa_{CO_2} is the arterial partial pressure of carbon dioxide and Pe_{CO_2} is the partial pressure of carbon dioxide in mixed expired gas (i.e., the mixture of CO_2-rich gas that enters the alveoli from the pulmonary capillaries and dead space gas, which is devoid of CO_2). Pe_{CO_2} increases during expiration, reaching a plateau at end-expiration. At end-expiration, the Pe_{CO_2} represents exhaled alveolar gas that has been in equilibrium with pulmonary capillary blood. In healthy individuals, the Pe_{CO_2} at end-expiration is equivalent to the Pa_{CO_2}.

Ventilation of the dead space is wasted ventilation, because only V_A participates in gas exchange. Therefore, as the metabolic rate and carbon dioxide production increase, V_A must increase to maintain an arterial P_{CO_2} of 40 mm Hg. The relationship among these variables is described by the alveolar carbon dioxide equation:

$$Pa_{CO_2} = CO_2 \text{ production}/\dot{V}_A$$

where Pa_{CO_2} is the partial pressure of carbon dioxide in the alveolus and $\dot{V}_A$ is alveolar ventilation. From this equation, one appreciates that the partial pressure of carbon dioxide in the alveolus is inversely proportional to alveolar ventilation.

The relationship described by the alveolar oxygen equation is similar:

$$Pa_{O_2} = O_2 \text{ consumption}/\dot{V}_A$$

However, this relationship is more complicated because Pa_{O_2} also is proportional to the fraction of inspired oxygen, the water vapor pressure, and the partial pressure of carbon dioxide in the alveolus (discussed later). The implications of the alveolar carbon dioxide and oxygen relationships are that (1) maintenance of a constant alveolar gas composition depends on a constant ratio of ventilation to metabolic rate; (2) if ventilation is too high (hyperventilation), alveolar P_{CO_2} will be low and alveolar P_{O_2} will be high; and (3) if ventilation is too low (hypoventilation), alveolar P_{CO_2} will be high and alveolar P_{O_2} will be low.

Mechanics of Breathing

Respiratory mechanics is the study of forces needed to deliver air to the lung and how these forces govern the volume and flow of gases. Mechanically, the respiratory system consists of two structures: the lungs and the chest wall. The lungs are elastic (spring-like) structures that are situated within another elastic structure, the chest wall. At end-expiration, with absent respiratory muscle activity, the inward recoil of the lung is exactly balanced by the outward recoil of the chest wall, representing the equilibrium position of the lung–chest wall unit. Normally, the recoil of the lung is always inward (favoring lung deflation), and the recoil of the chest wall is outward (favoring inflation); at high lung volumes, however, the chest wall also recoils inward (Fig. 15.5). The energy required to stretch the respiratory system beyond its equilibrium state (end-expiration during quiet breathing) is provided by the inspiratory muscles. With normal quiet breathing, gas flow out of the lung is usually accomplished by passive recoil of the respiratory system.

During a typical breath, inspiratory muscle contraction lowers the intrapleural pressure, which in turn lowers the intra-alveolar pressure. Once alveolar pressure becomes subatmospheric, air can flow from the mouth through the airways to the alveoli. At the end of inspiration, the inspiratory muscles are turned off, and the lungs and chest wall recoil passively back to their equilibrium states. This passive recoil of the respiratory system causes alveolar pressure to become positive throughout expiration until the resting position of the lung and chest wall are reestablished and alveolar pressure once again equals atmospheric pressure. During quiet breathing, pleural pressure is always subatmospheric, whereas alveolar pressure oscillates below and above zero (atmospheric) pressure (Fig. 15.6).

The major inspiratory muscle is the diaphragm. Others include the sternocleidomastoid muscles, the scalenus muscles, the parasternals, and the external intercostals. Diaphragm contraction results in expansion of the lower rib cage and compression of the intra-abdominal contents. The latter action results in expansion of the abdominal wall. The expiratory muscles consist of the internal intercostal muscles and the abdominal muscles. Expiratory flows can be enhanced by recruiting the expiratory muscles; this occurs during exercise or with cough.

To inflate the respiratory system, the inspiratory muscles must overcome two types of forces: the elastic forces imposed by the lung and the chest wall (elastic loads) and the resistive forces related to airflow (resistive loads). The elastic loads on the inspiratory muscles result from the respiratory system's tendency to resist stretch. The elastic forces are volume dependent; that is, the respiratory system becomes more difficult to stretch at volumes greater than the functional residual capacity (FRC) and more difficult to compress at volumes lower than the FRC. The elastic forces can be characterized by examining the relationship between lung volume and recoil pressure (Fig. 15.7). When either deflated or inflated, the lung and chest wall have characteristic recoil pressures. The slope of the relationship between lung volume and elastic recoil pressure of the chest wall or lung represents the

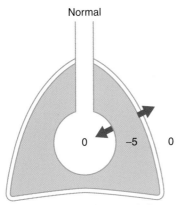

Fig. 15.5 Schematic diagram of the lung and chest wall at functional residual capacity (FRC). The *arrows* show that the expanding elastic force of the chest wall equals the collapsing elastic force of the lung. The intrapleural pressure is –5 at FRC because both forces are tugging on the pleural space in opposite directions.

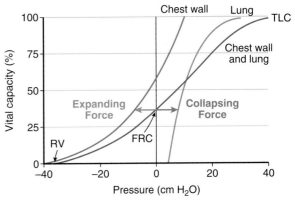

Fig. 15.7 Volume-pressure relationship of the respiratory system and its components, the lung and chest wall. Respiratory system recoil pressure at any volume is the sum of the lung and chest wall recoil pressures. Forces creating negative pressures expand the respiratory system, whereas forces creating positive pressures collapse the respiratory system. The slope of the volume-pressure curve represents the compliance of each structure. *FRC*, Functional residual capacity; *RV*, residual volume; *TLC*, total lung capacity.

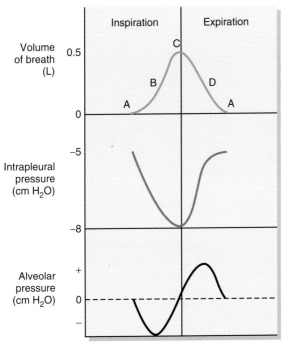

Fig. 15.6 Volume, intrapleural pressure, and alveolar pressure during a normal breathing cycle. The letters correspond to the various phases of the cycle: *A*, end-expiration; *B*, inspiration; *C*, end-inspiration; and *D*, expiration. Alveolar pressure is biphasic, with zero crossings at times of no flow (i.e., end-expiration and end-inspiration). Intrapleural pressure remains subatmospheric throughout.

compliance of each structure. The sum of the chest wall and lung recoil pressures represents the recoil pressure of the total respiratory system.

The elastic properties of the lung are related to two factors: the elastic behavior of collagen and elastin in the lung parenchyma and the surface tension in the alveolus at the air-liquid interface. Both factors contribute equally to lung elastic recoil. A surface-active substance called *surfactant* is produced by type II alveolar cells and lines the alveoli. This substance consists primarily of phospholipids. It lowers the surface tension of the air-liquid interface, making it easier to inflate the lung. The lungs are stiff (less compliant) and difficult to inflate in diseases that are characterized by a loss of surfactant (e.g., infant respiratory distress syndrome). Diseases such as pulmonary fibrosis, which

are characterized by excessive collagen in the lung, can make the lung stiff and difficult to inflate, whereas those such as emphysema, characterized by a loss of elastin and collagen, reduce lung recoil and increase lung compliance (Fig. 15.8). Normally, at FRC, it takes about 1 cm of water pressure (1 cm H_2O) to inflate the lungs 200 mL or to inflate the chest wall 200 mL. The lung and chest wall both need to be inflated to the same volume during inspiration, so 2 cm H_2O of pressure is required to inflate both to 200 mL. Therefore, normal respiratory system compliance is roughly 200/2 or 100 mL/cm H_2O and compliance of the lung or chest wall compliance is 200/1 or 200 mL/cm H_2O at volumes near FRC.

The second set of forces that the inspiratory muscles must overcome to inflate the lungs are flow-dependent forces; namely, tissue viscosity and airway flow resistance, the latter constituting the major component of the flow-dependent forces. Airway resistance during inspiration can be calculated by measuring inspiratory flow and the difference in pressure between the alveolus and the airway opening (ΔP_{A-ao}).

$$Resistance = \Delta P_{A-ao}/\dot{V}$$

The airflow velocity, the type of airflow (laminar or turbulent), and the physical attributes of the airway (radius and length) are the key determinants of airway resistance. Of the physical properties, the radius of the airways is the major factor. Resistance increases to the fourth power as the diameter decreases under conditions of laminar flow (streamline flow profile) and to the fifth power under conditions of turbulent flow (chaotic flow profile). Because airway diameter increases as lung volume increases, airway resistance decreases as lung volume increases (Fig. 15.9). Airway diameter also contributes to regional differences in airway resistance. Although the peripheral airways are narrower than the central airways, their total cross-sectional area is much greater than that of the central airways, as described earlier. Consequently, resistance to airflow of the peripheral airways is low relative to the central airways (see Fig. 15.3).

The type of airflow is another key determinant of airway resistance. Resistance is directly proportional to flow rate when flow is laminar. Resistance is much greater with turbulent flow because it is proportional to the square of the flow rate. The velocity of airflow determines,

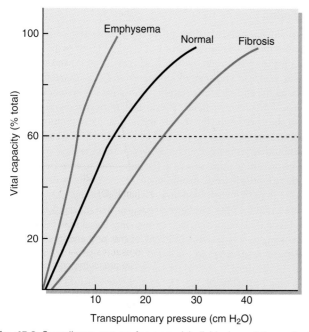

Fig. 15.8 Compliance curves for normal individuals and for patients with emphysema or pulmonary fibrosis. The transpulmonary pressure required to achieve a given lung volume is greatest for the patient with pulmonary fibrosis (notice the horizontal dashed line at 60% of the vital capacity). This increases the work of breathing.

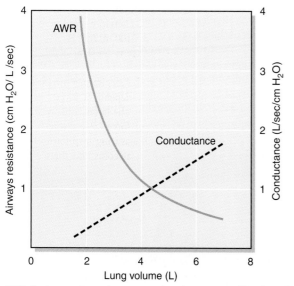

Fig. 15.9 As lung volume increases, the airways are dilated, and airways resistance (AWR) decreases. The reciprocal of resistance (conductance) increases as lung volume increases.

in part, whether the flow pattern is laminar or turbulent. Clinically, increased airway resistance can be seen in diseases associated with airway obstruction caused by an intrinsic mass, mucus within the airway, airway smooth muscle contraction, or extrinsic compression of the airways.

Lung elastic recoil also influences airway resistance and airflow. Decreased lung recoil increases resistance by promoting collapse of the small airways (E-Fig. 15.1). Normal resistance when breathing at FRC at low flow rates is in the range of 1 to 2 cm H_2O/L per second.

Distribution of Ventilation

The distribution of inhaled volume throughout the lung is unequal. In general, more of the inhaled volume goes to the bases of the lung than to the apex when the individual is inhaling while in an upright body position. This pattern of volume distribution leads to greater ventilation of the bases than at the apices. This inhomogeneity of ventilation results largely from regional differences in lung compliance. The alveoli at the lung apex are relatively more inflated at FRC than the alveoli at the lung base. The difference in alveolar distention from apex to base is related to pleural pressure differences from apex to base. The weight of the lung causes pleural pressure to be more negative at the apex and less negative at the base. The normal difference in pleural pressure from apex to base in an adult is about 8 cm H_2O (Fig. 15.10). Because the apical alveoli are more stretched at FRC, they are operating on a stiffer, less compliant region of their volume-pressure curve than the alveoli at the bases, making them more difficult to inflate than the basilar alveoli. Therefore, at the beginning of inspiration, more volume is directed toward the base than to the apex of the lung.

Control of Ventilation

Maintenance of adequate oxygenation and acid-base balance is accomplished through the respiratory control system. This system consists of the neurologic respiratory control centers, the respiratory effectors (muscles that provide the power to inflate the lungs), and the respiratory sensors. The respiratory center that automatically controls inspiration and expiration is located in the medulla of the brain stem. The respiratory center in the brain stem has an intrinsic rhythm generator (pacemaker) that drives breathing. The output of this center is modulated by inputs from peripheral and central chemoreceptors, from mechanoreceptors in the lungs, and from higher centers in the brain, including conscious control from the cerebral cortex. The respiratory center in the medulla is primarily responsible for determining the level of ventilation.

Carbon dioxide is the primary factor controlling ventilation. Carbon dioxide in the arterial blood diffuses across the blood-brain barrier, thereby reducing the pH of the cerebral spinal fluid and stimulating the central chemoreceptors. A change in $Paco_2$ above or below normal will increase or decrease ventilation, respectively. During quiet, resting breathing, the level of $Paco_2$ is thought to be the major factor controlling breathing. Only when the Pao_2 (i.e., the partial pressure of oxygen dissolved in the blood that is not bound to hemoglobin) falls substantially does ventilation respond significantly. Typically, Pao_2 needs to fall to less than 50 mm Hg before ventilation dramatically increases (Fig. 15.11). Low oxygen levels in the blood are not sensed by the respiratory center in the brain but are sensed by receptors in the carotid body. These vascular receptors are located between the internal and external branches of the carotid artery. Changes in Pao_2 are sensed by the carotid sinus nerve. Neural traffic projects to the respiratory center through the glossopharyngeal nerve, which serves to modulate ventilation. The carotid body also senses changes in $Paco_2$ and pH. Nonvolatile acids (e.g., ketoacids) stimulate ventilation through their effects on the carotid body.

The outcome of this complex respiratory control system is that variables such as Pao_2, $Paco_2$, and pH are held within narrow limits under most circumstances. The respiratory control center also can adjust tidal volume and frequency of breathing to minimize the energetic cost of breathing and can adapt to special circumstances such as speaking, swimming, eating, and exercise. Breathing can be stimulated by artificial manipulation of the Pco_2, Po_2, and pH. For example, ventilation is increased by rebreathing of carbon dioxide, inhalation of a concentration of low oxygen, or infusion of acid into the bloodstream.

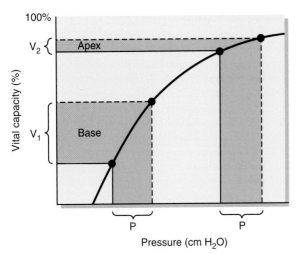

Fig. 15.10 Transpulmonary pressure and volume for lung units at the base and apex of the lung. Because pleural pressure is more negative at the apex of the lung, the alveoli in that region are stretched, placing them on a less compliant part of the volume-pressure curve. For a given change *(P)* in transpulmonary pressure during inspiration, the more compliant base inflates to a greater degree than the apex (V_1 and V_2, respectively).

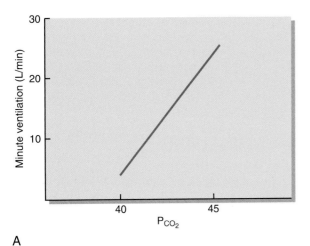

A

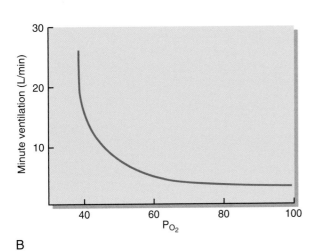

B

Fig. 15.11 (A) A rising partial pressure of carbon dioxide (P_{CO_2}) leads to a linear increase in minute ventilation. (B) The ventilatory response to hypoxemia is less sensitive and is clinically relevant only when the partial pressure of oxygen (P_{O_2}) has dropped significantly.

Perfusion

The pulmonary vascular bed differs from the systemic circulation in several respects. The pulmonary vascular bed receives the entire cardiac output of the right ventricle, whereas the cardiac output from the left ventricle is dispersed among several organ systems. Despite receiving the entire cardiac output, the pulmonary system is a low-resistance, low-pressure circuit. The normal mean systemic arterial pressure is about 100 mm Hg, whereas the normal mean pulmonary artery pressure is in the range of 15 mm Hg. The vascular bed can passively accommodate an increase in blood flow without raising arterial pressure by recruiting more vessels in the lung. During exercise, for example, there is little increase in pulmonary artery resistance despite a large increase in pulmonary blood flow. Hypoxic vasoconstriction, another feature unique to the pulmonary vascular system, regulates regional blood flow. This regulation aids in matching blood flow to ventilation by reducing flow to poorly ventilated regions of the lung.

Perfusion (Q̇) refers to the blood flow through an organ (i.e., the lung). In the upright individual, there is greater perfusion of the lung bases than of the apices (Fig. 15.12). In a low-pressure system such as the pulmonary circulation, the effects of gravity on blood flow need to be taken into account. The arterial-venous pressure difference usually provides the "driving" pressure for blood flow in the systemic circulation, but this is true only for certain regions of the lung. Pulmonary blood flow also needs to be considered in the context of alveolar pressure. Venous and arterial pressures are importantly affected by gravity, whereas alveolar pressure remains constant throughout the lung, assuming the airways are open. Therefore, as one descends from the apex to the base of the lung, arterial and venous pressures increase because of gravity but alveolar pressure remains constant.

At the apex, alveolar pressure may be greater than arterial pressure. This region of the lung is referred to as *zone 1*, and, in theory, it receives no blood flow. The alveolar pressure may be greater than arterial pressure, for example, in special circumstances such as hypovolemic shock, which lowers the arterial pressure, or with very high levels of positive end-expiratory pressure (PEEP), which increases alveolar pressure.

As one descends from the apex toward the midzone of the lung, arterial and venous pressures increase, whereas alveolar pressure remains

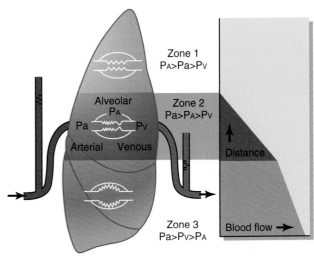

Fig. 15.12 Zonal model of blood flow in the lung. Because of the inter-relationship of arterial (Pa) and venous (Pv) vascular pressures and alveolar (PA) pressures, the lung base receives the most flow (see text for explanation). (From West JB, Dollery CT, Naimark A: Distribution of blood flow in isolated lung: relation to vascular and alveolar pressures, J Appl Physiol 19:713-724, 1964.)

constant. At some point, arterial pressure becomes greater than alveolar pressure. In this region, the driving pressure for blood flow is the arterial-alveolar pressure difference. This region is referred to as *zone 2* of the lung. Normally, zone 2 is very small because alveolar pressure is less than venous pressure in most of the lung. However, with high levels of PEEP, alveolar pressure becomes greater than venous pressure in more lung regions.

Further toward the base of the lung, the effects of gravity on arterial and venous pressures are more pronounced, venous pressure becomes greater than alveolar pressure, and the arterial-venous pressure difference provides the driving pressure for blood flow, as in the systemic circulation. This region is referred to as *zone 3* of the lung.

Normally, most of the lung is in zone 3, and most of the perfusion is to the lung base. This inequality in perfusion from apex to base is *qualitatively* similar to the inequality of ventilation from apex to base. However, blood flow increases from apex to base *more* than ventilation does, and this accounts for the small amount of ventilation-perfusion inequality that exists in the normal lung.

Gas Transfer

Oxygen and carbon dioxide are easily dissolved in plasma. Nitrogen is much less soluble and is not significantly exchanged across the alveolar-capillary interface. The driving force for the diffusion of a gas across a tissue barrier is the difference in partial pressure of the gas across the barrier. The partial pressure of oxygen in inspired room air entering the trachea is 150 mm Hg; this is derived from the equation, $P_{O_2} = (P_{atm} - P_{H_2O}) \times F_{IO_2}$, assuming that P_{atm} (atmospheric pressure) is 760 mm Hg, P_{H_2O} (the partial pressure of water vapor) is 47 mm Hg, and F_{IO_2} (the fraction of oxygen in inspired air) is 20.9%. In the alveolus, however, the partial pressure of oxygen is reduced to 100 mm Hg because the inspired V_T mixes with about 3 L of "oxygen-poor" air already in the lungs and is diluted by carbon dioxide moving into the alveolus from the pulmonary capillaries. The partial pressure of oxygen in the alveolus (P_{AO_2}) is set by the balance of these processes. Increasing minute ventilation increases the amount of oxygen added to the alveolus while lowering the P_{ACO_2}—the opposite result from hypoventilation. This reciprocal relationship between alveolar carbon dioxide and alveolar oxygen is described by the *alveolar gas equation*:

$$P_{AO_2} = [(P_{atm} - P_{H_2O}) \times F_{IO_2}] - (P_{ACO_2} / RER)$$

where RER is the respiratory exchange ratio, usually about 0.8.

The pressure gradient that drives diffusion of oxygen from the alveolus to the capillary is the difference between the alveolar P_{O_2} (100 mm Hg) and the arterial P_{O_2} (40 mm Hg) in the capillary blood entering the alveolus. By the time the blood leaves the alveolus, the P_{O_2} in the capillary blood has risen to 100 mm Hg. However, because small regions of ventilation-perfusion inequality and shunt exist in the normal lung, the P_{O_2} in the pulmonary veins from the lungs as a whole is usually about 90 mm Hg. Therefore, the difference between the alveolar and arterial partial pressures of oxygen, known as the *A-a gradient*, is typically about 10 mm Hg in health.

The pressure gradient that drives carbon dioxide from the mixed venous blood into the alveolus is the difference in partial pressure of carbon dioxide (45 mm Hg in mixed venous blood and 40 mm Hg in the alveolus). Despite the lower driving pressure for carbon dioxide compared with oxygen, the greater solubility of carbon dioxide allows complete equilibration between the alveolus and plasma during each respiratory cycle (Fig. 15.13).

Most of the oxygen contained in the blood is bound to hemoglobin; a small fraction is dissolved and measured as the P_{aO_2}. The amount of oxygen dissolved is about 3 mL/L in arterial blood, whereas the amount of oxygen bound to hemoglobin is about 197 mL/L, assuming a normal hematocrit. Each molecule of hemoglobin is capable of carrying four molecules of oxygen. The shape of the oxyhemoglobin association curve reflects the cooperative binding of oxygen to hemoglobin (Fig. 15.14). In general, the hemoglobin saturation is between 80% and 100% with P_{aO_2} values greater than 60 mm Hg and drops dramatically when the P_{aO_2} is less than 60 mm Hg. Factors that decrease the affinity of hemoglobin for oxygen include a reduction in blood pH, an increase in temperature, an increase in P_{aCO_2}, and an increase in the concentration of 2,3-diphosphoglyceric acid (2,3-DPG) (Fig. 15.15). These factors facilitate unloading of oxygen into tissues, which is seen as a shift of the oxyhemoglobin dissociation curve to the right. The oxygen-carrying capacity of hemoglobin is also affected by competitive inhibitors

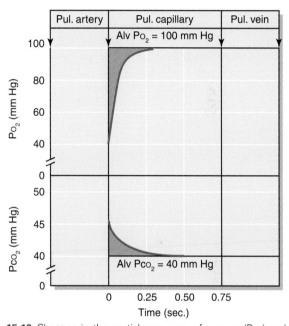

Fig. 15.13 Changes in the partial pressures of oxygen (P_{O_2}) and carbon dioxide (P_{CO_2}) as blood courses from the pulmonary artery through the capillaries and into the pulmonary veins. The diffusion gradient is greater for O_2 than for CO_2. However, equilibration of capillary and alveolar gas occurs for both molecules within the 0.75 second it takes for blood to traverse the capillaries. *Alv,* Alveolar; *Pul,* pulmonary.

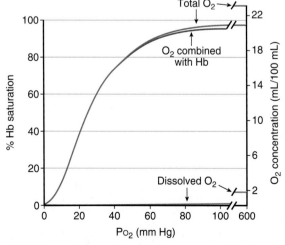

Fig. 15.14 The oxyhemoglobin dissociation curve. The bulk of the oxygen (O_2) is combined with hemoglobin (Hb). Little is dissolved in plasma. P_{O_2}, Partial pressure of oxygen.

for binding sites, such as carbon monoxide. Carbon monoxide has an affinity for hemoglobin that is 240 times greater than that of oxygen and preferentially binds to the hemoglobin molecule. However, this does not affect the amount of oxygen dissolved in the blood. Someone with carbon monoxide poisoning may have a normal Pao_2 but a very low blood oxygen content because of the high amount of desaturated hemoglobin.

About 5% of carbon dioxide in the blood is dissolved in plasma, and about 10% is bound to hemoglobin. However, carbon dioxide does not exhibit cooperative binding; therefore, the shape of the carbon dioxide–hemoglobin dissociation curve is linear. Carbon dioxide binds to the protein component of the hemoglobin molecule and to the amino groups of the polypeptide chains of plasma proteins to form carbamino compounds. About 10% of carbon dioxide is transported in this fashion. Most of the carbon dioxide is transported as bicarbonate ion: As carbon dioxide diffuses from metabolically active tissue into the blood, it reacts with water to form carbonic acid. This reaction primarily occurs in the red blood cells because

it is catalyzed by the enzyme carbonic anhydrase, which resides in those cells. Carbonic acid then dissociates to bicarbonate and hydrogen ion. Although there is more carbon dioxide dissolved in blood than oxygen, it is still a small fraction of the total carbon dioxide transported by blood.

Abnormalities of Pulmonary Gas Exchange

The arterial Po_2 and Pco_2 are determined by the degree of equilibration between the alveolar gas and capillary blood, which depends on four major factors: ventilation, matching of ventilation with perfusion, shunt, and diffusion. *Hypoxemia* refers to a reduction in the oxygen content of the blood and is determined by measuring the Po_2 of arterial blood. In contrast, *hypoxia* refers to a decrease in oxygen content of an organ, for example, myocardial hypoxia. Aberrations in the four factors listed can result in hypoxemia. A fifth cause of hypoxemia is a low inspired Po_2, which may occur at altitude.

Hypoventilation is defined as ventilation that is inadequate to keep Pco_2 from increasing above normal. Hypoxemia may occur when increased carbon dioxide in the alveoli displaces alveolar oxygen. As alveolar ventilation falls and $Paco_2$ rises, Pao_2 will have to fall. Administration of supplemental oxygen (i.e., increasing the Fio_2) can reverse hypoventilation-induced hypoxemia. When one is breathing room air, the difference between alveolar oxygen and arterial oxygen (A-a gradient) is normally about 10 mm Hg. Typically, this difference increases when hypoxemia is present. However, if the hypoxemia is caused by hypoventilation, the A-a gradient will be within normal limits. Causes of hypoventilation are varied and range from diseases or drugs that depress the respiratory control center to disorders of the chest wall or respiratory muscles that impair respiratory pump function. Disorders associated with hypoventilation include inflammation, trauma, or hemorrhage in the brain stem; spinal cord pathology; anterior horn cell disease; peripheral neuropathies; myopathies; abnormalities of the chest wall such as kyphoscoliosis; and upper airway obstruction. Administration of a higher Fio_2 alleviates the hypoxemia but does little to improve the elevated $Paco_2$.

The most common cause of hypoxemia in disease states is ventilation-perfusion mismatch. In regions where the ratio of ventilation $\dot{V}$ to perfusion $\dot{Q}$ is low, the blood receives little oxygen from the poorly ventilated alveoli. By contrast, in regions where $\dot{V}/\dot{Q}$ is high, the blood is well oxygenated but receives little additional oxygen despite the higher ventilation because the shape of the oxyhemoglobin dissociation curve plateaus at levels of high Pao_2. As a result, lung units with high $\dot{V}/\dot{Q}$ cannot completely correct for the low oxygen content of blood flowing past units with low $\dot{V}/\dot{Q}$. Thus, the oxygen uptake of the whole lung is lowered, causing hypoxemia. In the ideal lung, ventilation and perfusion would be perfectly matched (i.e., $\dot{V}/Q = 1$). However, the $\dot{V}/\dot{Q}$ normally ranges from 0.5 at the base to 3 at the apex, with an overall value of 0.8. If lung disease develops, ventilation-perfusion inequality may be amplified. If the $\dot{V}/\dot{Q}$ is less than 0.8, the A-a gradient is increased and hypoxia ensues. The $Paco_2$ is usually within the normal range but increases slightly at extremely low $\dot{V}/\dot{Q}$ ratios (Fig. 15.16). Typically, hypoxemia in diseases that affect the airways, such as chronic obstructive pulmonary disease (COPD), is caused by ventilation-perfusion mismatch. As with hypoxemia due to hypoventilation, administration of a higher Fio_2 improves hypoxemia by improving the Pao_2 in areas of *low* $\dot{V}/\dot{Q}$.

The third cause of hypoxemia is shunt. A right-to-left shunt occurs when a portion of blood travels from the right side to the left side of the heart without the opportunity to exchange oxygen and carbon dioxide in the lung. Right-to-left shunts can be classified as anatomic or physiologic. With an anatomic shunt, a portion of the blood bypasses the lung by traversing through an anatomic canal. In all healthy individuals, there

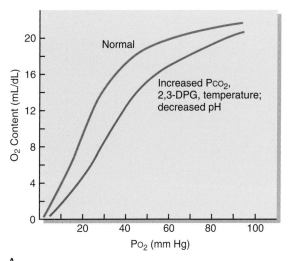

A

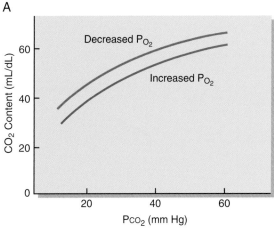

B

Fig. 15.15 (A) The various factors that decrease the oxygen affinity of hemoglobin are shown shifting the curve to the right. (B) The carbon dioxide dissociation curve is more linear than the oxyhemoglobin curve throughout the physiologic range. Increased partial pressure of oxygen in the arteries (Pao_2) shifts the curve to the right, decreasing the carbon dioxide content for any given arterial partial pressure of carbon dioxide ($Paco_2$) and thereby facilitating carbon dioxide off-loading in the lungs. The shift to the left at a lower Pao_2 facilitates carbon dioxide on-loading at the tissues. *2,3-DPG,* 2,3-Diphosphoglycerate.

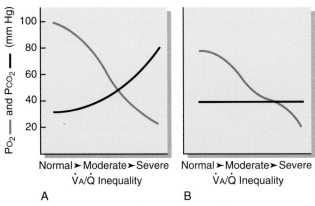

A   B

Fig. 15.16 (A) The effects of increasing inequality of alveolar ventilation and perfusion (decreasing $\dot{V}_A / \dot{Q}$) on the arterial partial pressures of oxygen (Po_2) and carbon dioxide (Pco_2) when cardiac output and minute ventilation are held constant. (B) The gas tensions change when minute ventilation is allowed to increase. Increased ventilation can maintain a normal arterial Pco_2 but can only partially correct the hypoxemia. (Modified from Dantzker DR: Gas exchange abnormalities. In Montenegro H, editor: Chronic obstructive pulmonary disease, New York, 1984, Churchill Livingstone, pp 141-160.)

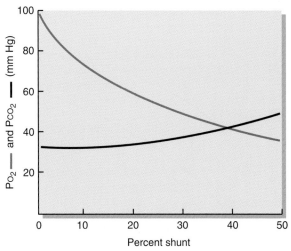

Fig. 15.17 The effects of increasing shunt on the arterial partial pressures of oxygen (Po_2) and carbon dioxide (Pco_2). The minute ventilation has been held constant in this example. Under usual circumstances, the hypoxemia would lead to increased minute ventilation and a fall in the Pco_2 as the shunt increased. (From Dantzker DR: Gas exchange abnormalities. In Montenegro H, editor: Chronic obstructive pulmonary disease, New York, 1984, Churchill Livingstone, pp 141-160.)

is a small fraction of blood in the bronchial circulation that passes to the pulmonary veins and empties into the left atrium, thereby reducing the Pao_2 of the systemic circulation. A smaller portion of the normal shunt is related to the coronary circulation draining through the thebesian veins into the left ventricle. Anatomic shunts found in disease states can be classified as intracardiac or intrapulmonary shunts. Intracardiac shunts occur when right atrial pressures are elevated and deoxygenated blood travels from the right atrium to the left atrium through an atrial septal defect or patent foramen ovale. Intrapulmonary anatomic shunts consist primarily of arteriovenous malformations or telangiectasias. With a physiologic right-to-left shunt, a portion of the pulmonary arterial blood passes through the normal vasculature but does not come into contact with alveolar air. This is an extreme example of ventilation-perfusion mismatch ($\dot{V}/\dot{Q} = 0$). Physiologic shunt can be caused by diffuse flooding of the alveoli with fluid, as seen in congestive heart failure or acute respiratory distress syndrome. Alveolar flooding with inflammatory exudates, as seen in lobar pneumonia, also causes a shunt. The fraction of blood shunted (Qs/Qt) can be calculated when the Fio_2 is 100% by the following equation:

$$Qs/Qt = (Cco_2 - Cao_2)/(Cco_2 - Cvo_2)$$

where Qs is the shunted blood flow, Qt is the total blood flow, Cco_2 is the end-pulmonary capillary oxygen content; Cao_2 is the arterial oxygen content; and Cvo_2 is the mixed venous oxygen content (amount of oxygen attached to hemoglobin in the blood returning from the body to right side of the heart).

If the shunt is severe enough, mechanical ventilation and PEEP are required to improve arterial oxygenation. At values less than 50% of the cardiac output, a shunt has very little effect on $Paco_2$ (Fig. 15.17). With shunting, the A-a gradient is elevated while the $Paco_2$ is within normal range or may be low. In contrast to hypoxemia due to hypoventilation or low $\dot{V}/\dot{Q}$, oxygen administration does not correct hypoxemia due to shunt because the shunted blood has no exposure to oxygen in the alveoli. However, the Pao_2 may increase somewhat because the higher Fio_2 improves oxygenation of blood traveling to low $\dot{V}/\dot{Q}$ areas that commonly coexist with shunt.

The fourth cause of hypoxemia is diffusion impairment. With normal cardiopulmonary function, the blood spends, on average, 0.75 second in the pulmonary capillaries. Typically, it takes only 0.25

second for the alveolar oxygen to diffuse across the thin alveolar capillary membrane and equilibrate with pulmonary arterial blood (see Fig. 15.13). However, if there is impairment to diffusion across this membrane, such as thickening of the alveolar capillary membrane by fluid, fibrous tissue, cellular debris, or inflammatory cells, it will take longer for the oxygen in the alveoli to equilibrate with pulmonary arterial blood. If the impediment to diffusion is such that it takes longer than 0.75 second for oxygen to diffuse, hypoxemia ensues, and the A-a gradient widens. Alternatively, if the time a red blood cell spends traversing the pulmonary capillary decreases to 0.25 second or less, hypoxemia may develop. Hypoxemia may be evident only during exercise in individuals with diffusion impairment because of the shortened red cell transit time. In these cases, the A-a gradient may be normal at rest but increases with exercise. With diffusion impairment, the $Paco_2$ usually is within the normal range. As with hypoxemia due to hypoventilation or ventilation-perfusion mismatch, administration of a higher Fio_2 improves hypoxemia due to impaired diffusion by raising the alveolar Po_2.

An additional cause of hypoxemia is low inspired oxygen. This may occur at high altitude: The Fio_2 is normal, but the Po_2 is low because the barometric pressure (P_{atm}) is low. Rarely, circumstances occur in which the Fio_2 is low (e.g., rebreathing air). Hypoxemia due to low inspired oxygen is associated with a normal A-a gradient and is usually accompanied by a low $Paco_2$. Supplemental oxygen corrects this form of hypoxemia. Finally, a low mixed venous Po_2 predisposes individuals to hypoxia (Fig. 15.18).

EVALUATION OF LUNG FUNCTION

Pulmonary function tests evaluate one or more major aspects of the respiratory system. Accurate measurements of lung volumes, airway function, and gas exchange require a pulmonary function laboratory. Pulmonary function tests are commonly used to aid in the diagnosis of disease and assess disease severity. In addition, they are helpful in monitoring the course of disease, assessing the risk for surgical procedures, and measuring the effects of varied environmental exposures (Table 15.1). The response to bronchodilators or other forms of treatment can also

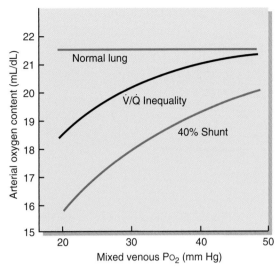

Fig. 15.18 The effects of increasing mixed venous partial pressure of oxygen (Po_2) on the arterial oxygen content under three assumed conditions: a normal lung, severe ventilation-perfusion inequality ($\dot{V}/\dot{Q}$), and the presence of a 40% shunt. For each situation, the patient is breathing 50% oxygen and the mixed venous Po_2 is altered, keeping all other variables constant. (From Dantzker DR: Gas exchange in the adult respiratory distress syndrome, Clin Chest Med 3:57-67, 1982.)

TABLE 15.1   **Indications for Pulmonary Function Testing**
Evaluation of signs and symptoms:
Shortness of breath
Exertional dyspnea
Chronic cough
Screening of at-risk populations
Monitoring of pulmonary drug toxicity
Follow-up after abnormal study results:
Chest radiograph
Electrocardiogram
Arterial blood gases
Hemoglobin
Preoperative assessment:
Assess severity
Follow response to therapy
Determine further treatment goals
Assess disability

be assessed with serial pulmonary function tests. Accurate interpretation of pulmonary function tests requires the appropriate reference standards. Variables that affect the predicted standards include age, height, gender, race, and hemoglobin concentration.

Spirometry, the simplest means of measuring lung function, can be performed in an office practice. A spirometer is an apparatus that measures inspiratory and expiratory volumes. Flow rates can be calculated from tracings of volume versus time. Typically, vital capacity (VC) is measured as the difference between a full inspiration to total lung capacity (TLC) and a full exhalation to residual volume (RV) (Fig. 15.19). Flow rates are measured after the patient is instructed to forcefully exhale from TLC to RV. Such a forced expiratory maneuver allows one to calculate the forced expiratory volume in 1 second (FEV_1) and the forced vital capacity (FVC) (Fig. 15.20). A value that is 80% to 120% of the predicted value is considered normal for FVC. Normally, people can exhale more

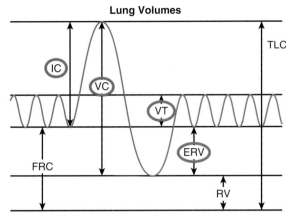

Fig. 15.19 Lung volumes and capacities. Although spirometry can measure vital capacity and its subdivisions *(red circles)*, calculation of residual volume (RV) requires measurement of functional residual capacity (FRC) by one of the following techniques: body plethysmography, helium dilution, or nitrogen washout. *ERV,* Expiratory reserve volume; *IC,* inspiratory capacity; *TLC,* total lung capacity; *VC,* vital capacity; *VT,* tidal volume.

than 75% to 80% of their FVC in the first second, and the majority of the FVC can be exhaled in 3 seconds. The ratio of FEV_1/FVC is normally greater than 0.80.

Spirometry can reveal abnormalities that are classified into two patterns: obstructive and restrictive. Obstructive impairments are defined by a low FEV_1/FVC ratio. Diseases that are characterized by an obstructive pattern include asthma, chronic bronchitis, emphysema, bronchiectasis, cystic fibrosis, and some central airway lesions. The reduction in FEV_1 (expressed as % predicted FEV_1) is used to determine the severity of airflow obstruction (E-Fig. 15.2). Peak expiratory flow rate (PEFR) can be measured as the maximal expiratory flow rate obtained during spirometry or when using a handheld peak flowmeter. The lower the PEFR, the more significant the obstruction. A peak flowmeter can be used at home or in the emergency department to evaluate the presence of obstruction. Severe asthma decompensation, for example, is usually associated with PEFRs of less than 200 L/minute (normal, 500 to 600 L/minute). At home, a low PEFR can alert the patient to seek medical attention.

A restrictive pattern is characterized by loss of lung volume. With spirometry, both the FVC and the FEV_1 are reduced, so the FEV_1/FVC ratio remains normal. The restrictive pattern must be confirmed by measurements of lung volumes. Lung volumes are measured by body plethysmography or by dilution of an inert gas such as helium. Lung volumes that can be measured with these techniques include FRC, TLC, and RV (see Fig. 15.19). As described earlier, FRC is the lung volume at which the inward elastic recoil of the lung equals the outward elastic recoil of the chest wall. Changes in FRC reflect abnormalities in lung elastic recoil. Diseases associated with increased elastic recoil (e.g., pulmonary fibrosis) are associated with a reduction in FRC, whereas those with decreased recoil (e.g., emphysema) are associated with an increase in FRC. TLC is the amount of air remaining in the thorax after a maximal inspiration. It is determined by the balance of the forces generated by the respiratory muscles to expand the respiratory system and the elastic recoil of the respiratory system. Restrictive lung disease is defined as a TLC less than 80% predicted, whereas values of TLC greater than 120% predicted are consistent with hyperinflation. The lower the % predicted TLC, the more severe the restrictive impairment.

Restriction may be caused by disorders of the lung, chest wall, respiratory muscles, or pleural space. Lung diseases that cause pulmonary

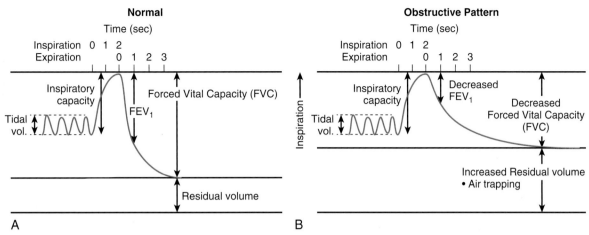

Fig. 15.20 Spirometry in a normal individual (A) and in a patient with obstructive lung disease (B). FEV_1 represents the forced expiratory volume in 1 second, and FVC represents the forced vital capacity. The FEV_1/FVC ratio is normally greater than 0.80. With obstruction, the FEV_1/FVC ratio is less than 0.70.

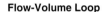

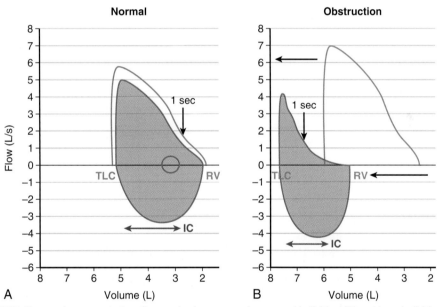

Fig. 15.21 The maximum expiratory flow and volume curve in a normal individual (A) and in an individual with obstructive lung disease (in this case, COPD) (B). Hyperinflation and air trapping *(arrows)* push the total lung capacity (TLC) and residual volume (RV) to the left (i.e., toward higher lung volumes). In addition, characteristic scalloping of the expiratory limb of the flow-volume curve develops. IC, Inspiratory capacity.

fibrosis cause a restrictive pattern because of the increased elastic recoil of the respiratory system. Diseases of the chest wall, such as kyphoscoliosis, obesity, or ankylosing spondylitis, can also cause restriction by reducing the elasticity of the chest wall. Weakness of the respiratory muscles causes restriction by reducing the force available to inflate the respiratory system. Myasthenia gravis, amyotrophic lateral sclerosis, diaphragm paralysis, and Guillain-Barré syndrome can be associated with weakness sufficient to cause restrictive lung disease. Finally, space-occupying lesions involving the pleural space, such as pleural effusions, pneumothorax, or pleural tumors, can cause restriction. Occasionally, RV and FRC may be elevated with no increase in TLC. This pattern is referred to as *air trapping* and can be seen with COPD or asthma.

The forced expiratory maneuver can be analyzed in terms of flow and volume by construction of a flow-volume loop (Fig. 15.21). Flow-volume loops are useful to identify obstructive and restrictive patterns. The characteristic appearance of obstructive impairment is concavity ("scooping") of the expiratory loop, whereas with restrictive impairments, the loops have a normal shape but are reduced in size. In addition, flow-volume loops are the primary means of identifying upper airway obstruction. Upper airway obstruction is characterized by a truncated (clipped) inspiratory or expiratory loop. A fixed obstruction produces clipping of both inspiratory and expiratory loops. Variable intrathoracic upper airway obstruction exhibits clipping of the expiratory loop, whereas variable extrathoracic obstruction exhibits clipping of the inspiratory loop (Fig. 15.22).

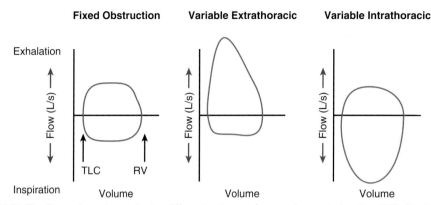

Fig. 15.22 The flow-volume loops display different patterns of upper airway obstruction. With fixed obstruction, both inspiratory and expiratory flows are reduced (clipped). With variable extrathoracic obstruction, only the inspiratory flows are clipped. With variable intrathoracic obstruction, only the expiratory flows are clipped. RV, Residual volume; TLC, total lung capacity.

Bronchoprovocation Testing

Bronchoprovocation testing is typically used to determine the presence or absence of hyperreactive airways disease. Some individuals with a clinical suspicion of asthma have normal expiratory flow rates and lung volumes. Bronchoprovocation testing in these individuals can be important to identify hyperreactive airways disease and support the diagnosis of asthma. Methacholine is a cholinergic agonist that causes bronchoconstriction. During the bronchoprovocation test, the subject inhales increasing concentrations of methacholine. Measurements of FEV_1, FVC, and specific airways conductance are obtained after the inhalation of each concentration until the maximal dose of methacholine has been administered. If the FEV_1 is reduced by 20% or more or the specific airways conductance is reduced by 40% or more, a diagnosis of hyperreactive airways disease is established. Patients with asthma demonstrate a fall in FEV_1 at considerably smaller doses than in normal individuals (Fig. 15.23).

Lung Diffusion Capacity

The diffusion of oxygen from the alveolus into the capillary can be assessed by measuring the diffusion capacity for carbon monoxide (D_{LCO}). To calculate the diffusion capacity for oxygen, one would need to know the alveolar volume and the partial pressures of oxygen in the alveolus and in the pulmonary capillary. Because it is not practical to measure the oxygen tension of pulmonary capillary blood, carbon monoxide is used rather than oxygen to assess diffusion capacity. Carbon monoxide diffuses across the alveolar capillary membranes much as oxygen does. However, carbon monoxide has the advantage of binding completely to hemoglobin. Therefore, the partial pressure of carbon monoxide in the pulmonary venous blood is negligible. The D_{LCO} is then measured as the rate of disappearance of carbon monoxide from the alveolus and is used as a surrogate for oxygen diffusion capacity.

The D_{LCO} measurement provides an overall assessment of gas exchange and depends on factors such as the surface area of the lung, the physical properties of the gas, perfusion of ventilated areas, hemoglobin concentration, and the thickness of the alveolar-capillary membrane. Therefore, an abnormal value may not only signify disruption of the alveolar-capillary membrane but may also be related to a reduction in surface area of the lung (pneumonectomy), poor perfusion (pulmonary embolus), or poor ventilation of alveolar units (COPD). A low D_{LCO} may be seen in interstitial lung diseases that alter the alveolar-capillary membrane or in diseases such as emphysema that destroy

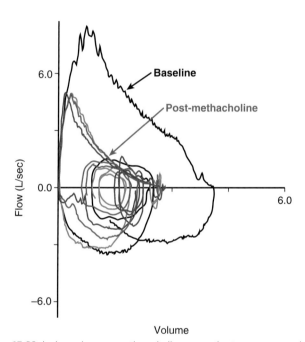

Fig. 15.23 In bronchoprovocation challenge, patients are exposed to increasing concentrations of an inhaled challenge (e.g., methacholine, histamine), followed by evaluation of the forced expiratory volume in 1 second (percentage of baseline value) or airways conductance. The FEV_1 falls by more than 20% (compared to baseline), and airways conductance by more than 40%, at lower concentrations of the challenge drug in individuals with asthma.

both alveolar septa and capillaries (E-Fig. 15.3). Anemia lowers the D_{LCO}. Most laboratories provide a hemoglobin correction for diffusion capacity. An increased D_{LCO} may be associated with engorgement of the pulmonary circulation by red blood cells or polycythemia.

Arterial Blood Gases

The measurement of Pao_2 and $Paco_2$ provides information about the adequacy of oxygenation and ventilation. This requires arterial blood sampling through arterial puncture or indwelling cannula (Table 15.2). Oxygenation also can be measured through noninvasive devices such as the pulse oximeter, which measures hemoglobin oxygen saturation, and through transcutaneous devices that measure Pao_2 and $Paco_2$. These devices are particularly useful for measuring oxygenation during exertion or sleep.

TABLE 15.2 **Normal Values for Arterial Blood Gases**
Partial pressure of oxygen (Pao$_2$): 104 − (0.27 × age)
Partial pressure of carbon dioxide (Paco$_2$): 36–44
pH: 7.35–7.45
Alveolar-arterial O$_2$ difference = 2.5 + (0.21 × age)

6-Minute Walk Distance

Often, alterations in oxygenation are not detected at rest but are unveiled during exertion. The 6-minute walk test is a standardized test in which the patient walks for 6 minutes while the oxygen hemoglobin saturation is measured. A decrease in saturation is abnormal and suggests impaired gas exchange capabilities, and a reduction in distance walked is a means of detecting deterioration of overall function due to lung disease. However, the 6-minute walk distance (6MWD) is primarily validated for following exercise capacity over time and in response to interventions. There is a "learning effect" that increases distance walked after the first attempt, and the minimal clinically important distance for this test is established as 30 meters. The 6MWD correlates well with peak oxygen consumption (VO$_2$ max) measured with maximal exercise testing.

In summary, pulmonary function tests, in conjunction with the history and physical examination, can be used to diagnose pulmonary disorders and assess severity and response to therapy, as illustrated in the flow diagram in E-Fig. 15.4.

EVALUATION OF LUNG DISEASE

Analysis of Exhaled Breath

Endogenously produced monoxides (nitric oxide and carbon monoxide) and volatile organic compounds (VOCs), collectively called the "volatolome," can be detected in the exhaled breath and may serve as biomarkers of pulmonary inflammation or cancer. Exhaled nitric oxide is elevated in asthma, and the US Food and Drug Administration has approved the test for exhaled nitric oxide for the diagnosis and evaluation of asthma exacerbations. The VOCs can be detected by gas chromatography or mass spectroscopy but more recently electronic "noses" have been developed that use changes in electrical resistance of polymers that bind VOCs to detect unique patterns of exhaled VOCs. These provide a "fingerprint" that may identify lung cancer, various pneumoconioses, obstructive sleep apnea, active pulmonary tuberculosis, and pulmonary hypertension. Cytokines and other similar compounds in the condensate phase of exhaled breath are being investigated for possible applications in inflammatory lung diseases (e.g., cystic fibrosis, bronchiectasis). Other nonpulmonary diseases such as malabsorption syndromes and *Helicobacter pylori* infection are also detected by analysis of exhaled breath.

Chest Radiography

Generally, the evaluation of a patient with lung disease begins with routine chest radiography and then proceeds to more specialized techniques such as computed tomography (CT) or magnetic resonance imaging (MRI). Ideally, the chest radiograph consists of two different films, a posteroanterior (PA) radiograph and a lateral radiograph (E-Fig. 15.5). Many pathologic processes can be identified on a PA chest radiograph, and the lateral view adds valuable information

about areas that are not well seen on the PA projection. In particular, the retrocardiac region, the posterior bases of the lung, and the bony structure of the thorax (e.g., the vertebral column) are better visualized on the lateral radiograph. The PA chest radiograph is obtained with the patient standing with his or her back to the x-ray beam and the anterior chest wall placed against the film cassette. The chest radiograph should be obtained while the patient takes the deepest breath possible. If the patient is too weak to stand or too sick to travel to the radiology department, the chest radiograph is performed at bedside (portable chest radiograph). The cassette is placed behind the patient's back while the patient is semi-supine in bed, and the x-ray beam travels from anterior to posterior (AP film). The quality of a portable film is not that of a standard PA film, but it still provides valuable information.

The examination of a chest radiograph should be systematic so that subtle abnormalities are not missed. It should include evaluation of the lungs and pulmonary vasculature, the bony thorax, the heart and great vessels, the diaphragm and pleura, the mediastinum, the soft tissues, and the subdiaphragmatic areas. Abnormalities that are visible on a chest radiograph include pulmonary infiltrates, nodules, interstitial markings, vascular abnormalities, masses, pleural effusions and thickening, cavitary lesions, cardiac enlargement, abnormal airway structure, and vertebral or rib fractures. In addition to the PA and lateral chest radiographs, the lateral decubitus projection is often used to identify the presence or absence of pleural effusion. The decubitus view is particularly useful in determining whether blunting of the costal phrenic sulcus is caused by freely flowing pleural fluid or related to pleural thickening. Chest radiography, in concert with a good history and physical examination, allows the clinician to diagnose chest disease in many circumstances.

Fluoroscopy

Fluoroscopic examination of the chest is useful for evaluating motion of the diaphragm. This technique is particularly helpful in diagnosing unilateral diaphragm paralysis. A paralyzed hemidiaphragm moves paradoxically when the patient is instructed to inhale or to forcefully sniff. However, fluoroscopy is limited when evaluating for bilateral diaphragm paralysis. Apparently normal descent of the diaphragm during inspiration, caused by compensatory respiratory strategies employed by the patient with bilateral diaphragm paralysis, leads to false-negative results. False-positive results are caused by paradoxical hemidiaphragm motion, which can be seen in as many as 6% of normal subjects during the sniff maneuver.

Ultrasonography

Point-of-care ultrasonography (POCUS) has improved clinical care by providing more focused and visual examinations of vital organs to aid in prompt diagnosis and management of diseases. In ultrasonography, sound waves in the frequency range of 3 to 10 MHz are reflected off internal tissues to produce images of viscera such as the liver, kidney, and heart. The air-filled lung cannot be imaged directly, but over the last decade, an understanding of various *artifacts* generated by ultrasound beams traversing normal and abnormal lung have led to increased application of ultrasound for imaging of the lung, particularly in the intensive care unit. Protocols are available to help with detecting lung consolidation, pulmonary edema, and volume responsiveness. Additionally, ultrasonography can rapidly and reliably detect a pneumothorax, pleural effusion, consolidation, and pulmonary edema with sensitivity and specificity similar to those of a chest radiograph (Fig. 15.24).

In addition to its diagnostic capabilities, ultrasound is routinely used in real time to direct invasive procedures, such as thoracentesis, pericardiocentesis, and placement of a pleural, central venous, or arterial catheter. Other applications of pulmonary ultrasound include assessment of volume status by imaging inferior vena cava collapsibility with respiration and assessment of right ventricular function. Two-dimensional B-mode ultrasound imaging of the diaphragm can be used to visualize diaphragm function during inspiration. Failure of the diaphragm to thicken by a minimum of 35% during inspiration when visualized from the infraaxillary view is indicative of diaphragm weakness.

Ultrasonography is noninvasive, rapidly and easily applied, relatively low-cost, readily portable to the bedside, and because it does not use radiation, safe for repeated use on a patient.

Computed Tomography

CT has many applications in pulmonary medicine and provides more detailed information about lung structure than chest radiography. With the use of this technique, cross sections of the entire thorax can be obtained, usually at 2- to 5-mm intervals. CT scanning allows visualization of airways up to the seventh generation and delineation of parenchymal anatomy, texture, and density. Image contrast can be adjusted to optimize visualization of the lung parenchyma, pleura, and

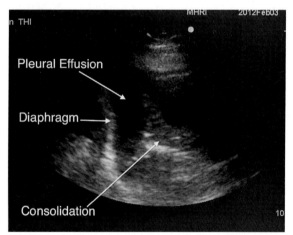

Fig. 15.24 Ultrasound image of the lung depicts the diaphragm, a pleural effusion, and an infiltrate.

mediastinal structures. The use of intravenous contrast material as part of the examination permits separation of vascular from nonvascular mediastinal structures. CT scans provide tremendous anatomic resolution when compared with chest radiography, but they expose the subject to about 70 times the radiation of a routine chest radiograph.

CT of the chest helps characterize pulmonary nodules and masses, distinguish between pleural thickening and pleural fluid, estimate the size of the heart and the presence of pericardial fluid, identify patterns of involvement of interstitial lung disease, detect cavities, and identify intracavitary processes such as mycetoma. It is also used to quantify the extent and distribution of emphysema, detect and measure mediastinal adenopathy for evaluating inflammatory diseases that involve mediastinal lymph nodes (e.g., sarcoidosis) and staging of lung cancer, and identify vascular invasion by neoplasm (Fig. 15.25). Newer generations of CT scanners are able to use multiple x-ray beams to create between 4 and 256 images simultaneously at a much faster rate (<10 seconds) than with the older models, which used only a single x-ray beam and detector. CT scans using much lower radiation doses are routinely advocated on a yearly basis for the early detection of lung cancer in older, high-risk smokers.

CT angiography allows for construction of three-dimensional images of the pulmonary vascular system. This imaging technique has emerged as the procedure of choice for identifying pulmonary embolism, supplanting pulmonary ventilation-perfusion scintigraphic lung scanning. The technique is used to identify pulmonary vascular abnormalities such as aortic dissection, pulmonary venous malformations, and aortic aneurysms. Additionally, three-dimensional construction of the airway and pulmonary parenchyma using CT images and specialized software has provided a means to electromagnetically guide a biopsy catheter through a bronchoscope (electromagnetic navigation bronchoscopy) to a distal pulmonary nodule or mass for biopsy. It could also be used to place a fiducial marker at the exact location of a lung cancer to accurately focus surgical or radiotherapy treatment.

Dynamic contrast-enhanced CT with single- or multi-detector scanner has been investigated as a modality to differentiate between a malignant and benign pulmonary nodule. First, baseline images are obtained using CT without contract enhancement. Subsequently, contrast is given over time while series of CT images are acquired. The difference time and contrast enhancement allow for evaluation of vascularity and blood flow patterns. Studies have confirmed high accuracy for differentiation.

High-resolution CT is a technique that generates thin (1-mm) anatomic slices to provide a high-contrast image of the pulmonary

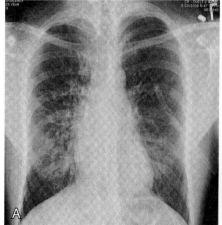
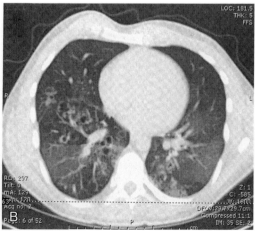

Fig. 15.25 Chest radiograph (A) and chest computed tomographic (CT) scan (B) of a patient with severe bronchiectasis. The abnormally dilated airways are better appreciated on the CT scan.

parenchyma. With high-resolution CT, a special reconstruction algorithm sharpens the soft tissue interfaces to provide superior visualization of the pulmonary parenchyma. This technique is used primarily to identify interstitial lung disease and bronchiectasis. It is extremely useful for identifying interstitial lung disease that may not be apparent on a plain chest radiograph, and it has supplanted bronchography in the diagnosis of bronchiectasis.

Magnetic Resonance Imaging

MRI is a tomographic technique that uses radio waves modified by a strong magnetic field to produce an image resulting from the resonation of protons in tissue water. The chief advantage of MRI is that it does not entail the use of ionizing radiation. The ability of MRI to image pulmonary parenchyma is limited because of the low proton density in air-filled regions of the lung, which therefore cannot generate MRI images, artifacts arising from multiple air-tissue interfaces, and respiratory motion artifacts. However, vascular structures and pulmonary perfusion are well imaged by MRI, especially with the use of intravenous contrast agents such as gadolinium chelates. Therefore, MRI is very useful in the study of aortic dissection and may have a role in the evaluation of pulmonary emboli and chronic thromboembolic pulmonary hypertension. Three-directional velocity-encoded MRI allows three-dimensional, time-resolved cine reconstruction of blood flow patterns and pressures and is used in cardiac imaging. It may also have a role in the measurement of pulmonary blood flow. Infiltrative pulmonary diseases and pulmonary edema increase proton density in the lung, allowing better definition by MRI of honeycombing in pulmonary fibrosis and pulmonary edema in acute respiratory distress syndrome (ARDS). The use of inhaled hyperpolarized inert gases such as helium-3 or xenon-129 offers the ability to quantify peripheral airspace size, measure gas flow in lobar and segmental bronchi, and detect regional differences in ventilation. Ongoing studies are being completed to establish its utility. It has promising applications in the evaluation of emphysema and asthma and after lung transplantation, including assessment of bronchodilator responsiveness. In particular, MRI is very useful in delineating extension of malignant pleural mesothelioma to adjacent chest wall tissue or diaphragm, where it is much superior to CT imaging because of superior contrast resolution.

Pulmonary Angiography

Pulmonary angiography entails placement of a catheter in the pulmonary artery, followed by rapid injection of a contrast agent. In the past, this was "gold standard" for diagnosis of pulmonary thromboembolic disease. Pulmonary angiography still can be useful for detection of congenital abnormalities of the pulmonary vascular tree, but CT and MRI have largely supplanted it.

Pulmonary Ventilation-Perfusion Scanning

Ventilation-perfusion ($\dot{V}/\dot{Q}$) scintigraphy utilizes radiopharmaceuticals such as technetium-99m as a noninvasive means to evaluate regional blood flow and ventilation. Therefore, it has been used in the past as an alternative to pulmonary angiography to detect pulmonary embolism. With the advent of CT angiography and its improvements over the years, $\dot{V}/\dot{Q}$ imaging is no longer favored for the initial evaluation of suspected pulmonary embolism. Additionally, alteration of regional blood flow (pulmonary vasoconstriction and shunt) due to lung diseases such as pneumonia or interstitial lung disease limits its diagnostic accuracy. The PIOPED study in 1990 investigated the diagnostic accuracy of a $\dot{V}/\dot{Q}$ scan for the diagnosis of pulmonary embolism. The study found that a $\dot{V}/\dot{Q}$ scan is useful when the clinical pretest probability is high but that it has poor diagnostic accuracy. Despite

its limitations, $\dot{V}/\dot{Q}$ scan still has utility in certain clinical scenarios. These scenarios include patients who have abnormal renal function, patients who are allergic to CT contrast, and patients with suspected chronic thromboembolic pulmonary hypertension (higher sensitivity compared to CT angiography). Quantitative lung perfusion scanning is also very useful preoperatively to assess the predicted postoperative lung function remaining after planned lobectomy or pneumonectomy. Therefore, it is used by thoracic surgeons to evaluate a patient's suitability for undergoing lobectomy or pneumonectomy for curative resection of lung cancer.

Positron Emission Tomography

Positron emission tomography (PET) detects metabolically active pulmonary nodules greater than 0.8 cm in diameter. It is helpful in assessing whether a nodule is benign or malignant. However, it does not distinguish between inflammation and malignancy. Therefore, assessment of multiple pulmonary nodules by PET is limited because of false-positive findings due to active granulomatous disease, such as previous exposure to tuberculosis, sarcoidosis, or fungal infestation; or to active infection, such as bacterial or viral pneumonia, bronchiolitis, or aspiration.

Dual-modality integrated PET-CT combines morphologic and functional imaging. The combination of PET and CT is helpful for localizing solitary metastatic lymph nodes in the hila and extrapulmonary locations, allowing better staging of lung cancer. In addition, PET-CT is helpful in planning radiation therapy for patients who have lung cancer associated with atelectasis.

Bronchoscopy

Fiberoptic bronchoscopy is used for diagnostic or therapeutic indications. It is most commonly performed to directly visualize the nasopharynx, larynx, vocal cords, and proximal tracheobronchial tree for diagnostic purposes. The procedure is performed by sedating the patient and providing local anesthesia with inhaled and instilled lidocaine. The bronchial mucosa is assessed for endobronchial masses, mucosal integrity, extrinsic compression, dynamic compression, and hemorrhage. The bronchoscope is equipped with a channel for passing a variety of instruments including biopsy forceps for sampling endobronchial lesions or lung tissue (transbronchial biopsy), and fine 19- to 22-gauge needles for transbronchial aspiration biopsy from lymph nodes or lung masses. Saline also can be instilled through the channel for bronchial washings or bronchoalveolar lavage. Bronchial washings and bronchoalveolar lavage can be analyzed for cytology, culture, and special stains. A bronchial brush is used to scrape the bronchial mucosa and harvest cells for cytology. Bronchoscopes can also be adapted with a terminal ultrasound probe to provide ultrasound images of the airways and neighboring tissues. This technique, called endobronchial ultrasound (EBUS) uses high acoustic frequencies, in the range of 20 MHz, to provide high-resolution images of proximal tissue and provides accurate positional guidance for needle aspiration of mediastinal lymph nodes. It is now routinely used to detect lung cancer metastasis to mediastinal lymph nodes and for the diagnosis of granulomatous disorders of the lymph nodes. A different radial ultrasound probe inserted through the working channel of a bronchoscope can facilitate confirmation of the position of a transbronchial biopsy forceps near a lung mass during transbronchial biopsy of a lesion in the periphery of the lung parenchyma. A newer technique called transbronchial lung cryobiopsy (TBLC) uses a probe that traverses the working channel of a bronchoscope into the periphery of the lung near the chest wall. The probe is rapidly cooled to freeze the adjacent lung tissue, which adheres to the probe and is fractured off, resulting in biopsy specimens that are larger and less susceptible to the crush artifact noted on routine forceps biopsies. This technique, though often complicated by serious hemorrhage, is in use for the diagnosis of interstitial lung disease with the hope that it will obviate the need for surgical biopsy.

Common therapeutic indications for bronchoscopy include retrieval of foreign bodies, suctioning of secretions, reexpansion of atelectatic lung by removing obstruction, detection and localization of hemoptysis, and assistance with difficult endotracheal intubations. In special centers, bronchoscopy is used to perform yttrium aluminum garnet (YAG) laser therapy, argon plasma coagulation therapy, and cryotherapy for endobronchial lesions. It is also used to guide placement of catheters for brachytherapy in lung cancer or guide placement of stents. Lasers produce a beam of light that can induce tissue vaporization, coagulation, and necrosis. Argon plasma coagulation therapy uses heat from ionized argon gas to debulk the tumor while simultaneously coagulating to stop bleeding. Cryotherapy probes induce tissue necrosis through hypothermic cellular crystallization and microthrombosis. Cryotherapy and electrocautery have been used to treat and relieve airway obstruction caused by benign tracheal bronchial tumors, polyps, and granulation tissue. The goal of endobronchial brachytherapy is to relieve airway obstruction from central tumors. This is typically used as an adjunct to conventional external-beam irradiation. Tracheobronchial stenting can be performed to manage airway compression associated with malignant tumors, tracheoesophageal fistulas, or tracheobronchomalacia. Bronchoscopy is generally a safe procedure with major complications, including significant bleeding, pneumothorax, and respiratory failure, occurring in 0.1% to 1.7% of patients.

PROSPECTUS FOR THE FUTURE

Continued refinement and evolution of techniques and methods currently used to assess pulmonary structure and function will enhance the ability to diagnose and treat individuals with lung disease. Although pulmonary function testing has been performed for decades, advances in equipment design and better standardization of methods will improve accuracy and reproducibility. Further development of noninvasive techniques used to measure changes in lung volume from body surface displacements may allow for assessment of pulmonary function in settings outside the pulmonary function laboratory. Analysis of exhaled gas for biomarkers has tremendous potential for early diagnosis of many lung diseases, especially cancer.

Great strides in assessing lung structure will evolve from advances in CT, PET, and MRI technology. CT volume-rendering techniques will provide images of the central airways, enabling "virtual bronchoscopy." This technique will be useful to guide biopsy site selection in conventional bronchoscopy and to allow visualization of airways distal to an endobronchial obstruction. Volumetric measurements of pulmonary nodules using CT segmentation techniques will allow more accurate calculation of nodule volume and better assessment of tumor doubling times. This, in concert with PET-CT, may provide more accurate means of determining the malignant potential of a solitary pulmonary nodule. Also, dynamic contrast-enhanced CT may help with differentiating between malignant and benign pulmonary nodules that would further improve the lung cancer screening process.

MRI may evolve into the preferred method for evaluating pulmonary emboli, mediastinal disease, and regional ventilation-perfusion matching. Velocity-encoded MRI is a promising modality for assessment of pulmonary vascular blood flow and pressures and may prove to be more accurate than current noninvasive methods. Lymph node–specific magnetic resonance contrast agents and the development of PET molecular tracers targeting tumor proteins and receptors may better differentiate enlarged lymph nodes caused by hyperplasia from those due to neoplasia. Finally, new insights into the function of the respiratory control centers in the cortex and brain stem may be attained from the use of functional MRI studies of the brain.

SUGGESTED READINGS

McCool FD, Hoppin FG Jr: Respiratory mechanics. In Baum GL, editor: Textbook of pulmonary diseases, Philadelphia, 1998, Lippincott-Raven, pp 117-130.

McCool FD, Tzelepis GE: Current clinical aspects of diaphragm dysfunction, N Engl J Med 366:932-942, 2012.

Miller WT: Radiographic evaluation of the chest. In Fishman AP, editor: Fishman's pulmonary diseases and disorders, New York, 2008, McGraw-Hill, pp 455-510.

Pellegrino R, Viegi G, Brusasco V, et al: Interpretative strategies for lung function tests, Eur Respir J 26:948-968, 2005.

Wagner PD: Ventilation, pulmonary blood flow, and ventilation-perfusion relationships. In Fishman AP, editor: Fishman's pulmonary diseases and disorders, New York, 2008, McGraw-Hill, pp 173-189.

Weibel ER: It takes more than cells to make a good lung, Am J Respir Crit Care Med 187:342-346, 2013.

West JB: Respiratory physiology: the essentials, ed 5, Baltimore, 1995, Williams & Wilkins.

West JB, Wagner PD: Pulmonary gas exchange, Am J Respir Crit Care Med 157:S82-S87, 1988.

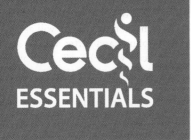

16

Obstructive Lung Diseases

Zoe G.S. Vazquez, Matthew D. Jankowich, Debasree Banerjee

INTRODUCTION

The obstructive lung diseases are a group of pulmonary disorders that result in dyspnea characterized by an obstructive pattern of expiratory airflow limitation on spirometry. These disorders include chronic obstructive pulmonary disease (COPD), asthma, cystic fibrosis (CF), bronchiectasis, and bronchiolar disorders. In some cases, these disorders overlap clinically (Fig. 16.1), sharing several features aside from the presence of expiratory airflow limitation. These features may include symptoms of wheezing and sputum production, chronic airway-centered inflammation, presence of airway structural changes resulting in remodeling of the airways, and episodic periods of temporarily worsened clinical status, known as exacerbations. However, the causes, locations, and patterns of airway inflammatory changes and remodeling, as well as the treatments, prognoses, and natural histories, are often significantly different, making clinical distinction among these disorders important.

COPD is characterized by abnormal airway inflammation and lung structure in response to an inhaled irritant (typically cigarette smoke), resulting in irreversible or incompletely reversible airflow limitation that is typically progressive over time. *Asthma* is distinguished from COPD by characteristic smooth muscle hyperreactivity and reversible airflow limitation, by its variable clinical course, and by its frequent association with atopy. These disorders are epidemic in the general population worldwide and account for a significant proportion of the morbidity and mortality associated with the obstructive lung diseases. *Bronchiectasis* is a permanent abnormal dilation of the bronchi that results in chronic cough, purulent sputum production, and hemoptysis. Bronchiectasis is caused by diverse conditions including CF, a genetic disorder resulting from mutations in the *CFTR* gene. The *bronchiolar disorders*, also called *small airways disorders*, result from inflammation and/or fibrosis of the small airways of the lung that leads to dyspnea. They may be difficult to diagnose because loss or obstruction of a majority of the small airways must occur before the appearance of expiratory airflow limitation on spirometry.

The basis for expiratory airflow obstruction varies among these disorders. The flow of air through the bronchial tree is directly proportional to the driving pressure and inversely proportional to the resistance. In obstructive lung disease, alterations in one or both of these processes may be present. Loss of lung elastic tissue, frequently present in COPD, results in decreased lung elastic recoil on expiration and therefore decreased driving pressure for expiratory airflow. By contrast, airflow limitation in asthma is primarily caused by smooth muscle contraction resulting in bronchoconstriction that increases airway resistance. Increases in airway resistance are also present in COPD and are related to small airway inflammation and fibrosis as well as small airway collapse due to decreased "tethering" of the airways in the setting of loss of surrounding lung elastic tissue. Mucus obstruction of airway lumens contributes to increased airway resistance in all the obstructive lung diseases.

Obstruction to airflow causes characteristic changes in lung volumes. The residual volume (RV) and functional residual capacity (FRC) are increased, whereas the total lung capacity (TLC) remains normal or is increased. Vital capacity, and particularly inspiratory capacity, is eventually reduced by the increase in RV. Several factors may contribute to the increase in FRC and RV in obstructive lung disease. Decreased lung elastic recoil in COPD increases the FRC because of reduced opposition to the outward force exerted by the chest wall. Loss of airway tone and decreased tethering by the surrounding lung in COPD, as well as bronchoconstriction and mucus plugging in acute asthma, allow airways to collapse at higher lung volumes and trap excessive air. Finally, under demands for increased minute ventilation (e.g., during exercise), the increased resistance to airflow may not allow the lungs to empty completely in the time available for expiration; this leads to so-called dynamic hyperinflation of the lungs as the volume of trapped air progressively increases while the inspiratory capacity is progressively limited. This phenomenon contributes to symptoms of chest tightness and dyspnea during exercise and results in exercise limitation, especially in COPD.

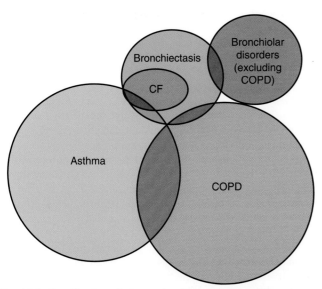

Fig. 16.1 Classification of obstructive lung diseases. Although most patients with chronic obstructive pulmonary disease (COPD) have small airways disease, the bronchiolar disorders do not overlap with COPD. *CF*, Cystic fibrosis.

TABLE 16.1 Features of Obstructive Lung Disease

Disorder	Clinical Features	Laboratory Findings
Chronic obstructive pulmonary disease	Chronic progressive dyspnea Cough, sputum production Periodic exacerbations	FEV_1/FVC <0.70 after bronchodilator use Often reduced D_{LCO}
Asthma	Episodic dyspnea, cough, and/or wheezing Nocturnal symptoms May have environmental trigger(s)	Variable airflow obstruction on spirometry Typically significant improvement in FEV_1 with bronchodilator use D_{LCO} normal or elevated Methacholine challenge shows airway hyperreactivity
Bronchiectasis	Chronic cough and purulent sputum production Hemoptysis	Chest radiograph: "tram track" shadows HRCT: dilated bronchi bigger than accompanying vessel, lack of tapering of bronchi, visible bronchi within 1-2 cm of lung border Sputum culture may grow *Haemophilus influenzae*, *Pseudomonas aeruginosa*, or atypical mycobacteria Laboratory evaluation may reveal specific etiology (e.g., decreased immunoglobulin levels in CVID)
Cystic fibrosis	Sinusitis, bronchiectasis, meconium ileus, malabsorption, infertility (in males, congenital absence of vas deferens)	Increased sweat chloride concentration, mutation in CFTR chloride channel, elevated fecal fat, abnormal nasal mucosal potential difference
Bronchiolar disorders	Progressive dyspnea Possible history of connective tissue disease, inflammatory bowel disease, lung transplantation, or hematopoietic stem cell transplantation	Fixed airflow obstruction on spirometry HRCT: mosaic attenuation pattern; centrilobular nodules; tree-in-bud opacities

CVID, Common variable immunodeficiency; *D_{LCO}*, diffusing capacity for carbon monoxide; *FEV_1*, forced expiratory volume in 1 second; *FVC*, forced vital capacity; *HRCT*, high-resolution computed tomography.

There are two major consequences of the changes in lung volume in obstructive lung disease. First, breathing at higher lung volumes requires a higher change in pressure to achieve a smaller change in lung volume, and this requirement increases the work of breathing. Second, larger lung volumes place the inspiratory muscles at a mechanical disadvantage. The diaphragm is flattened, decreasing its ability to change intrathoracic volume, and all the inspiratory muscle fibers are shortened, decreasing the tension they are able to exert to effect changes in lung volume. The combination of a higher work of breathing and mechanical disadvantages of the respiratory muscles caused by lung hyperinflation can lead to respiratory muscle fatigue and failure in the setting of an abrupt worsening of airway obstruction, as during an acute exacerbation of COPD or asthma.

In addition to the clinical history and physical examination, spirometry is a key step in the diagnostic work-up for a patient with suspected obstructive lung disease. Although spirometry is readily available and inexpensive, it is often underutilized, and as a consequence, obstructive lung diseases are underdiagnosed. Assessment of the clinical and spirometric response to a bronchodilator is a simple and helpful step in distinguishing asthma from COPD. Measurement of the diffusing capacity of the lungs for carbon monoxide (D_{LCO}) can also be helpful in separating asthma, which is characterized by a normal or elevated diffusing capacity, from COPD in which the diffusing capacity is often reduced by loss of surface area for gas exchange. More sophisticated testing, such as high-resolution chest computed tomography (HRCT), may be needed to help diagnose less common causes of obstructive lung disease (e.g., bronchiectasis).

The clinical features and laboratory findings associated with the various obstructive lung disorders are summarized in Table 16.1.

CHRONIC OBSTRUCTIVE PULMONARY DISEASE

Definition and Epidemiology

The Global Initiative for Chronic Obstructive Lung Disease (GOLD) currently defines COPD as a common preventable and treatable disease characterized by persistent airflow limitation that is usually progressive and associated with an enhanced chronic inflammatory response in the airways and lungs to noxious particles and gases. The presence of airflow limitation is established by spirometry: If the ratio of the forced expired volume in 1 second (FEV_1) to the forced vital capacity (FVC) is less than 0.70 after administration of a bronchodilator, airway obstruction is indicated. Although in the past COPD was defined by the presence of either *emphysema* (a pathologic enlargement of the distal air spaces) or *chronic bronchitis* (a clinical syndrome characterized by the presence of cough and sputum production for at least 3 months in each of 2 consecutive years), the current definition is based on the presence of airflow limitation and not on the presence of these entities. Both emphysema and chronic bronchitis may occur with or without the simultaneous presence of expiratory airflow limitation, and therefore these entities overlap with but are not synonymous with COPD. The current definition of COPD highlights the presence of persistent, reproducible expiratory airflow limitation and emphasizes the progressive nature of COPD and the presence of abnormal inflammation in the lungs and airways.

COPD is a common disorder in populations across the world. The Burden of Obstructive Lung Disease study, in a sample of adults from 12 countries, found that 10.1% had at least moderate airway obstruction (FEV_1/FVC <0.70 and FEV_1 <80% predicted) after administration of a bronchodilator. Prevalence rates for COPD are correlated with increasing age, lower socioeconomic status, and smoking. Although COPD is more prevalent in men than in women, the prevalence of

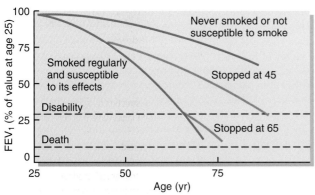

Fig. 16.2 Pattern of decline in forced expiratory volume in 1 second (FEV₁) with risks for morbidity and mortality from respiratory disease in a susceptible smoker compared with a normal patient and with a non-susceptible smoker. Although cessation of smoking does not replenish the lung function already lost in a susceptible smoker, it decreases the rate of further decline. (Data from Fletcher C, Peto R: The natural history of chronic airflow obstruction, BMJ 1:1645-1648, 1977.)

COPD in women has been increasing, and annual death rates for COPD have been steadily rising in both white and black women in the United States. COPD results in a significant economic burden in terms of health care expenditures and disability. In 2014, COPD accounted for 44.3 per 100,000 deaths in the United States. According to the World Health Organization, COPD is the fourth leading cause of death worldwide.

COPD is a complex disorder that results from a susceptibility to environmental factors brought about by a genetic predisposition. Cigarette smoking is the major environmental cause of COPD, although other factors may contribute, including outdoor air pollution, dust and fume exposure in the workplace, and indoor air pollution from use of biomass fuels for cooking and heat. Nonsmokers can and do develop COPD, highlighting the role of non–tobacco-related risk factors. A genetic predisposition is implied by the documentation of familial clusters of COPD. However, the only genetic disorder thus far definitively linked to COPD is α_1-antitrypsin deficiency resulting from mutations in *SERPINA1*, which accounts for approximately 1% to 2% of all COPD cases. Recent studies have highlighted other areas of the genome that are also associated with COPD susceptibility.

Several longitudinal studies have defined patterns of age-related decline in lung function and have documented the concept of age-related susceptibility to COPD. These studies showed that most adult nonsmoking men exhibit a decline in FEV₁ of 35 to 40 mL/year. This rate is increased to 45 to 60 mL/year in most cigarette smokers. However, the susceptible smoker may demonstrate losses of 70 to 120 mL/year (Fig. 16.2). This information allows the physician to project the rate of decrease of lung function in patients with COPD and to assess the effects of therapeutic interventions.

Pathology

Various structural changes have been observed in the airways and lungs of individuals with COPD. The current definition of COPD emphasizes the central role of chronic inflammation in the pathogenesis of COPD and in the development of pathologic lung and airway remodeling in the setting of COPD. Structural changes observed in COPD include emphysema and abnormalities of the small and large airways. There is increasing evidence that the small airways are the major site of airflow limitation and a central focus of pathology in COPD.

Emphysema in COPD

Emphysema is defined as a permanent enlargement of the air spaces distal to the terminal bronchioles (E-Fig. 16.1). This is caused by destruction of the lung parenchyma in the absence of significant fibrosis. These changes result in an abnormal acinus with limited capabilities for gas exchange. Based on thin gross lung sections, emphysema can be classified as either centrilobular or panlobular (E-Figs. 16.2 and 16.3). In centrilobular emphysema, the proximal part of the lobule (the respiratory bronchiole) is affected; this is the most common histologic feature observed in emphysema related to smoking. Panlobular emphysema is seen in α_1-antitrypsin deficiency.

α_1-Antitrypsin is a serine protease inhibitor that deactivates elastase molecules released by inflammatory cells that are capable of degrading connective tissue matrices. The observations that this enzyme was associated with emphysema and that emphysema could be reproduced in experimental models by the instillation of papain (a protease) into the lungs led to the hypothesis that emphysema is caused by an imbalance between protease and antiprotease systems in the lung. This theorized imbalance would favor proteolytic destruction of lung connective tissue, resulting in emphysema (the protease-antiprotease hypothesis). Research has focused on neutrophil elastase and its role in the destruction of lung elastin. Neutrophil elastase is the main target for inactivation by α_1-antitrypsin and has relatively unopposed effects. However, evidence for a primary role of this enzyme in cigarette smoke–induced emphysema is less clear, so the focus has broadened to include examination of the role of the matrix metalloproteinases (MMPs), produced by macrophages and other cells, in emphysema.

The inflammation induced by cigarette smoke is a trigger of the cycle of protease release and lung destruction resulting in emphysema (E-Fig. 16.4). Macrophages are activated by cigarette smoke and recruit neutrophils and other inflammatory cells to the lung, leading to the release of elastase and MMPs. The destruction of elastin and other connective tissue elements in the lungs by these proteases leads over time to the loss of elastic recoil and destruction of alveolar structures characteristic of emphysema.

Cigarette smoke contains many oxidant molecules capable of inducing oxidative stress in the lung. Oxidative stress has diverse effects, including the oxidative inactivation of antiproteases in the lung and the acetylation of specific histones in the chromatin of lung cells and macrophages, allowing the expression of various pro-inflammatory genes. Histone deacetylase activity is reduced in COPD, and this in turn may result in an inability to control the pro-inflammatory response in this condition. Pro-inflammatory gene expression promotes cytokine production and release, contributing to further inflammatory cell recruitment and activation. Systemic inflammation, triggered by ongoing pulmonary inflammation, may lead to nonpulmonary abnormalities associated with emphysema, including cachexia and skeletal muscle alterations. Finally, increased apoptosis of pneumocytes and endothelial cells has been observed in lungs with emphysema and could contribute to the loss of alveoli.

Understanding of emphysema pathogenesis has improved with the recognition that inflammation, oxidative stress, protease-antiprotease balance, and apoptosis are linked in a complex interaction induced by cigarette smoke. This improved understanding has broadened the range of potential therapies that may be effective in ameliorating the destructive process. To date, however, therapies targeted at molecular pathways involved in emphysema pathogenesis have not been successful in altering disease progression, with the possible exception of α_1-antitrypsin replacement therapy in individuals with α_1-antitrypsin deficiency.

α_1-Antitrypsin, an acute phase reactant, is produced primarily in the liver, from which it travels to the lung. By its effect on elastases in the lung, α_1-antitrypsin prevents the uncontrolled degradation of elastin in the lung parenchyma and protects against the development of emphysema. Individuals with the ZZ genotype of α_1-antitrypsin deficiency produce mutant forms of α_1-antitrypsin that have a tendency to inappropriately polymerize within the hepatocyte, leading to a deficiency in secreted α_1-antitrypsin and, in some cases, collateral damage to the liver caused by accumulation of intracellular misfolded, mutant α_1-antitrypsin. Patients who develop emphysema at a young age (<40 years) should be evaluated for this condition whether or not they smoke, as should patients with bronchiectasis and unexplained liver disease or cirrhosis. Testing shows reduced α_1-antitrypsin levels. Genotyping can reveal specific mutations (most commonly ZZ in severe deficiency). α_1-Antitrypsin supplementation has been used for patients with α_1-antitrypsin deficiency and appears to result in a decreased loss of lung density (surrogate for emphysema) by computed tomographic measurement.

Large and Small Airways Disease in COPD

Chronic bronchitis often coincides with emphysema in patients with COPD, but it may occur independently from either emphysema or COPD and is defined in clinical terms (described earlier). Cigarette smoking is the major cause, although exposure to pollutants such as dust and smoke may play a role. Pathologic findings are goblet cell hyperplasia, mucus hypersecretion and plugging, and airway inflammation and fibrosis (Fig. 16.3).

The disease mechanisms involved in the development of emphysema are also important in the pathogenesis of chronic bronchitis. However, in contrast to emphysema, chronic bronchitis is a disease of the large airways and not of the lung parenchyma. Therefore, the relationship of chronic bronchitis to airflow obstruction is less robust than for emphysema, and airflow limitation consistent with COPD in a patient with symptoms of chronic bronchitis may be more reflective of concomitant emphysema and small airways disease. Inflammation in chronic bronchitis leads to effects on the airway epithelium, including excess mucus production and impairment in mucociliary clearance.

Neurogenic stimuli are also important in the pathogenesis of airway obstruction in chronic bronchitis. The conducting airways are surrounded by smooth muscle, which contains adrenergic and cholinergic receptors. Stimulation of β_2-adrenergic receptors by circulating catecholamines dilates airways, whereas stimulation of airway irritant receptors constricts airways through a cholinergic mechanism by means of the vagus nerve. The irritant bronchoconstrictive pathways are normally present to protect against inhalation of noxious agents, but in pathologic states these pathways may contribute to airway hyperreactivity. A host of endogenous chemical mediators such as proteases, growth factors, and cytokines can also affect airway tone.

By definition, the predominant symptom in chronic bronchitis is sputum production. Bronchospasm may also be prominent. Recurrent bacterial airway infections are typical. As with patients with COPD, the evaluation of patients with chronic bronchitis should include pulmonary function tests and a chest radiograph in addition to standard laboratory testing.

Damage to the small airways (those less than about 2 mm in diameter) is integral to the pathogenesis of COPD. The small airways are the major site of resistance to airflow in COPD. Respiratory bronchiolitis, in which there is an accumulation of pigmented macrophages in and around the bronchioles (E-Fig. 16.5), may be an incidental finding in asymptomatic smokers without COPD. However, as COPD develops, other inflammatory cells are recruited to the small conducting airways, presumably in reaction to ongoing irritation from cigarette smoke or inhaled particles. With inflammation, the small airways in COPD can be affected by remodeling, leading to airway wall thickening and fibrosis, smooth muscle hypertrophy, and airway luminal narrowing, all of which contribute to airflow obstruction. Mucus plugs and inflammatory exudates can occlude the small airways, leading to increased resistance to airflow.

Recently, demonstration of profound decreases in small airway numbers and cross-sectional area in lungs of individuals with COPD has provided important evidence that loss of the small airways occurs with sufficient severity to result in detectable expiratory airflow limitation that characterizes COPD. Indeed, there is evidence that small airway loss may precede emphysema development in COPD.

Immune-mediated abnormalities are also seen at the level of the small airways in COPD. Lymphoid follicles may form around these airways in response to ongoing antigenic stimulation and bacterial infection, with a prominence of B cells and CD8+ T cells in more advanced COPD. These myriad changes at the small airway level contribute significantly to the physiologic abnormalities and altered local immune response in COPD.

Clinical Presentation

COPD related to chronic tobacco exposure is characterized by slowly progressive dyspnea that is first noticed during exertion but progresses over years until it is evident with minimal exertion (e.g., when dressing) or even at rest. Affected individuals complain of exercise intolerance and fatigue, and the disease eventually may lead to weight loss, depression, and anxiety as a result of increased work of breathing. Chronic cough can be present and is productive or dry, depending on the degree of mucus secretion (e.g., chronic bronchitis).

During the early stages of COPD, the physical examination may be normal. Normal examination results and the absence of symptoms often delay diagnosis. Inspection of the thorax and palpation may fail to reveal findings. As the disease progresses, the lungs may become hyperresonant to percussion, and auscultation may show diminished breath sounds with rhonchi or wheezes. The chest wall may begin to remodel, giving the patient the appearance of a "barrel chest." During the late stages of COPD, patients show evidence of increased work of breathing with use of accessory muscles, pursed-lip breathing, and weight loss. Skeletal muscle wasting may also become evident. Despite their respiratory insufficiency, some patients are able to sustain relatively

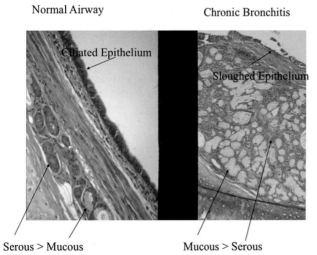

Normal Airway   Chronic Bronchitis

Ciliated Epithelium   Sloughed Epithelium

Serous > Mucous   Mucous > Serous

Fig. 16.3 Pathology of chronic bronchitis: Normally, airway submucosal serous glands outnumber mucous glands and the epithelium includes ciliated cells. In chronic bronchitis, mucous glands are more prevalent than serous glands and the epithelium is abnormal. (Courtesy Dr. Charles Kuhn.)

normal oxygen levels in blood until very late in the disease, leading to the classic clinical presentation of the "pink puffer." Other patients tend to retain carbon dioxide and diminish their work of breathing, resulting in chronic respiratory acidosis and, in extreme cases, polycythemia and cyanosis; this is the prototypical "blue bloater" phenotype. There is also an overlap of COPD with other respiratory disorders, such as obstructive sleep apnea, that may contribute to carbon dioxide retention.

Although COPD results in chronic, progressive dyspnea, periodic acute exacerbations are also characteristic. A rapid worsening of pulmonary function and an increased burden of respiratory symptoms such as dyspnea, cough, and sputum production characterize COPD exacerbations. Acute exacerbations are associated with various triggers, most importantly viral or bacterial respiratory infections, air pollution or other environmental factors, pulmonary embolism, and cardiac failure. Exacerbations are more common with increasing severity of COPD, with increasing age, and during the winter months. Exacerbations vary widely in severity. Severe exacerbations may lead to hospitalization, acute respiratory failure, and death. After an exacerbation, it may take weeks for the patient to return to a baseline level of function. Patients with frequent exacerbations of COPD experience an accelerated rate of decline in FEV_1. Patients who have experienced a COPD exacerbation are more likely to experience future exacerbations, suggesting that exacerbation is an important event in the natural history of COPD. On occasion, an exacerbation of COPD leading to acute respiratory failure is the first event leading to the diagnosis of COPD in an individual patient.

COPD is associated with a number of comorbid conditions, such as atherosclerotic heart disease, lung cancer, osteoporosis, and depression. These comorbidities may be related to smoking, to the chronic systemic inflammation present in patients with COPD, to the impaired quality of life resulting from COPD, or to treatments (e.g., corticosteroids) administered during the course of COPD. Monitoring for and appropriate management of these coexisting disorders is an important part of the ongoing assessment of patients with COPD.

As COPD progresses, the lung volumes increase (hyperinflation) and the diaphragms flatten, rendering inspiratory excursions inefficient. Tidal volume decreases and respiratory rate increases in an effort to decrease the work of breathing. In advanced disease, the cardiovascular system becomes affected as a result of the loss of vasculature in destroyed alveolar walls and vasoconstriction and vascular remodeling due to chronic hypoxia. With a limited area for blood flow, pulmonary vascular resistance is increased, leading to increased right ventricular afterload and development of pulmonary hypertension. This accelerates the development of right ventricular failure, which is referred to as cor pulmonale in the setting of lung disease. Right heart gallop, distended neck veins, hepatojugular reflux, and leg edema characterize cor pulmonale.

Diagnosis and Differential Diagnosis
Diagnosis
Pulmonary function tests, especially spirometry, are essential for the diagnosis of COPD. Classically, the diagnosis of COPD has been made using GOLD criteria, which defines COPD as an FEV_1/FVC ratio of less than 0.70 on post-bronchodilator spirometry. However, the American Thoracic Society (ATS)/European Respiratory Society (ERS) guidelines are coming into favor for diagnosing COPD. ATS/ERS defines COPD as FEV_1/FVC ratio less than the lower limit of normal based on the patient's sex and age. Although some degree of reversibility of the obstruction may be detected with bronchodilators, the obstructive defect is not entirely reversible in COPD. This characteristic and the consistent and progressive nature of the expiratory flow limitation

TABLE 16.2	GOLD Criteria
GOLD 1/mild COPD	$FEV_1 \geq 80\%$ predicted
GOLD 2/moderate COPD	$FEV_1 \geq 50\%$ but less than 80% predicted
GOLD 3/severe COPD	$FEV_1 \geq 30\%$ but less than 50% predicted
GOLD 4/very severe COPD	$FEV_1 < 30\%$ predicted

represent key features that help distinguish COPD from asthma, a major differential diagnostic consideration. The severity of disease and prognosis can be estimated by the FEV_1, as detailed in Table 16.2.

An FEV_1 of about 1 L (usually 50% predicted) suggests severe obstruction and, in the case of COPD, predicts a mean survival rate of 50% at 5 years. For a better predictor of mortality than FEV_1 alone, the BODE index can be used: body mass index, degree of obstruction as measured by FEV_1, modified Medical Research Council dyspnea score, and exercise capacity as denoted by 6-minute walk distance.

Lung volumes should be measured along with pulmonary function testing because the limitation to expired airflow and decreased elastic recoil lead to lung hyperinflation, as evidenced by increased RV, FRC, and, ultimately, TLC.

Destruction of alveoli decreases the surface area for gas exchange in emphysema. This loss of surface area, coupled with bronchial obstruction and altered distribution of ventilated air, results in ventilation-perfusion inequality or mismatch, a cause of hypoxemia. Hyperinflation leads to expansion of lung zone 1, the region of the lung in which alveolar pressure exceeds pulmonary arterial pressure. This process increases physiologic dead space because alveolar units ventilate areas that are not perfused. Hypercarbia can be avoided by increasing the minute ventilation, even with substantial ventilation-perfusion mismatching. However, eventually, the metabolic costs of increased ventilation become excessive, and respiratory muscles fatigue. Over time, chemoreceptors reset, allowing the level of partial pressure of carbon dioxide in arterial blood ($Paco_2$) to rise. Since $Paco_2$ is equal to alveolar partial pressure of carbon dioxide ($Paco_2$), the higher the $Paco_2$, the more CO_2 is exhaled with every breath, which increases the efficiency of ventilation. Significant individual variation is observed in relationship between the degree of mechanical impairment and in the magnitude of increase in $Paco_2$. Derangements in gas exchange can be detected by measuring arterial blood gases, by showing a decrease in Dl_{CO}, or by evaluating hemoglobin oxygen desaturation during exertion. The degree of decrease in Dl_{CO} correlates well with the radiologic extent of emphysema in COPD.

Chest radiography may fail to reveal abnormalities during the early stages of COPD, but in later stages, radiographic studies show hyperinflation, hyperlucency, flattening of the diaphragms, and bullous changes in lung parenchyma (E-Fig. 16.6). Pleural abnormalities, lymphadenopathy, and mediastinal widening are not characteristic of emphysema and should point to other diagnoses, such as lung cancer. Computed tomography is more sensitive than plain radiography because it allows for a more detailed evaluation of the lung parenchyma and surrounding structures. Computed tomography is useful in assessing the distribution of emphysema (E-Fig. 16.7) in patients for whom operative interventions such as lung volume reduction surgery are being contemplated (see later discussion). High-resolution CT is highly sensitive for the detection of occult emphysema and can reveal the pattern of emphysematous changes. Electrocardiography might show evidence of right ventricular strain. Echocardiography can reveal evidence of right ventricular hypertrophy or dilation and can often provide an estimate of pulmonary arterial pressures in patients with advanced COPD. A high blood hemoglobin level might reveal erythrocytosis in the setting of chronic hypoxemia, whereas increased white blood cell counts might suggest infection. The arterial blood gas analysis may show hypoxemia, hypercarbia, or both, whereas acidemia due to acute hypercarbia may be present during an exacerbation.

Differential Diagnosis

The differential diagnosis of COPD includes the other major obstructive lung disorders: asthma, bronchiectasis, and the bronchiolar disorders. Asthma can occur at any age and sometimes overlaps with COPD, such as in patients with childhood asthma who smoke as adults. However, patients with COPD are typically older than 40 years of age and have a lengthy smoking history, whereas patients with asthma often have a history of atopy, have more variable symptoms that are often worse at night, and typically have marked improvements in lung function after bronchodilator administration. Patients with asthma may have normal pulmonary function during periods in which their asthma is well controlled, whereas those with COPD demonstrate ongoing airway obstruction even during periods of relative clinical stability.

It can be difficult to distinguish COPD with chronic bronchitis from bronchiectasis, and HRCT is necessary to assess for the abnormal bronchial dilation that is diagnostic of bronchiectasis.

Bronchiolar disorders can also be difficult to distinguish from COPD but should be considered in patients with risk factors, such as connective tissue disease or occupational exposures. Again, more sophisticated testing, such as HRCT with inspiratory and expiratory views to demonstrate peripheral areas of gas trapping and centrilobular nodules consistent with mucus impaction of the small airways, or even lung biopsy, may be needed to diagnose bronchiolitis.

Nonpulmonary causes of dyspnea on exertion, such as congestive heart failure or coronary artery disease, should also be considered in the differential diagnosis of COPD.

Treatment and Prevention

Because a cure for COPD does not exist, the best approach to this condition is prevention. Most cases of COPD in the United States are caused by cigarette smoking. Therefore, an appropriate major emphasis has been placed on the development of community education programs that focus on smoking prevention and promote smoking cessation. Legislative measures banning smoking in various public settings and levying increased taxes on cigarettes have been used to diminish the effects of environmental or second-hand exposure to tobacco smoke and to discourage smoking. Although smoking cessation interventions are effective in only a minority of patients, smoking cessation decreases mortality in patients with COPD who do succeed in quitting.

Most patients who are successful at smoking cessation have had at least one prior failed attempt, so physicians should encourage smoking cessation with at least brief interventions at every opportunity, even in patients who have tried but failed to quit in the past. Long-term physician and group support increase the success of cessation attempts, and pharmacologic smoking cessation aides, including nicotine replacement with gum or transdermal patches, bupropion, and varenicline, may provide additional benefit. Although there is considerable interest in the potential benefits and risk of E-cigarettes, further study is required to define its role.

Pharmacologic Therapies

After a diagnosis of COPD is established, therapy is guided primarily by symptoms of dyspnea and frequency of exacerbations. Dyspnea is assessed using subjective scoring systems. Patients are considered to be higher risk if they have a high dyspnea score or if they have had either one hospitalization for COPD or two exacerbations not requiring hospitalization in the past year. Overall treatment is directed at avoiding complications such as exacerbations, relieving airflow obstruction

through use of bronchodilators, and providing supplemental oxygen to patients with hypoxemia. Commonly used inhaled bronchodilators include sympathomimetic agents (β_2-adrenoreceptor agonists) and anticholinergic agents. Ipratropium bromide, a short-acting anticholinergic agent, is effective at decreasing dyspnea and improving FEV_1 in COPD. Albuterol is the most commonly used β_2-agonist; its bronchodilator effect is rapid in onset and relatively short lived. In practice, a combination of albuterol and ipratropium is frequently prescribed because these agents produce greater benefits when used in combination than when used individually.

Short-acting agents are typically prescribed for patients with mild disease or intermittent symptoms on an as-needed basis. Short-acting bronchodilators can be delivered by metered-dose inhaler (MDI) or by nebulizer. The MDI offers advantages of portability and ease of administration and convenience. When used correctly with a spacer, MDIs are as effective as nebulizers in delivering the drug. Nebulization has no advantage over the use of MDIs in the long-term management of obstructive lung disease except in patients who are unable to use an MDI properly.

Long-acting bronchodilators are effective for maintenance therapy in patients who have at least moderate COPD. Long-acting agents include the long-acting β_2-agonists (LABAs), which are available in once- or twice-daily formulations, and the long-acting anticholinergic/muscarinic antagonists (LAMAs), which are administered once daily. There have been several large studies evaluating the efficacy of long-acting bronchodilators and inhaled corticosteroids (ICS) in COPD, as detailed in Table 16.3. Initiation of either a LABA or a LAMA is reasonable for patients with COPD who require a long-acting bronchodilator. In more advanced disease, there is some evidence of additional benefits from the combination of a LABA and a LAMA. Tachycardia, hypokalemia, and tremor are potential adverse effects of LABAs, whereas dry mouth and urinary retention may occur with LAMA administration.

Current data suggest that the chronic use of inhaled corticosteroids improves symptoms and decreases the frequency of exacerbations.

TABLE 16.3   Studies Evaluating the Efficacy of LABA, LAMA, and ICS

TORCH (2007): LABA/ICS vs ICS or LABA vs placebo	• n = 6112 • Length of study: 3 years • LABA/ICS associated with fewer COPD-related hospitalizations • No mortality benefit
INSPIRE (2007): LABA/ICS vs LAMA	• n = 1323 • Length of study: 2 years • No difference in exacerbation rates • More hospitalizations and deaths in LAMA group
UPLIFT (2008): LAMA vs placebo	• n = 5993 • Length of study: 4 years • No difference in decline of FEV_1
SPARK (2013): LAMA/LABA vs LAMA or LABA	• n = 2224 • Length of study: 64 weeks • LAMA/LABA was associated with fewer exacerbations than single agent
FLAME (2016): LABA/LAMA vs LABA/ICS	• n = 3362 • Length of study: 1 year • LABA/LAMA was associated with fewer COPD-related hospitalizations

Inhaled long-acting corticosteroids (e.g., beclomethasone, budesonide, fluticasone propionate) should be considered for individuals with COPD and a history of exacerbations but should not be used as monotherapy. Inhaled corticosteroids are less clearly effective in COPD than in asthma, and pneumonia occurs more frequently in patients with COPD treated with inhaled corticosteroids. Inhaled corticosteroids can be combined with LABAs; the combination salmeterol with fluticasone in patients with moderate to severe COPD was shown to improve health-related quality of life and to reduce exacerbations to a greater extent than either component alone.

Systemic use of corticosteroids is indicated during acute exacerbations, and intravenous corticosteroids are useful in the acute setting. Intravenous corticosteroids have also proved effective for the management of acute exacerbations of most obstructive lung diseases, including asthma (Fig. 16.4). Patients with acute exacerbations are usually transitioned from intravenous to oral steroids within 72 hours. While oral steroids were historically tapered over 14 days, more recent research suggests that a 5-day "burst" of steroids without a taper is noninferior to traditional tapering regimens. Other agents with anti-inflammatory capabilities, such as leukotriene inhibitors, are not indicated for treatment of COPD.

Theophylline, a methylxanthine, is a weak systemic sympathomimetic agent with a narrow therapeutic window. It is not a first-line drug in the treatment of COPD, although long-acting derivatives with improved safety profiles have been developed. Theophylline preparations have some anti-inflammatory activity and may provide additional bronchodilation in patients with COPD who do not respond adequately to inhaled β-agonists. When these preparations are used, blood concentrations should be maintained in the lower end of the therapeutic range (between 8 and 12 μg/mL). Toxicity is common at concentrations higher than 20 μg/mL. The metabolism of theophylline is decreased by many commonly used drugs (e.g., erythromycin), and toxic serum concentrations of theophylline can be reached quickly when these other drugs are administered unless the theophylline dose is adjusted appropriately. Toxic effects of theophylline may be observed in the gastrointestinal, cardiac, and neurologic systems. Severe theophylline toxicity can be fatal, and treatment with charcoal hemoperfusion may be required.

Phosphodiesterase type 4 (PDE4) inhibitors have been investigated for the treatment of COPD, and an oral PDE4 inhibitor was recently approved as add-on therapy for treatment of severe COPD with chronic bronchitis and a history of exacerbations. PDE4 inhibitors act to inhibit breakdown of cyclic adenosine monophosphate (cAMP), resulting in a weak bronchodilator effect (approximately 50 mL improvement in FEV_1); they should not be used as acute bronchodilators. However, roflumilast was demonstrated to reduce exacerbation rates in patients who had severe COPD with chronic bronchitis and a history of exacerbation in the prior year and were not using inhaled corticosteroids. Adverse effects include weight loss, nausea and loss of appetite, and an increase in psychiatric adverse reactions including suicidality.

Oxygen Therapy and Mechanical Ventilation

Continuous oxygen therapy has been shown to improve survival in patients with COPD and hypoxemia. Oxygen supplementation is recommended once the partial pressure of oxygen in arterial blood (Pao_2) drops below 55 mm Hg or the hemoglobin oxygen saturation decreases to 88%. Oxygen supplementation is indicated at higher levels of Pao_2 if end-organ damage, such as pulmonary hypertension, is present.

Oxygen therapy is frequently necessary for treatment of acute exacerbations of obstructive lung disease. In patients who hypoventilate chronically and therefore have an elevated $Paco_2$, elevating the inspired oxygen content may acutely worsen hypercarbia by inhibiting

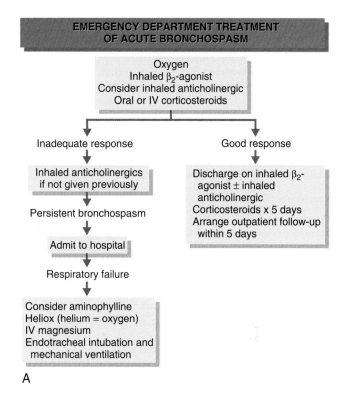

A

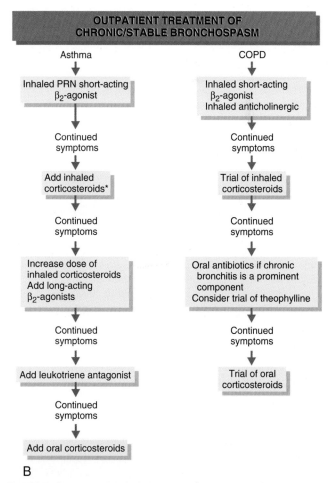

B

Fig. 16.4 Algorithms for the treatment of bronchospasm in patients in the emergency department (A) and in outpatients with stable disease (B). *IV,* Intravenous; *PRN,* as needed. *Leukotriene antagonists could be considered.

the hypoxic ventilatory drive and by promoting the dissociation of carbon dioxide from oxygenated hemoglobin (the Haldane effect). High-flow oxygen has been shown to be harmful in the setting of pre-hospital emergency treatment for COPD. Therefore, oxygen should be closely titrated to maintain normoxia and to avoid either hypoxemia or excessively elevated Pao_2. An oxygen saturation of 90% to 92% is a reasonable target in the absence of further data. During exacerbations of COPD leading to hypercarbic respiratory failure, noninvasive positive airway pressure ventilation has proved useful in reducing the work of breathing, alleviating diaphragm fatigue, and reducing the need for endotracheal intubation and mechanical ventilation.

Antibiotics

Exacerbations of airway obstruction may result most often from viral infections but also from bacterial infection. The most common bacterial pathogens in COPD are *Streptococcus pneumoniae, Haemophilus influenzae,* and *Moraxella catarrhalis.* Management of acute exacerbations with dyspnea and increased volume and purulence of mucus should include empiric administration of antibiotics, which have been shown to improve the success rate in exacerbation treatment. The role of chronic prophylactic antibiotic use in COPD is uncertain, and a trial of oral azithromycin resulted in a reduction in exacerbations but an increased risk of hearing loss. Immunization with influenza vaccines directed at specific epidemic strains reduces exacerbations of COPD. Pneumococcal vaccination is also recommended in patients with COPD.

Nonpharmacologic Therapies

Multiple airway clearance techniques aid in clearing of airway secretions, but their effectiveness in the management of emphysema and other obstructive lung diseases in adults is questionable. If needed, chest physiotherapy and postural drainage might be useful in patients with chronic bronchitis and increased sputum production. Few data support the use of specific mucolytics or expectorant agents for patients with COPD.

Patients with pulmonary disease of sufficient severity to compromise normal activities of daily living commonly demonstrate improved quality of life and less subjective dyspnea when enrolled in a comprehensive, high-quality pulmonary rehabilitation program. Pulmonary rehabilitation has not been shown to improve objective measures of pulmonary function, to affect the rate of decline in lung function, or to improve survival. However, it has been shown to improve the quality of life in motivated patients. An important part of pulmonary rehabilitation is nutritional assessment and careful attention to maintaining adequate nutrition. Malnutrition and cachexia are common in later stages of obstructive lung disease, and they result in decreased respiratory muscle strength and compromised immune function.

The role of surgery in COPD is generally limited. Bullectomy, lung volume reduction surgery (LVRS), and lung transplantation are all potentially effective surgical options for selected patients. Resection of nonfunctional areas of lung (e.g., bullectomy) may allow for compressed functional areas to expand and may improve symptoms, airflow, and oxygenation by improving ventilation-perfusion matching in a subgroup of patients. In addition, resection of bullae can decrease lung volumes, resulting in enhanced diaphragmatic function and decreased work of breathing. The best candidates for LVRS are those with predominantly upper lobe disease who have a low exercise tolerance despite rehabilitation and are without other major comorbidities. This subgroup may have reduced mortality after LVRS. In general, a high surgical mortality risk exists in patients referred for LVRS who have an FEV_1 or DLco of less than 20% predicted and in those who have more homogeneous distribution of emphysema. Patients with

high surgical risk may be candidates for endoscopic placement of endobronchial valves (EBV), which were FDA approved in 2018. EBVs are one-way valves that aim to deflate emphysematous regions of the lung by allowing air to flow out of but not into the affected alveoli.

Single or bilateral lung transplantation is an option for patients with end-stage airflow obstruction. The average survival after lung transplantation is 4 to 5 years. Rejection, viral infections, transplant-associated lymphoproliferative disease, and late occurrence of bronchiolitis obliterans remain significant problems, but the procedure can improve the quality of life in properly selected patients.

Palliative Care

Although the disease course can be unpredictable, discussion of end-of-life issues with the patient is an important component of longitudinal care as COPD progresses to an advanced stage. Preparation of advance directives regarding use of intensive care measures at the end of life may be desirable. Opioid narcotics can be highly effective for relieving dyspnea in patients with terminal complications of COPD.

Prognosis

COPD is a chronic and progressive disease with a variable and typically prolonged clinical course. As discussed previously, measurement of lung function (FEV_1 % predicted) has prognostic significance, and use of the multifactorial BODE index can improve prognostication compared with use of FEV_1 alone. Patients who have frequent exacerbations of COPD appear to have more rapid loss of lung function than those without exacerbations, suggesting that frequent exacerbations result in a worse clinical course.

At present, aside from smoking cessation and the addition of long-term oxygen therapy for patients with hypoxemia, interventions to improve survival in COPD are limited. No pharmacologic therapy for COPD has been definitively demonstrated to improve survival. In mild COPD, mortality is frequently related to comorbidities such as ischemic heart disease and lung cancer; in more advanced stages, a greater proportion of patients die from respiratory causes.

BRONCHIOLAR DISORDERS

Definition and Epidemiology

The bronchioles are defined as the small noncartilaginous airways (<2 mm in diameter). The bronchiolar disorders encompass a spectrum of diseases of widely varying causes primarily affecting these small airways. Bronchiolar disorders can be associated with cigarette smoking. For example, small airways disease contributes significantly to the syndrome of COPD. Respiratory bronchiolitis is also commonly found incidentally in smokers. However, bronchiolar disorders with etiologies other than cigarette smoking also exist. Bronchiolar disorders are associated with patchy inflammation and epithelial injury, fibrosis, mucoid impaction, or obliteration of the bronchioles (E-Fig. 16.8). These changes result in airflow limitation due to increased airway resistance.

Acute bronchiolitis related to respiratory syncytial virus infection is epidemic among infants and young children, but primary bronchiolar disorders, including infectious or postinfectious bronchiolitis, are rare in the adult general population and tend to affect specific patient populations.

Pathology

The pathology of the bronchiolar disorders is complex. A variety of terms are used to describe or classify the various histopathologic patterns of small airways disease, including *cellular bronchiolitis* (inflammatory cell infiltration of the small airway wall resulting in small airway narrowing), *follicular bronchiolitis* (formation of abundant lymphoid follicles in close apposition to the small airways, resulting in airway compression), *obliterative* or *constrictive bronchiolitis* (fibrosis surrounding the small airways resulting in narrowing of the affected airways), and *bronchiolitis obliterans* (formation of endoluminal fibrous lesions, sometimes called *Masson bodies*, obstructing the small airway lumen). The histopathologic pattern of small airways disease may suggest a likely underlying etiology; for example, follicular bronchiolitis is often, although not exclusively, seen in the context of Sjögren's syndrome.

Clinical Presentation

In general, the bronchiolar disorders manifest nonspecifically with dyspnea, which may be severe or progressive, and in some cases accompanied by cough or sputum production. The physical examination may reveal inspiratory squeaks or wheezes but may be surprisingly normal. The possibility of a bronchiolar disorder should be considered in particular settings. For example, bronchiolitis may complicate the course of rheumatoid arthritis, Sjögren's syndrome, or inflammatory bowel disease.

Diffuse panbronchiolitis is a rare idiopathic disorder most common in Japan that is characterized by cough with purulent sputum, sinusitis, and dyspnea. Recurrent respiratory infections with bacterial organisms such as *Pseudomonas aeruginosa* complicate the course of diffuse panbronchiolitis.

Bronchiolitis obliterans can be a clinical syndrome (in addition to a histopathologic term) that is associated with chronic allograft rejection after lung transplantation, graft-versus-host disease after allogeneic hematopoietic stem cell transplantation, and occupational toxin exposures. For example, occupational clusters of bronchiolitis obliterans have been described after exposure to diacetyl, a flavoring chemical used in the manufacture of microwave popcorn. Constrictive bronchiolitis can be seen in war veterans who were exposed to burn pits in Iraq or Afghanistan.

Diagnosis and Differential Diagnosis

In general, the bronchiolar disorders cause an obstructive pattern of expiratory airflow limitation on pulmonary function testing without evidence of reversibility. The bronchiolitis obliterans syndrome is diagnosed clinically by a decline in FEV_1 of 20% from a stable baseline value on serial testing after lung transplantation. HRCT is valuable in the diagnosis and assessment of the bronchiolar disorders. Characteristic findings on HRCT include centrilobular nodules or tree-in-bud opacities, reflecting impacted inflammatory exudates or sloughed epithelial cells in the bronchioles. A "mosaic attenuation" pattern, with decreased attenuation in geographic regions of lung reflecting areas of air trapping distal to obstructed bronchioles, is often seen on inspiration. CT scanning during the expiratory phase can confirm that this finding is caused by air trapping rather than decreased perfusion from pulmonary vascular disease. Lung biopsy may be of limited value because of the scattered, patchy nature of the abnormalities present in the bronchiolar disorders. The differential diagnosis includes COPD, which also causes poorly reversible obstruction on spirometry.

Treatment

Treatment of the bronchiolar disorders is challenging. Acute bronchiolitis typically resolves without treatment; bronchodilators and steroids are not clearly beneficial, although they are often prescribed. The bronchiolitis obliterans syndrome responds poorly to increased immunosuppression and is a frequent cause of death after lung transplantation. Azithromycin has been reported to increase FEV_1 in the

bronchiolitis obliterans syndrome. Macrolide antibiotics have also been reported to positively affect the clinical course of diffuse panbronchiolitis, possibly reflecting immunomodulatory or antifibrotic effects of these medications. Lung transplantation may be necessary in progressive bronchiolitis obliterans, and retransplantation has sometimes been performed in patients affected by the bronchiolitis obliterans syndrome after transplant rejection.

Prognosis

These disorders may be self-limited, as in acute bronchiolitis caused by respiratory syncytial virus, or relentlessly progressive and fatal, as in the bronchiolitis obliterans syndrome occurring after lung transplantation.

BRONCHIECTASIS

Definition and Epidemiology

Bronchiectasis (E-Fig. 16.9) is defined as an abnormal dilation of the bronchi (the large airways containing cartilage within their walls) resulting from inflammation and permanent destructive changes of the bronchial walls. The incidence of bronchiectasis is unknown, but it may affect more than 100,000 individuals in the United States and is more frequent in older age groups. There is likely a higher incidence of bronchiectasis in developing countries where there are lower childhood vaccination rates and a higher prevalence of pulmonary tuberculosis.

Pathology

Bronchiectasis may be localized to a bronchial segment or lobe of the lung, or it may be diffuse. The involved bronchi are abnormally dilated and demonstrate chronic inflammation within the bronchial wall with neutrophilic inflammation and bacterial colonization and infection in the bronchial lumen. The inflammation in bronchiectasis is associated with structural changes in the walls of the bronchi, including destructive changes affecting the elastic fibers, smooth muscle, and cartilage. As with COPD, there is also involvement of the small airways. Small airway obstruction leads to increased resistance to airflow that results in airflow obstruction despite the dilation of the larger airways. The classic pathologic classifications of bronchiectasis are *tubular* (the most common form, in which there is smooth dilation of the bronchi), *varicose* (dilated bronchi with indentations reminiscent of varicose veins), and *cystic* (end-stage bronchiectasis with dilated bronchi ending in sac-like structures resembling clusters of grapes).

Bronchiectasis is hypothesized to result from an environmental insult leading to bronchial damage in a susceptible host. This in turn leads to impaired infection clearance, bacterial colonization and infection or reinfection, ongoing inflammation of the airways, and further bronchial damage, creating a classic vicious cycle. An inciting infection, sometimes occurring in childhood, is thought to initiate the development of bronchial damage leading to bronchiectasis in many cases (postinfectious bronchiectasis). This may be a viral infection (e.g., measles), a necrotizing pneumonia (e.g., *Staphylococcus aureus* pneumonia), tuberculosis, or infection with an atypical mycobacteria (e.g., *Mycobacterium avium-intracellulare*). Because infections such as *M. avium-intracellulare* also complicate the course of bronchiectasis, determination of whether a mycobacterial infection was an initiator or a consequence of bronchiectasis may be difficult.

Localized bronchiectasis may also result from anatomic obstruction by an endobronchial foreign body, tumor, or broncholith or from extrinsic compression by lymphadenopathy. Right middle lobe syndrome, for example, results from narrowing of the right middle lobe bronchial orifice, often by lymph node enlargement in the setting of tuberculosis, which leads to localized bronchiectasis distal to the site of obstruction. Anatomic obstruction results in chronic or recurrent bacterial infections and inflammation leading to bronchial distortion and destruction over time.

Diffuse bronchiectasis can result from various impairments in host defenses that create a vulnerability to persistent or recurrent lung infection leading to bronchial damage. For example, bronchiectasis may occur with congenital defects that impair mucus clearance in the airways such as CF (discussed later) or primary ciliary dyskinesia, a rare inherited abnormality of the ciliary microtubules (the classic triad of sinusitis, situs inversus, and infertility is diagnostic of Kartagener's syndrome, a form of primary ciliary dyskinesia). Immunodeficiency states, such as hypogammaglobulinemia in combined variable immunodeficiency, may also result in bronchiectasis. α_1-Antitrypsin deficiency is also associated with bronchiectasis. Bronchiectasis also complicates certain connective tissue disorders such as rheumatoid arthritis.

Finally, bronchiectasis overlaps with the more common obstructive lung disorders, COPD and asthma. Certain patients with COPD also have bronchiectasis, often in the lower lobes. Allergic bronchopulmonary aspergillosis is a condition that occurs in asthmatics with hypersensitivity to aspergillus fungi. It is associated with central bronchiectasis, high levels of immunoglobulin E (IgE), and precipitins for *Aspergillus* species.

Clinical Presentation

Patients with bronchiectasis exhibit chronic cough and copious, sometimes foul-smelling sputum. The sputum produced may be greater in volume and purulence than with COPD or asthma. Shortness of breath and fatigue may also be present. Blood-streaked sputum is common, and massive hemoptysis may occur during the course of bronchiectasis. Localized crackles and clubbing may be present. Periodic exacerbations due to infection with bacterial pathogens, including *H. influenzae* and *P. aeruginosa*, are common. Nontuberculous mycobacterial colonization or infection may also occur. Pulmonary function tests typically show mild to moderate obstruction. Evidence of bronchial hyperresponsiveness may occur.

Diagnosis and Differential Diagnosis

Chest radiographs may be normal or may show increased interstitial markings. The classic finding is parallel lines in peripheral lung fields, described as "tram tracks," which represent thickened bronchial walls that do not taper from proximal to distal sites. However, HRCT is more sensitive for the detection of dilated airways and is the diagnostic test of choice in the evaluation of suspected bronchiectasis. Bronchiectasis on HRCT is diagnosed by demonstration of lack of airway tapering, airways that are larger in diameter than their accompanying blood vessel, and the presence of visible bronchi at the lung periphery (outer 1 to 2 cm of the lung). Bronchoscopy may be indicated in localized bronchiectasis to assess for endobronchial abnormalities or foreign body. Sputum can be cultured to assess for fungal or mycobacterial organisms that may be causative or for identification of specific bacterial pathogens during exacerbations. Once the diagnosis of bronchiectasis is established, investigation to determine the underlying cause, such as assessment of immunoglobulin levels to rule out combined variable immunodeficiency, is indicated.

The differential diagnosis includes chronic bronchitis and COPD, asthma, and, in the setting of hemoptysis and clubbing, lung cancer.

Treatment

Treatment of the underlying cause of the bronchiectasis should be undertaken if possible. An anatomic obstruction, such as from a foreign body or benign tumor, should be relieved. Atypical mycobacterial infection should be treated with an appropriate multidrug regimen in symptomatic patients after confirmation of the diagnosis with multiple smears and cultures. Allergic bronchopulmonary aspergillosis is typically treated with corticosteroids; addition of azole antifungals may also be beneficial. Bacterial exacerbations of bronchiectasis should be treated with a broad-spectrum antibiotic that is effective against the likely pathogens, such as amoxicillin or, in patients known to be colonized or infected by *Pseudomonas*, a fluoroquinolone. Aerosolized antibiotics are of benefit to suppress bacterial growth in bronchiectasis associated with CF and may be beneficial in non-CF bronchiectasis if *Pseudomonas* infection is present or if frequent exacerbations occur. Chronic administration of macrolide antibiotics has been shown to reduce inflammation and exacerbations in bronchiectasis but may also promote development of macrolide-resistant bacteria. Immunoglobulin supplementation may aid in the host defense against bacterial infection in individuals with hypogammaglobulinemia.

Airway clearance and postural drainage are the mainstays of treatment in bronchiectasis (discussed in further detail under CF). Bronchodilators may provide symptomatic relief. Massive hemoptysis should be managed with airway protection and identification of the bleeding site; bronchial artery angiography with embolization of the causative bleeding vessels can be life-saving. The role of surgery is mainly in resection of obstructing lesions that are causing distal bronchiectasis, in removal of a badly damaged isolated segment of bronchiectatic lung, and, on occasion, as a salvage therapy in resection of a site with uncontrolled hemorrhage.

Prognosis

The prognosis of patients with bronchiectasis is generally thought to be favorable, although deterioration of lung function over time has been shown to occur. Quality of life may be affected adversely, for example by chronic production of copious sputum or frequent exacerbations. Massive hemoptysis is an emergency situation that requires intensive management and may be fatal.

CYSTIC FIBROSIS

Definition and Epidemiology

CF is an autosomal recessive genetic disorder that results from mutations in the *CFTR* gene. CF affects about 30,000 children and adults in the United States and 70,000 worldwide. This disorder affects many organs, including the lungs, pancreas, and reproductive organs, although most mortality related to CF is due to lung disease. It is the most common lethal genetic disorder in the Caucasian population, with a carrier frequency of about 1 in 29, affecting 1 in 3300 live births. About 1000 new cases of CF are diagnosed each year. Although 75% of patients with CF are diagnosed during their first two years of life, some patients are not diagnosed until adulthood. The prognosis has improved significantly with recent advances in therapy. Before 1940, infants with CF rarely lived to their first birthday, but today more than half of the CF population in the United States is older than 18 years of age. Currently, the median predicted life span for a person with CF is about 37 years.

Pathology

CF results from pathogenic mutations in both alleles of a single gene, *CTFR*, which encodes the CF transmembrane conductance regulator (CFTR), a cAMP-regulated chloride channel that is present on the apical surface of epithelial cells (E-Fig. 16.10). The most common mutation is the ΔF508 mutation, a three-base-pair deletion that results in absence of the phenylalanine residue at the 508 position of the protein. However, more than 1900 mutations in CFTR have been identified to date. These mutations are categorized into five different classes based on their effects on CFTR. Class I and II mutations result in CFTR that is not present on the cell surface due to impaired translation or protein misfolding. Class III and IV mutations are associated with CFTR that is present on the cell surface but has abnormal function due to a gating defect or decreased conductivity. Class V mutations are associated with reduced expression of normally functioning CFTR.

Abnormal, reduced, or absent CFTR protein results in defective chloride transport and increased sodium reabsorption in airway and ductal epithelia; this leads to abnormally thick and viscous secretions in the respiratory, hepatobiliary, gastrointestinal, and reproductive tracts. The thick secretions do not easily clear from the airways, resulting in respiratory symptoms, and cause luminal obstruction and destruction of exocrine ducts in other organs, leading to exocrine organ fibrosis and dysfunction, including pancreatic damage.

Poor airway clearance predisposes CF patients to recurrent bacterial infection and eventual colonization with microorganisms such as *S. aureus* and *H. influenzae,* followed by *P. aeruginosa* in ensuing years. Persistent inflammation and infection cause bronchial wall destruction and bronchiectasis. Mucus plugging of small airways results in postobstructive cystic bronchiectasis and parenchymal destruction, progressive airflow obstruction, and eventually hypoxemia. The course of CF may additionally be complicated by the development of allergic bronchopulmonary aspergillosis or by nontuberculous mycobacterial infection. Colonization and infection with multidrug-resistant organisms such as the *Burkholderia cepacia* complex may occur in advanced CF, creating challenging management issues. The most common cause of death in CF is respiratory failure.

Clinical Presentation

Neonatal screening programs for CF exist nationwide in the United States to identify infants with possible CF who should undergo further testing (e.g., genotyping). Infants with CF may have meconium ileus or failure to thrive with steatorrhea. Salty-tasting skin may be noticed by caregivers. Patients with CF typically have chronic cough with thick sputum production, wheezing, and dyspnea. Pancreatic insufficiency and diabetes are common, and male patients may have azoospermia. Nasal polyps are often present, and clubbing is typical.

CF should be considered in the differential diagnosis of patients with unexplained chronic sinus disease, bronchiectasis, pancreatitis, malabsorption, or male infertility associated with absence of the vas deferens. Pulmonary function tests demonstrate hyperinflation and obstruction, with or without a bronchodilator response. Chest imaging studies show hyperinflation, bronchial wall thickening, and bronchiectasis.

Diagnosis and Differential Diagnosis

Measurement of the concentration of chloride in sweat (sweat test) is used to diagnose CF. The diagnosis is considered definitive if the clinical picture is consistent with CF and if the chloride concentration measured in a certified laboratory is greater than 60 mEq/L on at least two occasions. Genotyping can also confirm the diagnosis if known mutations are identified in both gene alleles and may be used if sweat testing is equivocal.

Treatment

The hallmark of CF treatment is aggressive airway hygiene. A typical airway clearance routine includes a series of therapies in the following order: First, patients use bronchodilators such as albuterol or ipratropium. Next, patients can use nebulized hypertonic (7%) saline to hydrate and loosen secretions, followed by aerosolized recombinant human deoxyribonuclease I (Dornase alfa) to decrease sputum viscosity. Then

patients should utilize a mechanical airway clearance technique. The specific technique is usually determined by patient preference. Available options include a vibratory vest, intrapulmonary percussive ventilation, or manual chest physiotherapy. The goal of the mechanical airway clearance techniques is to induce productive cough to clear mucous from the airways as much as possible. Lastly, patients can administer inhaled antibiotics (if applicable), such as tobramycin, colistin, or aztreonam, followed by inhaled steroids such as fluticasone propionate or budesonide.

Inhaled antibiotics are reserved for patients who are colonized with *Pseudomonas.* Inhaled tobramycin has been available as a nebulized solution since 1997 and as a dry powder inhaler since 2013. Inhaled tobramycin is typically prescribed as a 28-day course every other month. More recently, inhaled colistin and aztreonam have become available and can be used during tobramycin "off-months" or as alternatives to tobramycin if the patient is experiencing intolerable side effects or if their *Pseudomonal* resistance pattern warrants alternate therapy. Chronic anti-inflammatory therapy with azithromycin may be helpful in certain patients with CF.

Since 2012, there have been significant advancements in the treatment of CF due to the development of CFTR modulator drugs. As of 2019, there are three modulator therapies available, ivacaftor (Kalydeco®), lumacaftor/ivacaftor (Orkambi®), and tezacaftor/ivacaftor (Symdeko®). Ivacaftor is used in patients with class III genetic mutations. Ivacaftor binds CFTR causing the defective channel to remain open thus enabling chloride transport. In a large clinical trial, ivacaftor reduced sweat chloride by about 50%, increased FEV_1 by about 10%, and cut the incidence of pulmonary exacerbations in half. Ivacaftor can also be used in certain patients with class V mutations by increasing chloride transport through functioning CFTR to compensate for the reduced expression of these proteins.

Lumacaftor aids proper folding of CFTR and is used in combination with ivacaftor to treat patients who are homozygous for ΔF508 (class II mutation). Lumacaftor/ivacaftor was shown in clinical trials to improve FEV_1, increase BMI, and reduce pulmonary exacerbations. A common side effect of lumacaftor-ivacaftor is chest discomfort.

Tezacaftor can also be used in combination with ivacaftor in homozygous ΔF508 patients who cannot tolerate lumacaftor/ivacaftor due to side effects. In addition, tezacaftor/ivacaftor can also be used in patients with certain class II mutations other than ΔF508.

The first triple combination drug, Trikafta, was developed by adding elexacaftor to ivacaftor/tezacaftor. Trikafta was FDA approved in 2019 for patients with at least one ΔF508 mutation. It was shown to be superior to the other CF modulator therapies in improvement of lung function and quality of life as well as reduction in sweat chloride and frequency of exacerbations. As with other obstructive lung diseases, the ultimate therapy for patients with CF and end-stage lung disease is bilateral lung transplantation.

Prognosis

Although CF is still considered to be a fatal disease, significant advancements in therapy have led to considerable improvement in median survival time.

ASTHMA

Definition and Epidemiology

Asthma is described by the Global Initiative for Asthma as "a chronic inflammatory disorder of the airways in which many cells and cellular elements play a role. The chronic inflammation is associated with airway hyperresponsiveness that leads to recurrent episodes of wheezing, breathlessness, chest tightness, and coughing, particularly at night or in the early morning. These episodes are usually associated with widespread but variable airflow obstruction within the lung that is often reversible either spontaneously or with treatment."

The incidence of asthma is highest in children, but it affects all ages and occurs worldwide, with a preponderance of the disease in developed industrialized countries. Asthma affects millions of individuals worldwide. In the United States in 2017, 7.9% of the population (approximately 25,000,000 persons) were estimated to have asthma according to the Centers for Disease Control and Prevention. The prevalence of asthma has increased markedly over recent decades. Nevertheless, after rising in the late 20th century, the number of deaths from asthma has declined since 2000. Asthma death rates are higher in older age groups, females, and blacks.

Pathology

Underlying chronic airway inflammation is considered to be a major pathogenic feature of asthma. Patients with asthma have higher numbers of activated inflammatory cells within the airway wall, and the epithelium is typically infiltrated with eosinophils, mast cells, macrophages, and T lymphocytes, which produce multiple soluble mediators such as cytokines, leukotrienes, and bradykinins. Airway inflammation in asthma is typified by a type 2 helper T-cell (T_H2) response with predominantly eosinophilic inflammation, but some patients with severe asthma exhibit neutrophilic airway inflammation and cytokine production more characteristic of T_H1 inflammation.

The hallmark of asthma is airway hyperresponsiveness—a tendency of the airway smooth muscle to constrict in response to levels of inhaled allergens or irritants that would not typically elicit such a response in normal hosts. Inhaled allergens provoke airway mast cell degranulation by binding to and cross-linking IgE on the mast cell surface. Mast cell degranulation leads to the release of chemical mediators, which cause acute bronchoconstriction and thus increased airway resistance and wheezing as well as mucus hypersecretion (E-Fig. 16.11). Disruption of the continuity of the ciliated columnar epithelium and increased vascularity and edema of the airway wall also follow antigen exposure. In addition to allergens, factors such as stimulation of irritant receptors, respiratory tract infections, and airway cooling can provoke bronchoconstriction in asthmatic individuals. Airway cooling appears to be responsible for exercise-induced bronchoconstriction as well as some wintertime asthma attacks.

Asthma is associated with airway wall remodeling, which is characterized by hyperplasia and hypertrophy of smooth muscle cells (E-Fig. 16.12), edema, inflammatory infiltration, angiogenesis, and increased deposition of connective tissue components such as type I and type III collagen. This last effect leads not only to a thickening of the subepithelial lamina reticularis (E-Fig. 16.13) but also to an expansion of the entire airway wall. Airway remodeling may begin fairly early in the course of the disease. Whether inflammation leads to remodeling or whether these processes represent two independent manifestations of the disease is unknown. Pulmonary function does seem to decline at an accelerated rate in patients with asthma, and airway wall remodeling may play a role in this functional loss. Over time, airway wall remodeling may lead to irreversible airflow limitation, which can worsen the disease by rendering bronchodilator drugs less effective. In this way, airway wall remodeling may make the clinical distinction between asthma and COPD difficult.

The cause of asthma is unknown, but it is likely to be a polygenic disease influenced by environmental factors. Atopy is strongly linked to asthma. Exposure to indoor allergens such as dust mites, cockroaches, furry pets, and fungi is a significant factor; outdoor pollution and other irritants, including cigarette smoke, are also important.

Current concepts of asthma pathogenesis include a focus on impairment of the shift from a T_H2-predominant immunity to a T_H1 immune response early in life. Paradoxically, in the developed world, the perpetuation of T_H2 immune responses and the development of inappropriate allergic responses may be related to a relative lack of exposure of the immune system to appropriate infectious antigenic stimuli in childhood, the so-called hygiene hypothesis. Farming, for example, appears to be protective against the development of asthma and allergic disease, possibly in part because of the increased exposure to microbial antigens eliciting a T_H1 response. Increased exposure to other children (as in daycare settings) and less frequent use of antibiotics may also decrease asthma risk. On the other hand, asthma is common in poor urban settings in which there is heavy exposure to allergic antigens from dust mites and cockroaches. The timing and roles of particular environmental exposures in utero and in early life in the pathogenesis of asthma and allergic diseases remain to be fully elucidated, and there is no current theory that completely explains asthma pathogenesis or the recent increased incidence of asthma. The interplay of other aspects of modern life, such as changes in the microbiome, with regard to asthma propensity continues to be explored.

Several genetic polymorphisms have been associated with asthma, including variations in the β-adrenergic receptor leading to diminished responsiveness to β-agonists. Identification of other genetic polymorphisms that are important in asthma is a subject of ongoing research. Although asthma is more common in male children than in female children, the prevalence of asthma changes after puberty, and it is more common in adult women than in men. These facts, along with evidence of variation in asthma symptoms during the menstrual cycle and during pregnancy, suggest possible hormonal influences on asthma pathogenesis.

Asthma can be induced by workplace exposures in persons having no previous history of asthma (occupational asthma). Certain substances, such as isocyanates (used in spray paints) and Western red cedar wood dust, are provocative agents for the development of occupational asthma. Obesity has been linked to a higher incidence of asthma though the mechanisms by which obesity may influence asthma development remain unclear. Other potentiators of acute bronchospasm include viral infections, gastroesophageal reflux disease (GERD), and exposure to gases or fumes. These disorders may play a role in asthma development and may be targeted for therapy in some cases of asthma.

Clinical Presentation

Major symptoms of asthma are wheezing, episodic dyspnea, chest tightness, and cough. The clinical manifestations vary widely, from mild intermittent symptoms to catastrophic attacks resulting in asphyxiation and death. Although wheezing is not a pathognomonic feature of asthma, in the setting of a compatible clinical picture, asthma is the most common diagnosis. Often symptoms worsen at night or during the early hours of the morning. Other associated symptoms are sputum production and chest pain or tightness. Patients may exhibit only one or a combination of symptoms, such as chronic cough only (cough-variant asthma). Wheezing may occur several minutes after exercise (exercise-induced bronchoconstriction). Physical examination typically shows evidence of wheezing, although findings may be normal in between symptomatic periods. Rhinitis or nasal polyps may be present. In the case of an acute episode of bronchospasm or an exacerbation, the clinician may find that the patient has difficulty talking, is using accessory muscles of inspiration, has pulsus paradoxus, is diaphoretic, and has mental status changes ranging from agitation to somnolence. In patients with these findings, treatment should be immediate and aggressive.

Diagnosis and Differential Diagnosis

A diagnosis of asthma requires documentation of bronchial hyperreactivity and reversible airway obstruction. The history may provide sufficient documentation because most patients complain of characteristic periodic episodes of wheezing and other symptoms that respond to use of a bronchodilator. However, spirometry is recommended to assess formally for expiratory flow limitation, and reversibility is demonstrated by repeat spirometry after bronchodilator administration. At least 12% and 200 mL improvement in FEV_1 after bronchodilator use indicates reversibility. Because asthma is episodic, airflow limitation is variable and patients may exhibit symptoms at a time when spirometry cannot be performed. Peak expiratory flow measurements can be performed at home and may be helpful in establishing evidence of variability in expiratory flow.

Depending on the circumstances, formal testing for airway hyperactivity by bronchoprovocation challenge may be necessary. A stimulant with bronchoconstrictor activity, most commonly methacholine, is applied to the patient's airway. Methacholine, a synthetic form of acetylcholine, is preferred to histamine because there are fewer systemic side effects. Exercise can also be used to trigger an attack. Although most patients with or without asthma develop some degree of airflow limitation during bronchoprovocation testing, those with asthma develop airflow limitation at much lower doses. For a methacholine challenge, the concentration of methacholine required to produce a 20% decline in FEV_1 from baseline is reported. Although a positive bronchoprovocation challenge result is not by itself diagnostic of asthma, a negative result is helpful in ruling out asthma as a diagnosis.

Lung volume measurements may show hyperinflation during active disease, but the DLCO is typically normal or even elevated. During acute exacerbations of asthma, analysis of arterial blood gases is useful to determine gas-exchange status. A chest radiograph should be obtained if a concern for pulmonary infection exists, but routine chest radiography is not necessary. Fleeting or migratory infiltrates on chest radiographs in a patient with difficult asthma should suggest the possibility of allergic bronchopulmonary aspergillosis. Blood tests in asthma might reveal eosinophilia and increased levels of IgE. Skin tests might be useful to identify household products or other antigens that could precipitate asthma attacks in a specific patient.

The differential diagnosis includes tracheal disorders, respiratory tract tumors and foreign bodies, COPD, and bronchiectasis. In patients whose primary presenting complaint is chronic cough, the differential diagnosis includes other causes of chronic cough, such as GERD and postnasal drip. A major differential consideration in patients not responding to typical asthma treatment is vocal cord dysfunction.

Treatment

Simple, inexpensive peak expiratory flow meters can be used at home to monitor airflow obstruction. A diary should be maintained, and a clear written plan should be in place for using symptoms and peak flow information to intervene early in exacerbations and to tailor long-term therapy for optimal control of symptoms. Short-acting β-agonists are used for acute relief of symptoms such as wheezing. However, the cornerstone of maintenance therapy in all but mild intermittent asthma is administration of inhaled corticosteroids, which are highly effective in improving asthma control. Long-acting β-agonists may be added for additional symptomatic control as needed. LABAs should not be used as a monotherapy for asthma control because they do not control airway inflammation and increased mortality has been demonstrated with this therapeutic approach. However, these medications may be added to inhaled corticosteroids to provide additional symptom control.

Alternatively, leukotriene modifiers can be used in maintenance therapy, although they appear to be somewhat less effective than inhaled corticosteroids (see Fig. 16.4). Theophylline preparations may have additional benefit in some patients, but the narrow therapeutic window and modest efficacy of this drug limits its value. Recent evidence suggests that use of long-acting anticholinergics in patients with poor control on LABAs and inhaled corticosteroids may increase the time to exacerbation and provide additional bronchodilation. Oral or intravenous corticosteroids are used during acute asthma exacerbations. Long-term use of oral corticosteroids should be avoided, if possible, given the various side effects associated with chronic glucocorticoid administration.

Patients with severe refractory asthma who frequently require systemic corticosteroids might benefit from a monoclonal antibody therapy. Targets of monoclonal antibodies include IgE (omalizumab), IL-5 (mepolizumab, reslizumab), and IL-4 (dupilumab). Patients with poorly controlled asthma are candidates for anti-IgE therapy if they have elevated total IgE levels and positive allergy skin or radioallergosorbent testing (RAST). Patients are candidates for anti-IL-5 or anti-IL-4 therapy if they have peripheral eosinophilia.

Allergen avoidance is a reasonable measure in asthma, although the effects of specific interventions, such as mattress barrier protection to reduce dust mite exposure, appear limited. Treatment of associated conditions that may exacerbate asthma, such as allergic rhinitis and GERD, may be clinically beneficial and may aid in achieving asthma control. Bronchial thermoplasty is a new endoscopic technique in which radiofrequency energy delivered in a series of treatments is used to destroy airway smooth muscle. It has been shown to reduce exacerbations and improve quality of life in the months following treatment.

Acute severe asthma, or status asthmaticus, is an attack of severe bronchospasm that is unresponsive to routine therapy. Such attacks may be sudden (hyperacute asthma) and can be rapidly fatal, often before medical care can be obtained. In most cases, however, patients have a history of progressive dyspnea over hours to days, with increasing bronchodilator use. Treatment of status asthmaticus should be aggressive, including administration of nebulized bronchodilators and intravenous steroids. Heliox can be used in severe causes of asthma, which is a mixture of oxygen and helium (typically 70% helium and 30% oxygen) that promotes laminar flow rather than turbulent flow of gas through the airways. Continuous monitoring of blood oxygen saturation by pulse oximetry should be performed, often supplemented by arterial blood gas analysis to evaluate for hypercarbia. A rising $Paco_2$ in a patient with asthma is an ominous sign and may portend need for ventilatory support. Noninvasive ventilation has been used successfully to decrease the work of breathing and avoid the need for endotracheal intubation in patients with exacerbations of asthma, but intubation and mechanical ventilation are necessary for the management of respiratory failure in status asthmaticus. Mechanical ventilation of the patient with status asthmaticus can be extremely challenging and may require the use of paralytic agents to control the breathing pattern or even use of inhaled general anesthesia to relieve bronchospasm. Lastly, if a patient is unable to maintain adequate oxygenation with maximal ventilator support, extracorporeal membrane oxygenation (ECMO) can be considered.

Prognosis

The prognosis in most patients with asthma is excellent. Although there is no cure, most patients can achieve appropriate control of their asthma.

❖   For a deeper discussion on this topic, please see Chapter 81 ("Asthma"), Chapter 82 ("Chronic Obstructive Pulmonary Disease"), Chapter 83 ("Cystic Fibrosis"), and Chapter 84 ("Bronchiectasis, Atelectasis, Cysts, and Localized Lung Disorders") in *Goldman-Cecil Medicine*, 26th Edition.

SUGGESTED READINGS

Buist AS, McBurnie MA, Vollmer WM, et al: On behalf of the BOLD Collaborative Research Group: International variation in the prevalence of COPD (the BOLD Study): a population-based prevalence study, Lancet 370:741–750, 2007.

Burgel P-R, Bergeron A, de Blic J, et al: Small airways diseases, excluding asthma and COPD: an overview, Eur Respir Rev 22:131–147, 2013.

Decramer M, Janssens W, Miravitlles M: Chronic obstructive pulmonary disease, Lancet 379:1341–1351, 2012.

Global Initiative for Asthma: GINA report: global strategy for asthma management and prevention (updated 2012), Available at: http://www.ginasthma.org. Accessed August 29, 2014.

Global Initiative for Chronic Obstructive Lung Disease: Global strategy for the diagnosis, management, and prevention of chronic obstructive pulmonary disease (updated 2013), Available at: http://www.goldcopd.org. Accessed August 29, 2014.

Kim V, Criner GJ: Chronic bronchitis and chronic obstructive pulmonary disease, Am J Respir Crit Care Med 187:228–237, 2013.

King PT: The pathophysiology of bronchiectasis, Int J COPD 4:411–419, 2009.

McDonough JE, Yuan R, Suzuki M, et al: Small-airway obstruction and emphysema in chronic obstructive pulmonary disease, N Engl J Med 365:1567–1575, 2011.

Mogayzel PJ, Naureckas ET, Robinson KA, et al, and the Pulmonary Clinical Practice Guidelines Committee: Cystic fibrosis pulmonary guidelines: chronic medications for maintenance of lung health, Am J Respir Crit Care Med 187:680–689, 2013.

Pasteur MC, Bilton D, Hill AT: On behalf of the British Thoracic Society Bronchiectasis (Non-CF) Guideline Group: British Thoracic Society guideline for non-CF bronchiectasis, Thorax 65:i1–i58, 2010.

Ren CL, Morgan RL, Oermann C, et al: Cystic fibrosis pulmonary guidelines: use of cftr modulator therapy in patients with cystic fibrosis, Ann Am Thorac Soc, 2018.

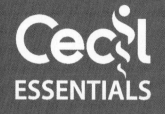

17

Interstitial Lung Diseases

Abhinav Kumar Misra, Matthew D. Jankowich, Barry S. Shea

OVERVIEW

The interstitial lung diseases (ILDs) are a heterogenous group of non-malignant and noninfectious lung diseases characterized by varying amounts of inflammation and/or fibrosis (scarring) of the lung parenchyma. The lung involvement in these disorders is often diffuse but can occur in a wide array of patterns. The disease process can involve any part of the anatomic lung interstitium, including that within the alveolar walls, the intra- and interlobular septa, and the airways. However, it can also involve the air spaces and airway lumens themselves, and therefore the term *interstitial* lung disease is somewhat misleading. *Diffuse parenchymal* lung disease (DPLD) is the more accurate name for this collection of disorders, but for the sake of convention, we will refer to them as ILDs throughout this chapter.

Well over 100 distinct ILDs have been described, and there is no universally accepted classification system. One useful way of approaching ILDs is to consider them as all belonging to one of three broad categories: (1) exposure-related ILDs, (2) ILDs attributable to systemic diseases, and (3) idiopathic ILDs (Table 17.1). Exposure-related ILDs can be broadly thought of as those ILDs caused by environmental and occupational exposures (e.g., hypersensitivity pneumonitis, pneumoconiosis), iatrogenic exposures (e.g., drug-induced ILD, radiation pneumonitis or fibrosis), or intentional exposures (e.g., cigarette smoking, inhalational drug use). The most common systemic diseases known to cause ILD are the connective tissue diseases (e.g., rheumatoid arthritis, systemic sclerosis, and polymyositis/dermatomyositis), but there are many others, including the vasculitides, amyloidosis, sarcoidosis, and a variety of genetic conditions (e.g., lysosomal storage diseases). Idiopathic ILDs are those for which a specific cause is unknown or not identified. Most of the idiopathic ILDs fall into a group of clinicopathologic entities known as the idiopathic interstitial pneumonias (IIPs), but there are some additional isolated ILDs that are also idiopathic (e.g., eosinophilic PNA, pulmonary alveolar proteinosis).

TABLE 17.1 Categories of Interstitial Lung Diseases

Idiopathic ILDs	Exposure-Related ILDs	Systemic Disease-Associated ILDs
Idiopathic interstitial pneumonias	Environmental and occupational exposures	Connective tissue diseases
Idiopathic pulmonary fibrosis (IPF)	Hypersensitivity pneumonitis (see Table 17.3)	Rheumatoid arthritis
Idiopathic nonspecific interstitial pneumonia (NSIP)	Pneumoconioses	Systemic sclerosis
Acute interstitial pneumonia (AIP)	Silicosis	Polymyositis and dermatomyositis
Cryptogenic organizing pneumonia (COP)	Asbestosis	Sjögren syndrome
Respiratory bronchiolitis–interstitial lung disease (RB-ILD)	Coal-worker's pneumoconiosis	Systemic lupus erythematosus
Desquamative interstitial pneumonia (DIP)	Berylliosis	Mixed connective tissue disease
Idiopathic lymphoid interstitial pneumonia (LIP)	Talc pneumoconiosis	Vasculitides
Idiopathic pleuroparenchymal fibroelastosis (IPPFE)	Hard metal pneumoconiosis	Granulomatosis with polyangiitis (GPA)
Eosinophilic pneumonia (acute and chronic)	Iatrogenic exposures	Microscopic polyangiitis (MPA)
Pulmonary alveolar proteinosis	Radiation-induced lung injury	Eosinophilic granulomatosis with polyangiitis (EGPA)
	Drug-induced lung injury (see Table 17.4)	Anti-glomerular basement membrane (anti-GBM) disease
	Antineoplastic therapies	Pauci-immune pulmonary capillaritis
	Biological agents	Sarcoidosis
	Cardiovascular drugs	Amyloidosis
	Antimicrobials	Lymphangioleiomyomatosis (LAM)
	Anti-inflammatory agents	Neurofibromatosis
	Intentional exposures	Hermansky-Pudlak syndrome
	Cigarette smoking	Inborn errors of metabolism
	Pulmonary Langerhans cell histiocytosis (PLCH)	Niemann-Pick disease
	Vaping associated pulmonary illness (VAPI)	Gaucher's disease
	Illicit drug use	
	"Crack lung"	
	Foreign body granulomatosis	
	Inhalational talcosis	

Because ILDs comprise a broad spectrum of disorders, the symptoms, exam findings, and physiologic, radiographic, and histologic abnormalities associated with them can vary greatly. Dyspnea on exertion and chronic cough are the two most common symptoms encountered in ILD patients, although these are nonspecific. These symptoms can often be insidious and progressive, and in many cases they can be present for months to years before a diagnosis is made. Exertional dyspnea can lead to exercise limitation, and in many cases patients, family members, and providers attribute such limitations to other factors, including aging, weight gain, and deconditioning. The presence of unexplained and gradually progressive dyspnea on exertion, with or without a persistent dry cough, should alert the clinician to the possibility of ILD. Other symptoms, such as wheezing, chest pain, hemoptysis, or constitutional symptoms are less common but can occur, and when present these symptoms may be clues to a specific diagnosis or class of ILDs. Most forms of ILD are chronic and progressive, but others can have more acute or subacute presentations and can be difficult to distinguish from infectious pneumonia. Waxing and waning symptoms can occur and are often associated with ILD caused by intermittent exposures. Some patients are asymptomatic and are diagnosed with ILD as an incidental finding on chest imaging done for other reasons (e.g., lung cancer screening).

Basic demographic factors such as age, sex, and race can provide some clues in determining potential causes of ILD. For example, idiopathic pulmonary fibrosis (IPF) is more common in men than in women and its incidence increases with age; it is only very rarely diagnosed in individuals under the age of 50 years. In contrast, connective tissue disease–associated ILD (CTD-ILD) tends to be more common in women and can occur often in young adults and even in the pediatric population. Inherited forms of ILD (Gaucher disease, Neiman-Pick disease) are also more likely in younger patients. Sporadic lymphangiomyomatosis (LAM) occurs almost exclusively in premenopausal women, sarcoidosis occurs more frequently in African Americans, and pulmonary Langerhans cell histiocytosis (LCH) is more common in young or middle-aged male smokers.

The history can further narrow the differential diagnosis for suspected ILD. Important factors to specifically query include rash, skin thickening, arthritis, myalgias or proximal muscle weakness, dysphagia, and Raynaud's phenomenon, any of which may suggest an underlying connective tissue disease. If a patient with ILD carries a known diagnosis of connective tissue disease, the work-up may be limited if imaging findings are typical of the pulmonary manifestations of that disease. A history of severe or poorly controlled asthma for a patient with radiographic infiltrates and constitutional symptoms should lead to consideration of eosinophilic granulomatosis with polyangiitis (EGPA), whereas a history of severe sinus disease should raise the possibility of granulomatosis with polyangiitis (GPA).

A detailed exposure history, including both domestic and occupational environmental exposures, is also important when evaluating a patient with ILD. For example, routine exposure to domestic birds, hot tubs, molds, or farming environments may suggest hypersensitivity pneumonitis. Home visits can also be informative here. Although the pneumoconioses due to asbestos and silica exposure are becoming much less common with modern safeguards and restrictions, these diseases continue to manifest long after exposure. High-technology manufacturing has particular hazards, such as beryllium exposure leading to berylliosis in susceptible individuals.

A medication exposure history is also important, and drug-induced ILD should be considered for all patients with diffuse lung disease seen on imaging. Smoking history is important because several ILDs are seen almost exclusively in cigarette smokers, including respiratory bronchiolitis–associated interstitial lung disease, desquamative interstitial pneumonia, and pulmonary LCH. Cigarette smoking and inorganic dust exposure also appear to be risk factors for the development of IPF. Acute and subacute ILD has also been described as a consequence of smoking or inhaling a variety of substances, including marijuana, synthetic cannabinoids, "crack" cocaine, and more recently electronic cigarettes.

Physical exam findings can also vary greatly. The most common finding is the presence of inspiratory crackles on lung exam, often most pronounced in the lung bases. Wheezing can be heard and can be a clue towards specific diagnoses (e.g., hypersensitivity pneumonitis), or it can be a sign of concomitant asthma or COPD. Some patients exhibit digital clubbing, focal enlargement of the terminal aspects of the fingers and/or toes with an unclear pathogenesis. Although this finding should prompt the clinician to suspect the presence of ILD, it can also be seen in other conditions, and it is of unknown significance. Exam findings of pulmonary hypertension with cor pulmonale (peripheral edema, loud P_2) can be seen in more advanced disease or can suggest the presence of a disorder known to cause both ILD and pulmonary vascular disease (e.g., systemic sclerosis). Similarly, extrapulmonary exam findings, such as synovitis, sclerodactyly, telangiectasias, mechanic's hands, muscle weakness, or lymphadenopathy can also provide important clues to a potential cause of ILD. In some cases the physical exam, including lung auscultation, can be entirely normal.

Pulmonary function testing (PFT) in ILDs generally reflects the pattern and severity of the disease process. Since most ILDs involve some combination of alveolar wall thickening and loss of functional air spaces, impaired gas exchange (reduced diffusion capacity for carbon monoxide, D_{LCO}) and evidence of restriction (reduced total lung capacity, TLC) are the most common abnormalities seen. The ratio of forced expiratory volume in 1 second to forced vital capacity (FEV_1/FVC) is generally preserved (i.e., no obstruction to airflow), although obstruction can also be seen when there is prominent airways involvement, such as with hypersensitivity pneumonitis, sarcoidosis, and lymphangioleiomyomatosis. An isolated reduction in the D_{LCO} may be the only obvious PFT abnormality in early or mild disease. In these cases the oxygen saturation may be normal at rest, but exercise oximetry may reveal the presence of exertional hypoxemia. Routine laboratory testing is often normal but some abnormalities, if present, can provide important clues to a specific diagnosis (e.g., peripheral eosinophilia, elevated serum creatinine). Detailed serologic testing to look for evidence of an underlying autoimmune or other systemic disease known to cause ILD is often performed.

Plain radiographs of the chest can provide evidence suggesting the presence of ILD, and in some cases can also help to establish a more definitive diagnosis, but high-resolution computed tomography (HRCT) of the chest provides much more detailed information and is almost always indicated in these cases. A variety of abnormalities can be seen on HRCT in ILD, including reticular, ground-glass, nodular, and consolidative opacities, mosaic attenuation, and honeycombing, and specific combinations and distributions of these abnormalities can often provide useful information when trying to determine a specific diagnosis. Certain HRCT patterns can often allow the diagnostic considerations to be significantly narrowed, and in some cases the HRCT pattern can be essentially pathognomonic for a particular disease. For example, a finding of bilateral, upper lung zone predominant peribronchovascular opacities with perifissural nodules and mediastinal and hilar lymphadenopathy would be highly suggestive of ILD due to sarcoidosis. Hypersensitivity pneumonitis (HP), pneumoconiosis, and lymphangioleiomyomatosis also tend to be upper lung zone predominant ILDs. Pulmonary LCH has a characteristic pattern of irregular nodules and thick-walled cysts in the mid to upper lung zones bilaterally, that when seen in a young-to-middle-aged active cigarette smoker can be viewed as confirmatory of the diagnosis. Other forms of ILD are often more pronounced in the lower lung zones, and there can be other features that suggest different diagnoses (e.g., honeycombing with IPF and subpleural sparing with NSIP). The presence of bilateral calcified pleural plaques can be strongly suggestive of asbestosis as the cause of ILD.

In many cases of ILD, a definitive diagnosis can be made on the basis of the medical history, physical exam, laboratory and physiological testing, and HRCT, often in the context of a multidisciplinary approach. However, in some cases this information is insufficient, and a lung biopsy is needed to obtain a lung tissue sample for histologic evaluation. Surgical lung biopsy (SLB), typically using a thoracoscopic approach, is the preferred method for evaluating most forms of ILD. Bronchoscopic transbronchial lung biopsy (TBLB) is less invasive but yields much smaller fragments of tissue, typically too small to allow appropriate examination of the lung architecture. TBLB is not recommended for the assessment of suspected IPF and many other forms of chronic fibrosing ILD, but it can be useful for diagnosing certain ILDs, most notably sarcoidosis and HP. Transbronchial lung cryobiopsy, which is less invasive than SLB but provides larger samples of lung tissue than those obtained with TBLB, is currently in use in many centers, but its exact role in tissue diagnosis of ILD remains unclear.

The lung's response to injury is relatively stereotyped, and particular biopsy patterns of injury, such as usual interstitial pneumonia or granulomatous inflammation, are seen in a variety of disorders. Interpretation of lung biopsy results must be done in the appropriate context and with incorporation of clinical and imaging data. For example, a biopsy result of usual interstitial pneumonia may carry a different prognosis in the setting of rheumatoid arthritis–associated ILD than in the setting of IPF.

Management of ILD depends on the specific disease, and treatments appropriate to specific entities are discussed throughout this chapter. Historically, pharmacologic therapy has largely consisted of glucocorticoids and other immunosuppressive agents, an approach that seems to be effective for those ILDs with a significant inflammatory component but is of unclear benefit when fibrosis predominates. More recently, antifibrotics have been developed that appear to be effective at slowing the progression of IPF and some other chronic fibrotic ILDs. Other key aspects of ILD management include exposure avoidance (particularly for exposure-related ILDs, such as HP, smoking-related ILD, and drug-induced ILD), supplemental oxygen, and pulmonary rehabilitation. Lung transplantation can be performed in patients who have advanced disease that is expected to severely limit life expectancy, but unfortunately many patients are not candidates for lung transplant due to age or other comorbidities. Even then there is a scarcity of suitable donor lungs available such that every year many patients die while on lung transplant waiting lists.

The remainder of this chapter is organized around the three broad categories of ILDs described above: idiopathic ILDs, exposure-related ILD, and ILDs due to systemic diseases.

IDIOPATHIC INTERSTITIAL LUNG DISEASES

Idiopathic Interstitial Pneumonias

The idiopathic interstitial pneumonias (IIPs) are a group of ILDs of unknown origin, each of which has distinct clinicopathologic features. For several decades, these conditions were generally considered to be different variations of idiopathic pulmonary fibrosis (IPF). However, with growing appreciation that the different radiographic and histologic patterns of disease had distinct clinical presentations, natural histories, and responses to treatment, they were formally reclassified as IIPs by the American Thoracic Society (ATS) and European Respiratory

TABLE 17.2 Idiopathic Interstitial Pneumonias (IIPs)

Major IIPs	
Chronic fibrosing	Idiopathic pulmonary fibrosis (IPF)
	Idiopathic nonspecific interstitial pneumonia (NSIP)
Acute/Subacute	Cryptogenic organizing pneumonia (COP)
	Acute interstitial pneumonia (AIP)
Smoking-related	Respiratory bronchiolitis–interstitial lung disease (RB-ILD)
	Desquamative interstitial pneumonia (DIP)
Rare IIPs	Idiopathic lymphoid interstitial pneumonia (LIP)
	Idiopathic pleuroparenchymal fibroelastosis (IPPFE)
Unclassifiable IIP	

Society (ERS) in 2002. This classification scheme was updated in 2013, at which time these entities were divided into major IIPs, rare IIPs, and unclassifiable IIPs (Table 17.2). The 6 major IIPs are IPF, idiopathic nonspecific interstitial pneumonia (NSIP), respiratory bronchiolitis–associated interstitial lung disease (RB-ILD), desquamative interstitial pneumonia (DIP), cryptogenic organizing pneumonia (COP), and acute interstitial pneumonia (AIP), and these can be further characterized as chronic fibrosing IPs (IPF and NSIP), smoking-related IPs (RB-ILD and DIP), and acute/subacute IPs (COP and AIP) (see Table 17.2). Rare IIPs include idiopathic lymphoid interstitial pneumonia (LIP) and idiopathic pleuroparenchymal fibroelastosis (PPFE). Some patients have idiopathic interstitial lung disease that does not meet criteria for any of these entities, and they are considered to have unclassifiable IIP.

Idiopathic Pulmonary Fibrosis

Definition, epidemiology, and pathogenesis. IPF has been defined in a consensus statement as a "specific form of chronic, progressive fibrosing interstitial pneumonia of unknown cause, occurring primarily in older adults, limited to the lungs, and associated with the histopathologic and/or radiologic pattern of usual interstitial pneumonia (UIP)." It is the most common of the IIPs, with an estimated incidence of 16.3 per 100,000 person years and prevalence of 42.7 per 100,000 people in the United States as of 2000, which translates to an estimated 89,000 individuals in the United States living with IPF at that time. The incidence of IPF appears to be increasing worldwide. There are likely many factors contributing to this increasing incidence, and one factor may be the overall aging of the world's population. Age is the single biggest risk factor for IPF, as many studies have shown that the incidence and prevalence increases steadily during each decade of life. It is only rarely diagnosed before the age of 50 years. Cigarette smoking has also been strongly associated with the development of IPF, as up to two thirds of IPF patients are current or former smokers. Other potential risk factors include exposure to inorganic and organic dusts and gastroesophageal reflux disease (GERD), the latter of which may lead to repetitive lung injury from recurrent microaspiration.

There is growing understanding of the role that genetics plays in IPF. Numerous genetic polymorphisms have been found to increase the risk of developing IPF. Most notably, a common polymorphism in the promoter region of the *MUC5B* gene has been found to confer a 5-fold and 18-fold increased risk of developing IPF when one or two copies of the risk allele are present, respectively. The fact that a family history of pulmonary fibrosis has also been increasingly recognized as an important risk factor for IPF also underscores the important genetic contribution to the disease. Some studies have suggested that up to 20% of cases may be familial (i.e., occurring in two or more first-degree relatives). The nomenclature of the familial form(s) of the disease is evolving; it has been referred to as familial IPF, familial pulmonary fibrosis (FPF), and familial interstitial pneumonia (FIP), the latter term reflecting the fact that in some cases the radiographic and/or histologic pattern of disease can be more suggestive of one of the other types of IIP rather than IPF. The familial form of the disease is often inherited in mendelian fashion, and specific causative mutations have been identified in 20% to 30% of these families, most commonly in the telomerase complex genes but also in the surfactant protein genes.

The pathogenesis of IPF is complex. Although it was for many years thought of as a disease driven by chronic inflammation, the paucity of inflammation seen on histologic sample from IPF lungs and the lack of response to aggressive anti-inflammatory therapy challenged this notion. It is now thought instead to be a disease characterized by aberrant or dysregulated wound-healing responses to repetitive lung injury. This current paradigm of IPF pathogenesis suggests that a complex interaction between host susceptibility (aging, genetics) and environmental factors (cigarette smoking, inhaled particulates, etc.) is ultimately what leads to the development of IPF. This shift in the understanding of IPF as being driven by aberrant wound-healing rather than chronic inflammation has also been important in leading to the discovery of effective therapies for this disease, as discussed below.

Pathology. The underlying histopathologic pattern found in the lungs of patients with IPF is called *usual interstitial pneumonia* (UIP). The characteristic histologic features of UIP include scar tissue deposition that is predominantly peripheral and patchy, with areas of fibrosis interspersed with areas with relatively normal lung (Fig. 17.1), along with fibroblastic foci, which are areas of active fibroblast proliferation and are thought to be the "leading edge" of fibrosis development. There is generally a paucity of inflammation, and in areas of more advanced fibrosis, microscopic honeycombing is often seen. Importantly, this UIP pattern can be seen in other disorders (e.g., connective tissue disease–related ILD and asbestosis), and therefore the diagnosis of IPF depends on not only identifying UIP, but also ruling out known causes of that histologic pattern (i.e., IPF is *idiopathic* UIP).

Clinical presentation. IPF is characterized by progressive accumulation of scar tissue in the lungs. As a consequence, patients typically present with insidious, gradually worsening dyspnea on exertion and a nonproductive cough. Symptoms are frequently present for 1 to 2 years before a diagnosis is made, although in some cases they can progress more slowly or more rapidly. Some patients with IPF are asymptomatic, and the disease is discovered because of abnormal physical exam findings or as an incidental finding on chest imaging studies done for other reasons (e.g., lung cancer screening).

Physical examination often reveals inspiratory crackles in the bases of both lungs, indicating the predominant site of scarring. Clubbing may exist, but extrapulmonary findings are generally absent. With increased scar deposition, the lungs become stiffer, as evidenced by decreased compliance. Pulmonary function tests show decreased lung volumes consistent with a restrictive process, and the D_{LCO} is generally reduced. Impaired oxygenation in IPF, initially with exercise and later at rest, often requires long-term oxygen supplementation.

The chest radiograph shows reticular opacities that are most predominant at the bases and the periphery of the lungs. HRCT allows better visualization of the lung and is useful in evaluating the extent and pattern of disease. The classic HRCT findings of IPF are bilateral, subpleural reticular opacities that are more pronounced in the lower lung zones, along with areas of radiographic honeycombing and traction bronchiectasis and bronchiolectasis (Fig. 17.2) in the absence of

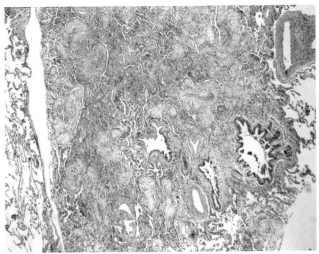

Fig. 17.1 Pulmonary fibrosis in idiopathic pulmonary fibrosis with usual interstitial pneumonia pathology that is adjacent to normal lung parenchyma. (Courtesy Dr. Charles Kuhn.)

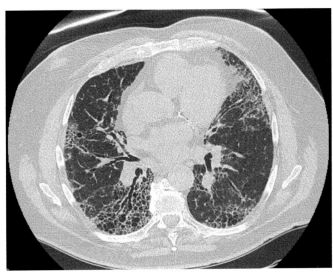

Fig. 17.2 Typical usual interstitial pneumonia (UIP) pattern of abnormality seen on chest computed tomography (CT) of a patient with IPF, demonstrating patchy, bilateral areas of subpleural reticulation, traction bronchiectasis and bronchiolectasis, and honeycombing.

significant ground-glass opacification, nodules, consolidation, or other features that suggest an alternative diagnosis. When these features are present on an HRCT in the absence of other abnormalities that suggest an alternative diagnosis (e.g., extensive ground-glass opacification, diffuse nodules or areas of consolidation), then a confident diagnosis of a UIP pattern can often be made without the need for a lung biopsy. In other cases when the HRCT pattern is not as definitive, a lung biopsy may be required to help distinguish UIP/IPF from other types of ILD.

Diagnosis and differential diagnosis. IPF is diagnosed on the basis of typical clinical, radiographic (HRCT), and if available, pathologic features (i.e., biopsy showing a UIP pattern). Other potential causes of ILD, such as connective tissue disease, hypersensitivity pneumonitis, and asbestosis, must be ruled out as best as possible by the history, examination, and selected laboratory testing. When an HRCT scan shows the typical UIP pattern described above (lower lung zone predominant, subpleural reticular opacities with areas of honeycombing) and no feature to suggest an alterative diagnosis, a diagnosis of IPF can be made without the need for a surgical lung biopsy. If honeycombing is absent on HRCT or atypical features such as ground-glass infiltrates, consolidation, diffuse nodules, or extensive air trapping are found, the radiographic diagnosis becomes less certain. In these cases, a lung biopsy may be indicated, and incorporation of the clinical, HRCT, and histologic information are then needed to make a diagnosis of IPF. Multidisciplinary discussion during the diagnostic process, with input from experienced clinicians, radiologists, and pathologists, is ideal.

Treatment. For decades there were no pharmacologic therapies that were proven to be helpful at slowing the progression of IPF. However, with improved understanding of IPF pathogenesis (described above), many novel therapies that target aberrant wound-healing responses have been studied in IPF. Two such therapies, pirfenidone (multiple mechanisms of action) and nintedanib (inhibits intracellular signaling of fibroblasts), have been shown in large randomized controlled trials to slow IPF progression by approximately 50%. In 2014, these drugs became the first ever to be approved by the US Food and Drug Administration (FDA) for treatment of IPF. Importantly, neither nintedanib or pirfenidone reverses established fibrosis or even completely stops the progression of the disease. Therefore, these treatments do not cure IPF, nor do they alleviate the symptoms of breathlessness or coughing, both of which can be debilitating. As such, the search for other potentially effective therapies for IPF is an area of intense ongoing investigation.

Because IPF is a progressive disease, even despite the availability of effective antifibrotic therapies, lung transplantation should be considered for patients with IPF. Many patients with IPF are not candidates for lung transplantation because of age, comorbidities, or other factors, but for those who are candidates, lung transplant may offer a chance at prolonged survival and improved quality of life. The median survival rate after lung transplant is only about 5.8 years, but this is steadily improving and still compares favorably to the expected survival of IPF patients at or near the top of lung transplant waiting lists, which is likely only weeks to months. Because of the unpredictable nature of disease progression in IPF, early referral for transplantation evaluation should be considered.

Prognosis. IPF is a progressive disease, and historically it has carried a poor prognosis. Median survival is often reported to be 2 to 3 years from the time of diagnosis. It is likely that the median survival will be prolonged in the era of antifibrotic therapy, but as stated, these therapies still do not cure the disease. There is considerable heterogeneity in the pace of progression in IPF, as the rate of lung function decline varies greatly between different individuals with the disease and even within any given patient over time. Furthermore, some patients with IPF experience acute or subacute respiratory deterioration in the absence of any clinically apparent superimposed cause (e.g., heart failure, pulmonary embolism, pneumonia). These episodes of acute deterioration are referred to as acute exacerbations of IPF and are associated with a very poor prognosis. HRCT findings include new ground-glass opacities and/or consolidation superimposed on the background of pulmonary fibrosis. Histologically, evidence of acute lung injury (i.e., diffuse alveolar damage) can be found on the background of UIP. These patients are often treated with high doses of steroids and/or other immunosuppressant medications, although data supporting such approaches are lacking. Mortality for IPF patients hospitalized with acute exacerbations is very high (50% to 90%).

Other Idiopathic Interstitial Pneumonias

The other major chronic fibrosing IIP is idiopathic nonspecific interstitial pneumonia (NSIP). This condition exhibits a histologic picture that is distinct from that of UIP/IPF and is characterized by diffuse, uniform infiltration of the lung interstitium with varying amounts of chronic (lymphoplasmacytic) inflammation and fibrosis, in contrast to the patchy, heterogenous pattern seen in UIP. It is sometimes characterized

as either cellular NSIP or fibrotic NSIP depending on the predominance of either inflammation or fibrosis, although it is not clear if these are truly distinct entities. As a clinical entity, idiopathic NSIP is not as well defined as IPF, and as a result it is not as well studied either. As with IPF, patients with idiopathic NSIP usually present with progressive dyspnea and cough, and HRCT typically reveals diffuse, bilateral, peripheral reticular opacities, although ground-glass opacities are often more prominent with NSIP and honeycombing is generally absent. In many instances, distinguishing between IPF and idiopathic NSIP by HRCT alone can be difficult. The prognosis for NSIP is much better than for IPF, with a 5-year survival rate of greater than 82% in one series. It may be responsive to immunosuppressive therapy, and although data are lacking, a trial period with such agents can be considered. Lung transplantation should be considered in these patients if they exhibit progressive disease. Importantly, the same NSIP histologic pattern may occur in other conditions, most notably connective tissue disorders (e.g., systemic lupus erythematosus, rheumatoid arthritis, polymyositis), and therefore the identification of a histologic pattern of NSIP should prompt a detailed search for these conditions, which occasionally can otherwise be occult.

Cryptogenic organizing pneumonia (COP) and acute interstitial pneumonia (AIP) are classified as acute/subacute IIPs. Patients with COP exhibit subacute onset of dyspnea and/or cough, often with associated constitutional symptoms. Radiographically, patients with COP typically have areas of air space consolidation, often multifocal and bilateral, that mimic infectious pneumonia. Concomitant ground-glass opacities are also common. Histologically, COP is characterized by patchy areas of organizing pneumonia, which is accumulation of granulation tissue (a loose collection of fibrin, fibroblasts, collagen, and inflammatory cells) within the distal air spaces (alveoli and alveolar ducts), with or without extension into the respiratory and terminal bronchioles (bronchiolitis obliterans). COP is generally very responsive to corticosteroid therapy, often with complete resolution, but it can also relapse when steroids are stopped. The histologic pattern of organizing pneumonia (OP) can be seen in a variety of conditions, specifically connective tissue diseases, acute/subacute hypersensitivity pneumonitis, inhalational exposures, and drug-induced ILD, so as with NSIP, a histologic finding of OP should prompt a thorough evaluation for known causes before it is classified as an idiopathic process.

Acute interstitial pneumonia (AIP) is an IIP that is characterized by the rapid onset and progression of dyspnea and hypoxemia. Symptoms and radiographic opacities develop over days to a few weeks, invariably leading to respiratory failure. Many patients report a prior illness suggesting an upper respiratory infection with constitutional symptoms. The histologic pattern shows diffuse alveolar damage with hyaline membrane formation with or without organization. These patients can therefore be thought of as having acute respiratory distress syndrome (ARDS) of unknown cause. Although a trial of high-dose steroids with or without additional immunosuppressants is generally recommended, data indicating efficacy for this approach are lacking. Mortality rates for AIP are high at approximately 50%. Most survivors have a good long-term prognosis, although in some instances they experience persistent severe lung fibrosis. Occult connective tissue disease—most notably polymyositis/dermatomyositis—can present with an acute respiratory illness that mimics AIP, and this association may account for the fact that some patients clearly improve with aggressive treatment.

Desquamative interstitial pneumonia (DIP) is a rare idiopathic pneumonia usually seen in younger individuals. It is associated in most cases with a history of cigarette smoking. Patients exhibit a progressive shortness of breath and bilateral infiltrates on chest radiographs. The HRCT pattern shows extensive ground-glass infiltrates, and a biopsy is often required for diagnosis. Tissue histologic findings show the accumulation of so-called smoker's macrophages, which contain yellow-brown pigment and fill the alveolar spaces, and some degree of interstitial inflammation and fibrosis.

Respiratory-bronchiolitis interstitial lung disease (RB-ILD) and DIP are classified as smoking-related IPs. Although these are classified as "idiopathic" ILDs, all cases of RB-ILD and the vast majority of cases of DIP are seen in cigarette smokers. RB-ILD and DIP are thought to represent a spectrum of illness, as both are characterized by abnormal accumulation of pigment-laden macrophages. The histologic finding of RB-ILD—accumulation of these macrophages in the lumens of the respiratory bronchioles—is considered a universal finding in active smokers and considered an asymptomatic/subclinical process. When the extent of macrophage accumulation becomes more extensive, involves the peribronchiolar air spaces, and/or causes symptoms or radiographic findings, it is referred to as RB-ILD. When the macrophage accumulation is even more extensive and involves the air spaces more diffusely, it is referred to as DIP. The prognosis for RB-ILD is generally excellent, with complete resolution occurring with smoking cessation alone. For DIP, the prognosis is more variable. Smoking cessation is still the mainstay of treatment, but many patients often also require treatment with corticosteroids. Some patients unfortunately develop progressive pulmonary fibrosis despite this approach. Very rare cases of DIP have been described in nonsmoking adults, although secondhand cigarette smoke and other inhalational exposures have been implicated.

Idiopathic lymphoid interstitial pneumonia (LIP) and idiopathic pleuroparenchymal fibroelastosis (PPFE) are classified as rare IIPs. LIP is characterized by extensive, relatively homogenous lymphoid infiltration of the interstitium, often with numerous lymphoid follicles. On HRCT, LIP is characterized by the combination of diffuse ground-glass opacity and frequently numerous thin-walled cysts. In many instances, LIP may be part of a spectrum of pulmonary lymphoproliferative disorders or true lymphoma. The vast majority of histologic LIP cases are associated with other conditions (e.g., connective tissue disease, HIV) and therefore are not truly idiopathic. Idiopathic pleuroparenchymal fibroelastosis (PPFE) is a relatively recently described entity characterized by dense, elastotic fibrosis of the pleura and subpleural lung parenchyma. HRCT typically shows patchy areas of subpleural, dense, plaque-like consolidation, often predominantly in the upper lung zones. Spontaneous pneumothorax is common. It is typically progressive and unresponsive to steroids or other immunosuppressive treatments. Idiopathic PPFE is still poorly understood, and the PPFE pattern has been described in a variety of conditions, including as a complication of both stem cell transplant and lung transplant. Additional rare histologic patterns of ILD have been described, such as acute fibrinous organizing pneumonia (AFOP) and bronchiolocentric pulmonary fibrosis and inflammation, but whether or not these represent distinct IIPs is still unclear. AFOP may exist along a clinical spectrum that includes AIP and COP, and bronchiolocentric patterns of ILD may be predominantly exposure-related. Lastly, there are some cases of IIP that, despite multidisciplinary discussion and review of clinical, HRCT, and histologic findings, do not fit into any of the clinicopathologic entities described above, and these are often referred to as unclassifiable IIP.

Other Idiopathic ILDs
Eosinophilic Pneumonia

Acute eosinophilic pneumonia (AEP) and chronic eosinophilic pneumonia (CEP) are two clinically distinct idiopathic forms of ILD characterized by eosinophilic infiltration of the lung parenchyma. AEP is typically characterized by fever, a nonproductive cough, and dyspnea that progresses over several days to weeks, often leading to acute respiratory failure. This disease typically affects male smokers between the ages of 20 and 40 years who are otherwise healthy. Chest imaging

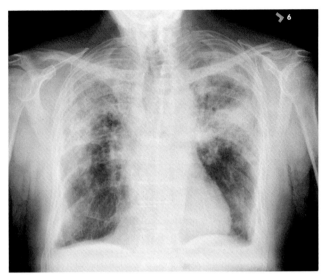

Fig. 17.3 Photographic negative of pulmonary edema in chronic eosinophilic pneumonia.

reveals diffuse bilateral pulmonary infiltrates. Eosinophilia is often not found in the peripheral blood initially but may occur 7 to 30 days after onset. Abundant eosinophils can be found in BAL fluid, and a level of greater than 25% of all nucleated cells is helpful in making the correct diagnosis. Although lung biopsy is typically not required to make the diagnosis, it can show eosinophilic infiltration with acute and organizing diffuse alveolar damage. Treatment with corticosteroids typically offers rapid and complete clinical and radiographic resolution without recurrence or residual sequelae.

Chronic eosinophilic pneumonia is an idiopathic disease predominantly of middle-aged women with a history of asthma. Also called *prolonged pulmonary eosinophilia*, this illness is characterized by a productive cough, dyspnea, malaise, weight loss, night sweats, and fever associated with progressive peripheral lung infiltrates that have been described as resembling the photographic negative of pulmonary edema on chest radiographs (Fig. 17.3). On presentation, most patients with chronic eosinophilic pneumonia have a peripheral eosinophilia of greater than 30% and BAL fluid eosinophilia. Histologic examination shows eosinophils and histiocytes in the lung parenchyma and interstitium, but minimal fibrosis. There is often histologic overlap with organizing pneumonia (OP). Spontaneous remissions have been reported, but respiratory failure can develop. Typically, treatment with corticosteroids is rapidly effective, but unlike AEP relapses are common and therefore prolonged therapy is often required.

Both AEP and CEP are diagnoses of exclusion, and other causes of eosinophilic lung infiltration must be ruled out, including fungal and parasitic infections, drug-induced ILD, connective tissue disease–ILD, EGPA, and hypereosinophilic syndrome (HES).

Pulmonary Alveolar Proteinosis

Pulmonary alveolar proteinosis (PAP) is a rare disorder in which lipoproteinaceous material accumulates within the alveoli due to impaired surfactant metabolism by alveolar macrophages. There are a variety of forms of PAP, which occurs more frequently in middle-aged patients and in current or former smokers. Primary PAP is due to impaired granulocyte-macrophage colony-stimulating factor (GM-CSF) signaling and can occur as an autoimmune disease due to neutralizing antibodies against GM-CSF, or as a hereditary disease due to mutations in GM-CSF receptor mutations. Secondary PAP occurs in conditions in which there is a functional impairment or decrease in the number of alveolar macrophages, as seen in various hematologic malignancies (e.g., leukemia), inhalation of toxic dusts (e.g., silica, aluminum), or after allogeneic bone marrow transplantation. PAP also has congenital forms that typically present in the neonatal period and are caused by various mutations that lead to dysregulated or defective surfactant production. Lung biopsy in PAP shows intra-alveolar accumulation of eosinophilic, acellular material staining positive with the periodic acid–Schiff (PAS) stain, which is consistent with surfactant.

Patients with PAP may be asymptomatic, or they may have progressive dyspnea on exertion, malaise, low-grade fever, and cough. Examination may reveal clubbing. The chest radiograph typically shows bilateral perihilar opacities. The CT scan may show diffuse ground-glass opacities with prominent thickening of the intralobular and interlobular septa, creating a pattern called "crazy paving," although this is a nonspecific finding that can be seen in many other forms or lung disease. The course of PAP may be complicated by opportunistic lung infection. BAL fluid can establish the diagnosis because it has a milky, opaque appearance. The fluid contains large, foamy alveolar macrophages and extracellular surfactant material that stains positive with PAS. Surgical or transbronchial lung biopsy may also be performed to establish the diagnosis if the BAL is nondiagnostic.

Asymptomatic patients with PAP and those with mild symptoms require no immediate treatment. Sequential whole lung lavage with warmed saline is indicated for patients with hypoxemia or severe dyspnea, and in up to 40% of patients it may be required only one time. Limited lobar lavage may be performed in milder disease. GM-CSF administration in patients with acquired PAP may be beneficial. Rituximab has been used in refractory PAP. The prognosis of auto-immune PAP is good, with excellent survival since the introduction of whole lung lavage.

EXPOSURE-RELATED ILDS

Environmental and Occupational Interstitial Lung Disease

Several environmental and occupational exposures may cause ILD, and these are generally classified as hypersensitivity pneumonitis (HP) and the pneumoconioses. Pneumoconioses are lung diseases resulting from the inhalation of mineral dusts, including silica, coal dust, or asbestos. HP is typically caused by the inhalation of organic dusts.

Hypersensitivity Pneumonitis

Definition and epidemiology. HP (also called *extrinsic allergic alveolitis*) is a relatively common ILD resulting from an abnormal immune response in the lungs to various inhaled agents, typically organic antigens. This immune response consists of both humoral and cellular components and causes a pattern of airway-centered inflammation and/or fibrosis. Potential antigens are diverse, ranging from bacterial, fungal, and animal proteins to low-molecular-weight chemicals that can act as haptens (Table 17.3). Host susceptibility seems to play an important role, because the vast majority of individuals subject to a particular exposure do not develop HP. The mechanisms contributing to host susceptibility are unclear but likely include genetic, environmental, and epigenetic factors. Although evocative descriptions have been given to occupational forms of this disease (e.g., paprika splitter's lung resulting from sensitivity to inhaled paprika dust contaminated with *Mucor stolonifer*), more routine exposures may occur in everyday life, such as hot tub water contaminated by mycobacterium avium complex (MAC), antigens from pet birds, or even common mold spores. The incidence and prevalence of HP are not well known and vary considerably based on many factors, such as geographic conditions, prevalent industries, and host mix. There is likely significant underdiagnosis of HP. For reasons that are unclear,

TABLE 17.3 Hypersensitivity Pneumonitis: Partial List of Common Etiologic Agents

Antigen	Source	Diseases
Bacteria	Moldy hay Sugar cane Compost Contaminated water	Farmer's lung, bagassosis, mushroom-worker's lung, humidifier lung, summer-type HP, composter's lung
Fungi	Moldy hay, cork, bark, cheese or wood dust Grains Compost Contaminated water or ventilation systems	Farmer's lung, suberosis, malt-worker's lung, maple bark-splitter's lung, humidifier lung, summer-type HP, composter's lung, sequoiosis, wood pulp-worker's disease, miller's lung
Mycobacteria	Contaminated water Metal cutting fluid	Hot tub lung, humidifier lung, swimming pool lung, machine-worker's lung
Animal proteins	Bird droppings, serum proteins, and feathers Pituitary powder Rat urine or serum proteins Fish meal	Pigeon breeder's lung, bird fancier's lung, feather duvet lung, duck fever, poultry-worker's lung, pituitary snuff-taker's lung, laboratory-worker's lung, fish meal-worker's lung
Chemicals	Isocyanates Anhydrides Bordeaux mixture	Chemical worker's lung, epoxy resin lung, vineyard-sprayer's lung

active cigarette smoking has been associated with a decreased risk of developing HP.

Pathology. Typical lung biopsy findings in HP demonstrate an airway-centered (i.e., bronchiolocentric) chronic inflammatory process involving the interstitium and air spaces, along with poorly formed granulomas containing multinucleated giant cells (Fig. 17.4). These findings are classically associated with the subacute form of the disease. In chronic HP there is generally considerable fibrosis and often features of fibrosing NSIP or UIP patterns in addition to areas of granulomatous and airway-centered inflammation. It is rare that lung biopsies are obtained in the acute form of HP, as it often resolves quickly, but histologic findings more associated with acute lung injury (along the diffuse alveolar damage organizing pneumonia (DAD-OP) spectrum) have been described in that setting.

Clinical presentation. HP can be classified as acute, subacute or chronic, although there can be considerable overlap between these forms. Acute HP usually presents with cough and dyspnea within hours after an intense exposure to a provocative antigen, often with prominent constitutional symptoms (e.g., fever, chills, malaise), and symptoms last for up to 24 hours. At the time of presentation, acute HP can be difficult to differentiate from bacterial or viral infection. Subacute HP is characterized by the gradual onset of cough and dyspnea, often with fatigue, anorexia, and weight loss, in response to prolonged lower level or intermittent antigen exposure. With intermittent exposure, symptoms of subacute HP may wax and wane. Chronic HP develops even more slowly than the subacute form, typically with insidious and gradually progressive cough and dyspnea and less variation in symptoms over time. Chronic HP is also thought to occur in response to sustained lower level antigen exposure, but it remains unclear if it represents the progression of prolonged, untreated subacute HP, or if subacute and chronic HP represent different host responses (inflammatory vs. fibrotic) to antigen-triggered immune-mediated lung injury.

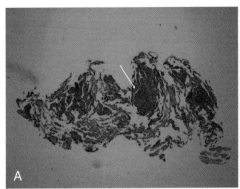
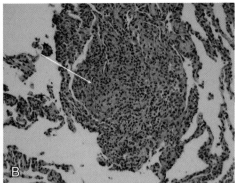

Fig. 17.4 (A) Poorly formed granulomas *(arrow)* in a patient with hypersensitivity reaction to a chemotherapy drug (low magnification). (B) Poorly formed granuloma *(arrow)* in a patient with a hypersensitivity reaction to a chemotherapy drug (high magnification).

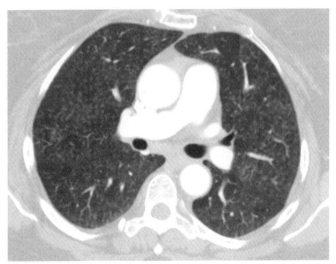

Fig. 17.5 CT image from a patient with hypersensitivity pneumonitis demonstrating diffuse, poorly formed, centrilobular nodules.

Tachypnea, hypoxemia, and diffuse inspiratory crackles are common physical exam findings in acute and subacute HP. Diffuse wheezes may also be present. Inspiratory crackles are also common in chronic HP, and these patients may also have digital clubbing. Hypoxemia with exertion may occur in earlier stages of chronic HP, with resting hypoxemia developing as the disease progresses. Pulmonary function tests usually show a restrictive pattern with abnormal gas exchange in subacute and chronic HP, although obstructive or mixed patterns are sometimes seen.

Chest radiographs in HP are characterized by nonspecific infiltrates, often in the middle and upper lung fields, although plain radiography may be normal in acute HP due to the fleeting nature of the disease. HRCT scanning is more sensitive than chest radiography and typically reveals ground-glass opacities, poorly formed centrilobular nodules (Fig. 17.5), and mosaic attenuation and air trapping patterns resulting from airway obstruction. Chronic HP may have architectural distortion with traction bronchiectasis and honeycombing and may be difficult to differentiate from IPF.

BAL findings are nonspecific but may demonstrate a lymphocytic alveolitis with a low CD4:CD8 ratio, although these findings seem to be less sensitive and specific for chronic compared to subacute disease. Patients with HP may have circulating IgG antibodies (serum precipitins) to the offending antigen, but these are not sufficiently sensitive nor specific for the diagnosis. The specific antigen may not be known or may not be tested for with standard test panels.

Diagnosis. An appropriate exposure, clinical history, BAL, and HRCT imaging findings can suggest the diagnosis, but a lung biopsy may be necessary for confirmation in some cases. Transbronchial biopsy has a relatively high yield for diagnosing subacute HP, but surgical lung biopsy is often required to differentiate chronic HP from other chronic fibrosing ILDs, such as IPF and NSIP.

Treatment and prognosis. For acute and subacute HP, clinical improvement often occurs with separation from the offending exposure, if it is identified. A typical clinical course of acute/subacute HP is improvement in the hospital setting (often with empiric antibiotics for presumed infection), followed by relapse when the patient returns to her or his prehospitalization environment. This waxing and waning pattern of illness can often be an important clue to the diagnosis of HP. The prognosis for acute and subacute HP is favorable, particularly if the offending antigen can be identified and the exposure eliminated. Corticosteroids can help relieve symptoms and accelerate recovery in subacute HP or in more severe cases of acute disease. Corticosteroids and/or other immunosuppressants are also often administered to patients with chronic HP, but data indicating efficacy are lacking. Even with aggressive immunosuppressive therapy, many patients with chronic HP continue to experience gradual worsening of their disease. The presence of fibrosis in HP is a poor prognostic indicator. In fact, chronic (fibrotic) HP often behaves similarly to IPF, with many patients progressing to lung transplantation or death from pulmonary fibrosis. As a result, there is great interest in the potential role of antifibrotic therapy for chronic HP. Identification of the offending antigen is of critical importance in HP, but even then antigen avoidance can be financially or psychologically challenging for patients in the setting of occupational, pet, or residential exposures.

Pneumoconioses

The pneumoconioses are fibroinflammatory lung diseases that result from the inhalation and accumulation of inorganic and mineral dusts in the lungs. The risk and extent of these diseases are related to the intensity and cumulative amount of exposure over time. Prevention of the pneumoconioses through occupational safeguards or, in the case of asbestos, legislative bans on use, is important because there are no effective treatments for these diseases.

Silicosis is caused by exposure to crystalline silica (silicon dioxide), which results in an inflammatory and fibrotic reaction and the formation of the characteristic silicotic nodule. Crystalline silica is abundant in nature, most commonly in the form of quartz, and is present in stone, sand, and concrete. Occupations with a higher likelihood of exposure to silica include mining, stone cutting, carving, polishing, foundry work, and abrasive clearing (e.g., sandblasting). Although exposure is usually chronic (over years), accelerated and acute disease manifestations have been described in the setting of heavier short-term exposures.

Acute silicosis is rare and the consequence of high-level silica exposure over a relatively short period of time. It is characterized by alveolar filling with silica dust and surfactant material, causing a pattern of disease that closely resembles pulmonary alveolar proteinosis (described above). Chronic silicosis results in simple nodular silicosis, and progressive massive fibrosis, which is characterized by extensive bilateral apical fibrosis resulting from the confluence of many silicotic nodules.

Patients with silicosis may have dyspnea or may be relatively asymptomatic but require further evaluation of an abnormal chest radiograph. Chest radiographs in uncomplicated silicosis show upper lobe nodular opacities, which may be subtle, whereas progressive massive fibrosis results in marked architectural distortion of the upper lobes (Fig. 17.6). Hilar node enlargement may be accompanied by "eggshell" nodal calcification. Pulmonary function tests in simple nodular silicosis may be normal or show a mixed obstructive or restrictive pattern, whereas progressive massive fibrosis is typically associated with severe restriction and hypoxemia. Patients with silicosis are at elevated risk for tuberculosis and should be screened for latent tuberculosis infection; there is also an association between silicosis and rheumatoid arthritis.

Coal worker's pneumoconiosis is an uncommon cause of pulmonary fibrosis, occurring in workers exposed to coal dust and graphite. Usually, the patients are exposed while working in underground mines. Coal worker's pneumoconiosis results in the formation of pigmented lesions in the lung surrounded by emphysema, called *coal macules*. Progressive massive fibrosis may subsequently occur. Most patients have chronic cough, which is usually productive, resulting from bronchitis related to coal exposure or to tobacco. The chest radiograph shows diffuse, small, rounded opacities. As with silicosis, there is an association with rheumatoid arthritis. Caplan's syndrome is the occurrence of multiple, large, sometimes cavitary lung nodules in association with rheumatoid arthritis after coal dust exposure.

Asbestosis results from chronic exposure to asbestos, which is a fibrous silicate used for insulation, for friction-bearing surfaces, and to strengthen materials. The inhaled asbestos fibers are deposited in the lungs, where the small fibers may be phagocytosed and cleared through lymphatics to the pleural space, but the longer fibers are often retained. Asbestos exposure typically leads to pleural disease characterized by pleural plaques, effusion, and fibrosis, but it does not necessarily affect the lung parenchyma. If it does, it is called *asbestosis*, with interstitial lung fibrosis resulting from asbestos exposure.

Asbestosis is characterized by a gradual onset of dyspnea. As with other pneumoconioses, the risk and severity of disease are related to the extent and duration of exposure. Asbestosis is often diagnosed after exposure has ceased, and disease progression may continue in the absence of ongoing exposure because of the reaction to retained asbestos fibers in the lung. The clinical presentation, pulmonary function tests, and imaging studies are similar to those for restrictive lung diseases such as IPF. However, the detection of significant pleural disease is useful in distinguishing this illness from other ILDs.

The diagnosis of asbestosis is made from the history of exposure and demonstration of concomitant pleural plaques and lower lobe predominant fibrotic changes on the chest radiograph or CT scan. In uncertain cases, the demonstration of asbestos in tissue specimens may be necessary. Asbestos bodies are the characteristic finding and consist of asbestos fibers coated by iron-containing (ferruginous) material. Asbestos exposure increases the incidence of malignancy, including lung carcinoma and mesothelioma, especially among people who also smoke. No specific treatment for asbestosis exists.

Berylliosis results from exposure to beryllium, a rare metal useful in modern, high-technology industries. Exposure to beryllium can lead to an acute chemical bronchitis and pneumonitis or chronic beryllium disease. Chronic beryllium disease is characterized by a granulomatous pneumonitis that is difficult to distinguish from sarcoidosis. The diagnosis is made by history of exposure, histologic examination, and laboratory confirmation using the beryllium lymphocyte proliferation test that is available at specialized centers. Corticosteroids may be useful in the treatment of berylliosis, but patients should avoid further exposure to beryllium.

Drug and Radiation-Induced ILD

A large number and variety of drugs can induce adverse reactions in the lung, often in the form of ILD (Table 17.4). These reactions vary in severity from self-limited hypersensitivity reactions to acute respiratory distress syndrome (ARDS) resulting in respiratory failure and even death. Together, this group of illnesses is often referred to as drug-induced lung injury (DILI). A high index of suspicion is needed to make the association between a drug and a pulmonary reaction, and a careful review of medications and other pharmacologic substances used by a patient is necessary in the setting of diffuse lung disease.

The clinical presentation of a drug-induced ILD is often nonspecific, with cough and dyspnea accompanied by radiographic

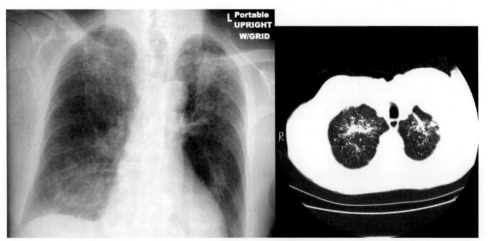

Fig. 17.6 Architectural distortion of the upper lobes in a patient with silicosis.

TABLE 17.4   Common Medications Associated With Drug-Induced Interstitial Lung Disease

Class	Drug	Class	Drug
Antineoplastic			Osimertinib
Cytotoxic agents	Bleomycin		Panitumumab
	Bortezomib		Rituximab
	Busulfan		Trametinib
	Carmustine		Trastuzumab
	Chlorambucil	Immune checkpoint inhibitors	Atezolizumab
	Cyclophosphamide		Avelumab
	Cytarabine		Durvalumab
	Docetaxel		Ipilimumab
	Doxorubicin		Nivolumab
	Etoposide		Pembrolizumab
	Fludarabine	Other Biologic Agents	Adalimumab
	Gemcitabine		Anakinra
	Hydroxyurea		Etanercept
	Ifosfamide		Infliximab
	Irinotecan		Tocilizumab
	Lomustine	Cardiovascular	Amiodarone
	Melphalan		Captopril
	Methotrexate		Flecainide
	Mitomycin-C		Hydralazine
	Oxaliplatin		Procainamide
	Paclitaxel		Quinidine
	Pemetrexed		Statins
	Procarbazine		Sotalol
	Temozolomide		Tocainide
	Thalidomide		
	Vinblastine	Antimicrobial	Daptomycin
Molecularly targeted agents	Bevacizumab		Nitrofurantoin
	Brigatinib		Sulfasalazine
	Erlotinib	Anti-inflammatory	Cyclophosphamide
	Ceritinib		Gold
	Cetuximab		Leflunomide
	Crizotinib		Methotrexate
	Dasatinib		Sulfasalazine
	Gefitinib		
	Imatinib		

opacities. Fevers can be present, and peripheral eosinophilia is sometimes found. Pulmonary function tests, if performed, usually reveal decreases in diffusion capacity and often show a restrictive pattern. ILD caused by medications usually does not produce a unique radiographic or histologic pattern of lung injury but may result in a variety of nonspecific reactions, including eosinophilic pneumonia, a hypersensitivity pneumonitis-type pattern, organizing pneumonia (OP), diffuse alveolar damage (DAD), nonspecific interstitial pneumonia (NSIP), and pulmonary fibrosis. Drug-induced systemic lupus erythematosus (SLE) can result in an acute pneumonitis, and pleural and pericardial effusions may also be present. Because the clinical presentation of patients with drug-induced ILDs lacks specificity, these are typically diagnoses of exclusion.

There are settings in which drug-induced lung disease may be especially relevant and should be strongly considered in the differential diagnosis. They include the use of antineoplastic therapy, patients with an acute SLE-like illness, and patients using specific agents known to induce pulmonary toxicity, such as methotrexate, amiodarone or nitrofurantoin. All types of antineoplastic therapy have been associated with lung toxicity and ILD, ranging

from classic cytotoxic agents (e.g., bleomycin, gemcitabine, taxanes), molecularly targeted therapies (e.g., tyrosine kinase inhibitors, EGFR inhibitors), and more recently immune checkpoint inhibitors (ICIs, e.g., nivolumab, pembrolizumab, ipilimumab). It has been estimated that up to 20% of patients receiving antineoplastic therapy develop some form of lung toxicity. Diagnosis of drug-induced ILD and identification of the offending medication can be challenging in patients receiving antineoplastic therapy because infection and chemotherapy-induced heart failure may result in similar symptoms and radiographic findings, and combination treatment with multiple agents (and radiation) is common. Biologic agents, such as tumor necrosis alpha (TNF-alpha) inhibitors and rituximab, have also rarely been associated with the development of drug-induced ILD. Because these drugs are often used to treat autoimmune conditions that are themselves associated with ILD (e.g., rheumatoid arthritis), in many cases it can be difficult to definitively assign a causal relationship between the drug exposure and the ILD. An online reference website (http://www.pneumotox.com) is available that tabulates the reported pulmonary toxicities of various drugs and is searchable by drug name and pattern of lung involvement.

Drug-induced ILD may be dose dependent, as with bleomycin, for which the risk of lung toxicity increases with cumulative doses exceeding 450 U. Amiodarone lung disease typically occurs with dosages greater than 400 mg per day. In other cases (e.g., with biologic or molecularly targeted therapies or immune checkpoint inhibitors) these reactions can be idiosyncratic and can occur either early or late in the treatment course. Synergistic lung toxicities may occur. For example, exposure to high levels of inspired oxygen may precipitate bleomycin lung injury and should be avoided if possible in exposed patients. Treatment of drug-induced ILD consists of discontinuation of the offending agent, glucocorticoids, and supportive care.

ILD can also be caused by ionizing radiation and is referred to as radiation-induced lung injury (RILI). There are two distinct types of RILI, radiation pneumonitis and radiation fibrosis, and these can occur in any patient undergoing thoracic irradiation for treatment of malignancy (e.g., lung or breast cancer, thoracic lymphoma). The main risk factors are the total dose of radiation delivered to the lung and volume of lung irradiated. Concurrent chemotherapy, particularly those that are known to sensitize tumors to radiation therapy, can also increase the risk of RILI. Interestingly, preexisting ILD also seems to confer an increased risk of RILI, suggesting that there may be host factors (e.g., genetics, prior environmental exposures) that predispose an individual to developing inflammatory or fibrotic reactions to a variety of insults to the lung.

Radiation pneumonitis usually develops within the first 3 months following irradiation, whereas radiation fibrosis typically presents much later (greater than 6 months). Symptoms are nonspecific and included dyspnea and a dry cough. Constitutional symptoms (fevers, malaise) may also be present. The physical exam typically reveals inspiratory crackles. Chest radiographs typically show hazy opacities in acute pneumonitis or reticulonodular opacities when fibrosis is present. HRCT imaging is generally done and provides more detailed information, demonstrating ground-glass opacities and areas of consolidation in radiation pneumonitis and reticular opacities, traction changes, and architectural distortion in the setting of radiation fibrosis. Although not always present, a "straight line effect"—the presence of radiographic or CT opacity that terminates abruptly, with a demarcation border that does not respect normal anatomic boundaries (Fig. 17.7)—is virtually pathognomonic for RILI. There are reports of RILI

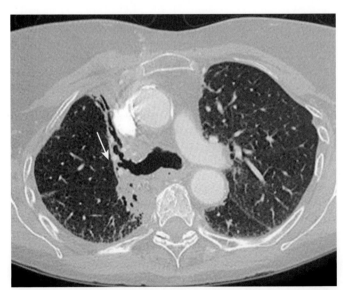

Fig. 17.7 CT image from a patient with lung fibrosis due to prior mediastinal radiation. There is a sharp demarcation between the fibrotic and normal lung *(arrow)* that crosses the major fissure, representing the "straight-line" effect.

occurring outside of the radiation field, but the mechanisms for more widespread lung injury after radiation are unknown. Bronchoscopy with BAL and/or lung biopsy can be helpful for ruling out infection or other processes (e.g., progression of cancer), but otherwise these modalities have little role in the diagnosis of RILI since the BAL fluid characteristics and histologic features are nonspecific.

Treatment of symptomatic, moderate-to-severe radiation pneumonitis typically consists of an extended course (4-6 weeks) of high-dose glucocorticoids, followed by gradual tapering. There can often be significant improvement in symptoms, lung function, and radiographic abnormalities in the subacute setting. However, those patients who develop radiation lung fibrosis generally do not improve, and corticosteroids (or other treatments) are generally ineffective.

Intentional Exposures
Cigarette Smoking

Cigarette smoking is well known to be the primary cause of chronic bronchitis and emphysema, collectively referred to as chronic obstructive pulmonary disease (COPD). It is also a risk factor for idiopathic pulmonary fibrosis (IPF), as described above. Although much less common than COPD, several types of ILD can also be directly caused by cigarette smoking, specifically respiratory bronchiolitis–interstitial lung disease (RB-ILD), desquamative interstitial pneumonia (DIP), and pulmonary Langerhans cell histiocytosis (PLCH). These are sometimes collectively referred to as smoking-related interstitial lung disease, and in many cases radiographic and histologic features of two of these entities can coexist. Despite their causal association with cigarette smoking, RB-ILD and DIP are also classified as idiopathic interstitial pneumonias (IIPs) and are discussed earlier in this chapter. Therefore, we will limit our discussion here to PLCH.

Pulmonary Langerhans cell histiocytosis

Definition and epidemiology. Pulmonary Langerhans cell histiocytosis (PLCH), formerly called *eosinophilic granuloma* or *pulmonary histiocytosis X,* is a rare ILD that is most common in middle-aged adults and seen almost exclusively in cigarette smokers. It is characterized by an abnormal infiltration of Langerhans cells, which are specific types of dendritic cells, into the lung parenchyma. Although a multisystem Langerhans cell disease related to clonal proliferation of Langerhans cells occurs in children, isolated pulmonary LCH in adult smokers does not appear to be a clonal neoplastic disorder.

Pathology. Pulmonary LCH results in the formation of cysts and nodules in the lungs. The accumulation of activated Langerhans cells results in stellate nodular infiltrates around the small airways, with eventual destruction and dilation of the airway walls, resulting in cystic changes in the lung parenchyma. Smoking may alter local immune signaling, attracting the Langerhans cells to the lungs, or it may cause local proliferation and increased survival of Langerhans cells in the lungs. Biopsy of the lung demonstrates multiple stellate lung nodules that may be cellular or fibrotic, containing Langerhans cells that stain for Cd1a and S100. Electron microscopy may reveal Birbeck granules, distinctive racquet-shaped structures in the Langerhans cells.

Clinical presentation. Patients may be asymptomatic or may exhibit constitutional symptoms, dyspnea on exertion, and cough, possibly with hemoptysis. Spontaneous pneumothorax may also occur. Pulmonary function tests show impaired diffusion capacity, and an obstructive or restrictive pattern may be seen. Chest imaging shows nodules that may be cavitary and cysts that predominate in the middle and upper lung zones. Classic HRCT findings are bilateral, mid and upper lung zone predominant, irregular nodules and "bizarre," thick-walled cysts (Fig. 17.8).

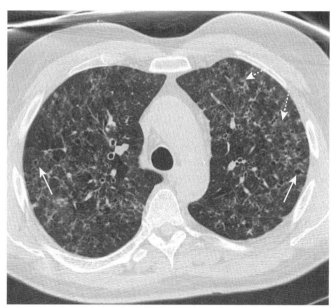

Fig. 17.8 CT image from a patient with pulmonary Langerhans cell histiocytosis (PLCH) demonstrating numerous thick-walled cysts *(solid arrows)* and irregularly shaped nodules *(dashed arrows)*.

Diagnosis and differential diagnosis. When the classic CT pattern described above is seen in a middle-aged cigarette smoker, PLCH can generally be diagnosed without the need for a lung biopsy. The differential diagnosis includes other cystic lung diseases, such as lymphangioleiomyomatosis (LAM), lymphocytic interstitial pneumonia (LIP), and Birt-Hogg Dubé syndrome, sarcoidosis, emphysema, and other smoking-related ILDs. The presence of coexisting emphysema or other smoking-related ILD (e.g., DIP) can sometimes confound the diagnosis on imaging alone.

Treatment and prognosis. The main treatment is tobacco cessation. Corticosteroids and cytotoxic agents are sometimes employed as adjunctive therapy. Lung transplantation may be considered in cases of advanced disease. In contrast to systemic LCH, pulmonary LCH is not a neoplastic disorder, and spontaneous regression may occur with smoking cessation. Although some patients have a benign course, others develop progressive disease or complications such as pulmonary hypertension, which may be fatal.

Other Exposures

Illicit drugs such as heroin and cocaine commonly produce adverse pulmonary reactions. Substances such as talc may be injected or inhaled inadvertently during the use of illicit drugs, resulting in pulmonary vascular or interstitial disease. Heroin use typically results in pulmonary edema or aspiration injury rather than ILD. Cocaine use can produce a variety of pulmonary effects, including organizing pneumonia, alveolar hemorrhage, and diffuse alveolar damage. "Crack lung" is a clinical diagnosis typified by dyspnea, hemoptysis, and pulmonary infiltrates occurring in the setting of crack cocaine use. Recently, the United States has seen an outbreak of acute ILD in the setting of electronic cigarette use or vaping, termed vaping-associated pulmonary illness (VAPI) or e-cigarette associated lung injury (EVALI). These cases have typically occurred in younger individuals and seem to be more common with the use of THC-containing e-cigarettes. A variety of patterns of lung injury have been seen, and many cases have been severe, with progression to ARDS and even death. The specific cause(s) of lung injury from e-cigarette use are currently unknown, but some cases have been linked to chemical additives (such as vitamin E acetate) in some e-cigarette products.

ILD DUE TO SYSTEMIC DISEASES

Interstitial lung disease can be a manifestation of a wide variety of systemic diseases (see Table 17.1), but by far the most common are the connective tissue disease (CTDs). Several vasculitides, which like CTDs are characterized by autoimmunity, also can cause ILD. Sarcoidosis is commonly thought of as a lung disorder, but it is in fact a multisystem disease that frequently involves the lung in a variety of different ways. In this chapter, we will discuss ILD associated with CTDs, the vasculitides, sarcoidosis, and lastly a more rare condition, lymphangioleiomyomatosis (LAM).

Connective Tissue Diseases

CTDs (also known as collagen vascular diseases, systemic rheumatic diseases) are a group of multisystem disorders characterized by dysregulation of the immune system (i.e., "autoimmunity") leading to inflammation and/or fibrosis of many different organ systems. ILD is a common manifestation of many CTDs, most notably systemic sclerosis (SSc), rheumatoid arthritis (RA), the idiopathic inflammatory myopathies (polymyositis/dermatomyositis; PM/DM), Sjögren's syndrome (SS), and mixed connective tissue disease (MCTD) (Table 17.5). Lung disease is a major cause of morbidity and mortality in these conditions. Chronic ILD is relatively uncommon in systemic lupus erythematosus (SLE), which usually is complicated by acute pneumonitis or diffuse alveolar hemorrhage. A finding of chronic ILD in a patient with SLE should prompt evaluation for MCTD or overlap syndromes (e.g., RA-SLE overlap).

Some patients presenting with ILD already have established CTD diagnoses, or the presence of CTD-ILD is discovered as a result of screening these high-risk patient populations. In other cases, a thorough history and physical examination may reveal abnormalities that strongly suggest an underlying CTD, such as inflammatory arthritis or joint deformities, myalgias or muscle weakness, sicca symptoms, esophageal dysmotility, Raynaud's phenomenon, rashes or other skin changes. In some cases, however, it appears that ILD can be the first sign of an otherwise occult CTD, with other manifestations of the disease not developing until months or even years later. This phenomenon of ILD preceding other CTD symptoms or signs is best described in RA and PM/DM, and the presence of an evolving CTD may be suspected based on the presence of circulating autoantibodies in the setting of ILD. For this reason, the evaluation of patients with newly diagnosed ILD typically involves routine serologic testing aimed at identifying evidence of occult CTD. Lastly, there are some patients with ILD who have circulating autoantibodies and/or clinical features that suggest a possible autoimmune process but do not meet criteria for any defined CTD. Terms that have been used to describe these entities include "lung-dominant" CTD, form fruste of CTD, or autoimmune-featured ILD. Recently, the term interstitial

TABLE 17.5 Frequency of Interstitial Lung Disease in Connective Tissue Diseases

Connective Tissue Disease	Incidence of ILD
Systemic sclerosis	50-60%
Rheumatoid arthritis	10-15%
Polymyositis/dermatomyositis	20-80%
Mixed connective tissue disease	50-60%
Sjögren's syndrome	10-20%
Systemic lupus erythematosus	5-10%

pneumonia with autoimmune features (IPAF) has been proposed, along with specific classification criteria, to better study and define this patient population. It remains to be seen whether the clinical course of those who could be classified as having IPAF more closely mimics that of defined CTD-ILD or that of the idiopathic interstitial pneumonias described above.

Lung biopsy is not typically indicated for the diagnosis of ILD in the setting of an established CTD, but when performed, the histologic patterns of ILD are similar to those seen with the IIPs. Nonspecific interstitial pneumonia (NSIP) is overall the most common histology associated with CTD-ILD, but usual interstitial pneumonia (UIP) and organizing pneumonia (OP) are also not uncommon. In some cases, there is a mix of histologic patterns (e.g. NSIP-OP overlap). HRCT patterns typically correspond to the histologic pattern.

Clinical manifestations of CTD-ILD are nonspecific but generally include exertional dyspnea and dry cough. CTD-ILD may be relatively asymptomatic, manifesting as an incidental finding on imaging or only detected as a consequence of aggressive screening with HRCT. Lung examination in patients with CTD-ILD may reveal bibasilar crackles, and pulmonary function tests often show a restrictive pattern with decreased diffusion capacity. If obstruction is identified on pulmonary function testing, airway manifestations of the connective tissue disorder, such as obliterative bronchiolitis in the setting of rheumatoid arthritis, must be considered. In the majority of cases of CTD-ILD, particularly with SSc and RA, the symptoms are chronic and slowly progressive, and this typically correlates with NSIP and/or UIP histologic and HRCT patterns of abnormality. More subacute symptoms can be seen with OP-like manifestations of CTD-ILD (often in RA or PM/DM). Importantly, acute fulminant presentations of CTD-ILD can also be seen, often with rapid progression to respiratory failure/ARDS. This is most often seen in PM/DM, where the histologic and HRCT patterns are often suggestive of diffuse alveolar damage (DAD) or a combination of DAD and OP, or in SLE, where DAD or capillaritis with DAH can be seen.

Other non-ILD forms of lung involvement can occur in CTD and may sometimes provide clues to the underlying diagnosis. The presence of pulmonary hypertension that does not seem to be attributable to the ILD itself is suggestive of SSc or MCTD, and the presence of pleural effusions suggests the possibility of SLE. Severe respiratory muscle weakness can occur in PM/DM and can contribute to dyspnea, PFT abnormalities, and respiratory failure. Lastly, pharyngeal muscle weakness (PM/DM) and/or esophageal dysfunction (SSc) can lead to recurrent aspiration.

Corticosteroids and other immunosuppressive drugs targeting the underlying disease process are generally considered the mainstay of treatment for CTD-ILD, although in most cases data from large, randomized controlled trials are lacking. Cyclophosphamide and mycophenolate have both been shown to be beneficial at slowing the progression of SSc-ILD, and smaller studies have suggested benefit to other treatment strategies in SSc and other CTDs (e.g., rituximab, azathioprine, calcineurin inhibitors, etc). In general, the likelihood of a response to immunosuppressive therapy seems to be somewhat determined by the pattern of ILD, similar to that seen in the IIPs (OP > cellular NSIP > fibrotic NSIP > UIP). As a group, CTD-ILDs are felt to be more responsive to treatment than IPF. However, because in many cases CTD-ILD can be predominantly a fibrotic process that is chronic and progressive (e.g., SSc-ILD and RA-ILD with a UIP pattern), there is a great deal of interest in using the newer antifibrotic agents developed for IPF in these patients, too. Indeed, a recent randomized controlled trial demonstrated

that the antifibrotic drug nintedanib was able to successfully slow the progression of SSc-ILD.

Vasculitides

The vasculitides represent a group of entities characterized by inflammation of blood vessel walls, leading to loss of vascular integrity, bleeding, and tissue ischemia. They include GPA, microscopic polyangiitis (MPA), EGPA, pauci-immune pulmonary capillaritis, anti–glomerular basement membrane (anti-GBM) disease, and CTD-associated vasculitis. Many of the vasculitides that affect the lungs are associated with circulating autoantibodies directed against neutrophil cytoplasmic antigens (i.e., antineutrophil cytoplasmic antibodies [ANCA]). Two major immunofluorescent patterns can be seen in ANCA testing: diffuse staining throughout the cytoplasm (cANCA) or perinuclear staining (pANCA). Specific antigens that ANCAs are directed against include proteinase 3 (PR3), typically causing the cANCA pattern, and myeloperoxidase (MPO), which typically causes the pANCA pattern.

GPA is a systemic necrotizing granulomatous vasculitis that often involves the small and medium-sized vessels of the upper airway, the lower respiratory tract, and the kidney. Although this triad is not always seen at initial presentation because only 40% of those affected have renal disease at that time, 80% to 90% of patients eventually develop glomerulonephritis. The most frequent manifestations of this illness are pulmonary, as highlighted by cough, chest pain, hemoptysis, and dyspnea. Constitutional symptoms such as fever and weight loss and symptoms due to involvement of the skin, eye, heart, nervous system, and musculoskeletal system are also common.

Chest imaging may show bilateral disease and infiltrates that evolve over the course of the illness. Lung nodules are common and may cavitate. Effusions and adenopathy are uncommon. Sinus films or CT scans can diagnose upper airway involvement. The diagnosis of GPA is supported by clinical findings and by circulating ANCAs, which are seen in 90% of patients. The remaining 10% of patients are ANCA negative. In ANCA-positive patients, antibodies are usually in a cANCA pattern and are directed against PR3; however, 10% to 20% may have pANCA patterns with anti-MPO antibodies.

Tissue biopsy at a site of active disease is usually needed to confirm a diagnosis of GPA. A renal biopsy is preferred because it is easier to perform and more often diagnostic. In the absence of renal involvement, a lung biopsy should be considered. Pathologically, GPA is characterized by small and medium-sized vessel necrotizing vasculitis and granulomatous inflammation. Special stains and cultures should be performed to exclude infections that can produce similar findings.

MPA is a form of systemic necrotizing small vessel vasculitis that universally affects the kidneys, whereas pulmonary involvement occurs in only 10% to 30% of patients. This rare condition has a prevalence of 1 to 3 cases per 100,000 people, but it is the most common cause of pulmonary-renal syndrome. MPA often is heralded by a long prodromal phase, characterized by constitutional symptoms followed by the development of rapidly progressive glomerulonephritis. In patients who develop lung involvement, diffuse alveolar hemorrhage (DAH) due to capillaritis is the most common manifestation. Joint, skin, peripheral nervous system, and gastrointestinal involvement also can be seen.

Seventy percent of patients with MPA are ANCA positive, and most are in a pANCA pattern with anti-MPO antibodies. Because pANCA/anti-MPO and cANCA/anti-PR3 antibodies can occur in MPA and GPA, these diseases cannot be distinguished based on their ANCA pattern. However, they can be distinguished pathologically because MPA is characterized by a focal, segmental necrotizing vasculitis affecting venules, capillaries, arterioles, and small arteries without clinical or pathologic evidence of necrotizing granulomatous inflammation. The absence or paucity of immunoglobulin localization in vessel walls distinguishes

MPA from immune complex–mediated small vessel vasculitis such as Henoch-Schönlein purpura and cryoglobulinemic vasculitis.

Treatments for GPA and MPA are similar. Combination therapy with corticosteroids and cyclophosphamide is the standard of care to induce remission. Plasma exchange is added in cases of severe disease and provides better renal outcomes. Azathioprine or methotrexate can be substituted for cyclophosphamide if remission is achieved. Rituximab may be used for induction of remission in place of cyclophosphamide or for relapsing disease.

EGPA (formerly known as Churg-Strauss syndrome) is characterized by the triad of asthma, hypereosinophilia, and necrotizing vasculitis. Many other organ systems, including the nervous system, skin, heart, and gastrointestinal tract, may be involved. The vasculitis can be associated with skin nodules and purpura. Although DAH and glomerulonephritis may occur, they are much less common than in the other small vessel vasculitides. Morbidity and mortality often result from cardiac or gastrointestinal complications or status asthmaticus and respiratory failure.

ANCAs are less helpful in the diagnosis of EGPA because only 50% of patients are ANCA positive. Anti-MPO antibodies are more commonly seen in these patients. Pathologically, a necrotizing small vessel vasculitis and an eosinophil-rich inflammatory infiltrate with necrotizing granulomas are seen. Most patients respond well to corticosteroids, but other immunosuppressants such as cyclophosphamide may be required for patients with refractory disorders.

Other causes of pulmonary capillaritis include the connective tissue diseases (particularly SLE), pauci-immune pulmonary capillaritis, and anti–glomerular basement membrane (anti-GBM) disease (i.e., Goodpasture's syndrome). Pauci-immune pulmonary capillaritis is characterized by neutrophilic infiltration of the alveolar septae with negative ANCA testing and no other systemic manifestations of vasculitis. Goodpasture's syndrome causes DAH associated with glomerulonephritis due to anti-GBM antibodies to the α_3 chain of type IV collagen that is also found in the lung basement membrane. More than 90% of patients with Goodpasture's syndrome have anti-GBM antibodies detectable in the serum. For those without circulating antibodies, the diagnosis may be confirmed by lung biopsy, although the kidney is the preferred site. Up to 40% may also be ANCA positive, primarily with anti-MPO antibodies. Pathologically, linear deposition of antibody along the alveolar or glomerular basement membrane is visible by direct immunofluorescence. The treatment of Goodpasture's syndrome is plasmapheresis and immunosuppression. The disease is fatal if left untreated.

Sarcoidosis

Definition and Epidemiology

Sarcoidosis is a multisystem granulomatous disorder of unknown cause. The lungs and thoracic lymph nodes are frequent sites of involvement. Sarcoidosis is relatively common, with a prevalence of 1 to 40 cases per 100,000 people worldwide. A higher incidence of sarcoidosis is reported among Scandinavian, German, and Irish individuals residing in northern Europe. In the United States, the prevalence rates of sarcoidosis are 10.9 cases per 100,000 white individuals and 35.5 cases per 100,000 African Americans, with women in both groups being more frequently affected. Because sarcoidosis may be asymptomatic, the true prevalence may be higher. Sarcoidosis typically occurs in individuals between 10 and 40 years old.

Pathology and Pathophysiology

Sarcoidosis is characterized by the formation in tissues of noncaseating granulomas that organize in an inner core of epithelioid histiocytes, CD4+ T lymphocytes, and giant cells, which are surrounded by a rim of lymphocytes, fibroblasts, and connective tissue (Fig. 17.9).

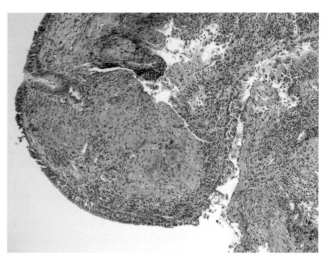

Fig. 17.9 Subepithelial noncaseating granuloma, which is characteristic of sarcoidosis, from an endobronchial biopsy.

Granulomas are found in the airways or lung parenchyma in more than 90% of patients with sarcoidosis. Granulomatous angiitis may also be found in the lungs. The upper respiratory system, lymph nodes, skin, and eyes are commonly involved. Virtually any other organ may be affected, including the liver, bone marrow, spleen, musculoskeletal system, heart, salivary glands, and nervous system.

The granulomas may be clinically silent or, if extensive, may disrupt normal organ structure and function. The cause of these lesions is unknown, but given the frequency of lung involvement, inhaled antigens ranging from bacteria (especially mycobacteria and *Propionibacterium*) to environmental substances have been hypothesized to trigger the onset of granulomatous inflammation. This inflammation may be self-limited or may be propagated, possibly by repeated exposure to the unknown antigen or because of defective immune regulation.

Familial susceptibility to sarcoidosis exists, and alleles of human leukocyte antigen (HLA) genes involved in antigen presentation and a mutation in the butyrophilin-like 2 gene *(BTNL2)*, a possible immunoregulatory gene, have been associated with susceptibility to sarcoidosis. A single causative antigen initiating granuloma formation may not exist, and sarcoidosis instead may represent a stereotypical inflammatory reaction to various antigens in a genetically susceptible host.

Sarcoidosis is associated with abnormal immune function as evidenced by cutaneous anergy and as exhibited in lung by an increased ratio of CD4+ to CD8+ T lymphocytes and increased concentrations of pro-inflammatory cytokines such as interferon-γ, interleukin-12, and tumor necrosis factor-α (TNF-α). These derangements can be detected in the bronchoalveolar lavage (BAL) fluid and are consistent with an imbalance in the production of type 1 (T_H1) and type 2 (T_H2) helper T-cell cytokines, favoring the production of the former and promoting persistent inflammation. Sarcoidosis may occur in the setting of immunomodulatory therapy, especially with interferon-α, or the immune reconstitution syndrome, occurring after initiation of antiretroviral therapy for human immunodeficiency virus (HIV) infection, highlighting the role of immune imbalances in the disorder.

Clinical Presentation

The clinical presentation of patients with sarcoidosis varies. The disease is frequently detected incidentally on routine chest radiographs of asymptomatic individuals. Others may have diverse acute or chronic symptoms. Patients may develop well-described acute syndromes such as Löfgren syndrome, which includes erythema nodosum, fever, arthritis, and hilar adenopathy, or uveoparotid fever (i.e., Heerfordt

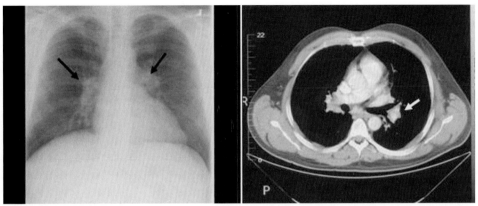

Fig. 17.10 Hilar adenopathy in a patient with sarcoidosis *(arrows)*. (A) Chest radiograph. (B) Chest computed tomography scan. (Courtesy Dr. Rafael L. Perez.)

syndrome), which exhibits the triad of uveitis, parotitis, and facial nerve palsy. Both syndromes are associated with better outcomes than for other clinical presentations of sarcoidosis.

In many cases, symptoms are vague and chronic, and they may include systemic symptoms such as low-grade fevers, fatigue, night sweats, or joint pains. Respiratory manifestations, including shortness of breath, wheezing, dry cough, and chest pain, occur in one third to one half of patients. Skin manifestations include erythema nodosum, plaques, nodules, and lupus pernio, a violaceous, often disfiguring, nodular lesion of the nose and cheeks. Ocular symptoms are also common, and the onset of uveitis may eventually lead to the diagnosis of sarcoidosis when granulomatous extraocular organ involvement is uncovered. Neurosarcoidosis may manifest with cranial nerve palsies or with headache in the setting of lymphocytic meningitis. Sarcoidosis can involve the heart, resulting in a cardiomyopathy. Arrhythmias and sudden cardiac death can occur as a result of the disruption of the conducting system by granulomatous infiltration. Pulmonary hypertension may result from pulmonary fibrosis or directly from granulomatous vasculitis.

In 90% of patients, the chest radiograph shows abnormalities that include bilateral hilar adenopathy (Fig.17.10), parenchymal opacities, or both. The radiographic changes characteristic of sarcoidosis have been classified as stages 0 through IV (Table17.6), but this staging system does not imply a typical chronologic progression. However, stage I patients have a better prognosis for resolution than those with more advanced stages of disease.

As in other ILDs, computed tomography (CT) is more sensitive for the detection of parenchymal abnormalities, and it more clearly demonstrates the extent of mediastinal adenopathy. Typical HRCT findings include bilateral, mid and upper lung zone predominant peribronchovascular opacities emanating from the hila, along with extensive micronodules that can be seen within the lung parenchyma and running along the interlobular septae, fissures, and pleural surfaces (Fig.17.11). Positron emission tomography (PET) or gallium-67 scans may reveal other sites of organ involvement.

Pulmonary function tests show restriction, obstruction, or mixed deficits. Liver involvement may cause mild elevation of transaminase levels, and cirrhosis and liver failure have been reported, although they are rare. Hypercalcemia and hypercalciuria may be detected and are caused by increased intestinal absorption of calcium as a result of increased conversion of vitamin D to its active form in sarcoid granulomas. Kidney stones may result from the abnormal calcium metabolism. Elevated levels of angiotensin-converting enzyme (ACE) are common but are not specific. The use of ACE levels in the diagnosis or management of sarcoidosis is controversial.

TABLE 17.6 Radiographic Staging of Sarcoidosis

Stage	Radiographic Findings
0	Normal radiograph
I	Adenopathy without parenchymal abnormality
II	Adenopathy and parenchymal disease
III	Parenchymal disease without lymphadenopathy
IV	End-stage fibrosis

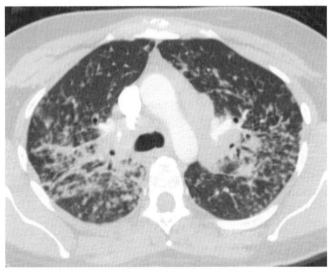

Fig. 17.11 CT image from a patient with sarcoidosis demonstrating bilateral, upper lung zone predominant peribronchovascular opacity and extensive micronodules.

Diagnosis

The diagnosis of sarcoidosis depends on a typical clinical, radiographic, and histologic picture and is a diagnosis of exclusion. Patients with classic syndromes such as the Löfgren syndrome or uveoparotid fever may not require biopsy; however, most patients require tissue biopsy of an affected organ. Tissue samples show noncaseating granulomas, but because this finding is nonspecific, careful attention should be given to ruling out other causes of granulomatous inflammation (e.g., mycobacterial infection) through stains and cultures.

Necrotizing granulomas have rarely been reported in sarcoidosis, but this finding should prompt an intense search for infection. In contrast to most ILDs, in which tissue diagnosis requires open lung biopsy, the granulomas in sarcoidosis can be identified in skin nodules or in lymph nodes. Due to frequent lung and lymph node involvement, bronchoscopy is commonly used to diagnose sarcoidosis. Results of bronchoscopy with transbronchial lung biopsy are positive for 50% to 60% of patients, but the procedure poses the risks of hemorrhage and pneumothorax. Because airway involvement is common, endobronchial biopsies may also demonstrate granulomas. However, there is increasing evidence that transbronchial needle aspiration of mediastinal and hilar lymph nodes using endobronchial ultrasound guidance may have a higher diagnostic yield for granulomas than conventional bronchoscopic techniques.

As mentioned above, sarcoidosis is a multisystem disease, so careful attention must be paid to potential signs and symptoms of extra-pulmonary involvement. After the diagnosis is made, all patients should have an ophthalmologic evaluation to assess for ocular involvement and an ECG to look for conduction abnormalities. Further cardiac testing, including Holter monitoring, echocardiography, or cardiac magnetic resonance imaging (MRI) should also be done depending on the presence of symptoms (e.g., palpitations) or ECG abnormalities. PET scanning can also be helpful for detecting active cardiac involvement from sarcoidosis. Additional imaging studies and/or tissue biopsies may be needed when symptoms or basic lab testing suggests other organ involvement (e.g., headaches, abnormal liver function tests, etc.).

Treatment

Corticosteroids are the mainstay of therapy, although they are not required in all patients with sarcoidosis because many patients are minimally symptomatic and may undergo spontaneous remission. Whether corticosteroids alter the disease course is uncertain. However, corticosteroid therapy should be considered in patients with extra-pulmonary organ involvement, respiratory symptoms, or evidence of progressive pulmonary disease. In patients with pulmonary involvement, oral prednisone at a dosage of 20 to 40 mg per day is typically initiated and maintained for a 4- to 6-week course before being slowly tapered over a course of 3 to 6 months. Some patients may experience remission with this treatment approach and may be managed off therapy for an extended period of time. For patients with disease that is refractory to corticosteroids, or for those who experience disease worsening when steroids are tapered, additional treatments should be considered. Methotrexate is the most commonly used steroid-sparing agent in sarcoidosis, but leflunomide, azathioprine, and mycophenolate have also been used. Anti TNF-α inhibitors (e.g., infliximab) can also be used for refractory disease, and there are some small studies to support this approach in individuals with refractory sarcoidosis or with extra-pulmonary involvement.

Prognosis

The course of sarcoidosis varies. Spontaneous remission is common, and death and disability occur rarely, making decisions regarding treatment initiation difficult. The acute sarcoidosis syndromes tend to remit and not recur. However, about one third of patients with sarcoidosis have chronic, progressive disease, and some patients develop pulmonary fibrosis or other end-organ damage.

Lymphangioleiomyomatosis
Definition and Epidemiology

Lymphangioleiomyomatosis is a rare, slowly progressive, multisystem disorder resulting in cystic interstitial lung disease and kidney angiomyolipomas that occurs in either a sporadic form or in association with tuberous sclerosis complex (TSC-LAM). Sporadic LAM occurs almost exclusively in women of childbearing age.

Pathology

The disease is characterized by extensive infiltration of the lungs and lymphatics with growths of smooth muscle–like lymphangioleiomyomatosis cells. Mutations in the *TSC1* or *TSC2* gene, which encodes tumor suppressor proteins that normally act as inhibitors of protein synthesis and cell growth, may result in tuberous sclerosis or lymphangioleiomyomatosis. Mutations in *TSC2* are associated with greater disease severity.

Clinical Presentation

Dyspnea and spontaneous pneumothorax are the most common presentations, with chylous pleural effusions and hemoptysis also occurring. These clinical presentations result from lung parenchymal destruction, airway narrowing, and lymphatic obstruction caused by the abnormal proliferation of the smooth muscle–like cells.

Imaging studies show an interstitial pattern with middle and upper lung predominance; multiple, thin-walled cystic lesions; and characteristically preserved lung volumes. Pleural effusion or pneumothorax may be seen on imaging. CT of the abdomen may reveal fat-containing kidney lesions consistent with angiomyolipomas. Pulmonary function tests typically show a progressive obstructive pattern, although mixed obstruction and restriction may also be seen.

Diagnosis

Although the clinical features coupled with characteristic imaging are often diagnostic, lung biopsy may be necessary in some cases. It demonstrates interstitial nodules composed centrally of spindle-shaped cells that stain for smooth muscle cell actin and for HMB-45, an antibody to the melanocytic glycoprotein 100, with staining involving the alveolar walls, lobular septa, venules, small airways, and pleura.

Treatment

Treatment involves management of pleural complications, including the use of pleurodesis to prevent recurrent pneumothorax or effusion, bronchodilator and oxygen therapy, and avoidance of pharmacologic estrogens, which may exacerbate the disease. Progesterones have been used in an attempt to modulate disease progression, but efficacy data are limited.

Because the products of the *TSC1* and *TSC2* genes normally act as inhibitors of the mammalian target of rapamycin (mTOR), pharmacologic mTOR inhibitors such as sirolimus and everolimus have been studied in lymphangioleiomyomatosis. Sirolimus stabilized lung function in lymphangioleiomyomatosis, and sirolimus and everolimus treatment resulted in angiomyolipoma shrinkage. Lung transplantation can be performed in patients with severe pulmonary dysfunction.

Prognosis

Lymphangioleiomyomatosis is a slowly progressive disease that can result in potentially fatal complications, especially respiratory failure.

SUMMARY

The interstitial lung diseases (ILDs), or *diffuse parenchymal lung diseases* (DPLDs), are a heterogenous group of nonmalignant and noninfectious lung diseases characterized by varying amounts of inflammation and/or fibrosis (scarring) of the lung parenchyma. ILDs manifest with a wide range of overlapping clinical presentations, radiographic findings, and histologic abnormalities. Because of the similarities shared by many ILDs and the rarity of most of these conditions, establishing a definitive diagnosis can often be difficult and requires the incorporation of a detailed history, physical exam, imaging, and histologic data. Although there is no universally accepted classification system for ILDs, it can be useful to think of these entities as falling into the three broad categories of exposure-related ILDs, ILDs attributable to systemic diseases, and idiopathic ILDs.

The treatment approach for ILDs generally revolves around treating the underlying illness (if present) and removal of offending exposures (if identified), as well as suppressing inflammation in those settings where inflammation is thought to play a prominent role. However, pulmonary fibrosis is a characteristic feature of many ILDs, and fibrosis often progresses despite these approaches. Fortunately, we are now starting to see the emergence of treatments that target the aberrant wound-healing processes that are thought to contribute to the development of lung fibrosis. Antifibrotic treatments are now available for idiopathic pulmonary fibrosis (IPF) that slow the progression of this otherwise fatal disease process, and these treatments may also be effective for other types of fibrotic ILD. However, until therapies are developed that can completely arrest—and ideally even reverse—fibrogenesis, lung transplantation remains the only option for a chance at prolonged survival for many patients afflicted with IPF and other ILDs.

SUGGESTED READINGS

Caminati A, Cavazza A, Sverzellati N, Harari S: An integrated approach in the diagnosis of smoking-related interstitial lung diseases, *Eur Respir Rev* 21(125):207–217, 2012.

Distler O, Highland KB, Gahlemann M, et al: Nintedanib for systemic sclerosis-associated interstitial lung disease, N Engl J Med 380(26):2518–2528, 2019.

Frankel SK, Schwarz MI: The pulmonary vasculitides, Am J Respir Crit Care Med 186(3):216–224, 2012.

Gupta N, Finlay GA, Kotloff RM, et al: Lymphangioleiomyomatosis diagnosis and management: high-resolution chest computed tomography, transbronchial lung biopsy, and pleural disease management. An official American Thoracic Society/Japanese Respiratory Society Clinical Practice Guideline, Am J Respir Crit Care Med 196(10):1337–1348, 2017.

King Jr TE, Bradford WZ, Castro-Bernardini S, et al: A phase 3 trial of pirfenidone in patients with idiopathic pulmonary fibrosis, N Engl J Med 370(22):2083–2092, 2014.

King Jr TE, Pardo A, Selman M: Idiopathic pulmonary fibrosis, Lancet 378(9807):1949–1961, 2011.

Lederer DJ, Martinez FJ: Idiopathic pulmonary fibrosis, N Engl J Med 378(19):1811–1823, 2018.

Mira-Avendano I, Abril A, Burger CD, et al: Interstitial lung disease and other pulmonary manifestations in connective tissue diseases, Mayo Clin Proc 94(2):309–325, 2019.

Raghu G, Remy-Jardin M, Myers JL, et al: Diagnosis of idiopathic pulmonary fibrosis. An official ATS/ERS/JRS/ALAT clinical practice guideline, Am J Respir Crit Care Med 198(5):e44–e68, 2018.

Richeldi L, du Bois RM, Raghu G, et al: Efficacy and safety of nintedanib in idiopathic pulmonary fibrosis, N Engl J Med 370(22):2071–2082, 2014.

Salisbury ML, Myers JL, Belloli EA, et al: Diagnosis and treatment of fibrotic hypersensitivity pneumonia. where we stand and where we need to go, Am J Respir Crit Care Med 196(6):690–699, 2017.

Spagnolo P, Rossi G, Trisolini R, et al: Pulmonary sarcoidosis, Lancet Respir Med 6(5):389–402, 2018.

Travis WD, Costabel U, Hansell DM, et al: An official American Thoracic Society/European Respiratory Society statement: update of the international multidisciplinary classification of the idiopathic interstitial pneumonias, Am J Respir Crit Care Med 188(6):733–748, 2013.

Vasakova M, Morell F, Walsh S, et al: Hypersensitivity pneumonitis: perspectives in diagnosis and management, Am J Respir Crit Care Med 196(6):680–689, 2017.

18

Pulmonary Vascular Diseases

Christopher J. Mullin, James R. Klinger

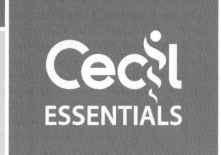

INTRODUCTION

Pulmonary vascular disease is a broad term for any disease that affects the blood vessels of the lungs. These diseases are a heterogeneous group of disorders with multiple causes, but most can be categorized as diseases of either pulmonary embolism or pulmonary hypertension. Some pulmonary vascular diseases, such as idiopathic pulmonary arterial hypertension (PAH), directly affect the pulmonary vessels, whereas other forms of pulmonary vascular disorders are compensatory responses to elevation of pulmonary venous pressure or recurrent hypoxia due to chronic heart and lung diseases. This chapter discusses pulmonary hypertension and pulmonary thromboembolism, with a focus on pulmonary arterial hypertension (PAH) and chronic thromboembolic pulmonary hypertension (CTEPH).

The normal pulmonary vasculature is a high-flow, low-resistance system with very high capacitance that can accept the entire output of the right ventricle with only slight increases in pressure. The right ventricle (RV) in health is well adapted to the pulmonary circulation and matches the cardiac output of the left ventricle with one fifth of the energy expenditure. However, the RV is unable to tolerate large increases in afterload, which occur acutely in the setting of pulmonary thromboembolism and more subacutely or chronically in pulmonary hypertension. As such, right ventricular function is important in the clinical manifestations, diagnosis, treatment, and prognosis of pulmonary vascular diseases.

❖ For a deeper discussion on this topic, please see Chapter 75, "Pulmonary Hypertension," in *Goldman-Cecil Medicine*, 26th Edition.

PULMONARY HYPERTENSION

Definition and Epidemiology

Normal pulmonary arterial pressure (PAP) in healthy adults at rest is about 25/10 mm Hg with a mean PAP (mPAP) of 14.3 mm Hg ± 3.0 mm Hg. Thus, mPAP above 20 mm Hg is two standard deviations above the mean and generally considered to be abnormal. However, mPAP increases slightly with age and is difficult to measure accurately due to limitations in normalizing intravascular pressure to atmospheric pressure. For these reasons, PH is usually defined as mPAP greater than or equal to 25 mm Hg. In 1998, the World Symposium on Pulmonary Hypertension proposed a classification of pulmonary hypertension that grouped diseases with similar pathologic and hemodynamic characteristics. In the most recent version of this classification (Table 18.1), PH is divided into five groups: (1) Pulmonary arterial hypertension (PAH), meant to infer disease of the pulmonary arteries, (2) pulmonary hypertension due to elevated pulmonary venous pressure caused by left-sided heart disease, (3) pulmonary hypertension due to chronic hypoxia or lung disease, (4) pulmonary hypertension

caused by chronic pulmonary emboli, and (5) pulmonary hypertension attributable to unclear or multifactorial mechanisms.

The most common types of pulmonary hypertension are WHO Groups 2 and 3. In one study, nearly 75% of adult cases of PH were due to left heart disease and 10% due to chronic lung disease. However, much of the attention on pulmonary vascular disease has focused on WHO Group 1 PAH. Despite representing a small minority of cases, PAH is the most severe form of pulmonary hypertension and often afflicts relatively young otherwise healthy individuals. Without treatment, median survival is about 3 years. In early registries, the peak incidence of PAH occurred in the fourth decade of life, but it can be seen at all ages and it affects women two to three times more frequently than men. The cause of PAH is unknown, but disease classification has been further subdivided into idiopathic PAH, heritable PAH, and associated PAH (APAH) in which PAH is associated with one of several diseases. Heritable PAH is caused primarily by mutations in the gene for bone morphogenetic protein receptor type 2 *(BMPR2)* representing nearly three quarters of the cases of familial PH and approximately 20% of patients with idiopathic PAH. Mutations in other related genes within the transforming growth factor-β family including (activin receptor-like kinase 1 [ALK1]) and endoglin (ENG) have also been described.

Idiopathic PAH is extremely rare with an incidence estimated at 1 to 10 in 1,000,000. However, APAH is not uncommon in patients with connective tissue disease, especially the limited cutaneous form of scleroderma and mixed connective tissue disease where it can be seen in up to 14% of patients. PAH also occurs in 2% to 3% of patients with portal hypertension and 0.5% of patients with HIV infection. It is also seen in patients exposed to methamphetamines, particularly the anorectic drug phentermine/fenfluramine, and is a common sequel of congenital heart diseases that result in significant left-to-right intracardiac shunt. Pulmonary veno-occlusive disease (PVOD) and pulmonary capillary hemangiomatosis (PCH) constitute a rare subgroup of PH that is characterized by vascular remodeling and occlusion of small pulmonary veins and venules, leading to severe hypoxia and in some cases interstitial edema.

Pulmonary Arterial Hypertension
Pathophysiology

Although the pathogenic mechanisms responsible for PAH are not well understood, the vascular remodeling associated with it has been well described. Prominent features include an obliterative vasculopathy characterized by medial vascular smooth muscle hypertrophy, adventitial thickening, and proliferation of pulmonary vascular endothelial cells. In situ thromboses of small pulmonary arteries and areas of perivascular inflammation are also frequently observed. Plexiform lesions consisting of abnormal proliferation of endothelial cells causing near complete obstruction of the vascular lumen of distal pre-acinar arterioles with areas of recanalization are considered pathognomonic of the

TABLE 18.1   World Health Organization Classification of Pulmonary Hypertension

Group 1: Pulmonary Arterial Hypertension (PAH)
- Idiopathic PAH
- Heritable PAH
- Drug- and toxin-induced
- PAH associated with:
  - Connective tissue disease
  - Human immunodeficiency virus infection
  - Portal hypertension
  - Congenital heart disease
  - Schistosomiasis

Long-term responders to calcium-channel blockers
PAH with overt features of venous/capillary involvement (pulmonary veno-occlusive disease or pulmonary capillary hemangiomatosis)
Persistent pulmonary hypertension of the newborn

Group 2: Pulmonary Hypertension Due to Left Heart Disease
- Heart failure with preserved left ventricular ejection fraction
- Heart failure with reduced left ventricular ejection fraction
- Valvular heart disease
- Congenital/acquired cardiovascular conditions leading to post-capillary PH

Group 3: Pulmonary Hypertension Due to Lung Diseases and/or Hypoxia
- Obstructive lung disease
- Restrictive lung disease
- Other lung diseases with mixed restrictive and obstructive pattern
- Hypoxia without lung disease
- Developmental lung diseases

Group 4: Pulmonary Hypertension Due to Pulmonary Arterial Obstructions
- Chronic thromboembolic pulmonary hypertension
- Other pulmonary artery obstruction: sarcoma, other malignant or nonmalignant tumors, arteritis without connective tissue disease, congenital pulmonary artery stenosis, parasites

Group 5: Pulmonary Hypertension With Unclear and/or Multifactorial Mechanisms
- Hematologic disorders: chronic hemolytic anemia, myeloproliferative disorders
- Systemic and metabolic disorders: sarcoidosis, pulmonary Langerhans cell histiocytosis, glycogen storage disease, Gaucher disease, neurofibromatosis
- Others: chronic renal failure with or without hemodialysis, fibrosing mediastinitis
- Complex congenital heart disease

Modified from Simonneau G, Montani D, Celermajer DS, et al. Haemodynamic definitions and updated clinical classification of pulmonary hypertension. Eur Respir J 2019; 53: 1801913.

 disease E-Fig. 18.1). In some cases, vascular remodeling extends into pulmonary capillaries and proximal pulmonary veins. These varied changes result in narrowing of the vascular lumen and are thought to contribute to the increase in pulmonary vascular resistance and pressure. In addition, numerous changes in vascular cell function have been described. Pulmonary vascular endothelial cells show decreased expression of vasodilators such as prostacyclin and nitric oxide and increased expression of pulmonary vasoconstrictors such as thromboxane and endothelin. Pulmonary vascular smooth muscle becomes hypertrophic and proliferative leading to muscularization of distal normally nonmuscularized vessels. Adventitial fibroblasts display an inflammatory phenotype that may induce changes in smooth muscle cell growth. Finally, the loss of distal pulmonary vessels due to abnormal apoptosis of pulmonary vascular endothelial cells is also likely to contribute to the pathogenesis of PAH. It is unclear if the obliterative vascular remodeling characteristic of PAH is the primary cause of the disease or a compensatory response to the increase in blood flow through the remaining vessels. A leading hypothesis is that PAH is caused by a double hit mechanism, the first being vascular injury resulting in loss of distal pulmonary vessels and the second being the deregulation of vascular repair mechanisms that lead to abnormal pulmonary vascular remodeling.

Clinical Presentation

The initial presentation of PAH is often subtle. Initial symptoms include dyspnea on exertion, fatigue or exertional lightheadedness. As the disease progresses, right ventricular failure causes peripheral edema, decreased appetite, ascites, and occasionally exertional chest pain. Severity of PAH is often classified by the degree of exercise impairment using a WHO modification of the New York Heart Association functional class as follows: class I, asymptomatic; class II, symptoms with normal activity; class III, symptoms with less than normal activity; and class IV, symptoms with any physical activity or at rest.

Chest radiographs may reveal prominent pulmonary arteries or right ventricular enlargement (E-Fig. 18.2). Pulmonary function test- ing usually shows normal spirometry, but diffusing capacity can be reduced reflecting the restricted circulation and decreased surface area available for gas exchange. Plasma brain natriuretic peptide levels rise as right ventricular pressure increases and a fall in oxygen saturation in response to exercise is often seen.

Diagnosis and Clinical Evaluation

The diagnosis of PAH depends on exclusion of other underlying heart or lung diseases that might cause pulmonary hypertension. Because PAH is

TABLE 18.2   **Medications for Treatment of Pulmonary Arterial Hypertension**

Drug Class	Drug Name	Route of Administration	Mechanism of Action
Endothelin receptor antagonist	Ambrisentan	Oral	Inhibits vasoconstriction by blocking endothelin
	Bosentan	Oral	
	Macintentan	Oral	
Phosphodiesterase type 5 inhibitor	Sildenafil	Oral, intravenous	Promotes vasodilation by delaying metabolism of intracellular cGMP
	Tadalafil	Oral	
Prostacyclin derivative	Epoprostenol	Intravenous, inhaled[a]	Promotes vasodilation by increasing intracellular cAMP
	Iloprost	Inhaled, intravenous infusion[a]	
	Treprostinil	Oral, inhaled, subcutaneous infusion, intravenous infusion	
Prostacyclin receptor agonist	Selexipag	Oral	Activates prostacyclin receptor
Soluble guanylyl cyclase stimulator	Riociguat	Oral	Promotes vasodilation by increasing cGMP synthesis

[a]Currently no commercial preparation available for this route of administration in the United States.

extremely rare in healthy individuals, every effort should be made to look for connective tissue disease, portal hypertension, HIV infection, congenital heart disease, chronic pulmonary emboli, or history of exposure to a potentially causative drug or toxin. Most patients should have pulmonary function testing to exclude obstructive or restrictive defects and measure oxygen saturation. Nocturnal hypoxemia from sleep-disordered breathing should be considered. A lung ventilation/perfusion scan should be done to exclude chronic pulmonary embolism and blood tests for screening for autoimmune disease, HIV, or liver dysfunction should be obtained. Left heart disease is usually evaluated by echocardiography, but in some patients, additional studies to assess coronary artery disease or infiltrative cardiomyopathies may be needed. Although rare, PCH and PVOD should be considered, the latter characterized by severe hypoxemia, decreased D_{LCO}, and a triad of centrilobular nodules and ground-glass opacities and thickened interlobular septa on high-resolution chest CT.

Transthoracic echocardiography is often the first step in excluding left-sided heart disease and when used with Doppler ultrasound can provide an estimate of pulmonary artery systolic pressure. In addition, it provides important information on right atrial and ventricular size and function and the relative degree of right- versus left-sided filling pressure by examining the position of the interatrial and interventricular septa. Finally, the presence of significant intracardiac shunts can often be detected.

Definitive diagnosis of PAH requires right heart catheterization to confirm increased mPAP and assess left-sided filling pressure via measurement of pulmonary artery occlusion pressure. Hemoglobin oxygen saturation should be measured in the superior or inferior vena cava, right atrium, and pulmonary artery to exclude significant left-to-right shunt. In patients with PAH, pulmonary vasoreactivity should be tested by administration of a short-acting selective pulmonary vasodilator such as inhaled nitric oxide or intravenous epoprostenol. A decrease in mPAP of 10 mm Hg or greater to a mPAP less than 40 mm Hg without a decrease in cardiac output is considered a positive response and identifies a small group of PAH patients who can often be treated successfully with a calcium-channel blocker.

Treatment

In the last 25 years, five classes of drugs have been approved for the treatment of PAH (Table 18.2). These drugs act primarily as semiselective pulmonary vasodilators, although antimitogenic properties that may slow pulmonary vascular remodeling have also been described. There are insufficient data to compare the relative efficacy of the different drug classes, but in general most treatment guidelines agree on several points: (1) In the absence of severe right heart failure, patients with a positive response to pulmonary vasodilator testing should be given a trial of calcium-channel blocker, usually nifedipine. (2) Patients with the greatest risk of death,

including those in WHO functional class IV, should be treated with continuous intravenous infusion of a prostacyclin derivative. (3) Patients with less advanced PAH such as those in functional class II or III should be treated with a combination of a phosphodiesterase type 5 inhibitor (PDE5) inhibitor and an endothelin receptor antagonist (ERA). Patients who are unable to tolerate this combination or who do not improve while taking it should be considered for treatment with soluble guanylate cyclase (sGC) stimulators in place of a PDE5 inhibitor or use of an inhaled or oral prostacyclin derivative or a prostacyclin receptor agonist.

Response to treatment is assessed by (1) symptomatic improvement as measured by change in functional class, (2) objective improvement in exercise capacity as assessed by 6-minute walk distance or cardiopulmonary exercise testing, (3) enhanced right ventricular function as assessed by echocardiogram or cardiac MRI and brain natriuretic peptide levels, and when necessary, (4) pulmonary hemodynamics assessed by repeat right heart catheterization.

Other interventions include supplemental oxygen to keep resting oxygen saturation greater than 90%, judicious use of diuretics to reduce peripheral edema and right ventricular overload, and a supervised exercise program such as pulmonary rehabilitation. The role of anticoagulation to prevent thrombosis in situ remains controversial, but some guidelines recommend low-level anticoagulation unless patients are at increased risk of bleeding. Patients who remain in or progress to functional class IV despite maximum medical therapy should be considered for lung transplantation. Current treatment guidelines also recommend consideration of referral of PAH patients to regional centers with experience in managing this disease.

OTHER TYPES OF PULMONARY HYPERTENSION

Pulmonary hypertension is a normal complication of any left-sided heart disease that increases pulmonary venous pressure such as left ventricular systolic or diastolic dysfunction or valvular heart disease. Pulmonary hypertension is also a common development of chronic lung disease, especially those that are associated with hypoxemia. These conditions have been called *secondary pulmonary hypertension* but now are usually referred to as WHO Group 2 and 3 PH (see Table 18.1). Hypoxic pulmonary vasoconstriction contributes to increased pulmonary vascular resistance in chronic or recurrent hypoxia. Longstanding hypoxia causes vascular remodeling that is similar to plexogenic pulmonary arteriopathy but does not include in situ thrombosis or formation of plexiform lesions (E-Fig. 18.3).

Due to the association of increased mortality when PH is present in patients with chronic heart and lung disease, there is considerable interest in using PAH medications for the treatment of WHO Groups 2 and 3. There is currently insufficient evidence to suggest that any of the currently available medications are beneficial in these other types of pulmonary hypertension. Considering their high costs and ability to worsen gas exchange and pulmonary edema formation, their use in patients who do not have Group 1 PAH is not recommended, and treatment should be directed at the underlying heart or lung disease.

PULMONARY THROMBOEMBOLISM

Definition and Epidemiology

Pulmonary thromboembolism refers to the passage of a clot from the venous system or the right ventricle into a pulmonary artery. Several other materials can embolize to the pulmonary arterial bed, including air, fat, amniotic fluid, tumor, or injected foreign bodies (e.g., talc). These embolic phenomena have different risk factors and clinical manifestations but occur much less commonly than venous thrombosis with pulmonary thromboembolism.

Pulmonary thromboembolic disease is a relatively common entity, with an incidence ranging from 400,000 to 650,000 cases per year in the United States. The deep veins of the femoral and popliteal systems of the lower extremities are the most common sources of venous thrombosis, but upper extremity thrombosis and right heart thrombi can also embolize to the lung. Predisposing factors for pulmonary embolism are the same as those for venous thrombosis and include venous stasis, hypercoagulability, and endothelial injury, as well as congenital or acquired prothrombotic disorders (e.g., activated protein C deficiency, factor V Leiden).

❖ For a deeper discussion on this topic, please see Chapter 75, "Pulmonary Hypertension," in *Goldman-Cecil Medicine*, 26th Edition.

Pathophysiology

An acute pulmonary thromboembolism can obstruct a branch of the pulmonary artery, resulting in an increased $\dot{V}/\dot{Q}$ ratio. This increases overall dead space ventilation, which can lead to inefficient excretion of carbon dioxide, potentially raising the partial pressure of carbon dioxide in arterial blood ($Paco_2$). Blood flow is shifted from the obstructed site to other areas, leading to $\dot{V}/\dot{Q}$ mismatch, shunting, and hypoxemia.

Right ventricular dysfunction is commonly encountered in acute pulmonary thromboembolism, occurring when a substantial portion of the pulmonary vascular bed is occluded and there is an acute increase in PAP. Approximately 5% of patients present with cardiogenic shock from right ventricular failure, and somewhere between 30% and 70% of normotensive patients will have right ventricular dysfunction on transthoracic echocardiography, which is associated with a worse prognosis.

Clinical Presentation and Diagnosis

Common symptoms of pulmonary thromboembolism include shortness of breath, chest pain, hemoptysis, and syncope. When the diagnosis of acute pulmonary embolism is suspected, risk factors such as recent immobilization or surgery, malignancy, or a prior history of venous thrombosis should be clinically documented, and a validated clinical scoring system, such as the Wells or Geneva score, can be used to assess the pretest probability of pulmonary embolism. The most common physical examination findings are tachycardia and tachypnea, and chest examination may be normal or may reveal isolated crackles or even diffuse wheezing. Edema of the extremities, especially if the edema is asymmetrical, may indicate venous thrombosis. Signs of right ventricular strain, such as an increased pulmonary component

Approach to diagnosis

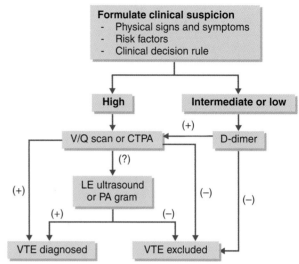

Fig. 18.1 A proposed diagnostic algorithm for the diagnosis of acute pulmonary embolism (PE). Clinical suspicion, often with the use of clinical decision rules, can determine if patients should proceed directly to an imaging study such as CT pulmonary angiography (CTPE) or ventilation-perfusion (V/Q) scan when the pretest probability is high. D-dimer testing is recommended in patients with a lower clinical suspicion for acute PE, where a negative D-dimer is a sensitive test and can exclude the diagnosis of venous thromboembolism (VTE).

of the second heart sound or a palpable right ventricular heave, can be observed in massive pulmonary embolus.

The electrocardiogram may show atrial tachyarrhythmias or evidence of right heart strain as shown by a new right bundle branch block or right ventricular strain pattern that mimics inferior myocardial infarction. The chest radiograph is often normal but may show atelectasis, isolated infiltrates, or a small pleural effusion, but in most cases, is not sufficiently sensitive to diagnose a pulmonary embolism.

Chest CT angiography is the main imaging modality used for the diagnosis of acute pulmonary embolism, although $\dot{V}/\dot{Q}$ scan and pulmonary angiography are used in certain clinical settings (Fig. 18.1). CT angiography provides a noninvasive, rapid, and sensitive way to detect pulmonary emboli (E-Fig. 18.4), and most diagnostic algorithms combine CT pulmonary angiography with clinical suspicion, D-dimer determination, and assessment of the lower extremities for deep vein thrombosis by CT or ultrasound.

However, for individuals with absolute or relative contraindications to CT angiography, the $\dot{V}/\dot{Q}$ scan provides an alternative approach. A *high-probability* $\dot{V}/\dot{Q}$ scan, characterized by multiple perfusion defects in areas of normal ventilation, is more than 90% accurate in diagnosing pulmonary embolism. A *normal* $\dot{V}/\dot{Q}$ scan excludes pulmonary embolism in essentially all cases. The test is less reliable when interpreted as *low, intermediate,* or *indeterminate* probability. In these circumstances, pulmonary embolism is observed in 4% to 66% of patients, and in these situations the diagnostic certainty depends on the pretest probability of pulmonary embolism. With improvements in CT angiography, pulmonary angiography is now performed very infrequently but could be considered when other tests are inconclusive, a high likelihood of pulmonary embolism exists, and there is a need for diagnostic certainty.

Risk Stratification and Treatment

Once acute pulmonary thromboembolism is diagnosed, risk stratification is essential to guide treatment decisions. This typically incorporates clinical appearance, vital signs, validated PE risk scores, and RV function assessed by imaging modalities and cardiac biomarkers. Acute PE that causes hemodynamic instability is referred to as massive PE or high-risk PE and warrants immediate consideration of reperfusion therapies. In acute PE patients who present without shock or hemodynamic instability, multimodal risk stratification is used to identify patients at low and intermediate risk, the latter typically defined by signs of RV dysfunction on CT or echocardiography, or elevated levels of troponin or B-type natriuretic peptide (BNP).

Treatment of acute PE centers on supportive care, systemic anticoagulation, and consideration of reperfusion therapy. Unless there are contraindications, systemic anticoagulation should be started after the diagnosis of acute PE is established. Intravenous unfractionated heparin or subcutaneous low-molecular-weight heparin (LMWH) are typically the preferred agents. For patients with a contraindication to anticoagulation, an inferior vena cava filter should be placed. Reperfusion therapies include systemic thrombolysis and surgical thrombectomy and are indicated in massive PE. The use of systemic thrombolytics in intermediate risk PE remains controversial and is not practiced routinely. Catheter-directed thrombolysis and catheter embolectomy are other available reperfusion therapies that are less well studied and not recommended for routine use.

After stabilization and clinical improvement, patients are transitioned to their long-term anticoagulation therapy. Options for anticoagulation include vitamin K antagonists such as warfarin, non–vitamin K oral anticoagulants (NOACs), such as apixaban or rivaroxaban, or LMWH. NOACs have increasingly become the preferred oral anticoagulant due to their safety profile and ease of use, but risks and benefits of each agent should be discussed with patients to allow for individualized decision making. Duration of anticoagulation for an acute pulmonary embolism is at least 3 months, after which extended therapy can be considered based on clinical risk factors (e.g. provoked vs. unprovoked event) and bleeding risk.

Chronic Thromboembolic Pulmonary Hypertension

Chronic thromboembolic pulmonary hypertension (CTEPH) is a distinct type of pulmonary hypertension, classified as WHO group 4 PH. CTEPH is characterized by incomplete or abnormal resolution of acute pulmonary thromboembolism such that residual emboli become organized and fibrotic. This develops in approximately 4% of patients after acute pulmonary embolism. However, nearly half of CTEPH cases occur in patients without a prior history of venous thromboembolism. The diagnosis of CTEPH requires precapillary pulmonary hypertension on RHC in the presence of chronic/organized flow limiting thrombi/emboli in the elastic pulmonary arteries after at least 3 months of effective anticoagulation (E-Fig 18.5). Unlike other forms of pulmonary hypertension, the mainstay of treatment is surgical. Pulmonary endarterectomy (PEA) is performed via median sternotomy with cardiopulmonary bypass, after which deep hypothermic circulatory arrest allows for visualization, identification of the dissection plane, and complete endarterectomy. PEA is often curative, and is associated with improved symptoms, hemodynamics, and survival.

In patients for whom PEA is not feasible, medical therapy with pulmonary vasodilators, namely riociguat, has been shown to be effective in improving hemodynamics and functional capacity. Balloon pulmonary angioplasty is an emerging therapeutic option for CTEPH patients with inoperable disease or in whom the risk-to-benefit ratio of PEA is not favorable.

PROSPECTUS FOR THE FUTURE

Numerous advances in our understanding of pulmonary vascular biology over the last 35 years have markedly enhanced understanding of the pathogenesis of pulmonary hypertensive disorders and have led to the development of therapies that slow disease progression, increase functional capacity, and increase quality of life. However, most pulmonary vascular diseases are not curable and result in decreased survival. New therapies designed to prevent the loss of healthy vessels and reverse vascular remodeling are needed before substantial gains in disease reversal and cure can be achieved. Cellular mechanisms that regulate endothelial apoptosis, angiogenesis, and perivascular inflammation appear to have potential as future therapeutic targets. Modulation of sex hormones, cellular bioenergetics, and epigenetic factors may be other promising approaches. Little is understood about the adaptive changes of the right ventricle to chronically increased afterload. Furthermore, studies are needed in the area of genetic predisposition to thromboembolic disease and vascular dysfunction leading to thrombus formation as well as the determination of appropriate follow-up evaluation for patients after acute PE and who might benefit from screening for chronic thromboembolic disease. Finally, national studies currently underway that seek to provide deep phenotyping of pulmonary vascular disease and establish national biobanks and patient registries should provide important tools to help investigators find more effective therapies for these devastating diseases.

SUGGESTED READINGS

Girerd B, Weatherald J, Montani D, Humbert M: Heritable pulmonary hypertension: from bench to bedside, Eur Respir Rev 26(145), 2017.

Humbert M, Guignabert C, Bonnet S, et al: Pathology and pathobiology of pulmonary hypertension: state of the art and research perspectives, Eur Respir J 53(1), 2019.

Klinger JR, Elliott CG, Levine DJ, et al: Therapy for Pulmonary Arterial Hypertension in Adults: Update of the CHEST Guideline and Expert Panel Report, Chest 155(3):565-586, 2019.

Konstantinides SV, Meyer G, Becattini C, et al, ESC Scientific Document Group: 2019 ESC Guidelines for the diagnosis and management of acute pulmonary embolism developed in collaboration with the European Respiratory Society (ERS), Eur Heart J 41:543-603, 2020.

Mullin CJ, Klinger JR: Chronic thromboembolic pulmonary hypertension, Heart Fail Clin 14(3):339-351, 2018.

Simonneau G, Montani D, Celermajer DS, et al: Haemodynamic definitions and updated clinical classification of pulmonary hypertension, Eur Respir J 53(1), 2019.

Stacher E, Graham BB, Hunt JM, et al: Modern age pathology of pulmonary arterial hypertension, Am J Respir Crit Care Med 186:261-272, 2012.

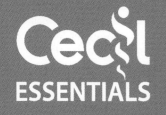

19

Disorders of the Pleura, Mediastinum, and Chest Wall

Eric J. Gartman, F. Dennis McCool

PLEURAL DISEASE

The pleura is a thin membrane that covers the entire surface of the lung, inner surface of the rib cage, diaphragm, and mediastinum. There are two pleural membranes: the visceral pleura, which covers the lung; and the parietal pleura, which lines the rib cage, diaphragm, and mediastinum. A layer of mesothelial cells lines both pleural surfaces. The closed space in between the surface of the lung and the chest cavity is called the *pleural space.* A small amount of fluid normally resides in this space and forms a thin layer between the pleural surfaces. Pleural fluid serves as a lubricant for the visceral and parietal pleurae as they move against each other during inspiration and expiration.

The blood vessels in the visceral pleura are supplied from the pulmonary circulation and have less hydrostatic pressure than the blood vessels in the parietal pleura, which are supplied by the systemic circulation. The pressure in the pleural space is subatmospheric during quiet breathing. Fluid is filtered from the higher-pressure vascular structures into the pleural space. The normal fluid turnover is about 10 to 20 mL per day, with 0.2 to 1 mL remaining in the pleural space. Pleural fluid usually contains a small amount of protein and a small number of cells that are mostly mononuclear cells. Although both parietal and visceral pleurae contribute to pleural fluid formation, most of the fluid results from filtration of the higher-pressure vessels supplying the parietal pleura.

After the fluid enters the pleural space, it is drained from the pleural space by a network of pleural lymphatics located beneath the mesothelial monolayer. The lymphatics originate in stomas on the parietal pleural surface. In abnormal circumstances of increased fluid production or impaired removal, fluid can accumulate in the pleural space. Factors that promote the entry of fluid into the pleural space include an increase in systemic venous pressure, an increase in pulmonary venous pressure, an increase in permeability of pleural vessels, and a reduction in pleural pressure. Conditions that increase hydrostatic pressure can be seen in congestive heart failure; changes in pleural membrane permeability can be seen in various inflammatory states or malignancy; and a reduction in pleural pressure can be seen with atelectasis. Occasionally, microvascular oncotic pressure may be sufficiently reduced to promote fluid entry into the pleural space in patients with hypoalbuminemia. Factors that block lymphatic drainage and interfere with the egress of fluid from the pleural space include central lymphatic obstruction and obstruction of lymphatic channels at the pleural surface by tumor.

Pleural Effusion

Pleural effusion is the accumulation of fluid in the pleural space. Pleural effusions usually are detected by chest radiography; however, the volume of fluid in the pleural space must exceed 250 mL to be visualized on a chest radiograph. When an effusion exists, there is blunting of the costophrenic angle on a posteroanterior chest film, which represents a fluid meniscus that can be detected posteriorly on the lateral chest radiograph, and fluid occasionally can be demonstrated in the minor or major fissures (E-Figs. 19.1 and 19.2). Apparent elevation or changes in the contour of the diaphragm on a posteroanterior chest film may signify a subpulmonic effusion, so called because it retains the general shape of the diaphragm without blunting the costophrenic angle; however, it is evident on the lateral film.

A decubitus chest radiograph can be obtained to determine whether the fluid is free flowing or loculated. Computed tomography (CT) of the chest provides better definition of the pleural space than plain radiography. Chest CT is particularly useful in defining loculated effusions and in differentiating pulmonary parenchymal abnormalities from pleural abnormalities, atelectasis from effusion, and loculated effusion from lung abscess or other parenchymal processes (E-Fig. 19.3). The edge of a parenchymal process usually touches the chest wall and forms an acute angle (0-90 degrees), whereas that of an empyema is usually an obtuse angle (90-180 degrees).

Thoracentesis is a procedure in which fluid is aspirated from the pleural space. To help minimize procedural complications and assist in needle placement, ultrasound or CT guidance should be used to direct the thoracentesis catheter into the pleural space.

Classifying pleural effusions as transudates or exudates greatly assists with the differential diagnosis. The approach to pleural effusions is outlined in E-Fig. 19.4. Further analysis of pleural fluid may provide a definitive diagnosis (e.g., malignancy); however, even without a definitive diagnosis, pleural fluid analysis can be useful in excluding possible causes of disease such as infection.

Transudates

Effusions that accumulate due to changes in oncotic and hydrostatic forces usually have a low protein content and are called *transudates* (Table 19.1). Congestive heart failure is the most common cause of a transudate, and the effusions are typically bilateral. If the effusion is unilateral, it involves the right hemithorax in most instances. Effusions due to heart failure almost universally are related to dysfunction of the left side of the heart, although they rarely can result from right heart failure (e.g., advanced pulmonary arterial hypertension).

Transudative effusions may be seen in cirrhosis, nephrotic syndrome, myxedema, pulmonary embolism, superior vena cava obstruction, and peritoneal dialysis. In patients with cirrhosis, the effusions are often right-sided, and the mechanism may be related to flow from the peritoneal space across diaphragmatic defects into the pleural space (i.e., hepatic hydrothorax). Transudative effusions are typically small to moderate sized and rarely require drainage to improve symptoms.

TABLE 19.1   Causes of Pleural Effusions

Conditions Associated With Transudates

Ascites
Cirrhosis
Congestive heart failure
Hypoalbuminemia
Intra-abdominal fluid
Malnutrition
Nephrotic syndrome
Peritoneal dialysis

Conditions Associated With Exudates

Asbestosis
Chylothorax
Collagen vascular disease
Complications of abdominal surgery
Dressler's syndrome (myocardial infarction, cardiotomy)
Drug-induced lupus
Empyema
Hemothorax
Infection
Intra-abdominal pathologic abnormalities (abscess)
Lymphedema
Malignancy (primary lung cancer, lymphoma, metastatic cancer)
Meigs' syndrome (benign ovarian tumor)
Myxedema
Pancreatitis
Parapneumonic causes (pneumonia, lung abscess, bronchiectasis)
Pulmonary embolism and infarction
Rheumatoid arthritis (pleurisy)
Ruptured esophagus
Subphrenic abscess
Systemic lupus erythematosus
Trauma
Uremia
Urinothorax
Miscellaneous sources

Modified from Light RW, Macgregor MI, Luchsinger PC, et al: Pleural effusions: the diagnostic separation of transudates and exudates, Ann Intern Med 77:507-513, 1972.

Exudates

Exudative effusions occur when there is an alteration in vascular permeability or pleural fluid resorption. They can be observed in inflammatory, infectious, or neoplastic conditions.

To distinguish an exudate from a transudate, one of three criteria must be fulfilled: (1) An exudate must have a pleural fluid–to-serum protein ratio greater than 0.5; (2) a pleural fluid–to-serum lactate dehydrogenase (LDH) ratio must be greater than 0.6; or (3) a pleural fluid LDH level must be greater than two thirds of the upper limit of normal (Table 19.2). When all three criteria are met, the sensitivity, specificity, and positive predictive value exceed 98% for defining an exudative effusion.

Measuring pleural fluid cholesterol may also help to distinguish an exudate from a transudate. Pleural fluid cholesterol is derived from degenerating cells within the pleural space and from vascular leakage due to increased permeability. A cholesterol level greater than 45 mg/dL is consistent with an exudative effusion.

Exudative effusions are commonly caused by infection. Parapneumonic effusion typically occurs in patients with bacterial pneumonia and can be further classified as an uncomplicated or complicated effusion.

TABLE 19.2   Differentiation of Exudative and Transudative Pleural Effusions

Characteristic	Exudate	Transudate
Pleural fluid–to-serum protein ratio	>0.5	<0.5
Pleural fluid LDH level	>⅔ of the upper limit of normal	<⅔ of the upper limit of normal
Pleural fluid–to-serum LDH ratio	>0.6	<0.6

LDH, Lactate dehydrogenase.
Modified from Light RW, Macgregor MI, Luchsinger PC, et al: Pleural effusions: the diagnostic separation of transudates and exudates, Ann Intern Med 77:507-513, 1972.

Uncomplicated parapneumonic effusions do not require drainage and respond to antibiotic therapy alone used for treatment of the underlying pneumonia. In contrast, complicated parapneumonic effusions do not respond to antibiotic therapy alone and require drainage to prevent the formation of an empyema. The transition from uncomplicated to complicated can occur extremely rapidly, within a 24-hour period in some cases.

Typically, an uncomplicated parapneumonic effusion has a pH level greater than 7.3, a glucose level greater than 60 mg/dL, and an LDH level less than 1000 IU/L. A pH level of less than 7.2 usually identifies a complicated effusion. However, this finding is not specific for infection, and the cause may be malignancy, rheumatoid arthritis, or trauma with esophageal disruption causing an associated reduction in pH level.

Complicated exudative effusions require drainage to avoid development of loculation, cutaneous fistulas, bronchopleural fistulas, or fibrothorax. The findings of pus or bacteria by Gram stain or culture confirms the diagnosis of empyema and requires immediate drainage. The injection of fibrolytic agents and DNase into the pleural space can augment full drainage of infected pleural effusions; however, treatment of complicated pleural effusions occasionally requires surgical intervention and lung decortication.

Primary tuberculosis in endemic areas may be associated with pleural effusion in up to 30% of patients. The effusion is caused by increased vascular permeability of the pleural membrane because of a hypersensitivity reaction, not direct infection. Typically, the pleural fluid is lymphocyte predominant and acid-fast stain and culture negative. Adenosine deaminase levels greater than 50 U/L may be helpful in identifying tuberculous pleural effusions. Tuberculous empyema is distinct from a tuberculous pleural effusion and can occur when there is an extension of infection from the thoracic lymph nodes into the pleural space or hematogenous spread of tuberculosis to the pleural space.

Malignant effusions are the second most common cause of exudative pleural effusions and confer a poor prognosis. Seeding of the parietal or visceral pleura with malignant cells can change vascular permeability and impede resorption, resulting in effusion formation. However, the finding of a pleural effusion in an individual with malignancy does not necessarily imply that there is a malignant process in the pleural space. Effusions in these individuals may be caused by atelectasis, postobstructive pneumonia, hypoalbuminemia, pulmonary emboli, or complications from irradiation or chemotherapy.

The most common cause of malignant effusion is lung cancer, followed by breast cancer and lymphoma. An effusion that is bloody suggests a malignant process; however, other causes of bloody pleural effusions include trauma, asbestos exposure, tuberculosis, collagen vascular disease, and thromboembolic disease. To confirm the diagnosis of malignancy, cytologic examination of the fluid is needed. Malignant cells can be seen in 60% of malignant effusions on the first thoracentesis. Sensitivity rises to 80% if three separate samples are obtained. If needed, a biopsy of the pleura may be useful in identifying a malignancy. Biopsies may be obtained via medical thoracoscopy, surgical video-assisted thoracoscopy or, less optimally, in a blinded fashion through a Cope or Abrams needle.

A low pleural fluid pH has prognostic and therapeutic implications for patients with malignant effusions. Patients with a low pleural fluid pH due to malignancy tend to have shorter survival times and poorer responses to chemical pleurodesis. Recurrent malignant pleural effusions may improve with chemical pleurodesis with talc or tetracycline derivatives, but effectiveness varies and a complete response is achieved in little more than 50% of patients. Alternatively, many patients with recurrent malignant effusions have tunneled indwelling pleural catheters placed, allowing intermittent drainage, relief of symptoms, and possibly mechanical pleurodesis over time.

Systemic inflammatory disorders such as rheumatoid arthritis and lupus erythematosus can be associated with exudative effusions. Rheumatoid pleural effusions are a common intrathoracic manifestation of rheumatoid disease and may be seen in as many as 5% of patients. Rheumatoid factor titers in pleural fluid are often greater than 1:320, and the pleural fluid glucose level is less than 60 mg/dL (or the pleural fluid–to-serum glucose ratio is less than 0.5). However, a low glucose level also may be found in complicated parapneumonic effusions or empyema, malignant effusion, tuberculosis pleurisy, lupus pleuritis, and esophageal rupture. In systemic lupus erythematosus, 15% to 50% of patients have pleural effusions, and the pleural fluid antinuclear antibody titer is greater than 1:160.

Measuring pleural fluid amylase concentrations may further refine the differential diagnosis for an exudative effusion. Finding a pleural amylase level greater than the upper limit of normal for serum amylase is consistent with acute pancreatitis, chronic pancreatic pleural effusion, esophageal rupture, or malignancy. Pancreatic disease is associated with pancreatic amylase isoenzymes, whereas malignancy and esophageal rupture are characterized by a predominance of salivary isoenzymes.

Pneumothorax

Pneumothorax is the accumulation of air in the pleural space. In this instance, pleural pressure becomes positive and there is compression of underlying lung. Patients with pneumothorax typically have acute onset of dyspnea. Findings include tachycardia, decreased breath sounds, decreased tactile fremitus, a pleural friction rub, subcutaneous emphysema, hyperresonance, and a tracheal shift to the opposite side.

The diagnosis can be made by obtaining an upright chest radiograph, and rapid assessment can be achieved with point-of-care ultrasound. Typically, the visceral pleura separates from the parietal pleura, and air can be seen between the visceral pleural lining and the rib cage. An end-expiratory radiograph increases the density of lung while reducing its volume, highlighting the difference between the lung parenchyma and the pleural gas.

Management of a significant pneumothorax usually requires insertion of a thoracostomy tube and suction followed by water-seal drainage. However, if the pneumothorax is small and the patient is not in distress, observation alone may be indicated. If there is not a continuing air leak, as from a bronchopleural fistula, the pleural air is reabsorbed into the blood with resolution of the pneumothorax.

A tension pneumothorax is a medical emergency that requires immediate decompression by placement of a chest catheter. A tension pneumothorax occurs when pleural pressure reaches levels sufficient to cause mediastinal shift, compression of the vena cava and heart, and hemodynamic compromise. This physiology implies an ongoing leak of air into the pleural space.

Pneumothorax is often associated with blunt or penetrating trauma. With penetrating trauma, air may leak into the pleural space through the chest wall or the lung. Mechanical ventilation has also been associated with pneumothorax. Patients with underlying lung disease receiving mechanical ventilation may acutely develop a pneumothorax. A sudden rise in peak airway pressures with a reduction in breath sounds can alert the clinician to this complication.

Pneumothorax may occur spontaneously or result secondarily from underlying lung disease. Typically, spontaneous pneumothorax occurs in tall, young, thin men, presumably a result of rupture of apical blebs. Underlying lung diseases that can be complicated by pneumothorax include emphysema, cystic fibrosis, granulomatous inflammation, necrotizing pneumonia, pulmonary fibrosis, and lung abscess. Catamenial pneumothorax occurs in women who have subpleural and diaphragmatic endometriosis, with rupture of the endometrial nodules at the time of menstruation causing pneumothorax.

Mesothelioma

Malignant mesotheliomas are neoplasms arising from the serosal membranes of the body cavities. Eighty percent of mesotheliomas originate in the pleura. Individuals usually are older than 55 years, and there is an association with asbestos exposure in the distant past. Symptoms include shortness of breath, chest pain, and weight loss.

The most common radiologic finding is a large, unilateral pleural effusion that may completely opacify the hemithorax. There may be circumferential pleural thickening, usually associated with various amounts of calcified pleural plaque and effusions. CT of the chest is the most accurate noninvasive method for assessing stage and progression of mesothelioma. Pleural fluid cytology frequently is insufficient for diagnosis, and the most efficient way of obtaining tissue is by CT-guided core biopsy or thoracoscopy.

The overall prognosis for patients with malignant mesothelioma is poor. No particular therapy has emerged as superior to supportive therapy alone in terms of survival.

MEDIASTINAL DISEASE

Lesion Location

The mediastinum is the central part of the thoracic cavity between the lungs that contains the heart and aorta, esophagus, trachea, lymph nodes, and thymus. The mediastinum is bordered by the two pleural cavities laterally, the diaphragm inferiorly, and the thoracic inlet superiorly. The mediastinal space can be divided into three compartments: anterior, middle, and posterior. The localization of mediastinal masses in one of these compartments assists in the differential diagnosis (Fig. 19.1).

The anterior mediastinal compartment is anterior to the pericardium and includes lymphatic tissue, the thymus, and the great veins. Lesions most commonly found in the anterior mediastinum are thymomas, germ cell tumors, lymphomas, intrathoracic thyroid tissue, and parathyroid lesions. Thymomas comprise 20% of mediastinal neoplasms in adults, and they are the most common anterior mediastinal primary neoplasm in adults. Symptoms due to myasthenia gravis may affect one third of patients with thymomas. Middle mediastinal lesions include tracheal masses, bronchogenic and pericardial cysts, enlarged lymph nodes, and proximal aortic disease (i.e., aneurysm or dissection). Posterior mediastinal masses include neurogenic tumors and cysts, meningocele, lymphoma, aneurysm of the descending aorta, and esophageal disorders such as diverticula and neoplasms.

Patients with systemic lymphoma often have mediastinal involvement, and 5% to 10% of patients with lymphoma have primary mediastinal lesions at clinical presentation. Mediastinal cysts can arise in the pericardium, bronchi, esophagus or stomach, thymus, and thoracic duct, and although benign, they can produce compressive symptoms. Lung cancer often presents with metastatic mediastinal adenopathy and is a sign of advanced stage.

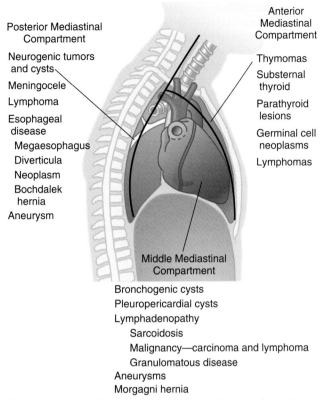

Fig. 19.1 Masses of the mediastinum and their anatomic locations.

Posterior Mediastinal Compartment
Neurogenic tumors and cysts
Meningocele
Lymphoma
Esophageal disease
Megaesophagus
Diverticula
Neoplasm
Bochdalek hernia
Aneurysm

Anterior Mediastinal Compartment
Thymomas
Substernal thyroid
Parathyroid lesions
Germinal cell neoplasms
Lymphomas

Middle Mediastinal Compartment
Bronchogenic cysts
Pleuropericardial cysts
Lymphadenopathy
Sarcoidosis
Malignancy—carcinoma and lymphoma
Granulomatous disease
Aneurysms
Morgagni hernia

Treatment of a mediastinal mass depends on the underlying pathology. Many require surgical resection, irradiation, chemotherapy, or careful monitoring over time.

Mediastinitis

Inflammation of the mediastinal structures can be acute or chronic. Acute mediastinitis is a rapidly progressive condition due to infection, and it most commonly complicates cardiothoracic surgical procedures or occurs as a result of trauma. Chest imaging studies may show a widening of the mediastinum, pneumothorax, or hydrothorax. Treatment requires microbiological identification, antibiotics, pleural drainage, and mediastinal evacuation.

Chronic mediastinitis (i.e., fibrosing mediastinitis) is a progressive illness that results from fungal or granulomatous infections, neoplasms, radiotherapy, occasionally drugs (such as methysergide), or it may be idiopathic. Patients usually remain asymptomatic until vascular, respiratory, or neurologic structures are affected; tracheobronchial narrowing is the most common manifestation. Diagnosis and treatment often require surgical intervention, although no treatment is highly successful.

CHEST WALL DISEASE

The chest wall is composed of the bony structures of the rib cage, the articulations between the ribs and the vertebrae, the diaphragm, and other respiratory muscles. Normal function of this ventilatory pump is needed to bring oxygen from the atmosphere into the body. A wide variety of chest wall and neuromuscular disorders can result in dysfunction of the ventilatory pump. These disorders typically result in a restrictive dysfunction characterized by a reduction in total lung capacity and vital capacity with a normal residual volume. Hypoventilation may ensue, resulting in hypercapnia, atelectasis, and hypoxemia.

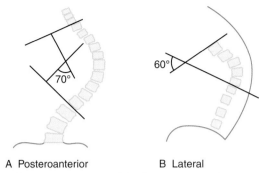

A Posteroanterior   B Lateral

Fig. 19.2 Schematic depiction of the lines constructed to measure the Cobb angle of scoliosis (A) and kyphosis (B).

Skeletal Disease

Kyphoscoliosis and ankylosing spondylitis are disorders that involve the spine and its articulations. Pectus excavatum involves the sternum, flail chest affects the ribs, and obesity adds to the soft tissue mass of the chest wall. These disorders primarily affect the respiratory system by stiffening its tissues. Of these disorders, kyphoscoliosis produces the most severe restrictive impairment, and ankylosing spondylitis and pectus excavatum cause little respiratory compromise.

Kyphoscoliosis refers to a group of disorders characterized by excessive spinal curvature in the lateral plane (i.e., scoliosis) and sagittal plane (i.e., kyphosis). The degree of curvature can be assessed by measuring the Cobb angle (Fig. 19.2). Greater degrees of spinal curvature are associated with greater restriction and an increased risk of respiratory failure (E-Fig. 19.5).

Kyphoscoliosis may be idiopathic, caused by neuromuscular disease, or associated with congenital vertebral malformations. Idiopathic kyphoscoliosis is the most common form, usually manifesting in late childhood or early adolescence and affecting females more than males (ratio of 4:1). It is thought to be a multigene condition with an autosomal or sex-linked inheritance pattern and variable phenotypic expression. A defect in the chromatin-remodeling gene (CHD7) has been associated with idiopathic kyphoscoliosis.

For a given degree of spinal deformity, individuals with kyphoscoliosis due to a neuromuscular disease have more respiratory impairment than those with idiopathic kyphoscoliosis. Factors that contribute to respiratory failure in patients with kyphoscoliosis include inspiratory muscle weakness, underlying neuromuscular disease, sleep-disordered breathing, and airway compression due to distortion of lung parenchyma and twisting of airways.

Treatment consists of general supportive measures such as immunizations against influenza and pneumococci, smoking cessation, maintenance of a normal body weight, supplemental oxygen, and treatment of respiratory infections. It is important to recognize nocturnal hypoventilation because it can be treated with noninvasive positive-pressure ventilation. This is typically delivered through a nasal or full face mask. Indications for instituting noninvasive ventilation include symptoms suggesting nocturnal hypoventilation, signs of cor pulmonale, nocturnal oxyhemoglobin desaturation, or an elevated daytime $Paco_2$.

Obesity

Obesity is a major health problem that affects children and adults throughout the world. Body fat usually constitutes 15% to 20% of body mass in healthy men and 25% to 30% of body mass in healthy women. In cases of obesity, the body fat content may increase by as much as 500% in women and 800% in men. The degree of obesity can be assessed by the body mass index, which is the ratio of body weight (BW) in kilograms to the square of the height (Ht) in meters (BW/Ht^2). Individuals with a BMI between 18.5 and 24.9 kg/m^2 are normal, and those with a BMI greater than 40 kg/m^2 are considered severely or morbidly obese.

Reductions in functional residual capacity and expiratory reserve volume are the most common pulmonary function abnormalities in obesity, whereas vital capacity and total lung capacity may be only minimally reduced. Obesity promotes breathing at low lung volumes, which reduces lung compliance and increases the work of breathing. A subgroup of individuals with obesity hypoventilate and become hypercapnic. When obesity is associated with hypoventilation, it is called the obesity-hypoventilation syndrome (i.e., Pickwickian syndrome). The mechanism underlying hypoventilation is unknown but may result from factors that reduce respiratory center chemosensitivity, such as hypoxia, sleep apnea, or adipokines such as leptin. The most important consequences of chronic hypoventilation are hypoxemia and pulmonary hypertension.

Nocturnal noninvasive positive-pressure ventilation can help to reverse these abnormalities. Weight loss is the optimal therapy, but it is not always attainable, and long-term weight loss maintenance is even more difficult. Pharmacotherapy or bariatric surgery should be considered for obese individuals who do not achieve weight control with conventional methods (i.e., diet, enhanced physical activity, and behavioral therapy).

Diaphragm Paralysis

The diaphragm separates the thorax from the abdomen and is the major muscle of inspiration. Diaphragm weakness or paralysis can involve one or both hemidiaphragms. Unilateral diaphragm paralysis is more common than bilateral diaphragm paralysis. The most frequent causes of unilateral paralysis include traumatic phrenic nerve injury, herpes zoster infection, cervical spinal disease, and compressive tumors. Patients may be asymptomatic, or the abnormality may be discovered as an incidental finding of an elevated hemidiaphragm on a chest radiograph (Fig. 19.3). The diagnosis is confirmed by seeing on fluoroscopy a paradoxical upward motion of the affected diaphragm during a vigorous sniff maneuver. There is no specific treatment for this disorder, but recovery after the initial injury occasionally occurs. When the patient has disabling symptoms and significant elevation of the diaphragm is seen on the chest radiograph, surgical plication of the diaphragm may provide some relief of symptoms.

Bilateral diaphragm paralysis is most often seen in the setting of a disease producing generalized muscle weakness or motor neuron disease such as amyotrophic lateral sclerosis. Pulmonary function test results are associated with severe restrictive impairments. When the patient assumes the supine position, there may be a further reduction (≤50%) in vital capacity. It is not surprising that orthopnea is an especially prominent symptom, and patients often have difficulty sleeping

in the supine position. Patients also complain of dyspnea when bending or lifting objects.

Bilateral diaphragm paralysis can be difficult to diagnose. Restriction evidenced by pulmonary function test results is nonspecific, as is the finding of low lung volumes on chest radiographs. Fluoroscopic sniff testing (i.e., diaphragm fluoroscopy) can yield false-negative and false-positive results. Measurement of transdiaphragmatic pressure is the gold standard, but it is somewhat invasive, requiring placement of catheters in the esophagus and stomach. Alternatively, B-mode ultrasound of the diaphragm in the zone of apposition is a very useful noninvasive means of diagnosing diaphragm paralysis, as it can directly assess the thickening of the diaphragm muscle (or lack thereof).

Treatment should address the underlying disease, which may or may not be reversible. If paralysis is idiopathic or caused by neuralgic amyotrophy (i.e., brachial plexus neuritis), more than 50% of individuals may recover. Phrenic nerve pacing may be used in patients with spinal cord injuries above C3, and noninvasive positive-pressure ventilation can be used to treat patients with nocturnal hypoventilation. Diaphragm plication is not indicated in patients with bilateral diaphragm paralysis.

PROSPECTUS FOR THE FUTURE

Numerous advances can be expected in treating individuals with pleural, mediastinal, and chest wall diseases. Progress in pleural fluid analysis using novel biomarkers and nucleic acid amplification tests may lead to more rapid and accurate diagnosis of tuberculous pleural effusions. Assays of pleural fluid tumor markers and chromosome analysis are promising developments for the differentiation of malignant from nonmalignant effusions. Mesothelioma remains resistant to traditional therapeutic approaches, but evolving technology centered on gene therapy may produce a new treatment modality.

Better visualization of mediastinal structures can be achieved as magnetic resonance imaging (MRI) evolves and becomes more routinely applied to examination of the chest. Molecular tracers targeting tumor receptors or proteins may be used with MRI and positron emission tomography imaging techniques to better differentiate malignant from benign mediastinal masses.

Noninvasive nocturnal ventilation remains a cornerstone of therapy for patents with chest wall and neuromuscular diseases, but compliance can be problematic. Continued evolution of techniques to deliver nocturnal noninvasive ventilation may improve compliance with treatment, and application of this technique to patients with obesity-hypoventilation syndrome may reduce morbidity and mortality for them.

Patients with diaphragm paralysis due to high cervical spinal cord lesions may benefit from advances in intramuscular diaphragm pacing. This technique may provide an alternative means of treating respiratory failure in these individuals and others with diaphragm paralysis.

For a deeper discussion on this topic, please see Chapter 92, ❖ "Diseases of the Diaphragm, Chest Wall, Pleura, and Mediastinum," in *Goldman-Cecil Medicine*, 26th Edition.

SUGGESTED READINGS

Brixey AG, Light RW: Pleural effusions occurring with right heart failure, Curr Opin Pulm Med 17:226-231, 2011.

Colice GE, Curtis C, Deslauriers J, et al: Medical and surgical treatment of parapneumonic effusions: an evidence-based guideline, Chest 18:1158-1171, 2000.

Davies HE, Davies RJ, Davies CW, BTS Pleural Disease Guideline Group: Management of pleural infection in adults: British Thoracic Society Pleural Disease Guideline 2010, Thorax 65: 2010.

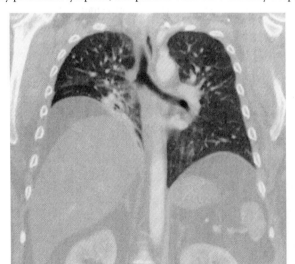

Fig. 19.3 Computed tomography of a patient with unilateral right hemidiaphragm paralysis and associated right lower lobe atelectasis.

Duwe BV, Sterman DH, Musani AI: Tumors of the mediastinum, Chest 128:2893-2909, 2005.

Gottesman E, McCool FD: Ultrasound evaluation of the paralyzed diaphragm, Am J Respir Crit Care Med 155:1570-1574, 1997.

Heffner JE, Klein JS: Recent advances in the diagnosis and management of malignant pleural effusions, Mayo Clin Proc 83:235-250, 2008.

Jankowich MD, Gartman EJ, editors: Ultrasound in the intensive care unit, New York, 2015, Humana Press.

Light RW: The undiagnosed pleural effusion, Clin Chest Med 27:309-319, 2006.

McCool FD, Tzelepis GE: Current clinical aspects of diaphragm dysfunction, N Engl J Med 366:932-942, 2012.

Rahman NM, Maskell NA, West A, et al: Intrapleural use of tissue plasminogen activator and DNase in pleural infection, N Engl J Med 365:518-526, 2011.

Stafanidis K, Dimopolous S, Nanas S: Basic principles and current applications of lung ultrasonography in the intensive care unit, Respirology 16:249-256, 2011.

Tzelepis GE, McCool FD: Nonmuscular diseases of the chest wall. In Grippi MA, et al, editors: Fishman's Pulmonary Diseases and Disorders, 5th ed, McGraw-Hill, 2015.

Yusen RD: Medical and surgical treatment of parapneumonic effusions: an evidence-based guideline, Chest 118:1158-1171, 2000.

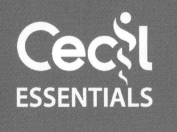

20

Respiratory Failure

Andrew E. Foderaro, Abhinav Kumar Misra

INTRODUCTION

The principle function of our lungs and respiratory system is gaseous exchange, absorption of oxygen and elimination of carbon dioxide produced by the body. Sudden inability to perform one or both of these functions leads to acute respiratory failure (ARF). Impairment of oxygen absorption will manifest as hypoxemia (arterial oxygen tension (Pao_2) <55-60 mm Hg) where impairment of carbon dioxide elimination (ventilation) is manifested by hypercapnia and respiratory acidosis (arterial carbon dioxide tension ($Paco_2$) >45 mm Hg). ARF is one of the most common causes for admission to an intensive care unit (ICU). The annual incidence of ARF in the United States is around 330,000 cases and carries significant short-term and long-term morbidity and mortality. Mortality rises with age, comorbidities, shock, or the presence of multiorgan failure. With an aging population in the United States the incidence of ARF is expected to rise.

PATHOPHYSIOLOGY

Respiratory failure can be classified as acute when derangements happen over hours to days or chronic when derangements occur more slowly over a longer period of time. Acute on chronic implies acute deterioration in someone with preexisting chronic respiratory failure. The respiratory system consists of two distinct parts: the lung (the gas exchanging organ) with the lung parenchyma and alveolar capillary interface, and the ventilatory pump comprising the lung and the chest wall (the respiratory muscles and airways that control ventilation).

Respiratory control is maintained by central neuronal respiratory centers in the medulla oblongata including the dorsal (DRG) and ventral respiratory groups (VRG). The DRG stimulates the diaphragm and intercostal muscles to contract causing inspiration and when activity ceases results in expiration. The VRG is involved in the forced inspiration and expiration through accessory muscles. The second respiratory center is located in the pons and consists of the pneumotaxic and apneustic center. These neurons are involved in control of rate and depth of breathing. Along with the central control there are peripheral chemoreceptors located in carotid bodies as well as aortic bodies constantly monitoring acidity and Pao_2 levels. Upon stimulation of respiratory muscles, the muscles contract generating a negative (subatmospheric) intrapleural pressure. This establishes a pressure gradient leading to flow of air towards alveoli where oxygen diffuses across the alveolar-capillary interface and forms oxyhemoglobin. The oxygen delivery to tissues is not only dependent on respiratory mechanics but also on hemoglobin and cardiac output.

Efficient gas exchange in our lungs is dependent on alveolar ventilation and pulmonary blood flow. This ratio is known as the ventilation-perfusion ($\dot{V}/\dot{Q}$) ratio. When there is alveolar ventilation without blood flow and thus without gas exchange this is referred to as dead space ventilation. Dead space consists of anatomic dead space (upper airway) as well as physiologic dead space (ventilation exceeding perfusion). In the case of physiologic dead space the $\dot{V}/\dot{Q}$ ratio is approaching infinity. Increased physiologic dead space ventilation can be seen when the alveolar-capillary interface is disrupted such as in emphysema, when pulmonary blood flow is reduced such as in low cardiac output, or when alveoli are overdistended due to positive-pressure ventilation. Alternatively, blood flow exceeding ventilation could lead to a portion of blood flow not partaking in gas exchange leading to intrapulmonary shunt. True shunt is when the $\dot{V}/\dot{Q}$ ratio is equal to 0. The fraction of cardiac output that does not partake in gas exchange is known as the shunt fraction, which is usually less than 10%. Increased shunt fraction can be seen when small airways are occluded (e.g., asthma), alveoli are collapsed (e.g., atelectasis), in alveolar filling diseases (e.g., pneumonia, pulmonary edema), or by bypassing the capillary bed (e.g., arteriovenous malformations).

Ideally, the oxygen that is present in the alveoli will equilibrate with the arterial blood. The difference between partial pressures of oxygen in alveolar space and arterial blood is known as the A-a gradient. This can be easily calculated with the help of the alveolar gas equation:

$$A\text{-}a \text{ gradient} = Pao_2 - Pao_2$$

$$Pao_2 = Pio_2 - (Paco_2/RQ)$$

Here, Pao_2 represents partial pressure of oxygen in the alveolar space, Pao_2 represents partial pressure of oxygen in the arterial blood, Pio_2 is partial pressure of oxygen in inhaled gas, $Paco_2$ is partial pressure of carbon dioxide in alveolar space, and RQ is the respiratory quotient (the ration of CO_2 production to O_2 consumption). In a healthy subject eating a mixed diet, the respiratory quotient is 0.8. Furthermore, $Paco_2$ can be replaced by partial pressure of carbon dioxide in arterial blood ($Paco_2$) as CO_2 diffuses efficiently.

$$P_AO_2 = FiO_2 (P_A - P_{H2O}) - (Paco_2/RQ)$$

FiO_2 is the fraction of oxygen, P_A is atmospheric pressure, and P_{H2O} is partial pressure of water vapor. Thus, for a normal healthy young person breathing room air at sea level the A-a gradient equation would be as follows:

$$A\text{-}a \text{ gradient} = [FiO_2 (P_A - P_{H2O}) - (Paco_2/RQ)] - Pao_2$$

$$A\text{-}a \text{ gradient} = [0.21 (760 - 47) - 40/0.8] - 90 = 10$$

Of note, the A-a gradient increases as a function of age. When patients are ventilated, their mean airway pressure needs to be added to atmospheric pressure to factor in the positive-pressure ventilation.

TABLE 20.1 Classification of Respiratory Failure

Organ System	Disease Entity
Respiratory	Upper airway obstruction
	Airway obstructive disease
	COPD
	Asthma
	Pulmonary parenchyma
	Pneumonia
	ARDS
	ILD flare
	Pulmonary hemorrhage
	Alveolar proteinosis
Pulmonary Vascular	Pulmonary thromboembolism
	Pulmonary hypertension
	Right-to-left intrapulmonary shunts
Cardiac	Cardiogenic pulmonary edema
	Right-to-left intracardiac shunts
Neuromuscular	Myasthenia gravis
	ALS
	Guillain-Barré syndrome
Central Nervous System	Decrease respiratory drive
	Sedative medications
	Opioids
	Brain stem insult
	Space occupying lesion
	CVA
	Trauma

TABLE 20.2 Mechanisms That Cause Lower Partial Pressure in the Arterial Blood (Pao_2)

Etiologies of Hypoxia	Observed A-a Gradient
Low inspired oxygen	Normal
Hypoventilation	Normal
Ventilation-perfusion mismatch	Elevated
Shunt	Elevated
Diffusion Impairment	Elevated

CLASSIFICATION OF RESPIRATORY FAILURE

There are several ways to classify respiratory failure. A brief classification based on organ system can be found in Table 20.1.

Type I Hypoxemic Respiratory Failure

Mechanisms that cause lower Pao_2 are listed in Table 20.2. The first two mechanisms, low inspired oxygen and hypoventilation, lead to low Pao_2 through low Pao_2, thus the A-a gradient is normal. It is usually easy to eliminate the first two mechanisms in the clinical setting. Hypoventilation can be ruled out if hypercarbia is not present on arterial blood gas as the elevated $Paco_2$ leads to increased $Paco_2$ and lower Pao_2 (see the alveolar gas equation above).

The other three mechanisms result in an elevated A-a gradient. $\dot{V}/\dot{Q}$ mismatch and shunt are essentially a part of the same spectrum with shunt reflecting the extreme version of $\dot{V}/\dot{Q}$ mismatch. Administering supplemental oxygen will improve Pao_2. Supplemental oxygen cannot correct hypoxemia induced by pure shunt because the blood is completely bypassing the alveoli either physically or functionally. Impaired diffusion is usually not clinically very important because oxygen transport across the alveolar-capillary interface is not diffusion limited even in individuals with preexisting interstitial disease.

Type II Hypercarbic Respiratory Failure

This represents incapability of the lungs to remove a sufficient amount of CO_2, due to either lower alveolar ventilation or, less commonly, higher production of carbon dioxide due to hyper-metabolic states such as sepsis, overfeeding, or fever. Minute ventilation is the product of respiratory rate and tidal volume. The dead space ventilation, both anatomic (in upper airways) and physiologic (areas where ventilation exceeds perfusion), does not take part in elimination of CO_2. Total alveolar ventilation is determined by the difference between total minute ventilation and dead space ventilation. As a result, both decreased tidal volume and increased dead space will lead to hypercarbia.

There are three major causes of ventilatory or hypercarbic failure: (1) Reduced central respiratory drive due to sedatives, drug overdoses or pathologic state of the medulla; (2) Mechanical defect in the chest wall (e.g., kyphoscoliosis, flail chest), disorders of the nerves or neuromuscular junctions such as myasthenia gravis, amyotrophic lateral sclerosis, or disorders of the respiratory muscles (e.g., myopathies); (3) Muscular fatigue usually seen when working against increased inspiratory load such as when hyperinflation is present or increased rate such that these muscles are no longer able to generate sufficient negative pleural pressure to maintain tidal volumes or required respiratory rate. Various etiologies of acute hypercarbic respiratory failure are summarized in Table 20.3.

TABLE 20.3 Causes of Hypercarbic Respiratory Failure

Etiology	Clinical Situation
Depressed CNS drive	Drugs: sedatives, opioids
	Brain stem/medulla lesions
	Sleep-disordered breathing
	Hypothyroidism
Neuromuscular transmission impairment	Spinal cord injury
	Phrenic nerve injury
	Demyelinating illness: ALS
	Neurotoxins: tetanus, botulism
	Neuromuscular junction disorders (e.g., myasthenia gravis, organophosphate poisoning)
	Muscle abnormalities: degenerative myopathies
Chest wall disease	Kyphoscoliosis
	Flail chest
	Obesity
	Pleural disruption: pneumothorax, pleural effusion
	Diaphragmatic rupture
Pulmonary disease	Upper airway obstruction
	Obstructive diseases
	Asthma
	COPD
	Alveolar filling process
	Pulmonary edema
	Atelectasis
	Pulmonary thromboembolism
	Bronchiectasis

Clinical Manifestations

Common clinical manifestations of acute respiratory failure include tachycardia, tachypnea, anxiety, and cyanosis. For a patient to have cyanosis they must have 3 to 5 g/dL of deoxygenated hemoglobin, which usually corresponds to 80% peripheral capillary oxygen saturation (Spo_2). Patients may not be tachypneic if they are medicated with sedatives or opioids. Altered mental state is also a common finding. In the setting of acute hypercarbia, patients may experience increased somnolence, headaches, slurred speech, and eventually coma.

Chest radiography is an essential tool and shows one of three findings: (1) Normal or relatively normal, in which case etiologies such as airway disorders, right-to-left shunts, pulmonary embolism, and neuromuscular disorders come to the forefront; (2) Focal infiltrates as are seen with pneumonia or aspiration; (3) Diffuse infiltrates as can be seen in acute respiratory distress syndrome (ARDS) and interstitial lung disease flares. Initial evaluation for suspected respiratory failure should also include blood gas testing evaluating for presence of hypoxia. If hypoxia is present, calculating the A-a gradient can help point us in the direction of etiologic process. If a patient is hypercarbic, is that enough to cause hypoxemia? In this case, A-a gradient should remain normal. If A-a gradient is elevated it is likely $\dot{V}/\dot{Q}$ that mismatch or shunt is playing a role. These are usually the most common causes of respiratory failure.

Principles of Management

The differential diagnoses for acute respiratory failure are extensive; hence the specific management strategies depend on correcting the underlying cause. As part of the initial management it should be ensured that the airway is patent and the patient is breathing and has stable circulation. Strategies to supplement oxygen and improve oxygenation and ventilation remain cornerstones of supportive care until the etiology resolves.

Oxygen Delivery Systems

A large number of oxygen delivery systems exist. Each of these systems is characterized by the mechanism of delivery, some of which limit the concentration of oxygen (FiO_2) that can be delivered. Normal inspiratory flow rate at rest is 15 L/min, which is intermixed with the flow provided by the O_2 delivery device. Nasal cannula is one of the most commonly and widely accepted delivery systems. These provide 1 to 6 L/min of 100% FiO_2, which is mixed with room air. At rest these can provide an FiO_2 of 24% to 40% (nasal cannula oxygen intermixed with room air). Even though this modality is widely accepted by patients, its use has limitations in the acute setting due to inability to achieve high concentrations of FiO_2. Standard face masks are reservoir systems with 100 to 200 mL of reservoir around the patient's face. These use 5 to 10 L of flow to provide 35% to 50% FiO_2 to patients, which is variable depending upon the flow rate at which the patient is actually breathing. These need a minimum flow of around 5 L to clear exhaled gases. When an air entrainment device is attached, the FiO_2 can be regulated regardless of the flow. Air entrainment works by creating a high velocity stream of gas by narrowing the outlet of the oxygen, creating a pull that leads to room air getting mixed with oxygen. The greater the flow, the greater the force to pull room air, therefore keeping FiO_2 constant. This phenomenon was earlier thought to be due to the Venturi effect, lending these masks the name Venturi masks or Venti masks. These masks provide 24% to 50% FiO_2 in a constant fashion irrespective of the flow rates.

Non-rebreather masks are another form of reservoir system with attached reservoir bags of 600 to 1000 mL. As long as the bag is inflated, patients breathe air primarily contained in the bag. The masks are equipped with one-way expiratory ports to allow expired air to leave but don't allow room air to mix with oxygen in the reservoir bag. In ideal settings these masks can provide high FiO_2 up to 100%; however, due to leaks because of inadequate seal the true FiO_2 is often closer to 80%.

TABLE 20.4 Physiologic Benefits of HFNC

Improved oxygenation
Decreased anatomic dead space
Decreased carbon dioxide generation
Generation of positive nasopharyngeal and tracheal airway pressure
Increased lung volumes
Improved work of breathing
Preconditioning of inspired gas (heated and humidified)
Better secretion clearance
Superior comfort
Reduced room air entrainment

High-Flow Nasal Cannula

High-flow nasal cannula (HFNC) can provide up to 40 to 60 L/min of heated and humidified gas. An oxygen blender connected to the circuit enables precise titration of FiO_2 ranging from 21% to 100%. In order to actually match this to alveolar FiO_2, flow from the HFNC should be equal to the patient's flow. HFNC also creates a flow-dependent clearance of carbon dioxide from upper airways. In randomized trials HFNC has been shown to generate positive airway pressure between 0.35 (mouth open) and 0.69 (mouth closed) cm H_2O of pressure for every 10 L/min of flow. This pressure is higher in the expiratory phase of respiration, almost behaving like positive end-expiratory pressure (PEEP). It helps in recruitment of alveoli and may be more pronounced in people with higher BMI. HFNC has been shown to improve lung compliance, reduce respiratory rate, and increase tidal volume by as much as 10%. The heated and humidified nature of inhaled gas leads to increased mucociliary clearance as shown in patients with bronchiectasis. Physiologic effects of HFNC are summarized in Table 20.4.

The principles and mechanism of action make HFNC a very promising oxygen delivery device. In multiple prospective observational studies, it has been associated with reduction in respiratory rate, heart rate, use of accessory muscles, and dyspnea scores in ICU patients and is often better tolerated than bilevel positive airway pressure ventilation devices. Parke and colleagues conducted a prospective randomized trial in ICU patients with mild to moderate hypoxemic ARF and demonstrated fewer desaturations and less need of noninvasive ventilation (NIV) compared to face masks. However, until recently the effect of HFNC on intubation rates and mortality was not known. In the FLORALI trial, HFNC was shown to have lower mortality and higher ventilator-free days, albeit in secondary analyses. In contrast to the FLORALI trial, results of the HOT-ER trial concluded that HFNC was not superior to conventional oxygen therapy, although the intubation rate in the HFNC group was lower at 5.5% versus 11.6% in the conventional oxygen therapy group but did not reach statistical significance ($P = 0.053$). In a meta-analysis HFNC was associated with a much lower rate of intubation and as such HFNC should be considered first-line therapy in patients for acute hypoxemic respiratory failure.

In other population groups, retrospective studies found no difference in mortality between HFNC and NIV in immunosuppressed patients with ARF. In patients with cancer and patients who had a lung transplant HFNC was associated with lower mortality and lower intubation rates when compared to conventional oxygen therapy. HFNC was ineffective as a rescue therapy when NIV and conventional oxygen therapy had failed, suggesting benefit of early use. In 2014, Maggiore and colleagues showed that HFNC at 50 L/min for 48 hours when applied to a high-risk patient population who passed a spontaneous breathing trial but had a Pao_2/FiO_2 ratio of less than 300 had much lower reintubation rates at 3.8% versus 21% (Venturi mask).

Expanding on this trial, in 2016 Hernandez et al. showed this to be true even in a lower-risk population with reintubation rates being 4.9% in HFNC compared to 12.2% in conventional therapy group. Number needed to treat to prevent 1 reintubation was 14. HFNC has not been shown to be superior to conventional therapy or NIV in postcardiac surgical patients or postabdominal surgery patients. It can be used as a preoxygenation tool during intubation.

Patients who are failing HFNC need to be promptly intubated for invasive mechanical ventilation. Delaying intubation for greater than 48 hours has been shown to be associated with increased mortality. Poor prognostic signs include persistent tachypnea, hypoxia, asynchronous breathing, acidosis with pH less than 7.25, nonpulmonary organ failure or hypotension.

Mechanical Ventilation

Until the 1950s the "iron lung" and other forms of negative-pressure ventilation were the most common forms of mechanical ventilation, especially outside of the anesthesia suite. However, during the polio epidemic in Europe in 1955, the mortality benefit as well as safety outside of anesthesia suites of invasive positive-pressure ventilation was demonstrated, leading to increased use of positive-pressure ventilation. In the 1980s, noninvasive ventilation began to be used for patients with chronic respiratory failure and eventually moved from the outpatient to the inpatient setting. Since then it has become increasingly popular with as much as a 400% increase in use compared to 20 years ago.

Noninvasive Ventilation

NIV is the provision of ventilatory assistance to the lung without use of invasive interface such as endotracheal intubation. NIV uses a variety of noninvasive interfaces including oronasal masks, full face masks, and nasal prongs. Success of NIV depends on the tolerability of the interface as well as the seal provided by the interface. There are essentially two modes of ventilation: constant positive airway pressure (CPAP) and bilevel positive airway pressure (BiPAP).

CPAP provides a constant positive pressure while the patient breathes spontaneously. The degree of ventilatory support provided by this mode is limited. It does not lead to an increase in tidal volumes. It does provide benefit in patients without obstructive lung disease such as obesity hypoventilation and patients with cardiogenic pulmonary edema. BiPAP provides two different pressures during different phases of respiration. During inspiration it provides a higher pressure called inspiratory positive airway pressure (IPAP) and during expiration it maintains a lower airway pressure, which it maintains constantly, called expiratory positive airway pressure (EPAP). The EPAP essentially is the same as CPAP, with IPAP providing a pressure difference that assists during inspiration and provides ventilatory support. Because both of these modalities raise mean airway pressure they help with alveolar recruitment to a certain degree and have a role in providing hemodynamic support to patients with heart failure.

NIV has distinct advantages over invasive mechanical ventilation. Importantly, it eliminates intubation and it eliminates the risk of upper airway trauma by intubation. In addition, it reduces patient discomfort, lowers risk of ventilator-associated pneumonia (VAP), and preserves airway clearance. Patients can be provided breaks from ventilation to allow communication and normal eating and drinking. There are multiple specific etiologies where NIV has become first-line therapy, which are discussed below. There are specific clinical situations where NIV is contraindicated and clinicians should move to invasive mechanical ventilation (IMV). These are summarized in Table 20.5.

TABLE 20.5	Contraindications for Noninvasive Ventilation (NIV)
Absolute Contraindications	**Relative Contraindications**
Cardiopulmonary arrest	Hemodynamically unstable
Facial surgery/trauma	Encephalopathy
Upper airway obstruction	Agitated or uncooperative
Vomiting	Unable to protect airway
Upper GI bleeding	Excessive secretions
	Multiple organ failure
	Swallowing impairment
	Inability to physically remove the mask

Hypercapnic respiratory failure. There are strong recommendations to use NIV in cases of acute COPD exacerbations with mild and moderate ARF with pH between 7.25 and 7.35 and $Paco_2$ of greater than 45 despite standard medical therapy. Early initiation of NIV has been shown to lower rates of intubation and the length of hospitalization as well as mortality. Though pH is the most important determinant, other clinical factors such as tachypnea, severity of dyspnea, and use of accessory muscles should also be considered. Although the mechanism of respiratory failure during asthma exacerbations resembles COPD exacerbation, the airway obstruction is less homogeneous and there is a higher risk of dynamic hyperinflation. Evidence to use NIV in this case is not as convincing. There is probably a narrow window to trial NIV and if respiratory failure does not improve to go ahead with invasive MV.

In patients with bronchiectasis such as cystic fibrosis patients, NIV has been shown to reduce the load on respiratory muscles as well as improve alveolar hypoventilation. NIV should be started if patients have hypercapnia either in the stable phase or during an exacerbation. It may be valuable supportive therapy as a bridge to lung transplantation. Similar to this patient population, in patients with neuromuscular disease respiratory pump impairment plays a pivotal role in alveolar hypoventilation. This usually presents initially as nocturnal hypoventilation, gradually getting worse as the disease progresses and leading to inspiratory muscle weakness, decreased chest wall compliance, and failure to clear secretions. Combining NIV with airway clearance therapies may delay intubation.

Hypoxemic respiratory failure. Several studies since the 1980s have looked at NIV in patients with cardiogenic pulmonary edema. Use of both forms of NIV (CPAP and BiPAP) have shown decreased mortality rate and decreased need for intubation in patients with ARF due to cardiogenic pulmonary edema and has been recommended as first-line therapy in the ATS 2017 guidelines. However, NIV should be used with caution in patients with acute coronary syndromes and cardiogenic shock because there is a slightly higher chance of myocardial infarction.

Guidelines recommend use of NIV in postsurgical patients who develop ARF. Use of both CPAP and BiPAP reduces intubation rates, nosocomial infections, as well as mortality once surgical complications have been ruled out.

Given the lower risk of VAP, NIV has been suggested in patients who are immune compromised with pooled analyses showing benefit and lower intubation risks. However, some studies have shown benefit of HFNC compared to NIV. In patients with ARF of unknown etiology NIV is not recommended. There are multiple disadvantages to consider, and the positive effects of NIV on alveolar recruitment are lost with any interruptions in therapy. NIV can mask clinical deterioration and delay intubations as well as cause lung injury if tidal volumes are too high. In patients with severe hypoxia with Pao_2/Fio_2 ratio of less than 150, use of NIV has been shown to have higher mortality.

TABLE 20.6   Risk Factors for Failure of NIV

Acute hypercarbic RF	Poor neurologic score: GCS <11
	Tachypnea: >35 breaths/min pH <7.25
	APACHE score >29
	Asynchronous breathing
	Excessive air leak
	Agitation
	Excessive secretions
	Poor tolerance
	Poor adherence to therapy
	No initial improvement within first 2 hrs of noninvasive ventilation
	No improvement in pH
	Persistent tachypnea, tachycardia
	Persistent hypercapnia
Acute hypoxic RF	Diagnosis of ARDS or pneumonia
	Age >40 yr
	Hypotension: systolic blood pressure <90 mm Hg metabolic acidosis: pH <7.25
	Low Pao_2/Fio_2 ratio <150
	Failure to improve oxygenation within first hour of noninvasive ventilation

Success of NIV is dependent on underlying disease. Disorders such as COPD exacerbation and cardiogenic edema are more responsive than hypoxemic respiratory failure of unknown etiology. Baseline severe acidosis (pH <7.25), severe hypoxia, respiratory distress with persistent high respiratory rate greater than 25, and nonpulmonary organ failure have been associated with NIV failure. Various risk factors for failure of NIV are summarized in Table 20.6.

Invasive mechanical ventilation. IMV is positive-pressure ventilatory assistance with the help of a tracheostomy or endotracheal tube connected to a ventilator. In the United States around 800,000 patients receive IMV annually. The fundamental operation of a ventilator involves four phases: (1) The trigger phase initiates the breath. This can be controlled by changing preset triggers such as flow or pressure in the circuit or by time (time-triggered) when the ventilation is completely controlled. (2) The target phase where the pressure or flow is maintained by the ventilator. (3) The cycling phase determines the end of the inspiratory phase. Once the variable—flow or pressure—reaches the preset value, the expiration phase starts. (4) The expiration phase is usually passive while maintaining a preset pressure (PEEP).

The simplest mode of ventilation is assist-control ventilation where the patient provides the initial trigger for a flow-targeted volume-cycled (volume assist-control ventilation, or VC) or pressure-targeted time-cycled (pressure assist control ventilation, or PC) ventilation. Both of these modes are usually on a simple feedback loop, so that if the patient's respiratory rate is too low then the ventilator will provide the set number of breaths per minute. When the patient's respiratory rate is higher, all breaths will be triggered by the patient and will get the set ventilatory assistance. Another simple mode is the pressure support mode (PS), where the patient triggers every breath. Apart from preset pressure assistance there is no cycling variable set and the patient controls the duration of the breath.

IMV is often lifesaving but it is fraught with complications. Many of these complications can be avoided and minimized. Initiation of IMV involves endotracheal intubation, which is a critical procedure. Prior to intubation patients need to be evaluated for factors that could indicate presence of a difficult airway. Preoxygenation is essential and use of rapid-sequence intubation with sedative and neuromuscular blocking agents increases the rate of successful intubation. Following placement of an endotracheal tube IMV is not well tolerated in most fully awake patients, hence the need for sedation. Sedation agents are associated with their own complications; for example, long-term use of benzodiazepines, especially in the form of continuous infusions, has been linked with delirium and poor long-term outcomes.

In addition to sedation-related complications, ventilators can provide 100% FiO_2, which can cause oxygen toxicity when used inappropriately. Hyperoxemia has been linked to poor outcomes in patients suffering from strokes or cardiac illness.

Positive-pressure ventilation can cause direct pressure-related injuries from three mechanisms: barotrauma, volutrauma, and atelectrauma. Barotrauma is an increase in pressure in the airways that can lead to alveolar or distal airway rupture leading to air leaks and pneumothorax or pneumomediastinum. Volutrauma can lead to overdistension of alveoli, causing alveolar-capillary interface disruption leading to inflammation. In the 1980s, the first studies showed diffuse parenchymal infiltrates from high inflation volumes. Atelectrauma occurs during the expiratory phase when small airways can collapse, especially in cases where lung compliance is markedly reduced. Repetitive opening and closing of alveoli and small airways can lead to damage to airway epithelium and inflammation.

Weaning From Ventilation

As the underlying cause of respiratory failure improves, attempts need to be made to get the patient off of MV as soon as possible. Determining when a patient can be removed from ventilation is challenging. In the ICU, several studies have shown bedrest negatively affects musculoskeletal, cardiovascular, and respiratory systems. Profound weakness is common in ICU patients, persists beyond hospitalization, and is linked with reduced post-ICU survival. Recent guidelines recommend liberation from MV using protocols for sedation and weaning and mobilizing patients as early as possible. Daily use of spontaneous breathing trials (SBT) has not only been shown to be safe but also shown to reduce weaning times from ventilation when compared to gradual lowering of ventilator settings. For a SBT to be successful, a patient needs to be able to spontaneously breathe with no or minimal ventilator support for at least 30 mins, not be apneic, not be persistently tachypneic (>35 breaths/min), and remain hemodynamically stable without increased work of breathing. Minimizing sedation agents have been shown to reduce duration of ventilation. Daily interruption of sedation as well as stopping sedation prior to SBT increase the chances of successful SBT. Risk factors for unsuccessful extubation are listed in Table 20.7.

TABLE 20.7   Risk Factors for Failed Extubation

Failure of two or more SBTs
Chronic heart failure
Weak cough
Stridor postextubation
Hypercarbia during SBT or after extubation $Paco_2$ >45
Age >65
APACHE score >12 on day of extubation
Pneumonia as cause of ARF

SPECIFIC CLINICAL SITUATION: ACUTE RESPIRATORY DISTRESS SYNDROME

ARDS is one of the most severe forms of hypoxemic respiratory failure. Based on several observational studies, the incidence of ARDS has been estimated to be about 7 per 100,000. In 2012 a panel of experts established the Berlin definition of ARDS. ARDS is characterized by acute hypoxic respiratory failure from acute diffuse inflammatory lung injury. This leads to increased vascular permeability, increased lung weight, and loss of aerated lung tissue, resulting in decreased lung compliance. The lung injury can be direct (e.g., inhalational injury or multifocal pneumonia) or indirect (e.g., pancreatitis or severe sepsis).

For a patient to be defined as having ARDS the onset must be within 1 week of a known clinical insult or new or worsening respiratory symptoms. Based on the degree of hypoxia, severity of ARDS was quantified as mild when Pao_2/Fio_2 ratio was between 200 to 300 mm Hg on PEEP of 5 or higher via invasive or noninvasive MV, moderate ARDS with a Pao_2/Fio_2 ratio less than 200 mm Hg, and severe with a Pao_2/Fio_2 ratio less than 100 mm Hg.

The majority of the cases of ARDS occur in the setting of predisposing clinical risk factors such as bacterial pneumonia, severe sepsis, severe trauma, drug or alcohol overdose, systemic inflammation (e.g., acute pancreatitis), and massive aspiration. These risk factors can be divided into those that cause direct lung injury and those that cause indirect lung injury likely via inflammatory cytokines. It is estimated that 30% to 40% of patients with severe sepsis will go on to develop ARDS. Direct inhalational injury, acute exacerbation of interstitial lung disease, burns, head trauma, and near-drowning are less common causes of ARDS.

ARDS is a complex and heterogeneous disorder with a pathophysiology that is only partially understood. During the initial phase, described as the exudative phase, after exposure to a risk factor, there is injury to the type I pneumocytes and disruption of the alveolar capillary interface. This leads to leakage of protein-rich plasma into the alveolar spaces, release of proinflammatory cytokines (e.g., IL1, IL8, TNF-α) and lipid mediators such as leukotriene B, and neutrophilic accumulation, resulting in predominantly dependent alveolar edema. Unlike cardiogenic edema, which is mostly due to hydrostatic forces, the alveolar fluid is rich in proteins leading to dysfunction of the surfactant activity and a proteolytic process. The process leads to diminished aeration, atelectasis, decreased lung compliance, intrapulmonary shunting, increased physiologic dead space, and significant hypoxemia. The chest radiograph at this stage shows diffuse bilateral alveolar and interstitial opacities that are nonspecific and difficult to distinguish from cardiogenic pulmonary edema, multifocal pneumonia or diffuse alveolar hemorrhage. As ARDS improves there is organization of alveolar exudates and a shift from neutrophilic to lymphocyte predominant pulmonary infiltrate. Type II pneumocytes proliferate and repair the alveolar basement membrane, differentiate into type I pneumocytes, and synthesize surfactant.

In most patients ARDS will resolve after the acute phase. Rarely, some patients enter a fibrotic phase. In these patients there is extensive interstitial fibrosis and disruption of normal pulmonary architecture as well as pulmonary vascular intimal changes predisposing them to pulmonary hypertension and right ventricular failure. This leads to a prolonged phase of decreased lung compliance and oxygenation and prolonged need for continued MV. This phase can last for weeks and is complicated by nonpulmonary organ dysfunction, deconditioning, and hospital-acquired infections.

General principles of management of ARDS patients include recognition and treatment of underlying causes and secondary illnesses. Patients with ARDS frequently require mechanical ventilation for support. Historically, these patients were ventilated with tidal volumes set at 12 to 15 mL/kg. However, in 2000 the ARDS Network published the results of their first study comparing tidal volumes of 6 mL/kg versus 12 mL/kg and revealed a 9% absolute reduction in mortality in the lower tidal volume group. Along with the mortality benefit, both ventilator-free days and organ failure–free days were also increased in the low tidal volume group. Currently the American Thoracic Society in conjunction with the European Respiratory Society recommends using lower tidal volumes of 4 to 8 mL/kg of predicted ideal body weight and lower inspiratory pressures (P_{plat} <30 mm Hg).

Further, although higher PEEP may improve alveolar recruitment, oxygenation, and prevent atelectrauma, there are risks of alveolar overdistension, increased intrapulmonary shunt, and hemodynamic effects. There have been multiple studies comparing high PEEP with lower PEEP, including studies from ARDS Network comparing average PEEP of 13 versus 8 with similar clinical outcomes. None of these studies showed evidence of barotrauma related to higher PEEP. In an individual patient meta-analysis from three randomized controlled trials, patients with moderate or severe ARDS (Pao_2/Fio_2 <200 mm Hg) had significant mortality benefit from higher PEEP while patients with mild ARDS did not have statistically significant benefit.

There have been multiple studies addressing fluid management in ARDS. The ARDS Network conducted a large multicenter randomized controlled trial looking at a liberal fluid strategy versus a conservative fluid strategy targeting lower intravascular pressures. Patients in the conservative group had a higher number of ventilator-free days, better oxygenation, and did not have a higher incidence of shock or need for dialysis. The 2010 ACURASYS trial looking at neuromuscular blockade for patients in moderate to severe ARDS showed a lower incidence of barotrauma and higher adjusted overall survival. However, the 2019 ROSE trial did not show a similar benefit between the two groups. From a physiological perspective, neuromuscular blockade needs to be administered when patient-ventilator desynchronies exist. However, some patients' ventilatory pattern predisposes them to ventilator-induced lung injury despite use of sedation strategies.

Rescue therapies need to be applied to patients in the setting of refractory hypoxia. Prone positioning was initially shown to improve oxygenation but not affect mortality in several small studies; however, in prespecified subgroup analyses of these studies, prone position for greater than 12 hours a day in patients with moderate to severe ARDS showed mortality benefit. This was subsequently confirmed in the PROSEVA trial, in which proning led to a mortality benefit in patients with severe ARDS. Hence, proning is recommended by ATS in patients with severe ARDS. Other rescue therapies such as inhaled nitric oxide can improve oxygenation in some patients. This therapy can also lead to loss of hypoxia-induced vasoconstriction in poorly ventilated portions of the lung, leading to worsening oxygenation. Extracorporeal membrane oxygenation (ECMO) refers to circulation of blood externally over a gas exchanger to oxygenate blood and eliminate carbon dioxide. This was first studied in the 1970s and did not show any benefit; however, mortality from ARDS at that time was close to 90% in both arms of the study. In 2009 the CESAR trial was published, which showed a mortality benefit in the treatment arm; however, 25% of the patients in the treatment arm ended up getting conservative management. There were no fixed ventilation protocols for patients in the control arm, therefore it was difficult to predict how much benefit was attributable to ECMO. Another randomized trial in 2018 did not show mortality benefit using ECMO versus reserving it as a rescue therapy with conventional lung-protective ventilation.

SUGGESTED READINGS

Acute Respiratory Distress Syndrome Network, et al: Ventilation with lower tidal volumes as compared with traditional tidal volumes for acute lung injury and the acute respiratory distress syndrome, N Engl J Med 342:1301-1308, 2000.

Brodie D, Bacchetta M: Extracorporeal membrane oxygenation for ARDS in adults, N Engl J Med 365:1905-1914, 2011.

Combes A, Hajage D, Capellier G, et al: Extracorporeal membrane oxygenation for severe acute respiratory distress syndrome, N Engl J Med 378:1965-1975, 2018.

Drake, MG: High-flow nasal cannula oxygen in adults: an evidence-based assessment, Ann Am Thorac Soc 15:145-155, 2018.

Fan E, Del Sorbo L, Goligher EC, et al: An official American Thoracic Society/European Society of Intensive Care Medicine/Society of Critical Care Medicine clinical practice guideline: mechanical ventilation in adult patients with acute respiratory distress syndrome, Am J Respir Crit Care Med 195:1253-1263, 2017.

Frat J-P, Ricard J-D, Coudroy R, et al: Preoxygenation with non-invasive ventilation versus high-flow nasal cannula oxygen therapy for intubation of patients with acute hypoxaemic respiratory failure in ICU: the prospective randomised controlled FLORALI-2 study protocol, BMJ Open 7:e018611, 2017.

Guérin C, Reignier J, Richard JC, et al: Prone positioning in severe acute respiratory distress syndrome, N Engl J Med 368:2159-2168, 2013.

Hernández G, Vaquero C, González P, et al. Effect of Postextubation High-Flow Nasal Cannula vs Conventional Oxygen Therapy on Reintubation in Low-Risk Patients: A Randomized Clinical Trial. JAMA 315(13):1354-1361, 2016.

Ischaki E, Pantazopoulos I, Zakynthinos S: Nasal high flow therapy: a novel treatment rather than a more expensive oxygen device, Eur Respir Rev 26:170028, 2017.

Maggiore SM, Idone FA, Vaschetto R, et al. Nasal high-flow versus Venturi mask oxygen therapy after extubation. Effects on oxygenation, comfort, and clinical outcome. Am J Respir Crit Care Med 190(3):282-288, 2014.

Mas A, Masip J: Noninvasive ventilation in acute respiratory failure, Int J Chron Obstruct Pulmon Dis 9:837-852, 2014.

Ouellette DR, Patel S, Girard TD, et al: Liberation from mechanical ventilation in critically ill adults: an official American College of Chest Physicians/American Thoracic Society clinical practice guideline: inspiratory pressure augmentation during spontaneous breathing trials, protocols minimizing sedation, and noninvasive ventilation immediately after extubation, Chest 151:166-180, 2017.

Parke RL, McGuinness SP, Eccleston ML. A preliminary randomized controlled trial to assess effectiveness of nasal high-flow oxygen in intensive care patients. Respir Care 56(3):265-270, 2011.

Pham T, Brochard LJ, Slutsky AS: Mechanical ventilation: state of the art, Mayo Clinic 92:1382-1400, 2017.

Rochwerg B, Brochard L, Elliott MW, et al: Official ERS/ATS clinical practice guidelines: noninvasive ventilation for acute respiratory failure, Eur Respir J 50:1602426, 2017.

Roussos C, Koutsoukou A: Respiratory failure, Eur Respir J Suppl 47:3s-14s, 2003.

Scala R, Pisani L: Noninvasive ventilation in acute respiratory failure: which recipe for success? Eur Respir Rev 27:180029, 2018.

Thompson BT, Matthay MA: The Berlin definition of ARDS versus pathological evidence of diffuse alveolar damage, Am J Respir Crit Care Med 187:675-677, 2013.

21

Transitions in Care From Pediatric to Adult Providers for Individuals With Pulmonary Disease

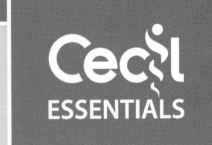

Kate E. Powers, Debasree Banerjee, Robin L. McKinney

INTRODUCTION

With advances in technology and pharmaceuticals, more than 90% of children born with life-shortening diseases will survive to adulthood. The transition of care from pediatric to adult providers is high risk, with the potential for poor clinical outcomes. There are few resources and limited formal education for pediatric and adult providers on transition of care for individuals with underlying pulmonary disease. This gap in knowledge among health care providers has significant effects on patient outcome, including accelerated progression of disease and increased health care cost.

The Society for Adolescent Health and Medicine defines transition in care as "the purposeful, planned movement from adolescents and young adults with chronic physical and medical conditions from child-centered to adult-oriented health care systems." Despite the recognized need for detailed and active measures to ensure the transfer of patient care, there are no standardized approaches for transition of care for individuals with underlying pulmonary disease. Many individuals experience gaps of care during the transfer phase of transition before definitively establishing care with an adult provider. These gaps in care are multifactorial including individual, cultural, geographic, logistic, and financial etiologies. Adolescents and young adults may lack the skill or neurocognitive development to fully assume management of their own care. This is further compounded by moving away from home, loss of insurance as a dependent, and lack of engagement of family or caretakers in adult practices. If not adequately planned for, parents' lack of legal right of their child at the age of majority significantly impacts care and consent in neurocognitively impaired individuals. Fragmented care may lead to poor health maintenance, decreased adherence to medical therapies, and avoidance of medical intervention in earlier stages of illness. An organized transition process establishes individual trust in new adult providers, especially for young adults with chronic disease. A smooth transition of health care allows for developmentally appropriate care in a system that can support the individual patient throughout life.

Our goal for this chapter is to illustrate successful methods to transition adolescents and young adults with underlying pulmonary disease and those chronically critically ill individuals into adult clinics utilizing specific pulmonary disease examples.

CYSTIC FIBROSIS AND OTHER MUCOCILIARY DISEASES

Cystic fibrosis (CF) is an autosomal recessive genetic multisystem disease with primary involvement occurring in the respiratory and gastrointestinal tracts. Mucus plugging, inflammation, and bacterial infections lead to lung damage with progressive small airway obstruction and lung scarring known as bronchiectasis that eventually contributes to worsening lung function and respiratory failure. In the gastrointestinal and hepatobiliary tracts as well as the exocrine pancreas, inspissation of viscous secretions leads to intestinal obstruction, cholestasis, and fat and protein malabsorption. CF affects approximately 30,000 individuals in the United States and 70,000 worldwide. It is the most common life-shortening inherited disease in Caucasians but impacts all races and ethnicities. CF is caused by mutations in a gene on chromosome 7 that encodes the CF transmembrane conductance regulator (CFTR) protein. The CFTR protein primarily functions as a chloride and bicarbonate receptor responsible for the movement of fluid into and out of epithelial cells lining the respiratory tract, biliary tree, intestines, vas deferens, sweat ducts, and pancreatic ducts. As of 2017, the median predicted survival is about 50 years. Improvement in survival has resulted from specialized care centers, early diagnosis, timely screening, therapies to optimize pulmonary function and nutrition as well as clinical care guidelines to standardize symptom-based treatments. Newly developed CFTR modulator therapies target the basic defect in CF and are now clinically available for more than 60% of the US CF population. Although modulator therapies cannot reverse existing disease, they have already further altered the CF-disease trajectory improving overall health, quality of life, and survival.

With improved survival into adulthood, successful transition and transfer of individuals from pediatric to adult CF programs is essential. A timeline for recommended CF-related milestones has been developed to support an individual with CF and his or her parent or support person through transition. CF R.I.S.E. (Responsibility. Independence. Self-care. Education.) is a transition resource that includes patient assessments and checklists, care team progress reports, and educational resource guides to optimize the transition process over time.

Specific educational goals are established by age: early school age (6-9 years old), late elementary and middle school (10-12 years old), early high school (13-15 years old), late high school (16-18 years old) and young adults (18-25 years old). Modules assist individuals with CF and their families to better understand the disease, CF-related care including medications and therapies, as well as planning for the future (Table 21.1).

Primary ciliary dyskinesia (PCD) is an autosomal recessive disease with more than 30 different genetic variants, characterized by congenital impairment of mucociliary clearance. These defects lead to ciliary immotility, ciliary dyskinesia or ciliary aplasia. Considerable variation exists in the clinical presentation of PCD, but most present in childhood with recurrent upper and lower respiratory infections. It is characterized by chronic cough, bronchiectasis, chronic rhinosinusitis, and recurrent otitis media. Individuals with PCD generally live an active

TABLE 21.1　Specific Educational Goals by Age

Milestones	6-9 Years Old	10-12 Years Old	13-15 Years Old	16-18 Years Old	18-25 Years Old
Understanding CF	Basics of CF	Many aspects of CF care	Most aspects of CF	All aspects of CF	Understands and learns about all adult-related CF care issues
Managing CF care					
Clinic visits	Able to answer some questions about general health status and symptoms with support person's input	Able to independently answer more questions	Independently answers most questions	Independently takes the lead including answering questions	Plans for and takes the lead
Health status	Begins to identify and report changes in symptoms or health to a parent/support person	Proactively identifies and reports changes in health and symptoms to parent/support person	Reports health/symptom changes to parents and care team	Implements recommended nutrition/ treatment changes after clinic and hospital visits	Implements recommended nutrition/ treatment changes after clinic and hospital visits
Coordination of care		Can report to care team all of the health care providers seen outside CF center	Can report to care team all of the health care providers seen outside CF center, reasons for and outcomes from those appointments	Works with parent to coordinate care with health care providers outside CF Center	Coordinates all care with health care providers outside CF center
Insurance and financial			Begins to watch parent/ support person order medication and supplies and starts to call for their own refills when needed	Monitors medications and supplies and calls in refills	Monitors medications and supplies, calls in refills, owns all medication and insurance-related management and reaches out to parent/ support person if questions arise
Transfer to adult care				Participates in key meetings and fills out paperwork associated with transfer	Participates in key meetings and fills out paperwork associated with transfer
Taking CF treatments and therapies					
Taking treatments	Begins taking steps towards remembering to take and carry pills and enzymes; Helps to set up nebulizer and airway clearance equipment; Takes and participates in all treatments with close oversight	Responsible for remembering to take and carry enzymes; Independently performs airway clearance with some oversight; Knows and sticks to treatment plan expectations	Independently administers enzymes and airway clearance; Responsible for following treatment plan in school and while on vacation with some supervision	Primarily responsible for taking all treatments with little parental supervision	Completely responsible for taking all treatments with little parental/support person supervision
Medication management		Begins tracking and sorting all medicines and proper storage plan for medicines	Tracks and sorts all medicines and tells parent when medicine is running low	Tracks and sorts all medications; demonstrates and calls for refills when medicine is running low	Responsible for tracking and sorting all medicines and identifying need for refills
Living with CF					
Planning for future	Pictures a future as an adult	Pictures a future and is able to talk about hopes and dreams	Begins to plan for future (big picture) and plan for how CF may impact future life plan and adulthood	Actively plans for future including college life, work, and/or living independently	Actively plans for future
Anxiety and depression	Aware of anxious or sad feelings and alerts a parent/support person	Can identify feelings of sadness and anxiety and bring to the attention of a parent/support person	Can identify warning signs of anxiety and depression and alert parent/support	Can identify warning signs of anxiety and depression and alert parent/support person	Can identify warning signs of anxiety and depression and alert parent/support person

TABLE 21.1	Specific Educational Goals by Age—cont'd				
Milestones	6-9 Years Old	10-12 Years Old	13-15 Years Old	16-18 Years Old	18-25 Years Old
Exercise	Participates in sports, exercise, or other health activities	Maintains an exercise routine/participates in sports of other healthy activities	Maintains an exercise routine/participates in sports or other healthy activities	Works with care team to develop an exercise routine	
Self-advocacy	Can answer very basic questions about CF from family, friends, and teachers	Has a short statement to answer basic questions about CF	More comfortable independently answering common questions from peers/others about CF	Able to answer questions from peers/others about CF	Able to answer questions from peers/others about CF
Support system	Understands the importance of a support system of peers with CF	Understands the importance of a support system and starts to develop a group of peers with CF	Understands the importance of and starts to develop a support system of peers with CF	Understands the importance of and utilizes a support system of peers with CF	Understands the importance of and utilizes a support system of peers with CF

life and have a normal lifespan. The rate of lung function decline is much slower than that with CF. Similar to CF, individuals with PCD benefit from implementation of a preventative airway clearance regimen to mobilize retained pulmonary secretions. Retained pulmonary secretions can be corrosive leading to chronic inflammation, recurrent infections, and bronchiectasis.

Bronchiectasis is a structural abnormality characterized by abnormal dilatation and distortion of the bronchial tree with resultant chronic obstructive lung disease. A range of pathophysiologic and disease processes other than CF contribute to bronchiectasis, and most include some combination of bronchial obstruction and infection. Bronchiectasis is frequently associated with atelectasis, emphysema, pulmonary fibrosis, and bronchial vasculature hypertrophy. Improving airway clearance and preventing further airway damage are the cornerstones of therapy. Prognosis and outcome in non-CF related bronchiectasis depends primarily on the underlying etiology. Prediction of outcomes is limited, but with early diagnosis and appropriate therapies, including a preventative airway clearance regimen, lung function in children can stabilize or improve over time. Non-CF related bronchiectasis typically progresses much more slowly than CF-related bronchiectasis and often improves if an airway clearance regimen is implemented to minimize retained pulmonary secretions.

Consensus guidelines for transitioning individuals with PCD or non-CF related bronchiectasis from pediatric to adult providers have not been established to date. Both benefit from continued implementation of a preventative airway clearance regimen to mobilize pulmonary secretions.

ASTHMA AND BRONCHOPULMONARY DYSPLASIA

Asthma and bronchopulmonary dysplasia (BPD) are two of the most common chronic lung diseases in pediatrics. While adult health care providers will likely have experience and be comfortable managing asthma, BPD is a disease that few will be familiar with. BPD results from premature birth with an incidence of 10,000 to 15,000 new cases annually in the United States.

In premature infants, the type II pneumocytes of the lung are underdeveloped and produce insufficient quantities of surfactant, a surface-active substance produced by specific alveolar epithelial cells that helps to decrease surface tension and prevent alveolar collapse. This disorder is called respiratory distress syndrome (RDS). The treatment of RDS is administration of exogenous surfactant and corticosteroids to enhance lung maturation. To sustain life while allowing maturation, mechanical ventilation and oxygen supplementation are required but contribute to the development of BPD.

BPD is defined as the need for 30% or greater oxygen and/or positive pressure at 36 weeks postgestational age (PGA) or discharge, in infants born before 32 weeks gestational age. The neonatal and pediatric provider is likely to be more familiar with the immediate sequela and morbidity associated with BPD than adult health care providers who may inherit an individual years after symptoms have become silent. Birth history is often overlooked by both pediatric and adult health care providers but may provide health information relevant well into adulthood. BPD is often clinically silent by age four, but there is increasing evidence that abnormal spirometry can be detected in early childhood and significantly contributes to adult diseases including chronic obstructive pulmonary disease (COPD) and asthma.

Recent studies challenge the traditional teaching that lung function continuously improves from birth until the third decade of life. Evidence suggests childhood illnesses such as BPD and asthma can contribute to lower-than-expected lung function. Given this lower-than-expected lung function, pathology such as COPD is more likely to occur earlier in life and potentially have a more severe course.

It is essential for pediatric providers to begin early with age-appropriate conversations on the management of asthma in preparation for transfer and transition of health care in adolescence and young adulthood. A minority of patients with moderate to severe childhood asthma will experience remission as they enter adulthood. The majority of individuals will have persistent symptoms. There is an association between severe asthma in childhood with decreased peak lung function and a more rapid decline of lung function compared to children without asthma that ultimately leads to COPD later in life. Pediatric and adult providers should be aware of these long-term outcomes, appropriately monitor lung function, and manage symptoms accordingly to try and prevent long-term lung remodeling leading to persistent disease.

DIFFUSE LUNG DISEASE (INTERSTITIAL LUNG DISEASE)

Diffuse lung disease (DLD) consists of a diverse group of disorders that impact the pulmonary parenchyma and interfere with gas exchange reflecting a spectrum of underlying pathology. These disorders are associated with extensive alteration of alveolar and airway architecture in addition to interstitial changes, therefore the term DLD is now preferred to ILD. Childhood interstitial lung disease (chILD) is still a term utilized when DLD is suspected based on clinical and radiologic features without an established etiology. Some conditions that cause DLD are similar in children and adults, they occur in different proportions, and certain diseases are unique to infants. All diseases are rare in childhood.

For many forms of DLD, treatment options are limited and often include medications with unproven efficacy and substantial side effects. Lung transplantation is an option for children with severe and progressive disease without a response to therapy. Consensus guidelines for transitioning individuals with DLD from pediatric to adult providers have not been established to date. Given the spectrum of underlying pathology and possible post–lung transplant status, individuals with DLD benefit from a focused transition of care.

INDIVIDUALS WITH TECHNOLOGY DEPENDENCE OR OTHER SPECIAL HEALTH CARE NEEDS

Children and youth with special health care needs (CYSHN) is defined as those who have one or more chronic physical, developmental, behavioral, or emotional condition requiring additional health and related services beyond that of children generally. Approximately 750,000 CYSHN transition into adulthood annually. While these individuals make up a small fraction of the pediatric patient population, they utilize the largest fraction of health care resources. Individuals with technology dependence include those who have tracheostomy dependence requiring part- or full-time mechanical ventilatory support.

Home oxygen therapy is often required in children with chronic respiratory conditions including CF, BPD, sleep-disordered breathing, sickle cell disease, pulmonary hypertension with and without congenital heart disease, and DLD. Despite a lack of empirical evidence regarding implementation, monitoring, and discontinuation of supplemental oxygen therapy, an expert panel through the American Thoracic Society published clinical practice guidelines in 2018. Optimal implementation includes age-appropriate oxygen equipment to maintain acceptable oxygen saturations according to age and respiratory condition and pulse oximetry.

Important steps to optimal transfer and transition include updating insurance status to reflect the coordination of special services with durable medical equipment companies and qualifying patients for certain state or national services. Adult providers frequently have a more patient-centered than family-centered approach to care than pediatric counterparts. Adolescence and young adulthood is often a time of educational transition with variation in access and medical support provided for children and youth with special health care needs. Lack of disease-specific education and few evidence-based guidelines may contribute to adult pulmonologists' limited expertise caring for an individual with technology dependence. General pediatric recommendations for improving transition include the preparation of a transition plan written in early adolescence starting at age 14. This plan includes individual patient and family perspectives, anticipated health care services the individual will need, and a financial plan. It should include preventative as well as disease-specific therapies and insurance coverage strategies for the transition period to decrease gaps of care.

IMPORTANCE OF A SUCCESSFUL TRANSITION

Data from 10 years ago suggested that more than 500,000 adolescents with special health care needs in the United States reach adulthood annually. As life expectancy for individuals with chronic lung disease, technology dependence or other special health care needs has increased, so has the need for a guided, structured transfer and transition of care and transition from pediatric to adult-focused care. The transition of individuals from pediatric to adult care should begin years before the actual transfer. The transition process should include individual- and family-specific education, patient understanding of disease including

TABLE 21.2	Multilevel Suggestions for Transition of Health Care
Patient level	Begin discussions of transition early in life
	Develop a road map in preparation for transition readiness, disease knowledge, and skills assessment to share with patients and families
	Create a personalized medical summary to ensure seamless continuity of care, especially where an electronic medical record is not shared by pediatric and adult programs
CF team level	Create an open and transparent dialogue between the pediatric and adult CF programs
	Develop a working transitional care policy at all levels of the multidisciplinary team (include input from patients and parents)
	Create a registry of eligible patients and a plan to discuss them periodically
	Identify outcome measures to monitor progress and success, including establishment of best practices and communication among pediatric and adult care teams
Institutional level	Seek institutional leadership buy-in
	Collaborate with other hospital programs focused on transition
	Invest in EMR systems with patient access to personal health records and built-in transition tools

rationale for therapies and overall prognosis, as well as a patient readiness assessment indicating if the patient can independently manage therapies and navigate the health care system.

The goals of a planned transition are to improve quality of life, maximize independence, and minimize interruption in care as a patient transfers from pediatric to adult primary and subspecialty care. A designated transition coordinator or champion allows for streamlined communication between health care providers and helps to ensure individual access to medications, interventions, and medical devices through to establishment of care with the adult provider. Although no single process for transition will work in all health care systems, it is essential that an approach that best meets the needs of patient populations and fits within the health care system constraints be established (Table 21.2).

Transition of health care is a complex process involving multiple factors for which a multidisciplinary care team will provide the best chance for success for the individual patient and family (Table 21.3).

Effective transition of care can prevent the deterioration of chronic health conditions while engaging the adolescent to become involved and take over their own care. Poor transition of care has been associated with missed health care visits, loss to follow-up, poor compliance with medications, and increased morbidities. All of these lead to increased emergency care utilization and worse outcomes. Research has identified obstacles that can make transition challenging, including the limited number of capable providers for adults, lack of individual readiness, cognitive disability, instability of mental health (anxiety/depression), and communication issues between pediatric and adult providers.

CF is an example of a chronic pulmonary disease in which much effort has been placed into implementing models to optimize the process of transition. The CF Foundation supported the training of additional providers and developed Adult Care Consensus Guidelines to provide goals and help standardize care. Research and

TABLE 21.3	**Multidisciplinary Care Team for Transition of Health Care**
Multidisciplinary Care Team	**Focus for Transition Assessment**
Physician/nurse practitioner	Supervising overall transfer and transition process
Registered nurse/care coordinator	Supporting communication of transfer and transition process
Registered dietician	Nutrition and supplementation knowledge, food insecurity risk
Clinic facilitator	Scheduling transfer; meet-and-greet adult team; supplying documents
Pharmacist	Medication knowledge
Behavioral psychologist	Mental/emotional strengths and any barriers to transition
Clinical social worker	Psychosocial strengths and any barriers to transition
Respiratory therapist	Airway clearance knowledge
Physical therapist	Physical activity knowledge as relates to airway clearance
Child life specialist	Age-appropriate disease education and tools for medication adherence

quality improvement projects have identified areas that can make transition a success:

- Make transition to adult care a gradual process.
- Remember that parents and caregivers also are going through a transition.
- Pediatric and adult care teams should work together to improve transition.

Developing a transition program is critically important and does not develop without committed individuals and institutions. Finally, there needs to be pediatric and young adult focused research to better establish guidelines for care that are applicable to this special population.

SUGGESTED READINGS

American Academy of Pediatrics Transition ECHO: https://www.aap.org/en-us/professional-resources/practice-transformation/echo/Pages/Transition.aspx.

CF R.I.S.E. Program materials: https://www.cfrise.com/.

A Consensus Statement on Health Care Transitions for Young Adults With Special Health Care Needs, Pediatrics 110(Suppl 3), 2002.

https://www.aap.org/en-us/Documents/practicesupport_preparing_adolescents_independent_living_webinar.pdf.

The Transition Readiness Assessment Questionnaire (TRAQ): www.rheumatology.org/Portals/0/Files/Transition-Readiness-Assessment-Questionnaire.pdf.

Preoperative and Postoperative Care

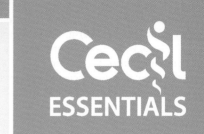

22

Preoperative and Postoperative Care

Kim A. Eagle, Kwame Dapaah-Afriyie, Arkadiy Finn

INTRODUCTION

More than 40 million people undergo noncardiac surgical procedures in the United States annually. A general medical and focused cardiovascular preoperative risk assessment involves evaluation of pertinent medical problems with an emphasis on those conditions that may become exacerbated in the perioperative period. Emerging evidence-based practices dictate that the physician should thoughtfully perform an individualized evaluation of the surgical patient to provide an accurate preoperative risk assessment, risk stratification, and modification of risk parameters that can then provide the framework for optimal perioperative risk reduction strategies.

The perioperative period is associated with hemodynamic changes due to surge in sympathetic activity, fluid shifts and their associated effect on the renin-angiotensin system (RAS), and effect of exposure to anesthetic agents.

Assessment of patients' functional status, exercise tolerance, and other preexisting comorbidities are core components of perioperative management. Patients younger than 50 years of age and having no significant medical comorbidities are at very low risk for developing perioperative complications. The increasing prevalence of medical conditions in the surgical patient warrants review of the perioperative approach to those conditions that may pose significant risk. This chapter reviews preoperative and postoperative cardiovascular and medical risk assessment that targets intermediate- to high-risk patients to strategically guide perioperative preventive therapies for optimal outcome.

CARDIAC DISEASE

Preoperative and Postoperative Cardiac Care

It is estimated that the incidence of cardiac complications after noncardiac surgical procedures is between 0.5% and 1%. In other words, 200,000 to 400,000 people will experience perioperative cardiac complications annually. Moreover, more than 25% of these patients will die. Patients who survive a postoperative myocardial infarction (MI) are twice as likely to die in the following 2 years as are patients with uneventful surgical procedures. Emerging evidence-based practices dictate that the physician should thoughtfully perform an individualized evaluation of the surgical patient to provide an accurate preoperative risk assessment, risk stratification, and modification of risk parameters that can then provide the framework for optimal perioperative risk reduction strategies. This section reviews preoperative and postoperative cardiovascular risk assessment that targets intermediate- to high-risk patients to strategically guide perioperative preventive therapies for optimal outcome.

IDENTIFICATION OF PATIENTS WITH ELEVATED RISK

The preoperative evaluation includes an assessment of the risk associated with the planned surgery or procedure. Low-risk procedures (e.g., colonoscopy, cataract surgery) are associated with a less than 1% risk of major adverse cardiovascular events (MACE) of death or MI. Those procedures with a MACE risk of 1% or greater are classified as conferring higher risk. Simple standardized preoperative screening questionnaires have been developed for the purpose of identifying patients at intermediate to high risk who may benefit from a more detailed clinical evaluation (Table 22.1).

TABLE 22.1 Standardized Preoperative Questionnaire[a]

1. Age, weight, and height
2. Are you
   a. Female and 55 years of age or older or male and 45 years of age or older?
   b. If yes, are you also 70 years of age or older?
3. Do you take anticoagulant medications ("blood thinners")?
4. Do you have or have you had any of the following heart-related conditions?
   a. Heart disease
   b. Heart attack within the last 6 months
   c. Angina (chest pain)
   d. Irregular heartbeat
   e. Heart failure
5. Do you have or have you ever had any of the following?
   a. Rheumatoid arthritis
   b. Kidney disease
   c. Liver disease
   d. Diabetes
6. Do you get short of breath when you lie flat?
7. Are you currently on oxygen treatment?
8. Do you have a chronic cough that produces any discharge or fluid?
9. Do you have lung problems or diseases?
10. Have you or any blood member of your family ever had a problem with any anesthesia other than nausea?
    a. If yes, describe
11. If female, is it possible that you could be pregnant?
    a. Perform pregnancy test
    b. Please list date of last menstrual period

[a]University of Michigan Health System patient information report. Patients who answer yes to any of questions 2 through 9 should receive a more detailed clinical evaluation.
From Tremper KK, Benedict P: Paper "preoperative computer," Anesthesiology 92:1212-1213, 2000.

Evaluation of such surgical patients should always begin with a thorough history and physical examination including a 12-lead resting electrocardiogram (ECG) in accordance with the American College of Cardiology/American Heart American (ACC/AHA) guidelines. A determination of the urgency of the surgery should be included in the history because truly emergent procedures are associated with unavoidably higher rates of morbidity and mortality.

Perioperative risk assessment begins with an assessment of the urgency of the noncardiac surgery; emergency surgery should not be delayed but may not allow for in-depth risk stratification. Preoperative testing should be done only for specific clinical conditions based on the history. Healthy patients of any age who are undergoing elective surgical procedures and have no coexisting medical conditions should not need any testing unless the degree of surgical stress could result in unusual changes from the baseline state. The history should focus on symptoms of occult cardiac disease.

PREOPERATIVE CARDIAC RISK ASSESSMENT

During the perioperative risk assessment of patients undergoing noncardiac surgery, there are active cardiac conditions that should be evaluated and treated in accordance with the ACC/AHA guidelines. These conditions include unstable coronary artery disease (CAD), decompensated heart failure, severe arrhythmia, and severe valvular disease (notably severe aortic stenosis and symptomatic mitral stenosis).

Assessment of exercise tolerance in preoperative risk stratification and precise prediction of in-hospital perioperative risk is most applicable in patients who self-report worsening exercise-induced cardiopulmonary symptoms, patients who may benefit from noninvasive or invasive cardiac testing regardless of the scheduled surgical procedure, and patients with known CAD or with multiple risk factors and the ability to exercise. For the prediction of perioperative events, "poor" exercise tolerance has been defined as inability to walk four blocks and climb two flights of stairs or as inability to meet a metabolic equivalent (MET) level of 4 (Table 22.2). Highly functional symptomatic patients (i.e., those who are able to achieve a functional capacity ≥4 METS

without symptoms, as when climbing a flight of stairs or running a short distance) rarely require noninvasive testing or intervention to lower the risk of noncardiac surgery.

If the patient has poor functional capacity or is symptomatic, physicians often use risk indices derived from empirical multivariable predictive models based on clinical assessment of risk factors to identify patients with elevated perioperative cardiac risk. Based on prospective comparison studies, the Revised Cardiac Risk Index (RCRI) is favored by many given its accuracy and simplicity (Table 22.3). A newer predictive model is the National Surgical Quality Improvement Program (NSQIP) risk calculator, which is based on multiple clinical predictors. The RCRI relies on the presence or absence of six identifiable predictive factors: high-risk surgery (suprainguinal vascular, intrathoracic, or intraperitoneal surgery), ischemic heart disease, congestive heart failure (CHF), cerebrovascular disease, diabetes mellitus (requiring insulin therapy), and renal failure (with a serum creatinine concentration >2.0 mg/dL). Each of the RCRI clinical predictors, if present, is assigned 1 point. The risk for cardiac events (i.e., MI, pulmonary edema, ventricular fibrillation or primary cardiac arrest, and complete heart block) can then be predicted. A patient with an RCRI score of 0 has an estimated risk of 0.4% to 0.5% for major cardiac complications; the risk is 0.9% to 1.3% for someone with a score of 1, 4% to 6.6% with a score of 2, and 9% to 11% with a score of 3 (Fig. 22.1). Cardiac risk particularly increases with the presence of two or more predictors and is greatest with three or more. The clinical utility of the RCRI is that it identifies patients who are at higher risk for cardiac complications and helps determine whether they may benefit from further risk stratification with noninvasive cardiac testing or from initiation of preoperative preventive medical management.

TABLE 22.2   Functional Status

Excellent (Activities Requiring >7 METS)
Carry 24 lb up eight steps
Carry objects that weigh 80 lb
Outdoor work (shovel snow, spade soil)
Recreation (ski, basketball, squash, handball, jog or walk 5 mph)

Moderate (Activities Requiring >4 but <7 METS)
Have sexual intercourse without stopping
Walk at 4 mph on level ground
Outdoor work (garden, rake, weed)
Recreation (roller-skate, dance, foxtrot)

Poor (Activities Requiring <4 METS)
Shower/dress without stopping, strip and make bed, dust, wash dishes
Walk at 2.5 mph on level ground
Outdoor work (clean windows)
Recreation (golf, bowl)

MET, Metabolic equivalent.
Modified from Hlatky MA, Boineau RE, Higginbotham MB, et al: A brief self-administered questionnaire to determine functional capacity (the Duke Activity Status Index), Am J Cardiol 64:651-654, 1989.

TABLE 22.3   Revised Cardiac Risk Index: Clinical Markers

1. High-risk surgical procedures
2. Ischemic heart disease
   a. History of myocardial infarction
   b. Current angina considered to be ischemic
   c. Requirement for sublingual nitroglycerin
   d. Positive exercise test
   e. Pathologic Q waves on ECG
   f. History of PTCA and/or CABG with current angina considered to be ischemic
3. Congestive heart failure
   a. Left ventricular failure by physical examination
   b. History of paroxysmal nocturnal dyspnea
   c. History of pulmonary edema
   d. S_3 gallop on cardiac auscultation
   e. Bilateral rales on pulmonary auscultation
   f. Pulmonary edema on chest radiography
4. Cerebrovascular disease
   a. History of transient ischemic attack
   b. History of cerebrovascular accident
5. Diabetes mellitus
   a. Treatment with insulin
6. Chronic renal insufficiency
   a. Serum creatinine concentration >2 mg/dL

CABG, Coronary artery bypass grafting; *ECG,* electrocardiogram; *PTCA,* percutaneous transluminal coronary angioplasty.
Modified from Lee TH, Marcantonio ER, Mangione CM, et al: Derivation and prospective validation of a simple index for prediction of cardiac risk of major noncardiac surgery, Circulation 100:1043-1049, 1999.

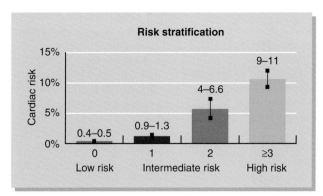

Fig. 22.1 Bar graph shows the predicted risk for cardiac events during surgery according to a patient's Revised Cardiac Risk Index score.

Preoperative Noninvasive Cardiac Testing for Risk Stratification

Evidence discourages widespread application of preoperative noninvasive cardiac testing for all patients. Rather, a selective approach based on clinical risk categorization appears to be both effective and cost-effective. No testing is recommended if it might delay surgical intervention for urgent or emergent conditions.

On a rare occasion, coronary revascularization offers the potential benefit of improving outcomes in high-risk patients—that is, patients with acute coronary syndromes, those with left main CAD, those with two-vessel coronary disease who have significant proximal left anterior descending artery stenosis (and either ischemia on noninvasive testing or reduced left ventricular ejection fraction), and those with three-vessel coronary vessel disease and an ejection fraction of less than 50%. Routine prophylactic coronary revascularization should not be performed in patients with stable CAD before noncardiac surgery. An RCRI score of 3 or higher in a patient with severe myocardial ischemia suggestive of left main or three-vessel disease should lead to consideration of coronary revascularization before noncardiac surgery in appropriate patients.

Noninvasive cardiac testing is most appropriate if it is anticipated that the patient will meet guidelines for initiation of additional medical therapy or coronary angiography and coronary revascularization in the event of a positive test. Noninvasive stress testing of patients with three or more clinical risk factors and poor functional capacity (<4 METS) who require vascular surgery is reasonable, provided that the result might change future management. When feasible, exercise stress testing is the modality of choice and offers the benefit of an objective assessment of functional capacity. Pharmacologic stress tests may be performed instead of exercise tests; they are typically reserved for patients with functional limitations.

Dobutamine echocardiography and nuclear perfusion testing for purposes of identifying patients at risk for perioperative MI or death have excellent negative predictive values (near 100%) but poor positive predictive values (<20%). Therefore, a negative study is reassuring, but a positive study is still only a weak predictor of a "hard" perioperative cardiac event. Which higher-risk patients are most likely to benefit from preoperative noninvasive cardiac testing and treatment strategies to improve outcomes is not well defined.

Preoperative Invasive Cardiac Testing for Risk Stratification

Recommendations for perioperative coronary angiography are similar to those for patients with suspected or known CAD in general and should conform to the ACC/AHA guidelines for coronary angiography. This procedure should be considered for patients who are at high risk for adverse outcomes based on the presence of unstable angina, angina refractory to medical treatment, high-risk results on noninvasive testing, or a nondiagnostic test in a high-risk patient undergoing high-risk noncardiac surgery. It should be considered on an individual basis for those with extensive ischemia revealed during noninvasive testing, for those at intermediate risk undergoing high-risk surgery for whom test results are nondiagnostic, for those convalescing from MI who require urgent noncardiac surgery, and for those with perioperative MI. In patients who have a high clinical risk (RCRI >3) and high-risk features on noninvasive cardiac testing, diagnostic cardiac catheterization should be considered (see Fig. 22.1).

PREOPERATIVE RISK MODIFICATION TO REDUCE PERIOPERATIVE CARDIAC RISK

Coronary Revascularization

Retrospective analyses of the Coronary Artery Surgery Study (CASS) registry and the Bypass Angioplasty Revascularization Investigation (BARI), along with prospective study of patients enrolled in the Coronary Artery Revascularization Prophylaxis (CARP) trial, have shown that prophylactic coronary revascularization with either coronary artery bypass grafting (CABG) or percutaneous coronary intervention (PCI) provides no short-term or mid-term benefit for patients without left main disease or multivessel CAD in the presence of poor left ventricular systolic function. Evidence is lacking to support elective coronary revascularization as a primary strategy for perioperative risk reduction in intermediate-risk patients undergoing major noncardiac surgery.

Recommendations for PCI are similar to those for patients with suspected or known CAD and should conform to the ACC/AHA guidelines. Recommendations by the AHA/ACC Society for Cardiovascular Angiography and Intervention, the American College of Surgeons, and the American Dental Association Science Advisory Committee are for a 30- to 45-day delay of surgery in patients taking thienopyridine dual antiplatelet therapy after bare-metal coronary stent placement and a 365-day wait after placement of a drug-eluting stent. Some studies indicate that the duration of dual antiplatelet therapy may be shortened to less than 1 year in selected patients receiving newer-generation stents (such as everolimus- or zotarolimus-eluting stents).

Currently, studies suggest that optimal medical therapy is the preferred strategy for intermediate- to high-risk patients with RCRI scores of 2 or higher who are without documented severe myocardial ischemia. As stated previously, the CARP trial demonstrated that preoperative coronary revascularization strategies to reduce perioperative cardiovascular risk did not offer significant benefit compared with excellent medical treatment in intermediate- to high-risk patients undergoing vascular surgery. However, high-risk patients with left main coronary stenosis, severe aortic stenosis, left ventricular ejection fraction of 20% or less, or unstable coronary symptoms were excluded from that trial. In many of these patients, coronary or valve surgery may be indicated on its own merit, without factoring in the noncardiac surgery. Therefore, coronary revascularization may be appropriate if diagnostic catheterization reveals left main disease or multivessel disease and depressed ejection fraction.

Using the information obtained from the composite algorithm (Fig. 22.2), a key decision is whether the risk for perioperative cardiac events is sufficiently low to proceed with surgery. For patients identified to be at high cardiac risk who are not candidates for coronary revascularization, the physician may decide to perform an operation that is thought to be less stressful such as a less extensive major plastic reconstruction, laparoscopic versus open procedures or alternative palliative procedures, or attempt to modify cardiac risk by additional intraoperative and perioperative therapies.

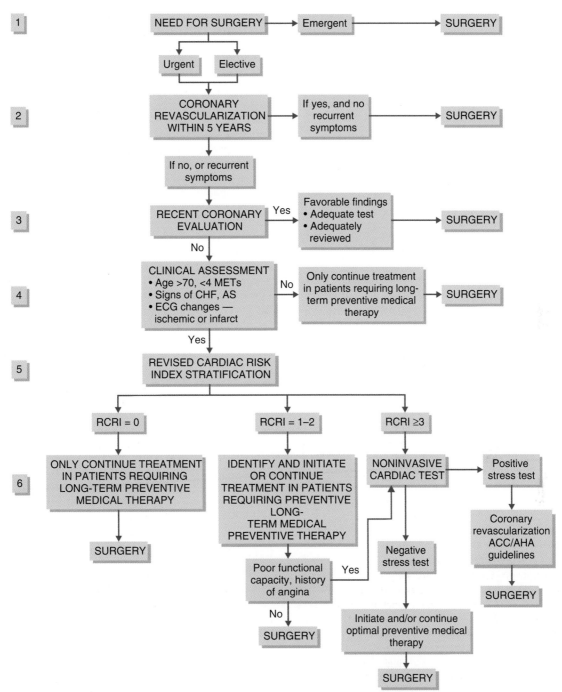

Fig. 22.2 Stepwise clinical evaluation algorithm for diagnostic cardiac catheterization. (1) Emergency surgery; (2) prior coronary revascularization; (3) prior coronary evaluation; (4) clinical assessment; (5) Revised Cardiac Risk Index; (6) risk modification strategies. Preventive medical therapy includes β-blocker and statin therapy. *ACC,* American College of Cardiology; *AHA,* American Heart Association; *AS,* aortic stenosis; *CHF,* congestive heart failure; *ECG,* electrocardiogram; *MET,* metabolic equivalent; *RCRI,* Revised Cardiac Risk Index.

β-Adrenergic Antagonists

There is uncertainty about the effectiveness and safety of perioperative β-blockade in patients undergoing noncardiac surgery. The ACC/AHA guidelines focusing on recommendations for perioperative β-blocker therapy limit class I recommendations to patients undergoing surgery who are already receiving β-blockers to treat angina, symptomatic arrhythmias, or hypertension. Class IIb recommendations are given for the initiation of β-blocker therapy prior to surgery in those with

intermediate- or high-risk myocardial ischemia noted on preoperative noninvasive stress testing (level of evidence C) and patients with three or more RCRI risk factors (level of evidence B).

The Perioperative Ischemic Evaluation (POISE) trial addressed the benefit versus risk of perioperative β-blockade. The POISE trial randomized 8351 intermediate- to high-risk patients older than 45 years of age to receive either a long-acting oral metoprolol succinate (metoprolol CR) or placebo in the perioperative period. The results showed that the incidence of cardiac death, nonfatal MI, or cardiac arrest was reduced in the metoprolol group compared with placebo. However, there was an increased incidence of mortality and stroke in the metoprolol group compared with the placebo group. Stroke was associated with perioperative hypotension, bleeding, atrial fibrillation, and a history of stroke or transient ischemic attack. The POISE trialists highlighted the importance of a clear risk and benefit assessment for the initiation of preoperative β-blockers (see Fig. 22.2).

Preexisting β-blockade should be continued because withdrawal might increase perioperative mortality. If β-blockers are newly initiated in appropriately selected higher-risk patients undergoing noncardiac surgery, they should be carefully titrated and not abruptly initiated on a high-dose regimen in order to avoid hypotension or bradycardia.

HMG-CoA Reductase Inhibitors (Statins)

Prospective and retrospective evidence supports the perioperative prophylactic use of 3-hydroxy-3-methylglutaryl–coenzyme A (HMG-CoA) reductase inhibitors (statins) for reduction of perioperative cardiac complications in patients with established atherosclerosis. Statins should be continued in patients who are already on statin therapy and undergoing noncardiac surgery. A class IIa indication is assigned to the use of statins for patients undergoing vascular surgery with or without clinical risk factors.

Angiotensin-Converting Enzyme Inhibitors

Angiotensin-converting enzyme inhibitors (ACEIs) and angiotensin II–receptor blockers (ARBs) are frequently prescribed for the management of hypertension, CHF, chronic renal failure, and ischemic heart disease. Evidence supports the discontinuation of these agents for 24 hours before noncardiac surgery because of adverse circulatory effects after induction of anesthesia in patients on these medications (hypotension) that may result in the need for vasopressin agonists for management of the ensuing refractory hypotension.

Oral Antithrombotic Agents

Evidence-based recommendations regarding perioperative use of aspirin, clopidogrel, other antiplatelet agents, or combination therapy to reduce cardiac risk currently lack clarity. A substantial increase in perioperative bleeding and transfusion requirement in patients receiving dual antiplatelet therapy has been observed. The discontinuation of clopidogrel for 5 days and aspirin for 5 to 7 days before major surgery to minimize the risk of perioperative bleeding and transfusion must be balanced with the potentially increased risk for an acute coronary syndrome, especially in high-risk patients including those with recent coronary stent implantation. If clinicians elect to withhold aspirin before surgery, it should be restarted as soon as possible postoperatively, especially after vascular graft procedures. (See further information on anticoagulants and surgery later in chapter.)

POSTOPERATIVE CARDIAC RISK ASSESSMENT

Monitoring for Myocardial Infarction

Although there are no standard criteria for their diagnosis, most perioperative MIs occur within the first 3 days after noncardiac surgery. Although an ECG is recommended in the setting of signs or symptoms suggestive of myocardial ischemia, MI, or arrhythmia in the postoperative period, the usefulness of postoperative screening with ECGs is uncertain. Measurement of serum cardiac biomarkers should be reserved for patients at high risk and for those who demonstrate ECG changes, symptoms of myocardial ischemia, new arrhythmias, unexplained shortness of breath, or hemodynamic evidence of cardiovascular dysfunction.

NONCARDIAC SURGERY IN PATIENTS WITH SPECIFIC CARDIOVASCULAR CONDITIONS

Valvular Heart Disease

All patients undergoing noncardiac surgery should be assessed especially for aortic stenosis by physical examination and by two-dimensional echocardiography for any suspicious murmur. Symptomatic *severe* stenosis represents an active cardiovascular condition that should be evaluated and managed before elective surgery is undertaken. Appropriately selected patients can be managed with valve replacement or valvuloplasty as a bridge to noncardiac surgery.

Less is known about the perioperative risks associated with mitral stenosis and mitral regurgitation in patients undergoing noncardiac surgery. Usually, a preoperative history and physical examination, chest radiograph, or ECG provides clues to the diagnosis, which can be confirmed by echocardiography. Accurate diagnosis may help optimize intraoperative anesthetic strategies, choice of pharmacologic interventions and invasive monitoring, and postoperative medical management. Patients with severe mitral stenosis are likely to benefit from balloon mitral valvuloplasty or surgical intervention before high-risk surgery.

Patients with aortic or mitral valvular regurgitation benefit from volume control and afterload reduction. In aortic insufficiency, it is thought that faster heart rates are better tolerated than slow ones because slow heart rates lead to increased diastolic filling and can exacerbate left ventricular volume overload.

Arrhythmias and Conduction Defects

Ventricular and atrial arrhythmias historically are recognized as predictors of perioperative cardiac complications. Therefore, identification of a preoperative arrhythmia warrants a careful evaluation for the presence and severity of underlying ischemic heart disease, cardiomyopathy, or other conditions that may contribute to perioperative complications. In general, asymptomatic arrhythmias or conduction defects warrant only observation and maintenance of an optimal metabolic state.

Congestive Heart Failure and Left Ventricular Dysfunction

CHF has been identified as a significant marker of cardiac risk in noncardiac surgery. Every effort should be made to identify the etiology of CHF and optimally control it preoperatively because it is a known risk factor for postoperative cardiac complications. Close monitoring of volume status is needed to avoid perioperative decompensation. Intravenous inotropic agents, vasodilators, or both may be useful for a short duration in the perioperative period to prevent or treat CHF, depending on the situation.

RENAL DISEASE

Renal dysfunction affects critical excretory and synthetic functions required for homeostasis. The major ensuing clinical effects include hypertension, volume overload, and electrolyte derangements.

Hypertension

A well-controlled blood pressure is desirable to reduce perioperative cardiovascular complications. The goal is to have blood pressure within an acceptable range based on current guidelines. Non-urgent procedures should be delayed for adequate BP control to be attained.

The stress response in the perioperative period does increase the incidence of so-called "white coat hypertension." These patients do not require aggressive lowering of blood pressure that can result in reduced perfusion to the brain and kidneys, resulting in cerebrovascular accidents and acute kidney injury, respectively.

Antihypertensives (Medications)

- ACEIs, ARBs, and renin antagonists' effect on the RAS have been associated with intraoperative hypotension and should be held on the day of surgery. These can be resumed within 48 hours based on patients' blood pressure, volume status, and renal function
- Diuretics should ideally be held in the perioperative period except in patients with evidence of volume overload. The need for patients to be NPO and associated volume losses during surgery usually result in hypovolemia. Diuretics often need to be adjusted perioperatively to reduce risk of acute kidney injury.
- α-Blockers and β-blockers should not be stopped abruptly except in patients who are hypotensive. These medications are associated with rebound hypertension when stopped abruptly. Doses should rather be reduced and holding parameters instituted in cases of hypotension in order to prevent hypertensive crisis associated with rebound hypertension.
- Calcium-channel blockers and vasodilators can be stopped abruptly if not required for optimization of blood pressure.

Acute Kidney Injury

Refer to the Kidney Disease: Improving Global Outcomes (KDIGO) classification of acute kidney injury (AKI).

Kidney injury can be due to prerenal, intrarenal or postrenal etiologies. Perioperative AKI occurs in about 1% of patients, but risk is much higher in patients having vascular and/or cardiac procedures and in patients with chronic kidney disease, cirrhosis, and heart failure. AKI in the perioperative period is often due to fluid losses, fluid shifts to other body compartments, and/or activation of the RAS. It is essential for the etiology of preoperative AKI to be elucidated and addressed before proceeding with elective surgery. It is critical to maintain euvolemia, while aiming to keep electrolytes—especially serum potassium, magnesium, and sodium—within normal limits.

Management

Prerenal AKI patients typically respond to IVF and measures to ensure adequate renal perfusion by preventing hypotension.

Intrarenal AKI patients require consultation from nephrology colleagues to ensure adequate and timely management to prevent progression of the underlying AKI condition and for initiation of renal replacement therapy if needed.

Postrenal insufficiency is due to obstructive uropathy typically due to BPH, urethral stenosis or calculi. Renal ultrasound or CT of the abdomen and pelvis provides information about the nature and severity of the obstruction. Consultation from urology colleagues is often required.

In all patients with AKI, maintaining adequate renal perfusion by keeping spontaneous bacterial peritonitis (SBP) greater than 110 mm Hg is critical, and avoidance of potential nephrotoxins is essential.

Chronic Kidney Disease (CKD)

Refer to the KDIGO classification for staging.

The majority of the perioperative complications are of cardiac etiology. As much as possible, euvolemic status needs to be attained before surgical procedures are performed. Patients on dialysis need to be dialyzed at least 24 hours before the planned procedure. Patients on peritoneal dialysis who require laparotomy often need temporary conversion to hemodialysis to maintain required volume status and address electrolyte abnormalities.

For non–dialysis dependent patients, adequate renal perfusion needs to be maintained and potential nephrotoxins avoided to prevent worsening of CKD.

Nephrotic Syndrome

Maintenance of adequate volume status and renal perfusion is important. Diuretic doses may need to be adjusted. For patients on corticosteroids (prednisone >5 mg daily) for the management of this condition, it should be assumed that their hypothalamic-pituitary-adrenal (HPA) axis is at least partially compromised. Stress dose corticosteroids given as hydrocortisone 100 mg IV every 8 hours, with a transition to an oral regimen in 24 to 48 hours, and then continuing with the usual dose during the perioperative period is usually an appropriate plan.

Renal Transplant Medicine

Immunosuppressive medications should be continued perioperatively. For patients who are unable to take oral medications such as cyclosporine, IV cyclosporine should be given; the dose required is a third of the oral dose.

Monitoring of drug serum levels is essential in view of potential drug-drug interactions.

HEPATIC DISEASE

Acute and chronic liver diseases (Fig. 22.3) can lead to hepatic dysfunction that may worsen perioperatively because of anesthetic agents and hemodynamic effects of a surgical procedure. The major

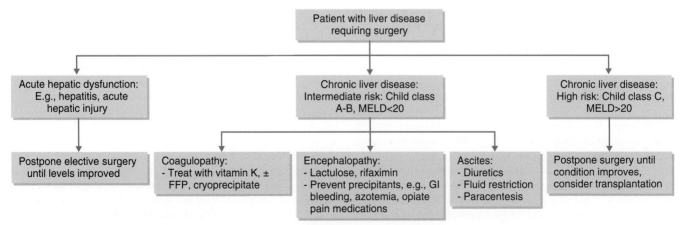

Fig. 22.3 Approach to preoperative risk stratification and interventions in patients with liver disease.

concerns are drug-induced hepatotoxicity, precipitating decompensation of liver cirrhosis and/or development of fulminant liver failure. Perioperative management involves treatment of the complications of liver disease, including coagulopathy, ascites, encephalopathy, and malnutrition.

- Elective procedures in patients with asymptomatic hepatic dysfunction should be postponed pending additional evaluation and reassessment of operative risk.
- Patients with acute hepatic inflammation or hepatocellular and/or cholestatic injury should have elective procedures postponed until there is evidence of recovery.
- Patients with chronic liver disease with preserved hepatic function require close monitoring although their operative risk is minimal.

Cirrhosis is a chronic liver disease, which results in impaired synthetic and metabolic functions.

SBP antibiotic prophylaxis is required for patients with low ascitic fluid protein levels (<1 g/L) for the duration of hospitalization perioperatively. Additional indications for SBP prophylaxis include prior history of SBP and patients with evidence of upper gastrointestinal blood loss.

Patients with ascites due to portal hypertension who may require therapeutic paracentesis will need albumin infusion if more than 5 L is drained to reduce risk for AKI, and the rapid reaccumulation of ascitic fluid.

Diuretic regimens should be adjusted as needed to help maintain required volume status and to keep serum electrolytes within normal limits.

Precipitants of hepatic encephalopathy in patients with cirrhosis need to be avoided as much as possible. Elective procedures in patients who are encephalopathic should be postponed while their clinical condition is managed with the aid of a hepatologist.

Coagulopathy is one of the primary features of chronic advanced liver disease. The etiology is often multifactorial, including hepatic synthetic dysfunction, thrombocytopenia, malnutrition, and the effect of cholestasis on vitamin K absorption. The following measures should be taken to address coagulopathy in the perioperative period.

1. Vitamin K supplementation with or without fresh-frozen plasma (FFP) is often used to correct coagulopathy before surgery. Use of FFP is mainly limited to instances where massive blood transfusion (>4 units) raises concern for dilutional coagulopathy.
2. Cryoprecipitate can address hypofibrinogenemia if serum fibrinogen is less than 100 mg/dL.
3. Platelet transfusion can be used to attain a desired serum platelet level depending on the type of surgical procedure, greater than 50,000 μL for most surgical interventions, but greater than 100,000 μL for neurosurgical procedures.
4. NR values tend to be elevated due to hepatic dysfunction, but this does not confer any antithrombotic properties due to the concept of rebalanced hemostasis. Patients who require deep vein thrombosis (DVT) prophylaxis should still receive subcutaneous heparin or other pharmacologic interventions to reduce DVT risk.

The Model for End-Stage Liver Disease (MELD) and Child-Pugh score/classification (also referred to as Child criteria) have been used for risk assessment of patients with liver disease. The MELD score is calculated using total bilirubin, international normalized ratio (INR), and serum creatinine. This results in four MELD levels, with scores greater than 25 indicating highest mortality risk. Child-Pugh scores are calculated using five clinical measures: total bilirubin, serum albumin, prothrombin time (PT), ascites, and hepatic encephalopathy. The scoring of these clinical measures results in classification of patients in Child class A, B, or C. Patients in class C have the highest mortality risk.

More recently, the integrated MELD score (iMELD), which incorporates serum sodium level for MELD scores less than 12, has been adapted and has been shown to have a better prognostic strength compared with the MELD or Child-Pugh scores.

Surgery is contraindicated in patients with Child-Pugh class C, high MELD/iMELD score (>20), acute hepatitis, severe coagulopathy, or severe extrahepatic manifestations of liver disease (e.g., acute renal failure, hypoxia). Avoid surgery, if possible, in patients with a MELD score of greater than or equal to 18 or Child-Pugh class B unless they have undergone a thorough preoperative evaluation and preparation.

- Use sedatives and neuromuscular blocking agents cautiously.
- Optimize nutrition and medical therapy for cirrhotics:
  - Correct coagulopathy with vitamin K with or without FFP to achieve an INR less than 1.6.
  - The goal platelet count is greater than 50 to 100×10^3/L. This may vary depending on the type of surgical procedure.
  - Address ascitic fluid volume to reduce risk of abdominal wall herniation, wound dehiscence, and compartment syndrome.
- Postoperatively, emphasis should be placed on:
  - Signs of acute liver failure, including worsening jaundice, encephalopathy, and ascites.
  - Monitoring for and correction of renal dysfunction and/or electrolyte abnormalities.
  - Some patients may require IV tranexamic acid to address postoperative bleeding due to the altered fibrinolytic system.

PULMONARY DISEASE

The major components of effective preoperative care are measures to prevent or reduce perioperative complications including pulmonary infections, exacerbation of underlying pulmonary disease, hypoxic hypercarbic respiratory episodes, and avoidance of pulmonary embolism.

For asymptomatic patients there is generally no need for preoperative chest radiographs or pulmonary function tests (PFTs). Preoperative PFTs are, however, essential in patients who are scheduled to have lung resection procedures to help predict postoperative lung function.

Patients with unexplained dyspnea need to be evaluated before having surgical procedures that require general anesthesia.

A combined cardiopulmonary risk index is proposed for risk stratification of pulmonary complications. Pulmonary risk factors have been added to the Goldman Cardiac Risk Index; patients with a combined score of greater than 4 points (of a total of 10) are 17 times more likely to develop complications. These pulmonary risk factors include the following:

- Obesity (i.e., body mass index >27 kg/m²)
- Cigarette smoking within 8 weeks of surgery
- Productive cough within 5 days of surgery
- Diffuse wheezing within 5 days of surgery
- FEV_1/FVC ratio less than 70% and $Paco_2$ greater than 45 mm Hg

In the preoperative history and physical exam, patients should be screened for obstructive sleep apnea (OSA). Adequate management of OSA is critical to prevent cardiopulmonary and neurovascular complications. The commonly used tool is the STOP-BANG score. A formal sleep study is needed in high-risk patients who are scheduled for elective procedures.

COPD/Bronchial Asthma

Patients with these conditions should have their treatment regimen optimized and be instructed to continue with their medications up to the morning of their procedures. Patients with features of exacerbation should be started on systemic corticosteroids. Planned procedures should be rescheduled if possible.

HPA axis suppression should be assumed to be present in patients who have received systemic steroids for more than 3 weeks in the past 6 months. These patients should receive stress-dose coverage perioperatively.

There is no role for prophylactic perioperative use of antibiotics. Elective procedures should be cancelled in patients with active infections.

Obstructive Sleep Apnea

Patients require CPAP (continuous positive airway pressure) perioperatively. Blood gas monitoring is required.

Smoking cessation does reduce pulmonary complications and should be encouraged several weeks before planned elective procedures.

Breathing exercises including use of incentive spirometry are worthwhile risk-reduction measures that should be used.

Postoperative management is based on:
- Appropriate use of antibiotics to treat infections
- Use of high-dose steroids of management of flare-up of underlying lung diseases
- Maintenance of adequate oxygenation.

Prevention of Venous Thromboembolism

In patients undergoing major orthopedic surgery such as hip and knee joint replacement, venous thromboembolism (VTE) prophylaxis with low-molecular-weight heparin (LMWH), adjusted dose warfarin, apixaban, rivaroxaban or aspirin should be initiated postoperatively and continued for a period of up to 35 days. Placement of inferior vena cava filters is unlikely to offer added benefit to patients with contraindications to thromboprophylaxis. Patients undergoing nonorthopedic surgeries should be risk stratified for VTE and those at high risk receive prophylaxis with LMWH or low-dose unfractionated heparin. See American College of Chest Physicians guidelines in the suggested readings section.

ENDOCRINE DISEASE

Diabetes Mellitus

Diabetes mellitus is a common condition requiring preoperative management because uncontrolled diabetes is associated with hyperglycemic crises, infection, reduced wound healing, and increased mortality. Optimal perioperative glucose targets vary but generally fall between 80 to 180 mg/dL. Evaluation includes known complications of diabetes including neuropathy, chronic kidney disease, and heart disease. Hemoglobin A_{1C} measurement will correlate with recent (1-3 months) blood glucose levels and may be helpful with assessment of hyperglycemia risk. Oral and noninsulin injectable medications are generally continued until the morning of surgery at which time they are temporarily discontinued. Long-acting basal insulin is continued but may require dose reduction by 20% to 30% if a fasting period is required. Withholding of long-acting insulin in type 1 diabetics may result in onset of ketoacidosis and should be avoided. Short-acting insulin doses may be reduced or temporarily eliminated depending on oral intake restrictions. Intraoperative and postoperative monitoring of blood glucose via fingerstick (every 2-4 hours) will help identify occurrence of hypo- or hyperglycemia. Long- and short-acting insulin should be used to treat and prevent hyperglycemia while being mindful of the patient's insulin sensitivity to avoid hypoglycemia. Transition back to home regimen may begin when the patient is clinically stable, resumes steady oral intake and no further procedures/operations are planned (see Chapter 68).

Thyroid Disease

Hypo- and hyperthyroidism are each associated with worsening of associated symptoms, morbidity, and even death. Although routine laboratory screening is not recommended, evaluation should be done when symptoms of thyroid dysfunction are noted in patient assessments. Mild to moderate hypothyroidism should be treated with preoperative oral levothyroxine. Treatment of severe hypothyroidism including myxedema coma include IV levothyroxine and IV liothyronine and postponement of elective surgery until thyroid hormone levels are stable. Untreated hyperthyroidism may result in postoperative thyroid storm, which is characterized by tachycardia, confusion, fever, and cardiovascular collapse. Patients with thyrotoxicosis should be treated with β-blockers and antithyroid medications preoperatively (see Chapter 65).

Adrenal Insufficiency and Long-Term Corticosteroid Use

The adrenal glands produce cortisol and various catecholamines in response to stimulation from the HPA axis. Patients receiving long-term exogenous corticosteroids (20 mg daily of prednisone or equivalent for >3 weeks) are considered at risk of adrenal insufficiency due to HPA axis suppression. Because surgery is a state of induced stress, an IV corticosteroid regimen (intravenous hydrocortisone 50-100 mg and up to three times daily) is required with a plan to taper to routine doses based on hemodynamic response (see Chapter 66).

HEMATOLOGIC DISEASE

Screening for disorders of bleeding hemostasis includes questions identifying episodes of bleeding diathesis, medications posing high bleeding risk, and family history of hemophilia or other inherited bleeding disorders. Patients with liver disease, end-stage renal disease, and collagen vascular disease may have higher perioperative bleeding risk. Commonly obtained laboratory testing includes PT, INR, activated prothrombin time (aPTT), and platelet count.

Management of anticoagulants and antithrombotics in the perioperative setting is a frequent concern given their frequent use in clinical practice. Perioperative risk of bleeding and thromboembolic events should be evaluated because not all surgical procedures require discontinuation of anticoagulation (Table 22.4). In situations of high risk of bleeding, the vitamin K antagonist warfarin is held 5 days prior to the planned procedure. Direct oral anticoagulants such as apixaban, dabigatran, and rivaroxaban may be discontinued within 24 to 48 hours of the procedure depending on overall bleeding risk and renal function. In situations of high risk of thromboembolism due to interruption of therapy, bridging therapy may be provided with heparin infusion or LMWH injection until oral therapy may be safely resumed (Table 22.5). Perioperative management of antithrombotics, such as aspirin, clopidogrel, and other P2Y12 inhibitors should be based upon the indications for antithrombotic use and the type of surgery to be performed as noted in the section on cardiologic disease.

Preoperative anemia is associated with an increase in postoperative transfusion, morbidity, and mortality. A target preoperative hemoglobin is not well established and may depend on the expected blood loss, but most patients will likely tolerate levels as low as 7 g/dL. Screening, work-up, and optimization of anemia should occur with enough lead time to allow for correction and optimization prior to elective surgical procedures.

INFECTIOUS DISEASE

Surgical site infections (SSIs) complicate up to 20% of operations leading to significant morbidity and mortality. SSIs occur within 30 days of surgery and are defined as affecting the superficial, deep or organ/space

TABLE 22.4	Risk Factors for Bleeding and Thrombosis in the Anticoagulated Patient		
	INDICATIONS FOR ANTICOAGULATION THERAPY[a]		
	Atrial Fibrillation	**Mechanical Heart Valve**	**VTE**
High-risk features for periprocedural bleeding: Consider interruption of therapy	Procedure-related bleeding risk: Consult surgeon or surgical society guidelines for procedure bleeding risk classification. Common high-risk procedures include: vascular surgery, pacemaker lead extraction, kidney biopsy, radical hysterectomy, total hip replacement, and many others. Patient-related bleed risk increased if: Major bleed or intracranial hemorrhage <3 months; thrombocytopenia or abnormal platelet function (uremia and aspirin use); supratherapeutic INR; history of periprocedural bleeding		
High-risk features for perioperative thromboembolism: Consider bridging therapy	• CHADS2-Vasc 7+ • CVA/TIA/VTE <3 months prior • Rheumatic valvular heart disease	• Mitral valve prosthesis • CVA/TIA <6 months prior • Cage-ball or tilting disk aortic valve prosthesis	• VTE <3 months prior • Severe thrombophilia (protein C or S deficiency, antiphospholipid syndrome, history of recurrent thrombosis when off anticoagulation)

CHADS2-VASC, Clinical prediction rule for estimating the risk of stroke in patients with nonrheumatic atrial fibrillation.
[a]Decisions on bridging therapy are clinically based—evaluate thrombotic risk balanced by patient bleeding risk, consider additional information, and use clinical judgement.

TABLE 22.5	Interruption of Therapy and Bridging of Anticoagulation	
	Anticoagulant Class	
	Vitamin K Antagonists • Warfarin	Direct Oral Anticoagulants (DOACs) • Dabigatran • Apixaban • Rivaroxaban
Interruption of therapy	• INR 2.0-3.0, discontinue 5 days prior to procedure • INR 1.5-1.9, discontinue 3-4 days prior to procedure	• Dependent on creatinine clearance • If renal function is normal, stop 1-2 days prior to surgery
Bridging therapy	• Therapeutic UFH or LMWH • Start UFH when INR <2 • UFH: Stop >4 hours prior to procedure • LMWH: Stop 12-24 hours prior to procedure • LMWH use and dosing must be renally adjusted	• Therapeutic UFH or LMWH • Start UFH when INR <2 • UFH: Stop >4 hours prior to procedure • LMWH: Stop 12-24 hours prior to procedure • LMWH use and dosing must be renally adjusted
Reinitiation of therapy	• Restart at patient's regular dose • Timing is procedure specific: consult with surgeon (most within 24 hours)	• Will render patient therapeutically anticoagulated within hours • Discuss timing of reinitiation with surgeon/proceduralist (most within 24 hours)
Special considerations	• Postprocedure bridging therapy may be considered in patients with moderate or high risk • Discontinue bridging therapy once INR >2.0	• Inability to take PO: may use UFH or LMWH • Obviates need for DVT prophylaxis • Special caution in setting of spinal anesthesia due to risk of hematoma formation

LMWH, Low-molecular-weight heparin; *UFH,* unfractionated heparin.

areas of the wound. Patient risk factors for SSIs include age, nutritional status, and diabetes while operative risk factors include initial contamination of surgical wound, operative technique, and many others. Perioperative care is focused on prevention through the implementation of care bundles (small sets of straightforward evidence-based interventions) including preoperative antibiotics, hair removal, avoidance of hypothermia, and glycemic control. Preoperative antibiotic coverage should include *Staphylococcus aureus* for clean wounds and expand to cover other organisms depending on wound type and risk of contamination. Skin decontamination with topical agents such as chlorhexidine has become routine but may not confer benefit in all patients.

NEUROLOGIC DISEASE

Neurologic conditions that may become exacerbated in the perioperative period include neuromuscular diseases, Parkinson's disease, and stroke.

Neuromuscular Diseases

Conditions such as myasthenia gravis, amyotrophic lateral sclerosis (ALS), and muscular dystrophies predispose patients to a variety of complications. Myasthenia gravis, an autoimmune disease affecting acetylcholine receptors at the neuromuscular junction that leads to skeletal muscle weakness, may worsen acutely in the perioperative period. Respiratory insufficiency or failure due to myasthenic crisis requires assessment of inspiratory function by measuring the negative inspiratory force at the bedside.

Dysphagia, which accompanies many neuromuscular diseases, may lead to aspiration pneumonitis/pneumonia. Swallow evaluation is necessary in the perioperative setting to mitigate this risk in patients with ALS, which is characterized by motor neuron degeneration and may be complicated by postoperative aspiration pneumonia and respiratory failure. Patients with muscular dystrophies are at risk for cardiac arrhythmias and may require cardiac rhythm monitoring. Malignant hyperthermia syndrome is a rare inherited condition presenting as perioperative muscle rigidity, fever, and cardiac arrhythmias.

Parkinson's Disease

Parkinson's disease is a common neurodegenerative disorder associated with dyskinesia, dysphagia, dysmetria, and loss of function. Missed doses of levodopa, a common therapy for Parkinson's, may result in fever, dysautonomia, and worsening of Parkinson's disease symptoms. Levodopa therapy should be continued without interruption if possible, depending on the clinical situation. Patients with Parkinson's disease may require longer rehabilitation following surgical procedures.

Stroke

Perioperative stroke incidence is low but carries a high rate of mortality and morbidity. Most perioperative strokes are embolic in mechanism. Risk factors include history of stroke, diabetes mellitus, hypertension, atrial fibrillation, and advanced age. Addressing modifiable risk factors and appropriate management including use of aspirin and statin therapy for known intracranial atheromatous disease should be pursued. In high-risk patients with atrial fibrillation, perioperative bridging of anticoagulation therapy should be considered to minimize risk of stroke.

RHEUMATOLOGIC DISEASE

Autoimmune conditions such as rheumatoid arthritis and lupus are commonly treated with medications aimed at reducing the activity of the immune system. Disease-modifying antirheumatic drugs such as methotrexate, azathioprine, mycophenolate mofetil, which are used in a range of rheumatic conditions, may be continued in the perioperative period. Biologic agents such as adalimumab, infliximab, and other similar agents are thought to raise the risk of perioperative infection and should be held perioperatively. In addition, surgery should ideally be scheduled for the end of the dosing cycle.

SPECIAL NEEDS OF THE GERIATRIC PATIENT

One third of inpatient surgeries in the United States are performed on adults older than age 65. Patients in the geriatric population have a greater risk of perioperative morbidity and mortality. Geriatric preoperative risk assessment should focus on function, cognition, and evaluation of medications, in addition to the systems-based approach in this chapter. Impairment of activities of daily living (ADLs) is directly associated with increased postoperative mortality. Screening for function may be performed with a variety of scales developed for this purpose. Gait speed and the timed Up and Go test are useful objective assessments. Underlying cognitive impairment is an independent risk factor for postoperative delirium. Cognition may be evaluated with the Mini-Cog scale or Montreal Cognitive Assessment. Identification of concerns in the patient's functional status and/or cognition preoperatively may lead to reevaluation of the surgical management plan. Postoperatively, strategies should focus on physical rehabilitation and measures to reduce risk of delirium including minimal use of medications that promote delirium, frequent reorientation, multicomponent interventions, and judicious use of antipsychotic medications.

Review of medications with a view toward postoperative complications should especially include antihypertensives (hypotension), diuretics (volume depletion), diabetes medications (hypo- or hyperglycemia), antithrombotic agents (bleeding or thrombosis), benzodiazepines, opiates, and other sedative hypnotics (sedation and delirium). Indications for each medication should be reviewed and assessment of the risks and benefits should be performed.

SUMMARY

The success of standardized evidence-based preoperative and postoperative risk reduction strategies in patients undergoing noncardiac surgery depends on collaborative teamwork and careful communication among the surgeons, the anesthesiologist, the patient's primary care physician, and the consultant.

The risk for a perioperative cardiac complication varies with the severity of the surgical procedure and with RCRI stratification. A systematic, stepwise approach for preoperative cardiac risk assessment in patients undergoing noncardiac surgery facilitates a decision as to whether the risk for perioperative cardiac events is sufficiently low to proceed with the surgery. The patient's comorbid conditions and risk factors must be assessed for risk of exacerbation and steps taken to reduce risk to the patient in the perioperative period. Postoperatively, close monitoring of the patient's condition is required. Patients who develop complications after the operation will require timely and appropriate interventions by the surgical and medical teams. Finally, cardiac and medical perioperative care are evolving fields and practitioners must strive to keep their knowledge and practices current through literature review and guideline awareness.

For a deeper discussion on this topic, please see Chapters 403, "Preoperative Evaluation," and 405, "Postoperative Care and Complications," in *Goldman-Cecil Medicine*, 26th Edition.

SUGGESTED READINGS

Auerbach A, Goldman L: Assessing and reducing the cardiac risk of noncardiac surgery, *Circulation* 113:1361–1376, 2006.
Boersma E, Kertai MD, Schouten O, et al.: Perioperative cardiovascular mortality in noncardiac surgery: validation of the Lee cardiac risk index, *Am J Med* 118:1134–1141, 2005.
Doherty JU, Gluckman TJ, Hucker WJ, et al.: 2017 ACC expert consensus decision pathway for periprocedural management of anticoagulation in patients with nonvalvular atrial fibrillation: a report of the American College of Cardiology Clinical Expert Consensus Document Task Force, *J Am Coll Cardiol* 69:871–898, 2017.
Falck-Ytter Y, Francis CW, Johanson NA, Curley C, Dahl OE, Schulman S, et al.: Prevention of VTE in orthopedic surgery patients: Antithrombotic Therapy and Prevention of Thrombosis, 9th ed: American College of Chest Physicians Evidence-Based Clinical Practice Guidelines, *Chest* 141(Suppl 2):e278S–325S, 2012 Feb.
Fleisher LA, Fleischmann KE, Auerbach AD, et al.: 2014 ACC/AHA guideline on perioperative cardiovascular evaluation and management of patients undergoing noncardiac surgery: a report of the American College of Cardiology/American Heart Association task force on practice guidelines, *J Am Coll Cardiol* S0735- 1097(14), 2014, 05536-3.
Hassan SA, Hlatky MA, Boothroyd DB, et al.: Outcomes of noncardiac surgery after coronary bypass surgery or coronary angioplasty in the Bypass Angioplasty Revascularization Investigation (BARI), *Am J Med* 110: 260–266, 2001.
Kristensen SD, Knuuti J, Saraste A, et al.: 2014 ESC/ESA guidelines on non-cardiac surgery: cardiovascular assessment and management: the joint task force on non-cardiac surgery: cardiovascular assessment and management of the European Society of Cardiology (ESC) and the European Society of Anesthesiology (ESA), *Eur Heart J* 35(35):2382–2431, 2014.
McFalls EO, Ward HB, Moritz TE, et al.: Coronary-artery revascularization before elective major vascular surgery, *N Engl J Med* 351:2795–2804, 2004.
POISE Study Group: Effects of extended-release metoprolol succinate in patients undergoing non-cardiac surgery (POISE trial): a randomized controlled trial, *Lancet* 371:1839–1847, 2008.
Rechenmacher SJ, Fang JC: Bridging anticoagulation: primum non nocere, *J Am Coll Cardiol* 66:1392–1403, 2015.

SECTION V

Renal Disease

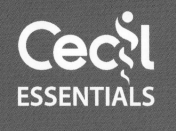

23

Renal Structure and Function

Orson W. Moe, Javier A. Neyra

INTRODUCTION

The kidney maintains the composition and quantity of body fluids, and kidney failure is manifested by dysfunction of multiple organs. Chronic kidney disease is approaching epidemic proportions worldwide, and acute kidney injury affects a very high percentage of hospital admissions and ambulatory patients, with high rates of morbidity and mortality. The etiologies of these conditions are very diverse and often geographically specific. In addition to loss of glomerular filtration and tubular function, kidney diseases include hypertension, urolithiasis, and a host of electrolyte disorders that do not affect the glomerular filtration rate (GFR) but nonetheless cause significant morbidity and mortality. To understand these conditions, a thorough knowledge of the anatomy and function of the kidney is requisite.

Approximately 25% of the cardiac output is distributed to the kidneys, where the blood is continuously cleansed of toxins. In addition to excretion, the kidney is an important metabolic organ and a source of endocrine molecules. Renal failure represents a disruption of all of these functions. Selected aspects of renal structure and function are reviewed briefly in this chapter to set the foundation for the subsequent chapters that deal with specific renal diseases.

RENAL STRUCTURE

Macroscopic Anatomy

The kidneys are seated against the posterior wall of the abdomen in the retroperitoneal space, rendering them readily accessible for percutaneous biopsy. The lower poles may be palpable on deep inspiration in a lean individual. Each human kidney weighs about 120 to 170 g; is about 11 cm long, 6 cm wide, and 3 cm thick; and is endowed with approximately 1 million nephrons with interindividual variations. The "kidney size" commonly referred to in clinical sonographic reports is actually the cephalocaudal renal length, which is not an accurate surrogate for renal volume and mass and may be influenced by patients' body habitus. Despite this caveat, renal length is an acceptable clinical surrogate of renal volume.

The kidney is surrounded by a fibrous capsule (anteriorly, Gerota fascia and posteriorly, fascia retro renalis). The renal arteries enter the kidney and the renal vein and ureters leave the kidney in the renal pelvis. The bisected surface consists of the lighter-colored outer *cortex* and the darker inner *medulla* (Fig. 23.1A). A sample from a clinical biopsy typically originates from the cortex in the lower pole. The medulla is divided into outer and inner regions, and the outer medulla is subdivided into outer and inner stripes. The medulla has multiple conical contours, called *pyramids*, with their apices abutting on the renal pelvis as papillae. The contact points of the renal pelvis with the renal papillae are cup-like structures called *calyces*. Interpolated between the pyramids are centripetal extensions of cortical tissue called *columns of Bertin* (see Fig. 23.1A).

Renal Circulation

Each kidney receives blood from a single renal artery, although supernumerary arteries are present in up to one third of individuals. Just before or after the renal artery enters the kidney, it divides into interlobar arteries that pass between the pyramids of the kidney radially up the columns of Bertin (see Fig. 23.1A). The interlobar arteries further divide into arcuate arteries, which arch along the corticomedullary junction (see Fig. 23.1B). Arcuate arteries give rise to cortical ascending arteries, which bring blood to the glomeruli. Afferent arterioles ramify into glomerular capillaries, distributing blood to individual glomeruli. Features of the renal circulation are summarized in Table 23.1.

The glomerular capillary is the site for glomerular ultrafiltration. Even though the efferent arteriole is downstream from the glomerular capillary, it is not a venule because it has arteriolar walls and is upstream of the second capillary system surrounding the tubules. The peritubular capillaries provide oxygen and nutrients for the kidney, collect the fluid and solutes reabsorbed by tubules to return into the circulation, and deliver the solutes to be secreted by tubule into the tubule fluid. The peritubular capillaries surrounding the cortical and juxtamedullary nephrons originate from the efferent arterioles of cortical and juxtamedullary glomeruli, respectively. In certain pathologic settings, peritubular capillary flow or integrity can be disrupted, decreasing oxygenation and promoting ischemic injury.

The vessels that run parallel to loops of Henle are called *vasa recta* (see Fig. 23.1D) because of their long, straight structures. Blood from the peritubular capillaries is returned to the circulation by a venous system that mirrors the architectural structure of the arterial supply: interlobular vein, arcuate vein, interlobar vein, and renal vein. The parallel countercurrent nature of the vasculature provides the basis for the very high medullar tonicity, which allows urine concentration but also direct arteriovenous diffusion of oxygen, giving rise to the very low oxygen tension in the medulla. This low oxygen tension renders the kidney prone to ischemic injury, which is one of the most common causes of acute kidney injury (see Chapter 29).

Renal Nerves

The capsules of the kidney and the ureters have pain fibers derived from splanchnic nerves. This explains the costovertebral angle pain that occurs when the kidneys are inflamed and during renal colic during kidney stone passage. The renal parenchyma does not have pain fibers but is richly innervated with sympathetic nerves that enter the renal parenchyma with the renal artery. The sympathetic nerves

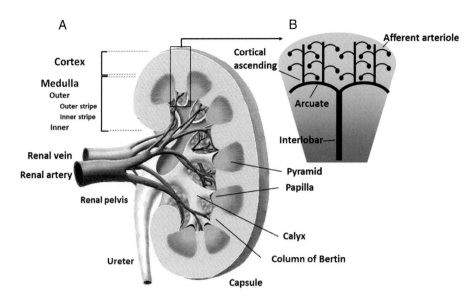

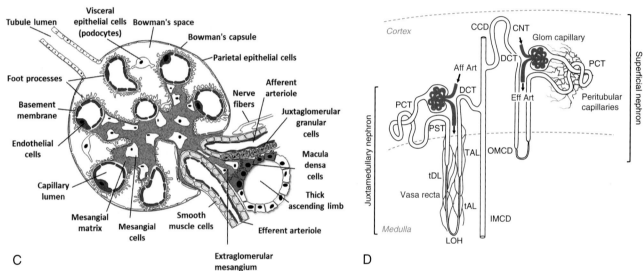

Fig. 23.1 (A) Gross anatomy of the kidney. (B) Schematic representation of the vasculature within a column of Bertin. (C) Structural components of the glomerulus. (D) Schematic representation of a superficial and a juxtamedullary nephron based on the location of their glomeruli. The tubules are intimately intertwined with the capillary system. The peritubular capillaries come off the efferent arteriole leaving the glomerular capillary. The capillaries that bathe the long descending and ascending limbs of the Henle loop are called the vasa recta due to their straight nature. The tubular segments are named axially: *CCD,* Cortical collecting duct; *CNT,* connecting tubule; *DCT,* distal convoluted tubule; *IMCD,* inner medullary collecting duct; *LOH,* loop of Henle; *OMCD,* outer medullary collecting duct; *PCT,* proximal convoluted tubule; *PST,* proximal straight tubule; *TAL,* thick ascending limb; *tAL,* thin ascending limb; *tDL,* thin descending limb.

TABLE 23.1	**Characteristics of the Renal Circulation**
Feature	**Implications**
Few or no anastomoses	Very prone to regional disruption of blood supply
Among the highest blood flow rates per gram of tissue	Lowest oxygen extraction (lowest arteriovenous O_2 difference)
Functional arteriovenous shunts	Solutes and gases (e.g., O_2) can diffuse directly from artery to vein without passing through capillaries
Two capillary systems in tandem	The two capillaries serve completely different functions, in the glomeruli and tubules in sequence

abut on the arterioles (see Fig. 23.1C), stimulate renin release, decrease renal blood flow, and promote renal retention of sodium (Na^+). Renal sympathetic denervation has been proposed as a novel treatment of resistant hypertension using radiofrequency energy delivered via an intrarenal arterial catheter radially to disrupt the nerve fibers on the renal artery, but thus far the data have not been conclusive.

Walk the Nephron

The functional unit of the kidney is the nephron. Each human kidney has approximately 1 million nephrons. Approximately 30% of these have their glomeruli situated deep in the cortex and are referred to as *juxtamedullary nephrons*; the rest are in the outer cortex and are referred to as *superficial nephrons*. Each nephron is a glomerulus followed by a tubule that ends in the renal pelvis. The surrounding capillaries and the interstitial space are important functional components of the nephron.

Glomerulus

The glomerulus consists of the glomerular vasculature (arterioles and capillaries) supported by the mesangium (mesangial cells and matrix) inside Bowman's capsule (parietal and visceral epithelial cells) (see Fig. 23.1C). The visceral cells of Bowman's capsule are the podocytes, so named because of their numerous "foot processes." The smooth muscle layers of the afferent and efferent arterioles are critical in determining arteriolar tone. The glomerular capillary contacts the mesangium on one side and is separated from the foot processes of the podocytes on the opposite side by the glomerular basement membrane (GBM). The glomerulus filters large volumes of water and small solutes while retaining most of the proteins and all of the cells in the blood. The glomerular filtration barrier is a tripartite structure composed of the capillary endothelium, the GBM, and the podocyte slit diaphragm.

Lining the inside of the GBM is a single layer of fenestrated endothelial cells. The fenestrations (50 to 100 nm in diameter) provide a barrier to negatively charged large molecules in the blood. The GBM contains laminin, type IV collagen, entactin (nidogen), and proteoglycans that restrict movement of large molecules (e.g., albumin) from the capillary into Bowman's space. The GBM contains dense negative charges due to glycoproteins with sialic acid residues that restrict the passage of anionic plasma solutes. It can be the site of deposition of immunocomplexes that cause glomerulonephritis (e.g., membranous glomerulonephritis, membranoproliferative glomerulonephritis, lupus nephritis). Autoantibodies against the GBM cause severe inflammation and loss of filtration. Autoantibodies against a podocyte membrane glycoprotein (M-type phospholipase A2 receptor, PLA2R) can cause antibody-mediated primary membranous nephropathy. The epithelial layer consists of podocytes and the parietal epithelium, which is flat and squamous with few organelles. At the vascular pole, the parietal epithelium is contiguous with a completely different epithelium—the proximal convoluted tubule.

On the visceral side of Bowman's space are the podocytes, which constitute part of the filtration barrier. These cells have a highly interdigitating system of foot processes that rest against the basement membrane. The podocyte cell bodies lie within the extracellular matrix. The spaces between foot processes are filtration slits of approximately 40 nm in diameter bridged by slit diaphragms, which are also negatively charged, contributing to the containment of middle-size negatively charged particles in the capillary. In the last decade, there have been momentous advances in identifying the components of the slit diaphragm complex and understanding their functions. A full discussion is not possible here, but major slit diaphragm–associated proteins include nephrin, podocin, neph-1/2/3, FAT-1, R-cadherin, catenin, CD2AP, ZO-1, and α-actinin 4. Mutations of many of these genes cause congenital proteinuric kidney disease (see Chapter 26).

Tubules

The parietal epithelium of Bowman's capsule becomes the renal tubule (see Fig. 23.1D) as it leaves the glomerulus. The renal tubule is a prototypical polarized epithelium. Its salient characteristics are summarized

in Fig. 23.2. A simple cylinder would not suffice in terms of surface area for transport. In the luminal apical membrane, surface amplification is achieved either by protrusions or by a more extensive form of protrusions called the *brush border* in the proximal tubule. Between cells are structures called *tight junctions*. Although they are called tight junctions, some are truly tight (with high resistance to solute and charge movement), whereas others are quite leaky to solutes. In addition to resistance, these complexes also regulate whether the junction is more permeable to one ion type compared with another selective permeability. On the other side of the tight junction is the intercellular space, which is contiguous with the interstitial space. The basolateral cell membrane on the interstitial-capillary side amplifies its surface area by infoldings into the cell and interdigitations between two cells.

The movement of a solute can be through a cell (transcellular transport) or around the cell (paracellular transport) (see Fig. 23.2A). Solute transport is an energy-consuming process that requires metabolic fuels. There are many kinds of transport proteins (see Fig. 23.2B). ATPases directly couple hydrolysis of adenosine triphosphate (ATP) to transport. Cotransporters (or symporters) move two solutes in the same direction, and countertransporters (antiporters) move two different solutes in opposite directions. Channels function as protein-lined "holes" that allows specific solutes to permeate. Different transporters can also be coupled together to form a new transport system. Finally, there are proteins that protrude outside the cell in the junctional area to provide a conduit for paracellular transport.

Specialized Structures
Interstitium

The space between the tubules and peritubular capillaries constitutes about 5% to 10% of renal volume and harbors interstitial fibroblasts and dendritic cells. In diseases such as interstitial nephritis (see Chapter 27), the interstitium is full of inflammatory cells, which elaborate cytokines and chemokines that profoundly affect filtration and tubular function. The resident fibroblasts are stellate cells with projections that physically contact tubules and capillaries, provide scaffold support, and secrete and maintain matrix. These cells, when stimulated by cytokines, can transform into myofibroblasts and contribute to interstitial fibrosis, a common pathobiologic feature of kidney disease. Some specialized fibroblasts in the deep cortex are sensors of oxygen and producers of circulating erythropoietin. The dendritic cells are antigen-presenting cells that express major histocompatibility complex (MHC) class II molecules. They are in intimate communication with the renal parenchyma, constantly sampling and responding to the local antigenic environment. Dendritic cells are involved with innate and adaptive immunity and are major players in immunologic homeostasis and diseases of the renal parenchyma.

Juxtaglomerular Apparatus

A unique feature of the nephron is that each thick ascending limb traverses back to and engages in physical contact with its parent glomerulus. The tubular cell at the point of contact is different from the rest of the thick ascending limb and is called the *macula densa*. The tripartite structure comprising the macula densa, the afferent and efferent glomerular arterioles, and the extraglomerular mesangium, a special part of the mesangium that protrudes outside the glomerulus, is called the *juxtaglomerular apparatus* (JGA) (see Fig. 23.1C). The JGA is an important structure in the maintenance of GFR by tubuloglomerular feedback and regulation of afferent arteriole resistance and is the site of endocrine renin production.

Organelles Such as Mitochondria and Endoplasmic Reticulum

The kidney is second to the heart in mitochondrial content and oxygen consumption per unit mass. In addition to their role as the

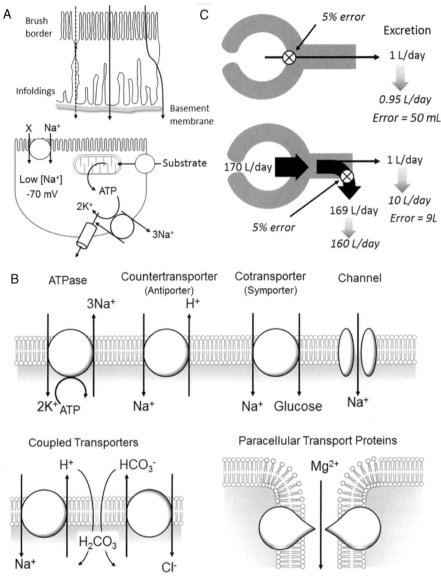

Fig. 23.2 (A) *Top*, Transcellular and paracellular transport of solutes. Solute transport is an energy-consuming process that requires metabolic fuels; a sodium cotransporter and a sodium-potassium countertransporter are shown. (B) Transport proteins. *Top*, Adenosine triphosphatases (ATPases) directly couple ATP hydrolysis to transport. Cotransporters (symporters) move two solutes in the same direction (e.g., Na^+-glucose cotransporter or sodium-glucose linked transporter [SGLT]), and countertransporters (antiporters) move two different solutes in opposite directions. Channels function as protein-lined "holes" that allow specific solutes to permeate. *Lower left*, Different transporters can be coupled together to form a new transport system. *Lower right*, Proteins that protrude outside the cell in the junctional area provide a conduit for paracellular transport. (C) Comparison of a pure filtration (or secretion) design *(top)* and a filtration-reabsorption design *(bottom)*. See text for details.

power generator of a cell, mitochondria serve many roles as regulatory, synthetic, and adaptive functions in the cell. Mitochondria are under complex regulation and undergo a plethora of abnormalities in many kidney diseases. Mitochondria-targeted therapeutics are emerging with the notion that maintenance of mitochondria health can prevent pathogenesis and progression of chronic kidney disease. The endoplasmic reticulum (ER) helps maintain the quality of proteins through the unfolded protein response (UPR) pathway, and ER dysfunction with maladaptive UPR activation is named ER stress. ER stress is now known to be present in a wide variety of kidney diseases, and modulators of ER stress will assume important therapeutic roles.

RENAL FUNCTION

Excretory Function

Renal excretion of a substance can be mediated and modified by one or a combination of three processes: filtration, secretion, and reabsorption. Fig. 23.2C compares two designs—pure filtration (or secretion) and filtration-reabsorption—and their implications in terms of demands on regulation. The filtration-reabsorption mechanism allows high filtration rates to be achieved, and the coupling with reabsorption prevents loss of valuable fluid and electrolytes. This design also enables economy in transport mechanisms through adaptive targeting of key solutes while allowing the rest to be excreted. However, there is a price to be paid for this configuration. Consider the excretion of 1 L/day by pure filtration (or secretion). If there is a 5% error (reduction in filtration or secretion), only 0.95 L/day will be excreted—a difference of 50 mL. Compare this to a filtration-reabsorption mechanism wherein 170 L/day is filtered and 169 L/day is reabsorbed, resulting in the same 1 L/day excretion. A 5% error (reduction) in reabsorption would result in reabsorption of 160 L/day and excretion of 10 L/day, with an absolute error of 9 L. One consequence of a filtration-reabsorption design is that regulation has to have exquisite fidelity, and even small errors are not tolerated.

Filtration

Filtration occurs exclusively at the glomerulus. The GFR, measured as volume per unit time, has been the standard quantitative surrogate for overall kidney function, although there are many disturbances of renal function that are not associated with a decrease in GFR (e.g., nephrotic syndrome, tubulopathies, renovascular hypertension, kidney stones). Numerically, GFR can be conceptualized as an equation:

$$GFR = K_f \times (\Delta P - \Delta \Pi)$$

where the ultrafiltration coefficient, K_f, is equal to the surface area for filtration multiplied by the hydraulic permeability; the hydrostatic driving force, ΔP, is the pressure gradient between the glomerular capillary and Bowman's space, which drives fluid to go into Bowman's space to form urine; and the osmotic driving force, $\Delta \Pi$, is the osmotic pressure gradient between the glomerular capillary and Bowman's space, which holds fluid back in the capillary and slows down filtration.

Many renal diseases affect the determinants of GFR. Glomerular disease (see Chapter 26) decreases K_f by affecting both the filtration surface area and the hydraulic permeability. Changes in ΔP are commonly involved in diseases that reduce GFR. Changes in renal blood flow and more importantly in afferent and efferent arteriolar resistances can drastically affect ΔP and GFR. Functional changes in ΔP, such as pre-renal failure from hypovolemia, hepatorenal syndrome (see Chapter 29), or intra-abdominal hypertension can radically lower GFR simply by hemodynamic changes without any structural glomerular lesions.

Reabsorption

High GFR, which is required to maintain a high metabolic rate, can be sustained only if there is high reclamation to maintain intravascular volume and prevent circulatory collapse. Tubular reabsorption thwarts the loss of valuable solutes and allows for finer tuning of the water and solutes not reabsorbed. The resulting tubular contents are excreted. In the mammalian kidney, tubular reabsorption assumes critical roles in the regulation of excretion of many solutes (Table 23.2). A universal mechanism of reabsorption is energy-dependent transepithelial transport, which is mostly Na^+ dependent but can be Na^+ independent. The proximal tubules participate in the reabsorption of all solutes, but some solutes are sequentially reabsorbed by the proximal and distal segments; in these cases, the generic design tends to be high-capacity reabsorption proximally and more of a high-gradient reabsorption for fine tuning distally. The axial difference can occur within the same nephron segment (e.g., early vs. late proximal tubule) or across different segments (e.g., proximal vs. distal nephron segments).

Secretion

Secretion is an ancient mode of excretion that is found in lower-order organisms. Although the human nephron is not primarily secretory in nature, a number of solutes are still handled by secretion. For example, the renal excretion of potassium (K^+), hydrogen ions (H^+), and uric acid involves secretion. Many organic cations and anions are secreted by the proximal tubule, and so are many exogenous toxins such as xenobiotics. The secretion of creatinine by organic cation transporters in the proximal tubule is the reason why creatinine clearance overestimates GFR. The secretion of furosemide by organic cation transporters in the proximal tubule is why response to this drug is attenuated in settings of renal hypoperfusion and/or proximal tubular damage such in acute kidney injury.

Integrated Models of Excretion

The modes of excretion are coordinated in a precise, complex, and concerted fashion to effect excretion with exquisite accuracy (see Table 23.2). The kidney is capable of a large range of urinary tonicity (<50 to 1200 mOsm), depending on the need of the organism to excrete or conserve electrolyte-free water. Water is filtered at the glomerulus and is handled isotonically in the proximal tubule. At the lumen of the distal convoluted tubule, urine is maximally dilute as a consequence of low water permeability throughout the thick ascending limb of Henle. The subsequent fate of the urine determines whether there is electrolyte-free water excretion (dilute urine), achieved by low water permeability of the collecting duct, or electrolyte-free water conservation (concentrated urine), effected by the action of antidiuretic hormone (ADH), which renders the collecting tubule permeable to water.

Na^+ homeostasis basically occurs via filtration-reabsorption; it is regulated by changes in effective arterial blood volume (EABV) mediated by neurohormonal afferent signals (e.g., renin-angiotensin-aldosterone system [RAAS]) that act directly on tubules. In the proximal tubule, Na^+ reabsorption is also regulated by peritubular physical factors. K^+ undergoes an interesting sequence in which the filtered load is largely reabsorbed in the proximal tubule and the thick ascending limb; the final determinant of excretion is secretion by the collecting duct, for which aldosterone and distal Na^+ delivery are major regulators.

Only Ca^{2+} that is not bound to plasma protein is filtered; it is reabsorbed largely via paracellular pathways in the proximal tubule and thick ascending limb and via transcellular pathways in the distal convoluted tubule.

A massive amount of bicarbonate (HCO_3^-) is filtered and must be reclaimed to forestall catastrophic acidosis. H^+ secretion provides the mechanism for HCO_3^- reclamation as well as acid excretion, with the H^+ being carried by urinary buffers such as ammonia.

Metabolic Function

The kidney is a major metabolic organ. It consumes a wide range of fuels, regulates plasma levels of metabolic substrates, and is a major source of gluconeogenesis. Metabolic substrates such as amino acids, glucose, organic anions, and fatty acids are converted to ATP, the universal energy unit for all cells (see Fig. 23.2A). ATP is directly hydrolyzed by proteins such as Na^+/K^+-ATPase to create a low intracellular Na^+ concentration ($[Na^+]$) and a negative interior cell voltage, thus translating the chemical energy into chemical gradients. About 80% to 90% of the oxygen consumption of the kidney can be attributed to Na^+ transport. For example, a protein such as the Na^+-glucose cotransporter (sodium-glucose linked transporter [SGLT], see Fig. 23.2B) on the proximal tubule luminal membrane, couples the movement of Na^+ ions to glucose molecule (carrying a net positive charge). The low cell $[Na^+]$ and negative voltage energize glucose uptake, allowing the proximal tubule to capture most of the filtered glucose that otherwise would be lost in the urine. In normal physiology, this glucose reclamation is beneficial to conserve calories. The pharmacologic inhibition of Na^+-coupled glucose reabsorption (SGLT-2 inhibitors) leads to low glycosuric threshold and creation of a "glucose sink" to control glycemia. Surprisingly, many additional beneficial cardiovascular and renal effects have been observed with SGLT-2 inhibitors that are not explained by glycemic control.

TABLE 23.2   Solute Excretion

Solute	Filtration	Reabsorption	Secretion	Fe (%)	Regulation
Water	Yes	Yes	No	0.3-6.0	Responds primarily to body tonicity but also EABV.
					ADH is the major regulator of collecting duct water permeability.
Na^+	Yes	Yes	No	0.2-2.0	Responds to EABV.
					Reabsorption is stimulated by sympathetic nerves, angiotensin II, aldosterone; inhibited by atrial natriuretic peptides, dopamine, uroguanylin.
K^+	Yes	Yes	Yes	5-20	Responds to total body potassium status.
					Secretion is controlled primarily by aldosterone and distal Na^+ delivery.
Ca^{2+}	Yes	Yes	No	2-10	Responds to serum ionized $[Ca^{2+}]$ and body need for calcium.
					Major calciotropic hormones include parathyroid hormone, vitamin D, and calcitonin.
					Renal epithelia directly respond to ionized calcium via the calcium sensing receptor.
Mg^{2+}	Yes	Yes	No	3-5	Responds to total body magnesium status and requirements.
					Paracrine regulation is via epidermal growth factor.
HCO_3^-	Yes	Yes	Yes	0.1-0.5	Most bicarbonate reabsorption is to reclaim the filtered load.
					Responds to systemic acid-base status, which can be mediated by direct sensing by the renal epithelia or via hormonal actions (e.g., angiotensin II, endothelin).
					Bicarbonate can also be secreted in the collecting duct when alkali excretion is required.
Phosphate	Yes	Yes	No	5-20	Responds to serum phosphate concentration and body phosphate status.
					Reabsorption primarily resides in the proximal tubule and is regulated by parathyroid hormone and fibroblast growth factor-23.
Glucose	Yes	Yes	No	0.2-0.5	The proximal tubule reclaims almost all filtered glucose except when the filtered load exceeds reabsorptive capacity.
					The cortical proximal tubule performs gluconeogenesis from other organic substrates.
Uric acid	Yes	Yes	Yes	10-50	Major routes of uric acid clearance are (1) renal excretion and (2) intestinal secretion and uricolysis.
					Handling of both secretion and reabsorption in the proximal tubule is complex, and regulatory mechanisms are unclear.
Creatinine	Yes	No	Yes	1.0-1.2	Filtered at the glomerulus and secreted by the proximal tubule.
					The contribution of the tubules to creatinine clearance increases when GFR declines.

ADH, Antidiuretic hormone; *EABV,* effective arterial blood volume; *FE,* fractional excretion under normal physiology.

TABLE 23.3   Some Endocrine Hormones Elaborated by the Kidney

Hormone	Source	Function	Drugs
Renin	JGA	Converts angiotensinogen to angiotensin I as an integral part of the renin-angiotensin-aldosterone system	Renin inhibitor ACE inhibitor Angiotensin receptor blocker Mineralocorticoid receptor blocker
$1,25(OH)_2$ vitamin D	Mostly proximal tubule	Converts the precursor 25(OH) vitamin D to its active form, $1,25(OH)_2$ vitamin D	25-Hydroxyvitamin D 1,25-Dihydroxyvitamin D Synthetic vitamin D analogues
Erythropoietin	Renal interstitial cells	Stimulates erythropoiesis in the bone marrow	Recombinant human erythropoietin Glycosylated recombinant human erythropoietin Other "EPO mimetic" erythropoiesis-stimulating agents

ACE, Angiotensin-converting enzyme; *JGA,* juxtaglomerular apparatus.

The amount of filtered organic molecules far exceeds the metabolic consumption by the kidney. Very large amounts of organic metabolic substrates are passively filtered daily; these substrates are not meant to be excreted, but the high GFR and lack of retention at the glomerular capillaries obligate their presence in the glomerular urine. In the proximal tubule, the bulk of the filtered organic molecules are reclaimed from the urine and returned to the systemic circulation. Several thousands of millimoles of amino acids, glucose, and organic cations and anions are retrieved each day by the kidney from the urine.

Metabolic and Endocrine Function

The kidney rivals the liver as a gluconeogenic organ that sustains circulating blood glucose levels. Although there is no doubt that this is a critical physiologic function, there are no clinical examples of hypoglycemia stemming purely from lack of renal gluconeogenesis.

In addition to the prominent and more obvious roles in solute and water balance, the kidney also is an important endocrine organ. The autocrine and paracrine substances elaborated by the kidney are important for both intrarenal and systemic regulation. Although this subject is not addressed fully here, three of these substances are highlighted because they represent important pharmacologic targets (Table 23.3).

Renin

As the initiating component of the RAAS, renin is important for maintenance of the circulation. The RAAS permits the kidney to have a constant GFR in the face of low and fluctuating salt intake, a property that is vital for terrestrial existence. Renin is produced by the JGA (see earlier discussion). Despite the benefits and importance of the RAAS in physiology, its continuous and excessive activation in many disease states appears to be maladaptive and contributes to kidney and cardiovascular injury. Pharmacologic blockade of RAAS pathways at various levels has proved beneficial in animal disease models and human clinical studies, and agents to block RAAS signaling are now in clinical use, with others under development (see Table 23.3).

Vitamin D

1α-Hydroxylase (cytochrome P-450 isoenzyme 27B1) is found primarily in the proximal tubule, where the major body defense for maintaining phosphate homeostasis is localized. The kidney is one of the most important organs for maintaining calcium and phosphate homeostasis, not just as the major controller of external balance but as an elaborator of systemic factors such as vitamin D and the Klotho protein. Conversion of the precursor 25(OH)-hydroxyvitamin D to its active form, 1,25(OH)$_2$dihydroxyvitamin D, is achieved not exclusively but substantially in the kidney and is mediated by 1α-hydroxylase. Vitamin D deficiency is an important complication in chronic kidney disease. Replacement of vitamin D is efficacious in reducing the complications of chronic kidney disease.

Erythropoietin

Erythropoietin, which is produced mainly in the kidney, stimulates erythropoiesis. The erythropoietin-producing cells are strategically located in the cortical interstitium to sense the balance between oxygen delivery and consumption. The current model suggests that upregulation of renal erythropoietin production (mainly by anemia and hypoxia) occurs via an increase in the number of latent erythropoietin-producing cells. The mechanism of erythropoietin deficiency in kidney disease is not well known, although it does not simply involve destruction of erythropoietin-producing interstitial cells. One possible mechanism is decreased renal oxygen consumption as a consequence of reduced GFR; this results in higher renal tissue oxygen tension and suppression of erythropoietin production. Another theory is direct inhibition of the erythropoietin-producing cells by inflammatory cytokines. Others have proposed transdifferentiation of erythropoietin-producing cells into myofibroblasts and a decrease in the number of interstitial cells that can be recruited to produce erythropoietin.

The use of erythropoiesis-stimulating agents (ESAs) has revolutionized the treatment of anemia associated with chronic kidney disease, but because of incomplete understanding of erythropoietin and erythropoietin receptor biology, the clinical outcome is far from ideal due to inability to tailor the optimal hematocrit for individual patients and uncertainty about possible extra-erythropoietic effects of erythropoietin. The new class of hypoxia-inducible factor prolyl hydroxylase inhibitors as ESAs increases endogenous erythropoietin production.

SUGGESTED READINGS

Kaissling B, Le Hir M: The renal cortical interstitium: morphological and functional aspects, Histochem Cell Biol 130:247-262, 2008.

Maezawa Y, Cina D, Quaggin SE: Glomerular cell biology, Waltham, 2013, Academic Press, pp 721-757.

Moe OW, Giebisch G, Seldin DW: Logic of the kidney. In Lifton RP, Somio S, Glebisch GH, et al, editors: Genetic diseases of the kidney, New York, 2009, Elsevier, pp 39-73.

Reiser J, Sever S: Podocyte biology and pathogenesis of kidney disease, Annu Rev Med 64:357-366, 2013.

24

Approach to the Patient With Renal Disease

Rajiv Agarwal

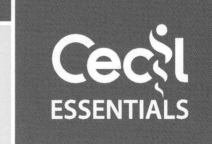

INTRODUCTION

Chronic kidney disease (CKD) is commonly defined as having an estimated glomerular filtration rate (GFR) of less than 60 mL/min/1.73 m² for at least 3 months. Most patients with CKD are seen in the outpatient setting, and at first consultation an important objective is to uncover the cause of CKD. In the long term the objectives of care are the preservation of kidney and cardiovascular function and the prevention of the long-term complications of CKD. Once kidney function deteriorates to the extent that it can no longer sustain an appropriate quality of life the objective of care evolves to the provision of renal replacement therapy. In some patients, discussion may be about withholding the provision of renal replacement therapy. In contrast to the clinical approach to patients with CKD, most patients with acute kidney injury (AKI) are hospitalized. The focus of their care also starts with accurate determination of the cause of AKI, but over a period of days to weeks it is important to reverse the kidney failure if possible, replace kidney function if needed, and manage the many potential adverse consequences of AKI. Thus, the approach to the care of patients with AKI and CKD are largely non-overlapping and are discussed separately.

Distinction of AKI From CKD

Because of the widespread use of automated systems for serum chemistry analysis, an elevated serum creatinine concentration is the most common initial manifestation of kidney disease. This test is performed as a screen for renal function abnormalities in most metabolic panels; in most cases, an elevated serum creatinine concentration reflects reduced filtration function of the kidney. After ensuring that intravascular volume is appropriate, the approach to the patient depends on whether kidney failure is acute or chronic. Accordingly, the initial step in evaluating an elevated serum creatinine level is to assess the time course and duration of the changes to distinguish AKI from CKD.

A careful history, physical examination, and laboratory evaluation, including imaging studies, are all fundamental to this process. The highest priority is to address acute volume depletion, bleeding, and other causes of intravascular volume loss. Evidence of chronicity may be discovered by searching the records for prior abnormalities of serum creatinine, albuminuria or proteinuria, abnormal urine sediment, or anatomic features such as the presence of multiple cysts in both kidneys discovered on an ultrasound or CT scan. Similarly, a call to the primary care doctor may provide clues to suggest the presence of kidney disease at an earlier time. In the United States, electronic medical record systems are ubiquitous and deep knowledge of this electronic record is often essential to discover the onset date of CKD.

Small kidney size, as assessed by ultrasound, can be highly suggestive of CKD. The size of the kidney depends on the height of the patient, but in general, a kidney length on ultrasound images of less than 9 cm in an adult male is considered small. The presence of normal-sized or even large kidneys does not exclude the diagnosis of CKD. In fact, it is common in patients with diabetic nephropathy for kidneys to be 11 or 12 cm long. Radiography of clavicles or hands is not commonly performed but may demonstrate renal osteodystrophy and suggest the presence of CKD.

Anemia is common in both AKI and CKD and therefore is not a differentiating feature. However, the presence of secondary hyperparathyroidism points toward CKD. Rarely, if the initial evaluation is unrevealing, a kidney biopsy may be required to distinguish AKI from CKD and to define the etiology of injury.

APPROACH TO THE PATIENT WITH CHRONIC KIDNEY DISEASE

If the elevated creatinine concentration is thought to be chronic in nature, the history and physical examination should focus initially on detection of diabetes mellitus and hypertension, the two most common causes of CKD. In all cases, the evaluation also includes laboratory testing of renal function, serum electrolytes, complete blood count, testing for albuminuria, and microscopic urine sediment analysis. Kidney ultrasound is almost always obtained early in the evaluation to eliminate ureteral or bladder obstruction, a cause of reversible renal failure. In addition, the ultrasound provides important information about kidney size, symmetry, and echogenicity. Kidney biopsy may be needed in some patients, but parenchymal scarring is common in many forms of CKD so the biopsy may not be diagnostic.

Because diabetes and hypertension are common causes of kidney disease, it is important to recognize the associated presentations. To establish a likely diagnosis of diabetic nephropathy, a long-standing history of documented diabetes mellitus is typical. An eye exam that notes diabetic retinopathy often goes hand-in-hand with diabetic nephropathy; however, the absence of diabetic retinopathy does not rule out CKD due to diabetes mellitus. Albuminuria and large kidneys on ultrasound are often seen. However, as many as a third of patients with CKD due to type 2 diabetes mellitus do not have albuminuria. In patients with diabetes mellitus or hypertension, the urinary sediment is usually unremarkable, so the presence of red blood cells (RBCs) casts or a significant number of dysmorphic erythrocytes should initiate a careful evaluation for other causes of CKD.

In cases of hypertensive nephrosclerosis, established hypertension typically antedates the diagnosis of renal failure for many years, and the presence of hypertensive retinopathy or cardiovascular disease (e.g., left ventricular hypertrophy) is common. Proteinuria is typically minimal or absent (<2 g/day), and the kidneys are symmetrically small on ultrasound.

Although hypertension and type 2 diabetes mellitus are common, among patients with CKD it is important not to assume that diabetes and hypertension are always the cause of CKD. The diagnosis of hypertension or diabetes mellitus as the cause of CKD requires that no other identifiable cause of kidney disease is apparent after a thorough evaluation. Notably, in individuals with hypertension, genes such as *APOL1* have been identified that appear to be associated with a greater risk of renal disease, and genetic analysis may emerge as one approach to identify those most at risk so that strategies for prevention can be tested in the future.

Once a diagnosis of CKD is established, ongoing evaluation is required, because those with CKD are at increased risk for complications such as hypertension, metabolic bone disease, anemia, hyperkalemia, and metabolic acidosis. Furthermore, the initial diagnosis of CKD may be modified over time, such as by the discovery of RBC casts in a patient with diabetes mellitus. AKI may be superimposed on CKD. The assessment of hypertension requires an accurate assessment of blood pressure. Measurements of three readings after quiet rest at intervals of 1 minute using an oscillometric device is now recommended; auscultatory methods utilizing Korotkoff sounds are no longer recommended. If hypertension or volume overload becomes difficult to manage, the dietary intake of sodium can be estimated by 24-hour urine collection. The number of medications prescribed to patients with CKD is substantial, which calls for monitoring for medication adherence. The latter, for instance, may provide clues to lack of control of BP. For a more detailed approach and slightly different opinion on the measurement of the arterial blood pressure, see Chapter 12.

History and Examination

The signs and symptoms of CKD depend on the stage at presentation. Early in the clinical course, nonspecific fatigue is typical, and there may be no discernable clues to CKD on examination, highlighting the need for laboratory screening. As filtration rate declines, the signs and symptoms of CKD become more common and may include pedal edema, facial puffiness, flank pain, polyuria, nocturia, and hypertension. Symptoms referable to uremia, such as nausea, dysgeusia, and vomiting, tend to occur late and should not be relied on to make a diagnosis of early CKD.

Sometimes the manifestations of the primary disease predominate. For example, the presence of fever, arthralgia, and rash in a young woman with renal failure and active urinary sediment is highly suggestive of lupus nephritis; or intravenous drug use, cardiac murmur, vegetations on cardiac valve, and positive blood culture should alert to a possible diagnosis of endocarditis-associated glomerulonephritis. A family history of deafness, hematuria, and CKD can point to the diagnosis of Alport's syndrome; or a history of cerebral hemorrhage due to a ruptured aneurysm may suggest underlying polycystic kidney disease.

Medication history should focus on exposure to nephrotoxins, including long-term use of nonsteroidal anti-inflammatory drugs (NSAIDs), lithium, exposure to cisplatin, and recent escalation of the dose of diuretics. Some nonprescription drugs can lead to CKD (e.g., cocaine-induced glomerulonephritis, Ma Huang–induced ephedrine kidney stones).

Past medical history may clue in to possible etiologies; for example, diabetic retinopathy to diabetic nephropathy; recurrent urinary tract infection to renal calculi; and hepatitis C, infective endocarditis, or Wegner's granulomatosis to glomerulonephritis.

Physical examination can reveal the presence of anemia, skin rash (such as in endocarditis, Fabry's disease, Henoch-Schönlein purpura, or cryoglobulinemia), rales, pericardial or pleural friction rub, pedal edema, abdominal bruit, or enlarged kidneys. Retinal examination is of particular importance and may reveal diabetic retinopathy or changes associated with hypertension; in a patient with rapid deterioration of renal function, retinal examination may show cholesterol emboli or septic emboli, pointing to the existence of cholesterol emboli or bacterial

endocarditis as possible causes. Rectal examination to assess prostate enlargement in men and pelvic examination in women may point to clues to urinary tract obstruction such as a tumor or neurogenic bladder. Examination of the muscle mass is important when interpreting serum creatinine concentration (see later discussion).

The assessment of blood pressure is particularly important. Often, blood pressure is elevated in the clinic but normal at home (*white coat hypertension*). Occasionally, the blood pressure is elevated at home but not in the clinic (*masked hypertension*). In patients who complain of orthostatic symptoms but appear to have normal or high blood pressure in the clinic, home blood pressure measurements or 24-hour ambulatory blood pressure monitoring may be required. The latter may reveal very low blood pressure with orthostatic symptoms, and antihypertensive therapy may need to be modified.

The overall condition of the patient and level of functional status is important in deciding therapies. For example, transplantation may be an option for a patient with correctable cardiovascular disease and dialysis for someone with calcified iliac arteries where kidney transplant may not be possible. However, the physician and the patient's family may share the decision to forego renal replacement in an elderly person with advanced dementia and poor functional status.

Assessment of Kidney Function

Knowledge of both the severity of renal impairment and the rate of change in renal function is important in managing CKD. Rapid deterioration of kidney function over a few weeks to a few months may not reflect native renal disease progression; rather, it may reflect superimposed volume depletion (e.g., escalation in the dose of diuretics), exposure to nephrotoxins (e.g., NSAID use), or urinary tract obstruction. Alternatively, rapid progression of kidney disease may be seen in certain disease states such as malignant hypertension, crescentic glomerulonephritis, microangiopathic hemolytic anemia (thrombotic thrombocytopenic purpura, scleroderma), vasculitides (lupus nephritis, Wegener's granulomatosis), atheroembolic renal disease, or multiple myeloma. In general, a slower progression of decline in kidney failure is anticipated in patients with CKD caused by polycystic kidney disease, hypertension, or diabetes mellitus.

Serum creatinine is the most commonly measured of kidney functions. Along with the assessment of albuminuria, it is an important component for staging CKD (Fig. 24.1). If estimated GFR is less than 60 mL/min/1.73 m² for 3 months or longer, kidney disease is said to be chronic.

Notably, serum creatinine concentration does not rise to above the population threshold of normal (about 1.3 mg/dL in men and 1.1 mg/dL in women) until approximately 40% of kidney function is lost. In earlier stages of kidney disease, serum creatinine is maintained in the normal range by enhanced tubular secretion of creatinine. This process of creatinine secretion requires cationic transporters, and drugs that compete with creatinine secretion (e.g., cimetidine, triamterene, trimethoprim) may cause elevation of serum creatinine without depressing true GFR. A clinical clue to an impairment in cationic transport of creatinine is the lack of rise in blood urea nitrogen despite an increase in serum creatinine concentration.

With advanced kidney failure, the magnitude of absolute changes in serum creatinine concentration may be more rapid. The relationship between serum creatinine and GFR is nonlinear, accelerating as the GFR declines. This means, for example, that an increase in serum creatinine concentration from 3 to 3.5 mg/dL is associated with a lesser decline in GFR than is a change from 1 to 1.5 mg/dL. Specific knowledge of the baseline level of serum creatinine is important; for example, change from 0.6 to 1.2 mg/dL is still within the normal range in an adult man but actually reflects an approximately 57% loss of GFR.

Prognosis of CKD by GFR and Albuminuria Categories: KDIGO 2012			Persistent albuminuria categories Description and range		
			A1	**A2**	**A3**
			Normal to mildly increased	Moderately increased	Severely increased
			<30 mg/g <3 mg/mmol	30–300 mg/g 3–30 mg/mmol	>300 mg/g >30 mg/mmol
GFR categories (ml/min/1.73 m²) Description and range	**G1**	Normal or high	≥90		
	G2	Mildly decreased	60–89		
	G3a	Mildly to moderately decreased	45–59		
	G3b	Moderately to severely decreased	30–44		
	G4	Severely decreased	15–29		
	G5	Kidney failure	<15		

Green: Low risk (if no other markers of kidney disease, no CKD); Yellow: moderately increased risk; Orange: high risk; Red: very high risk.

Fig. 24.1 Chronic kidney disease (CKD) nomenclature used by the Kidney Disease Improving Global Outcomes (KDIGO) consortium. CKD is defined as abnormalities of kidney structure or function, present for 3 months or longer, with implications for health. CKD is classified on the bases of cause, glomerular filtration rate (GFR), and albuminuria. (From KDIGO: 2012 clinical practice guideline for the evaluation and management of chronic kidney disease, Kid Intl Suppl 3:18, 2013. Available at http://www.kdigo.org/clinical_practice_guidelines/pdf/CKD/KDIGO_2012_CKD_GL.pdf. Accessed June 1, 2014.)

The relationship between GFR and serum creatinine is best interpreted at steady state and not when the GFR is changing rapidly. For example, bilateral nephrectomy in a patient with previously normal kidney function (as might occur in a patient with renal cell carcinoma) results in a drop in GFR from 100 to 0 mL/min. However, serum creatinine would be expected to increase by only about 1 mg/dL/day, and a plateau may not be achieved before 1 week. This delay reflects the fact that the generation of creatinine is insufficient to saturate the volume of distribution of creatinine. A plateau will be reached more rapidly if the rate of creatinine generation is increased, the volume of distribution of creatinine is small, or residual renal function is substantial. Given these variables, it is important to be aware that serum creatinine may be a poor marker of GFR in non–steady-state conditions. Similarly, among patients with end-stage renal disease receiving renal replacement therapy although the laboratory may report eGFR (estimated GFR), this is a poor estimate of GFR given that the creatinine is being removed by extracorporeal means.

There also are several conditions in which serum creatinine may be falsely low in relation to the GFR. Because creatinine generation is dependent on muscle mass, low creatinine generation occurs in diseases associated with sarcopenia, such as motor neuron diseases (amyotrophic lateral sclerosis), wasting illnesses (advanced cancer, tuberculosis, cardiac cachexia), and even malnutrition. Visual examination of muscle mass (thighs, arms, temporal muscles) may therefore be important in the interpretation of serum creatinine concentrations. Other conditions associated with low creatinine generation include cirrhosis and advanced age. Creatinine generation is reduced in sepsis, and kidney function may be worse than is detectable by estimation of GFR through measurement of serum creatinine.

Among patients with severe CKD (e.g., GFR <20 mL/min), creatinine is secreted and urea is absorbed by the tubule. Tubular secretion of creatinine is fortuitously balanced by tubular reabsorption of urea, making measurements of urea clearance and creatinine clearance useful in estimating true GFR. An average of creatinine and urea clearance closely approximates true GFR in such situations.

At steady state—that is, when the patient is neither gaining nor losing weight—the 24-hour urine urea nitrogen measurement can be used to estimate dietary protein intake. In addition to its excretion in urine, nitrogen is lost through the gut, through the skin, and, as non-urea nitrogen, through the kidney in proportion to body weight. It is estimated that 31 mg/kg/day of non-urea nitrogen is excreted in this fashion. Dietary protein intake can be calculated as 6.25 g protein per gram of total daily nitrogen excretion. Accordingly, the formula for dietary protein intake in grams per day is (urine urea nitrogen + 0.031 × body weight in kg) × 6.25.

Although urea by itself is less useful to assess kidney function, it can be helpful in conjunction with the serum creatinine measurement. Urea is reabsorbed by the tubule in sodium-avid states. The normal ratio of urea to creatinine is 10:1. In states of volume depletion such as diuretic use, diarrhea, sweat losses, or third spacing (e.g., leakage of fluid outside the vascular compartment such as in peritoneal cavity [ascites] or pleural space [pleural effusion]), the urea-to-creatinine ratio may be greater than 20:1. Sometimes, ratios greater than 20:1 are also seen in catabolic states (e.g., long-bone fracture, corticosteroid use, burns, sepsis), increased gut protein load (upper gastrointestinal bleeding, high-protein diet), or obstructive uropathy. In contrast, creatinine may rise disproportionally more than urea, for example in advanced cirrhosis, low-protein diets, or states associated with the use of cationic transport inhibitors (e.g., cimetidine).

For many decades, the assessment of creatinine clearance by a 24-hour urine collection has been the mainstay of assessing renal function. However, given that creatinine may be secreted (and not just filtered), this test may overestimate GFR. Furthermore, voiding outside the collection jug is common and may lead to errors in estimating GFR. Although a 24-hour urine collection is not routinely recommended to assess renal function, it may still be useful for estimating GFR in sarcopenic individuals and in those with advanced liver disease. Creatinine clearance can be easily calculated as the urinary flow rate (in mL/min) times the ratio of urinary creatinine to plasma creatinine. A timed collection is needed. Creatinine excretion approximates 15 mg/kg/day. Although this rate is variable (the coefficient of variation from day to day over 28 days on a standard diet varies from 6% to 22%) and depends on meat intake, it can be used to estimate whether urine has been grossly undercollected or overcollected.

Usually, GFR is estimated through the use of equations that account for age in years, race, sex, and serum creatinine. The Modification of Diet in Renal Disease (MDRD) equation uses a creatinine measurement (Scr) that has been calibrated to an isotope dilution mass spectrometry standard:

$$GFR \ [in \ mL/min/1.73 \ m^2] = 175 \times (Scr)^{-1.154}$$
$$\times (Age)^{-0.203} \times 0.742 \ [if \ female] \times 1.212 \ [if \ black]$$

A newer equation, called the Chronic Kidney Disease Epidemiology Collaboration (CKD-EPI) equation, is less likely to estimate GFR as low if the GFR is higher than 60 mL/min/1.73 m². This equation is more complicated:

$$GFR \ [60 \ ml/min/1.73 \ m^2] = 141 \times min(Scr/k, 1)^{\alpha}$$
$$\times max(Scr/k, 1)^{-1 \triangleright 209} \times 0.993^{Age}$$
$$\times 1.018 \ [if \ female] \times 1.159 \ [if \ black]$$

where Scr is serum creatinine (in mg/dL), κ is 0.7 for females and 0.9 for males, α is −0.329 for females and −0.411 for males, *min* indicates the minimum of Scr/κ or 1, and *max* indicates the maximum of Scr/κ or 1. Several calculators to estimate GFR using the CKD-EPI equation or the MDRD equation are available on the World Wide Web or as applications for personal devices.

Assessment of Albuminuria

The assessment of albuminuria is fundamental because it may point to the cause of the CKD. Furthermore, the severity of albuminuria is directly associated with an accelerated progression of CKD and cardiovascular disease. As a result, albuminuria is now used to stage CKD (see Fig. 24.1).

Albumin excretion rate is normally less than 10 mg/24 hr, and an excretion rate of 30 mg/24 hr or higher is considered abnormal and moderately increased. An albumin excretion rate of 300 mg/24 hr or higher is considered severely increased. Albuminuria can be more conveniently assessed by measuring the ratio of urine albumin and urine creatinine concentrations in a spontaneously voided urine specimen. Given that the creatinine excretion rate averages 1 g/day, an albumin-to-creatinine ratio of 30 mg/g creatinine or higher is considered abnormal and moderately increased; a ratio of 300 mg/g creatinine is considered severely increased.

An albumin excretion rate higher than 2200 mg/24 hr (which corresponds to approximately 3000 mg protein/24 hr) is considered nephrotic. Such a degree of albuminuria/proteinuria is often accompanied by edema, hypoalbuminemia, and hyperlipidemia. The combination of these disorders is referred to as the *nephrotic syndrome* and

reflects a profound disorder of glomerular permselectivity. Common causes of nephrotic syndrome in adults are diabetic nephropathy, focal segmental glomerulosclerosis, membranous nephropathy, and amyloidosis. Among children, minimal change nephropathy and focal segmental glomerulosclerosis are important causes of nephrotic syndrome.

Assessment of Blood Pressure

Hypertension is a common accompaniment of CKD, yet the evaluation of hypertension often is performed poorly. Current management of hypertension is directed most often to management of blood pressure measurements obtained during clinic visits. Measurement of BP during clinic visits therefore should be accurately performed. At present, measurement of three readings of BP in the nondominant arm, after seated rest for 5 minutes, is the standard of care. The average of the three readings is used to make clinical decisions regarding the management of hypertension. Despite accurate measurements of BP in the clinic, BP may be falsely higher in the clinic (*white coat hypertension*) or lower in the clinic (*masked hypertension*) compared with 24-hour ambulatory blood pressure measurements. At present, in the United States, the latter technique is mostly limited to research or to management of hypertension in a few difficult cases. However, home blood pressure recordings self-measured by the patient twice daily for about 1 week every month can help diagnose and manage hypertension more effectively. Self-performance of these measurements may promote adoption of a more healthful diet and better medication adherence by the patient, as well as reducing therapeutic inertia on the part of the physician.

An important cause of poor control of BP in patients with or without CKD is poor medication adherence. Pill burden directly relates to nonadherence with medications, and patients with CKD are often prescribed multiple medications. Thus, the assessment of adherence to medications should be a routine part of assessment.

Assessment of Dietary Sodium Intake

At steady state, when body weight is neither increasing nor decreasing, the dietary sodium intake can be judged by 24-hour urine collection. To establish adequacy of urine collection, the measurement of urine creatinine in 24-hour urine sample is important. The creatinine excretion rate in an adequately collected specimen should approach 1 g/day for women and 1.5 g/day for men. Dietary potassium and protein intake can be monitored similarly. Measurement of urine urea nitrogen in the 24-hour urine sample can reveal the adequacy of dietary protein intake. Dietary sodium restriction can improve blood pressure, can enhance the biologic actions of inhibitors of the renin-angiotensin system, and may protect the heart, blood vessels, and kidneys independent of improvement in blood pressure.

Microscopic Urinalysis

Microscopic urinalysis at initial evaluation and on an ongoing basis can reveal vital information about the health of the kidney. Evaluation should be performed by centrifugation of at least 12 mL of a freshly voided specimen. Cells, casts, crystals, and other elements can corroborate the diagnosis of the cause of CKD. Examples are shown in Figs. 24.2 through 24.5. (See also E-Fig. 29.1 and Table 29.3.)

Renal Imaging

Bladder ultrasonography is a tool that can be used to assess residual urine volume. The wide availability of this tool allows diagnosis of bladder outlet obstruction without the need to catheterize the patient.

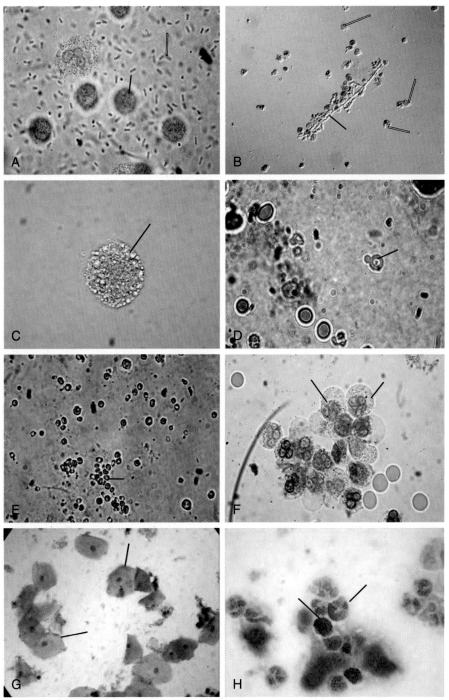

Fig. 24.2 Cells often found in urine of patients with kidney disease. (A) Sternheimer-Malbin–stained urine sediment (100× objective) in a patient with urinary tract infection. *Solid line* shows a leukocyte and *hollow line* indicates bacteria. (B) Sternheimer-Malbin–stained urine sediment (40×) in a patient with fungal urinary tract infection. *Solid line* shows a pseudohypha and *hollow lines* indicate leukocytes. (C) Unstained urine sediment (40×) shows an oval fat body in a patient with nephrotic syndrome. (D) Sternheimer-Malbin–stained urine sediment (100×) in a patient with immunoglobulin A (IgA) nephropathy. *Solid line* shows an acanthocyte characterized by outpouching of the red blood cell (RBC) membrane. (E) Sternheimer-Malbin–stained urine sediment (40×) in a patient with IgA nephropathy shows many acanthocytes *(solid line)*. When acanthocytes constitute more than 5% of the RBCs, their presence is considered significant. (F) Sternheimer-Malbin–stained urine sediment (100×) in a patient with recovering acute tubular necrosis (ATN). *Solid lines* indicate glitter cells. The granules of these leukocytes have a Brownian motion and appear to glitter under the microscope. These cells can be seen in large numbers during the recovery stage of ATN and in patients with urinary tract infection. (G) Sternheimer-Malbin–stained urine sediment (40×) shows numerous squamous cells, indicating poor collection technique. (H) Hansel-stained urine sediment (100×) shows eosinophils that can be seen in patients with allergic interstitial nephritis, cholesterol emboli, or, sometimes, urinary tract infection.

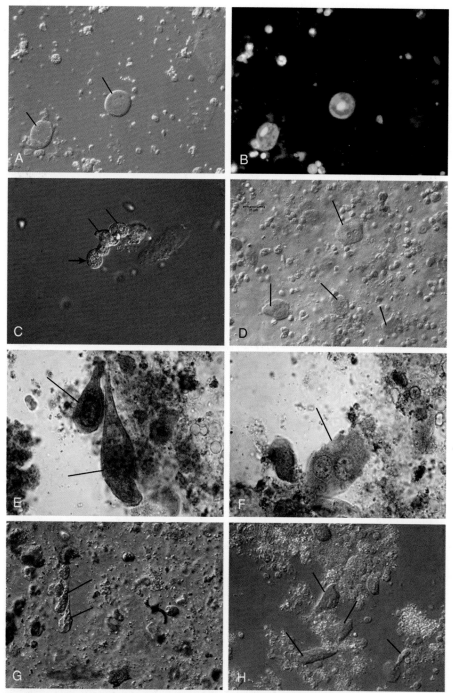

Fig. 24.3 Tubular cells often found in urine of patients with acute kidney injury. (A) Unstained urine sediment (40× objective) in a patient recovering from acute tubular necrosis (ATN). *Solid lines* show intact renal tubular epithelial cells. (B) Same specimen as in A but stained with acridine orange-propidium iodide and viewed with a triple excitation band fluorescence filter (triple-cube). Red cells are dead and green cells are live. Both tubular cells appear viable. Smaller cells are leukocytes. (C) Unstained urine sediment (40×) shows several renal tubular cells that appear monomorphic (as in images A and B), indicating acute tubular injury. The *arrow* indicates a binucleate tubular cell. (D) Unstained urine sediment (40×) shows several renal tubular cells *(solid lines)* that appear dysmorphic. Instead of being round, the cells are angular. Furthermore, these cells are multinucleated, indicating failure of the cell to divide. Large numbers of dysmorphic renal tubular cells are often seen if the acute tubular injury is substantial. (E) Unstained urine sediment (100×) shows two tear-drop-shaped dysmorphic renal tubular epithelial cells *(solid lines)*. Because the patient had jaundice, the cells appear to have a color despite lack of staining. (F) Unstained urine sediment (100×) shows one dysmorphic, binucleate renal tubular epithelial cell *(line)*. This is the same patient as in E. (G) Unstained urine sediment (40×) shows severe ATN. No dirty-brown granular casts were seen, but the tubular cells were dysmorphic *(lines)*. The large amount of granular debris and absence of casts suggests failure to form Tamm-Horsfall protein and more severe tubular injury. This patient also had jaundice, as is evident from the yellow hue. (H) Unstained urine sediment (40×) shows dysmorphic renal tubular epithelial cells (triangular, cigar-shaped, and polygonous), often multinucleated as denoted by *lines*.

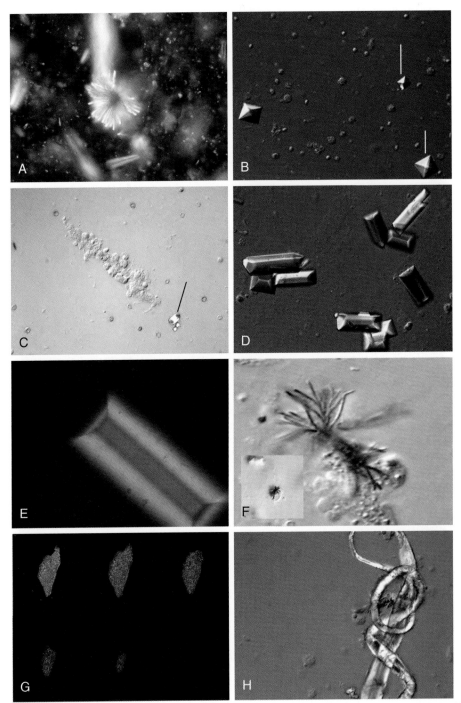

Fig. 24.4 Crystals commonly found in urine sediment. All images were made with the use of polarized light and a diffusion interference contrast microscope. (A) Uric acid crystals (40× objective). (B) Calcium oxalate dihydrate crystals *(white lines)* (40×). Large numbers are seen in patients with ethylene glycol poisoning. (C) Calcium oxalate monohydrate crystals *(solid line)* (40×). (D) Magnesium ammonium phosphate crystals, or triple phosphate crystals, are often found in patients with a complicated urinary tract infection (40×). (E) Coffin-lid appearance of magnesium ammonium phosphate crystals (100×). (F) Bilirubin crystals in a patient with acute tubular necrosis and obstructive jaundice (100×). Inset shows 40× view of the bilirubin crystals. (G) Calcium phosphate crystals (40×) in a patient with tumor lysis syndrome. Sequential images *(left to right, top to bottom)* show dissolution of the crystals within a few minutes after urine was acidified by adding 2% perchloric acid. (H) Fiber artifact in the urine is of no clinical significance.

Renal ultrasonography is the most accurate way of determining kidney size. It is commonly performed to detect renal masses, cysts, and evidence of obstruction characterized by dilatation of the pelvicalyceal system and to evaluate the size and shape of the kidneys. The presence of small kidneys (i.e., <9 cm on both sides) suggests the presence of scarring and therefore CKD. However, kidneys that are larger, typically in the range of 11 to 13 cm, are often seen in conjunction with CKD due to diabetes mellitus, amyloidosis, and multiple myeloma.

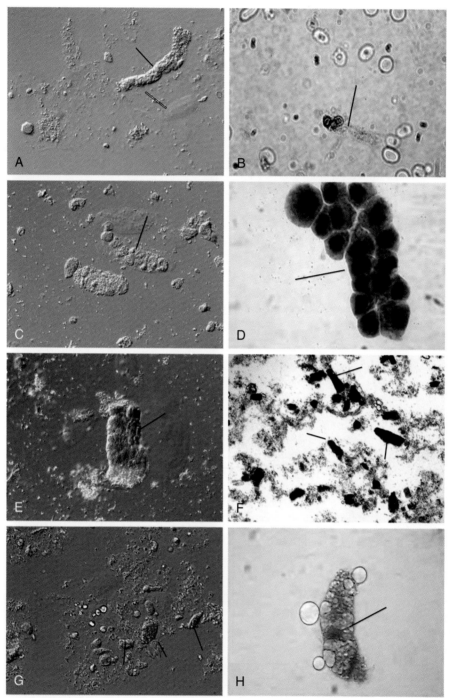

Fig. 24.5 Casts in urine. (A) Unstained urine sediment (40× objective) in a patient with glomerulonephritis. *Solid line* shows a granular cast, and *hollow line* shows a hyaline cast. (B) Sternheimer-Malbin–stained urine sediment (40×). The *solid line* points to an erythrocyte cast in a patient with immunoglobulin A nephropathy. (C) Unstained urine sediment (40×) shows several renal tubular cells and an epithelial cell cast *(solid line)* indicating acute tubular injury. (D) Papanicolaou-stained urine sediment *(solid line)* (100×) shows an epithelial cell cast in an otherwise stable patient with diabetic nephropathy. (E) Unstained urine sediment (40×) shows bilirubin-stained granular cast *(solid line)* indicating renal inflammation in a patient with liver disease. (F) Unstained urine sediment (10×) shows dirty-brown granular casts *(solid line)* indicative of acute tubular necrosis (ATN). (G) Unstained urine sediment (40×) shows severe ATN. No dirty-brown granular casts were seen, but the tubular cells *(solid lines)* were dysmorphic and multinucleated. (H) Sternheimer-Malbin–stained urine sediment (40×) shows a fatty cast *(solid line)* in a patient with nephrotic syndrome.

Therefore, the presence of small kidneys is not required to make a diagnosis of CKD.

The echogenicity of the kidneys is compared with that of liver parenchyma. Typically, the kidneys are less echogenic than the liver. Increased echogenicity of the kidneys suggests the presence of scarring and therefore CKD. Renal ultrasonography can also easily detect the presence of cysts in the kidneys and therefore is a useful technique to detect polycystic kidney disease.

Pulsed Doppler imaging is often used to calculate the resistive index by estimating the systolic and diastolic Doppler velocities in the renal cortex. A resistive index greater than 0.8 suggests that interventional procedures to revascularize the kidney would be unlikely to benefit the patient in terms of improving blood pressure or protecting the long-term decline in kidney function. If the two kidneys differ in size by 1.5 cm, it suggests the presence of renovascular disease in an adult. In children, reflux nephropathy or congenital abnormalities are more common causes of asymmetric kidney size.

Computed tomography (CT) of the kidney is often helpful to evaluate complex cysts. In contrast to simple cysts, complex cysts are suspicious for the presence of malignancy, and CT can evaluate them better than ultrasonography. Likewise, CT is important for evaluating renal masses, stones, retroperitoneal conditions (e.g., hemorrhage, tumor, abscess), and renal vein thrombosis. In morbidly obese people, CT is often used to guide kidney biopsy. The use of contrast agents to assess vascular lesions of the kidney may be not be possible if kidney function is compromised due to fear of precipitating AKI. Limiting the volume of the contrast agent and volume repletion before radiocontrast administration may minimize renal injury.

Although *intravenous pyelography* can image the structures in the kidney, contrast CT has taken the place of classic intravenous pyelography in many centers because of the risk of inducing nephrotoxicity in patients with CKD. In contrast, *retrograde pyelography* is often used by urologists to define the site and nature of obstruction within the ureter and the pelvis. In addition, during the procedure, ureteric stones can be removed with the use of a basket device.

Magnetic resonance imaging (MRI) is useful for imaging of the vasculature and therefore for the diagnosis of renal vein thrombosis and renal artery stenosis. Gadolinium-based contrast agents are often used for MRI because of their paramagnetic properties. These agents should be avoided if the GFR is less than 30 mL/min/1.73 m^2, because in such patients they have been implicated in causing a disabling and untreatable condition called *nephrogenic systemic fibrosis*. It is now believed that the risk of this disabling condition is directly related to the release of free gadolinium from gadolinium-based contrast agents. Stable macrocyclic agents that minimize the release of free gadolinium after administration such as gadoterate acid and godobutrol are preferred over the older gadolinium-based contrast agents. MRI cannot be performed in patients who have metallic implanted devices with magnetic properties such as pacemakers, artificial joints, or aneurysmal clips. Although nonferrous surgical metal can distort an MRI image, most are safe within the strong magnetic field of an MRI machine. Research now reveals that MRI examination after a total joint replacement is not only possible, but adjusting pulse sequences and parameters often can provide accurate information on soft tissue tissues and causes of joint failure.

After injection of a small amount of radioactive substance, *radionuclide imaging* can be performed to assess renal perfusion and function of the kidneys. One advantage of this technique is that it can assess kidney function and perfusion simultaneously for each kidney. It therefore allows diagnosis of renal artery stenosis, especially when it is performed before and after administration of angiotensin-converting enzyme (ACE) inhibitors.

Renal arteriography is the reference standard for the diagnosis of renal artery stenosis. It involves direct injection of a radiocontrast dye into the renal arteries. In patients with CKD, contrast injection can be limited and carbon dioxide can be injected to avoid nephrotoxicity. This technique is also useful for assessing vascular malformations in the kidney and for making a diagnosis of polyarteritis nodosa. In the latter condition, renal arteriography can detect the presence of microaneurysms.

APPROACH TO THE PATIENT WITH ACUTE KIDNEY INJURY

The initial approach to patients with AKI focuses on the following factors: (1) the evaluation of risk or susceptibility to renal injury, (2) the cause(s) of the AKI, (3) the severity of injury, and (4) the presence of distant organ effects or consequences. In all cases, it is important to evaluate and optimize intravascular volume early in the course, because this is a readily addressable factor that can prevent or minimize further injury.

Evaluation of Risk or Susceptibility to Renal Injury

The risk factors for AKI include, first and foremost, prior existence of CKD; CKD can easily be detected by a low estimated GFR or the presence of albuminuria. Other common risk factors for AKI include advanced age, diabetes mellitus, hypertension (especially when treated with inhibitors of the renin-angiotensin system), chronic liver disease or cirrhosis, and multiple myeloma.

Causes of AKI

AKI is a challenging medical problem, and a careful and stepwise approach to evaluation is essential. This approach is guided by knowledge of the causes of injury, which can be divided into five major groups: ischemia, toxins, obstruction, inflammation, and infection.

Ischemia can be caused by volume loss from the gastrointestinal system (vomiting or diarrhea), the skin (sweating, burns), or the kidneys (diuretics, Addison's disease, and solute diuresis). Comparing the body weight of the patient with those weights recorded in the medical record can be valuable. A substantial decrease in body weight may point toward volume depletion as a possible cause of AKI. Third-space fluid losses, as observed in patients with ascites, pancreatitis, or ileus, can make the diagnosis of volume depletion challenging because such patients may not have an overall loss in body weight. Ischemia is a common cause of AKI due to poor perfusion associated with significant blood loss or sepsis or both. In the setting of ischemia, glomerular hypoperfusion is aggravated when patients are taking inhibitors of the renin-angiotensin system.

Nephrotoxins can be divided into two major groups: endogenous and exogenous. The endogenous toxins include paraproteins, myoglobin, hemoglobin, uric acid (e.g., in tumor lysis syndrome), and bile acids. Exogenous toxins include contrast agents, aminoglycosides, vancomycin, chemotherapeutic agents such as cisplatin, and NSAIDs.

Inflammation can involve the glomerular, interstitial, and vascular compartments. Inflammation of these structures produces glomerulonephritis, interstitial nephritis, and vasculitis, respectively.

Infection is an important cause of injury to the nephron. Infection-associated AKI is often diagnosed in the intensive care unit, where early sepsis can manifest as a fall in urine output followed by an increase in serum creatinine, confirming AKI. The causes of AKI in the setting of sepsis are often multifactorial and include ischemia, direct tubular dysfunction due to sepsis, and concomitant administration of drugs such as nephrotoxic antibiotics (commonly, high doses of vancomycin) and procedures (radiocontrast imaging), often performed to reverse sepsis.

Therefore, declines in urine volume, especially in the intensive care unit, should lead to a diligent search for a focus of infection.

Urinary tract obstruction is often a reversible cause of renal injury and therefore important to diagnose. Although urine output is frequently reduced with obstruction, partial obstruction may be associated with an increase in urine output. Renal ultrasound is useful to diagnose hydronephrosis; urinalysis may reveal hematuria or infection or may be bland. Left untreated, renal atrophy may ensue.

In many ways, the severity of injury is best assessed at the bedside. Oliguric renal failure (100-400 mL urine/24 hr) or anuric renal failure (<100 mL urine/24 hr) has a worse prognosis than nonoliguric renal failure (>400 mL urine/24 hr). A low fractional excretion of sodium or, if the patient is taking diuretics, a low fractional excretion of urea may suggest volume depletion as the likely cause. Fractional excretion of any substance is simply calculated as the ratio of the clearance of the analyte in question to the clearance of creatinine. However, a low fractional excretion of urea or sodium may have causes other than volume depletion. For example, because of the heterogeneous nature of nephronal injury, contrast-induced injury, sepsis, or burns often result in a low fractional excretion of sodium despite intrinsic renal failure.

Intrinsic renal injury can be detected by examining the urine sediment. The classic manifestation of acute tubular necrosis (ATN) is the presence of dirty-brown granular casts. However, in severe AKI, there may be a large amount of amorphous granular material without cast formation (see Figs. 24.3 and 24.5). This occurs because severe AKI may result in failure to produce the Tamm-Horsfall protein that is now called uromodulin, leading to no formation of casts. In the absence of dirty-brown granular casts, a diagnosis of acute tubular injury can still be made based on the presence of dysmorphic epithelial cells in the urine. These epithelial cells, under hypoxic conditions, transform from the round, fried-egg appearance of the tubular cell to angular cells taking the shape of triangles or teardrops (see Fig. 24.3). A normal sediment, on the other hand, suggests minimal or no kidney injury.

The individual elements that can be seen in the urine and may be of diagnostic importance are as follows: dysmorphic RBCs, sterile pyuria manifested by white blood cells (WBCs) in the urine without bacteria, urinary tract infection characterized by both WBCs and bacteria in the urine, dysmorphic tubular cells suggesting ATN, intact renal tubular cells suggesting recovery from AKI, bubble cells, glitter cells, and oval fat bodies (see Figs. 24.2 and 24.3).

Budding yeast in a patient with diabetes may suggest the need to remove a long-standing indwelling catheter. Uric acid crystals in large amount suggest tumor lysis syndrome, calcium oxalate crystals may suggest ethylene glycol poisoning, and magnesium ammonium phosphate (triple phosphate) crystals may suggest infection with urease-positive organisms (see Fig. 24.4).

Casts can occur in various forms, such as RBC, WBC, epithelial cell, granular, hyaline, and dirty-brown granular casts. They can also occur in various shapes, such as broad and narrow casts. Examples of these are demonstrated in Fig. 24.5.

Severity of Injury

The severity of injury needs to be assessed, as well as its relationship to the preexisting state of kidney health. Severe injury is required for AKI to be manifested when the kidney is otherwise healthy. Little damage is needed to produce a severe injury if CKD preexists. More important, however, is the response to injury. It remains unclear why certain individuals have low GFR and others with the same extent of injury do not. This likely reflects the protective nature of responses that can result in poor or better GFR.

Presence of Distant Organ Effects on Consequences

End-organ manifestations of AKI include pulmonary edema or acute respiratory distress syndrome, uremic encephalopathy as alteration of mental status or asterixis, and uremic pericarditis or pleuritis manifested as pericardial or pleural friction rub. Although pulmonary edema is still a common manifestation of uremia, uremic serositis and encephalopathy are now rare.

For a deeper discussion on this topic, see Chapter 106, "Approach ❖ to the Patient with Renal Disease," in *Goldman-Cecil Medicine*, 26th Edition.

SUGGESTED READINGS

Agarwal R, Delanaye P: Glomerular filtration rate: when to measure and in which patients?, Nephrol Dial Transplant. https://doi.org/10.1093/ndt/gfy363.

Earley A, Miskulin D, Lamb EJ: et al: Estimating equations for glomerular filtration rate in the era of creatinine standardization: a systemic review, Ann Intern Med 156:785–795, 2012.

Gansevoort RT, Matsushita K, van der Velde M, et al: Lower estimated GFR and higher albuminuria are associated with adverse kidney outcomes: a collaborative meta-analysis of general and high-risk population cohorts, Kidney Int 80:93–104, 2011.

Maroni BJ, Steinman TI, Mitch WE: A method for estimating nitrogen intake of patients with chronic renal failure, Kidney Int 27:58–65, 1985.

Perazella M, Coca S, Kanbay M, et al.: Diagnostic value of urine microscopy for differential diagnosis of acute kidney injury in hospitalized patients, Clin J Am Soc Nephrol 3:1615–1619, 2008.

Perrone RD, Madias NE, Levey AS: Serum creatinine as an index of renal function: new insights into old concepts, Clin Chem 38:1933–1953, 1992.

Pickering TG, Miller NH, Ogedegbe G, et al.: Call to action on use and reimbursement for home blood pressure monitoring: a joint scientific statement from the American Heart Association, American Society Of Hypertension, and Preventive Cardiovascular Nurses Association, Hypertension 52:10–29, 2008.

Pickering TG, Shimbo D, Haas D: Ambulatory blood-pressure monitoring, N Engl J Med 354:2368–2374, 2006.

25

Fluid and Electrolyte Disorders

Biff F. Palmer

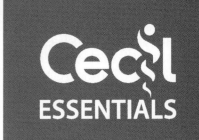

NORMAL VOLUME HOMEOSTASIS

In the average adult, the total body water is equal to 50% to 60% of body weight: 60% for men and 50% for women because of extra body fat, which is water free. Thus, in an average 70-kg male, total body water is 42 kg or 42 L, while in an average 70-kg female, total body water is 35 kg or L. Of the total body water, approximately two thirds is located intracellularly while one third is located extracellularly. Of the extracellular fluid (ECF) volume, only one fourth is located within the intravascular space. In a 70-kg man with a total body water of 42 L, 28 of these liters will be located intracellularly, while only 14 L are located in the ECF, and only 3.5 L are located in the extracellular intravascular compartment.

ECF volume is determined by the balance between sodium intake and excretion. Under normal circumstances, wide variations in salt intake lead to parallel changes in renal salt excretion, such that ECF volume and total body salt is maintained within narrow limits. This relative constancy of ECF volume is achieved by a series of afferent sensing systems, central integrative pathways, and both renal and extrarenal effector mechanisms acting in concert to modulate sodium excretion by the kidney (Table 25.1).

The concentration of sodium chloride (NaCl) in the plasma is regulated by renal water handling. The maintenance of plasma tonicity is achieved by sensing and effector mechanisms that differ from those that regulate volume. However, the systems that regulate volume and plasma tonicity do work in concert. For example, if the baroreceptors of the body detect that ECF volume is low, the kidney will respond by retaining NaCl. This will transiently lead to an increase in the tonicity of the ECF that will stimulate arginine vasopressin (AVP) release, causing renal water retention and expansion of the ECF volume.

Osmolality and Tonicity

Osmolality is defined as the number of particles per kilogram of solution. Plasma osmolality can be directly measured in an osmometer or can be calculated using the following equation:

$$\text{Calculated osmolality} = (Na^+ \times 2) + \text{glucose}/18 + \text{BUN}/2.8$$

where Na^+ is the sodium ion concentration and BUN is the blood urea nitrogen level.

The osmolar gap is the difference between the measured and calculated osmolality and is normally less than 10 mOsm/L. A higher value indicates the accumulation of an unmeasured substance such as ethanol, methanol, ethylene glycol, and acetone.

It is important to distinguish osmolality from tonicity. Whereas *osmolality* refers to all particles, *tonicity* describes whether the particles are effective or ineffective osmoles. Effective osmoles such as Na^+, glucose, or mannitol cannot penetrate cell membranes and thus can lead to changes in cell volume. Ineffective osmoles such as urea and alcohols are ineffective osmoles because they pass freely into and out of cells and are unable to effect changes in cell volume. As an example, chronic kidney disease patients with BUN levels greater than 100 mg/dL have no cellular shifts of fluid due to the urea. The plasma osmolality is high, but plasma tonicity is normal.

HYPONATREMIA

Hyponatremia is one of the most common electrolyte abnormalities encountered in clinical practice. Increasing age, medications, various disease states, and administration of hypotonic fluids are among the known risk factors for the disorder. Although hyponatremia is most commonly a marker of hypo-osmolality, there are three general causes of hyponatremia not associated with a hypo-osmolar state (Fig. 25.1). The first of these is pseudohyponatremia. This condition occurs in the setting of hyperglobulinemia or hypertriglyceridemia in which plasma water relative to plasma solids is decreased in blood leading to less Na^+ in a given volume of blood.

The second cause involves true hyponatremia but with elevations in the concentration of an effective osmole. Clinical examples include hyperglycemia as seen in uncontrolled diabetes or rarely hypertonic infusion of mannitol used in the treatment of cerebral edema. Increased plasma glucose concentration raises serum osmolality, which pulls water out of cells and dilutes the serum Na^+. For every 100-mg/dL rise in glucose or mannitol the serum Na^+ will quickly fall by 1.6 mEq/L. The increased tonicity will also stimulate thirst and AVP secretion, both of which contribute to further water retention. As the plasma osmolality returns towards normal, the decline in serum Na^+ will be 2.8 mEq/L for every 100-mg/dL rise in glucose. The net result is a normal plasma osmolality but a low serum Na^+.

The third cause of hyponatremia in the absence of a hypo-osmolar state is the addition of an isosmotic (or near isosmotic) non-Na^+ containing fluid to the extracellular space. This situation typically occurs during a transurethral resection of the prostate or during laparoscopic surgery when large amounts of a non-conducting flushing solution containing glycine or sorbitol are reabsorbed systemically.

The presence of hypotonic hyponatremia implies that water intake exceeds the ability of the kidney to excrete water. Because the normal kidney can excrete 20 to 30 L of water per day, the presence of hyponatremia with normal renal water excretion implies the patient is drinking at least those volumes of water. This condition is referred to as *primary polydipsia*. Urine osmolality will be less than 100 mOsm/L in this setting. Hyponatremia in association with a maximally dilute urine can also result from more moderate fluid intake combined with extremely limited solute intake, a condition often referred to as "beer potomania" syndrome.

TABLE 25.1 Sensors and Effectors That Determine Osmoregulation and Volume Regulation

Factor	Osmoregulation	Volume Regulation
What is sensed	Plasma osmolality	Effective arterial volume (EAV)
Sensors	Hypothalamic osmore-ceptors	Low and high pressure baroreceptors
Effectors	Arginine vasopressin (AVP), Thirst	Aldosterone, Angiotensin II, Sympathetic nerves
What is effected	Urine osmolality, Thirst	Urine Na$^+$ excretion

In the absence of primary polydipsia, hypotonic hyponatremia results when water intake exceeds the renal capacity for water excretion due to an inappropriately concentrated urine (some value >100 mOsm/L). The effective arterial blood volume (EAV) must be defined in this setting. Decreased EAV causes baroreceptor stimulation of AVP secretion and leads to decreased distal delivery of filtrate to the tip of the loop of Henle, accounting for the inability to maximally dilute the urine. If EAV is low, ECF volume can be low in the volume-depleted patient (hypovolemic hyponatremia) or can be high in the edematous patient (hypervolemic hyponatremia). A normal EAV points to euvolemic causes of hyponatremia (isovolemic hyponatremia).

Approximately two thirds of diagnosed hyponatremia cases are acquired in the hospital, where the common practices of monitoring daily fluid intake, patient weight, and Na$^+$ levels normally allow prompt diagnosis. Administration of hypotonic fluids in the postoperative period is a risk factor for acute iatrogenic hyponatremia, particularly because AVP levels remain increased several days after surgical procedures. Iatrogenic cases can be prevented by close monitoring of electrolytes and urine output and by fluid restriction and avoidance of solutions with low-Na$^+$ content; this approach applies particularly to elderly patients.

In neurosurgical patients, the syndrome of inappropriate antidiuretic hormone secretion (SIADH) and cerebral salt wasting (CSW) are two potential causes of hyponatremia. Distinguishing between these two disorders can be challenging because there is considerable overlap in the clinical presentation. The primary distinction lies in the assessment of the EAV. SIADH is a volume-expanded state due to AVP-mediated renal water retention. CSW is characterized by a contracted EAV resulting from renal salt wasting. Making an accurate diagnosis is important because the therapy of each condition is quite divergent. Vigorous salt replacement is indicated in patients with CSW, and fluid restriction is the treatment of choice in patients with SIADH.

Common causes of hyponatremia outside the hospital setting include overhydration, diarrhea, vomiting, CNS infection, extreme exercise, liver failure, renal failure, congestive heart failure, drugs, SIADH, and combinations of these and other factors. Thiazide diuretics are the most common cause of drug-induced hyponatremia. Hyponatremia typically develops in the first 2 weeks of drug initiation and is most likely to occur in elderly women and during the summer months because of the increased ingestion of hypotonic fluids when it is hot. Concomitant use of nonsteroidal anti-inflammatory drugs (NSAIDs) and selective serotonin reuptake inhibitors (SSRIs) can further increase the risk of thiazide-induced hyponatremia.

Treatment of Hyponatremia

Symptoms of hyponatremia include nausea and malaise, which can be followed by headache, lethargy, muscle cramps, disorientation, restlessness, and obtundation. When treating a patient with hyponatremia,

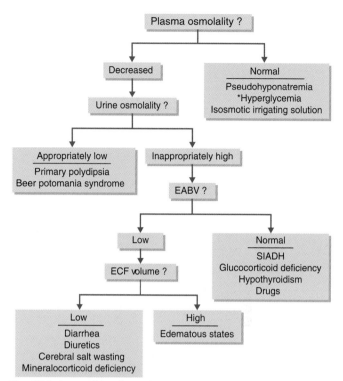

Fig. 25.1 Approach to the patient with hyponatremia. Assessment of effective arterial blood volume (EAV) is key to understanding the mechanism of renal NaCl retention and whether it is primary or in response to a low EAV. By definition, EAV is the arterial volume sensed by the kidney. Thus, if the kidney is working normally and it is retaining NaCl, EAV must be low, and if a normally functioning kidney is excreting large amounts of NaCl, the EAV is large. The physical examination is the most reliable way to assess EAV. The presence or absence of edema and orthostatic changes in blood pressure and pulse are particularly useful findings indicative of EAV. Laboratory tests are also useful in the assessment of EAV. Collection of a spot urinary sample for Na$^+$, Cl$^-$, and creatinine allows calculation of the fractional excretion of Na$^+$ or fractional excretion of Cl$^-$ using the following equations: FE$_{Na}$ (%) = [(urine Na$^+$ × plasma creatinine)/(plasma Na$^+$ × urine creatinine)] × 100 FE$_{Cl}$ (%) = [(urine Cl$^-$ × plasma creatinine)/(Plasma Cl$^-$ × urine creatinine)] × 100. If these parameters are low (<0.5 to 1%), a low EAV is indicated. Other findings suggestive of a low EAV include an increase in the blood urea nitrogen (BUN)/creatinine ratio (>20:1), increased serum uric acid concentration (due to increased proximal tubular reabsorption), and increased hematocrit and serum albumin concentration secondary to hemoconcentration. *Osmolality can be normal or increased with hyperglycemia.

the Na$^+$ concentration should be raised at the rate at which it fell. In patients with chronic hyponatremia (>48 hours duration), the serum Na$^+$ concentration has fallen slowly. Neurologic symptoms are generally minimal, brain size is normal, and the number of intracellular osmoles is decreased. Sudden return of ECF osmolality to normal values will lead to cell shrinkage and possibly precipitate osmotic demyelination. This complication can be avoided by limiting correction to less than 10 to 12 mEq/L in 24 hours and to less than 18 mEq/L in 48 hours. In a patient whose serum Na$^+$ concentration has decreased rapidly (<48 hours), neurologic symptoms are frequently present, and there is cerebral edema. In this setting, there has not been enough time to remove osmoles from the brain, and rapid return to normal ECF osmolality merely returns brain size to normal.

In general, the development of hyponatremia in the outpatient setting is more commonly chronic in duration and should be corrected slowly. By contrast, hyponatremia of short duration is more likely to be

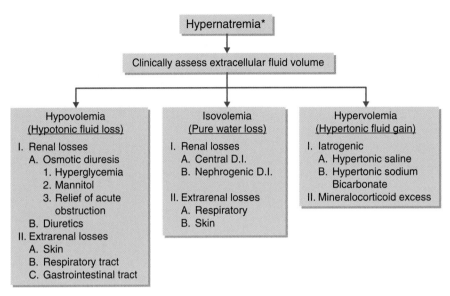

*All are associated with impairment of thirst or access to water

Fig. 25.2 Approach to the patient with hypernatremia.

encountered in hospitalized patients receiving intravenous free water. Use of "ecstasy," exercise-induced hyponatremia, or patients with primary polydipsia can also lead to acute hyponatremia and if symptomatic may similarly require rapid correction.

HYPERNATREMIA

Hypernatremia is a relatively common problem, particularly among the elderly and critically ill. Hypernatremia always indicates hypertonicity and shrinkage of cells. It is an independent risk factor for mortality in the ICU setting.

The initial approach to any patient with hypernatremia is to determine why there has been inadequate intake of water (Fig. 25.2). Hypernatremia is rare in conscious patients who have free access to water because of the extreme sensitivity of the thirst mechanism. Usually there is inadequate water intake due to an alteration in the level of consciousness so that patients become unaware of thirst or cannot adequately communicate the need for water or there is restricted access to water. Only rarely is there a specific lesion of the thirst center. A reduced sensation of thirst occurs in otherwise normal individuals as a feature of increasing age.

The next step is to search for the presence of accelerated water loss or increased Na+ gain, both of which will increase the likelihood of a patient developing hypernatremia. This can be accomplished by clinical assessment of EAV. Hypovolemic hypernatremia results from fluid losses in which the Na+ concentration is less than the plasma concentration. Hypervolemic hypernatremia can be due to iatrogenic administration of hypertonic NaCl or hypertonic NaHCO₃ or from mineralocorticoid excess.

Pure water loss, whether from mucocutaneous routes or from the kidneys, causes isovolemic hypernatremia. Because two thirds of pure water loss is sustained from within cells, patients will not become clinically volume depleted unless the water deficit becomes substantial. Insensible losses from the respiratory tract or skin result in concentrated urine. Inappropriate water loss by the kidney, whether from central or nephrogenic diabetes insipidus, results in dilute urine. Although renal water loss can lead to hypernatremia in patients with impaired thirst or access to water, most patients with diabetes insipidus have neither of these defects and typically present with polyuria, polydipsia, and a normal serum sodium concentration.

Evaluation of Polyuria and Polydipsia

Polyuria can be the result of an osmotic diuresis or a water diuresis. In turn, a water diuresis may result from inappropriate water loss as in either central or nephrogenic diabetes insipidus or may represent appropriate water loss as in primary polydipsia. The clinical setting and urine osmolality help to differentiate between these processes (Fig. 25.3).

Osmotic diuresis causing polyuria is often evident from the clinical setting. Poorly controlled glucose levels in a patient with diabetes mellitus, administration of mannitol to a patient with increased intracranial pressure, and high-protein enteral feedings (urea diuresis) are all examples in which polyuria is the result of osmotic diuresis. Urine osmolality greater than 300 mOsm/L) in the polyuric patient is suggestive of solute or osmotic diuresis.

After excluding the presence of osmotic diuresis, one must then discriminate between the causes of water diuresis. In patients with central diabetes insipidus, the onset of symptoms is characteristically abrupt in nature, whereas patients with nephrogenic diabetes insipidus typically have a more gradual onset of symptoms. Patients with primary polydipsia are more vague in dating the onset of their symptoms. Both nephrogenic and central diabetes insipidus are characterized by severe and frequent nocturia, a feature that is typically absent in patients with primary polydipsia. Patients with central diabetes insipidus seem to have a predilection for ice water, which is not typically described in the other two conditions. A serum Na+ concentration less than 140 mEq/L is suggestive of primary polydipsia because these patients tend to be in mild positive water balance. By contrast, a value greater than 140 mEq/L is more suggestive of either central or nephrogenic diabetes insipidus because these patients tend to be in mild negative water balance. Finally, urine osmolality will increase in response to water deprivation in primary polydipsia but show no response in diabetes insipidus. Central and nephrogenic diabetes insipidus are distinguished by the change in urine osmolality following subcutaneous administration of AVP (increased in central with no change in nephrogenic).

Treatment of Hypernatremia

Signs and symptoms of hypernatremia include lethargy, weakness, fasciculations, seizures, and coma. Increased ECF osmolality initially causes cell shrinkage within the brain. In response, cells generate

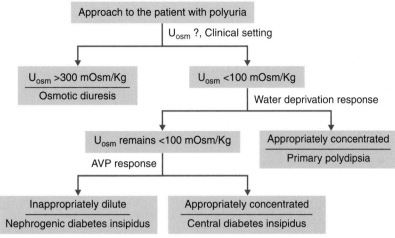

Fig. 25.3 Approach to the patient with polyuria. *AVP,* Arginine vasopressin; *U,* urine.

intracellular osmoles, which pull water back into the cells, returning brain size to normal. If extracellular osmolality is returned rapidly to normal, the extra intracellular osmoles will pull water into the brain cells, resulting in cerebral edema. Thus, in general, hypernatremia should be corrected slowly by water administration at a rate that leads to half correction in 24 hours. The water deficit can be estimated from the following formula:

$$\text{Water deficit} = \text{Current body water (0.6 in men and 0.5 in women} \times \text{body weight)} \times \left[\left([Na^+]_{plasma}/140\right) - 1\right]$$

Calculation of the amount of water to give must add insensible losses and any ongoing losses from the urinary and gastrointestinal tract. This formula also does not include the volume of isotonic saline required in those patients who may be concomitantly volume depleted. Careful monitoring of the serum Na^+ is required to ensure the rate of correction is appropriate.

HYPOKALEMIA

Hypokalemia is a common clinical disorder. Decreases in total body K^+ are usually due to gastrointestinal or renal losses whereas hypokalemia in the setting of normal total body K^+ is due to cell shift. In most cases, the cause can be determined by history, measurement of blood pressure, examination of acid-base balance, and measurement of urinary K^+ levels.

Cellular Shift With Normal Total Body Potassium

In the absence of physical and historical evidence of gastrointestinal or renal K^+ losses, either a redistribution of K^+ at the cellular level or laboratory error will account for a low serum K^+. Spurious causes of hypokalemia can be seen in leukemia patients with leukocyte counts of 100 to 250,000 $\times$ 10^9/L, in which still-viable leukocytes extract K^+ from the serum in the sample tube. Interestingly, some patients with acute myeloid leukemia develop kidney K^+ wasting due to increased urinary excretion of lysozyme. This protein increases the luminal electronegativity in the collecting duct, providing a greater driving force for K^+ secretion.

The regulation of K^+ distribution between the intracellular and extracellular space is referred to as internal K^+ balance. Although the kidney is ultimately responsible for maintenance of total body K^+, factors that modulate internal balance are important in the disposal of acute K^+ loads. A large potassium meal could potentially double

extracellular K^+ were it not for the rapid shift of the K^+ load into cells. The kidney cannot excrete K^+ rapidly enough in this setting to prevent life-threatening hyperkalemia. Thus, it is important that this excess K^+ be rapidly shifted and stored in cells until the kidney has successfully excreted the K^+ load. The major regulators of K^+ shift into cells are insulin and catecholamines.

Insulin excess, whether given exogenously in a patient with diabetes mellitus or endogenous secretion as seen in a normal person given a high glucose load, will lower the serum K^+. β-Adrenergic agonists used in the treatment of bronchospasm or in treating premature labor will cause similar K^+ shifts. In the setting of an acute myocardial infarction, hypokalemia may result as a sequela of high circulating epinephrine levels and might predispose to arrhythmias in this clinical setting. Other clinical disorders resulting in intracellular sequestration of K^+ are treatment of megaloblastic anemia with vitamin B_{12}, hypothermia, and barium poisoning. Hypokalemic periodic paralysis is inherited in an autosomal dominant pattern and is characterized by episodic hypokalemia resulting in muscle weakness. An acquired form of the disorder is seen in thyrotoxic patients, who are often of Japanese or Mexican descent.

Decreased Total Body Potassium

In the absence of cell shift, low serum K^+ can result from inadequate dietary intake, extrarenal losses through the gastrointestinal tract or skin, or renal losses. The urinary K^+ concentration serves as a useful guide in discerning between these possibilities. A urine K^+ concentration of less than 20 mEq/L is suggestive of extrarenal losses, whereas a urine concentration of greater than 40 mEq/L suggests renal K^+ losses. A limitation of a random value is the degree of urinary concentration. A urine K^+ concentration of 40 mEq/L may be an appropriate response in a hypokalemic patient with maximally concentrated urine due to decreased water intake. By the same token, a random urine value of less than 15 mEq/L may represent renal K^+ wasting if obtained in the setting of water diuresis.

The transtubular potassium gradient (TTKG) is a method designed to overcome the limitations of a random urine K^+ concentration in the evaluation of a dyskalemic patient:

$$TTKG = U_{potassium} \times Serum_{osmolality}/Serum_{potassium} \times U_{osmolality}$$

The formula estimates the ratio of K^+ in the lumen of the cortical collecting duct to that in the peritubular capillaries at a point where tubular fluid is isotonic relative to plasma. While still often used, the

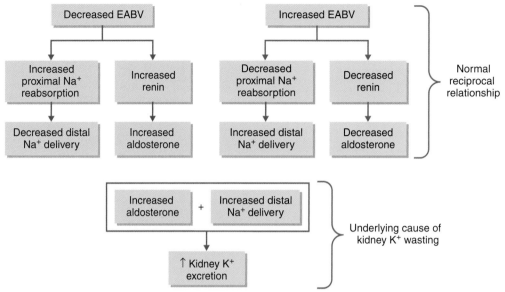

Fig. 25.4 The relationship between effective arterial volume and distal Na⁺ delivery in determining renal K⁺ excretion.

assumptions on which the formula is based have been called into question. For this reason, a urine K⁺ to creatinine ratio is now the preferred way to assess renal K⁺ handling. A ratio of less than 13 mEq K⁺/g creatinine or less than 2.5 mEq K⁺/mmol creatinine is considered an appropriate response to gastrointestinal potassium loss, remote use of diuretics, decreased dietary intake, and potassium shift into cells. Higher values suggest an inappropriate response of the kidney.

Inadequate dietary intake is an unusual cause of hypokalemia. Clinical situations associated with extreme K⁺-deficient diets include anorexia nervosa, crash diets, alcoholism, and intestinal malabsorption. Increased renal K⁺ excretion owing to magnesium deficiency (which is often present in these clinical situations) may contribute to the observed hypokalemia.

Extrarenal Potassium Losses

Sweat, with its low concentration of K⁺, is an unusual cause of K⁺ depletion. However, during physical training sweat losses can become substantial and K⁺ depletion may result. Gastrointestinal syndromes are the most common clinical disorders of extrarenal K⁺ losses. Diarrhea leads to fecal K⁺ wastage and is associated with a normal anion gap acidosis. Acidosis will result in K⁺ redistribution out of cells, leading to a degree of hypokalemia that is not as severe as the degree of total body K⁺ depletion.

Renal Potassium Losses

Increased distal delivery of Na⁺ and water and increased mineralocorticoid activity can each stimulate renal K⁺ secretion. Under normal physiologic conditions, these two determinants are inversely regulated by EAV (Fig. 25.4). Decreases in EAV are associated with increased aldosterone secretion but lower distal delivery of Na⁺ and water secondary to enhancement of reabsorption in the proximal nephron. It is for this reason that renal K⁺ excretion is relatively independent of volume status. It is only under pathophysiologic conditions that distal Na⁺ delivery and aldosterone become coupled. In this setting, renal K⁺ wasting will occur. This coupling can be due to a primary increase in mineralocorticoid activity or a primary increase in distal Na⁺ delivery. The term *primary* means that the changes are not secondary to changes in EAV. The causes of hypokalemia, grouped according to the physiologic determinants of renal K⁺ excretion, are given in Fig. 25.5.

Primary Increase in Mineralocorticoid Activity

Increases in mineralocorticoid activity can be due to primary increases in renin secretion, primary increases in aldosterone secretion, or increases in a non-aldosterone mineralocorticoid or increased mineralocorticoid-like effect. In all of these conditions, ECF volume is expanded and hypertension is typically present. The differential diagnosis for the patient with hypertension, hypokalemia, and metabolic alkalosis rests on the measurement of plasma renin activity and plasma aldosterone levels.

Primary Increase in Distal Sodium Delivery

Conditions that give rise to primary increases in distal Na⁺ delivery are characterized by normal or low ECF volume. Blood pressure is typically normal. Increases in distal Na⁺ delivery are most frequently due to diuretics that act proximal to the cortical collecting duct. Increased delivery can also be the result of non-reabsorbed anions such as bicarbonate as with active vomiting or a type II proximal renal tubular acidosis. Ketoanions (β-hydroxybutyrate and acetoacetate) and the Na⁺ salts of penicillins are other examples. The inability to reabsorb these anions in the proximal tubule results in increased delivery of Na⁺ to the distal nephron. Because these anions also escape reabsorption in the distal nephron, a more lumen-negative voltage develops and the driving force for K⁺ excretion into the tubular fluid is enhanced. Disorders of hypokalemia due to primary increases in distal Na⁺ delivery can best be categorized by the presence of metabolic acidosis or metabolic alkalosis.

Clinical Presentation

The most important clinical manifestations of hypokalemia occur in the neuromuscular system. Low serum K⁺ leads to cell hyperpolarization that impedes impulse conduction and muscle contraction. Typically, a flaccid paralysis develops in the hands and feet that moves proximally to eventually include the trunk and respiratory muscles. Death may occur from respiratory insufficiency. A myopathy may also occur that can evolve to rhabdomyolysis (muscle cell lysis) and acute kidney injury. Hypokalemia can also lead to smooth muscle dysfunction including paralytic ileus. Changes in electrocardiogram (ECG) include ST depression, T-wave flattening, and an increase in

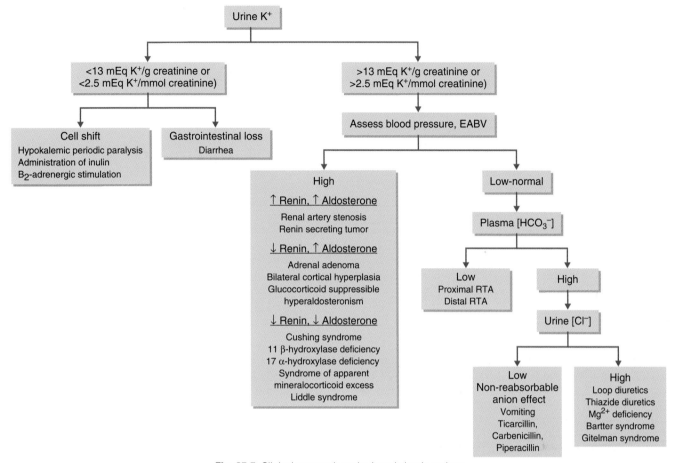

Fig. 25.5 Clinical approach to the hypokalemic patient.

the amplitude of the U wave. Patients treated with cardiac glycosides are at increased risk for premature ventricular contractions, and supraventricular and ventricular tachyarrhythmias, when hypokalemic.

Hypokalemia also causes a renal concentrating defect due both to a decrease in the medullary gradient and resistance of the cortical collecting tubule to AVP. This leads to polyuria and polydipsia. Prolonged hypokalemia can also lead to tubulointerstitial nephritis and renal failure (kaleopenic nephropathy). Because insulin release is regulated partially by serum K^+, hypokalemia can lead to glucose intolerance.

Treatment of Hypokalemia

The serum K^+ levels can at times be misleading as to the degree of deficit because a normal or even increased K^+ level can occur with significant total body K^+ depletion. In the absence of significant K^+ shifts, a decline in the serum K^+ from 4 to 3 mEq/L generally is associated with a deficit of 300 to 400 mEq intracellular K^+ per 70 kg body weight. A serum K^+ concentration of 2 mEq/L reflects a deficit of roughly 600 mEq. Despite these guidelines, the serum K^+ level should be monitored frequently during replacement therapy.

K^+ can be given orally or intravenously as the potassium chloride (KCl) salt. Potassium bicarbonate or citrate can be given if there is concomitant metabolic acidosis. The safest way to administer KCl is orally. KCl can be given in doses of 100 to 150 mEq/day. Liquid KCl is bitter tasting and, like the tablet, can be irritating to the gastric mucosa. The microencapsulated or wax-matrix forms of KCl are better tolerated.

Intravenous administration of K^+ may be necessary if the patient cannot take oral medications or if the K^+ deficit is large and is resulting in cardiac arrhythmias, respiratory paralysis, or rhabdomyolysis.

Intravenous KCl should be given at a maximum rate of 20 mEq/hour and maximum concentration of 40 mEq/L. Higher concentrations will result in phlebitis. Replacement of KCl in dextrose-containing solutions can lower the serum K^+ further secondary to insulin release. Thus, saline solutions are preferred. Depending on the specific cause, additional therapy of chronic hypokalemia involves the use of K^+-sparing diuretics such as amiloride, spironolactone or triamterene. These agents must be used cautiously in patients with renal insufficiency or in patients with other disorders that impair renal K^+ excretion.

HYPERKALEMIA

Like the hypokalemic disorders, a high serum K^+ can occur in the setting of normal or altered body stores of K^+. The body has a marked ability to protect against hyperkalemia. This includes regulatory mechanisms that will excrete excess K^+ quickly and mechanisms that will redistribute excess K^+ into cells until it is excreted. All causes of hyperkalemia therefore involve abnormalities in these mechanisms.

Pseudohyperkalemia is an in vitro phenomenon due to the mechanical release of K^+ from cells during the phlebotomy procedure, specimen processing, or in the setting of marked leukocytosis and thrombocytosis. (As noted above, with certain leukemias with high WBC counts, extraction of K^+ from the serum by cells in the sample tube can result in spurious hypokalemia.)

Excessive Dietary Intake

In the presence of normal renal and adrenal function, it is difficult to ingest enough K^+ in the diet to produce hyperkalemia. Rather, dietary intake of K^+ as a contributor to hyperkalemia is usually observed in the setting of impaired kidney function. Dietary sources particularly enriched with K^+ include melons, citrus juice, and commercial salt substitutes containing K^+.

Cellular Redistribution

Cellular redistribution is a more important cause of hyperkalemia than of hypokalemia. Tissue damage is probably the most important cause of hyperkalemia due to redistribution of K^+ out of cells. This can be due to rhabdomyolysis, trauma, burns, massive intravascular coagulation, and tumor lysis (either spontaneous or following treatment). The effect of metabolic acidosis to cause K^+ exit from cells is dependent upon the type of acid present. Mineral acidosis (NH_4Cl or HCl) by virtue of the relative impermeability of the chloride anion results in the greatest efflux of K^+ from cells. By contrast, organic acidosis (lactic or β-hydroxybutyric) results in no significant efflux of K^+. Increased osmolality as in uncontrolled diabetes causes K^+ to move out of cells. In fact, it is the hypertonic state as well as insulin deficiency that accounts for hyperkalemia often seen in patients with diabetic ketoacidosis who are total body K^+ depleted. β-Adrenergic blocking agents can interfere with the disposal of acute K^+ loads. Other drugs that can result in hyperkalemia include the depolarizing muscle relaxant succinylcholine and severe digitalis poisoning.

Decreased Renal Excretion of Potassium

Decreased renal excretion of K^+ can occur because of one or more of three abnormalities: a primary decrease in distal delivery of salt and water, abnormal cortical collecting duct function, and a primary decrease in mineralocorticoid levels.

Primary Decrease in Distal Delivery (Acute and Chronic Kidney Disease)

Acute decreases in glomerular filtration rate (GFR), as occur in acute kidney injury, lead to marked decreases in distal delivery of salt and water that may secondarily decrease distal K^+ secretion. When acute kidney injury is oliguric, distal delivery of NaCl and volume are low and hyperkalemia is a frequent problem. When kidney injury is nonoliguric, however, distal delivery is usually sufficient and hyperkalemia is unusual. Decreased distal Na^+ delivery is a risk factor for hyperkalemia in patients with decompensated congestive heart failure. In chronic kidney disease patients, hyperkalemia is unusual until the GFR falls to less than 10-20 mL/min. The occurrence of hyperkalemia with a GFR of greater than 10 mL/min should raise the question of decreased aldosterone levels or a specific lesion of the cortical collecting duct.

Primary Decrease in Mineralocorticoid Activity

Decreased mineralocorticoid activity can result from disturbances that originate at any point along the renin-angiotensin-aldosterone system. Such disturbances can be the result of a disease state or be due to effects of various drugs. Hyperkalemia most commonly develops when one or more of these drugs are administered in a setting where the renin-angiotensin-aldosterone system is already impaired. One common example is the use of angiotensin-converting enzyme inhibitors (ACEI) or angiotensin-receptor blockers (ARB) in patients with diabetes mellitus with hyporeninemic hypoaldosteronism.

Distal Tubular Defects

Certain interstitial renal diseases can affect the distal nephron specifically and lead to hyperkalemia in the presence of only mild decreases in GFR and normal aldosterone levels. Amiloride and triamterene inhibit Na^+ transport, which makes the luminal potential more positive and secondarily inhibits K^+ secretion. A similar effect occurs with

trimethoprim and accounts for the development of hyperkalemia following the administration of the antibiotic trimethoprim-sulfamethoxazole. Spironolactone and eplerenone compete with aldosterone and thus block the mineralocorticoid effect.

Clinical Presentation

Hyperkalemia leads to depolarization of the resting membrane because the potential across cell membranes is in part determined by the ratio of intracellular to extracellular K^+. The heart is particularly sensitive to this depolarizing effect. The progressive changes of hyperkalemia on the electrocardiogram are peaking of T waves, widening of the PR and QRS interval, development of a sine wave pattern, and eventually ventricular fibrillation and asystole. In general, ECG changes appear at a serum K^+ of 6 mEq/L with acute onset of hyperkalemia, whereas the ECG may remain normal up to a concentration of 8 to 9 mEq/L with chronic hyperkalemia. Hyperkalemia can also cause neuromuscular manifestations such as ascending paralysis and eventual flaccid quadriplegia. Hyperkalemia also decreases ammonia availability to act as a buffer for distal H^+ secretion. This effect impairs bicarbonate regeneration, leading to the development of a normal anion gap metabolic acidosis.

Treatment of Acute Hyperkalemia

The immediate treatment of life-threatening hyperkalemia is the administration of calcium, usually in the form of calcium gluconate or calcium chloride. ECG changes such as increasing PR interval or a widening QRS complex warrant treatment with calcium. Glucose and insulin therapy will shift K^+ into cells. Acute administration of glucose without insulin can potentially worsen hyperkalemia in patients with diabetes mellitus by raising extracellular osmolality and causing K^+ to shift into the extracellular space. $NaHCO_3$ administration through expansion of the ECF space results in dilution of the serum K^+. Additionally, K^+ is shifted into cells whenever concomitant metabolic acidosis is corrected. Inhalation of β_2-agonists such as albuterol or parenteral use of salbutamol can cause significant K^+ shifts into cells.

The effects of calcium, bicarbonate, glucose and insulin, and β_2-agonist therapy will provide immediate relief of acute toxicity but will not decrease total body K^+. Measures to reduce total body K^+ include the administration of K^+ binding drugs and dialysis.

Treatment of Chronic Hyperkalemia

After review of the patient's medication profile, drugs that can impair renal K^+ excretion should be discontinued if possible. Nonsteroidal anti-inflammatory drugs, either prescribed or those over-the-counter, are common offenders in this regard. Patients should be placed on a low K^+ diet with specific counseling against the use of K^+-containing salt substitutes. Diuretics are particularly effective in minimizing hyperkalemia. In patients with an eGFR less than 30 mL/min, thiazide diuretics can be used, but loop diuretics are required with more severe renal insufficiency. In chronic kidney disease patients with metabolic acidosis (bicarbonate concentration < 22 mEq/L), $NaHCO_3$ should be given. K^+-binding drugs can be utilized when hyperkalemia is refractory to the approaches outlined above. Sodium polystyrene sulfonate (Kayexalate) has been available for over 50 years but is poorly tolerated and has been linked to gastrointestinal toxicity. Patiromer and sodium zirconium cyclosilicate (ZS-9) are new K^+-binding drugs that are well tolerated when used chronically and can maintain normokalemia in the setting of renin-angiotensin-aldosterone system inhibitors.

METABOLIC ACIDOSIS

Metabolic acidosis is diagnosed by a low pH, a reduced HCO_3^- concentration, and respiratory compensation resulting in a decrease in the

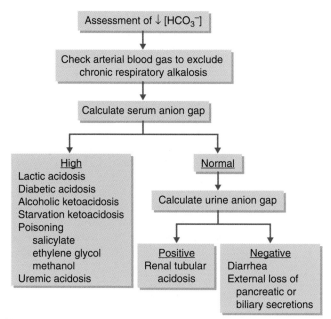

Fig. 25.6 Approach to the patient with a reduced serum HCO_3^- concentration.

partial pressure of carbon dioxide (Pco_2). A low HCO_3^- concentration alone is not diagnostic of metabolic acidosis because it also results from the renal compensation to chronic respiratory alkalosis. Measurement of the arterial pH differentiates between these two possibilities. The pH is low in hyperchloremic metabolic acidosis and high in chronic respiratory alkalosis. The clinical approach to a patient with a low serum HCO_3^- concentration is given in Fig. 25.6.

After confirming the presence of metabolic acidosis, calculation of the serum anion gap is a useful step in determining the differential diagnosis of the disorder. The anion gap is equal to the difference between the plasma concentrations of the major cation (Na^+) and the major measured anions ($Cl^- + HCO_3^-$).

$$Anion\ gap = (Na^+) - (Cl^-) - (HCO_3^-)$$

The normal value of the anion gap is approximately 12 ± 2 mEq/L. Most of the unmeasured anions consist of albumin; therefore, the normal anion gap changes in the setting of hypoalbuminemia (normal anion gap is approximately three times the serum albumin in g/dL). Because the total number of cations must equal the total number of anions, a fall in the serum HCO_3^- concentration must be offset by a rise in the concentration of other anions. If the anion accompanying excess H^+ is Cl^-, the fall in the serum HCO_3^- concentration is matched by an equal rise in the serum Cl^- concentration. The acidosis is classified as a normal gap or hyperchloremic metabolic acidosis. By contrast, if excess H^+ is accompanied by an anion other than Cl^-, the fall in HCO_3^- is balanced by a rise in the concentration of the unmeasured anion. The Cl^- concentration remains the same. In this setting, the acidosis is said to be a high anion gap metabolic acidosis.

A useful method for differentiating extrarenal from renal causes of metabolic acidosis is to measure urinary NH_4^+ excretion. Extrarenal causes of metabolic acidosis are associated with an appropriate increase in net acid excretion, primarily reflected by high levels of urinary NH_4^+ excretion. By contrast, net acid excretion and urinary NH_4^+ levels are low in metabolic acidosis of renal origin. Unfortunately, measurement of urinary NH_4^+ is not a test that is commonly available in clinical medicine. However, the amount of urinary NH_4^+ can be indirectly assessed by calculating the urinary anion gap (UAG).

$$UAG = (UNa^+ + UK^+) - UCl^-$$

Under normal circumstances, the UAG is positive, with values ranging from 30 to 50. Metabolic acidosis of extrarenal origin is associated with a marked increase in urinary NH_4^+ excretion and, therefore, a large negative value will be obtained for the UAG. If the acidosis is of renal origin, urinary NH_4^+ excretion will be minimal and the UAG will usually be positive.

The UAG can be misleading when other unmeasured ions are excreted. For example, increased urinary excretion of sodium keto acid salts in diabetic and alcoholic ketoacidosis and urinary excretion of sodium hippurate and sodium benzoate in toluene exposure can keep the UAG positive despite an appropriate increase in urinary ammonium excretion. Increased urinary excretion will also be missed when NH_4^+ is excreted with an anion other than Cl^- such as β-hydroxybutyrate or hippurate. In these settings, calculation of the urine osmolal gap is used as an indirect measure of ammonium excretion. The urine osmolal gap is the difference between the measured and the calculated urine osmolality:

$$Urine\ osmolal\ gap = calculated\ urine\ osmolality\ (mOsmol/kg)$$
$$= (2 \times [Na^+ + K^+]) + [urea\ nitrogen\ in$$
$$mg/dL]/2.8 + [glucose\ in\ mg/dL]/18$$

The urine osmolal gap normally ranges from approximately 10 to 100 mOsmol/kg. Because NH_4^+ salts are generally the only other major urinary solute that contribute significantly to the urine osmolality, values appreciably greater than 100 mOsmol/kg reflect increased excretion of NH_4^+ salts.

Urine pH cannot reliably differentiate acidosis of renal origin from that of extrarenal origin. For example, an acid urine pH does not necessarily indicate an appropriate increase in net acid excretion. With a significant reduction in the availability of NH_4^+ to serve as a buffer, only a small amount of distal H^+ secretion will lead to a maximal reduction in urine pH. In this setting, the pH of the urine is acid but the quantity of H^+ secretion is insufficient to meet daily acid production. By contrast, alkaline urine does not necessarily imply a renal acidification defect. In conditions where availability of NH_4^+ is not limiting, distal H^+ secretion can be massive and yet the urine remains relatively alkaline because of the buffering effects of NH_4^+.

Hyperchloremic or Normal Anion Gap Metabolic Acidosis

Hyperchloremic (normal anion gap metabolic) acidosis can be of renal or extrarenal origin. Metabolic acidosis of renal origin is the result of abnormalities in tubular H^+ transport. Metabolic acidosis of extrarenal origin is most commonly caused by gastrointestinal losses of HCO_3^-. Other causes include the external loss of biliary and pancreatic secretions and ureteral diversion procedures. Fig. 25.7 provides a clinical approach to metabolic acidosis of renal origin.

Renal Origin

Proximal renal tubular acidosis (type II). The diagnosis of proximal RTA is suspected in a patient with a normal anion gap acidosis, hypokalemia, and an intact ability to acidify the urine to a pH of less than 5.5 while in a steady state. In the steady state, the serum HCO_3^- concentration is usually in the range of 16 to 18 mmol/L. Proximal RTA can be an isolated finding but most commonly is accompanied by generalized dysfunction of the proximal tubule (Fanconi syndrome). The urine anion gap is positive because proximal tubular dysfunction also impairs ammoniagenesis.

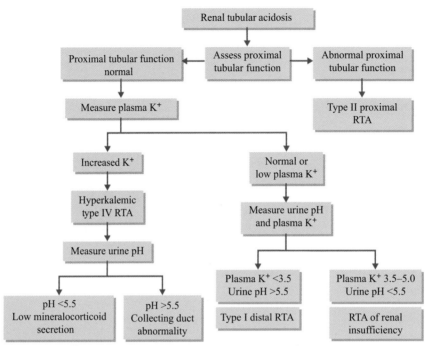

Fig. 25.7 Approach to the patient with acidosis of renal origin.

Proximal RTA is not associated with nephrolithiasis or nephrocalcinosis. However, osteomalacia can develop because of chronic hypophosphatemia and/or deficiency in the active form of vitamin D. Osteopenia may also be present because of acidosis-induced demineralization of bone. The treatment of patients with proximal RTA is difficult. Correction of the acidosis is often not possible even with large amounts of HCO_3^- (3 to 5 mmol/kg daily) because exogenous alkali is rapidly excreted in the urine. In addition, such therapy leads to accelerated renal K^+ losses. Use of a thiazide diuretic to induce enough volume depletion to lower the GFR and thus decrease the filtered load of HCO_3^- may increase the effectiveness of alkali therapy. Potassium-sparing diuretics may limit the degree of renal K^+ wasting. Once therapy is initiated, close monitoring is required to guard against severe electrolyte derangements. Acetazolamide and topiramate can cause metabolic acidosis due to inhibitory effects on carbonic anhydrase.

Hypokalemic distal renal tubular acidosis (type I). The diagnosis of distal RTA should be considered in a patient with hyperchloremic normal gap acidosis, hypokalemia, and an inability to lower the urine pH maximally. A urine pH greater than 5.5 in the setting of systemic acidosis is consistent with distal RTA. The urinary anion gap is positive. The systemic acidosis tends to be more severe than in patients with a proximal RTA with serum HCO_3^- concentrations as low as 10 mmol/L. Hypokalemia can also be severe and cause musculoskeletal weakness and symptoms of nephrogenic diabetes insipidus. Patients frequently manifest nephrolithiasis and nephrocalcinosis. This predisposition to renal calcification results from the combined effects of increased urinary Ca^{2+} excretion due to acidosis-induced bone mineral dissolution, a persistently alkaline urine pH, and low urinary citrate excretion.

Correction of the metabolic acidosis in distal RTA can be achieved by administration of alkali in an amount equal to daily acid production (usually 1 to 2 mmol/kg per day). In patients with severe K^+ deficits, correction of the acidosis with HCO_3^- can transiently cause further lowering of the extracellular K^+ concentration and result in symptomatic hypokalemia. In this setting, the K^+ deficit should be corrected prior to correcting the acidosis. Potassium citrate is the preferred form of alkali for those patients with persistent hypokalemia or with calcium stone disease.

Hyperkalemic distal renal tubular acidosis (type IV). A type IV RTA should be suspected in a patient with a hyperchloremic normal gap metabolic acidosis associated with hyperkalemia. The urinary anion gap is slightly positive, indicating little to no NH_4^+ excretion in the urine. Patients in which the disorder is caused by a defect in mineralocorticoid activity typically have a urine pH of less than 5.5, reflecting a more severe defect in NH_3 availability than in H^+ secretion. In patients with structural damage to the collecting duct, the urine pH may be alkaline, reflecting both impaired H^+ secretion and decreased urinary NH_4^+ excretion. The syndrome occurs most often in association with mild-to-moderate renal insufficiency; however, the magnitude of hyperkalemia and acidosis are disproportionately severe for the observed degree of renal insufficiency (Table 25.2). The primary goal of therapy is to correct the hyperkalemia. In many instances, lowering the serum K^+ will simultaneously correct the acidosis by restoring renal NH_4^+ production, thereby increasing the buffer supply for distal acidification.

Renal tubular acidosis of renal insufficiency. Patients with chronic kidney disease initially develop a hyperchloremic normal gap metabolic acidosis associated with normokalemia as the GFR falls below 30 mL/min. With more advanced chronic kidney disease (GFR < 15 mL/min), the acidosis changes to predominately an anion gap metabolic acidosis reflecting a progressive inability to excrete phosphate, sulfate, and the Na^+ salts of various organic acids. At this stage, the acidosis is commonly referred to as *uremic acidosis*.

Correction of the metabolic acidosis in patients with chronic kidney disease is achieved by treatment with $NaHCO_3$ 0.5 to 1.5 mmol/kg/day beginning when the HCO_3^- level is less than 22 mmol/L. Metabolic acidosis needs to be aggressively treated because it can contribute to metabolic bone disease, increase catabolism, and contribute to the progressive loss of kidney function.

Extrarenal Origin of Metabolic Acidosis

Diarrhea. Loss of HCO_3^- in intestinal secretions beyond the stomach leads to the development of metabolic acidosis. Volume loss signals the kidney to increase the reabsorption of salt. Renal retention of NaCl

TABLE 25.2 Causes of Hyperkalemic Distal (Type IV) Renal Tubular Acidosis

I. Mineralocorticoid deficiency
  A. Low renin, low aldosterone
    1. Diabetes mellitus
    2. Drugs
      a. Nonsteroidal antiinflammatory agents
      b. Cyclosporin, tacrolimus
      c. β-blockers
  B. High renin, low aldosterone
    1. Adrenal destruction
    2. Congenital enzyme defects
    3. Drugs
      a. Angiotensin-converting enzyme inhibitors
      b. Angiotensin II receptor blockers
      c. Heparin
      d. Ketoconazole
II. Abnormal cortical collecting duct
  A. Absence or defective mineralocorticoid receptor
  B. Drugs
    1. Spironolactone, eplerenone
    2. Triamterene
    3. Amiloride
    4. Trimethoprim
    5. Pentamidine
  C. Chronic tubulointerstitial disease

TABLE 25.3 Causes of Lactic Acidosis

I. Type A (tissue underperfusion and or hypoxia)
  A. Cardiogenic shock
  B. Septic shock
  C. Hemorrhagic shock
  D. Acute hypoxia
  E. Carbon monoxide poisoning
  F. Anemia
II. Type B (absence of hypotension and hypoxia)
  A. Hereditary enzyme deficiency (glucose 6-phosphatase)
  B. Drugs or toxins
    1. Phenformin, metformin
    2. Cyanide
    3. Salicylate, ethylene glycol, methanol
    4. Propylene glycol
    5. Linezolid
    6. Propofol
    7. Nucleoside reverse transcriptase inhibitors: stavudine, didanosine
  C. Systemic disease
    1. Liver failure
    2. Malignancy

combined with the intestinal loss of $NaHCO_3$ generates a hyperchloremic normal gap metabolic acidosis. Net acid excretion markedly increases due to increases in urinary excretion of NH_4^+. Hypokalemia due to gastrointestinal losses and the low serum pH both stimulate the synthesis of NH_3 in the proximal tubule. The increase in availability of NH_3 to act as a urinary buffer allows for a maximal increase in H^+ secretion by the distal nephron. Urine pH during chronic diarrheal states may be persistently greater than 6.0 due to the large increase in buffer capacity.

A patient who presents with hypokalemic hyperchloremic metabolic acidosis with a urine pH greater than 5.5 could have either a diarrheal state or a hypokalemic (type I) distal RTA. Although the clinical history would be the easiest way to distinguish between these two possibilities, in a patient with surreptitious laxative abuse this may not be helpful. Determination of the urinary anion gap is the best way to distinguish between them. In diarrhea, urine pH is high because of the large amount of NH_4^+ in the urine. This would be reflected by a negative urinary anion gap because most of the NH_4^+ is excreted in the urine as NH_4Cl. In hypokalemic distal RTA the urine pH is high because of the inability to secrete H^+ in the distal nephron. Urinary excretion of NH_3 is very low and the urinary anion gap is positive.

Ileal conduits. Surgical diversion of the ureter into the intestine may lead to the development of a hyperchloremic normal gap metabolic acidosis due to systemic reabsorption of NH_4^+ and Cl^- from the urinary fluid and exchange of Cl^- for HCO_3^- through activation of the Cl^-/HCO_3^- exchanger on the intestinal lumen. The main determinants for this complication are the length of time the urine is in contact with the bowel and the total surface area of bowel exposed to urine.

Anion Gap Metabolic Acidosis
Lactic Acidosis

Lactic acidosis is generated whenever an imbalance develops between the production and utilization of lactic acid. The accumulation of a nonchloride anion accounts for the increase in anion gap. Severe exercise and grand mal seizures are examples in which lactic acidosis can develop because of increased production. The short-lived nature of the acidosis in these conditions suggests that a concomitant defect in lactic acid utilization is present in most conditions of sustained and severe lactic acidosis. Type A lactic acidosis is characterized by disorders in which there is underperfusion of tissue or acute hypoxia. Such disorders include patients with cardiopulmonary failure, severe anemia, hemorrhage, hypotension, sepsis, and carbon monoxide poisoning. Type B lactic acidosis occurs in patients with a variety of disorders that have in common the development of lactic acidosis in the absence of overt hypoperfusion or hypoxia (Table 25.3).

D-Lactic Acidosis

D-Lactic acidosis is a unique form of metabolic acidosis that can occur in the setting of small bowel resections or in patients with a jejunoileal bypass. These short bowel syndromes create a situation in which carbohydrates that are normally reabsorbed in the small intestine are delivered in large amounts to the colon. In the presence of colonic bacterial overgrowth, these substrates are metabolized into D-lactate and absorbed into the systemic circulation. Accumulation of D-lactate produces an anion gap metabolic acidosis in which the serum lactate is normal because the standard test for lactate is specific for L-lactate. These patients typically present after ingestion of a large carbohydrate meal with neurologic abnormalities consisting of confusion, slurred speech, and ataxia. Ingestion of low-carbohydrate meals and antimicrobial agents to decrease the degree of bacterial overgrowth are the principal treatments.

Diabetic Ketoacidosis

Diabetic ketoacidosis is a metabolic condition characterized by the accumulation of acetoacetic acid and β-hydroxybutyric acid resulting from insulin deficiency and a relative or absolute increase in glucagon concentration. The degree to which the anion gap is elevated will depend on the rapidity, severity, and duration of the ketoacidosis as well as the status of the ECF volume. Although an anion gap acidosis is the dominant disturbance in diabetic ketoacidosis, a hyperchloremic normal gap acidosis is often present in the earliest stages of ketoacidosis when extracellular volume is near normal.

Confirmation of the presence of ketoacids can be achieved with use of nitroprusside tablets or reagent strips. However, this test can be misleading in assessing the severity of ketoacidosis because it only detects the presence of acetone and acetoacetate and does not permit reaction with β-hydroxybutyrate. Treatment of diabetic ketoacidosis involves the use of insulin and intravenous fluids to correct volume depletion. Deficiencies in K^+, Mg^{2+}, and phosphate are common and, therefore, these electrolytes are typically added to intravenous solutions.

Alcoholic Ketoacidosis

Ketoacidosis develops in patients with a history of chronic ethanol abuse, decreased food intake, and often a history of nausea and vomiting. The presence of alcohol withdrawal, volume depletion, and starvation markedly increases the levels of circulating catecholamines and results in the peripheral mobilization of fatty acids that is much larger in magnitude than that typically found with starvation alone. The metabolism of alcohol leads to an increase in the $NADH:NAD^+$ ratio causing a higher β-hydroxybutyrate to acetoacetate ratio. The nitroprusside reaction may be diminished by this redox shift despite the presence of severe ketoacidosis. Glucose administration leads to the rapid resolution of the acidosis because stimulation of insulin release leads to diminished fatty acid mobilization from adipose tissue as well as decreased hepatic output of ketoacids.

Ethylene Glycol and Methanol Poisoning

Ethylene glycol and methanol poisoning are characteristically associated with the development of a severe anion gap metabolic acidosis. Together with the appearance of the anion gap, an osmolar gap also becomes manifest and is an important clue to the diagnosis of ethylene glycol and methanol poisoning. Metabolism of ethylene glycol by alcohol dehydrogenase generates various acids, including glycolic, oxalic, and formic acids. Ethylene glycol is a component of antifreeze and solvents and is ingested by accident or as a suicide attempt. The initial effects of intoxication are neurologic and begin with drunkenness but can quickly progress to seizures and coma. If left untreated, cardiopulmonary symptoms such as tachypnea, noncardiogenic pulmonary edema, and cardiovascular collapse may appear. Twenty-four to 48 hours after ingestion, patients may develop flank pain and acute kidney injury, which are often accompanied by abundant calcium oxalate crystals in the urine.

Methanol is also metabolized by alcohol dehydrogenase and forms formaldehyde, which is then converted to formic acid. Methanol is found in a variety of commercial preparations such as shellac, varnish, and de-icing solutions. As with ethylene glycol ingestion, methanol is ingested by accident or as a suicide attempt. Clinically, methanol ingestion is associated with an acute inebriation followed by an asymptomatic period lasting 24 to 36 hours. At this point, abdominal pain caused by pancreatitis, seizures, blindness, and coma may develop. The blindness is due to direct toxicity of formic acid on the retina. Methanol intoxication is also associated with hemorrhage in the white matter and putamen that can lead to the delayed onset of a Parkinson-like syndrome. Lactic acidosis is also a feature of methanol and ethylene glycol poisoning and contributes to the elevated anion gap.

In addition to supportive measures, the therapy for ethylene glycol and methanol poisoning is centered on reducing the metabolism of the parent compound and accelerating the removal of the alcohol from the body. Fomepizole (4-methylpyrazole) is now the agent of choice to inhibit the enzyme alcohol dehydrogenase and prevent formation of toxic metabolites.

Salicylate Poisoning

Aspirin (acetylsalicylic acid) poisoning leads to increased lactic acid production. The accumulation of lactic, salicylic, keto, and other organic acids account for the development of an anion gap metabolic acidosis. At the same time, salicylate has a direct stimulatory effect on the respiratory center. Increased ventilation lowers the Pco_2, contributing to the development of a respiratory alkalosis. Children primarily manifest an anion gap metabolic acidosis with toxic salicylate levels, whereas a respiratory alkalosis is most evident in adults.

In addition to conservative management, the initial goal of therapy is to correct systemic acidemia and to increase the urine pH. By increasing systemic pH, the ionized fraction of salicylic acid will increase and as a result, there will be less accumulation of the drug in the central nervous system. Similarly, an alkaline urine pH will favor increased urinary excretion because the ionized fraction of the drug is poorly reabsorbed by the tubule. At serum concentrations of greater than 80 mg/dL or in the setting of severe clinical toxicity, hemodialysis can be used to accelerate the removal of the drug from the body.

Pyroglutamic Acidosis

Pyroglutamic acidosis is a cause of anion gap metabolic acidosis accompanied by alterations in mental status ranging from confusion to coma. Reported cases occur in critically ill patients receiving therapeutic doses of acetaminophen, a setting in which glutathione levels are reduced because of acetaminophen metabolism and oxidative stress associated with critical illness. The diagnosis of pyroglutamic acidosis should be considered in patients with unexplained anion gap metabolic acidosis and recent acetaminophen ingestion.

METABOLIC ALKALOSIS

The pathogenesis of metabolic alkalosis involves both the generation and maintenance of this disorder. The generation of metabolic alkalosis refers to the addition of new HCO_3^- to the blood because of either loss of acid or gain of alkali. New HCO_3^- may be generated by either renal or extrarenal mechanisms. Because the kidneys have an enormous capacity to excrete HCO_3^-, even vigorous HCO_3^- generation may not be enough to produce sustained metabolic alkalosis. To maintain a metabolic alkalosis, the capacity of the kidney to correct the alkalosis must be impaired or the capacity to reclaim HCO_3^- must be enhanced.

Clinical Consequences of Metabolic Alkalosis

Metabolic alkalosis is generally considered a benign condition; however, a high blood pH can result in a number of effects that decrease tissue perfusion. Increases in blood pH (alkalemia) cause respiratory depression and decrease tissue oxygen delivery through the Bohr effect and vasoconstriction. Alkalosis should be aggressively corrected in critically ill patients in whom perfusion of the heart and brain is essential.

Approach and Treatment of Metabolic Alkalosis

Metabolic alkalosis is best approached according to the mechanism of maintenance because correction of the maintenance mechanism leads to correction of the metabolic alkalosis. If EAV can be restored with saline, the metabolic alkalosis is easily corrected. Several conditions are poorly responsive to the administration of NaCl. Metabolic alkalosis in these conditions is generally maintained by a combination of increased mineralocorticoid levels along with high distal Na^+ delivery and hypokalemia. The distinction between these entities relies on assessment of EAV (Table 25.4).

Decreased EAV: Saline Responsive

Gastrointestinal acid loss. Loss of acid, as occurs with vomiting or nasogastric suction, is a common cause of metabolic alkalosis maintained by volume contraction. The loss of gastric acid generates a metabolic alkalosis, while the loss of NaCl in the gastric fluid leads

TABLE 25.4 Classification of Metabolic Alkalosis According to Mechanism, Cause, and Response to Administration of Saline

Effective Arterial Volume (EAV)	Low	Low	High
Urine Cl⁻ concentration (mEq/L)	<15	>15	>15
Response to saline	Corrects (saline responsive)	No correction (saline resistant)	No correction (saline resistant)
Maintenance	Low EAV	Low EAV + high distal Na⁺ delivery and mineralocorticoid effect	High distal Na⁺ delivery and mineralocorticoid effect

Etiology	Gastrointestinal acid loss
	  Vomiting/nasogastric suction
	  Congenital chloridorrhea
	  Villous adenoma
	  Post-hypercapneic alkalosis
	Diuretics
	Non-reabsorbable anions
		Primary increase in distal delivery of Na⁺
		  Active diuretic use (loop and thiazide)
		  Mg²⁺ deficiency
		  Bartter syndrome
		  Gitelman syndrome
			Primary increase in mineralocorticoid or mineralocorticoid like effect
			  Conn's syndrome
			  Liddle syndrome
			  Glucocorticoid-suppressible hyperaldosteronism

TABLE 25.5 Treatment of Various Saline-Resistant Causes of Metabolic Alkalosis

DECREASED EAV		INCREASED EAV	
Cause	Treatment	Cause	Treatment
Thiazide and loop diuretics	Discontinue drug, replete EAV	Renin secreting tumor	Remove tumor
Mg²⁺ deficiency	Replete Mg²⁺ deficit	Primary hyperaldosteronism	Remove tumor, spironolactone for BAH
Gitelman syndrome	Amiloride, triamterene, or spironolactone, K⁺ supplements, Mg²⁺ supplements	Glucocorticoid suppressible hyperaldosteronism	Dexamethasone
Bartter syndrome	Amiloride, triamterene, or spironolactone, K⁺ supplements, Mg²⁺ supplements in some	Liddle syndrome	Amiloride or triamterene

BAH, Bilateral adrenal hyperplasia; *EAV*, effective arterial blood volume.

to volume contraction. During active vomiting, the plasma HCO₃⁻ concentration tends to be higher than the threshold for reabsorption in the proximal nephron. The resultant bicarbonaturia leads to increased excretion of $NaHCO_3$ and $KHCO_3$, resulting in further total body Na⁺ depletion and development of K⁺ depletion. During this active phase, urine Cl⁻ is less than 15 mEq/L, in the presence of high urine Na⁺, high urine K⁺, and a urine pH of 7 to 8. When the patient stops vomiting, equilibrium is established such that bicarbonaturia stops but a metabolic alkalosis is maintained by the volume contraction, K⁺ depletion, and reduction in GFR. Of these factors, decreased EAV is clearly the main factor in maintenance of metabolic alkalosis. At this time, urine Na⁺ and Cl⁻ are both low. Administration of NaCl results in bicarbonaturia and the metabolic alkalosis is corrected.

Diuretics. Thiazide and loop diuretics are another common cause of metabolic alkalosis. These diuretics lead to metabolic alkalosis generated in the distal nephron by the combination of high aldosterone levels and enhanced distal delivery of Na⁺. If diuretics are stopped and the patient is maintained on a low-salt diet, the alkalosis will be maintained despite the fact that distal delivery is no longer increased. In this setting, patients tend to be volume contracted and K⁺ deficient. Once again, the contraction of EAV is the major factor leading to the maintenance of metabolic alkalosis. Saline infusion in this setting corrects the metabolic alkalosis.

Decreased EAV: Saline Resistant

In some forms of metabolic alkalosis, the alkalosis is maintained by decreased EAV, but because other maintenance factors are also present, the alkalosis is not completely saline responsive. In these patients,

saline infusions may improve the metabolic alkalosis but will not completely correct it. In general, these patients may have a low EAV but typically do not have a low urine Cl⁻. Continued use of thiazide or loop diuretics, magnesium deficiency, Gitelman syndrome, and Barrter syndrome are examples of this condition. The treatment of various causes of metabolic alkalosis is summarized in Table 25.5.

Increased EAV: Saline Resistant

The last type of metabolic alkalosis is not maintained by decreased EAV, but rather is maintained by high mineralocorticoid levels (in the presence of maintained distal delivery of Na⁺) and K⁺ deficiency. The most common cause of this saline-resistant alkalosis is a primary increase in mineralocorticoid levels not related to volume contraction. The mechanism of the generation of the alkalosis described above, enhanced Na⁺ delivery with high mineralocorticoid activity, is also responsible for maintenance of the metabolic alkalosis in this setting. In addition, K⁺ deficiency, which also occurs in this setting, exacerbates the tendency to alkalosis.

The preferred treatment of metabolic alkalosis in patients with volume expansion and primary mineralocorticoid excess is to remove the underlying cause of the persistent mineralocorticoid activity. When this is not possible, therapy is directed at blocking the actions of the mineralocorticoid at the level of the kidney.

RESPIRATORY ALKALOSIS

Primary respiratory alkalosis results from hypocapnia and is defined by an arterial partial pressure of carbon dioxide ($Paco_2$) of less than 35

TABLE 25.6 Compensation in Acid-Base Disorders

Disorder	Compensatory Changes
Acute respiratory acidosis	For every 10 mm Hg rise in P_{CO_2} the HCO_3^- increases by 1 mEq/L
Chronic respiratory acidosis	For every 10 mm Hg rise in P_{CO_2} the HCO_3^- increases by 3.5 mEq/L
Acute respiratory alkalosis	For every 10 mm Hg fall in P_{CO_2} the HCO_3^- decreases by 2 mEq/L
Chronic respiratory alkalosis	For every 10 mm Hg decrease in P_{CO_2} the HCO_3^- decreases by 5 mEq/L
Metabolic acidosis	1.2 mm Hg decrease in P_{CO_2} for each 1 mEq/L fall in HCO_3^- $P_{CO_2} = HCO_3^- + 15$ P_{CO_2} = last digits of pH
Metabolic alkalosis	P_{CO_2} increases by 0.7 for each mEq/L HCO_3^-

mm Hg in the setting of alkalemia. Primary respiratory alkalosis must be differentiated from secondary hypocapnia, which is a compensatory mechanism in the setting of primary metabolic acidosis.

Etiology

Respiratory alkalosis is the most frequent acid-base disturbance encountered. It is particularly common in hospitalized patients, where it can be the initial clue to the presence of gram-negative sepsis. Hepatic failure is a common and important cause of primary hypocapnia. The severity of hypocapnia correlates with the level of blood ammonia and has prognostic significance. The presence of respiratory alkalosis can be an important clue to the presence of salicylate intoxication. High progesterone levels (pregnancy) can also cause respiratory alkalosis.

Clinical Manifestation of Respiratory Alkalosis

Mild respiratory alkalosis causes lightheadedness, palpitations, and paresthesias of the extremities and the circumoral area. Acute hypocapnia decreases cerebral blood flow and causes binding of free calcium to albumin in the blood. Thus, patients with acute respiratory alkalosis might present clinically in a similar way to patients with hypocalcemia, manifesting positive Chvostek and Trousseau signs. Patients with ischemic heart disease might occasionally develop cardiac arrhythmias, ischemic electrocardiographic changes, and even angina pectoris during acute hypocapnia.

Diagnosis

The diagnosis of respiratory alkalosis is made by evaluating the patient's history, performing a physical exam, and obtaining laboratory data including a blood gas analysis. Tachypnea or Kussmaul breathing can be detected on physical exam and may be the first clue to the presence of a primary respiratory alkalosis or a compensatory respiratory mechanism in the setting of a primary metabolic acidosis. Changes in serum electrolytes can aid in the diagnosis of respiratory alkalosis. An acute fall in P_{CO_2} causes a HCO_3^--Cl^- shift in red blood cells and accounts for the small initial compensatory response in acute respiratory alkalosis in which the HCO_3^- concentration falls by 2 mEq/L for every 10 mm Hg decrease in P_{CO_2}. Table 25.6 provides the expected compensatory responses for acid-base disorders.

In chronic respiratory alkalosis, the renal HCO_3^- reabsorptive capacity decreases and there is a transient HCO_3^- diuresis. This process takes 2 to 3 days to become fully manifest. Once a new steady state is achieved, the HCO_3^- concentration will have decreased by 5 mEq/L

for each 10 mm Hg fall in P_{CO_2}. A higher or lower value for the plasma HCO_3^- concentration suggests the presence of an additional metabolic disorder.

To defend ECF volume in the setting of increased urinary loss of $NaHCO_3$, the kidney retains NaCl. These changes are reflected in the serum electrolytes of patients with chronic respiratory alkalosis in which the Cl^- is typically increased with respect to the serum Na^+ concentration. Another characteristic finding is an increase of 3 to 5 mEq/L in the serum anion gap. The increased gap is due to the greater fixed negative charge on serum albumin as well as an increase in serum lactate concentration. Lactate production is increased due to a stimulatory effect of high pH on phosphofructokinase, the rate-limiting step in the glycolytic pathway.

Treatment

Primary respiratory alkalosis is treated by correcting the underlying cause. A patient with anxiety-hyperventilation syndrome should be treated by providing reassurance. Rebreathing into a paper bag or any other closed system will cause the P_{CO_2} to increase with each breath taken and lead to a partial correction of hypocapnia and improvement of symptoms. In the rare case where there is no response to conservative management, sedatives can be used. In mechanically ventilated patients, the P_{CO_2} can be increased by either raising the inspired CO_2 tension or by increasing the dead space of the ventilator circuit. Correction of respiratory alkalosis may prove helpful in correcting arrhythmias in patients with underlying coronary disease. In contrast, caution is warranted in raising the P_{CO_2} in patients with brain injury because cerebral perfusion may increase and cause further worsening of intracranial pressure. Respiratory alkalosis frequently develops as a complication of hypoxia. Administration of oxygen or return to lower altitudes can reverse the respiratory alkalosis that develops in this setting.

RESPIRATORY ACIDOSIS

Respiratory acidosis develops because of ineffective alveolar ventilation. This acid-base disorder, which is also called primary hypercapnia, needs to be differentiated from secondary hypercapnia, which develops as a compensatory mechanism in the setting of primary metabolic alkalosis. Primary hypercapnia is clinically recognized by the presence of $Paco_2$ levels of greater than 45 mm Hg on arterial blood gas analysis. However, $Paco_2$ levels of less than 45 mm Hg might still be indicative of respiratory acidosis if a primary metabolic acidosis is not adequately compensated by alveolar ventilation.

Etiology of Respiratory Acidosis

The development of respiratory acidosis is usually multifactorial. Major causes of CO_2 retention include diseases or malfunction within any element of the respiratory system, including the central and peripheral nervous systems, the respiratory muscles, the thoracic cage, the pleural space, the airways, and the lung parenchyma. The following six factors should be considered in the differential diagnosis of acute and chronic respiratory acidosis: inhibition of the medullary respiratory center, disorders of the chest wall and the respiratory muscles, airway obstruction, disorders affecting gas exchange across the pulmonary capillary, increased CO_2 production, and mechanical ventilation.

Clinical Manifestations of Respiratory Acidosis

Hypercapnic encephalopathy is a clinical syndrome that usually starts with irritability, headache, mental cloudiness, apathy, confusion, anxiety, restlessness, and can progress to asterixis, transient psychosis, delirium, somnolence, and coma. Papilledema and other manifestations of increased intracranial pressure that are collectively named *pseudotumor cerebri* are occasionally observed in patients with either acute or chronic hypercapnia. The increase in intracranial pressure is in part due to cerebral vasodilation resulting from acidemia. Acute respiratory acidosis is typically more symptomatic than acute metabolic acidosis because CO_2 diffuses and equilibrates across the blood-brain barrier much more rapidly than does HCO_3^-, resulting in a more rapid fall in cerebral spinal fluid and cerebral interstitial pH. Severe hypercapnia can also lead to decreased myocardial contractility, arrhythmias, and peripheral vasodilatation, particularly when the blood pH falls to less than 7.1.

Diagnosis

The diagnosis of primary respiratory acidosis is made by the presence of acidemia and hypercapnia on arterial blood gas analysis. Changes in the serum chemistries can aid in the diagnosis of respiratory acidosis. Acute hypercapnia is associated with a shift of HCO_3^- out of red blood cells in exchange for Cl^-; a process termed the *red cell HCO_3^--C^- shift*. Acutely, the plasma HCO_3^- concentration increases by 1 mmol/L for each 10 mm Hg elevation in $Paco_2$. After 24 to 48 hours of hypercapnia proximal tubular cells increase H^+ secretion, resulting in accelerated HCO_3^- reabsorption. The retention of $NaHCO_3$ leads to slight expansion of the ECF compartment and causes increased renal excretion of NaCl to return volume back to normal. The net effect is increased serum HCO_3^- and decreased Cl^- concentration. In chronic respiratory acidosis, there is a 3.5 mEq/L increase in HCO_3^- for each 10 mm Hg elevation in $Paco_2$. Higher or lower plasma HCO_3^- concentrations suggest the presence of mixed respiratory and metabolic acid-base disorders.

Treatment of Respiratory Acidosis

The mainstay of treatment in respiratory acidosis is to recognize and treat the underlying cause whenever possible. Patients with acute respiratory acidosis are primarily at risk of hypoxemia rather than hypercapnia or acidemia. Thus, immediate therapeutic efforts should focus on establishing and securing a patent airway to provide adequate oxygenation. In patients with status asthmaticus, a lower ventilatory rate and peak inspiratory pressure may be required to minimize barotrauma to the lung but at the expense of a persistently higher Pco_2. Small amounts of $NaHCO_3$ can help prevent excessive falls in blood pH in this setting. The downside of such therapy is that infusion of $NaHCO_3$ can result in increased CO_2 production, causing a further increase in Pco_2 when ventilation cannot be increased.

Excessive oxygen should be avoided in patients with chronic respiratory acidosis because it may lead to worsening hypoventilation. When mechanical ventilation is required, care should be taken to lower the $Paco_2$ carefully and slowly because there is the risk of overshoot alkalemia due to the presence of a high HCO_3^- (post-hypercapneic metabolic alkalosis). The kidneys must excrete the HCO_3^- in order to normalize the acid-base status. This excretion will not occur when EAV is reduced either because of salt depletion owing to restricted intake or diuretic therapy or a salt retentive state such as heart failure and cirrhosis. Correction of the superimposed metabolic alkalosis can usually be achieved with saline and discontinuation of loop diuretics if they are being utilized. In edematous patients with heart failure, this may not be possible, and acetazolamide may be needed to correct the alkalosis.

SUGGESTED READINGS

Palmer BF: Approach to fluid and electrolyte disorders and acid-base problems, Primary Care 35:195–213, 2008.

Palmer BF: Diagnostic approach and management of inpatient hyponatremia, J Hospital Med 5:S1–S5, 2010.

Palmer BF: Managing hyperkalemia caused by inhibitors of the renin-angiotensin-aldosterone system, N Engl J Med 351:585–592, 2004.

Palmer BF: Metabolic acidosis. In Feehally J, Floege J, Tonelli M, Johnson RJ, editors: Comprehensive clinical nephrology, ed 6, Philadelphia, 2019, Elsevier, pp 149–159.

Palmer BF: A physiologic based approach to the evaluation of a patient with hyperkalemia, Am J Kidney Ds 56(2):387–393, 2010.

Palmer BF: A physiologic-based approach to the evaluation of a patient with hypokalemia, Am J Kidney Ds 56:1184–1190, 2010.

Palmer BF: Respiratory acid-base disorders. In Mount D, Sayegh M, Singh Ajay, editors: Core concepts in the disorders of fluid, electrolytes and acid-base balance, New York, 2013, Springer, pp 297–306.

Palmer BF: Respiratory alkalosis, Am J Kidney Ds 60:834–838, 2012.

Palmer BF, Alpern RJ: Metabolic alkalosis, J Am Soc Nephrol 8:1462–1469, 1997.

Palmer BF, Clegg DJ: Electrolyte and acid-base disorders in patients with diabetes mellitus, N Engl J Med 373:548–559, 2015.

Palmer BF, Clegg DJ: Electrolyte disturbances in patients with chronic alcohol-use disorder, N Engl J Med 377:1368–1377, 2017.

Palmer BF, Clegg DJ: Physiology and Pathophysiology of Potassium Homeostasis: Core Curriculum 2019; Am J Kidney Ds 74:682–695, 2019.

Palmer BF, Clegg DJ: Salicylate toxicity, N Engl J Med 382:2544–2555, 2020.

Palmer BF, Clegg DJ: The use of selected urine chemistries in the diagnosis of kidney disorders, Clin J Am Soc Nephrol 14:306–316, 2019.

26

Glomerular Diseases

Sanjeev Sethi, An S. De Vriese, Fernando C. Fervenza

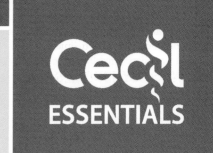

INTRODUCTION

Glomerular injury or disease can manifest as hematuria, proteinuria, hypertension, fluid retention, and a reduction in the glomerular filtration rate. Traditionally, glomerular diseases have been grouped according to clinical presentation, including asymptomatic microscopic hematuria, the nephritic syndrome, the nephrotic syndrome, rapidly progressive glomerulonephritis (RPGN), and chronic glomerulonephritis. An alternative classification of glomerular diseases is according to the histologic pattern on kidney biopsy, such as minimal change disease (MCD), membranoproliferative glomerulonephritis (MPGN), membranous nephropathy, and focal segmented glomerulosclerosis (FSGS). However, many glomerular diseases can manifest with more than one constellation of signs and symptoms and show more than one histologic pattern on renal biopsy. In addition, a particular clinical presentation or histologic pattern can be caused by different underlying disease processes. Great progress has been made in unraveling the molecular causes of glomerular diseases. For instance, autoantibodies against the phospholipase A_2 receptor or thrombospondin-7A receptor have been associated with membranous nephropathy. In the future, the etiologic approach to the classification of glomerular diseases will undoubtedly be expanded. As such, a condition can be more accurately described by combining the different approaches (e.g., antiphospholipase A_2 receptor antibody–associated membranous nephropathy presenting with nephrotic syndrome).

CLINICAL PRESENTATION

A detailed history and careful physical examination, with particular attention to the time of symptom onset, help to clarify the differential diagnosis of suspected glomerular disease. Blood pressure and fluid status should be recorded. Urine microscopy is a critical element of this assessment, and it may reveal hematuria, typically with dysmorphic red blood cells and casts. Hematuria due to glomerular disease is painless and the urine is often brown or cola-colored rather than bright red; clots are rare. The differential diagnosis should be made with other causes of brown urine, including hemoglobinuria, myoglobinuria, and specific foods or drug dyes (e.g., beetroot). Normal red blood cell excretion is 3 or fewer red blood cells per high power field or less than 8000 red blood cells per milliliter of uncentrifuged urine. To distinguish glomerular from nonglomerular hematuria, a freshly voided urinary sediment can be examined microscopically. With nonglomerular hematuria, the erythrocytes are normocytic, have a biconcave appearance, and a regular shape. In glomerular hematuria, the erythrocytes are microcytic, lack a biconcave disc appearance, and are irregularly shaped (dysmorphic). Usually 50% or more of the erythrocytes are dysmorphic and red blood cell casts may also be seen (active urinary sediment). Glomerular hematuria is generally seen throughout the voiding process and can be increased by vigorous exercise or fever. Terminal hematuria (hematuria confined to the last few milliliters of a void) is a feature of bladder disease.

Quantitative evaluation of the degree of urinary protein excretion is essential. In adults, urinary total protein excretion is less than 150 mg/24 h, and urinary albumin excretion is less than 20 mg/24 h. Persistent albumin excretion of 30 to 300 mg/24 h is termed microalbuminuria. Albumin excretion above 300 mg/24 h, the level at which the standard dipstick becomes positive, reflects overt proteinuria. Levels above 3.5 g/24 h are considered to be nephrotic-range proteinuria. It should be recognized that nephrotic-range proteinuria (>3.5 g/24 h) and nephrotic syndrome (>3.5 g/24 h and serum albumin <3.5 g/dL by bromocresol green method or <3.0 g/dL by bromocresol purple method) are not synonymous. This distinction is particularly important when the kidney biopsy reveals FSGS. Patients with full-blown nephrotic syndrome most likely have primary FSGS, whereas patients with nephrotic-range proteinuria often have FSGS due to a secondary process.

A 24-hour urine collection remains the gold standard, but it is cumbersome to perform, is often collected incorrectly, and does not provide a rapid result. The accuracy of the urine collection should be assessed by simultaneously quantifying urinary total protein and creatinine excretion. If urinary creatinine excretion is within 15% of the expected value (expected creatinine excretion in 24 hours = [140 − age in years] × weight in kg × 0.2 [× 0.85 if female]), the collection can generally be regarded as accurate. A protein-to-creatinine ratio measured on a 24-hour urine collection is a useful alternative. Using the protein and creatinine concentration available from the readings on the 24-hour urine collection, calculate the urine protein to creatinine ratio (UPCR). Then, multiply the calculated UPCR by the expected 24-hour urine creatinine excretion (as per the above-mentioned formula) to estimate the magnitude of protein in the collection.

The above-mentioned approach assumes that the patient's 24-hour urine creatinine excretion is appropriate for their body size. If this relationship is altered by malnutrition, muscle wasting, limb-loss, body-building or unusual habitus, then as carefully as possible a complete and accurate 24-hour urine collection must be obtained. For vegetarians, the expected 24-hour urine creatinine excretion should be reduced by about one third. Random "spot" or first morning UPCR should not be used to estimate proteinuria. Such values are inherently highly variable due to variation in protein excretion during the day and differences in urinary creatinine excretion based on age, gender, and lean body (muscle) mass.

Glomerular proteinuria can be classified as transient or hemodynamic (functional) (e.g., fever, exercise induced, orthostatic) or as persistent (fixed). Although functional proteinuria is benign, fixed nephrotic-range proteinuria usually results from glomerular diseases. Total proteinuria greater than 1 g/24 h in a patient with a negative urine dipstick (which detects only albumin) suggests that the proteinuria is caused by light chains or low-molecular-weight proteins (e.g., retinol-binding protein, α_1-microglobulin).

CLINICAL SYNDROMES

Asymptomatic Microscopic Hematuria

Glomerular hematuria can occur with or without subnephrotic range proteinuria. Renal function parameters and blood pressure are typically normal.

Glomerular diseases commonly presenting with asymptomatic hematuria include IgA nephropathy, Alport syndrome, and thin glomerular basement disease.

Nephrotic Syndrome

Nephrotic syndrome is defined as persistent urinary total protein excretion greater than 3.5 g/24 h, accompanied by a serum albumin concentration less than 3.5 g/dL. Edema, hyperlipidemia, and lipiduria (i.e., doubly refractile fat bodies) are common but are not required for the diagnosis.

Complications of the nephrotic syndrome include hypogammaglobulinemia, vitamin D deficiency due to loss of vitamin D–binding protein, and iron deficiency anemia due to hypotransferrinemia. Thrombotic complications from loss of antithrombin III such as renal vein thrombosis may occur, especially in patients with greater protein loss (>10 g/24 h) and serum albumin levels less than 2 g/dL. Patients with severe nephrotic syndrome are particularly susceptible for acute renal failure when there is superimposed volume depletion, sepsis or use of nephrotoxic agents such as nonsteroidal anti-inflammatory drugs (NSAIDs).

Management of patients with nephrotic syndrome includes diuretics to control edema, regulation of blood pressure (angiotensin-converting enzyme inhibitors [ACEIs] and angiotensin-receptor blockers [ARBs] are preferred), limitation of the intake of protein to between 0.8 and 1 g/kg/day and sodium to less than 4 g/day, and control of lipid levels. Anticoagulation should be considered for patients at increased risk, especially if the nephrotic syndrome is caused by membranous nephropathy or amyloidosis.

Glomerular diseases commonly presenting with nephrotic syndrome include MCD, FSGS, membranous nephropathy, HIV-associated nephropathy, amyloidosis and diabetic nephropathy.

Nephritic Syndrome

The nephritic syndrome is defined by oliguria, edema, hypertension, proteinuria (usually <3.5 g/24 hr), and abnormal urinalysis with dysmorphic red blood cells or red blood cell casts. Glomerular diseases commonly presenting with nephritic syndrome include infection-related glomerulonephritis, IgA nephropathy, and C3 glomerulopathy.

Rapidly Progressive Glomerulonephritis

RPGN is a clinical syndrome characterized by progressive loss of kidney function with a time course of days to months in a patient with active urinary sediment (see Chapter 24 and E-Fig. 29.1 and Table 29.3). Patients may have oliguria. Most of the pulmonary-renal syndromes manifest in this fashion, and the pathologic corollary is often a focal, necrotizing, crescentic glomerulonephritis. When RPGN is suspected, renal biopsy with immunofluorescence studies is extremely helpful.

Linear deposition of immunoglobulin G (IgG) points to Goodpasture disease or anti–glomerular basement membrane (anti-GBM)–mediated glomerulonephritis. Immunoglobulins and complement suggest systemic lupus erythematosus (SLE), cryoglobulinemia, immunoglobulin A (IgA) nephropathy, or postinfectious glomerulonephritis. Negative or weak immunofluorescence (pauci-immune) findings usually indicate an antineutrophil cytoplasmic autoantibody (ANCA) vasculitis (Fig. 26.1).

Chronic Glomerulonephritis

Patients can be presumed to have chronic glomerulonephritis in the setting of a slowly progressive loss of renal function over the course of months or years, accompanied by persistent glomerular hematuria. Proteinuria is usually in the subnephrotic range. Hypertension is nearly always present. Renal ultrasound usually shows small kidneys with increased echogenicity.

Glomerular diseases often presenting as chronic glomerulonephritis include IgA nephropathy, C3 glomerulopathy, and Alport syndrome.

PRIMARY PODOCYTOPATHIES

Minimal Change Disease

MCD is defined by a renal biopsy with no significant glomerular abnormalities on light microscopy, negative immunoglobulin and complement deposition on immunofluorescence, and widespread foot

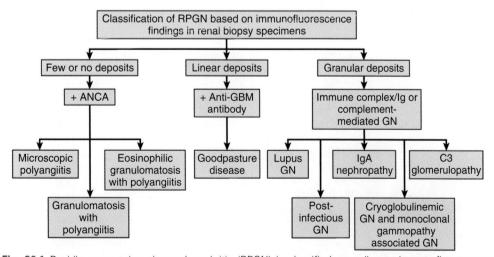

Fig. 26.1 Rapidly progressive glomerulonephritis (RPGN) is classified according to immunofluorescence microscopy findings in renal biopsy specimens. *ANCA,* Antineutrophil cytoplasmic autoantibody; *GBM,* glomerular basement membrane; *GN,* glomerulonephritis; *IgA,* immunoglobulin A.

process effacement on electron microscopy (Fig. 26.2). MCD is the most common cause of nephrotic syndrome in children and accounts for up to 20% of adults with primary nephrotic syndrome.

The pathogenesis of MCD is unknown. The association with Hodgkin lymphoma suggests that MCD may be a consequence of T-lymphocyte abnormalities, with T cells producing a lymphokine that is toxic to glomerular epithelial cells. Most cases of MCD are idiopathic, although drugs (e.g., NSAIDs), hematologic malignancies (mainly Hodgkin lymphoma), and thymoma are well-recognized causes of secondary MCD. Concomitant interstitial nephritis suggests drugs (e.g., NSAIDs) as the likely cause of MCD.

In children, MCD usually manifests with nephrotic syndrome of acute onset. Hematuria, hypertension, or impaired renal function is unusual and suggests another diagnosis. When nephrotic syndrome occurs in a child with normal urinalysis results, the diagnosis is MCD until proven otherwise, and treatment with high-dose corticosteroid therapy can be started, often without the need of a renal biopsy.

More than 90% of children achieve complete remission after 4 to 8 weeks of treatment. Children who do not respond to corticosteroid therapy should undergo a renal biopsy. Adolescents and adults also respond to high-dose corticosteroids (>80%), but the response is slower, and treatment for 16 weeks or more may be required to achieve remission. Therapy usually is continued for 4 to 8 weeks after remission.

Among patients who have a response to corticosteroids, about 25% have a long-term remission. However, up to 25% of the patients have frequent relapses, and up to 30% become steroid dependent. For these patients, alternative therapies aiming to minimize corticosteroid toxicity include alkylating agents, antimetabolites, calcineurin inhibitors (cyclosporine or tacrolimus), and rituximab (a chimeric human-murine monoclonal antibody that targets the CD20 antigen expressed on B cells). Although these agents may allow a lower corticosteroid dose, some patients respond poorly or not at all, and their use may be complicated by significant side effects. Noncompliance is always a concern, especially in young patients.

Focal Segmental Glomerulosclerosis

FSGS is not a specific disease entity, but a lesion, caused by a wide variety of conditions. The common pathophysiologic element is podocyte injury and depletion leading to glomerular scarring (Fig. 26.3). FSGS accounts for less than 15% of cases of idiopathic nephrotic syndrome in children and up to 25% in adults. In African Americans, FSGS is often associated with the presence of the G1 and G2 polymorphisms in the *APOL1* gene. Hypertension is found in 30% to 50% of patients with FSGS, and microscopic hematuria occurs in 25% to 75% of cases. Up to 30% of those with FSGS have impaired renal function.

The pathogenesis of idiopathic or primary FSGS is unknown. A circulating permeability factor has been demonstrated in some patients. The soluble urokinase-type plasminogen activator receptor (suPAR) has been identified as a potential marker because levels are elevated in two thirds of cases of primary FSGS and levels are higher in renal transplant recipients with recurrent FSGS. However, suPAR levels do not distinguish primary from secondary FSGS, and serum levels increase with reductions in the glomerular filtration rate. Further research is needed to define the role of serum suPAR in primary FSGS.

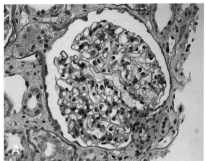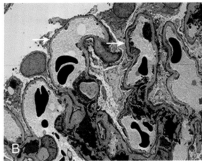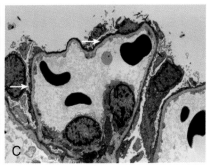

Fig. 26.2 Minimal change disease. (A) Light microscopy shows a normal-appearing glomerulus (periodic acid–Schiff, ×40). (B and C) Electron microscopy shows diffuse foot process effacement *(arrows)* (B, ×2500; C, ×4200). Immunofluorescence studies were negative for immune deposits.

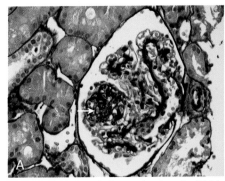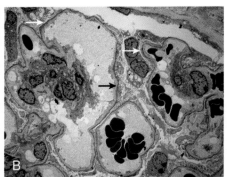

Fig. 26.3 Focal segmental glomerulosclerosis. (A) Light microscopy shows segmental sclerosis *(arrow)* with segmental consolidation of the glomerular capillary tufts and visceral epithelial cell hypertrophy over the segmentally sclerosed tufts (silver methenamine, ×40). (B) Electron microscopy shows diffuse foot process effacement *(arrows)* of the visceral epithelial cells (×1850). Immunofluorescence studies were negative for immune deposits.

Secondary causes of FSGS include genetic mutations in podocyte genes, human immunodeficiency virus (HIV) infection, drugs, sickle cell disease, vesicoureteral reflux, obesity, unilateral renal agenesis, remnant kidneys, and aging (Table 26.1). Five histologic variants of FSGS have been described according to the Columbia classification: classic (or Not Otherwise Specified), perihilar, cellular, tip, and collapsing. However, this classification is based on LM examination only and does not take into account the degree of foot process effacement on EM. This classification has potential prognostic significance, but it should not be used as a tool to differentiate the different pathophysiologic forms of FSGS. The collapsing variant, which has the worst prognosis, is more common in African Americans and patients with HIV infection.

Spontaneous remission of proteinuria is uncommon (<5% of cases). Treatment of the primary forms consists of prolonged (>4 months) high-dose corticosteroid therapy (prednisone, 1 mg/kg/day), but there is no study comparing this approach with other forms of therapy. However, if patients are going to respond to corticosteroids, proteinuria starts to decrease soon after the start of treatment, and those who show no significant reduction (>30%) in proteinuria after 2 to 3 months of prednisone at 1 mg/kg/day (maximum 80 mg/day) are unlikely to respond, and corticosteroid therapy should be tapered and discontinued. For patients who respond to corticosteroids but undergo relapse, alternative therapy includes the use of cytotoxic drugs alone or in combination with corticosteroids, calcineurin inhibitors, and possibly rituximab. Patients with limiting side effects or contraindications to corticosteroids (e.g., obesity) can be treated with a calcineurin

inhibitor as first-line therapy. Similarly to treatment with corticosteroids, if patients are going to respond to a calcineurin inhibitor, proteinuria starts to decrease soon after the start of treatment. For patients with secondary forms of FSGS, treatment should target the cause.

In all patients, treatment with an ACEI or ARB, alone or in combination, may substantially reduce proteinuria and prolong renal survival. Patients who have a non–nephrotic-range proteinuria have the best renal survival (>80% at 10 years). In patients who continue to have a high degree of proteinuria (>10 g/day), end-stage renal disease (ESRD) typically develops over 5 to 20 years. Idiopathic FSGS may recur in a transplanted kidney.

Membranous Nephropathy

Membranous nephropathy is the leading cause of nephrotic syndrome in white individuals. It occurs in persons of all ages and races but is most often diagnosed in middle age, with the incidence peaking during the fourth and fifth decades of life. The male-to-female ratio is about 2:1. Most patients have nephrotic syndrome, normal renal function, and no hypertension. Microscopic hematuria may be detected in about one third of patients.

Autoantibodies against the phospholipase A_2 receptor (PLA_2R) and thrombospondin-7A in podocytes are found in about 70% and less than 5% of patients with the primary form of the disease, respectively. Recently, three new antigens have been discovered in primary membranous nephropathy. These include neural epidermal growth factor-like 1 protein (NELL-1), semaphorin 3B (Sema3B), and protocadherin 7 (PCDH7). Secondary membranous nephropathy is caused by autoimmune diseases (e.g., SLE, autoimmune thyroiditis), infection (e.g., hepatitis B virus [HBV], hepatitis C virus [HCV]), drugs (e.g., penicillamine, NSAIDs), and solid malignancies (e.g., colon cancer, lung cancer). A subset of patients with membranous nephropathy is associated with accumulation of exostosin 1 (EXT1) and exostosin 2 (EXT2) in the glomerular basement membrane. Autoimmune disease is common in this group of patients, and EXT1/EXT2 may represent the target antigen in secondary (autoimmune) membranous nephropathy.

On light microscopy, capillary walls may appear thickened, and methenamine silver stain shows subepithelial projections ("spikes") along the capillary walls. Immunofluorescence microscopy shows marked granular deposition of IgG and C3 along the capillary walls, and subepithelial deposits are seen on electron microscopy (Fig. 26.4). Staining for IgG subclasses may help to differentiate primary from secondary membranous nephropathy. IgG1, IgG2 and IgG3 tend to be highly expressed in lupus membranous nephropathy (class V lupus nephritis), whereas IgG1 and IgG4 tend to be highly expressed in primary membranous nephropathy. IgG4 staining tends to be absent in the immune deposits of membranous nephropathy secondary to malignancy.

Up to one third of the patients with membranous nephropathy undergo spontaneous remission, and another one third of patients

TABLE 26.1 Causes of Focal Segmental Glomerulosclerosis
Primary (Idiopathic) FSGS
• Attributed to a circulating permeability factor
Secondary FSGS
• Genetic mutations in podocyte genes
• Viral: HIV-associated nephropathy, parvovirus B19, simian virus 40, cytomegalovirus
• Drug induced: heroin, interferon (α, β, γ), pamidronate, sirolimus, calcineurin inhibitors
• Adaptive: reduced nephron mass or glomerular adaptation, unilateral renal agenesis, obesity-related glomerulopathy, basement membrane defects healing phase of focal proliferative glomerulonephritis, body building, sickle cell anemia, hypertensive nephrosclerosis, thrombotic microangiopathy, aging kidney
• Other causes: hemophagocytic syndrome

FSGS, Focal segmental glomerulosclerosis; *HIV,* human immunodeficiency virus.

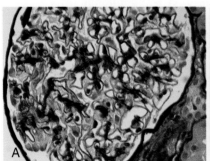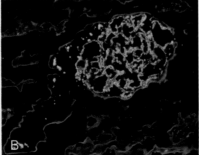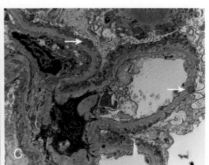

Fig. 26.4 Membranous nephropathy. (A) Light microscopy shows thickened glomerular basement membranes (×60). (B) Immunofluorescence study shows granular immunoglobulin G deposition along the capillary walls (×20). (C) Electron microscopy shows subepithelial electron-dense deposits (arrows) (×15,000).

undergo partial remission. Initial therapy should include angiotensin II receptor blockade, a low-salt diet (<4 g/day), a low-protein diet (0.8 to 1 g/kg/day), and lipid control. If spontaneous remission occurs, it usually does so within the first 12 to 24 months.

Early treatment should be given to patients with severe nephrotic syndrome (e.g., proteinuria >10 g/24 h) and high or increasing anti-PLA$_2$R antibody titers, while conservative therapy is continued in asymptomatic patients, who maintain proteinuria at less than 4 g/24 h and have low or decreasing anti-PLA$_2$R antibody titers.

Rituximab has recently garnered attention as a potential breakthrough in the treatment of membranous nephropathy. A recent multicenter randomized controlled trial of rituximab versus cyclosporine in patients with severe membranous nephropathy (MENTOR) revealed that rituximab is not inferior to cyclosporine in inducing complete or partial remission of proteinuria but is superior in maintaining long-term remission of proteinuria and will likely become the first-line therapy for the treatment of membranous nephropathy.

The probability of renal survival is more than 80% at 5 years and about 60% at 15 years. Patients with an accelerated course should be evaluated for superimposed anti-GBM disease, acute interstitial nephritis, or renal vein thrombosis.

IMMUNE-COMPLEX GLOMERULONEPHRITIS

Infection-Related Glomerulonephritis

Poststreptococcal glomerulonephritis (PSGN) is a classic form of acute glomerulonephritis that develops 1 to 4 weeks after a pharyngitis or skin infection with specific (nephritogenic) strains of group A β-hemolytic streptococci. It typically occurs in children and usually has a benign course. More recently, however, infection-related glomerulonephritis has been recognized to have a broader spectrum, affecting elderly and immunocompromised patients and associated with different bacteria, particularly staphylococci. Unlike classic PSGN, the variant occurs when the infection is still active and has an unfavorable prognosis. The term *infection-related GN* is often used to include both PSGN and GN occurring in the setting of a concurrent infection.

Infection-related glomerulonephritis manifests clinically with the abrupt onset of nephritic syndrome. In patients with PSGN, cultures are usually negative, but elevated titers of antistreptolysin O (ASO), antistreptokinase, antihyaluronidase, and anti-deoxyribonuclease (anti-DNAse B) antibodies may provide evidence of recent streptococcal infection. Activation of the alternative complement pathway is reflected by low C3 complement levels. C4 levels are usually normal or mildly decreased. Other nephrologic conditions associated with low complement are C3 glomerulopathy, lupus nephritis, cryoglobulinemic glomerulonephritis, fibrillary glomerulonephritis, IgG4-mediated renal disease, and cholesterol emboli (Table 26.2).

Renal biopsy typically shows diffuse glomerular hypercellularity and infiltration of polymorphonuclear leukocytes, monocytes, or macrophages on light microscopy. Immunofluorescence shows granular deposition of IgG, C3, and occasionally immunoglobulin M (IgM). On electron microscopy, characteristic dome-shaped subepithelial deposits ("humps") can be seen along the GBM (Fig. 26.5).

Treatment is supportive and aims to minimize fluid overload, optimize blood pressure control, and eradicate ongoing infection. For children, the prognosis is excellent, with most patients recovering renal function in 1 to 2 months. Some patients have persistent microscopic hematuria, proteinuria, hypertension, and renal dysfunction and are said to have *atypical, persistent,* or *resolving* PSGN. Some of these patients have mutations or autoantibodies to proteins in the alternative complement cascade and as such represent patients with C3 glomerulopathy.

Immunoglobulin A (IgA) Nephropathy

IgA nephropathy (formerly called Berger disease) is the most common form of primary glomerulopathy. On light microscopy, mesangial proliferation is seen, along with mesangial deposition of IgA on immunofluorescence and electron-dense deposits in the mesangium on electron microscopy (Fig. 26.6).

Patients may have episodes of macroscopic hematuria accompanying an intercurrent upper respiratory tract infection (synpharyngitic) or have asymptomatic hematuria, with or without proteinuria, detected on routine urinalysis. Proteinuria is common, but nephrotic syndrome occurs in less than 10% of cases and raises the possibility of a primary podocytopathy (e.g., MCD) superimposed on the IgA nephropathy.

The pathogenesis of IgA nephropathy has been linked to galactose-deficient IgA1 (GD-IgA1) molecules and increased formation of anti–GD-IgA1 autoantibodies, with deposition of IgG or IgA anti–GD-IgA1 immune complexes in the mesangium, resulting in activation of complement and cytokine cascades. Secondary causes of IgA nephropathy include chronic liver disease, celiac disease, dermatitis herpetiformis, and ankylosing spondylitis.

In up to 60% of the patients, IgA nephropathy has a benign clinical course, and patients maintain proteinuria of less than 500 mg/24 h and preserved renal function. However, progression to ESRD occurs in up to 40% of patients over 10 to 25 years. Clinical predictors of progression include proteinuria greater than 1 g/24 h, hypertension, presence of crescents on renal biopsy, and impaired renal function at diagnosis. Any degree of proteinuria carries a worse prognosis for a patient with IgA nephropathy. IgA nephropathy frequently recurs after renal transplantation, but loss of the allograft from recurrent disease is uncommon.

The use of angiotensin II system blockade and high-dose corticosteroids has been beneficial in slowing or halting progression of renal disease. Henoch-Schönlein purpura is the systemic form of IgA nephropathy. The prognosis is generally good for children but varies in adults.

In patients with normal renal function, treatment is supportive only. Patients with persistent proteinuria greater than 1 g/24 h and/or progressive renal failure should be considered for treatment with high-dose corticosteroids with or without cytotoxic medication.

Membranoproliferative Glomerulonephritis

MPGN is not a specific disease entity but a pattern of glomerular injury resulting from predominantly subendothelial and mesangial deposition of immune complexes or complement factors and their products. On light microscopy, mesangial hypercellularity, endocapillary proliferation, and capillary wall remodeling with double-contour formation are characteristic, and they result in a lobular accentuation of the glomerular tufts. Immunofluorescence microscopy shows immunoglobulins or complement factors, depending on the underlying cause of MPGN. Electron microscopy typically shows mesangial and subendothelial deposits, and, less commonly, intramembranous and subepithelial deposits (Fig. 26.7).

Based on a recent proposal, MPGN can be classified as immune complex mediated or complement mediated. Immune complex–mediated MPGN shows immunoglobulin and complement factors on immunofluorescence

TABLE 26.2 Glomerular Diseases Associated With Hypocomplementemia

Acute lupus nephritis
C3 glomerulopathy (C3 glomerulonephritis and dense deposit disease)
Cholesterol emboli
Cryoglobulinemic glomerulonephritis
Postinfectious glomerulonephritis
IgG4-related nephropathy
Fibrillary glomerulonephritis

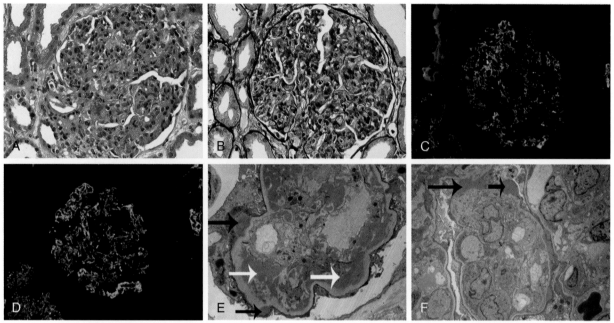

Fig. 26.5 Postinfectious glomerulonephritis. (A and B) Light microscopy shows diffuse endocapillary prolif-erative glomerulonephritis. Notice the prominent neutrophil infiltration in the glomerular capillaries (A, hema-toxylin and eosin; B, silver methenamine; both ×40). (C and D) Immunofluorescence studies show granular immunoglobulin G and C3 deposition along the capillary walls (both ×20). (E and F) Electron microscopy shows subendothelial deposits *(white arrows)* and subepithelial humplike deposits *(black arrows)*. The sub-endothelial deposits likely result from circulating immune complexes that are deposited along the glomerular capillary walls and drive the inflammatory response (E, ×5800). The subepithelial deposits likely represent in situ immune complex formation (F, ×2850).

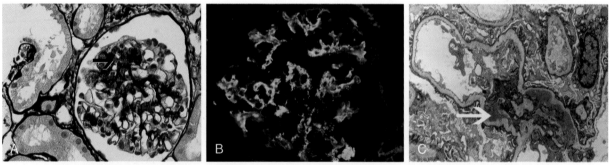

Fig. 26.6 Immunoglobulin A (IgA) nephropathy. (A) Light microscopy shows mesangial hypercellularity *(black arrow)* (silver methenamine, ×40). (B) Immunofluorescence microscopy shows bright mesangial IgA staining. (C) Electron microscopy shows large mesangial electron-dense deposits *(arrow)* (×7860).

microscopy. Complement-mediated MPGN shows complement factors and a lack of significant immunoglobulin on immunofluorescence microscopy (Fig. 26.8). Immune complex/Ig–mediated MPGN results from chronic infections, autoimmune diseases, and monoclonal gammopathies. Complement-mediated MPGN is caused by genetic or acquired dysregulation of the alternative pathway of complement (C3 glomerulopathy) and can be further subclassified as C3 glomerulonephritis and dense deposit disease (DDD) based on electron microscopy examination.

Immune complex–mediated MPGN precipitated by an infection is most commonly caused by HCV (i.e., cryoglobulinemic glomerulonephritis). The clinical presentation varies and can include nephrotic and nephritic features. In patients with cryoglobulinemic MPGN, the levels of C3, C4, and CH50 are persistently low, reflecting activation of classical complement pathway. Patients with C3 glomerulonephritis or DDD may have a persistently low level of C3 but a normal level of C4. A C3 nephritic factor is found in many cases. C3 nephritic factor

is an autoantibody to alternative pathway C3 convertase, resulting in persistent breakdown of C3.

The absence of well-designed studies based on the current insights in the pathogenesis of MPGN make it impossible to give strong treatment recommendations. From a practical point of view, patients with MPGN due to chronic infections (e.g., HCV, endocarditis), autoimmune disease, and plasma cell dyscrasias (monoclonal gammopathy) should undergo treatment of the underling disease. Patients with normal kidney function, no active urinary sediment, and non–nephrotic-range proteinuria can be treated conservatively with angiotensin II blockade to control blood pressure and reduce proteinuria, because the long-term outcome is relatively benign in this setting. Follow-up is required to detect early deterioration in kidney function. Patients with C3 glomerulonephritis or DDD with proteinuria greater than 1000 mg/24 h and/or abnormal kidney function but not rapidly progressive disease, and who do not have a genetic mutation leading to factor H deficiency, can be considered for additional treatment

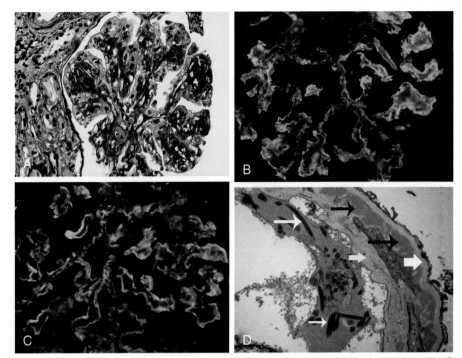

Fig. 26.7 Immune complex–mediated membranoproliferative glomerulonephritis due to hepatitis C virus infection. (A) Light microscopy shows a membranoproliferative pattern of injury with mesangial expansion, endocapillary proliferation, double-contour formation along the capillary walls, and lobular accentuation of the glomerular tufts (silver methenamine, ×40). (B and C) Immunofluorescence microscopy shows bright capillary wall staining for immunoglobulin M (B, ×40) and for C3 (C, ×40). (D) Electron microscopy shows capillary wall thickening and a double-contour formation due to accumulation of subendothelial electron-dense deposits *(black arrows)*, cellular elements, and new basement membrane formation (i.e., duplication) *(yellow arrow)* that produces the double contour. The *thick white arrow* indicates the old basement membrane, and fibrin tactoids *(white arrows)* in glomerular capillary loops indicate a prothrombotic state (×1350).

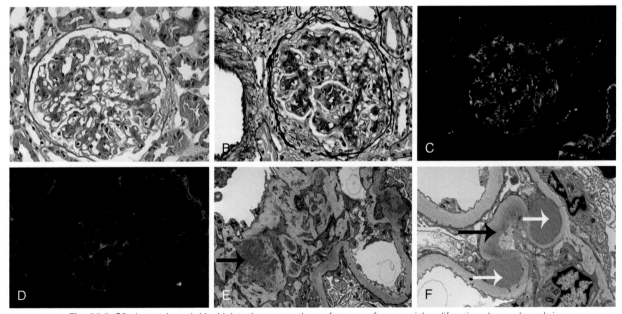

Fig. 26.8 C3 glomerulonephritis. Light microscopy shows features of mesangial proliferative glomerulonephritis (A, periodic acid–Schiff, ×40) and membranoproliferative glomerulonephritis (B, silver methenamine stain, ×40) in the same biopsy. Immunofluorescence microscopy shows bright granular mesangial and capillary wall staining for C3 (C) and negative staining for immunoglobulin G (D). (E) Electron microscopy shows a large accumulation of smudgy mesangial deposits *(arrow)* (×10,000). (F) Electron microscopy shows subendothelial deposits *(black arrow)* and subepithelial humplike deposits *(white arrows)* (×150,000). The subepithelial deposits sometimes make it difficult to distinguish C3 glomerulonephritis from postinfectious glomerulonephritis. However, C3 glomerulonephritis may not show Ig (as in this case), and the term *atypical postinfectious glomerulonephritis* sometimes is applied in cases of C3 glomerulonephritis with subepithelial humplike deposits.

with mycophenolate mofetil plus oral corticosteroids. Patients who have advanced renal insufficiency and severe tubulointerstitial fibrosis of renal biopsy are unlikely to benefit from immunosuppressive therapy.

Lupus Nephritis

Lupus nephritis occurs in up to 50% to 70% of patients with SLE and is associated with a poor prognosis. Proteinuria is the most common

TABLE 26.3 Abbreviated International Society of Nephrology/Renal Pathology Society 2003 Classification of Lupus Nephritis

Type	Morphologic Class	Renal Manifestation
I	Minimal mesangial lupus nephritis	Normal urinary sediment
I	Mesangial proliferative lupus nephritis	Low-grade hematuria and/or proteinuria Normal renal function
III	Focal lupus nephritis	Active sediment, proteinuria <3 g/1.73 m²/day
IV	Diffuse lupus nephritis	Nephritic and nephrotic syndromes Hypertension; progressive renal failure
V	Membranous lupus nephritis	Nephrotic syndrome
VI	Advanced sclerosing lupus nephritis	Inactive urinary sediment Chronic renal failure

Modified from Weening JJ, D'Agati VD, Schwartz MM, et al: The classification of glomerulonephritis in systemic lupus erythematosus revisited, J Am Soc Nephrol 15:241-250, 2004.

initial manifestation, and it is often in the nephrotic range and accompanied by a decline in renal function. Urinalysis does not always reflect the severity of the glomerular lesion, and kidney biopsy is indicated in those with proteinuria or active urinary sediment, or both, because the type of renal lesion influences the therapeutic decisions. The International Society of Nephrology/Renal Pathology Society (ISN/RPS) classification of lupus nephritis recognizes six morphologic classes of renal involvement (Table 26.3). However, patients may migrate from one class to another spontaneously or after treatment.

Immunofluorescence typically shows glomerular deposition of IgG, IgM, IgA, C1q, and C3 (i.e., full-house pattern). On electron microscopy, tubuloreticular inclusions are common within glomerular and vascular endothelial cells. Electron-dense deposits sometimes show fingerprint-like substructures) (Fig 26.9). Histologic lesions correlate with the prognosis; classes III and IV have the worst prognosis (see Fig 26.9). Other manifestations of SLE include acute and chronic tubulointerstitial nephritis and glomerular capillary thrombi in patients with antiphospholipid antibodies.

Three guidelines for the management of lupus nephritis have been published recently by the American College of Rheumatology, the Kidney Disease-Improving Global Outcomes (KDIGO) working group, and the Joint European League Against Rheumatism and European Renal Association–European Dialysis and Transplant Association (EULAR/ERA-EDTA). For class I lupus nephritis, the prognosis is excellent, and no immunosuppression is required. Patients with class II lupus nephritis and proteinuria less than 1 g/24 h should be treated as dictated by the extrarenal clinical manifestations of lupus. Patients with class II lupus nephritis and proteinuria greater than 3 g/24 h should be treated with corticosteroids or calcineurin inhibitors.

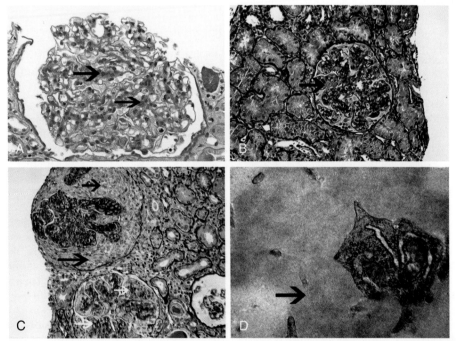

Fig. 26.9 Light microscopy (A to C) and electron microscopy (D) are used to identify lupus nephritis. (A) Mild mesangial proliferative glomerulonephritis (International Society of Nephrology/Renal Pathology Society [ISN/RPS] class II) has mesangial hypercellularity *(arrows)* (periodic acid–Schiff, ×40). (B) Diffuse endocapillary proliferation with cryoglobulins in the glomerular capillaries, identified as pale, silver-negative material *(arrow)* (silver methenamine, ×20). (C) In diffuse proliferative glomerulonephritis (ISN/RPS class IV), the glomerulus on top shows a large cellular crescent *(black arrows)*, and the glomerulus at the bottom shows diffuse endocapillary proliferation *(white arrows)* (silver methenamine, ×20). (D) Electron-dense deposits have fingerprint substructures *(arrow)* (×46,000).

TABLE 26.4   Cryoglobulins and Associated Diseases

Cryoglobulinemia Type	Immunoglobulin Class	Associated Diseases
I. Monoclonal immunoglobulins	M > G > A > BJP	Myeloma, Waldenström macroglobulinemia
II. Mixed cryoglobulins with monoclonal immunoglobulins	M/G ≫ G/G	Sjögren syndrome, Waldenström macroglobulinemia, lymphoma, essential cryoglobulinemia
III. Mixed polyclonal immunoglobulins	M/G	Infection, SLE, vasculitis, neoplasia, essential cryoglobulinemia

A, IgA; *BJP,* Bence Jones protein (κ light chain); *G,* IgG; *M,* IgM; *SLE,* systemic lupus erythematosus.

Patients with class III or IV lupus nephritis should undergo induction therapy with corticosteroids plus cyclophosphamide or mycophenolate mofetil because both are considered equivalent. Pure class V (membranous) lupus nephritis usually has a benign prognosis, and initial therapy should be supportive. However, patients with progressive or persistent nephrotic-range proteinuria should be treated with corticosteroids plus an additional immunosuppressive agent (e.g., cyclosporine, tacrolimus, mycophenolate mofetil or rituximab). Patients with ESRD should be considered for renal transplantation because there is a low rate of recurrence in the transplanted kidney.

Cryoglobulinemic Glomerulonephritis

Cryoglobulins are immunoglobulins that precipitate at low temperatures and redissolve on rewarming. Cryoglobulinemia usually leads to a systemic inflammatory syndrome with weakness, arthralgias or arthritis, palpable purpura, peripheral neuropathy, and glomerulonephritis. Serum levels of C4 are typically low due to activation of complement by the classical pathway. The disease mainly involves small to medium-sized blood vessels and causes vasculitis due to cryoglobulin-containing immune complexes.

Cryoglobulinemia is classified as type I, II, or III on the basis of immunoglobulin composition. It can be idiopathic or occur in association with autoimmune diseases (see Fig. 26.11B), malignancy, or infection (Table 26.4). HCV infection is the most common cause of cryoglobulinemia.

Renal disease occurs in 20% to 60% of patients with cryoglobulinemia and manifests as proteinuria, microscopic hematuria, nephrotic syndrome, or renal impairment. Hypertension is common and may be severe, particularly in the setting of acute nephritic syndrome. The cryocrit values correlate poorly with disease activity. On light microscopy, renal biopsy specimens show an immune complex–mediated membranoproliferative pattern of injury, and on electron microscopy, diffuse, dense subendothelial deposits with a microtubular or crystalline appearance may be seen occluding the capillary loops.

Treatment targets the underlying pathologic process to minimize or eliminate the associated cryoglobulinemia. Patients with active HCV infection, for example, should receive antiviral therapy when possible, and those with a monoclonal gammopathy should receive appropriate antimyeloma therapy. Immunosuppressive therapy (including the use of rituximab) with or without plasmapheresis should be considered for patients with a rapidly progressive, organ- or life-threatening course, regardless of the cause of the mixed cryoglobulinemia. Overall, the renal prognosis is usually good, with few patients progressing to ESRD. The long-term outcome reflects the underlying process.

Fibrillary Glomerulonephritis and Immunotactoid Glomerulopathy

Fibrillary glomerulonephritis and immunotactoid glomerulopathy are uncommon disorders, being present in 0.5 to 1% of native kidney biopsies. Fibrillary glomerulonephritis is by far more common, accounting for approximately 85% to 90% of cases. The identification of the protein DnaJ heat shock protein family (Hsp40) member B9 (DNAJB9) in the glomeruli of patients with fibrillary glomerulonephritis but not in those with immunotactoid glomerulopathy has established that the two are distinct, pathogenically unrelated disease entities (Fig. 26.10). In approximately one third of patients with fibrillary glomerulonephritis a history of malignancy, monoclonal gammopathy or autoimmune disease can be documented. By contrast, immunotactoid glomerulopathy is more frequently associated with chronic lymphocytic leukemia and related B-cell lymphomas or multiple myeloma.

In fibrillary glomerulonephritis, light microscopic findings are nondiagnostic and variable, showing patterns that may be seen in other glomerulonephritides. Immunofluorescence microscopy is positive for IgG, C3, and usually both kappa and lambda (i.e., polyclonal) light chains. Electron microscopy shows random fibrillar deposits in the mesangium and glomerular capillary walls that are clearly distinct from those seen in amyloidosis. The fibrils are larger than those in amyloidosis (16 to 24 nm in fibrillary glomerulonephritis and 30 to 50 nm in immunotactoid glomerulopathy (with microtubular formation) versus 10 nm in diameter in amyloidosis).

The presenting clinical features of fibrillary glomerulonephritis and immunotactoid glomerulopathy are similar to those in other forms of glomerular disease, including hypertension, hematuria, proteinuria, and abnormal renal function.

No therapies have been clearly shown to be beneficial for either fibrillary glomerulonephritis or immunotactoid glomerulopathy. Patients with an associated malignancy, monoclonal gammopathy or autoimmune disease, may benefit from treatment of the underlying disorder.

Pauci-Immune Glomerulonephritis: Antineutrophil Cytoplasmic Antibody–Associated Vasculitides

The ANCA-associated vasculitides (AAVs) are a group of three heterogeneous syndromes: granulomatosis with polyangiitis (GPA, formerly Wegener's granulomatosis), microscopic polyangiitis (MPA), and eosinophilic granulomatosis with polyangiitis (EGPA, formerly Churg-Strauss syndrome). The unifying feature is a necrotizing small vessel vasculitis with a predilection for the kidneys, lungs, and peripheral nervous system that occurs in association with autoantibodies against antigens in the cytoplasm of neutrophils (i.e., myeloperoxidase [MPO] and proteinase 3 [PR3]).

Approximately 75% of the patients with GPA are PR3-ANCA positive, and 20% are MPO-ANCA positive, whereas about 50% of patients with MPA are MPO-ANCA positive and about 40% are PR3-ANCA positive. Necrotizing granulomatous inflammation, which affects the upper and lower respiratory tract and frequently precedes other disease manifestations, is characteristic of GPA but not MPA. EGPA is characterized by asthma and eosinophilia in addition to features of small vessel vasculitis such as mononeuritis multiplex. AAV is the most common cause of a RPGN in patients older than 60 years. AAV is associated with signs and symptoms ranging from limited renal disease to RPGN and pulmonary-renal syndrome (Table 26.5). Renal biopsy is characterized by a focal, necrotizing, and crescentic glomerulonephritis with pauci-immune immunofluorescence (Fig. 26.11).

Patients with newly diagnosed severe AAV vasculitis can be treated with a combination of high-dose corticosteroids and cyclophosphamide or high-dose corticosteroids and rituximab. The PEXIVAS trial

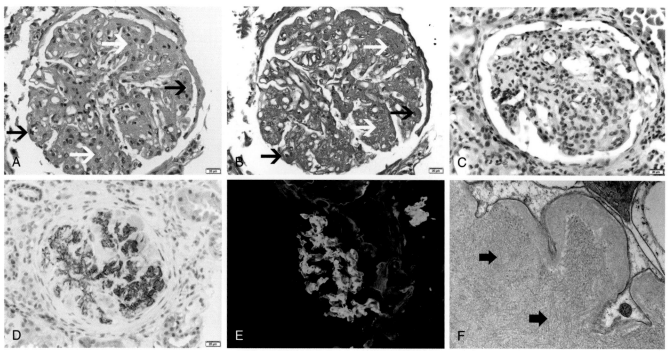

Fig. 26.10 Fibrillary glomerulonephritis. (A-B) Light microscopy showing mesangial expansion with increase in cellularity *(white arrow)* and thickened capillary walls *(black arrow)* (A, hematoxylin and eosin ×40; B, periodic acid–Schiff stain ×40). (C) Congo red stain is negative (×40). (D) Immunohistochemistry for DNAJB9 is positive. (E) Immunofluorescence studies show IgG staining in the mesangium and along capillary walls, and (F) electron microscopy shows fibrillary deposits *(thick arrows)* along the capillary walls (×30000).

TABLE 26.5 Signs and Symptoms of Antineutrophil Cytoplasmic Autoantibody Vasculitis

Abdominal pain and gastrointestinal bleeding
Cutaneous purpura, petechiae, nodules, ulcerations, and necrosis
Facial pain, necrotizing (hemorrhagic) sinusitis, and septal perforation
Hematuria, proteinuria, and renal failure
Hemoptysis and pulmonary infiltrates or nodules
Muscle and pancreatic enzymes in blood
Myalgias and arthralgias
Peripheral neuropathy (mononeuritis multiplex)

showed that addition of plasma exchange in patients with pulmonary hemorrhage, respiratory compromise, or severe renal failure (i.e., serum creatinine >5.5 mg/dL) is of no benefit. The prognosis for AAV varies. Those with severe renal failure have the worst prognosis, and even after successful therapy AAVs have a relapse rate of 30% to 50% in the first 5 years. In patients with renal involvement, rising ANCA titers are predictors of relapse. Patients with GPA or who are PR3-ANCA positive or presenting with relapsing disease are at higher risk for future relapses.

Anti–Glomerular Basement Membrane Antibody–Mediated Glomerulonephritis

Anti-GBM antibody–mediated glomerulonephritis (anti-GBM GN, formerly called Goodpasture disease) is a pulmonary-renal syndrome caused by circulating anti-GBM antibodies. On immunofluorescence staining of biopsy specimens, a linear pattern of IgG staining is seen along the GBM and alveolar basement membrane (Fig. 26.12) using antibodies directed against the α3 chain of type IV collagen (COL4A3

protein). Patients usually have RPGN and various degrees of pulmonary hemorrhage.

The treatment of anti-GBM GN is based on high-dose pulse methylprednisolone (1 g/day for 1 to 3 days) followed by corticosteroids (prednisone, 1 mg/kg/day up to 80 mg daily) in combination with oral cyclophosphamide (2 to 3 mg/kg/day up to 200 mg daily, adjusted for age and creatinine level) and plasma exchange. The prognosis is predicted in part by the percentage of circumferential crescents on the renal biopsy specimen, oliguria, and the need for dialysis. Those with an initial serum creatinine level less than 5.0 mg/dL have a 90% probability of renal survival at 5 years; but those with 100% circumferential crescents and on dialysis do not recover renal function, and immunosuppressive regimens should be avoided except in the case of pulmonary hemorrhage.

Anti-GBM GN rarely recurs. Patients with ESRD are candidates for renal transplantation after the antibody has disappeared (6 to 12 months).

GLOMERULAR DISEASES CAUSED BY PLASMA CELL DYSCRASIAS

Amyloidosis

Amyloidosis is characterized by systemic extracellular deposition of randomly arranged fibrils 8 to 12 nm in diameter that stain positive with Congo red (i.e., orange-green birefringence with polarized light) or thioflavin T. Several processes, including malignancy, genetic mutations, and aging, can produce at least 24 amyloidogenic proteins. With renal deposition, amyloid in biopsy specimens appears as pale, amorphous, extracellular deposits that are periodic acid–Schiff (PAS) and methenamine silver stain negative (Fig. 26.13).

The affinity for kidney compared with other target organs varies according to the type of amyloid protein. Renal manifestations include proteinuria, nephrotic syndrome, and renal failure. Affected patients typically have large kidneys on ultrasound, but the diagnosis depends

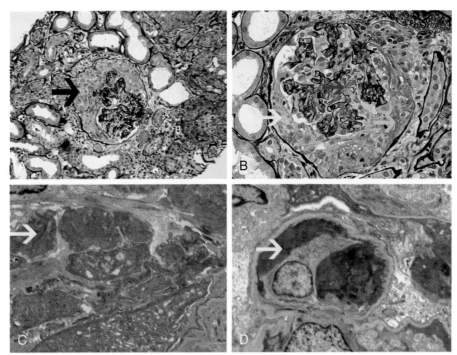

Fig. 26.11 Crescentic glomerulonephritis in a patient with MPO-ANCA associated vasculitis. (A and B) Light microscopy and silver methenamine staining show a large cellular crescent *(black arrow)* with fibrinoid necrosis *(blue arrow)*, hemorrhage into the Bowman capsule *(yellow arrow)*, and collapse of capillary tufts (A, ×20; B, ×40). (C and D) Electron microscopy shows fibrinoid necrosis (i.e., necrotizing lesion) in the Bowman space *(white arrow)* and capillary loops *(short white arrow)* (both, ×11100).

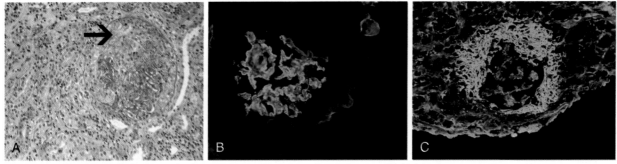

Fig. 26.12 Anti–glomerular basement membrane–mediated disease. (A) Light microscopy shows a large, circumferential crescent *(arrow)*, with collapse of the glomerular capillary tufts and many infiltrating neutrophils in the crescent (periodic acid–Schiff, ×20). Immunofluorescence microscopy shows linear staining for anti–immunoglobulin G antibody (B) along the glomerular capillary walls and bright staining for fibrinogen in the Bowman tuft (C), indicating crescent formation and fibrinoid necrosis (both, ×40).

on demonstration of amyloid deposits. After amyloid is detected, typing should be performed when possible because treatments vary according to the protein involved. The most common approach to amyloid typing involves immunofluorescence or immunohistochemistry, but genetic testing and liquid chromatography mass spectrometry are also helpful for high-resolution amyloid typing.

Treatment of amyloidosis depends on the origin of the amyloidogenic protein. In patients with amyloid light chain (AL) amyloidosis, antimyeloma therapy can be beneficial. In selected cases, bone marrow transplantation has led to resolution of the disease. Secondary amyloid A (AA) amyloidosis is most common in patients with rheumatoid arthritis, inflammatory bowel disease, chronic infection, or familial Mediterranean fever. Treatment of AA amyloidosis is directed at the underlying inflammatory process with antimicrobials or anti-inflammatory medications.

Light Chain Deposition Disease

Light chain deposition disease is a paraprotein-associated disorder. The peak incidence is in the sixth decade of life, and men are affected more commonly than women. Approximately 30% to 50% of patients with light chain deposition disease have multiple myeloma. Most have a detectable monoclonal protein (usually κ light chain) in the serum or urine, but no hematologic abnormality is identified in about 10% of cases. The clinical presentation is very heterogeneous and can vary from mild renal dysfunction, proteinuria without nephrotic syndrome, to clinically overt acute renal failure. Fanconi syndrome, characterized by normoglycemic glycosuria, aminoaciduria, and phosphaturia, is the classic presentation. Immunoglobulin deposits in other organs may result in myriad of associated clinical symptoms.

Renal biopsy specimens show acellular, eosinophilic mesangial nodules that stain strongly positive with PAS, often mimicking diabetes

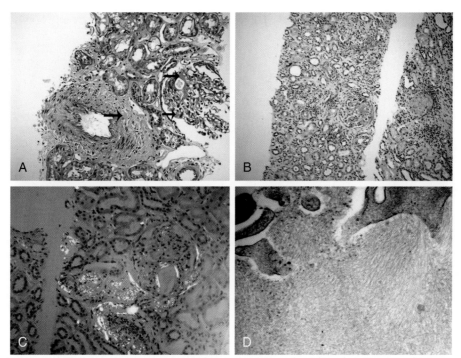

Fig. 26.13 Amyloidosis. (A) Light microscopy shows amyloid deposits characterized by mesangial expansion *(small arrows)* with material negative for staining. The material is also seen in vessel walls, where the *arrow* points to vascular deposits (periodic acid–Schiff stain, ×20). (B) Congo red staining is positive for amyloid and shows reddish-brown material in the glomeruli, interstitium, and vessel walls (×10). (C) Amyloid deposits show apple green to orange-yellow birefringence under polarized light (×20). (D) Electron microscopy shows randomly oriented amyloid fibrils. The fibrils measured 9 nm thick (×49,000).

mellitus. The deposited monoclonal proteins do not form fibrils and are Congo red negative. Immunofluorescence microscopic findings are diagnostic, with diffuse linear immunoglobulin light chain deposition (κ in 80% of cases) along the GBM and tubular basement membranes. On electron microscopy punctate powdery granular electron dense deposits are seen along the GBM and TBM (Fig. 26.14).

Encouraging results have emerged with the use of anti-plasma cells targeted therapy and autologous stem cell transplantation. Unless remission is achieved after chemotherapy, the disease will recur in the kidney allograft.

FIBRILLARY GLOMERULONEPHRITIS AND IMMUNOTACTOID GLOMERULOPATHY

See section on immune-complex glomerulonephritis.

GLOMERULONEPHRITIS ASSOCIATED WITH VIRAL INFECTIONS

Hepatitis B

HBV-mediated glomerular disease usually manifests as membranous nephropathy, especially in children. The diagnosis of HBV-mediated glomerular disease requires detection of the virus in the blood and the exclusion of other causes of glomerular diseases.

HBV-mediated glomerular disease usually has a favorable prognosis, with a high spontaneous remission rate in children, but it is often progressive in adults. Patients with HBV infection and glomerulonephritis should receive antiviral therapy (e.g., entecavir) as recommended by standard clinical practice guidelines for management of HBV infection. Those with severe vasculitis or RPGN may be candidates for immunosuppressive therapy in combination with antiviral

therapy. Rituximab treatment of patients who are positive for HBV has been associated with fatal acute hepatitis. Rituximab is therefore contraindicated in patients with chronic HBV unless antiviral therapy is also given and in patients with an active hepatitis flare.

Hepatitis C

See the section on cryoglobulinemic glomerulonephritis.

HIV-Associated Nephropathy

Patients with HIV infection can have many forms of kidney injury due to sepsis, co-infection with HBV or HCV, nephrotoxic drugs, and use of antiretroviral agents. HIV-associated nephropathy (HIVAN) is a clinicopathologic entity characterized by nephrotic-range proteinuria and a collapsing form of FSGS, often with microcystic tubular dilation. On electron microscopy, tubuloreticular inclusions (i.e., interferon fingerprints) may be seen within the glomerular and vascular endothelial cells.

HIVAN occurs almost exclusively in patients of African descent when CD4 levels are low. It is thought to be caused by infection and subsequent expression of HIV viral genes in podocytes. The onset of proteinuria is typically acute. Proteinuria can be greater than 10 g/day, and renal insufficiency can progress rapidly.

THROMBOTIC MICROANGIOPATHIES

Thrombotic microangiopathy is characterized by thrombocytopenia, microangiopathic hemolytic anemia, and microvascular occlusion, resulting in various degrees of organ dysfunction. Markers of hemolysis include low haptoglobin levels, increased levels of lactate dehydrogenase and unconjugated bilirubin, and a high reticulocyte count. Schistocytes are seen in peripheral blood smears.

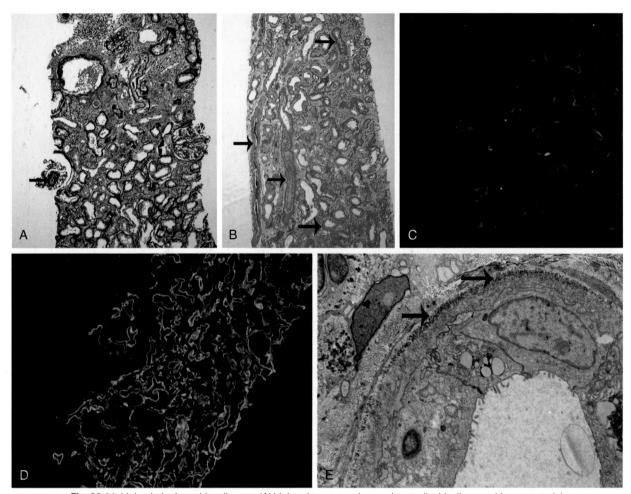

Fig. 26.14 Light chain deposition disease. (A) Light microscopy shows glomeruli with silver-positive mesangial nodules *(arrow)* and thickened tubular basement membranes (silver methenamine, ×10). (B) Periodic acid–Schiff staining shows thickened, wavy tubular basement membranes *(arrow)* (×10). Immunofluorescence studies found negative staining for λ light chains (C) and bright staining for κ light chains (D) along the tubular basement membranes (both ×10). (E) Electron microscopy shows granular, punctate, electron-dense deposits *(arrows)* along the tubular basement membranes (×5800).

The quintessential forms of thrombotic microangiopathy include hemolytic uremic syndrome (HUS) and thrombotic thrombocytopenic purpura (TTP). Although previously thought to represent different manifestations of the same disease, these disorders are distinct clinically and mechanistically. In adults, predominant neurologic involvement suggests a diagnosis of TTP, and predominant renal involvement points to HUS. In most cases, the clinical presentations are very similar, making it difficult to distinguish between HUS and TTP on clinical grounds alone. Other causes of thrombotic microangiopathy include malignant hypertension, drugs (e.g., cocaine, quinidine, ticlopidine), autoimmune diseases (e.g., SLE, scleroderma, antiphospholipid antibody syndrome), malignancy, HIV infection, and antibody-mediated rejection.

Kidney biopsy in HUS and TTP reveals microthrombi in glomerular capillaries and arterioles, and mesangial expansion with loose granular material, called *mesangiolysis*, may be seen in HUS and TTP and in malignant hypertension or autoimmune diseases (Fig. 26.15). Malignant hypertension and autoimmune diseases may also show thickening and intimal fibrosis of arteries and onion-skinning (i.e., laminated deposition of basement membrane–type material) of the vessel walls. Thrombi are common and may occlude the vascular lumen.

Hemolytic Uremic Syndrome

Two subtypes of HUS are recognized: a sporadic or diarrhea-associated form (D+ HUS) and an atypical or non–diarrhea-associated form (D− HUS). D+ HUS is the most frequently encountered form, and it is linked strongly to ingestion of meat contaminated with enterohemorrhagic *Escherichia coli* or other infectious agents. The bacterium produces a Shiga-like toxin that binds to a glycolipid receptor on renal endothelial cells and triggers activation of the alternative complement cascade, leading to endothelial damage. Therapy for D+ HUS is supportive. Children with D+ HUS have a good prognosis (90% recover renal function), but older patients have increased mortality rates and unfavorable long-term renal survival.

Atypical or D− HUS represents 10% to 15% of the cases of HUS and is more common in adults. The disease results from genetic mutations or autoantibodies against complement factors or complement factors regulating proteins (i.e., C3, factor B, factor H, factor I, MCP, CFHR1, and CFHR3) that control the activity of C3 convertase of the alternative complement pathway. The resulting defective control of C3 convertase leads to widespread activation of the complement cascade.

The complement inhibitor eculizumab has been approved for the treatment of patients with atypical HUS. Eculizumab and plasma infusion may also be considered in the treatment of children with D+ HUS and severe central nervous system involvement such as seizures, stroke, or coma.

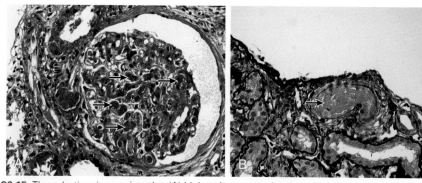

Fig. 26.15 Thrombotic microangiopathy. (A) Light microscopy shows multiple, small thrombi *(arrows)* in glomerular capillaries in the setting of hemolytic uremic syndrome (Masson trichrome, ×40). (B) Light microscopy shows a thrombus *(arrow)* in a small artery in the setting of scleroderma (silver methenamine, ×20).

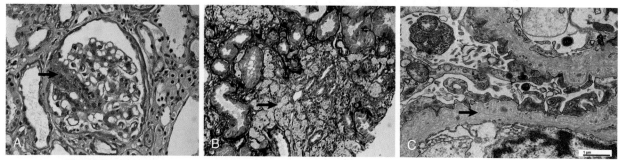

Fig. 26.16 Alport syndrome. (A) Light microscopy shows focal segmental glomerulosclerosis *(arrow)* (periodic acid–Schiff, ×40). (B) Light microscopy shows numerous foam cells *(arrow)* in the interstitium (silver methenamine, ×40). (C) Electron microscopy shows thickening of the glomerular capillary walls with multiple lamellations of basement membrane material *(arrow)* and formation of the classic basket-weave appearance (×212,000).

Thrombotic Thrombocytopenic Purpura

TTP results from mutations in the von Willebrand factor (VWF)–cleaving protease (ADAMTS13) or development of an autoantibody against ADAMTS13. ADAMTS13 cleaves large multimers of VWF, and abnormalities or deficiency of ADAMTS13 activity affects VWF function. Patients can have acute or chronic (i.e., relapsing) TTP. Microthrombi rich in large VWF multimers develop in the arterioles and capillaries of the brain and other organs.

Genetic or acquired forms of ADAMTS13 deficiency can be treated by plasma infusion or exchange to supply functional protease. Plasma exchange should be initiated promptly, based on findings of microangiopathic hemolytic anemia and thrombocytopenia without evidence of other causes of thrombotic microangiopathy (e.g., scleroderma, malignancy, antiphospholipid syndrome). Treatment should not await test results for the levels or activity of ADAMTS13.

DISEASES WITH GLOMERULAR BASEMENT MEMBRANE ABNORMALITIES

Alport Syndrome

Alport syndrome is an inherited disorder of basement membranes. In more than one half of patients, the disease results from a mutation in the *COL4A5* gene that codes for the α5 chain of type IV collagen (α5[IV]). The mutation in *COL4A5* disables a developmental switch in the GBM collagen that retains its embryonic phenotype and results in a friable GBM.

Alport syndrome is frequently associated with sensorineural hearing loss and ocular abnormalities (e.g., lenticonus of the anterior

lens capsule). Patients characteristically have persistent or intermittent hematuria and usually have mild proteinuria, which progresses with age and may reach nephrotic range in up to 30%. The disease is X-linked in approximately 85% of patients, but autosomal recessive and autosomal dominant patterns of inheritance have been described.

In virtually all male patients, the syndrome progresses to ESRD, often before the age of 30 years. The disease is usually mild in heterozygous women, but some develop ESRD, usually after the age of 50 years. The rate of progression to ESRD is fairly constant among affected men within individual families, but it varies markedly from family to family. The degree of deafness correlates with the rate of progression to ESRD.

On light microscopy, the glomerular changes are nonspecific. Diagnostic features are usually seen on electron microscopy. At an early stage, thinning of the GBM may be the only visible abnormality and may suggest thin basement membrane disease. With time, the GBM thickens, and the lamina densa splits into several irregular layers that may branch and rejoin, producing a characteristic basket-weave appearance (Fig. 26.16).

Immunohistochemical studies of type IV collagen show the absence of α3(IV), α4(IV), and α5(IV) chains from the GBM and distal tubular basement membrane. This abnormality occurs only in patients with Alport syndrome and is diagnostic. In families with an unquestionable diagnosis, evaluation of patients with newly diagnosed hematuria can be limited to kidney ultrasound and urinary tract examination in most cases. If a defined mutation has been previously identified, molecular diagnosis of affected men or gene-carrying women is possible. In other cases, confirmation of the diagnosis can be obtained by examination of skin biopsy by immunofluorescence for the expression of the α5(IV)

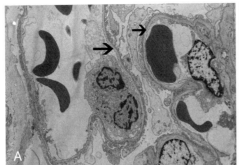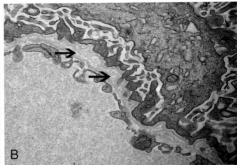

Fig. 26.17 (A) In thin glomerular basement membrane nephropathy, electron microscopy shows glomerular basement membranes *(arrows)* that are 198 nm thick (×5800). (B) Alport syndrome. Electron microscopy showing thickened glomerular capillary walls with lamellations and disorganization of the glomerular basement membranes (×30000). Arrows point to thin glomerular basement membranes in A and to the lamellations in B.

chain. Absence of the α5(IV) chain from epidermal basement membrane is diagnostic of X-linked Alport syndrome and may avoid a renal biopsy. Direct sequencing of the *COL4A5* gene can help to diagnose patients in whom a clear diagnosis cannot be made based on clinical findings and histologic methods or to identify the carrier state in asymptomatic female members of X-linked Alport syndrome families.

No specific treatment is available for Alport syndrome. Tight control of blood pressure and moderate protein restriction are recommended to retard the progression of renal disease, but the benefit is unproven. Patients with Alport syndrome are phenotypic knockouts for the α3(IV) chain. Consequently, kidney transplantation carries a 5% to 10% risk of subsequent anti-GBM GN due to the introduction of an intact α3(IV) chain with the transplanted kidney and subsequent generation of auto-antibodies to the antigen present in the intact α3(IV) chain of the transplanted kidney.

Thin Glomerular Basement Membrane Nephropathy

Thin glomerular basement membrane nephropathy, also known as benign familial hematuria, is a relatively common condition characterized by isolated glomerular hematuria and associated with the renal biopsy finding of an excessively thin GBM. It is usually transmitted as an autosomal dominant disease. Heterozygous mutations in the *COL4A3* or *COL4A4* genes have been described in numerous patients with thin glomerular basement membrane nephropathy, indicating a genetically heterogeneous condition.

The usual clinical presentation is isolated, persistent hematuria that is first detected in childhood. In some patients, hematuria is intermittent and may not manifest until adulthood. On light microscopy, glomeruli appear normal, and immunofluorescence microscopy shows no immunoglobulin or complement deposition. Electron microscopy shows diffuse thinning of the GBM (Fig. 26.17). In adults, a GBM thickness less than 250 nm strongly suggests thin GBM disease.

The condition is usually benign and requires no specific treatment. However, a few patients have progressive renal disease that leads to ESRD.

FABRY'S DISEASE

Fabry's disease is an X-linked recessive inborn error of glycosphingolipid metabolism caused by deficient activity of the lysosomal enzyme α-galactosidase A, which results in the progressive accumulation of neutral glycosphingolipids (predominately globotriaosylceramide, particularly in the vascular endothelial cells of the kidney and heart.

Early manifestations of the disease include angiokeratoma, episodic pain crises, and hypohidrosis. With time, progressive

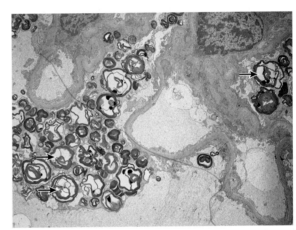

Fig. 26.18 Fabry's disease. Electron microscopy shows visceral epithelial cells (i.e., podocytes) with numerous multilamellated structures called *myelin bodies* or *zebra bodies (arrows)* that are made of glycosphingolipids (×4800).

globotriaosylceramide accumulation in the microvasculature in the kidney, heart, and brain leads to clinical manifestations such as proteinuria, renal failure, cardiac arrhythmias, and strokes, resulting in early death during the fourth and fifth decades of life of affected men.

Light microscopy reveals vacuolated glomerular cells, especially podocytes. Electron microscopy shows enlarged podocytes lysosomes filled with osmiophilic, granular to lamellated membrane structures (i.e., zebra bodies) (Fig. 26.18). Enzyme replacement therapy can lead to significant improvement of neuropathic pain, but the beneficial effects on the severity or progression of other disease manifestations are less clear.

DIABETIC NEPHROPATHY

Diabetic nephropathy accounts for more than 50% of patients on dialysis in the United States. In type 1 diabetes mellitus, nephropathy usually manifests 10 to 15 years after the initial diagnosis; and a similar natural history is likely for patients with type 2 diabetes mellitus. The main risk factors include a positive family history of diabetic nephropathy, hypertension, and poor glycemic control. The risk may be greater in some racial groups (e.g., Pima Indians, African Americans).

The pathogenesis is complex. Increased glycosylation of proteins with accumulation of advanced glycosylation end products that

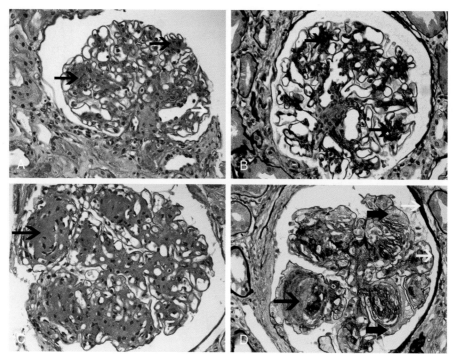

Fig. 26.19 Light microscopy shows diabetic glomerulosclerosis. (A and B) Early diabetic nodule formation *(arrows)*. (C and D) Well-formed Kimmelstiel-Wilson lesions result from mesangial expansion *(thin black arrows)*. The nodules are periodic acid–Schiff and silver methenamine positive. The glomerular capillary lumen is distended by formation of small microaneurysms *(thick black arrows)*. The glomerular basement membrane and Bowman capsule *(white arrows)* are thickened (A and C, periodic acid–Schiff; B and D, silver methenamine; all ×40).

cross-link with collagen and glomerular hyperfiltration with hypertension are important. Microalbuminuria (i.e., urinary albumin excretion >30 but <300 mg/24 h) is the initial manifestation of diabetic nephropathy. With time, microalbuminuria may evolve into overt proteinuria (>300 mg/24 h), with the degree of proteinuria correlating roughly with the renal prognosis.

After overt proteinuria develops, progression to ESRD is relentless, although rates of decline vary among patients. For patients with type 1 diabetes, there is a strong correlation (95%) between the development of nephropathy and other signs of diabetic microvascular compromise (e.g., diabetic retinopathy), but the correlation is weaker for patients with type 2 diabetes. Hypertension is almost universal among patients with proteinuria. It is difficult to control and usually requires at least three antihypertensive agents.

On renal biopsy, early signs of diabetic nephropathy include glomerular hypertrophy and thickening of the GBM. As the disease progresses, arteriolar hyalinosis, arteriosclerosis, and progressive mesangial expansion (i.e., diffuse diabetic glomerulosclerosis) and nodular formations (i.e., Kimmelstiel-Wilson nodules) develop (Fig. 26.19). For patients with a history of diabetes longer than 10 years and retinopathy, a renal biopsy may not be necessary. However, renal biopsy is indicated for patients with an atypical course of the disease (e.g., nephrotic syndrome), those with less than 10 years of type 1 diabetes, or patients with rapid loss of renal function.

Treatment with ACEIs or ARBs slows progression of diabetic nephropathy and should be used in all patients with albuminuria, even if normotensive. Tight glycemic control (i.e., glycated hemoglobin <7.0%) may also retard progression of diabetic nephropathy. Target systolic blood pressure should be less than 125 mm Hg, but this may be difficult to achieve and may require multiple medications and a strict low-salt diet.

SUGGESTED READINGS

De Vriese AS, Glassock RJ, Nath KA, et al: A proposal for a serology-based approach to membranous nephropathy, J Am Soc Nephrol 28(2):421–430, 2017.

De Vriese AS, Sethi S, Nath KA, et al: Differentiating primary, genetic, and secondary FSGS in adults: A clinicopathologic approach, J Am Soc Nephrol 29(3):759–774, 2018.

Kashtan CE: Alport syndrome: Achieving early diagnosis and treatment, Am J Kidney Dis S0272-6386(20)30734-4, 2020.

Kitching AR, Anders HJ, Basu N, et al: ANCA-associated vasculitis, Nat Rev Dis Primers 6(1):71, 2020.

McAdoo SP, Pusey CD: Anti-glomerular basement membrane disease, Clin J Am Soc Nephrol 12(7):1162–1172, 2017.

Noris M, Remuzzi G: Atypical hemolytic-uremic syndrome, N Engl J Med 361(17):1676–1687, 2009.

Ortiz A, Germain DP, Desnick RJ, et al: Fabry disease revisited: Management and treatment recommendations for adult patients, Mol Genet Metab 123(4):416–427, 2018.

Roccatello D, Saadoun D, Ramos-Casals M, et al: Cryoglobulinaemia, Nat Rev Dis Primers 4(1):11, 2018.

Sethi S, Fervenza FC: Membranoproliferative glomerulonephritis—a new look at an old entity, N Engl J Med 366(12):1119–1131, 2012.

Vivarelli M, Massella L, Ruggiero B, et al: Minimal change disease, Clin J Am Soc Nephrol 12:332–345, 2017.

27

Major Nonglomerular Disorders of the Kidney

Nilum Rajora, Shani Shastri, Pooja Koolwal, Ramesh Saxena

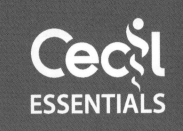

INTRODUCTION

Nonglomerular structures of the kidney include blood vessels, tubules, and interstitium. The tubulointerstitial compartment comprises 80% of kidney parenchyma, with most of the volume accounted for by tubules, interstitial cells, extracellular matrix, and interstitial fluid. Although primary glomerular and vascular diseases are associated with significant tubulointerstitial changes, the clinical presentations are dominated by injury of the glomeruli and the vasculature, and are discussed in Chapters 26 and 28.

Primary tubulointerstitial disorders are characterized by structural and functional abnormalities predominantly involving kidney tubules and the interstitium and are associated with a myriad of clinical presentations based on the principal structure involved: acute tubulointerstitial nephritis, characterized by sudden onset and a rapid decline in kidney function; chronic tubulointerstitial nephropathy, characterized by a more protracted clinical course; cystic diseases with kidney cysts and kidney failure; nephrolithiasis with pain, hematuria, and sometimes acute kidney injury (AKI). This chapter will cover primary tubulointerstitial disorders of the kidney.

ACUTE INTERSTITIAL NEPHRITIS

Definition, Epidemiology, and Pathology

Acute interstitial nephritis (AIN), also called *tubulointerstitial nephritis*, is characterized by inflammation and edema of the kidney interstitium; glomeruli and vessels are distinctly normal. AIN is associated with an acute, rapid decline in kidney function and is a common cause of AKI. AIN is seen in 1% to 3% of kidney biopsies, but if biopsy is done in the setting of AKI with clinical suspicion for AIN, 15% to 27% of biopsies show AIN.

On gross examination, the kidneys are pale and swollen. Histologically, the hallmarks of AIN include interstitial edema and infiltration of the interstitium with inflammatory cells comprising lymphocytes, monocytes, plasma cells, eosinophils, and macrophages (E-Figs. 27.1 and 27.2). This inflammation can progress to fibrotic changes in 7 to 10 days. Immunofluorescence studies typically are unrevealing. Tubular basement membrane immune deposits can be seen in cases of AIN associated with some drug-induced tubulointerstitial nephritis, immunoglobulin G4 (IgG4)–associated nephritis, membranous nephropathy, membranoproliferative glomerulonephritis, lupus nephritis, Sjögren syndrome, and other autoimmune diseases.

Any drug can cause AIN but frequently used therapeutic drugs merit particular emphasis. Common causes of AIN are shown in Table 27.1. They include antibiotics, allopurinol, mesalamine, nonsteroidal anti-inflammatory drugs (NSAIDs), proton pump inhibitors, and chemotherapeutic agents. Other causes of AIN include infections, autoimmune disorders, tubulointerstitial nephritis and uveitis

syndrome, snakebite, and herbal supplements. Nephrotoxicity of novel biologic agents used in cancer therapy is increasingly being recognized (see Table 27.1). Several of these drugs are associated with AIN. In many such cases, autoimmunity rather than drug sensitivity is the basis of tubulointerstitial inflammation.

Clinical Presentation

In most cases, AIN begins abruptly with a decrease in kidney function within days of exposure to the offending agent. However, AIN may ensue after several weeks of the exposure in some cases. Characteristic clinical manifestations include rash, fever, and eosinophilia. Modest proteinuria (usually <1 g/day) or hematuria may be observed, and oliguria is uncommon. A high index of suspicion is required for diagnosis because these features may be absent.

Diagnosis and Differential Diagnosis

When evaluating a patient with a recent decline in kidney function, the diagnosis of AIN is suggested by a history of exposure to the known offending agents coupled with typical clinical features. In addition to identifying elevated serum creatinine levels, a urinalysis can detect the characteristic findings of white blood cells, red blood cells, and white blood cell casts in urine. Identification of eosinophils in urine with Hansel or Wright stains is highly suggestive, but their absence does not rule out AIN. Moreover, eosinophils in urine can be observed in other diseases, including cholesterol embolism, urinary tract infections, parasitic disorders, and glomerulonephritis.

Unfortunately, there is currently no noninvasive test that reliably diagnoses drug-induced AIN. Kidney biopsy should be considered when the diagnosis is not obvious. Besides tubular injury, other histologic features may suggest the underlying disease that is associated with AIN. IgG4-related AIN has presence of tubular basement membrane immune complex deposits and an increase in IgG4-positive plasma cells in the interstitium. Sarcoidosis associated AIN may also have granulomas on biopsy, and AIN related to systemic lupus erythematosus (SLE) may also show diffused immune complex deposits on immunofluorescence. A definitive diagnosis of AIN requires a kidney biopsy, although most times it is not necessary for management when clinical features are highly suggestive.

Treatment and Prognosis

Treatment of patients with AIN consists of removal of the offending drug and management of the underlying infection or autoimmune process. The role of corticosteroids in limiting the inflammatory process is controversial, but early use (within 7 to 14 days) may decrease the duration of AIN and protect kidney function. When indicated, the usual approach includes high-dose intravenous methylprednisolone (250 mg consecutively for 3 days), followed by oral prednisone (1 mg/kg) tapering over 4 to 6 weeks. Patients who are intolerant or resistant

TABLE 27.1 Causes of Acute Interstitial Nephritis

Cause	Examples
Antibiotics	Penicillin
	Cephalosporin
	Sulfa drugs
	Ciprofloxacin
	Rifampin
Nonsteroidal anti-inflammatory drugs	Naproxen
	Ibuprofen
	Diclofenac
	Celecoxib
Diuretics	Thiazides
	Furosemide
	Triamterene
Other drugs	Cimetidine
	Proton pump inhibitors
	Phenytoin
	Allopurinol
Chemotherapeutic agents	Ifosfamide
	Interferon
	Sorafenib
	Sunitinib
	Adriamycin
	Ipilimumab
	Carboplatin
	Bevacizumab
Systemic infections	Legionnaires disease
	Leptospirosis
	Streptococcal infection
	Cytomegalovirus infection
Primary kidney infections	Acute bacterial pyelonephritis
Autoimmune disorders	Sarcoidosis
	Sjögren syndrome

TABLE 27.2 Clinical Findings That Suggest Chronic Interstitial Nephritis

Hyperchloremic metabolic acidosis (out of proportion to the degree of kidney injury)
Hyperkalemia (out of proportion to the degree of kidney injury)
Reduced maximal urinary concentrating ability (e.g., polyuria, nocturia)
Partial or complete Fanconi syndrome (e.g., phosphaturia, bicarbonaturia, aminoaciduria, uricosuria, glycosuria)
Modest proteinuria (<2 g/day)
Anemia
Hypertension

infiltration within the interstitial compartment (E-Fig. 27.3). The infiltrates are typically less conspicuous compared with AIN, and there is more interstitial fibrosis. In earlier stages of CIN, glomeruli are usually spared, but with progression, glomerular abnormalities such as segmental and global sclerosis can develop.

Clinical Presentation and Laboratory Findings

Patients with CIN are usually asymptomatic until they develop overt chronic kidney disease (CKD). The features are nonspecific and include fatigue, lack of appetite, nausea, vomiting, hypertension, and sleep disturbances, and other laboratory and clinical findings may develop, as listed in Table 27.2. CIN can also cause proximal or distal tubular dysfunction, which can lead to defects in acidification of the urine, partial or complete Fanconi syndrome and decreased concentrating ability. Laboratory data for these patients may show elevated levels of creatinine, proteinuria, hematuria, glycosuria, and pyuria. Due to the destruction of erythropoietin-producing interstitial cells, anemia, associated fatigue, and decreased exercise tolerance are common as CIN progresses.

Diagnosis and Differential Diagnosis

The histologic findings of CIN are nonspecific, and the differential diagnosis can be extensive, as shown in Table 27.3. Repeated injuries from drugs, toxins, radiation nephritis, and reflux nephropathy can result in a similar histologic picture. The most common cause of CIN is chronic NSAID use. Other causes include infections, immune-mediated disorders, drug reactions, hematologic disorders, chronic urinary tract obstruction, and urinary reflux. Some metabolic disorders and exposure to heavy metals can also lead to CIN. The clinical importance, distinguishing features, causes, and management of several forms of CIN are discussed in the following sections.

Analgesic Nephropathy

Analgesic nephropathy is the prototype CIN, and it occurs commonly worldwide. This disorder is caused by long-term ingestion of aspirin in various combinations with phenacetin, caffeine, or acetaminophen. In its most severe form, analgesic nephropathy is associated with papillary necrosis.

The cumulative amount of phenacetin-acetaminophen combination required to cause CIN is estimated to be at least 2 to 3 kg. Although initially thought to be exclusively associated with phenacetin-containing combinations, all analgesics, including acetaminophen, aspirin, and NSAIDs, are capable of inducing CIN.

Analgesic nephropathy is most commonly detected in women in the sixth and seventh decades of life. Patients with analgesic nephropathy may have elevated serum creatinine, modest proteinuria, sterile pyuria, and anemia. Occasionally, patients develop flank pain and gross hematuria, suggesting papillary necrosis. Diagnosis is supported

to steroids may benefit from mycophenolate mofetil (500 to 1000 mg twice daily).

Most cases of drug-related AIN resolve after removal of the offending drug. In tubulointerstitial nephritis and uveitis syndrome, both the ocular and kidney changes respond to a brief course of corticosteroids, but the disease can relapse. The overall prognosis depends on the duration of the AIN; a longer interval between onset of AIN and drug withdrawal can lead to irreversible kidney damage. Because of the rapid transformation of interstitial cellular infiltrates into fibrosis, up to 40% of patients may not fully recover baseline kidney function, and about 10% of the patients may become dialysis dependent.

CHRONIC INTERSTITIAL NEPHRITIS

Chronic interstitial nephritis (CIN) is a clinicopathologic diagnosis. Prolonged exposure to a causative agent initiates an indolent inflammatory process, and CIN can lead to permanent kidney damage over months to years before it manifests clinically. Patients usually have a gradual decline in kidney function. CIN is common and accounts for 15% to 30% of all cases of end-stage renal disease (ESRD).

Pathology

Histologically, CIN shows tubular atrophy, flattened epithelial cells, tubule dilation, interstitial fibrosis, and areas of mononuclear cell

TABLE 27.3   Conditions Associated With Chronic Interstitial Nephritis

Associated Conditions	Examples
Hereditary diseases	Karyomegalic interstitial nephritis
Metabolic disturbances	Hypercalcemia, nephrocalcinosis
	Hyperuricemia
	Hyperoxaluria
	Hypokalemia
	Cystinosis
Drugs and toxins	Analgesics, nonsteroidal anti-inflammatory drugs
	Lead
	Nitrosoureas
	Cisplatin
	Calcineurin inhibitors
	Lithium
	Chinese herbs
	Olanzapine
Immune-mediated diseases	Granulomatosis with polyangiitis (Wegener's granulomatosis)
	Sjögren syndrome
	Systemic lupus erythematosus
	Vasculitis
	Sarcoidosis
	Crohn's disease
Hematologic disease or malignancy	Multiple myeloma
	Sickle cell disease
	Lymphoma
Infection	Chronic pyelonephritis
	Xanthogranulomatous pyelonephritis
	Hepatitis
	Epstein-Barr virus
	HIV
Obstruction	Tumors
	Stones
	Bladder outlet obstruction
	Vesicoureteral reflux
Miscellaneous disorders	Mesoamerican nephropathy
	Radiation nephritis
	Hypertensive arterionephrosclerosis
	Renal ischemic disease

by a history of heavy analgesic use, and computed tomography (CT) may reveal microcalcifications at the papillary tips.

Treatment of analgesic nephropathy is supportive and includes discontinuation of analgesic use. Long-term follow-up studies are characterized by progression to ESRD requiring renal replacement therapies. A high incidence of uroepithelial cancers is also observed in patients with long-term analgesic use.

Chinese Herb Nephropathy and Balkan Endemic Nephropathy

Chinese herb nephropathy (CHN) and Balkan endemic nephropathy (BEN), also called *aristolochic acid nephropathy* (AAN), are chronic tubulointerstitial kidney diseases associated with urothelial carcinoma. The clinical expression and pathologic lesions observed at different stages of CHN and BEN are strikingly similar except for the higher prevalence of CHN among women and familial clustering of BEN. Both have been linked to exposure to the nephrotoxin and carcinogen aristolochic acid. It has been suggested that the terms *CHN* and *BEN* should be abandoned and replaced by the term *AAN*.

Aristolochic acid is a major component of *Aristolochia*-containing herbal remedies and is commonly prescribed in China and other Asian countries. AAN was first reported in 1993 in Belgium in young women taking aristolochic acid–containing Chinese herbs for weight reduction, and the finding has been confirmed by many others. BEN was described 50 years ago in farming villages in the Balkan area, where there is dietary exposure to aristolochic acid through the contamination of flour prepared from locally grown wheat.

Unique features of AAN include clustering of the cases among adults in endemic areas and close association with upper urinary tract carcinomas. About 50% of the affected patients develop transitional cell carcinomas; aristolochic acid induces DNA damage with a distinct molecular signature. Unfortunately, no effective specific treatment for AAN is available. Management is supportive with regular monitoring for urothelial malignancy.

Heavy Metals

Heavy metals such as cadmium, lead, and chromium can cause CIN, and exposure usually represents an environmental toxin. Cadmium exposure occurs with tobacco smoke and contaminated water and food. Lead exposure occurs from contact with lead-based paint and lead-contaminated dust and soil. Chromium is used to increase the hardness and corrosion resistance of alloy steel, and chromium exposure can occur when industrial plant employees work with alloy steels, dyes, paints, inks, and plastics. Proximal tubules are the principal site of accumulation and injury, but other nephron segments also can be injured.

Heavy metal nephrotoxicity ranges from mild tubular dysfunction to advanced CKD. The extent of kidney damage depends on the nature, dose, route, and duration of exposure. With chronic exposure, changes consistent with CIN are observed on kidney biopsy. The best-characterized clinical feature of heavy metal kidney toxicity is the Fanconi syndrome, which results from proximal tubule damage. These patients have low-molecular-weight proteinuria, aminoaciduria, bicarbonaturia, glycosuria, and phosphaturia. Other clinical findings of lead toxicity include gout from decreased urate excretion in proximal tubules, hemolytic anemia, encephalopathy, and neuropathy.

Other than supportive care, no specific treatment is available for heavy metal–associated kidney disease. Chelating agents may be used in acute poisoning, but no randomized clinical trials have proved the efficacy of chelation on clinical outcomes.

Sarcoidosis

Sarcoidosis is a chronic, multisystem, inflammatory disease of unknown origin. It is characterized by noncaseating, epithelioid granulomas in affected organs, leading to organ dysfunction. The severity and diversity of the clinical manifestations related to sarcoidosis depend on the extent of the infiltrating granulomatous lesions. Granulomatous tubulointerstitial nephritis is observed in approximately 20% of patients with sarcoidosis and responds well to steroid therapy. Sarcoidosis is described in details elsewhere.

Corticosteroid therapy is effective in the acute setting and in advanced tubulointerstitial nephritis. Treatment includes prednisone (1 mg/kg/day) for 6 to 12 weeks followed by taper. Some patients with granulomatous tubulointerstitial nephritis may require long-term treatment with steroids to preserve kidney function, although the side effects of steroids limit their use in advanced kidney disease. The efficacy of corticosteroid-sparing agents such as mycophenolate mofetil or azathioprine for sarcoid-related interstitial nephritis requires further investigation.

Radiation Nephritis

Radiation exposure is a significant cause of CKD, and radiation nephritis develops in most patients if they are exposed to more than

23 Gy. Ionizing radiation directly damages all molecules, including DNA, and initiates cellular synthesis of reactive oxygen species, which cause secondary tissue damage. Hydroxyl radicals are generated within milliseconds of tissue exposure. Oxidative stress and other factors may play additional roles over time, and patients may develop severe kidney injury and impaired function 6 to 12 months (or longer) after exposure. Histopathologically, early and late changes can be seen that include cell swelling, mesangiolysis, variable tubular injury, tubular atrophy, glomerular scarring, and increased mesangial matrix.

The diagnosis is usually based on a history of radiation exposure and the clinical findings of kidney injury. Treatment is supportive.

Sickle Cell Disease

CKD is relatively common in patients with sickle cell disease, an inherited hematologic disorder characterized by hemolytic anemia and vascular occlusion by sickled red cells. Under normal conditions, the renal medullary zone is characterized by low oxygen tension, acidic pH, and high osmolality, which can predispose to increased blood viscosity and red blood cell sickling. This increases the likelihood of local ischemia and infarction of the kidney microcirculation. In the vasa recta, vascular occlusion can interfere with the countercurrent exchange system in the inner medulla, resulting in a defect in the urine-concentrating mechanism.

Patients may have nocturia or polyuria and can develop gross hematuria due to papillary necrosis resulting from medullary ischemia and infarction. The sloughed papillae can obstruct urinary tract outflow, leading to obstructive nephropathy and kidney failure. Another abnormality associated with sickle cell disease is proteinuria, a consequence of glomerular hyperfiltration that results from reduction in nephron mass.

The treatment of sickle cell nephropathy focuses on primary management of the hematologic disorder. Tubular dysfunction may require potassium and bicarbonate supplementation to treat hypokalemia and acidosis, and those with ESRD are treated with dialysis and renal transplantation.

Lithium

Lithium is a monovalent cation, which is freely filtered through the glomeruli. Up to 80% of filtered lithium is reabsorbed in the proximal tubule, and a small fraction is reabsorbed in the distal nephron through the epithelial sodium channel ($E_{Na}C$). Lithium causes dysregulation of the aquaporin water channel and $E_{Na}C$ expression in the cortical collecting duct. The most common manifestation of kidney disease associated with lithium is CIN manifesting as a chronic, insidious decline in kidney function. The course of kidney disease after discontinuation of lithium is highly unpredictable, with no reliable clinical clues to identify those destined for recovery or progression.

Lithium also is associated with nephrogenic diabetes insipidus, which can occur in up to 40% of patients as early as 8 weeks after lithium initiation. Other tubular dysfunctions associated with lithium include water diuresis, natriuresis, and metabolic acidosis. Lithium-associated nephrogenic diabetes insipidus can be treated with $E_{Na}C$ blockade by amiloride.

Mesoamerican Nephropathy

Mesoamerican nephropathy, now formally designated as CKD of nontraditional causes, is an emerging form of progressive CKD identified in the last two decades. It is primarily seen in agricultural workers (usually in sugarcane or cotton plantations) in Central America. A similar nonproteinuric CKD has been described in South Asia and Sri Lanka as well. The most significant risk factor is prolonged, strenuous physical labor in hot and humid climates. Other risk factors include male gender, low body mass, consumption of high-fructose beverages, exposure to heavy metals from soil, nephrotoxins or NSAIDs and infectious diseases such as leptospirosis and hantavirus infections. Pesticide exposure alone does not appear to increase risk. Pathogenesis is not yet clearly understood; however, current hypothesis suggests that repeat episodes of heat stress and dehydration lead to activation of renin-angiotensin-aldosterone system, vasopressin and polyol-fructokinase pathway causing increased oxidative stress and recurrent AKI, eventually leading to tubulointerstitial nephritis. Moreover, heat exposure and consequent dehydration can enhance tubular reabsorption of toxins and potentially enhance toxin-mediated kidney injury. Furthermore, heat exposure can result in heat stroke or low grade rhabdomyolysis that can exacerbate kidney injury.

Patients are usually young or middle-aged men, normotensive, have minimal edema, and may describe symptoms of dysuria or nocturia. Laboratory data are notable for elevated creatinine, hypokalemia, hypomagnesemia, hyperuricemia, and urinalysis is often unremarkable with no hematuria and minimal (if any) proteinuria. Abdominal ultrasound shows small kidneys with cortical thinning. Diagnosis requires appropriate clinical context and kidney biopsy. Histologic features show tubulointerstitial damage, glomerulosclerosis, and chronic glomerular ischemia. Treatment is supportive and further efforts should be directed to preventing disease progression.

Urinary Tract Obstruction

Urinary tract obstruction is a common cause of AKI and CKD. When kidney function is normal at baseline, unilateral or partial obstruction anywhere along the urinary tract may be asymptomatic, with no discernable change in kidney function or urine output. Bilateral urinary tract obstruction, however, can lead to acute and chronic kidney injury and ESRD. It is important to address this possibility early in the clinical course of unexplained kidney injury or uremia.

Obstruction to urine flow causes an increase in ureteral intraluminal pressure. Over time, nephron tubules are injured, and the resulting changes in thromboxane A_2 and angiotensin levels decrease renal blood flow. Tubular damage leads to urinary concentrating defects, renal tubular acidosis (RTA), and hyperkalemia. If complete obstruction is not relieved, ischemia and nephron loss decrease the glomerular filtration rate.

Common causes of obstructive nephropathy are shown in Table 27.4. Among elderly men, benign prostatic hypertrophy is of particular concern. Overall, the clinical presentation depends on the cause, site, and time course of obstruction. Patients with obstructive nephropathy may present with decreased urine output associated with suprapubic pain (i.e., bladder distention from ureteral obstruction), renal colic (i.e., nephrolithiasis), urinary tract infections, fever, AKI, hypertension, and hematuria. Pain resulting from stretching of the urinary collecting system is the most common presenting symptom. Acute ureteral obstruction usually results in severe flank pain that typically radiates to the groin and is referred to as *renal colic*. Patients with complete bladder outlet obstruction develop AKI and anuria. Patients with incomplete or intermittent bladder outlet obstruction have urinary hesitancy, dribbling, urgency, decreased urine stream, nocturia, and polyuria. These patients are usually pain free. Tubular injury from obstruction causes decreased urinary concentrating capability leading to polyuria.

The physical examination should include palpation of the kidney and bladder, as well as a rectal, pelvic, and prostate assessment. The patient may have an enlarged and palpable bladder, enlarged prostate, costovertebral tenderness, groin pain, hypertension, or gross hematuria. The mainstays of the initial evaluation include measurement of the postvoid residual volume of the bladder (>125 mL is considered

TABLE 27.4 Causes of Urinary Obstruction

Cause	Examples
Congenital urinary tract malformation	Meatal stenosis
	Ureterocele
	Posterior urethral valves
	Urethral atresia
	Phimosis
	Megaureter–prune belly syndrome
Intraluminal obstruction (urethra and bladder outlet)	Phimosis
	Urethral strictures
	Benign prostate hyperplasia
	Pelvic tumor
	Anticholinergic drugs
	Neurogenic bladder
	Tuberculosis
	Radiation
	Trauma
	Calculi
	Blood clots
	Papillary necrosis (sickle cell disease, diabetes mellitus)
Extrinsic compression	Pelvic tumors
	Prostatic hypertrophy
	Retroperitoneal fibrosis or tumors
Acquired anomalies	Urethral strictures
	Neurogenic bladder
	Intratubular precipitates
	Bladder mass or stones

significant and may indicate obstruction) and ultrasound or CT scan of kidneys and urinary tract to evaluate the kidneys, ureters, and bladder for distention or other abnormalities.

The initial goals of therapy are to manage volume status, electrolyte abnormalities, infection, and other complications of obstructive nephropathy and to relieve the obstruction as soon as possible to prevent further damage to the kidney parenchyma. If urinary obstruction is suspected, a catheter should be placed in the bladder to address possible bladder outlet obstruction. If a large postvoid residual volume (>125 mL) is detected, the urinary catheter should remain in place while the cause is ascertained. Occasionally, relief of obstruction is associated with a large postobstructive diuresis that may be sufficient in degree to cause volume depletion and hypotension.

If the obstruction is acute, complete recovery of kidney function can be expected. If the anatomic site of the urinary tract obstruction is above the bladder, more sophisticated approaches to drainage (e.g., percutaneous nephrostomy tube placement) may be required to relieve obstruction.

CYSTIC KIDNEY DISEASES

Kidney cysts are fluid-filled tubular structures lined by a polarized epithelium. They result from defects in the structure and function of renal tubular epithelial cells. Kidney cysts can be solitary or multiple, simple or complex. Cystic kidney disease can be developmental, hereditary or acquired that develops in patients with CKD. Cystic diseases can be localized to kidneys or have systemic manifestations. Depending on the underlying cause of cysts, age of presentation can vary from prenatal to later in life. Cystic kidney diseases are also important causes of ESRD.

Several cellular and molecular mechanisms involved in cystogenesis have been uncovered in recent years. An algorithm for evaluation of kidney cysts is outlined in E-Fig. 27.4.

Simple Cysts

Simple cysts are most common. Widespread use of ultrasonography and CT has resulted in frequent detection of kidney cysts. They are usually unilateral, solitary, well-defined structures, but they can be multiple and bilateral. They tend to be more common among older adults and are often benign, incidental findings on radiographic imaging. Sonography reveals a thin-walled, fluid-filled cavity with no septations or calcifications. The diameter varies between 0.5 and 1.0 cm, but a few may be as large as 3 to 4 cm in diameter.

Diagnosis: Simple cysts are usually asymptomatic but occasionally may result in a palpable abdominal mass, infection, back pain, or hematuria. Differentiation of simple cysts from cysts associated with genetic disorders is based on the cystic pattern, age at detection, and family history.

Treatment: In the absence of symptoms, no treatment is required for simple cysts. If the kidney cyst becomes infected, causes pain, or leads to renin-mediated hypertension, percutaneous drainage is often the first step in further evaluation and management.

Complex Cysts

Differentiation of simple from complex cysts is usually made radiographically. When in doubt, histologic examination is required to exclude malignancy, but imaging is sensitive and specific, and it suffices in most cases. The distinction between complex and simple cysts is important in monitoring the need for intervention because simple cysts are usually benign, whereas complex cysts have a higher risk of malignancy and other complications. In a simple cyst, complications such as hemorrhage or infection can result in the development of features of more complex cysts, including calcification, septa, irregular borders, and multilobularity.

Initial evaluation of kidney cyst includes ultrasonography and, if ultrasound is equivocal, triphasic CT is done to characterize the cyst. If the characteristics of a cyst in terms of size, nodularity, mural enhancement, or septations change over time, the likelihood of malignancy increases.

To help with diagnosis and management, the Bosniak classification of kidney cysts was introduced in 1986 and has been revised since then. This classification, which includes four categories with several important subcategories, based on triphasic CT findings, is described in Table 27.5. Category I and category II cysts are benign. Category II F cysts have a range of reported malignancy rates of 0 to 38% so requires follow-up. The risk increases to almost 50% for category III cysts. Category III and IV renal cysts are considered to be renal carcinoma unless proven otherwise, and they are usually surgically resected. While the current Bosniak classification of kidney cysts predicts likelihood of cancer, it does not assess the aggressiveness of the tumor. With the technological innovations and advancement of knowledge, new proposal for further revision of Bosniak classification was made in 2019.

Acquired Cystic Kidney Disease in CKD

Acquired cystic kidney disease (ACKD) is a disease consequent from long-term CKD. It is defined by three or more cysts per kidney in a patient with CKD or ESRD. The prevalence of ACKD increases with the duration of dialysis, reaching 87% after 10 years of dialysis. Patients of male gender, older age, with history of heart disease, larger kidneys, and kidney calcifications are more likely to develop ACKD.

TABLE 27.5 Bosniak Renal Cyst Classification Scheme

Category	Description
I. Simple cyst	A benign simple cyst with a thin wall and no septa, calcifications, or solid components.
II. Minimally complicated	A benign cystic lesion with a few thin septa. The wall or septa may contain fine calcifications or short segment of a slightly thickened calcification. (This category also includes uniformly high-attenuating lesions that are less than 3 cm in diameter, well marginated, and nonenhancing.)
IIF. Complicated	Well-marginated cysts but more complicated than category II. They have multiple thin septa or minimal smooth thickening of the septa or wall and may contain calcifications that may be thick and nodular. (This category also includes totally intrarenal, nonenhancing high-attenuating lesions that are more than 3 cm in diameter.)
III. Indeterminate	Indeterminate cystic masses that have thickened, irregular, or smooth walls or septa. These lesions are enhancing on computed tomography. Between 40% and 60% of lesions are malignant (e.g., cystic renal cell carcinoma, multiloculated cystic renal cell carcinoma). The remaining lesions are hemorrhagic, chronic, infected cysts or multiloculated cystic nephroma and are benign.
IV. Malignancy	On computed tomography, they have characteristics of category III cysts and contain enhancing soft tissue components that are adjacent to and independent of the wall or septum on the cyst. Between 85% and 100% of lesions are malignant; evaluation and surgical excision are recommended.

Neither the cause of the underlying ESRD nor the mode of dialysis influences the progression of ACKD. It has been postulated that damage to the kidney parenchyma in CKD increases local growth factors levels that promote hypertrophy and cyst generation in the remaining nephrons. In some cases, increased levels of growth factors and mutated genes (e.g., *ERBB2*) may cause the malignant transformation of cysts, the primary clinical concern in 3% to 7% of ACKD patients.

ACKD-related cyst formation is limited to the kidneys and is an incidental finding on radiographic imaging. Patients with ACKD are usually asymptomatic but may develop infectious or bleeding complications. ACKD can be differentiated from hereditary causes of cystic renal disease by presence of CKD or ESRD and the absence of any other clinical findings.

Patients with ACKD do not require specific treatment. Cysts are managed based on the Bosniak category as discussed in the section on renal cell carcinoma (RCC). Routine screening for ACKD among dialysis patients is contentious but is recommended for patients during their pretransplantation evaluation. Kidney transplant recipients with ACKD should get yearly kidney ultrasound because of higher risk of malignancy due to exposure to immunosuppression and longer life expectancy.

Hereditary Cystic Kidney Diseases

The most common inherited cystic kidney diseases are the polycystic kidney diseases (PKDs), including autosomal dominant and autosomal recessive forms of PKD. Other hereditary cystic renal diseases include autosomal dominant tubulointerstitial kidney disease, Von Hippel–Lindau disease (VHLD), and tuberous sclerosis. In the inherited disorders, several mutations have been associated with cyst formation. In PKD, the cysts are not connected to the urinary drainage system, and cellular secretion results in cyst enlargement. Mutation of any of the tubular epithelial–related genes such as *PKD1*, *PKD2*, and mucin-1 *(MUC1)* can result in disruption of normal ciliary function, resulting in cyst formation from over-proliferation of tubular epithelium and increased fluid secretion.

Polycystic Kidney Disease

PKD consists of two main form of monogenetic cystic kidney disease: autosomal dominant polycystic kidney disease (ADPKD) and autosomal recessive polycystic kidney disease (ARPKD). Patients with PKD develop multiple fluid-filled cysts in both kidneys and sometimes in other organs as well. Cysts usually form in the distal segment of the nephron and collecting ducts from outgrowths of kidney epithelial cells, abnormal fluid secretion, and altered cell-matrix interaction. Once the cysts are formed, they detach from the tubules and

TABLE 27.6 Extrarenal Manifestations of ADPKD

Organ Involved	Manifestations
Liver	Polycystic liver disease
Brain	Intracranial aneurysms
Vascular	Thoracic aortic dissection
	Coronary artery aneurysm
Cardiac	Valvular heart disease
	Mitral valve prolapse and regurgitation
	Tricuspid valve prolapse and regurgitation
Other	Pancreatic cyst
	Seminal vesicle cyst
	Colonic and duodenal diverticula

progressively increase in size, compressing nearby nephrons, interstitium, and vessels. Injury to adjacent kidney structures leads to inflammation and fibrosis.

Autosomal Dominant Polycystic Kidney Disease

Definition and epidemiology. ADPKD is the most common cause of cystic renal disease and an important cause of ESRD. The monogenetic, progressive disorder is characterized by multiple cysts in kidneys and other organs, including the liver and pancreas. The incidence of ADPKD is 1 case in 400 to 1000 live births, and between 300,000 and 600,000 Americans are affected by the disease.

Pathology and pathogenesis. Mutations in the *PKD1* and *PKD2* genes are responsible for about 85% and 15% of ADPKD cases, respectively, and there is evidence for important modifier genes. *PKD1* is located on chromosome 14 and encodes the protein polycystin 1 (PC1), which functions as a membrane receptor. *PKD2* is located on chromosome 4 and encodes polycystin 2 (PC2), which functions as a calcium-permeable cation channel (E-Fig. 27.5). PC1 and PC2 regulate intracellular calcium homeostasis and signaling pathways involved in tubular morphogenesis and cell-cell interactions. PC1 and PC2 also are integral membrane proteins of cilia, including the primary cilia of renal tubular cells. ADPKD is now classified under the new class of diseases called *ciliopathies.* In addition to renal tubules, PC1 and PC2 proteins are found in diverse cell types, including bile ducts, endothelial cells, and neurons. Consequently, ADPKD patients with mutated PC1 or PC2 proteins often have extrarenal manifestations (Table 27.6).

TABLE 27.7 Ultrasonography Criteria of ADPKD

Age	Number of Cysts
Positive family history	
<30 years	≥2 unilateral or bilateral
	≥3 cysts unilateral or bilateral
30-39 years	≥2 cysts in each kidney
40-59 years	≥4 cysts in each kidney
>60 years	
No family history	>10 cysts in each kidney
16-40 years	

In the kidney, increase in cyst size and number over time damages adjacent renal architecture and causes CKD and renin-mediated hypertension. Total kidney volume increases continuously and is associated with progressive decline of kidney function. Higher rates of kidney enlargement are associated with a more rapid decrease in kidney function.

Clinical presentation. ADPKD is a multisystem disease. The clinical presentation may range from no symptoms to an array of systemic manifestations, including polycystic liver disease, which is detected in about 80% of adults. Cardiac valvular abnormalities and cerebral aneurysms are key noncystic features of ADPKD, and familial clustering of cases occurs. Cerebral aneurysms are observed in about 8% of patients with ADPKD, but the incidence increases to 20% among those with a positive family history of cerebral aneurysm or subarachnoid hemorrhage. ADPKD patients, with positive family history of cerebral aneurysm or sudden death of unknown cause, should be screened for cerebral aneurysm.

Most patients with ADPKD develop cysts before the age of 30, but CKD can be delayed to beyond the fourth decade. Patients with the *PKD2* mutation have later onset and slower progression of the disease than patients with the *PKD1* mutation. Kidney survival associated with *PKD2* mutations is about 20 years longer than that associated with *PKD1* mutations. Besides the cysts, other kidney manifestations of APKD include urinary concentrating defects, hypertension, and nephrolithiasis. Twenty percent of patients with ADPKD can develop uric acid and calcium oxalate nephrolithiasis and may have renal colic, obstructive nephropathy, or urinary tract infection.

Diagnosis. ADPKD is usually diagnosed by imaging of the kidneys. The finding of three or more cysts (unilateral or bilateral) in those younger than age 30, two or more cysts in each kidney in those between 40 and 59 years of age, and four or more cysts in each kidney in patients older than 60 years is sufficient to make diagnosis of ADPKD (Table 27.7). Absence of more than two cysts in individuals older than 40 years of age makes ADPKD very unlikely. Genetic testing is usually not required for an individual with a positive family history if other diagnostic criteria for ADPKD are met, but other family members should be screened with ultrasound of kidneys.

Treatment. Total kidney volume correlates with disease manifestation of PKD. No specific treatment is available to prevent the growth of kidney or liver cysts. Tolvaptan, a vasopressin receptor 2 inhibitor, has been recently approved to slow progression of kidney disease in PKD. Given the high cost and side effect profile of the drug, it should only be given to select patients with ADPKD who will likely benefit most from it. Due to hepatotoxicity, use of tolvaptan requires close monitoring of liver enzymes. Other interventions include enhanced hydration; maintenance of healthy weight; decrease in sodium, protein, and caffeine intake; and treatment of hypertension and dyslipidemia, which may delay the progression of renal disease. Renin-mediated hypertension is a common complication of ADPKD, and it contributes to an increased incidence of cardiovascular mortality and faster progression to ESRD. The main and most effective therapy remains control of hypertension by angiotensin-converting enzyme inhibitors or angiotensin-receptor blockers to achieve a target blood pressure of less than 125/75 mm Hg. Dual blockade with angiotensin-converting enzyme inhibitors and angiotensin-receptor blockers does not provide any additional benefit and increases risk of hyperkalemia.

Renal cyst enlargement can cause pain, and cysts can be complicated by infection or bleeding that warrants specific intervention. Surgical decompression is usually reserved for patients who fail conservative management. If ESRD occurs, patients are treated with renal replacement therapy, including dialysis and kidney transplantation. Preemptive management of intracranial aneurysms is important but controversial.

Prognosis. The time of onset and rate of progression of ADPKD varies from patient to patient, even within the same family. Risk factors for progressive CKD include increases in kidney cyst volume, a *PKD1* gene mutation, and uncontrolled hypertension. Other risk factors include male gender, diagnosis of ADPKD before 30 years of age, hypertension before 35 years of age, concurrent diabetes mellitus, and hematuria. About 45% of the patients with ADPKD develop ESRD by 60 years of age, but they have a better prognosis than patients with ESRD from other causes.

Autosomal Recessive Polycystic Kidney

Definition and epidemiology. ARPKD also is classified under the ciliopathies. ARPKD is characterized by diffuse dilation of the collecting ducts and congenital hepatic fibrosis. The estimated incidence of ARPKD is 1 case in 20,000 live births.

Pathogenesis. Mutations in *HNF1B* and the polycystic kidney and hepatic disease 1 gene *(PKHD1)* are responsible for ARPKD. *PKHD1* is a large gene located on chromosome 6. More than 300 mutations have been identified at different loci of the *PKHD1* gene. Fibrocystin (i.e., polyductin) is the product of *PKHD1* and is expressed in the primary cilia of the thick ascending limb, in cortical and medullary ducts in the kidney, and in hepatic bile ducts. It has an important role in the terminal differentiation of kidney and biliary ductules.

Clinical presentation. ARPKD, phenotypically, is highly variable. Patients with ARPKD may be diagnosed at different ages, but those with a more severe phenotype present in utero or at birth because they develop enlarged kidneys, oligohydramnios, pulmonary hypoplasia, Potter facies (flattened nose, recessed chin, epicanthal folds, and low-set ears), and deformities of the spine and limb. Neonates usually have kidney enlargement and kidney failure, and older patients have liver disease, including portal hypertension, hepatosplenomegaly, variceal bleeding, and hepatic fibrosis.

Differential diagnosis. The initial diagnosis is usually suspected on the basis of kidney imaging with antenatal or infantile ultrasound. Abdominal ultrasound shows bilateral enlarged kidneys with multiple cysts. Fetal imaging shows oligohydramnios, pulmonary hypoplasia, and Potter syndrome. Although molecular diagnostic analysis is the gold standard for diagnosing ARPKD, it is difficult to perform due to the high level of heterogeneity of the *PKHD1* gene.

Treatment and prognosis. No treatment is available for ARPKD, and genetic testing is usually not performed outside of research scenarios. Most deaths occur in utero or at the time of birth, and of those with ARPKD who survive birth, 20% to 30% die within the first year of life. Neonates have more kidney manifestations, and older patients have more liver disease manifesting as portal hypertension, hepatosplenomegaly, and bleeding esophageal or gastric varices. The likelihood of patients being alive without ESRD increases with older age at presentation due to their more benign phenotypes. Due to autosomal recessive inheritance, recurrence risk of ARPKD in subsequent pregnancies of parents of an ARPKD child is 25%.

Juvenile Nephronophthisis and Autosomal Dominant Tubulointerstitial Kidney Disease

Definition and epidemiology. Nephronophthisis (NPHP) and autosomal dominant tubulointerstitial kidney disease (ADTKD) are hereditary forms of cystic kidney disease. Both produce bilateral cysts at the corticomedullary junction of the kidney and are associated with progressive CKD and ESRD. They are clinically and pathologically indistinguishable, and they are separated only by the age of onset and mode of inheritance.

NPHP is an autosomal recessive cystic kidney disease, and the median age of onset of renal disease is 11.5 years. ADTKD has an autosomal dominant pattern of inheritance, and the median age of onset of renal disease is 28.5 years. NPHP is more common than ADTKD and is the most common cause of ESRD in the first 3 decades of life.

Pathogenesis. Several genes are associated with the NPHP and ADTKD phenotypes. Functional defects of any of the proteins associated with these genes can lead to ciliary dysfunction and development of multiple cysts. Mutations in at least three genes—*MUC1, REN,* and *UMOD* encoding mucin-1, renin, and uromodulin, respectively—can lead to ADTKD. *UMOD* gene mutation is the most common mutation and patients with this mutation develop gout at an early age along with CKD. NPHP is caused by mutations in at least 20 genes encoding proteins that are associated with cilia, basal bodies, and centromeres. Mutation of *NPHP1* is the most common mutation, reported in approximately 20% of the patients, whereas other mutations contribute to less than 3% each.

Clinical presentation. The three clinical forms of NPHP are based on the onset of ESRD: an infantile form with a median onset at 1 year of age, a juvenile form with a median onset at 13 years of age, and an adolescent form with a median onset at 19 years of age. Some children may present with extrarenal symptoms: retinitis pigmentosa (Senior-Løken syndrome), mental retardation, cerebellar ataxia, bone anomalies, or liver fibrosis. Situs inversus and ventricular cardiac septal defect can also be present in the infantile form of NPHP. In patients with ADTKD, symptoms usually develop in the fourth or fifth decade of life and include hematuria, infection or nephrolithiasis. ESRD develops between the ages of 50 and 70 years.

Differential diagnosis. The diagnosis of NPHP or ADTKD is based mainly on clinical features. Medullary cysts, a low urinary specific gravity, and absence of significant proteinuria may suggest either disease. Genetic testing is available for several gene mutations and can be applied based on the age at presentation. Siblings can be screened by kidney ultrasound and urine concentration test results. Kidney biopsy is usually not indicated because the findings of interstitial fibrosis and tubular atrophy are nonspecific.

Treatment and prognosis. No specific treatment is available for NPHP or ADTKD, and treatment is mainly supportive. The time of onset of ESRD varies between 30 and 60 years, depending on the type of mutation. Sodium supplementation for salt wasting, allopurinol for gout, and dialysis or renal transplantation for ESRD are part of supportive care. NPHP and ADTKD do not recur after renal transplantation.

Medullary Sponge Kidney

Medullary sponge kidney (MSK), also known as Lenarduzzi-Cacchi-Ricci disease, is a relatively uncommon cystic disorder. It usually occurs sporadically, but familial cases have been reported. MSK is characterized by ectasia and cystic dilation of medullary and papillary collecting ducts, resulting in a spongy appearance of the kidney on imaging. MSK is associated with urinary acidification and concentration defects, a high risk of nephrocalcinosis and kidney stones, and a moderate risk of urinary infections and CKD. The prevalence of MSK is 1 case in 5000 persons in the general population, and 15% to 20% of patients with nephrolithiasis have MSK.

No clear genetic basis for MSK has been established. MSK is usually detected between the ages of 30 and 50 years. Most patients with MSK are asymptomatic and may have incidental findings on imaging. The clinical course is benign and is usually not associated with ESRD.

When suspected, CT urography has replaced intravenous urography as the imaging study of choice for the diagnosis of MSK. There is retention of contrast media in renal pyramids and cystic collecting ducts, giving the appearance of blush or diffused linear striations. Nephrocalcinosis is common in patients with MSK but is not required to make the diagnosis of MSK. CT imaging may help in excluding papillary necrosis, ADPKD, obstruction, or pyelonephritis.

TUBEROUS SCLEROSIS

Definition and Epidemiology

Tuberous sclerosis complex (TSC) (i.e., Bourneville disease) is an autosomal dominant genetic disorder that affects adults and children. TSC causes benign tumors to form in multiple organ systems, including the skin, brain, and kidneys. TSC is often characterized by related neurologic disorders such as epilepsy and mental retardation.

The prevalence of TSC in the general population is approximately 1 in 10,000 and 50% to 65% of cases are sporadic. Because TSC has an autosomal dominant pattern of inheritance, there is a 50% risk of siblings being affected. Genetic counseling is important for affected families. The overall diagnosis and management of TSC is discussed in Chapter 115.

Pathology

TSC is caused by inactivating mutations in the *TSC1* or *TSC2* genes, located on chromosome 9, and chromosome 16, adjacent to the *PKD1* gene, respectively. They, respectively, encode the hamartin and tuberin proteins, which together form a complex that regulates specific cellular growth, motility, and migration of cells. Inactivating mutations of the *TSC1* or *TSC2* genes result in disruption of these processes and may cause unrestricted growth of cells and tumorigenesis.

TSC conveys a lifetime risk of 2% to 3% for RCC. Kidney tumors are usually bilateral and occur at an early age. More commonly, the tumors are benign angiomyolipomas, composed of abnormal, thick-walled vessels, smooth muscle cells, and adipose tissue, seen in about 80% of patients with TSC by the age of 10 years. These benign kidney tumors often require no treatment. However, they can grow, become locally invasive, and cause bleeding, pain, and hypertension.

Conclusive guidelines for surveillance are unavailable, but annual magnetic resonance imaging of kidney and brain lesions is suggested until the age of 21 years and then every 2 to 3 years to monitor their growth. Patients with progressive lesions should have yearly imaging. If the angiomyolipomas become locally invasive or cause bleeding, surgical intervention is needed.

Mutations in the *TSC1* or *TSC2* gene cause constitutive activation of mTOR. Everolimus, an inhibitor of mTOR, has been approved for the treatment of patients with TSC-associated subependymal giant cell astrocytomas, who are not surgical candidates.

VON HIPPEL–LINDAU DISEASE

VHLD is an autosomal dominant disease that affects multiple organ systems. It is caused by germline mutations in *VHL*, a tumor suppressor gene located on chromosome 3. This mutation predisposes to RCC and to tumor formation in other organs, including the eyes, cerebellum, spinal cord, adrenal glands, epididymis, and pancreas. VHLD

TABLE 27.8 TNM Staging System of Renal Cell Carcinoma

Primary Tumor (T)

TX	Primary tumor cannot be assessed
T0	No evidence of primary tumor
T1	**Tumor <7 cm and limited to the kidney**
T1a	Tumor <4 cm and limited to the kidney
T1b	Tumor >4 cm but <7 cm and limited to the kidney
T2	**Tumor >7 cm and limited to the kidney**
T2a	Tumor >7 cm but <10 cm and limited to the kidney
T2b	Tumor >10 cm and limited to the kidney
T3	**Tumor extends into major veins or perinephric tissues but not into the ipsilateral adrenal gland and not beyond Gerota fascia**
T3a	Tumor grossly extends into the renal vein or its segmental branches, or tumor invades perirenal and/or renal sinus fat but not beyond Gerota fascia
T3b	Tumor grossly extends into the vena cava below the diaphragm
T3c	Tumor grossly extends into the vena cava above the diaphragm or invades the wall of the vena cava
T4	**Tumor invades beyond Gerota fascia, including contiguous extension into the ipsilateral adrenal gland**

Regional Lymph Nodes (N)

NX	Regional lymph nodes cannot be assessed
N0	No regional lymph node metastasis
N1	Metastasis in regional lymph node(s)

Distant Metastasis (M)

M0	No distant metastasis
M1	Distant Metastasis

Anatomic Stage/Prognosis Groups

Stage	T	N	M
Stage I	T1	N0	M0
Stage II	T2	N0	M0
Stage III	T1 or T2	N1	M0
	T3	N0 or N1	M0
Stage IV	T4	Any N	M0
	Any T	Any N	M1

affects approximately 1 in 40,000 births, and about 7000 patients are affected in the United States. There is an important association with pheochromocytoma in some patients with VHLD that warrants consideration.

RCC occurs in up to 70% of patients with VHLD. It is usually bilateral and the clear cell type. RCC affects younger patients with a mean age at presentation of 26 years. For a high-risk patient, the diagnosis of VHLD is suggested by central nervous system or retinal hemangioblastoma, RCC, or pheochromocytoma. These patients should be referred for detailed assessment. When indicated, genetic testing can be performed to assess possible mutations of the *VHL* gene.

KIDNEY TUMORS

Each year, approximately 74,000 new cases of renal cancer are diagnosed and 15,000 deaths from RCC are reported in the United States. Most cases are sporadic, but there is an association between RCC and VHLD and tuberous sclerosis that has helped to explain the cellular mechanisms involved.

RCC originates from renal epithelial cells and accounts for 85% of renal cancers. Based on histology, the five subtypes are clear cell, papillary (chromophilic), oncocytoma, collecting duct (Bellini duct), and chromophobe RCC. Clear cell carcinoma is the most common subtype and accounts for about 75% to 85% of all cases.

The classic triad of symptoms of flank pain, hematuria, and a palpable flank mass is uncommon (10%). About 50% of cases are identified

as a result of an incidental finding on radiographic imaging. Other clinical symptoms are nonspecific and include fatigue, anemia, and weight loss. Paraneoplastic syndromes associated with RCC include erythrocytosis (due to overproduction of erythropoietin), hypercalcemia (due to excess parathyroid hormone–related peptide), hepatic dysfunction (Stauffer syndrome), and cachexia.

The initial diagnosis of RCC is usually made by imaging. Unlike simple cysts, which are anechoic, round, and smooth walled, RCC is more likely to be a septate, irregular, thick-walled mass. When RCC is suspected, additional evaluation by CT urography or magnetic resonance imaging is usually required, along with complete staging and evaluation for metastases (Table 27.8). Biopsy is usually reserved, to confirm the diagnosis for medical treatment, for the patients who are not surgical candidates.

When possible, the primary treatment of localized RCC is surgical resection, which usually includes complete or partial nephrectomy. Locally advanced or metastatic RCC is treated medically with chemotherapy and immunomodulatory therapy with interleukin-2. Newer therapies include tyrosine kinase inhibitor (Sunitinib) and two immune checkpoint inhibitors, nivolumab and ipilimumab.

The prognosis for RCC depends primarily on the clinical stage at the time of presentation as assessed by the tumor-node-metastasis (TNM) criteria. TNM stages I through III have a better prognosis than TNM stage IV (metastatic) RCC. Poor prognostic factors include a lower Karnofsky performance status, elevated lactate dehydrogenase level, low hemoglobin level, and hypercalcemia. With documented metastases, the 1-year survival rate is 12% to 71%, and the 3-year survival rate is 0% to 31%, but in the past decade with availability of newer drugs, survival has improved (see Chapter 59).

NEPHROLITHIASIS

Nephrolithiasis is a major public health problem. It imposes a substantial burden on human health and considerable financial expenditure for the nation. Calcium-containing stones are the most common stones, comprising approximately 80% of all stones. Uric acid, struvite, and cysteine stones are less common, accounting for approximately 9%, 10%, and 1% of all stones, respectively, but have high recurrence rates.

Epidemiology

The prevalence of stones has been substantially increasing. National Health and Nutrition Examination Survey (NHANES) demonstrated an increase in self-reported prevalence of kidney stones in the United States from 3.2% in 1976 to 1980, to 8.8% in 2007 to 2010, to 10.1% in 2014. Moreover, the incidence of kidney stones is also increasing and is estimated to be approximately 0.5% in North America and Europe. Diet and lifestyle factors likely play significant roles in the changing epidemiology.

Nephrolithiasis increases with age. It is more common in men than in women; however, in the last 2 decades, the male to female ratio has changed from 3:1 to about 2:1. Comparison of NHANES data over time showed prevalence of kidney stones was stable in males but increased in females, with the most significant increase noted in females of childbearing age. Epidemiologic studies have noted a relationship between nephrolithiasis and metabolic syndrome, and the magnitudes of this association were greater for women compared with men. This may be one plausible explanation for the increasing incidence of kidney stones among women. The prevalence is higher in Caucasian males, intermediate in Hispanic and Asian males, and less frequent in black males. The highest risk of stone formation has been reported in men in the United Arab Emirates and Saudi Arabia and has been attributed to genetic and environmental factors. Stone recurrence is common with the relapse rate of kidney stones being 50% in 5 to 10 years and 75% in 20 years. Risk factors associated with recurrent stone formation include younger age of onset, positive family history, underlying medical conditions, and urinary infections. The Recurrence of Kidney Stone (ROKS) nomogram provides a clinical tool to estimate the risk of recurrence in first-time symptomatic stone formers. It uses participants' characteristics at baseline to estimate recurrence at varying times, thus identifying those who may benefit from dietary and medical interventions. An electronic version of the ROKS nomogram is available at https://qxmd.com/calculate/calculator_3/roks-recurrence-of-kidney-stone-2014.

Pathogenesis

Stone formation occurs as a result of supersaturation of urinary solutes, expressed as the ratio of solute concentration in urine to its known solubility. A ratio of greater than 1 indicates that urine is supersaturated with the given substance and promotes crystallization, whereas a ratio of less than 1 inhibits crystallization. Low urine volume increases supersaturation of all solutes, thereby promoting stone formation. Urine pH influences free ion activity. The main determinants for crystallization vary for different stones: low urine volume and high urinary calcium and oxalate concentration promote calcium oxalate crystals, whereas alkaline urine and high urinary calcium concentrations promote calcium phosphate crystals. Acidic urine is the main determinant for uric acid crystals, and for cystine crystals it is high urinary cystine concentration and acidic urine. Urine contains substances such as citrate, pyrophosphate, magnesium, Tamm-Horsfall glycoprotein, glycosaminoglycans, osteopontin, and calgranulin that can inhibit

TABLE 27.9 Medications Associated With Stone Formation	
Mechanism	**Medication**
Hypocitraturia	Acetazolamide
	Zonisamide
	Vitamin C
	Topiramate
Hypercalciuria	Vitamin D
	Antacids
	Theophylline
	Nifedipine
Hyperuricosuria	Probenecid
	Aspirin
Precipitation within the tubule	Indinavir
	Atazanavir
	Acyclovir
	Sulfadiazine
	Triamterene
	Guaifenesin/ephedrine

crystal aggregation in urine. Of these, citrate is the only inhibitor that can be measured and modified in clinical settings; thus, it is a focus of therapeutic intervention.

Clinical Presentation

Patients are often asymptomatic, and calculi are detected as an incidental finding on imaging studies. Flank pain with or without gross hematuria is the most common presentation. Pain can vary in intensity from mild to severe and is classically abrupt in onset, paroxysmal, waxing and waning. Other associated symptoms include dysuria, urgency, nausea, and vomiting. Location of pain is suggestive of site of obstruction and may vary as the stone migrates. Upper ureteral obstruction (as in the ureteropelvic region) can cause flank pain, while lower ureteral obstruction can cause pain to radiate to the ipsilateral testes or labium. Some patients may pass gravel, more typical with uric acid stones. Complications associated with nephrolithiasis include obstruction, hydronephrosis, infection, and AKI from obstructive uropathy in the setting of bilateral obstruction or unilateral obstruction in case of the solitary kidney. Conditions that can mimic renal colic include ectopic pregnancy in women, bleeding within the kidney leading to formation of clots, hemorrhagic cysts, loin pain hematuria syndrome, and malingering.

Diagnosis

Detailed history is crucial and should include age at the first episode, number of stones, bilateral or unilateral stones, frequency of stone formation, type of stone if known, type and number of surgical interventions, family history of stone disease, and any associated infections. Certain clues elucidated on history may point towards a systemic etiology for nephrolithiasis; for example, patients with malabsorptive states may be predisposed calcium oxalate stones. History should also include detailed dietary habits, including amount of fluid intake, dietary sodium, protein, oxalate, and calcium intake to determine the potential cause or contributors of stone formation. Certain medications can potentiate stone formation and are shown in Table 27.9. Except during an acute episode of stone passing, most patients will have a normal physical examination. However, physical examination may sometimes reveal findings of systemic condition such as presence of tophi in patients with hyperuricosuria and uric acid stones.

Laboratory testing should include complete metabolic profile and uric acid. Hypokalemia and metabolic acidosis are suggestive of RTA.

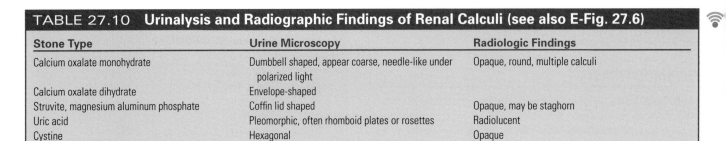

TABLE 27.10	Urinalysis and Radiographic Findings of Renal Calculi (see also E-Fig. 27.6)	
Stone Type	**Urine Microscopy**	**Radiologic Findings**
Calcium oxalate monohydrate	Dumbbell shaped, appear coarse, needle-like under polarized light	Opaque, round, multiple calculi
Calcium oxalate dihydrate	Envelope-shaped	
Struvite, magnesium aluminum phosphate	Coffin lid shaped	Opaque, may be staghorn
Uric acid	Pleomorphic, often rhomboid plates or rosettes	Radiolucent
Cystine	Hexagonal	Opaque

TABLE 27.11	Treatment Modalities for Different Nephrolithiasis Risk Factors	
Urinary Abnormality	**Dietary Change**	**Medication**
Hypercalciuria	Adequate dietary calcium intake Reduce animal protein intake Reduce sodium intake to <2 g/day	Thiazide diuretic
Hyperoxaluria	Adequate dietary calcium intake Avoid high oxalate foods	Consider vitamin B_6 (Pyridoxine)
Hyperuricosuria	Reduce purine intake	Allopurinol
Hypocitraturia	Increase fruit and vegetable intake Reduce animal protein intake	Potassium citrate (alkali)
Low urine volume	Increase fluid intake Goal urine output is >2-2.5 L per day.	

If hypercalcemia is noted, parathyroid hormone should be checked to assess for primary hyperparathyroidism. A careful urinalysis should be performed, and certain findings may point toward a specific diagnosis (Table 27.10 and E-Fig. 27.6). Uric acid crystals are formed in acidic urine, whereas calcium phosphate and struvite crystals are formed in alkaline urine. High urine specific gravity is suggestive of inadequate fluid intake. In patients with suspected struvite stones, urine culture should be obtained. Retrieving the stone for chemical analysis is essential to help identify the type of stone and thus guide therapy. All patients should strain their urine and retrieve any stone. A 24-hour urine collection is the cornerstone of evaluation in patients with nephrolithiasis and includes urine volume, pH, calcium, magnesium, potassium, uric acid, citrate, oxalate, sodium, urea nitrogen, ammonium, sulfate, phosphate, and creatinine (to assess the completeness of the collection). Preferably two collections should be done in outpatient settings when the patients are consuming their usual diet. Because individuals tend to change their dietary habits after an acute episode, the collection should be performed 6 weeks after an episode of renal colic. Urine collection should be repeated periodically to assess the impact of dietary changes and therapeutics.

Noncontrast helical CT has replaced intravenous urography (or intravenous pyelogram) as the diagnostic test of choice for evaluation of kidney stones. CT can detect both radiopaque and radiolucent stones with high sensitivity and specificity. Ultrasound can also detect radiolucent and radiopaque stones in kidneys but may miss ureteral stones. Ultrasound has a role in evaluating stones in pediatric and pregnant patients.

Treatment

Small (<4 mm), nonobstructive stones can be managed conservatively because they have a good chance passing spontaneously. With increase in stone size there is a progressive decrease in the spontaneous passage rate from 55% for stones smaller than 4 mm, to 35% for 4- to 6-mm stones, and 8% for stones greater than 6 mm, respectively.

During an acute colic episode, pain management is essential and can be controlled with use of NSAIDs or narcotics. Patients should be instructed to increase their fluid intake in order to increase their urine output to at least 2 liters per day to hasten stone passage. α-1 Adrenergic-receptor blockers and calcium-channel blockers can be used to facilitate stone passage. α-1 Adrenergic-receptor blockers decrease ureteral smooth muscle tone as well as frequency and force of peristalsis, whereas calcium-channel blockers suppress smooth muscle contraction and reduce ureteral spasm. Presence of any signs of urinary tract infection, inability to take oral fluids, or obstruction of a single functioning kidney requires hospitalization. In the presence of AKI, anuria, or sepsis with an obstructive stone, urgent urologic consultation should be obtained. Urology consult should also be obtained for stones larger than 10 mm, failure of conservative management, and presence of anatomic abnormalities that would prevent passage of the stone. Type of surgical intervention is determined by stone size, type, location, and presence of infection. For proximal ureteral stones, both shock-wave lithotripsy and ureteroscopy are first-line therapy. Shock-wave lithotripsy is most effective for smaller (<10 mm) calculi. For mid- or distal ureteral stones, ureteroscopy is first-line therapy. Shock-wave lithotripsy has lower morbidity and lower complication rates compared to ureteroscopy; however, the latter has a greater stone-free rate with a single procedure. Percutaneous nephrolithotomy is recommended for larger (>20 mm) or complex calculi (e.g., staghorn calculi).

Prevention of Stones

General measures to prevent recurrent stones include increasing fluid intake to greater than 2 to 2.5 L/day and limiting dietary sodium intake to less than 2 g/day and protein intake to 0.8 to 1 g/day. Dietary calcium restriction is not recommended because calcium in food binds to oxalate in the bowel and reduces urinary excretion of the highly lithogenic oxalate. On the other hand, additional calcium supplements in between meals should be avoided in patients with calcium stones.

Specific Types of Stones

Specific treatment modalities may be implemented when the metabolic risk factors for stone formation are identified (Table 27.11).

TABLE 27.12 Principle Risk Factors for Formation of Calcium Stones

Low urinary volume
High urinary oxalate
High urinary calcium
Low urinary citrate
Dietary factors
    Low dietary intake of fluids, calcium, phytates, potassium
    High intake of oxalates, sodium, protein, sucrose
Medical conditions: obesity, metabolic syndrome, diabetes mellitus, primary hyperparathyroidism, gout, medullary sponge kidneys

Calcium Stones

Approximately 80% of stones are calcium stones, most of which are composed primarily of calcium oxalate, mixed oxalate and phosphate, and less often, pure calcium phosphate. Calcium oxalate supersaturation is not pH-dependent in the physiologic range whereas alkaline urine promotes calcium phosphate supersaturation. The pathophysiologic mechanisms for calcium kidney stone formation are complex, diverse, and can be associated with a number of metabolic derangements (Table 27.12).

Hypercalciuria. Hypercalciuria is the most common metabolic abnormality found in recurrent calcium stones formers, detected in 30% to 60% of adults with nephrolithiasis. It is defined as calcium excretion 250 mg/day or greater in women and 300 mg/day or greater in men. It is most often familial or idiopathic. Gut calcium absorption is increased in persons with idiopathic hypercalciuria, but serum calcium values remain unchanged as the absorbed calcium is promptly excreted. There are three primary pathophysiologic mechanisms for hypercalciuria. (1) Increased intestinal calcium absorption (absorptive hypercalciuria), which is the most common abnormality. (2) Enhanced calcium mobilization from bone (resorptive hypercalciuria), which leads to urinary loss of bone calcium. This can be seen in patients with primary hyperparathyroidism, immobilization, and metastatic tumors. (3) Decreased renal calcium reabsorption (renal leak), the pathogenesis of which is unclear and is thought to be due to a primary defect in renal tubular absorption of calcium. High sodium intake results in decrease in proximal sodium reabsorption. The ensuing urinary sodium excretion results in physiologic increase in calcium excretion, thus promoting stone formation. High animal protein intake can lead to increased acid load, causing calcium release from bones and resulting in increased urinary calcium excretion. Moreover, acidosis resulting in decreased tubular calcium reabsorption and depletion of urinary citrate.

Thiazide diuretics are commonly used to decrease urine calcium excretion in recurrent calcium stone formers. They are effective in treating hypercalciuria and reducing stone recurrence regardless of the underlying pathophysiologic mechanism. They cause volume contraction-induced increased proximal tubule calcium absorption. Thiazides can cause hypokalemia-induced hypocitraturia; therefore they should be supplemented with potassium. Potassium citrate has an advantage over other agents because it because it provides both potassium and citrate.

Hyperoxaluria. Hyperoxaluria (>45 mg/day in women and 55 mg/day in men) is detected in 10% to 50% of calcium stone formers. Hyperoxaluria increases calcium oxalate supersaturation and thus promotes calcium oxalate stone formation. Hyperoxaluria can result from increased dietary intake, increased gastrointestinal absorption of oxalate, or overproduction of oxalate as a result of an inborn error in metabolism. Foods known to increase urinary oxalate excretion include rhubarb, spinach, potatoes, beetroot, most nuts, chocolate,

tea, raspberries, figs, plums, and high amounts of vitamin C. Enteric hyperoxaluria occurs in patients with malabsorption of fat, which leads to binding of dietary calcium to excessive enteric fat, and subsequent increase in absorption of free oxalate in the colon. This is commonly seen in patients with chronic diarrhea, inflammatory bowel diseases, celiac disease, and intestinal resection or after bariatric surgery. In patients with enteric hyperoxaluria, cholestyramine can be used to bind bile acids and oxalate; however, it is not always well tolerated. Other concomitant stone risk factors include low urine volume, acidic urine, and hypocitraturia. Rarely, hyperoxaluria is caused by inborn errors in metabolism such as primary hyperoxaluria, a rare autosomal recessive genetic disorder of oxalate synthesis. Type 1 primary hyperoxaluria is more common and often presents in childhood with nephrolithiasis, nephrocalcinosis, and kidney failure. Type II primary hyperoxaluria has a milder course with similar clinical manifestations.

Treatment measures include a low-oxalate diet and increased calcium intake with meals to bind intestinal oxalate and prevent its absorption. Patients should be advised to avoid excessive vitamin C (>500 mg/day). In addition, for patients with enteric hyperoxaluria, measures to reduce steatorrhea such as low-fat diet, cholestyramine, and administration of medium-chain triglycerides should be instituted. Liver transplant is the definitive therapy for patients with primary hyperoxaluria. Pyridoxine, which promotes conversion of glyoxylate to glycine, may reduce oxalate production in patients with type 1 primary hyperoxaluria. *Oxalobacter formigenes*, a colonic bacteria that uses oxalate for cellular metabolism, has been shown to be associated with a decreased risk of recurrent calcium oxalate stone formation, presumably because the bacterium degrades oxalate, prevents its absorption, and thus promotes excretion. However, a randomized control trial comparing use of *Oxalobacter formigenes* to placebo in patients with primary hyperoxaluria did not show reduction in urinary oxalate levels.

Hypocitraturia. Citrate, an endogenous inhibitor of calcium stone formation, is the only inhibitor that is measured and can be modified in clinical settings. It is a tricarboxylic acid that mostly stems from endogenous oxidative metabolism, freely filtered through the glomerulus and actively reabsorbed in the proximal tubule. Citrate binds to urinary calcium to form a soluble complex and thus prevents precipitation of calcium with oxalates or phosphates. Citrate also directly inhibits crystal aggregation. Hypocitraturia, defined by citrate concentration of less than 325 mg/day, can be a consequence of metabolic acidosis, high protein intake, carbonic anhydrase inhibitors, hypokalemia, or as an idiopathic disorder. Fall in tubular fluid pH results in conversion of trivalent citrate anion into the divalent anion, which is more easily reabsorbed via the sodium-citrate cotransporter in the luminal membrane. In addition, acidosis results in increased cell citrate utilization and upregulation of proximal renal tubular reabsorption of citrate leading to hypocitraturia.

Both potassium and sodium alkali supplementation can effectively raise urinary pH and citrate. However, potassium citrate is more effective in preventing calcium stone formation compared to sodium citrate because the sodium load can worsen hypercalciuria. Required dose for potassium citrate is 15 to 25 mmol two or three times a day. One potential concern with alkali therapy is the risk of calcium phosphate stone formation. In addition, among patients with reduced kidney function, serum potassium needs to be monitored closely for hyperkalemia.

Calcium Phosphate Stones

Calcium phosphate stone formation is a result of hypercalciuria, hypocitraturia, and persistently alkaline urine. Calcium phosphate stones can be seen in conditions causing distal RTA (inherited defects,

---

secondary to autoimmune conditions or idiopathic), with use of carbonic anhydrase inhibitors such as acetazolamide (which reduces bicarbonate reabsorption in the proximal tubule), or with use of antiepileptic drugs that have carbonic anhydrase inhibitory activity such as topiramate and zonisamide. In patients with distal RTA, correction of the systemic acidosis with oral alkali (usually potassium citrate or potassium bicarbonate) is recommended with the goal of increasing serum bicarbonate level and urinary citrate excretion. Administration of alkali to maintain the serum bicarbonate level with the risk associated with a higher urine pH should be balanced. Urinary pH should be monitored closely on alkali therapy and not increased above 7 (because of increased risk for precipitating calcium phosphate crystals). A thiazide diuretic can be added to lower urinary calcium if stone formation persists, even if the urine calcium is in the "normal" range or when low bone density is present. Among patients with stone disease due to the administration of medications, discontinuation of the medication, if feasible, will prevent new stone formation.

Uric Acid Stones

The three major urinary abnormalities causing uric acid precipitation are low urinary pH (urine pH <5.5), low urine volume, and hyperuricosuria (defined as uric acid excretion >800 mg/day in men and >750 mg/day in women). Acidic urine is a more important risk factor for uric acid stones than hyperuricosuria. In low urinary pH the relatively soluble urate gets converted into insoluble uric acid, thereby facilitating lithogenesis. Excessive acid load (high animal protein diet) or chronic bicarbonate loss in patients with chronic diarrhea can result in low urinary pH, thus increasing the propensity for uric acid stone formation. Increased incidence of uric acid stones can be seen in patients with insulin resistance and type 2 diabetes mellitus and has been linked to impaired ammonia synthesis resulting in reduced urinary pH. Hyperuricosuria may be seen in certain clinical conditions such as myeloproliferative disorders, tumor lysis syndrome, and rare genetic disorders of uric acid synthetic pathway or mutations in renal uric acid transporters.

Alkaline therapy along with increasing urine volume is the most effective treatment of uric acid stones. Potassium citrate 30 to 80 mmol in divided doses is prescribed to maintain urine pH greater than 6.5 to 7. Raising the urinary pH to greater than 7 may result in calcium phosphate precipitation and should be avoided. Other measures to decrease uric acid excretion and raise urinary pH include low animal protein and low purine diet. In situations where marked hyperuricosuria persists despite dietary measures, xanthine oxidase inhibitors such as allopurinol at doses of 100 to 300 mg/day can be prescribed.

Struvite Stones

Struvite stones or triple phosphate stones are composed of magnesium ammonium phosphate and calcium carbonate-apatite. They can grow rapidly and if left untreated can fill the entire renal pelvis (i.e., staghorn calculi) and may lead to CKD and ESRD. These stones result from chronic urinary tract infections with urea-splitting organisms (Table 27.13), which increase the urine pH by generating ammonium to produce stones composed of ammonium-magnesium-phosphate.

The cornerstone of treatment for struvite stones includes early surgical removal of the bacteria-laden stones and eradicating the infection with antibiotics. Also, it is important to define and treat any metabolic abnormality. Acetohydroxamic acid, a urease inhibitor, is the only drug approved for the treatment of infectious kidney stones; however, its use is limited by its side effects such as headache, thrombophlebitis, tremor, nausea, vomiting, rash, abdominal discomfort, anemia, and reticulocytosis. This treatment should only be used if other measures are ineffective. Medical management alone for struvite stones is rarely successful and is not recommended unless patients are too ill for surgery or refuse stone removal.

TABLE 27.13   Urease-Producing Bacteria
Most species of *Proteus* and *Providencia*
Corynebacterium
Klebsiella
Pseudomonas
Serratia
Haemophilus
Staphylococcus

Cystine Stones

Cystinuria is the most common of the rare hereditary kidney stone diseases and is caused by an autosomal recessive defect in renal transport of amino acid cystine. Mutations of one of the two subunits of the amino acid transporter in the kidney leads to defective renal tubular reabsorption of dibasic amino acids such as cystine, arginine, lysine, and ornithine. Cystine stones are the main complication of this defect due to the low solubility of cystine in urine. Characteristic hexagonal cystine crystals can be seen on urine sediment (see Table 27.10). Cystinuria is diagnosed by family history of stones, stone formation at a young age, mildly radiopaque stones, and measurement of urinary cystine excretion. Patients with cystinuria excrete 250 to 1000 mg of cystine per day (normal is approximately 30 mg/day). Treatment must be aimed at decreasing the urinary cystine concentration by increasing urine volume to greater than 4 liters per day, reducing sodium intake, and alkalinizing the urine (urine pH >6.5) with potassium citrate or sodium bicarbonate and by decreasing animal protein intake. Persistence of urine cystine excretion greater than 250 mg/L, cystine crystals on urine sediment, and failure to elevate pH to greater than 7.0 despite conservative measures may require initiation of thiol-derivatives such as D-penicillamine and α-mercaptopropionylglycine (tiopronin). These drugs split cystine molecules into two cysteines and produce a highly soluble disulfide compound; however, their use may be limited by their side effect profile.

SUGGESTED READINGS

Badr M, El Koumi MA, Ali YF, et al: Renal tubular dysfunction in children with sickle cell haemoglobinopathy, Nephrology (Carlton) 18:299–303, 2013.

Bergman C, Guay-Woddford LM, et al.: Polycystic kidney disease, Nat Rev Dis Primers 50:1–24, 2018. 4.

Bosniak MA: The current radiological approach to renal cysts, Radiology 158:1–10, 2012.

Chen Z, Prosperi M, Bird VY. Prevalence of kidney stones in the USA: the National Health and Nutrition Evaluation Survey. Nov 26, 2018.

Cornec-Le Gall E, Audrezet MP, Chen JM, et al: Type of PKD1 mutation influences renal outcome in ADPKD, J Am Soc Nephrol 24:1006–1013, 2013.

Crino PB, Nathanson KL, Henske EP: The tuberous sclerosis complex, N Engl J Med 355:1345–1356, 2006.

Katabathina VS, Kota G, Dasyam AK, et al: Adult renal cystic disease: a genetic, biological, and developmental primer, Radiographics 30:1509–1523, 2010.

Khan SR, Pearle MS, Robertson WG, et al: Kidney stones, Nat Rev Dis Primers, 2016.

Moe OW: Kidney stones: pathophysiology and medical management, Lancet 367:333–344, 2006.

Moe OW, Pearle MS, Sakhaee K: Pharmacotherapy of urolithiasis: evidence from clinical trials, Kidney Int 79:385–392, 2011.

Perazella MA, Markowitz GS: Drug-induced acute interstitial nephritis, Nat Rev Nephrol 6:461–470, 2010.

Perazella MA, Shirali AC: Nephrotoxicity of cancer immunotherapies: past, present and future, JASN 29:2039–2052, 2018.

Pfau A, Knauf F: Update on nephrolithiasis: core curriculum, AKJD, 2016.

Rule AD, et al.: The ROKS Nomogram for predicting a second symptomatic stone episode, JASN, 2014.

Silverman SG, Pedrosa I, Ellis JH, et al: Bosniak classification of cystic renal masses, version 2019: an update proposal and needs assessment, Radiology 292:475–488, 2019.

Torres VE, Chapman AB, Devuyst O, et al: Tolvaptan in patients with autosomal dominant polycystic kidney disease, N Engl J Med 367:2407–2418, 2012.

Whelan TF: Guidelines on the management of renal cyst disease, Can Urol Assoc J 4:98–99, 2010.

Worcester EM, Coe FL: Calcium kidney stones, N Engl J Med 363:954–963, 2010.

Zeisberg M, Kalluri R: Physiology of the renal interstitium, CJASN 10(10):1831–1840, 2015.

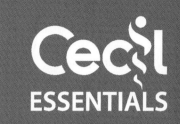

28

Vascular Disorders of the Kidney

Abdallah Geara, Jeffrey S. Berns

INTRODUCTION

The spectrum of vascular disorders of the kidneys is broad as a result of high renal blood flow and the intimate relationship between blood supply and fundamental glomerular and tubular functions. In this chapter, emphasis is placed on the clinical manifestations of hypertension, chronic kidney disease (CKD), end-stage kidney failure, and the many other causes of acute kidney injury (AKI).

RENAL VASCULAR ANATOMY

With a volume of around 150 mL each, the kidneys compromise less than 1% of the body mass and yet receive 20% to 25% of the cardiac output. The renal arteries arise directly from the aorta and enter the renal hilum. The right renal artery passes anterior to the inferior vena cava (IVC) and is longer than the left renal artery. In up to 30% of the population, accessory renal arteries arise from the aorta to provide blood to portions of one or both kidneys, which may become important when evaluating patients for renovascular hypertension.

The renal arteries give rise to segmental, interlobar, and arcuate arteries (Fig. 28.1). Arcuate arteries course along the corticomedullary junction and give rise to interlobular arterioles, which extend outward into the cortex before branching into afferent arterioles, from which the glomerular capillary tufts arise. The postglomerular efferent arterioles from more superficial glomeruli form a capillary network in the renal cortex, and those extending from glomeruli nearer the cortical-medullary junction (i.e., juxtamedullary glomeruli) form capillaries that extend deeper into the medulla in association with thin, descending and ascending loops of Henle as the vasa recta. The vasa recta provide the sole blood supply for the renal medulla, making this portion of the kidney particularly susceptible to ischemic injury. Venules from the ascending vasa recta and the cortical capillary network empty into the renal veins.

The left renal vein returns to the IVC anterior to the aorta and inferior to the inferior mesenteric artery, which may rarely cause compression of this vein, causing what is known as the "nutcracker syndrome," typically presenting with hematuria with or without left flank pain. The left gonadal vein also empties into the left renal vein, and a left varicocele may be evident if the renal vein is occluded by thrombosis or tumor involvement. The right renal vein is much shorter and empties directly into the IVC. The right gonadal vein empties directly into the IVC rather than into the right renal vein.

We categorize vascular diseases of the kidney based on the blood vessels typically involved (glomerulonephritis is addressed in Chapter 26):

- Main renal artery and segmental branches: Renovascular disease, fibromuscular dysplasia (FMD), aortic dissection, thromboembolic diseases and large and medium vessels vasculitis.

- Interlobular arterioles and glomerular arterioles: Hypertensive nephrosclerosis, atheroembolic disease, preeclampsia, scleroderma renal crisis, thrombotic microangiopathy (TMA) and antiphospholipid antibody syndrome (APS).
- Renal veins: Renal vein thrombosis (RVT).

RENOVASCULAR DISEASE

Any process that narrows the lumen of the main or branch renal arteries sufficiently can elicit a humoral response mediated by increased renin release from the ipsilateral kidney, which leads to increases in circulating angiotensin II and aldosterone levels. Activation of the renin-angiotensin-aldosterone system increases systemic blood pressure and renal arterial perfusion pressure and single nephron glomerular filtration rate (GFR) beyond the stenosis. This is mediated through angiotensin II-mediated preferential efferent arteriolar vasoconstriction that counterbalances the increase in resistance imposed by narrowing of the main or branch arteries.

Hemodynamically significant renal artery stenosis (RAS) requires a reduction in lumen diameter of at least 50% to 60%. In the stenotic kidney, a decrease in the glomerular capillary pressure results in activation of the renin-angiotensin-aldosterone system, systemic vasoconstriction mediated by angiotensin II, and increased renal sodium and fluid reabsorption, resulting in elevation of systemic blood pressure. If the contralateral kidney has no stenosis, the increased systemic blood pressure increases sodium excretion by that kidney (i.e., pressure natriuresis). Thus, clinically, a patient with unilateral renal artery stenosis and two functioning kidneys has hypertension secondary to angiotensin II-mediated systemic vasoconstriction without significant hypervolemia. Because hypertension in this setting is maintained by increased vasoconstriction due to angiotensin II, treatment is aimed at blocking the synthesis or effect of the elevated angiotensin II levels with an angiotensin-converting enzyme (ACE) inhibitor or angiotensin-receptor blocker (ARB).

If the arteries to both kidneys are narrowed, pressure natriuresis does not occur, and hypertension is maintained chronically by the resulting intravascular volume expansion rather than by increased total peripheral resistance. Treatment with diuretics becomes more important in this circumstance. The latter situation also occurs when there is only a single functioning kidney that has stenosis or when an initially normal contralateral kidney suffers microvascular damage from long-standing hypertension (Fig. 28.2).

The pathophysiology of hypertension with RAS is such that its treatment may also compromise kidney function and reduce the GFR. If the kidney contralateral to the one with hemodynamically significant RAS has normal function, lowering the systemic blood pressure maintains the kidney with the stenosis in a hemodynamically compromised

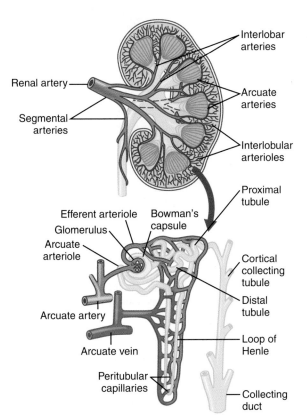

Fig. 28.1 *Top:* Cross-section of the human kidney showing renal arteries and veins. *Bottom:* Schematic of the microcirculation of each nephron. (From Guyton AC, Hall JE: Textbook of medical physiology, ed 11, 2016, Saunders, Chapter 26, 323-333.)

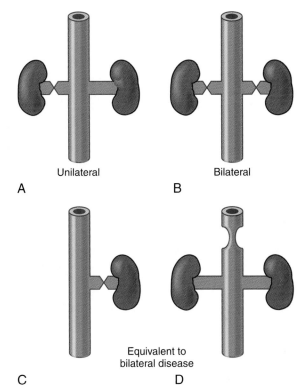

Fig. 28.2 Anatomy of renal artery stenosis. Renal artery stenosis may be unilateral (A), bilateral (B), or unilateral with a solitary kidney (C). Aortic disease may serve functionally as bilateral renal artery stenosis (D).

state. However, this may not be detectable by measurement of the serum creatinine concentration because of the normally functioning contralateral kidney. A decline in the GFR may, however, be evident if there is underlying dysfunction of the contralateral kidney, as is often the case in long-standing hypertension, diabetes, or vascular disease. When a solitary functioning kidney or both kidneys are affected (i.e., bilateral RAS), AKI may result when ACE inhibitor or ARB treatment is initiated.

Atherosclerotic Renovascular Disease
Clinical Presentation

Atherosclerosis is the primary cause of RAS in adults, although any process that narrows one or both renal arteries may cause renal ischemia; others are discussed later in this chapter. Atherosclerotic renovascular disease is a common form of secondary hypertension, affecting up to 5% of patients with hypertension. Atherosclerotic RAS rarely occurs in patients younger than 40 years, and it is more common in men, white individuals, smokers, diabetics, and patients with atherosclerotic disease in other arterial systems. The prevalence of RAS increases to between 10% to 45% in patients with other atherosclerotic risk factors such as coronary artery disease, peripheral vascular disease, and aortic disease.

RAS should be suspected in patients with refractory hypertension or new-onset hypertension in patients older than 50 years, particularly if they have overt risk factors for atherosclerotic RAS (Table 28.1). Evaluation should always begin with a thorough history and physical examination, including attention to blood pressure and pulse amplitude in each extremity. A significant discrepancy between extremities may indicate peripheral vascular disease and increase the likelihood of RAS. An abdominal bruit is detected in about 50% of subjects but

TABLE 28.1 **Clinical Findings of Atherosclerotic Renovascular Disease**
Onset of new, severe hypertension or sudden worsening of chronic hypertension at >55 years of age
Accelerated, resistant, or malignant hypertension
Unexplained atrophic kidney or size discrepancy >1.5 cm between kidneys
Sudden, unexplained ("flash") pulmonary edema
Unexplained chronic kidney disease in an individual with atherosclerotic vascular disease elsewhere
Development of acute kidney injury or worsening of chronic kidney disease after starting an ACE inhibitor or ARB

ACE, Angiotensin-converting enzyme; *ARB,* angiotensin II–receptor blocker.

is not specific for RAS. Edema is not typically found unless significant CKD or another edematous condition also exists.

Laboratory evaluation may reveal hypokalemia (K^+ <3.5 mEq/L) or metabolic alkalosis (HCO_3^- >28 mEq/L) due to secondary hyperaldosteronism, although neither may be present. A reduced GFR with an elevated serum creatinine concentration may be found, but a normal serum creatinine concentration does not rule out hemodynamically significant RAS. Plasma renin activity and aldosterone concentrations may be elevated, but their measurement is of limited clinical utility in assessing hypertensive patients for RAS or in making therapeutic decisions. Urinalysis results are usually normal, although low-grade proteinuria (usually <1 g/day) from long-standing hypertension may be seen.

Diagnosis

Standard renal ultrasound imaging may suggest the presence of underlying RAS if it reveals a significant discrepancy in kidney size or if both are smaller than normal, because kidney size diminishes over time after prolonged ischemia. *Renal ultrasound with Doppler analysis* provides information about flow velocity in the renal arteries that may be helpful in detecting hemodynamically significant RAS. However, *renal duplex ultrasonography* is technically demanding, particularly in obese patients. Since at any given center, the sensitivity, specificity, and positive and negative predictive values of renal duplex ultrasonography are likely to be unknown, its clinical utility is mainly when positive for RAS; a negative test is not informative in patients with high clinical suspicion. Serial measurement of the kidney size and measurement of the renal resistive index ([peak systolic velocity − end-diastolic velocity] divided by peak systolic velocity) are helpful in assessing the potential benefit of revascularization. A high resistive index reflects an advanced degree of likely irreversible intrinsic kidney damage.

Computed tomography (CT) with intravenous iodinated contrast (i.e., CT angiography [CTA]) permits high-resolution evaluation of the arterial vasculature and can be a very useful diagnostic imaging study, particularly in patients with normal or near-normal kidney function. Its use is limited in patients with more significantly impaired kidney function due to the risk of contrast-induced AKI. Some newer CT imaging machines have a higher resolution and better tissue reconstruction allowing the visualization of RAS with lower amounts of contrast exposure.

Magnetic resonance angiography (MRA) with intravenous contrast is also useful for detecting RAS. Gadolinium administration to patients with advanced kidney disease (GFR <15 to 30 mL/min) may be contraindicated because of the risk of nephrogenic systemic fibrosis, although this appears to be much less of a concern with newer nonionic linear and macrocyclic gadolinium contrast agents. Overall, CTA and MRA appear to have similarly high sensitivity and specificity in the assessment of patients with atherosclerotic RAS. In RAS secondary to FMD, CTA and MRA are less sensitive because the disease involves the more distal part of the renal artery.

A *functional renal nuclear medicine test* might seem pathophysiologically ideal to detect RAS that is impacting kidney perfusion. Nuclear imaging has been used with various isotopes to assess isotopic uptake and excretion by each kidney before and after the administration of a short-acting ACE inhibitor (e.g., captopril). However, due to the high prevalence of baseline asymmetry of blood flow in patients with CKD and inability to accurately diagnose RAS when it is bilateral, radionuclear tests have fallen out of favor due to limited specificity and sensitivity for the diagnosis of RAS and are not commonly used any longer to assess for the presence of RAS or to determine whether RAS might be amenable to revascularization.

The most sensitive and specific test—but also the most invasive—is *renal arteriography*, which remains the gold standard for the detection of RAS. An advantage of arteriography is that angioplasty and stenting can be performed during the procedure (discussed later) if indicated. Because of the frequent occurrence of accessory renal arteries, an aortogram must be performed rather than selective renal angiography to ensure that all vessels are visualized. This also allows for detection of aortic atherosclerotic disease.

Treatment

Patients with atherosclerotic RAS typically have coexistent cerebrovascular, coronary, and peripheral vascular disease as the result of a long history of multiple risk factors such as cigarette smoking and hyperlipidemia. Clinicians should recognize this high cardiovascular risk and understand that long-term outcomes for patients with atherosclerotic RAS are often determined by coexisting atherosclerotic disease of the cerebral, cardiac, or peripheral vascular circulations. The absolute risk of developing end-stage renal disease (ESRD) is increased for patients

with atherosclerotic RAS compared with those without RAS, especially in patients with bilateral RAS or RAS of a solitary kidney.

As with atherosclerotic disease in other arterial circulations, atherosclerotic RAS should prompt efforts for intensive lipid lowering, use of aspirin, smoking cessation, and control of hypertension and diabetes mellitus.

Intervention for atherosclerotic RAS remains controversial despite several randomized clinical trials designed to investigate the benefits and risks of medical management compared with angioplasty and renal artery stenting. Small clinical studies have suggested that renal artery angioplasty and stenting may improve blood pressure control in selected cases of atherosclerotic RAS, but identifying which patients may benefit has been problematic, and many have little or no improvement in blood pressure or are not able to significantly reduce the number of required antihypertensive medications. Two major randomized, controlled clinical trials of treatment of RAS with angioplasty did not demonstrate significant clinical benefit in terms of blood pressure control, kidney function, or mortality for most patients with atherosclerotic RAS, although both have been criticized for selection bias (excluding some high-risk patients with recurrent flash pulmonary edema and patients whose doctors felt they were likely to benefit from revascularization) and recruiting significant numbers of low-risk patients who were not on optimal medical therapy.

Renal artery angioplasty and stenting carry a risk of acute worsening of kidney function due to atheroembolic disease, contrast nephropathy, or in-stent thrombosis, among other technical complications, and the procedures may lead to irreversible, progressive kidney dysfunction and ESRD. Decisions to correct atherosclerotic RAS with angioplasty and stenting or surgery must be made on a case-by-case basis, considering:

- Underlying kidney function and pace of kidney function loss, if any.
- Severity and duration of hypertension: persistence of uncontrolled HTN after optimal medical therapy, intolerance to optimal medical therapy, and the short duration of blood pressure elevation prior to the diagnosis of RAS.
- Atherosclerotic disease in other vascular beds and life expectancy based on age and other comorbid conditions.
- Flash pulmonary edema.

There is no role for angioplasty alone without stenting in most patients with atherosclerotic RAS due to the high risk of recurrent stenosis.

Medical management of hypertension in patients with atherosclerotic RAS must take into consideration other comorbid conditions. Use of an ACE inhibitor or ARB and diuretics is often very effective, but patients treated with these agents must be monitored closely for further compromise of their kidney function.

Fibromuscular Dysplasia

FMD is a nonatherosclerotic, noninflammatory disease that causes RAS. FMD typically affects young women more than other groups but men and older age groups can be affected. The cause is not established, but it is thought to be a developmental defect. FMD is responsible for 35% to 50% of renovascular hypertension in children and 5% to 10% of renovascular hypertension in adults.

FMD most commonly affects the renal arteries (bilaterally in about 35% of affected patients), but carotid and vertebral arteries can also be affected.

Classification of FMD is based on the histologic layer of the artery involved (i.e., intima, media, or adventitia) (Table 28.2). Medial fibroplasia with a mural aneurysm is the most common cause of FMD in adults (70% of cases). It consists of alternating fibromuscular ridges and aneurysmal segments in the distal two thirds of the renal artery and has a classic string-of-beads appearance on angiography (Fig. 28.3). Perimedial fibroplasia of the outer one half of the media produces severe multifocal stenosis and causes about 15% of FMD in adults. Because histologic specimens are rarely obtained, FMD is classified by the angiographic appearance with multifocal disease identified as FMD involving the media and unifocal disease as FMD of the intima and/or adventitia.

Medial subtypes of FMD usually have a benign course and are responsive to angioplasty. The intimal subtype may have a higher likelihood of ischemic events and multiorgan system involvement. Symptoms are usually precipitated by stenosis, but FMD may rarely cause dissection or macroaneurysms that require intervention. Although CTA or MRA may be useful in the detection of FMD in the main renal arteries and main branch arteries, arteriography is necessary for detection of stenosis in smaller arteries.

Treatment for FMD depends on the severity of complications. Pharmacologic treatment alone may be adequate to control hypertension in many patients, with an ACE inhibitor or ARB the antihypertensives of choice. Intervention with angioplasty (with or without stenting) or surgery should be considered for patients with severe or difficult to control hypertension or declining kidney function. Angioplasty without stenting is successful in many patients, but recurrent stenosis is not uncommon, and new stenosis from FMD may develop at other sites. For this reason, regular monitoring of blood pressure and serum creatinine levels is essential, and many patients require imaging studies to detect new or recurrent lesions.

TABLE 28.2 Histologic Classification of Fibromuscular Dysplasia

Subtype	Percentage of All Cases (%)	Radiologic Appearance
Medial fibroplasia	60-70	String of beads with aneurysms
Perimedial fibroplasia	15	String of beads without large aneurysms
Medial hyperplasia	5-15	Smooth tubular stenosis
Intimal fibroplasia	1-2	Focal or smooth stenosis
Adventitial fibroplasia	<1	Focal or smooth tubular stenosis

Aortic Dissection

Aortic dissection occurs after disruption of the intimal layer of the aorta and propagation of blood flow that dissects along the wall of the aorta, producing a false lumen and compression of the true aortic lumen. Aortic dissection is classified by the site of origin (i.e., DeBakey classification) or the segment of the aorta involved (i.e., Stanford classification). DeBakey type I and II dissections originate in the ascending aorta, and type III dissections originate in the descending aorta. Stanford type A refers to dissections involving the ascending aorta, and type B refers to all others not involving the ascending aorta.

Major branch vessels of the aorta, including the renal arteries, may become obstructed or occluded as a result of extension of the dissection. Aortic dissection frequently compromises the renal arteries (the left more commonly than the right) when it extends into the abdominal aorta and causes renal failure in approximately 20% of patients with type B dissections. When disease is extensive enough to cause AKI, vascular compromise to the intestinal and cerebral vasculature and severe aortic regurgitation often contribute to the high mortality rate.

Aortic dissection most frequently affects older patients (>50 years of age) with coexistent vascular risk factors such as hypertension, smoking, and atherosclerosis. Men are affected more commonly than women. Occasionally, a genetic connective tissue defect such as Marfan syndrome or Ehlers-Danlos syndrome type IV (about 5% of cases) causes aortic dissection, and these conditions should be considered in younger patients (<40 years of age).

AKI occurs in about 20% of patients diagnosed with acute type B aortic dissection and is an independent predictor of in-hospital mortality. Trauma or procedures (e.g., aortic catheterization) can also cause dissection of the aorta or renal artery. Isolated, spontaneous renal artery dissection may rarely occur, most commonly in the setting of polyarteritis nodosa (PAN) or FMD. Segmental arterial mediolysis is another uncommon condition of unknown origin that is characterized by vacuolar degeneration of smooth muscle cells in the arterial media, which leads to disruption of the arterial medial layer, vessel dissection, hemorrhage, and ischemia. Segmental arterial mediolysis can affect abdominal visceral arteries and virtually any other arterial system.

The most frequent symptom during aortic dissection is chest pain, which may be described as a ripping sensation. Isolated loss of pulse in one or more extremities may provide a clinical clue, and the number of

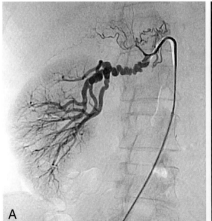
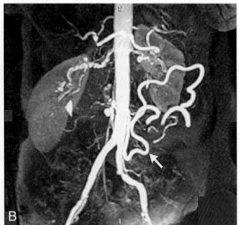

Fig. 28.3 (A) Typical medial fibroplasia (i.e., string-of-beads appearance) on an angiogram of a right renal artery. (B) Gadolinium-enhanced magnetic resonance angiography in the same patient, revealing bilateral medial fibroplasia of the renal arteries and a large marginal artery of Drummond *(arrow)*, indicates that there is disease of the superior mesenteric artery. (From Slovut DP, Olin JW: Fibromuscular dysplasia, N Engl J Med 350:1862-1871, 2004.)

arteries involved correlates with the severity of dissection. A common clue to the diagnosis on a routine chest radiograph is a widened mediastinum, with or without a pleural effusion (most often on the left).

After the diagnosis of aortic dissection is established, evaluation of renal artery involvement is best undertaken noninvasively to minimize further vascular injury. Contrast-enhanced CT, magnetic resonance imaging, or MRA usually provide images capable of confirming or excluding renal involvement, although each modality carries the same limitations as outlined for the evaluation of RAS. Transesophageal echocardiography is useful for establishing the diagnosis of aortic dissection, but it does not provide information about the aorta below the diaphragm. Renal duplex ultrasonography may be useful for evaluating renal perfusion in the setting of aortic dissection, but it is not recommended for the initial investigation of aortic dissection.

Aortic dissection is a hypertensive emergency that requires aggressive reduction of blood pressure; systolic blood pressure should be maintained between 100 and 120 mm Hg. Antihypertensive medications that reduce the rate of increase in blood pressure during the cardiac cycle, such as β-adrenergic receptor blockers, have a theoretical benefit in managing aortic dissection by reducing the rate of progression.

Surgical treatment options for renal involvement due to aortic dissection depend on individual circumstances, and careful evaluation by an experienced vascular surgeon is recommended. Thoracic aortic dissection requires surgical repair due to the high mortality rate if left untreated, but isolated abdominal aortic disease may be medically managed.

Thromboembolic Disease

Systemic arterial emboli, typically originating from the left atrium or left ventricle in patients with atrial fibrillation, infectious endocarditis, cardiac valvular disease, or atrial myxoma, may cause acute obstruction of the renal arteries. Rarely, a paradoxical embolus may occur from the venous system through an atrial septal defect.

Symptoms of acute renal ischemia and infarction include flank pain, gross hematuria, and fever. Laboratory findings are nonspecific but include an elevated level of lactate dehydrogenase (LDH), hematuria, and leukocytosis. A definitive diagnosis can be based on the finding of a focal nonenhancing region on contrast-enhanced CT. Imaging studies are necessary to differentiate renal artery embolic disease from renal artery dissection.

The renal mass affected by a renal artery embolus is usually not large enough to reduce kidney function so that dialysis is necessary, although some worsening of kidney function may be observed. The diagnosis of renal infarction is rarely made early enough to initiate treatment with intra-arterial thrombolysis or thrombectomy, and it is questionable whether the risks and marginal benefit of these procedures warrant aggressive treatment except in patients where the occlusion is affecting the main renal artery and is addressed soon after occurrence. Therapy should instead address the underlying source of renal emboli with symptomatic treatment of pain as necessary. Systemic anticoagulation may be indicated to reduce the risk of further thromboembolic events.

Large and Medium-Sized Vessel Vasculitis

Systemic vasculitides such as temporal (giant cell) arteritis and Takayasu's arteritis affect primarily large and medium-sized arteries. PAN and Kawasaki disease affect primarily medium-sized and smaller arteries. These vasculitides are not associated with antineutrophil cytoplasmic antibodies (ANCAs) and do not typically cause glomerulonephritis. They are distinguished from ANCA-associated vasculitides that involve smaller blood vessels and more commonly cause glomerulonephritis.

Takayasu's arteritis and giant cell arteritis are typically associated with a granulomatous vasculitis of the aorta and its branches. Giant cell arteritis typically involves the carotid, vertebral, and temporal arteries, and renal involvement is rare. Both occur much more commonly in women than men. Takayasu's arteritis is usually diagnosed in patients younger than 50 years of age, whereas giant cell arteritis is diagnosed in those 50 years of age or older.

Involvement of the main renal arteries occurs in about 40% of patients with Takayasu's arteritis, producing areas of stenosis with renal ischemia or renal infarction. Common clinical features are constitutional symptoms, claudication, bruits, and hypertension. Pulses are often diminished or absent in one or more extremities, and a blood pressure discrepancy more than 10 mm Hg in the limbs is common. The diagnosis of Takayasu's arteritis is most often made on clinical grounds along with typical angiographic or other imaging findings. Corticosteroids are the primary treatment modality. The stenotic lesions are usually reversible when corticosteroid therapy is given during the early phase of the disease before the lesions becomes fibrotic and irreversible. About half of patients have chronic, persistent or corticosteroid-dependent disease and require therapy with additional or alternative immunosuppressants such as azathioprine, mycophenolate, methotrexate, leflunomide or cyclophosphamide. More recently targeted immunosuppression with antagonists of interleukin-6 (such as tocilizumab) and blockers of the tumor necrosis factor alpha (TNFα) pathway (such as infliximab or etanercept) may be effective in helping maintain remission.

PAN is a medium-sized or small vessel vasculitis with no gender predilection that predominantly occurs in adults between 40 and 60 years of age. It is an idiopathic systemic necrotizing vasculitis. Some cases may be secondary to hepatitis B virus infection, hepatitis C virus infection, or hairy cell leukemia. Peripheral neuropathy in the form of mononeuritis multiplex is one of the most frequent findings with PAN.

PAN affects the main renal arteries and renal interlobar arteries (less commonly, the arcuate and interlobular arteries) with a necrotizing vasculitis that typically produces microaneurysms of the intrarenal arteries. They can be seen on arteriograms in 40% to 90% of patients with renal involvement. Renal ischemia leads to loss of kidney function and renin-mediated hypertension. Low-grade proteinuria and hematuria may be seen, but the finding of acute glomerulonephritis indicates some other disorder. Renal infarction may occur, and rarely, a renal artery aneurysm may cause renal artery dissection or rupture.

The diagnosis is made on clinical grounds and by arteriography. There are no confirmatory serologic tests; PAN is not an ANCA-associated vasculitis. Arteriography appears to be superior for diagnosis compared with CTA and MRA. Progressive renal disease is not typical but may occur. Treatment with corticosteroids and immunosuppressive drugs is effective in reducing disease severity and mortality.

Kawasaki disease is an arteritis associated with the mucocutaneous lymph node syndrome that affects mostly medium-sized and small arteries, although the aorta may also be involved. It is primarily a self-limited disease of infants and young children. Renal involvement is extremely rare.

Hypertensive Nephrosclerosis

Chronic hypertension in susceptible individuals may lead to development of proteinuria, CKD, and ESRD. Hypertensive nephrosclerosis is cited as a cause of CKD and ESRD in African Americans at a much higher rate than white individuals, even with similar levels of blood pressure control and despite good control.

The renal manifestations of chronic hypertension include renal arterial and arteriolar intimal thickening and luminal narrowing with medial hypertrophy and fibroblastic intimal thickening of arteries and deposition of hyaline-like material (plasma proteins) in the walls of arterioles. Glomeruli show global and focal glomerulosclerosis; the former likely results from glomerular ischemia and the latter from increased intracapillary pressure and compensatory hypertrophy and injury in response to nephron loss. Wrinkled glomerular basement membranes due to glomerular ischemia are seen on electron microscopy. Chronic interstitial nephritis with tubular atrophy and interstitial fibrosis is another manifestation of chronic ischemic tubular injury seen with hypertensive nephrosclerosis, particularly in patients with other disorders such as diabetes mellitus, atheroembolic disease, and atherosclerotic RAS.

The overall risk of hypertensive nephrosclerosis with progressive CKD is low in the general hypertensive population, and most patients with hypertensive nephrosclerosis have mild hypertension. The risk is greater for those who have had poorly controlled hypertension and for those of African descent, who are at particularly high risk for hypertensive nephrosclerosis. Polymorphisms in the gene that encodes for apolipoprotein L1 (*APOL1*) is found more commonly in African Americans compared with European Americans and strongly associated with the risk of hypertensive nephrosclerosis. A diagnosis of hypertensive nephrosclerosis as the cause of otherwise unexplained CKD is much less likely to be made in white patients compared with black patients, particularly in the absence of long-standing, severe hypertension or a history of malignant hypertension.

The diagnosis of hypertensive nephrosclerosis is typically made clinically based on a history of long-standing hypertension that precedes development of proteinuria and CKD in the absence of other causes. Kidney biopsy is rarely performed except when other disorders are suggested clinically or by laboratory evaluation. The urinary sediment is typically bland, with only low-grade proteinuria (<1 g/day). Symmetrical loss of renal cortical thickness is commonly found on renal ultrasound.

Pharmacologic treatment of severe hypertension reduces the risk for progression of CKD to ESRD in many patient populations, providing further evidence for the causative role of hypertension. The optimal blood pressure for patients with hypertensive nephrosclerosis has not been determined. For black patients, this was best addressed by the African American Study of Kidney Disease (AASK) trial, which examined more than 1000 African Americans with long-standing hypertension, slowly progressive CKD, and low-grade proteinuria. Subjects were allocated to treatment with ramipril, metoprolol, or amlodipine to a blood pressure goal of 125/75 mm Hg or 140/90 mm Hg. The mean rate of change in GFR and the rate of other secondary outcomes were similar in the two groups, suggesting that lowering blood pressure to less than 140/90 mm Hg does not provide further benefit in slowing CKD progression in black patients with hypertensive nephrosclerosis. However, there was a trend favoring the lower blood pressure goal for patients with higher baseline proteinuria.

Lower blood pressure goals may also be appropriate for patients with other comorbid conditions such as diabetes mellitus. Besides affecting CKD progression, blood pressure control reduces the risk of heart failure and stroke. Most patients with hypertensive nephrosclerosis and CKD require multiple antihypertensive medications to control blood pressure, typically including a thiazide or thiazide-like diuretic (when GFR is well preserved) and a loop diuretic (as the GFR declines to less than 25 to 30 mL/min), along with an ACE inhibitor or ARB, calcium-channel blocker, and β-blocker.

Atheroembolic Disease

Atheroembolic disease is the result of cholesterol embolization from atherosclerotic plaques, most commonly from the aorta and typically dislodged during an invasive arterial procedure such as cardiac catheterization, aortic angiography, cardiac surgery, or surgery on the aorta. Cholesterol emboli may occur spontaneously or may be precipitated by systemic anticoagulation, such as with heparin, or during systemic administration of thrombolytic agents. Because patients must have underlying atherosclerosis, the incidence increases with age, and atheroembolic disease rarely occurs before 40 years of age.

As the result of systemic embolization from atheromatous plaques, cholesterol crystals lodge in small arterial vessels, including the arcuate or interlobular arteries of the kidneys. Cholesterol emboli frequently involve other organs, and the pattern of organ involvement depends in part on whether disrupted plaque is in the ascending or descending aorta. The extremities are commonly affected with digital ischemia and gangrene, the skin with livedo reticularis, and the gastrointestinal tract with intestinal ischemia, but any organ can be affected. Embolization from the ascending aorta can cause cardiac ischemia, and emboli arising from the ascending aorta or carotid arteries (e.g., after carotid endarterectomy) can cause stroke.

Cholesterol embolization to the eye may be recognized by finding Hollenhorst plaques on funduscopic examination, which are whitish yellow flecks at retinal arteriole bifurcations. They are often asymptomatic but may cause retinal ischemia with usually transient visual field defects.

Patients with atheroembolic disease may have fever, eosinophilia, eosinophiluria, and hypocomplementemia, particularly acutely. Laboratory findings include an elevated erythrocyte sedimentation rate and elevated levels of amylase or liver enzymes. The widespread systemic clinical and laboratory manifestations of atheroemboli can lead to a clinical picture suggesting systemic vasculitis.

The typical pattern of renal atheroembolic disease is a decline in kidney function that first becomes apparent 3 or more days after an inciting procedure or other event. The degree of acute and chronic kidney injury that follows is determined by the magnitude of the embolic burden, whether atheroembolism is a one-time or ongoing process, and the degree of inflammation induced by the plaque material. Many patients have stabilization of the process after the initial insult, whereas others progress with various patterns and tempos to advanced CKD and ESRD. Cholesterol embolization also may cause severe hypertension due to acute renal ischemia leading to renin release.

Diagnosis of renal atheroembolic disease is usually made clinically in the appropriate setting, but for some patients, a kidney biopsy is needed to confirm the diagnosis and exclude others. Because the fixation process washes out the cholesterol crystals from the renal biopsy sample, the pathologic examination reveals a typical needle-shaped disruption in the arterial lumen surrounded by reactive inflammatory and fibrous intimal proliferation leading to a luminal occlusion and distal ischemic injury.

There is no specific treatment for cholesterol emboli. Because an inflammatory reaction typically results from the emboli, some physicians advocate corticosteroids, but their use is unproved for preventing further atheroembolism or progression of kidney failure. Avoidance of anticoagulation has been recommended to prevent dissolution and embolization of thrombus that may overlie an atheromatous plaque. Statin therapy is recommended for most patients for treatment of their underlying atherosclerotic disease, but it has not been shown to influence the renal manifestation of atheroemboli. Treatment with ACE inhibitors or ARBs may be effective for hypertension control in the acute setting, but worsening kidney function may limit their use. Dialysis may be necessary if AKI and ESRD develop.

Preeclampsia

Preeclampsia is characterized by the new onset of sustained hypertension (blood pressure ≥140/90 mm Hg) and proteinuria (>300 mg/day) that develops after 20 weeks' gestation in a previously normotensive woman. Although hypertension and proteinuria are the principal features of preeclampsia, it is a systemic vascular disease that may also cause central nervous system symptoms (e.g., visual disturbances, headache, altered mental status), abdominal pain, nausea and vomiting, liver dysfunction, thrombocytopenia, pulmonary dysfunction, impaired fetal growth, nephrotic-range proteinuria, and AKI. If grand mal seizures develop without other explanation, a diagnosis of eclampsia is made. The HELLP syndrome, characterized by *h*emolysis, *el*evated *l*iver enzymes, and a *l*ow *p*latelet count, may be a manifestation of severe preeclampsia, although some consider it to be a separate disorder. It is also associated with increased maternal and fetal mortality. History of hypertension and CKD are risk factors for preeclampsia. Other major risk factors are nulliparity, preeclampsia in previous pregnancy, multifetal gestation, autoimmune disease, and family history of preeclampsia.

Preeclampsia should be distinguished from other hypertensive conditions that can occur during pregnancy, including preexisting hypertension that occurs before 20 weeks' gestation and persists after delivery, preeclampsia superimposed on preexisting chronic hypertension, and gestational hypertension (i.e., new-onset hypertension after 20 weeks' gestation without proteinuria or other related manifestations).

Progress has been made in understanding the pathogenesis of preeclampsia, and maternal and placental or fetal factors have been implicated. Abnormal development of placental vasculature in early pregnancy is thought to lead to some degree of placental hypoperfusion that releases antiangiogenic factors into the maternal circulation, disturbing the delicate balance of angiogenic and antiangiogenic factors. This causes systemic endothelial dysfunction in the mother that leads to hypertension, proteinuria, and other manifestations of the disease.

Soluble FMS-related tyrosine kinase 1 (sFLT1) is a placenta-derived circulating antiangiogenic factor that appears to play a central role in the pathogenesis of preeclampsia. It antagonizes the proangiogenic effects of vascular endothelial growth factor (VEGF) and placental growth factor (PGF) by binding to them and preventing interaction with their receptors. Soluble endoglin (sENG), another antiangiogenic factor that is widely expressed on vascular endothelium, is thought to be an important mediator of preeclampsia. Endothelial dysfunction in preeclampsia is associated with increased sensitivity to vasopressor agents, including angiotensin II, systemic vasoconstriction, and reduced fibrinolytic function.

Kidney biopsy findings include glomerular endothelial cell swelling (i.e., endotheliosis) and occlusion of the capillary lumen with ischemia. These findings are also seen with other microangiopathic disorders, although fibrin thrombi in glomerular capillaries are less commonly seen than with other causes. Foot process effacement is not usually seen.

The only effective treatment for preeclampsia is delivery of the fetus and placenta. The timing of delivery must take into account gestational age, severity of preeclampsia, presence or absence of systemic features, and status of the fetus and mother. Proper obstetric care is essential to balance the risk to the mother against the risk for prematurity of the fetus. In high-risk pregnancies, low-dose aspirin is started in the second and third trimester to reduce the risk of developing preeclampsia.

Treatment of mild hypertension in women with preeclampsia should be avoided because it does not treat the underlying disease process, alter the course of disease, or reduce clinical sequelae. In the absence of clinical manifestations other than proteinuria, it is usually unnecessary to start antihypertensive medications unless the systolic blood pressure is greater than 150 mm Hg or the diastolic blood pressure is higher than 100 mm Hg. Labetalol and hydralazine, both of which can be given intravenously or orally, are often recommended as first-line therapy for acute management. For chronic treatment, methyldopa or labetalol are often recommended initially, with extended-release nifedipine added if necessary. Diuretics and dietary sodium restriction usually are avoided unless the patient has pulmonary edema.

The risk profile of these medications is poorly defined in pregnancy. ACE inhibitors, ARBs, and direct renin inhibitors are contraindicated during pregnancy because of the risk of fetal abnormalities. Magnesium sulfate is used in severe cases of preeclampsia to reduce the risk of seizures, but it does not treat other manifestations of the disease or reduce maternal or fetal mortality rates.

Most manifestations of preeclampsia begin to improve shortly after delivery, but in some women, hypertension, proteinuria, and other manifestations may persist for several weeks or months before resolving completely. Because preeclampsia is a risk factor for future hypertension, kidney disease, and cardiovascular events, continued medical follow-up is essential.

Scleroderma Renal Crisis

Systemic sclerosis (i.e., scleroderma) is an idiopathic connective tissue disorder associated with deposition of collagen and other extracellular matrix proteins that produces inflammation and fibrosis of the skin and internal organs. Proliferative endovascular lesions may lead to obliteration of the vascular internal lumina and renal ischemia, with hypertension, increased renin activity, and elevated levels of angiotensin II and aldosterone.

AKI and rapidly worsening hypertension in patients with scleroderma is called *scleroderma renal crisis*. It occurs in approximately 5% to 10% of patients with scleroderma, typically within the first few years after onset and primarily in those with systemic rather than localized cutaneous scleroderma who also have progressive skin and cardiac involvement. Subclinical renal involvement with mild proteinuria, hypertension, and elevated serum creatinine concentration occurs much more frequently. Scleroderma renal crisis occasionally develops before the clinical diagnosis of scleroderma has been made.

Scleroderma renal crisis is often associated with rapid and severe loss of kidney function, oliguria, hypertensive encephalopathy, and heart failure. Microangiopathic hemolytic anemia (MAHA) may also occur. Low-grade proteinuria is often present but the urinalysis is not usually otherwise "active" (red blood cells, casts, etc.). About 10% of patients with scleroderma renal crisis do not have hypertension. This occurs more commonly among patients being treated with ACE inhibitors or high-dose corticosteroids.

Anti–RNA polymerase III antibodies are strongly associated with the risk of scleroderma renal crisis and have been suggested as markers for scleroderma renal crisis. Other risk factors include diffuse and rapidly progressive skin involvement and high-dose glucocorticoid use.

Renal biopsy may reveal interlobular artery involvement with intimal thickening, endothelial cell proliferation, and edema with obliteration of the vessel lumen with concentric onion-skinning of the wall of arterioles. Fibrinoid necrosis occurs in afferent arterioles with intravascular fibrin accumulation extending into the glomeruli, often with ischemic collapse, but without features of glomerulonephritis.

Activation of the renin-angiotensin-aldosterone system appears to play an important role in the progression of the disease. Before the advent of ACE inhibitors and hemodialysis, scleroderma renal crisis was fatal in about 75% of patients at 1 year. ACE inhibitor therapy has reduced this 1-year mortality rate to less than 15%. Captopril is often recommended as the ACE inhibitor of choice due to its short half-life and ease of dose titration. If the diagnosis of scleroderma renal crisis is made before advanced renal failure is established, ACE inhibition may halt or reverse the decline in renal function. Some experts recommend continuing ACE inhibitors even if kidney function declines and temporary dialysis is necessary, citing an increased chance of renal recovery, which has been described in scleroderma renal crisis patients even after 18 to 24 months of dialysis dependence. ACE inhibitors are not useful for prevention of scleroderma renal crisis, and their use in this setting has been associated with a poorer outcome, including greater risk of requiring permanent dialysis if renal crisis occurs. Use of ACE inhibitors rather than ARBs is recommended because of the long track record of success with ACE inhibitors in this disease. Patients with ESRD secondary to scleroderma renal crisis have a high mortality on dialysis, poor dialysis access maturation, and reduced allograft survival following renal transplantation.

THROMBOTIC MICROANGIOPATHY OF THE KIDNEY

TMA is a pathologic lesion secondary to various distinct pathogenic mechanisms leading to endothelial injury, microvascular thrombosis, and MAHA. These syndromes each lead to organ dysfunction due to microvascular thrombosis, but each syndrome has distinct clinical, pathophysiologic, and epidemiologic features. AKI is commonly seen in TMA due to the propensity of the glomerular endothelium to damage.

The traditional classification of TMA into thrombotic thrombocytopenic purpura (TTP) and hemolytic uremic syndrome (HUS) has undergone evolution and currently TMAs are subclassified based on the underlying pathogenic process (Fig. 28.4 and Table 28.3). Although many processes cause microvascular endothelial injury, renal involvement from these disorders affects the vasculature at different levels. Renal involvement by HUS and TTP primarily affects the glomeruli, whereas scleroderma often extends to the interlobular arteries, and malignant hypertension more often affects the afferent arterioles. However, there is significant overlap and similar histologic features among these diseases, making careful clinical evaluation essential for accurate determination of the cause.

Thrombotic Thrombocytopenic Purpura

TTP is characterized by MAHA and thrombocytopenia. Patients may also have fever, AKI, and neurologic impairment. Purpura is only rarely observed, and it is not necessary to make the diagnosis. TTP occurs with a female-to-male ratio of 4:3 and a peak incidence in the third and fourth decades of life. MAHA and thrombocytopenia manifesting similar to TTP may occur in response to some drugs (e.g., ticlopidine, cyclosporine, tacrolimus), after stem cell transplantation, in association with human immunodeficiency virus (HIV) infection, and in patients with malignant hypertension, sepsis, disseminated intravascular coagulation, or advanced cancers.

TTP is caused by a deficiency or reduced activity of ADAMTS13 (a disintegrin-like and metalloproteinase with thrombospondin-1–like domains). ADAMTS13 is a plasma protease that normally cleaves von Willebrand factor (VWF) and limits the extent of intravascular thrombosis (Fig. 28.5). Microthrombi composed primarily of platelets and VWF accumulate in the vascular bed of multiple organs, leading to a MAHA. Deficiency in ADAMTS13 may be acquired, caused by anti-ADAMTS13 autoantibodies (mostly immunoglobulin G [IgG]), or, much less commonly, genetic.

Other laboratory abnormalities are manifestations of the MAHA and include thrombocytopenia; an elevated LDH concentration, indirect bilirubin concentration, and reticulocyte count; and a low haptoglobin concentration. Coagulation laboratory test results (e.g., prothrombin time, activated partial thromboplastin time, fibrinogen level) are typically normal, although levels of fibrin split products may be elevated. AKI, microscopic hematuria, and low-grade proteinuria are frequently detected.

Without treatment, TTP has a mortality rate of about 90%, with most deaths occurring within 3 months of the onset of symptoms. Treatment with plasma infusion can normalize ADAMTS13 levels, reducing intravascular hemolysis and mortality rates. Plasmapheresis and replacement with fresh-frozen plasma has the advantage of removing inhibitory autoantibodies in addition to normalizing ADAMTS13 levels because of the large volume of plasma that can be infused.

ADAMTS13 activity must be assayed before therapy is initiated to obtain accurate results, but treatment should not be delayed for the results to return. The severity of ADAMTS13 deficiency (<5%) predicts future relapse, although those with severe deficiency are just as likely to respond initially to plasmapheresis as those with a mild deficiency. Patients with MAHA due to other causes not associated with ADAMTS13 deficiency usually have a minimal response to plasmapheresis or plasma infusion. Patients with HUS do not have abnormalities in ADAMTS13 levels or function.

Hemolytic-Uremic Syndrome
Shiga Toxin-Producing *Escherichia coli*

Gastrointestinal tract infection with the Shiga-toxigenic *Escherichia coli* (STEC) strain O157:H7 produces a diarrheal illness that is complicated in about 15% of cases by a MAHA with intraglomerular thrombosis and AKI. STEC-HUS most commonly affects infants and children, although adults may also be affected. Cases are often clustered because of outbreaks of *E. coli* O157:H7, with peaks occurring in summer and autumn. *E. coli* is endemic in the gastrointestinal tract of cattle, and cases are often tracked to undercooked meat, exposure to bovine fecal matter, animal exposure, or other contaminated food products. In May 2011, an outbreak of STEC-HUS in Germany was tracked back to fenugreek sprouts grown from contaminated seeds. The pathogenic agent, *E. coli* O104:H4, was particularly virulent with 30% of infected patients, mostly adults, developing HUS.

Shiga-toxigenic bacterial strains commonly produce a prodrome of painful, bloody diarrhea, which precedes the development of HUS by 2 to 12 days (median, 3 days). Shiga toxin is directly thrombogenic in the renal vasculature. Although intravascular coagulation in STEC-HUS is usually limited to the kidney, the heart, gastrointestinal tract, and central nervous system may also be affected.

Laboratory abnormalities in HUS include elevated creatinine levels, anemia, schistocytes on the peripheral smear, elevated reticulocyte count, and thrombocytopenia. In contrast to disseminated intravascular coagulation, fibrinogen levels are normal or high, and the prothrombin time is normal or only slightly prolonged. Fresh stool should be sent for culture of *E. coli* O157:H7, which can aid in tracing the source of an outbreak. Stool studies should also be performed for patients without diarrhea because *E. coli* O157:H7 may rarely cause HUS in the absence of intestinal symptoms. If *E. coli* O157:H7 is not detected, culture for other Shiga-toxigenic organisms should be pursued.

The pathologic renal lesions of HUS include vessel wall thickening with endothelial cell swelling and intraglomerular thrombosis with platelet- and fibrin-rich thrombi. Fragmentation of red blood cells may be seen in the renal vasculature and within the vessel wall.

Treatment of STEC-HUS is supportive, including adequate volume repletion with isotonic intravenous fluids, transfusion for severe anemia, and avoidance of other nephrotoxic agents (e.g., nonsteroidal anti-inflammatory drugs, aminoglycoside antibiotics, iodinated contrast). Platelet transfusion is not recommended because it may worsen the ongoing microvascular thrombosis. Antibiotic treatment of patients with bloody diarrhea is controversial. Corticosteroids, anticoagulation (e.g., aspirin, heparin), thrombolytic agents, and plasma administration have proved ineffective for the treatment of STEC-HUS. In very severe cases, especially with central nervous system involvement, eculizumab (a complement pathway inhibitor) can be used.

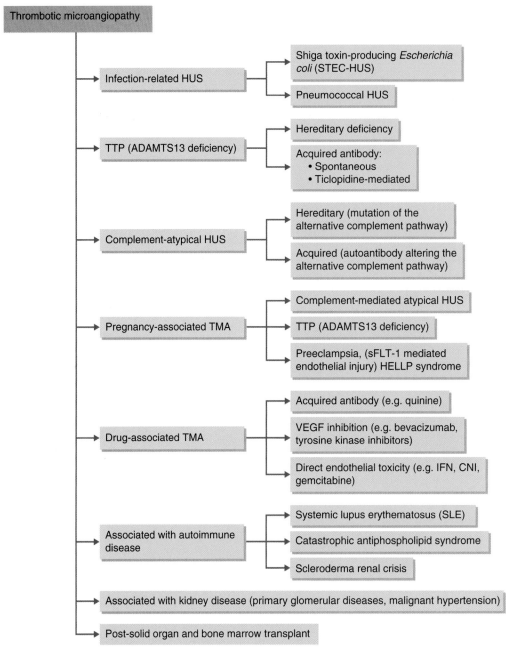

Fig. 28.4 Thrombotic microangiopathy (TMA). *CNI,* Calcineurin inhibitor; *HELLP,* hemolysis, elevated liver enzymes, and a low platelet count; *HUS,* hemolytic uremic syndrome; *IFN,* interferon; *sFLT-1,* soluble fms-like tyrosine kinase-1; *TTP,* thrombotic thrombocytopenic purpura; *VEGF,* vascular endothelial growth factor.

With supportive care alone, most patients with STEC-HUS recover with normalization of renal function or only mild residual CKD, although about 25% may develop advanced CKD or ESRD over the next 1 to 2 decades of life. Risk for CKD is increased with cortical necrosis and involvement of more than 50% of glomeruli identified on renal biopsy. The risk for complications and death increases with age, with the mortality rate increasing from about 5% to 10% for children to about 30% for adults.

Complement-Mediated Atypical HUS

The alternative complement pathway is the amplification loop of the complement system. Dysregulation of this pathway due to either hereditary or acquired causes may lead to complement-mediated endothelial damage and atypical HUS (aHUS). Mutations of genes for

components of the alternative complement pathway, including C3, factor B, regulators of factor H (CFH/CFHR fusions), factor I, and CD46, have been implicated. These mutations have an incomplete penetrance and frequently a triggering factor such as infection or pregnancy precedes the onset of clinical manifestations. In some childhood forms of complement-mediated aHUS, an acquired autoantibody against factor H can be detected and gastrointestinal prodrome is often reported. Failure to detect a genetic maturation or autoantibody does not rule out this disease because it is likely that not all responsible causes have been identified.

Complement-mediated aHUS historically has had a very poor prognosis with high likelihood of ESRD and death. The disease frequently recurs in a renal allograft with the recurrence rate depending on the underlying mutation, with the highest risk for CFH, CFB,

TABLE 28.3 Pathogenesis, Clinical/Diagnostic Characteristics, and Management of Main Thrombotic Microangiopathic Syndromes

	Pathogenesis	Clinical Characteristics	Diagnostic Characteristics	Management
Shiga toxin–producing *Escherichia coli* (STEC-HUS)	Enteric infection with Shiga toxin–producing pathogen (*E. coli* O157; *E. coli* O104)	All age groups with peak incidence in children for the *E. coli* O157 pathogen. Enteric prodrome is common (5% do not have diarrhea)	Fibrin predominates intravascular thrombi. Swollen endothelial cells. STEC isolated in the stool	Supportive. No role for plasma exchange. Possible role for eculizumab in severe CNS involvement. Antibiotics (controversial)
TTP	ADAMTS 13 deficiency (hereditary or acquired autoantibody). Ticlopidine-induced autoantibody	Other affected family members if hereditary. In women with predisposition presents clinically in the 2nd and 3rd trimester of pregnancy. No diarrheal prodrome. Neurologic symptoms predominate	Low ADAMTS 13 activity (<10%). VWF predominates intravascular thrombi. Absence of swollen endothelial cells	Plasma exchange. Immunosuppression (e.g. rituximab for acquired autoantibody). Stop ticlopidine
Complement-mediated aHUS	Dysregulation of the alternative complement pathway: Hereditary or acquired (anti-FH Ab)	Diarrhea can be present (30% at presentation). Hereditary disease has incomplete penetrance. Trigger (e.g., infection, pregnancy) often identified. High recurrence in kidney allograft	C3 can be low (normal levels do not exclude the disease). ADAMTS13 activity >10%. Negative genetic and autoantibody testing does not exclude the diagnosis	Eculizumab. Partial response to plasma exchange. Liver transplant may be considered
Pneumococcal HUS	Neuraminidase-mediated exposure of the endothelium antigens leading to endothelial injury	Mainly children <2 years. Frequently associated with pneumonia and empyema	Positive Coombs test	Supportive care. Treatment of the infection
Quinine-induced TMA	Autoantibodies against GP Ib/IX or IIb/IIIa	Not dose related. Can occur early (after single exposure) or late (up to 10 years after exposure)	ADAMTS13 activity ≥10%	Supportive. Plasma exchange not effective

ADAMTS3, A disintegrin and metalloproteinase with thrombospondin-1–like domains; *anti-FH Ab,* anti-factor H antibody; *CNS,* central nervous system; *GP,* glycoprotein platelets; *HUS,* hemolytic uremic syndrome; *TMA,* thrombotic microangiopathy; *TTP,* thrombotic thrombocytopenic purpura; *VWF,* von Willebrand factor.

and C3 mutations and the lowest with CD46 mutations. Eculizumab is a humanized monoclonal antibody that binds with high affinity to complement protein C5 and prevents the generation of C5a, C5b, and the terminal complement complex C5b-9. In patients with complement-mediated HUS, eculizumab inhibits complement-mediated TMA. It is used both to treat the disease and to prevent recurrence after kidney transplantation. Because complement components are mainly produced by the liver, a combined liver kidney transplant can be curative.

Malignancy-Associated TMA

In patients with a cancer diagnosis, TMA can be due to the cancer or its therapy. Disseminated malignancy can produce embolic tumor cells leading to endothelial damage and erythrocytes shearing. It has a very poor prognosis. TMA has also been described with cancer therapeutic agents that interfere with the VEGF pathway such as bevacizumab and tyrosine-kinase inhibitors (e.g., sunitinib). The VEGF pathway is upregulated in the majority of human tumors and it is thought to be important for expanding neovascularization of the tumor. In the kidney glomeruli, VEGF is produced locally by podocytes and endothelial cells express tyrosine kinase VEGF receptors. A disruption of this balance will lead to endothelial injury and TMA. Clinically, most patients present with hypertension and proteinuria. In rare cases, a severe

systemic TMA can develop, often associated with use of higher doses of the cancer therapeutic agents. Most of these disorders are reversible after stopping the medication.

Other chemotherapeutic agents associated with TMA include gemcitabine, mitomycin C, vincristine, and proteasome inhibitors (e.g., bortezomib, carfilzomib, and ixazomib). Gemcitabine-related TMA is directly related to the cumulative dose. Usually treated conservatively, in severe cases with persistent TMA eculizumab therapy may be considered.

In patients receiving an allogenic bone marrow transplant, TMA occurs in 10% to 40% of patients and is considered a manifestation of graft versus host disease (GVHD) or radiation therapy. Therapy for this form of TMA is controversial and mainly directed toward treating GVHD, although eculizumab may be tried.

Pregnancy-Related TMA

Pregnancy acts as a trigger for both TTP and complement-mediated aHUS. TTP occurs mainly during the second and third trimester of pregnancy. Normal pregnancy is associated with an augmentation of VWF antigen release leading to TTP in patients who are already predisposed by a congenital or acquired ADAMTS13 deficiency.

Pregnancy-related aHUS occurs in the postpartum period. Delivery acts as a triggering factor for aHUS in patients with certain genetic

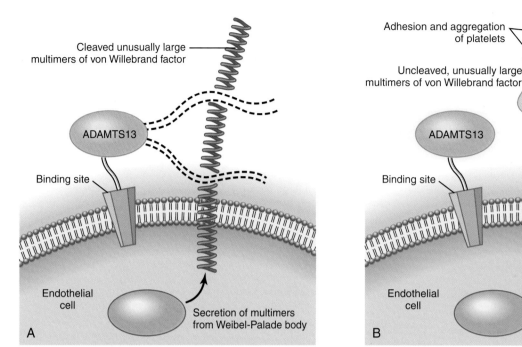

Fig. 28.5 Relation between ADAMTS13 activity, excessive adhesion and activation of platelets, and thrombotic thrombocytopenic purpura. (A) In normal subjects, ADAMTS13 (i.e., von Willebrand factor–cleaving metalloprotease) molecules attach to binding sites on endothelial cell surfaces and cleave unusually large multimers of von Willebrand factor as they are secreted by stimulated endothelial cells. The smaller von Willebrand factor forms that circulate after cleavage do not induce the adhesion and aggregation of platelets during normal blood flow. (B) Absent or severely reduced activity of ADAMTS13 in patients with thrombotic thrombocytopenic purpura prevents timely cleavage of unusually large multimers of von Willebrand factor as they are secreted by endothelial cells. The uncleaved multimers induce the adhesion and aggregation of platelets in flowing blood. (From Moake JL: Thrombotic microangiopathies, N Engl J Med 347:589-600, 2002.)

mutations of the alternative complement pathway. Historically the outcomes were very poor, with more than 75% of patients developing ESRD. Eculizumab is an effective therapy and can be used during pregnancy.

The HELLP syndrome is a TMA of the liver sinusoids that can have a presentation similar to TTP or aHUS. Although rare, AKI can occur due to an acute tubular necrosis type of injury that is rapidly reversible with recovery from the HELLP syndrome.

ANTIPHOSPHOLIPID ANTIBODY SYNDROME

Antiphospholipid antibodies (APAs) refer to autoantibodies such as lupus anticoagulants or IgG or immunoglobulin M (IgM) anticardiolipin antibodies or anti-β_2-glycoprotein that interfere with phospholipid-binding proteins and in vitro phospholipid-dependent clotting assays such as the partial thromboplastin time. Because not all lupus anticoagulants cause prolongation of the partial thromboplastin time, other tests of the coagulation system, such as the dilute Russell viper venom time, may need to be obtained. The diagnosis of APS is based on the occurrence of arterial or venous clotting events or fetal loss during pregnancy after 10 or more weeks' gestation or multiembryonic losses before 10 weeks' gestation in the setting of laboratory detection of an APA. Lupus anticoagulant and anticardiolipin antibodies are detectable in up to 10% of healthy populations, and their presence alone is insufficient for a diagnosis of APS. Apolipoprotein H (apo H, formerly β_2-glycoprotein 1) is the main antigenic target of anticardiolipin antibodies.

In the absence of an underlying autoimmune disease, the syndrome is referred to as primary APS. Secondary APS occurs when associated with other diseases such as systemic lupus erythematosus (SLE). APAs are detectable in 30% to 50% of patients with SLE, and renal involvement is often observed in this setting.

The procoagulant effect of APAs may result from interference with the anticoagulant apo H, inhibition of fibrinolysis, direct endothelial injury, accelerated atherosclerosis, and activation of platelet, monocyte, and endothelial cells. Renal involvement occurs in about 25% of patients with primary APS and can occur in patients with SLE or other causes of APS. Thrombosis may occur throughout the renal vasculature, including main or branch renal arteries, arterioles, glomeruli, and veins. These findings resemble those found in other diseases associated with a TMA. Focal atrophy of the cortex in association with interstitial fibrosis may be observed due to resulting ischemia.

The renal manifestations of APS vary. Some patients have mild proteinuria with preserved kidney function, and others develop severe hypertension, nephrotic-range proteinuria, and AKI or CKD. Renal arterial thrombosis can cause infarction, acute onset of flank pain, hematuria, and decreased kidney function. RVT may be silent or, if acute and complete, may manifest with sudden flank pain and reduced kidney function. Pathologic changes seen on renal biopsy of patients with primary APS are small vessel vaso-occlusive disease with fibrous intimal hyperplasia of interlobular arteries, recanalizing thrombi in arteries and arterioles, focal cortical atrophy, and TMA. Other manifestations of APS include thrombocytopenia, hemolytic anemia, and a prolonged activated partial thromboplastin time in the absence of heparin therapy. It is worth noting that a high prevalence of APAs has been reported in ESRD patients undergoing hemodialysis, with dialysis access thrombosis as a main manifestation.

Long-term warfarin anticoagulation with a target international normalized ratio (INR) between 2 and 3 is indicated for patients with primary or secondary APS and prior deep vein thrombosis, arterial thrombosis, or recurrent spontaneous abortion. Because warfarin is contraindicated during pregnancy, heparin with or without low-dose aspirin (81 mg) is necessary until the end of pregnancy.

Treatment of APA-positive patients in the absence of prior clinical events is controversial because of the high false-positive rate for the tests. Aspirin therapy for primary prevention in patients persistently positive for APAs has been advocated but not proved. Plasmapheresis, prednisone, and hydroxychloroquine have been advocated for the treatment of TMA due to APS and should be considered in severe cases.

RENAL VEIN THROMBOSIS

RVT is uncommon, occurring mostly in association with malignancy, but it also is a consequence of nephrotic syndrome, abdominal surgery or trauma, pancreatitis, and genetic or acquired hypercoagulable states. Most malignancy-associated RVT is caused by renal cell carcinoma with venous invasion, often with spreading to the contralateral kidney, which may cause bilateral renal vein occlusion.

The nephrotic syndrome is associated with a risk for venous thrombosis throughout the circulation, including RVT. The RVT risk in patients with nephrotic syndrome correlates with severity of proteinuria and hypoalbuminemia; patients with a serum albumin concentration of less than 2 g/dL and/or proteinuria more than 10 g/day are at particular risk. Some studies have documented an incidence of RVT as high as 30% among patients with nephrotic syndrome, but most cases are not clinically apparent. Patients with membranous nephropathy seem to be at greatest risk for RVT for reasons that are not known, but RVT can also occur with nephrotic syndromes due to focal segmental glomerular sclerosis, membranoproliferative glomerulonephritis, minimal change disease, and diabetic kidney disease. Hypercoagulability is thought to result from loss of the antithrombotic protein antithrombin III in urine, although other factors such as increased procoagulant factors and platelet activation may also be involved.

RVT may manifest with symptoms attributable to renal cell carcinoma, such as flank pain, gross hematuria, nausea, anorexia, or lower extremity swelling. In male patents, left renal vein occlusion may cause a left varicocele, a result of the venous drainage of the left gonadal vein. In patients without a malignancy, symptoms of RVT depend on the acuity of the thrombosis. Acute, complete thrombosis may manifest with hematuria, flank pain, abdominal distention, and acute renal failure. RVT in adults usually occurs gradually because of collateral venous drainage return; in this setting, symptoms of AKI are uncommon, although proteinuria and creatinine levels may be mildly elevated. In these cases of chronic RVT, patients will typically come to clinical attention for pulmonary embolus.

Because patients often do not have symptoms, RVT is likely more common than reported in the literature. Some have suggested CT screening of asymptomatic, high-risk patients, particularly those with membranous nephropathy and severe proteinuria and hypoalbuminemia.

The standard method for diagnosis is renal venography, but because it has the risks of clot dislodgment, bleeding, and use of iodinated contrast, less invasive methods are commonly used. Contrast-enhanced CT venography appears to have a relatively high sensitivity and specificity, although it carries some risk for contrast nephropathy. Magnetic resonance imaging using gadolinium-based contrast or time-of-flight sequencing without contrast may also be useful. Renal Doppler ultrasound is useful, but it is operator dependent and has lower sensitivity than CT venography.

Treatment with systemic anticoagulation is recommended in the absence of contraindications. Most clinicians maintain anticoagulation for 6 to 9 months, similar to the approach for nonrenal deep vein thrombosis and pulmonary embolism. The long-term recurrence risk is low if the underlying predisposition is successfully treated, and patients are unlikely to require indefinite anticoagulation. Direct intravenous thrombolysis or operative thrombectomy may be considered in severe cases, particularly if the RVT is a source of pulmonary emboli or is causing AKI. Prophylactic anticoagulation in high-risk patients, such as those with severe membranous nephropathy (serum albumin concentration <2.8 g/dL) should be considered for appropriate candidates.

For a deeper discussion on this topic, please see Chapter 116, ❖ "Vascular Disorders of the Kidney," in *Goldman-Cecil Medicine*, 26th Edition.

SUGGESTED READINGS

ASTRAL Investigators, Wheatley K, Ives N, Gray R, et al.: Revascularization versus medical therapy for renal-artery stenosis, *N Engl J Med* 361(20):1953, 2009.

Barbour T, Johnson S, Cohney S, et al: Thrombotic microangiopathy and associated renal disorders, *Nephrol Dial Transplant* 27:2673–2685, 2012.

Brocklebank V, Wood KM, Kavanagh D: Thrombotic microangiopathy and the kidney, *Clin J Am Soc Nephrol* 13(2):300–317, 2018 Feb 7.

Cooper CJ, Murphy TP, Cutlip DE, Jamerson K, et al.: CORAL Investigators. Stenting and medical therapy for atherosclerotic renal-artery stenosis, *N Engl J Med* 370(1):13, 2014.

Fattori R, Cao P, De Rango P: et al: Interdisciplinary expert consensus document, on management of type B aortic dissection, *J Am Coll Cardiol* 61:1661–1678, 2013.

Friedman DJ, Pollak MR: Genetics of kidney failure and the evolving story of APOL1, *J Clin Invest* 121:3367–3374, 2011.

Jennette JC, Nachman PH: ANCA glomerulonephritis and vasculitis, *Clin J Am Soc Nephrol* 12(10):1680–1691, 2017 Oct 6.

Krüger T, Conzelmann LO, Bonser RS: et al: Acute aortic dissection type A, *Br J Surg* 99:1331–1344, 2012.

Maynard SE, Thadhani R: Pregnancy and the kidney, *J Am Soc Nephrol* 20:14–22, 2009.

Noris M, Mescia F, Remuzzi G: STEC-HUS, atypical HUS and TTP are all diseases of complement activation, *Nat Rev Nephrol* 8:622–633, 2012.

Ruiz-Irastorza G, Crowther M, Branch W, et al: Antiphospholipid syndrome, *Lancet* 376:1498–1509, 2010.

Sadler JE: Von Willebrand factor, ADAMTS13, and thrombotic thrombocytopenic purpura, *Blood* 112:11–18, 2008.

Scolari F, Ravani P: Atheroembolic renal disease, *Lancet* 375:1650–1660, 2010.

Shanmugam VK, Steen VD: Renal disease in scleroderma: an update on evaluation, risk stratification, pathogenesis and management, *Curr Opin Rheumatol* 24:669–676, 2012.

Specks U, Merkel PA, Seo P, et al: Efficacy of remission-induction regimens for ANCA-associated vasculitis, *N Engl J Med* 369:417–427, 2013.

Textor SC, Misra S, Oderich GS: Percutaneous revascularization for ischemic nephropathy: the past, present, and future, *Kidney Int* 83:28–40, 2013.

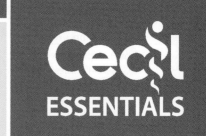

29

Acute Kidney Injury

Mark A. Perazella, Jeffrey M. Turner

DEFINITION

Acute kidney injury (AKI) is a syndrome defined as an abrupt decrease in glomerular filtration rate (GFR) sufficient to promote the retention of nitrogenous waste products (blood urea nitrogen [BUN] and creatinine); disturb the regulation of extracellular fluid volume, electrolyte balance, and acid-base homeostasis; and impair drug excretion. Importantly, even mild abnormalities in kidney structure and function are associated with other end-organ complications and increased mortality.

AKI includes a spectrum of clinical conditions. The numerous causes of AKI vary based on individual comorbidities (and risk for AKI) and whether kidney injury develops in the outpatient setting or in hospital. The incidence of AKI is rising, and its complications include progression to more severe kidney failure, need for renal replacement therapy (RRT), chronic kidney disease (CKD), and death. Several consensus groups have produced definitions and diagnostic criteria for AKI. Table 29.1 describes the diagnostic criteria for the Risk, Injury, Failure, Loss, and End-stage renal disease (ESRD) (RIFLE); Acute Kidney Injury Network (AKIN); and Kidney Disease: Improving Global Outcomes (KDIGO) classifications.

In 2004, the RIFLE classification was put forth to standardize the definition of AKI. Changes in serum creatinine concentration (over 7 days), reductions in estimated glomerular filtration rate (eGFR), and urine output parameters were used in this diagnostic system. The Risk (R), Injury (I), and Failure (F) categories were applicable to AKI, whereas the Loss (L) and ESRD (E) categories were CKD stages. In 2007, the AKIN group modified the RIFLE criteria definition of AKI by adding an absolute increase in serum creatinine of only 0.3 mg/dL, eliminating the eGFR criteria, and changing the time frame for AKI to develop (to 48 hours, compared with the 7 days for RIFLE diagnosis). Focusing on AKI, the AKIN criteria replaced the R, I, and F categories from the RIFLE criteria with stages 1, 2, and 3 and eliminated the L and E categories. In 2012, the KDIGO group combined parts of the RIFLE and AKIN criteria to capture AKI with increased sensitivity.

Understanding of the pathophysiology underlying development of AKI has advanced, and better diagnostic tools have moved the field forward. However, specific directed therapies remain limited for the most common forms of AKI. Although technical advances in RRT and supportive care have improved, patients commonly develop other end-organ disease in the setting of AKI. More concerning is the relatively high mortality rate associated with AKI, particularly when it develops in the hospital setting and requires RRT. E-Table 29.1 shows some of the clinically important outcomes associated with AKI.

ETIOLOGY

In most cases, more than one process contributes to AKI, but for ease of classification, three broad categories (Fig. 29.1) are used: (1) *prerenal AKI*, the result of a decrease in renal blood flow and perfusion of the kidney; (2) *intrinsic AKI*, the result of disease affecting one of the renal parenchymal compartments; and (3) *postrenal AKI*, the result of obstruction to urinary flow anywhere along the urinary tract starting from the renal calyces/pelves and involving the ureters, bladder, or urethra.

The most common form of AKI is due to prerenal physiology, particularly in the outpatient setting, but also in the hospital. Postrenal AKI is more common in elderly men with prostatic hyperplasia, patients with bladder dysfunction, and patients with certain malignancies. Intrinsic AKI may be due to a vascular process, glomerular disease, interstitial disease, or tubular injury. The most common intrinsic AKI is an entity known as *acute tubular necrosis* (ATN), or more recently *acute tubular injury* (ATI), which is histologically more accurate. This is a clinical syndrome characterized by an abrupt and sustained decline in GFR due to an acute ischemic injury, nephrotoxic insult, or a combination of both. The clinical recognition of ATN is based primarily on exclusion of prerenal and postrenal causes of AKI, as well as other causes of intrinsic AKI (glomerulonephritis [GN], acute interstitial nephritis [AIN], and vasculitis). Once other intrinsic causes of AKI are excluded, it is reasonable to conclude ATN is the cause or major contributor to AKI. Although the name *acute tubular necrosis* is not an entirely valid histologic description of the lesion, the term will be utilized as it is part of the language of clinical medicine.

EPIDEMIOLOGY

AKI occurs more commonly in hospitalized patients as compared to the community setting. Community-acquired AKI defined by various step-wise increases in serum creatinine has an incidence of approximately 1%. Nearly half of the patients involve AKI superimposed on CKD. Prerenal AKI accounts for approximately 70% of cases, obstructive uropathy approximately 17%, and intrinsic AKI from various etiologies approximately 11% of the AKI cases. In contrast, hospital-acquired AKI has an incidence ranging from 4.9% to 7.2%. The incidence of AKI is higher in intensive care unit (ICU) admissions, approximating 30%. CKD, older age, and other comorbidities are important risk factors for AKI. Prerenal AKI remains the most common cause, followed by intrinsic AKI from nephrotoxic medications and ischemic ATN.

TABLE 29.1	**Classification of Acute Kidney Injury**	
Stage	Serum Creatinine Increase Within 7 Days	Urine Output
Kidney Disease: Improving Global Outcomes (KDIGO) Classification (2012)		
1	1.5-1.9 times baseline *or* ≥0.3 mg/dL within 48 hr	<0.5 mL/kg/hr × 6-12 hr
2	2-2.9 times baseline	<0.5 mL/kg/hr × ≥12 hr
3	3 times baseline *or* an increase in the serum creatinine to ≥4 mg/dL with an absolute increase ≥0.3 mg/dL within 48 hr or 1.5 times baseline within 7 days *or* initiation of RRT *or* in patients aged <18 yr, eGFR decreased to <35 mL/min/1.73 m²	<0.3 mL/kg/hr × ≥24 hr
Acute Kidney Injury Network (AKIN) Classification (2007)		
1	1.5-1.9 times baseline *or* ≥0.3 mg/dL within 48 hr	<0.5 mL/kg/hr × 6-12 hr
2	2-2.9 times baseline	<0.5 mL/kg/hr × ≥12 hr
3	3 times baseline *or* increase in serum creatinine ≥4 mg/dL with an increase ≥0.5 mg/dL *or* initiation of RRT	<0.3 mL/kg/hr × ≥24 hr *or* anuria ≥12 hr
RIFLE Classification (2004)		
Risk	1.5-1.9 times baseline *or* GFR decrease >25%	<0.5 mL/kg/hr × 6 hr
Injury	2-2.9 times baseline *or* GFR decrease >50%	<0.5 mL/kg/hr × 12 hr
Failure	3 times baseline *or* GFR decrease >75% *or* serum creatinine ≥4 mg/dL with an increase ≥0.5 mg/dL	<0.3 mL/kg/hr × 24 hr *or* anuria × 12 hr
Loss	Complete loss of renal function for >4 wk	
ESRD	End-stage renal disease >3 mo	

eGFR, Estimated glomerular filtration rate; *GFR*, glomerular filtration rate; *RRT*, renal replacement therapy.

DIAGNOSTIC EVALUATION

History and Physical Examination

Evaluation of the patient with AKI should be methodical and systematic to ensure that potentially reversible causes are diagnosed and treated expeditiously to preserve kidney function and limit development of permanent kidney injury, as depicted in Table 29.2. Part of the difficulty in arriving at a correct diagnosis is that several potential causes of AKI often coexist. Emphasis is placed on thorough analysis of available data and examination of the sequence of deterioration in kidney function and urine volume in relation to the chronologies of the potential causes of AKI.

Knowledge of the natural history of the various causes of AKI also is critical. The evaluation should include a thorough patient history and chart review to identify risk factors for prerenal AKI (e.g., vomiting, diuretics, diarrhea, heart failure, cirrhosis); potential nephrotoxic drugs (prescribed or over-the-counter, including alternative/complementary medications); risk factors for prostate disease, cervical cancer, or bladder cancer; and symptoms of urinary tract obstruction (e.g., prostatism, overflow incontinence, anuria). Some of the important chart review data are presented in E-Table 29.2. The urine volume is less than 400 mL/day with oliguric AKI, less than 100 mL/day with oligo-anuric AKI, and less than 50 mL/day with anuric AKI. Normal urine output does not exclude the diagnosis of AKI: Nonoliguric AKI (>400 mL/day) can be associated with nephrotoxic AKI and partial urinary obstruction. Wide variation in daily urine output also suggests AKI due to partial urinary tract obstruction. Anuria has a limited differential diagnosis, suggesting complete urinary obstruction, a vascular catastrophe, or severe cortical necrosis.

A thorough physical exam is critical in patients with AKI, and particular attention should be given to determining the patient's volume status. Reduced body weight, hypotension, an orthostatic fall in blood pressure (BP), or flat neck veins may be present in patients with prerenal AKI or ischemic ATN caused by true volume depletion. On the other hand, the presence of edema, pulmonary rales, or an S₃ gallop signals venous congestion from cardiac dysfunction that can be the cause of cardiorenal syndrome. Alternatively, edema, ascites, and asterixis

suggest acute liver dysfunction or cirrhosis, which can be the cause of AKI due to hepatorenal syndrome. It is important to differentiate these disorders, because their appropriate therapies differ. Some individuals can have signs of increased total body water in the form of edema, while simultaneously having signs of reductions in their intravascular volume in the form of hypotension and weak pulses. In these individuals, invasive intravascular monitoring may be helpful. This includes measurement of cardiac filling pressures or central venous pressures with an indwelling catheter. In addition, recent research has shown that noninvasive techniques including respiratory variations in systolic blood pressure, pulse pressure, calculated stroke volume, or the collapsibility of the inferior vena cava measured on bedside ultrasound are also useful methods for volume assessment that do not require the placement of a vascular catheter.

Evidence of systemic disease also should be sought. Findings may include signs of pulmonary hemorrhage indicative of a vasculitis or Goodpasture's syndrome, skin rash as a manifestation of systemic lupus erythematosus, atheroemboli, vasculitis, cryoglobulins, or AIN, as well as joint disease making lupus or rheumatoid arthritis a consideration.

Basic Laboratory Tests

Laboratory tests are directed by the differential diagnosis that is postulated after a complete history, chart review, and physical examination have been performed. Basic tests include a complete blood count to assess for anemia (microangiopathic or immune-mediated) and thrombocytopenia (thrombotic thrombocytic purpura [TTP], hemolytic-uremic syndrome [HUS], and disseminated intravascular coagulation [DIC]). Other tests to evaluate the cause of AKI include various serologic measurements (antinuclear antibody [ANA], antineutrophil cytoplasmic antibodies [ANCA], anti–glomerular basement membrane antibody [anti-GBM], anti–double-stranded DNA antibodies [anti-dsDNA], and hepatitis B and C viral serologies), complement levels, cryoglobulin levels, blood cultures, serum lactate dehydrogenase (LDH) and haptoglobin measurements, serum and urine immunoelectrophoresis, and serum free light chain assay.

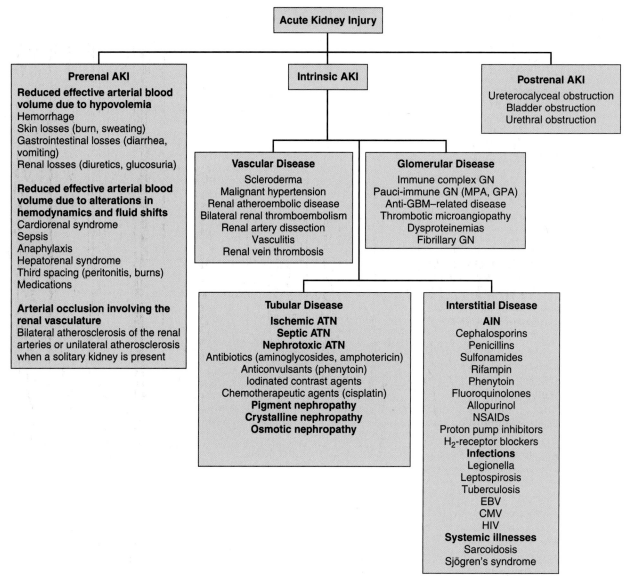

Fig. 29.1 Common causes of acute kidney injury (AKI). *AIN,* Acute interstitial nephritis; *ATN,* acute tubular necrosis; *CMV,* cytomegalovirus; *EBV,* Epstein-Barr virus; *GBM,* glomerular basement membrane; *GN,* glomerulonephritis; *GPA,* granulomatosis with polyangiitis; H_2, histamine 2; *HIV,* human immunodeficiency virus; *HUS,* hemolytic uremic syndrome; *MPA,* microscopic polyangiitis; *NSAIDs,* nonsteroidal anti-inflammatory drugs; *TTP,* thrombotic thrombocytopenic purpura.

TABLE 29.2   **Diagnostic Approach to the Patient With Acute Kidney Injury**
1. Record review (see E-Table 29.2); special attention to evidence of recent reduction in glomerular filtration rate and sequence of events leading to deterioration of kidney function to determine possible causative factors
2. Physical examination, including evaluation of hemodynamic status
3. Urinalysis and urine microscopy with thorough sediment examination
4. Determination of urinary indices, including fractional excretion of sodium and urea
5. Catheterization and measurement of postvoid residual urine volume if outlet obstruction is suspected
6. Fluid challenge in cases of suspected prerenal AKI
7. Radiologic studies, particular as dictated by the clinical setting (e.g., ultrasonography to look for obstruction)
8. Kidney biopsy

AKI, Acute kidney injury.

TABLE 29.3 Urinalysis and Microscopic Examination of the Urine Sediment

Test	Prerenal	Vasculitis	GN	ATN	AIN	Postrenal
Specific gravity	High	Normal/high	Normal/high	Isosmotic	Isosmotic	Isosmotic
Dipstick blood	Negative	Positive	Positive	±	±	Negative
Dipstick protein	Negative	Positive	Positive	Negative	±	Negative
Urine sediment examination	Negative, hyaline casts	RBC casts, dysmorphic RBCs	RBC casts, dysmorphic RBCs	Granular casts, RTECs	WBC casts, eosinophils	Negative, sometimes WBCs/RBCs

AIN, Acute interstitial nephritis; *ATN,* acute tubular necrosis; *GN,* glomerulonephritis; *RBCs,* red blood cells; *RTECs,* renal tubular epithelial cells; *WBCs,* white blood cells.

Urinalysis and Urine Microscopy

Urinalysis is a key component of the diagnostic evaluation of AKI, as summarized in Table 29.3. It is important to evaluate urine specific gravity (SG), as well as the presence of blood (or heme), protein, or leukocyte esterase.

A very high urine SG typically suggests prerenal AKI, whereas isosthenuria (SG = 1.010) indicates intrinsic AKI (e.g., ATN). A thorough microscopic examination of the spun urine sediment, with quantification of the urinary elements, adds essential information to the case. Bland urine with no blood or protein and few to no cells or casts favors a diagnosis of prerenal AKI. Vascular causes of AKI have a variable urine tonicity and sometimes hematuria (isomorphic or dysmorphic red blood cells [RBCs]) and granular casts. GN exhibits variable urine tonicity, positive blood and protein on the dipstick, RBCs, and RBC casts. ATN shows isotonic urine with variable protein and variable heme on urine dipstick (heme is positive with rhabdomyolysis and hemolysis). Renal tubular epithelial cells (RTECs), RTEC casts, and fine or coarse pigmented granular casts (sometime muddy brown E-Fig. 29.1) may be present on the sediment examination.

Urine in patients with postrenal AKI is typically isotonic and bland unless there is associated infection (pyuria), nephrolithiasis (hematuria), or concomitant ATN (RTECs, RTEC casts, granular casts).

With certain processes, crystals may be indicative of the underlying cause of AKI. For example, calcium oxalate crystals may suggest enteric hyperoxaluria or ethylene glycol intoxication, uric acid crystals may point to acute urate nephropathy, and various other crystals may indicate a drug-induced form of AKI (see Figs. 24.2, 24.3, and 24.4).

Urinary Indices

Spot urine chemistry testing (sodium, creatinine, and urea), along with plasma samples (sodium, creatinine, and BUN), has been used to evaluate renal tubular function in the setting of AKI, primarily to distinguish prerenal AKI from ATN. These measures allow the clinician to calculate fractional excretion of sodium (FE_{Na}) and fractional excretion of urea (FE_{Urea}); they are thought to be more accurate indicators than urine sodium concentration, which is less than 10 to 20 mEq/L with prerenal AKI and greater than 20 mEq/L with ATN.

The ratio of the clearance of sodium (Na) to that of creatinine (Cr) is calculated as a percentage:

$$FE_{Na} = (U_{Na}/P_{Na}) \times P_{Cr}/U_{Cr} \times 100$$

where U and P are the concentrations in urine and plasma, respectively. Likewise, the ratio of urea clearance to creatinine clearance is

$$FE_{Urea} = (U_{Urea}/P_{Urea}) \times (P_{Cr}/U_{Cr}) \times 100$$

The rationale for the use of these indices is that the ratio of urine to plasma creatinine concentrations (U_{Cr}/P_{Cr}) provides an index of the fraction of filtered water excreted. Assuming that all of the creatinine filtered at the glomerulus is excreted into the urine, any increment in the concentration of creatinine in urine over that in plasma must result from the removal of water.

In prerenal AKI, because of the increased stimulus for salt and water retention, U_{Cr}/P_{Cr} typically is considerably greater than it is in ATN; moreover, FE_{Na} is less than 1%, and urine sodium concentrations are characteristically low. In contrast, in AKI due to ATN, the nephrons excrete a large fraction of their filtered sodium and water, resulting in a lower U_{Cr}/P_{Cr}, higher urine sodium concentrations, and a higher FE_{Na} (E-Table 29.3). An important clinical exception to this finding is that FE_{Na} can be high (>1% to 2%) with prerenal AKI in the setting of diuretic therapy. To counter this effect, calculation of FE_{Urea} has been used: An FE_{Urea} less than 35% favors a diagnosis of prerenal AKI and an FE_{Urea} greater than 50% favors ATN.

Interpretations of these tests, therefore, must be made in conjunction with other assessments of the patient, because clinically important exceptions to these generalizations exist. As an example, prerenal AKI can manifest with an elevated FE_{Na} or FE_{Urea} in the setting of glycosuria, metabolic alkalosis, bicarbonaturia, salt-wasting disorders, or CKD. Similarly, ATN with low FE_{Na} and FE_{Urea} occurs with pigmenturia, sepsis, radiocontrast injury, severe heart or liver failure, and nonoliguric ATN.

Renal Imaging

If either prerenal AKI or ATN is the likely cause of AKI, and if the clinical setting does not require the exclusion of another cause, then no further diagnostic evaluation is required. Further assessment may be necessary if the diagnosis is uncertain, especially if the clinical setting suggests other possibilities (e.g., obstruction, vascular accident); if clinical findings make the diagnosis of prerenal AKI or ATN unlikely; or if oliguria persists without a good reason. When indicated, diagnostic renal imaging is important in the evaluation of AKI. Retroperitoneal ultrasonography of the kidneys, ureters, and bladder is the first test used because it is readily available, noninvasive, free of radiation exposure, and fairly accurate.

Ultrasonography provides information about kidney size (large, normal, or small) and the parenchyma (normal or increased echogenicity), the status of the pelvis and urinary collecting system (normal or hydronephrotic), and the presence of structural abnormalities (e.g., stones, masses, enlarged lymph nodes). In the setting of AKI, this test can rapidly confirm or exclude the presence of hydronephrosis (E-Fig. 29.2) and a diagnosis of obstructive uropathy. Interrogation of the renal arteries by Doppler ultrasonography provides important information about renal blood flow and renal artery stenosis; however, this test is highly operator dependent.

Computed tomography (CT) of the retroperitoneum provides important information about the cause of postrenal AKI (e.g., tumor, stones, retroperitoneal fibrosis) when ultrasound findings are negative or inconclusive. CT angiography can also accurately diagnose renal artery disease and renal infarction, but there is a risk of nephrotoxicity in those patients with underlying acute or chronic kidney disease. *Magnetic resonance (MR) imaging* does not add much to CT scanning except in the diagnosis of retroperitoneal fibrosis. *Gadolinium MR* angiography can safely provide important information about renal artery stenosis or thrombosis, but it should be used cautiously in patients with AKI or stage 4 or greater CKD. Nephrogenic systemic fibrosis can develop in these patients, especially with nonionic or linear gadolinium contrast agents and in the setting of inflammation.

Radionuclide tests are used to assess the presence or absence of renal blood flow, differences in flow to the two kidneys, and excretory (secretory) function. However, these studies have limited utility in AKI and have reduced accuracy in quantitating absolute rates of flow.

Kidney Biopsy

When prerenal AKI, ATN, and obstructive uropathy are unlikely, percutaneous kidney biopsy is sometimes required to determine the cause of AKI and to direct appropriate therapy. Reasonable criteria to support use of kidney biopsy include absence of an obvious cause of AKI such as hypotension or nephrotoxin exposure and prolonged oliguria, usually for more than 2 to 3 weeks. Other potential indications include evaluation for myeloma-related kidney disease in an elderly patient with unexplained AKI; extrarenal manifestations of systemic diseases such as systemic lupus erythematosus, rheumatoid arthritis, or vasculitis; and determination of whether AIN is present in patients receiving a potential culprit drug.

Kidney tissue should be thoroughly examined with the use of light microscopy, immunofluorescence staining, and electron microscopy to facilitate an accurate diagnosis. This ensures a diagnosis of the cause of AKI in most patients. However, kidney biopsy should be employed judiciously to avoid complications such as traumatic renal arteriovenous malformation, severe bleeding requiring transfusion or embolization, other organ injury (liver, spleen, bowel), and nephrectomy for intractable bleeding.

Future Tests for AKI

The limitations of currently available tests to estimate GFR and kidney injury have led to proteomics-based studies to identify novel biomarkers of AKI. The hope is that novel biomarkers will improve the diagnosis and prognosis of AKI. For example, early AKI diagnosis would permit implementation of appropriate preventive strategies and treatment regimens to abrogate permanent loss of kidney function. In patients who develop AKI, biomarker concentrations demonstrate changes earlier than serum creatinine concentrations and appear to distinguish between prerenal AKI, ATN, and other glomerular disorders, which may allow directed interventions and avoidance of potentially harmful therapies. One such example is aggressive intravenous fluid therapy in patients with ATN, which risks volume overload and other end-organ consequences. Finally, biomarkers may allow clinicians to better predict outcomes such as worsening kidney function, RRT requirement, and mortality in patients with hospital-acquired AKI.

CLINICAL PRESENTATION, DIFFERENTIAL DIAGNOSIS, AND MANAGEMENT OF AKI

Prerenal AKI

Prerenal AKI is primarily the result of inadequate blood flow to the kidneys. Renal blood flow approximates more than 1 L/minute, which is necessary to maintain GFR, preserve oxygen delivery, and sustain ion transport and other energy-requiring processes. Therefore, normal kidney function depends on adequate perfusion; a significant reduction in renal perfusion diminishes filtration pressure and lowers GFR.

Volume Depletion

Both "true" and "effective" hypovolemia activate several neurohormonal vasoconstrictor systems as mechanisms to protect circulatory stability. The substances released include catecholamines from the sympathetic nervous system, endothelin from the vasculature, angiotensin II from the renin-angiotensin system (RAS), and vasopressin. They raise BP through arterial and venous constriction but also can constrict afferent arterioles and reduce GFR, especially when systemic BP is inadequate to maintain renal perfusion pressure.

Structural lesions in the renal arterial and arteriolar tree can also reduce perfusion and promote prerenal AKI. Kidney adaptive responses are stimulated to counterbalance diminished renal perfusion in these circumstances. These adaptive processes include the myogenic reflex, which is activated by low distending pressures sensed in the renal baroreceptors and causes afferent arteriolar vasodilatation. Prostaglandins (e.g., PGE_2, PGI_2), nitric oxide, and products from the kallikrein-kinin system modify the effects of these vasoconstrictors on the afferent arteriole. Importantly, disturbance of the balance between afferent vasodilatation and efferent vasoconstriction can disrupt intrarenal hemodynamics and precipitate AKI.

Medications

The balance of vasoconstricting and vasodilating processes may be altered by medications such as nonsteroidal anti-inflammatory drugs (NSAIDs) and selective cyclooxygenase 2 (COX2) inhibitors. These drugs act to cause prerenal AKI through inhibition of vasodilatory prostaglandins in patients who require prostaglandin effects to maintain renal perfusion. Despite its vasoconstrictor properties, angiotensin II acutely preserves glomerular filtration pressure and GFR in states of reduced renal perfusion by constricting the efferent arteriole more than the afferent arteriole. This salutary effect in part explains the GFR reduction that occurs when a patient who is dependent on angiotensin II to constrict the efferent arteriole is treated with an ACE inhibitor or an angiotensin II receptor blocker (ARB).

Cardiorenal Syndrome

The cardiorenal syndrome (CRS) is an umbrella term that encompasses a number of coexistent cardiac or kidney derangements. Although there are five subtypes of CRS, hospital-acquired AKI due to CRS is most often of the type 1 variety. Reduced cardiac output, arterial underfilling, elevated atrial pressures, and venous congestion, independently or in combination, can impair the renal circulation and reduce GFR, thereby causing a form of prerenal AKI. These processes stimulate neurohumoral adaptations such as activation of the sympathetic nervous system and RAS and increases in vasopressin and endothelin-1, in an attempt to preserve perfusion to vital organs. However, these adaptations enhance salt and water retention and systemic vasoconstriction, which ultimately promote or exacerbate prerenal AKI by two mechanisms: (1) They increase cardiac afterload and further reduce cardiac output and renal perfusion, and (2) they increase central venous pressure, renal venous pressure, and/or intra-abdominal pressure, ultimately lowering GFR.

AKI in patients with heart failure is often caused by CRS type 1, but certainly these patients can also suffer true prerenal AKI from overzealous diuresis or from ischemic or nephrotoxic ATN. Prerenal AKI from true volume depletion is responsive to judicious administration of intravenous fluids and diuretic withdrawal, making it easy to recognize. It is sometimes more difficult to distinguish CRS type 1 from ATN because the processes often coexist.

Identification of AKI in the setting of heart failure is clinically relevant because reduced GFR is generally associated with a worse prognosis. Therapy is directed at improving cardiac function, especially in patients with low cardiac output, and relieving pulmonary and renal congestion. Small to moderate increases in serum creatinine (0.5 mg/dL) that occur in the setting of effective therapy for venous congestion in acute heart failure are acceptable and typically lead to improved long-term outcomes at 30 days and beyond. Loop diuretics are part of the central treatment strategy for relieving venous congestion; however, these agents can directly stimulate maladaptive neurohormonal responses, transiently worsening kidney function after their introduction. Patients with congestive heart failure often have some degree of diuretic resistance. Strategies to overcome this resistance include combination therapy with thiazide diuretics and rarely device-driven ultrafiltration. With advanced AKI, RRT is required to treat uremia, metabolic complications, and volume overload. Therapies for end-stage cardiac failure include cardiac transplantation and placement of a left ventricular assist device for long-term destination therapy or as a bridge to transplantation.

Hepatorenal Syndrome

A strong physiologic interplay also occurs between liver disease and kidney impairment. Patients with advanced, decompensated cirrhosis or fulminant acute hepatic failure develop a unique form of prerenal AKI called hepatorenal syndrome (HRS). The International Ascites Club diagnostic criteria for HRS include (1) the presence of cirrhosis and ascites, (2) serum creatinine levels higher than 1.5 mg/dL, (3) no improvement in kidney function after at least 48 hours of diuretic withdrawal and volume expansion with albumin, (4) absence of shock, (5) no nephrotoxic drug exposure, and (6) absence of parenchymal kidney disease. There are two subtypes of HRS based on rapidity and severity of kidney impairment. Type 1 HRS is characterized by rapidly progressive renal failure, defined by doubling of the initial serum creatinine concentration (to >2.5 mg/dL in <2 weeks). Type 2 HRS is characterized by moderate kidney failure (serum creatinine increase from 1.5 to 2.5 mg/dL). The hallmark of HRS is profound renal vasoconstriction in the setting of systemic and splanchnic arterial vasodilatation. The hemodynamic changes that occur in HRS are summarized in E-Fig. 29.3.

There is no test that is specific for the diagnosis of HRS, and diagnosis requires exclusion of other causes of AKI. The main differential diagnoses of type 1 HRS are prerenal AKI and ATN, which have an acute onset with progressive deterioration of kidney function. Recognition of prerenal AKI is typically easier, because it responds to intravenous fluids (albumin and saline), whereas HRS type 1 and ATN are more difficult to differentiate. Distinguishing ATN from HRS is crucial, because therapies for these two forms of AKI are very different, as are their prognoses and outcomes. For HRS, midodrine and octreotide, vasopressin (or its analogue terlipressin outside of the United States), or norepinephrine is used, whereas ATN requires primarily supportive therapy with initiation of RRT if necessary. Liver (or combined liver-kidney) transplantation is the definitive therapy for HRS.

Intrinsic AKI

Intrinsic AKI reflects kidney injury that arises from a process that damages one of the compartments of the renal parenchyma. To simplify the approach, kidney disease is organized into anatomic sites of injury in the vasculature, glomerulus, tubules, and interstitium.

Vascular Disease

Intrinsic AKI may result from vascular disease in large or medium-sized arteries, small arteries, and arterioles within the renal parenchyma and veins draining the kidneys. Bilateral renal artery thrombosis superimposed on underlying high-grade stenoses, significant cardiac or aortic thromboembolism occluding the renal arteries, or dissection of the renal arteries may cause AKI. With acute presentations, the clinical features often include flank or abdominal pain, fever, hematuria, and oligo-anuria or anuria. Therapy with thrombolytics may reverse acute thrombosis and thromboembolism and restore renal blood flow with early diagnosis. Percutaneous angioplasty with stent placement can noninvasively correct significant underlying renal artery stenosis. Renal artery dissection often requires surgical repair, but at times stent placement may suffice. Vasculitis of large renal vessels (e.g., Takayasu's arteritis, giant cell arteritis) is an extremely rare cause of AKI.

Induction of AKI by renal atheroemboli occurs less commonly than before due to changes in techniques that now include more commonly inserting the catheter into the radial artery for cardiac procedures as opposed to the more traditional method of inserting the catheter into the femoral artery to approach the heart, and perhaps due to the use of softer wires during vascular procedures. Cholesterol crystal embolization is caused most often by invasive vascular procedures in patients with atherosclerotic disease that disrupt the fibrous cap on the ulcerated plaque. However, thrombolytic therapy and therapeutic anticoagulation can also precipitate embolization in patients who have a significant burden of renal artery or aortic plaque. When it occurs, atheromatous material may lodge in interlobar, arcuate, or interlobular arteries in the kidneys. In addition to AKI, clinical manifestations include abrupt onset of severe hypertension, livedo reticularis, digital or limb ischemia, abdominal pain from pancreatitis or bowel ischemia, gastrointestinal bleeding, muscle pain, central nervous system symptoms such as focal neurologic deficits, confusion, amaurosis fugax, and retinal ischemic symptoms. Peripheral eosinophilia, hypocomplementemia, elevated sedimentation rate, and eosinophiluria variably accompany the syndrome. Treatment is primarily preventive by avoiding the factors known to precipitate atheroembolization. BP control, treatment with statins, amputation of necrotic limbs, aggressive nutrition, avoidance of anticoagulation (to reduce the risk for further embolization), and RRT for severe AKI may improve the dismal prognosis associated with this syndrome. Steroids and iloprost are sometimes used, but their therapeutic role is uncertain.

AKI from vasculitis involving the medium and small vessels has been described with classical polyarteritis nodosa. It is either idiopathic or secondary to hepatitis B antigenemia and manifests with severe hypertension and AKI. Renal arteriography demonstrating beading in the arterial tree of the kidney (and other organs) is diagnostic. Scleroderma is a disorder characterized by arterial and arteriolar narrowing due to deposition of mucinous material. Scleroderma renal crisis manifests as AKI and severe hypertension, often malignant, in a patient with a disease flare. Urinalysis and urine microscopy may be bland or may show cellular activity. Fibrinoid necrosis with ischemic injury occurs in the kidney. ACE inhibitors effectively control BP and improve AKI.

Rarely, AKI may develop in the setting of renal vein thrombosis, a well-known complication of nephrotic syndrome. Imbalance of anticoagulant substances lost in the urine and procoagulant substances produced by the liver leads to a hypercoagulable state and renal vein thrombosis. AKI is thought to develop from raised intrarenal pressures and reduced kidney perfusion. Therapy includes acute thrombolysis and chronic anticoagulation as well as treatment of the underlying glomerular lesion (often membranous nephropathy) and reduction in proteinuria.

Glomerular Disease

A number of glomerular diseases can cause AKI, and the more common entities are reviewed here. Acute proliferative GN may be broadly classified as (1) immune complex disease, (2) pauci-immune disease, or (3) anti-GBM–related disease. They are all characterized by glomerular cell proliferation and necrosis, polymorphonuclear cell infiltration, and, with severe injury, epithelial crescent formation (E-Fig. 29.4). Acute proliferative GN manifests with hypertension and edema formation and with laboratory results pertinent for hematuria and proteinuria, described as *nephritic sediment*. Examination of the urine sediment classically reveals dysmorphic RBCs and RBC casts (see Figs. 24.2 and 24.3). Therapy is directed at the underlying cause, with supportive measures and RRT as necessary.

TTP and HUS are two of the more common causes of thrombotic microangiopathy, which is marked by platelet deposition and endothelial injury with thrombosis of arterioles and glomerular capillaries. AKI results from severe glomerular damage with profound ischemia and necrosis. The thrombotic microangiopathies may manifest with nephritic sediment. Patients with HUS may have severe AKI, or it may be mild, as in patients with TTP. Microangiopathic hemolytic anemia and thrombocytopenia are key features. Therapy often includes modulation of the immune system with plasma exchange or eculizumab, in addition to supportive measures.

The dysproteinemias, which deposit monoclonal immunoglobulin light or heavy chains (or both) in the kidney, may also promote glomerular lesions. The type, metabolism, and packaging of the immunoglobulin determine which type of glomerular lesion develops: light or heavy chain deposition disease, amyloidosis, or one of the fibrillary GNs. The immunoglobulin deposition diseases often manifest with nephrotic proteinuria and AKI, rarely with hematuria.

Light chain deposition disease, heavy chain deposition disease, and light/heavy chain deposition disease cause nodular glomerular lesions. Amyloidosis is also associated with the formation of acellular glomerular nodules. The fibrillary GNs (fibrillary and immunotactoid) may be associated with mesangial expansion or glomerular nodules. More commonly, they appear as a mesangial proliferative, mesangiocapillary, or membranous lesion, sometimes with formation of epithelial crescents. These diseases can be distinguished by electron microscopy. Light and heavy chain diseases produce granular deposits, whereas amyloidosis appears as haphazard fibrils in the 8- to 12-nm size range. Fibrillary GN has fibrils in the 20- to 30-nm range, and immunotactoid GN shows fibrils in the 30- to 50-nm range with organized microtubular fibrils. In addition, positive immunohistochemistry staining for DNAJB9 is highly specific for fibrillary GN.

Tubular Disease

Acute tubular necrosis. ATN is the most common form of hospital-acquired intrinsic AKI, accounting for more than 80% of AKI episodes. It is classically divided into ischemic ATN, which makes up almost 50% of the cases, nephrotoxic ATN, and combinations of both. In many instances, ATN results from multiple insults acting together to injure the kidney. The end result of either ischemic or toxic insult is tubular cell injury and death. E-Table 29.4 outlines the important factors underlying the pathogenesis of ATN.

Ischemic ATN. Ischemic ATN is, for the most part, an extension of severe and uncorrected prerenal AKI. Prolonged renal hypoperfusion causes tubular cell injury, which persists even after the underlying hemodynamic insult resolves and may be associated with ischemia-reperfusion injury. Intraoperative and postoperative hypotension impairs renal perfusion and occurs relatively frequently after cardiac and vascular surgical procedures. Ischemic, nephrotoxic, and

multifactorial ATN are common on the medical wards and in the ICU. Risk for ischemic ATN is increased by the comorbidities these patients possess. Sepsis and septic shock, severe intravascular volume depletion, cirrhotic physiology, and cardiogenic shock are examples of situations that confer high risk for development of ischemic ATN. Employment of vasopressors to restore BP may further reduce renal perfusion and exacerbate ischemia. In some cases, ischemic ATN is so profound that cortical necrosis (ischemic atrophy of the renal cortex) develops.

Nephrotoxic ATN. Nephrotoxic ATN occurs when exogenous substances injure the tubules, primarily through direct toxic effects but also through perturbations in intrarenal hemodynamics or a combination of these factors. In the past, organic solvents and heavy metals (e.g., mercury, cadmium, lead) were a frequent cause of ATN. Since then, many potentially toxic medications have been synthesized and observed to cause tubular injury by multiple mechanisms.

Aminoglycosides cause proximal tubular injury. AKI rarely develops within the first week of therapy, and injury initially manifests with subtle changes in urine concentrating ability and increased RTECs and granular casts in the urine sediment. The antifungal agent amphotericin B induces AKI through two distinct mechanisms: destruction of cellular membranes through sterol interactions and vasoconstriction-induced tubular ischemia. ATN develops in a dose-dependent fashion and manifests with increasing serum creatinine levels and RTECs and granular casts in the urine. Liposomal and lipid complex formulations are less nephrotoxic but can precipitate AKI in high-risk patients.

Radiocontrast material is a common cause of AKI because it is so widely used with imaging procedures. AKI develops in patients with underlying risk factors such as CKD (estimated GFR <30 mL/min), especially diabetic nephropathy, "true" or "effective" intravascular volume depletion, advanced age, and exposure to other nephrotoxins. The incidence of AKI may be 25% and approaches 50% in patients with underlying risk factors. ATN occurs from both ischemic tubular injury (prolonged decrease in renal blood flow) and direct toxicity (osmotic cellular injury, oxidative stress, inflammation). Large radiocontrast volumes increase risk, whereas low-osmolar and iso-osmolar radiocontrast agents are less nephrotoxic than high-osmolar material.

The antiviral agents cidofovir and tenofovir, once they have entered the cell from the peritubular blood via the human organic anion transporter 1 on the basolateral membrane, cause AKI through disruption of mitochondrial and other cellular functions. Several chemotherapeutic agents, including the platinum-based drugs, ifosfamide, mithramycin, imatinib, pentostatin, and pemetrexed, cause ATN through direct toxic effects. As with other nephrotoxins, part of their ability to induce ATN resides in the renal handling by the kidneys (transport through tubular cells) as they are being excreted. In addition, zoledronate, the polymixins, high-dose vancomycin, foscarnet, and deferasirox also cause nephrotoxic ATN. Vancomycin may cause a unique form of AKI known as cast nephropathy. Also, the combination of vancomycin plus piperacillin-tazobactam increases risk for AKI. AKI prevention is best achieved by judicious prescription of these drugs to high-risk patients, appropriate dose adjustments, avoidance of superimposed volume depletion, and close monitoring with early markers of injury such as urine microscopy.

Pigment nephropathy. Pigment nephropathy represents the nephrotoxic renal tubular effects of endogenously produced substances. The most common examples are overproduction of heme moieties in serum that are eventually filtered at the glomerulus and excreted in urine. With severe rhabdomyolysis, the heme pigment released from muscle is myoglobin. AKI develops in the setting of myoglobinuria from the combination of direct myoglobin tubular toxicity (in an acid urine), volume depletion, and obstructing myoglobin casts. Therapy includes intravenous fluids (the addition of bicarbonate is questionable), supportive care, and sometimes RRT. Most patients recover kidney function to near-baseline.

Massive intravascular hemolysis from various causes (e.g., immune-mediated, microangiopathic) is associated with hemoglobinuria, which induces tubular injury by promoting the formation of reactive oxygen species and by reducing renal perfusion through inhibition of nitric oxide synthesis. Therapy is directed at the primary cause, with intravenous fluids and supportive care. Most patients ultimately recover kidney function.

Crystalline nephropathy. AKI may result from crystal deposition in distal tubular lumens after massive rises in uric acid or therapy with certain medications. Risk factors for AKI due to crystal deposition are underlying kidney disease and intravascular volume depletion. Acute uric acid nephropathy from urate crystal deposition and tubular obstruction develops in patients with massive tumor lysis syndrome.

Drugs such as sulfadiazine promote intratubular deposition of sulfa crystals in acid urine, whereas acyclovir crystal deposition occurs after large, rapid intravenous doses of the drug, and atazanavir and indinavir crystal deposition occurs in the setting of volume contraction and urine pH higher than 5.5. Ciprofloxacin can cause AKI due to intratubular crystal deposition when administered in excessive doses, primarily in patients with unrecognized kidney disease and those with alkaline urine. In addition, methotrexate or large doses of intravenous vitamin C (producing oxalate) can cause AKI due to intratubular crystal deposition.

Weight loss therapies such as bariatric surgery with small bowel bypass and orlistat, through induction of malabsorption, cause enteric hyperoxaluria and calcium oxalate crystal deposition, an entity known as acute oxalate nephropathy (E-Fig. 29.5). Sodium phosphate–containing bowel purgatives have also been associated with AKI due to acute phosphate nephropathy, an entity characterized by calcium phosphate intratubular crystal deposition.

Diagnosis of crystalline nephropathy is based on a history of exposure to a culprit agent or an underlying disease state associated with excessive crystal production (see Fig. 24.4).

Osmotic nephropathy. Osmotic nephropathy is a little known entity that can promote AKI through the induction of proximal tubular swelling, cell injury, and occlusion of intratubular lumens. The hyperosmolar and unmetabolizable nature of substances such as sucrose, dextran, mannitol, the sucrose excipient of intravenous immune globulin, and hydroxyethylstarch underlies the pathophysiology of this kidney lesion. Cells develop severe swelling with cytoplasmic vacuoles that form due to accumulation of the offending substance within intracellular lysosomes, disturbing cellular integrity and occluding tubular lumens. AKI results from this abnormal tubular process when patients with underlying kidney disease or other risk factors for kidney injury (e.g., intravascular volume depletion, older age) receive these hyperosmolar substances. AKI is dose related and may require RRT. Although most patients recover from AKI, CKD can result. Therapy is primarily supportive, along with avoidance of further exposure to these agents.

Interstitial Disease

Interstitial disease develops in the setting of infection with certain agents, systemic diseases, infiltrative malignancies, and exposure to some medications. Of these, drug-induced disease is by far the most common entity (E-Table 29.5), especially in the hospitalized patient. The syndrome of AIN is characterized by AKI and a variety of clinical findings. The clinical presentation varies based on the offending agent and the host response. As an example, β-lactam antibiotics frequently

cause the classic triad of fever, maculopapular skin rash, and eosinophilia. Arthralgias, myalgias, and flank pain may also occur. Aside from causing AKI, NSAIDs can rarely lead to allergic or extrarenal manifestations such as fever, rash, or eosinophilia.

Urinalysis may reveal dipstick-positive (trace to 1+) protein, blood, and leukocyte esterase. Urine microscopy may be bland (≈20%), but more often, the urine sediment demonstrates white blood cells (WBCs), RBCs, WBC casts, and granular casts. Wright or Hansel stain may reveal eosinophils in the urine, but neither of these tests is sensitive or specific for AIN. The urine cytokine TNF-alpha and IL9 appear to possess excellent sensitivity and specificity for diagnosing AIN.

The diagnosis is best confirmed by kidney biopsy. A cellular infiltrate consisting of lymphocytes, monocytes, eosinophils, and plasma cells is typically present; interstitial edema and fibrosis vary based on the time of drug exposure (E-Fig. 29.6). Tubulitis, or invasion of lymphocytes into the tubular cells, is frequently part of AIN. Granuloma formation and interstitial inflammation occur with certain drugs such as anticonvulsants and sulfonamides, systemic diseases such as sarcoidosis, tubulointerstitial nephritis with uveitis, and idiopathic granulomatous interstitial nephritis. The glomeruli and vasculature are spared until very late in the disease. If kidney biopsy is not possible, gallium scanning or positron emission tomography of the kidneys may help with diagnosis, especially when the differential diagnosis is primarily between AIN and ATN.

Early diagnosis of AIN, coupled with rapid drug withdrawal before advanced tubulointerstitial fibrosis develops, maximizes successful renal recovery. Corticosteroid therapy is controversial but may reduce the duration of AKI and perhaps improve recovery of kidney function in patients with severe AKI if it is used early (within 2 weeks of diagnosis).

Before development of antibiotics and other drugs that have been associated with AIN, interstitial infection was the major cause of tubulointerstitial nephritis. Microbial agents such as staphylococci, streptococci, mycoplasma, diphtheroids, and legionella are well-described causes of AIN. Several viral agents including cytomegalovirus, Epstein-Barr virus, human immunodeficiency virus (HIV), Hantaan virus, parvovirus, and rubeola also are associated with AIN. In addition, infectious agents that cause rickettsial diseases, leptospirosis, and tuberculosis also invade the renal interstitium.

The renal interstitium is the target of a number of systemic illnesses. Sarcoidosis causes a lymphocyte-dominant AIN, which can be associated with noncaseating granulomas. AKI and urine sediment containing WBCs and WBC casts point to this disease, along with other systemic findings. Steroids reduce the severity of AIN, but CKD is a potential long-term complication. Systemic lupus erythematosus is more commonly associated with various forms of proliferative GN; AIN may coexist with glomerular disease, or, in rare instances, it may be present in isolation. The interstitial inflammatory lesion is caused by immune complex deposition in the tubulointerstitium. AIN usually responds to the cytotoxic therapy given for lupus nephritis. Sjögren's syndrome also causes a lymphocyte-dominant AIN; it appears to be another immune complex–mediated disease of the renal interstitium.

Patients with HIV infection may develop interstitial disease that appears immune related. Diffuse infiltrative lymphocytosis syndrome (DILS) is a Sjögren-like syndrome associated with multivisceral infiltration of CD8-positive T lymphocytes. DILS appears to be a host-determined response to HIV. Immune reconstitution inflammatory syndrome (IRIS) is another multivisceral disease characterized by an interstitial infiltrate. This disease occurs when combination antiretroviral therapy reconstitutes the immune system in the setting of a previous or occult opportunistic infection. An exuberant immune reaction results in T cell infiltration of several organs, including the kidneys, which develop AIN. Therapy involves treatment of the opportunistic infection. Occasionally, corticosteroids are required to suppress the inflammatory response.

Infiltration of the kidney by cancer is an uncommon cause of AKI. Autopsy studies confirm a high rate of asymptomatic renal infiltration. The malignancies most often associated with interstitial infiltration are the lymphomas and leukemias. Lymphomatous infiltration of the kidney parenchyma can occur in the form of discrete nodules or diffuse interstitial infiltration. Lymphoma may cause massive kidney enlargement (nephromegaly) and AKI. Leukemic infiltration also causes nephromegaly, AKI, and, rarely, renal potassium wasting from either tubulointerstitial damage or lysozyme production. Successful treatment of the underlying malignancy typically improves the infiltrative lesion; however, irradiation of the kidneys may provide additional benefit. Exclusion of obstructive uropathy from bulky retroperitoneal lymph node disease is also required.

Postrenal AKI

AKI can develop when obstruction to urine flow occurs along the genitourinary system (E-Table 29.6). The process causing postrenal AKI is called *obstructive uropathy*, whereas the dilated urinary collecting system identified on imaging is termed *hydronephrosis*. Tubular defect with AKI that results from urinary obstruction is called *obstructive nephropathy*. AKI can develop only when obstruction is bilateral, involving both ureters or the bladder, or unilateral in a person with a single functioning kidney. Importantly, either complete or partial obstruction can cause AKI. In general, complete obstruction is associated with more severe AKI and hypertension, intravascular volume overload, hyperkalemia, metabolic acidosis, and hyponatremia.

A wide variety of disorders, originating anywhere from the renal calyces to the urethra, can cause AKI due to urinary obstruction. The most common causes of obstructive uropathy in the upper urinary tract are stones and retroperitoneal disease; in the lower tract, at the level of the bladder and below, prostatic hyperplasia and bladder dysfunction most often obstruct urinary flow. Obstructive uropathy should be considered in many patients with AKI, especially those with a history suggesting risk. A history of nephrolithiasis or certain cancers, along with flank pain, suggests upper tract disease; a history of prostate or bladder disease, together with symptoms of prostatism and urinary retention, points to lower tract obstruction. A directed physical examination of the flanks, suprapubic area, and prostate for flank tenderness, a palpable bladder, or prostatic enlargement is required. Large residual urine demonstrated on straight catheterization of the bladder bespeaks lower tract obstruction.

Ultrasonography of the kidneys and retroperitoneum is the most appropriate initial test to evaluate the patient with AKI and possible urinary tract obstruction. The sensitivity and specificity of renal ultrasonography for the detection of urinary obstruction are approximately 90%. Several processes blunt dilatation of the collecting system and the formation of hydronephrosis, including acute obstruction of less than 48 to 72 hours' duration, severe intravascular volume depletion superimposed on obstruction, and retroperitoneal disease involving the kidneys and ureters that encases the collecting system. If ultrasonographic findings are equivocal or negative but high suspicion for urinary obstruction persists, a CT scan may provide more information. One of the major benefits of CT imaging is the ability to detect stones, tumor, enlarged lymph nodes, and other processes causing obstruction despite the absence of hydronephrosis. As last resort, if obstruction as the cause of AKI is still considered likely, retrograde pyelography may provide a diagnosis of upper tract obstruction.

Therapy for AKI due to obstructive uropathy requires rapid diagnosis and intervention to relieve the obstructive process. Delayed interventions, especially in patients with complete obstruction,

compromise recovery of kidney function. Upper urinary tract obstruction requires either retrograde ureteral stent placement or nephrostomy tube insertion when it is caused by severe retroperitoneal disease such as ureteral or bladder cancer. Relief of lower tract obstruction with a bladder catheter, a suprapubic tube (rarely), or a nephrostomy tube is the first step in treatment. Electrolyte and fluid management also are required to ensure patient safety in developing postobstructive diuresis. It is a phenomenon that occurs primarily in patients with bilateral, complete obstruction and is characterized by large urine volumes after relief of obstruction. Postobstructive diuresis is physiologic in that excess sodium and water are being excreted from the hypervolemic patient, but impaired tubular function (sodium and water) may lead to excessive diuresis and volume depletion. In this setting, judicious fluid repletion is required to avoid iatrogenic postobstructive diuresis as well as underresuscitation and hypotension.

COMPLICATIONS OF AKI

Considering the normal functions of the kidneys, it is not surprising that a number of metabolic complications develop in the setting of AKI. Hyperkalemia is a potentially life-threatening complication that often requires urgent intervention. Hyperkalemia disturbs the magnitude of the action potential in response to a depolarizing stimulus. The electrocardiogram (ECG) is a better guide to therapy than a single measurement of potassium concentration. The sequential ECG changes observed in hyperkalemia are peaked T waves, PR prolongation, QRS widening, and a sine wave pattern. The presence of any of these ECG changes mandates prompt therapy.

Metabolic acidosis is common in AKI. However, it is usually well tolerated and does not require therapy unless arterial pH declines to less than 7.1. Hyperkalemia and severe metabolic acidosis not responsive to medical therapy are indications for initiation of RRT. Hypocalcemia is a common but asymptomatic finding and usually does not require therapy. Significant hyperphosphatemia may occur but often can be managed with oral phosphate binders. Anemia typically does not require treatment unless it is severe, is symptomatic, or contributes to cardiac dysfunction. Uremic manifestations of AKI are listed in E-Table 29.7. They may be subtle findings, or they may be obvious and life-threatening, requiring urgent RRT.

Importantly, infectious complications are the main cause of death because of the immune compromise, edema with end-organ dysfunction and skin breakdown, and numerous indwelling catheters in these patients.

GENERAL MANAGEMENT OF AKI

Management of AKI begins with identification of the cause and pathogenesis of the inciting process. In addition, the complications associated with AKI need to be recognized and rapidly treated to avoid serious adverse events. Prerenal AKI requires optimization of renal perfusion by repletion of intravascular volume in those who are volume depleted and correction of heart failure, liver failure, and other "effective" causes of reduced intravascular volume. Intrinsic AKI requires directed therapy of the disturbed kidney compartment. Management of postrenal AKI mandates early intervention to relieve obstruction and preserve kidney function.

Most consequences of AKI are managed initially with conservative measures. These include interventions to correct hypovolemia or hypervolemia, improvement of hemodynamics, and correction of hyponatremia, hyperkalemia, metabolic acidosis, and hyperphosphatemia. Conversion of patients from oliguric to nonoliguric AKI makes management easier but does not improve outcomes in terms of morbidity or mortality. Manifestations of severe uremia and the other consequences of AKI, as listed in E-Table 29.7, may necessitate RRT if conservative measures are unsuccessful or incompletely reverse the complication. Despite significant research efforts in recent years to determine if earlier versus later initiation of RRT improves outcomes in those with AKI, mixed results amongst the various studies has left clinicians with no clear consensus on this topic. Therefore, the timing of RRT initiation is often individualized to each clinical scenario based on a number of factors including the severity of metabolic disturbances, the likelihood of rapid renal recovery in subsequent hours and days, and the preferences of both the treating clinician and the patient and his or her surrogates.

Hospital-based RRT, which includes primarily acute hemodialysis and continuous renal replacement therapies (CRRTs), is required in certain patients with AKI. Continuous therapies, which can be employed only in the ICU, include continuous venovenous hemofiltration, hemodialysis, hemodiafiltration, slow low-efficiency dialysis, and extended daily dialysis. Emergent indications include severe hyperkalemia, uremic end-organ damage (e.g., pericarditis, seizure), refractory metabolic acidosis, and severe volume overload including pulmonary edema. Although the data do not support a cutoff BUN value to initiate RRT, it is sensible to initiate therapy before severe uremic complications develop. Intractable volume overload with anasarca complicated by skin breakdown is another potential indication. Acute hemodialysis is the modality most commonly employed to treat the consequences of AKI. However, critically ill patients who are hemodynamically unstable benefit most from continuous therapies. CRRT allows more precise control of volume, uremia, acid-base disturbances, and electrolyte disorders with less hemodynamic instability. CRRT also allows aggressive nutritional support. Peritoneal dialysis is rarely used for AKI but is a reasonable modality.

OUTCOME AND PROGNOSIS OF AKI

Despite the significant advances in supportive care and RRT technology, acute and long-term complications, including mortality, remain common. The mortality associated with AKI in the hospital setting depends on the patient's severity of illness and burden of organ dysfunction. As the number of failed organs increases from 0 to 4, the mortality rate associated with AKI increases from less than 40% to more than 90%. Also, in-hospital mortality increases with AKI that develops in the medical or surgical ICU. Long-term outcomes for

patients with AKI include increased risk for death (compared with hospitalized patients without AKI). Furthermore, patients with CKD who have a prehospitalization eGFR lower than 45 mL/min/1.73 m^2 who develop RRT-requiring AKI have a much higher mortality rate than patients with CKD not complicated by AKI. On the whole, all forms of AKI, including the RRT-requiring forms, appear to be associated with an increased risk for development of new CKD, progression of CKD, ESRD, and death.

For a deeper discussion on this topic, please see Chapter 112, "Acute Kidney Injury," in *Goldman-Cecil Medicine*, 26th Edition .

SUGGESTED READINGS

Bellomo R, Ronco C, Kellum JA: Acute kidney injury, *Lancet* 380:756–766, 2012.
Coca SG, Yusuf B, Shlipak MG, et al.: Long-term risk of mortality and other adverse outcomes after acute kidney injury: a systematic review and meta-analysis, *Am J Kidney Dis* 53:961–973, 2009.
Cruz DN, Ricci Z, Ronco C: Clinical review: RIFLE and AKIN—time for reappraisal, *Crit Care* 13:211, 2009.
Haase M, Bellomo R, Devarajan P, et al.: Accuracy of neutrophil gelatinase-associated lipocalin (NGAL) in diagnosis and prognosis in acute kidney injury: a systematic review and meta-analysis, *Am J Kidney Dis* 54:1012, 2009.
Hertzberg D, Ryden L, Pickering JW, et al.: Acute kidney injury-an overview of diagnostic methods and clinical management, *Clin Kidney J* 10(3):323–331, 2017.
Hsu RK, Hsu CY: The role of acute kidney injury in chronic kidney disease, *Semin Nephrol* 36(4):283–292, 2016.
Hsu RK, McCulloch CE, Dudley RA, et al.: Temporal changes in incidence of dialysis-requiring AKI, *J Am Soc Nephrol* 24:37–42, 2013.
KDIGO: 2012 clinical practice guideline for acute kidney injury. Chapter 2.5: Diagnostic approach to alterations in kidney function and structure, *Kid Intl Suppl* 2:33–36, 2012.
Mehta RL, Kellum JA, Shah SV, et al.: Acute Kidney Injury Network: report of an initiative to improve outcomes in acute kidney injury, *Crit Care* 11:R31, 2007.
Moreau R, Lebrec D: Acute kidney injury: new concepts, *Nephron Physiol* 109:73–79, 2008.
Perazella MA: The urine sediment and a biomarker of kidney disease, *Am J Kidney Dis* 66(5):748–755, 2015.
Rosner NH, Perazella MA: Acute kidney injury in the cancer patient, *N Engl J Med* 376(18):1770–1781, 2017.
Uchino S, Kellum J, Bellomo R, et al.: Acute renal failure in critically ill patients, *JAMA* 294:813–818, 2005.

30

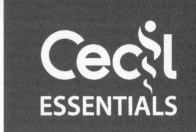

Chronic Kidney Disease

T. Alp Ikizler, Anna Marie Burgner, Beatrice P. Concepcion

DEFINITION AND EPIDEMIOLOGY

Chronic kidney disease (CKD) is defined as persistent abnormalities of kidney structure or function. Markers of kidney damage *or* glomerular filtration rate (GFR) less than 60 mL/1.73 m^2 per minute must be present to meet the diagnostic criteria of CKD. The CKD spectrum includes patients with a normal GFR and kidney damage characterized by proteinuria or electrolyte abnormalities, to elevated serum creatinine, representing a decrease in GFR, to kidney failure or end-stage renal disease (ESRD). Additionally, these must be present and persistent for at least 3 months to differentiate CKD from acute kidney injury (AKI). According to the Kidney Disease Improving Global Outcomes (KDIGO) 2012 guidelines, CKD is classified based upon the underlying cause of kidney disease, GFR category, and albuminuria category. There are six GFR category levels ranging from normal or high (G1 ≥90 mL/min/1.73 m^2) to kidney failure (G5 <15 mL/min/1.73 m^2), and three albuminuria category levels based upon severity (Table 30.1). The rationale for these classification domains is because of differences in observed risk of health consequences and prognosis depending upon each domain's severity.

CKD is a worldwide public health problem. In the United States, the prevalence of CKD is estimated to affect 14.8% of the population, and most have mildly decreased GFR with mild to moderate increased albuminuria (Fig. 30.1). Yet, many people with CKD will progress to ESRD and require maintenance dialysis or kidney transplantation. The crude rate of new ESRD patients in the United States was relatively stable from 2000 to 2010 but started rising again in 2011; however, the United States Renal Data System (USRDS) reported in 2016 that the standardized incidence rate has appeared to plateau (348.2 per million population) (E-Fig. 30.1). Trends in overall prevalence of ESRD suggest a continuing increase in the numbers of patients requiring care, although in 2016 the increase was only 3%—the lowest rate recorded since the inception of the USRDS (E-Fig. 30.2). Care of the ESRD patient is costly, accounting for $35.4 billion (7.2%) of the U.S. Medicare budget in 2016. In addition to concern about progression to ESRD, decreased GFR and proteinuria have each been increasingly recognized as independent risk factors for cardiovascular disease and death. Thus, diagnosis of CKD will identify those at risk not only for kidney function loss but also for decreased survival.

The most common causes of ESRD include diabetes mellitus (40%), hypertension (28%), glomerulonephritis (6% to 7%), and cystic or congenital conditions (2% to 3%). During the evaluation of CKD, every attempt should be made to arrive at the specific cause of kidney disease. Kidney biopsy is the most specific tool to reach a definitive diagnosis and guides treatment, informs prognosis, and determines suitability for kidney transplantation. However, the procedure itself has potential complications, and clinical information, including present, past, and family histories, serology, examination of the urine sediment, and kidney imaging may be sufficient to provide a conclusive diagnosis.

PATHOLOGY

To ensure adequate solute, water, and acid-base balance, the surviving nephrons must adjust by increasing their filtration and excretion rates. Patients with CKD, especially more advanced stages, are vulnerable to edema formation and severe volume overload, hyperkalemia, hyponatremia, and azotemia. During progressive kidney disease, sodium balance is maintained by increasing fractional excretion of sodium by the nephrons. Acid excretion is maintained until late stages of CKD, when the GFR falls to less than 30 mL per minute. Initially, increased tubular ammonia synthesis provides an adequate buffer for hydrogen in the distal nephron. Later, a significant decrease in distal bicarbonate regeneration results in hyperchloremic metabolic acidosis. Further nephron loss leads to retention of organic ions such as sulfates, which results in an anion gap metabolic acidosis. Metabolic acidosis appears to contribute to progression of CKD, and correction by base supplementation may be a potential treatment, although large multicenter randomized clinical trials are lacking.

Once GFR has decreased to below a critical level, CKD tends to progress to ESRD, regardless of the initial insult. Fig. 30.2 shows how risk factors may interact with pathophysiologic mechanisms to accelerate CKD progression. Detailed studies have elucidated interrelated mechanisms, including glomerular hemodynamic responses to nephron loss, proteinuria, and proinflammatory responses. Activation of the renin-angiotensin-aldosterone system (RAAS) pathway and increased transforming growth factor-β (TGF-β) also contribute to kidney fibrosis. Interventions that reduce intraglomerular pressure, such as protein restriction and the use of angiotensin-converting enzyme (ACE) inhibitors or angiotensin-receptor blockers (ARBs), help attenuate progression of kidney disease and further support the importance of glomerular hemodynamics and RAAS in progressive kidney disease.

CLINICAL PRESENTATION

General Features of Uremic Syndrome

Evidence of kidney disease commonly presents not with overt signs or symptoms, but first as abnormalities on laboratory or other diagnostic tests. Patients with CKD may not have symptoms until advanced stages where the GFR is less than 15 mL per minute. *Uremia* is a syndrome that affects every organ system. Uremic syndrome is likely the consequence of many factors, including retained molecules, deficiencies of important hormones, and metabolic abnormalities, rather than the effect of a single uremic toxin (E-Fig. 30.3). Among these toxins, urea can cause symptoms of fatigue, nausea, vomiting, and headaches. Its breakdown product (cyanate) can result in carbamylation of lipoproteins and peptides, leading to multiple organ dysfunctions. Guanidines, byproducts of protein metabolism, are increased and can inhibit α$_1$-hydroxylase activity within the kidney leading to secondary hyperparathyroidism.

TABLE 30.1 Categories of Glomerular Filtration Rate and Albuminuria in CKD

Category	GFR (mL/1.73 m²/min)	Terms
G1[a]	≥90	Normal or high
G2[a]	60-89	Mildly decreased
G3a	45-59	Mildly to moderately decreased
G3b	30-44	Moderately to severely decreased
G4	15-29	Severely decreased
G5	<15	Kidney failure

	AER	ACR		
Category	(mg/24 hours)	(mg/g)	(mg/mmol)	Terms
A1	<30	<30	<3	Normal to mildly increased
A2	30-300	30-300	3-30	Moderately increased
A3	>300	>300	>30	Severely increased

ACR, Albumin-to-creatine ratio; AER, albumin excretion rate; GFR, glomerular filtration rate.
[a]G1 and G2 alone, without other evidence of kidney damage, do not meet the criteria for CKD.

				Albuminuria categories			
				A1	**A2**	**A3**	
				Normal to mildly increased	Moderately increased	Severely increased	
				<30 mg/g <3 mg/mmol	30-300 mg/g 3-30 mg/mmol	>300 mg/g >30 mg/mmol	**Total**
GFR categories (ml/min/1.73 m²)	**G1**	Normal to high	≥90	54.9	4.2	0.5	59.6
	G2	Mildly decreased	60–89	30.2	2.9	0.3	33.5
	G3a	Mildly to moderately decreased	45–59	3.6	0.8	0.3	4.7
	G3b	Moderately to severely decreased	30–44	1.0	0.4	0.2	1.7
	G4	Severely decreased	15–29	0.13	0.10	0.15	0.37
	G5	Kidney failure	<15	0.01	0.04	0.09	0.13
			Total	89.9	8.5	1.6	100

Fig. 30.1 Distribution of CKD in the United States by GFR and albuminuria categories.

β_2-microglobulin accumulation in patients with ESRD has been associated with neuropathy, carpal tunnel syndrome, and amyloid infiltration of the joints. Finally, certain protein-bound solutes such as indoxyl sulfate and the conjugates of p-cresol, may confer cardiovascular toxicity by affecting leukocyte, endothelial, and vascular smooth muscle cell function. Major manifestations of uremia are summarized in Fig. 30.3.

Cardiovascular

In addition to hypertension, cardiovascular disorders are common in patients with CKD. More than 60% of patients with ESRD who start dialysis have echocardiographic manifestations of left ventricular hypertrophy, dilation, and systolic or diastolic dysfunction. Metabolic consequences of CKD, including accelerated atherogenesis, contribute to metastatic calcification in the myocardium, cardiac valves, and arteries. Arrhythmias, including those resulting in sudden death, may be caused by electrolyte abnormalities, cardiac structural changes or ischemic cardiovascular disease. Pericarditis can occur in patients with uremia before they start dialysis, as well as in ESRD patients receiving inadequate dialysis.

Gastrointestinal

Gastrointestinal disturbances are among the earliest and most common signs of the uremic syndrome. Patients describe a metallic taste and loss of appetite. Later, they experience nausea, vomiting, and weight loss, and those with severe uremia may also experience stomatitis and enteritis. There may be gastrointestinal bleeding caused by gastritis, peptic ulceration, and arterial venous malformations in the setting of platelet dysfunction.

Neurologic

Central nervous system (CNS) manifestations are frequent in advanced CKD and characterized predominantly by changes in cognitive function and sleep disturbances. Lethargy, irritability, asterixis, seizures, and frank encephalopathy with coma are late manifestations of uremia and are usually avoided by timely initiation of kidney replacement therapy. Peripheral neurologic manifestations appear as a progressive symmetrical sensory neuropathy in a glove-and-stocking distribution. Patients have decreased distal tendon reflexes and loss of vibratory perception. Peripheral motor impairment can result in restless legs, footdrop, or wristdrop. The majority of these neurologic manifestations reverse with maintenance dialysis or kidney transplantation.

Musculoskeletal

Alterations in calcium and phosphate homeostasis, with hyperparathyroidism and disturbance of vitamin D metabolism, are also common. Hypocalcemia and secondary hyperparathyroidism are the result of phosphate retention and the lack of α_1-hydroxylase activity in the failing

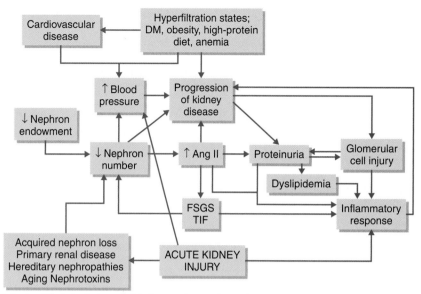

Fig. 30.2 A simplified depiction of risk factors interacting with pathophysiologic mechanisms to accelerate chronic kidney disease progression. *DM,* Diabetes mellitus; *FSGS,* focal segmental glomerulosclerosis; *TIF,* tubulointerstitial fibrosis. (Adapted from Taal MW, Brenner BM: Predicting initiation and progression of chronic kidney disease: Developing renal risk scores. Kidney Int 70:1694-1705, 2006.)

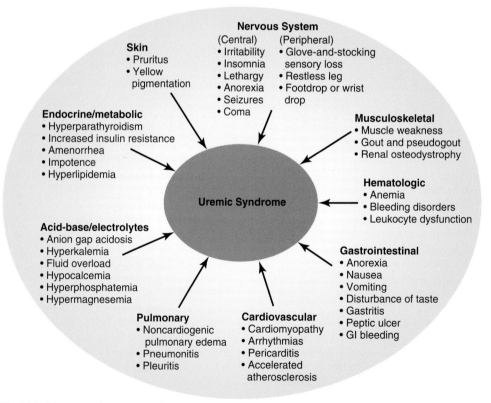

Fig. 30.3 Diagrammatic summary of the major manifestations of the uremic syndrome. *GI,* Gastrointestinal.

kidney, with consequent deficiency of the most active form of vitamin D. Over time, maladaptive parathyroid hypertrophy (i.e., tertiary hyperparathyroidism) leads to bone disease and tissue calcification.

Hematologic and Immunologic

Erythropoietin (EPO), a hormone produced by the kidney that regulates erythrocyte production, becomes progressively deficient as CKD progresses. EPO and iron deficiency are common causes of anemia in CKD. Administration of synthetic EPO results in correction of anemia, improved quality of life and anemia-related symptoms, and decreased dependence on blood transfusions. Caution must be exercised because higher doses of EPO resulting in elevations of the serum hemoglobin to more than 13 g/dL may be associated with a higher risk for adverse cardiovascular events. Bleeding disorders, primarily from defects in platelet adherence and aggregation, are common in patients with uremia. Uremic bleeding can be generally controlled with cryoprecipitate, desmopressin, conjugated estrogens, treatment of anemia, and dialysis.

Defects occur in both the humoral and cellular immune systems in patients with CKD. Although the leukocyte count is normal and appropriately responsive in advanced CKD, patients are generally immunosuppressed and susceptible to infections. This may be due to functional abnormalities of polymorphonuclear leukocytes, lymphocytes, and other cellular host defenses. Additionally, patients with CKD may have a variable immune response to vaccination.

Endocrine and Metabolic

Thyroid function testing may be less reliable in uremia. Common laboratory findings include an increased triiodothyronine resin uptake, a low triiodothyronine level resulting from the impaired conversion of thyroxine to triiodothyronine peripherally, and normal thyroxine levels. Thyroid-stimulating hormone levels are usually normal.

A deranged pituitary-gonadal axis can result in sexual dysfunction exhibited by impotence, decreased libido, amenorrhea, sterility, and uterine bleeding. Patients have decreased plasma levels of testosterone, estrogen, and progesterone, with normal or increased levels of follicle-stimulating hormone, luteinizing hormones, and prolactin. Pregnancy is uncommon in female patients who have a GFR of less than 30 mL per minute.

Lipid abnormalities are also common in CKD. They are most consistent with type IV hyperlipoproteinemia, with a marked increase in plasma triglycerides and less of an increase in total cholesterol. The activity of lipoprotein lipase is decreased in uremia, with a reduction in the conversion of very-low-density lipoprotein to low-density lipoprotein and thus hypertriglyceridemia. The treatment of choice is the hydroxymethylglutaryl–coenzyme A reductase (HMG-CoA) inhibitor class of drugs, especially in CKD patients not yet on maintenance dialysis, because of their pluripotent effects on inflammation and atherosclerosis.

Electrolytes

Hyperkalemia occurs in patients with CKD as a result of decreased renal clearance of potassium, intracellular to extracellular shifts of potassium in the setting of metabolic acidosis related to kidney failure, and the concomitant use of medications such as RAAS blockers. The primary method of treatment is dietary reduction of potassium but may also include use of loop diuretics or potassium-binding medications. Hypokalemia is much less common in CKD but may occur in the setting of very poor nutritional intake or use of high-dose potassium-wasting diuretic medications.

Skin

Uremic hue, a yellowish skin color, is likely the result of retained liposoluble pigments, such as lipochromes and carotenoids. Uremic hue usually responds to dialysis, control of hyperparathyroidism, improved calcium and phosphate balance, and, occasionally, ultraviolet rays. Nail findings of uremia include the half-and-half nail, characterized by red, pink, or brownish discoloration of the distal nail bed, pale nails, and splinter hemorrhages. Other common signs and symptoms include pruritus, and ecchymoses due to disorders of bleeding. Calciphylaxis, or calcific uremic arteriolopathy, results in painful skin calcification and is often seen in patients with uncontrolled hyperparathyroidism. Use of warfarin is suggested to be a risk factor for this condition.

DIAGNOSIS

Comprehensive care of kidney disease includes screening, diagnosing, and treating CKD and complications of CKD to prevent CKD development and progression (E-Fig. 30.4). Screening for CKD is recommended in patients with high-risk comorbid disease, including diabetes mellitus and hypertension and those with a family history of kidney disease. The diagnosis of chronic kidney disease requires demonstrating evidence of kidney damage that has been persistent for at least 3 months. Imaging abnormalities may be consistent with kidney damage, but more commonly this is shown by detection of albuminuria or by reductions in the clearance of toxins by the kidney. Albuminuria may be detected in a spot collection of urine and is best when reported as an albumin-to-creatinine ratio (ACR). In general, an ACR of 30 mg/g or greater confirmed on repeat sample and without evidence of urinary infection raises concern for a diagnosis of CKD and warrants additional investigation.

Measurement of clearance of toxins by the kidney is most often estimated as the glomerular filtration rate (eGFR). Initial assessment should be performed using a serum creatinine-based estimating equation. These include the Modification of Diet in Renal Disease (MDRD) Study Equation and the Chronic Kidney Disease Epidemiology Collaboration (CKD-EPI) equation. Each of these has limitations and cautions regarding application of its results, and a detailed overview can be found in the KDIGO 2012 Clinical Practice Guidelines. Another serum biomarker, cystatin C, may be considered and integrated into another estimating equation for patients who have an eGFR 45-59 mL/min/1.73 m^2 and who may not have albuminuria or kidney imaging abnormalities to confirm evidence of CKD.

Once a diagnosis of CKD is established, management goals include (1) prevention of progression of CKD, (2) identifying and treating symptoms and complications of CKD, and (3) preparing patients for renal replacement therapy (RRT) where appropriate.

TREATMENT

Prevention of Progression

In addition to treatment of the specific underlying cause of kidney disease, methods used to slow progression of CKD include optimal control of hypertension, diabetes, and other cardiovascular disease risk factors (i.e., tobacco cessation), use of medications that block the RAAS pathway, diet modifications, avoidance of nephrotoxins, and addressing potentially reversible causes of acute kidney injury in the setting of CKD.

Management of Hypertension and Diabetes

Several controlled trials have conclusively confirmed that treatment of hypertension attenuates the rate of progression of kidney disease. The present recommendation is to target blood pressure to lower than 130/80 mm Hg in patients with diabetes or kidney disease. However, the evidence supporting this recommendation in CKD is limited and there is debate suggesting a higher target may be acceptable. Medications that block the production or effect of angiotensin II prevent the progression of CKD above and beyond control of hypertension in patients with proteinuria. Dihydropyridine calcium-channel blockers have not been shown to be as beneficial as ACE inhibitors or ARBs in slowing CKD progression.

For patients with diabetes mellitus, adequate glycemic control has been shown to prevent progression of CKD. Recommended goal glycosylated hemoglobin (A_{1c}) measures are less than 7% irrespective of a concurrent diagnosis of CKD, although this level of glycemic control warrants caution due to hypoglycemic risk (see Chapter 68). ACE inhibitors and ARBs may be considered in patients with diabetes and proteinuria, but without hypertension, to slow CKD progression. More recently, use of sodium-glucose cotransporter-2 (SGLT2) inhibitors have shown beneficial effects on kidney outcomes mainly in patients

TABLE 30.2   Drug Dosages in Chronic Kidney Disease

Major Dosage Reduction	Minor or No Reduction	Avoid Usage
Antibiotics		
Aminoglycosides	Erythromycin	
Penicillin	Nafcillin	Nitrofurantoin
Cephalosporins	Clindamycin	Nalidixic acid
Sulfonamides	Chloramphenicol	Tetracycline
Vancomycin	Isoniazid, rifampin	
Quinolones	Amphotericin B	
Fluconazole	Aztreonam, tazobactam	
Acyclovir, ganciclovir	Doxycycline	
Foscarnet		
Imipenem		
Others		
Digoxin	Antihypertensives	Aspirin
Procainamide	Benzodiazepines	Sulfonylureas
H_2 antagonists	Quinidine	Lithium carbonate
Meperidine	Lidocaine	Acetazolamide
Codeine	Spironolactone	NSAIDs
Propoxyphene	Triamterene	Phosphate-containing bowel-preparation agents

NSAIDs, Nonsteroidal anti-inflammatory drugs.

with type 2 diabetes and established atherosclerotic cardiovascular disease. Several other studies suggested that treatment with glucagon-like peptide-1 (GLP-1) receptor agonists could also have beneficial effects on kidney outcomes in patients with type 2 diabetes.

Diet

Dietary protein restriction is advocated to slow progression of CKD. Several meta-analyses indicate that reduced protein diets may be modestly beneficial to slow CKD progression, but the largest clinical trial, the MDRD study, did not show a significant benefit. The recommended dietary protein intake in advanced CKD is 0.60 g/kg per day with at least 50% of the protein being of high biologic value. The present consensus is that aggressive dietary management in patients with CKD, with proper restriction of sodium, potassium, phosphorus, and protein intake under the supervision of a dietician, may reduce progression of CKD, albeit to a small extent.

Avoidance of Toxic Drug Effects

Many drugs that are excreted by the kidney should be avoided, or their doses should be reduced, as shown in Table 30.2. Drugs may injure the kidney in many ways, including direct toxicity leading to acute tubular necrosis, induction of interstitial nephritis, or development of urinary crystals that obstruct the kidney. Common classes of medications that injure the kidney include antibiotics, specifically aminoglycosides; nonsteroidal anti-inflammatory drugs, including cyclo-oxygenase-2 (COX-2) inhibitors; and antiretroviral medications. Over-the-counter herbal medications, including aristolochic acids, may cause CKD. Others, such as St. John's Wort, may interact with kidney transplant medications and should be avoided. Iodinated radiocontrast agents can cause acute worsening of kidney function, especially in patients with CKD. Iso-osmolar contrast agents are less toxic than high-osmolar agents. Patients at high risk for contrast-induced kidney injury should receive adequate hydration, and the volume of the contrast should be minimized. The magnetic resonance imaging (MRI) contrast agent gadolinium, has been associated with the severe fibrotic skin condition of nephrogenic systemic fibrosis in patients with advanced CKD.

Reversible Causes of Acute Deterioration in Kidney Function

The rate of decline in GFR for individual patients is generally log linear. Accordingly, plotting 1/serum creatinine against time usually predicts the rate at which a specific patient will reach ESRD (E-Fig. 30.5). When such a patient suddenly shows acute worsening of kidney function, the differential diagnosis should be considered and investigated, as described in Chapter 29.

Care for the Patient With End-Stage Renal Disease

As CKD progresses to kidney failure, preparation is needed for RRT. Patients with moderate CKD should be referred to a nephrologist for co-management, including evaluation of risk for CKD progression, estimation of timing until initiation of RRT, and education related to RRT. Late referral (<3 months before ESRD) is associated with a higher risk for death after initiation of RRT.

Renal Replacement Therapies

For patients who are suspected to progress to ESRD, discussions to inform patients and their family about available options of RRT should occur early and be paired with an assessment of the expectations and values of the patient. Options include kidney transplantation, dialysis or medical management without dialysis, sometimes referred to as conservative care. In suitable candidates, kidney transplantation is encouraged because it allows a better quality of life, increased survival rate, and greater chance for rehabilitation. In 2016, 87.3% of incident individuals began renal replacement therapy with hemodialysis (HD), 9.7% started with peritoneal dialysis (PD), and 2.8% received a preemptive kidney transplant. Kidney transplants may be from either deceased or living donors. In the United States in 2016, 20,161 kidney transplants were performed, 28% of which were from living donors. There are two types of dialysis, hemodialysis and peritoneal dialysis. The distribution of patients receiving various modalities differs in other countries. Maintenance dialysis is initiated when the patient displays signs of uremia, usually when eGFR is 10 mL per minute or less and there are no apparent reversible causes of kidney failure. However, maintenance dialysis may be started at any time when complications of ESRD, such as volume overload and hyperkalemia, cannot be controlled medically.

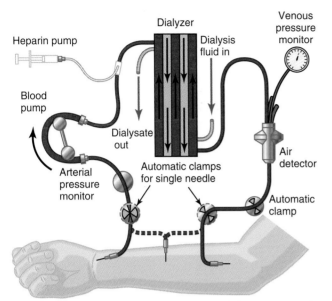

Fig. 30.4 Essential components of a dialysis delivery system that, together with the dialyzer, make up an *artificial kidney*. In isolated ultrafiltration, no dialysis fluid is used (bypass mode). Also shown is the apparatus for using a single needle for inflow and outflow of blood from the patient. (From Keshaviah PR: Hemodialysis monitors and monitoring. In Maher JF [ed]: Replacement of renal function by dialysis, 3rd ed. Boston, Kluwer Academic Publishers, 1989. Reprinted by permission of Kluwer Academic Publishers.)

Hemodialysis

As illustrated in Fig. 30.4, blood is pumped from a vascular access into tubing that leads to a large number of capillaries bundled together in a dialyzer (E-Fig. 30.6). The capillaries are made up of semisynthetic materials and are semipermeable, capable of allowing exchange of small molecules. Moving in the opposite direction to blood is a dialysate solution that is passing through outside the capillaries, thus allowing countercurrent exchange. This solution contains sodium chloride, bicarbonate, and varying concentrations of potassium. Diffusion through the membrane allows low-molecular-weight substances such as urea and organic acids to move across according to the concentration gradient. Fluid is removed by *ultrafiltration*, which is achieved by applying transmembrane hydrostatic pressure across the dialyzer.

In the setting of ESRD, an average patient undergoing *intermittent* maintenance hemodialysis requires 4 hours of dialysis 3 times a week. Common complications during hemodialysis include hypotension and muscle cramping. Avoiding excessive fluid weight gain can minimize these complications.

Access for hemodialysis. The recommended access for hemodialysis is a permanent access such as an arteriovenous fistula (AVF) or arteriovenous graft (AVG), rather than an indwelling catheter. Although the goal is for more than 70% of prevalent hemodialysis patients to use an AVF or AVG for dialysis access (http://www.healthypeople.gov/2020/), many patients continue to use catheters, especially at the time of initiation of maintenance hemodialysis. Temporary catheters are placed into the internal jugular, subclavian, or femoral veins similar to other central venous lines. Permanent catheters have a cuff around the outer wall of the tubing and tunnel under the chest wall skin for some distance before entering the internal jugular vein. Catheters have higher rates of infection and a higher risk for mortality compared with AVF and AVG.

Peritoneal Dialysis

In peritoneal dialysis, the peritoneal capillaries act as a semipermeable membrane like a hemodialysis dialyzer. This technique has several advantages over hemodialysis because it allows independence from the long time spent in dialysis units, it does not require as stringent dietary restrictions, and more patients return to full-time employment. In continuous ambulatory peritoneal dialysis, dialysate of 2- to 3-L volumes is instilled through a peritoneal catheter (E-Fig. 30.7) into the peritoneal cavity for varying amounts of time and exchanged 4 to 6 times daily. In continuous cyclic peritoneal dialysis, the patient is connected to a machine referred to as a *cycler* that allows inflow of smaller volumes of dialysate with shorter dwell time overnight while the patient sleeps. Modifications in this regimen can be made to fit a patient's lifestyle and still achieve adequate clearance of toxins and removal of fluid. Ultrafiltration is achieved through increasing dextrose concentration in the dialysate. Two major drawbacks of peritoneal dialysis are peritonitis and difficulty in achieving adequate clearances in patients with excess body mass. Peritonitis can be treated with intraperitoneal antibiotics. Additionally, a slow deterioration occurs in the permeability of the peritoneal membrane, especially after one or more peritonitis episodes, leading to inadequate dialysis and, ultimately, the need to change the modality of RRT.

Kidney Transplantation

Kidney transplantation is the preferred modality of RRT. In suitable candidates, it provides patients with superior survival and a better quality of life compared to remaining on maintenance dialysis. It is also a more cost-effective long-term treatment option compared to maintenance dialysis. The variety of available immunosuppressive therapies, including calcineurin inhibitors (cyclosporine and tacrolimus), mammalian target of rapamycin (mTOR) inhibitors (sirolimus and everolimus), mycophenolate mofetil/mycophenolic acid, and novel agents such as belatacept have resulted in excellent short- and long-term graft survival.

Types of kidney transplants. Kidney transplant donors may be deceased or living and, among those living, may be related or unrelated. The majority of deceased donation occurs after brain death but can also occur after cardiac death. Deceased donor 1-year and 5-year graft survival is 93% and 75%, and a living donor is 98% and 85%, respectively.

There is an effort to increase living donation because the deceased donor supply is inadequate, resulting in prolonged waiting times for recipient candidates on the deceased donor waiting list. The advantages and disadvantages of living versus deceased donor transplantation are summarized in Table 30.3. The use of kidney paired donation and/or desensitization allows for transplantation of recipients with potential donors who are blood group or immunologically incompatible. Kidney paired donation utilizes exchange algorithms to bypass incompatibility by matching blood group or human leukocyte antigen (HLA)-incompatible recipient-donor pairs with other incompatible pairs, resulting in each donor donating a kidney to the other person's intended recipient. On the other hand, desensitization utilizes antibody-directed therapy such as plasmapheresis or intravenous immunoglobulin to reduce donor-specific HLA antibodies or blood group antibodies in recipients to prevent acute rejection despite blood group or HLA incompatibility. As a means of expanding the supply of deceased donor kidneys and reducing deceased donor waiting times, kidneys from marginal donors such as those of advanced age or with comorbid conditions such as hypertension and cerebrovascular disease are utilized in selected recipients who would benefit from earlier transplantation. In addition, increased Public Health Service risk donors, such as those who have a history of intravenous drug abuse, are increasingly being utilized. In the setting of negative nucleic acid testing, the absolute risk of transmission of hepatitis C, human immunodeficiency virus, and hepatitis B virus from these donors is less than 1%.

TABLE 30.3 Comparison of Donor Sources for Kidney Transplantation

Advantages	Disadvantages
Living Donor	
Waiting time for transplant reduced	Small potential postoperative risks for the donor
Sequelae of long-term dialysis avoided	Small potential long-term risk of kidney function decline in the donor
Elective surgical procedure	Requirement of a willing, medically suitable donor
Better early graft function with shorter hospitalization	
Better short-term and long-term success	
Deceased Donor	
Availability to any recipient	Waiting time variable
Availability of other organs for combined transplants (i.e., kidney-pancreas transplant)	Operation performed urgently
Availability of vascular conduits for complex vascular reconstruction	Higher rates of delayed or slow graft function
	Short-term and long-term success not as good as from a living donor

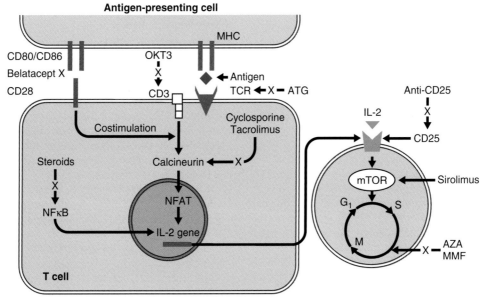

Fig. 30.5 Pathways of T-cell activation and site of action of immunosuppressive agents. *ATG*, Antithymocyte globulin; *AZA*, azathioprine; *IL*, interleukin; *MHC*, major histocompatibility complex; *MMF*, mycoplasma membrane fraction; *MTOR*, mammalian target of rapamycin; *NFAT*, nuclear factor of activated T cells; *TCR*, T-cell receptor.

Immunosuppressant drug therapy. Achieving adequate immunosuppression while minimizing drug toxicity and the risk of infection is at the heart of the success of kidney transplantation. All protocols for immunosuppression aim to inhibit the T lymphocyte, targeting different sites or pathways in the 3-signal model of T-cell activation and proliferation. The mechanisms of action of commonly used immunosuppressants is illustrated in Fig. 30.5. Additionally, antibody-directed therapy is usually employed in those who require desensitization due to preexisting HLA or blood group antibodies.

Induction immunosuppression is administered at the time of transplant and the immediate postoperative period in the form of high-dose steroids, with or without a T lymphocyte–depleting agent such as antithymocyte globulin or a nondepleting agent such as basiliximab (an interleukin-2 inhibitor). *Maintenance immunosuppression* is initiated postoperatively and is composed of at least two drugs, with or without corticosteroids. In the United States, the most common regimen at the time of discharge from the hospital after a transplant is tacrolimus, mycophenolate, and prednisone.

The hepatic cytochrome P-450 system is essential for cyclosporine, tacrolimus, and mTOR inhibitor metabolism. Significant changes in the levels of these drugs may occur when patients start or discontinue taking any of several drugs that can induce or inhibit this system. Therefore, evaluation for drug-drug interactions is critical to prevent toxic or even subtherapeutic effects of either the immunosuppressant drug or the other prescribed therapy. *Cyclosporine* exerts its activity by initially binding to cyclophilin. The cyclosporine-cyclophilin complex subsequently inhibits calcineurin, a calcium-dependent phosphatase that dephosphorylates nuclear factor of activated T cells (NFAT). The inhibition of NFAT dephosphorylation prevents transcription of T-cell activation genes. Side effects of cyclosporine include hypertension, hyperkalemia, hypomagnesemia, exacerbation of gout, dyslipidemia, hypertrichosis, and gingival hypertrophy. *Tacrolimus* has a mechanism of action and side-effect profile like those of cyclosporine. However, it binds to FK-binding protein instead of cyclophilin. It also has additional problems of hyperglycemia and an increased tendency toward neurotoxicity. Rather than causing hypertrichosis, it causes alopecia. Both cyclosporine and tacrolimus can cause calcineurin inhibitor nephrotoxicity, and this is often related to afferent arteriolar vasoconstriction leading to decreased glomerular blood flow. Nephrotoxicity can be acute or chronic and ultimately may contribute to chronic allograft nephropathy and graft loss.

Mycophenolate mofetil or *mycophenolic acid* specifically inhibits T-lymphocyte and B-lymphocyte proliferation by interfering with purine synthesis and thus DNA synthesis. Side effects include leukopenia, anemia, and upper and lower gastrointestinal symptoms.

Sirolimus and *everolimus* bind to FK-binding protein and subsequently inhibit mTOR, thus blocking the phosphorylation of *p70(s6)* kinase and the eukaryotic initiation factor 4E–binding protein, PHAS-I. This action leads to the dampening of cytokine and growth factor activity on T, B, and nonimmune cells. The major side effects are thrombocytopenia, proteinuria, impaired wound healing, and dyslipidemia. mTOR inhibitors can also cause mouth ulcerations, lymphedema, and pneumonitis.

Due to the persistence of episodes of rejection and graft loss over time, novel immunosuppressive agents continue to be developed. Most recently, *belatacept*, a fusion protein that inhibits T-cell activation by blocking the CD80 and CD86 sites on antigen presenting cells, has been shown to confer superior long-term graft function compared to a cyclosporine-based maintenance regimen. This is despite an increased risk of developing early severe acute rejection episodes. Belatacept is administered intravenously and its most serious adverse effect is an increased incidence of post-transplant lymphoproliferative disorder (PTLD) compared to cyclosporine. It is therefore contraindicated in recipients who have not been exposed to Epstein-Barr virus because these patients are at an already higher risk for PTLD at baseline.

Acute rejection. Clinically, acute rejection is detected by a rise in serum creatinine or the development of new proteinuria. In severe cases, graft tenderness and oliguria can occur. *Acute cellular rejection* occurs when T lymphocytes recognize foreign antigens, especially when presented in association with class II histocompatibility antigens. This prompts lymphocyte activation and subsequent invasion of the tubulointerstitium, and in severe cases the blood vessel wall, by activated cytotoxic lymphocytes, resulting in tubulitis and/or endothelialitis. This type of rejection is usually treated with high-dose steroids with or without antithymocyte globulin depending on the severity of the rejection and the initial response to steroid therapy. *Acute humoral rejection* usually occurs in the presence of preexisting or de novo donor-specific HLA antibodies and manifests in the transplanted kidney as microvascular inflammation with or without C4d staining on immunofluorescence. This type of rejection is usually treated with intravenous immune globulin and plasmapheresis, with or without B-cell directed therapy.

Post-transplantation infection. Infection is second only to cardiovascular disease as the leading cause of mortality in kidney transplant recipients. Prophylaxis is used immediately after kidney transplantation to prevent opportunistic infections such as *Pneumocystis jirovecii* pneumonia, cytomegalovirus infection, herpes simplex virus infection, and *Candida* infections. In addition to common community-acquired bacterial and viral infections, kidney transplant recipients are also susceptible to numerous viral, fungal, and other opportunistic infections that normally do not cause severe illness in the immunocompetent host.

Post-transplantation malignant disease. Immunosuppression increases the risk for developing malignant disease. Skin cancer (mostly squamous cell) has the highest incidence in transplant recipients compared with all other types of malignancy. With continuous surveillance and aggressive management, metastasis from skin cancers is rare. Transplant recipients are also at increased risk for developing non-Hodgkin lymphoma and Kaposi sarcoma. In addition to age-appropriate screening, cancer surveillance should be an essential part of post-transplantation care.

PROGNOSIS

The prognosis of CKD varies depending upon the underlying cause, its severity at presentation, and the response to therapy. Yet, it is important to recognize that CKD in general is a significant risk factor for cardiovascular disease and death. Mortality from cardiovascular disease in CKD patients, especially those with stage 3 to 5 disease, is 3.5 times that of an age-matched population (E-Fig. 30.8) and accounts for more than 50% of the deaths in ESRD patients. Research to understand the underlying mechanisms and final pathway, as well as those specific to patients with unique characteristics, will be necessary to advance our efforts to reduce related risks and cure kidney disease.

SUGGESTED READINGS

Abbate M, Remuzzi G: Progression of renal insufficiency: mechanisms. In Massry SG, Glassock RJ, editors: *Massry and Glassock's textbook of nephrology*, 4th ed, Philadelphia, 2001, Lippincott, Williams & Wilkins, pp 1210–1217.

Coresh J, Selvin E, Stevens LA, et al.: Prevalence of chronic kidney disease in the United States, JAMA 298:2038–2047, 2007.

Durrbach A, Francois H, Beaudreuil S, et al.: Advances in immunosuppression for renal transplantation, Nat Rev Nephrol 6:160–167, 2010.

Fishman JA, AST Infectious Disease Community of Practice: Introduction: infection in solid organ transplant recipients, Am J Transplant(Suppl 4)S3–6, 2009.

Halloran PF: Drug therapy: immunosuppressive drugs for kidney transplantation, N Engl J Med 351:2715–2729, 2004.

Kidney Disease: Improving Global Outcomes(KDIGO) CKD Work Group: KDIGO 2012 clinical practice guideline for the evaluation and management of chronic kidney disease, Kidney Inter Suppl 3:1–150, 2013.

Luke RG: Chronic renal failure. In Goldman L, Bennett JC, editors: Cecil textbook of medicine, 21st ed, Philadelphia, 2000, WB Saunders, pp 571–577.

National Kidney Foundation: KDOQI clinical practice guidelines and clinical practice recommendations for diabetes and chronic kidney disease, Am J Kidney Dis 49(2 Suppl 2):S12–S154, 2007.

Sarafidis P, Ferro CJ, Morales E, et al. SGLT-2 inhibitors and GLP-1 receptor agonists for nephroprotection and cardioprotection in patients with diabetes mellitus and chronic kidney disease. A consensus statement by the EURECA-m and the DIABESITY working groups of the ERA-EDTA, Nephrology Dialysis Transplantation 34:208–230, 2019.

Sarnak MJ, Levey AS, Schoolwerth AC, et al.: Kidney disease as a risk factor for development of cardiovascular disease: A statement from the American heart association councils on kidney in cardiovascular disease, high blood pressure research, clinical cardiology, and epidemiology and prevention, Circulation 108:2154–2169, 2003.

U.S. Renal Data System, USRDS 2018 Annual Data Report: Atlas of chronic kidney disease and end-stage renal disease in the United States, National Institutes of Health, Bethesda, MD, 2018, National Institute of Diabetes and Digestive and Kidney Diseases.

Vincenti F, Rostaing L, Grinyo J, et al.: Belatacept and long-term outcomes in kidney transplantation, N Engl J Med 374(4):333–343, 2016.

Voora S, Adey DB: Management of kidney transplant recipients by general nephrologists: core curriculum 2019, Am J Kidney Dis 73(6):866–879, 2019.

Gastrointestinal Disease

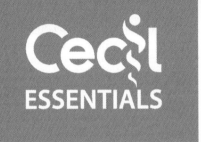

31

Common Clinical Manifestations of Gastrointestinal Disease: Abdominal Pain

Charles M. Bliss, Jr.

DEFINITION AND EPIDEMIOLOGY

Abdominal pain is a frequent manifestation of intra-abdominal disease. However, abdominal pain is difficult to localize or grade because the sensation of pain often is colored by emotional and physical factors. Abdominal pain may be classified as acute or chronic. Acute pain occurs suddenly and more often suggests serious physiologic alterations. Chronic pain may be present for several months; although it does not mandate immediate attention, chronic pain may lead to prolonged evaluation. According to a recent survey of 71,812 patients, 25% of the respondents reported abdominal pain within the past week. Appropriate evaluation of abdominal pain requires knowledge of pain mechanisms, close attention to history and physical examination findings, and recognition of important accompanying symptoms as well as awareness of the strengths and weaknesses of the tests that might be used.

PHYSIOLOGY

Abdominal pain results from stimulation of receptors specific for thermal, mechanical, or chemical stimuli. Once these receptors are excited, pain impulses travel through sympathetic fibers. Abdominal pain can be characterized as somatic or visceral. Somatic pain originates from the abdominal wall and parietal peritoneum, whereas visceral pain originates in internal organs and from the visceral peritoneum. Two types of neurons carry pain: *A fibers*, which have rapid conduction, and *C fibers*, which have slow conduction. Most visceral neurons are of the C type, and the pain resulting from their stimulation tends to be variable with regard to sensation and localization. In contrast, both A and C fibers originate from the parietal peritoneum and abdominal wall, and somatic pain tends to be sharp and distinctly localized.

Because of this pattern of innervation, abdominal viscera are not sensitive to cutting, tearing, burning, or crushing. However, visceral pain results from stretching of the walls of hollow organs or of the capsule of solid organs, as well as from inflammation or ischemia.

CAUSES OF ABDOMINAL PAIN

Multiple intra-abdominal and extra-abdominal disorders can produce abdominal pain. Distinguishing acute from chronic symptoms is helpful. The approach varies with each specific cause, but acute abdominal pain usually demands prompt intervention.

CLINICAL PRESENTATION

History

The differential diagnosis of abdominal pain, whether acute or chronic, requires thorough history taking with regard to pain characteristics, location and radiation, timing, and the presence of any accompanying symptoms. Recognition of characteristic patterns is essential to narrowing the differential diagnosis.

Pain location often indicates the organ responsible for the problem. For instance, epigastric pain is usually typical of peptic ulcer or dyspepsia, whereas right upper quadrant pain is more suggestive of cholecystitis and other biliary disorders. Early in the course of illness, pain may be perceived in one location and subsequently felt in another; this pattern of progression may be suggestive of specific pain syndromes. In acute cases, abdominal pain tends to be sharp and severe. The pain of a perforated viscus is intense, and the pain from a dissecting aneurysm may be described as tearing or crushing. Chronic pain may be less severe; pain from irritable bowel or dyspepsia is constant and dull, and the pain of chronic peptic ulcer is described as gnawing or hunger pain. The pattern of pain relief is helpful for diagnosing some conditions. The physician should also inquire about whether the pain is steady or intermittent and whether it occurs at night. For nocturnal pain, a distinction should be made between pain that awakens the patient and pain that is felt when the patient wakes up for other reasons.

Table 31.1 outlines characteristics, location, and radiation of pain for a few common acute and chronic abdominal conditions.

Physical Examination

Examination of the abdomen provides valuable clues to the diagnosis, but the examination should start with the general appearance of the patient. A patient who is writhing in bed and unable to find a comfortable position may be suffering from obstruction. In contrast, a patient lying with the lower extremities flexed and avoiding any motion may be suffering from peritonitis because movement makes peritoneal pain worse. Abdominal distention indicates obstruction or ascites. Visual inspection for peristalsis is helpful for the diagnosis of small bowel obstruction, but this sign is present only in the early stages. Focal areas of distention may indicate hernias; notice should also be taken of any scars from prior surgeries.

Auscultation should be performed in several areas to evaluate the timbre and pattern of bowel sounds and to search for bruits or hums. Absence of bowel sounds suggests ileus, whereas the presence of hyperactive, high-pitched sounds may indicate obstruction. Multiple bruits

TABLE 31.1	Key Abdominal Pain Syndromes		
Condition	**Type**	**Location**	**Radiation**
Acute Abdominal Pain			
Appendicitis	Crampy, steady	Periumbilical, RLQ	Back
Cholecystitis	Intermittent, steady	Epigastric, RUQ	Right scapula
Pancreatitis	Steady	Epigastric, periumbilical	Back
Perforation	Sudden, severe	Epigastric	Entire abdomen
Obstruction	Crampy	Periumbilical	Back
Infarction	Severe, diffuse	Periumbilical	Entire abdomen
Chronic Abdominal Pain			
Esophagitis	Burning	Retrosternal	Left arm, back
Peptic ulcer	Gnawing	Epigastric	Back
Dyspepsia	Bloating, dull	Epigastric	None
IBS	Crampy	LLQ, RLQ	None

IBS, Irritable bowel syndrome; *LLQ,* left lower quadrant; *RLQ,* right lower quadrant; *RUQ,* right upper quadrant.

alert the examiner to the possibility of significant vascular disease, suggesting ischemia.

The abdomen should be palpated gently, starting in an area away from the pain. The examiner searches for areas of localized tenderness and rebound as well as for masses and enlarged organs. Percussion is performed to identify the size of organs or to determine the presence of ascites. Pain on percussion of the abdomen indicates peritoneal reaction, as does severe rebound tenderness.

A rectal examination is important for identifying a rectal tumor in the case of colon obstruction or tenderness high in the rectum in acute appendicitis. A pelvic examination should be performed in women to rule out pelvic inflammatory disease, or masses.

ACUTE ABDOMEN

The evaluation of a patient with an acute abdomen is a challenge in medical practice. The acute abdomen is caused by sudden inflammation, perforation, obstruction, or infarction of an intra-abdominal organ. The urgent question to be answered is whether immediate surgery is needed; a quick but complete evaluation is necessary to avoid undue delay in intervention for patients who require surgery. The physician must assess for abdominal tenderness, rebound, and guarding. Early surgical consultation should be obtained, even in doubtful cases, rather than awaiting confirmation of the diagnosis via laboratory or radiologic studies. However, many extra-abdominal conditions such as pneumonia, myocardial infarction, nephrolithiasis, and metabolic disorders can cause acute abdominal pain.

In some instances of the acute abdomen in its early stages, there are few findings. The examiner should be aware that patients with benign chronic conditions may have severe pain at presentation that is out of proportion to any physical findings. The context provided by the medical history, particularly previous abdominal surgery, is very valuable. Indeed, a patient with sudden crampy pain and abdominal distention may have an intestinal obstruction caused by adhesions or an incarcerated hernia. Therefore, examination of the entire patient, looking for jaundice, skin lesions, evidence of prior surgery, or evidence of chronic liver disease, is important.

In evaluating a patient with acute abdominal symptoms, a complete blood cell count with differential, a urinalysis, and measurements of serum amylase, lipase, bilirubin, and electrolytes are necessary components of the laboratory examination. Additional studies may be done but usually do not aid in the rapid decision making required. An elevated white blood cell count may indicate inflammatory disease, and extremely high values are typical of acute intestinal ischemia. An elevated serum amylase concentration usually indicates acute pancreatitis, although a perforated ulcer or mesenteric thrombosis can also cause hyperamylasemia.

Radiographic examination with an abdominal film is important to reveal the intra-abdominal gas pattern, and an upright film that includes the diaphragm or a left lateral decubitus film may identify intra-abdominal air suggesting perforation of a hollow viscus. Ultrasonography can be helpful in the diagnosis of acute cholecystitis or appendicitis. Computed tomography (CT) scans have become more helpful with technologic improvements in scanners; early CT scans allow prompt diagnosis of sometimes unsuspected abdominal diseases. Examination with a radiopaque medium should be used judiciously, especially if surgery is anticipated. E-Figs. 31.1 through 31.4 are CT images of appendicitis, diverticulitis, pancreatitis, and ulcerative colitis, respectively.

CHRONIC ABDOMINAL PAIN

In the evaluation of chronic abdominal pain, it can be challenging to distinguish between organic pain resulting from a specific pathologic process and functional pain. The location and characteristics of pain, as already discussed, serve as important guides, as do other accompanying symptoms. The presence of postprandial nausea and vomiting suggests chronic peptic ulcer, disorders of gastric emptying, or outlet obstruction. Documentation of weight loss mandates the search for an organic cause, such as inflammatory bowel disease or celiac disease. If anorexia accompanies weight loss, particularly in elderly patients, cancer must be excluded. If no cancer can be found and all objective tests are normal, the possibility of chronic depression must be entertained.

The most frequent causes of chronic abdominal pain are functional. Dyspepsia is characterized by chronic intermittent epigastric discomfort, sometimes accompanied by nausea or bloating. These symptoms are not always relieved by acid suppression and may be the result of an underlying motor disorder. Furthermore, when *Helicobacter pylori* is found in a patient with dyspeptic symptoms, its eradication may not necessarily lead to the resolution of symptoms. Controversy exists regarding the most effective strategy for the treatment of dyspepsia when *H. pylori* organisms are found in the absence of peptic ulcer disease.

Irritable bowel syndrome (IBS) is a very common disorder. Estimates are that 15% of Americans suffer from IBS on a regular basis and that 40% to 50% of referrals to gastroenterologists are related to IBS. The syndrome consists of abdominal distention, flatulence, and disordered bowel function. There are two important variants of IBS: constipation predominant IBS (IBS-C) is characterized by pain in the setting of constipation, and diarrhea predominant IBS (IBS-D) involves pain in the setting of diarrhea. IBS with both diarrhea and constipation is sometimes denoted as IBS mixed. The abdominal pain of IBS tends to be in the left lower quadrant, but it can be located elsewhere or be more generalized. Any patient with weight loss, anemia, nocturnal symptoms, steatorrhea, or onset of symptoms after age 50 years should be evaluated carefully for organic disease because these symptoms are not associated with IBS.

The Rome criteria, developed for research studies, may be helpful in the diagnosis of IBS. These criteria include pain that is associated with change in bowel habits, relieved with defecation, or accompanied by distention or bloating. Patients are reassured, counseled, and treated with anticholinergic agents and stool softeners. Although serotonin (5-HT) agonists such as alosetron and

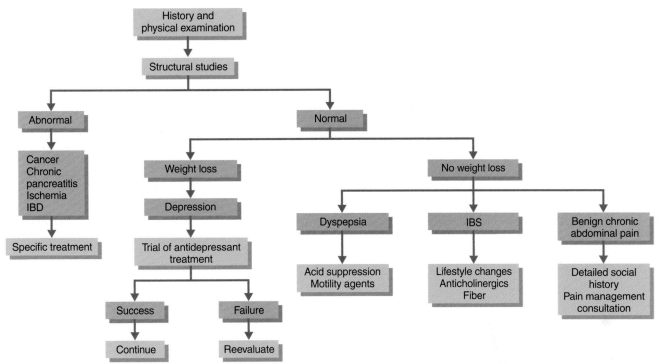

Fig. 31.1 Approach to the patient with chronic abdominal pain. *IBD,* Inflammatory bowel disease; *IBS,* irritable bowel syndrome.

tegaserod showed promise initially, they have been relegated to limited use due to unacceptable side effects. Eluxadoline, which targets opioid receptors, has been helpful in some cases of IBS-D in controlling pain and diarrhea in patients who have failed loperamide. Linaclotide causes increased secretion of chloride and bicarbonate into the intestinal lumen via a cyclic guanosine monophosphate (cGMP) pathway. This pathway also may be responsible for relief of visceral pain in patients with IBS-C. However, its use has been limited by unacceptable side effects, though a lower 72 mcg dose is now available. A new member of this class, plecanatide, has shown promise in initial studies but has not yet proved to be more effective than linaclotide. Tenapanor is a member of a new class of small molecule medications that act by inhibiting transport of sodium from the lumen of the large intestine, leading to improvements in constipation and pain in patients with IBS-C. This medication is still in the process of study but has been approved by the FDA. It represents a new method of treatment.

The more challenging clinical problem is *functional abdominal pain syndrome.* This term describes a condition in which the pain has been present for months or years. The complaints of pain often are not related to eating, defecation, or menses, unlike other causes of chronic pain. The patient is most likely to be a woman who has undergone numerous examinations and diagnostic studies with negative findings and, in many cases, surgical operations without any relief. Lengthy or repeated diagnostic work-ups are counterproductive and only convince the patient that one more test is what is needed to determine the source of the pain. The physician must establish that organic disease is not present and must also realize that the pain is real. These patients are not malingerers despite the fact that the pain does not fit any familiar pattern. Depression may be the result rather than the cause of the pain.

Management of chronic abdominal pain is demanding and requires as much tact, diplomacy, and compassion as scientific knowledge. An effort should be made to inquire about social factors, including history

of physical and sexual abuse, particularly in women. Psychiatric evaluation may be necessary, but the suggestion for such a consultation may be interpreted by the patient as evidence that the physician believes "the pain is in my head." Referral to a competent pain management specialist is helpful in some cases. This approach offers the possibility of providing relief with nerve blocks if the pain is localized or with other pain-relieving devices. If this approach fails, referral to a psychologist or psychiatrist may be acceptable to the patient.

Because of the challenges involved with chronic pain treatment, especially in light of the current issues with opioids, new approaches using less traditional methods are being tried.

A new study done in the Netherlands showed that use of tetrahydrocannabinol, one of the active substances in marijuana, is not effective in the treatment of chronic pain from prior surgery or chronic pancreatitis.

Fig. 31.1 presents a practical approach to chronic abdominal pain.

For further information, please see Chapter 128, "Functional Gastrointestinal Disorders," in *Goldman-Cecil Medicine,* 26th Edition.

SUGGESTED READINGS

Almario CV, Ballal ML, Chey WD, et al: Burden of gastrointestinal symptoms in the United States: results of a nationally representative survey of over 71,000 Americans, Am J Gastroenterol 113:1701–1710, 2018.

Brenner DM, Fogel R, Dorn SD, et al: Efficacy, safety, and tolerability of plecanatide in patients with irritable bowel syndrome with constipation: results of two phase 3 randomized clinical trials, Am J Gastroenterol 113:735–745, 2018.

Brenner DM, Sayuk GS, Gutman CR, et al: Efficacy and safety of eluxadoline in patients with irritable bowel syndrome with diarrhea who report inadequate symptom control with loperamide: RELIEF phase 4 study, Am J Gastroenterol 114:1502–1511, 2019.

Chang L, Lembo A, Sultan S: American gastroenterological association institute technical review on the pharmacological management of irritable bowel syndrome, Gastroenterology 147:1149–1172, 2014.

Chey WD, Lembo AJ, Rosenbaum DP: Tenapanor treatment of patients with constipation-predominant irritable bowel syndrome: a phase 2, randomised, placebo-controlled efficacy and safety trial, Am J Gastroenterol 112:763–774, 2017.

De Vries M, van Rijckevorsel DCM, Vissers KCP, et al: Tetrahydrocannabinol does not reduce pain in patients with chronic abdominal pain in a phase 2 placebo-controlled study, Clin Gastroenterol Hepatol 15:1079–1086, 2017.

Lacy BE, Chey WD, Cash BD, et al: Eluxadoline efficacy in IBS-D patients who report prior loperamide use, Am J Gastroenterol 112:924–932, 2017.

Schoenfeld P, Lacey BE, Chey WD, et al: Low dose linaclotide (72 μg) for chronic idiopathic constipation: a 12-week, randomized, double-blind, placebo-controlled trial, Am J Gastroenterol 113:105–114, 2017.

Shah ED, Kim HM, Shoenfeld P: Efficacy and tolerability of guanylate cyclase-c agonists for irritable bowel syndrome with constipation and chronic idiopathic constipation: a systematic review and meta-analysis, Am J Gastroenterol 113:329–338, 2018.

Sperber AD, Drossman D: The functional abdominal pain syndrome, Aliment Pharmacol Ther 33:514–524, 2011.

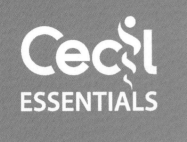

32

Common Clinical Manifestations of Gastrointestinal Disease: Gastrointestinal Hemorrhage

Waihong Chung, Abbas Rupawala

INTRODUCTION

Gastrointestinal bleeding (GIB) is a major cause of morbidity, accounting for over 844,000 emergency department visits and 513,000 hospitalizations in the United States in 2014. GIB also accounts for over 2.2 million days of productivity loss and $5 billion in direct cost annually. Despite increasing costs of care, mortality due to GIB has declined in recent years in part due to increased rates of endoscopy and improved endoscopic therapy. GIB can result from a variety of etiologies (Table 32.1), its presentation can vary greatly depending on age and comorbidity, and its clinical course can evolve rapidly over time and in response to treatment. It is, therefore, essential to apply a systematic approach to the management of all cases of suspected GIB. We advocate a four-step approach that can be encapsulated by a simple mnemonic *PRET*: *P*rioritize, *R*esuscitate, *E*valuate, and *T*reat.

APPROACH TO PATIENTS WITH GASTROINTESTINAL BLEEDING

Prioritize

The first step in the approach to GIB is to prioritize and triage patients based on acuity and severity of blood loss. The objective of this step is to guide the pace of evaluation and ensure that the patient is managed in a timely and cost-effective manner.

GIB can be broadly classified as overt GIB, when patients present with hematemesis, coffee-ground emesis, melena, or hematochezia (Table 32.2), and occult GIB, when symptoms of overt bleeding are absent but patients are anemic with heme (occult blood) positive stools. In addition to symptoms of bleeding, patients may also present with some combination of weakness, dizziness, lightheadedness, shortness of breath, postural changes in blood pressure or pulse, cramping abdominal pain, and diarrhea. Intuitively, overt GIB likely represents faster or higher volume blood loss; thus, patients presenting with overt GIB should be prioritized to receive an expedited work-up in the emergency room or in the inpatient setting. Meanwhile, patients with occult GIB, who are otherwise asymptomatic, may be evaluated safely and more efficiently in the outpatient setting.

GIB can also be classified into acute GIB, arbitrarily defined as bleeding duration of less than 3 days, and chronic GIB. The authors, however, find this classification less useful in guiding prioritization because it fails to convey the difference in severity between protracted or continual occult GIB versus ongoing or recurrent overt GIB.

Resuscitate

The second step is to resuscitate and stabilize the patient's hemodynamic parameters and to alleviate symptoms. The objective of this step is to prevent and reverse the complications of blood loss and restore end-organ perfusion. It is worth emphasizing that adequate resuscitation is *the most important step* in the management of GIB and must take priority over the subsequent steps of evaluation and treatment.

In cases of overt GIB, the resuscitative effort should follow the basic principle of airway, breathing, and circulation. Airway management and respiratory support should be considered in patients presenting with massive or recurrent hematemesis as well as those with altered mental status to minimize risk of aspiration. Restoration of normal circulatory function should be achieved by rapid infusion of an isotonic crystalloid fluid, such as normal saline or lactated Ringer's solution. Concerns regarding volume overload and pulmonary edema in patients with heart failure or renal failure should not delay initiation of fluid resuscitation but may necessitate the use of positive-pressure ventilation. A restrictive transfusion threshold of hemoglobin less than 7 g/dL has been shown to improve survival (95% vs. 91%) and decreased rebleeding (10% vs. 16%) compared to a threshold of 9 g/dL. This is especially true in cirrhotic patients presenting with suspected variceal bleeding where over-transfusion may increase portal hypertension, bleeding and mortality.

In cases of occult GIB, resuscitation should aim at relieving the symptoms of anemia. Those with severe, symptomatic anemia and signs of end-organ ischemia, such as angina or renal insufficiency, may be transfused. Those with nonsevere symptoms of anemia, such as weakness, fatigue, exercise intolerance, or exertional dyspnea, can receive oral or parenteral iron replacement therapy.

Evaluate

The third step is performing a focused history and physical exam and obtaining relevant laboratory and imaging tests (Table 32.3). The goal of this step is to localize the potential bleeding site and identify the most likely etiology of the bleed.

From a diagnostic and therapeutic perspective, it is most useful to distinguish GIB into upper GIB (UGIB), historically defined as bleeding emanating from a source proximal to the ligament of Treitz, and lower GIB (LGIB). LGIB can be further subdivided into small bowel bleeding, originating proximal to the terminal ileum, and colonic bleeding. UGIB has traditionally been considered to account for 76% to 82% of GIB cases and is associated with a significantly higher emergency room to hospital admission rate (78% vs. 40%) as well as in-hospital mortality (1.5% vs. 0.5%) compared to LGIB. Patients with suspected UGIB should, therefore, be managed more aggressively, including offering an early endoscopy within 24 hours of presentation, while those with self-limiting LGIB may be observed clinically. Up to 15% of patients presenting with presumed LGIB may have UGIB. The term *obscure*

TABLE 32.1   Common Etiologies of GIB

Source	Associated Clinical Features	Management
Upper Gastrointestinal Tract		
Esophagitis/esophageal ulcer	Reflux, dysphagia, odynophagia	Acid suppression, antireflux surgery
Esophageal cancer	Dysphagia, weight loss	Chemoradiation, surgery
Gastroesophageal varices/portal gastropathy	Chronic liver disease, portal hypertension	Octreotide, endoscopic therapy, antibiotics
Mallory-Weiss tear	Repeated retching, vomiting, alcoholics	Supportive care, endoscopy
Gastritis/gastric ulcer/duodenitis/duodenal ulcer	NSAIDs, alcohol, *Helicobacter pylori*, epigastric pain	Hold NSAIDs, treat *H. pylori*, acid suppression, endoscopic therapy
Gastric cancer	Early satiety, weight loss, abdominal pain	Surgery, chemotherapy
Gastric antral vascular ectasia	Cirrhosis, systemic sclerosis	Endoscopic therapy
Angioectasias	Painless bleeding, may be present throughout GI tract, aortic stenosis (Heyde syndrome)	Endoscopic therapy
Cameron lesion	Hiatal hernia	Surgery for hiatal hernia repair
Dieulafoy lesion	Cardiovascular disease, chronic kidney disease, NSAIDs, alcohol	Endoscopic therapy
Aortoenteric fistula	History of open abdominal aortic aneurysm repair, sentinel bleed, large-volume bleeding	Surgery
Hemobilia	History of biliary tract instrumentation, biliary malignancy	Repeat endoscopy, vascular interventional radiology (VIR), surgery
Hemosuccus pancreaticus	Pancreatic pseudocyst, pancreatic tumor	VIR
Lower Gastrointestinal Tract		
Diverticular bleed	Diverticulosis, painless hematochezia in older patients	Endoscopic therapy, VIR
Infectious colitis	History of exposure, diarrhea, abdominal pain	Treat underlying infection
Inflammatory bowel disease	History of colitis, diarrhea, abdominal pain, fever, tenesmus	Treat underlying inflammation
Ischemic colitis	History of profound hypotension, abdominal pain, followed by bleeding	Supportive care, surgery
Angioectasia	Obscure overt or occult bleeding	Endoscopic therapy
Radiation-induced telangiectasia	Pelvic radiation	Endoscopic therapy
Meckel's diverticulum	Painless hematochezia in younger patients	Surgery
Colorectal cancer	Weight loss, change in bowel habits, anemia	Surgery, chemotherapy
Colon polyp	Painless hematochezia	Endoscopic resection
Post-polypectomy bleed	Recent colonoscopy with polypectomy	Endoscopic therapy
Hemorrhoidal bleed	Hematochezia with bowel movement	Supportive care, surgery, banding
Stercoral ulcer	Severe constipation	Supportive care, treat constipation

TABLE 32.2   Definitions of Overt GIB

Hematemesis

Vomiting of bright red blood or partially digested blood that resembles coffee grounds.

Source of bleeding is likely to be proximal to the ligament of Treitz.

Consider swallowed blood from nasopharynx (e.g., epistaxis) or the respiratory tract (hemoptysis).

Melena

Passing of black, tarry, and usually foul-smelling stool, representing digested blood.

Source of bleeding is likely to be in the upper gastrointestinal tract, the small bowel, or occasionally the proximal colon.

As little as 50-100 mL of blood can result in melena.

Hematochezia

Passing of bright red blood or maroon stool per rectum.

Source of bleeding is likely to be in the lower gastrointestinal tract (small bowel and colon).

10-15% of severe UGIB with brisk bleeding may present with hematochezia.

GIB, which was previously used interchangeably with small intestinal bleeding, is now reserved to describe cases of overt or occult GIB where the bleeding source is not readily identified after complete evaluation of the entire GI tract including the small bowel.

Signs and symptoms that are strongly predictive of an UGIB include the presence of bright red blood or coffee-ground emesis as well as a markedly elevated blood urea nitrogen (BUN)-to-creatinine ratio in a patient without chronic kidney disease. Melena refers to black, tarry, foul-smelling stools formed as a result of blood being altered by gastric acid, digestive enzymes, and intestinal bacteria. Although the presence of melena is often indicative of UGIB, it can also be seen in cases of small intestinal as well as right-sided colonic bleed. The use of naso-gastric lavage for ruling out UGIB has largely fallen out of favor due to its poor negative likelihood ratio and its association with significant patient discomfort.

A critical decision point in the evaluation step is assessing the odds of variceal bleeding being the etiology, as it is a serious gastrointestinal emergency that is associated with a high (>30%) mortality rate and is managed somewhat differently than other etiologies of GIB. Any patients with known varices, acute alcoholic hepatitis, or cirrhosis of any etiologies, especially those with signs and symptoms of portal

TABLE 32.3 Key Information in the Evaluation of GIB

History	Physical Exam	Laboratory Test
• Nature of bleeding (hematemesis, melena, hematochezia)	• Vital signs	• Complete blood count
• Other gastrointestinal symptoms	• Presence of gross blood in oropharynx	• Basic metabolic panel
• Systemic (cardiopulmonary, constitutional, and other) symptoms	• Presence of abdominal tenderness	• Hepatic function panel
• Medications: NSAIDs, corticosteroids, bisphosphonates, anticoagulants, and antiplatelets	• Digital rectal exam	• Prothrombin Time/INR
• Illicit drug and alcohol exposure		• Blood type and cross match
• Surgical history		
• Past medical history		
• Peptic ulcer disease		
• *Helicobacter pylori* infection and treatment		
• Gastrointestinal bleed		
• Chronic liver disease		
• Inflammatory bowel disease		
• Malignancy		
• Pelvic radiation		
• Recent endoscopic interventions (e.g., polypectomy)		

hypertension as evident by the presence of *caput medusa*, jaundice, splenomegaly, and/or ascites on exam as well as coagulopathy and thrombocytopenia on laboratory tests, should be managed as a potential variceal hemorrhage.

Older patients and those with significant comorbidities, continued bleeding, and hemodynamic instability are also at higher risk of poor outcomes and should be managed more aggressively and monitored in the intensive care setting. Prognostic scores such as the Glasgow-Blatchford score, Rockall scale, and AIMS65 score may help identify high-risk patients in need of more urgent evaluation and treatment.

Treat

The fourth step in the management of GIB is to confirm the location and etiology of bleeding and to deliver treatment both locally and systemically. The goal of this step is to achieve adequate hemostasis and minimize the risk of rebleeding. A comprehensive treatment plan for GIB may consist of up to six components that can be summarized by another simple mnemonic *CAMPER*: Coagulopathy, Acid suppression, Medical therapy, Preprocedural preparation, Endoscopy, and Rescue technique.

Coagulopathy

Coagulopathy should be addressed in any patient presenting with overt GIB. In general, pharmacologic anticoagulation and antiplatelets should be held, unless otherwise contraindicated due to another medical condition such as recent vascular stent placement, until hemostasis is achieved. In patients presenting with hemodynamically significant

GIB, reversal of warfarin using intravenous vitamin K as well as inactivated 4-factor prothrombin complex concentrate (PCC) should be considered. Fresh frozen plasma has fallen out of favor due to its higher risk of adverse reactions and volume overload but may be an option when PCC is not available. Patients on direct oral anticoagulants do not typically require reversal due to their shorter half-life, although the use of antifibrinolytic agents can be considered in those with significant comorbidities or worsening bleeding symptoms. Specific reversal agents for the direct oral anticoagulants are reserved for those at imminent risk of death from bleeding. Cirrhotic patients are not necessarily hypocoagulable despite the elevated INR due to impaired synthesis of both anticoagulants and procoagulants. Platelet transfusion should be considered in those with a platelet level less than 50,000/μL but has limited benefit in individuals continuing on antiplatelet agents. Desmopressin can be considered in patients with uremic platelet dysfunction or von Willebrand disease.

Acid Suppression

Acid suppression with an intravenous proton pump inhibitor (PPI) should be initiated on admission in patients with suspected UGIB. It primarily helps with clot stabilization and is associated with reduced rates of high-risk stigmata identified on endoscopy, the need for endoscopic therapy in patients with peptic ulcer bleeding, and the risk of ulcer rebleeding. The optimal dose of preprocedure PPI has not been determined, although intermittent PPI therapy was found to be comparable to continuous therapy in patients with endoscopically treated high-risk bleeding ulcers.

Medical Therapy

Medical therapy plays an important role in the management of GIB in cirrhotic patients. Prophylactic antibiotics, intravenous ceftriaxone or a quinolone, may be administered to any cirrhotic patients with GIB for 7 days to decrease the risk of bacterial infections and mortality. Vasoactive medications, such as octreotide, terlipressin, and vasopressin, should be initiated as soon as possible in any patients presenting with suspected variceal bleeding and continued for 3 days if the etiology is confirmed on endoscopy.

Preprocedural Preparation

Preprocedural preparation is essential to achieving adequate endoscopic hemostasis while minimizing procedure-related complications. Prokinetic agents, such as erythromycin or metoclopramide, should be considered in patients presenting with ongoing or recurrent hematemesis in order to clear the stomach of food and blood clots, which may obscure potential bleeding sources and increase the risk of aspiration. Similarly, adequate colon cleansing using a polyethylene glycol-based solution until the colon is clear of stool and blood clots is preferred prior to colonoscopy and associated with higher cecal intubation rate, improved diagnostic yield, and lower risk of perforation.

Endoscopy

Endoscopy serves a diagnostic and therapeutic role in the management of GIB after adequate resuscitation. Urgent upper endoscopy should be performed within 12 hours of hospitalization in any patients with suspected variceal bleeding, and early upper endoscopy within 24 hours of hospitalization is recommended in patients with nonvariceal overt UGIB. Patients with ulcers and stigmata of recent bleeding may need endoscopic therapy to reduce risk of rebleeding. Examples of endoscopic hemostatic techniques include epinephrine injection, contact thermal coagulation for visible vessels, as well as through-the-scope clip and over-the-scope clip as methods to achieve physical tamponade of a bleeding site. In cases of variceal bleeding, band ligation and injection of sclerosing agents for esophageal varices and injection of cyanoacrylate and other tissue glue in gastric varices can be performed. Other techniques include argon plasma coagulation for superficial vascular lesions and hemostatic topical powders as temporizing measures. The optimal timing of colonoscopy for overt LGIB is less well defined. Urgent colonoscopy, defined variably as within 12 to 24 hours of hospitalization, may improve diagnostic yield but does not improve rebleeding risk, need for surgery, or length of stay compared to elective colonoscopy. In general, it is reasonable to prioritize patients with ongoing or recurrent overt LGIB for an inpatient colonoscopy whereas those with self-limiting bleed may be evaluated electively. Hemodynamically unstable patients with suspected LGIB should also undergo upper endoscopy to rule out a brisk UGIB. Presence of blood in terminal ileum may be indicative of a proximal or small bowel bleeding source. Video capsule endoscopy (VCE) is a valuable tool for diagnosing a small bowel bleeding source, especially when performed within 72 hours of index bleeding episode. Patients with occult GIB should undergo endoscopy and colonoscopy, followed by VCE if necessary, electively once they are medically optimized. Enteroscopy techniques such as push, balloon, or spiral enteroscopy can be used for diagnosis and treatment of small bowel pathology detected on capsule endoscopy. Computed tomography (CT) and magnetic resonance (MR) enterography techniques have largely replaced fluoroscopy and can be used to diagnose small bowel pathology when VCE is not available.

Rescue Technique

Rescue techniques are sometimes necessary, for both diagnostic and therapeutic purposes, in patients who fail endoscopic management or are unable to tolerate endoscopy. CT angiography or multidetector row CT is a reasonable first-line imaging test to facilitate localization of GIB in patients presenting with hemodynamically significant overt GIB. Angiography relies on active bleeding and may be falsely negative in cases of intermittent bleeding. Tagged red blood cell scintigraphy, although less readily available and more logistically cumbersome than CT angiography, is ideally suited for evaluation of intermittent, obscure GIB because of its higher sensitivity and the ability to perform repeated scans after initial injection of tagged cells. Super-selective angiographic embolization can be successful in achieving immediate hemostasis in many cases of GIB, including large penetrating duodenal ulcers, small bowel tumor bleed, and colonic diverticular bleed. In cases of uncontrollable variceal bleeding, balloon tamponade or esophageal stenting can be used as a bridge to more definitive treatment such as transjugular intrahepatic portosystemic shunt (TIPS) or balloon-occluded retrograde transvenous obliteration (BRTO) for esophageal and gastric varices, respectively. Hemostatic spray consists of an inorganic powder that may be used endoscopically in cases of severe ulcer or cancer-related bleeding or other nonvariceal bleeding where directed therapy may not be possible. Ultimately, surgery may be necessary in a small proportion of patients with severe or recurrent bleeding, such as bleeding associated with tumors, perforated ulcers, recurrent ulcer bleeding or severe colitis that is refractory to endoscopic or interventional radiologic therapies.

SUGGESTED READINGS

ASGE Standards of Practice Committee, et al.: The role of endoscopy in the management of suspected small-bowel bleeding, *Gastrointest Endosc* 85:22–31, 2017.

Gerson LB, Fidler JL, Cave DR, Leighton JA: ACG clinical guideline: diagnosis and management of small bowel bleeding, *Am J Gastroenterol* 110:1265–1287, 2015.

Hwang JH, Fisher DA, Ben-Menachem T, et al.: The role of endoscopy in the management of acute non-variceal upper GI bleeding, *Gastrointest Endosc* 75:1132–1138, 2012.

Kim BS, Li BT, Engel A, et al.: Diagnosis of gastrointestinal bleeding: A practical guide for clinicians, *World J Gastrointest Pathophysiol* 5:467–478, 2014.

O'Leary JG, Greenberg CS, Patton HM, Caldwell SH: AGA clinical practice update: coagulation in cirrhosis, *Gastroenterology* 157:34–43, 2019.

Stanley AJ, Laine L: Management of acute upper gastrointestinal bleeding, *BMJ* 364:l536, 2019.

Strate LL, Gralnek IM: ACG clinical guideline: management of patients with acute lower gastrointestinal bleeding, *Am J Gastroenterol* 111:459–474, 2016.

Villanueva C, Colomo A, Bosch A, et al.: Transfusion strategies for acute upper gastrointestinal bleeding, *N Engl J Med* 368:11–21, 2013.

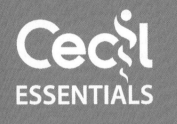

33

Common Clinical Manifestations of Gastrointestinal Disease: Malabsorption

Brisas M. Flores, Sharmeel K. Wasan

DEFINITION AND EPIDEMIOLOGY

The main purpose of the gastrointestinal (GI) tract is to digest and absorb major nutrients (fats, carbohydrates, and proteins), essential micronutrients (vitamins and trace minerals), water, and electrolytes. Impaired absorption of these nutrients is defined as malabsorption. Under normal conditions, the digestion and absorption of nutrients requires both mechanical and enzymatic breakdown of food. Mechanical processes include chewing, gastric churning, and the to-and-fro mixing in the small intestine. Enzymatic hydrolysis is initiated by intraluminal processes requiring salivary, gastric, pancreatic, and biliary secretions and is completed at the intestinal brush border. The final products of digestion are then absorbed through the intestinal epithelial cells and transported into the portal circulation. The coordinated regulation of gastric emptying, normal intestinal progression, and the presence of adequate intestinal surface area are all important factors. The human gut microbiome, which comprises the communities of microorganisms that inhabit the GI tract, has been recognized to play an important role in nutrient utilization as well. From birth, interactions between the microbiota and the intestinal mucosa contribute to maturation of the host immune system. Disruptions to the homeostasis between the microbiota and the host immune system can lead to increased inflammation and decreased absorption.

Most dietary components can be absorbed anywhere along the length of the small intestine, but there are important exceptions in which absorption is limited to specific areas (e.g., vitamin B_{12} and cholesterol are absorbed only in the terminal ileum). Diseases associated with diffuse mucosal involvement, such as celiac disease, can lead to impaired absorption of many nutrients, whereas diseases affecting only the terminal ileum can lead to decreased vitamin B_{12} absorption. Bile acids are necessary for fat absorption; they undergo an enterohepatic circulation with release into bile and reabsorption from the terminal small intestine. Diseases interfering with this mechanism deplete the bile acid pool and can lead to fat malabsorption. Water and electrolytes are absorbed primarily by the colon. In addition, there is caloric salvage of much of the carbohydrate from indigestible fiber through bacterial enzymatic activity in the colon. The following sections discuss normal assimilation of the major nutrients and the approach to evaluation of patients with suspected malabsorption.

DIGESTION AND ABSORPTION OF FAT

Dietary fat is composed predominantly of triglycerides ($\approx$95%) with long-chain fatty acids (16- and 18-carbon molecules). In animal fat, the constituent fatty acids are mostly saturated (e.g., palmitic acid, stearic acid), whereas those of vegetable origin are rich in unsaturated fatty acids (i.e., having one or more double bonds in the carbon chain, such as oleic and linoleic acids). Fats are insoluble in water (hydrophobic),

and digestion begins with a process of emulsification, wherein larger fat droplets are dispersed in the aqueous medium of the lumen. In the proximal small intestine, bile salts from liver and pancreatic enzymes are released into the intestinal lumen; there, they mix with and bind to the surface of these globules, where colipase activity results in the release of fatty acids and a monoglyceride. These are taken up as mixed micelles with bile salts, and these hydrophobic particles cross the unstirred water layer that overlies the epithelial brush border.

Within the cell, fatty acids are resynthesized into triglycerides, and, together with cholesterol and phospholipids, they are packaged into chylomicrons and very-low-density lipoproteins to be exported via lymphatic channels. Bile salts remain in the intestinal lumen, are recycled into new micelles, and are finally reabsorbed in the terminal ileum with 95% efficiency. Most dietary lipids are absorbed in the jejunum, together with the fat-soluble vitamins A, D, E, and K. It is recommended that dietary fat account for no more than 35% of calories because higher levels are associated with increased risk of cardiac disease, obesity, and some cancers. The recommended intake is 20% to 35% of daily dietary intake.

DIGESTION AND ABSORPTION OF CARBOHYDRATES

Most dietary carbohydrates consist of starch (a glucose polymer) and the disaccharides sucrose and lactose, but only monosaccharides are absorbed. Salivary and pancreatic amylases release oligosaccharides from starch. The final hydrolysis to glucose monomers occurs at the brush border and includes disaccharide hydrolysis by sucrase and lactase. Glucose and galactose are actively transported in conjunction with sodium, whereas fructose absorption occurs by facilitated diffusion. About one half of dietary energy is derived from carbohydrate, with a nutritional goal of 45% to 65% and an increased component of insoluble fiber (i.e., that which is indigestible by mammalian enzymes but variably broken down by colonic bacteria).

DIGESTION AND ABSORPTION OF PROTEINS

Dietary proteins are the major source for amino acids and the only source for the essential amino acids. Digestion starts in the stomach with pepsins secreted by the gastric mucosa, but most of the hydrolysis is accomplished by pancreatic enzymes in the proximal small bowel. The pancreas secretes the proteases trypsin, elastase, chymotrypsin, and carboxypeptidase as inactive proenzymes. Enterokinase (more properly, enteropeptidase) is secreted by the intestinal brush border; it splits trypsinogen to its active form, trypsin, which in turn converts the other proenzymes to their active forms. The products of luminal brush border peptidase digestion consist of amino acids and oligopeptides, which are transported across the epithelial cell. The transfer of most amino acids is sodium dependent and takes place in the proximal small bowel. Dietary requirements for amino acid nitrogen are met with about 10% to 35% of calories from protein.

MECHANISMS OF MALABSORPTION

The term *maldigestion* refers to defective hydrolysis of nutrients, whereas *malabsorption* refers to impaired mucosal absorption. In clinical practice, however, *malabsorption* refers to all aspects of impaired nutrient assimilation. Malabsorption can involve multiple nutrients, or it can be more selective. Therefore, the clinical manifestations of malabsorption are highly variable. The complete process of absorption consists of a *luminal phase*, in which various nutrients are hydrolyzed and solubilized; a *mucosal phase*, in which further processing takes place at the brush border of the epithelial cell with subsequent transfer into the cell; and a *transport phase*, in which nutrients are moved from the epithelium to the portal venous or lymphatic circulation. Impairment in any of these phases can result in malabsorption (Table 33.1).

Luminal Phase

Digestion is accomplished for the most part by pancreatic enzymes, particularly lipase, colipase, and trypsin; the gastric digestive enzymes do not play a major role. As a consequence, chronic pancreatitis can result in malabsorption, particularly for fat and protein. Deficiency in bile salts also contributes to fat malabsorption and may result from cholestatic liver disorders (impaired secretion of bile), bacterial overgrowth (resulting in luminal bile salt deconjugation), or ileal disease or resection with loss of effective enterohepatic circulation of the bile acids. The major part of the luminal phase of digestion occurs in the duodenum and the proximal jejunum.

Mucosal Phase

Mucosal disease is a more common cause of malabsorption. It can result from diffuse small intestinal diseases such as celiac disease or Crohn's disease, or from a decrease in surface area (e.g., after surgical resection for small bowel infarction). The net effect is a smaller effective mucosal surface and a relative loss of mucosal absorption. Selective defects in an otherwise normal intestine may result in specific entities such as lactase deficiency or abetalipoproteinemia.

Transport Phase

After absorption, nutrients leave the cells through venous or lymphatic channels. Consequently, malabsorption may be associated with mesenteric venous obstruction, lymphangiectasia, or lymphatic obstruction due to malignancy or infiltrative processes such as Whipple disease.

The absorptive process can be impaired at many stages. For example, patients with subtotal gastrectomy or bariatric surgery often experience malabsorption. There are resultant defects at all phases: impaired gastric churning, premature emptying, and impaired mixing (in the jejunum) of food with bile and pancreatic enzymes. The impaired mixing is a consequence of anatomic changes (gastrojejunostomy bypassing the duodenum) and reduced production of pancreatic enzymes (because cholecystokinin and secretin release is blunted when gastric contents bypass the duodenum). Moreover, stasis may lead to bacterial overgrowth in the afferent loop with changes in the bile acids needed for fat absorption. Another example of manifold mechanisms is diabetes mellitus, which may lead to delayed gastric emptying, abnormal intestinal motility, bacterial overgrowth, and pancreatic exocrine insufficiency.

CLINICAL PRESENTATION

The clinical manifestations of malabsorption are usually nonspecific, particularly in the early stages. A change in bowel movements, usually with diarrhea, and weight loss despite adequate food intake may occur in more severe cases. Usually, however, patients have relatively mild symptoms such as bloating and flatulence. Clinical manifestations related to a specific micronutrient deficiency can occur. For example, iron deficiency anemia may be the only manifestation of celiac disease

TABLE 33.1 Pathophysiologic Mechanisms in Malabsorption		
Luminal Phase	**Mucosal Phase**	**Transport Phase**
Reduced nutrient availability	Extensive mucosal loss (resection or infarction)	Vascular conditions (vasculitis; atheroma)
Cofactor deficiency (pernicious anemia; gastric surgery)	Diffuse mucosal disease (celiac disease)	Lymphatic conditions (lymphangiectasia; irradiation; nodal tumor, cavitation, or infiltrations)
Nutrient consumption (bacterial overgrowth)	Crohn's disease; irradiation; infection; infiltrations; drugs: alcohol, colchicine, neomycin, iron salts	
Impaired fat solubilization	Brush border hydrolase deficiency (lactase deficiency)	
Reduced bile salt synthesis (hepatocellular disease)	Transport defects (Hartnup cystinuria; vitamin B_{12} and folate uptake)	
Impaired bile salt secretion (chronic cholestasis)	Epithelial processing (abetalipoproteinemia)	
Bile salt inactivation (bacterial overgrowth)		
Impaired cholecystokinin release (mucosal disease)		
Increased bile salt losses (terminal ileal disease or resection)		
Defective nutrient hydrolysis		
Lipase inactivation (Zollinger-Ellison syndrome)		
Enzyme deficiency (pancreatic insufficiency or cancer)		
Improper mixing or rapid transit (resection; bypass; hyperthyroidism)		

Modified from Riley SA, Marsh MN: Maldigestion and malabsorption. In Feldman M, Scharschmidt BF, Sleisenger MH, editors: Sleisenger and Fordtran's Gastrointestinal and Liver Disease: Pathophysiology/Diagnosis/Management, ed 6, Philadelphia, 1998, WB Saunders, pp 1501-1522.

in some patients. Muscle wasting and edema result from protein malabsorption. Nutritional anemia, caused by deficiencies of iron, folate, and vitamin B_{12}, contributes to fatigue. Bleeding tendency (e.g., ecchymosis) may be attributed to prolonged prothrombin time resulting from vitamin K deficiency related to fat malabsorption. Bulky, oily stools are the hallmark of steatorrhea resulting from fat malabsorption, whereas bloating (abdominal distention) and soft diarrheal movements occur as a result of carbohydrate malabsorption. Signs associated with malabsorption are presented in Table 33.2.

DIAGNOSIS

Malabsorption can be caused by a large number of disorders, some of the more common of which are listed in Table 33.2. The cause of malabsorption can often be determined by a very detailed patient history. However, because the clinical symptoms are varied, more specific

assays of albumin, cobalamin, iron, cholesterol, calcium, folic acid, and prothrombin time are useful to support the diagnosis of malabsorption. These tests are helpful in assessing the severity of malabsorption, but they are not specific for the differential diagnosis. Many tests are available in the work-up of malabsorption; those that have been most useful clinically are discussed in the following sections (Fig. 33.1).

Fecal Fat Analysis

If fat malabsorption is suspected, the simplest qualitative method for detecting fat in stool is microscopic examination with Sudan staining of a drop of stool. Sensitivity varies anywhere from 80% to 99%, but the test is quick and easy. The result correlates well with the quantitative measurement of fecal fat when moderate to severe steatorrhea is present. To quantify fat, stool is collected for three consecutive days while the patient is on a diet containing 60 g to 100 g of fat per day, and the specimen is analyzed for fat content. If the fecal fat amount is

TABLE 33.2   Signs Associated With Malabsorption Syndromes

Signs	Associated Syndromes
Gastrointestinal	
Mass	Crohn's disease, lymphoma, tuberculosis, glands
Distention	Intestinal obstruction, gas, ascites, pseudocyst (pancreatic), motility disorder
Steatorrheic stool	Mucosal disease, bacterial overgrowth, pancreatic insufficiency, infective or inflammatory, drug induced
Extraintestinal	
Skin	
Nonspecific	Pigmentation, thinning, inelasticity, reduced subcutaneous fat
Specific	Blisters (dermatitis herpetiformis), erythema nodosum (Crohn's disease), petechiae (vitamin K deficiency), edema (hypoproteinemia)
Hair	
Alopecia	Gluten sensitivity
Loss or thinning	Generalized inanition, hypothyroidism, gluten sensitivity
Eyes	
Conjunctivitis, episcleritis	Crohn's disease, Behçet's syndrome
Paleness	Severe anemia
Mouth	
Aphthous ulcers	Crohn's disease, gluten sensitivity, Behçet's syndrome
Glossitis	Deficiencies of vitamin B_{12}, iron, folate, niacin
Angular cheilosis	Deficiencies of vitamin B_{12}, iron, folate, B complex
Dental hypoplasia (pitting, dystrophy)	Gluten sensitivity
Hands	
Raynaud's phenomenon	Scleroderma
Finger clubbing	Crohn's disease, lymphoma
Koilonychia	Iron deficiency
Leukonychia	Inanition
Musculoskeletal	
Monoarthropathy and polyarthropathy	Crohn's disease, gluten sensitivity, Whipple disease, Behçet's syndrome
Back pain (osteomalacia, osteoporosis, sacroiliitis)	Crohn's disease, malnutrition, gluten sensitivity
Muscle weakness (low potassium, magnesium, vitamin D; generalized inanition)	Diffuse mucosal disease, bacterial overgrowth, lymphoma
Nervous System	
Peripheral neuropathy (weakness, paresthesias, numbness)	Vitamin B_{12} deficiency
Cerebral (seizures, dementia, intracerebral calcification, meningitis, pseudotumor, cranial nerve palsies)	Whipple disease, gluten sensitivity, diffuse lymphoma

From Riley SA, Marsh MN: Maldigestion and malabsorption. In Feldman M, Scharschmidt BF, Sleisenger MH, editors: Sleisenger and Fordtran's Gastrointestinal and Liver Disease: Pathophysiology/Diagnosis/Management, ed 6, Philadelphia, 1998, WB Saunders, pp 1501-1522.

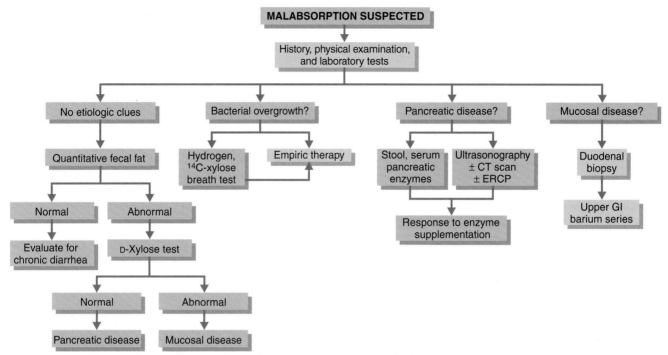

Fig. 33.1 Approach to the patient with suspected malabsorption. *CT,* Computed tomography; *ERCP,* endoscopic retrograde cholangiopancreatography; *GI,* gastrointestinal. (Modified from Riley SA, Marsh MN: Maldigestion and malabsorption. In Feldman M, Scharschmidt BF, Sleisenger MH, editors: Sleisenger and Fordtran's Gastrointestinal and Liver Disease: Pathophysiology/Diagnosis/Management, ed 6, Philadelphia, 1998, WB Saunders, pp 1501-1522.)

greater than 7 g per day, it is suggestive of fat malabsorption. Patients with steatorrhea (excess fat in the stool) often have results with greater than 20 g per day. Values ranging from 7 to 14 g per day are suggestive of fat malabsorption, but values should be interpreted judiciously as diarrheal illnesses can also produce these results. This test is cumbersome and nonspecific, but it offers an accurate quantification of fecal fat excretion provided fat consumption is appropriate. Near-infrared reflectance spectroscopy may produce similar results, but this is not often utilized in the United States.

Tests of Pancreatic Exocrine Function

Aspiration of duodenal contents for evaluation of bicarbonate and enzyme output after stimulation of the pancreas may be the best index of pancreatic exocrine function. However, the test is invasive, time-consuming, and performed only in a few specialized centers. The measurement of pancreatic enzymes (i.e., fecal elastase 1) in the stool is simple and provides helpful laboratory evidence for the diagnosis of moderate to severe pancreatic insufficiency. Pancreatic calcifications seen on abdominal films or computed tomography (CT) scans indicate the presence of chronic pancreatitis. Magnetic resonance cholangiopancreatography (MRCP) and endoscopic retrograde cholangiopancreatography (ERCP) can help outline abnormal duct anatomy and may supplement CT scanning for diagnostic purposes to evaluate the sequelae of chronic pancreatitis. However, normal findings on pancreatography do not exclude the presence of pancreatic exocrine insufficiency.

Small Intestinal Biopsy

Whereas the gross appearance of the mucosa during upper GI endoscopy can provide some clues regarding the presence of a disease causing malabsorption, biopsy of the small intestinal mucosa is a key diagnostic test for diseases that affect the cellular phase of absorption.

In some diseases, the histologic features are diagnostic; in others, the findings may be highly suggestive (Table 33.3). Several tissue samples should be taken from the duodenal bulb and from the distal duodenum to enhance the diagnostic accuracy.

Imaging Studies

In patients with malabsorption, barium studies of the small bowel are usually nonspecific. Occasionally, however, distinct anatomic changes are seen, such as in jejunal diverticulosis, lymphoma, Crohn's disease, strictures, or enteric fistulas. Also, there may be a distinctive barium pattern of thin-walled, dilated loops suggestive of celiac disease. CT and magnetic resonance enterography provide a more detailed imaging of the small intestine and are more sensitive in identifying abnormalities such as active bowel inflammation, mesenteric stranding and edema, strictures, fibrofatty proliferation of the mesentery, and fistula formation.

Wireless capsule endoscopy is a noninvasive method that permits direct visualization of the small bowel mucosa and can provide a more detailed evaluation of small bowel disease compared with radiographic studies. However, capsule endoscopy should be avoided in patients in whom a stricture is suspected because of the risk of retention. The detection of mucosal lesions by the capsule endoscopy can often be followed by deep enteroscopy (double-balloon endoscopy, single-balloon endoscopy, or spiral enteroscopy), allowing for tissue biopsy, tattoo placement before surgery, balloon dilatation, and foreign body retrieval.

Schilling Test

Vitamin B_{12} is an essential micronutrient, and its absorption requires several steps. First, the ingested vitamin binds to salivary R-factor protein. In the stomach, gastric parietal cells secrete intrinsic factor, which mixes with the ingested meal. In the duodenum, pancreatic trypsin

TABLE 33.3 Utility of Small Bowel Biopsy Specimens in Malabsorption

Findings Often Diagnostic

Whipple disease
Amyloidosis
Eosinophilic enteritis
Lymphangiectasia
Primary intestinal lymphoma
Giardiasis
Abetalipoproteinemia
Agammaglobulinemia
Mastocytosis

Findings Abnormal But Not Diagnostic

Celiac disease
Systemic sclerosis
Radiation enteritis
Bacterial overgrowth syndrome
Tropical sprue
Crohn's disease

Data from Trier JS: Diagnostic value of peroral biopsy of the proximal small intestine. N Engl J Med 285:1470, 1971.

hydrolyzes the R-protein, freeing the vitamin to bind with intrinsic factor. The vitamin B_{12}–intrinsic factor complex is then absorbed by specific receptors that are found only on enterocytes in the distal ileum. Malabsorption of vitamin B_{12} can occur because of lack of intrinsic factor (e.g., pernicious anemia, gastric resection), pancreatic insufficiency, bacterial overgrowth, or ileal resection or mucosal disease (e.g., Crohn's disease).

The Schilling test quantifies vitamin B_{12} absorption using radiolabeled vitamin B_{12} as a marker. The test may be expanded to several stages to amplify its diagnostic spectrum. In stage 1, after the injection of 1000 µg of unlabeled vitamin B_{12} to saturate hepatic storage, the patient ingests 0.5 µg of radiolabeled vitamin. Urine is then collected for the measurement of radioactivity; reduced radioactivity suggests B_{12} malabsorption. The test is repeated (stage 2) with the addition of oral intrinsic factor to the ingested vitamin B_{12}. If urinary excretion of the radiolabel is corrected, pernicious anemia is diagnosed. If malabsorption is still present, the patient is given a short course of oral antibiotics (stage 3), and the test is repeated; correction of radiolabeled B_{12} excretion establishes bacterial overgrowth. If the test result remains abnormal, oral pancreatic enzymes are given (stage 4) and the test is repeated; correction of the abnormality at this stage implies pancreatic deficiency. Finally, if all these interventions fail, ileal disease or absence of transcobalamin protein is determined by other diagnostic tests, including assessment for intrinsic factor antibodies or *Helicobacter pylori* infection. This long outline serves merely as an example of an algorithm of clinical analysis; the usual routine in clinical settings is to administer parenteral vitamin B_{12} while the etiology is delineated by other modalities.

D-Xylose Test

The D-xylose test serves as an indicator of mucosal absorption in the proximal small bowel and is used to determine whether defects in the epithelium of the intestine are responsible for malabsorption. D-Xylose is a 5-carbon monosaccharide that is transported across the intestinal mucosa largely by passive diffusion. In this test, the subject ingests 25 g of D-xylose, and urine is collected for the next 5 hours. Healthy subjects excrete more than 4.5 g of D-xylose in 5 hours (or ≥20% of

the ingested load). Excretion of a lower amount of D-xylose suggests abnormal absorption. However, an abnormally low (false-positive) result may occur in the presence of impaired renal excretory function, gastroparesis, massive peripheral edema, ascites, aspirin, neomycin, indomethacin, and glipizide. Abnormal results can also be seen in the presence of bacterial overgrowth as a result of bacterial degradation of D-xylose in the lumen, but this "pseudomalabsorption" may be corrected after treatment with antibiotics serving as a therapeutic trial.

Breath Tests

Breath tests rely on bacterial degradation of luminal compounds, which releases metabolic byproduct gases (e.g., hydrogen, methane, carbon dioxide) that can be measured in the exhaled breath. In the case of disaccharidase deficiency, a specific disaccharide (e.g., lactose) that is orally ingested but not properly absorbed in the small intestine is delivered to the colon, where bacterial fermentation liberates metabolites; hydrogen gas is the marker assayed in the breath. In the presence of bacterial overgrowth of the small intestine, orally ingested glucose ferments in the proximal small bowel (instead of being absorbed), resulting in increased hydrogen in the breath; here, the timing of exhaled hydrogen aids in the diagnosis. The measurement of radioactive carbon dioxide in the breath after ingestion of a nutrient labeled with carbon 14 (^{14}C) has been used to estimate the malabsorption of fat or bile acids and for measurement of bacterial overgrowth (^{14}C-xylose).

Summary

The overlap of symptoms and the large number of diagnostic tests available for evaluation of malabsorption necessitate the use of a systematic approach and a rational algorithm (see Fig. 33.1). The most accurate test for fat malabsorption remains the 72-hour fecal fat analysis; however, the test is difficult to carry out in clinical practice. Surrogate screening for steatorrhea is done with the qualitative stool fat examination (Sudan stain) and measurement of serum carotene. If the stool fat content is normal, the patient may still have selective impairment of absorption of a specific carbohydrate. This latter condition should be suspected if the primary symptoms are cramps, flatulence, and diarrhea. The most common example of carbohydrate malabsorption is lactose intolerance; specific tests include the oral lactose tolerance test, but measurement of breath hydrogen is more sensitive and more specific.

More generally, an *osmotic gap in fecal water* suggests a dietary (rather than a secretory) cause of the diarrhea related to luminal short-chain fatty acids or carbohydrates. The osmotic gap is calculated by the following formula:

$$\text{Osmotic gap} = \text{Plasma osmolality} - [2 \times (\text{fecal } [Na^+] + \text{fecal } [K^+])]$$

The osmotic gap is not calculated by directly measuring stool osmolality, because it increases with time in the specimen container. In addition, luminal osmolality is equal to serum osmolality because the colon cannot establish a gradient against the serum concentration of solutes.

When fat malabsorption is demonstrated (>7 g/24 hours, or increased qualitative stool fat and decreased serum carotene), a D-xylose absorption-excretion test should be performed next. A normal D-xylose test result makes diffuse mucosal disease unlikely and suggests maldigestion, principally pancreatic enzyme or bile salt deficiency. Clues to chronic pancreatitis include a history of alcohol abuse or previous episodes of pancreatitis. Unusual causes of pancreatic malabsorption, such as cystic fibrosis, microlithiasis, or drug toxicity, require specific testing and a detailed history. Serum enzyme tests and abdominal imaging (plain films or, with much greater sensitivity, abdominal CT scans) can be obtained next to identify pancreatic disease. If the urinary D-xylose excretion is abnormal, the breath hydrogen test may be used to diagnose bacterial overgrowth using glucose for the carbohydrate load. If no bacterial overgrowth is present, a mucosal biopsy should be performed (see Table 33.3). Imaging studies of the small bowel may be helpful on occasion.

If the cause of malabsorption remains unclear, other considerations should include parasitic infection, such as *Giardia lamblia*, or ascariasis involvement of the pancreatic duct (more common in undeveloped countries). These diagnoses require a careful stool examination for ova and parasites or fecal antigen studies.

TREATMENT

The specific treatment of malabsorption depends on identification of the underlying condition. Occasionally, therapeutic trials for treatable conditions should be instituted, such as a gluten-free diet for celiac disease, pancreatic enzyme replacement for pancreatic exocrine malfunction, metronidazole for *G. lamblia* infection, or broad-spectrum antibiotics for suspected bacterial overgrowth. Parenteral nutrition may have a role in maintaining adequate nutritional status. Treatment modalities are discussed in later chapters focusing on specific diseases. Two disorders, celiac disease and bacterial overgrowth, are discussed here as illustrative of the pathophysiology.

Celiac Disease

Celiac disease (also called celiac sprue, nontropical sprue, or gluten-sensitive enteropathy) is characterized by intestinal mucosal injury resulting from gluten-related immunologic damage in persons genetically predisposed to this condition. The prevalence is estimated at about 1% in Western countries and has notably been rising across the world over the past 20 years. There is about an 80% concordance rate in monozygotic twins and less than 20% concordance rate in dizygotic twins. The prevalence of the disease among relatives of patients with celiac disease is approximately 10%. There is a strong association of celiac disease with human leukocyte antigen (HLA) class II molecules, particularly HLA-DQ2 and HLA-DQ8. However, in Western countries about 40% of the population possess either HLA-DQ2 or DQ8, notably different than the estimated celiac disease prevalence of 1%.

The disease is induced by exposure to storage proteins found in grain plants such as wheat (which contains gliadin), barley, and rye and their products. Oats are implicated, not because of gliadin, but because of contamination with wheat during packaging and transportation. The exposure initiates a cellular immune response that results in mucosal damage, particularly in the proximal intestine. Results of investigations suggest that an enzyme, tissue transglutaminase, may be the autoantigen of celiac disease.

Clinical Presentation

Celiac disease can manifest with the classic constellation of symptoms and signs of a malabsorption syndrome. Not uncommonly, however, the manifestation is atypical, with nonspecific GI symptoms such as bloating, chronic diarrhea (with or without steatorrhea), flatulence, lactose intolerance, or deficiencies of a single micronutrient (e.g., iron deficiency anemia). Extraintestinal complaints such as depression, weakness, fatigue, arthralgias, osteoporosis, or osteomalacia may predominate. A number of diseases, including dermatitis herpetiformis, type 1 diabetes mellitus, autoimmune thyroid disease, and selective

immunoglobulin A (IgA) deficiency, are found in significant association with celiac disease.

Diagnosis

Celiac disease is a leading consideration in every patient with the malabsorption syndrome. It should be included as well in the differential of atypical manifestations, such as iron deficiency anemia, metabolic bone disease, neuropsychiatric symptoms, and intestinal lymphoma. Fiberoptic or capsule endoscopy may show the typical features of broad and flattened villi; with the former instrument, tissue can be sampled for histologic analysis. Intestinal biopsy is the most valuable test in establishing the diagnosis. The spectrum of pathologic changes ranges from normal villous architecture with an increase in mucosal lymphocytes and plasma cells (the infiltrative lesion) to partial blunting or total villous flattening. Although abnormal biopsy findings are not specific, they are highly suggestive, particularly because most other conditions that can mimic celiac disease (e.g., Crohn's disease, gastrinoma, lymphoma, tropical sprue, graft-versus-host disease, immune deficiency) may be distinguished clinically. A clinical response to a gluten-free diet establishes the diagnosis and precludes the need, in adults, to document healing by repeated biopsies. Serologic blood tests (antigliadin, antiendomysial, antireticulin, and tissue transglutaminase IgA antibodies) are helpful in screening of patients with atypical symptoms and asymptomatic relatives of patients with celiac disease. HLA genotyping has a high negative predictive value but low positive predictive value and is not routinely ordered.

Treatment

Strict, lifelong adherence to a gluten-free diet is the only treatment for celiac disease. Specific nutritional supplementation should be provided to correct deficiencies, particularly those of iron, vitamins, and calcium. A clinical response may be seen within a few weeks. Follow-up monitoring with serologic testing should be done after 3 to 6 months in the first year and then yearly thereafter in stable patients clinically responding to a gluten-free diet. Repeat biopsies should be considered for those who are seronegative or have persistent symptoms despite a gluten-free diet. The long-term prognosis is excellent for patients who adhere to the diet, although there may be a slight increase in the incidence of malignancies, particularly lymphoma.

Nonresponsive and Refractory Celiac Disease

Patients with ongoing symptoms more often than not are not truly adhering to a gluten-free diet. There may also be presence of an additional disease process, such as inflammatory bowel disease, microscopic colitis, lactose intolerance, pancreatic insufficiency, and ulcerative jejunitis.

Patients with persistent celiac disease activity despite adherence to a strict gluten-free diet for 12 months are deemed to have refractory celiac disease (RCD). Type 1 RCD is characterized by normal intraepithelial lymphocytes and a polyclonal T-cell receptor population. Type 2 RCD is described as having aberrant intraepithelial lymphocytes with monoclonal T-cell receptors. The overall prognosis for type 1 RCD is good, with a 5-year survival rate of 80%. Type 2 RCD, on the other hand, has a 5-year mortality rate of 50%. Type 2 RCD is strongly associated with ulcerative jejunitis and enteropathy-associated T-cell lymphoma (EATL). MR enterography, CT enterography, capsule endoscopy, and device-assisted enteroscopy may all be helpful in the diagnosis. PET CT is useful in diagnosing associated malignancy. Treatment options for type 2 RCD include azathioprine, steroids, methotrexate, cyclosporine, alemtuzumab, cladribine or fludarabine with or without autologous stem cell transplant.

Bacterial Overgrowth Syndrome

The proximal small bowel normally contains fewer than 10^4 bacteria per milliliter of fluid, with no anaerobic *Bacteroides* organisms and few coliforms. Overgrowth of luminal bacteria can result in diarrhea and malabsorption by a number of mechanisms, including (1) deconjugation of bile salts, which leads to impaired micelle formation and impaired uptake of fat; (2) patchy injury to the enterocytes (small intestinal epithelial cells); (3) direct competition for the use of nutrients (e.g., uptake of vitamin B_{12} by gram-negative bacteria or the fish tapeworm *Diphyllobothrium latum*); and (4) stimulated secretion of water and electrolytes by products of bacterial metabolism, such as hydroxylated bile acids and short-chain (volatile) organic acids.

Conditions Associated With Bacterial Overgrowth

The most important factors maintaining the relative sterility of the upper gut are gastric acidity, peristalsis, and intestinal immunoglobulins (IgA). Conditions that impair these functions can result in bacterial overgrowth. Impaired peristalsis may be caused by motility disorders (e.g., scleroderma, amyloidosis, diabetes mellitus) or by anatomic changes (e.g., surgically created blind loops, obstruction, jejunal diverticulosis). Achlorhydria, pancreatic insufficiency, and hypogammaglobulinemia are also associated with bacterial overgrowth but uncommonly result in clinical steatorrhea. One should have particular suspicion for bacterial overgrowth in patients with chronic pancreatitis and associated diabetes mellitus, low zinc levels, and opiate use with ongoing weight loss or steatorrhea despite enzyme replacement therapy.

Diagnosis

Direct culture of jejunal aspirate is the most definitive diagnostic test, but it is invasive, uncomfortable, and costly. The ^{14}C-xylose breath test is an accurate and sensitive laboratory test; measurement of breath hydrogen after an oral challenge with glucose is simpler but not as sensitive or as specific. Adding methane to the hydrogen breath test may capture up to 20% to 30% of the population who produce methane as the byproduct of carbohydrate fermentation. An empirical therapeutic trial with antibiotics is an acceptable alternative to diagnostic testing.

Treatment

When appropriate, specific therapy, such as surgery for intestinal obstruction, should be provided. More commonly, patients are treated with antibiotics, most appropriately those that are effective against aerobic and anaerobic enteric organisms. Rifaximin, amoxicillin-clavulanate, quinolone, metronidazole with a cephalosporin or trimethroprim-sulfamethoxazole are suitable agents. A single course of therapy for 7 to 10 days may be therapeutic for months. In other patients, intermittent therapy (1 week of every 4) or even an extended period of continuous therapy may be effective, although data are limited.

MALABSORPTIVE THERAPY

Cardiovascular disease and other consequences of obesity have reached epidemic proportions in the United States, and one approach to this problem has been the deliberate induction of malabsorption (primarily of fats) to reduce a patient's lipid levels and body mass index. Medications used for this purpose include bile acid–binding resins, such as cholestyramine and colestipol, and the lipase inhibitors orlistat (Xenical) and ezetimibe (Zetia). Surgical treatment (bariatric operations) usually consists of gastric partition combined with some degree of small intestinal bypass, which induces significant weight loss by several proposed mechanisms, including malabsorption, improved nutrient deposition, and enhanced satiety. Recent data suggest that the malabsorption itself contributes less to overall weight loss from bariatric surgery than the latter two mechanisms and that it is fat malabsorption, rather than carbohydrate or protein malabsorption, that predominates. Please refer to Chapter 69 to review obesity in more detail.

SUGGESTED READINGS

Bai JC, Ciacci C; World Gastroenterology Organisation Global Guidelines: Celiac Disease February 2017. J Clin Gastroenterol. 2017 Oct;51(9):755-768. Erratum in: J Clin Gastroenterol. 2019 Apr;53(4):313.

Dye CK, Gaffney RR, Dykes TM, et al: Endoscopic and radiographic evaluation of the small bowel in 2012, *Am J Med* 125:1228.e1–1228.e12, 2012.

Forsmark CE: Management of chronic pancreatitis, *Gastroenterology* 144:1282–1291, 2013.

Goulet O, Ruemmele F: Causes and management of intestinal failure in children, *Gastroenterology* 2(Suppl 1):S16–S28, 2006.

Lee AA, Baker JR, Wamsteker EJ, Saad R, DiMagno MJ: Small intestinal bacterial overgrowth is common in chronic pancreatitis and associated with diabetes, chronic pancreatitis severity, low zinc Levels, and opiate use, *Am J Gastroenterol* 114(7):1163–1171, 2019.

Mueller K, Ash C, Pennisi E, et al: The gut microbiota: introduction, *Science* 336:1245, 2012.

Nasr I, Nasr I, Campling H, Ciclitira PJ. Approach to patients with refractory coeliac disease. F1000Res. 2016 Oct 20;5. pii: F1000 Faculty Rev-2544. eCollection 2016. Review.

Shannahan S, Leffler DA: Diagnosis and updates in Celiac disease, *Gastrointest Endosc Clin N Am* 27(1):79–92, 2017.

Siddiqui I, Ahmed S, Abid S: Update on diagnostic value of breath test in gastrointestinal and liver diseases, *World J Gastrointest Pathophysiol* 7(3):256–265, 2016.

34

Common Clinical Manifestations of Gastrointestinal Disease: Diarrhea

Ronan Farrell, Sean Fine

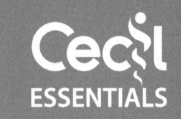

DEFINITION

Diarrhea can range from a mild self-limiting illness to a chronic debilitating disease. Although many definitions of diarrhea exist, the most clinically relevant definition is the passage of a greater number of stools of decreased form from a patient's baseline. The average number of bowel movements for a normal adult can range from three per day to three per week. Therefore, it remains crucial to establish through history a normal, baseline bowel habit prior to making the diagnosis. Once a diagnosis is made, diarrhea is initially classified into acute or chronic. Acute diarrhea has a duration of less than 4 weeks and is commonly infectious, whereas chronic diarrhea is diagnosed when symptoms have been ongoing for more than 4 weeks.

PATHOPHYSIOLOGY

Each day, as we consume water and food, the fluid ingested is added to the many secretions produced in our body, including salivary, pancreatic, and biliary secretions. Approximately 9 L of fluid eventually enters the small bowel, of which 90% is absorbed, leaving 1 L of fluid to pass into the colon. Ninety percent of this fluid is absorbed in the colon, leaving 100 mL to be excreted each day in feces. Any disease process in the gut that interferes with the absorption of water or the excretion of electrolytes can result in excess water in the gut lumen and diarrhea. The colon can overcome excess water excreted into its lumen by absorbing up to 4000 mL/24 hr, although 100 mL of excess water beyond this compensation is enough to cause diarrhea.

EVALUATION OF ACUTE DIARRHEA

The majority of acute diarrheal illnesses are infectious in nature. Acute infectious diarrhea can have an abrupt onset with clinical features including cramps, fevers, vomiting, bloody stools, and urgency. Outbreaks can be found in groups of people who travel or work closely together (daycare centers, nursing facilities, college dorms, hospital wards). For these reasons, it is important to take a detailed travel and exposure history from all patients who present with acute diarrhea. Most cases of infectious diarrhea are self-limiting, requiring only supportive treatment, and do not require further investigation. However, infants, elderly, immunosuppressed, and pregnant patients are at a greater risk for potential complications and may need closer attention to hydration status and electrolyte disturbances in a hospital setting. Other indicators of severe disease that may warrant a more robust clinical evaluation (Table 34.1) and treatment include diarrhea lasting longer than 72 hr, fever, bloody or mucoid stools, severe abdominal pain or signs of sepsis.

Acute Infectious Diarrhea

Clinically, acute infectious diarrhea can be classified into milder noninflammatory diarrhea and the more severe inflammatory diarrhea (Table 34.2). Noninflammatory diarrhea is usually a mild illness but can still result in severe electrolyte disturbances. These microorganisms act by disrupting the absorptive or secretory mechanisms of the small bowel and do not typically invade the mucosa, thus fecal leukocytes are usually absent. Noninflammatory acute diarrhea is mostly caused by viral illness such as rotavirus and norovirus. These viral illnesses are passed easily from person to person and can occur in large outbreaks. Symptoms can last 2 to 3 days before fully resolving. Bacteria that act in a similar way include Enterotoxigenic *Escherichia coli* and *Vibrio cholera*. Enterotoxigenic *Escherichia coli* is a common cause of travelers' diarrhea than can last up to 7 days. *Vibrio cholera* is less common in industrialized nations and can present with extreme diarrhea and can cause large epidemics in countries with unclean drinking water or poor sanitation.

Noninflammatory acute diarrhea caused by bacteria that use preformed toxin to mediate small bowel mucosal disruption is commonly referred to as "food poisoning." These bacteria use preformed toxin to mediate mucosal disruption that leads to an abrupt onset of illness, almost within 6 hours of eating contaminated food. *Staphylococcus aureus* is typically found in stale dairy products or processed meats. *Clostridioides perfringens* forms a toxin that is heat-labile and therefore found in meats that have not been reheated or cooked properly, whereas *Bacillus cereus* is classically implicated in acute diarrheal illness after eating reheated rice.

Protozoal infections are a rare cause of noninflammatory acute diarrhea. Giardia, a protozoal infection, can present as an acute illness often with abdominal bloating but is more commonly associated with chronic diarrhea and found in hikers who drink stream water. Cryptosporidia is a waterborne and self-limiting diarrhea but can also cause chronic diarrhea in the immunocompromised. It is important to note that although the above infectious agents may be implicated, often no diagnosis is found in self-limiting noninflammatory diarrhea and extensive investigation can be avoided.

Inflammatory diarrhea is caused by microorganisms that invade or release toxins that disrupt the intestinal barrier. This leads to the presence of elevated numbers of fecal leukocytes. These acute diarrheal illnesses are usually less voluminous and associated with bloody diarrhea, high fevers, cramping, and tenesmus. Risk factors include food consumption and preparation of undercooked meats, vegetables, and dairy products. In the United States, *Salmonella* and *Campylobacter jejuni* are the two most commonly isolated bacterial agents. Both are associated with undercooked poultry and stale, unpasteurized dairy products. *Shigella* is an invasive bacteria that can result in grossly bloody diarrhea. Enteroinvasive and enterohemorrhagic *Escherichia coli*, found in undercooked meats or raw produce, can also cause bloody diarrhea. *Yersinia enterocolitica* is associated with undercooked pork and may present as a "pseudo-appendicitis" from mesenteric adenitis. When acute diarrhea is the presenting symptom in pregnant women, *Listeria monocytogenes* found in unpasteurized dairy products should always be considered in the differential diagnosis. *Vibrio parahaemolyticus* is commonly found in brackish water or in coastal areas and in contaminated shellfish.

Although rare, and usually only in the immunosuppressed, cytomegalovirus can cause invasion and ulceration of the colon resulting in inflammatory diarrhea. *Entamoeba histolytica* is a parasite that can cause severe diarrhea. It is found mostly in tropical countries with poor sanitation and may also seed to liver and brain resulting in abscess formation.

Another rare form of infectious diarrhea is Whipple disease, caused by the actinomycete *Tropheryma whipplei*, which causes malabsorption that results in weight loss, diarrhea, joint pain, and cognitive problems. Tropical sprue also causes malabsorption and is found in tropical climates of the Caribbean, South America, and Asia. The causative organism has not been identified, but symptoms respond to antibiotic treatment and therefore are highly suspected to be infectious.

Clostridioides difficile infection (CDI) is a common cause of severe hospital-acquired diarrheal infection resulting in a pseudomembranous colitis. *Clostridioides difficile* can colonize the human GI tract but usually does not cause clinical symptoms unless the normal gut flora is altered, therefore allowing *C. difficile* to grow uncontrolled. CDI should be considered in all hospitalized patients that develop diarrhea

or have a history of antibiotic use. Other high-risk patients include the elderly, immunosuppressed patients, and patients with inflammatory bowel disease. CDI can result in large, voluminous, watery diarrhea, usually with significant leukocytosis, that can be a major cause of morbidity and mortality. Testing for CDI is commonly done using molecular tests for the toxins associated with CDI such as polymerase chain reaction and is highly sensitive but does not differentiate between colonization and infection. This can result in high false-positive testing; therefore, it is important to only send CDI testing in patients with symptoms of infectious diarrhea. This will increase the positive predictive value of the test.

Treatment

Volume depletion is the main consideration when evaluating a person with acute diarrhea. By evaluating the volume status of patients and their ability to maintain adequate oral intake, a decision can be made whether to treat with oral rehydration or if admission to hospital and intravenous fluids are needed. The objective of rehydration and electrolyte replacement is to prevent hypotension and electrolyte disturbances that can be a major cause of morbidity and mortality, especially in the elderly and very young. For most people with acute diarrhea, fluid replacement can be achieved with sports drinks and eating saltine crackers. Some people with more severe disease or the elderly and infants may require a more balanced commercially available oral rehydration solution. In patients with mild illness, who are afebrile and do not have bloody diarrhea, symptomatic relief agents such as loperamide or diphenoxylate can be used to reduce the volume of diarrhea. These antimotility drugs reduce gut motility, therefore allowing slower passage of water through the gut and allowing greater reabsorption of fluid. Another class of agents that can be used are antisecretory drugs such as bismuth subsalicylates.

The decision to treat with antibiotics is a common one faced by physicians who are evaluating patients with acute diarrhea. In the community, most diarrheal illnesses are viral and therefore empiric treatment with antibiotics is not recommended. In a returning traveler who is being evaluated for diarrhea, the severity of the illness will guide treatment. Mild travelers' diarrhea should not be treated with antibiotics. Antibiotics have been shown to be effective in reducing the duration of moderate to severe travelers' diarrhea by 1 to 3 days when compared to no treatment. Moderate to severe travelers' diarrhea

TABLE 34.1 Diagnostic Evaluation of Acute Severe Diarrhea

Lab	Complete blood count, basic metabolic panel, C-reactive protein, blood cultures
Stool studies	*Salmonella, Shigella, Campylobacter, Yersinia*, enterohemorrhagic *Escherichia coli* and *Clostridioides difficile*
Imaging	1. Radiograph abdomen for evaluation of intra-abdominal free air or toxic megacolon 2. Computed tomography for signs and symptoms of peritonitis or if there is sustained fever or bacteremia despite treatment with appropriate antibiotics

TABLE 34.2 Acute Diarrhea Lasting Less Than 2 Weeks

Noninflammatory		Inflammatory	
Mild watery diarrhea Disruption of small bowel transport Fecal leukocytes (-)		Severe bloody diarrhea Invasion and destruction of gut mucosa Fecal leukocytes (+)	
Preformed toxin "food poisoning"	*Staphylococcus aureus* *Bacillius cereus* *C. perfringens*	Bacterial	*Campylobacter* *Salmonella* *Shigella* *E. coli* *Clostridioides difficile* *Vibrio parahaemolyticus*
Viral	Norovirus Rotavirus	Viral	Cytomegalovirus (CMV)
Bacterial	*Escherichia coli* *Vibrio cholera*	Parasitic	*Entamoeba histolytica*
Parasitic	Giardia Cryptosporidium Cyclospora		

includes patients with fever, abdominal pain, bloody stool, and sepsis. The most common pathogen identified in travelers' diarrhea is enterotoxigenic *Escherichia coli*, followed by *Campylobacter jejuni*, *Shigella*, and *Salmonella*. Fluoroquinolones, such as ciprofloxacin, are the antibiotics of choice for most cases of travelers' diarrhea. Rifaximin also has been shown to be as effective as ciprofloxacin for noninvasive travelers' diarrhea. However, the resistance of *Campylobacter* to fluoroquinolones is increasing, and in such cases, treatment with a macrolide such as azithromycin should be used. Antibiotics should be avoided in enterohemorrhagic *Escherichia coli* because there may be an increased risk of hemolytic-uremic syndrome related to increased release of Shiga-like toxin.

The recommended treatment of initial CDI is with oral vancomycin or fidaxomicin for 10 days. Patients who have a repeat CDI should be treated with oral vancomycin therapy using a tapered and pulsed regimen. Finally, patients who have more than one recurrence of CDI should be considered for fecal microbiota transplant. Although numerous studies and meta-analyses have been performed on the benefits of probiotics in CDI, currently there is insufficient evidence to recommend their use for the primary prevention of CDI.

CHRONIC DIARRHEA

Chronic diarrhea can be defined as an increase in stool frequency, reduced consistency, and duration longer than 4 weeks. Patient symptoms may include loose stools, increased stool frequency, change of consistency or incontinence. These symptoms can be disabling, and patients will often describe a fear of leaving the house or avoiding long trips without immediate access to a toilet. Though acute diarrhea is commonly infectious in nature, the differential diagnosis of chronic diarrhea is vast and includes intestinal inflammation, colonic neoplasia, malabsorption due to small bowel mucosal disorders, maldigestion due to pancreatic insufficiency, motility disorders, and functional bowel disorders.

Evaluation of Chronic Diarrhea

A thorough history is essential in narrowing down the diagnosis in chronic diarrhea. History should focus on travel and exposures, stool characteristics, prior surgeries, current medications, and over-the-counter supplements. Infectious causes of chronic diarrhea are uncommon in the United States but should be considered in newly arrived immigrants, returned travelers, and people with exposure to farm animals or unclean drinking water. The characteristics of the patient's stool should be described because the presence of blood may suggest

malignancy or inflammatory bowel disease (IBD), oily or sticky stools may suggest malabsorption or maldigestion, and watery stools point to an osmotic or secretory process. Associated symptoms such as fevers, abdominal pain, bloating, and cramps should be noted, as should the relationship of defecation to meals and periods of fasting. Nocturnal symptoms and weight loss can strongly suggest an organic etiology. In patients who are of colon cancer screening age or have alarm features, endoscopic evaluation should be performed. Alarm features include microcytic anemia, bloody diarrhea, fevers, weight loss, nocturnal symptoms, or family history of IBD or colorectal cancer. It is helpful to classify chronic diarrhea into inflammatory, watery or fatty (Table 34.3).

Laboratory Testing

Routine laboratory testing can be used to provide clues to the etiology or severity of chronic diarrhea. A microcytic anemia may point towards chronic blood loss or iron malabsorption seen in an inflammatory process. Macrocytic anemia may point towards a vitamin B_{12} deficiency that can be seen in IBD or in patients who have had small bowel or gastric resection.

Leukocytosis, elevated inflammatory markers such as C-reactive protein, and fecal calprotectin can be seen in inflammatory diarrhea. Serology testing for antitissue transglutaminase antibodies can be performed to rule out celiac disease. Finally, hormone-secreting tumors are rare and should only be tested for in highly selected patients.

Further Evaluation of Chronic Diarrhea

Due to clustering of symptoms, one of the most practical tasks facing a physician in evaluating chronic diarrhea is to try and make the distinction between functional and organic etiologies.

Irritable bowel syndrome (IBS) is common and can present with an array of symptoms that can include diarrhea, bloating, cramping, and abdominal pain associated with defecation. The Rome IV consensus, formed by a worldwide committee to set criteria for the diagnosis of functional gastrointestinal disorders, may help establish the diagnosis. The most recent criteria focuses on abdominal pain in relation to defecation, change in frequency or change in consistency of stool (Table 34.4). The majority of patients who present with classic symptoms of IBS do not need further diagnostic testing and the focus should be on treatment through diet or available medicines approved for IBS.

When a specific etiology is strongly suspected in the work-up of chronic diarrhea that has no confirmatory testing or testing may be invasive or expensive, an empirical trial of treatment may be pursued. Examples include patients with a history of small bowel resection or

TABLE 34.3	**Causes of Chronic Diarrhea**			
	Watery Diarrhea		**Inflammatory Diarrhea**	**Fatty Diarrhea**
Osmotic	**Secretory**		• IBD: Crohn's disease, ulcerative colitis	**Malabsorption**
• Osmotic laxatives: Lactulose, magnesium sulphate (milk of magnesia), polyethylene glycol (Miralax)	• IBD: Crohn's disease, ulcerative colitis		• Diverticulitis	• Celiac disease
	• Microscopic colitis		• Pseudomembranous colitis	• Whipple's disease
	• Hyperthyroidism		• Ischemic colitis	• Short bowel syndrome
• Carbohydrate malabsorption (lactase deficiency)	• Medication		• Radiation colitis	• Mesenteric ischemia
	• Bacterial toxins		• Bacterial infection: tuberculosis, yersiniosis	• Small intestinal bacterial overgrowth
	• Irritable bowel syndrome		• Viral infection: cytomegalovirus, herpes simplex	**Maldigestion**
	• Neoplasm: colon carcinoma, lymphoma		• Parasitic infection: strongyloides	• Exocrine pancreatic insufficiency
	• Bile acid malabsorption		• Neoplasm: colon carcinoma, lymphoma	• Reduced bile acid secretion (primary biliary cholangitis)
	• Neuroendocrine tumors			

IBD, Inflammatory bowel disease.

TABLE 34.4	**Criteria for Diagnosis of IBS**

Recurrent abdominal pain on average at least 1 day/week in the last 3 months, associated with two or more of the following:
Related to defecation
Associated with change in the frequency of stool
Associated with a change in stool consistency

TABLE 34.5 Chronic Watery Diarrhea

	Osmotic	Secretory
Stool volume (L/day)	<1 L	>1 L
Effect on fasting	Reduced	Continued
Fecal osmotic gap	>100 mOsm/kg	<50 mOsm/kg
pH	Usually <5	Usually >6

cholecystectomy who may be empirically treated for bacterial overgrowth or started on a bile acid binder. In such patients who fail empiric treatment or in which the diagnosis remains broad and elusive, a colonoscopy with biopsies should be performed.

Chronic Inflammatory Diarrhea

Chronic inflammatory diarrhea typically presents with bloody diarrhea associated with abdominal pain. Any disease process that can disrupt or inflame the mucosa of the gut should be considered, including infections, inflammatory bowel disease, ischemia, neoplasm or radiation enteritis. Direct visualization with colonoscopy is the best next diagnostic step. Biopsies should be taken to characterize the inflammation. Ischemic colitis should be suspected in elderly patients with underlying vascular disease and a recent hypotensive episode. Characteristic findings on colonoscopy show rectal sparing that is not seen with ulcerative colitis and well-demarcated, segmental inflammation, usually in the watershed area of the splenic flexure. Inflammatory bowel disease, which includes both Crohn's disease or ulcerative colitis, is a more common cause of chronic inflammatory diarrhea. Crohn's disease can involve any part of the GI tract and the presentation may not include bloody diarrhea and can be more varied. Typical symptoms include abdominal pain, weight loss, and diarrhea. However, oral ulcers, fistulous openings or perianal disease in the setting of chronic inflammatory diarrhea are also strong indicators pointing towards Crohn's disease. During colonoscopy, the terminal ileum should be evaluated for ulcers and strictures, which would be consistent with Crohn's disease. In contrast, ulcerative colitis involves only the colon. Clinical presentation and severity are dependent on the location and extent of colonic involvement. When the rectum or rectosigmoid region is involved, patients can present with mild intermittent bloody diarrhea, rectal urgency, and tenesmus. Rarely, patients with isolated severe rectal inflammation may also present with constipation and an inability to pass stools. Pancolitis and left-sided colitis typically have more profound presentations with severe abdominal pain, fevers, anemia, and frequent bloody diarrhea.

Chronic Watery Diarrhea

Chronic watery diarrhea should be subdivided into secretory and osmotic types, based on fecal osmotic gap. The fecal osmotic gap is calculated as 290 mOsm/kg − 2 × (stool Na + stool K). When the calculated fecal osmotic gap is greater than 100 mOsm/kg, it is consistent with osmotic diarrhea, while a gap of less than 50 mOsm/kg is suggestive of a secretory etiology of diarrhea such as infection, inflammation, or circulating secretagogues (Table 34.5).

Osmotic diarrhea may be caused by magnesium ingestion or malabsorption of carbohydrates. Both result in water retention in the lumen of the gut and therefore a high osmotic gap. High magnesium concentration in the stool is commonly seen in patients who use laxatives or high doses of antacids. For this reason, it is important to review medication lists. Lactose intolerance due to lactase deficiency or ingestion of other poorly absorbed sugars can also pull water into the lumen of the gut, resulting in diarrhea. As these malabsorbed carbohydrates

ferment, the stool becomes more acidic. Therefore, a pH less than 7.0 can point to excess carbohydrates in the stool. Common dietary sugar substitutes that cause osmotic diarrhea include sorbitol and high-fructose corn syrup. For this reason, osmotic diarrhea should disappear with fasting.

Secretory diarrhea can result from any process that impairs or disrupts the absorption of salt and water in the gut. Often an overlap of secretory and inflammatory diarrhea may be seen.

Although rare in developed countries, infectious organisms can cause chronic diarrhea and should be ruled out, especially in returned travelers. Parasites such as *Cryptosporidium*, *Microsporidia*, *Cyclospora*, and *Giardia* can all cause chronic secretory diarrhea. Testing of stool for ova and parasites should be performed if there is a travel history or recent immigration from a high-risk area. Giardia testing using ELISA is recommended in all patients with chronic diarrhea.

More commonly, mucosal disease as seen in IBD or structural disease as seen in short bowel syndrome or neoplasm is the cause of chronic secretory diarrhea. Imaging with small bowel radiograph or computerized tomography (CT) should be used to assess for tumors, strictures, fistulas or inflammation. Further examination with colonoscopy should be performed for direct visualization and biopsies of the mucosa.

Microscopic colitis is characterized by chronic watery diarrhea and is commonly seen in women older than 60 years old, although men and women of any age can be affected. Typical symptoms include more than 10 watery stools/day that can be accompanied by abdominal cramping and even mild weight loss. Nocturnal symptoms are common. There are two subtypes of microcytic colitis, lymphocytic and collagenous. The cause of microscopic colitis is unknown but there is a strong association with other autoimmune diseases and certain medications such as proton pump inhibitors and nonsteroidal anti-inflammatory drugs. Direct visualization with colonoscopy typically shows no mucosal inflammation, so biopsies of the left and right colon are needed to make this histologic diagnosis. Budesonide is recommended as first-line treatment for microscopic colitis; however, this medication may be cost prohibitive, and alternative treatments include bismuth subsalicylate or aminosalicylates.

Patients who are post cholecystectomy or have ileal disease or resection may have bile acid malabsorption. This can result when excess bile acid is passed into the colon resulting in electrolyte absorption impairment. In such cases, a trial of bile acid–sequestering resins should be tried.

Peptide-secreting neuroendocrine tumors are rare and should only be investigated when the work-up has been unrevealing for chronic diarrhea. Plasma peptides such as gastrin and vasoactive intestinal peptide (VIP) can be used to help diagnose Zollinger-Ellison syndrome or VIPoma respectively. Elevated levels of gastrin can be seen in patients taking acid suppressing medications such as proton pump inhibitors; however, in Zollinger-Ellison syndrome, gastrin levels are often 10 times the upper limit of normal. CT, MRI, or endoscopic ultrasound of the liver and pancreas should be performed to identify tumors. Zollinger-Ellison syndrome can have characteristic multiple gastric ulcers seen on endoscopy whereas VIPoma can have profound hypokalemia when electrolytes are checked.

Carcinoid syndrome is characterized by secretory diarrhea resulting from the release of excess serotonin from a neuroendocrine tumor. Serotonin syndrome should be suspected in patients with unexplained chronic diarrhea who have symptoms such as flushing of the skin, wheezing, and heart murmurs. Urine should be tested for elevated 5-HIAA.

Chronic Fatty Diarrhea

Chronic fatty diarrhea or steatorrhea can often be described as oily, floating, or sticky stool. Such characteristic stool often implies malabsorption or maldigestion from pancreatic or small bowel mucosal disease. In many cases the cause of fatty diarrhea may be obvious, such as a patient with chronic pancreatitis or severe biliary disease. In other cases, the etiology may not be so obvious and Sudan stain of fecal smear or fecal fat concentration can be obtained. A high concentration of fat in the stool greater than 9.5 g/100 g suggests maldigestion as seen in exocrine pancreatic insufficiency and lack of bile. A low concentration of fecal fat can be seen in mucosal disease that results in the malabsorption of fat and carbohydrates together (see below). CT or MRI of the pancreas, biliary system, and small bowel should be obtained to further assess structural disease and pancreatic disease.

Malabsorption of fat and carbohydrates can result in excess fluid being pulled into the lumen of the gut, therefore diluting the concentration of fecal fat. Such conditions include celiac disease, short bowel syndrome, and small intestine bacterial overgrowth (SIBO). Celiac disease is caused by gluten intolerance and is mainly seen in people of European descent. Presentation can vary from iron deficiency anemia and weight loss to mild abnormalities in liver function tests. Testing for antitissue transglutaminase antibodies with an IgA level can be used to screen for the disease. If suspicions remain high despite negative serologic testing, endoscopy with duodenal biopsies can be performed for definitive diagnosis. The treatment is complete gluten

avoidance. SIBO results when the small bowel is colonized by excessive microbes. Patients with motility disorders such as gastroparesis or structural disease such as blind intestinal loops are at risk. SIBO should be considered in such patients who complain of bloating, abdominal pain, and chronic diarrhea. Hydrogen breath testing can be used to confirm the diagnosis. Treatment with a course of antibiotics can be initiated following a positive test.

Maldigestion is seen in patients who have insufficient amounts of bile to break down fats, such as in primary biliary cholangitis or exocrine pancreatic insufficiency due to lack of pancreatic enzymes. In such cases, measuring stool chymotrypsin and stool elastase can be performed to confirm suspicions of this disorder. In other cases, imaging with MRI, CT or endoscopic ultrasound should be obtained to confirm pancreatic disease. Patients who are strongly suspected of having pancreatic insufficiency are best served with a trial of pancreatic enzymes and evaluating their response.

SUGGESTED READINGS

Camilleri M, Sellin JH, Barrett KE: Pathophysiology, evaluation, and management of chronic watery diarrhea, Gastroenterology 152(3):515–532.e2, 2017.

Riddle MS, DuPont HL, Connor BA: ACG clinical guideline: diagnosis, treatment, and prevention of acute diarrheal infections in adults, Am J Gastroenterol 111(5):602–622, 2016.

Schiller LR, Pardi DS, Sellin JH: Chronic diarrhea: diagnosis and management, Clin Gastroenterol Hepatol 15:182–193, 2016.

Shane AL, Mody RK, Crump JA, et al: 2017 Infectious diseases society of america clinical practice guidelines for the diagnosis and management of infectious diarrhea, Clin Infect Dis 65(12):e45–e80, 2017.

Smalley W, Falck-Ytter C, Carrasco-Labra A, et al.: AGA clinical practice guidelines on the laboratory evaluation of functional diarrhea and diarrhea-predominant irritable bowel syndrome in adults (IBS-D), Gastroenterology 157(3):851–854, 2019.

Steffen R, Hill DR, DuPont HL: Traveler's diarrhea: a clinical review, JAMA 313(1):71–80, 2015.

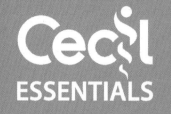

35

Endoscopic and Imaging Procedures

Andrew Canakis, Christopher S. Huang

INTRODUCTION

Since Mikulicz first used a prototype esophagoscope to visualize the lumen of the esophagus in 1880, physicians have been attempting to peer into every portion of the gastrointestinal (GI) tract in an attempt to understand disease and to restore their patients to health. This goal has become more achievable than ever, thanks to the wide variety of both invasive and noninvasive endoscopic and imaging procedures that are currently available. This chapter reviews the various endoscopic and radiographic procedures currently in use, including their indications and basic information regarding their performance.

GASTROINTESTINAL ENDOSCOPY

Gastrointestinal endoscopy is the primary modality for directly visualizing the GI tract, as well as obtaining tissue samples to establish definitive diagnoses. Moreover, a wide variety of therapeutic maneuvers can be performed endoscopically to deal with a host of disease processes, such as hemostasis for bleeding ulcers or varices, resection or ablation of neoplastic tissue, dilation or stenting of strictures, and removal of bile duct stones, to name just a few.

Over the years, endoscopes have evolved from early rigid designs with limited capabilities to more sophisticated flexible instruments with advanced imaging capabilities, specialized features for therapeutic maneuvers, and different designs to enable examination of specific areas of the GI tract and biliopancreatic systems. Endoscopes come in varying lengths and diameters ranging from 3.1 mm to 15 mm (Fig. 35.1) and consist of a control handle, insertion tube, and connector section that attaches to the light source and image processing units. The control handle comprises dials that deflect the scope tip in all directions, as well as buttons for suction, air/water insufflation, and image capture. The control handle also includes the entry port to the "working channel" that runs down the length of the insertion tube, through which a wide array of accessories such as biopsy forceps, snares, and balloon dilators can be passed. The tip of the insertion tube houses a charge-coupled device for color image generation, a light guide illumination system, and an objective lens, which may be oriented for forward viewing, side viewing, or oblique viewing, depending on the type of endoscope.

Technologic advances continue to improve the quality of endoscopic imaging, such as the recent introduction of high-definition instruments, magnification endoscopy (from baseline of 30 to 35× to up to 150×), and enhanced imaging technologies such as narrow band imaging (NBI) and multiband imaging.

GI endoscopy can be performed in dedicated endoscopy suites or at a patient's bedside in emergency situations. After positioning the patient appropriately and providing sedation, if necessary, the lubricated endoscope is passed through the intended orifice and advanced

manually by the endoscopist. The angulations of the GI lumen are navigated by deflecting the endoscope tip and by applying torque to the instrument shaft (i.e., rotating the shaft along the long axis of the instrument). Endoscopy is generally safe, with complications that include bleeding (0.3% to 1% after colonoscopic polypectomy), perforation (0.05% in general, but 0.1% to 0.5% after polypectomy), and sedation-associated hypotension and hypoxia (1% to 5%). Death related to endoscopic procedures is exceedingly rare (0% to 0.01%).

Esophagogastroduodenoscopy

Esophagogastroduodenoscopy (EGD), often referred to as *upper endoscopy*, is performed with a *gastroscope* and allows the endoscopist to visualize the esophagus, stomach, and duodenum to its third and sometimes fourth portions (Fig. 35.2). Common indications for EGD include evaluation of upper GI symptoms (such as dyspepsia, heartburn, nausea, vomiting, dysphagia and odynophagia), screening for and surveillance of Barrett esophagus, screening for gastroesophageal varices, suspected upper GI bleeding (acute or chronic), and investigation of malabsorptive diarrhea (e.g., celiac sprue or protein-losing enteropathy). A partial list of the therapeutic interventions that can be performed during EGD include the treatment of esophageal varices; dilation of esophageal strictures, rings, and webs; removal or ablation of neoplastic tissue; hemostasis therapy for upper GI bleeding; and the placement of palliative stents for malignant obstruction of the esophagus, pylorus, or duodenum.

Enteroscopy

Examination of the small intestine beyond the ligament of Treitz is not feasible with a standard gastroscope. More recently, greater strides have been made to gain direct visualization of the 6 m or so of the small intestine. *Push* enteroscopy using a long (>200 cm) endoscope allows the endoscopist to both image and biopsy or cauterize lesions in the small intestine, but due to looping of the endoscope and tortuosity of the small intestine, advancing this instrument beyond the first 50 cm of jejunum can be difficult. Balloon-assisted enteroscopy is a newer technique that provides endoscopic access to most of the small bowel. Double balloon enteroscopy (DBE) was initially introduced in 2001 and has emerged as the primary modality for extensive examination of the small bowel. This method employs balloons, incorporated into overtubes or the endoscope itself, to permit pleating of the small bowel onto the endoscope. By inflating and deflating the balloons in sequence, the enteroscope can be advanced through extremely long stretches of small intestine. Combining an anterograde (through the mouth) and retrograde (through the anus) approach may potentially allow for complete examination of the entire small intestine. However, its use is limited to high volume tertiary centers due to its technical difficulties and long procedure times. As a result, single balloon

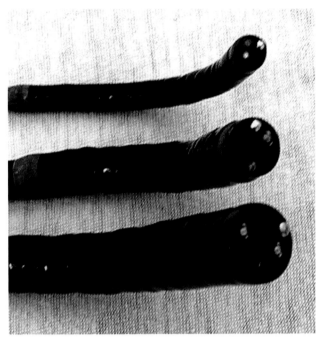

Fig. 35.1 Endoscopes used for upper GI endoscopy. Endoscopes of varying sizes are available for use in different situations. The uppermost endoscope (6-mm diameter) can be used for unsedated endoscopy. The middle endoscope (9-mm diameter) is used for standard diagnostic endoscopy. The lowermost endoscope (12-mm diameter) is used for therapeutic endoscopy, such as the placement of enteral stents. (Courtesy of Brian C. Jacobson.)

enteroscopy (SBE) was developed in 2007 as a means to shorten procedure times, though the chances of total enteroscopy are limited by its single balloon design. A meta-analysis comparing DBE and SBE found that both modalities had similar diagnostic/therapeutic yields, adverse events, and failure rates.

Spiral enteroscopy represents a different technique that utilizes rotational energy of a spiral overtube device that retracts the small bowel over the scope, allowing for deep enteroscopy. Recently, the novel use of a motorized spiral endoscope was developed as a means to improve scope maneuverability, decrease procedure times, and limit the cumbersome nature of balloon enteroscopy (which often requires two operators). Through the use of a foot-switch-operator motor, an overtube equipped with spiral-shaped fins can smoothly advance through the small bowel. Additionally, the system is equipped with high-definition imaging and a 3.2-mm channel that may offer versatile diagnostic and therapeutic modalities in the near future.

Intraoperative enteroscopy is the final means for obtaining visualization of the entire small bowel, although this is obviously the most invasive approach and is now uncommonly performed given the development of device-assisted enteroscopy procedures. In this procedure, a surgeon will make an incision in the patient's abdomen and then pleat the small bowel onto the enteroscope while the endoscopist visualizes the lumen. Once a lesion is identified, the surgeon may elect to proceed directly to a resection of the affected segment of small intestine if the lesion is not amenable to endoscopic treatment.

Video Capsule Endoscopy

The desire to obtain visualization of the GI lumen in the least invasive way has resulted in the development of video capsule endoscopy, the use of pill-sized wireless cameras that the patient swallows (E-Fig. 35.1 and Video 35.1). Currently, capsule endoscopes are available for the

evaluation of the esophagus, small intestine, and the colon. Capsule endoscopes are swallowed or deployed endoscopically and transmit images wirelessly to a data recorder as they travel through a patient's GI tract, without the need for sedation. At the end of the study, the data recorder allows for stored images to be uploaded into a computer for viewing while the capsule is ultimately passed in the patient's stool. The esophageal capsule is helpful in patients being screened for esophageal varices or individuals with suspected complications of acid reflux, such as reflux esophagitis or Barrett esophagus. The small bowel capsule has become the gold standard for visualizing the small intestine, most commonly for the purpose of investigating obscure GI bleeding (E-Figs. 35.2 and 35.3 and Videos 35.2 and 35.3) and suspected inflammatory bowel disease (E-Figs. 35.4 and 35.5). Colon capsule endoscopy (CCE) is typically used in patients with a prior colonoscopy failure or suspected lower GI bleeding and may even offer a role in monitoring disease activity in inflammatory bowel disease (IBD) patients. Recent technologic advancements in second-generation CCE now offers clinicians with high-resolution, nearly 360-degree views of the colon with adaptive frame rates that improve battery life and visualization during rapid motions. Additionally, its adjunctive software can estimate polyp size and provide flexible spectral imaging color enhancement to further differentiate neoplastic versus non-neoplastic lesions. Although rare, the main potential complication of capsule endoscopy is retention within the small bowel, usually at a site of pathology.

Sigmoidoscopy and Colonoscopy

Flexible sigmoidoscopy allows visualization of the rectum, sigmoid colon, and descending colon to the level of the splenic flexure. Enemas are given before the procedure to clear stool from the distal colon. Because sigmoidoscopy is generally a brief procedure and not particularly painful, sedation is typically not necessary, making it a convenient tool for colorectal cancer screening. Sigmoidoscopy may also be useful for evaluating symptoms such as chronic diarrhea and rectal bleeding suspected to be arising from the distal colon or rectum, as well as assessing response to therapy in patients with inflammatory bowel disease involving the rectosigmoid colon.

Colonoscopy allows direct visualization of the entire large bowel and the terminal ileum. Bowel cleansing for colonoscopy requires the ingestion of osmotically active solutions, such as polyethylene glycol, coupled with a clear liquid diet for 24 hours before the procedure. Colonoscopy can be more uncomfortable for the patient than sigmoidoscopy due to stretching and distension of the colon, so sedation and analgesia are typically provided. Colonoscopy has become widely performed as a first-line colorectal cancer screening test because of its ability to not only detect early cancers but also *prevent* colon cancer (through the removal of premalignant polyps). Other indications for colonoscopy include evaluation of chronic diarrhea, iron deficiency anemia, overt and occult GI blood loss, and assessing inflammatory bowel disease, including surveillance for dysplasia. Therapeutic interventions possible during colonoscopy include polypectomy, endoscopic mucosal resection of neoplastic lesions, thermal ablation of vascular ectasias, decompression of colonic dilation associated with pseudo-obstruction, stenting of malignant obstruction, and control of lower GI bleeding.

Endoscopic Retrograde Cholangiopancreatography

Endoscopic retrograde cholangiopancreatography (ERCP) is a combined endoscopic and radiographic procedure for imaging and intervening within the biliary and pancreatic ducts. A *duodenoscope* is a specially designed instrument for use during ERCP that includes an imaging lens oriented on the side of the endoscope's tip (as opposed to the front), allowing a direct view of the ampulla of Vater on the medial wall of the second

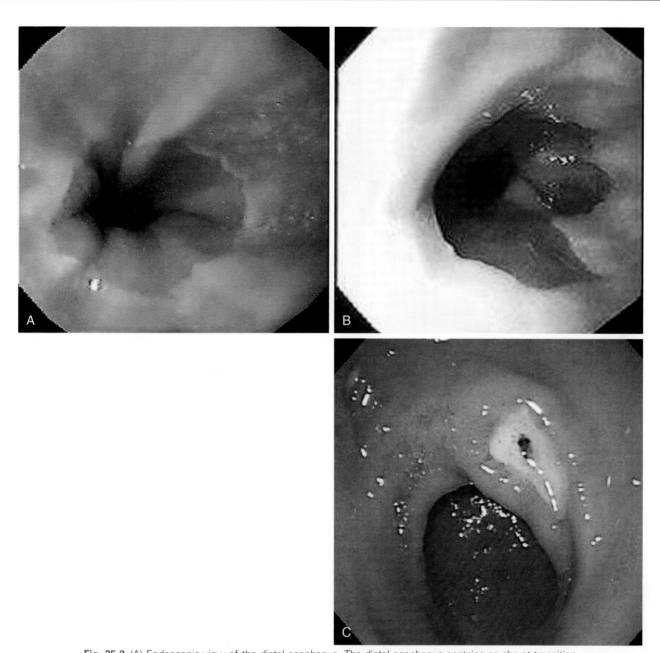

Fig. 35.2 (A) Endoscopic view of the distal esophagus. The distal esophagus contains an abrupt transition between its squamous-lined mucosa and the columnar-lined mucosa of the stomach. (B) Endoscopic view of Barrett esophagus, in which the squamous epithelium of the distal esophagus is replaced by columnar-lined epithelium. Evident in this view is a tongue of columnar-lined mucosa extending proximally into the esophagus. (C) Endoscopic view of a gastric ulcer. A yellow-based ulceration with a pigmented spot is visualized on the gastric wall at the transition between the corpus and the antrum. (Courtesy of M. Michael Wolfe.)

portion of the duodenum. An adjustable instrument *elevator* located at the tip of the duodenoscope helps the endoscopist guide a catheter and other accessories into the duct of interest. Contrast is then injected through the catheter, filling the duct, and fluoroscopic images are obtained (Fig. 35.3). Indications for ERCP include evaluation and treatment of bile duct obstruction due to benign or malignant causes (e.g., bile duct stones, strictures, and bile duct or pancreatic malignancies), cholangitis, postoperative or traumatic bile leaks and pancreatic duct leaks, and transpapillary drainage of pseudocysts. Therapeutic interventions possible during ERCP include sphincterotomy (an incision through the sphincter of Oddi using a catheter with an electrocautery cutting wire), removal of bile duct stones, and placement of biliary or pancreatic duct stents to alleviate signs and symptoms of obstruction or to promote healing of duct leaks. ERCP

carries a significant (5%) risk for complications, including pancreatitis, postsphincterotomy bleeding, and perforation. Therefore, ERCP should only be performed when therapeutic benefits are anticipated.

Choledochoscopy and *pancreatoscopy* are techniques in which an endoscope 3 mm or less in diameter is passed through the accessory channel of a duodenoscope and into the bile or pancreatic ducts. The use of this small endoscope permits direct visualization of ductal abnormalities, guides electrohydraulic lithotripsy of large stones, and allows for direct sampling of ductal lesions.

Endoscopic Ultrasound

Endoscopic ultrasound (EUS) or endosonography is performed with an endoscope containing an ultrasound transducer in its tip. Because

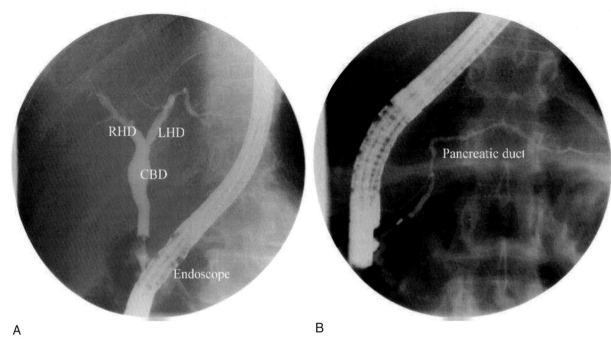

A
B

Fig. 35.3 Endoscopic retrograde cholangiopancreatography (ERCP). (A) Normal cholangiogram. Contrast injected into the biliary tree during ERCP demonstrates the intraductal anatomy of the common bile duct *(CBD)*, right hepatic duct *(RHD)*, left hepatic duct *(LHD)*, and smaller intrahepatic biliary radicals. (B) Normal pancreatogram. Contrast injected into the pancreatic duct during ERCP defines the intraductal anatomy throughout the length of the pancreas. (Courtesy of Brian C. Jacobson.)

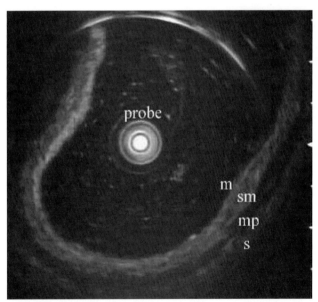

Fig. 35.4 Endoscopic ultrasound of the gastrointestinal wall. A 12-MHz ultrasound probe, passed through the accessory channel of an endoscope, demonstrates the normal layers of the rectal wall. The mucosa *(m)* appears as a superficial, hyperechoic *(white)* band and a deeper hypoechoic *(black)* band. The submucosa *(sm)* appears as the next hyperechoic layer. The muscularis propria *(mp)* appears hypoechoic, and the serosa *(s)* appears as the outermost, hyperechoic layer. (Courtesy of Brian C. Jacobson.)

this transducer can be placed within the GI lumen, high-resolution images of the bowel wall can be obtained, revealing distinct layers that correspond to the mucosa, submucosa, muscularis propria, and serosa (Fig. 35.4). This technique allows the endoscopist to stage tumor depths and determine the layer of origin of subepithelial masses. In addition, EUS can image beyond the gastrointestinal tract wall, providing sonographic images of adjacent structures within the mediastinum and upper abdomen, including the pancreas, liver, gallbladder, mesenteric vessels, lymph nodes, and adrenal glands. High-frequency EUS catheter probes can be passed through the accessory channel of a duodenoscope and into the biliary and pancreatic ducts to provide sonographic images of small tumors and stones. They can likewise be used through a standard endoscope to evaluate diminutive subepithelial lesions and stage obstructing esophageal cancers. Fine-needle aspiration (FNA) as well as core biopsy can be performed under EUS guidance and is the preferred approach to obtaining a tissue diagnosis in many circumstances (e.g., pancreatic masses or cysts, subepithelial lesions of the GI tract, and intra-abdominal or paraesophageal lymphadenopathy). Technologic advancements such as elastography and contrast-enhanced harmonic EUS have further enhanced the diagnostic capability of EUS, particularly in terms of distinguishing malignancy from benign processes. Furthermore, EUS-guided vascular access provides a unique modality for portal vein sampling and portal pressure measurements. However, EUS is more than just a diagnostic modality, and the spectrum of EUS-guided therapies is rapidly expanding. Therapeutic maneuvers that can be performed via EUS guidance include transluminal drainage of pseudocysts and walled-off pancreatic necrosis, pancreatic cyst ablation, celiac axis neurolysis, fiducial (technical) placement into solid tumors to guide stereotactic radiotherapy, and achieving bile duct access or biliary drainage (when initial attempts at ERCP have failed or surgically altered anatomy precludes standard ERCP.)

"Second Space" and "Third Space" Endoscopy

Recent advancements in endoscopic techniques and equipment have led to the development of so-called "second-space" and "third-space" endoscopy procedures within the peritoneal cavity and intramural/submucosal tissue planes, respectively.

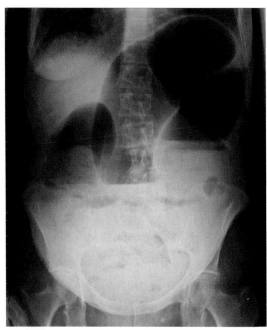

Fig. 35.5 Upright plain radiograph of the abdomen. Air in dilated loops of colon and air-fluid levels can be seen in this patient with a sigmoid volvulus. (Courtesy of Brian C. Jacobson.)

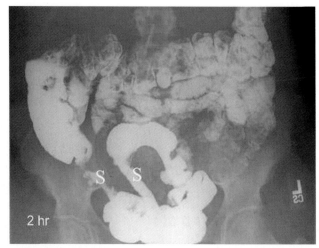

Fig. 35.6 Small bowel follow-through. Ingested barium defines the contours of the small and large bowel lumen. A long stricture *(S)* of the terminal ileum can be seen in this patient with Crohn's disease. (Courtesy of Brian C. Jacobson.)

Natural orifice transluminal endoscopic surgery (NOTES) is an evolving, minimally invasive field that combines endoscopic and surgical approaches to access the peritoneal cavity. Through the use of an endoscope, a clinician can access a desired target or organ through a transgastric, transcolonic, transvaginal or transurethral approach. Examples of NOTES procedures include cholecystectomy, appendectomy, sleeve gastrectomy, hysterectomy, and hernia repair.

The success and promise of NOTES procedures has led to the development of "third space" endoscopic interventions within the intramural tissue planes of the gastrointestinal tract. Such procedures include full-thickness resection of subepithelial tumors of the GI tract, as well as peroral endoscopic myotomy (POEM) to treat achalasia and esophageal motility disorders. By utilizing submucosal endoscopy, the POEM procedure consists of four steps involving a mucosal incision, submucosal tunneling, subsequent myotomy, and finally mucosal closure through the placement of clips or sutures. POEM has become a very popular modality in treating achalasia, due to its long-term efficacy, lack of abdominal incisions, and rapid recovery.

The same principles and techniques of POEM have been used in the treatment of pyloric dysfunction in patients with gastroparesis in what is known as gastric POEM (G-POEM). Lately, there has been a growing body of evidence proposing that pyloric dysfunction may indeed be a significant contributor to the pathogenesis and symptomatic effects related to gastroparesis. In this context, the need for an alternative, more effective, and minimally invasive therapeutic modality that can target a subset of patients who exhibit pyloric dysfunction has emerged. G-POEM has shown promise, but further long-term and head-to-head studies are needed to see if this modality can emerge as first-line therapy.

NONENDOSCOPIC IMAGING PROCEDURES

Plain Abdominal Radiographs

Plain abdominal radiographs include upright, supine, and lateral decubitus films obtained with standard radiograph equipment and without the use of contrast agents. Plain films are most useful in the initial evaluation of abdominal pain or nausea and vomiting, particularly when perforation or obstruction is suspected, and they may reveal evidence of a pneumoperitoneum, dilated bowel loops and air-fluid levels, excessive amounts of stool, or displacement of bowel loops. These findings are indicative of a perforation, obstruction or ileus, constipation or fecal impaction, and volvulus or organ enlargement, respectively (Fig. 35.5). Calcifications, such as those seen in chronic pancreatitis and gallstone disease, may also be visible on these radiographs.

Contrast Studies

Contrast agents such as barium or the water-soluble diatrizoate (e.g., Gastrografin) can be administered by mouth or rectum to detect mucosal abnormalities (ulcerations and masses), strictures, herniations, diverticula, and abnormal peristalsis. Contrast agents can be used alone *(single contrast)* or with the instillation of air or ingestion of gas-forming agents *(double contrast)*. The former method is more useful for detecting obstructing lesions and motility disturbances, whereas the latter method aids in detecting more subtle findings such as small ulcerations or polyps.

A *video esophagogram* (also known as modified barium swallow) entails the filming of a patient's oral cavity and pharynx during the ingestion of contrast materials of various thicknesses and textures. This imaging modality permits careful assessment of a patient's ability to manipulate a food bolus, swallow effectively, and avoid aspiration events. A video esophagogram is indicated for evaluating patients with oropharyngeal dysphagia and recurrent aspiration pneumonia. A standard *barium esophagogram* (barium swallow) focuses attention on the esophagus during the ingestion of a bolus of contrast. This study can detect esophageal rings, webs, strictures, and motility problems that endoscopy might miss. A barium esophagogram may be useful for evaluating esophageal dysphagia, either as a complementary test to endoscopy, or when endoscopy is contraindicated.

An *upper GI series* includes serial radiographic images as an ingested contrast agent travels through the esophagus, stomach, and duodenum. This study can define gastric abnormalities, such as masses, ulcerations, and mucosal thickening. It is indicated in evaluating abdominal pain and suspected gastric outlet obstruction. If radiographic imaging continues as the contrast agent traverses the jejunum and ileum, the study is called a *small bowel follow-through* (Fig. 35.6). Indications for a small bowel follow-through include suspected small bowel obstruction or partial obstruction from any cause, suspected small bowel mucosal diseases such as Crohn's disease, and obscure GI blood loss (although this has been

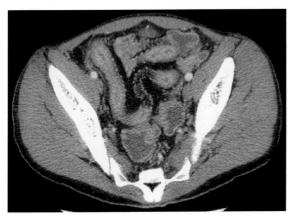

Fig. 35.7 Computed tomography enterography. A long segment of inflamed terminal ileum is demonstrated in this patient with Crohn's disease. (Courtesy of Christopher S. Huang.)

largely replaced by video capsule endoscopy). During this more involved procedure, a radiologist will obtain multiple films, including *spot films*, or close-up views of regions that appear abnormal. Fluoroscopy can be used to follow a contrast agent during the journey through the small bowel. Attention is paid not only to structural findings but also to the length of time required for contrast to reach and enter the colon. For more detailed small bowel images, *enteroclysis* can be performed. This method requires the infusion of concentrated contrast directly into the small bowel through a nasojejunal tube placed under fluoroscopic guidance. Because of its invasive nature, as well as the availability of better small bowel imaging techniques, enteroclysis is now rarely performed.

Single- and double-contrast barium enemas can detect colonic strictures, diverticula, polyps, and colonic ulcerations, and they can be therapeutic in reducing a sigmoid volvulus. Double-contrast barium enema may be used for colorectal cancer screening as a stand-alone test or in conjunction with flexible sigmoidoscopy, or it may be used to visualize the proximal colon when colonoscopy cannot be completed for various reasons. However, it is now infrequently used for these purposes given its relatively poor sensitivity, as well as availability of computed tomography colography ("virtual colonoscopy," discussed later). In general, the upper GI series and barium enema have been superseded by upper endoscopy and colonoscopy because the endoscopic procedures offer increased sensitivity for detecting mucosal abnormalities, the ability to obtain mucosal biopsies, and the potential for resection of identified lesions.

Transabdominal Ultrasound

Ultrasonography is often the first imaging study obtained in the evaluation of suspected biliary colic, jaundice, and abnormal liver tests. Its use of sound waves to create an image obviates the need for radiation exposure, and the addition of Doppler techniques permits the assessment of vascular flow. Ultrasound can detect parenchymal abnormalities, such as fatty liver or cirrhosis, focal masses or cysts, ascites, biliary ductal dilation, gallstones, and large vessel thromboses. It may detect thickening of the gut wall and areas of intussusception. Ultrasound is also used to guide needle placement for biopsies or fluid aspiration. Ultrasound cannot penetrate bone or air, preventing its use as a more general diagnostic tool for the GI tract.

Computed Tomography, Computed Tomography Enterography, and Computed Tomography Colography

Computed tomography (CT) uses computer-aided reconstruction of multiple radiographic images obtained in a circular or helical course around a patient's vertical axis. Internal organs are visualized based

on their inherent tissue densities compared with their surroundings. The GI lumen is usually opacified by having the patient drink an oral contrast agent. In addition, intravenous contrast agents can be administered to highlight regions with increased blood flow, thereby improving detection of pathologic lesions, such as tumors and areas of active inflammation. CT can detect parenchymal lesions, such as tumors, cysts, and abscesses, as well as define the size, shape, and characteristics of parenchymal organs, such as the liver and spleen. Vascular abnormalities, such as perigastric varices or large vessel thromboses, and intra-abdominal fluid, such as ascites, can also be seen with CT. The caliber and contour of the GI tract wall are demonstrated by CT, aiding in the diagnosis of inflammatory lesions, such as colitis, diverticulitis, and appendicitis. CT can also be used to guide needle biopsies of abdominal masses and to place electrodes into tumors for ablative therapies such as radiofrequency ablation. The use of CT to guide placement of drainage catheters has made possible the percutaneous treatment of intra-abdominal abscesses, pseudocysts, and pancreatic necrosis.

CT enteroclysis and *CT enterography* are two emerging techniques developed to provide better images of the small intestine. CT enteroclysis uses a nasojejunal tube to deliver contrast into the small intestine, whereas CT enterography uses an orally ingested low-density intraluminal contrast to distend the lumen and highlight the small intestinal mucosa (Fig. 35.7). With the advancement of this technology and its ability to reconstruct images in multiple planes, both luminal and extraluminal information can be obtained.

CT can also be used to obtain high-resolution images of the colon. CT colonography, or *virtual colonoscopy*, makes use of special image reconstruction software to create accurate visualization of the colonic lumen, provided that the patient has completed a bowel-cleansing regimen identical to that used for colonoscopy (although techniques that do not require such preparation are being developed). These CT images are 70% to 90% sensitive for detecting polyps or masses within the colon, helping to determine which patients need therapeutic colonoscopy. CT colonography is considered an acceptable option for colorectal cancer screening in average risk individuals but is primarily used to complete colonic visualization in the setting of an incomplete colonoscopy (due to technical reasons or obstructing pathology).

Magnetic Resonance Imaging and Magnetic Resonance Cholangiopancreatography

Similar to CT, magnetic resonance imaging (MRI) provides multiple cross-sectional images of the abdomen and pelvis. These images are created using powerful field magnets to orient small numbers of nuclei within the body in such a way as to produce a measurable magnetic moment. MRI therefore avoids radiation exposure but requires the patient to lie nearly motionless, and often within a small enclosed tube, for prolonged periods. MRI can visualize parenchymal lesions such as masses and cysts and may better characterize abnormalities seen on CT, such as hemangiomas, hepatic focal nodular hyperplasia, and fatty liver. MRI is also helpful in better characterizing perirectal abscesses and fistulas in Crohn's disease. Special rectal MRI probes or coils can provide detailed images of rectal cancer used for tumor staging, as well as evaluate the anal sphincters in patients with fecal incontinence.

MRI of the biliary and pancreatic ducts (*magnetic resonance cholangiopancreatography*, MRCP) is a noninvasive method that can detect ductal dilation, strictures, stones (Fig. 35.8), pancreatic parenchymal changes in chronic pancreatitis, and congenital ductal abnormalities, such as pancreas divisum. *Magnetic resonance angiography* is a magnetic resonance method for visualizing blood vessels and serves as an important noninvasive tool for evaluating patients with suspected mesenteric ischemia, vasculitis, and other vascular anomalies.

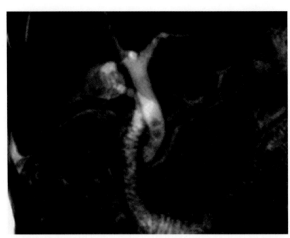

Fig. 35.8 Magnetic resonance cholangiopancreatography. Several stones are visualized within the common bile duct, appearing as hypointense filling defects on T2-weighted images. (Courtesy of Christopher S. Huang.)

Visceral Angiography

Angiography is an invasive technique whereby a catheter is introduced into a blood vessel, and intravascular contrast is injected during fluoroscopic imaging to visualize the vessel's lumen. Visceral angiography is used for evaluating mesenteric vessels in the setting of GI bleeding and suspected mesenteric ischemia. For GI bleeding, angiography is sensitive enough to detect 1 to 1.5 mL per minute of blood loss. Once the site of bleeding has been localized, the radiologist can infuse vasopressin (a vasoconstrictor) or embolize the vessel using tiny coils or gelatin sponges to ensure hemostasis. In the setting of mesenteric ischemia, angiography permits localization of a vascular stenosis or obstruction, followed by possible therapeutic interventions (e.g., balloon angioplasty, stent placement, infusion of vasodilators and thrombolytics). Other indications for angiography include the placement of transjugular intrahepatic portosystemic shunts (TIPS) in cirrhotic patients with intractable variceal bleeding or refractory ascites and for chemoembolization of liver tumors.

Radionuclide Imaging

Technetium-99m (^{99m}Tc) is currently the major radionuclide used in GI imaging. Its 6-hour half-life and ready availability make it ideal for clinical use. ^{99m}Tc is used to label various substances for use in several imaging techniques. ^{99m}Tc-sulfur colloid scanning and ^{99m}Tc-labeled red blood cell scanning are two distinct methods that can be used to detect active GI bleeding. The latter uses the patient's own blood cells to carry the radionuclide throughout the body. These methods can detect as little as 0.05 to 0.4 mL per minute of blood loss. However, localization of the site of bleeding is less accurate with these methods compared with angiography. ^{99m}Tc scans are often performed before angiography to document ongoing bleeding before subjecting a patient to the more invasive, less sensitive study. A ^{99m}Tc-labeled red blood cell scan can also be used to diagnose a hepatic hemangioma with an almost 100% positive predictive value.

Cholescintigraphy using ^{99m}Tc-iminodiacetic acid (IDA) analogs is the most commonly performed liver study in nuclear medicine. The radionuclide is taken up by the liver, is excreted into bile, and passes through the biliary tree into the gallbladder and duodenum. Failure to visualize the gallbladder during a hepatobiliary IDA scan may indicate cholecystitis secondary to cystic duct obstruction by a gallstone. Meckel's diverticulum can be a source of abdominal pain and bleeding, but it can be difficult to visualize with standard endoscopic and radiographic imaging. The agent ^{99m}Tc-pertechnetate has a high affinity for gastric mucosa and is therefore used to demonstrate the presence of this congenital anomaly.

Gastric emptying studies are useful for the evaluation of patients with suspected gastroparesis. Patients are given a ^{99m}Tc-sulfur colloid-labeled standardized meal (consisting of liquid egg whites, toast, jam/jelly, and water) and are imaged at 0, 1, 2, and 4 hours after meal ingestion. Gastric retention of greater than 10% at 4 hours is highly sensitive and specific for delayed gastric emptying.

Radionuclide imaging studies are also useful for the detection, staging, and monitoring of certain neoplasms such as neuroendocrine tumors (NETs). Most well-differentiated NETs express somatostatin receptors and can therefore be detected with radiolabeled somatostatin analogues such as 111-In pentetreotide and 68-Ga DOTATATE.

PROSPECTUS FOR THE FUTURE

Through continued technologic advances, improvements in both endoscopic and radiologic image quality and resolution will also continue. In addition, the gastrointestinal lumen will no longer be regarded as a boundary to therapeutic endoscopy. Examples of expected innovations include the following:

- *The continued expansion of endoscopic procedures beyond the walls of the GI tract*, providing a less invasive approach to treatment of diseases traditionally managed surgically.
- "Second-space" and "third-space" endoscopy techniques are likely to be refined further, and bariatric endoscopy techniques are likely to become more widely performed.
- Further development of computer-aided diagnosis (or "artificial intelligence") for colonoscopy with automated polyp detection and characterization.

SUGGESTED READINGS

ASGE Technology Committee, Aslanian HR, Sethi A, et al.: ASGE guideline for endoscopic full-thickness resection and submucosal tunnel endoscopic resection, *VideoGIE* 4(8):343–350, 2019.

Byrne MF, Jowell PS: Gastrointestinal imaging: Endoscopic ultrasound, *Gastroenterology* 122:1631–1648, 2002.

DiSario JA, Petersen BT, Tierney WM, et al.: Enteroscopes, *Gastrointest Endosc* 66:872–880, 2007.

Fletcher JG, Huprich J, Loftus EV, et al.: Computerized tomography enterography and its role in small-bowel imaging, *Clin Gastroenterol Hepatol* 6:283–289, 2008.

Gore RM, Levine MS: *Textbook of gastrointestinal radiology*, ed 2, Philadelphia, 2000, Saunders.

Mishkin DS, Chuttani R, Croffie J, et al.: ASGE Technology Status Evaluation Report: Wireless capsule endoscopy, *Gastrointest Endosc* 63:539–545, 2006.

Muguruma N, Tanaka K, Teramae S, Takayama T: Colon capsule endoscopy: toward the future, *Clin J Gastroenterol* 10(1):1–6, 2017.

Riff BP, DiMaio CJ: Exploring the small bowel: update on deep enteroscopy, *Curr Gastroenterol Rep* 18(6):28, 2016.

Schneider M, Höllerich J, Beyna T: Device-assisted enteroscopy: A review of available techniques and upcoming new technologies, *World J Gastroenterol* 25(27):3538–3545, 2019.

Shah SL, Perez-Miranda M, Kahaleh M, Tyberg A: Updates in Therapeutic Endoscopic Ultrasonography, *J Clin Gastroenterol* 52(9):765–772, 2018.

Thrall JH, Ziessman HA: *Nuclear Medicine: The Requisites*, ed 2, St. Louis, 2000, Mosby.

36

Esophageal Disorders

Harlan Rich, Zilla Hussain, Neal D. Dharmadhikari

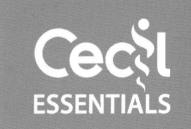

INTRODUCTION

The esophagus is a muscular tube that serves as conduit for the passage of solids and liquids into the stomach. It averages 23 to 25 cm in length and descends from the pharynx, at the lower border of the cricoid cartilage, to the stomach, at the cardiac orifice. Its descent is generally vertical and follows anterior to the vertebral column through the diaphragm and into the abdomen.

The esophagus is made up of four strata: mucosa, submucosa, muscularis externa, and adventitia. The stratified squamous nonkeratinized mucosa also contains the lamina propria and smooth muscle muscularis mucosae. Esophageal cardiac glands, in the lamina propria, produce mucous secretions that coat the lining of the esophagus. The submucosal layer contains esophageal glands, mucous and serous cells, and the Meissner, or submucosal, plexus. The muscularis externa is composed of an inner circular and outer longitudinal muscle layer. The upper third is mostly skeletal muscle innervated by the vagus nerve, while the lowest third is predominantly smooth muscle innervated by the enteric nervous system. The middle third is a mix of both skeletal and smooth muscle. The Auerbach, or myenteric, plexus is located between the inner circular and outer longitudinal layers. The outermost layer of the esophagus is the adventitia. A serosal layer covers the short segment of the abdominal esophagus across the diaphragm to the gastric cardia.

Sphincters are found at each end of the esophagus: the upper esophageal sphincter (UES) and the lower esophageal sphincter (LES). The UES is composed of three striated skeletal muscles: cricopharyngeus, thyropharyngeus, and cranial cervical esophagus. It maintains a degree of muscular activity at rest and relaxes during swallowing, vomiting, or belching. Opening of the UES occurs both via relaxation of these muscles and the pulling open of the sphincter via the superior and inferior hyoid and posterior pharyngeal muscles. The LES is a zone of circular, smooth muscle that maintains tonic contraction at rest and relaxes during swallowing, vomiting, and belching. The LES is supported by a functional external sphincter composed of the right crus of the diaphragm, which surrounds the esophagus as it enters the abdomen. Together, the LES and the functional external sphincter contribute to a high-pressure zone, preventing the regurgitation of gastric contents. Relaxation of the LES occurs when vagal efferent impulses activate myenteric neurons that release nonadrenergic, noncholinergic neurotransmitters, predominantly nitric oxide, and vasoactive intestinal polypeptide.

Swallowing requires the synchronization of voluntary and involuntary processes. Food mixes with saliva in the mouth and then is pushed back into the oral pharynx by the tongue. Once food enters the oral pharynx the glottis closes, protecting the airway. The bolus is then pushed to the esophagus where the UES is located. The UES relaxes, allowing food to enter the esophagus and then immediately closes, preventing the regurgitation of food. The bolus spends 8 to 13 seconds in the esophagus. Primary peristaltic waves, activated by central sequential firing mechanisms in the striated esophagus, and a latency gradient through the smooth muscle esophagus activated by vagal impulses, allow the bolus to travel through the esophagus. The pressure created by these waves ranges from 40 to 180 mm Hg. The pressure varies by the bolus's location in the esophagus, consistency, volume, and temperature. The LES relaxes and peristaltic waves push the bolus into the stomach.

SYMPTOMS OF ESOPHAGEAL DISEASE

Heartburn and regurgitation are two of the most common symptoms of esophageal disease and are defining features of gastroesophageal reflux disease (GERD). Heartburn is described as a burning sensation in the chest but can also be described as chest pain. Regurgitation is the sensation of food or liquid moving up and down the esophagus or as a sour taste in the mouth.

Dysphagia describes difficulty swallowing and can be characterized by trouble initiating a swallow or a bolus of material feeling stuck in the neck or chest while swallowing. The etiology of dysphagia can be mechanical or functional in nature. Odynophagia is pain with swallowing. Globus sensation is the feeling of something "stuck" or "tightness" in the esophagus. This symptom may be unrelated to swallowing, separating it from dysphagia.

Chest pain can be a manifestation of esophageal disease, but cardiac disease should always be considered. Chest pain related to cardiac disease, or angina, can have characteristics similar to those associated with esophageal-related chest pain. A careful history and physical examination with appropriate diagnostic studies can help distinguish the etiology of chest pain.

DIAGNOSTIC STUDIES OF THE ESOPHAGUS

Radiology

Barium esophagography, a video fluoroscopic procedure, can be used to assess dysphagia and can diagnose structural abnormalities in the esophagus or altered motility. When performed with a speech therapist (a modified barium swallow), it can be used to study the swallowing mechanism in more detail. A timed barium esophagogram can be used to assess esophageal emptying.

Computed tomography (CT) and magnetic resonance imaging (MRI) can often be used to define anatomy further and assess disease outside the lumen and beyond the mucosa. Positron emission tomography (PET) can be used to evaluate the esophagus but is typically used to evaluate malignant pathology when there is concern for metastasis.

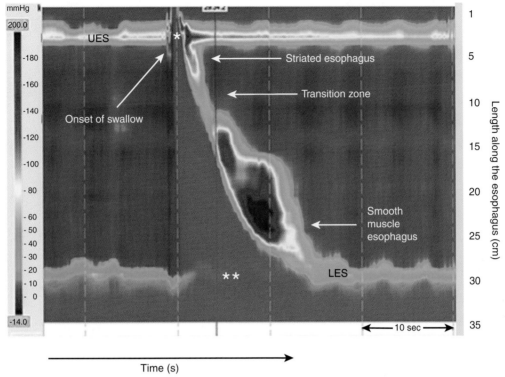

Fig. 36.1 High-resolution manometry (HRM) of normal esophageal peristalsis. HRM catheter consisting of 36 pressure sensors is inserted via the nares into the stomach to provide a complete physiologic pressure map of the hypopharynx, upper esophageal sphincter (UES), esophagus, lower esophageal sphincter (LES) and stomach. The Y-axis represents with sensor location; whereas the X-axis represents time. The color variation represents the different pressures along the length of the catheter at a given time and location. The resting UES and LES are shown as horizontal color bands. The relaxations of the UES (*) and LES (**) are shown as decreases in pressures (corresponding to approximately 20 mm Hg on color-pressure bar). The LES opens shortly after the UES relaxes with the onset of a wet swallow. Esophageal primary peristalsis is shown as a diagonal color band running from the UES to the LES. The onset of the swallow is seen on HRM as the high pressure contraction in the proximal, striated esophagus, followed by a lower pressure segment corresponding to the transition zone and a subsequent increase in pressure in the smooth muscle esophagus.

Endoscopy and Endoscopic Imaging

Esophagogastroduodenoscopy (EGD, upper endoscopy) allows for a direct visualization of the mucosal surface of the esophagus, stomach, and duodenum. An endoscope is a flexible fiberoptic tube with a camera that can be used for the diagnosis, screening, monitoring, and treatment of various pathologies. Endoscopes have additional channels through which a variety of endoscopic tools (i.e., forceps, dilators, injection needles, hemostatic tools) can be used to sample or treat the visualized area.

Endoscopic ultrasound (EUS) incorporates an ultrasound probe on the end of an endoscope. This ultrasound allows for imaging and biopsy across the wall of the esophagus and other nearby anatomical structures.

Manometry

Esophageal manometry is a physiologic evaluation of esophageal contractile function. High-resolution manometry is the diagnostic gold standard for the diagnosis of motility disorders. It utilizes a catheter lined with 20 to 36 pressure sensors at 1-cm intervals that is inserted via the nasal passage to the gastric body. The sensors record and compute the frequency and pressures of esophageal peristaltic waves and LES and UES function. The high-resolution manometry pressures are used to generate esophageal pressure topographies represented by color-coded, pressure-space-time plots. These objective metrics are applied to the Chicago Classification to diagnose esophageal motility disorders (Fig. 36.1).

Esophageal pH Monitoring

Esophageal wireless pH monitoring and catheter-based reflux testing are diagnostic tools used to study reflux disease. The wireless pH capsule is typically positioned 5 cm above the LES. The capsule measures the pH at the site for 24 to 48 hours in the ambulatory setting. The data are then reported as a percentage of the day the pH remains below 4. A combined impedance-pH probe measures acid and non-acid reflux as well as the direction of transit of a food or fluid bolus.

STRUCTURAL DISORDERS

Cricopharyngeal Bars

A cricopharyngeal bar is a radiographic finding consisting of a prominent posterior indentation of the esophagus at the level of the cricopharyngeus that is often asymptomatic but can contribute to dysphagia. The prominence is thought to be due to muscle spasm or impairment of muscle compliance at the UES. Cricopharyngeal bars can be managed via surgical and nonsurgical interventions. Nonsurgical options include dilation at the site or injection of botulinum toxin. Surgical management technique occurs via cricopharyngeal myotomy.

Diverticula

Diverticula of the esophagus are outpouchings contained within layers of the esophageal wall. True diverticula involve all layers to the esophageal wall, whereas false diverticula are limited to the submucosa and mucosa.

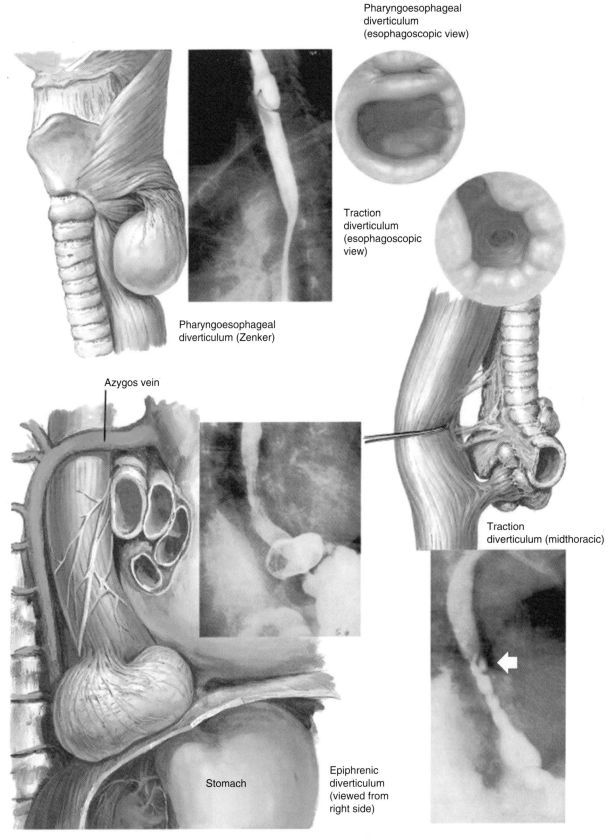

Fig. 36.2 Esophageal diverticula.

All diverticula are further categorized by their location. They are classified as proximal or pharyngoesophageal (Zenker's and Killian-Jamieson) diverticula, mid-esophageal or traction or parabronchial diverticula, and epiphrenic diverticula. The prevalence of Zenker's diverticula (ZD) ranges from 0.01% to 0.11%, and the majority of patients are diagnosed in their sixth to eighth decades of life. The prevalence of the other types of diverticula are unknown but are far less common than Zenker's diverticula (Fig. 36.2).

ZD forms in the Killian triangle, an area of sparse musculature bordered by the cricopharyngeus and thyropharyngeus muscles in the posterior pharyngeal wall. As a result of diminished compliance of the cricopharyngeus muscle and the UES, the hypopharynx is exposed to increased intra-bolus pressures while swallowing, causing the ZD to form. ZD are false diverticula. Parabronchial diverticula are likely associated with mediastinal fibrosis, which is often due to inflammation of the mediastinum caused by other pathology (i.e., fungal infections, tuberculosis). Traction on the esophageal wall causes these diverticula to form. Long-standing distal esophageal obstruction can lead to the formation of pulsion diverticula either through anatomic abnormalities or motility disorders. Diffuse esophageal spasm has been associated with parabronchial diverticula, whereas achalasia has been associated with epiphrenic diverticula. The latter two are true diverticula.

Patients with ZD often present with oropharyngeal dysphagia but can also suffer from complete esophageal obstruction. Classically, these patients will complain of dysphagia with regurgitation and halitosis. Parabronchial and epiphrenic diverticula are most often asymptomatic and diagnosed as incidental findings on imaging. The complications of these diverticula are typically related to their underlying disorders (i.e., motility disorders).

Diverticula are diagnosed using barium swallow, endoscopy, and computed tomography. Manometry can also be used to diagnose underlying motility issues that contribute to diverticula formation.

Symptomatic ZD should be treated. Smaller ZD can be treated with cricopharyngeal myotomy alone. Larger ZD may need additional interventions, including diverticulum suspension or diverticulectomy. Endoscopic cricopharyngeal myotomy is an alternative to surgical approaches. Parabronchial and epiphrenic diverticula are most successfully addressed by treating the underlying disorder (i.e., motility disorders or strictures). They can also involve extended myotomy and diverticulectomy.

Rings and Webs

Esophageal rings are areas of narrowing in the esophageal lumen. An "A" ring is a muscular ring found in the upper part of the phrenic ampulla at the area of highest pressure in the LES and is defined by smooth muscle hypertrophy with normal surface epithelium. A "B" (or Schatzki) ring is a mucosal ring at the squamocolumnar junction with squamous epithelium above the ring and columnar epithelium below. This ring can lead to luminal narrowing and dysphagia. Their etiology and pathophysiology are poorly understood.

Patients with Schatzki ring often complain of dysphagia to solid food that is chronic and intermittent. The diameter of the ring is inversely associated with the incidence and symptoms. A barium swallow with a full column technique is the best modality to diagnose Schatzki rings. An endoscope can visualize Schatzki rings but can miss rings with larger diameters.

The treatment of all esophageal rings is mechanical dilation. This can be performed with Savary dilators or radial expanding balloon dilators. There is a high rate of reoccurrence after treatment and a scant 11% of patients are symptom free after 3 years. However, repeated dilations can be performed without increasing the complication rate.

An esophageal web is a thin, membranous tissue covered with squamous epithelium that reduces the size of the esophageal lumen. The webs can be congenital or acquired. Congenital webs are rare. Acquired esophageal webs are associated with Plummer-Vinson syndrome (iron deficiency anemia, glossitis, koilonychia, and esophageal/pharyngeal carcinoma).

Patients with esophageal webs will present with dysphagia. The webs are diagnosed by barium swallow or endoscopy. Lifestyle modifications are encouraged to reduced symptoms, but some patients must be treated with mechanical dilation similar to the treatment for Schatzki rings.

Malignancy

Esophageal cancer is the seventh most common cancer and the sixth leading cause of cancer-related mortality worldwide. The five-year survival rate after diagnosis is 15% to 20%. The incidence of esophageal cancer varies by region. In developed countries, the incidence of squamous cell cancer (SCC) has fallen and adenocarcinoma has become the leading type. However, SCC remains more prevalent worldwide. The major risk factors for developing SCC are alcohol and tobacco use. There are other carcinogens which, similar to alcohol and tobacco, are thought to lead to inflammation and dysplasia. Tobacco is a moderate risk factor for the adenocarcinoma. Obesity and body mass index remain the strongest risk factors for the development of esophageal adenocarcinoma. Obesity can predispose patients to GERD and Barrett esophagus, which also cause adenocarcinoma. The progression of gastrointestinal reflux disease to adenocarcinoma is described in a subsequent section (Fig. 36.3).

With esophageal cancer, patients often complain of progressive dysphagia and weight loss. Depending on the progression of symptoms, they may also present with anemia or other symptoms. The treatment of esophageal cancer depends on progression and staging but can involve chemotherapy, radiation, surgery, and/or palliative measures.

Hiatal Hernias

A hiatal hernia results in abdominal contents, such as the stomach, becoming displaced above the diaphragm. Hiatal hernias are subcategorized into four types: type I (sliding hiatal hernia), type II (paraesophageal hernia; the proximal stomach protrudes up through the diaphragm along the distal esophagus), type III (a combination of type I and type II), and type IV (herniation of other abdominal organs). Sliding hiatal hernias are the most common variety. Types II through IV are considered variations of paraesophageal hernias (Fig. 36.4).

Sliding hernias are a result of laxity in the phrenoesophageal membrane, a membrane that anchors the esophagus to the diaphragm. This results in a widening of the hiatal tunnel, allowing the gastric cardia to herniate into the thorax. Increasing age and obesity often contribute to the decreasing elasticity of the phrenoesophageal membrane. Paraesophageal hernias are caused by defects in this membrane.

Hernias may be diagnosed by plain film, barium swallow studies, cross-sectional imaging, and endoscopy. Asymptomatic hiatal hernias rarely need to be treated. If a type I hiatal hernia is associated with GERD, then medical or surgical treatment should be considered. The course of treatment would focus on treating the symptoms of GERD. Paraesophageal hernias (type II-IV) are prone to complications including volvulus, obstruction, incarceration, and perforation and should be treated expediently because continued enlargement will lead to worsening symptoms and complications.

GASTROESOPHAGEAL REFLUX DISEASE AND SEQUELAE

A consensus (the Montreal consensus, specifically) amongst a panel of world experts defined GERD as "a condition which develops when the reflux of stomach contents causes troublesome symptoms and/or complications." This definition includes symptomatic syndromes and syndromes with esophageal injury but does not include functional heartburn.

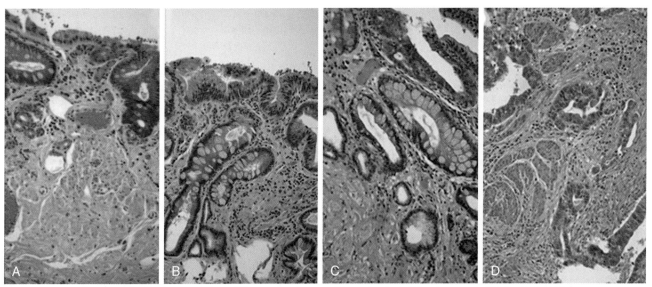

Fig. 36.3 Histologic progression of Barrett esophagus with no dysplasia (A) to low-grade (B) dysplasia, high-grade dysplasia (C), and esophageal adenocarcinoma (D).

Pathophysiology and Symptoms

The pathophysiology of GERD is determined by numerous factors including gastric acid–esophageal mucosa interaction, incompetence of the gastroesophageal junction, decrease in esophageal mucosal defenses, and altered sensory mechanisms that interpret the symptoms.

Numerous modalities can be used to help diagnose and manage GERD, but often history is enough to diagnose and begin treatment. The symptoms that are characteristic of GERD include heartburn and regurgitation. Chest pain can also be a presenting symptom but should be distinguished from cardiac chest pain. Patients can also present with less common, atypical symptoms such as dysphagia, dyspepsia, epigastric pain, bloating, nausea, and belching.

Diagnosis

The diagnosis of GERD is established using history of symptoms, objective testing (endoscopy and esophageal pH monitoring), and patient responsiveness to therapy. A proton pump inhibitor (PPI) trial is a method that may be used to diagnose GERD in patients with typical symptoms without concerning features that may include dysphagia, odynophagia, weight loss, anemia, nausea, or vomiting. A lack of response to PPIs does not exclude the diagnosis of GERD, and atypical symptoms are not as reliable at predicting response. Therefore, objective testing with endoscopy or esophageal pH monitoring should be considered in patients who do not respond to PPIs.

Endoscopy provides direct visualization of the esophageal lumen and evaluation of the esophageal mucosa in patients with suspected GERD. It can demonstrate objective findings suggestive of GERD such as erosive esophagitis, strictures, and Barrett esophagus. Not all symptomatic patients will have evidence of erosions or mucosal damage, which can limit the diagnostic specificity of endoscopy. Endoscopy allows for biopsy of the mucosa, which is helpful in screening for Barrett esophagus, but can also aid in establishing another diagnosis. Eosinophilic esophagitis may have a similar presentation and biopsy can be used to differentiate between GERD without erosions and eosinophilic esophagitis. Biopsy is not recommended to diagnose GERD in patients with heartburn and normal endoscopy.

Esophageal pH monitoring with or without impedance may objectively demonstrate the presence of abnormal esophageal acid exposure, non-acid reflux, reflux frequency, and symptoms associated with reflux.

Management

Lifestyle modifications are a part of the initial therapy for GERD. Patients are counseled on behaviors that may improve symptoms and recommendation of avoidance of foods that trigger symptoms. Weight loss is advised for overweight and obese patients. Weight gain, even in patients with normal BMI, can provoke new GERD symptoms. Other behavior modifications include tobacco cessation, raising the head of the bed, and avoiding recumbent position for at least 2 hours after a meal. The common foods that can trigger heartburn and regurgitation include coffee, alcohol, chocolate, fatty foods, citrus, and spicy foods. It is important that all lifestyle modifications be tailored to each patient's symptoms and disease course.

When lifestyle modifications fail, medical interventions should be attempted. Medications that can treat GERD include antacids, histamine-receptor antagonists (H2 blockers), and PPIs. Patients often utilize over-the-counter antacids to provide symptom relief of GERD. These antacids work to neutralize gastric hydrochloric acid and inhibit pepsin. With the advent of H2 blockers and PPIs, antacid use has declined, but a smaller cohort of patients will continue using them for heartburn. H2 blockers reversibly bind to histamine H2 receptors, preventing histamine released during a meal from binding to receptors on ECL and parietal cells. PPIs are superior to H2 blockers because they essentially irreversibly block the hydrogen-potassium ATPase that secretes hydrochloric acid from the gastric parietal cells. They have been shown to contribute to esophageal healing and have decreased relapse rates when compared to H2 blockers. In addition, PPIs have also been shown to be superior for heartburn relief.

Surgical options can be considered for GERD or esophagitis refractory to medical therapy, when patients suffer side effects of medical therapy, exhibit noncompliance, or need correction of a concomitant large hiatal hernia. The surgical options for treatment include laparoscopic fundoplication or bariatric surgery. Laparoscopic fundoplication involves "wrapping" the fundus of the stomach around the end of the esophagus to help repair and provide support to the LES. Bariatric surgery with gastric bypass in obese patients with GERD can also be used to treat GERD.

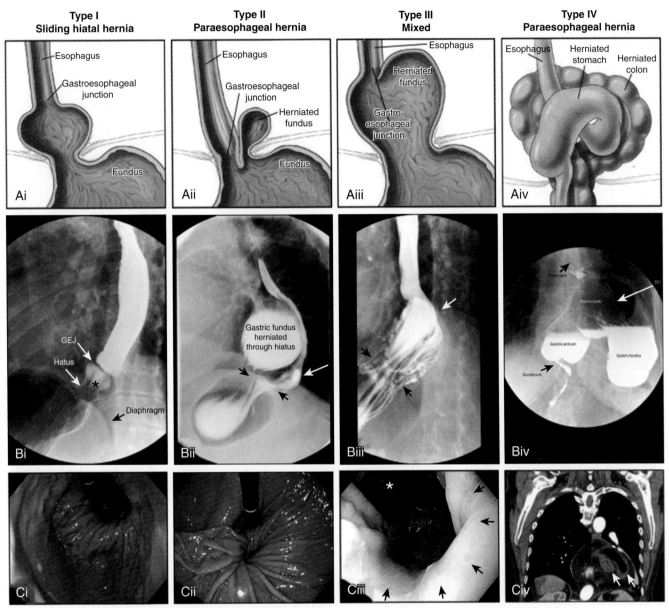

Fig. 36.4 Anatomic drawings (row A), barium contrast radiography (row B), and computed tomographic (iv) views (row C) of Type I or sliding hiatal hernia (column 1), Type II PEH (column 2), Type III PEH (column 3), and Type IV PEH (column 4). Pane Bi: *, sliding hiatal hernia. Pane Bii: True paraesophageal hernia adjacent to GEJ. Separation between GEJ and diaphragm noted, consistent with a small adjacent hiatal hernia. *White arrow:* Barium tablet present. *Black arrows:* Widened hiatus. Pane Biii: *White arrow:* Gastroesophageal junction. *Black arrows:* Widened diaphragmatic hiatus. Pane Biv: Herniated, intrathoracic stomach with herniation of duodenum. This stomach is flipped in an organoaxial rotation. Pane Ci: Sliding hiatal hernia. Pane Cii: Separate PEH present, herniated through laxity in phrenoesophageal membrane. Lax diaphragmatic hiatus also present. Pane Ciii: Image taken from the diaphragmatic hiatus *(black arrows)*. Herniation of GEJ noted with large adjacent fundus/PEH *(white asterisk)*. Pane Civ: Coronal computed tomography (CT) image of an intrathoracic stomach with herniated loops of colon *(white arrows)*. GEJ, Gastroesophageal junction; *PEH,* paraesophageal hernia.

Extraesophageal Manifestations of GERD

GERD contributes to several extraesophageal manifestations including respiratory, laryngopharyngeal, and dental symptoms. Respiratory symptoms include pulmonary disease (asthma, idiopathic pulmonary fibrosis, bronchitis, etc.), cough, wheezing, and shortness of breath. Laryngeal symptoms present as hoarseness, throat pain, globus, choking, postnasal drip, laryngeal and tracheal stenosis, and laryngospasm. Dental erosions can also be a result of GERD.

Non-GERD causes of extraesophageal manifestations should be considered prior to associating the symptoms with GERD. Diagnostic tools are

unable to provide reliable evidence of causality between GERD and extraesophageal symptoms. In addition, PPIs have not shown a clear therapeutic benefit in the treatment of these symptoms. The diagnosis of GERD, as described previously, can help with the association, but the presence or absence of GERD cannot reliably establish it as cause of extraesophageal symptoms. Clinicians often rely on symptom association analysis to find a temporal association between reflux symptoms and other symptoms.

Acid suppression with a PPI is still used to treat extraesophageal symptoms when typical GERD symptoms are present. When typical GERD symptoms are not present, reflux monitoring is considered prior to starting a PPI trial. Surgery is not generally considered in PPI nonresponders because the available data show no benefit in patients who have surgery.

Barrett Esophagus

Barrett esophagus (BE) is defined as the presence of at least 1 cm of metaplastic columnar epithelium in the tubular esophagus and can be described as either long-segment BE (>3 cm) or short-segment BE (<3 cm). It can further be described using the Prague classification system, which uses the circumferential extent of BE and the extent of the longest visualized segment.

BE can develop from long-standing GERD. The diagnosis of GERD is associated with a 10% to 15% risk of developing Barrett esophagus. The risk factors for developing BE are chronic GERD (>5 years), age greater than 50, male gender, tobacco use, central obesity, and Caucasian race. BE can progress to dysplasia and esophageal adenocarcinoma. The risk factors for progression include advancing age, central obesity, tobacco use, and lack of NSAID, PPI, or statin use. The majority (>90%) of patients diagnosed with BE do not die of esophageal adenocarcinoma. The risk of progression from BE to cancer is determined by the amount of dysplasia (nondysplastic is 0.2% to 0.5% risk per year, low-grade dysplasia is 0.7% risk per year, high-grade dysplasia is 7% per year).

Screening for BE should be considered in men with chronic GERD (>5 years) and/or weekly symptoms of reflux who have two additional risk factors: age greater than 50 years, Caucasian, central obesity, history of smoking, or first-degree relative with BE or adenocarcinoma. Although the progression of BE to adenocarcinoma is rare in females, they should still be screened based on the presence of the aforementioned risk factors. The endoscopist should take at least eight random biopsies to maximize yield on histology to look for intestinal metaplasia. The pathology from the biopsies is confirmed by two pathologists making the diagnosis. Alternative screening modalities include balloon cytology.

BE is treated with chemoprevention, endoscopic therapy, or surgery. All patients with BE should receive once-daily PPI for chemoprevention. Endoscopic treatment is not required in the absence of dysplasia. At initial diagnosis, if nodularity is observed in the suspected segment, the patient should undergo endoscopic mucosal resection as a diagnostic and therapeutic procedure. Endoscopic ablative therapy is used in patients with low-grade and high-grade dysplasia. Ablative techniques include radiofrequency ablation and the lesser used cryotherapy. Recurrence rates appear to be similar across different ablative modalities. Endoscopic ultrasound can also be used to evaluate the depth of invasion of nodules and adenocarcinoma, guiding definitive therapy. Antireflux surgery can be used in patients with poor control of reflux symptoms on PPI.

Endoscopic surveillance is continued to monitor for stability or progression of BE. The surveillance intervals are determined by the level of dysplasia from 3 to 5 years for patients without dysplasia, to as often as every 3 months for patients with high-grade dysplasia treated endoscopically. Surveillance endoscopy will collect four-quadrant biopsies at 2-cm intervals in patients without dysplasia and 1-cm interval in patients with prior dysplasia. Any visible abnormalities are also sampled. Virtual or chemical chromoendoscopy may enhance the yield of surveillance.

MOTILITY DISORDERS

Achalasia

Achalasia is a primary esophageal motor disorder defined as aperistalsis in the esophageal body and relaxation failure of the LES resulting in increased tone in the LES. The pathophysiology of achalasia is related to the loss of inhibitory innervation in the esophagus. Primary achalasia is caused by the failure of distal inhibitory neurons (ganglion cells) in the esophageal myenteric plexus. Denervation can also occur within the extraesophageal vagus nerve or dorsal motor nucleus of the vagus. Cholinergic innervation has also been found to remain intact and

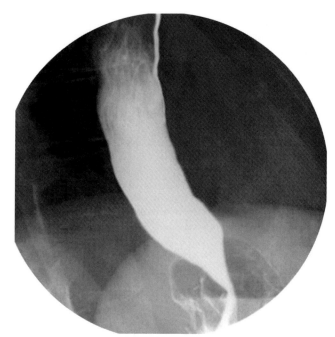

Fig. 36.5 Barium contrast radiography demonstrating narrowing at the esophagogastric junction with a bird-beak appearance and a dilated distal esophagus with retained contrast and an air-fluid level.

could possibly contribute to the increase in LES pressure. The denervation is thought to be an autoimmune process with increasing evidence, suggesting that genetic susceptibility and latent human herpes simplex virus 1 may also play a role. This is considered primary achalasia and is idiopathic by definition.

Dysphagia to solids and liquids is the classic presentation, but patients may also suffer from regurgitation, heartburn, and chest pain. Initial work-up of achalasia includes a barium swallow and/or endoscopy. A barium swallow can show esophageal dilation with a bird-beak narrowing around the gastroesophageal junction (Fig. 36.5). An endoscopy allows observation of esophageal dilation, a high-pressure LES, and the possibility of retained food in the esophagus and helps to exclude causes of secondary achalasia. The "gold standard" for the diagnosis of achalasia is high-resolution esophageal manometry. Manometry can record aperistalsis in the distal esophagus and absent LES relaxation. High-resolution manometry has defined subsets of patients with achalasia, using the Chicago Classification, who have different responses to treatment and prognoses. Type I, or classic achalasia, shows aperistalsis, incomplete or absent LES relaxation, and high resting LES pressure. Type II shows panesophageal pressurization with swallows and type III shows spastic lumen obliterating contractions of the distal esophagus with 20% or more of swallows.

The goal of treating achalasia is to promote esophageal emptying and decrease LES pressure. The initial (and most effective) treatment options include pneumatic dilation or laparoscopic surgical (Heller) myotomy. Pneumatic dilation is an endoscopic approach used to treat achalasia, involving the use of balloons to dilate the LES, theoretically breaking the fibers within. The number and the degree of dilations are determined by progression of symptom relief. Surgical (Heller) myotomy can provide a permanent solution by cutting the LES, allowing for food and liquid to pass through freely. In patients who are poor candidates for definitive therapy, endoscopy can be used to inject botulinum toxin into the gastroesophageal junction, which inhibits acetylcholine release from nerves. Acetylcholine is responsible for increased LES tone, especially when there is denervation of the inhibitory nerves. Botulinum toxin will thereby reduce the tone of the LES. If botulinum toxin therapy fails, pharmacologic therapy with nitrates and calcium-channel blockers may be considered, but the effects do not provide long-term treatment. The newest approach to treatment, POEM (Per Oral Endoscopic Myotomy), uses an endoscope to tunnel below the esophageal mucosa to perform a myotomy from within, without the need for surgical incisions.

Diffuse Esophageal Spasm

Diffuse esophageal spasm (DES) is defined by uncoordinated contractions in the esophagus. Esophageal manometry provides the most specific description of the spasms. Specifically, the Chicago Classification defines DES as 20% or greater premature contractions (<4.5 seconds) with normal LES relaxation. Patients often present with dysphagia and chest pain. Similar to achalasia, DES is likely related to a decrease in inhibitory innervation. This is often observed on barium swallow.

Pharmacologic therapy has been ineffective in reliably treating DES. Pneumatic dilation of the LES or the esophageal body may alleviate some of the symptoms, but botulinum toxin is used to a better effect.

VARIANT FORMS OF ESOPHAGITIS

Eosinophilic Esophagitis

Eosinophilic esophagitis (EoE) is (likely) an allergen-mediated eosinophilic-dominant inflammation of the esophageal mucosa and is diagnosed when esophageal biopsies in symptomatic patients show 15 or greater eosinophils per high-power microscopic field. When assessing for EoE, two to four esophageal biopsies should be taken from the proximal and distal esophagus. Endoscopy can visualize fixed esophageal rings in the lumen, which are characteristic, but not diagnostic, of EoE. These rings are often referred to as trachealization of the esophagus. Other features include white eosinophilic exudates, longitudinal furrows, edema, diffuse esophageal narrowing, strictures, and lacerations secondary to the endoscope.

When EoE is diagnosed, a PPI response should be tested. Following an 8-week PPI trial, a repeat endoscopy and biopsy should be performed. If symptoms and eosinophilia have resolved then PPI-responsive esophageal eosinophilia (PPI-REE) is diagnosed. PPI-REE may be associated with GERD. If symptoms and eosinophilia persist, then EoE is diagnosed.

The goal of treatment for EoE is improvement in symptoms and decrease in esophageal inflammation. The first-line pharmacologic therapy is 8 weeks of swallowed topical corticosteroids (fluticasone or budesonide). If symptoms do not improve or rapid improvement is needed, then systemic corticosteroids (i.e., prednisone) can be used. Conversely, a specific elimination diet can also be used as initial therapy prior to the administration of topical corticosteroids. When medical and dietary therapy fail, then esophageal dilation is considered in patients with strictures.

Pill-Induced Esophagitis

Pill-induced esophagitis results in direct esophageal mucosal injury due to a pill. Patients will complain of heartburn, chest pain, odynophagia, and dysphagia. Common medications that can cause this include: tetracycline, doxycycline, clindamycin, aspirin, nonsteroidal anti-inflammatory drugs (NSAIDs), bisphosphonates, potassium chloride, quinidine preparations, iron compounds, emepronium, alprenolol, and pinaverium.

Complications include stricture, esophageal hemorrhage, and perforation. Cessation of the offending agent is often enough to treat the condition with eventual mucosal healing.

ESOPHAGEAL INFECTIONS

Infections of the esophagus are rare in immunocompetent patients. Immunocompromised individuals are typically affected, including patients on immunosuppressive medications, chemotherapy, and patients suffering from AIDS. In patients with AIDS, infectious esophagitis is more prevalent as the CD4 count declines, especially with counts below 100. The most common symptom of infectious esophagitis is odynophagia often associated with dysphagia, chest pain, and gastrointestinal bleeding. Coinfection is common and treatment is targeted by etiology. Maintenance suppressive therapy with antifungal or antiviral agents may need to be initiated in patients with AIDS.

The most common cause of infectious esophagitis is *Candida*. It typically presents with dysphagia and odynophagia, but oral thrush in patients has a high positive predictive value for esophageal candidiasis. On endoscopy, friable white patches overlying the mucosa are visualized and fungal hyphal forms are seen on histology. Patients are typically treated successfully with oral fluconazole whereas intravenous fluconazole or an echinocandin is used in patients unable to tolerate oral therapy.

Cytomegalovirus (CMV) esophagitis occurs in severely immunocompromised patients. These patients present almost identically to patients with candida esophagitis except without oropharyngeal thrush. Endoscopy reveals large (>10 cm), shallow ulcers in the middle to distal parts of the esophagus. The margins are distinct and the ulcers are often described as "punched-out." Histopathologic examination of mucosal and submucosal biopsies from the ulcer edges and bases can accurately diagnose CMV esophagitis. Histology will reveal large endothelial cells or fibroblasts with large, dense inclusion bodies. CMV esophagitis is treated with intravenous ganciclovir, foscarnet (intravenous) or valganciclovir (intravenous or oral).

Another cause of infectious esophagitis is herpes simplex virus (HSV). HSV-1 is typically the offending strain, but HSV-2 can also be a cause. HSV esophagitis is often seen in immunosuppressed individuals but can affect healthy adults. The endoscopic appearance of HSV esophagitis is multiple, small, superficial ulcers in the distal esophagus. More advanced or aggressive infections can reveal large confluent ulcers, pseudomembranous or denuded epithelium. Viral cultures can grow HSV-1 and occasionally HSV-2. The quantitative polymerase chain reaction for HSV-1 has a high sensitivity when tested in biopsy samples. Histopathologic examination reveals large intranuclear Cowdry type-A inclusion bodies along with ballooning degeneration and multinucleated giant cells. HSV esophagitis is treated with acyclovir (oral or intravenous) or valacyclovir (oral).

ESOPHAGEAL TRAUMA AND EMERGENCIES

Perforation of the Esophagus

Perforation of the esophagus can be due to numerous etiologies. The most common cause is iatrogenic but can occur due to trauma, caustic injury, malignancy, or severe vomiting. Iatrogenic perforation is often related to instrumentation from endoscopy, nasogastric tube insertion, intubation, or dilation. Boerhaave syndrome describes the spontaneous rupture of the esophagus following severe vomiting.

The most common presenting symptom is pain, which can vary depending on location of the perforation. Patients may also present with symptoms of shock or systemic infection. A physical exam can reveal palpable crepitus in the neck or chest related to subcutaneous emphysema.

Esophageal perforation should be diagnosed and treated promptly. A chest radiograph can suggest perforation by revealing mediastinal air, pleural effusion, pneumothorax, and subdiaphragmatic air. The diagnosis can be confirmed with computed tomography, Gastrografin imaging or emergency endoscopy.

The treatment of esophageal perforation starts with adequate resuscitation and early antibiotics, if needed. The perforation can be repaired surgically or by endoscope. Surgery is indicated in unstable patients or patients with abdominal esophageal perforations. An endoscope can be used to place stents or clips. Perforations can be treated conservatively as well with medical management. This includes no oral intake for at least 7 days, parenteral nutrition, empiric antibiotics (consider antifungals), and management of complications (i.e., drainage of abscesses).

Foreign Bodies and Food Impaction

Ingestion of foreign bodies can be accidental or intentional. Symptoms depends on the object's size, shape, consistency, and location, but some patients will remain asymptomatic. Food can also become lodged in the esophagus and present with similar symptoms to foreign bodies. Food impaction is normally the result of an underlying disease process including peptic stricture, Schatzki ring, EoE, or malignancy.

Foreign bodies and food can result in complete obstruction of the esophagus. Patients will present with inability to handle secretions and severe chest pain. If the obstruction does not resolve spontaneously, emergent endoscopy is often required to resolve the obstruction. Occasionally, glucagon can be administered intravenously when food impaction is suspected prior to endoscopic intervention. Glucagon relaxes the LES and esophageal smooth muscle allowing for spontaneous passage of the bolus.

Mallory-Weiss Tear

A Mallory-Weiss tear is a mucosal or submucosal tear near the gastroesophageal junction. It results from anything that may cause a rapid increase in intra-abdominal pressure and gastric herniation. It is most often described in the setting of retching or vomiting but can also occur as a result of increased strain or forceful coughing.

Patients present with hematemesis and/or melena. They will often report excessive retching or vomiting, but the tear can also occur without this history. Endoscopy is used to diagnose a tear and rule out other causes of an upper gastrointestinal bleed.

Supportive therapy involves treating the underlying disorder and reducing instances of vomiting and retching. A Mallory-Weiss tear can be massive but is rarely fatal. Endoscopic therapies for ongoing bleeding include use of epinephrine, which can be injected locally to reduce bleeding. Cauterization, clipping, and ligation can also be used to control the site of bleeding. Patients with persistent bleeding may undergo angiographic intervention or, in rare instances, surgical intervention.

SYSTEMIC AND OTHER ILLNESSES

Scleroderma

Progressive systemic sclerosis can affect any part of the gastrointestinal tract, but more often involves the esophagus. The progressive loss of smooth muscle, collagen deposition, and fibrosis in the esophageal wall can cause reduced or absent peristalsis, GERD, and a patulous LES. Manometry is used to diagnose the esophageal disease, whereas endoscopy can be used to evaluate for complications.

Dermatologic Disorders

A wide variety of dermatologic disorders can affect the esophagus. These disorders include pemphigus vulgaris, bullous pemphigoid, erythema multiforme, Behçet's syndrome, lichen planus, dermatitis herpetiformis, and toxic epidermolysis necrosis/Stevens-Johnson syndrome. The treatment of the underlying disorder is most effective in treating the esophageal involvement and often involves glucocorticoids.

SUGGESTED READINGS

Ajani JA, D'Amico TA, Bentrem DJ, et al: Esophageal and esophagogastric junction cancers, version 2.2019, NCCN clinical practice guidelines in oncology, J Natl Compr Canc Netw 17(7):855–883, 2019.

Dellon ES, Gonsalves N, Hirano I, et al: ACG clinical guideline: evidenced based approach to the diagnosis and management of esophageal eosinophilia and eosinophilic esophagitis (EoE), Am J Gastroenterol 108(5):679–692, 2013.

Kahrilas PJ, Bredenoord AJ, Fox M, et al: The Chicago Classification of esophageal motility disorders, v3.0, Neurogastroenterol Motil 27(2): 160–174, 2015.

Shaheen NJ, Falk GW, Iyer PG, Gerson LB, American College of Gastroenterology: ACG clinical guideline: diagnosis and management of Barrett's esophagus, Am J Gastroenterol 111(1):30–50, 2016.

Vakil N, van Zenten SV, Kahrilas P, et al: The Montreal definition and classification of gastroesophageal reflux disease: a global evidence-based consensus, Am J Gastroenterol 101(8):1900–1920, 2006; quiz 1943.

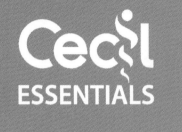

37

Diseases of the Stomach and Duodenum

Alma M. Guerrero Bready, Akwi W. Asombang, Steven F. Moss

INTRODUCTION

The process of digestion begins in the mouth, with mastication. The ingested food bolus is then propelled into the esophagus, passes through the lower esophageal sphincter (LES), and enters the stomach. The stomach can hold between 1.5 and 2 L of food, which allows for intermittent feeding. While in the stomach, food is further broken down through a series of chemical and mechanical reactions into smaller particles (chyme) that travel through the pyloric channel into the beginning of the small intestine, the duodenum. This chapter reviews the normal anatomy and physiology of the stomach and duodenum and discusses the most common disease processes affecting these two organs.

ANATOMY

Anatomy of the Stomach

The stomach is a hollow organ with a superior dome-like structure on the lateral aspect (the fundus) (Fig. 37.1). The outer edge along the dome and down to the end of the stomach is called the greater curvature. On the other side is the lesser curvature. The stomach is made up of four parts: the cardia, fundus, corpus, and the pylorus. The stomach is connected proximally to the distal esophagus by the LES, a circular smooth muscle structure under parasympathetic and sympathetic control. The LES acts as a valve to prevent gastric contents from traveling in a retrograde fashion into the esophagus, thus preventing gastroesophageal reflux. The most proximal region of the stomach is the cardia, which is the area between the LES and the fundus. Below the fundus is the gastric body (also known as the corpus), which has characteristic longitudinal folds or ridges (rugae). This gastric body is where food is mainly mixed and broken down. Below a prominent circular fold (the *angulus incisura*), is the antrum, which leads into the pyloric channel. The antrum holds food until it is ready to be released through the pylorus (a circular structure made up of smooth muscle) into the duodenum. A hiatal hernia occurs when part of the stomach is pushed upward through a weakness in the diaphragm into the chest.

The stomach is innervated and controlled by both the sympathetic nervous system, via the celiac plexus, and by the parasympathetic nervous system, which is supplied by the anterior and posterior trunks of the vagus nerve. The arterial supply for the stomach originates from the celiac trunk (Video 37.1).

Anatomy of the Duodenum

Immediately past the pylorus, the duodenum bends posteriorly to become a retroperitoneal structure and curves around the head of the pancreas in a C-shape and then re-emerges into the peritoneal cavity to join the second portion of the small intestine, the jejunum (see Fig. 37.1). The duodenum can be divided into four parts: superior (first part, or bulb), descending (second part), horizontal (third part), and ascending (fourth part). Within the descending duodenum is the ampulla of Vater, where the biliary system and the pancreatic duct unite to drain their secretions into the duodenum via the major duodenal papilla.

Similar to the stomach and the rest of the digestive tract, the duodenum is innervated by both the parasympathetic and sympathetic nervous system. The blood supply to the first half of the duodenum is from projections of the celiac trunk and to the second half of the duodenum by the superior mesenteric artery. It is this transition point that demarcates the progression from foregut to midgut.

HISTOLOGY

Histology of the Stomach

The walls of the stomach and duodenum, like the rest of the digestive system, are composed of four layers: the mucosa, submucosa, muscularis externa, and serosa. In the stomach, the mucosa is formed by a layer of simple columnar epithelial cells that invaginate to create gastric pits. These extend into millions of gastric glands that secrete gastric acid and other products. The depth and function of the gastric pits and glands differ between the various regions of the stomach. Below the mucosa is the submucosa, which houses dense connective tissue and lymphocytes, plasma cells, arterioles, venules, lymphatics, and the submucosal plexus (Meissner plexus). Deeper to this layer is the muscularis externa, which provides the contractions needed for the stomach to churn chyme. This muscle layer contains the inner oblique, middle circular, and outer longitudinal smooth muscle layers. In addition, it contains the myenteric neural plexus (Auerbach plexus). The outermost layer of the stomach is a continuation of the visceral peritoneum called the serosa.

Histology of the Duodenum

The duodenal wall is also comprised of the mucosa, submucosa, muscularis externa, and serosa. However, in the case of the duodenum, the epithelial cells contain microvilli and are arranged such that the surface of the duodenum has projections of epithelial cells called villi that are flanked by intestinal glands, called crypts of Lieberkühn. Villi and microvilli serve to increase the absorptive surface of the duodenum. In addition to its primarily absorptive function, the submucosa of the duodenum contains Brunner glands, which secrete an acid-neutralizing solution that protects the rest of the digestive tract from the effects of the acidic gastric juices.

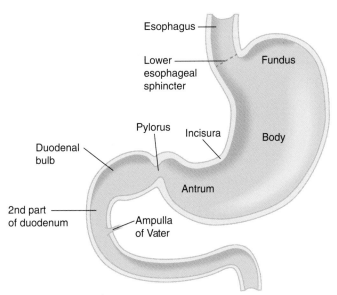

Fig. 37.1 Normal gastroduodenal anatomy.

GASTRODUODENAL SECRETIONS

Gastric secretions are responsible for breaking down food macromolecules into nutrients that can be absorbed in the gut. Gastric secretions are finely coordinated in a sophisticated system of feedback loops that ensure the balance between an acidic environment to break down food (created by parietal cells secreting hydrochloric acid) and a protective environment that defends the integrity of the gastric lumen. The latter is achieved by secretion of a bicarbonate-rich water/electrolyte/mucus solution from surface mucosal cells that buffers the gastric acid, to prevent autodigestion of the gastric epithelial cells and glands. Gastric secretions also function to protect the digestive tract from pathogenic microorganisms and aid in the absorption of calcium, iron, and vitamin B_{12}.

Parietal Cells
Acid Secretion
Gastric juice is primarily made up of hydrochloric acid (HCl), which is secreted by parietal cells at a concentration of 160 mmol/L. Parietal cells are mostly located in the gastric fundus and body, and they are stimulated to release HCl through three major pathways.

Histamine is released by specialized neuroendocrine cells called enterochromaffin-like (ECL) cells, and it is the major stimulant of H+ ion secretion. Histamine acts on H2 receptors, to activate adenylate cyclase leading to increased level of intracellular cAMP. This results in activation of the proton pumps (H+, K+-ATPases), located on the apical surface of the cell, to promote the release of HCl into the gastric lumen (Fig. 37.2).

Acetylcholine (Ach), which is released from nerve endings following vagal stimulation, also promotes acid secretion by acting on the M3 receptor on the basal aspect of parietal cells This increases intracellular Ca++, which also stimulates acid release into the stomach lumen via the apical proton pump (see Fig. 37.2).

Gastrin promotes acid release in two distinct ways (see Fig. 37.2). Gastrin is released from G cells in the antrum in response to food (especially protein) and also in response to the neural release of gastrin-related peptide, stimulated by gastric distension. Gastrin circulates in the bloodstream and may directly bind CCK2/gastrin receptors in parietal cells, stimulating the release of H+. Of greater functional consequence during feeding, gastrin also stimulates acid secretion indirectly by binding similar CCK2/gastrin receptors in ECL cells to

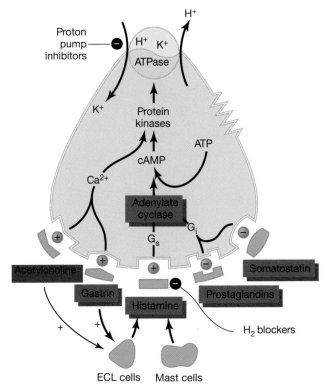

Fig. 37.2 Stimuli and mechanisms of gastric acid secretion by the parietal cell.

promote the release of histamine, which in turn acts on H2 receptors on parietal cells, as previously mentioned.

Acid secretion is inhibited by somatostatin, which is released by D cells in the gastric antrum and fundus. D cells are stimulated to secrete somatostatin when there is a high concentration of H+ ions in the gastric lumen, and they are inhibited by ACh. Somatostatin inhibits acid secretion by decreasing cAMP levels in parietal cells and by inhibiting gastrin release from G cells (see Fig. 37.2).

Intrinsic Factor
In addition to being the key cell for acid secretion, parietal cells also secrete intrinsic factor, a glycoprotein that plays a critical role in vitamin B_{12} absorption. Intrinsic factor is released from parietal cells under the same stimuli as H+ ions and binds vitamin B_{12} in the alkaline environment of the duodenum. This binding ultimately enables vitamin B_{12} absorption via specific receptors in the terminal ileum.

Chief Cells
Chief cells are zymogenic cells located deep in the gastric pits that secrete the pro-enzyme pepsinogen. Pepsinogen is converted into the active form, pepsin, under the acidic conditions created by gastric juices. Pepsin aids in digestion by breaking down proteins into peptides and amino acids, which, as mentioned above, aid in the release of gastrin as well as CCK.

Protective Factors
Gastroduodenal cells are at a high risk for damage given the very low pH of gastric juices, but these cells are well protected by several mechanisms that prevent autodigestion. The first line of defense is a mucosal barrier that consists of a thick, alkaline, aqueous mucus and HCO_3^--rich fluid that serves to lubricate the mucosa and neutralize acid at the epithelial level. This mucus is secreted in the stomach by mucus-producing cells located at the neck of gastric pits and in the

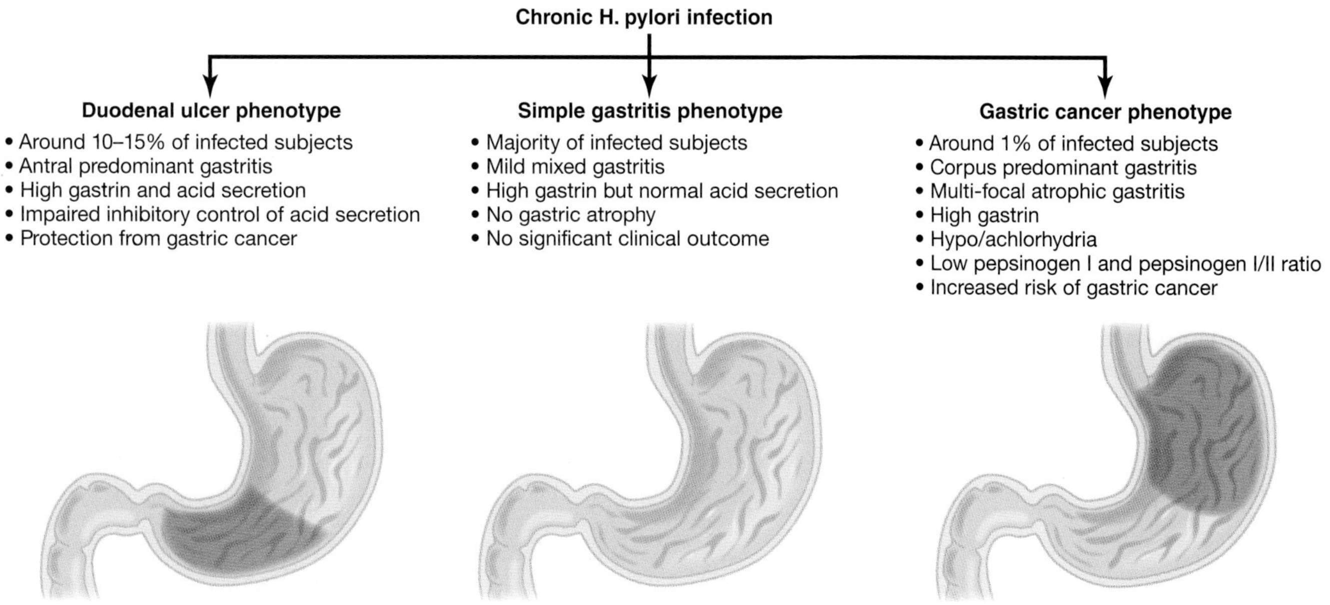

Chronic H. pylori infection

Duodenal ulcer phenotype	Simple gastritis phenotype	Gastric cancer phenotype
• Around 10–15% of infected subjects • Antral predominant gastritis • High gastrin and acid secretion • Impaired inhibitory control of acid secretion • Protection from gastric cancer	• Majority of infected subjects • Mild mixed gastritis • High gastrin but normal acid secretion • No gastric atrophy • No significant clinical outcome	• Around 1% of infected subjects • Corpus predominant gastritis • Multi-focal atrophic gastritis • High gastrin • Hypo/achlorhydria • Low pepsinogen I and pepsinogen I/II ratio • Increased risk of gastric cancer

Fig. 37.3 Diverse pathologic and clinical consequences of *H. pylori*. Acid secretory status and ultimately clinical outcome are dependent upon the extent and degree of gastric inflammation in response to *H. pylori* infection. (From Amieva MR, El-Omar EM. Host-bacterial interactions in *Helicobacter pylori* infection. Gastroenterology. 2008;134:306-23.)

duodenum by mucus-producing goblet cells. Additionally, the lipid bilayer and tight junctions of the apical epithelial cell membranes serve to protect the mucosa from H+ ions diffusing into the stomach wall, thus preserving mucosal integrity. A rich submucosal blood supply enables rapid drainage of H+ ions from the mucosa and neutralizes H+ ions intravascularly with HCO_3^- and proteins. Of note, prostaglandins promote blood flow, mucus secretion, and stimulation of HCO_3^- secretion, thus prostaglandins play an important role in gastric mucosal defense.

GASTRODUODENAL MOTILITY

The physiology of gastric motility and emptying can be understood via two major gastric geographic regions. As food enters the stomach, it increases gastric intraluminal pressure, causing the fundus and proximal body to relax reflexively (a process called accommodation) in order to allow space to store recently ingested food. The proximal stomach, however, also has characteristic tonic contractions, which aid in downstream gastric emptying.

Distally in the stomach, high-pressure peristaltic contractions by the lower gastric body and the antrum grind food and liquefy it into chyme. Once food particles reach a small enough size, they are propelled through the pylorus and into the duodenum.

Gastroduodenal motility is coordinated through intrinsic and extrinsic neural and hormonal signals. Neuronal control originates from the enteric nervous system and the sympathetic and parasympathetic nervous system via gastric mechanoreceptors, whereas certain hormones, such as gastrin and cholecystokinin, serve to relax the proximal stomach and create contractions in the distal stomach.

A series of negative feedback loops initiated by the presence of chyme within the duodenum inhibit further gastric emptying into the duodenum.

PEPTIC ULCER DISEASE

Definition and Epidemiology

A peptic ulcer is a defect or defects in the mucosal layer of the stomach or duodenum measuring at least 5 mm in diameter that penetrates into the muscularis mucosa. Lesions that are smaller than 5 mm or more superficial to the muscularis mucosa are classified as erosions. Men and women are at equal risk for developing peptic ulcer disease (PUD), and in the United States the lifetime risk of suffering from PUD is about 5% to 10%.

Gastric acid plays an important role in the digestion of food. PUD development is the result of an imbalance of gastric acid and other noxious substances in the gastric lumen relative to gastric protective functions. Some persons with PUD do secrete excessive amounts of gastric acid, particularly in duodenal ulcer disease, where depletion of antral somatostatin by *Helicobacter pylori* leads predictably to gastrin and acid hypersecretion (Fig. 37.3). However, most people with PUD have normal-to-low acid secretion, suggesting that a defect in mucosal defense is the major pathophysiologic culprit.

The two most common causes of PUD are *H. pylori* infection and the use of nonsteroidal anti-inflammatory drugs (NSAIDs). These two factors compromise mucosal defense mechanisms and predispose patients to peptic ulcers. They work synergistically to increase the risk of PUD when both factors are present. The risk of developing PUD increases with age, and, given that the prevalence of *H. pylori* has been decreasing in the general population and the use of NSAIDs has been increasing among older persons, the incidence of PUD has been decreasing in younger age groups (who tend to have low rates of NSAID use and *H. pylori* infection), and increasing in persons 65 years of age and older.

Other factors also modulate the risk of developing PUD. For example, smoking impairs ulcer healing, increases the risk of recurrence, and is associated with a higher PUD-related mortality. Similarly, there is an association between PUD development and concomitant use of high-dose corticosteroids with NSAIDs, though there is no evidence that corticosteroids alone cause PUD.

Less common causes of PUD include hypersecretory states such as Zollinger-Ellison syndrome, Crohn's disease, vascular insufficiency, viral infection, radiation therapy, and cancer therapy. Development of PUD may also be influenced by other factors such as stress, personality type, alcohol consumption, occupation, and diet, though these play a relatively minor role compared with the effects of *H. pylori* infection and NSAID usage.

Additionally, certain chronic diseases are positively correlated with PUD. These include chronic obstructive pulmonary disease, systemic mastocytosis, cirrhosis, and uremia.

Given that PUD is a complex disease resulting from diverse pathophysiologic processes, this chapter focuses on the different etiologic agents and mechanisms individually, after considering the shared clinical features.

Clinical Presentation

The clinical presentation of PUD varies depending on the location and severity of the ulcer. Uncomplicated PUD typically presents as sharp, burning, nonradiating epigastric abdominal pain. In duodenal ulcers the pain tends to occur 2 to 3 hours after the ingestion of food or at night, when the stomach is empty. The opposite is often true of gastric ulcers. Patients with duodenal ulcers tend to present with weight gain because the ingestion of food relieves symptoms, whereas patients with gastric ulcers tend to be food averse and are more likely to present with weight loss. Older patients (>60 years) may report no pain at all at the time of presentation and may instead present with nonspecific complaints, such as confusion, restlessness, abdominal distention, and falls. In pregnant patients, symptoms are often fairly mild and might even improve as the pregnancy progresses. They may also present as abnormal patterns of nausea and vomiting of pregnancy, such as nocturnal vomiting or worsening of vomiting in the third trimester. Most patients with PUD present after several weeks or months of symptoms, unless there is a complication that necessitates urgent medical care.

Diagnosis

The diagnosis of PUD requires clinical suspicion in patients with the appropriate clinical presentations. Physical exam may determine focal epigastric tenderness.

Contrast imaging with a barium upper GI series used to be the primary method of diagnosis but is now supplanted by the widespread availability of upper gastrointestinal endoscopy, now considered the "gold standard" for diagnosis because it permits direct visualization of the ulcer or ulcers.

In addition to providing a diagnosis of PUD, endoscopy also enables tissue sampling by biopsy to evaluate for malignancy and *H. pylori* infection. Furthermore, endoscopy can be therapeutic, providing curative hemostasis in patients with acute life-threatening GI bleeding secondary to PUD.

Causes of Peptic Ulcer Disease

There are several conditions associated with the development of ulcer disease; these may be present in isolation or coexist with each other. Identifying specific causes is important to prevent recurrences.

Helicobacter pylori

H. pylori is a flagellated gram-negative bacillus that colonizes the gastric epithelium of half of the world's population. This bacterium is responsible for over 80% of duodenal ulcers and at least half of all cases of gastric ulcers. However, only a fraction of patients with *H. pylori* infection

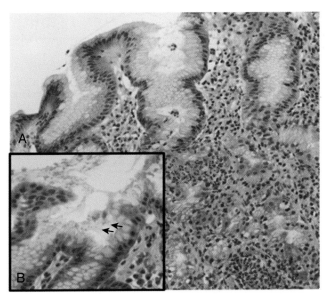

Fig. 37.4 (A) Gastric biopsy (hematoxylin and eosin stain) showing gastric mucosa with intense inflammatory infiltrate including clusters of neutrophils infiltrating gastric pit and surface epithelium and lymphocytes and plasma cells in the lamina propria. At high power (B) *H. pylori* organisms can be seen faintly *(arrows)* adjacent to surface epithelial cells. (Courtesy of Murray Resnick, MD, PhD, Adjunct Professor of Pathology and Laboratory Medicine, Warren Alpert Medical School, Providence, RI.)

develop PUD. *H. pylori* infection is also a strong risk factor for PUD and malignancy (adenocarcinoma and mucosa-associated lymphoid tissue [MALT] lymphoma), as well as a cause of iron deficiency anemia and immune thrombocytopenic purpura (ITP). Infection is transmitted via the fecal-oral route and typically occurs during childhood. *H. pylori* infection tends to persist throughout the lifetime of the host if left untreated, despite a strong gastric inflammatory response and both cell-mediated and humoral immune system recognition.

Rates of *H. pylori* infection differ globally, with highest prevalence in the developing world. In the United States, infection rates are 10% to 15% in persons under 12 years old and 50% to 60% in persons older than 60 years. There is increased prevalence in persons with lower socioeconomic status, increased household crowding and, in the United States, higher prevalence in immigrants from the developing world.

H. pylori has several unique characteristics enabling gastric colonization. *H. pylori* can survive in gastric acid by producing urease, which catalyzes the conversion of urea (which is present in gastric juice) into ammonia, thus neutralizing *H. pylori*'s microenvironment. *H. pylori*'s flagella allow the organism to move fluidly through the stomach's viscous mucous layer toward gastric epithelial cells, where *H. pylori* uses a series of adhesins and receptors to attach and chronically infect its host. At the gastric epithelium, *H. pylori* induces an inflammatory response consisting of neutrophils, leukocytes, plasma cells, and macrophages. Neutrophilic infiltration of the gastric epithelium causing chronic gastritis is a hallmark of *H. pylori* infection, easily recognizable in gastric biopsies (Fig. 37.4).

Determinants of pathogenicity include the location of infection within the stomach, *H. pylori* genomic heterogeneity, and differences in host response. For example, infections that are most predominant in the antrum are more strongly associated with duodenal ulcers and increased acidity due to depletion of antral somatostatin-producing cells leading to uninhibited gastrin secretion. In contrast, *H. pylori* colonization of the corpus is correlated with gastric ulcers, gastric adenomas, and decreased acid production due to inflammation-mediated inhibition of parietal cell secretion and subsequent parietal cell loss resulting in atrophic gastritis (see Fig. 37.3). This latter pattern of gastric inflammation is most common in persons residing in Southeast Asia, South America, and certain regions of Central, Eastern, and Southern Europe.

Additionally, *H. pylori's* ability to produce lipopolysaccharide, leukocyte-activating factors, specific adhesins and vacuolating toxins, and a type IV bacterial secretory system contribute to its virulence. Strains with more of these pathogenic factors have been associated with more severe disease states. The most important of those pathogenic markers is cytotoxin-associated gene *(cagA)*, a marker of the presence of the type IV secretory system, which is associated with acute gastritis, peptic ulcers, and gastric cancer. This multigene *H. pylori* system serves as a "molecular syringe" functioning to insert certain *H. pylori* proteins directly into host epithelial cells to activate pro-inflammatory and pro-oncogenic signaling pathways.

Diagnosis of *H. pylori*

In persons with clinical manifestations of *H. pylori*, eradication of the infection leads to improved outcomes. Because eradication of *H. pylori* from asymptomatic patients has not yet been shown to significantly prevent disease, *H. pylori* diagnostic testing is generally reserved for those patients with certain *H. pylori*–associated diseases or conditions such as PUD, uninvestigated dyspepsia without alarm symptoms, unexplained iron deficiency anemia, idiopathic thrombocytopenic purpura, early gastric cancer, and low-grade MALT lymphoma. It is remarkable that 80% of patients with low-grade MALT lymphoma and *H. pylori* infection will be cured by *H. pylori* eradication.

There are two categories of diagnostic tests for *H. pylori*: invasive and noninvasive. Noninvasive tests include urea breath test and stool antigen test, and the invasive tests are performed on endoscopic biopsies by histology, rapid urease test, and culture. The sensitivity of these tests, however, is decreased by proton pump inhibitors (PPIs), antibiotics, and bismuth compounds. Blood tests for the presence of *H. pylori* antibodies are relatively inaccurate and no longer recommended. They are particularly poor at monitoring the outcome of treatment because they may remain positive months to years after successful eradication.

For the urea breath test, patients must stop taking PPIs 2 weeks prior to the test. They ingest urea in which the carbon atoms are labeled with either radioactive carbon-14 or nonradioactive carbon-13. If present, *H. pylori* hydrolyzes the urea into ammonia. The presence of a labeled carbon atom in exhaled CO_2 indicates active *H. pylori* infection, and with a 95% specificity and sensitivity, it is the best choice for test of cure.

The stool antigen test detects fecal antigens by immunoassay. Proton pump inhibitors must be stopped 2 weeks prior to the test, but it is a good test for both detection and eradication, though their sensitivity and specificity are slightly lower than the urea breath test.

Invasive tests all require endoscopic biopsies. The *H. pylori* can be visualized histologically (especially if immunohistochemistry or other special stains are used) and the presence of chronic active gastritis, a hallmark of *H. pylori* infection, noted. Additionally, the biopsy can be tested with a rapid urease test, which detects pH changes in the urea-rich test matrix when the *H. pylori* derived urease converts urea to ammonia. Biopsies may also be used to culture *H. pylori*; however, this is a relatively costly and time-consuming process that is currently rarely used. The major advantage of this method is that it allows testing for antibiotic resistance of individual strains. This is an increasingly important focus of research and likely to be important in clinical practice, too, due to the emergence of multiply antibiotic-resistant *H. pylori*.

Given the increasing incidence of antibiotic resistance in *H. pylori*, a test of cure 4 weeks after the end of treatment and 2 weeks after cessation of PPI treatment with a stool antigen or breath tests is recommended to confirm eradication of *H. pylori*.

Treatment of *H. pylori*

Treatment consists of combination therapy with antibiotics and acid inhibitors to guarantee adequate antibiotic coverage and to ensure penetration of the antibiotics into the gastric mucosa (Fig. 37.5). Additionally, the duration of therapy must be long enough to ensure eradication.

The increasing rates of antibiotic resistance, especially to clarithromycin and levofloxacin, make it imperative that providers ask patients about any prior macrolide antibiotic exposures, because prior exposure is associated with likely resistance. They have also spurred efforts to measure local antibiotic resistance rates.

The treatment options are bismuth quadruple therapy, which consists of a PPI, bismuth, tetracycline, and metronidazole for 14 days, and clarithromycin triple therapy, which consists of a PPI, clarithromycin, and amoxicillin or metronidazole for 14 days. Given the increasing rates of clarithromycin resistance, however, clarithromycin triple therapy is falling out of favor and should only be used in regions where it is known that *H. pylori* clarithromycin resistance rates are less than 15% and in patients with no history of macrolide exposure. Otherwise, bismuth quadruple therapy is the current therapy of choice with an expected cure rate of 80% to 90%.

If a patient fails initial treatment, then second-line therapy for that patient should avoid any antibiotics that were previously taken by the patient. If the patient failed first-line bismuth quadruple therapy, salvage therapy should contain either clarithromycin or levofloxacin depending on local antimicrobial resistance patterns and the patient's prior antibiotic exposures. If the patient failed clarithromycin triple therapy, bismuth quadruple therapy should be tried next. Other "salvage" options in cases of recurrent failure include regimens containing rifabutin and dual regimens of high-dose amoxicillin and high-dose PPIs.

H. pylori infection treatment is complete only after eradication has been confirmed with a test of cure, as outlined above.

NSAID-Induced PUD

NSAIDs are a class of drugs that are very useful in the treatment of pain, arthritis, and inflammatory diseases; however, their use can be limited by their side effect profile. Upper GI side effects are dose dependent and include PUD and GI bleeds. Side effects are also more common in patients with certain risk factors, such as age older than 65 years, past history of PUD, heart disease, and concomitant therapy with antiplatelet agents, corticosteroids, and anticoagulants. There is synergism between *H. pylori* infection and chronic NSAID use in terms of PUD risk.

NSAID-induced PUD accounts for approximately 100,000 hospital admissions annually, and about 25% of persons on chronic NSAID therapy will develop PUD. Chronic NSAID users who have the above-mentioned risk factors have a 9% risk of having a serious adverse event, while those who do not have risk factors only have a 0.4% risk. Thus, before starting a patient on chronic NSAIDs, it is important to evaluate their risk factors and consider alternative therapies, if appropriate.

Mechanism of Injury

Half of people taking NSAIDs will develop NSAID-induced gastropathy consisting of superficial mucosal hemorrhages and erosions. These asymptomatic erosions are usually found incidentally during upper endoscopies performed for other reasons and are mainly concentrated in the gastric antrum. Most cases of NSAID gastropathy will not progress to PUD.

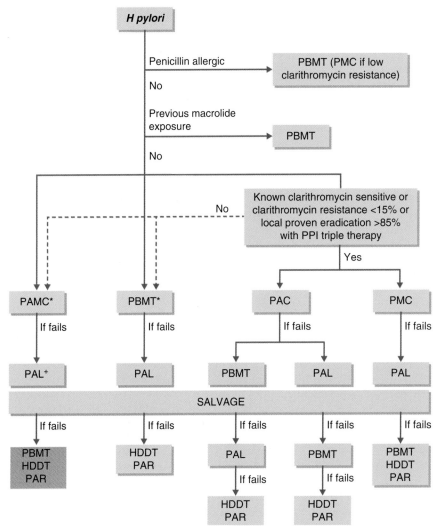

Fig. 37.5 *H. pylori* eradication therapy algorithm. *PAC,* Clarithromycin-based PPI triple therapy with amoxicillin; *PAL,* levofloxacin-based therapy; *PAMC,* concomitant non-bismuth quadruple therapy; *PAR,* rifabutin containing therapy; *PBMT,* PPI/bismuth/metronidazole/tetracycline quadruple therapy; *PMC,* clarithromycin-based PPI triple therapy with metronidazole; *HDDT,* high-dose dual therapy. (From Fallone CA, Moss SF, Malfertheiner P. Reconciliation of recent *Helicobacter pylori* treatment guidelines in a time of increasing resistance to antibiotics. Gastroenterology 2019;157:44-53.)

Once ingested and exposed to gastric acid, NSAIDs become weak acids and are able to cross the lipid bilayer membranes of gastric epithelial cells. There, they lose a hydrogen atom and become trapped intracellularly, disrupting normal cell function. This leads to decreased cellular integrity and increased cellular permeability leaving gastric epithelial cells vulnerable to topical injury, hemorrhages, erosions, and cell death.

Additionally, NSAIDs also inhibit the arachidonic acid pathway, which is crucial for the synthesis of prostaglandins (PGs) that protect gastric epithelial cells, and for mucosal integrity. The synthesis of PGs is catalyzed by cyclooxygenases (COX). The COX-1 isoform is constitutively expressed in the GI tract independent of external factors. In contrast, COX-2 is largely inducible, promoting PG synthesis under the influence of inflammatory mediators that are present in pro-inflammatory states. PGs play a very important role in gastric mucosal protection by increasing mucus and bicarbonate production, increasing blood flow to the gastric mucosa, and promoting epithelial cell repair and turnover after injury. Inhibition of PG synthesis by NSAIDs leaves epithelial cells vulnerable to unopposed injury from gastric acid and pepsin. Aspirin exposes patients to PUD in a similar way. It acetylates COX-1, thus irreversibly inhibiting it.

The more common NSAIDs, such as ibuprofen, naproxen, diclofenac, and aspirin, are nonselective COX inhibitors. Selective COX-2 inhibitors, such as celecoxib and valdecoxib, were developed with the aim of reducing gastric toxicity by primarily acting at sites of inflammation, thus leaving COX-1 function intact. Though the COX-2 inhibitors have fewer GI side effects, they have been associated with increased cardiovascular events such as myocardial infarctions and strokes. The COX-2 inhibitors that are still on the market now carry a black box warning.

Prevention and Therapy of NSAID-Induced PUD

Prevention and treatment of NSAID-induced PUD can be divided into three categories: primary prevention, treatment, and secondary prevention.

Prior to prescribing chronic NSAIDs, providers should assess a patient's risk for NSAID-induced adverse side effects, such as history of ulcers and GI bleeding, age older than 65 years, concomitant *H. pylori* infection, and co-prescription with antiplatelet agents, steroids, and anticoagulants.

Those patients with risk factors for developing NSAID-induced PUD should receive co-therapy with a gastroprotective agent. Currently there are several treatment options, including H2 receptor antagonists (H2RAs), synthetic prostaglandins, and PPIs. PPIs remain the co-treatment of choice because they are most efficacious in this regard and generally very well tolerated.

H2RAs work by blocking histamine 2 receptors in parietal cells, thus decreasing acid production. However, in clinical trials their effects on NSAID ulcer prevention have been very limited.

Prostaglandins such as misoprostol work similarly to endogenous prostaglandins in the protection of the stomach and duodenal lining. Unfortunately, prostaglandins are poorly tolerated due to their side effect profile, which includes diarrhea and abdominal pain.

PPIs inhibit the H+/K+-ATPase in parietal cells, hence reducing acid secretion into the gastric lumen. Prescription of PPIs together with NSAIDs significantly reduces GI-related NSAID complications with a 10% to 15% absolute risk reduction in ulcer formation and ulcer-related bleeding in high-risk patients taking nonselective NSAIDs. It must be noted, though, that recent studies have shown that selective COX-2 inhibitors plus a PPI provide better GI protection compared to a nonselective NSAID plus PPI.

With the widespread overuse of chronic PPIs in recent years (principally for GERD and dyspepsia), several likely adverse side effects of PPIs have come to light. These include increased risk of micronutrient deficiencies such as hypomagnesemia, iron and vitamin B_{12} deficiency, and GI-related infections, such as *Clostridioides difficile* infection (CDI) and small intestinal bacterial overgrowth (SIBO). Additionally, PPI use has been associated with increased incidence of osteoporosis and bone fractures and acute interstitial nephritis. More controversially, associations of chronic PPI usage with chronic kidney disease, cerebrovascular disease, upper GI cancers, and dementia have been reported in some studies, though almost entirely from observational cohorts. Better controlled prospective studies are needed to clarify any causal link between PPIs and these side effects. However, given these potential side effects, patients should be evaluated individually for PPI co-prescription with NSAIDs, and the lowest effective doses should be used when prescribing long-term in primary prophylaxis.

H. pylori infection in the setting of chronic NSAID has been shown to increase the risk of PUD, more specifically for duodenal ulceration. The risk for developing ulcers in *H. pylori* positive patients starting chronic NSAID therapy is higher during the first few months after starting therapy. Therefore, *H. pylori* testing, and treatment is recommended prior to starting chronic NSAID use.

Treatment of NSAID-related ulcers is more straightforward. First and foremost, the offending NSAID or aspirin should be discontinued if medically possible in order to allow endogenous protective prostaglandins to be formed. Subsequently, acid secretion should be suppressed with standard doses of PPIs (or H2RAs or misoprostol). In patients who require NSAID therapy but have a history of PUD, risk factors should be assessed, and COX-2 inhibitors should be used preferentially, along with co-therapy with a PPI if there are no cardiovascular contraindications to COX-2 inhibitor therapy.

Patients with cardiovascular risk factors for whom aspirin is required for secondary prevention of myocardial infarction cannot stop aspirin therapy. In this case, cardiovascular protection outweighs the benefit of aspirin cessation for PUD treatment. These patients must be tested for *H. pylori*, if they have not been previously tested, and they should be treated if they test positive. Additionally, these patients must remain on PUD prophylaxis with either a PPI or misoprostol.

Zollinger-Ellison Syndrome

PUD generally occurs in patients with normal or near normal rates of acid secretion. However, a rare cause of PUD is the Zollinger-Ellison syndrome (ZES), in which PUD is the direct result of severe acid hypersecretion due to gastrin-producing G-cell tumors, called gastrinomas. These tumors are generally located in the pancreas or the duodenum, and patients with ZES typically present with recurrent, multiple, refractory ulcers as well as PUD-related complications, esophagitis, and diarrhea. Individuals with ZES generally do not have concomitant *H. pylori* infection or use NSAIDs therapy. This condition will be discussed in further detail later in the chapter.

Stress-Induced Ulcers

Critically ill ICU patients are at increased risk of developing stress ulcers that lead to increased risk of clinically significant GI bleeding. The risk is higher in burn victims, those with significant injury, cranial trauma, shock, and mechanical ventilation. Endoscopically, stress-related mucosal damage is found in 60% to 100% of patients recently admitted to the ICU. Stress ulcers are typically multiple and shallow. They usually present with hematemesis or melena in the ICU patient.

ICU patients are predisposed to stress ulcers due to decreased splanchnic vascular perfusion and impaired microcirculation due to hypovolemia, shock, and low cardiac output leading to gut ischemia and injury. Additionally, they are often subject to pro-inflammatory states, associated with decreased innate mucosal defenses.

Prevention of stress ulcers with acid suppression through prophylactic treatment with PPIs or H2RAs has been common practice for the past four decades. Recently, the side effect profile of these agents has been evaluated against the risk of stress ulcer bleeds. Serious side effects of PPIs and H2RAs in the ICU setting include increased rate of nosocomial infections, such as ventilator-associated pneumonia and CDI. Consequently, stress ulcer prophylaxis should be reserved only for those patients at high risk for life-threatening GI bleeding such as patients with a history of GI bleeding within the past 12 months, greater than 48 hours of mechanical ventilation, spinal or traumatic brain injuries, and patients with coagulopathies.

Idiopathic Ulcers

Ulcers that appear to arise spontaneously with no known cause are called idiopathic ulcers. Idiopathic PUD (IPUD) prevalence varies by geographic location and has a prevalence of about 15% in developed countries as compared to around 80% in developing countries. With the advent of increased *H. pylori* treatment, the incidence of non–*H. pylori* idiopathic ulcers has increased dramatically, mainly in Asian countries. Idiopathic ulcers, similar to *H. pylori* ulcers, have a slightly higher likelihood of being located in the duodenum.

Diagnosis of idiopathic ulcers requires exclusion of all known causes of PUD such as missed *H. pylori* infection, surreptitious use of ulcerogenic medications, certain systemic diseases such as Crohn's disease, eosinophilic gastroenteritis, vasculitis, ZES, and other infections besides *H. pylori* that may lead to ulcers such as cytomegalovirus (CMV), herpes simplex virus (HSV), tuberculosis (TB), and syphilis.

IPUD carries an increased risk of ulcer recurrence when compared with other etiologies. One study concluded that recurrence rates for *H. pylori*–positive, NSAID-induced, and IPUD-related ulcers were 4.1%, 11.7%, and 23.2%, respectively.

Treatment consists of PPI administration for 4 to 8 weeks, or longer in the case of complicated disease. After PPI administration, it is important to monitor patients clinically. If there is recurrence, maintenance therapy is reasonable.

General PUD Treatment

As highlighted above, the single most important treatment option for PUD is to tailor therapy based on ulcer etiology. Generally, ulcers will heal with antisecretory treatment with a PPI. Uncomplicated duodenal ulcers, specifically those associated with *H. pylori* infection, will heal with 14 days of PPI treatment, which is part of *H. pylori* treatment itself. Complicated ulcers, however, necessitate a longer treatment of 8 to 12 weeks. NSAID-induced ulcers should be treated for a minimum of 8 weeks if the NSAID is stopped. Idiopathic ulcers must be evaluated as previously mentioned. Patients with ZES will need treatment as outlined later.

Maintenance Treatment

In addition to detailed evaluation of the etiology of ulceration for each individual patient and treatment according to the root cause of PUD (i.e., *H. pylori* infection, NSAIDs, ZES), some patients will require maintenance therapy to prevent ulcer recurrence.

After eliminating risk factors for PUD, patients with the following high-risk characteristics may benefit from antisecretory therapy with a PPI: (1) giant ulcer (>2 cm) and age older than 50 or multiple comorbidities, (2) *H. pylori*–negative ulcer disease, (3) non-NSAID disease, (4) refractory peptic ulcers defined as ulcers that do not heal after 12 weeks of PPI treatment, (5) *H. pylori* eradication failure, (6) recurrent peptic ulcer, (7) continued NSAID use. Maintenance therapy regimens include either an H2RA or a PPI at the lowest possible therapeutic dose. The risks of chronic PPIs versus the likelihood of developing PUD should be reviewed periodically.

Special Considerations

Patients that require dual antiplatelet therapy, specifically aspirin and clopidogrel, for treatment after cardiac catheterization, unstable angina, NSTEMI or stroke tend to be co-treated with PPIs to reduce GI side effects. Both PPIs and clopidogrel are metabolized by CYP2C19, leading to concerns that PPIs may decrease the efficacy of clopidogrel and lead to catastrophic events. This risk, however, has been assessed by various systematic reviews and, although the research obviously shows that PPIs decrease the risk of GI events, it has not demonstrated a clear adverse effect on patients on clopidogrel.

Additionally, new anticoagulants, such as dabigatran, rivaroxaban, apixaban, and edoxaban, are becoming more commonly used in patients who need long-term anticoagulation. Though research on these drugs and GI bleeding as it relates specifically to PUD is lacking, these drugs are linked to increased risk of GI bleeding overall and likely lead to increased bleeding in patients with PUD.

Surgery

The efficacy of nonsurgical ulcer treatment has increased dramatically with the discovery of *H. pylori* eradication treatment and antisecretory therapy. As a result, surgery is rarely used to treat PUD. It is an important therapeutic option, however, for patients with complications, such as gastric outlet obstruction, bleeding and perforation.

Complications of PUD

The most common complications of PUD include bleeding, perforation, and obstruction, with bleeding being the most common and obstruction being the least common.

Bleeding

GI bleeding accounts for half a million hospitalizations per year and about $5 billion in annual costs in the United States. Upper GI bleeds (UGIBs) make up half of those hospitalizations and carry a significant mortality rate of up to 7.4%. Peptic ulcers are the most frequent cause of UGIBs, making up about a third of all cases.

Bleeding ulcers present with the classic symptoms of an UGIB and vary depending on the severity of the bleed. In chronically bleeding UGIB, patients present with occult blood in the stool and possibly iron deficiency anemia. When the bleed is acute, patients will have coffee-ground emesis and melena (black and tarry stool); however, a patient with a brisk UGIB may present with hematemesis and, possibly, hematochezia with hypotension. Treatment of bleeding ulcers includes fluid resuscitation, blood transfusions when hemoglobin levels fall below 7 g/dL or below 8 g/dL in patients with existing cardiovascular disease or who are symptomatic, intravenous PPI therapy (which should be switched to oral therapy as soon as the patient tolerates oral medications), and an esophagogastroduodenoscopy (EGD) within 24 hours of admission. If the patient has high-risk clinical features, such as hemodynamic instability or hematemesis, EGD should be performed within 12 hours of admission. Endoscopic intervention is dictated by the features of the bleeding ulcer. Typically, endoscopic interventions, such as injections, sclerotherapy, or clips, are employed if there is active bleeding from the ulcer, or if there is a clot adherent to the ulcer. In active bleeding, combination therapy such as injected epinephrine followed by the application of clips produces improved outcomes over a single modality. Hospital discharge is dependent on the patient's clinical status, but it is typically after 3 days of hospitalization for patients with high-risk bleeds.

Perforation

Perforation of a peptic ulcer accounts for 2% to 10% of ulcer complications. Perforation happens when an ulcer penetrates the full thickness of the stomach or duodenal wall. It should be suspected if a patient develops sudden, severe abdominal pain. On physical examination, the patient will have exquisite abdominal pain and tenderness, guarding, and, potentially, signs of peritonitis such as rebound tenderness. Upright chest and abdominal radiographs will show free peritoneal air under the diaphragm; however, if they do not, and the clinical suspicion for perforation is high, the next most useful imaging modality, if the perforation happened within the previous 6 hours, is ultrasound. After 6 hours have elapsed, CT may provide diagnostic value.

Patients with an abdominal perforation need to be treated for hemodynamic instability and receive antibiotics targeting enteric bacteria. Additionally, they should undergo an emergent surgical evaluation. Risks of surgery must be weighed against the individual patient's risk of perforation-related mortality. However, nonoperative management is appropriate only for a small number of patients, and the most effective treatment remains surgical repair of the perforation.

Gastric Outlet Obstruction

Though much less common than UGIB and perforation, gastric outlet obstruction (GOO) is a serious complication of a peptic ulcer located at the pylorus. Though PUD historically accounted for the majority of cases of obstruction, the incidence of GOO in PUD has declined as treatment for PUD has steadily improved. Currently, the leading cause of GOO is malignancy, therefore malignancy must be ruled out by endoscopy in all cases.

The precise etiology of GOO is unknown; however, it is more prevalent in patients with duodenal or pyloric ulceration. Causes of GOO secondary to PUD are likely multifactorial, from inflammatory-related causes such as spasm, edema, and pyloric dysmotility in the acute setting to more chronic causes such as scarring and fibrosis as the ulcer heals.

Patients with GOO present with early satiety, nausea, bloating, vomiting, and weight loss. On physical exam, patients will have stigmata of dehydration, abdominal distention, and a succussion splash. At presentation, patients should undergo gastric decompression to clear the gastric contents, and electrolyte abnormalities must be evaluated and treated along with IV rehydration.

Radiographic imaging will demonstrate an enlarged gastric bubble and dilated proximal duodenum on abdominal radiographs. Computed tomography of the abdomen will generally show gastric distention and retained chyme in the gastric cavity with an associated fluid level (Fig. 37.6).

Ultimately, patients must undergo EGD for diagnostic and possible therapeutic purposes (Fig. 37.7). Endoscopic biopsies must be obtained from the site of obstruction to evaluate for malignancy and from the antrum and body to determine if there is underlying *H. pylori* infection. If PUD is suspected, antisecretory IV treatment with a PPI must be initiated to promote healing of the ulcer and alleviation of the obstruction. Oral alimentation must be introduced slowly, as tolerated by the patient. Patients with refractory obstruction who fail conservative treatment may be treated endoscopically with balloon dilation, endoscopic stent placement, or even surgery. Additionally, patients should receive treatment for *H. pylori* and other causes of PUD, if indicated.

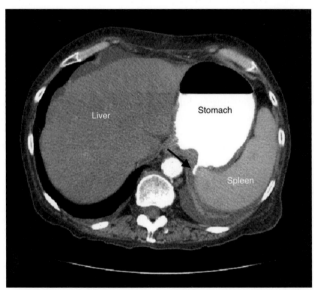

Fig. 37.6 Transverse view of an abdominal CT demonstrating a gastric outlet obstruction with significant narrowing at the distal stomach *(arrow)*. This has caused gastric distention with retained fluid in the stomach and a visible fluid level. (From Mönkemüller, et al. Gastrointestinal Endoscopy 2012;75:463-465.)

ZOLLINGER-ELLISON SYNDROME

Definition and Epidemiology

ZES is a rare condition that results from ectopic gastrin secretion due to a neuroendocrine tumor, called a *gastrinoma*. This leads to elevated levels of basal acid secretion in the stomach. Symptoms such as multiple or *H. pylori*–negative duodenal ulcers, recurrent ulcers, refractory ulcers, esophagitis, and unexplained diarrhea should raise clinical suspicion of ZES. Gastrinomas are primarily located in the duodenum (60% to 80%) or pancreas (10% to 14%) in an area known as the "gastrinoma triangle." They are also rarely found in other areas such as the stomach, liver, bile duct, and ovary. ZES tends to present in patients between 45 and 50 years old, and there is a slight male predominance with an estimated male to female ratio of 2:1 to 3:2. The diagnosis is often delayed due to low clinical suspicion.

Although the majority of ZES cases develop sporadically, 10% to 54% of ZES cases are found in patients with multiple endocrine neoplasia type 1 (MEN1). Multiple endocrine neoplasia type 1 is an autosomal dominant genetic disorder, usually of the *menin* gene located on chromosome 11q13. In addition to gastrinomas, patients with MEN1 also have increased incidence of parathyroid hyperplasia, pancreatic endocrine tumors, pituitary adenomas, and adrenal adenomas. Therefore, patients diagnosed with ZES must be screened for MEN1.

Pathophysiology of ZES

The main pathologic characteristic of ZES is excessively elevated levels of circulating gastrin, secreted autonomously from gastrinomas. Unlike physiologic gastrin production, gastrin release from gastrinomas is not subject to regular inhibitory feedback loops. This unregulated acid secretion causes excessive acid secretion that eventually leads to peptic ulceration in 90% of people with ZES. Exaggerated gastrin levels also act as trophic factors for ECL and parietal cells resulting in hypertrophic gastric rugae that are visible on endoscopy.

Clinical Presentation

In addition to an elevated risk of PUD, as detailed above, a third of patients may present with unexplained diarrhea, which can sometimes lead to electrolyte imbalances such as hypokalemia, steatorrhea, and weight loss. Diarrhea may be the sole clinical manifestation in about 20% of patients. Diarrhea occurs when the high acid load reaches the small intestine causing direct enterocyte damage, inactivation of pancreatic lipase, and precipitation of bile acids, which interferes with micelle formation.

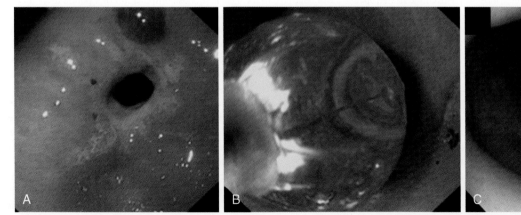

Fig. 37.7 Endoscopic appearance of gastric outlet obstruction due to a pyloric channel stricture. (A) Pyloric channel stricture. (B) Endoscopic view of balloon dilation of the pyloric stricture. (C) Post-procedure view of the pylorus after successful balloon dilation. (From Kochhar et al. Gastrointestinal Endoscopy 2018;8:899-908.)

Other manifestation of ZES include esophageal syndromes from gastric acid hypersecretion, such as dysphagia, esophagitis, esophageal ulceration, strictures, or even perforation. In fact, reflux esophagitis may occur in up to 40% of patients with ZES.

Diagnosis

As in the diagnosis of other rare diseases, the most important factor in diagnosing ZES is having a high index of suspicion for ZES in patients that present with classic symptoms, as detailed above. These classic symptoms, however, may be hard to discern in the age of ubiquitous PPI use because these antisecretory agents may mask ZES symptoms. Diagnosis of ZES requires the presence of hypergastrinemia and hyperchlorhydria.

Initially, patients with suspected ZES should be evaluated by obtaining a fasting gastrin level and obtaining a gastric pH. A low gastric pH in conjunction with high gastrin levels is characteristic because, in achlorhydric states, gastrin will be appropriately elevated but so will pH. Because PPIs also affect the gastric pH, PPIs must be discontinued for at least 1 week prior to testing. PPI discontinuation in patients with ZES incurs serious risks and should be done only after careful evaluation of the risks and benefits of PPI withdrawal for diagnostic purposes under the supervision of experienced practitioners. Some case reports have described serious health complications of ZES that developed just 48 hours after PPI withdrawal.

Gastrin levels greater than ten times the upper limit of normal (ULN) with a gastric pH less than 2 establishes the diagnosis of ZES. However, most patients with ZES will have equivocal gastrin levels. A secretin stimulation test can help make the diagnosis in this case.

The secretin stimulation test takes advantage of the paradoxical increase in gastrin secretion after the administration of secretin in patients with gastrinomas. Similar to gastrin and gastrin pH levels, the secretin test must be obtained while the patient is not under antisecretory therapy. Gastrin levels are obtained before and after the administration of 2 U/kg of secretin. The test is positive if gastrin levels increase at least 120 pg/mL with secretin administration.

After the diagnosis of ZES is made, all patients must be screened for MEN1 by measuring calcium, parathyroid hormone (PTH), and MEN1 germline mutation testing. In addition, first-degree relatives of patients with MEN1 also must be screened. Because a majority of gastrinomas are malignant, it is critical to attempt to localize the gastrinoma with the purpose of tumor resection.

A useful imaging modality for localizing gastrinomas is a somatostatin-receptor scintigraphy (SRS) scan combined with CT scan, but other modalities such as CT, MRI, and ultrasonography may also be used. In experienced hands, upper endoscopy with endoscopic ultrasound (EUS) has similar sensitivity to SRS (74% and 75% respectively) and can be helpful in determining the location of the gastrinoma.

Treatment of ZES

After ruling out other causes of hypergastrinemia (such as pernicious anemia or PPI-induced hypergastrinemia, in which the high gastrin occurs secondary to *low* acid secretion), the most important treatment goal for ZES is reduction and normalization of acid secretion, which can be achieved through PPI therapy. To control acid secretion in ZES, PPIs typically need to be taken at elevated doses, sometimes double the standard dose or higher. PPI treatment must be titrated to achieve a basal acid output (BAO) that is less than 10 mmol/hour the hour preceding the next scheduled dose. When patients are unable to take oral medications, IV PPI therapy must be administered to control acid secretion. In extreme cases, vagotomy may be performed to decease acid secretion.

Surgery can sometimes uncover a hitherto unrecognized primary tumor. Additionally, it allows for evaluation of tumor grade and stage and removes the source of the ectopic gastrin production. Regardless, surgery significantly improves survival rates in patients with ZES. Gastrinomas tend to metastasize via a hematogenous route primarily to the lymph nodes, followed by the liver. Up to 50% of patients will have liver metastases at presentation.

GASTRITIS

Gastritis is a general term that is used to describe inflammation in the gastric mucosa. Gastric inflammation can be caused by a variety of conditions, most commonly *H. pylori* infection and NSAID gastritis (more strictly in the latter case termed *gastropathy*, because inflammation is rather mild). Gastritis can be acute or chronic and may be secondary to other infectious causes, autoimmune disorders, drugs, and ischemia. Every effort should be made to identify the cause of gastritis, though many times a specific diagnosis may not be identifiable.

Atrophic gastritis is a histopathologic entity of glandular loss that results from chronic inflammation. It can be divided into two major types: multifocal (secondary to environmental factors, *H. pylori*, specific diets) or corpus predominant (autoimmune) gastritis. This section will focus on the corpus predominant subtype, autoimmune metaplastic atrophic gastritis (AMAG).

AMAG is a chronic inflammatory gastritis caused by autoantibodies against intrinsic factor and the parietal cells in the fundus and body. It has a prevalence of 2% with a female to male ration of 3:1, and it is more common in persons with other autoimmune diseases, specifically diabetes mellitus and autoimmune thyroid disease. AMAG increases the risk of intestinal-type gastric adenocarcinoma and gastric carcinoid tumors. Patients typically present with nonspecific GI symptoms and are generally diagnosed relatively late in their disease, once they have hematologic manifestations, such as macrocytic anemia due to vitamin B_{12} deficiency (pernicious anemia). Due to the inability to absorb vitamin B_{12}, these patients may present with concomitant neurologic and psychiatric symptoms, though this happens in less than 10% of cases. On biopsy, patients will have gastric body mucosal atrophy as well as ECL hyperplasia in the setting of hypochlorhydria (and resultant hypergastrinemia). Treatment consists of vitamin B_{12} supplementation and surveillance for associated diseases.

Infectious gastritis may be caused by infections other than *H. pylori*, such as CMV, *Mycobacterium avium-intracellulare*, enterococcal infections, HSV, as well as parasitic and fungal infections. Treatment for infectious gastritis involves treatment of the specific microbe causing damage to the gastric mucosa.

Eosinophilic gastritis (EG) is a part of a continuum of eosinophil-associated gastrointestinal disorders (EGIDs). It is associated with systemic eosinophilia in about 75% of patients with EGID. In EG, there is an eosinophilic infiltration, which rarely includes all layers of the gastric wall. There is mucosal involvement in 60% of cases, muscular involvement in 30% of cases, and subserosal involvement in 10% of cases. Diagnosis is difficult, given the varying locations of infiltration, and the nonspecific appearance of the stomach on EGD. Eosinophilic gastritis may be a cause of GOO. Treatment includes systemic steroids; however, there has been some success treating patients with elemental diets free of allergenic foods.

Ménétrier's disease is a very rare condition associated with hypertrophy of the gastric mucosa primarily in the body of the stomach. Histologically, there is proliferation of the gastric glands with cystic dilation of the basilar portion. The etiology of the disease is unknown, and the diagnosis is difficult to make. Diagnosis generally necessitates

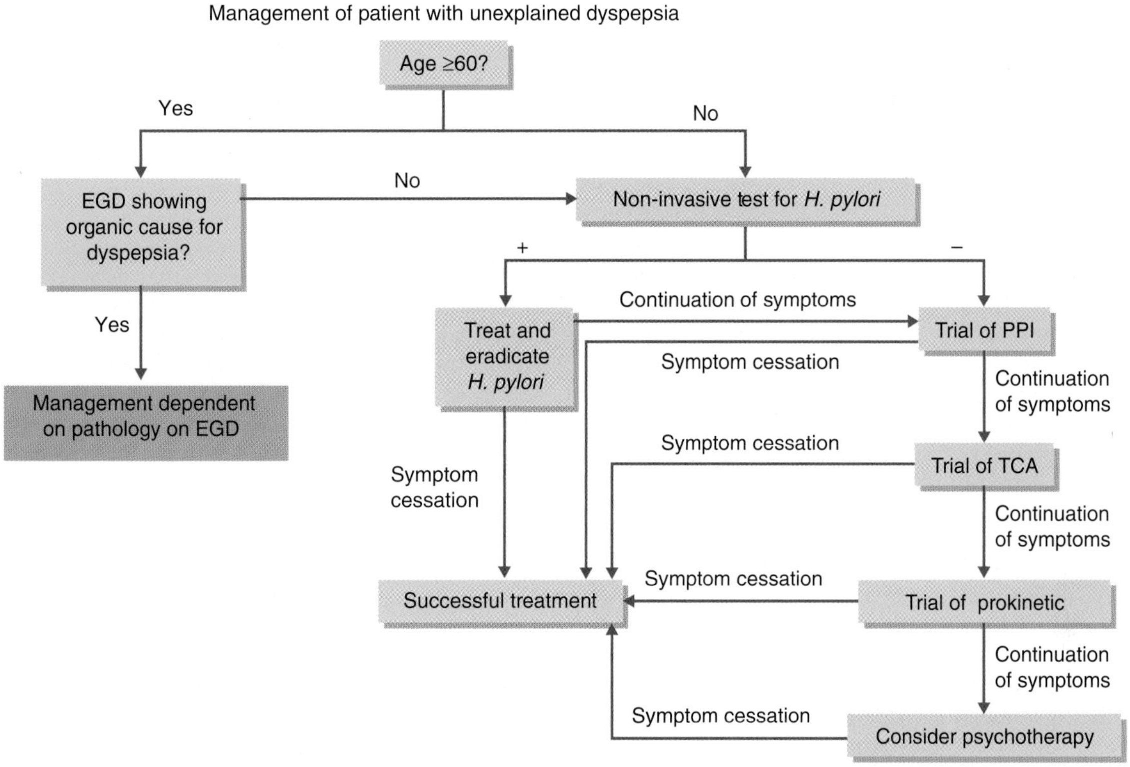

Management of patient with unexplained dyspepsia

Fig. 37.8 Guideline for management of patients with dyspepsia. *EGD*, Esophagogastroduodenoscopy; *TCA*, tricyclic antidepressant. (Adapted from Moayyedi PM, Lacy BE, Andrews CN, Enns RA, Howden CW, Vakil N. ACG and CAG Clinical Guideline: Management of Dyspepsia. Am J Gastroenterol. 2017;112:988-1013.)

evaluation of the gross appearance of the gastric mucosa during endoscopy along with the characteristic constellation of symptoms. Clinically, there is associated nausea, vomiting, anemia, hypochlorhydria, and peripheral edema secondary to hypoalbuminemia.

Lymphocytic gastritis is another rare disorder characterized by mucous and gastric epithelium infiltration by T cells. It is associated with celiac disease, *H. pylori* gastritis, collagenous colitis, and Ménétrier's disease.

FUNCTIONAL (NONULCER) DYSPEPSIA

When a patient presents with a constellation of symptoms similar to that of PUD or gastritis without evidence of ulceration on EGD, they are said to have *nonulcer dyspepsia (NUD)*. Nonulcer dyspepsia is a diagnosis of exclusion. The etiology of NUD is not well understood; however, patients with NUD may have impaired gastric mucosal integrity, dysmotility, dysregulation of the gut-brain axis, or sensory dysfunction. Psychosocial factors and psychiatric disorders such as depression and anxiety, however, are very strongly associated with NUD. NUD affects 10% to 30% of the world's population.

Specific diagnostic criteria include bothersome postprandial fullness, early satiety, epigastric pain, or epigastric burning, in addition to a lack of evidence of an organic or structural explanation of the symptoms on EGD, imaging, or laboratory studies. Patients older than 60 years of age should have an EGD to evaluate for possible malignancy. Depending on individual clinical symptoms, some patients may benefit from motility studies to evaluate for dysmotility and gastroparesis (Fig. 37.8).

Unfortunately, treatment for NUD is limited and therapeutic modalities have not been well studied. Some (about 1 in 10) dyspeptic patients with NUD who test positive for *H. pylori* may respond to H.

pylori eradication even if they do not have evidence of PUD on endoscopy. Antisecretory therapy with a PPI or H2RA is recommended for *H. pylori*–negative patients and those that have been successfully treated for *H. pylori* who continue to have symptoms. Tricyclic antidepressants are recommended for patients that continue to be symptomatic despite *H. pylori* eradication and antisecretory therapy. Further treatment options include prokinetics, such as cisapride and domperidone, though these are not available in the United States. Patients who do not respond to therapy and have ongoing, bothersome symptoms may benefit from psychological therapies, the most common being cognitive behavioral therapy.

CYCLIC VOMITING SYNDROME

Cyclic vomiting syndrome (CVS) is an idiopathic condition that presents both in children and adults with the mean age of presentation of 37 years in the adult population. The etiology of CVS is largely unknown, but it has been observed to be triggered in patients with chronic cannabis use, migraine headaches, and by certain foods (which typically also trigger migraine headaches). Characteristically, patients present with bouts of vomiting lasting hours to days with absence of vomiting between episodes. Adult patients will commonly report alleviation of symptoms while taking hot showers or baths.

Diagnosing CVS is difficult, and many years may elapse before a clear diagnosis is made. Clinicians may often misdiagnose patients with recurrent infectious gastroenteritis or other self-limiting causes of vomiting. Specific criteria for diagnosis include (1) stereotypical bouts of acute vomiting lasting less than 1 week, (2) three or more episodes in the prior year and two in the past 6 months, occurring at least 1 week apart, (3) absence of vomiting between episodes. The diagnosis of CVS must be made only after excluding other possible diagnoses.

In the acute setting, therapy is supported with IV fluids, antiemetics, and slow reintroduction of food as tolerated by the patient. Antiemetics taken prior to the attack during the prodromal period may prevent or reduce the longevity of symptoms. Maintenance therapy consists of avoidance of triggers and, if appropriate, psychosocial treatment. When a patient presents with CVS in the setting of cannabis use, cannabis use must be stopped.

RAPID GASTRIC EMPTYING

Rapid gastric emptying, also known as *dumping syndrome*, is a debilitating condition manifesting in postprandial gastrointestinal and vasomotor symptoms that occur following esophageal, gastric, or bariatric surgery. It is due to premature delivery of food into the small intestine. Postsurgical rapid gastric emptying occurs in 25% to 50% of cases with 5% to 10% of patients experiencing debilitating symptoms; however, this diagnosis is also correlated with diabetes mellitus, and idiopathic cases have also been reported. Rapid gastric emptying can be divided into two categories, early and late dumping syndrome, of which the early variation is most common. It is defined as less than 30% retention of gastric contents within 1 hour of solid meal ingestion.

In early rapid gastric emptying, hyperosmolar food is delivered to the small intestine triggering the release of vasoactive substances such as neurostatin, vasoactive intestinal peptide (VIP), and glucose modulators such as incretins, insulin, and glucagon. This results in gastrointestinal symptoms such as early satiety, pain, diarrhea, nausea, cramps, and bloating, vasomotor symptoms such as hypotension, and sympathetic nervous system response such as facial flushing, palpitations, and diaphoresis within 30 minutes of meal ingestion.

The symptoms of late gastric emptying are a result of hyperinsulinemia and subsequent reactive hypoglycemia. Hyperinsulinemia occurs secondary to an increased release of incretins in response to undigested carbohydrates in the small intestine. Symptoms, including diaphoresis, tremulousness, decreased concentration, and altered levels of consciousness, occur 1 to 3 hours postprandially. Early and late gastric emptying may be present in isolation, but they frequently coexist.

Diagnosis of rapid gastric emptying primarily relies on a high clinical suspicion in patients with typical clinical symptoms of rapid gastric emptying. Other diagnostic modalities include oral glucose tolerance test and radionuclide scintigraphy.

First-line treatment includes lifestyle modifications to reduce the amount of food taken per meal, eating at more frequent intervals, and separating solid from liquid food ingestion. Additionally, it can be helpful to lie down after meals and decrease carbohydrate and lactose ingestion. Early consultation with a dietitian is important to ensure that an adequate nutritional status is maintained. When lifestyle modification methods fail to alleviate symptoms, pharmacologic options include acarbose, guar gum, or symptomatic treatment with loperamide, tincture of opium, and other methods of pain control. Octreotide, which inhibits the secretion of vasoactive agents, may also be helpful.

GASTROPARESIS

Gastroparesis occurs when there is delayed gastric emptying into the small intestine, causing a characteristic constellation of symptoms. It is most commonly seen in diabetics, postsurgical patients, and those on chronic scheduled opioid therapy. A third of cases are idiopathic, and women are more likely than men to develop this disorder. Up to 30% to 50% of patients with type 1 diabetes have delayed gastric emptying, as do 15% to 30% of patients with type 2 diabetes.

Diabetic gastroparesis is better understood than idiopathic gastroparesis. The etiology of diabetic gastroparesis is similar to that of diabetic neuropathy with possible denervation of the vagus nerve causing a delay in gastric emptying. Additionally, patients with diabetes-related gastroparesis have been found to have decreased numbers of interstitial cells of Cajal (ICCs), the pacemaker cells of the GI tract, as well as decreased levels of nitric oxide release from enteric neural cells. Although patients with idiopathic gastroparesis also have decreased numbers of ICCs, the cause of idiopathic gastroparesis is less well understood, though enterovirus infections have been implicated.

Clinically, patients experience early satiety, abdominal distension, nausea, vomiting, anorexia, and malnutrition. Though all patients with gastroparesis experience nausea, patients with diabetes tend to have more severe and more frequent episodes of vomiting when compared to those with idiopathic gastroparesis. Patients with idiopathic gastroparesis are more likely to have severe postprandial fullness and early satiety.

Some patients with idiopathic gastroparesis are misdiagnosed as having nonulcer dyspepsia, therefore a high index of suspicion is key to the diagnosis. After gastric outlet obstruction has been ruled out, the timing of gastric emptying may be evaluated with gastric emptying scintigraphy, breath testing, or a wireless motility capsule. It is very important that patients refrain from taking prokinetic or gastroparetic agents prior to these studies.

Treatment takes a stepwise approach beginning with dietary modifications (small, spaced out meals), improving glucose control in diabetic patients, and adding prokinetic agents. More invasive procedures such as gastric pacemakers may be tried in severe cases.

GASTRIC VOLVULUS

Gastric volvulus is a rare condition that affects both adult and pediatric patients, where the stomach rotates at least 180 degrees along its transverse or longitudinal axis causing gastric inlet or outlet obstruction. In extreme cases, gastric volvulus may cause strangulation, necrosis, and perforation; therefore it is considered a surgical emergency. The mortality rate for acute gastric volvulus ranges between 15% to 20%, whereas it is 0% to 13% for chronic cases. Rotation of the stomach is generally caused by paraesophageal hernias, structural abnormalities (such as neoplasms), adhesions, and gastric ligamentous laxity (Fig. 37.9).

Clinically, presentation varies depending on acuity and degree of obstruction. Borchardt triad of acute abdominal pain, severe retching without vomiting, and inability to place a gastric tube is present in 70% of cases with acute gastric volvulus. If the volvulus is severe enough to cause strangulation and necrosis, hematemesis may be seen. Patients with chronic gastric volvulus may present with vague symptoms such as abdominal pain, dysphagia, and bloating. These may be misdiagnosed as other upper GI disorders.

Given the rarity and nonspecific presentation of gastric volvulus, diagnosis is often done while investigating other causes for the patient's symptoms. Evidence of gastric outlet obstruction with an interruption, such as two pockets of air-fluid levels, is seen on radiographs. Additionally, given the correlation with esophageal hernias, these can also be seen on radiographs and should increase index of suspicion for gastric volvulus. These patients typically have subsequent abdominal CT scans that show abnormal location of the antrum and evidence of GOO.

Treatment can be divided into three categories: conservative, endoscopic, or surgical. In the acute setting, patients must be treated and

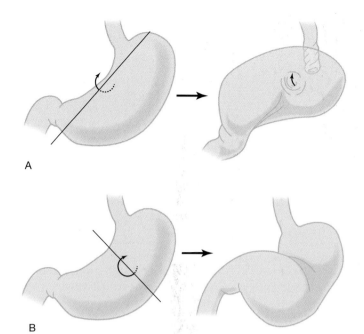

Fig. 37.9 The two major types of gastric volvulus. (A) Organoaxial volvulus, in which there is anterior rotation about the cardiopyloric axis, resulting in an upside-down stomach with the greater curve on top and the lesser curve on the bottom. Obstruction may occur at the gastroesophageal junction and the pyloroantral area. (B) Mesenteroaxial volvulus, in which there is anterior rotation about an axis perpendicular to the cardiopyloric axis. The greater curve remains on the bottom. (From Tsang, Tat-Kin et al. Endoscopic reduction of gastric volvulus: The alpha-loop maneuver Gastrointestinal Endoscopy 1995; 42: 244-248.)

stabilized. Conservative therapy consists of placing a gastric tube and laying patients in the prone position. It is generally reserved for stable patients with viable stomach tissue at the time of presentation. An endoscopic approach affords therapeutic and diagnostic value because it can assess the condition of the gastric mucosa and may sometimes lead to resolution of the volvulus with insufflation. Critically ill patients with evidence of tissue compromise generally must undergo surgery to relieve the volvulus and resect damaged tissue. Surgery also repairs gastric perforations and hiatal hernias. Patients generally undergo a gastropexy (fixation of the stomach to the anterior abdominal wall) to prevent future episodes.

SUGGESTED READINGS

Cook D, Guyatt G: Prophylaxis against gastrointestinal bleeding in hospitalized patients, N Engl J Med 378:2500–2516, 2018.

Crowe SE: Helicobacter pylori Infection, N Engl J Med 380:1158–1165, 2019.

Laine L, Jensen DM: Management of patients with ulcer bleeding, Am J Gastroenterol 107:345–360, 2012.

Lanas A, Chan FKL: Peptic ulcer disease, Lancet 530:613–624, 2017.

Moayyedi PM, Lacy BE, Andrews CN, Enns RA, Howden CW, Vakil N: ACG and CAG clinical guideline: management of dyspepsia, Am J Gastroenterol 112:988–1013, 2017.

Murugesan SV, Varro A, Pritchard DM: Review article: Strategies to determine whether hypergastrinemia is due to Zollinger-Ellison syndrome rather than a more common benign cause, Aliment Pharmacol Ther 29:1055–1068, 2009.

Siddique O, Ovalle A, Siddique AS, Moss SF: Helicobacter pylori infection: an update for the internist in the age of increasing global antibiotic resistance, Am J Med 131:473–479, 2018.

38

Inflammatory Bowel Disease

Talha A. Malik, Michael F. Picco, Francis A. Farraye

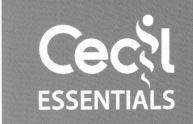

INTRODUCTION

Inflammatory bowel disease (IBD) comprises two chronic disorders: ulcerative colitis (UC) and Crohn's disease. The diagnosis of IBD is based on review of clinical, endoscopic, radiologic, and histologic data. Although the cause of these two diseases has yet to be defined, new and emerging targeted anti-inflammatory treatments hold great promise in helping to reduce morbidity and improve the quality of life of individuals with IBD.

UC is characterized by chronic inflammatory changes that involve the colonic mucosa in a continuous superficial fashion, typically starting in the rectum and extending proximally. Depending on the extent of the disease, UC can be divided into proctitis (rectum only), proctosigmoiditis (rectum and sigmoid), left-sided colitis (extending to the splenic flexure), and pancolitis (inflammation extends proximal to the splenic flexure). This classification is significant for both prognosis and therapy. Unlike UC, Crohn's disease can involve any segment of the gastrointestinal tract from the mouth to the anus, often in a discontinuous fashion. It is characterized by transmural chronic inflammation, which results in complications such as abscesses, fistulas, and strictures.

Historical Perspective

Ulcerative colitis was first described in ancient Greece by Hippocrates as a condition characterized by chronic diarrhea and bloody stools. In 1859, Samuel Wilks, a British physician, described "ulcerative colitis" as a discrete disease entity.

In 1913, the British physician Kennedy Dalziel first described patients with transmural inflammation of the small and large intestines. Subsequently, in 1932, Dr. Burrill Crohn, Dr. Leon Ginzburg, and Dr. Gordon Oppenheimer published papers describing a condition that caused inflammation of the terminal ileum and which they called regional or terminal ileitis. This disease entity later began to be referred as Crohn's disease.

The first breakthrough that established IBD as the major intestinal autoimmune disease occurred in the 1950s when it was demonstrated that symptoms in patients with both UC and Crohn's disease responded to corticosteroids. In the 1980s, traditional immune modulators, mainly thiopurines, were used as first-line steroid sparing agents. In 1997, Targan and colleagues published findings from the "Crohn's Disease cA2 Study" that looked at the efficacy of infliximab, a biologic antibody against tumor necrosis factor (TNF) cA2 in the induction of remission in luminal Crohn's. This began the era of biologics. During the first decade of the 21st century, biologics given intravenously or as subcutaneous injections emerged as the most effective therapeutic agents used to induce and maintain remission in moderate to severe UC and Crohn's disease. Since then, new oral agents are now available and effective in the treatment of patients with IBD.

EPIDEMIOLOGY

There is variation in the incidence and prevalence of UC and Crohn's disease across the globe based on geographic region, particular environment, immigration trends, and ethnic group. In the past, UC was generally considered to be slightly more common. However, this trend has changed with the rising incidence of Crohn's disease. It is estimated that there are more than 2 million people with IBD in North America. The annual incidence in North America of both UC and Crohn's disease is estimated to be between 0 to 20 per 100,000 persons. The estimates for prevalence of UC and Crohn's disease in North America are 35 to 250 per 100,000 and 25 to 300 per 100,000, respectively. The incidence and prevalence of IBD reflect the interplay of complex genetic and environmental factors that contribute to these disorders. For example, both diseases are more common in northern climates and among white individuals, particularly among populations of European descent living in North America, South Africa, and Australia. Although incidence rates of IBD are lowest among Hispanic and Asian populations, IBD can occur in any ethnic or racial group from anywhere in the world. The cause of IBD remains unknown, but it is believed to result from a combination of genetic, immunologic, infectious, and environmental factors. In addition, research points toward a relationship between the human microbiome and dysfunction of the immune system in patients with IBD.

UC and Crohn's disease can occur at any age, but the peak age of onset for UC is between 30 and 40 years of age and for Crohn's disease it is between 20 and 30 years. There is another peak, especially for UC, between 60 and 70 years of age based on studies in several European cohorts. The incidence and prevalence of UC and Crohn's disease appear to be similar in North American men and women.

RISK FACTORS AND PATHOPHYSIOLOGY

IBD is likely a result of an uncontrolled immune-mediated inflammatory response in genetically predisposed individuals to an environmental trigger that interacts with the intestinal flora and primarily affects the alimentary tract.

Approximately 5% to 20% of patients with IBD have a first-degree relative with the disease, and first-degree relatives of IBD patients have about a 10- to 15-fold increased risk for developing IBD, predominantly with the same disease as the proband. A positive family history is more frequently observed in patients with Crohn's disease compared with UC, suggesting that genetic factors are more important in the etiology of Crohn's disease. The lifetime risk of developing IBD in first-degree relatives has been estimated at 5% in Crohn's disease and about 2% in UC among non-Ashkenazi Jewish populations and 8% and 5% within Ashkenazi Jewish populations, respectively.

Through genome-wide association studies (GWAS), over 200 genetic loci have been identified as being associated with IBD. However, there is little diagnostic utility in clinical practice of these genetic variants due to their overall low incidence in IBD populations. With increasingly diverse populations being studied, this may change. Examples of single nucleotide polymorphisms (SNPs) associated with Crohn's include sequences in the *NOD2*, IL23-receptor and the *ATG16L1* genes. It is thought that *NOD2* variants may predict more complicated disease, mainly in European patients with stricturing ileal and penetrating disease. IL-12 variants may be associated with risk for early surgery.

Additionally, other genes associated with IBD that have been identified through GWAS include *IRGM, LRRK, FUT2, CARD9, TNFSF15, FCG2RA, NKX2-3, PTPN2, ZNF365, ECM1, STAT3*, and *IL10R* among others. As mentioned, these variants have little diagnostic or therapeutic utility in clinical practice at this time due to lack of replication of associations noted in small studies.

Profound alterations in mucosal immunology have been demonstrated in patients with IBD. In the normal immunologic state of the intestine, activated lymphoid tissue is abundant within the mucosal compartment. This state has been described as controlled or physiologic inflammation, and it likely develops in response to constant encounters with antigenic substances (derived from host microbial flora or dietary and environmental sources) that have crossed the epithelial barrier from the luminal environment. Indeed, one of the main functions of the intestinal immune system is to discriminate noxious or harmful substances and organisms from nonharmful ones. As a result, a large and well-maintained network of many different mucosal immune cells exists, including cells involved in reducing immune responses (regulatory cells) and those involved in activating immune responses. In IBD, this homeostatic balance, or immune tolerance, is dysregulated, resulting in overactivation of the immune system.

In the past, it was thought that inflammation in Crohn's was predominantly mediated by T_H1 cells and in UC it was primarily mediated by T_H2 cells; there is now considerable evidence that each of their pathogeneses is more complex and nuanced, whereby both types of T helper cells appear to play a role. Furthermore, there is recent evidence that T_H17 cells produce pro-inflammatory cytokines that facilitate inflammation in IBD, the most notable of which appear to be IL-6 and IL-17. Moreover, IL-23R is expressed in high numbers on T_H17 cells and has been postulated to play a key role in propagation of inflammation in both UC and Crohn's disease.

Overall, the immune mechanisms mediating inflammation in IBD are complex and work through significant interactions with environmental triggers, the genome, and the gut microbiome to produce active disease necessitating the need for a personalized approach to management.

As alluded to, environmental factors also are believed to play a role in the pathogenesis of IBD because the disease is more common in industrialized countries. Moreover, the frequency has increased in countries as they become more industrialized. It has been postulated that poor sanitation, food contamination, and crowded living conditions are associated with helminthic infection, which leads to regulatory T-cell conditioning and stimulation of IL-10 and transforming growth factor-β production by mononuclear cells, thereby preventing intestinal inflammation.

The only environmental factor clearly associated with IBD is tobacco smoking. Tobacco seems to be protective against UC, with an older age of onset in former smokers. Among UC patients, smoking cessation may cause an exacerbation. Moreover, studies have shown that tobacco smokers with UC may have a milder disease course, require less immune suppression, and have a reduced need for surgery.

Conversely, Crohn's disease is associated with a more aggressive disease course. Tobacco consumption is associated with a 2-fold increase in the risk of development of Crohn's disease and an earlier age of onset. Passive smoking may also increase the risk. Smoking leads to more frequent exacerbations of Crohn's disease, an increased need for immunosuppression and surgery, as well as a higher risk of postresection recurrence. Not all studies demonstrate these associations, suggesting a gene-environment interaction of tobacco and IBD with the divergent effects on UC and Crohn's disease not well understood.

Diet may also play a role. There is observational evidence that patients with Crohn's disease consumed a much higher quantity of refined sugars represented by sugar, candy, and sweetened foods like cakes and cookies prior to their diagnosis. Subsequently, it was suggested that high sugar intake itself could also interact with intestinal flora and produce pro-inflammatory intestinal agents. In addition to increased intake of refined sugars, newly diagnosed patients with IBD consumed less dietary fiber, raw fruit, and vegetables when compared to healthy controls. A systematic review of past epidemiologic surveys and case control studies performed in Japanese patients suggested an association between increased consumption of animal meat in addition to carbohydrates as potential risk for development of Crohn's disease. The researchers hypothesized that Western dietary patterns may be responsible for the increased occurrence of IBD in Japan.

Study of the relationship between obesity and IBD is especially important because of credible molecular evidence that links adipose tissue physiology to intestinal inflammation. However, it is still not entirely clear whether this link translates into a causal or clinically meaningful association between obesity and Crohn's disease.

Recently, there has been interest in understanding the association between cannabis and IBD. There are no credible epidemiologic data suggesting that cannabis plays a role in the development of IBD or its management. However, studies are ongoing.

Medications suggested to be potential risk factors for the development of IBD include, most importantly, nonsteroidal anti-inflammatory drugs (NSAIDs). NSAIDs have also been implicated in exacerbating existing disease. Other medications potentially linked to development of IBD include oral contraceptives, hormone replacement therapy, and antibiotics, but evidence for these is not as strong as with NSAIDs.

Mycobacterium avium subspecies *paratuberculosis* has been linked to Crohn's disease but this association has not been confirmed. Similarly, associations between *Salmonella*, *Campylobacter*, and measles virus have been reported to increase the risk of IBD, but not proven.

Poor hygiene (lack of sanitation), especially early in life, may protect against the development of IBD. Other potential associations include stress, anxiety, depression, disruptive sleep pattern, and sedentary lifestyle. Although provocative, these associations have not been confirmed in well-designed prospective studies.

CLINICAL PRESENTATION

Intestinal Manifestations
Ulcerative Colitis

UC is characterized by chronic inflammation of the mucosal surface that involves the rectum and extends proximally through the colon in a continuous manner. The extent and severity of colonic inflammation determine prognosis and presentation (insidious vs. acute onset). Most patients initially exhibit diarrhea, abdominal pain, urgency to defecate, rectal bleeding, and the passage of mucus per rectum. At presentation, approximately 40% to 50% of patients have proctitis or proctosigmoiditis, 30% to 40% have left-sided colitis (disease extending to the splenic flexure), and the remaining 20% to 25% have pancolitis. Though data are variable, depending on the cohort, it has been observed that up to 50% of patients diagnosed with proctitis or proctosigmoiditis will progress to more extensive disease by 25 years of follow-up.

The typical clinical course of UC is one of chronic intermittent exacerbations followed by periods of remission. A disease flare may be suggested by the development of diarrhea, hematochezia, and abdominal pain, with dehydration, fever, and tachycardia suggesting more severe disease. Elevated fecal calprotectin, erythrocyte sedimentation rate (ESR) or C-reactive protein (CRP) level may also indicate a flare. Anemia commonly occurs and is caused by chronic blood loss from the involved colonic mucosa as well as bone marrow suppression from the systemic inflammatory process. Perforation can occur in patients with severe or fulminant colitis, especially those taking corticosteroids, and in the setting of toxic megacolon. Toxic megacolon is characterized by gross dilation of the large bowel associated with fever, abdominal pain, dehydration, tachycardia, and bloody diarrhea.

Crohn's Disease

The clinical presentation of Crohn's disease depends on the section of gastrointestinal tract involved and the type of inflammation. Crohn's disease can involve any portion of the gastrointestinal tract; the most common site is ileocecal/ileocolonic (40% of patients), followed by isolated small bowel disease mostly affecting the terminal ileum (30%), and isolated colonic involvement (25%). The remaining sites of Crohn's disease are rarely (5%) affected in isolation and include the esophagus, stomach, and duodenum.

Symptoms in Crohn's disease often include right lower quadrant abdominal pain, fever, weight loss, diarrhea, and sometimes a palpable inflammatory mass on physical exam. Hematochezia may be present with colonic involvement but is less common than in UC. The symptoms can often be present for months or years before a diagnosis is made, and in children, growth retardation may be the sole presenting sign. In contrast to UC, the inflammation in Crohn's disease is transmural and can result in deep ulcerations and the formation of fistulous tracts. Fistulas may form between different segments of bowel (e.g., enteroenteric, enterocolonic) or between bowel and skin (enterocutaneous), bowel and bladder (enterovesicular), or rectum and vagina (rectovaginal). Over time, as many as 30% to 40% of patients will develop perianal involvement with fissures, fistulas or abscesses.

Chronic inflammation can cause fibrosis and stricture formation, which in turn may result in partial or complete intestinal obstruction with the patient complaining of abdominal pain, distention, nausea, and vomiting. Strictures can also lead to stasis with subsequent small intestinal bacterial overgrowth. Small bowel disease may lead to vitamin D deficiency. Extensive ileal mucosal disease may lead to malabsorption of vitamin B_{12} (resulting in a megaloblastic anemia and neurologic side effects if not corrected) and malabsorption of bile salts (resulting in diarrhea induced by unabsorbed bile salts and potential fat-soluble vitamin deficiency). Depletion of the bile salt pool can lead to the formation of gallstones. Weight loss may result from generalized malabsorption caused by loss of absorptive surfaces. Chronic fat malabsorption leads to luminal binding of free fatty acids to calcium; this allows oxalate, which normally is poorly absorbed because it complexes to calcium in the gut lumen, to be absorbed in the colon. The increase in oxalate absorption increases the risk for urinary calcium oxalate stone formation. Patients with an ileostomy or chronic volume loss from diarrhea are also at increased risk for uric acid stones.

Extraintestinal Manifestations

Although both UC and Crohn's disease primarily involve the bowel, they are also associated with inflammatory manifestations in other organ systems. This reflects the systemic nature of these disorders

TABLE 38.1 **Extraintestinal Manifestations of Inflammatory Bowel Disease**
Skin
Pyoderma gangrenosum
Erythema nodosum
Sweet syndrome
Hepatobiliary
Primary sclerosing cholangitis
Cholelithiasis
Autoimmune hepatitis
Musculoskeletal
Seronegative arthritis
Ankylosing spondylitis
Sacroiliitis
Ocular
Uveitis
Episcleritis
Miscellaneous
Hypercoagulable state
Autoimmune hemolytic anemia
Amyloidosis

(Table 38.1). Extraintestinal manifestations can occur in parallel or independently of disease activity and they can become more difficult to treat than the bowel disease itself.

The most common extraintestinal manifestation is arthritis, which is seen in about 9% to 50% of patients and is divided into two major types: axial and peripheral. Axial arthropathy consists of sacroiliitis or ankylosing spondylitis and does *not* parallel activity of bowel disease. Ankylosing spondylitis occurs in 5% to 10% of IBD patients and manifests with low back pain and stiffness that is usually worse during the night, in the morning, or after inactivity. Sacroiliitis alone (without ankylosing spondylitis) is common in IBD (up to 20% of patients) but in many cases is asymptomatic. Peripheral arthropathy is divided into type 1 and type 2. Type 1 peripheral arthropathy affects peripheral large joints. It is an asymmetric, seronegative, oligoarticular, nondeforming arthritis that may involve the knees, hips, wrists, elbows, and ankles. This peripheral arthropathy usually parallels disease activity. Peripheral arthropathy type 2 involves typically metacarpal phalangeal (MCP) joints, is typically symmetrical, and does *not* parallel disease activity.

Liver complications of IBD include both parenchymal and biliary tract diseases. Parenchymal diseases include fatty liver, pericholangitis, and chronic active hepatitis. Pericholangitis, also known as small-duct sclerosing cholangitis, is the most common of these diseases. It usually is asymptomatic, identified only by abnormalities in alkaline phosphatase and γ-glutamyl transpeptidase (GGT) on laboratory tests and histologically by portal tract inflammation and bile ductule degeneration. Small-duct sclerosing cholangitis may progress to cirrhosis.

Biliary tract disease includes an increased incidence of gallstones and primary sclerosing cholangitis (PSC). PSC is a chronic cholestatic liver disease marked by fibrosis of the intrahepatic and extrahepatic bile ducts. It occurs in 1% to 4% of patients with UC and less often in those with Crohn's disease. Overall, about 70% of patients with PSC have UC. Fibrosis leads to strictures of the bile ducts, which in turn may lead to recurrent cholangitis (with fever, right upper quadrant pain, and jaundice) and progression to cirrhosis. In addition, about 10% of patients develop cholangiocarcinoma. Medical or surgical

TABLE 38.2　Differentiating Features of UC and Crohn's Disease

	Ulcerative Colitis	Crohn's Disease
Site of involvement	Involves colon only	Any area of the gastrointestinal tract
	Rectum almost always involved	Rectum usually spared
Pattern of involvement	Continuous	Skip lesions
Diarrhea	Bloody	Usually nonbloody
Severe abdominal pain	Rare	Frequent
Perianal disease	No	In 30% of patients
Fistula	No	Yes
Endoscopic findings	Erythematous and friable	Aphthoid and deep ulcers
	Superficial ulceration	Cobblestoning
Radiologic findings	Tubular appearance resulting from loss of haustral folds	String sign of terminal ileum
		RLQ mass, fistulas, abscesses
Histologic features	Mucosal involvement only	Transmural
	Crypt abscesses	Crypt abscesses, granulomas (about 30%)
Smoking	Protective	Worsens course
Serology	pANCA more common	ASCA more common

ASCA, Anti–Saccharomyces cerevisiae antibodies; *pANCA,* perinuclear antineutrophil cytoplasmic antibody; *RLQ,* right lower quadrant.

therapy for IBD does not modify the course of PSC and most patients progress to cirrhosis and may require liver transplantation.

The two classic dermatologic manifestations that can be associated with IBD are pyoderma gangrenosum and erythema nodosum. Pyoderma gangrenosum occurs in about 5% of patients and is characterized by a discrete ulcer with a necrotic base, usually on the legs. The ulcer may spread and become large and deep, destroying soft tissues. Pyoderma is unrelated to disease activity. Treatment is usually with systemic or intralesional steroids, or both. Other treatment options include dapsone, cyclosporine, and anti-TNF agents. Erythema nodosum occurs in 10% of IBD patients, usually with peripheral arthropathy, and produces raised, tender nodules, usually over the anterior surface of the legs. Erythema nodosum responds to treatment for the underlying bowel disease. A less common dermatologic manifestation of IBD is Sweet syndrome or acute febrile neutrophilic dermatosis. This condition is characterized by the sudden onset of fever, leukocytosis, and tender, erythematous, well-demarcated papules and plaques that show dense neutrophilic infiltrates on histologic examination.

Ocular manifestations of IBD include uveitis and episcleritis. They occur in 1% to 5% of patients. Uveitis (or iritis) is an inflammatory condition of the anterior chamber that produces blurred vision, photophobia, headache, and conjunctival injection that may not parallel disease activity. Local therapy includes corticosteroids and atropine. Episcleritis is typically associated with disease activity. It produces burning eyes and scleral injection without vision deficits and is treated with topical corticosteroids.

DIAGNOSIS AND DIFFERENTIAL DIAGNOSIS

The diagnosis of IBD is based on a constellation of clinical features and endoscopic, radiographic, and histologic findings. Laboratory tests are not specific and usually demonstrate inflammation (leukocytosis) and anemia when the disease is active. Perinuclear antineutrophil cytoplasmic antibody (pANCA) is positive in up to 70% of patients with UC but is uncommon in patients with Crohn's disease, whereas anti–*Saccharomyces cerevisiae* antibodies (ASCA) are common (up to 60%) in Crohn's disease but not typically found in UC (Table 38.2). Additional markers, mainly for Crohn's disease, have improved the sensitivity and specificity of serologic testing, including antibodies to OmpC (*Escherichia coli* outer membrane porin C) and antibodies to bacterial flagellins CBir1, FlaX, and A4-Fla2. Due to lack of sensitivity

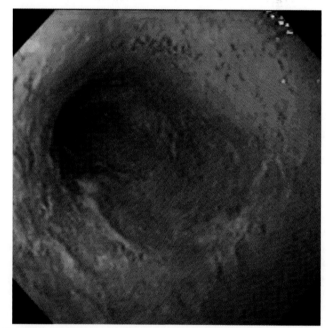

Fig. 38.1 Endoscopic image of ulcerative colitis demonstrates diffuse inflammation characterized by erythema, edema, friability, and hemorrhage.

and specificity, laboratory testing is of limited value and should not be used to make a diagnosis of IBD.

Colonoscopy findings in patients with UC are nonspecific, typically revealing granular mucosa, decreased vascular markings, exudate, and superficial ulcerations (Fig. 38.1) typically beginning in the rectum. In more severe cases, the mucosa is friable, with deeper ulcerations. Patients with long-standing severe disease can develop pseudopolyps, which represent islands of normal tissue in regions of previous ulceration. In Crohn's disease (Fig. 38.2), endoscopic examination may show aphthoid erosions, deep linear or stellate ulcers, edema, erythema, exudate, and friability with intervening areas of normal mucosa (skip lesions). However, a diagnosis of indeterminate colitis is made in 10% to 15% of patients because of an overlap of findings. For example, colonic Crohn's disease may produce superficial continuous rectal involvement similar to that seen in UC. Similarly, chronic UC

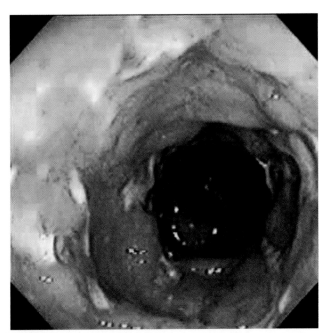

Fig. 38.2 Endoscopic image of Crohn's disease demonstrates linear ulcers in areas of otherwise normal mucosa.

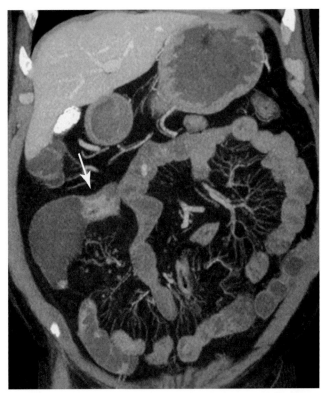

Fig. 38.3 Computed tomographic enterography shows inflammatory stricture *(arrow)* and small bowel wall thickening in a patient with Crohn's disease.

can infrequently result in inflammation of the terminal ileum, called backwash ileitis, usually when severe disease of the cecum or ascending colon is present. In many patients with indeterminate colitis, repeated examination is necessary, or complications may develop that help identify the disease form.

Several types of radiologic studies can be used to diagnose IBD. In Crohn's disease, the most sensitive radiographic test to diagnose small bowel disease is CT or MR enterography. On traditional small bowel radiography, segments of edematous bowel appear thickened next to uninvolved mucosa, a characteristic pattern referred to as *cobblestoning*. Tight, long strictures in the small bowel can be identified and are called a *string sign*. Cross-sectional imaging with computed tomographic (CT) enterography and magnetic resonance enterography (MRE) has replaced traditional small bowel radiography. Cross-sectional imaging can identify bowel wall thickening with surrounding inflammation, as well as intra-abdominal abscesses and fistulas (Figs. 38.3 and 38.4). A characteristic finding on cross-sectional imaging in Crohn's disease is infiltration of the mesentery with fat, commonly known as *creeping fat*.

Video capsule endoscopy allows for direct visualization of the small bowel mucosa where erosions or ulcerations of the small bowel may be found (Fig. 38.5). Patients with known or suspected strictures should be evaluated for risk of capsule retention before undergoing capsule endoscopy.

Mucosal biopsies in IBD reveal acute and chronic inflammation with infiltration by plasma cells, neutrophils, lymphocytes, and eosinophils; focal ulcerations; crypt architectural distortion; and crypt abscesses (Figs. 38.6 and 38.7). The presence of chronic inflammation distinguishes IBD from other types of acute self-limited colitis like enteric infection. In Crohn's disease, the inflammation is transmural and more commonly focal. Granulomas are found in 25% to 30% of histologic specimens in Crohn's disease. The presence of granulomas is not required but can assist in making the diagnosis of Crohn's disease in the right clinical setting (Fig. 38.8). Granulomas are not diagnostic because they can be found in many other diseases, such as Behçet's disease, tuberculosis, *Yersinia* infection, gastrointestinal and hepatic sarcoidosis, and lymphoma.

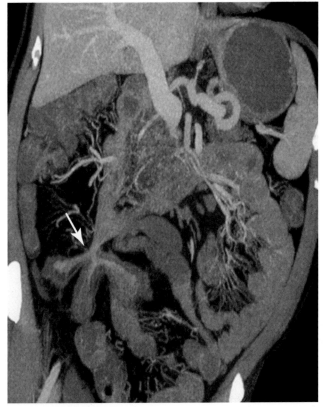

Fig. 38.4 Computed tomographic enterography shows extensive Crohn's disease with fistula *(arrow)*.

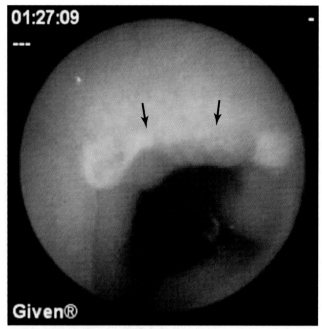

Fig. 38.5 Video capsule endoscopic image shows ulcerated stenosis in a patient with Crohn's disease *(arrows)*.

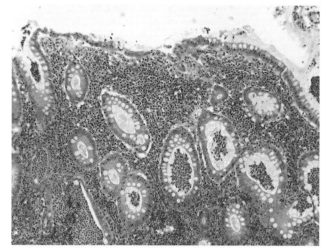

Fig. 38.7 Mucosal biopsy specimen demonstrates crypt branching and a crypt abscess characteristic of ulcerative colitis (hematoxylin and eosin stain).

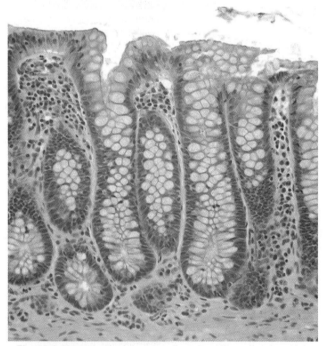

Fig. 38.6 Normal colonic mucosa (hematoxylin and eosin stain).

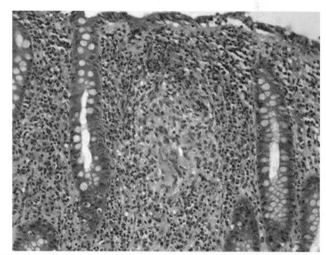

Fig. 38.8 Colonic biopsy specimen demonstrates a chronic inflammatory infiltrate with a granuloma in a patient with Crohn's colitis (hematoxylin and eosin stain).

The differential diagnosis of IBD includes infectious colitis, ischemic colitis, radiation enteritis, enterocolitis induced by nonsteroidal anti-inflammatory drugs, diverticulitis, appendicitis, gastrointestinal malignancies, and irritable bowel syndrome. In patients with acute onset of bloody diarrhea, infectious causes that must be excluded with stool testing include *Salmonella enteritidis, Shigella* species, *Campylobacter jejuni, Escherichia coli* O157, and *Clostridioides difficile. Clostridioides difficile* is more common among patients with IBD. Among the infectious causes, *Yersinia enterocolitica* can mimic Crohn's disease because the pathogen causes ileitis, mesenteric adenitis, fever, diarrhea, and right lower quadrant abdominal pain. *Mycobacterium tuberculosis*

infection, strongyloidiasis, and amebiasis must be excluded in high-risk populations, because these infections can mimic IBD, and treatment with corticosteroids can lead to disseminated infection and death.

TREATMENT

Treatment of IBD follows a systematic, standardized, and evidence-based approach. It relies on first identifying the type of IBD, then categorizing severity of disease, and then identifying a management goal, which now encourages a "treat to target" approach and focuses on endoscopic improvement and healing. Next, a therapeutic agent is selected incorporating data from well-designed clinical studies and also patient tolerability and overall safety, convenience, and preference. Furthermore, the treatment of IBD includes a focus on employing more aggressive and effective "top down" strategies by using biologic and newer oral agents earlier in the course in selected patients with moderate to severe disease. Maximizing the efficacy of current therapies now includes achieving therapeutic levels of these drugs when possible in the attempt to achieve endoscopic healing rapidly and thus improve long-term outcomes.

TABLE 38.3   Treatment Options

Disease Severity	Ulcerative Colitis	Crohn's Disease
Mild	Oral and topical 5-ASA compounds Budesonide MMX	Budesonide EC Elemental diet
Moderate	Oral and topical 5-ASA compounds Oral steroids or budesonide MMX Azathioprine, 6-MP Infliximab, adalimumab, golimumab Vedolizumab Tofacitinib Ustekinumab	Oral steroids or budesonide EC Azathioprine, 6-MP Methotrexate Infliximab, adalimumab, certolizumab pegol Vedolizumab Ustekinumab
Severe	Intravenous steroids Cyclosporine Infliximab, adalimumab, golimumab Vedolizumab Tofacitinib Ustekinumab Surgery	Intravenous steroids Methotrexate Infliximab, adalimumab, certolizumab vedolizumab Ustekinumab Surgery

5-ASA, 5-Aminosalicylic acid; *6-MP*, 6-mercaptopurine.

Patients with mild or moderate disease can be managed as outpatients. Patients with severe or fulminant disease—with abdominal pain, fever, tachycardia, anemia, and leukocytosis—require hospital admission and multidisciplinary team management. Because IBD is a chronic recurrent illness, treatment is centered on controlling the acute attack with induction of remission, followed by maintenance of remission. Treatment options for UC and Crohn's disease are summarized in Table 38.3.

In brief, treatment agents for IBD broadly include nontargeted immune suppressants such as corticosteroids, topical anti-inflammatories including 5-aminosalicylic acid (mesalamine) and related agents, antibiotics, and traditional immunomodulators including thiopurine analogs (azathioprine, 6-MP) that inhibit replication of inflammatory cells by inducing cell death or apoptosis and methotrexate, which inhibits replication of inflammatory cells by inhibiting cell division or mitosis.

Newer approved biologic and oral agents work variably by targeting effector pro-inflammatory cytokines such as TNF-alpha and IL-12/23, targeting immune cell function such as the JAK-STAT enzyme pathway or inhibiting cell trafficking such as the alpha-4/beta7 adhesion inhibition.

5-Aminosalicylic Acid (Mesalamine)

The 5-aminosalicylates are given either orally or topically (suppository/enema) or as a combined regimen. They are safe and effective for treatment (i.e., induction of remission) of mild to moderate UC and for maintenance of remission. The efficacy of the 5-aminosalicylic acid (5-ASA) agents in induction or maintenance of remission in Crohn's disease has not been demonstrated. This class of anti-inflammatory medications includes sulfasalazine (Azulfidine) at a dose of 4 to 6 g/day in divided doses. This drug consists of 5-ASA linked to a sulfapyridine moiety; the 5-ASA is released after bacterial lysis of the azo bond in the distal small bowel and colon. Side effects, including headache, nausea, and skin reactions, require discontinuation of sulfasalazine in about 30% of patients. Reversible oligospermia may occur with sulfasalazine.

Rare serious side effects include pleuropericarditis, pancreatitis, agranulocytosis, interstitial nephritis, and hemolytic anemia may occur with sulfasalazine and 5-ASA. Patients who take sulfasalazine need folic acid supplementation.

Derivatives of oral 5-ASA compounds include mesalamine (Pentasa, 4 g/day in divided doses; Delzicol, 2.4 g/day in divided doses; Asacol HD, 2.4 to 4.8 g/day in divided doses; Lialda, 2.4 to 4.8 g once daily; Apriso, 1.5 g once a day), olsalazine (Dipentum, 1 to 2 g/day in divided doses), and balsalazide (Colazal, 6.75 g/day in divided doses; Giazo 3.3 g/day in divided doses). Topical forms of mesalamine (Canasa suppositories, 1000 mg once daily; Rowasa enemas, 4 g once nightly) are commonly used because of a more favorable side effect profile.

Corticosteroids

Corticosteroids may be used topically, orally, or intravenously. They are effective for controlling active inflammatory disease but not for maintaining remission and should act as a bridge to maintenance therapy. They are not indicated for maintenance therapy. They are indicated for moderate or severe disease in patients with UC for whom treatment with 5-ASA has failed. The most commonly used agents are parenteral methylprednisolone for severe/fulminant disease requiring hospitalization at doses of 45 to 60 mg intravenously daily and for outpatients, oral prednisone, started in doses between 40 and 60 mg/day. Patients typically improve rapidly, and the medication is usually tapered down slowly (i.e., by 5 to 10 mg/week) until discontinuation. Patients who do not improve after 1 week of oral treatment and those with more severe disease are best treated in the hospital with intravenous corticosteroids.

Controlled trials have shown that budesonide EC (Entocort EC) is more effective than placebo or oral 5-ASA and has similar efficacy to prednisolone for the induction of remission in Crohn's disease of the terminal ileum (level of evidence I, A). Entocort EC (9 mg given once daily as three 3-mg pills) undergoes extensive first-pass hepatic metabolism and is approved for inducing and maintaining remission of ileal and ileocolonic Crohn's disease (level of evidence III, A) with decreased corticosteroid side effects. Budesonide MMX (Uceris 9 mg given once daily) has an extended release that targets the colon and is approved for the treatment of mild to moderate UC but should not be used as maintenance therapy. Corticosteroids have numerous side effects with long-term use.

Traditional Immunomodulators

The traditional immunomodulators used in IBD include azathioprine (Imuran) and its active metabolite, 6-mercaptopurine (6-MP) (Purinethol), as well as methotrexate and cyclosporine. Metabolism of azathioprine and 6-mercaptopurine is based on the enzyme thiopurine methyl transferase (TPMT). TPMT should be measured in each patient before starting therapy to determine starting dose to minimize toxicity and maximize efficacy. Hematologic monitoring for drug toxicity on therapy is essential. Azathioprine and 6-MP are effective therapies for maintaining remission in both Crohn's disease and UC and are used primarily as corticosteroid-sparing agents. They have a slow onset of action (weeks to months) and consequently are not used to induce remission. Side effects include pancreatitis, nausea, abnormal liver enzymes, bone marrow suppression, opportunistic infections, and an increased risk of lymphoma and nonmelanoma skin cancer.

Methotrexate can be used for induction (25 mg subcutaneously once weekly) and maintenance of remission (15 to 25 mg subcutaneously once weekly) in active Crohn's disease; the side effect profile includes bone marrow suppression, mucositis, interstitial pneumonitis, and with long-term use, cirrhosis. Folic acid should be given with methotrexate to reduce the risk of mucositis. Methotrexate has been studied as a primary treatment for UC and was not found to be effective. Intravenous cyclosporine (2 mg/kg/day given over 24 hours) is used as a rescue medicine and, in severe UC refractory to intravenous steroids, as a *bridge* treatment to one of the above immunomodulators or biologic agents. Given the potential for both short-term and long-term side effects, as well as the need for close follow-up, patients needing these medications are best managed by gastroenterologists.

Previously used as primary therapy for IBD, azathioprine/6-mercaptopurine and methotrexate are now more commonly used in combination with newer more effective biologic therapies, especially anti-TNF agents.

Biologic Agents

Biologics are a class of medications that target specific aspects of the immune system. The first such agent to be used in IBD was infliximab (Remicade), a chimeric monoclonal antibody to TNF-α, which has been shown to be effective in the treatment of both moderate to severe Crohn's disease, including fistulizing disease, and UC (level of evidence I, A). Anti-TNF agents that are administered subcutaneously include adalimumab (Humira) and golimumab (Simponi), which are fully human monoclonal antibodies, and certolizumab pegol (Cimzia), which is a humanized anti-TNF antibody Fab fragment. Adalimumab, certolizumab pegol, and infliximab are indicated for the treatment of patients with moderate to severe Crohn's disease. Adalimumab, infliximab, and golimumab are approved to treat moderate to severe UC. These agents can be associated with adverse reactions including infusion reactions (infliximab), delayed-type hypersensitivity reaction, and with development of anti-drug antibodies resulting in reduced effectiveness.

Natalizumab (Tysabri), a humanized anti–α_4-integrin antibody, blocks inflammatory cell migration and adhesion and is approved for the treatment of moderate to severe Crohn's disease in patients who have had an inadequate response to, or are unable to tolerate, conventional Crohn's disease therapies including inhibitors of TNF-α. Due to its link with progressive multifocal leukoencephalopathy (PML) and approval of a more gut selective agent, vedolizumab, it is now rarely used. Vedolizumab (Entyvio), a humanized monoclonal antibody to α4β7 integrin, is approved for the treatment and maintenance of both Crohn's and UC.

Ustekinumab, a monoclonal antibody against the P40 subunit of IL-12 and IL-23, is approved for the induction and maintenance of remission in moderate to severe Crohn's and UC.

Tofacitinib, an oral small molecule that inhibits Janus kinase (JAK) enzymes, is approved for treatment of moderate to severe UC in patients intolerant of or who have not responded to anti-TNFs. Because of the potent effects these biological drugs and oral agents have on the immune system, careful patient selection and monitoring for complications are necessary. Reactivation of latent tuberculosis and other serious infections have been reported with the anti-TNF agents. Other rare but serious complications include non-Hodgkin's lymphoma, exacerbation of congestive heart failure, abnormal complete blood count (CBC) and liver function test results, venous thrombosis, and demyelinating disease. Natalizumab is associated with rare cases of progressive multifocal leukoencephalopathy caused by the human JC virus.

Future biologic agents with alternative mechanisms of action are being developed. These include several selective IL-23 inhibitors such as risankizumab, mirikizumab, guselkumab, and brazikumab. These biologics selectively target the P19 subunit of the interleukin-23 (IL-23) cytokine, thus being more selective than ustekinumab (Stelara), which inhibits the P40 components of both IL-12 and IL-23. A theoretical advantage of IL-23 selectivity is thought to be reduced potential side effects related to targeting of IL-12, including risk of carcinogenesis suggested in some animal studies.

Additional JAK inhibitors (filgotinib, upadacitinib) are being examined for their role in treatment of IBD. Etrolizumab, a beta7 inhibitor, and ontamalimab, a MadCAM-1 ligand inhibitor, are inhibitors of cell trafficking that are in clinical trials. Ozanimod (RPC1063), an oral agent that acts as a selective agonist and modulator of sphingosine phosphate receptor subtypes 1 and 5, thus inhibiting lymphocyte trafficking to sites of inflammation, is also being tested for its efficacy in UC and Crohn's disease.

The availability of these biologic agents has changed the approach to the management of IBD. The emphasis now has shifted from treating symptoms alone and maintaining clinical remission to treating to a target of endoscopic remission. Endoscopic remission or mucosal healing (as it is typically referred to) is defined as the absence of mucosal ulceration or erosion. The finding of ulceration in the lining of the bowel is associated with higher likelihood of disease flare in asymptomatic patients. Achieving endoscopic remission has been associated with better long-term patient outcomes including longer sustained clinical remissions, lower rates of hospitalization and, in some studies, lower rates of surgery. In this paradigm, after a therapy has been started, an asymptomatic patient will undergo an evaluation 6 to 9 months later to look for evidence of endoscopic remission or ongoing intestinal inflammation. If persistent or significant disease is present, then treatment is typically optimized or changed to try to achieve endoscopic remission. This treat to target approach continues to undergo further study.

Other Agents

Other agents for the treatment of IBD include antibiotics, probiotics, antidiarrheal agents, bile salt resin binders, and nutritional support.

Although used widely in the past for luminal Crohn's, antibiotics are now less commonly employed in routine treatment of patients with luminal Crohn's disease. Current use of antibiotics in active Crohn's is largely limited to treatment of pyogenic complications and in perianal disease. Metronidazole may prevent postoperative recurrence in some patients with luminal Crohn's but adverse effects typically limit its usefulness. There is some evidence for the efficacy of a novel enteric form of rifaximin in mild to moderately active luminal Crohn's disease. The role of antibiotics in UC is unclear, and further studies are required. However, intravenous antibiotics may be used in the initial treatment of severe, toxic, or fulminant colitis when infection is a concern. Antibiotics are useful to treat bacterial overgrowth that can be associated with Crohn's disease.

Probiotics are viable nonpathogenic organisms considered to be food products that after ingestion may prevent or treat intestinal diseases and have been explored in the treatment of IBD. There is some evidence for their efficacy in pouchitis (see later) and UC but no clear benefit in Crohn's disease has been noted thus far. Additional studies are ongoing.

Antidiarrheal agents and bile salt resin binders have no effect on IBD inflammation but can be used as adjuncts for management of diarrhea in patients with IBD, but antidiarrheal agents should be used cautiously during exacerbations of colitis because they may precipitate toxic megacolon. The main role of antidiarrheal medications involves controlling diarrhea in patients who have undergone previous resections. Patients with Crohn's disease who have had less than 100 cm of terminal ileum removed can develop a bile salt malabsorptive state, during which bile salts enter the colon and cause a secretory diarrhea. Bile salt resin binders such as cholestyramine are an effective treatment in these cases. When patients have undergone one or more extensive resections amounting to more than 100 cm of ileum, the bile salt pool is depleted and fat malabsorption develops. These patients may require a low-fat diet supplemented with medium-chain triglycerides and antidiarrheal agents, but bile salt resin binders should not be used.

Nutritional support is an important adjunctive aspect in the management of IBD. However, the role of nutrition as a primary treatment has been limited to patients with small bowel Crohn's disease, especially in children. These patients may achieve and maintain remission with total parenteral nutrition or elemental diets after prolonged periods (at least 4 weeks) and potentially avoid the need for corticosteroids. Many patients with Crohn's disease or UC experience weight loss during exacerbations of their illness and need caloric supplements. Vitamins and minerals can be given orally as a multivitamin with folic acid. Vitamin B_{12} should be supplemented parenterally in patients who have extensive ileal disease or an ileal resection. Patients taking corticosteroids require supplemental calcium and vitamin D, and individuals with extensive small bowel involvement can also develop malabsorption of fat-soluble vitamins (A, D, E, and K), iron, and, rarely, trace minerals. A low-fiber diet may be necessary in patients with active disease or strictures. There is some observational evidence to suggest effectiveness of the specific carbohydrate diet (SCD) in patients with IBD but it is very restrictive in nature; therefore, it is not being widely recommended until further research becomes available.

More studies on diet as a treatment for IBD are needed. Complementary and alternative medicines are used frequently by patients with IBD and it is important that treating clinicians ask about their use.

Surgical Management

Surgical intervention is indicated for patients with complications such as obstruction, perforation, fibrotic stricture, massive gastrointestinal hemorrhage, or toxic megacolon or who are not responsive to medical treatment. The other main indication for surgical treatment is the presence of dysplasia or cancer. For patients with UC, regardless of the extent of disease, the entire colon must be removed. Historically, the initial operation for UC was a total proctocolectomy and Brooke ileostomy, but ileal pouch–anal anastomosis has become the procedure of choice in most patients. In this operation, the colon is removed and the small bowel is constructed into a reservoir (ileal pouch) that is anastomosed to the anus or a short segment of the rectum, allowing defecation through the anus. Complications include the development of inflammation of the rectum (cuffitis) or pouch (pouchitis), fecal incontinence, reduced fertility, and need for reoperation. Surgery is not curative in Crohn's disease. Many surgical procedures in patients with Crohn's disease are performed to manage complications of the disease, including segmental resection, stricturoplasty, fistulectomy, and abscess drainage.

PROGNOSIS

Approximately two thirds of patients with UC have at least one relapse in the 10 years after their diagnosis. About 20% to 30% of patients with extensive UC will require colectomy within their lifetime. Only 5% of individuals with proctitis undergo colectomy by 10 years after diagnosis. In contrast, more than 60% of Crohn's patients require surgery within the 10 years after their diagnosis although these data are based on patients treated in the pre-biologic era. The rate of recurrence in Crohn's disease is high, with 70% of patients having an endoscopic recurrence within 1 year after surgery and 50% having a symptomatic recurrence within 4 years. Predictors of a severe course in Crohn's disease include stricturing or penetrating disease and perianal disease.

The risk for colon cancer is increased in patients with UC, and its magnitude is related to the extent and duration of disease. The colon cancer risk is increased 10- to 20-fold after 8 to 10 years of disease in pancolitis, and after 15 to 20 years in left-sided colitis. The cumulative incidence of colorectal cancer is 2.5% after 20 years and 7.6% after 30 years of disease. Proctitis is not associated with an increased risk of colorectal cancer. In colonic Crohn's disease, the risk of colorectal cancer is equivalent to that in patients with UC of similar extent and duration. Patients with isolated small bowel Crohn's disease are not at increased risk for colorectal cancer. The rates of small bowel carcinoma and lymphoma are increased in patients with Crohn's disease but the absolute risk is very low.

Surveillance for dysplasia and colon cancer among patients with UC and Crohn's disease colitis should be performed by colonoscopy 8 to 10 years after the onset of symptoms. Surveillance examinations are performed every 1 to 3 years. Proctitis does not require endoscopic surveillance, but colonoscopy should be performed 8 years after diagnosis to look for evidence of proximal spread of the disease. Patients with IBD and PSC appear to have a particularly increased risk for colon cancer, and yearly surveillance is recommended after the initial diagnosis of PSC. UC associated with PSC may have minimal or no symptoms, so all patients with PSC should undergo colonoscopy with biopsy to look for evidence of UC. The classic approach for UC surveillance has been to take a minimum of 33 "random" mucosal biopsy samples during the colonoscopic examination, in addition to targeted samples of visible lesions. The use of chromoendoscopy (spraying of the colon surface with indigo carmine or methylene blue dye during colonoscopy) increases the detection of dysplastic lesions in patients with UC and has replaced the performance of random biopsies in some societal guidelines. Polypoid dysplasia entirely removed by polypectomy in the colon can be managed with continued surveillance colonoscopy. Colectomy is indicated in patients with unresectable dysplasia or evidence of colorectal cancer.

As understanding of the etiologic and pathophysiologic aspects of IBD increases, major advances in diagnosis and treatment are anticipated. These will be based on better use of molecular, genetic, and serologic tests to differentiate among the subtypes of disease; earlier and more targeted use of biologic agents to manage inflammation; and improvements in the detection and prevention of colorectal cancer in those at risk.

SUGGESTED READINGS

Abraham BP, Quigley EMM: Probiotics in inflammatory bowel disease, Gastroenterol Clin North Am 46(4):769–782, 2017.

Ananthakrishnan AN: Epidemiology and risk factors for IBD, Nat Rev Gastroenterol Hepatol 12(4):205–217, 2015.

Damas OM, Garces L, Abreu MT: Diet as adjunctive treatment for inflammatory bowel disease: review and update of the latest literature, Curr Treat Options Gastroenterol 17(2):313–325, 2019.

De Souza HSP, Fiocchi C, Iliopoulos D: The IBD interactome: an integrated view of aetiology, pathogenesis and therapy, Nat Rev Gastroenterol Hepatol 14(12):739–749, 2017.

Feuerstein JD, Cheifetz AS: Crohn disease: epidemiology, diagnosis, and management, Mayo Clin Proc 92(7):1088–1103, 2017.

Feuerstein JD, Moss AC, Farraye FA: Ulcerative colitis, Mayo Clin Proc 94(7):1357–1373, 2019.

Johnson CM, Dassopoulos T: Update on the use of thiopurines and methotrexate in inflammatory bowel disease, Curr Gastroenterol Rep 20(11):53, 2018.

Laine L, Kaltenbach T, Barkun A, McQuaid KR, Subramanian V, Soetikno R: SCENIC guideline development panel. SCENIC international consensus statement on surveillance and management of dysplasia in inflammatory bowel disease, Gastrointest Endosc 81(3):489–501, 2015.

Lichtenstein GR, Loftus EV, Isaacs KL, Regueiro MD, Gerson LB, Sands BE: ACG clinical guideline: management of crohn's disease in adults, Am J Gastroenterol 113(4):481–517, 2018.

Ma C, Panaccione R, Khanna R, Feagan BG, Jairath V: IL12/23 or selective IL23 inhibition for the management of moderate-to-severe Crohn's disease? Best Pract Res Clin Gastroenterol 38–39, 2019.

Malik TA: Inflammatory bowel disease: historical perspective, epidemiology and risk factors, Surg Clin North Am 95(6):1105–1122, 2015.

McGovern DP, Kugathasan S, Cho JH: Genetics of inflammatory bowel diseases, Gastroenterology 149(5):1163–1176, 2015.

Rubin DT, Ananthakrishnan AN, Siegel CA, Sauer BG, Long MD: ACG clinical guideline: ulcerative colitis in adults, Am J Gastroenterol 114(3):384–413, 2019.

Weisshof R, El Jurdi K, Zmeter N, Rubin DT: Emerging therapies for inflammatory bowel disease, Adv Ther 35(11):1746–1762, 2018.

Windsor JW, Kaplan GG: Evolving epidemiology of IBD, Curr Gastroenterol Rep 21(8):40, 2019.

39

Diseases of the Pancreas

David R. Lichtenstein, Pushpak Taunk

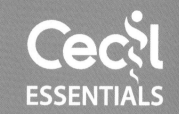

ACUTE PANCREATITIS

Definition and Epidemiology

Acute pancreatitis is an acute inflammatory process of the pancreas that may also involve peripancreatic tissues and remote organ systems. It is one of the leading causes of hospitalization for patients with gastrointestinal disorders in the United States, with more than 275,000 admissions annually. This translates into an overall incidence of 5 to 30 cases per 100,000 people in the general population. The aggregate cost of acute pancreatitis is more than $2.6 billion per year and the overall case fatality is roughly 5%. Approximately 80% of patients admitted with acute pancreatitis have mild, self-limited disease.

Pathology

The pancreas is located in the retroperitoneum and has exocrine and endocrine functions (Fig. 39.1) derived from the pancreatic acinus and the pancreatic islet, respectively. As an exocrine gland, the pancreas participates in normal digestion and nutrient absorption. The enzymes secreted by the pancreas digest starch (i.e., amylase), fats (i.e., lipase), and protein (i.e., trypsin and other proteolytic enzymes). Within acinar cells, proteolytic digestive enzymes are synthesized and packaged separately in the Golgi region into condensing vacuoles and transported in an inactive form referred to as zymogens to the apical portions of the cell. When stimulated, they are discharged into the central ductule of the acinus by exocytosis.

Normal physiology involves secretion of inactive enzymes into the duodenum, where they are converted to an active form by enterokinase, a brush border enzyme secreted by small bowel enterocytes. Trypsinogen conversion to active trypsin is the trigger enzyme that subsequently converts the other zymogens to active enzymes (E-Fig 39.1).

The pathogenesis of acute pancreatitis remains incompletely understood. Based on experimental models, the initiating event appears to involve intra-acinar activation of trypsin from trypsinogen, resulting in acute intracellular injury, pancreatic autodigestion, and the potential for profound systemic complications after activated enzymes are leaked into the bloodstream. The acinar cell injury results in a systemic inflammatory response that involves multiple cytokines, including platelet activating factor, tumor necrosis factor-α (TNF-α), and various interleukins. Initiating events may include obstruction of the pancreatic duct (e.g., gallstones, pancreatic tumor), overdistention of the pancreatic duct (e.g., from endoscopic retrograde cholangiopancreatography [ERCP]), reflux of biliary or duodenal juices into the pancreatic duct, changes in permeability of the pancreatic duct, ischemia of the organ, and toxin-induced cholinergic hyperstimulation (Fig. 39.2).

During the initial hospitalization for acute pancreatitis, reasonable attempts to determine the cause are appropriate, particularly those that

may affect acute management. The cause of acute pancreatitis is readily identified in 70% to 90% of patients after an initial evaluation consisting of the history, physical examination, focused laboratory testing, and routine radiologic studies. Gallstones account for 45%, alcohol for 35%, miscellaneous causes for 10%, and idiopathic causes for 10% to 20% of acute pancreatitis cases (Table 39.1).

Gallstone Pancreatitis

Among patients with gallstones, the incidence of acute pancreatitis is about 0.17% per year. Gallstones increase the relative risk of pancreatitis 25- to 35-fold. Gallstone pancreatitis is more common in women than men. It is theorized that gallstone passage causes transient obstruction of the pancreatic duct, precipitating acute pancreatitis. Acute gallstone pancreatitis should be suspected when associated with a transient elevation in liver-associated enzymes, particularly alanine aminotransferase (ALT) levels greater than 150 IU/L. Most stones pass spontaneously from the ampulla and do not require intervention (discussed later).

Alcoholic Pancreatitis

Acute alcoholic pancreatitis is the second most common cause of pancreatitis in the United States. Approximately 10% of individuals with an alcohol use disorder develop attacks of pancreatitis that are indistinguishable from other forms of acute pancreatitis. Prolonged alcohol use (four to five drinks daily over a period of more than 5 years) is required for alcohol-associated pancreatitis. The type of alcohol does not affect risk, and binge drinking in the absence of long-term, heavy alcohol use infrequently precipitates acute pancreatitis. Alcoholics with acute pancreatitis most commonly have underlying chronic disease. However, some have true acute alcoholic pancreatitis because not all patients progress to chronic pancreatitis, even with continued alcohol use. The mechanism of pancreatic injury, the genetic and environmental factors that influence its development in alcoholics, and the reason only a small proportion of alcoholics develop pancreatitis are unclear (see "Chronic Pancreatitis").

Hypertriglyceridemia

Hypertriglyceridemia is the third most identifiable cause of pancreatitis, and serum triglyceride levels greater than 1000 mg/dL may precipitate attacks of acute pancreatitis. Patients may have lactescent (milky) serum owing to increased concentrations of chylomicrons. Both primary and secondary disorders of lipoprotein metabolism are associated with hypertriglyceridemic pancreatitis. Although the exact pathogenesis of hypertriglyceridemic pancreatitis is unclear, the release of free fatty acids by lipase may damage pancreatic acinar cells or capillary endothelium. The main treatment modalities for initial management of hypertriglyceridemia are apheresis with therapeutic plasma

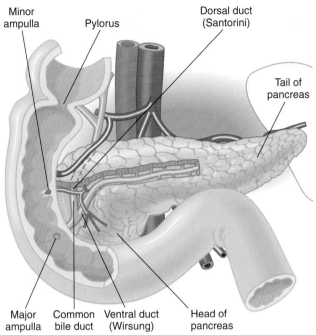

Fig. 39.1 Normal anatomy of the pancreas.

exchange and insulin. Lowering serum triglyceride levels to less than 200 mg/dL can prevent pancreatitis and is typically done with a combination of diet and medications.

Drug-Related Pancreatitis

Drugs appear to cause fewer than 5% of all cases of acute pancreatitis, although hundreds of medications have been implicated. The drugs most strongly associated with acute pancreatitis are azathioprine, 6-mercaptopurine, didanosine, valproic acid, angiotensin-converting-enzyme inhibitors, eluxadoline, and mesalamine. Though there are several potential pathogenic mechanisms of drug-induced pancreatitis, the most common is a hypersensitivity reaction. This tends to occur 4 to 8 weeks after starting the drug and is not dose related. On re-challenge with the drug, pancreatitis recurs within hours to days. The second mechanism is the presumed accumulation of a toxic metabolite that may cause pancreatitis, typically after several months of use. Pancreatitis caused by drugs is usually mild and self-limited.

Heredity

Hereditary causes of pancreatitis include mutations in the genes encoding cationic trypsinogen *(PRSS1)*, pancreatic secretory trypsin inhibitor (serine protease inhibitor Kazal type 1 *[SPINK1]*), cystic fibrosis transmembrane conductance regulator *(CFTR)*, chymotrypsin

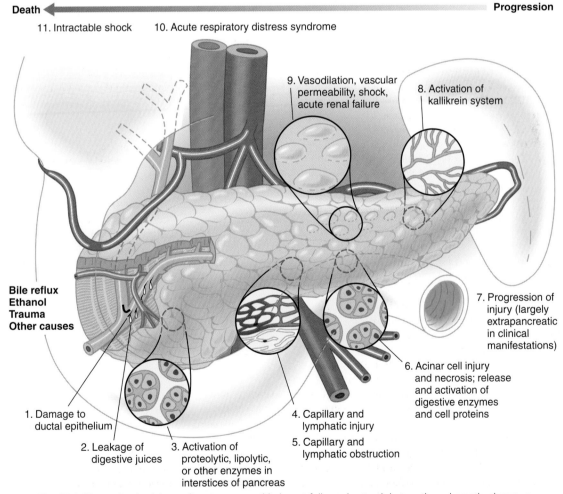

Fig. 39.2 The pathophysiology of acute pancreatitis is not fully understood, but as the schematic shows, a cascade of events seems likely, beginning with the release of toxic substances into the parenchyma and ending with shock and death. Damage to the ductal epithelium or acinar cell injury may result from bile reflux, increased intraductal pressure, alcohol, or trauma. (Modified from Grendell JH: The pancreas. In Smith LH Jr, Thier SO, editors: Pathophysiology: the biological principles of disease, ed 2, Philadelphia, 1985, WB Saunders, p 1228.)

TABLE 39.1 Causes of Acute Pancreatitis

Obstruction
Gallstones
Tumors: ampullary or pancreatic tumors
Parasites: *Ascaris* or *Clonorchis* species
Developmental anomalies: pancreas divisum, choledochocele, annular pancreas
Periampullary duodenal diverticula
Hypertensive sphincter of Oddi
Afferent duodenal loop obstruction

Toxins
Ethyl alcohol
Methyl alcohol
Scorpion venom: excessive cholinergic stimulation causes salivation, sweating, dyspnea, and cardiac arrhythmias; seen mostly in the West Indies
Organophosphorus insecticides

Drugs
Definite associations (documented with rechallenges): azathioprine or 6-mercaptopurine, valproic acid, estrogens, tetracycline, metronidazole, nitrofurantoin,
  pentamidine, furosemide, sulfonamides, methyldopa, cytarabine, cimetidine, ranitidine, sulindac, dideoxycytidine
Probable associations: thiazides, ethacrynic acid, phenformin, procainamide, chlorthalidone, L-asparaginase

Metabolic Disorders
Hypertriglyceridemia, hypercalcemia, end-stage renal disease

Trauma
Accidental: blunt trauma to the abdomen (e.g., car accident, bicycle)
Iatrogenic: postoperative, endoscopic retrograde cholangiopancreatography

Infectious Diseases
Parasitic: ascariasis, clonorchiasis
Viral: mumps, rubella, hepatitis A, hepatitis B, hepatitis C, coxsackievirus B, echovirus, adenovirus, cytomegalovirus, varicella virus, Epstein-Barr virus, human
  immunodeficiency virus
Bacterial: mycoplasma, *Campylobacter jejuni*, tuberculosis, *Legionella* species, leptospirosis

Vascular Disorders
Ischemia: hypoperfusion (e.g., postcardiac surgery) or atherosclerotic emboli
Vasculitis: systemic lupus erythematosus, polyarteritis nodosa, malignant hypertension

Idiopathic Disorders
Accounts for 10–30% of patients with pancreatitis
Up to 60% have occult gallstone disease (e.g., biliary microlithiasis, gallbladder sludge)
Less common causes: sphincter of Oddi dysfunction, mutations in the cystic fibrosis transmembrane regulator

Miscellaneous Disorders
Penetrating peptic ulcer
Crohn's disease of the duodenum
Pregnancy-associated disorders
Pediatric associations: Reye's syndrome, cystic fibrosis
Autoimmune pancreatitis

C (i.e., caldecrin) *(CTRC)*, the calcium-sensing receptor *(CASR)*, and claudin-2. Aside from acute pancreatitis, mutations in these genes may increase the risk of development of diabetes and pancreatic cancer.

The role of genetic testing in idiopathic acute pancreatitis is controversial. Diagnosis of these genetic disorders contributes little to direct management because specific therapy is unavailable. Similarly, inadvertent disclosure of the results of genetic testing protects patients' health care insurance but may impact other financial decisions such as disability and life insurance. However, identification of an underlying genetic cause may obviate the need for further testing, allow more informed family planning, and enable better surveillance for complications, including pancreatic cancer. The decision to pursue genetic testing is one that should be made only with the advice and involvement of an experienced counselor.

Neoplasia

Primary pancreatic ductal adenocarcinoma, ampullary tumors, metastasis to the pancreas, and intraductal papillary mucinous neoplasms are uncommon causes of acute pancreatitis. The mechanism of pancreatitis is presumably secondary to obstruction of the pancreatic duct. These causes should be considered for patients older than 40 years. Pancreatitis has been reported in up to 10% of patients with pancreatic cancer (see Chapter 58).

Smoking

Smoking was once thought to be a risk factor due to its synergism with alcohol. However, studies have suggested that cigarette smoking is an independent risk factor for acute and chronic pancreatitis by mechanisms that are unclear.

Autoimmune Pancreatitis

Autoimmune pancreatitis (AIP) is a benign disease representing two distinct but overlapping immune-mediated inflammatory conditions of the pancreas referred to as type 1 and type 2 AIP. Type 1 is the classic and more common form of AIP. It is characterized histologically by a periductal lymphoplasmacytic infiltrate, storiform fibrosis, obliterative phlebitis, and abundant immunoglobulin G4 (IgG4) immunostaining (>10 IgG4-positive cells per high-power field).

The most common manifestation of AIP is obstructive jaundice, which closely mimics pancreatic cancer with focal enlargement of the pancreatic head. AIP can also manifest as acute pancreatitis in up to 15% to 30% of individuals, and about 5% of patients evaluated for acute or chronic pancreatitis have AIP. AIP has a peak incidence in the sixth or seventh decades of life and tends to affect men twice as often as women. Serum IgG4 levels are elevated to more than two times the upper limit of normal in most patients. Computed tomography (CT) typically demonstrates diffuse enlargement of the pancreas with delayed (rim) enhancement and a diffusely irregular, attenuated main pancreatic duct. More than 60% of individuals have clinical and histologic involvement of other organs, including the biliary tree, retroperitoneum, lacrimal and salivary glands, lymph nodes, periorbital tissues, kidneys, thyroid, lungs, meninges, aorta, breast, prostate, pericardium, and skin. Although a majority of patients initially respond to glucocorticoids, a significant portion of patients relapse once glucocorticoids are discontinued. Immunomodulator drugs have been used in those that fail steroids, relapse or cannot be weaned off steroids.

A less common form of AIP (type 2 AIP) has a similar clinical and radiographic presentation in the pancreas, but in contrast to type 1 disease, it requires histologic confirmation of an idiopathic duct centric pancreatitis lesion. Other hallmarks of type 1 disease are absent such that IgG4 levels are normal and other organs are not involved. Type 2 AIP is similarly steroid responsive but unlike type 1 disease, relapse is uncommon.

Pancreas Divisum

At approximately 4 weeks' gestation, the dorsal pancreas forms as an evagination from the duodenum, and shortly thereafter, the ventral pancreas forms from the hepatic diverticulum (E-Fig. 39.2). At approximately the eighth intrauterine week of life, the ventral pancreas rotates posterior to the duodenum and comes to rest posterior and inferior to the head portion of the dorsal pancreas with associated fusion of the main ducts. If fusion is incomplete, the duct of Wirsung drains only the ventral pancreas through the major ampulla, and the duct of Santorini drains the bulk of the pancreas (i.e., dorsal pancreas) through the relatively small accessory (minor) ampulla. This anomaly, called *pancreas divisum*, occurs in 5% to 10% of the general population and is associated with acute and chronic pancreatitis.

Theories suggest that pancreatitis results from relative outflow obstruction of the main dorsal duct through the small accessory ampulla. Endoscopic papillotomy, stent placement across the minor papilla, and surgical sphincteroplasty are therapeutic maneuvers that may reduce the incidence of recurrent pancreatitis by increasing drainage through the accessory papilla. While there are studies that appear to show an association between pancreas divisum and pancreatitis, there is controversy as to whether pancreas divisum is truly a cause of acute recurrent pancreatitis.

Clinical Presentation

The hallmark of acute pancreatitis is persistent abdominal pain. In atypical cases, patients may have unexplained organ failure or postoperative ileus. The onset of pain is typically sudden, severe, and worse when supine. Pain is usually located in the upper abdomen and may radiate to the back, chest, and flanks. Nausea and vomiting are common. Physical examination usually reveals severe upper abdominal tenderness that is sometimes associated with guarding.

Pancreatic enzymes, vasoactive substances (e.g., kinins), and other toxic substances (e.g., elastase, phospholipase A_2) are liberated by the inflamed pancreas and extravasate along fascial planes in the retroperitoneal space, lesser sac, and peritoneal cavity. These materials cause chemical irritation and contribute to the development of ileus, chemical peritonitis, third-space losses of protein-rich fluid, hypovolemia, and hypotension. The toxic molecules may reach the systemic circulation by lymphatic and venous pathways and contribute to subcutaneous fat necrosis and end-organ damage, including shock, renal failure, and respiratory insufficiency (i.e., atelectasis, effusions, and acute respiratory distress syndrome [ARDS]). Grey Turner sign (i.e., ecchymosis of the flank) or Cullen sign (i.e., ecchymosis in the periumbilical region) may be associated with hemorrhagic pancreatitis.

Metabolic problems, which are common in severe disease, include hypocalcemia, hyperglycemia, and acidosis. Hypocalcemia is most commonly caused by concomitant hypoalbuminemia. Other mechanisms include complexing of calcium to released free fatty acids, protease-induced degradation of circulating parathyroid hormone (PTH), and failure of PTH to release calcium from bone.

Acute pancreatitis is associated with a variety of local and vascular complications, including local spread of inflammation to contiguous organs. The most common include peripancreatic fluid collections, pseudocyst formation, obstruction of the duodenum or bile duct, and exocrine or endocrine insufficiency. Less common complications include pancreatic fistula formation, vascular thrombosis (i.e., splenic, portal and superior mesenteric veins), colonic necrosis, and development of an arterial pseudoaneurysm. Trypsin can activate plasminogen to plasmin and induce clot lysis. However, trypsin also can activate prothrombin and thrombin and produce thrombosis leading to disseminated intravascular coagulation.

Acute peripancreatic fluid collections are pools of peripancreatic fluid confined by normal peripancreatic fascial planes without a definable wall encapsulating the collection. These fluid collections occur during the first 4 weeks after interstitial pancreatitis. When a localized acute peripancreatic fluid collection persists beyond 4 weeks, it is likely to develop into a pancreatic pseudocyst.

Pancreatic pseudocysts (E-Fig. 39.3) are encapsulated fluid collections with well-defined inflammatory walls and are usually located outside the pancreas with minimal or no necrosis. They occur a minimum of 4 weeks after the onset of acute pancreatitis. Although most pseudocysts remain asymptomatic, presenting symptoms may include abdominal pain, early satiety, nausea, and vomiting due to compression of the stomach or gastric outlet. Rapidly enlarging pseudocysts may rupture, hemorrhage, obstruct the extrahepatic biliary tree, erode into surrounding structures, and become infected.

The term *acute necrotic collection* describes a nonorganized accumulation of heterogeneous fluid and necrotic material in the setting of necrotizing pancreatitis. The necrosis may involve the pancreatic parenchyma or peripancreatic tissue, or both. Walled-off pancreatic necrosis is a mature, encapsulated collection of pancreatic or peripancreatic necrosis that usually occurs more than 4 weeks after the onset of necrotizing pancreatitis.

Abdominal compartment syndrome is diagnosed when the intra-abdominal pressure exceeds 20 mm Hg and there are signs of new respiratory, renal, or vascular organ failure. Intra-abdominal hypertension typically occurs early and is the result of pancreatic inflammation and fluid third spacing. Abdominal compartment syndrome is associated with mortality rates ranging up to 50% to 75% in various reports. Suggested treatment includes analgesics, sedation, nasogastric tube decompression, and fluid restriction. If these measures do not result in improvement, percutaneous catheter decompression followed if unsuccessful by a surgical laparotomy is recommended. The ability of this approach to improve outcomes is the focus of ongoing research.

Diagnosis and Differential Diagnosis

The diagnosis of acute pancreatitis is based on a combination of clinical, biochemical, and radiologic factors. A diagnosis of acute pancreatitis requires two of the following three features: abdominal pain characteristic of acute pancreatitis; serum amylase or lipase levels, or both, at least three times the upper limit of normal; and characteristic findings of acute pancreatitis on imaging.

Elevated serum amylase levels may occur in a wide variety of other conditions, including bowel perforation, intestinal obstruction or ischemia, acute appendicitis, cholecystitis, tubo-ovarian disease, and renal failure. Serum amylase levels may be normal in patients with hypertriglyceridemia or alcohol-induced acute pancreatitis. Serum lipase is preferred because it is more sensitive and specific than serum amylase for the diagnosis of acute pancreatitis. The serum lipase level remains normal in some nonpancreatic conditions associated with an elevated serum amylase level, including macroamylasemia (i.e., formation of large molecular complexes between amylase and abnormal immunoglobulins), salivary gland disorders, and tubo-ovarian disease, but it may similarly rise in appendicitis, renal disease, and cholecystitis. The serum lipase concentration is more sensitive than that of amylase because it remains elevated longer and may be diagnostic even for patients seeking medical attention several days after symptom onset. Repeated measurements of serum pancreatic enzymes have little value in assessing clinical progress, and the magnitude of serum amylase or lipase elevation does not correlate with the severity of pancreatitis.

Contrast-enhanced computed tomography (CECT) or magnetic resonance imaging (MRI) of the pancreas should be used for patients whose diagnosis is unclear or who fail to improve within the first 48 to 72 hours after hospital admission. Imaging findings supporting acute pancreatitis include pancreatic enlargement, peripancreatic inflammatory changes, and extrapancreatic fluid collections. Imaging does not exclude the diagnosis of acute pancreatitis because the pancreas appears normal in 15% to 30% of those with mild disease. CECT is also useful for assessing disease severity based on the presence and extent of complications such as pancreatic necrosis and acute peripancreatic fluid collections. Pancreatic imaging should be performed after adequate fluid resuscitation to minimize the risk of contrast-induced nephrotoxicity.

MRI is preferred for patients with a contrast allergy and renal insufficiency because T2-weighted images without gadolinium contrast can similarly diagnose pancreatic necrosis. Early imaging (within 72 hours of symptom onset) can underestimate the existence and extent of pancreatic necrosis. Gallstone pancreatitis should be suspected in patients with transient elevation in liver function test results, particularly a serum ALT level elevated more than 3-fold. Transabdominal ultrasonography should be performed in all patients with acute pancreatitis when considering a diagnosis of gallstone pancreatitis.

Prognosis

The distinction between interstitial and necrotizing acute pancreatitis has important prognostic implications (Fig. 39.3). *Interstitial pancreatitis* is characterized by an intact microcirculation and uniform enhancement of the gland on CECT. *Necrotizing pancreatitis* is characterized by disruption of the pancreatic microcirculation so that large areas (>3 cm or >30%) of pancreatic parenchyma do not enhance on CECT. Approximately 20% to 30% of patients with acute pancreatitis have necrotizing pancreatitis.

The finding of pancreatic necrosis predicts a more severe course, particularly infection in the necrotic pancreatic tissue, also called *infected necrosis*. Infection is a strong determinant of the severity of illness and accounts for a large percentage of the deaths from acute pancreatitis. Infected necrosis develops in 30% to 50% of patients with acute necrotizing pancreatitis but not in those with interstitial disease. Infected necrosis should be suspected in patients with persistent systemic inflammatory response syndrome (SIRS) or organ dysfunction. The diagnosis can be made if extraluminal gas is seen on CECT. More commonly, CT-guided needle aspiration is obtained for Gram stain and culture of necrotic material, or antibiotics are given empirically based on clinical suspicion after appropriate cultures are obtained. Antibiotics that penetrate pancreatic tissue, including cephalosporins, carbapenems, quinolones, and metronidazole, are used for treatment of infected necrosis.

Risk assessment should be performed for all patients to stratify the severity of illness. The current classification includes mild, moderate, and severe forms. Mild acute pancreatitis, the most common form, is characterized by the absence of organ failure and pancreatic necrosis. Mild pancreatitis usually does not require pancreatic imaging, and patients recover within several days with restoration of normal pancreatic function and gland architecture. Patients with mild acute pancreatitis account for 80% of all attacks and less than 5% of the overall mortality rate.

Moderately severe pancreatitis is characterized by local complications and/or transient organ failure over a time period of less than 48 hours. Local complications include pancreatic necrosis (with or without infection) and acute peripancreatic fluid collections or pancreatic pseudocysts. Death from moderately severe pancreatitis is much less common than in cases of severe pancreatitis.

Severe acute pancreatitis is defined by persistent organ failure extending for more than 48 hours. Severe acute pancreatitis occurs in 15% to 20% of patients. Most individuals with persistent organ failure have underlying necrotizing disease. The respiratory, cardiovascular, and renal systems are most commonly affected. Early deaths (within the first week) are most often the result of multiple organ failure caused by the release of inflammatory mediators and cytokines. Late deaths are more likely to result from local or systemic infection. The risks of infection and death correlate with disease severity and pancreatic necrosis. The overall mortality approaches 30% among patients with persistent organ failure.

Despite the importance of recognizing severe disease, most patients are initially admitted to the hospital without necrosis or organ failure, and methods to predict individuals more likely to progress to severe disease during the initial several days of hospitalization have been defined. A combination of clinical assessment, scoring systems, serum markers, and CECT scanning provides the most useful prognostic information (Table 39.2). Regardless of the prognostic factor chosen, there are significant limitations in predicting disease severity.

Clinical predictors of a poor outcome include severe comorbid illnesses, older age (≥60 years), obesity, and long-term, heavy alcohol use. Laboratory findings associated with increased mortality include blood urea nitrogen elevation (>20 mg/dL) on admission or a rise during the first 24 hours of admission, hemoconcentration from third spacing of fluids reflected by an elevated hematocrit of 44 or greater on admission, and serum markers reflecting a robust systemic inflammatory response, such as a C-reactive protein level greater than

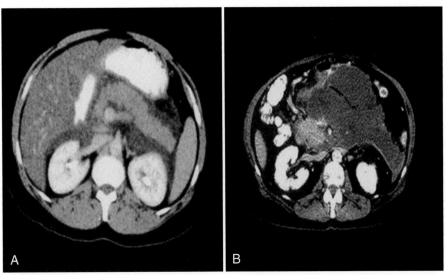

Fig. 39.3 Contrast-enhanced computed tomography demonstrates interstitial pancreatitis (A) and necrotizing pancreatitis (B).

TABLE 39.2 Predictors of Severe Pancreatitis

Criteria	Prognostic Indicators
Signs[a]	Heart rate: >90 beats/min
	Temperature: >38° C or <36° C
	White blood cell count: >12,000 or <4,000 cells/μL or >10% bands
	Respiratory rate >20 beats/min or $Paco_2$ <32 mm Hg
Patient characteristics	Comorbid illnesses
	Age >55 yr
	Obesity (BMI >30 kg/m^2)
Laboratory values	BUN level of 20 mg/dL or higher and any rise in BUN during the first 24 hr of admission associated with increased mortality
	Serum creatinine >1.8 mg/dL within first 24 hr
	Hemoconcentration with Hct ≥44 on admission or failure of Hct to decrease in first 24 to 48 hr with volume resuscitation predicts severe pancreatitis
	Serum marker reflecting a systemic inflammatory response, CRP >150 mg/dL
Imaging findings	Pleural effusion
	Pancreatic necrosis
	Acute extrapancreatic fluid collections
Scoring systems	
Ranson's criteria	Eleven prognostic indicators, including five available on admission (age >55 yr, WBC >16,000/mm^3, glucose >200 mg/dL, LDH >350 IU/L, AST >250 U/L) and six measured at the end of the first 48 hr (Hct decreased >10, BUN >5 mg/dL, Po_2 <60 mm Hg, base deficit >4 mEq/L, serum calcium <8 mg/dL, estimated fluid sequestration >6 L); mortality rate of 10–20% for three to five signs and >50% for six or more signs
Acute Physiologic and Chronic Health Evaluation (APACHE II) system	Calculated by assigning points based on age, heart rate, temperature, respiratory rate, mean arterial pressure, Pao_2, pH, potassium, sodium, creatinine, Hct, WBC, GCS, and previous health status
Bedside Index for Severity of Acute Pancreatitis (BISAP)	Five variables available in initial 24 hr: BUN >25 mg/dL, impaired mental status (GCS score <15), finding of SIRS, age >60 yr, and pleural effusion on imaging. Each variable adds 1 point to the total score, and scores of 3, 4, and 5 correspond to mortality rates of 5.3%, 12.7%, and 22.5%, respectively.

AST, Aspartate aminotransferase; *BMI,* body mass index; *BUN,* blood urea nitrogen; *CRP,* C-reactive protein; *GCS,* Glasgow Coma Scale; *Hct,* hematocrit; *LDH,* lactate dehydrogenase; *SIRS,* systemic inflammatory response syndrome; *WBC,* white blood cells.
[a]SIRS predisposes to multiple organ dysfunction and pancreatic necrosis. SIRS is defined by two or more of these criteria persisting for more than 48 hours.

150 mg/dL (sensitivity of 80%, specificity of 76%, positive predictive value of 67%, and negative predictive value of 86%). Imaging studies predicting a severe outcome include a pleural effusion seen on chest radiography within the first 24 hours or pancreatic imaging identifying necrosis. Unfortunately, CT evidence of severe acute pancreatitis lags

behind clinical findings, and an early CT study can underestimate the severity of the disorder.

Severe pancreatitis is predicted by organ dysfunction, including shock (systolic blood pressure <90 mm Hg), respiratory failure (Pao_2 ≤60 mm Hg), and acute renal injury (creatinine >2.0 mg/L after rehydration). SIRS predisposes to multiple organ dysfunction and pancreatic necrosis.

Well-established scoring systems include Ranson's criteria, Acute Physiologic and Chronic Health Evaluation II (APACHE II), APACHE combined with scoring for obesity (APACHE-O), the Glasgow Scoring System, and Bedside Index for Severity of Acute Pancreatitis (BISAP). With increasing scores, the likelihood of a complicated, prolonged, and fatal outcome increases. Unfortunately, because these scoring systems have a high false-positive rate (i.e., in many patients with high score, severe pancreatitis does not develop), they are not universally used. During the first 48 to 72 hours, a rising hematocrit or BUN, persistent SIRS after fluid resuscitation or the presence of pancreatic or peripancreatic necrosis on cross-sectional imaging constitute evidence of evolving severe pancreatitis.

Treatment

Early steps in the management of patients with acute pancreatitis can decrease severity, morbidity, and mortality (Fig. 39.4). Prevention of complications depends largely on monitoring, vigorous hydration, and early recognition of pancreatic necrosis and choledocholithiasis. Patients with multiorgan dysfunction and those with predicted development of severe disease are at greatest risk for adverse outcomes and should be treated when possible in a care unit with intensive monitoring capability and multidisciplinary input.

Supportive Care

Patients with acute pancreatitis are treated supportively with aggressive intravenous hydration, parenteral analgesics, and bowel rest. Supplemental oxygen is recommended initially for all patients. Nasogastric tube suction is indicated for symptomatic relief in patients with nausea, vomiting, and ileus. No specific treatments are effective in limiting systemic complications. Agents that put the pancreas to rest (e.g., somatostatin, calcitonin, glucagon, H_2-receptor antagonists) and enzyme inhibitors (e.g., aprotinin, gabexate mesylate) have not been shown to lower disease-related morbidity and mortality.

Antibiotics

Antibiotic therapy is no longer recommended for patients with sterile necrosis due to the lack of proven benefit. For patients with suspected infected necrosis, appropriate antibiotics are initiated before the confirmatory diagnosis, with the initial choice taking into consideration the likely pathogenic organisms and the ability of the antimicrobials to penetrate into necrotic pancreatic tissues. After culture results are available, the antibiotics can be tailored appropriately.

Fluid Management

Vigorous fluid resuscitation is important for maintaining the microcirculation and perfusion of the pancreas during the early phase of acute pancreatitis. Early aggressive intravenous hydration during the first 12 to 24 hours after the onset of symptoms translates into a potential benefit of reduced pancreatic necrosis and organ failure. Vigorous fluid therapy is of little value after 24 hours. Crystalloid, the preferred intravenous fluid, is administered at an initial rate of 250 to 500 mL/hour or 5 to 10 mL/kg/hr with a preceding bolus infusion for individuals with severe volume depletion. Lactated Ringer's solution may be the preferred crystalloid replacement because in one comparative study, it reduced the incidence of inflammatory markers by more than 80% compared with normal saline infusion. Goal-directed fluid therapy is recommended for patients with acute pancreatitis. Goal-directed therapy is defined as titration of intravenous fluids every few hours to specific clinical and biochemical targets of perfusion (e.g., heart rate, blood pressure, urine output, BUN, and hematocrit). Caution must be used for the elderly and those with underlying cardiovascular or renal impairment.

Analgesia

Despite the theoretical concern that narcotic analgesia may result in sphincter of Oddi spasm and worsening pancreatitis, there is no evidence to support withholding narcotics from patients with acute pancreatitis. The physician should consider liberal use of patient-controlled analgesia, although this approach has not been compared prospectively with on-demand analgesia. There is no evidence to indicate superiority of a specific opiate. Patients administered repeated doses of narcotic analgesics should have oxygen saturation monitored due to risks of unrecognized hypoxia.

Nutritional Care

Patients with mild acute pancreatitis can begin oral feeding within 24 hours of admission without waiting for resolution of pain or normalization of serum pancreatic enzyme levels. Early introduction of a low-fat solid diet is as safe as the traditional approach of progressive advancement from a clear liquid diet and is associated with a shorter length of hospital stay.

For patients with predicted severe pancreatitis or small bowel ileus, early introduction of oral intake may not be tolerated due to postprandial abdominal pain, nausea, and vomiting. These individuals can have nutrition introduced as nasoenteric or nasogastric feeding. Enteral feeding is preferable to total parenteral nutrition (TPN) because it is less expensive than TPN and is associated with a reduction in systemic infection, need for surgical intervention, organ failure, and mortality. Enteral feeding is usually well tolerated, even by patients with an ileus. Nasogastric feeding offers a safe alternative to nasojejunal feeding because it appears to be equally safe and effective. Parenteral nutrition should be reserved for patients who cannot achieve sufficient caloric intake through the enteral route or those in whom enteral access cannot be maintained.

Management of Recurrence and Necrosis

Gallstone pancreatitis. The risk of gallstone pancreatitis (see also Chapter 45) recurrence is as high as 50% to 75% within 6 months of the initial episode, and cholecystectomy before discharge is recommended for patients with mild attacks of pancreatitis. Cholecystectomy performed during the initial admission for patients with suspected biliary pancreatitis is associated with substantial reductions in mortality and gallstone-related complications, readmission for recurrent pancreatitis, and pancreaticobiliary complications. Cholecystectomy is often delayed in patients with severe pancreatitis to allow for better exposure of the ductal anatomy at the time of surgery. Urgent ERCP (Video 39.1) with identification and clearance of bile duct stones is recommended for patients with documented choledocholithiasis on imaging, cholangitis or strong evidence of ongoing biliary obstruction, as suggested by imaging and laboratory data. Biliary sphincterotomy leaving the gallbladder in situ is considered an effective alternative for those who are not candidates for cholecystectomy.

Acute fluid collections and pseudocysts. Acute peripancreatic fluid collections do not require any specific therapy, other than supportive therapy that is standard for acute pancreatitis. Most remain sterile and are reabsorbed spontaneously during the first several weeks after the onset of acute pancreatitis. When a localized acute peripancreatic fluid collection persists beyond 4 weeks, it is likely to develop into a pancreatic pseudocyst. While patients with asymptomatic pseudocysts should be followed, for those who are symptomatic, pseudocyst drainage should be considered. Indications for pseudocyst drainage include suspicion of infection or progressive

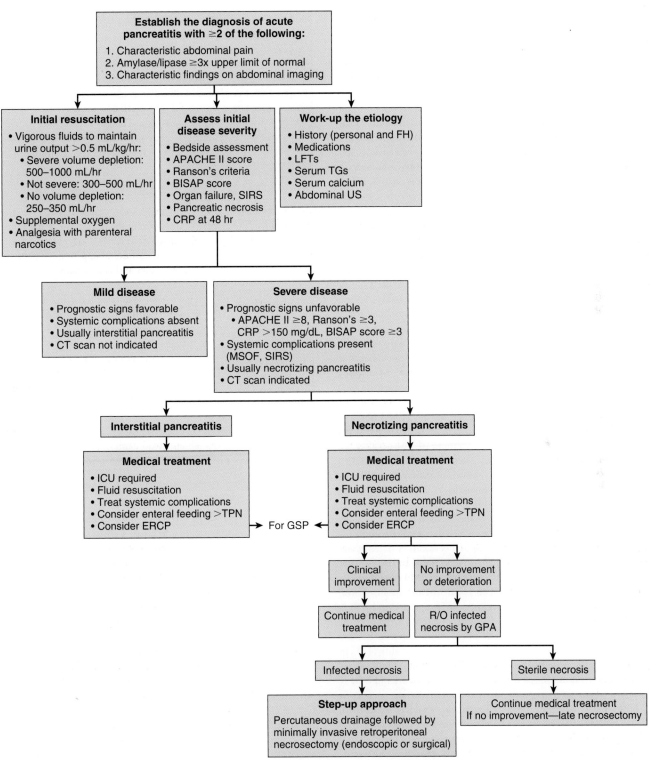

Fig. 39.4 Management algorithm for acute pancreatitis. Some of the guidelines, such as the diagnostic utility of the C-reactive protein (CRP) level, require further validation. Antibiotic use, including the type and duration of treatment, continues to be examined, and these suggested approaches will likely be modified by the findings of future studies. *APACHE II,* Acute Physiologic and Chronic Health Evaluation II; *BISAP,* Bedside Index for Severity of Acute Pancreatitis; *CT,* computed tomography; *ERCP,* endoscopic retrograde cholangiopancreatography; *FH,* family history; *GPA,* CT-guided percutaneous aspiration; *GSP,* gallstone pancreatitis; *ICU,* intensive care unit; *LFTs,* liver function tests; *MSOF,* multiple system organ failure; *R/O,* rule out; *SIRS,* systemic inflammatory response syndrome; *TGs,* triglycerides; *TPN,* total parenteral nutrition; *US,* ultrasound.

enlargement with associated symptoms including biliary obstruction, abdominal pain, early satiety, and nausea and vomiting due to stomach compression or gastric outlet obstruction. In symptomatic patients, if the pseudocyst is mature and encapsulated, treatment can involve endoscopic, surgical, or percutaneous drainage. Based on available expertise, endoscopic ultrasound (EUS) guided drainage is preferred with cystogastrostomy or cystoduodenostomy.

Sterile pancreatic and extrapancreatic necrosis. Sterile pancreatic necrosis usually is treated with supportive medical care during the first several weeks, even in patients with multiple organ failure. After the acute pancreatic inflammatory process has subsided and coalesced into an encapsulated structure (e.g., walled-off pancreatic necrosis), débridement may be required for intractable abdominal pain, vomiting caused by extrinsic compression of stomach or duodenum, biliary obstruction, failure to thrive or persistent systemic toxicity. Débridement is delayed for at least 4 to 6 weeks after the onset of pancreatitis and can be performed by a combination of endoscopic, radiologic, and surgical techniques. Asymptomatic pancreatic necrosis does not warrant intervention, regardless of the extent and location.

Infected pancreatic and extrapancreatic necrosis. The development of infection in the necrotic collection is the main indication for therapy. The development of fever leukocytosis and increasing abdominal pain suggests infection of the necrotic tissue. A CT scan may reveal evidence of air bubbles in the necrotic cavity.

Infected pancreatic necrosis is best treated with drainage or débridement, or both. Routine CT-guided fine-needle aspiration to diagnose infected necrosis is not recommended given that clinical and imaging signs are accurate in the majority of patients. In addition, there is a high false-negative rate of the samples. Thus, débridement warrants consideration when infected necrosis is suspected, even if infection is not documented. The consensus is that the best outcomes are achieved when invasive interventions are delayed for a minimum of 4 weeks after the onset of disease to allow liquefaction of necrotic tissues and a fibrous rim to form around the necrosis (i.e., walled-off pancreatic necrosis). This delay makes drainage end débridement easier and reduces the risk of complications or death. Patients with infected necrosis are initially treated with broad-spectrum antibiotics and medical support to allow encapsulation of the necrotic collections, which may facilitate intervention and reduce complications of bleeding and perforation. When there is dramatic clinical deterioration, patients are not stable and delay is not feasible, and early intervention with a percutaneous drain is required.

Traditional management of infected pancreatic necrosis has been open surgical necrosectomy with closed irrigation by indwelling catheters, necrosectomy with closed drainage without irrigation, or necrosectomy and open packing. The open surgical approaches are associated with a high morbidity (34% to 95%) and mortality (11% to 39%) rates. A more conservative step-up approach using percutaneous catheter drainage as the initial treatment has gained favor, and a delay in invasive treatment is now standard. The step-up approach consists of antibiotic administration, percutaneous drainage as needed, and after a delay of several weeks, minimally invasive débridement, if required. This approach is superior to traditional open necrosectomy with respect to the risk of major complications or death. If the percutaneous approach fails, it is followed by a less invasive, video-assisted retroperitoneal débridement (VARD) or endoscopic transluminal drainage with or without necrosectomy, provided expertise is available.

CHRONIC PANCREATITIS

Definition and Epidemiology

Chronic pancreatitis is characterized by inflammation, fibrosis, and irreversible loss of acinar (exocrine) and islet (endocrine) cell function.

TABLE 39.3 Causes of Chronic Pancreatitis (TIGAR-O)
Toxic-Metabolic
Alcohol
Tobacco
Hypercalcemia
Hypertriglyceridemia
Chronic renal failure
Idiopathic
Early onset
Late onset
Tropical
Genetic
Autosomal dominant-cationic trypsinogen (PRSS1)
Autosomal recessive-CFTR, SPINK1, chymotrypsin C
Autoimmune
Isolated (types 1 and 2)
Syndromic (Sjögren's, inflammatory bowel disease, primary biliary cholangitis)
Recurrent Acute Pancreatitis
Postnecrotic severe acute pancreatitis
Post-irradiation
Ischemic vascular
Obstructive
Benign-pancreas divisum, sphincter of Oddi dysfunction, post-traumatic pancreatic duct stricture
Neoplastic-pancreatic ductal adenocarcinoma, IPMN, ampullary tumor

CFTR, Cystic fibrosis transmembrane conductance regulator; *IPMN,* intraductal papillary mucinous neoplasia; *PRSS1,* serine protease 1; *SPINK1,* serine peptidase inhibitor Kazal type 1.

This disorder contrasts with acute pancreatitis, which is usually nonprogressive. The two conditions may overlap because recurrent attacks of acute pancreatitis may lead to chronic pancreatitis, and individuals with chronic pancreatitis may experience exacerbations of acute pancreatitis. The annual incidence of chronic pancreatitis ranges from 5 to 12 cases per 100,000 people, and the prevalence is about 50 cases per 100,000 people.

Pathology

Chronic pancreatitis can be classified using a system termed "TIGAR-O," which refers to *t*oxic-metabolic, *i*diopathic, *g*enetic, *a*utoimmune, *r*ecurrent and severe acute pancreatitis, and *o*bstructive (Table 39.3). The most common cause of chronic pancreatitis is chronic alcoholism, accounting for 45% to 65% of cases. Alcohol can cause episodes of acute pancreatitis, but at the time of the initial attack, structural and functional abnormalities often indicate underlying chronic pancreatitis. Because most alcohol users do not develop pancreatitis, the presumption is that unidentified genetic, dietary, or environmental influences must coexist with alcohol use. Smoking is a causal, dose-dependent risk factor for chronic pancreatitis. The effect of smoking is synergistic with alcohol consumption and contributes profoundly to the development and progression of the disease.

Twenty percent of US patients with chronic pancreatitis have no immediately demonstrable cause. Gallstone pancreatitis, the major cause of acute pancreatitis, rarely leads to chronic pancreatitis. Calcific pancreatitis is a major cause of chronic pancreatitis in South India and other parts of the tropics. Autoimmune pancreatitis, genetic mutations (*CFTR, SPINK1, PRSS1, CTRC, CASR*), obstruction (e.g., tumors, sphincter of Oddi dysfunction, pancreas divisum), hypertriglyceridemia, and hypercalcemia are potential causes of cases initially labeled idiopathic.

Clinical Presentation

Most patients with chronic pancreatitis experience episodic or continuous pain. Occasionally, patients exhibit exocrine or endocrine insufficiency in the absence of pain. Other patients are asymptomatic and are found to have chronic pancreatitis incidentally on imaging.

The pain of chronic pancreatitis is typically epigastric, often radiates to the back, is occasionally associated with nausea and vomiting, and may be partially relieved by sitting upright or leaning forward. The pain is often worse 15 to 30 minutes after eating. Early in the course of chronic pancreatitis, the pain may occur in discrete attacks; as the condition progresses, the pain tends to become continuous.

The pain of chronic pancreatitis is poorly understood. Possible causes include inflammation of the pancreas, increased intrapancreatic pressure, neural inflammation, and extrapancreatic causes, such as stenosis of the common bile duct and duodenum.

Glucose intolerance occurs with some frequency in chronic pancreatitis, but overt diabetes mellitus usually manifests late in the course of disease. Diabetes in patients with chronic pancreatitis is different from typical type 1 diabetes in that the pancreatic alpha cells, which produce glucagon, are also affected, increasing the risk of hypoglycemia.

Clinically significant endocrine or exocrine insufficiency (i.e., protein and fat deficiencies) does not occur until more than 90% of pancreatic function is lost. Steatorrhea usually occurs before protein deficiencies because lipolytic activity decreases faster than proteolysis. Mild pancreatic exocrine insufficiency (PEI) may take the form of abdominal bloating or malabsorption of fat-soluble vitamins (A, D, E, K) and vitamin B_{12}, although clinically symptomatic vitamin deficiency is uncommon. Because reduced vitamin D absorption can result in osteoporosis, osteopenia, and fractures, periodic assessment of vitamin D levels and bone densitometry are recommended. More severe PEI may lead to overt malabsorption and weight loss.

Diagnosis and Differential Diagnosis

Because direct biopsy of the pancreas has considerable risk, the diagnosis of chronic pancreatitis is typically based on indirect tests of pancreatic structure and function. Marked structural changes usually correlate with severe functional impairment. In early chronic pancreatitis, however, mild abnormalities of pancreatic function can precede the morphologic changes seen on imaging. Studies of pancreatic structure may remain normal even with advanced deterioration of pancreatic function.

Laboratory evaluations of serum pancreatic enzymes, such as amylase and lipase, are frequently normal in the setting of well-established chronic pancreatitis, even during painful exacerbations. Serum pancreatic enzymes neither confirm nor exclude the diagnosis.

Tests of Function

Function tests assess pancreatic secretory reserve of ductal function or acinar function by measuring secretion of bicarbonate ions (HCO_3^-) or digestive enzymes, respectively. Direct tests (e.g., secretin stimulation) involve stimulation of the pancreas through the administration of hormonal secretagogues. Indirect tests measure the consequences of pancreatic insufficiency, and although more widely available, the results usually are not abnormal until enzyme output has declined by more than 90%. Thus they are insensitive to early pancreatic insufficiency.

Clinicians have preferentially relied on noninvasive methods to circumvent the challenges associated with direct pancreatic function tests. Clinically available indirect tests of pancreatic function include analyses of fecal fat, fecal elastase, and serum trypsin.

The secretin stimulation test takes advantage of the normal response of pancreatic ductular cells to secrete HCO_3^- in response to physiologic and exogenously administered secretin. The observation that HCO_3^- production is impaired early in the course of chronic pancreatitis led to the use of this test to diagnose early-stage disease (sensitivity of 95%). The test involves oral placement of a double-lumen gastroduodenal catheter for aspiration and quantitative measurement of pancreatic enzyme and HCO_3^- production before and after stimulation with intravenous secretin. This test is primarily performed for patients with suspected chronic pancreatitis who have chronic abdominal pain but negative or equivocal results of imaging studies. Peak pancreatic fluid HCO_3^- concentrations of less than 80 mEq/L represent pancreatic insufficiency. The secretin stimulation test has been infrequently used in clinical practice because the study is labor intensive and is associated with discomfort. Endoscopic collection methods have simplified pancreatic fluid collection and made the test more suitable for clinical use.

The 72-hour fecal fat determination is sometimes used for detection of steatorrhea (fecal fat >7 g/24 hours), but the test is not specific for pancreatic exocrine insufficiency. The test also lacks sensitivity because steatorrhea occurs only in advanced chronic pancreatitis. Because the quantitative fecal fat test is inconvenient, unpleasant for patients, and prone to laboratory error, a qualitative assay is used preferentially in clinical practice to assess for malabsorption.

Determination of fecal elastase is the most commonly used noninvasive indirect test for the diagnosis of pancreatic exocrine insufficiency. Elastase, a protease synthesized by pancreatic acinar cells, is useful for evaluating insufficiency because it is stable in stool, unaffected by pancreatic enzyme replacement, and correlates well with stimulated pancreatic function test results. Moderate to severe exocrine insufficiency is based on fecal elastase values of less than 200 µg/g of stool. False-positive results can be seen with diarrheal illnesses, due to a dilutional effect.

Tests of Structure

Imaging findings with CT scan, ultrasound, and MRI may show changes of chronic pancreatitis include ductal abnormalities (e.g., dilation, stones, irregular beaded walls, and side branch ectasia), parenchymal abnormalities (e.g., calcification, inhomogeneity, atrophy), gland contour changes, and pseudocysts (E-Fig 39.4). Imaging studies are often normal or inconclusive in the early stages of disease (see E-Fig. 39.4). CT imaging and MRI are also helpful in identifying complications of chronic pancreatitis including pseudocysts, portosplenic venous thrombosis, arterial pseudoaneurysms, and pancreatic duct fistulas.

CT scanning is often considered the preferred initial test for diagnosis of chronic pancreatitis. Magnetic resonance cholangiopancreatography is a noninvasive diagnostic imaging modality that provides visualization of the pancreatic parenchyma similar to CT scanning but with improved duct imaging resulting in a greater sensitivity for diagnosis of chronic pancreatitis. MRI pancreatic duct images are similar to those obtained by ERCP but without the risk of precipitating acute pancreatitis. Stimulation of the pancreas using IV secretin enhances main and side branch pancreatic duct visualization, which may improve the diagnostic accuracy for chronic pancreatitis. ERCP provides reliable structural information about the pancreatic ductular system including ductal dilation, strictures, abnormal side branches, communicating pseudocysts, and ductal stones and fistulas. ERCP is highly effective for visualizing these ductal and duct-related findings, with a sensitivity for the diagnosis of chronic pancreatitis of 71% to 93% and a specificity of 89% to 100%. The major limitation of ERCP is the development of procedure-related acute pancreatitis in up to 5% of patients. Thus, ERCP should not be used for diagnostic purposes but instead be reserved for patients with established chronic pancreatitis when endoscopic therapy is recommended (discussed later).

Endoscopic ultrasound (EUS) as a diagnostic imaging study for chronic pancreatitis relies on quantitative and qualitative parenchymal tissue and ductal findings. EUS appears to be equally or more sensitive than other tests of structure and function. An international consensus panel proposed the Rosemont criteria for diagnosing chronic pancreatitis. Major criteria include hyperechoic foci with shadowing that indicates pancreatic duct calculi and parenchymal lobularity with honeycombing. Minor criteria include cysts, a dilated main duct (≥3.5 mm in diameter), irregular pancreatic duct contour, dilated side branches (≥1 mm in diameter), hyperechoic duct wall, parenchymal strands, nonshadowing hyperechoic foci, and lobularity with noncontiguous lobules. In the absence of any of these criteria, chronic pancreatitis is unlikely, whereas with detection of four or more criteria, the disease is likely, even when other imaging and pancreatic function tests may still be normal.

Treatment
Malabsorption
Treatment of PEI is best achieved with pancreatic enzyme replacement therapy (PERT). Most commercial preparations consist of pancreatin, which is the shock-frozen powdered extract of porcine pancreas containing lipase, amylase, trypsin, and chymotrypsin.

In order to treat malabsorption due to PEI, it is necessary to provide approximately 10 percent of the normal pancreatic enzyme output. This translates into approximately 30,000 international units (IU) or the equivalent 90,000 United States Pharmacopeia units (USP) of lipase per meal. For most patients, the recommended dose depends on the size and nature of the meal (i.e., fat content), residual pancreatic function, and therapeutic goals (i.e., elimination of steatorrhea, reduction in the abdominal symptoms of maldigestion, or improvement in nutrition). Due to residual pancreatic lipase secretion and physiologic gastric lipase secretion, it is appropriate to begin therapy with 40,000 to 50,000 USP of lipase with each meal and one half of that amount with snacks. Administration of acid-stable, encapsulated microspheres or microtablets filled with pancreatic enzymes has greatly increased the efficacy of enzyme supplementation. Enzyme preparations should be taken with meals. If more than one capsule/tablet per meal must be taken, it may be beneficial to take one part of the dose at the beginning and the rest during the meal.

Other factors may accentuate steatorrhea, including concomitant small bowel bacterial overgrowth, which can occur in up to 25% of patients with chronic pancreatitis. Bacterial overgrowth may be caused by hypomotility due to pancreatic inflammation or chronic use of narcotic analgesics.

Pain
The greatest challenge in treating chronic pancreatitis is controlling abdominal pain. Pain may improve over time, but the course is not predictable and improvement may take years. Therapy targets the mechanisms responsible for pancreatic pain, including pancreatic hyperstimulation, ischemia, obstruction of ducts, inflammation, and neuropathic hyperalgesia. Pain can develop in the early stages of chronic pancreatitis before morphologic changes can be demonstrated on imaging studies. Patients with chronic pancreatitis are at increased risk for pancreatic cancer, which may cause a change in the pain pattern, and extrapancreatic causes of pain must always be considered.

Pain management should proceed in a stepwise fashion and begin with lifestyle modifications such as alcohol and tobacco abstinence, a low-fat diet, and pancreatic enzyme supplementation, followed by a sequentially more aggressive and invasive approach for symptomatic failures, although it should be recognized that placebo alone is effective for up to 30% of patients. Several approaches can be considered for chronic pain relief.

1. Tobacco and alcohol abstinence. Abstention may decrease the frequency of painful attacks and reduce the likelihood of pancreatic function deterioration and development of pancreatic cancer.
2. Analgesics. Most patients with chronic pain require analgesics. Nonopioid analgesics such as acetaminophen and nonsteroidal anti-inflammatory drugs are used as initial treatment. If possible, the use of opioids should be avoided due to the risk of abuse, tolerance, and addiction. When deemed necessary, weak opioids (e.g., tramadol or codeine) are initially prescribed before escalation to stronger opioids (e.g., morphine, oxycodone, fentanyl) for poorly controlled pain. The risk of dependence to opioids is not known in this setting; however, patients with previous addictive behaviors such as substance use with alcohol or tobacco are at greater risk for analgesic dependence and addiction. Safe opioid prescribing practices are necessary with close monitoring of patients' symptoms and adherence to a well-defined plan that includes a patient agreement, regular follow-up, urine drug testing, and query of the state's online prescription monitoring program.
3. Secretion suppression. Oral pancreatic enzyme replacement, somatostatin analogue, and enteral nutrition are proposed treatments to blunt pain by reducing pancreatic secretion. These therapies are of unproven benefit and not routinely recommended as adjuncts to pain therapy. When PERT is initiated for pain management, the non–enteric-coated pancrelipases (i.e., pancreatic enzyme preparations) are preferred because the enteric-coated preparations theoretically release their enzymes further down the intestine, away from the stimulatory cholecystokinin (CCK) enterocytes.
4. Neural transmission modification. Gabapentinoids, including pregabalin, have been used effectively to treat neuropathic pain disorders, including diabetic neuropathy and neuropathic pain of central origin. Based on the finding that pancreatic pain is accompanied by similar alterations of central pain processing, studies suggest a benefit with pregabalin as an adjuvant treatment to decrease pain associated with chronic pancreatitis. Similarly, tricyclic antidepressants, selective serotonin reuptake inhibitors, and serotonin-norepinephrine reuptake inhibitors can be administered on a trial basis.
5. Neuroablative techniques such as celiac plexus blockade can be performed by injection of a local anesthetic and a steroid into the region of the celiac ganglia. This can be accomplished through endoscopic (i.e., EUS) or percutaneous radiologic guidance. The results are disappointing with a pain reduction in a minority of individuals (15% to 50%) that is not durable with pain reduction or relief of up to 1 to 6 months.
6. Antioxidants. Oxidative stress can cause direct pancreatic acinar cell damage through several pathways. Supplementation with antioxidants, such as selenium, vitamins C and E, and methionine, may relieve pain and reduce oxidative stress. In a randomized trial, the reduction in the number of painful days per month was higher for the patients who received antioxidants compared with those who received placebo (7.4 vs. 3.2 days). Patients who received antioxidants also were more likely to become pain free (32% vs. 13%).
7. Endoscopic decompression. Endoscopic decompression of the pancreatic duct is an option for obstruction caused by strictures, stones, or sphincter of Oddi dysfunction. Endoscopic therapies include pancreatic sphincterotomy, stricture dilation, stone

removal with intracorporeal or extracorporeal shock wave lithotripsy, and temporary plastic stent placement. Complete or partial pain relief is reported for approximately 50% to 80% of carefully selected patients during follow-up extending as long as 3 to 4 years.

8. Surgery. Surgical pancreatic ductal drainage, usually with lateral pancreaticojejunostomy (i.e., Puestow procedure), can be offered to those with a dilated (>6 mm in diameter) main pancreatic duct. Pain reduction is reported by approximately 80% of patients. This procedure is safe and has an operative mortality rate of less than 5%; however, only 35% to 60% of patients are free of pain at the 5-year follow-up. Individuals with nonobstructed, nondilated pancreatic ductal systems with disease predominating in the pancreatic head may be offered resection of the focally diseased portion of the gland with a pancreaticoduodenectomy or a duodenum-preserving pancreatic head resection also referred to as a Frey or Beger procedure. Highly selected patients with diffuse pancreatic parenchymal disease refractory to other forms of therapy may benefit from a total pancreatectomy with islet cell autotransplantation.

Management of Complications

The complications of chronic pancreatitis include pseudocysts, pancreatic fistulas, biliary obstruction, pancreatic cancer, small bowel bacterial overgrowth, and isolated gastric varices due to splenic vein thrombosis.

Pancreatic fistulas. Pancreatic fistulas occur as a result of duct disruption resulting in localized fluid collections, ascites, or pleural effusions. Treatment consists of bowel rest, endoscopic pancreatic duct stenting, and administration of a somatostatin analogue. Surgical intervention may be needed if this conservative approach is unsuccessful.

Vascular complications. The splenic vein courses along the posterior surface of the pancreas, where it can be affected by inflammation from pancreatitis or malignancy that leads to thrombosis. Splenic vein thrombosis can result in isolated fundal gastric varices. Splenectomy is usually curative for patients who develop bleeding from gastric varices.

Pseudoaneurysm formation is a complication of acute and chronic pancreatitis. Affected vessels, including the hepatic, splenic, pancreaticoduodenal, and gastroduodenal arteries, lie close to the pancreas. CT or MR imaging shows the pseudoaneurysm as a cystically dilated vascular structure in or adjacent to the pancreas. EUS with Doppler imaging can show blood flow within the pseudoaneurysm. Mesenteric angiography permits confirmation of the diagnosis and provides a means of therapy because selective embolization of the pseudoaneurysm can be accomplished during the procedure. Surgery for bleeding pseudoaneurysms is difficult and associated with high morbidity and mortality rates.

Biliary and duodenal obstruction. Symptomatic obstruction of the bile duct or duodenum, or both, develops in a few patients with chronic pancreatitis. Postprandial pain and early satiety are characteristic of duodenal obstruction, whereas pain and cholestasis (sometimes with resultant cholangitis) suggest a bile duct stricture. These complications most commonly result from inflammation or fibrosis in the head of the pancreas or an adjacent pseudocyst.

Endoscopic stenting may be attempted for bile duct strictures, but they are often refractory and typically require prolonged treatment. Endoscopic failures can be treated with surgical biliary decompression. The importance of decompression is underscored by the observation that it can reverse secondary biliary fibrosis associated with bile duct obstruction.

CARCINOMA OF THE PANCREAS

Definition and Epidemiology

Pancreatic ductal adenocarcinoma (PDAC) is the fourth leading cause of cancer-related death in the United States, with approximately 45,000 new cases diagnosed annually (see also Chapter 58). The peak incidence of PDAC occurs in the seventh decade of life. There is a modest male-to-female predominance (relative risk of 1.4:1), and blacks have a 30% to 40% higher incidence of PDAC than white individuals in the United States.

Many environmental factors have been implicated as increasing the risk for pancreatic cancer. Cigarette smoking is the most consistent factor, with the increased risk attributed to the aromatic amines found in cigarette smoke. Other risk factors include obesity, lack of physical activity, and diabetes mellitus. Studies evaluating the relationship between diet and pancreatic cancer are inconclusive. A Western diet (i.e., high intake of fat and meat, particularly smoked or processed meats) has been linked to the development of pancreatic cancer in many studies. Chronic pancreatitis also increases the risk of PDAC (relative risk as high as 13-fold), particularly in those individuals with hereditary pancreatitis and tropical pancreatitis. Epidemiologic studies have failed to find a consistent association between alcohol or coffee consumption and the development of pancreatic cancer.

Up to 10% of patients with pancreatic cancer have a family history of the disease, but most cannot be identified with a known genetic disorder. Recognized genetic disorders that predispose to pancreatic cancer include hereditary pancreatitis (*PRSS1* gene), hereditary nonpolyposis colorectal cancer, familial adenomatous polyposis, hereditary breast and ovarian cancers (*PALB2* and *BRCA2* genes), Peutz-Jeghers syndrome (*STK11* gene), familial atypical mole melanoma syndrome (*CDKN2A* gene), ataxia telangiectasia (*ATM* gene), and the Von Hippel–Lindau syndrome (*VHL* gene). Screening to detect precancerous lesions or early cancers should be considered for individuals with a cumulative predicted risk of PDAC greater than 5% or relative risk (RR) of 5 or greater (having ≥2 relatives with PDAC including ≥1 a first degree, or having a germline mutation of a predisposing gene and ≥2 relatives with PDAC or ≥1 a first degree, or Peutz–Jeghers syndrome even in the absence of a family history) and eligible for a possible pancreatic resection after discussion of the risks and benefits of such screening. Although imaging surveillance of high-risk family cohorts is practiced at some centers of expertise, there is no consensus about the optimal methods or frequency of pancreatic cancer screening. Screening with EUS and/or MRI can be considered but has not been shown to improve survival rates.

Pathology

More than 95% of malignant neoplasms of the pancreas arise from the exocrine pancreas. The term *pancreatic cancer* usually refers to ductal adenocarcinoma of the pancreas, representing 85% to 90% of all pancreatic neoplasms. *Exocrine pancreatic neoplasm* is a more inclusive term that includes neoplastic pancreatic ductal and acinar cells and their stem cells (e.g., pancreatoblastoma). Other, less common exocrine cancers include adenosquamous carcinomas, squamous cell carcinomas, signet ring cell carcinomas, and undifferentiated carcinomas. Neoplasms arising from the endocrine pancreas (i.e., islet cell or neuroendocrine tumors) comprise no more than 5% of pancreatic neoplasms.

Pancreatic cancers are composed of several distinct elements, including pancreatic cancer cells, tumor stroma, and stem cells. The precursor lesion of pancreatic cancer is pancreatic intraepithelial neoplasia, which progresses from mild dysplasia (PanIN grade 1) to more severe dysplasia (PanIN grades 2 and 3) and eventually to invasive carcinoma.

TABLE 39.4	**Definitions of Pancreatic Ductal Adenocarcinoma Treatment Categories**
Resectable	No evidence of tumor spread outside the pancreas
	No involvement of the superior mesenteric artery (SMA), celiac, or common hepatic artery (CHA)
	No invasion of the superior mesenteric vein (SMV) or portal vein (PV)
Metastatic	Evidence of spread to other organs (typically liver, lung, or peritoneum)
Borderline resectable	Tumor abutment (<50% of vessel circumference) of celiac, SMA or CHA
	Involvement but patent SMV or PV or short-segment occlusion with option for reconstruction
Locally advanced	Arterial encasement (>180 degrees or 50% of vessel circumference) of SMA, celiac or CHA
	SMV/PV occlusion without ability to surgically reconstruct

Clinical Presentation

The clinical manifestations of pancreatic carcinoma may be nonspecific and are often insidious. The clinical presentation is dependent to a great extent on tumor location and stage. PDAC localized to the head of the pancreas (70% to 80%) are more frequently symptomatic than those located in the body or tail (20% to 30%). Most PDAC has reached an advanced stage by the time of diagnosis. Common presenting signs and symptoms of pancreatic cancer include jaundice, weight loss, and abdominal pain. The pain is usually constant, with radiation to the back. Because most cancers begin in the pancreatic head, patients may exhibit obstructive jaundice or a large, palpable gallbladder (i.e., Courvoisier's sign).

Painless jaundice is the most common manifestation in patients with a potentially resectable and curable lesion. Anorexia, nausea, and vomiting may also occur, along with emotional disturbances such as depression. Less common manifestations include superficial thrombophlebitis (i.e., Trousseau sign), acute pancreatitis, diabetes mellitus, ascites, paraneoplastic syndromes (e.g., Cushing's syndrome), hypercalcemia, gastrointestinal bleeding, splenic vein thrombosis, and a palpable abdominal mass.

Diagnosis and Staging

The goal of imaging in the evaluation of suspected pancreatic carcinoma is to establish the diagnosis with a high degree of certainty and to determine resectability in patients who are otherwise candidates for operative resection. The diagnosis of pancreatic cancer is frequently suggested by a pancreatic mass seen on imaging studies. Evidence of a dilated pancreatic duct, hepatic metastases, invasion of vessels, or a dilated common bile duct in the setting of biliary obstruction may also be found. The imaging appearance may be impossible to distinguish from benign causes of pancreatic masses such as focal pancreatitis or autoimmune pancreatitis. Pancreas protocol triple phase (i.e., arterial, late arterial, and venous phases) cross-sectional multidetector CT scanning is the best initial study to diagnose and stage pancreatic cancer by identifying a mass lesion and assessing for liver metastasis or vascular invasion. CT is reported to have a sensitivity of 90% to 97% for identifying PDAC, although it is less sensitive for diagnosing small (<2 cm) lesions, with a sensitivity of 65% to 75%. CT is not sensitive for detecting nodal metastases. MRI is an alternative imaging modality that has similar accuracy to CT scanning for the diagnosis and staging of PDAC. EUS is superior to CT and MRI for detecting small lesions of the pancreas and should be performed when there is strong suspicion of PDAC despite the absence of a mass lesion by other imaging modalities. EUS-guided fine-needle aspiration (sensitivity of 85% to 90% and specificity approaching 100%) is recommended when histologic confirmation will alter management such as confirming malignancy in unresectable disease prior to initiating palliative care, confirming

a potentially resectable tumor prior to neoadjuvant therapy, and for a suspected mass not visible on cross-sectional imaging.

The imaging techniques are highly accurate for recognizing unresectable disease, but they are somewhat limited for identifying resectable disease because occult metastases (<1 cm in diameter) may be on the surface of the liver or peritoneum. Staging laparoscopy may reduce morbidity and cost from open surgical tumor resection; it should be considered for patients with the highest likelihood of occult metastatic disease (i.e., those with tumors of the body or tail of the pancreas) who appear to have potentially resectable disease by CT (one half of whom have occult peritoneal metastases), those with large (>3 cm) primary tumors, those for whom imaging suggests occult metastatic disease, and those with a very high initial CA 19-9 level (>1000 units/mL).

The use of tumor markers to diagnose carcinoma of the pancreas has yielded disappointing results. The tumor marker CA 19-9 has a sensitivity of 70% to 80% and a specificity of 85% to 95% for diagnosing selected patients already exhibiting signs and symptoms that suggest pancreatic cancer. However, for early-stage cancers, CA 19-9 has limited sensitivity. Use of CA 19-9 requires the Lewis blood group antigen, which is absent in 5% to 10% of the population. The greatest utility for CA 19-9 is to identify occult metastasis in patients with seemingly resectable tumors, for monitoring patients after apparently curative surgery, and for following those receiving chemotherapy for advanced disease. Rising CA 19-9 levels suggest recurrent disease even in the absence of radiographically detectable lesions.

Treatment

Dividing patients with PDAC into resectable, borderline resectable, locally advanced, and metastatic categories is clinically useful (Table 39.4).

Resectable Disease

Unfortunately, only 10% to 20% of carcinomas in the head of the pancreas and rare cancers of the body and tail are resectable for cure. Current criteria for resectability include the absence of distant metastases and the absence of tumor involvement of major arteries (superior mesenteric, celiac, and common hepatic). Venous involvement requires vascular patency and criteria for resectability will depend on the surgeon's experience and ability to perform vascular reconstruction.

Universal preoperative ERCP for patients with biliary obstruction is not recommended due to lack of proven benefit and the potential to increase adverse events. Selective use of ERCP with biliary stent placement is recommended for those patients with biliary obstruction and a clinical presentation of either cholangitis, intractable pruritus, marked hyperbilirubinemia, or when surgery is delayed for neoadjuvant therapy. Technical success of ERCP is achieved in over 90% of such patients with an acceptable complication rate of under 5%. At the time of stent placement, ERCP tissue sampling techniques can confirm a diagnosis of pancreatic malignancy (sensitivity of 30% to 60% and specificity 100%).

The standard operation for pancreatic cancer of the head or uncinate process is the Whipple procedure (i.e., pancreaticoduodenectomy). Whipple resection consists of removal of the pancreatic head, distal common bile duct, gallbladder, duodenum, proximal jejunum, gastric antrum, and regional lymph nodes. Reconstruction requires pancreaticojejunostomy, hepaticojejunostomy, and gastrojejunostomy. The pylorus-preserving version of the Whipple procedure leaves the stomach intact. The surgical mortality rate for this procedure is approximately 3% when performed by experienced pancreatic surgeons. Adjuvant therapy is indicated in all patients following resection of PDAC, irrespective of the pTNM stage, as it improves progression-free and overall survival rates.

Locally Advanced and Borderline Resectable

The term *borderline resectable* is reserved for patients with focal tumor abutment of the visceral arteries (celiac, superior mesenteric artery [SMA], or common hepatic), defined as contact of the tumor with less than one half circumference of the vessel wall, or short-segment occlusion of the superior mesenteric vein (SMV) or SMV–portal vein confluence. The latter is considered a relative rather than absolute contraindication to curative resection as some surgeons are performing resection with vascular reconstruction for selected individuals under these circumstances. Also, for tumors of the tail of the pancreas, encasement of the splenic vein does not necessarily obviate resectability. Locally advanced disease refers to individuals with unresectable cancer due to arterial encasement (>180° or >50% vessel circumference) of SMA, celiac or common hepatic arteries or SMV/PV occlusion without an option for reconstruction.

The use of preoperative neoadjuvant chemoradiation therapy in an effort to convert patients with unresectable borderline or locally advanced disease to a resectable status has increased the overall resection rate, but no difference in survival has been demonstrated.

Metastatic or Unresectable Disease

Although practice varies across institutions, most surgeons consider a pancreatic cancer to be categorically unresectable if there is extrapancreatic involvement, including extensive peripancreatic lymphatic extension, nodal involvement beyond the peripancreatic tissues, or distant metastases (e.g., liver, peritoneum, omentum, extra-abdominal sites). Other indications of unresectability include vascular encasement (i.e., tumor contact with more than one-half of the vessel's circumference), or direct involvement of the superior mesenteric artery, aorta, celiac artery, or hepatic artery, as defined by the absence of a fat plane between the tumor and these structures on CT imaging.

Patients with metastatic or inoperable pancreatic cancer should be offered treatment with multidisciplinary input based on goals of care, patient preferences, performance status (PS) and social support systems. If protocol enrollment is not available or is declined, conventional systemic chemotherapy should be offered because it provides benefit improving disease-related symptoms and overall survival.

- Patients under age 75 years with an ECOG PS 0 to 1 and bilirubin less than 1.5 mg/dL should be offered FOLFIRINOX or gemcitabine plus nab-paclitaxel;
- Patients with an ECOG PS 2 and bilirubin less than 1.5 ULN should be offered gemcitabine plus nab-paclitaxel or gemcitabine;
- Patients with an ECOG PS 0 to 2 and bilirubin 1.5 ULN or greater or comorbidities should be offered gemcitabine; and

- Patients with an ECOG PS 3 to 4 should be offered best supportive care.

For patients with inoperable cancers and poor performance status, palliative interventions to alleviate jaundice, pain, and intestinal obstruction often become the focus of therapy. When advanced disease is observed operatively, the surgeon must determine whether to perform additional palliative surgery. Biliary bypass is indicated in patients with obstructive jaundice. Duodenal bypass is indicated when features suggest impending gastric outlet obstruction. Alternative palliative endoscopic approaches are available for patients not undergoing exploratory surgery.

Prognosis

Carcinoma of the pancreas accounts for approximately 5% of cancer deaths in the United States. The overall prognosis is poor because less than 20% of patients are alive beyond the first year after diagnosis, and only 7% survive to the fifth year. Although 15% to 20% of patients have resectable disease at initial diagnosis, most have locally advanced or metastatic cancer. Median survival is 8 to 12 months for patients with locally advanced unresectable disease and 3 to 6 months for those with metastases at diagnosis.

A Whipple resection for pancreatic head cancers is the only chance for cure; however, the median survival after surgery is 15 to 20 months. Five-year survival after margin negative (R0) pancreaticoduodenectomy is approximately 25% to 30% following node-negative resection and 10% for node-positive disease. The overall 5-year survival rate is 10% to 25%, and up to 50% of those who survive 5 years ultimately die of recurrent cancer. Poor prognostic factors include a high tumor grade, a large tumor, high levels of CA 19-9 before and after surgery, tumor-positive surgical margins, and lymph node metastases.

For a deeper discussion of these topics, please see Chapter 135, ❖ "Pancreatitis," and Chapter 185, "Pancreatic Cancer," in *Goldman-Cecil Medicine*, 26th Edition.

SUGGESTED READINGS

Baron TE, DiMaio CJ, Wang AY, et al: American Gastroenterological Association Clinical Practice update: management of pancreatic necrosis, Gastroenterology 158:67–75, 2020.

Fogel EL, Shahda S, Sandrasegaran K, et al: A multidisciplinary approach to pancreas cancer in 2016: a review, Am J Gastroenterol 112:537–554, 2017.

Forsmark CE: Management of chronic pancreatitis, Gastroenterology 144:1282–1291, 2013.

Gardner TB, Adler DG, Forsmark CE: ACG clinical guideline: chronic pancreatitis, Am J Gastroenterol, 2020.

Hidalgo M: Pancreatic cancer, N Engl J Med 362:1605–1617, 2010.

Paulson AS, Cao HS, Tempero MA, et al: Therapeutic advances in pancreatic cancer, Gastroenterology 144:1316–1326, 2013.

Singh VK, Yadav D, Garg PK: Diagnosis and management of chronic pancreatitis: a review, JAMA 322:2422–2434, 2019.

Tenner S, Baillie J, DeWitt J, et al: American College of Gastroenterology guideline: management of acute pancreatitis, Am J Gastroenterol 108:1400–1415, 2013.

Vege SS, DiMagno MJ, Forsmark CE, et al: Initial medical treatment of acute pancreatitis: American Gastroenterological Association Institute Technical review, Gastroenterology 154:1103–1139, 2018.

Whitcomb DC: Genetic risk factors for pancreatic disorders, Gastroenterology 144:1292–1302, 2013.

Yadav D, Lowenfels AB: The epidemiology of pancreatitis and pancreatic cancer, Gastroenterology 144:1252–1261, 2013.

Diseases of the Liver and Biliary System

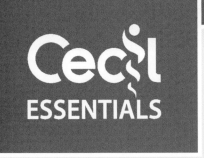

40

Laboratory Tests in Liver Diseases

Michael B. Fallon, Ester Little

INTRODUCTION

The liver is a large and complex organ, involved in major metabolic, secretory, and nutritional functions. It plays a central role in glucose homeostasis, synthesis and secretion of bile, and synthesis of lipoproteins and plasma proteins, including clotting factors and vitamin storage (vitamins B_{12}, A, D, E, and K). It is also the site of biotransformation, detoxification, and excretion of a multitude of endogenous and exogenous compounds.

Given the diversity of the liver roles, the clinical manifestation of liver diseases is varied and can be quite subtle. The first step in evaluating a patient with liver disease is the clinical history, and signs of liver disease can also be seen on physical exam (e.g., jaundice, dark urine, light colored stools, gastrointestinal bleeding, spider angiomas, palmar erythema, hepatomegaly, splenomegaly, ascites, and asterixis). The history and physical findings guide the initial set of laboratory tests ordered.

LIVER CHEMISTRY TESTS

The most widely used tests to evaluate the liver are aspartate and alanine aminotransferases (AST and ALT), alkaline phosphatase (ALP), gamma glutamyl transpeptidase (GGT), bilirubin, albumin, and prothrombin time. They are commonly referred to as "liver function tests." However, this is misleading because (1) they do not accurately reflect the function of the liver, (2) abnormal levels can indicate diseases affecting other organs, and (3) they may be normal in patients with advanced liver disease. A better terminology is liver chemistry tests. These tests reflect patterns of abnormalities seen in liver and biliary cell injury.

Patterns of Abnormalities in Liver Chemistry Tests

There are primarily three patterns of abnormalities in liver chemistry tests: one that reflects damage of the hepatocytes or hepatocellular damage (AST and ALT), one that reflects cholestasis and damage of the biliary cells (ALP and GGT), and one when patients have isolated elevation in bilirubin.

The tests are interpreted based on limits of normality and may vary between different laboratories. However, for ALT, it is now recognized that the limit of normality should be the same for all, and many professional societies have included the following levels in their guidelines: normal ALT ranges from 29 to 33 units/L in adult men and 19 to 25 units/L in adult women. Table 40.1 depicts the most common liver chemistry tests and the disease processes associated with each set of tests.

Hepatocellular Damage

ALT and AST are intracellular enzymes that catalyze the transfer of the α-amino group of aspartate or alanine to the α-keto group of ketoglutaric acid, resulting in formation of pyruvate or oxaloacetic acid, respectively. Vitamin B_6 is required to carry out this reaction. In the presence of cell injury or death, AST and ALT are released into circulation. ALT is found predominantly in hepatocytes and is more specific, whereas AST is also found in the heart, lungs, kidney, pancreas, brain, and skeletal muscle.

In most hepatocellular disorders (i.e., viral hepatitis, autoimmune hepatitis, hemochromatosis, Wilson's disease and some drug-induced liver injury) ALT is higher than or equal to AST. However, in alcoholic liver disease this ratio is reversed. A ratio greater than 2 is seen in 70% and greater than 3 in 96% of the patients with known alcoholic liver disease. Chronic and heavy alcohol consumption leads to vitamin B deficiency. The effect of vitamin B_6 deficiency is more prominent on ALT than AST activity, causing the increase in AST/ALT ratio. Not uncommonly, the AST is also higher than ALT in patients with nonalcoholic fatty liver disease (NAFLD), mimicking alcoholic liver disease.

The magnitude of elevation in aminotransferases also helps identify the possible cause of liver damage. Marked elevation, above 15 times the upper limit of normality (ULN), is seen in acute viral hepatitis, acetaminophen toxicity, hypoxic hepatopathy (shock, ischemia, hypoxemia) or acute bile duct obstruction. More modest elevations, usually 10 to 15 times the ULN, are seen in alcoholic hepatitis, autoimmune hepatitis, Wilson's disease, Budd-Chiari, and malignant infiltration of the liver (usually from breast cancer, small cell lung cancer, lymphoma, melanoma). In patients with chronic viral hepatitis, ALT and AST levels are rarely above 10 times the ULN, except during exacerbations of chronic hepatitis B. Elevations less than four times the ULN are more commonly seen in nonalcoholic fatty liver disease, hemochromatosis, α1-antitrypsin deficiency, celiac disease, and thyroid disease. Once the liver damage has progressed to cirrhosis, the elevation in aminotransferases is mild and can be normal. Conversely, ALT and AST can be massively elevated in diseases not related to the liver, such as rhabdomyolysis and heat stroke. In addition to acetaminophen, multiple medications can cause elevation in the aminotransferases at different levels of magnitude, including diclofenac, fluoxetine, isoniazid, ketoconazole, lisinopril, phenytoin, rifampin, ritonavir, and statins.

The rate at which the AST and ALT levels decrease as the patient improves can also help in identifying the cause. More rapid decline suggests ischemia or resolution of an acute biliary obstruction.

Cholestasis

The tests that indicate cholestasis and biliary cell damage are ALP and GGT. Serum ALP comprises a group of isoenzymes derived from the liver, intestine, bone, and placenta. The liver isoenzyme (ALP-1) is present in the mucosal cells lining the bile ducts and increases in response to bile duct damage from inflammation or obstruction. In these circumstances,

TABLE 40.1 Liver Chemistry Tests

Liver Chemistry Test	What It Reflects	Associated Diseases
Aspartate aminotransferase and alanine aminotransferase	Hepatocellular damage	Viral hepatitis, autoimmune hepatitis (AIH), alcoholic hepatitis, hemochromatosis, ischemic hepatitis, Budd-Chiari syndrome, α1-antitrypsin deficiency, Wilson's disease, and drugs
Alkaline phosphatase and γ-glutamyl transpeptidase	Cholestasis, biliary cell damage, and infiltrative processes	Primary biliary cholangitis (PBC), primary sclerosing cholangitis (PSC), familial cholestatic syndromes, AIDS cholangiopathy, cholestasis of pregnancy, biliary obstruction by stones or cancer, drugs, sarcoidosis, amyloidosis, and malignancy infiltration
Isolated bilirubin elevation	Increased production and impaired uptake, conjugation or excretion of bilirubin	Hemolysis, Gilbert, Crigler-Najjar, Dubin-Johnson, and Rotor syndromes
Decreased albumin and prolonged prothrombin time	Impaired synthetic liver function	Liver failure, severe acute hepatitis, and advanced liver disease with cirrhosis

GGT and 5′-nucleotidase (5′-NT) are simultaneously released. Thus, an elevation of ALP without elevation of GGT and 5′-NT indicates a nonhepatic cause. Fractionation of the different ALP isoenzymes by electrophoresis can be useful in determining alternative sources.

ALP does not differentiate intrahepatic from extrahepatic cholestasis. Examples of disorders that cause *intrahepatic cholestasis* are primary biliary cholangitis (PBC), primary sclerosing cholangitis (PSC), infections (AIDS cholangiopathy), familial cholestatic syndromes, cholestasis of pregnancy, total parenteral nutrition, ischemic cholangiopathy, liver allograft rejection, congestive hepatopathy (liver congestion secondary to right-sided heart failure), some medications (amiodarone, anabolic steroids, amoxicillin clavulanate, carbamazepine, estrogens, naproxen, phenytoin, rifampin), and infiltrative diseases (sarcoidosis, amyloidosis, malignant infiltration of the liver). Causes of *extrahepatic cholestasis* include bile duct stones or tumors, diverticulum of the ampulla of Vater, chronic pancreatitis, and pancreatic cancer.

ALP is frequently below normal range in patients with Wilson's disease, particularly those presenting with acute liver failure, in whom bilirubin is disproportionally elevated compared to alkaline phosphatase.

GGT is very nonspecific, and in addition to liver diseases it can be elevated in pancreatic diseases, myocardial infarction, renal failure, alcoholism, chronic obstructive pulmonary disease, and from several medications. As noted above, 5′-NT would not be elevated in these conditions.

Isolated Bilirubin Elevation

Patients with both hepatocellular diseases and cholestasis frequently also have bilirubin elevation secondary to leakage of bilirubin into the serum. However, some patients have elevated bilirubin with normal ALT, AST, ALP and GGT, which is termed *isolated bilirubin elevation*. In such cases, the first step is to fractionate the bilirubin to determine if it is caused by an elevation in the unconjugated (indirect) or conjugated (direct) bilirubin. An increase in *unconjugated bilirubin* results from overproduction (hemolysis), impaired uptake (Gilbert's disease) or impaired conjugation (Crigler-Najjar syndrome). An increase in *conjugated bilirubin* is due to decreased excretion in the bile ducts (Dubin-Johnson and Rotor syndromes) or leakage of the pigment from hepatocytes into serum.

More detailed discussion on cholestasis and isolated elevation of bilirubin can be found in Chapter 41.

LIVER SYNTHETIC FUNCTION

Albumin

From 300 g to 500 g of albumin is distributed in body fluids, and the adult liver synthesizes 15 g of albumin per day. Serum albumin concentration reflects the rate of synthesis, degradation, and volume of distribution. The synthesis of albumin is influenced by several factors including nutritional status, serum oncotic pressure, hormones, and cytokines.

The half-life of albumin in serum is 14 to 20 days. Low albumin is seen in prolonged liver dysfunction or acute liver impairment, and a decrease in albumin concentration reflects a reduction in albumin synthesis.

Hypoalbuminemia does not always reflect liver synthetic dysfunction. Several other conditions may decrease albumin, including malnutrition, nephrotic syndrome, protein losing enteropathy, and systemic inflammation.

Coagulation Factors and Prothrombin Time

The liver is the major site for the synthesis of 11 coagulation factors, including factors I, II, V, VII, IX, X, XII, and XIII. Deficiency in clotting factors occurs in more severe or more advanced stages of liver diseases. These factors can be measured individually or indirectly by determining the prothrombin time (PT).

The PT is dependent on factors II, V, VII and X, all of which are synthesized in the liver. Prolonged PT is not specific to liver diseases and can be seen in several congenital or acquired disorders. When these conditions are excluded, a prolonged PT is usually secondary to deficiency of vitamin K (inadequate dietary intake, prolonged obstructive jaundice, intestinal malabsorption or prolonged broad spectrum antibiotic use) or by poor utilization of vitamin K because of advanced liver disease. The administration of a single parenteral dose of vitamin K normalizes the PT in cases of vitamin K deficiency.

The magnitude of the prolongation of PT reflects the severity of the liver disease; however, PT does not correlate with the coagulation status or the risk of bleeding in patients with cirrhosis. In fact, in patients with cirrhosis there is also a decrease in synthesis of anti-hemostatic factors, and some patients become relatively hypercoagulable and have an increased risk of clot formation, despite having prolonged PT. This is an important and frequently misunderstood concept.

Gamma Globulins

Elevation of individual gamma globulins can be suggestive of specific liver diseases. Some examples include elevation of immunoglobulin G (IgG) in patients with autoimmune hepatitis, elevation of immunoglobulin M (IgM) in PBC, and elevation of immunoglobulin A (IgA) in patients with alcoholic cirrhosis. IgG4-related disease is an autoimmune phenomenon in which increased IgG4 levels cause dysfunction in multiple organs, including bile ducts (IgG4-related cholangiopathy).

Specific Markers of Liver Diseases

Specific laboratory tests are required for the diagnosis of some liver diseases.

- **α1-Antitrypsin (α1AT):** it can be quantified and, if decreased, the A1AT phenotype can be determined
- **Autoimmune hepatitis:** antinuclear antibody (ANA), anti–smooth muscle antibody (ASMA), anti–liver/kidney microsomal antibody type 1 (anti-LKM1)

- **Primary biliary cholangitis:** antimitochondrial antibody (AMA)
- **Hemochromatosis:** iron panel (serum iron, total iron binding capacity, transferrin saturation and ferritin) and HFE gene mutations
- **Wilson's disease:** serum ceruloplasmin and urinary copper levels
- **Viruses:** different viruses (e.g., hepatitis A, B, C, D, E, Epstein-Barr virus, cytomegalovirus, and herpes virus) that cause hepatitis are detected using polymerase chain reaction.

Biomarkers of Liver Fibrosis

Liver biopsy is the "gold standard" for evaluation of liver histopathology. Although the complications are few, it is an invasive test and the need for less invasive means to evaluate fibrosis led to several studies in search of surrogate markers for hepatic fibrosis. Many such tests combine clinical and serum markers and have been validated in specific populations, particularly chronic hepatitis C and nonalcoholic fatty liver disease. Caution is needed when using the results in other patient populations. In addition, serum markers are not liver specific and concurrent sites of inflammation may contribute to deranged serum levels.

These tests are used to differentiate patients with more significant stages of fibrosis and cirrhosis (stages 3 and 4), from those with minimal or no fibrosis (stages 0 and 1). The stages are based on the METAVIR score and range from 0 to 4, where stage 4 corresponds to cirrhosis.

Examples of such tests include the following:

- **APRI Score** is based on the AST and platelet count (AST elevation/platelet count) × 100. It has been mostly studied in patients with HCV, HCV and HIV co-infection, alcoholic liver disease, and NAFLD.
- **FibroSure or FibroTest** uses the measurement of α2-macroglobulin, α2-globulin, γ-globulin, apolipoprotein A1, GGT, and total bilirubin. It also utilizes the patient's age and sex. The results classify the patients as having mild fibrosis, indeterminate fibrosis or significant fibrosis. It has been better studied in patients with HCV and has a better specificity than sensitivity.
- **HepaScore** utilizes the combination of bilirubin, GGT, hyaluronic acid, α2-macroglobulin, age, and sex. Its performance is similar to the FibroTest.

- **FIB 4 index** combines platelet count, ALT, AST, and age. Better studied in HCV and NAFLD.
- **NAFLD fibrosis score** considers the patient's age, body mass index, blood glucose, aminotransferases, platelet count, and albumin.

Other panel tests have included products of collagen synthesis or degradation, enzymes involved in matrix biosynthesis or degradation, extracellular matrix glycoproteins, and proteoglycans/glycosaminoglycans.

The routine use of these panels in clinical practice is not clearly established and some suggest their use in combination with image modalities.

Image tests applying mechanical waves and measuring their propagation speed through liver tissue using ultrasound and MRI have become more readily available. They have been studied in a broader spectrum of liver diseases and have better sensitivity and specificity than the serologic tests. Nevertheless, at this point none of these tests fully substitute for liver biopsy.

SUGGESTED READINGS

Gao Y, Zheng J, Liang P, et al: Liver fibrosis with two-dimensional US shear-wave elastography in participants with chronic hepatitis B: a prospective multicenter study, Radiology 289:407–415, 2018.

Newsome PN, Cramb R, Davison SM, et al: Guidelines on the management of abnormal liver blood tests, Gut 67:6–19, 2018.

Northup PG, Caldwell SH: Coagulation in liver disease: a guide for the clinician, Clin Gastroenterol Hepatol 11:1064–1074, 2013.

Poynard T, De Ledinghen V, Zarski JP, et al: Relative performances of FibroTest, Fibroscan, and biopsy for the assessment of the stage of liver fibrosis in patients with chronic hepatitis C: a step toward the truth in the absence of a gold standard, J Hepatol 56:541–548, 2012.

Rockey D, Caldwell SH, Goodman ZD, et al: AASLD position paper: liver biopsy, Hepatology 49:1017–1044, 2009.

Sebastiani G, Halfon P, Castera L, et al: Comparison of three algorithms of non-invasive markers of fibrosis in chronic hepatitis C, Aliment Pharmacol Ther 35:92–104, 2012.

Tapper EB, Saini SC, Sengupta N: Extensive testing or focused testing of patients with elevated liver enzymes, J Hepatol 66:313–319, 2017.

41

Jaundice

Mohanad T. Al-Qaisi, Mashal Batheja, Michael B. Fallon

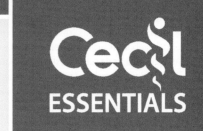

INTRODUCTION

Jaundice is the condition of yellowish pigmentation of the skin, the conjunctival membranes over the sclera, and other mucous membranes that is caused by elevated serum bilirubin levels (hyperbilirubinemia). The term jaundice is derived from *jaune*, the French word for "yellow," and the condition is also known as *icterus* (Greek for "yellow"). Normal serum bilirubin levels range from 0.5 to 1.0 mg/dL, and plasma bilirubin concentrations typically must exceed 2.5 mg/dL before jaundice becomes evident clinically.

Although jaundice is commonly due to liver and biliary tract disease, it has many causes, so it is not surprising that the diagnosis and management of jaundice have challenged clinicians for centuries. In most cases, jaundice or hyperbilirubinemia per se is not a pathologic condition but rather a sign of one or more illnesses originating from or affecting the liver and blood. However, there is one notable exception: In newborns, high bilirubin levels can lead to pathologic cerebral changes. In this condition, which is known as *kernicterus* (*kern* is the German word for "nucleus"), persistent elevation of unconjugated bilirubin leads to its deposition in the cerebral basal ganglia (or nuclei). This process can be prevented and treated and therefore merits special recognition to prevent damage to the developing brain.

BILIRUBIN METABOLISM

Hyperbilirubinemia can be classified based on the three phases of hepatic bilirubin metabolism: uptake, conjugation, and excretion into the bile (the rate-limiting step). In addition, jaundice can be classified into prehepatic, hepatic, and posthepatic causes (Table 41.1). Although the approaches are complementary, the latter classification may be more useful for the practicing clinician.

The main source of bilirubin is the hemoglobin released from senescent red blood cells, and the liver serves as its primary site of metabolism and excretion. Abnormalities at any step in bilirubin production, metabolism, or excretion can lead to an increase in the serum bilirubin and clinical jaundice. Under normal conditions, human red blood cells have a lifespan of about 120 days. As they age, erythrocytes are broken down and removed from the circulation by phagocytes. Most bilirubin (80%) is derived from the breakdown of hemoglobin released from these cells; the remainder is derived from ineffective erythropoiesis in the bone marrow and from catabolism of myoglobin and hepatic hemoproteins such as the cytochrome P-450 isoenzymes. The normal rate of bilirubin production is approximately 4 mg/kg body weight per day (E-Fig. 41.1).

As erythrocytes are destroyed within the reticuloendothelial system, free hemoglobin is ingested by macrophages and then split into heme and globin moieties. The heme ring is cleaved by the enzyme microsomal heme oxygenase to form biliverdin (*verde* = "green"), which is then converted to the tetrapyrrole pigment bilirubin by the cytosolic enzyme biliverdin reductase. This unconjugated (or "indirect") bilirubin is released into the plasma, where it is tightly bound to albumin. Because unconjugated bilirubin is insoluble in water, it cannot be excreted in urine or bile. However, it is permeable across lipid-rich environments and therefore can traverse the blood-brain barrier and the placenta.

The unconjugated bilirubin-albumin complex is transported to the liver. Once in the space of Disse, this complex dissociates; unconjugated bilirubin is transported across the basolateral plasma membrane of liver cells and attaches to intracellular binding proteins (ligandins). It is then conjugated with glucuronic acid by the enzyme uridine diphosphate glucuronyl transferase (UDP-GT) to form bilirubin monoglucuronide and diglucuronide, making the molecule water soluble. This conjugated (or "direct") bilirubin is excreted into bile via active transport across the canalicular membrane by means of a multispecific canalicular transport protein. In healthy persons, most bilirubin circulates in its unconjugated form with less than 5% of circulating bilirubin appearing in its conjugated form. If biliary excretion of conjugated bilirubin is impaired, it can exit the basolateral membrane and reenter the circulation, causing an increase in plasma levels. Because conjugated bilirubin is water soluble and less tightly bound to albumin than its unconjugated form, it is readily filtered by the glomerulus and appears in the urine, giving it a dark color (choluria). Once in bile, bilirubin enters the intestine, where bacteria convert it to colorless tetrapyrroles (urobilinogens) that are excreted in feces. Up to 20% of urobilinogen is reabsorbed and undergoes enterohepatic circulation or excretion in urine.

LABORATORY MEASUREMENT OF BILIRUBIN

The *van den Bergh reaction*, which is the most commonly used test for detecting bilirubin in biologic fluids, combines bilirubin with diazotized sulfanilic acid to form a colored compound. The direct-reacting fraction is roughly equivalent to conjugated bilirubin and the indirect-reacting fraction (total minus direct fraction) to unconjugated bilirubin. This characteristic provides a means for classifying jaundice into two categories: unconjugated hyperbilirubinemia and conjugated hyperbilirubinemia.

UNCONJUGATED HYPERBILIRUBINEMIA

Mechanisms that cause unconjugated hyperbilirubinemia include overproduction, impaired hepatic uptake, and decreased conjugation

TABLE 41.1 Classification of Jaundice and Representative Causes

Prehepatic Causes
Predominantly unconjugated hyperbilirubinemia
Hemolysis (e.g., sickle cell disease, autoimmune hemolytic anemia, mechanical cardiac valve with accelerated red cell destruction)
Microbe-induced hemolysis (malaria, leptospirosis)
Ineffective erythropoiesis (e.g., megaloblastic anemias)
Hematoma resolution

Hepatic Causes
Unconjugated hyperbilirubinemia
Decreased hepatic uptake
  Therapeutic drugs that interfere with bilirubin uptake (e.g., rifampin, metformin, methimazole, propylthiouracil, clopidogrel, sulfamethoxazole/trimethoprim)
  Herbal medicines (e.g., *Teucrium viscidum*, kava-kava, chaparral, greater celandine)
  Hyperthyroidism
  Diminished uptake and decreased cytosolic binding proteins (e.g., newborn or premature infants)
  Shunting of blood away from the liver (portal hypertension or surgical shunt)
Decreased conjugation due to limited glucuronyl transferase activity
  Gilbert syndrome
  Crigler-Najjar syndrome types I and II
  Neonatal jaundice
  Breast-milk jaundice
  Drug-induced inhibition (e.g., chloramphenicol)
Predominantly conjugated hyperbilirubinemia
Impaired hepatic excretion
  Familial cholestasis (Dubin-Johnson syndrome, Rotor syndrome, benign recurrent cholestasis, cholestasis of pregnancy)
  Hepatocellular injury from infiltrative disorders, hemochromatosis, α_1-antitrypsin deficiency, lymphoma, sarcoidosis, extensive metastases)
  Liver cirrhosis
  Hepatitis
  Drug-induced cholestasis (chlorpromazine, erythromycin estolate, isoniazid, halothane, and many others)
  Primary biliary cirrhosis
  Congestive heart failure
  Sepsis

Posthepatic Causes
Extrahepatic biliary obstruction
  Common bile duct obstruction from gallstones
  Benign and malignant tumors of the pancreas
  Tumors of bile ducts (cholangiocarcinoma) and ampulla of Vater
  Biliary strictures (postsurgical, gallstone-related, primary sclerosing cholangitis)
  Congenital disorders (biliary atresia, cystic fibrosis)
  Infectious cholangiopathy
  Chronic pancreatitis (fibrosis of the head of the pancreas)

of bilirubin. These disorders are not usually associated with significant hepatic disease.

Etiology of Hyperbilirubinemia

There are many potential causes of hyperbilirubinemia, and the major categories are summarized in Table 41.1. It is helpful to consider them mechanistically as conditions affecting the balance of bilirubin production, liver metabolism, and excretion. The classic cause of bilirubin overproduction is hemolysis, whereas the most common cause of impaired bilirubin uptake and metabolism is cirrhosis or other liver disease (viral hepatitis, drugs, hepatotoxins or ischemia). Bile duct obstruction due to cancer (classically cholangiocarcinoma or pancreatic head cancer), stones, or strictures is the most common cause of obstructive jaundice. Because multiple mechanisms are often involved in an individual patient, the evaluation of jaundice can be complex.

Prehepatic Jaundice

Prehepatic jaundice is associated with excessive bilirubin production (Fig. 41.1), which most often results from hemolysis (intravascular or extravascular), resolution of large hematomas, or mechanical injury to red cells, as in disseminated intravascular coagulation (see Chapter 48). Certain genetic diseases can lead to increased red cell lysis and therefore hemolytic jaundice. Sickle cell anemia is the classic cause, but others include glucose 6-phosphate dehydrogenase deficiency and hereditary spherocytosis. Infectious diseases also can cause hemolysis, either directly (e.g., malaria) or indirectly (e.g., autoimmune injury). Jaundice resulting from hemolysis is characteristically mild in degree, and serum bilirubin levels rarely exceed 5 mg/dL in the absence of coexisting hepatic disease. Ineffective erythropoiesis, which may be significantly increased in megaloblastic anemia, also leads to mild jaundice.

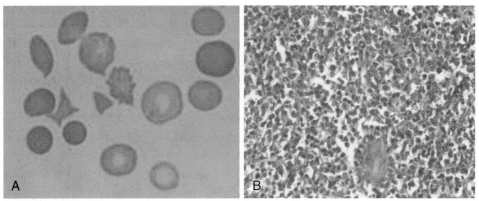

Fig. 41.1 Hemolytic anemia associated with lymphoma. (A) Blood smear shows the destroyed red blood cells. (B) Lymphoma.

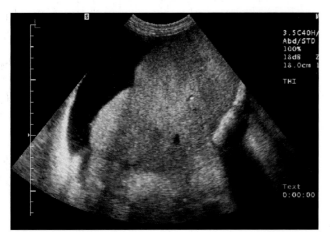

Fig. 41.2 Ultrasound image shows a cirrhotic liver with atrophy, irregular contours, and ascites.

Hemolysis should be considered in the evaluation of unconjugated hyperbilirubinemia and evaluated by examination of the peripheral blood smear (and, in some cases, the bone marrow smear and biopsy) as well as measurements of the reticulocyte count, haptoglobin, lactate dehydrogenase (LDH), erythrocyte fragility, and Coombs testing as indicated.

Hepatic or Hepatocellular Jaundice

Typically, considerable reserve exists within the liver, so jaundice of hepatocellular origin can be indicative of significant injury or dysfunction. The differential diagnosis is broad because the liver is susceptible to many different forms of injury (Fig. 41.2). The most common categories are viral hepatitis, exposure to toxins (e.g., alcohol, carbon tetrachloride, amanita, and increasingly herbs and supplements), medications (INH, antibiotics), autoimmune disorders (e.g., autoimmune hepatitis, primary biliary cholangitis [PBC], primary sclerosing cholangitis [PSC]), and liver tumors (primary or metastatic). Impaired hepatic uptake of bilirubin can be a cause of unconjugated hyperbilirubinemia. When present, it is typically caused by competition for bilirubin uptake by drugs such as rifampin. Removal of the competing agent usually leads to resolution of the jaundice.

Impaired Conjugation

Another common cause of unconjugated hyperbilirubinemia is Gilbert syndrome, a benign disorder that affects up to 7% of the population. This represents a normal variant that is not associated with intrinsic liver disease. Rather, it typically manifests during the second or third decade of life as mild unconjugated hyperbilirubinemia that is exacerbated by fasting or physical stress. Most of those affected have a total bilirubin level of less than 3 mg/dL, mostly of the unconjugated (indirect) fraction. The underlying genetic variant responsible is a homozygous abnormality in the TATAA element of the promoter region of the UDP-GT gene that results in lower enzymatic levels. The diagnosis is strongly suggested by unconjugated hyperbilirubinemia in the setting of normal hepatic enzyme levels, no known liver disease, and no evidence of hemolysis. Liver biopsy usually is not indicated, and therapy is not warranted. However, the bilirubin level does decrease significantly with phenobarbital administration. It is important to be aware of this common cause of unconjugated hyperbilirubinemia so that the patient can be reassured and more costly or invasive tests can be avoided. Although Gilbert syndrome has generally been thought to have a benign course, sometimes people with this condition might be at an increased risk of developing gallstones. On the other hand, patients with Gilbert syndrome might be at a lower risk to develop cardiovascular disease, because unconjugated bilirubin has antioxidant properties that may offer some protective effect and mitigate progression of atherosclerosis.

Crigler-Najjar syndrome is another cause of unconjugated hyperbilirubinemia in which the bilirubin levels may be much higher due to a genetically determined decrease or absence of UDP-GT activity. Conjugation may also be impaired by mild, acquired defects of UDP-GT induced by drugs such as chloramphenicol.

NEONATAL JAUNDICE

About 50% of term and 80% of preterm babies develop jaundice, which usually appears 2 to 4 days after birth and resolves spontaneously after 1 to 2 weeks. Most jaundice in newborn infants occurs for two main reasons. First, the enzymatic and transport pathways responsible for bilirubin metabolism are relatively immature and are unable to conjugate bilirubin as efficiently or as quickly as in adults. Second, bilirubin production is increased. Of those two mechanisms, the major defect is in bilirubin conjugation, which may cause mild to moderate unconjugated hyperbilirubinemia between the second and fifth days of life lasting until day 8 in normal births or about day 14 in premature births. This neonatal jaundice is usually harmless, and no specific therapy is required other than close observation.

More severe pathologic unconjugated hyperbilirubinemia can occur in neonates and usually is caused by a combination of hemolysis secondary to blood group incompatibility and defective conjugation. This neonatal jaundice is a serious condition that requires immediate attention because severe hyperbilirubinemia can lead to permanent neurologic damage (kernicterus). Phototherapy provided by conventional lighting or a fiberoptic light is the treatment of choice; it reduces neonatal jaundice (as assessed by serum bilirubin levels) compared with no treatment. Low-threshold compared with high-threshold phototherapy reduces neurodevelopmental impairment and hearing loss and reduces serum bilirubin on day 5 in infants with extremely low birth weight. However, it increases the duration of phototherapy, and it has no effect on mortality or on the rate of exchange transfusion. Close phototherapy, compared with distant light-source phototherapy, reduces the duration of phototherapy in infants with hyperbilirubinemia. If jaundice does not improve with phototherapy, other causes of neonatal jaundice should be assessed.

CONJUGATED HYPERBILIRUBINEMIA

Conjugated hyperbilirubinemia is associated with impaired formation or excretion of *all components* of bile, a situation termed *cholestasis*. The two major mechanisms of conjugated hyperbilirubinemia are defective excretion of bilirubin from hepatocytes into bile (intrahepatic cholestasis) and mechanical obstruction to the flow of bile through the bile ducts.

Impaired Hepatic Excretion (Intrahepatic Cholestasis)

Intrahepatic cholestasis can result from a wide range of conditions, including those that impair canalicular transport (e.g., certain drugs, circulating inflammatory cytokines during sepsis) and those that cause destruction of the small intrahepatic bile ducts. PBC, for example, is a chronic, progressive liver disease that occurs primarily in women and is characterized by the indolent destruction and subsequent disappearance over time of small lobular bile ducts. The gradual decrease in the number of bile ducts leads to progressive cholestasis, portal inflammation, fibrosis, and eventually cirrhosis. A similar loss of intrahepatic ducts can occur as a result of chronic rejection after liver transplantation.

Drug-induced cholestasis is increasingly common, and immune-mediated or idiosyncratic mechanisms can be the underlying cause. In some cases, there is associated hepatitis with significant cell injury (this can lead to hepatocellular damage and elevations in alanine aminotransferase [ALT] and aspartate aminotransferase [AST]). Representative drugs include, but are not limited to, nitrofurantoin, oral contraceptives, anabolic steroids, erythromycin, cimetidine, gold salts, chlorpromazine, prochlorperazine, imipramine, sulindac, tolbutamide, ampicillin, and other penicillin-based antibiotics. Given the broad access to drugs in Western societies and the unpredictable nature of the adverse liver effects, a high index of suspicion for drug-induced cholestasis is required. Drug-induced liver injury is generally considered a diagnosis of exclusion, after a thorough evaluation has ruled out other viral, autoimmune, and metabolic etiologies.

Intrahepatic cholestasis of pregnancy (ICP), also known as idiopathic jaundice of pregnancy, is a cholestatic disorder that is characterized by pruritus in the absence of a skin rash and elevation of aminotransferases (often up to 100 IU/L), alkaline phosphatase, 5-nucleotidase, and total and direct bilirubin concentrations. Total levels of bilirubin rarely exceed 6 mg/dL. The levels of γ-glutamyl transpeptidase are normal or only modestly elevated. ICP occurs in the second or third trimester of pregnancy and usually resolves spontaneously within 2 to 3 weeks after delivery. The diagnosis is suggested by the combination of pruritus and abnormal liver function tests with exclusion of other causes such as gallstones or intrinsic liver disease. ICP is associated with a higher risk for adverse perinatal outcome, including preterm birth, meconium passage, and fetal death.

The cause of ICP is not fully defined, but genetic, hormonal, and environmental factors are all likely to be involved. There is a high incidence of ICP in Chile and some other areas, and studies of potential genetic contributors are underway. Because adverse outcomes appear to occur predominantly after 37 weeks gestation, management by an experienced obstetrics team and consideration of early delivery are warranted. Ursodeoxycholic acid may be effective in ameliorating maternal pruritus and improving liver function test results; however, no medication has yet been shown to reduce the risk to the fetus.

The hemophagocytic syndrome, also known as hemophagocytic lymphohistiocytosis (HLH), is an uncommon hyperinflammatory disorder caused by severe hypercytokinemia. It manifests as fever, splenomegaly, and jaundice, with hemophagocytosis in the bone marrow and other tissues pathologically. Primary or familial HLH, also called familial erythrophagocytic lymphohistiocytosis, is a heterogeneous autosomal recessive disorder that has been found to be more prevalent with parental consanguinity. Secondary HLH is associated with malignancy, immunodeficiency, and infection, especially viral infection. In HLH, there is an inherent defect of natural killer cells and cytotoxic T cells, so they are unable to cope effectively with the infectious agent or antigen. Liver biopsies in HLH reveal sinusoidal dilation with hemophagocytic histiocytosis.

Postoperative jaundice typically occurs 1 to 10 days after surgery and has an incidence of approximately 15% after heart surgery and 1% after elective abdominal surgery. It is multifactorial in origin, with increased bilirubin load from bleeding and blood transfusions as well as impaired bilirubin conjugation and secretion caused by inflammatory cytokines. It typically resolves fully over time.

In hepatocellular disease, all three steps of hepatic bilirubin metabolism are impaired. Excretion, the rate-limiting step, is usually most affected, leading to predominantly conjugated hyperbilirubinemia.

Jaundice can be profound in acute hepatitis (see Chapter 42) without adverse prognostic implications. In chronic liver disease, however, persistent jaundice usually implies irreversible decrease in hepatic function and a poor prognosis.

Posthepatic Jaundice

Posthepatic jaundice, also called obstructive jaundice, results from a complete or partial obstruction of intrahepatic or extrahepatic bile ducts (Fig. 41.3 and E-Fig. 41.2). The most common causes are gallstones in the common bile duct and tumors of the pancreatic head. Not infrequently, the first sign of pancreatic cancer is jaundice. Other causes include strictures of the common bile duct resulting from prior surgery or passage of gallstones. Primary sclerosing cholangitis should be considered in the setting of jaundice and biliary strictures that may be seen on imaging studies (magnetic resonance cholangiopancreatography [MRCP] or endoscopic retrograde pancreatography [ERCP]). Less common causes include congenital biliary atresia, pancreatitis, pancreatic pseudocysts, and parasites such as liver flukes (e.g., *Clonorchis sinensis*, *Dicrocoelium dendriticum*, *Opisthorchis viverrini*).

Mirizzi syndrome is an uncommon cause of posthepatic jaundice observed in 0.7% to 1.4% of patients after cholecystectomy. This syndrome is caused by extrinsic compression from an impacted stone in the cystic duct that impinges on and obstructs the common bile duct (see Table 41.1). Portal hypertensive biliopathy (or vascular biliopathy) is characterized by anatomic and functional abnormalities of the intrahepatic, extrahepatic, and pancreatic ducts in patients with portal hypertension associated with extrahepatic portal vein obstruction or, less frequently, cirrhosis. These morphologic changes, consisting of dilatation and stenosis of the biliary tree, are caused by extensive venous collaterals that develop in an attempt to decompress the portal

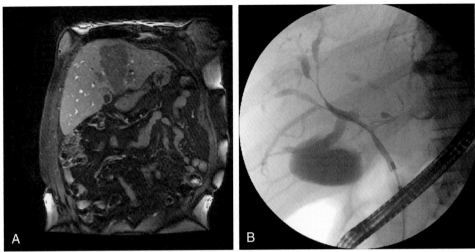

Fig. 41.3 Hepatocellular carcinoma compressing the bile ducts. (A) Sagittal view of computed abdominal tomography scan. (B) Endoscopic retrograde cholangiopancreatography demonstrates multiple strictures of the bile ducts.

venous blockage. The condition is usually asymptomatic until it has progressed to a more advanced stage such as biliary cirrhosis.

Immunoglobulin G4 (IgG4)–related sclerosing disease has recently been recognized as a distinct disease entity that can affect the bile ducts, gallbladder, pancreas, and other sites. Most cases of IgG4-related pancreatobiliary disease are associated with elevated serum IgG4 levels, extensive IgG4-positive plasma cells, and infiltration of lymphocytes into various organs, which leads to fibrosis. Several established systems are used to diagnose IgG4 disease; they rely on a combination of imaging findings of the pancreas, bile duct, and other organs; serologic findings; pancreatic histologic findings; and response to corticosteroid therapy.

CLINICAL APPROACH TO THE EVALUATION OF JAUNDICE

The differential diagnosis of jaundice is broad, thus a thorough history and physical examination along with judicious use of laboratory and imaging studies are necessary to define its underlying etiology. Jaundice appears as yellowing of the skin and sclera. Other conditions may mimic this presentation (e.g., carotenemia, Addison's disease, quinacrine ingestion), but scleral and mucosal discolorations are absent in these conditions. In hypercarotenemia, for example, the yellowish-orange coloration typically involves only the palms of the hands and soles of the feet.

An elevated serum bilirubin level, usually higher than 3 mg/dL, confirms the clinical impression of jaundice. The most important initial step is to define whether the jaundice is predominantly caused by an elevation of unconjugated or conjugated bilirubin. If jaundice is primarily the result of unconjugated bilirubin, evaluation for hemolysis and other conditions with shortened red blood cell survival is required. In patients with elevated conjugated bilirubin, the clinical challenge lies in determining whether biliary obstruction or impaired hepatic excretion is responsible (see Chapter 40).

In cholestatic jaundice caused by biliary obstruction, the alkaline phosphatase level is typically increased to more than three times normal, whereas serum transaminases are usually elevated less than 5-fold to 10-fold (E-Fig. 41.3; see Chapter 40). Patients with cholestasis may also develop pruritus and malabsorption of fat and fat-soluble vitamins (vitamins A, D, E, and K). More specific causes of biliary obstruction are suggested by recurrent abdominal pain and nausea (gallstones) or epigastric pain radiating to the back with weight loss and gallbladder distention (carcinoma of the pancreatic head). In complete biliary obstruction, conjugated hyperbilirubinemia is prominent and usually peaks at about 30 mg/dL in the absence of renal failure. Eosinophilia may accompany drug-induced jaundice. Inquiring about the use of drugs known to cause cholestasis, serologic testing for antimitochondrial antibody in suspected PBC, and ERCP or MRCP to evaluate PSC may be helpful.

In jaundice produced by hepatocellular disease (see Chapters 40 and 42), serum transaminases are characteristically elevated more than 10-fold and alkaline phosphatase levels are less than three times normal. Evidence of hepatocellular damage is commonly associated and includes a prolonged prothrombin time, hypoalbuminemia, and clinical features of hepatic dysfunction (palmar erythema, spider angiomas, gynecomastia, and ascites). A careful evaluation includes inquiry about the use of drugs known to cause hepatocellular injury, alcohol, risk factors for viral hepatitis, and preexisting liver disease. More selected laboratory studies, such as serologic testing for hepatitis, are usually required (see Chapter 42).

A diagnostic approach to jaundice is outlined in E-Fig. 41.3. If extrahepatic obstruction is suspected, noninvasive studies such as ultrasound or computed tomography should be used to determine whether bile ducts are dilated. If dilated ducts are found on noninvasive imaging, then direct cholangiography (either endoscopic or radiologic) provides the most reliable approach to management and potential treatment of cholestatic jaundice. If intrahepatic cholestasis is suggested clinically and extrahepatic obstruction is excluded by noninvasive means or by direct cholangiography, then the emphasis is placed on further laboratory testing to define the specific cause. Liver biopsy is sometimes required to define a specific histologic diagnosis, rule out other causes of disease, and assess the degree of injury and fibrosis.

For a deeper discussion on this topic, please see Chapter 138, "Approach to the Patient with Jaundice or Abnormal Liver Tests," in *Goldman-Cecil Medicine*, 26th Edition.

SUGGESTED READINGS

Berk PD: Approach to the patient with jaundice or abnormal liver tests. In Goldman L, Ausiello D, editors: Cecil textbook of medicine, ed 22, Philadelphia, 2004, Saunders, pp 897–905.

Pathak B, Sheibani L, Lee RH: Cholestasis of pregnancy, Obstet Gynecol Clin North Am 37:269–282, 2010.

Suárez V, Puerta A, Santos LF, et al.: Portal hypertensive biliopathy: a single center experience and literature review, World J Hepatol 5:137–144, 2013.

Trauner M, Wagner M, Fickert P, et al.: Molecular regulation of hepatobiliary transport systems: clinical implications for understanding and treating cholestasis, J Clin Gastroenterol 39(4 Suppl 2):S111–S124, 2005.

Vlachou PA, Khalili K, Jang HJ, et al.: IgG4-related sclerosing disease: autoimmune pancreatitis and extrapancreatic manifestations, Radiographics 31:1379–1402, 2011.

Woodgate P, Jardine LA: Neonatal jaundice, Clin Evid (Online) Epub Sep 15, 2011. Available at: http://www.ncbi.nlm.nih.gov/pubmed/21920055. Accessed September 19, 2014.

42

Acute and Chronic Hepatitis

Nayan M. Patel, Jen Jung Pan, Michael B. Fallon

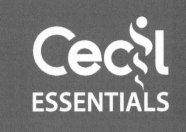

INTRODUCTION

The term *hepatitis* denotes inflammation of the liver. It is applied to a broad category of clinicopathologic conditions that result from the damage produced by viral, toxic, metabolic, pharmacologic, or immune-mediated injury to the liver.

ACUTE HEPATITIS

Acute hepatitis implies a recent-onset inflammatory condition lasting less than 6 months. It can culminate either in complete resolution of the liver damage with return to normal function and structure or rapid progression of the acute injury toward extensive necrosis and a fatal outcome. Depending on the etiology, some may also progress to develop a chronic hepatitis. The most common causes of acute hepatitis are viral hepatitis (hepatitis A through E) and nonviral causes such as drug-induced liver injury, alcohol, toxins, autoimmune hepatitis, and Wilson's disease.

Acute Viral Hepatitis

Five hepatotropic viruses cause classic acute viral hepatitis (Table 42.1), but other viruses, including cytomegalovirus, herpesviruses, and Epstein-Barr virus can also cause liver injury. All of the hepatotropic viruses are ribonucleic acid (RNA) viruses except hepatitis B virus (HBV), which has a deoxyribonucleic acid (DNA) genome.

Hepatitis A virus (HAV) is a nonenveloped, single-stranded RNA virus classified in the Picornaviridae family and in the *Hepatovirus* genus. It is stable at moderate temperature and low pH, allowing the virus to survive in the environment and be transmitted by the fecal-oral route. The course is generally self-limited and does not lead to chronic infection.

Hepatitis E virus (HEV) belongs to the genus *Hepevirus* in the Hepeviridae family and has four genotypes. HEV1 and HEV2 are restricted to human beings and are transmitted via contaminated water in developing countries. HEV1 occurs mainly in Asia, whereas HEV2 occurs in Africa and Mexico. HEV3 and HEV4 infect human beings, pigs, and other mammalian species and are responsible for sporadic cases of autochthonous hepatitis E in both developing and developed countries. HEV3 has a worldwide distribution. HEV4 mostly occurs in Southeast Asia. While typically self-limited, acute liver failure and hepatic decompensation can occur in patients who are pregnant, malnourished, or have preexisting liver disease. Additionally, patients with solid organ transplants can develop a chronic HEV infection.

HBV is a small DNA virus that belongs to the Hepadnaviridae family. Approximately 250 million persons are carriers of HBV worldwide; of these, 75% reside in Asia and the Western Pacific. Both acute and chronic HBV infection can occur. Chronic hepatitis B infection is a major cause of hepatocellular carcinoma worldwide and can occur without cirrhosis because of integration of HBV DNA into hepatocytes.

Hepatitis C virus (HCV) is a single-stranded positive-sense RNA virus that belongs to the Flaviviridae family and has been classified as the sole member of the genus *Hepacivirus*. Approximately 74 million people are infected with HCV worldwide and 2.4 million in the United States. HBV has eight genotypes (labeled A through H), and HCV has six genotypes (1 through 6). Both HBV and HCV viruses are transmitted parenterally. HBV is present in virtually all body fluids and excreta of carriers. Transmission occurs most commonly through blood and blood products, contaminated needles, and sexual contact. Historically, HCV was the main cause of post-transfusion hepatitis before 1992. It is currently the most common cause of hepatitis among intravenous drug users. The Centers for Disease Control and Prevention now recommends one-time screening of persons born between 1945 and 1965 for hepatitis C because of the high prevalence of the disease in this birth cohort.

Hepatitis D virus (HDV) is classified in a separate genus of the Deltaviridae family. It is a small, defective RNA virus that can propagate only in an individual who has coexistent HBV infection, either after simultaneous transmission of the two viruses or via superinfection of an established HBV carrier. HDV has at least eight genotypes, four of which (genotypes 5 through 8) seem to be of exclusively African origin. Of the 250 million chronic carriers of HBV worldwide, more than 15 million have serologic evidence of exposure to HDV. Like HBV, HDV is transmitted via the parenteral route through exposure to infected blood or body fluids. Because there is evidence for sexual transmission, people with high-risk sexual activity are at increased risk for infection.

Clinical and Laboratory Manifestations

Acute viral hepatitis typically involves an asymptomatic incubation period from exposure to the first appearance of symptoms. This can be weeks to months depending on the type of viral hepatitis. Next a prodromal phase lasting several days that is characterized by constitutional and gastrointestinal symptoms including malaise, fatigue, anorexia, nausea, vomiting, myalgia, and headache occurs. A mild fever may be present (Fig. 42.1). Clinical manifestations of hepatitis A depend on the age of the host: fewer than 30% of infected young children showed symptomatic hepatitis, whereas about 80% of infected adults had severe acute hepatitis with remarkably elevated serum aminotransferases (Fig. 42.2). Arthritis and urticaria resembling serum sickness, attributed to immune complex deposition, are present in 5% to 10% of cases of acute hepatitis B and C. Taste and smell alterations may also occur. Jaundice soon appears, with bilirubinuria and acholic (pale) stools, which are often accompanied by an improvement in the patient's sense of well-being. The liver is usually tender and enlarged; splenomegaly is found in about one fifth of patients. Notably, many patients with acute viral hepatitis are asymptomatic or have symptoms without jaundice (anicteric hepatitis). In such instances, medical attention often is not sought.

TABLE 42.1   Characteristics of Acute Viral Hepatitides

	Hepatitis A	Hepatitis B	Hepatitis C	Hepatitis D	Hepatitis E
Causative agent	27–28 nm RNA virus Nonenveloped	42 nm DNA virus Enveloped	55–65 nm RNA virus Enveloped	36–43 nm RNA virus Enveloped	27–34 nm RNA virus Nonenveloped
Transmission	Fecal-oral	Blood-borne, sexual, percutaneous, perinatal	Similar to HBV; vertical and sexual route uncommon	Similar to HBV	Similar to HAV; transfusion; vertical transmission
Incubation period (days)	15–50	30–180	14–180	Similar to HBV	15–60
Onset	Acute	Acute, insidious	Insidious	Acute, insidious	Acute, insidious
Fulminant disease (%)	0.01–0.5	1	<0.1	5–20	1–2
Chronic hepatitis	No	Yes	Yes	Yes/No	Yes/No
Treatment	Supportive	Nucleos(t)ide analogues; IFN-α	DAA ± ribavirin	IFN-α	Supportive; ribavirin
Prophylaxis	Hygiene; immune globulin, vaccine	Similar to HAV	Hygiene	Hygiene, HBV vaccine	Hygiene, vaccine

DAA, Direct-acting antiviral; HAV, hepatitis A virus; HBV, hepatitis B virus; IFN-α, interferon-α.

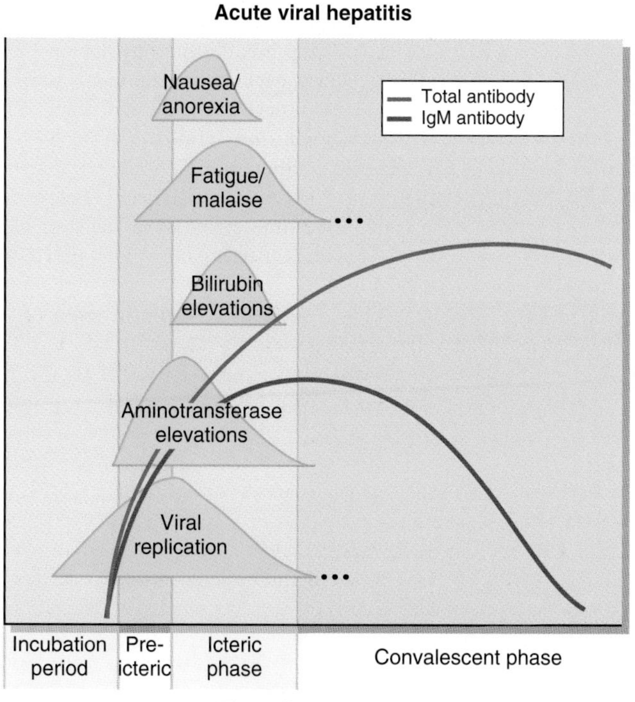

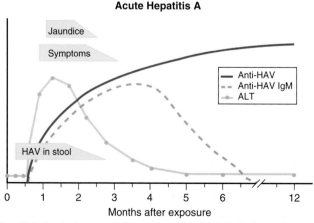

Acute viral hepatitis

Fig. 42.1 Typical clinical, laboratory, and serological course in acute self-resolving viral hepatitis. IgM, Immunoglobulin M.

Acute Hepatitis A

Fig. 42.2 Serologic course of acute hepatitis A. ALT, Alanine aminotransferase; HAV, hepatitis A virus; IgM, immunoglobulin M.

Alanine aminotransferase (ALT) and aspartate aminotransferase (AST) are released from acutely damaged hepatocytes, and serum levels can rise to 20-fold or more above normal. An elevated serum bilirubin level (>2.5 to 3 mg/dL) results in jaundice and is defined as icteric hepatitis. Values higher than 20 mg/dL are uncommon and correlate in a general way with the severity of disease. Elevations in serum alkaline phosphatase (ALP) are usually limited to three times normal levels except in cases of cholestatic hepatitis. A complete blood cell count most commonly shows mild leukopenia with atypical lymphocytes. Anemia and thrombocytopenia may also be present. The icteric phase of acute viral hepatitis may last days to weeks and is followed by gradual resolution of symptoms and laboratory values.

Diagnosis

Acute viral hepatitis can be diagnosed either directly, by detecting the nucleic acids of the infecting virus, or indirectly, by demonstrating an immune response in the host (Tables 42.2 and 42.3). Epstein-Barr virus and cytomegalovirus hepatitis are part of the differential diagnosis and also may be diagnosed by the appearance of specific antibodies of the immunoglobulin M (IgM) class.

In acute hepatitis B, hepatitis B surface antigen (HBsAg) and e antigen (HBeAg) are present in serum. Both are usually cleared within 3 months in acute self-limited infection, but HBsAg may persist in some patients with uncomplicated disease for 6 months to 1 year. Clearance of HBsAg is followed after a variable period by the emergence of antibodies against hepatitis B surface antigen (anti-HBs), which confers long-term immunity. Antibodies against hepatitis B core antigen (anti-HBc) and e antigen (anti-HBe) appear in the acute phase of the illness, but neither provides immunity. During the serologic window period, anti-HBc IgM, a marker of active viral replication suggesting recent infection, may be the only evidence of HBV infection (Fig. 42.3).

Every patient who is HBsAg positive should be tested for antibodies against HDV (anti-HDV IgG), which persist even after the patient has cleared HDV infection. Active HDV infection is now confirmed by the detection of serum HDV RNA with sensitive real-time polymerase chain reaction (PCR) assays. However, because of the variability of the genome sequence, assays of HDV RNA can produce false-negative results. Testing of anti-HDV IgM antibodies still has a role in patients who test negative for HDV RNA but have clinical features of HDV-related liver disease. While there is no diagnostic feature, suspicion for active HDV co-infection should be higher in acute liver failure from acute HBV infection.

Acute hepatitis C can be detected within 2 weeks after exposure with the use of a sensitive PCR assay for HCV RNA. Serum antibodies

---

TABLE 42.2   Serologic Markers of Viral Hepatitis

Agent	Marker	Definition	Significance
HAV	Anti-HAV IgM	IgM antibody to HAV	Marker of acute or recent infection
	Anti-HAV IgG	IgG antibody to HAV	Marker of acute or previous infection; post vaccination; confers protective immunity
HBV	HBsAg	Hepatitis B surface antigen	The presence of HBsAg indicates that the person is infectious
	HBeAg	Hepatitis B e antigen	Transiently positive in acute infection; may persist in chronic infection; reflection of active viral replication and high infectivity
	Anti-HBs	Antibody to surface antigen	Marker of acute self-limited infection; post vaccination; confers protective immunity
	Anti-HBe	Antibody to e antigen	Transiently positive in convalescence; positive in chronic infection before seroconversion; usually a reflection of low infectivity
	Anti-HBc IgM	IgM antibody to core antigen	Marker of acute or exacerbation of chronic infection
	Anti-HBc IgG	IgG antibody to core antigen	Appears at the onset of symptoms in acute infection and persists for life; not seen in vaccinees without prior infection
HCV	Anti-HCV	Antibody to HCV	Marker of acute and chronic infection; does not provide immunity
HDV	Anti-HDV IgM	IgM antibody to HDV	Positive in acute infection, negative in past infection but persists in a large proportion of patients with chronic infection
	Anti-HDV IgG	IgG antibody to HDV	Positive in all individuals exposed to HDV, and persists long-term, even after viral clearance
HEV	Anti-HEV IgM	IgM antibody to HEV	Marker of acute or recent infection[a]
	Anti-HEV IgG	IgG antibody to HEV	Marker of chronic or previous infection[a]

HAV, Hepatitis A virus; *HBV*, hepatitis B virus; *HCV*, hepatitis C virus; *HDV*, hepatitis D virus; *HEV*, hepatitis E virus; *IgG*, immunoglobulin G; *IgM*, immunoglobulin M.
[a]Serologic testing is unreliable, and seroconversion might never occur in immunosuppressed persons.

TABLE 42.3   Interpretation of Diagnostic Markers in Hepatitis B

	HBsAg	HBeAg	Anti-HBc IgM	Anti-HBc IgG	Anti-HBs	Anti-HBe	Blood HBV DNA
Acute infection	+	+	+	+	–	+/–	High
Acute self-limited infection	–	–	+	+	+	+/–	–
Vaccinated	–	–	–	–	+	–	–
Chronic infection							
HBeAg positive	+	+	–	+	–	–	High
HBeAg negative	+	–	–	+	–	+	Low
Immune escape	+	–	–	+	–	+	High
Occult infection	–	–	–	+	–	+/–	Very low
Reactivation of chronic infection	+	+	+/–	+	–	+/–	High

anti-HBc IgG, Immunoglobulin G antibody against hepatitis B core antigen; *anti-HBc IgM*, immunoglobulin M antibody against hepatitis B core antigen; *anti-HBe*, antibody against hepatitis B e antigen; *anti-HBs*, antibody against hepatitis B surface antigen; *HBeAg*, hepatitis B e antigen; *HBsAg*, hepatitis B surface antigen; *HBV DNA*, hepatitis B virus deoxyribonucleic acid.

---

to HCV develop within 12 weeks after exposure, or within 4 to 5 weeks after biochemical abnormalities are discovered. Importantly, these are not neutralizing antibodies and do not confer immunity (Fig. 42.4). At onset of symptoms, 30% of patients will be missed if checked by serum enzyme immunoassay (EIA) for HCV antibody alone.

Commercial EIAs for hepatitis E to detect both IgM and IgG class antibodies are also available but may lack sensitivity and specificity. Diagnosis of HEV infection should be established by PCR assays in immunosuppressed patients, because serologic testing is unreliable, and seroconversion might never occur.

Complications

Cholestatic hepatitis. In some patients, most commonly during HAV infection, a prolonged but self-limited period of cholestasis (total bilirubin >10 mg/dL) occurs that is characterized by marked conjugated hyperbilirubinemia, elevation of ALP, and pruritus. Further investigation may be required to rule out biliary obstruction (see Chapters 40, 41, and 45).

Relapsing hepatitis. For unknown reasons, up to 10% of patients can experience a relapse of HAV infection after an initial resolution. This is characterized by biochemical relapse, but often milder clinical symptoms, and will typically resolve spontaneously.

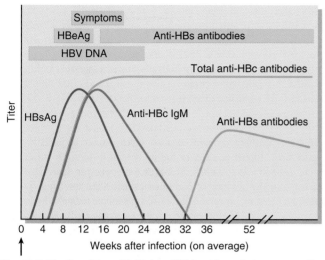

Fig. 42.3 Kinetics of hepatitis B virus (HBV) markers during acute self-resolving hepatitis B. The *arrow* indicates infection. *HBc,* Hepatitis B core; *HBeAg,* hepatitis B e antigen; *HBs,* hepatitis B surface; *HBsAg,* hepatitis B surface antigen; *IgM,* immunoglobulin M.

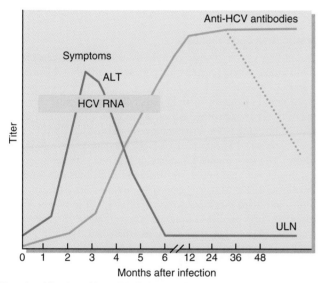

Fig. 42.4 Kinetics of hepatitis C virus markers during acute self-resolving hepatitis C. *ALT,* Alanine aminotransferase; *ULN,* upper limit of normal.

Fulminant hepatitis. Massive hepatic necrosis occurs in fewer than 1% of patients with acute viral hepatitis; it leads to a devastating and often fatal condition called acute liver failure. This condition is discussed in detail in Chapter 43.

Chronic hepatitis. Hepatitis A does not progress to chronic liver disease, although occasionally it has a relapsing course. Persistence of elevated levels of ALT and AST, viral antigens, or nucleic acids beyond 6 months in patients with hepatitis B or C suggests evolution to chronic hepatitis, although slowly resolving acute hepatitis may occasionally exhibit such test abnormalities for up to 12 months with eventual complete resolution. About 60% of organ transplant recipients infected with HEV fail to clear the virus and go on to develop chronic hepatitis. Chronic hepatitis is considered in detail later in this chapter.

Rare complications. Acute viral hepatitis may rarely be followed by aplastic anemia, which tends to affect mostly male patients and results in a mortality rate greater than 80%. Pancreatitis, myocarditis, pericarditis, pleural effusion, and neurologic complications including

Guillain-Barré syndrome, aseptic meningitis, and encephalitis have also been reported. Extrahepatic manifestations such as cryoglobulinemia and glomerulonephritis are associated with hepatitis B and C, and polyarteritis nodosa is associated with hepatitis B. These manifestations are more common in patients who fail to clear acute HBV or HCV and develop chronic hepatitis.

Management

Unless complicated by fulminant hepatitis, cases of acute hepatitis A, B, and E are usually self-limited and are managed by supportive care including rest, maintenance of adequate hydration and dietary intake, and avoidance of alcohol use. Hospitalization may be needed for patients who cannot tolerate oral intake and for those with evidence of deteriorated liver function, such as hepatic encephalopathy or coagulopathy.

In general, hepatitis A and E may be regarded as noninfectious after 3 weeks, whereas hepatitis B is potentially infectious to sexual contacts throughout its course, although the risk is low once HBsAg has been cleared. Studies of antiviral therapy in acute hepatitis B have not shown clear benefit, although some experts advocate the use of nucleos(t)ide analogues, specifically in the setting of acute liver failure due to hepatitis B. Treatment of acute hepatitis C is not always needed because 20% to 50% of patients will spontaneous clear the virus. This typically occurs within 6 months of the time of infection. If a decision is made to initiate treatment, current guidelines suggest monitoring HCV RNA for 12 to 16 weeks before starting treatment to allow for possible spontaneous clearance. Because of the safety and efficacy of direct acting antivirals (DAAs), the same regimen of medication for chronic hepatitis C is recommended for acute HCV.

Prevention

In patients with hepatitis A or E, both feces and blood contain virus during the prodromal and early icteric phases. General hygiene measures should include handwashing by contacts and careful handling, disposal, and sterilization of excreta, contaminated clothing, and utensils. HAV vaccination is appropriate for children older than 12 months of age, travelers to endemic areas, individuals with immunodeficiency or chronic liver disease, and those with high-risk behaviors or occupations. HAV vaccination is preferred over immunoglobulin for postexposure prophylaxis, based on results from randomized trials. With the availability of two candidate vaccines, one of which is already licensed for use in China, HEV prevention through vaccination is now a realistic possibility.

HBV is rarely transmitted by body fluids other than blood; however, it is highly infectious, and strict adherence to universal precautions is mandatory. Efforts at preventing hepatitis B have involved the use of hepatitis B immunoglobulin (HBIG) and recombinant HBV vaccines. Prophylaxis with HBIG after blood or mucosal exposure should be given within 7 days along with HBV vaccine. Preventive vaccination is currently recommended for high-risk individuals—health care professionals, patients undergoing hemodialysis, patients with chronic liver disease, residents and staff of custodial care institutions, and sexually active homosexual men—and is advocated universally for children. In the United States, the first hepatitis B vaccination is recommended to be given within 12 to 24 hours of birth.

No accepted prevention strategies other than universal precautions are available for HCV, and serum immunoglobulin is not useful for postexposure prophylaxis. The advent of widespread blood product screening for hepatitis C has made such infection after transfusion a rarity.

Alcoholic Liver Disease

Alcohol abuse continues to be a major cause of liver disease in the Western world. The three major pathologic findings resulting from alcohol abuse are fatty liver, alcoholic hepatitis, and cirrhosis. These findings are not mutually exclusive and may all be present in the same patient. The first two conditions are potentially reversible. Alcoholic cirrhosis is discussed in Chapter 44.

Mechanism of Injury

The mechanisms of liver injury caused by alcohol are complex. Ethanol and its metabolites, acetaldehyde and nicotinamide adenine dinucleotide phosphate, are directly hepatotoxic and cause a large number of metabolic derangements. Induction of cytochrome P-450 (i.e., CYP2E1) stimulates reactive oxidant species and cytokine pathways, particularly tumor necrosis factor-α (TNF-α). These are critical in initiating and perpetuating hepatic injury, as well as causing fibrosis through stellate cell activation. Excess alcohol leads to increased intestinal permeability, and the resultant endotoxemia from bacterial lipopolysaccharide leads to hepatic inflammation from upregulation of TNF-α.

Hepatotoxic effects from alcohol vary considerably among individuals based on dose, duration, drinking patterns, sex, ethnicity, genetic factors, and comorbidities that may affect the liver. The amount of alcohol ingested is the most important risk factor for the development of alcoholic liver disease. Women have a lower threshold of injury than men and have decreased amounts of gastric alcohol dehydrogenase as compared to men. The risk of cirrhosis is increased in men who drink greater than 60 to 80 grams of alcohol daily and women who drink more than 20 grams of alcohol daily. Malnutrition and other forms of chronic liver disease may potentiate the toxic effects of alcohol on the liver.

Clinical and Pathologic Features

Alcoholic fatty liver may manifest as incidentally discovered hepatomegaly or elevated aminotransferase levels on screening blood tests. Vague discomfort in the right upper quadrant of the abdomen may be the only symptom. Jaundice is rare, and aminotransferases are only mildly elevated (<5 times normal). Liver biopsy shows either diffuse or centrilobular fat occupying most of the hepatocytes.

Alcoholic hepatitis is a distinct entity characterized by acute hepatic inflammation that carries a high morbidity and mortality in its most severe form. It is characterized on liver biopsy by the histologic triad of Mallory bodies, infiltration by polymorphonuclear leukocytes, and a network of interlobular connective tissue surrounding hepatocytes and central veins (pericellular, perivenular, and perisinusoidal fibrosis). Patients with alcoholic hepatitis may be asymptomatic, or they may be extremely ill with hepatic failure. Other common symptoms are anorexia, nausea, vomiting, weight loss, and abdominal pain. For those with fever, infection needs to be ruled out. Rapid onset of jaundice is commonly present and may be pronounced, with cholestatic features that require differentiation from biliary tract disease (see Chapters 40, 41, and 45). Physical examination may reveal cutaneous signs of chronic liver disease, including spider angiomas and palmar erythema. In addition, gynecomastia, parotid enlargement, testicular atrophy, and loss of body hair may be found. The presence of ascites and hepatic encephalopathy can occur. Aminotransferases are only moderately increased (200 to 400 U/L) in alcoholic hepatitis compared with other forms of acute hepatitis. The ratio of AST to ALT almost always exceeds 2:1, in contrast to viral hepatitis, in which the aminotransferases are usually increased in parallel. The white blood cell count may be strikingly increased.

Diagnosis

A history of excessive and prolonged alcohol intake is frequently difficult to obtain from patients with alcoholic liver disease. However, historical, clinical, and biochemical features of alcoholic hepatitis are often sufficient to establish the diagnosis. Many patients suspected or found to imbibe alcohol excessively may have causes in addition to alcohol contributing to liver disease (e.g., chronic viral hepatitis). Therefore, when other causes of liver disease are suggested, and alcohol intake is uncertain, appropriate serologic testing and a liver biopsy may be needed to establish a diagnosis.

Treatment

Complete abstinence from alcohol is the most important step. Meticulous supportive care, including enteral feeding for those with severe anorexia, is the cornerstone of treatment for acute alcoholic hepatitis. In the absence of contraindications (i.e., infection, gastrointestinal bleeding, or renal failure), some patients with alcoholic hepatitis may benefit from treatment with corticosteroids. A calculated discriminant function (DF) value greater than 32 (where DF = 4.6 × [prothrombin time (in seconds) − control (in seconds)] + total bilirubin [in mg/dL]) may identify a subgroup of patients who are more likely to benefit from the use of corticosteroids, but these patients have advanced liver disease and a high mortality rate. Similarly, a Model for End-stage Liver Disease (MELD) score greater than 21 predicts a 90-day mortality of 20%. Pentoxifylline, an oral TNF-α antagonist, was shown to reduce the risk of renal failure but not mortality in a single randomized trial but has not shown benefit in other trials.

Complication and Prognosis

Alcoholic fatty liver disease completely resolves with cessation of alcohol intake. Alcoholic hepatitis can also resolve, but it commonly progresses either to cirrhosis, which may already be present at the time of initial diagnosis, or to hepatic failure and death. The development of encephalopathy, ascites, acute kidney injury, and gastrointestinal bleeding from varices often complicates alcoholic hepatitis (see Chapter 44). Patients with a DF greater than 32 have a high risk of death. The Lille model combines six reproducible variables (age, renal insufficiency, albumin, prothrombin time, bilirubin, and evolution of bilirubin at day 7) and is highly predictive of death at 6 months and helps guide corticosteroid therapy if initiated. A score greater than 0.45 predicts a 6-month survival rate of 25%, compared with 85% survival when the score is less than 0.45.

Drug-Induced Liver Injury

Drug-induced liver injury (DILI) refers to liver injury caused by drugs or other chemical agents and represents a special type of adverse drug reaction. More than 1000 medications and supplements are known to cause hepatotoxicity. Antibiotics remain the drugs most commonly responsible for DILI in the United States and Europe; the annual incidence of antibiotic-associated DILI is 1 in 10,000 to 100,000 individuals.

DILI may be classified by the pattern of liver injury observed. *Acute hepatocellular injury* is characterized by elevated levels of serum ALT and minimal elevations of serum ALP. *Cholestatic injury* is characterized by a disproportionately elevated level of ALP, which is synthesized and released by injured bile ducts. Liver injury that has both hepatocellular and cholestatic features is called *mixed liver injury*. DILI can also be classified into two broad categories, predictable and unpredictable, depending on the hepatotoxins involved. Predictable hepatotoxins, such as acetaminophen and carbon tetrachloride, cause dose-dependent liver injury. Acetaminophen is now the leading cause of life-threatening acute liver failure in the United States and Europe. Unpredictable hepatotoxins cause DILI in a so-called idiosyncratic fashion. Idiosyncratic reactions are difficult to predict and are not dose dependent. They generally tend to occur within the first 3 months of initiating a medication. They occur relatively rarely in individuals with unique genetic and environmental characteristics.

Clinical and Laboratory Manifestations

DILI symptoms are similar to those associated with viral hepatitis and include malaise, anorexia, nausea and vomiting, right upper quadrant abdominal pain, jaundice, acholic stools, and dark (tea-colored) urine. Patients with cholestatic DILI may also have pruritus. Fever and rash, hallmarks of hypersensitivity, may be present with DILI caused by certain drugs such as anticonvulsants and sulfamethoxazole-trimethoprim. Cholestatic or mixed hepatitis related to amoxicillin-clavulanic acid (Augmentin) may develop shortly after the drug has been stopped, usually within 2 to 3 weeks. Nitrofurantoin (Macrobid) characteristically causes a chronic hepatitis after many weeks, months, or even years of therapy and is often associated with the presence of serum antinuclear antibodies (ANA).

Diagnosis

The diagnosis of DILI is challenging because of the lack of specific or uniform clinical features or laboratory tests in the majority of cases. A high level of suspicion for DILI is essential for diagnosis, as is the exclusion of other possible causes of liver injury. Generally, DILI occurs within the first 3 months of initiation of a medication but can occur after longer periods. The Russel-Uclaf Causality Assessment Method (RUCAM) provides objective and consistent assessment but can be cumbersome for routine clinical use. Moreover, a study conducted by Grant and Rockey suggested that expert opinion outperforms RUCAM in making a diagnosis of DILI. There is definitely a need for a simple, accurate, and reproducible method for diagnosing DILI.

Hepatitis E appears to be a small but important alternative diagnosis for suspected DILI. Of 318 patients in the multicenter U.S. Drug-Induced Liver Injury Network (DILIN) with suspected drug hepatotoxicity, 9 (3%) were found to be positive for HEV IgM.

Treatment

The mainstay of management of DILI is withdrawal of the offending agent and supportive care, which is usually sufficient in cases of mild to moderate DILI. Rechallenge of the implicated drug should be avoided. Specific therapies are available for some types of DILI. Timely administration of N-acetylcysteine (NAC) for acetaminophen overdose can be lifesaving. NAC may also improve outcomes of patients with early acute liver failure from etiologies other than acetaminophen. Corticosteroids are probably ineffective for DILI from most drugs; however, a short course of steroids is sometimes used for treatment of immune-mediated DILI with the manifestations of rash, fever, and eosinophilia. Ursodeoxycholic acid is safe and may possibly hasten the resolution of jaundice and pruritus.

Complication and Prognosis

With supportive care and discontinuation of the offending drug, mild to moderate DILI usually resolves rapidly. Cholestatic liver injury may take many weeks and even months to completely resolve. Occasionally, cholestatic DILI can progress to permanent bile duct injury with so-called vanishing bile duct syndrome. Patients may develop progressive liver injury or develop acute liver failure manifesting with encephalopathy and coagulopathy, and may need liver transplantation.

CHRONIC HEPATITIS

Chronic hepatitis is defined as a sustained inflammatory process in the liver lasting longer than 6 months. On initial presentation, chronic hepatitis can be difficult to differentiate from acute hepatitis on clinical or histologic criteria alone. Except for hepatitis A, acute viral hepatitis, especially that caused by HBV or HCV, can ultimately lead to chronic hepatitis. Nonalcoholic steatohepatitis (NASH) is now the most frequent cause of chronic hepatitis in the United States and Western Europe. Several drugs can cause chronic hepatitis including methyldopa, isoniazid, minocycline, propylthiouracil, and hydralazine. In contrast to acute hepatitis, an etiologic agent is sometimes difficult to identify in cases of chronic hepatitis. The pathogenesis of these idiopathic forms may represent quiescent autoimmune disease, undetected past DILI or NASH, antibody-negative viral infection, or misdiagnosed cholestatic liver injury (e.g., primary biliary cirrhosis [PBC], primary sclerosing cholangitis [PSC]).

Chronic Viral Hepatitis

In Western countries, acute HBV infection usually occurs in adults; 5% to 10% of patients fail to clear the virus and develop chronic hepatitis. In other areas, vertical transmission and childhood acquisition is common. Children who are infected within 2 years of birth have a much higher rate of chronic hepatitis B. HBV infection without evidence of any liver damage may persist, resulting in asymptomatic hepatitis B carriers. In Asia and Africa, many such carriers appear to have acquired the virus from infected mothers during infancy (vertical transmission).

Patients who are HBsAg and HBeAg positive and have high blood HBV DNA (>20,000 IU/mL), coupled with elevated serum aminotransferases, are in a high replicative phase (see Table 42.3). In contrast, patients in a low replicative phase are HBsAg and anti-HBe positive, have low blood HBV DNA (<20,000 IU/mL), and have near-normal or normal aminotransferase levels. These patients likely have HBV with precore and/or core promoter mutation. Patients infected with HBV in a high replicative phase are at high risk for cirrhosis and hepatocellular carcinoma. Such patients, and those who have already progressed to early cirrhosis, are the primary candidates for antiviral therapy.

Currently, eight drugs are approved for the treatment of adults with chronic hepatitis B in the United States, including interferon-α and its pegylated form and six nucleos(t)ide analogues (lamivudine, telbivudine, adefovir dipivoxil, tenofovir disoproxil, entecavir, and tenofovir alafenamide). The primary aim of therapy is to eliminate or permanently suppress HBV and thus reduce the activity of hepatitis and slow or limit the progression of liver disease. It is important to start therapy with a nucleos(t)ide analogue that has a high genetic barrier to resistance, such as entecavir or tenofovir, as first-line therapy. Long-term follow-up studies have shown interferon-based therapy increases HBsAg seroclearance over time. HBsAg seroclearance is less common in patients who are treated with nucleos(t)ide analogues rather than interferon-based therapy. All patients with chronic HBV are at risk for hepatocellular carcinoma and should undergo screening based on age, sex, and ethnicity. The risk of hepatocellular carcinoma decreases with decreasing viral load.

In patients with HBV and HDV coinfection, the fate of HDV is determined by the host response to HBV, which in more than 95% of adults results in viral clearance. By contrast, HDV superinfection of an individual with chronic hepatitis B usually results in chronic HDV infection. Treatment with nucleos(t)ide analogues is not effective in reducing HDV replication. The accepted practice for treatment of chronic HDV infection is weekly pegylated interferon for at least 48 weeks. In patients with a high concentration of HBV DNA, the addition of a potent nucleos(t)ide analogue to inhibit HBV replication is logical, but long-term effectiveness has yet to be defined.

Chronic hepatitis C develops in up to 75% of individuals who are acutely exposed to HCV (Fig. 42.5). Approximately 1.6% of the United States population (4.1 million people) are positive for antibodies to HCV (anti-HCV), and 2.4 million of them have chronic infection. Up

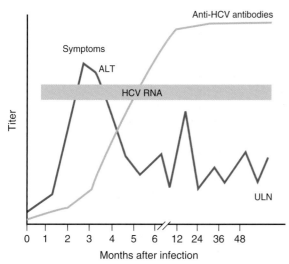

Fig. 42.5 Kinetics of hepatitis C virus (HCV) markers during acute hepatitis C that evolves toward chronic infection. *ALT,* Alanine aminotransferase; *ULN,* upper limit of normal.

to 20% of HCV cases progress to cirrhosis, usually within 20 to 30 years after infection. HCV has six major genotypes, of which genotype 1 is the most common in the United States, followed by genotypes 2 and 3. The genotype helps determine the treatment regimen and duration of therapy. The goal of antiviral therapy is to achieve a sustained virologic response (SVR12) or cure, defined as an undetectable HCV RNA level 12 weeks after treatment discontinuation. The current medications for hepatitis C are very effective and achieve cure in 98% to 99% of treatment naïve patients. These newer second-generation direct-acting antivirals target HCV replication, and have dramatically increased cure rates, shortened treatment duration, and minimized side effects. These medications work via novel mechanisms of action that target HCV enzymes needed for replication such as NS5B polymerase, NS3/4 protease, and the HCV protein NS5A. Pegylated interferon-α and ribavirin are now historical medications for treatment of chronic hepatitis C, where patients were treated for 24 or 48 weeks with SVR rates of 50% and a high incidence of side effects.

Among organ transplant recipients, the consumption of game meat, pork products, or mussels may result in HEV infection, which is most commonly asymptomatic without jaundice. About 60% of such infections become chronic, and up to 10% of patients progress to cirrhosis. Treatment includes careful reduction in immunosuppression, which results in viral clearance in 30% of patients on ribavirin monotherapy.

Autoimmune Hepatitis

Autoimmune hepatitis (AIH) has several clinical forms that share typical histologic findings including significant hepatic inflammation with a preponderance of plasma cells and fibrosis. Type 1, or classic, AIH is characterized by the presence of hypergammaglobulinemia, as well as the autoantibodies ANA or anti–smooth muscle antibodies (ASMA) in up to 80% of cases. Type 2 AIH is characterized by the presence of anti–liver/kidney microsomal antibodies (anti-LKM1) and the absence of ANA and ASMA. The type 1 variant can affect people of any age or gender, whereas the less common type 2 variant primarily affects girls and young women. A third type of AIH with antibodies to soluble liver antigen or liver-pancreas antigen (anti-SLA/LP) is no longer considered a unique entity because these antibodies may be found in type 1 and 2 variants as well. There are also uncommon overlap variants of AIH that have features of both AIH and other liver diseases such as PBC or PSC.

There are no pathognomonic features of AIH, and the diagnosis is made by a combination of factors. A simplified diagnostic algorithm that includes the presence of autoantibodies, hypergammaglobulinemia, typical liver histology, and absence of viral hepatitis has proved useful in identifying patients with AIH. Extrahepatic manifestations such as amenorrhea, rashes, acne, vasculitis, thyroiditis, and Sjögren's syndrome are common. Evidence of hepatic failure and the presence of chronic disease on liver biopsy are often discernable at the time of diagnosis. Indications for treatment include abnormal liver function tests and significant hepatic inflammation on biopsy.

Corticosteroids are the mainstay of treatment, typically in combination with azathioprine as a steroid-sparing agent. This regimen is efficacious in most patients (>80%) and in many instances prolongs survival.

Nonalcoholic Fatty Liver Disease

Nonalcoholic fatty liver disease (NAFLD) has a spectrum of presentations from simple steatosis, which usually does not progress to advanced liver disease, to NASH, which may exhibit or lead to cirrhosis. It is the most common cause of abnormal liver function tests among adults in the United States and Western Europe. NAFLD is commonly seen in people with central obesity, hypertension, diabetes, and hyperlipidemia, although it can be observed in persons with normal weight as well. Insulin resistance plays a central role in the pathophysiology of NAFLD. Estimates indicate that about 80 to 100 million Americans have NAFLD; of these, 18 million have NASH and almost 20% have signs of advanced disease (i.e., bridging fibrosis, cirrhosis) on histologic examination.

Liver biopsy is the "gold standard" for diagnosis of NASH. The NAFLD Activity Score has been developed and represents the sum of scores for steatosis, lobular inflammation, and hepatocyte ballooning that are typically seen on liver biopsy. It ranges from 0 to 8, with a score of 5 or higher considered diagnostic of NASH. Liver biopsy is invasive, costly, and can cause complications including a small mortality risk (0.01% to 0.1%). The use of liver biopsy has declined with newer noninvasive assessments of liver fibrosis and steatosis. Liver biopsy predominantly is used when there is diagnostic uncertainty to the etiology of disease. Radiologic imaging studies based on ultrasound and MRI can determine fibrosis by measuring liver stiffness with transient elastography technology and can also estimate the degree of steatosis.

Currently, this is no FDA-approved treatment available for NASH. Clinical trials of agents that therapeutically target the development of hepatic steatosis and fibrosis are underway and have shown beneficial effects on hepatic fibrosis. However, weight reduction with a goal of 5% to 7% of body weight loss and regular exercise are associated with biochemical and histologic improvement and are important components of therapy. Vitamin E and pioglitazone have been shown to improve hepatic inflammation in nondiabetic patients with NASH, but they are not routinely recommended because of questions regarding long-term safety and side effects.

Genetic and Metabolic Hepatitis

Hemochromatosis is an autosomal recessive genetic disorder that causes low levels of the iron regulatory hormone hepcidin causing defective sensing of iron stores and leads to excessive absorption of iron from the digestive tract. In the United States, about 1 of every 250 Caucasians have the condition; however, clinical expression is variable. Elevated ferritin and transferrin saturation values are typically used to screen patients with evidence of chronic liver disease and guide the need for further genetic testing. Most patients with hemochromatosis are homozygous for the C282Y mutation in the *HFE* gene, and a subset of individuals who are heterozygous for both C282Y and the H63D mutation may also develop iron overload. Iron overload is very uncommon among those who are homozygous for the H63D mutation. Genetic mutations in a number of other proteins involved in iron sensing have also been associated with iron overload but are not routinely tested in clinical practice.

Hemochromatosis is a systemic disease that causes iron deposition in parenchymal cells in various organs including the liver, heart, pancreas, and pituitary glands. Patients may develop liver cirrhosis and cancer, heart failure, diabetes mellitus, hypogonadism, and arthralgias. A high index of suspicion is required to detect the disorder in early stages. The standard treatment for hemochromatosis is therapeutic phlebotomy. For patients who cannot undergo phlebotomy, chelation therapy may be offered.

Wilson's disease is an autosomal recessive genetic disorder that results from mutations in the *ATP7B* gene located on chromosome 13. These mutations result in excessive accumulation of copper in a number of organs, most notably the liver, cornea, and brain. The prevalence of the disease is approximately 1 in 30,000 live births in most populations. Wilson's disease can occur at any age. Measurement of the 24-hour urine copper excretion, slit lamp examination of corneas for Kayser-Fleischer rings, and direct measurement of hepatic copper confirm the diagnosis. Patients should receive lifelong chelation treatment with either penicillamine or trientine. Zinc may be used to maintain stable copper levels in the body.

α_1-*Antitrypsin deficiency* (AAT) is an autosomal recessive genetic disorder of chromosome 14 that causes retention of AAT in the liver, resulting in liver damage. AAT is a protease inhibitor of the proteolytic enzyme elastase. The normal gene product is designated as PiM, and the deficiency variants are PiS (50% to 60%) and PiZ (10% to 20%). The most common carrier phenotypes are PiMS and PiMZ, and the disease phenotypes are PiZZ, PiSS, and PiSZ. Low serum AAT and diastase-positive staining of hepatocellular AAT inclusions on liver biopsy support the diagnosis. Phenotypic testing in the serum has been the traditional gold standard for the diagnosis. However, genotypic testing is now available and widely used. Lung disease results from a loss of protective effects in patients with low levels of circulating AAT. AAT replacement therapy is an option for those with lung disease but is not useful for patients with liver disease.

For a deeper discussion on this topic, please see Chapters 139, "Acute Viral Hepatitis," and 140, "Chronic Viral and Autoimmune Hepatitis," in *Goldman-Cecil Medicine*, 26th Edition.

SUGGESTED READINGS

Asselah T, Marcellin P: Interferon free therapy with direct acting antivirals for HCV, Liver Int 33(Suppl 1):93–104, 2013.

Feldman M, Friedman LS, Brandt LJ: Sleisenger and Fordtran's gastrointestinal and liver disease-2 Volume Set,ed 10, 2015, Chapters 78-82.

Grant LM, Rockey DC: Drug-induced liver injury, Curr Opin Gastrointesterol 28:198–202, 2012.

Hughes SA, Wedemeyer H, Harrison PM: Hepatitis delta virus, Lancet 378:73–85, 2011.

Jeong SH, Lee HS: Hepatitis A: clinical manifestations and management, Intervirology 53:15–19, 2010.

Kamar N, Bendall R, Legrand-Abravanel F, et al: Hepatitis E, Lancet 379:2477-2488, 2012.

Liaw YF: Impact of therapy on the outcome of chronic hepatitis B, Liver Int 33(Suppl 1):111–115, 2013.

43

Acute Liver Failure

Anil Seetharam, Michael B. Fallon

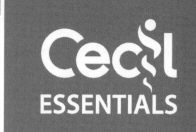

DEFINITIONS

Acute liver failure (ALF) is an infrequent condition characterized by rapid deterioration of liver function resulting in altered mentation and coagulopathy in individuals without preexisting liver disease. A widely accepted working definition includes International Normalized Ratio (INR) greater than 1.5 and any degree of altered mentation (encephalopathy) in a subject without preexisting cirrhosis and illness of less than 26 weeks' duration. Associated multisystem organ dysfunction and encephalopathy with chance for brainstem herniation mandate prompt recognition and transfer to an intensive care unit (ICU). Though etiologic specific treatment and supportive measures can be employed, liver transplantation remains the only chance for cure in those who do not spontaneously recover.

PATHOGENESIS

ALF develops as a result of severe, unrelenting inflammation with hepatocyte necrosis and collapse of the liver's architectural framework. This feature contrasts with the changes of cirrhosis and complications of portal hypertension that dominate chronic liver disease (see Chapter 44). ALF may result from infection with hepatotropic viruses A, B, C, D, or E (see Chapter 42) or from herpes simplex virus (HSV). Additionally, dose-dependent or idiosyncratic exposure to hepatotoxins such as acetaminophen, isoniazid, halothane, valproic acid, or mushroom toxins (*Amanita phalloides*) can produce ALF. Reye's syndrome, a disease that predominantly affects children, and acute fatty liver of pregnancy often resemble ALF; and are characterized by microvesicular fatty infiltration and little hepatocellular necrosis. Rare causes of ALF include: Wilson's disease, hepatic ischemia, autoimmune hepatitis, and malignancy (E-Figs. 43.1 and 43.2).

CLINICAL PRESENTATION

The clinical presentation includes progressive jaundice and hepatic encephalopathy without clinical evidence of underlying chronic liver disease. Other common but nonspecific symptoms include nausea, vomiting, loss of appetite, right upper abdominal pain from hepatomegaly, fever, fatigue, dark urine, and clay-colored stools. Typically, the features of impaired hepatic synthetic and metabolic function predominate, with portal hypertension much less common compared to patients with established cirrhosis.

DIAGNOSIS

The clinical presentation of ALF can be dramatic, with jaundice and advanced systemic manifestations as the first indication of a severe and potentially life-threatening illness. A thorough medical history is essential and focused on potential exposure to viruses and hepatotoxins, pregnancy, an event associated with hypotension, and clues to suggest autoimmune causes.

Early laboratory testing should focus on assessing the severity of hepatic dysfunction and on detection of possible acetaminophen exposure, for which specific antidote treatment must be promptly initiated. Further specialized laboratory testing is designed to identify specific viral causes—with tests for anti–hepatitis A immunoglobulin M (IgM), hepatitis B surface antigen (HBsAg), anti–hepatitis B core antigen (anti-HBc) IgM, hepatitis D antigen, anti–hepatitis C antibody and/or hepatitis C virus RNA, anti–hepatitis E IgM, anti-varicella IgM, and herpes simplex IgM—or other causes (e.g., ceruloplasmin level or autoimmune markers). Acute fatty liver of pregnancy may progress to ALF in the peripartum period; however, a pregnancy test should be performed in all females of childbearing age because viral illnesses (HSV, hepatitis E) may have a more severe course in pregnancy.

A negative serum acetaminophen level does not exclude acetaminophen overdose because the drug is rapidly cleared from the blood. Importantly, acetaminophen overdose accounts for approximately 50% of all cases of ALF and 20% of all cases of presumed indeterminant causes in Western countries. Small quantities of acetaminophen (or acetaminophen-containing compounds) may precipitate ALF in the context of consistent alcohol use due to constitutive activation (by ethanol) of cytochrome pathways creating toxic acetaminophen metabolites.

Imaging of the liver including ultrasound with Doppler may be utilized to assess liver architecture and blood flow into/out of the liver. Though not obligatory, a liver biopsy may be considered to assess for etiology; biopsy is often performed via the transjugular route secondary to coagulopathy and acuity of illness.

TREATMENT

Treatment of ALF is largely supportive, because specific treatment for the underlying cause of liver failure is often not available. However, many processes that result in widespread liver cell necrosis and ALF are transient events, and liver cell regeneration with recovery of liver function often occurs if patients survive the initial insult. Acetaminophen toxicity and hypotension causing hepatic necrosis are representative. In contrast, ALF resulting from viral hepatitis or idiosyncratic drug-induced liver injury (DILI) typically has a longer time course and an uncertain prognosis. In either case, meticulous supportive treatment in an intensive care unit setting has been shown to improve survival. Patients with ALF should be treated in centers with experience with this disease and with a liver transplantation program. Numerous systemic complications can result from ALF, and each must be thoroughly identified and treated (Table 43.1). As liver failure progresses,

TABLE 43.1	**Management of Selected Problems in Fulminant Hepatic Failure**	
Organ System	**Pathogenesis**	**Supportive Measures**
Hepatic encephalopathy	Diminished hepatocyte function	Identification of treatable causes (e.g., hypoglycemia, drugs used for sedation, sepsis, gastrointestinal bleeding, electrolyte imbalance, decreased Po_2, increased Pco_2)
		Lactulose and rifaximin
Cerebral edema	Systemic and local inflammation and circulating neurotoxins, including arterial ammonia	Elevate head of bed 20–30 degrees
		Hyperventilate (Pco_2 reduction)
		ICP monitor placement
		Mannitol
Renal	Prerenal kidney injury from diminished effective circulating volume, acute tubular necrosis, or functional leading to acid/base/electrolyte imbalance	Continuous renal replacement therapy
Cardiovascular	Low systemic vascular resistance	Intravenous resuscitation with normal saline and changed to half-normal saline containing 75 mEq/L sodium bicarbonate if acidotic
	Diminished central vascular tone compromises peripheral tissue oxygenation	Vasopressor support to maintain a mean arterial pressure of at least 75 mm Hg or a cerebral perfusion pressure of 60–80 mm Hg
Hematologic	Concomitant reduction in levels of both procoagulant and natural anticoagulant proteins, in conjunction with elevation of factor VIII (FVIII) and Von Willebrand factor, resulting in reduced thrombin generation capacity	Vitamin K 10 mg IV × 1
		Fresh-frozen plasma, platelets, and rFVIII generally reserved for active bleeding or need for invasive procedure
		Acid suppression to prevent luminal GI tract bleeding
Infectious	Immune dysfunction	Surveillance cultures of blood, urine, and tracheal aspirate when applicable
		Low threshold to initiate broad-spectrum antibiotic and antifungal therapy

a syndrome of multisystem organ failure can result; this can include encephalopathy, coagulopathy, infection, and renal failure.

Hepatic encephalopathy is often the first and most dramatic sign of liver failure. The precise pathogenesis of hepatic encephalopathy in ALF remains unclear and is likely multifactorial; however, it differs from that associated with chronic liver disease or portal hypertension in two important aspects. First, it often responds to therapy only when liver function improves, and second, it is frequently associated with hypoglycemia or cerebral edema, two other potentially treatable causes of coma. Therapy for hepatic encephalopathy in ALF differs slightly from the principles outlined in Chapter 44. Use of lactulose may be considered (orally or through a nasogastric tube) but should be discontinued if there is no significant improvement in mentation. Rifaximin, a nonabsorbable antibiotic, can be given as an adjunct orally or per tube. Intubation is often necessary to protect the airway from aspiration and to allow ventilation in patients with advanced encephalopathy.

Cerebral edema, the pathogenesis of which is unknown, is a leading cause of death in ALF. Differentiation between cerebral edema and hepatic encephalopathy can be difficult, and computed tomography of the head is often unreliable as observable architectural changes of edema may lag behind clinical progression. Measurement of intracranial pressure (ICP) can be considered, although it is associated with complications including bleeding. The goal is to maintain an ICP of less than 20 mm Hg while maintaining a cerebral perfusion pressure (calculated as mean arterial pressure minus ICP) greater than 60 mm Hg. Supportive measures to limit ICP elevation include: control of agitation, head elevation of 20 to 30 degrees, hyperventilation, systemic vasopressors to maintain mean arterial pressure, administration of mannitol, barbiturate-induced coma, and urgent liver transplantation.

As hepatic synthetic function deteriorates, *hypoglycemia* can occur as a result of impaired hepatic gluconeogenesis and insulin degradation. All patients at risk should receive 10% glucose IV infusions with frequent monitoring of blood glucose levels. Other metabolic abnormalities commonly occur, including hyponatremia, hypokalemia, respiratory alkalosis, and metabolic acidosis. Therefore, frequent

monitoring of blood electrolytes and pH is indicated. Renal replacement therapy may be employed to regulate acid/base/electrolyte balance, with continuous modes preferred over intermittent hemodialysis.

Bleeding occurs frequently and is commonly caused by gastric erosions in the setting of impaired synthesis of clotting factors and prolonged prothrombin times. All patients should receive vitamin K and prophylactic gastric acid suppression. Fresh-frozen plasma administration is reserved for when clinically significant bleeding occurs or if major procedures, including ICP monitoring and central line placement, are performed. Studies in ALF have found a concomitant and proportional reduction in plasma levels of both procoagulants and natural anticoagulant proteins, in conjunction with a significant elevation in plasma levels of factors-VIII (FVIII) and Von Willebrand factor, resulting in an overall efficient, albeit reduced, thrombin generation capacity in comparison with healthy controls. Global hemostasis as assessed with thromboelastography (TEG) may be normal by several compensatory mechanisms, even in patients with markedly elevated INR.

Up to 80% of patients with ALF develop infection at some point in their illness; both bacterial (≈80% of infections) and fungal (≈20% of infections) have been implicated. Patients are at higher risk for infection as a result of impaired immunity resulting from liver failure and the need for invasive monitoring. Severe infection may occur without fever or leukocytosis. Therefore, frequent cultures are recommended and warranted with abrupt changes in status, and there should be a low threshold for beginning antibiotic therapy.

Although often employed to guide evaluation, no single prognostic model discriminates those who will spontaneously recover and those who will require transplant. The United States Acute Liver Failure Group (ALFSG) prospectively enrolled over 1900 subjects with ALF managed with and without transplantation and aimed to develop a model for ALF to predict transplant-free survival at 21 days. Clinical demographics and laboratory parameters were collected at enrollment and recorded serially up to 1 week. Variables of prognostic value adopted in the predictive model included: admission coma grade, liver failure etiology and vasopressor requirement, as well as admission INR and bilirubin values. The model correctly predicted outcome in 66.3% of subjects, slightly outperforming historic King's College Criteria and the Model for End-stage Liver Disease (MELD) score.

Liver transplantation (see Chapter 44) has been performed with success in patients with ALF and is the treatment of choice for patients who appear unlikely to recover spontaneously. Because of high risk of abrupt clinical deterioration, the optimal approach is for potential candidates to be transferred to transplantation centers before significant complications develop (e.g., coma, cerebral edema, hemorrhage, infection). ALF subjects who meet transplant program criteria for listing in the United Sates are granted status 1A, placing them at the highest priority on the waiting list.

PROGNOSIS

Etiology of ALF and the degree of hepatic encephalopathy are key determinants of prognosis. Patients with ALF resulting from acetaminophen overdose or viral hepatitis A or B have a better survival rate than do patients with Wilson's disease or those with indeterminate etiology. The short-term survival rate for patients with ALF in coma is 20% without liver transplantation.

Currently, ALF accounts for approximately 8% of all liver transplants, as per data from the Scientific Registry of Transplant Recipients (SRTR) with 1-year survival rates of 84% in the United States. Patients who survive without transplantation also have an excellent prognosis because liver tissue usually regenerates normally regardless of the cause of ALF.

SUGGESTED READINGS

Bernal W, Wendon J: Acute liver failure, N Engl J Med 369(26): 2525–3, 2013.

Koch DG, Tillman H, Durkalski V, Lee WM, Reuben A: Development of a model to predict transplant-free survival of patients with acute liver failure, Clin Gastroenterol Hepatol 14(8):1199–1206, 2016.

Lee WM, Larson AM, Stravitz RT: AASLD position paper: the management of acute liver failure—update 2011. Available at: http://www.aasld.org/practiceguidelines/Documents/AcuteLiverFailureUpdate2011.pdf.

44

Cecil ESSENTIALS

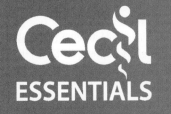

Cirrhosis of the Liver and Its Complications

Shivang Mehta, Michael B. Fallon

LIVER CIRRHOSIS

Definition

Cirrhosis is a slowly progressive disease that is characterized by formation in the liver of fibrous and scar tissue that eventually replaces normal hepatocytes and impairs portal blood flow. Fibrosis can be a self-perpetuating result of many initial processes, including infectious, inflammatory, toxic, metabolic, genetic, and vascular insults that lead to liver damage. Most of the clinical features of cirrhosis develop as a result of portal hypertension, hepatocellular dysfunction, or altered cellular differentiation.

Etiology

Alcoholic liver disease, nonalcoholic steatohepatitis (NASH), and hepatitis C virus infection are the most common causes of cirrhosis in industrialized nations; hepatitis B virus is the major cause in Asia and in most of Africa. There are many other significant causes of cirrhosis, including biliary cirrhosis (primary and secondary), autoimmune hepatitis, inherited diseases (e.g., α_1-antitrypsin deficiency), and drug-induced injury, that require specific evaluation. However, a significant number of patients with cirrhosis at presentation have no readily identifiable cause. These cases are referred to as idiopathic or cryptogenic in origin, and it remains a diagnosis of exclusion. Common and uncommon conditions that may lead to cirrhosis are listed in Table 44.1. Chronic active hepatitis, nonalcoholic fatty liver disease (NAFLD)/NASH, and α_1-antitrypsin deficiency are discussed in Chapter 42.

Pathology

The typical sequence of events that leads to development of cirrhosis involves significant hepatocyte injury followed by ineffective repair that results in hepatic fibrosis. The injury can be acute or chronic in nature, depending on the mechanism. The fibrotic response to injury leads to development of nodules surrounded by fibrous tissue that consist of foci of regenerating hepatocytes, formation of fibrovascular membranes, rearrangement of blood vessels, and finally cirrhosis. This disruption of the normal hepatic lobular architecture distorts the vascular bed and contributes to development of portal hypertension and intrahepatic shunting. On gross morphology, cirrhosis can be referred to as macronodular (>3 mm regenerating nodules), commonly seen as a result of chronic active hepatitis, or micronodular (<3 mm regenerating nodules) a typical feature of alcoholic cirrhosis or cirrhosis of mixed origin.

Clinical Presentation

Symptoms of liver cirrhosis are often nonspecific in the early stages and include fatigue, malaise, weakness, weight change, anorexia, and nausea. With progression of portal hypertension or loss of hepatocytes, increased abdominal girth, sexual dysfunction, altered mental status, and gastrointestinal bleeding may be noted. Physical findings depend on the stage at presentation. Table 44.2 highlights the pathogenic mechanisms underlying these diverse signs and symptoms.

Diagnosis

Owing to significant reserves of liver function, patients with cirrhosis are often asymptomatic and the diagnosis is established incidentally at the time of physical examination or laboratory testing. Alternatively, patients abruptly experience specific life-threatening complications of cirrhosis, most notably variceal bleeding, ascites, spontaneous bacterial peritonitis, and hepatic encephalopathy (HE). If cirrhosis is suspected on clinical grounds, the diagnosis can be made reliably by a combination of clinical, laboratory, and radiologic findings in most cases. Although liver biopsy is still considered the "gold standard" for accurate diagnosis, new noninvasive modalities to estimate fibrosis have come to the forefront. The predominant modalities utilized to assess fibrosis non-invasively are FibroSure, FibroScan (ultrasound with shear wave elastography), and magnetic resonance elastography (MRE). With these advances, biopsy is now done more often to assess the stage and severity of disease, assign prognosis, and monitor the response to treatment.

Laboratory Findings

Hepatocellular dysfunction leads to impaired protein synthesis (hypoalbuminemia), hyperbilirubinemia, low levels of blood urea nitrogen (BUN), and elevated serum ammonia levels. Portal hypertension causes hypersplenism, which results in anemia, thrombocytopenia, and leukopenia. Patients with ascites often develop dilutional hyponatremia as a result of avid renal retention of sodium (Na^+) and water. The liver enzymes alanine aminotransferase (ALT) and aspartate aminotransferase (AST) are good markers of active hepatocyte necrosis, whereas elevations of alkaline phosphatase and bilirubin out of proportion to ALT and AST suggest intrahepatic or extrahepatic biliary obstruction. FibroSure is a laboratory test that consists of a panel comprising total bilirubin, GGT, α2-macroglobulin, haptoglobin, and apolipoprotein A1 corrected for age and sex to provide a surrogate for advanced fibrosis validated in populations with hepatitis B and C.

Radiology

Various radiologic modalities including ultrasound (with and without Doppler imaging of the portal and hepatic venous vasculature), computed tomography, and magnetic resonance imaging have complementary profiles in the evaluation of suspected cirrhosis. Findings supportive of the diagnosis of cirrhosis include relative enlargement of the left hepatic and caudate lobes as a result of right lobe atrophy, surface nodularity, and features of portal hypertension such as ascites, intra-abdominal varices, and splenomegaly.

TABLE 44.1 Common Causes of Cirrhosis

Alcohol abuse
Nonalcoholic steatohepatitis
Viral hepatitis (chronic hepatitis B, C, and D)
Cardiac cirrhosis
Chronic right-sided heart failure
Constrictive pericarditis
Drug-induced liver injury (DILI)
Autoimmune hepatitis
Primary biliary cirrhosis
Hemochromatosis (primary and secondary)
Wilson's disease
α_1-Antitrypsin deficiency

TABLE 44.2 Clinical Features and Pathogenesis of Cirrhosis

Signs and Symptoms	Pathogenesis
Constitutional	
Fatigue, anorexia, malaise, weakness, weight loss	Liver synthetic or metabolic dysfunction
Cutaneous	
Spider angiomas, palmar erythema	Altered estrogen and androgen metabolism
Jaundice	Decreased bilirubin excretion
Caput medusae	Portosystemic shunting due to portal hypertension
Endocrine	
Gynecomastia, testicular atrophy, decreased body hair in men	Altered estrogen and androgen metabolism
Decreased libido, virilization, and menstrual irregularities in women	
Gastrointestinal	
Abdominal pain	Hepatomegaly, hepatocellular carcinoma
Abdominal swelling	Ascites due to portal hypertension
Gastrointestinal bleeding	Variceal hemorrhage due to portal hypertension
Hematologic	
Anemia, leukopenia, thrombocytopenia	Hypersplenism secondary to portal hypertension
Ecchymosis	Decreased synthesis of coagulation factors
Neurologic	
Altered sleep pattern, somnolence, confusion, asterixis	Hepatocellular dysfunction: inability to metabolize ammonia to urea

Transient elastography (FibroScan) is a newer noninvasive modality that provides an indirect measure of liver fibrosis and cirrhosis by calculating liver stiffness. Abnormal liver stiffness suggests underlying fibrosis; in the presence of clinical and laboratory features of cirrhosis, this finding may obviate the need for diagnostic liver biopsy in some patients. Other modalities include ultrasound with shear wave velocity (50 Hz), which uses velocity within the liver to determine stiffness. MRE is an addition to imaging provided by MR that incorporates acoustic vibrations across the entire liver to determine liver stiffness. It is currently the most accurate noninvasive modality but is limited by availability and cost. Biopsy is more invasive and is usually reserved for situations in which the results of noninvasive studies are indeterminate or the cause of the liver disease is in doubt.

COMPLICATIONS OF CIRRHOSIS

The major sequelae of cirrhosis are illustrated diagrammatically in Fig. 44.1 and can be categorized broadly into features of hepatocellular dysfunction and portal hypertension. The pathophysiologic interrelationships among these complications are described in the following sections.

Hepatocellular Dysfunction

The loss of hepatocyte mass that occurs in cirrhosis results in impaired synthesis of many important proteins, which in turn leads to hypoalbuminemia, deficient production of vitamin K–dependent coagulation factors, and diminished capacity for hepatic detoxification (see Chapters 40 to 43 for details). In addition, there is a decline in the capacity for conjugation and excretion of bilirubin.

Portal Hypertension

Under normal circumstances, the portal circulation is a low-pressure system with only small changes in pressure as blood flows from the portal vein, through the liver, and into the inferior vena cava. The hepatic venous pressure gradient (HVPG), which reflects sinusoidal pressure, is the gradient between the wedged hepatic venous pressure and the free hepatic venous pressure measured by direct catheterization. Normal HVPG values range between 3 and 5 mm Hg. In cirrhosis, the distortion of hepatic architecture by fibrous tissue and regenerative nodules, along with an increased intrahepatic vascular tone, leads to increased resistance to portal venous flow and resultant portal hypertension. Portal hypertension is defined as an HPVG greater than 5 mm Hg, and clinically significant complications typically develop at values greater than 10 mm Hg.

Although cirrhosis is the most important cause of portal hypertension, any process that increases resistance to portal blood flow through the presinusoidal, sinusoidal, or hepatic venous outflow tracts may result in portal hypertension (Table 44.3). In addition, cirrhosis is associated with increased cardiac output, which leads to greater splanchnic blood flow, further aggravating portal hypertension. It is important to recognize that the HVPG is reliably increased only in sinusoidal portal hypertension.

With sustained portal hypertension, portosystemic collaterals are formed that have the benefit of decreasing portal pressures at the expense of bypassing the liver. Major sites of collateral formation include the gastroesophageal junction, retroperitoneum, rectum, and falciform ligament of liver (abdominal and periumbilical collaterals). Clinically, the most important collaterals are those connecting the portal to the azygos vein through the dilated and tortuous vessels (varices) in the submucosa of the gastric fundus and esophagus.

VARICEAL HEMORRHAGE
Definition and Pathology

Varices are abnormally large veins that are most commonly recognized near the gastroesophageal junction or the stomach wall. Gastroesophageal varices usually develop when the portal pressure

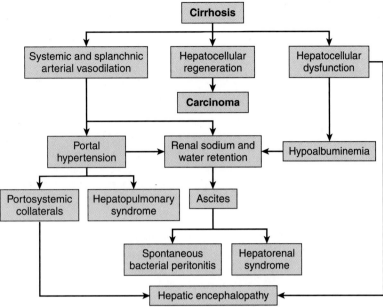

Fig. 44.1 Interrelationships among the complications of cirrhosis.

TABLE 44.3 Causes of Portal Hypertension

Increased Resistance to Flow

Presinusoidal

Extrahepatic
  Portal or splenic vein occlusion
Intrahepatic
  Schistosomiasis
  Congenital hepatic fibrosis
  Sarcoidosis

Sinusoidal

Cirrhosis (many causes)
Alcoholic hepatitis

Postsinusoidal

Extrahepatic
  Budd-Chiari syndrome
  Cardiac causes: constrictive pericarditis
Intrahepatic
  Veno-occlusive disease

Increased Portal Blood Flow

Splenomegaly not caused by liver disease
Arterioportal fistula

gradient (HVPG) exceeds 10 mm Hg, and the risk for variceal rupture increases when the gradient is higher than 12 mm Hg. Bleeding occurs most commonly from large varices in the esophagus when high tension in the walls of these vessels leads to rupture. Among gastric varices, fundal varices have the highest rate of bleeding and may bleed with portal pressure gradients of less than 12 mm Hg.

Clinical Presentation

Variceal bleeding usually manifests as painless hematemesis, melena, or hematochezia, which typically leads to hemodynamic compromise due to higher portal pressures. Bleeding is further aggravated by impaired hepatic synthesis of coagulation factors and thrombocytopenia from hypersplenism.

Treatment

The management of gastroesophageal varices includes prevention of initial bleeding (primary prophylaxis), treatment of acute variceal hemorrhage, and prevention of rebleeding (secondary prophylaxis) (Fig. 44.2). If varices are large, primary prophylaxis is commonly undertaken with nonselective β-adrenergic receptor blocking (NSBB) agents such as propranolol and nadolol. Surveillance for varices using esophagogastroduodenoscopy (EGD) is advocated only if endoscopic band ligation (EBL) is the initial treatment modality. EGD is recommended every 2 to 8 weeks until obliteration of varices, then in 3 to 6 months, after which surveillance can be done every 6 to 12 months. Periodic EBL is also effective if the patient has contraindications or intolerance to β-blockers. Isosorbide mononitrate therapy should not be used for prophylaxis because it has been shown to increase adverse events. EBL and NSBB should not be used in combination to prevent first variceal bleed.

When varices are present, 5% to 15% of patients experience an initial episode of bleeding annually, and this episode carries a significant mortality risk of 7% to 15% at 6 weeks. Management includes stabilization (airway, breathing, and circulation) and blood transfusions to maintain a hemoglobin level of 7 to 8 g/dL. Combined pharmacologic and endoscopic therapy is the current standard for control of bleeding and is superior to either therapy alone. Prophylactic intravenous antibiotics should be administered early because they reduce the risk for infection, rebleeding, and death.

Current pharmacologic therapy consists of octreotide, a somatostatin analogue, which is widely used because of a good safety profile. This agent is best instituted before endoscopic examination. Endoscopic therapy includes EBL or sclerotherapy or both. EBL is the preferred modality given the lower incidence of adverse effects and complications. In patients with gastric variceal hemorrhage, endoscopic variceal ablation with cyanoacrylate glue is superior to EBL, although this therapy is not approved in the United States. Balloon tamponade (Sengstaken-Blakemore tube, Linton tube, or Minnesota tube) or esophageal stenting have been used as temporary measures reserved only for cases in which endoscopic therapy has failed in the setting of massive hemorrhage. A recent meta-analysis in limited studies for esophageal stenting versus

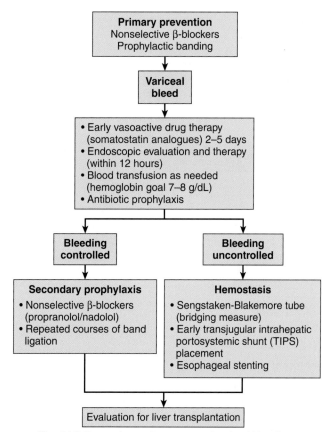

Fig. 44.2 Prevention and treatment of variceal bleeding.

TABLE 44.4	Classification of Ascites	
SAAG High (>1.1 g/dL)	**SAAG Low (<1.1 g/dL)**
Cirrhosis	Peritoneal carcinomatosis
Alcoholic hepatitis	Peritoneal tuberculosis
Chronic hepatic congestion	Pancreatic and biliary disease
Right ventricular heart failure	Nephrotic syndrome
Budd-Chiari syndrome	
Constrictive pericarditis	
Massive liver metastases	
Myxedema	
Mixed ascites	

SAAG, Serum-ascites albumin gradient.

balloon tamponade revealed esophageal stenting to have improvement in bleeding control despite issues with stent migration. Also, there is evidence that early (within 72 hours of admission) placement of a transjugular intrahepatic portosystemic shunt (TIPS) in a subset of patients with advanced liver disease improves survival after bleeding. The most common side effect of the TIPS is postprocedural encephalopathy.

Recommendations for secondary prophylaxis to prevent rebleeding include a combination of nonselective β-blockers (propranolol and nadolol) and variceal obliteration through repeated courses of EBL. In patients who undergo TIPS, the patency must be assessed using Doppler ultrasound on a regular basis.

Prognosis

Overall, the frequency and mortality rates from variceal bleeding appear to be decreasing in the United States over the past 2 decades. However, variceal hemorrhage is life-threatening, and after an initial episode the risk of rebleeding approaches 60% with a mortality rate of approximately 33% if secondary prophylaxis is not instituted.

ASCITES

Definition and Pathology

Ascites represents the accumulation of excess fluid in the peritoneal cavity. Although cirrhosis is the most common cause of ascites, there are also other important causes (Table 44.4). The precise sequence of events leading to the development of cirrhotic ascites remains debated.

Diagnosis

Physical examination is relatively insensitive for detection of small volumes of ascites, but bulging flanks, shifting dullness, and evidence of portal hypertension (e.g., distended veins over the abdominal wall

and caput medusae) become evident with increasing amounts of fluid. Abdominal ultrasound is both sensitive and specific and is widely used in screening. When fluid is present, abdominal paracentesis is the quickest and most direct approach for confirmation of the presence of fluid in the abdominal cavity and initial characterization of the cause. In addition to standard measures such as cell count, the serum-ascites albumin gradient (SAAG), which is proportional to the sinusoidal portal pressure, is calculated as follows:

$$SAAG = (Serum\ albumin\ concentration) \\ - (Ascitic\ fluid\ albumin\ concentration)$$

An elevated SAAG (>1.1 g/dL) correlates well with portal hypertension as the likely cause of fluid accumulation (see Table 44.4).

Clinical Presentation

Patients usually report increasing abdominal girth, fullness of the flanks, and weight gain with or without peripheral edema. Ascites becomes clinically detectable with fluid accumulation greater than about 500 mL. Shifting dullness to percussion is the most sensitive clinical sign of ascites, but about 1500 mL of fluid must be present for reliable detection.

Treatment

Management of cirrhotic ascites depends on the cause. Patients with high SAAG (>1.1 g/mL), which is used as a surrogate measure for elevated portal pressures, usually respond to salt restriction (<2 g/day) and diuretics to stimulate renal Na^+ loss. The administration of spironolactone, an aldosterone antagonist, supplemented with a loop diuretic (e.g., furosemide), is effective in about 90% of patients. Diuresis should be monitored closely because aggressive diuretic therapy may result in electrolyte disturbances (e.g., hyponatremia, hypokalemia) and hypovolemia, leading to impaired renal function and potentially precipitating HE. Water restriction is implemented when the serum sodium concentration is less than 120 to 125 mEq/L.

Prognosis

Refractory ascites occurs in up to 10% of patients with cirrhosis and is defined as the persistence of tense ascites despite maximal diuretic therapy (spironolactone, 400 mg/day, and furosemide, 160 mg/day) or the development of azotemia or electrolyte disturbances at submaximal doses of diuretics. Treatment includes repeated large-volume paracentesis and colloid volume expansion with albumin (6 to 8 g/L of fluid removed), TIPS placement in appropriate candidates, and eventually liver transplantation (Fig. 44.3). Peritoneovenous shunts are rarely used and are reserved for patients who are not candidates for paracentesis, TIPS, or transplantation.

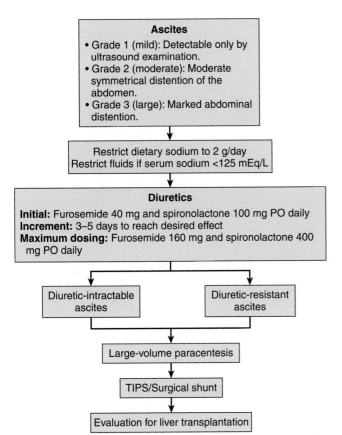

Ascites
- Grade 1 (mild): Detectable only by ultrasound examination.
- Grade 2 (moderate): Moderate symmetrical distention of the abdomen.
- Grade 3 (large): Marked abdominal distention.

↓

Restrict dietary sodium to 2 g/day
Restrict fluids if serum sodium <125 mEq/L

↓

Diuretics
Initial: Furosemide 40 mg and spironolactone 100 mg PO daily
Increment: 3–5 days to reach desired effect
Maximum dosing: Furosemide 160 mg and spironolactone 400 mg PO daily

↓

Diuretic-intractable ascites | Diuretic-resistant ascites

↓

Large-volume paracentesis

↓

TIPS/Surgical shunt

↓

Evaluation for liver transplantation

Fig. 44.3 Management of ascites in cirrhosis. *TIPS,* Transjugular intrahepatic portosystemic shunt.

SPONTANEOUS BACTERIAL PERITONITIS

Definition and Pathology

Cirrhotic patients may develop infection of ascitic fluid in the absence of an obvious source of contamination or surgically treatable source, a condition known as acute spontaneous bacterial peritonitis (SBP). The exact mechanism of contamination of the ascitic fluid is unclear. Factors such as bacterial overgrowth, altered motility, and increased intestinal permeability causing transient translocation of bacteria into the bloodstream and eventual seeding of the peritoneal fluid may contribute. The microbiology of SBP includes most commonly *Escherichia coli* and Enterobacteriaceae *(Klebsiella)*. Gram-positive organisms such as *Streptococcus (viridans), Enterococcus,* and *Pneumococcus* species may also be found. With the use of prophylactic antibiotics for SBP there has been a shift to gram-positive organisms being isolated. Anaerobes are uncommon, and a single organism is isolated on culture in most cases; the presence of multiple organisms suggests bowel perforation or other causes of peritonitis.

Clinical Presentation

Clinical features may include fever, abdominal pain, and signs of peritoneal irritation, particularly in advanced cases. Often, early infection is clinically silent or manifests with worsening of HE, diarrhea, ileus, or renal insufficiency.

Diagnosis

Diagnostic paracentesis should be considered in any patient with cirrhotic ascites who deteriorates clinically. The diagnosis of SBP is highly likely if a high concentration (>250 cells/mm³) of polymorphonuclear leukocytes (PMNs) is present in the ascitic fluid, and this finding

should prompt empiric therapy while blood and ascitic fluid culture results are pending. The use of rapid bedside diagnostic methods such as leukocyte esterase reagent strips is not routinely recommended in view of their low sensitivity. However, inoculation of both aerobic and anaerobic blood culture bottles with the first samples of peritoneal fluid retrieved at bedside significantly increases the yield of capturing potential pathogens.

Treatment

Patients are usually treated with intravenous third-generation cephalosporin (e.g., ceftriaxone, 2 g every 24 hours); quinolones, in particular ciprofloxacin, are routinely used in the United States, provided that the patient does not have prior exposure and is not in overt shock. Response to treatment is usually seen within 72 hours; therapy is continued for a minimum of 5 days and can extend up to 14 days. Repeat peritoneal fluid analysis may be done if recovery is delayed or to ensure that the ascitic fluid is sterile after treatment. The administration of intravenous albumin on day 1 (1.5 g/kg) and day 3 (1 g/kg) has been shown to decrease the incidence of renal dysfunction and to improve short-term survival in SBP.

Prognosis

There is a high rate of recurrence, up to 70% within 1 year, and the 1-year mortality rate with a prior episode of SBP is 50% to 70%. Long-term antibiotic prophylaxis is indicated to reduce the recurrence rate to approximately 20%. Short-term prophylaxis should be considered for patients with cirrhosis and ascites who are hospitalized with upper gastrointestinal bleeding. Common prophylactic regimens for SBP include fluoroquinolones (ciprofloxacin, 500 mg/daily; norfloxacin, 400 mg/day) and trimethoprim-sulfamethoxazole (1 double-strength tablet daily). Long-term antibiotic prophylaxis can lead to infection with resistant extended-spectrum β-lactamase (ESBL)-producing organisms or methicillin-resistant *Staphylococcus aureus* (MRSA).

HEPATORENAL SYNDROME

Definition and Pathology

Hepatorenal syndrome (HRS) is a form of functional renal failure that occurs in the presence of significant hepatic synthetic dysfunction and ascites. Three mechanisms of kidney dysfunction have been proposed: splanchnic arterial vasodilation, renal arterial vasoconstriction, and cardiac dysfunction.

Clinical Presentation and Diagnosis

Patients with HRS typically have advanced ascites and other manifestations of cirrhosis but are not otherwise symptomatic. However, some patients may notice decreased urine output or signs of encephalopathy. There is no single laboratory or imaging study that can be used alone to diagnose HRS. However, the 5-year probability of developing HRS in patients with cirrhosis and ascites is 40%, and HRS develops in approximately 30% of cirrhotic patients who are admitted with SBP. Therefore, a high clinical suspicion is warranted along with a systematic approach to diagnosis based on fulfillment of certain criteria.

The International Club of Ascites (ICA) developed updated diagnostic criteria incorporating new definitions of acute kidney injury (AKI) in 2015:

1. Cirrhosis with ascites
2. Diagnosis of AKI according to ICA-AKI criteria: 50% increase in the serum creatinine level from baseline which is known or presumed to have occurred within the 7 days prior *OR* Rise of 0.3 mg/dL (26.4 μmol/L) in the serum creatinine level in less than 48 hours

3. Lack of response after at least 2 days of diuretic withdrawal and volume expansion with albumin (1 g/kg of body weight/day, to a maximum of 100 g/day)
4. Absence of shock
5. Lack of current or recent treatment with nephrotoxic drugs
6. Absence of parenchymal kidney disease as indicated by protein-uria of more than 500 mg/day, microhematuria (>50 red blood cells/high-power field), or abnormal renal US findings

HRS has two types, HRS-AKI type 1 and HRS-CKD (chronic kidney disease) type 2. HRS-AKI is characterized as an increase in serum creatinine 0.3 mg/dL or greater within 48 hrs or 50% or greater from baseline value according to ICA consensus document *and/or* urinary output 0.5 mL/kg body weight or less for longer than 6 hours. HRS-CKD is defined as eGFR less than 60 mL/min per 1.73 m^2 for 3 months or greater in the absence of other (structural) causes.

Typically, the kidneys are histologically normal and can regain normal function in the event of recovery of liver function (e.g., after liver transplantation). Severe cortical vasoconstriction has been demonstrated angiographically, and such vasoconstriction reverses when these kidneys are transplanted into patients who do not have cirrhosis.

Treatment and Prognosis

The mortality rate is high in HRS, and so prevention is important. In all patients with cirrhosis, precipitating factors (e.g., diuretics, lactulose, nonsteroidal anti-inflammatory drugs, angiotensin-converting enzyme inhibitors) should be avoided if possible. Patients should be promptly diagnosed and treated for any signs of SBP, and colloid (albumin) should be administered if rising creatinine levels are observed. Prevention of variceal bleeding should also be optimized by primary and secondary prophylaxis.

Studies have shown an increased mortality rate with AKI among hospitalized cirrhotic patients. Several medical therapies are currently under review, including use of terlipressin, a vasopressin V_1 receptor analogue, in combination with albumin for type 1 HRS. Other studies have evaluated the combination of octreotide and midodrine (an α-adrenergic agonist) and intravenous albumin. Placement of TIPS has also been reported to stabilize or even improve renal function, mainly in patients with HRS-CKD. However, a significant limitation of TIPS is the possibility of worsening hepatic function in decompensated cirrhosis. Liver transplantation has become the accepted treatment for HRS because it is the only known therapeutic intervention that reverses the process. It is limited by rapid progression of HRS and lack of available organs.

HEPATIC ENCEPHALOPATHY

Definition

HE is a complex, reversible neuropsychiatric syndrome that occurs in patients with chronic liver disease, portal hypertension, or portosystemic shunting. HE is also seen in patients with acute liver failure. HE develops in about 30% to 45% of cirrhotic patients, and when it is present, the survival probability is approximately 23% at 3 years.

Pathophysiology

The pathogenesis of HE in the setting of cirrhosis is thought to be multifactorial and may differ in acute and chronic liver disease. Contributors include the inadequate hepatic removal of potential endogenous neurotoxins, altered permeability of the blood-brain barrier, and abnormal neurotransmission. Elevation of blood ammonia levels, derived from both amino acid deamination and bacterial hydrolysis of nitrogenous compounds in the gut, has been the best studied factor, but its specific role in the pathogenesis of HE remains uncertain. Many other potential contributors to HE have been investigated,

including increased tone of the inhibitory GABAA/benzodiazepine neurotransmitter system, activation of the astrocytic 18-kDa translocator protein (PTBR), production of endogenous benzodiazepine-like compounds, altered cerebral metabolism, zinc deficiency, increase in serotonin levels, upregulation of H1 receptors, altered melatonin production, and deposition of manganese in the basal ganglia.

Clinical Presentation

The clinical features of HE include disturbances of higher neurologic function such as intellectual and personality disorders, dementia, inability to copy simple diagrams (constructional apraxia), disturbance of consciousness, disturbances of neuromuscular function (asterixis, hyperreflexia, myoclonus), and, rarely, a Parkinson-like syndrome and progressive paraplegia. One of the earliest manifestations of overt HE is alteration of the normal sleep-wake cycle.

Diagnosis

There is no laboratory or imaging study that allows a specific diagnosis of HE. Rather, it is a clinical syndrome. Blood levels of ammonia are commonly measured, but elevated levels are neither sensitive nor specific for HE. Neuropsychometric and neurocognitive tests such as the Portosystemic Encephalopathy Syndrome Test (PSET) and the earlier Stroop Color-Word Test evaluate the patient's attention, concentration, fine motor skills, and orientation and have been shown to be highly specific for the diagnosis of HE, but they are reasonably labor intensive. Therefore, a smartphone-based application known as EncephalApp was created incorporating the Stroop test that is validated for use in detection of covert/minimal HE. It is imperative that reversible causes of neurologic dysfunction, such as hypoglycemia, subdural hematoma, meningitis, and drug overdose, be considered and excluded early in the differential diagnosis of altered mental status in patients with cirrhosis.

Classification of Hepatic Encephalopathy

There are three major types of HE: type A (Acute), which is associated with acute liver failure; type B (Bypass), which is associated with portosystemic shunts in the absence of liver disease; and type C (Cirrhosis), which is associated with liver cirrhosis and is subdivided into episodic, persistent, and minimal types.

HE has been further graded based on the West Haven Criteria from 0 to 4. A new nomenclature, termed the Spectrum of Neurocognitive Impairment in Cirrhosis (SONIC) classification, has been proposed to improve recognition of earlier forms of HE that require specialized testing for detection and to facilitate research studies. Patients are divided into those who are unimpaired, those with covert HE, and those with overt HE (Table 44.5).

Treatment

Treatment of HE starts with identifying and addressing any precipitating factors (Table 44.6), reducing and eliminating substrates for the generation of nitrogenous compounds, and preventing ammonia absorption from the bowel. Protein restriction was considered to be important in preventing excess ammonia production in the past; however, studies have demonstrated that dietary restriction of protein is not of significant benefit. Short-term protein restriction may be considered for patients with severe encephalopathy, but long-term restriction is associated with worsening malnutrition. Treatment with formulas rich in branched-chain amino acids has shown no benefit in improving encephalopathy or mortality.

Nonabsorbable disaccharides (e.g., lactulose) are the mainstay treatment of HE. These agents are fermented to organic acids by colonic bacteria, processes that lower stool pH and trap NH_4^+ in the colon, thereby decreasing absorption. In addition, the cathartic effect

TABLE 44.5 Clinical Stages of Hepatic Encephalopathy as Defined by the West Haven Criteria and the Proposed Sonic Classification

	WEST HAVEN CRITERIA		SONIC			
Grade	Intellectual Function	Neuromuscular Function	Classification	Mental Status	Special Tests	Asterixis
0	Normal	Normal	Unimpaired	Not impaired	Normal	Absent
Minimal	Normal examination findings. Subtle changes in work or driving	Minor abnormalities of visual perception or on psychometric or number tests	Covert HE	Not impaired	Abnormal	Absent
1	Personality changes, attention deficits, irritability, depressed state	Tremor and incoordination				
2	Changes in sleep-wake cycle, lethargy, mood and behavioral changes, cognitive dysfunction	Asterixis, ataxic gait, speech abnormalities (slow and slurred)	Overt HE	Impaired	Abnormal	Present (absent in coma)
3	Altered level of consciousness (somnolence), confusion, disorientation, and amnesia	Muscular rigidity, nystagmus, clonus, Babinski sign, hyporeflexia				
4	Stupor and coma	Oculocephalic reflex, unresponsiveness to noxious stimuli				

SONIC, Spectrum of Neuro-Cognitive Impairment in Cirrhosis.
Modified from Nevah MI, Fallon MB: Hepatic encephalopathy, hepatorenal syndrome, hepatopulmonary syndrome, and systemic complications of liver disease. In Feldman M, Friedman LS, Brandt LJ, editors: Sleisenger and Fordtran's gastrointestinal and liver disease, ed 9, Philadelphia, 2010, Saunders.

TABLE 44.6 Hepatic Encephalopathy: Precipitating Factors

Gastrointestinal bleeding
Increased dietary protein
Constipation
Infection
Central nervous system depressant drugs (benzodiazepines, opiates, tricyclic antidepressants)
Deterioration in hepatic function
Hypokalemia: most often induced by diuretics
Azotemia: most often induced by diuretics
Alkalosis: most often induced by diuretics
Hypovolemia: most often induced by diuretics

of lactulose eliminates ammonia and other nitrogenous compounds. Patients are usually directed to achieve two to three soft stools per day as the goal of lactulose therapy. Reduction and elimination of nitrogenous compound substrates can also be achieved by administering enemas and using nonabsorbable antibiotics such as rifaximin in patients who do not tolerate or respond to lactulose. Rifaximin (Xifaxan), 550 mg PO twice daily, is approved by the US Food and Drug Administration for the treatment of HE and has a favorable side effect profile; however, cost is the limiting factor. Other agents that affect intestinal motility and ammonia generation are being evaluated, including acarbose and probiotics.

HEPATOPULMONARY SYNDROME AND PORTOPULMONARY HYPERTENSION

The effects of cirrhosis and portal hypertension on the pulmonary circulation manifest as two distinct disorders, hepatopulmonary syndrome (HPS) and portopulmonary hypertension (PoPH).

Hepatopulmonary Syndrome

HPS occurs in 5% to 30% of patients with cirrhosis and is a progressive disease. It is characterized by gas exchange abnormalities (increased alveolar-arterial gradient and hypoxemia) resulting from intrapulmonary vascular dilation. The vascular dilation leads to vascular remodeling and angiogenesis, resulting in impaired oxygen transfer from the alveoli to the central stream of red blood cells within capillaries. Usually, this functional intrapulmonary right-to-left shunt significantly improves with the administration of 100% oxygen. HPS also has been reported in cases of hepatic venous outflow obstruction without cirrhosis.

Diagnosis

HPS is diagnosed based on high clinical suspicion and measurement of a widened alveolar-arterial oxygen gradient on room air in the presence or absence of hypoxemia. The gradient is calculated by analyzing arterial blood gases. HPS is graded from mild, in which the arterial partial pressure of oxygen (Pao$_2$) is greater than 80 mm Hg) to very severe (Pao$_2$ <50 mm Hg). Intrapulmonary shunting is demonstrated by contrast echocardiography, in which agitated saline is injected into a peripheral vein during the performance of two-dimensional echocardiography. Delayed appearance of microbubbles in the left cardiac chambers (more than three to six cardiac cycles after injection) indicates intrapulmonary vasodilation. Early visualization of microbubbles in the left cardiac chambers indicates intracardiac shunting. Other tests, including chest radiography, computed tomography, and pulmonary function tests, are performed to exclude intrinsic cardiopulmonary disorders.

Clinical Presentation

Clinical features range from subclinical abnormalities in gas exchange to profound hypoxemia causing significant dyspnea. Classically in HPS, the dyspnea is worse on standing and improves when the patient lies down (orthodeoxia and platypnea, respectively). Patients may also have marked nocturnal hypoxemia.

Screening and Treatment

Screening by pulse oximetry typically targets patients with values lower than 96% at rest on room air for further evaluation; however, recent data suggest that this may not be an appropriate screening tool. Currently, there is no established medical therapy for HPS. Recent evaluation of newer agents such as sorafenib showed no significant improvement. Liver transplantation remains the only option and reverses HPS in most patients. The use of TIPS to treat HPS is not established.

Prognosis

HPS carries a mortality rate of up to 40% in 2.5 years.

Portopulmonary Hypertension

PoPH is defined as the presence of pulmonary arterial hypertension in the setting of portal hypertension.

Diagnosis and Pathology

The diagnosis of PoPH is based entirely on results of right heart catheterization. The diagnostic values include a mean pulmonary arterial pressure greater than 25 mm Hg at rest or 30 mm Hg with exercise, a pulmonary capillary wedge pressure lower than 15 mm Hg, and a pulmonary vascular resistance greater than 240 dynes, all in the presence of portal hypertension or liver disease or both. PoPH is graded according to the mean pulmonary artery pressure, from mild (>25 to 35 mm Hg) to moderate (35 to 50 mm Hg) to severe (>50 mm Hg). Patients with mild PoPH do not appear to have increased operative risk. Moderate PoPH carries a high intraoperative risk and should be medically managed before transplantation. Severe PoPH is generally considered a contraindication to surgery. The exact mechanisms of PoPH are poorly understood. Histologically, it has characteristics similar to those of pulmonary hypertension.

Clinical Presentation

The most common symptom of PoPH is dyspnea on exertion, but many cirrhotic patients with PoPH are asymptomatic.

Treatment

In addition to symptomatic treatment (oxygen for dyspnea and diuretics for volume overload), the medical management of PoPH is similar to that for pulmonary arterial hypertension. The drugs most commonly used in treatment for PoPH are prostacyclins (intravenous, inhaled or subcutaneous), oral treatments including phosphodiesterase inhibitors, and endothelin receptor antagonist.

If moderate PoPH responds to therapy, liver transplantation may be considered. However, it has not been established whether successful liver transplantation reliably reverses PoPH. Liver transplantation is contraindicated in severe PoPH because of high transplant-related morbidity and mortality. However, there were no dedicated randomized clinical trials of these therapies until the PORTICO trial. The PORTICO trial was a double-blind, placebo-controlled, multicenter study of macitentan, an endothelin receptor antagonist. Macitentan showed improved pulmonary vascular resistance without hepatotoxicity. More novel agents are being studied.

Prognosis

Untreated PoPH carries high rates of morbidity and mortality; the mean survival time from diagnosis is 15 months. A study on the U.S.-based Registry to Evaluate Early and Long-term Pulmonary Arterial Hypertension Disease Management (REVEAL) showed a 5-year survival rate of 40% from the time of diagnosis in patients with PoPH.

HEPATOCELLULAR CARCINOMA

Epidemiology

Liver cancer is the fifth most common cancer in men and the seventh most common in women worldwide; HCC is the most common type of liver cancer. In the United States, approximately 90% of liver cancers are HCC, and cholangiocarcinomas account for most of the rest. In other areas of the world, including sub-Saharan Africa, China, Japan, and Southeast Asia, HCC is one of the most frequent malignancies and is an important cause of mortality, particularly among middle-aged men.

Etiology

HCC often arises from a cirrhotic liver, and it is closely associated with chronic viral hepatitis. Hepatitis B virus DNA has been shown to integrate into the host cell genome, where it may disrupt tumor suppressor genes and activate oncogenes. In areas of high prevalence, vaccination to prevent infection with hepatitis B virus has reduced the incidence of HCC. The exact pathophysiologic mechanisms leading to tumor genesis in patients with other causes of cirrhosis (e.g., hemochromatosis, alcohol, hepatitis C viral infection) remain poorly understood. Risk factors for the development of HCC and its clinical manifestations are listed in (Table 44.7).

Diagnosis

Table 44.8 lists currently used imaging techniques for detection of HCC and the most common findings. A tissue specimen may be necessary to confirm the diagnosis in some cases, but it is not needed if characteristic clinical and radiologic features are present, especially if they are accompanied by a rise in serum α-fetoprotein levels. The Hepatic Carcinoma Early Detection Screening (HES) algorithm for early detection of HCC was developed and has been validated in the Veterans affairs (VA) cohort. The algorithm includes patient's age, ALT level, platelet count, and current and rate of change to AFP level. It has shown an improvement in early detection in patients with cirrhosis in comparison to AFP alone.

Staging

Although many staging systems for HCC are in use, the Barcelona Clinic Liver Cancer (BCLC) system is most commonly used.

Treatment

Patients with well-compensated cirrhosis may undergo surgical resection or liver transplantation, with a 5-year survival rate of up to 70%. Nonsurgical options include percutaneous ethanol injection, transarterial chemoembolization (TACE), and radiofrequency ablation. The first-line treatment for many years was Sorafenib (a receptor tyrosine kinase angiogenesis inhibitor) for use in patients with unresectable HCC. However, recently another agent was approved, lenvatinib, which works by the same mechanism, and both have been shown to prolong survival of these patients. Second-line agents have also been approved, which include regorafenib, cabozantinib, and nivolumab.

Prognosis

In patients with widespread, multifocal disease and in those with vascular invasion, the prognosis is poor, with a 5-year survival rate of 5% to 6%. Accordingly, emphasis is placed on prevention of viral hepatitis and other causes of liver disease and on screening by ultrasound of those who are at higher risk, including patients with known cirrhosis.

TABLE 44.7 Hepatocellular Carcinoma

Associations
Chronic hepatitis B infection
Chronic hepatitis C infection
Hemochromatosis (with cirrhosis)
Cirrhosis (alcoholic, cryptogenic)
Aflatoxin ingestion, Thorotrast exposure
α_1-Antitrypsin deficiency
Androgen administration

Common Clinical Presentations
Abdominal pain
Abdominal mass
Weight loss
Deterioration of liver function

Unusual Manifestations
Bloody ascites
Tumor emboli (lung)
Jaundice
Hepatic or portal vein obstruction
Metabolic effects
Erythrocytosis
Hypercalcemia
Hypercholesterolemia
Hypoglycemia
Gynecomastia
Feminization
Acquired porphyria

Clinical and Laboratory Findings
Hepatic bruit or friction rub
Serum α-fetoprotein >400 ng/mL

TABLE 44.8 Imaging Characteristics of Hepatocellular Carcinoma

Ultrasonography
Mass lesion with varying echogenicity but usually hypoechoic

Dynamic Computed Tomography
Arterial phase: tumor enhances quickly
Venous phase: quick de-enhancement of tumor relative to parenchyma

Magnetic Resonance Imaging
T1-weighted images: hypointense
T2-weighted images: hyperintense
After gadolinium administration, tumor increases in intensity

VASCULAR DISEASE OF THE LIVER

Disorders of the hepatic vasculature are uncommon and include portal vein thrombosis (PVT), hepatic vein thrombosis (Budd-Chiari syndrome), and veno-occlusive disease. Affected patients usually have portal hypertension with or without associated liver dysfunction, which may mimic the presentation of cirrhosis.

Portal Vein Thrombosis
Definition and Etiology

Thrombosis of the portal vein may develop after blunt abdominal trauma, umbilical vein infection, neonatal sepsis, intra-abdominal inflammatory diseases (e.g., pancreatitis), or hypercoagulable states, and in association with cirrhosis. Myeloproliferative diseases (including polycythemia vera, essential thrombocytosis, and myelofibrosis) are now being recognized as possible causes of PVT. One study observed that as many as 25% to 65% of patients with splanchnic vein thrombosis in the absence of cirrhosis had a myeloproliferative disease. The Janus kinase 2 (JAK2) mutation is a marker for myeloproliferative disease and is often checked in patients with PVT. The disease produces the manifestations of portal hypertension, but the liver histology is usually normal.

Diagnosis

The diagnosis is established by angiography, but noninvasive imaging modalities such as Doppler ultrasonography, computed tomography, and magnetic resonance imaging may reveal thrombus, collateral circulation near the porta hepatis, and splenomegaly. In long-standing PVT, tortuous venous channels develop within the organized clot, leading to cavernous transformation.

Treatment

In acute PVT, thrombolysis may be attempted, but anticoagulation with warfarin remains the mainstay of therapy. In most patients, recanalization of the thrombus occurs within 6 months after initiation of anticoagulation. Recommendations for duration of anticoagulation after an acute event vary and are usually 3 to 6 months. Long-term anticoagulation may be used in cases of chronic thrombosis, especially when associated with hypercoagulable states.

Concern exists that anticoagulation may precipitate hemorrhage from varices that arise as a consequence of portal hypertension; however, studies have not shown an increased risk for variceal bleeding in anticoagulated patients with chronic PVT. In fact, studies suggest a role for prophylactic anticoagulation (enoxaparin) for prevention of PVT and hepatic decompensation in cirrhosis. If variceal hemorrhage occurs, it is best managed with endoscopic obliteration. Prophylaxis with β-blockers to prevent variceal bleeding may decrease the portal pressure, potentially propagating thrombus, and therefore is not usually recommended. If endoscopic treatment fails, surgical management with portosystemic shunting may be attempted, but this approach is often difficult because of the absence of suitable patent vessels. The use of TIPS has also been studied in nonocclusive PVT and may be beneficial in establishing patency of the portal vein for future interventions such as liver transplantation in lieu of anticoagulation only.

Budd-Chiari Syndrome
Definition and Etiology

Occlusion of the major hepatic veins or the inferior vena cava, especially in the intrahepatic and suprahepatic segments, causes Budd-Chiari syndrome. Most cases are associated with hematologic disease (e.g., polycythemia vera, paroxysmal nocturnal hemoglobinuria, essential thrombocytosis, other myeloproliferative disorders), pregnancy, oral contraceptive use, tumors (especially HCC), or other causes of a hypercoagulable state (e.g., factor V Leiden mutation, protein C and S deficiency). Abdominal trauma and congenital webs of the vena cava are also related to Budd-Chiari syndrome. About 20% of cases are idiopathic, but many of these patients prove to have early, subclinical myeloproliferative disease or genetic mutations associated with a hypercoagulable state.

Clinical Presentation

Budd-Chiari syndrome can manifest acutely, possibly in association with acute liver failure, or it can manifest as a subacute or chronic illness. Acute disease produces right upper quadrant abdominal pain, hepatomegaly, ascites, and jaundice, whereas the subacute or chronic form produces primarily portal hypertension. Elevation of serum bilirubin and transaminase levels may be mild, but liver function is often poor, with profound hypoalbuminemia and coagulopathy.

Diagnosis

The diagnosis can be established noninvasively with Doppler ultrasonography, which shows decreased or absent hepatic vein blood flow, and computed tomography, which shows delayed or absent contrast filling of the hepatic veins and hypertrophy of the caudate lobe. Magnetic resonance angiography may also demonstrate these findings. Hepatic venography is especially useful if the results of noninvasive imaging are inconclusive. Venography often shows an inability to catheterize and visualize the hepatic veins; the characteristic spider-web pattern of collateral vessels may also be demonstrated, and the inferior vena cava may appear compressed owing to hepatomegaly or an enlarged caudate lobe. On liver biopsy, centrilobular congestion, hemorrhage, and necrosis (nutmeg liver) are seen, with cirrhosis developing in patients with chronic obstruction.

Treatment

Treatment should be individualized and is dependent on the mode and severity of presentation and the potential cause of the disease. Supportive therapy to relieve ascites and edema (e.g., dietary sodium restriction, diuretics) and chronic anticoagulation may be considered for patients with chronic Budd-Chiari syndrome in whom methods to decompress congestion are not feasible. Thrombolysis followed by anticoagulation is most useful in patients with acute forms of the disease. In selected patients (such as those with venous webs or strictures or single-vessel thrombosis), angioplasty with or without stent placement may be used. Decompressive modalities are most useful before the development of cirrhosis and include transjugular intrahepatic portacaval and side-to-side portacaval shunts. In patients with cirrhosis, liver transplantation followed by continued anticoagulation is often considered the best option.

Veno-Occlusive Disease
Definition and Etiology

Hepatic veno-occlusive disease, also called sinusoidal obstruction syndrome, often occurs after cytoreductive therapy and before bone marrow transplantation but may also follow exposure to other drugs or herbal preparations (e.g., azathioprine, pyrrolizidine alkaloids). Endothelial cell injury leads to obstruction at the level of the hepatic venules and the sinusoids.

Clinical Presentation

The disease is characterized by jaundice, painful hepatomegaly, and fluid retention. Clinical manifestations can be rapidly progressive and lead to multiorgan dysfunction and death in 20% to 25% of patients.

Diagnosis

The diagnosis is clinically suspected when weight gain, epigastric or right upper quadrant abdominal pain, and jaundice develop within the first 3 to 4 weeks after bone marrow transplantation. Laboratory abnormalities include hyperbilirubinemia, elevated transaminases, and, in severe cases, profound synthetic dysfunction. Doppler abdominal ultrasonography may reveal ascites, reversal of portal vein flow, and an elevated hepatic artery resistance index. Liver biopsy is diagnostic and is usually obtained with use of the transjugular approach. The advantages of this approach compared with the percutaneous route include the ability to measure the hepatic venous pressure gradient (which is typically elevated in veno-occlusive disease) and a lower incidence of bleeding.

Treatment

Mild forms of the disease may favorably respond to supportive therapy alone. In moderate to severe disease, treatment has been attempted with tissue plasminogen activator and heparin, antithrombin III, prostaglandin E_1, and glutamine plus vitamin E, although the efficacies of these treatments have not been clearly established. Defibrotide (a mixture of porcine-derived single-stranded phosphodiester oligonucleotides) has been evaluated as a potential treatment option for severe veno-occlusive disease; however, evidence for efficacy has been mixed.

LIVER TRANSPLANTATION

MELD Score

The Model for End-stage Liver Disease (MELD) score was originally calculated based on the serum creatinine concentration, prothrombin time (International Normalized Ratio), and bilirubin level and has been used to predict short-term mortality in cirrhosis and to prioritize patients awaiting liver transplantation. However, in 2016 an adjustment was made to the MELD score to include the serum sodium, now commonly referred to as the MELD-Na. The MELD-Na score ranges from 6 to 40. Higher scores are associated with more advanced disease and increased predicted mortality. Patients are typically considered for liver transplantation when the MELD-Na score reaches 15.

Prognosis

Liver transplantation is a highly successful procedure in patients with progressive, advanced, and otherwise untreatable liver disease. Advances in surgical techniques and supportive care, the use of cyclosporine and tacrolimus for immunosuppression, and careful selection of patients have all contributed to the excellent results of liver transplantation. Between 70% and 80% of patients undergoing liver transplantation survive at least 5 years, usually with good quality of life. The most common indication for liver transplantation in the United States is chronic liver disease resulting from alcohol. Other liver diseases for which transplantation is commonly performed include cirrhosis from NAFLD, hepatitis C virus, autoimmune hepatitis, primary biliary cirrhosis, and primary sclerosing cholangitis. Patients with hepatitis B are candidates for liver transplantation if they can be given hepatitis B immunoglobulin or nucleoside analogues to help prevent recurrence. Excellent results have also been obtained in selected patients with acute liver failure (see Chapter 43). Liver transplantation for malignant hepatobiliary disease has been less successful because of recurrent disease in the transplanted liver.

For a deeper discussion on this topic, please see Chapter 144, "Cirrhosis and Its Sequelae," in *Goldman-Cecil Medicine*, 26th Edition.

SUGGESTED READINGS

Angeli Paolo, Garcia-Tsao G, Nadim MK, Parikh CR. News in pathophysiology, definition and classification of hepatorenal syndrome: a step beyond the international Club of ascites (ICA) consensus document, J Hepatol 71(4):811–822, 2019.

Garcia–Tsao G, Abraldes JG, Berzigotti A, Bosch J. Portal hypertensive bleeding in cirrhosis: Risk stratification, diagnosis, and management: 2016 practice guidance by the American Association for the study of liver diseases, Hepatology 65(1):310–335, 2017.

Kamath PS, Kim W: The model for end-stage liver disease (MELD), Hepatology 45:797–805, 2007.

Kim WR, Biggins SW, Kremers WK, et al: Hyponatremia and mortality among patients on the liver-transplant waiting list, N Engl J Med 359(10):1018–1026, 2008.

Krowka MJ, Miller DP, Barst RJ, et al: Portopulmonary hypertension: a report from the US-based REVEAL registry, Chest 141:906–915, 2012.

Runyon BA: Management of adult patients with ascites due to cirrhosis: update 2012, AASLD Practice Guideline, AASLD 3(1):5–8, 2012.

Valla DC: Thrombosis and anticoagulation in liver disease, Hepatology 47:1384–1393, 2008.

Villa E, Cammà C, Marietta M, et al: Enoxaparin prevents portal vein thrombosis and liver decompensation in patients with advanced cirrhosis, Gastroenterology 143:1253–1260, 2012.

45

Disorders of the Gallbladder and Biliary Tract

Stacie A. F. Vela, Michael B. Fallon

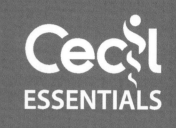

INTRODUCTION

The gallbladder and biliary tract transport bile from the liver into the intestines, a process central to digestion of fat and absorption of lipids and fat-soluble vitamins. Gallbladder and biliary tract diseases are among the most common and costly of all digestive disorders. This chapter examines the principal gallbladder and biliary tract disorders, focusing on cholelithiasis. The reader is referred to Chapter 41 for a detailed discussion of bilirubin metabolism and the diagnostic approach to jaundice and to Chapter 35 for a review of the various imaging techniques used to study the biliary tract.

NORMAL BILIARY ANATOMY AND PHYSIOLOGY

Fig. 45.1 outlines the basic anatomy of the liver and biliary tract. The liver produces 500 to 1500 mL of bile per day. The secretory product of individual hepatocytes contains bile acids, phospholipids, and cholesterol, which are transported across the apical membrane and into the canalicular space between cells. These canaliculi merge to form larger intrahepatic bile ducts and then the common hepatic duct. During fasting, tonic contractions of the sphincter of Oddi, located in the region of the ampulla of Vater, divert about one half of the bile through the cystic duct into the gallbladder, where it is stored and concentrated by water resorption. Cholecystokinin, which is released after food enters the small intestine, causes the sphincter of Oddi to relax, allowing delivery of a timed bolus of bile into the intestine. Bile acids are present in millimolar concentrations. They are detergent molecules that possess both fat-soluble and water-soluble moieties. Cholesterol is secreted by the liver to the intestine, where it undergoes fecal excretion (see E-Fig. 41.1 in Chapter 41). In the intestinal lumen, bile acids solubilize dietary fat and promote its digestion and absorption. Bile acids are, for the most part, efficiently reabsorbed by the small intestinal mucosa, particularly in the terminal ileum. They are then recycled to the liver for re-excretion, a process termed *enterohepatic circulation*.

GALLBLADDER DISORDERS

Gallstones (Cholelithiasis)

Gallstone formation constitutes a significant health problem, affecting 10% to 15% of the adult population. Complications from gallstones are a leading cause for hospital admissions related to gastrointestinal problems. In the United States, gallstone disease leads to more than 750,000 cholecystectomies annually, making this the most common elective abdominal surgery, with estimated costs of $6.5 billion per year. Gallstones are of two types: 75% are made of cholesterol, and 25% are pigmented stones (black or brown). The latter are composed of calcium bilirubinate and other calcium salts. The risk factors for cholelithiasis are shown in Table 45.1.

Pathogenesis of Cholelithiasis

The three main factors that lead to cholesterol gallstone formation are cholesterol supersaturation of bile, nucleation, and gallbladder hypomotility. These are influenced by both genetic background and intestinal factors (Fig. 45.2).

The liver is the most important organ in regulating total-body cholesterol stores. Once it is secreted, cholesterol, which is insoluble in water, is solubilized in bile through the formation of mixed micelles with bile acids and phospholipids. In most individuals, there is more cholesterol in bile than can be maintained in stable solution. This is even more pronounced in the setting of insulin resistance. As bile becomes supersaturated, microscopic cholesterol molecules aggregate into coalescent vesicles that crystallize, a process referred to as *nucleation*. The gradual deposition of additional layers of cholesterol leads to the appearance of macroscopic stones. Factors that influence nucleation include bile transit time, gallbladder contraction, bile composition (concentrations of cholesterol, phospholipids, and bile salts), and presence of bacteria, mucin, and glycoproteins, which can act as a nidus to initiate cholesterol crystal formation. The interplay between *pronucleating* and *antinucleating* factors in the gallbladder may determine whether cholesterol gallstones will form from supersaturated bile. Gallbladder sludge is a super-concentrated mixture of bile acids, bilirubin, cholesterol, mucus, and proteins that exhibits various degrees of fluidity and is prone to precipitate into a semisolid or solid form.

The pathophysiologic factors leading to pigment stone formation are less well understood; however, increased production of bilirubin conjugates (hemolytic states), increased biliary calcium (Ca^{2+}) and bicarbonate (HCO_3^-) levels, cirrhosis, and bacterial deconjugation of bilirubin to a less soluble form are all associated with pigment stone formation. Black pigment stones, which are composed primarily of calcium bilirubinate, are formed in sterile bile in the gallbladder and are common in chronic hemolytic states, in cases of cirrhosis, and in patients with ileal resection. Their brown pigment counterparts, composed primarily of calcium salts, are formed in the bile ducts and are seen in the setting of infection of the biliary tract.

Many of the recognized predisposing factors for cholelithiasis and gallbladder sludge can be understood in terms of the pathophysiologic scheme outlined previously:

1. Biliary cholesterol saturation is increased by insulin resistance, estrogens, multiparity, oral contraceptives, obesity, rapid weight loss, and terminal ileal disease, which decreases the bile acid pool.
2. Nucleation is enhanced by biliary parasites, recurrent bacterial infection of the biliary tract, altered intestinal microbiome, and antibiotics such as ceftriaxone, which has a proclivity to concentrate and crystallize with calcium in the biliary tree. Total parenteral nutrition and blood transfusions also promote bile pigment accumulation and *gelfaction* of sludge.

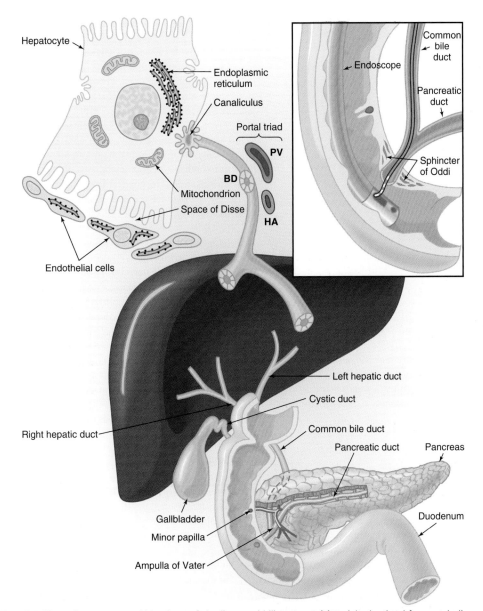

Fig. 45.1 Normal anatomy and histology of the liver and biliary tract. Materials destined for metabolism or excretion by the liver (such as unconjugated bilirubin) enter the sinusoidal bed and cross the endothelial barrier and the space of Disse. Unconjugated bilirubin is taken up by the hepatocyte, conjugated with glucuronide to become water soluble, and excreted into bile across the canalicular membrane of the hepatocyte. The canaliculi empty into bile ductules (BD), which lead to the interlobular (small), septal (medium), and large intrahepatic bile ducts and finally to the main branches of the common bile duct. The portal areas, or portal triads, are composed mainly of portal vein (PV), hepatic artery (HA), and BD branches. During fasting, tonic contraction of the sphincter of Oddi, located in the region of the ampulla of Vater, diverts about one half of the bile through the cystic duct into the gallbladder, where it is stored and concentrated to be released later during meal times. Disease at any level of the biliary tree can lead to cholestasis and obstructive jaundice. The *inset* shows an endoscopic retrograde cholangiopancreatography procedure. See Figs. 45.5, 45.6, and 45.7 for radiographic depictions in specific biliary tract disorders.

3. Bile stasis is caused by gallbladder hypomotility (resulting from pregnancy, somatostatin, or fasting), bile duct strictures, choledochal cysts, biliary parasites, and total parenteral nutrition.

Clinical Manifestations of Gallstones

Gallstones develop at some point in 10% to 20% of Americans. Between 50% and 60% of these individuals remain asymptomatic, but about one third develop biliary colic or chronic cholecystitis, and 15% develop acute complications. The natural history of gallstone disease is outlined in Fig. 45.3. Obstruction of the biliary tract at any level by stones or sludge is the underlying cause of the clinical manifestations of gallstone disease. Obstruction by gallstones can occur at the level of the cystic duct, common hepatic duct, common bile duct, or ampulla of Vater (see Figs. 45.1 and 45.3). Symptoms arise from contraction of the gallbladder during transient obstruction of the cystic duct by gallstones, and persistent obstruction of the cystic duct leads to superimposed inflammation or infection of the gallbladder (i.e., acute cholecystitis). Obstruction of the distal common bile duct may result image

TABLE 45.1	Risk Factors for Cholelithiasis

Primary
Age
Obesity
Female sex
Rapid weight loss
Ethnic background (e.g., Native American)

Secondary
Drugs: oral contraceptives, ceftriaxone, octreotide, thiazide diuretics
Pregnancy
Diabetes mellitus
Low socioeconomic status
Sedentary lifestyle
Total parenteral nutrition
Hemolysis
Cirrhosis
Crohn's disease
Biliary parasites (e.g., *Clonorchis sinensis*)
Terminal ileum resection

in abdominal pain, cholangitis (infection of the biliary tract), or pancreatitis (resulting from pancreatic duct obstruction). The presence of a large stone in the cystic duct can cause common bile duct obstruction and is referred to as *Mirizzi syndrome*. Common conditions to consider in the differential diagnosis of gallstone disease are listed in Table 45.2.

Asymptomatic Gallstones

Most gallstones, up to 75%, are clinically "silent," and they are often uncovered as an incidental finding during abdominal ultrasound performed for another reason. The risk of developing symptoms is low, averaging 2% to 3% per year, 10% at 5 years, and 1% to 2% per year with major complications. Expectant management is an appropriate choice for the general population. Prophylactic cholecystectomy should be considered in those groups who are at increased risk for the development of complications, including (1) patients with diabetes, who have a greater morbidity and mortality from acute cholecystitis; (2) patients with a calcified (porcelain) gallbladder, large gallbladder polyps, or large stones (>3 cm), which are associated with an increased risk for gallbladder carcinoma; (3) patients with sickle cell anemia, in whom hepatic crises may be difficult to differentiate from acute cholecystitis; (4) children with gallstones, because they frequently develop symptomatic disease; and (5) Native Americans, who are predisposed to gallbladder cancer in the setting of gallstones.

Symptomatic Gallstones and Biliary Colic

Symptomatic cholelithiasis is defined by gallbladder pain in the presence of gallstones. *Biliary colic* refers to the constellation of symptoms experienced when the gallbladder contracts against outlet obstruction. Classically, biliary colic starts as a steady ache in the epigastrium or right upper quadrant; it has a sudden onset, reaches a plateau of intensity over a few minutes, and then subsides gradually over 30 minutes to several hours. Referred pain may be felt at the tip of the scapula or right shoulder. Nausea and vomiting may occur, but fever and a palpable mass (signs of acute cholecystitis) are not evident. Other symptoms, such as dyspepsia, fatty food intolerance, bloating and flatulence, heartburn, and belching, may occur in patients with gallstones; however, these symptoms are nonspecific and frequently occur in individuals with normal gallbladders.

Gallstones are best demonstrated by transabdominal ultrasonography; therefore, it is recommended as the initial test to evaluate cholelithiasis. The sensitivity and specificity of ultrasound are greater than 90%, but accuracy drops to 20% for visualization of stones within the common bile duct. This limitation has been overcome by endoscopic ultrasonography (EUS) (Video 45.1) and magnetic resonance cholangiopancreatography (MRCP), both of which have an accuracy of 90% to 95% for detecting cholelithiasis and common bile duct stones. Computed tomography, often done in the emergency department for evaluation of abdominal pain, can identify presence of gallstones but is not as reliable or cost-effective as ultrasound. Oral cholecystography is no longer used for the routine evaluation of gallstones.

If gallbladder removal is indicated, laparoscopic cholecystectomy has replaced open cholecystectomy as the treatment of choice for recurrent biliary pain. Open cholecystectomy is typically reserved for selected high-risk patients (e.g., prior abdominal surgery with adhesions, obesity, cirrhosis). If choledocholithiasis is suspected, laparoscopic cholecystectomy may be accompanied by perioperative endoscopic retrograde cholangiopancreatography (ERCP) (see Fig. 45.1 inset and Chapter 35) or intraoperative cholangiography. Factors that may predict the presence of choledocholithiasis include jaundice, pancreatitis, abnormal liver test results, and bile duct dilation.

Cholecystectomy relieves biliary pain in virtually all patients with gallstone disease and prevents the development of future complications. Dissolution of cholesterol gallstones by orally administered chenodeoxycholic acid or ursodeoxycholic acid is successful in highly selected patients but is slow and costly and requires lifelong administration. Alternative methods to eliminate gallstones, including contact dissolution and fragmentation of stones, are used rarely.

Acute Cholecystitis

Acute cholecystitis refers to distention, edema, ischemia, inflammation, and secondary infection of the gallbladder. This typically results from obstruction of the cystic duct by gallstones or, less commonly, from gallbladder cancer or sludge. The clinical hallmark of acute cholecystitis is the acute onset of upper abdominal pain that lasts for several hours. The pain gradually increases in severity and typically localizes to the epigastrium or right hypochondrium with radiation to the right lumbar, scapular, and shoulder area. Nausea and vomiting, anorexia, and low-grade fever are common. Unlike biliary pain, the pain of acute cholecystitis does not subside spontaneously. The findings on physical examination in patients with acute cholecystitis may include inspiratory arrest on palpation of the right upper quadrant (Murphy sign), fever, and, less commonly, mild jaundice or a palpable gallbladder.

Complications of acute cholecystitis include emphysematous cholecystitis (in people with diabetes, older adults, and individuals who are immunosuppressed), empyema, gangrene, and perforation of the gallbladder. Gallbladder perforation may occur directly into the peritoneum ("free") or through a cholecystenteric fistula with gallstone migration and bowel obstruction (gallstone ileus). Mirizzi syndrome is the occurrence of profound jaundice resulting from extrinsic compression of the bile duct by an impacted stone in the cystic duct at the gallbladder neck.

The diagnostic approach for suspected acute cholecystitis is similar to that for biliary pain. A transabdominal ultrasound study that demonstrates gallstones, along with pericholecystic fluid, gallbladder wall thickening, and localized tenderness when the ultrasound probe is placed over the gallbladder (ultrasonographic Murphy sign), provides strong supportive evidence for acute cholecystitis. Ultrasound is safe and widely available and has emerged as the initial test of choice because it is noninvasive as well as cost-effective. Radionuclide scanning after intravenous administration of technetium-99m–labeled

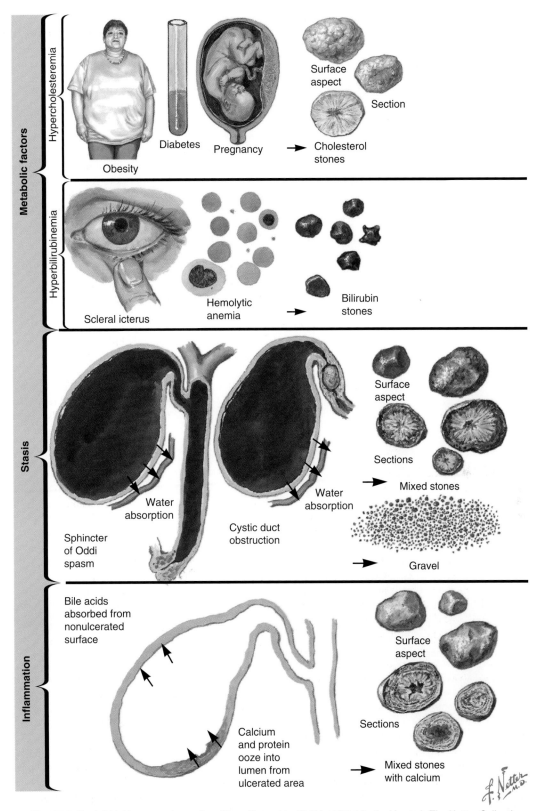

Fig. 45.2 Cholelithiasis: stone formation. (From Reynolds JC, Ward PJ, Martin JA, et al. *The Netter Collection of Medical Illustrations*, 2nd edition, Volume 9, Digestive System, Part III: Liver, Biliary Tract, and Pancreas. Elsevier, 2016, Plate 2-13, Page 116.)

diisopropyl iminodiacetic acid (DISIDA) or hepatobiliary iminodiacetic acid (HIDA) is also accurate. If the gallbladder fills with the isotope, acute cholecystitis is highly unlikely; if contrast material enters the bile duct and duodenum without gallbladder visualization, acute cholecystitis is strongly supported.

Because of the high risk for recurrent acute cholecystitis, most patients need to undergo cholecystectomy, which is often performed within the first 24 to 48 hours after presentation or, less often, 4 to 8 weeks after an acute episode (Fig. 45.4). Cholecystostomy may be performed for patients who have a high operative risk. Antibiotics are

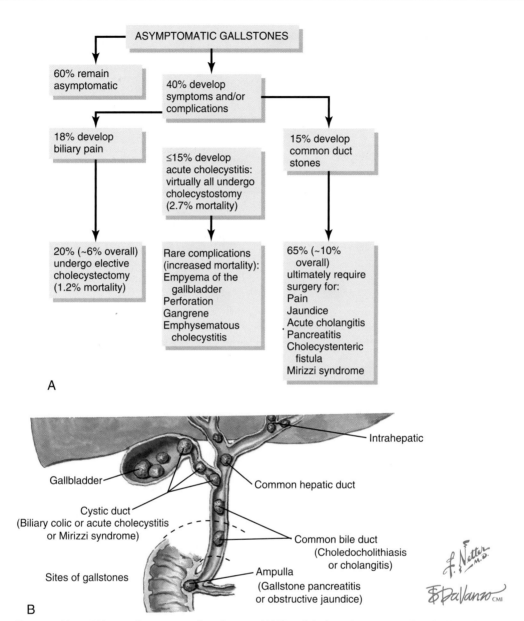

Fig. 45.3 Natural history of asymptomatic gallstones. (A) The clinical syndromes associated with gallstones are shown, and the numbers represent the approximate percentage of adults who develop one or more of these symptoms or complications over a 15- to 20-year period. Over this period, about 30% of individuals with gallstones undergo surgery. (The risk for developing complications of gallstones varies considerably among series. The figures shown represent those derived from more recent studies.) (B) Clinical manifestations of symptomatic gallstones. Locations of blockages associated with various conditions are indicated. (Part B from Reynolds JC, Ward PJ, Martin JA, et al. *The Netter Collection of Medical Illustrations*, 2nd edition, Volume 9, Digestive System, Part III: Liver, Biliary Tract, and Pancreas. Elsevier, 2016, Plate 2-14, Page 117.)

typically used when fever or leukocytosis is present. Expectant management is reserved for patients with uncomplicated disease who are not good operative candidates and those in whom the diagnosis is not clear.

Acalculous Cholecystitis

Acalculous cholecystitis is an acute inflammatory condition in patients without gallstones. It accounts for approximately 5% of all cases of acute cholecystitis and carries higher morbidity and mortality rates than acute calculous cholecystitis. Acalculous cholecystitis is classically associated with the triad of prolonged fasting, immobility, and hemodynamic instability, such as may occur in critically ill patients, especially if they have required total parenteral nutrition or blood transfusions. Gallbladder ischemia and stasis are considered important

in the pathogenesis. It is also seen in patients with AIDS, often in association with cytomegalovirus or *Cryptosporidia* infection. Abdominal pain, fever, and leukocytosis in a patient with the classic triad along with ultrasonographic features of a thickened gallbladder wall and a positive Murphy sign in the absence of gallstones raise suspicion for this entity. As in acute cholecystitis, the gallbladder is not visualized on HIDA scanning. Management includes administration of antibiotics and cholecystectomy. If the patient is seriously ill, the gallbladder can be drained percutaneously as a temporizing measure that can bridge the patient to surgery. If a patient is not a candidate for cholecystectomy, some specialized centers have expertise in endoscopically placing a lumen opposing metal stent directly from the stomach or duodenum into the gallbladder for drainage.

TABLE 45.2   Differential Diagnosis of Cholelithiasis

Peptic ulcer disease
Gastroesophageal reflux disease
Nonulcer dyspepsia
Irritable bowel syndrome
Sphincter of Oddi dysfunction
Hepatitis and perihepatitis (Fitz-Hugh–Curtis syndrome)
Hepatic abscess
Nephrolithiasis
Pyelonephritis
Perinephric abscess
Pneumonia
Angina pectoris
Pancreatitis
Ruptured ectopic pregnancy
Appendicitis

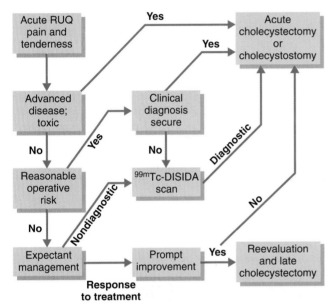

Fig. 45.4 Algorithm for management of right upper quadrant (RUQ) pain and tenderness in patients with suspected acute cholecystitis. This scheme is based on a policy of early operation (conventional or laparoscopic) for appropriate patients and use of cholecystostomy (operative or percutaneous) for patients who are poor operative risks. *99mTc-DISIDA*, Technetium-99m–labeled diisopropyl iminodiacetic acid.

Chronic Cholecystitis

Chronic cholecystitis is a term used by pathologists to describe chronic inflammatory cell infiltration of the gallbladder on histopathology. Chronic cholecystitis is thought to be an evolving inflammatory process, caused by repeated episodes of low-grade gallbladder obstruction over a period of days to years resulting in recurrent mucosal trauma and inflammation. The symptoms are those of biliary colic without clinical features of acute cholecystitis. Gallstones are the causative agent in most patients. However, there is little correlation between the number of gallstones and the degree of gallbladder wall inflammation. In approximately 12% of patients with chronic cholecystitis, there are no demonstrable stones. The diagnosis is made in a patient with gallstones who has the clinical signs and symptoms with no other obvious cause. Transabdominal ultrasound is the best initial test, and EUS may be used to demonstrate microlithiasis (gallstones ≤3 mm) if gallstones

are not seen on initial imaging. The treatment is laparoscopic cholecystectomy, but conversion to open cholecystectomy is required in up to 5% of cases.

Gallbladder Polyps

Gallbladder polyps are outgrowths of the gallbladder mucosal wall that are seen in up to 5% of normal subjects undergoing gallbladder ultrasonography. Most of these lesions are not neoplastic but are hyperplastic or represent lipid deposits (cholesterolosis). The differential diagnosis includes cholesterol polyps, adenomyomatosis, inflammatory polyps, adenomas, and gallbladder cancer. Factors associated with increased risk of malignancy include age greater than 60 years, size greater than 1 cm, presence of gallstones, and increased size on subsequent imaging. Cholecystectomy is indicated if one or more of these risk factors are present or if the patient has biliary symptoms. Polyps that are smaller than 1 cm should be monitored with periodic ultrasound examination.

Gallbladder Carcinoma

Gallbladder carcinoma is relatively uncommon but has a high case fatality rate. The incidence and mortality are higher in Latin American countries (e.g., Chile) and in Southeast Asia. Carcinoma of the gallbladder often produces advanced disseminated disease with weight loss, jaundice, pruritus, and a large right upper quadrant mass. Symptoms may resemble those of acute or chronic cholecystitis, particularly if the tumor is small. Risk factors include gallbladder polyps, porcelain gallbladder, choledochal cysts, gallstones, and anomalous pancreaticobiliary junction. Although early-stage tumors can be treated surgically, most cases are diagnosed at an advanced stage and are incurable.

Gallbladder Dyskinesia

Gallbladder dyskinesia is a disorder caused by abnormal motility or contraction of the gallbladder in the absence of gallstones resulting in symptoms of biliary colic. Laboratory studies and abdominal imaging findings are usually normal. HIDA scanning may show a decreased gallbladder ejection fraction, or there may be reproducible pain with administration of cholecystokinin (CCK). Cholecystectomy commonly shows acalculous cholecystitis.

BILIARY TRACT DISORDERS

Choledocholithiasis

In Western countries, most stones found in the common bile duct (choledocholithiasis) originate in the gallbladder. Up to 15% of individuals with cholelithiasis develop choledocholithiasis (Fig. 45.5). Less commonly, stones may form de novo in the biliary tree. Common bile duct stones may be asymptomatic (30% to 40%), or they may produce biliary colic and jaundice. Two major complications are acute cholangitis and acute pancreatitis. The diagnosis is supported by the results of liver function tests and abdominal imaging. Transabdominal ultrasound is the initial imaging modality of choice; it has a sensitivity of 20% to 90% for detection of a stone and 55% to 90% for detection of dilation of the common bile duct. EUS and MRCP have replaced ERCP for diagnosis of bile duct stones; the sensitivity and specificity are 94% and 95%, respectively, for EUS and 93% and 94% for MRCP. ERCP is reserved for therapeutic interventions.

Acute Cholangitis

Acute (suppurative) cholangitis is a life-threatening infection of the biliary tract that can occur as a result of choledocholithiasis. The biliary tree is usually a sterile environment. In the setting of obstruction, migration of bacterial pathogens can cause severe infection with a mortality rate up to 30%. The classic clinical manifestations are abdominal

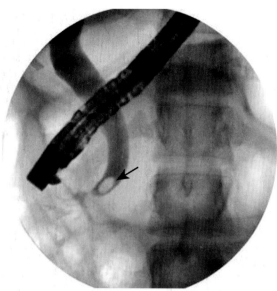

Fig. 45.5 Cholangiogram obtained on endoscopic retrograde cholangiopancreatography demonstrates a common bile duct stone.

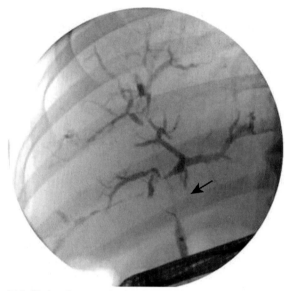

Fig. 45.6 Cholangiogram obtained on endoscopic retrograde cholangiopancreatography demonstrates a Klatskin tumor at the bile duct bifurcation.

pain, jaundice, and fever (Charcot's triad). It is important to note that clinical findings may be absent or atypical in elderly or immunosuppressed patients. Cholangitis can be mild, moderate, or severe and, if severe, rapidly lead to sepsis, shock, and death. Diagnosis is based on a compatible clinical and laboratory picture (abnormal liver function test results and leukocytosis) together with radiologic or endoscopic evidence of common bile duct stones.

Treatment of acute cholangitis includes administration of broad-spectrum antibiotics and prompt removal of stones, typically with ERCP and sphincterotomy (Video 45.2). The timing of ERCP should be planned based on the severity of illness. Cholecystectomy is subsequently performed after the patient has been stabilized.

Gallstone Pancreatitis

Biochemical evidence of pancreatic inflammation complicates choledocholithiasis and acute cholecystitis in up to 30% and 15% of patients, respectively. There are two proposed mechanisms by which gallstones may induce pancreatitis: reflux of bile into the pancreatic duct due to transient obstruction of the ampulla and obstruction at the ampulla secondary to stones or edema. Evaluation of the biliary tree with transabdominal ultrasound, MRCP, or endoscopic ultrasound should be performed in the setting of gallstone pancreatitis to evaluate for choledocholithiasis. Laboratory testing alone can be misleading because edema of the head of pancreas during pancreatitis can cause cholestasis. If choledocholithiasis is confirmed, ERCP with sphincterotomy should be performed. Considering that gallstone pancreatitis recurs in 25% of patients, a cholecystectomy should be performed once the patient has recovered clinically from an attack of pancreatitis.

Biliary Neoplasms

Cholangiocarcinoma and cancer of the ampulla of Vater are uncommon in the United States. Cholangiocarcinoma can arise at any level of the biliary system and is classified as intrahepatic (25%) or extrahepatic (75%). It is more common in older men, occurring predominantly in men 50 to 70 years of age. Risk factors include primary sclerosing cholangitis (PSC), choledochal cysts, chronic ulcerative colitis, liver flukes, and recurrent pyogenic cholangitis (Oriental cholangiohepatitis). Patients with these cancers usually have unremitting painless jaundice, although necrosis and sloughing of the tumor can cause intermittent biliary obstruction and the appearance of occult fecal blood.

Cholangiocarcinoma located at the bifurcation of the extrahepatic bile duct (50% of cases) is known as a *Klatskin tumor* (Fig. 45.6). Surgical cure is possible in only a small proportion of patients with cholangiocarcinoma. If the tumor is unresectable, palliative biliary drainage may be indicated. Recently, liver transplant has also become an option for carefully selected patients with localized, but unresectable disease.

Nonmalignant Causes of Biliary Obstruction
Biliary Strictures

Benign biliary strictures usually result from surgical injury or chronic pancreatitis. Biliary strictures resulting from surgical injury may cause symptoms even years after the initial injury. Early diagnosis is important because strictures that partially obstruct are clinically asymptomatic and can cause secondary biliary cirrhosis. Biliary stricture should be suspected in any patient with a history of surgery of the right upper quadrant or chronic pancreatitis who has persistently elevated levels of serum alkaline phosphatase and γ-glutamyl transpeptidase. Endoscopic balloon catheter dilatation with or without stenting or surgical repair is useful in selected patients.

Other Causes of Biliary Obstruction

Structural abnormalities such as choledochal cysts, Caroli's disease (congenital segmental intrahepatic bile duct dilation), and duodenal diverticula may cause bile duct obstruction, often with secondary choledocholithiasis resulting from bile stasis. Hemobilia, with intermittent bile duct obstruction by blood clots, may be caused by hepatic injury, neoplasms, or hepatic artery aneurysms. Biliary parasites should always be considered as a cause of biliary obstruction in the appropriate epidemiologic setting. *Ascaris lumbricoides* is a common cause of cholangitis and jaundice in South America, Africa, and the Indian subcontinent. *Clonorchis sinensis* is the etiologic agent of Oriental cholangiohepatitis in Korea and Southeast Asia and in immigrants to the United States. The liver fluke *Fasciola hepatica* is a leading cause of biliary strictures and cholangitis worldwide, most commonly in the Bolivian Andes.

Primary Sclerosing Cholangitis

PSC is an idiopathic condition of nonmalignant, nonbacterial, chronic inflammatory fibrosis and obliteration of the intrahepatic and

ERCP is an effective treatment of cholestasis in selected patients. Most patients with advanced PSC eventually progress to end-stage liver disease, and evaluation for liver transplantation is appropriate in advanced disease. One third of patients with PSC will develop cholangiocarcinoma; therefore, thorough clinical and laboratory studies (liver function tests and cancer markers such as CA 19-9) and radiologic follow-up are warranted.

Sphincter of Oddi Dysfunction

Sphincter of Oddi dysfunction is a benign disorder that can lead to noncalculous obstruction of the flow of bile or pancreatic juice at the level of the pancreaticobiliary junction. Patients typically have unexplained biliary-type abdominal pain with or without elevated results on liver function tests and with or without bile duct dilation. In a selected group of patients, endoscopic or surgical sphincterotomy is of value. Identifying those who would benefit can be challenging and controversial because sphincter of Oddi dysfunction can be difficult to discern from functional abdominal pain.

For a deeper discussion of this topic, please see Chapter 146, "Diseases of the Gallbladder and Bile Ducts," in *Goldman-Cecil Medicine*, 26th Edition.

Acknowledgment

The authors gratefully acknowledge the work of Matthew P. Spinn, who contributed this chapter to the previous edition.

SUGGESTED READINGS

Adeel S, Khan AS, Dageforde LA: Cholangiocarcinoma, Surg Clin North Am 99(2):315–335, 2019.

Hyun JJ, Kozarek RA: Sphincter of Oddi dysfunction: sphincter of Oddi dysfunction or discordance? What is the state of the art in 2018? Curr Opin Gastroenterol 34(5):282–287, 2018.

Pezzilli R, Zerbi A, Campra D, Capurso G, Golfieri R, Arcidiacono PG, et al: Consensus guidelines on severe acute pancreatitis, Dig Liver Dis 47(7):532–543, 2015.

Sulzer JK, Ocuin LM: Cholangitis, Surg Clin North Am 99(2):175–184, 2019.

Tazuma S, Unno M, Igarashi Y, Inui K, Uchiyama K, Kai M, et al: Evidence-based clinical practice guidelines for cholelithiasis 2016, J Gastroenterol 52(3):276–300, 2017.

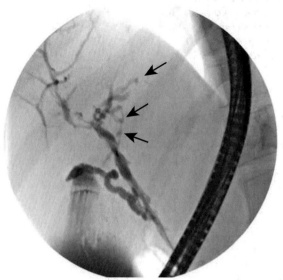

Fig. 45.7 Cholangiogram obtained on endoscopic retrograde cholangiopancreatography demonstrates the characteristic beading of the intrahepatic and extrahepatic bile ducts in a patient with primary sclerosing cholangitis.

extrahepatic bile ducts. It most commonly occurs in young men (two thirds of patients are younger than 45 years of age), often in association with ulcerative colitis. Approximately 70% of patients with PSC have ulcerative colitis. The clinical spectrum of PSC is broad, ranging from asymptomatic patients with abnormal liver enzyme levels (typically an elevated alkaline phosphatase concentration) to patients with recurring episodes of fever, chills, abdominal pain, and jaundice. The diagnosis of PSC is made by MRCP or ERCP, which show characteristic changes (beading) of the intrahepatic and/or extrahepatic bile duct (Fig. 45.7).

No proven therapy exists for PSC, although ursodeoxycholic acid and methotrexate are being used in some centers. Other forms of therapy include prophylactic antibiotics for prevention of recurrent bacterial cholangitis, treatment of pruritus, and repletion of fat-soluble vitamins. Endoscopic dilatation of a dominant biliary stricture during

Hematologic Disease

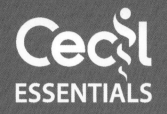

46

Hematopoiesis and Hematopoietic Failure

Eunice S. Wang, Nancy Berliner

HEMATOPOIESIS

Hematopoiesis is the process of formation and development of blood cells. The constituents of peripheral blood arise by a complex and carefully regulated process of ontogeny. The pluripotent hematopoietic stem cell (HSC) maintains itself by self-renewal and undergoes multilineage differentiation to generate the appropriate numbers and types of cells in the circulating blood compartment (Table 46.1). The hematopoietic system is unique in that it is constantly undergoing this full cycle of maturation by which a primitive cell develops into a variety of highly specialized end-stage cells, all of which have different lifespans and occur in different quantities.

The bone marrow must have the capacity to produce cells to compensate for the normal rapid turnover of hematopoietic cells resulting from senescence, normal use, and migration into tissue spaces. It must have a reserve capacity to produce additional cells in response to unusual demands that arise from bleeding, infection, or other stresses. Understanding the repeated cycle of cellular ontogeny and self-renewal that meets these challenges provides important insights into normal and pathologic mechanisms in hematology.

Hematopoietic Tissues

Hematopoiesis commences in the embryonic yolk sac, in which early erythroblasts in blood islands form the first hemoglobinized cells. After 6 weeks' gestation, the fetal liver begins producing primitive lymphocytoid cells, megakaryocytes, and erythroblasts, and the spleen becomes a secondary site of erythropoiesis. Hematopoiesis then shifts to its definitive long-term site in the bone marrow, the principal site for lifelong hematopoiesis in the normal host.

Early in life, all fetal bones contain regenerative bone marrow, but the marrow becomes progressively replaced by fat with age. In adults, active marrow resides only in the axial skeleton (i.e., sternum, vertebrae, pelvis, and ribs) and in the proximal ends of the femur and humerus. Consequently, bone marrow samples, which are needed for many hematologic diagnoses, are usually obtained from the iliac crest or sternum. Under pathologic conditions that stress the capacity of the marrow space, as seen in diseases associated with marrow fibrosis (e.g., chronic myeloproliferative diseases) or in severe inherited hemolytic anemia (e.g., thalassemia major), extramedullary hematopoiesis may be reestablished in sites of fetal hematopoiesis, especially the spleen.

Stem Cell Theory of Hematopoiesis

All mature hematopoietic cells are hypothesized to originate from a small population of pluripotent stem cells. Comprising less than 1% of all cells in the bone marrow, these cells bear no distinctive morphologic markings and are best defined by their unique functional properties.

Stem cells have two distinctive characteristics. First, they are highly resilient and productive, capable of continuously replenishing huge numbers of granulocytes, lymphocytes, and erythrocytes throughout life. The demand for a continuous, fluctuating supply of blood cells requires a hematopoietic system capable of producing large numbers of selected cells in a short time. For example, overwhelming infection by invading microorganisms triggers the release of neutrophils, whereas hypoxia or acute blood loss leads to increased red blood cell production. Second, HSCs represent a self-renewing cell population that is able to maintain its numbers while providing a continued supply of progenitor cells of many different lineages.

Despite their vast proliferative potential, under normal conditions, most HSCs are quiescent, and few cells undergo expansion or differentiation at any one time. However, their ability to proliferate is striking. Studies with lethally irradiated mice have demonstrated the ability of a few transplanted cells (i.e., spleen colony-forming unit [CFU-S] cells) to regenerate multilineage hematopoiesis.

The signals regulating the differentiation of pluripotent stem cells into committed progenitors are unknown. Data suggest that the first step in lineage commitment is a stochastic (chance) event; subsequent stages of maturation are hypothesized to occur under the influence of growth factors, or cytokines (Table 46.2). Cytokines act on different cells through specific cytokine receptors. Receptor activation induces signal-transduction pathways that lead to changes in gene transcription and eventual cell proliferation and differentiation. These growth factors also act as survival factors for the developing hematopoietic cells by preventing *apoptosis* (i.e., programmed cell death). This process occurs in the cellular milieu of the bone marrow, where hematopoiesis depends in part on the nonhematopoietic cells (i.e., fibroblasts, endothelial cells, osteoblasts, and fat cells) that make up that microenvironment. Research in HSC biology has focused on how these cells are regulated by growth factors, unique cell surface ligands, and key interactions between stem cells and the surrounding microenvironmental cells (i.e., mesenchymal stromal cells, adipocytes, immune cells) within specialized marrow regions termed *stem cell niches*.

Hematopoietic Differentiation Pathway

Hematopoiesis has been hypothesized to proceed along a tightly regulated hierarchy (Fig. 46.1) governed by effects of intrinsic transcription factors and cytokines in the bone marrow microenvironment. As more primitive cells mature under the influence of specific regulatory cytokines, they undergo several cell divisions and become *progenitor cells* committed to one lineage. They also lose their self-renewal capacity. Morphologically, these cells are transformed from nonspecific blast-like cells into cells that can be identified by their color, shape, and granular and nuclear content. Functionally, they acquire distinguishing cell surface receptors and responses to specific signals.

Maturing granulocytes and erythroid cells undergo several more cell divisions in the bone marrow, whereas lymphocytes travel to the thymus and lymph nodes for further development. Megakaryocytes cease cellular

TABLE 46.1   Normal Values for Peripheral Blood Cells

Cell Type and Size	Mean	Range
Hemoglobin	Women: 14 g/dL	Women: 12-16 g/dL
	Men: 15.5 g/dL	Men: 13.5-17.5 g/dL
Hematocrit	Women: 41%	Women: 36-46%
	Men: 47%	Men: 41-53%
Reticulocyte count	60,000/μL (1%)	35,000-85,000/μL (0.5-1.5%)
Mean corpuscular volume		80-100 fL
Platelet count	250,000/μL	150,000-400,000/μL
Total white blood cell count	7400/μL	4500-11,000/μL
Neutrophils	4400/μL (40-60%)	1800-7700/μL
Lymphocytes	2500/μL (20-40%)	1000-4800/μL
Monocytes	300/μL (<5%)	200-950 (4-11%)

TABLE 46.2   Cytokines and Their Activities

Acronym	Name	Effects on Hematopoiesis (and Possible Clinical Applications)
EPO	Erythropoietin	Stimulation of proliferation and maturation of erythroid progenitors; produced by the kidney in response to anemia and hypoxia; important clinically for treatment of anemia associated with low EPO levels (e.g., renal failure, anemia of chronic disease)
G-CSF	Granulocyte colony-stimulating factor	Stimulation of proliferation and maturation of granulocytes; more broad-based effect because also increases release of stem cells in peripheral blood; clinically important for treatment of neutropenia and mobilization of stem cells for transplantation
GM-CSF	Granulocyte-monocyte colony-stimulating factor	Proliferation of granulocyte and monocyte precursors; role unclear in steady-state hematopoiesis (mice deficient in GM-CSF gene still develop normally and no major perturbation of hematopoiesis up to 12 weeks of age)
TPO	Thrombopoietin	Proliferation of megakaryocytes; clinical studies of recombinant TPO were discontinued due to auto-antibody formation in individual patients
M-CSF	Monocyte colony-stimulating factor	Proliferation of monocytes
IL-2	Interleukin-2	Proliferation of T cells
IL-3	Interleukin-3 (multi–colony-stimulating factor)	Proliferation of granulocytes, monocytes; broad-based effects, appearing to increase the proliferation of stem cells; not in use clinically, differentiation of basophils and eosinophils from primitive hematopoietic stem cells
IL-4	Interleukin-4	Proliferation of B cells, differentiation of basophils and eosinophils
IL-5	Interleukin-5	Proliferation of T cells, B cells; proliferation and differentiation of eosinophils, differentiation of basophils and eosinophils
IL-11	Interleukin-11	Proliferation of megakaryocytes; undergoing clinical testing
LIF	Leukemia inhibitory factor	Proliferation of stem cells and megakaryocytes
SCF	Stem cell factor (kit ligand)	Proliferation of progenitor cells; broad-based effects on multiple lineages

division but continue with nuclear replication. Eventually, these cells are released from the marrow as fully functional erythrocytes, mast cells, granulocytes, monocytes, eosinophils, macrophages, and platelets.

Pluripotent Stem Cells

The pluripotent HSC is morphologically indistinguishable and is best identified by its expression of the cell differentiation antigen, CD34,

and by its ability to form pluripotent colonies in vitro. Under the influence of interleukin-1 (IL-1), IL-3, IL-6, FMS-like tyrosine kinase 3 (FLT3), and a specific stem cell factor (KIT ligand [KITLG], or steel factor), this cell matures into a myeloid-lineage stem cell (i.e., granulocyte-erythrocyte-macrophage-megakaryocyte colony-forming unit [CFU-GEMM] cell) or a lymphoid-lineage stem cell. In the presence of granulocyte-macrophage colony-stimulating factor (GM-CSF) and

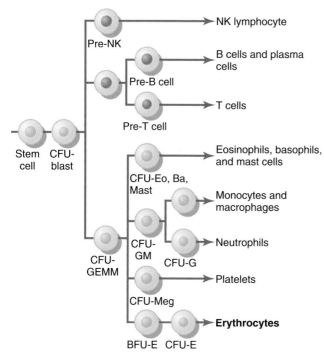

Fig. 46.1 Development of bone marrow cells. *Ba,* Basophil; *BFU,* blast-forming unit; *CFU,* colony-forming unit; *E,* erythroid; *Eo,* eosinophil; *G,* granulocyte; *GEMM,* granulocyte-erythrocyte-macrophage-megakaryocyte; *GM,* granulocyte-macrophage; *Meg,* megakaryocyte; *NK,* natural killer.

TABLE 46.3 **Differential Diagnosis Of Pancytopenia**
Primary bone marrow disorders
• Aplastic anemia
• Congenital aplastic anemia syndromes
• Fanconi anemia
• Shwachman-Diamond syndrome
• Congenital dyskeratosis
• Acquired aplastic anemia
• Hypocellular myelodysplastic syndrome
• Myelofibrosis
• Paroxysmal nocturnal hemoglobinuria
• Acute leukemias: acute lymphocytic leukemia, acute myeloid leukemia
• Hairy cell leukemia
Systemic diseases with secondary bone marrow effects
• Metastatic solid tumor to marrow
• Autoimmune disorders: systemic lupus erythematosus, Sjögren's syndrome
• Nutritional deficiencies: vitamin B_{12}, folate, alcoholism
• Infections: overwhelming sepsis from any cause, viruses, brucellosis, ehrlichiosis (mycobacteria)
• Storage diseases: Gaucher's disease, Niemann-Pick disease
• Anatomic defects: hypersplenism

IL-3, the myeloid stem cell further differentiates into daughter cells of its named lineages (see Fig. 46.1). The lymphopoietic stem cell becomes a pre-B cell or a prothymocyte (pre-T cell) and leaves the marrow for further maturation.

Erythroid Lineage

Primitive erythroid precursors arising from the myeloid stem cell are called burst-forming unit–erythroid cells. These cells then differentiate into erythroid colony-forming unit (CFU-E) cells, which are the committed progenitor cells of erythrocytes. CFU-E cells express receptors for erythropoietin (EPO), an 18-kD molecule produced by renal interstitial cells in response to low oxygenation states or anemia. EPO upregulates proliferation of CFU-E cells and promotes their maturation into proerythroblasts and reticulocytes, which begin to synthesize hemoglobin (see Table 46.2).

Granulocyte and Monocyte Lineages

Human GM-CSF acts early in the hematopoietic pathway to regulate maturation of the CFU-GEMM stem cell. Differentiation of this myeloid precursor into specific committed progenitors occurs under the direction of granulocyte CSF (G-CSF) and monocyte CSF (see Table 46.2). Granulocyte CFU cells undergo sequential transformation into easily recognizable myeloblasts, myelocytes, and eventually early polymorphonuclear neutrophils with their characteristic polysegmented nuclei. Monocyte CFU cells, in contrast, retain a single nucleus as they mature from monoblasts to promonocytes to monocytes and sometimes to macrophages.

Other Lineages

Eosinophils and basophils develop from CFU-GEMM cells under the influence of IL-5 and IL-3 plus IL-4, respectively. The acquisition of their specific granular contents helps in distinguishing their precursors from those of early monocytes.

The development of platelets is morphologically distinct from the other lineages. CFU-GEMM cells differentiate into megakaryocyte CFU cells, so named because the cells cease cell division early but not nuclear replication. Megakaryocytes are the only cells in the body with the capacity to double their DNA content (i.e., endomitosis). Over the course of several cell cycles, the maturing megakaryocyte eventually acquires several times the nuclear content of other cells in preparation for its eventual dissolution into platelets with a fraction of the cytoplasm of other hematopoietic cells. Two growth factors, thrombopoietin (TPO) and IL-11, increase platelet counts by promoting megakaryocyte development (see Table 46.2).

Stem Cell Plasticity

Provocative data have challenged the conventional paradigm of hierarchical HSC differentiation. Laboratory evidence has demonstrated that HSCs can be induced to dedifferentiate into more immature progenitors that have the ability to cross lineages and transdifferentiate into myriad non-lymphohematopoietic cells such as vascular endothelial precursors, myocytes, hepatocytes, gastrointestinal epithelial cells, and neurons. This plasticity of HSCs constitutes an intrinsic property of adult stem cells and/or fusion of hematopoietic cells with other tissue cells and supports further investigation of adult HSCs as a dynamic, renewable resource for tissue repair and regeneration.

PRIMARY HEMATOPOIETIC FAILURE SYNDROMES

Diseases of the HSC that disrupt the normal regulated pattern of stem cell development can result in underproduction of mature progeny (i.e., aplastic anemia), overproduction of mature progeny (i.e., chronic myeloproliferative disease), or failed differentiation with the production of excess immature forms (i.e., myelodysplasia and acute leukemia). *Hematopoietic failure,* defined as the inability of HSCs to produce normal numbers of mature blood cells, manifests clinically as peripheral pancytopenia (i.e., decreased production of all blood cell lineages).

Although marrow dysfunction producing pancytopenia can result from several hematologic and nonhematologic causes (Table 46.3), primary bone marrow failure disorders are characterized by a profound impairment of the ability of the HSC to replenish the stem cell pool. Marrow failure syndromes can arise from intrinsic HSC defects including germline inherited disposition and age-related clonal hematopoietic mutational events. In other cases, marrow failure disorders are the result of extrinsic damage to normal HSCs. The treatment modalities for primary hematopoietic failure disorders include exogenous growth factor administration, immunosuppressive therapy, and allogeneic stem cell transplantation.

Growth Factors in Clinical Use

Discovery of the factors that influence normal hematopoiesis led to important therapeutic applications for patients with defects in hematopoietic cell production. The finding that committed hematopoietic cells of each lineage can be stimulated to proliferate and differentiate by specific cytokines (see Table 46.2) has been therapeutically useful. Advances in DNA technology led to the synthesis and purification of recombinant human (rh) proteins with similar biologic activity in vivo. Administration of these products to patients enabled successful manipulation of mature cells in the peripheral blood. For example, exogenous EPO has become a mainstay in the management of anemia caused by renal failure, chemotherapy, and marrow failure syndromes. The use of G-CSF or GM-CSF in patients with febrile neutropenia and documented infection or sepsis after chemotherapy or radiation therapy has reduced hospital stays and shortened the period of high infection risk. Administration of GM-CSF is thought to improve host immune responses to fungal infections. High-dose G-CSF also is routinely used to mobilize CD34$^+$ marrow stem cells into the peripheral blood for collection before and after stem cell transplantation in patients with delayed stem cell engraftment (discussed later).

Early trials of TPO growth factors to stimulate platelet production were halted because of development of antihuman TPO antibodies in some patients, leading to severe thrombocytopenia. Second-generation thrombopoietic agents bearing no structural resemblance to TPO but designed to bind and activate the TPO receptor are in clinical use. Romiplostim is a recombinant Fc-peptide fusion protein termed a peptibody that when given as a weekly subcutaneous injection can increase platelet counts, decrease platelet transfusion requirements, and improve quality of life for patients with refractory chronic immune-mediated thrombocytopenia. Eltrombopag is an orally available, small, organic TPO agonist that increases platelet counts and decreases bleeding in similar patients. The clinical utility of eltrombopag when added to immunosuppressive regimens for treatment of aplastic anemia supports its role as an activator of HSC production.

Hematopoietic Stem Cell Transplantation
Types of Transplantations

Improved understanding of HSC biology has fostered the development of techniques to manipulate these cells for therapeutic purposes. The antitumor effects of most chemotherapeutic drugs and radiation therapy are dose dependent, and both cause the major dose-limiting toxicity of myelosuppression. Several modes of stem cell transplantation have been developed.

In *autologous transplantation*, the patient's bone marrow or peripheral blood stem cells (PBSCs) are collected during remission after high-dose chemotherapy or G-CSF administration. These cells are cryopreserved, thawed, and reinfused. This approach incurs a higher risk of relapse as a result of reinfusion of a stem cell product that may remain contaminated with tumor cells and is generally considered therapeutically equivalent to administration of multiple cycles of high-dose chemotherapy with noncurative intent.

In *allogeneic stem cell transplantation (alloSCT),* abnormally functioning hematopoietic bone marrow is eradicated and replaced with normal bone marrow or stem cells from a compatible source either from a related or unrelated donor. High-dose chemotherapy with or without total body irradiation is used to destroy the patient's marrow, followed by infusion of new stem cells that engraft and restore normal hematopoiesis. Treatment-related mortality and morbidity occurs due to infectious complications during cytopenic periods and development of *graft-versus-host disease (GVHD),* an autoimmune phenomenon in which intact lymphocytes in the transplanted marrow attack the host tissues. Despite improvements in supportive care and immunomodulatory therapy, mortality rates associated with transplant remain in the range of 10% to 30% even in younger patients. To mitigate the risk of GVHD, all potential donors and patients are tested for compatibility of human leukocyte antigen (HLA) and major and minor histocompatibility complex (MHC) proteins expressed on all cells. Three major HLA class I antigens (i.e., A, B, and C) and three MHC class II antigens (i.e., DP, DQ, and DR) have been identified. The HLA gene loci are tightly linked on chromosome 6 and are almost always inherited on a single cluster of genes, or *haplotype.* All children are a half-match (i.e., haploidentical) to each of their parents, and full siblings have a 25% probability of being HLA identical to one another. HLA-matched, nonrelated transplants have higher rates of GVHD than transplants from HLA-matched, related donors as a result of other minor HLA incompatibilities. Patients who receive an HLA-mismatched stem cell transplantation risk acute GVHD, marrow rejection, and fatal marrow aplasia. Morbidity and mortality rates associated with non–HLA-compatible transplants can be prohibitive. Patients younger than 50 years are considered the best candidates for this intensive therapy, although this is changing in the setting of newer supportive modalities.

It is now believed that the immunologic effects of transplanted allogeneic cells are as important as or more important than cytoreduction in effecting cure of hematologic malignancies. Evidence indicates that the excellent response of patients to alloSCT may largely be related to the active suppression of the patient's original (residual) or relapsing disease by donor immune cells from the newly transplanted donor graft, referred to as the *graft-versus-leukemia (GVL) effect.* Studies have documented that donor lymphocyte infusions (DLI) can restore remission in patients with early evidence of relapse after alloSCT for chronic myelogenous leukemia. Conversely, procedures that minimize the reactivity between donor and host increase disease relapse. For example, there is an increased rate of relapse among patients who undergo syngeneic (identical twin) stem cell transplantation and patients who receive T-cell–depleted marrow in an attempt to reduce GVHD.

Recognition of the immunologic benefits of alloSCT has led to the development of *reduced intensity* (also known as *non-myeloablative*) allogeneic stem cell transplants. These transplants are now standard of care in adult patients otherwise ineligible for traditional myeloablative transplantation regimens due to age (>55 years old) other comorbidities, or without fully HLA-matched donors available. Conditioning and immunosuppressive regimens are administered in doses sufficient to permit donor stem cell engraftment without aggressive cytoreduction. These so-called "mini" transplants result in chimeric marrows (i.e., part patient and part donor) and are not characterized by significant periods of cytopenias or hematopoietic compromise. Most responding patients convert to a fully donor-derived marrow over time. The use of newer immunosuppressive regimens has also allowed patients to receive transplants from related family members who are only 50% HLA matched (so called *haplotype identical* or *haploidentical* transplants). Almost all patients have compatible half-matched parents, siblings, children, or even grandchildren, thereby allowing for multiple family members to serve as donors. Although feasible and well tolerated in many patients, haploidentical transplants are associated with an enhanced risk of relapsed disease due to reduced GVL effects and therefore are best utilized for those with optimal disease control at time of the procedure. Although historically used in the treatment of primary malignant stem cell disorders such as leukemia, the therapeutic potential of alloSCT is now increasingly being employed for patients with nonmalignant hematologic conditions (e.g., aplastic anemia, sickle cell anemia, congenital immunodeficiencies), solid tumors (e.g., renal cell carcinoma, melanoma), and particularly autoimmune diseases (e.g., amyloidosis, systemic lupus, multiple sclerosis).

Hematopoietic Stem Cell Sources

Historically, alloSCT has employed donor bone marrow stem cells aspirated from the posterior iliac crest and intravenously infused after myeloablation and immunosuppressive therapy. The process of engraftment or reconstitution of normal hematopoietic function takes several weeks. Patients often require almost daily platelet and red blood cell transfusions, and they are hospitalized during this period of prolonged neutropenia to minimize life-threatening bacterial, viral, and fungal infections. Other complications include severe mucositis, hemorrhagic cystitis, GVHD, relapsed disease, and graft failure.

The discovery that high-dose G-CSF treatment mobilizes large numbers of CD34+ hematopoietic progenitor and stem cells from bone marrow sites into circulating blood (i.e., 10-fold to 15-fold increase over baseline levels) has led to the routine use of PBSCs collected by apheresis procedures in place of bone marrow stem cells for allogeneic transplantation. Compared with marrow-derived stem cells, PBSCs engraft more rapidly after myeloablation. Patients receiving allogeneic PBSC transplants have decreased neutrophil recovery time, lower transfusion requirements, fewer inpatient hospital days, and similar rates of acute GVHD and long-term survival outcomes as traditional marrow-transplanted patients. Because PBSC collections often contain 3-fold to 4-fold more CD34+ stem cells and 10-fold more lymphoid cells than harvested marrow grafts, higher rates of chronic GVHD may occur.

Umbilical cord blood (UCB) stem cells constitute a rich source of immature CD34+ HSCs. In the past, the less stringent HLA-compatibility requirements for UCB HSC matches has allowed the use of these transplants as a therapy for patients lacking fully compatible HLA-matched donors. Although still considered experimental, some transplantation centers have reported long-term outcomes after UCB HSC transplants similar to those for conventional marrow or peripheral PBSC transplants for primary hematologic diseases. However, the relatively limited numbers of CD34+ stem cells found in harvested UCB units accounts for a much slower hematopoietic recovery after the procedure and a statistically higher risk for nonengraftment compared with other stem cell sources. For this reason, UCB transplantation procedures have been limited to pediatric patients and smaller adults or to adult patients for whom there is more than one HLA-compatible UCB unit.

Aplastic Anemia
Definition and Epidemiology

Aplastic anemia (AA) is a rare disorder characterized by pancytopenia with a markedly hypocellular bone marrow. This disease was first described in 1888 by Paul Ehrlich, who observed that autopsy bone marrow specimens from a young woman who died of severe anemia and neutropenia were extremely hypoplastic. Later studies demonstrated that patients with severe AA possessed only a fraction of normal pluripotent stem cell numbers despite normal functional marrow stromal cells and normal or even elevated levels of stimulatory cytokines. The incidence of AA ranges from 1 to 5 cases per million people in the general population. It occurs predominantly in young adults (20 to 25 years old) and older adults (60 to 65 years old). The incidence is 3-fold higher in developing countries (e.g., Thailand and China) compared

with industrialized Western nations (e.g., Europe and Israel), a fact that is not explained by differences in drug or radiation exposure.

Etiology

AA arises as either an inherited disorder or an acquired syndrome or as an idiopathic phenomenon. A small number of cases occur in the context of a congenital bone marrow failure disorder, including Fanconi anemia, Schwachman-Diamond syndrome, and dyskeratosis congenita. The most common of these, Fanconi anemia, is an autosomal recessive disorder arising from mutations in genes encoding DNA repair proteins. The known causes of acquired AA are numerous (Table 46.4) and range from myeloablative radiation exposure to common viruses and medications. Prior bone marrow toxicity from drugs, chemicals (e.g., benzene, cyclic hydrocarbons found in petroleum products, rubber, glue, insecticides, chemical dyes), or radiation predisposes to AA because these agents directly injure proliferating and differentiating HSCs by inducing DNA damage. In contrast, cytotoxic chemotherapy, especially with alkylating agents, and radiation therapy target all rapidly cycling cells and often induce reversible bone marrow aplasia. Despite these many causes, most cases of AA are idiopathic.

The etiology of both acquired and congenital AAs appear to be mechanistically linked through abnormal telomere maintenance. Telomeres are repeated nucleotide sequences that cap and protect chromosome ends from degradation. Cell division leads to normal telomere erosion; when telomeres reach a critically short length, cells cease to proliferate, senesce, and undergo apoptosis, often with accompanying DNA damage and genomic instability. Telomerase enzyme in normal HSCs preserves long telomeres and promotes quiescence and a prolonged cellular lifespan. Patients with autosomal dominant dyskeratosis congenita have mutations in the genes for telomerase complexes, predisposing to premature aging and enhanced marrow failure in the setting of accelerated telomere shortening. One third of patients with acquired AA also have short telomeres, likely due to a combination of genetic, environmental, and epigenetic factors.

Autoreactive host lymphocytes can destroy normal hematopoiesis in AA. Bone marrow stromal cells and cytokine levels in patients with AA are normal. The fact that AA also occurs in diseases of immune dysregulation and after viral infections further suggests an immune-mediated mechanism for the disease. One hypothesis is that drug or viral antigens presented to the immune system trigger cytotoxic T-cell responses that persist and destroy normal stem cells. Only 1 in 100,000 patients develops severe AA as an idiosyncratic drug reaction. Whether these individuals have a genetically predisposed sensitivity to common exposures (e.g., nonsteroidal anti-inflammatory drugs, sulfonamides, Epstein-Barr virus) is unknown.

TABLE 46.4 Causes of Acquired Aplastic Anemia

Drugs (dose related): chemotherapeutic agents, antibiotics (chloramphenicol, trimethoprim-sulfamethoxazole)

Idiosyncratic causes (many unproved): chloramphenicol, quinacrine, nonsteroidal anti-inflammatory drugs, anticonvulsants, gold, sulfonamides, cimetidine, penicillamine

Toxins: benzene and other hydrocarbons, insecticides

Viral infection: hepatitis, Epstein-Barr virus, human immunodeficiency virus (HIV)

Immune disease: graft-versus-host disease in immunodeficiency, hypogammaglobulinemia

Paroxysmal nocturnal hemoglobinuria (PNH)

Radiation exposure

Pregnancy

Clinical Presentation

The clinical onset of AA can be insidious or abrupt. Patients often complain of symptoms related to their cytopenias: weakness, fatigue, dyspnea, or palpitations resulting from anemia; gingival bleeding, epistaxis, petechiae, or purpura caused by low platelet counts; or recurrent bacterial infections caused by low or nonfunctioning neutrophils. In some cases, patients will report recent upper respiratory syndrome. Results of the physical examination may be normal or characterized by ecchymoses and bleeding complications. Patients with congenital AA may have various abnormalities.

Diagnosis and Differential Diagnosis

Diagnostic confirmation of AA requires bone marrow biopsy to confirm hypocellularity and to rule out other marrow processes. Normal bone marrow cellularity ranges from 30% to 50% up to age 70 years and is less than 20% after 70 years of age (E-Fig. 46.1A). In contrast, bone marrow cellularity in patients with AA usually ranges from 5% to 15%, with increased fat accumulation and few or no hematopoietic cells and primarily plasma cells and lymphocytes (see E-Fig. 46.1B). In AA, hematopoietic progenitor and precursor cells are morphologically normal but number less than 1% of normal levels, and they are markedly dysfunctional, with a decreased ability to form differentiated progenitor cell colonies in vitro. A hypocellular marrow with evidence of increased blasts, dysplastic hematopoietic cells (e.g., pseudo-Pelger-Huët abnormalities, micromegakaryocytes) (E-Fig. 46.2), and clonal cytogenetically abnormal cells in the peripheral blood or marrow are diagnostic of acute leukemia or myelodysplasia, not AA. In young patients, a diagnosis of Fanconi anemia is made by demonstrating enhanced sensitivity of cultured cells to mitomycin or diepoxybutane-induced chromosomal damage on special testing. Although patients with AA typically have a low reticulocyte count from low red blood cell production and a paucity of blood cells (E-Fig. 46.3A) and macrocytic red cells (see E-Fig. 46.3B) on the peripheral blood smear, these features are nondiagnostic because patients with other primary marrow disorders may exhibit similar findings.

Treatment and Prognosis

Treatment of AA is based on the severity of disease and clinical characteristics. Patients with mild cytopenias can be monitored expectantly. However, patients with severe AA based on peripheral blood cell counts (defined as a neutrophil count <500/μL, platelet count <20,000/μL, anemia with corrected reticulocyte count <1%, and marrow cellularity of 5% to 10%) have a poor median survival of 2 to 6 months without treatment. Because most of these patients die of overwhelming infections, supportive care with broad-spectrum antibiotics, antifungal agents, and antiviral agents is warranted for those with advanced neutropenia. Red blood cell and platelet transfusions can help patients who are profoundly symptomatic.

Current therapeutic approaches to AA focus on replacing the defective HSCs by stem cell transplantation and controlling an overactive immune response with HSC activation. All young patients with severe AA and an HLA-compatible bone marrow donor should be considered for alloSCT, which offers the best chance for definitive cure. Conditioning regimens for those AA patients with congenital abnormalities must be carefully considered prior to alloSCT. Although long-term survival is excellent for patients younger than 30 years transplanted from a sibling donor (75% to 90%), morbidity due to the transplant itself and the management of long-term complications are continuing problems. Outcomes for patients older than 40 years or patients without any HLA-matched related donor are poor.

The presumed immune mechanisms for drug-induced aplasia have led to immunosuppressive approaches to the treatment of AA in older patients, those without a compatible donor and/or otherwise ineligible for alloSCT. Treatment of AA with traditional chemotherapy such as high-dose cyclophosphamide usually has proved too toxic. However, immunosuppressive therapy (IST) using a combination of anti-thymocyte globulin (ATG) and cyclosporine (a specific T-cell inhibitor) restores marrow function and independence from red blood cell or platelet transfusions in up to 70% of patients with a 5-year survival of 90%. Side effects of ATG include anaphylaxis and serum sickness as a result of foreign antigens in the antisera and are usually self-limited. Eltrombopag is an oral TPO mimetic drug originally developed for its ability to stimulate platelet production by binding to MPL receptors on megakaryocytes. In vitro data suggested that administration of high doses of exogenous TPO also could stimulate proliferation and maintenance of HSCs expressing TPO receptors in spite of high levels of endogenous TPO in AA patients. Treatment of refractory severe AA patients with eltrombopag led to hematologic responses in 44% of patients. Subsequently, eltrombopag was added to frontline ATG and cyclosporine (CSA) for newly diagnosed AA and resulted in overall response rates of 80% to 94% after 6 months with excellent long-term survival. Complete hematologic responses occurred in numerous patients with markedly improved marrow cellularity and numbers of measured hematopoietic stem and progenitor cells. This three-drug combination (ATG, CSA, and eltrombopag) has now become the standard of care for up-front treatment of severe AA patients.

Because endogenous cytokine production is usually high in patients with AA, the routine use of growth factors such as G-CSF, EPO, or stem cell factor typically is ineffective. Despite high endogenous TPO levels in AA patients with refractory disease, long-term administration of eltrombopag as maintenance therapy with or without other immunosuppression (ATG, CSA) may have some effect in long-term sustained blood cell counts. Patients who survive initial treatment of AA remain at increased risk for the emergence of other primary hematologic disorders, such as myelodysplasia, leukemia, and paroxysmal nocturnal hemoglobinuria (PNH). A proportion of AA patients also may relapse with loss of hematologic responses over time. Recurrence may warrant retreatment with ATG, androgens, and newer immunosuppressive agents.

Paroxysmal Nocturnal Hemoglobinuria
Definition, Epidemiology, and Etiology

PNH is a rare disease characterized by intravascular hemolysis, venous thrombosis, and bone marrow failure. The disease arises from expansion of pluripotent HSCs containing a somatic mutation in the phosphatidylinositol glycan complementation class A (*PIGA*) gene. Loss of *PIGA*, which codes for a membrane lipid moiety (i.e., glycosyl phosphatidylinositol [GPI]), produces abnormal hematopoietic cells deficient in dozens of proteins that are normally attached to the cell surface by the GPI anchor. Disease manifestations of PNH result from lack of the GPI-linked proteins (CD55 and CD59) that usually protect red blood cells and platelets from complement-mediated attack. Loss of CD55 or CD59 leads to increased immune destruction of blood cells. The release of hemoglobin from broken red cells causes disease symptoms, specifically sudden irregular episodes of passing dark colored urine. The name "paroxysmal nocturnal hemoglobinuria" arises from the observation that dark urine occurs more frequently at night or in the early morning because the urine has been concentrated over night during sleep. In reality, hemolysis in this disorder is a continuous process and does not occur solely at night but during the day as well when it may not be as obvious to patients or clinicians.

Blood cells arising from abnormal PNH clones can have complete (type III cells) or partial (type II cells) GPI deficiency. The degree of GPI deficiency is associated with the severity of the clinical symptoms. GPI-deficient cells typically coexist in the marrow with various populations of normal GPI-expressing cells (type I cells). Small numbers of abnormal PNH clones in patients with AA or myelodysplastic syndrome (MDS) suggest significant overlap in the causes of these three diseases. This led to reclassification of PNH as classic PNH disease and PNH in the setting of another specified bone marrow disorder. Suppression of normal hematopoiesis by the host immune system directly or indirectly by a preceding or coexistent disorder appears to provide a marrow environment favoring selective expansion of PNH stem cell clones and their deficient blood cell progeny over normal hematopoiesis.

Clinical Presentation

Patients are typically younger individuals with varying chronic complaints of abdominal pain, dysphagia, erectile dysfunction and impotence (in men), and intense lethargy due to smooth muscle dystonia resulting from depletion of circulating nitric oxide levels by free hemoglobin. Not all affected patients exhibit symptoms. Despite the continuous hemolysis, patients may experience acute exacerbations intermittently or frequently during periods of infection, trauma, and stress that may be difficult to manage. In addition to hemolysis, individuals with PNH are susceptible to recurrent potentially life-threatening thromboses and acute as well as chronic renal disease.

Diagnosis and Differential Diagnosis

The diagnosis of PNH is typically made by identification of complete or partial GPI protein deficiency on red cells and granulocytes. Usually this is determined by the loss of CD59, CD55, CD16, or CD24 expression in a clonal population. Laboratory tests reveal ongoing, low-grade intravascular hemolysis with increased lactate dehydrogenase levels correlating with severity of hemolysis and symptoms. Cytopenias, particularly anemia, often render patients transfusion dependent with ongoing hemoglobinuria due to the release of free plasma hemoglobin from intracellular compartments. About 15% of PNH patients have spontaneous resolution of disease without long-term sequelae, suggesting that *PIGA* mutations may appear transiently and disappear spontaneously in normal hematopoietic cell populations for unknown reasons.

Treatment

Eculizumab is a humanized monoclonal antibody that binds with high affinity to the complement protein C5, preventing terminal complement-mediated intravascular hemolysis in patients with PNH. Eculizumab therapy decreases hemolysis and hemoglobinuria, reduces requirements for red blood cell transfusions, improves chronic renal failure, and is associated with significant improvement in quality of life and survival for PNH patients. The incidence of life-threatening thrombotic events is decreased by more than 80%, likely contributing to the significant improvement in overall survival. Although this agent is associated with a theoretical increased risk for meningococcal infections due to complement-mediated blockade, the long-term safety and efficacy of sustained eculizumab therapy administered for more than 5 years appear to outweigh the potential risks of prolonged treatment. A recently developed longer-acting version of eculizumab offers patients who require lifelong therapy with this complement inhibitor increased convenience with less frequent outpatient administration. Newer agents targeting different stages of the complement pathway are currently in clinical investigation for PNH and other complement-activated hemolytic anemias. Other treatment for PNH includes supportive care with transfusions, iron and folic acid supplementation, and alloSCT in selected patients for curative intent. Documented venous thrombosis is treated with lifelong full anticoagulation.

Prognosis

Despite advances in treatment and adequate anticoagulation, PNH remains a life-threatening disease. Venous thrombosis involving the cerebral and intra-abdominal veins occurs in about one half of patients and is the cause of death for up to one third, although the cause of the increased thrombotic risk is not entirely understood. Other causes of morbidity and mortality are side effects of progressive AA and a 5% long-term risk for leukemic transformation. Historically, the median survival from diagnosis is 10 to 15 years, with one third of patients dying within 5 years of the diagnosis. Whether long-term eculizumab therapy can change the natural history of disease is unknown and is the goal of an international registry of PNH patients.

Myelodysplastic Syndrome
Definition and Epidemiology

MDS is a biologically heterogeneous group of marrow disorders characterized by ineffective and disordered hematopoiesis in one or more of the major myeloid cell lines: erythroid cells, neutrophils and their precursors, and megakaryocytes. Patients have one or more cytopenias despite normal or increased numbers of hematopoietic cells in the bone marrow. Disordered maturation is accompanied by increased intramedullary apoptosis, which contributes to the decreased release of mature cells into the periphery. Primary MDS is predominantly a disease of elderly persons and occurs in about 1 of 500 patients between the ages of 60 and 75 years.

Etiology

Prior exposure to radiation therapy, myelotoxic chemotherapy, and organic chemicals such as benzene and formaldehyde has been linked to the development of what is termed "secondary" MDS. This disorder may occur at any age and comprises 10% to 15% of all diagnosed MDS cases. Therapy-related MDS is defined as MDS arising months to years after prior chemotherapy involving any cytotoxic agent but particularly alkylating agents and anthracyclines, ionizing radiation, radiolabeled antibody therapy, or alloSCT for any cancer or noncancer-related condition. Because therapy-related MDS typically evolves swiftly to more aggressive disease, these cases have been reclassified with therapy-related AML and treated accordingly (see Chapter 47).

Although the remaining majority of cases of MDS were previously thought to be idiopathic, emerging data have demonstrated that age-related clonal hematopoiesis underlies the development of MDS in many older individuals. Extensive genomic analyses of peripheral blood samples in otherwise healthy individuals have identified certain clonal molecular abnormalities, such as *DNMT3A*, *TET2*, and *ASXL1* mutations, present in hematopoietic cells several years prior to the development of overt hematologic disorders or even abnormal blood counts. Individuals who present with a single cytopenia and at least one clonal mutation in an otherwise normal marrow by morphology or who have a clonal marrow karyotype have been designated to have *CCUS (clonal cytopenia of unknown significance)*. Increased number of mutations and specific mutations have been associated with increased risk of evolution to hematologic malignancy with highest risk seen in patients with two or more mutations, *RUNX1*, *JAK2V617F*, or *p53* mutations. The ideal management of these individuals, a proportion of whom will inevitably develop myeloid malignancies, is not certain but many physicians will choose to monitor these patients closely with intermittent blood cell counts. MDS is also considered a precursor syndrome with an overall risk of transformation to acute myeloid leukemia (AML) of 25% to

30%. It is now clear that progression from clonal myeloid HSC injury to multilineage hematopoietic failure and enhanced myeloblast growth reflects a continuum of disease ranging from clonal hematopoiesis to MDS and subsequent AML (see Chapter 47).

Clinical Presentation

Most patients with MDS are referred for evaluation of an incidental finding of peripheral cytopenia. Symptomatic patients usually exhibit findings related to the secondary effects of cytopenias: bleeding and bruising caused by thrombocytopenia, infection caused by leukopenia, or fatigue and dyspnea related to anemia. Physical examination is usually unremarkable, although 25% or more of patients may have splenomegaly. In some patients with MDS, development of skin lesions with fever (i.e., acute febrile neutrophilic dermatosis [Sweet syndrome]) may herald the transformation of MDS into acute leukemia. The disease course of MDS varies widely based on specific prognostic information (see later) including number and severity of cytopenias and karyotypic abnormalities. Although lower-risk MDS patients may live normal lifespans, most patients will eventually die prematurely of cytopenia-related complications, marrow failure, or evolution to AML with a median survival ranging from months to less than 2 years in the highest risk disease.

Diagnosis and Differential Diagnosis

Diagnosis of MDS requires evidence of dysplasia of at least 10% of marrow myeloid hematopoietic cells or 5% to 19% marrow blasts, the presence of peripheral cytopenia in one or more myeloid lineages, and absence of other known causes for the cytopenia. The World Health Organization (WHO) also defines MDS in any marrow regardless of morphology, which contains pathognomonic karyotypic abnormalities, for example, aberrations in chromosome 5 and 7, or 3 or greater aberrations (complex karyotype).

Morphologic evidence of dysplastic changes diagnostic of MDS often require specialized hematopathology review. Review of the peripheral blood smear may show characteristic morphologic abnormalities in addition to cytopenias. Erythroid cells are usually macrocytic, often with basophilic stippling. Neutrophils are often hypogranular and hypolobulated with a characteristic bilobed nuclear morphology called *pseudo-Pelger-Huët abnormality*. This anomaly should be anticipated when automated differential cell counts report unusually large numbers of bands. The bone marrow in MDS is usually normocellular or hypercellular, although 10% of patients may have a hypocellular marrow. Dysplastic changes usually occur in all three cell lines. Erythroid cells appear megaloblastic, with multinucleated cells or asynchronous nuclear-cytoplasmic development. Extremely small micromegakaryocytes and agranular megakaryocytes also may be seen. The myeloid series shows poor maturation with a left shift to earlier hypogranulated myeloid forms. Although elevated numbers of myeloid blasts are common, increasing blast numbers indicate progression to acute leukemia. Electron microscopy of the marrow shows cellular changes (i.e., prominent nuclear chromatin, cytoplasmic vacuoles, and blebs) characteristic of increased apoptosis (see examples in E-Fig. 46.4).

In the past, MDS was classified based on dysplastic marrow morphology and percentage of blasts as one of five subtypes: refractory anemia (RA), refractory anemia with ringed sideroblasts (RARS), refractory anemia with excess blasts (RAEB), refractory anemia with excess blasts in transformation (RAEBT), and chronic myelomonocytic leukemia (CMML). Later, these five subtypes were expanded to eight subtypes, with recognition of multilineage dysplasia as an important feature (e.g., refractory cytopenia with multilineage dysplasia, refractory cytopenia with multilineage dysplasia and ringed sideroblasts) and the reclassification of CMML

as myeloproliferative-myelodysplastic syndrome (MPN/MDS) (Table 46.5). MDS with an isolated 5q− cytogenetic abnormality was established as a distinct clinical syndrome. Therapy-related MDS/AML is defined as evidence of marrow dysplasia after prior chemotherapy, radiation therapy, or other myeloablative therapy. Although MDS patients with refractory anemia and excess blasts or refractory cytopenia with multilineage dysplasia usually fare poorly, morphologic classification of MDS correlates only approximately with overall survival.

The natural history and treatment of some MDS subtypes is more closely associated with specific cytogenetic and molecular abnormalities, demanding that careful molecular studies be performed during initial evaluation. For example, MDS characterized by deletion of the short arm of chromosome 7 (7p−) or complex cytogenetic abnormalities such as monosomy 7 or trisomy 8 often have mutations in the p53 tumor suppressor genes and universally poor clinical outcomes. In contrast, patients with MDS featuring an isolated deletion in the long arm of chromosome 5 (i.e., 5q− syndrome) are predominantly older women with a refractory macrocytic anemia, normal or elevated platelet counts, and an overall better clinical prognosis. These patients often live for several years with intermittent red blood cell transfusions, have a low risk of leukemic transformation, and often respond to therapy with lenalidomide (see later).

For the one third to one half of patients with cytopenia and myeloid dysplasia with normal marrow karyotype, the diagnosis of MDS should be one of exclusion after other potential causes of marrow failure and pancytopenia have been evaluated (see Table 46.3). MDS should never be diagnosed in acute disease states, during chronic hospitalization, or within 6 months of known myelotoxic therapy including irradiation or chemotherapy for any cancer or noncancer-related indication(s). Other causes such as vitamin B_{12} or folate deficiency, chronic alcohol use, over-the-counter medications or supplements, and infections including human immunodeficiency virus (HIV) infection should be considered. Patients with possible MDS and a hypocellular bone marrow should also be evaluated for AA and/or PNH.

Prognosis

Although several risk classification systems have been developed to predict outcomes of MDS patients, accurate prediction of MDS prognosis remains a work in progress. The original classification (WHO) was developed by an international working group to be employed at initial disease detection and partitions patients based on age, cytopenias, karyotype, and marrow blasts into different risk categories (see Table 46.5). Based on criticism that the original classification relies only on characteristics of patients at disease onset and includes cases now considered to be acute myeloid leukemia, another WHO classification–based prognostic scoring system (WPSS) was devised emphasizing morphology, karyotype, and transfusion dependence at any time during the MDS disease course (Table 46.6). The International Prognostic Scale (IPSS) divides MDS patients into five new risk categories and was validated to predict for overall survival and leukemic evolution for MDS at any follow-up time (Table 46.7). To further complicate things, data derived from multiple international databases and encompassing 7012 patients was analyzed to generate yet another new classification system, the Revised International Prognostic Scoring System (R-IPSS) including more comprehensive karyotypic abnormalities (Table 46.8). In general, using any of these systems, MDS patients can be divided into three general risk categories: low, intermediate (low to high), or high to very high-risk disease and treated accordingly.

Whole-genome sequencing of untreated MDS samples has revealed that at least 78% of patients carry one or more oncogenic

TABLE 46.5 World Health Organization Classification of Myelodysplastic Syndromes

Class	Definition
Refractory anemia	Blood: anemia, no or rare blasts BM: erythroid dysplasia only, <5% blasts, and <15% ringed sideroblasts
Refractory anemia with ringed sideroblasts (RARS)	Blood: anemia, no blasts BM: ≥15% ringed sideroblasts, erythroid dysplasia only, <5% blasts
Refractory cytopenia with multilineage dysplasia (RCMD)	Blood: cytopenias (bicytopenia or pancytopenia), no or rare blasts, <1 × 10⁹/L monocytes BM: dysplasia in ≥10% of the cells of two or more myeloid cell lines, <5% blasts, no Auer rods, <15% ringed sideroblasts
Refractory cytopenia with multilineage dysplasia and ringed sideroblasts (RCMD-RS)	Blood: cytopenias (two or more), no or rare blasts, no Auer rods, and <1 × 10⁹/L monocytes BM: dysplasia in ≥10% of the cells of two or more myeloid cell lines, <5% blasts, ≥15% ringed sideroblasts, no Auer rods
Refractory anemia with excess blasts type 1 (RAEB-1)	Blood: cytopenias, <5% blasts, no Auer rods, <1 × 10⁹/L monocytes BM: unilineage or multilineage dysplasia, 5-9% blasts, no Auer rods
Refractory anemia with excess blasts type 2 (RAEB-2)	Blood: cytopenias, 5-19% blasts, Auer rods ± <1 × 10⁹/L monocytes BM: unilineage or multilineage dysplasia, 10-19% blasts, ± Auer rods
Myelodysplastic syndrome–unclassified (MDS-U)	Blood: cytopenias, no or rare blasts, no Auer rods BM: unilineage dysplasia in one myeloid line, <5% blasts, no Auer rods
MDS associated with isolated del(5q)	Blood: anemia, usually normal or increased platelet count, <5% blasts BM: normal to increased megakaryocytes with hypolobulated nuclei, <5% blasts, isolated cytogenetic abnormality of deletion 5q, no Auer rods

BM, Bone marrow.

TABLE 46.6 World Health Organization Classification-Based Prognostic Scoring System (WPSS) for Myelodysplastic Disorders

Factor	SCORINGᵃ			
	0	1	2	3
WHO category	RA, RARS, 5q–	RCMD, RCMD-RS	RAEB-1	RAEB-2
Karyotypeᵇ	Good	Intermediate	Poor	—
Transfusion requirementᶜ	No	Regular	—	—

5q–, Myelodysplastic syndrome with isolated del(5q) and marrow blasts less than 5%; *MDS,* myelodysplastic syndrome; *RA,* refractory anemia; *RARS,* refractory anemia with ringed sideroblasts; *RCMD,* refractory cytopenia with multilineage dysplasia; *RCMD-RS,* refractory cytopenia with multilineage dysplasia and ringed sideroblasts; *RAEB-1,* refractory anemia with excess of blasts type 1; *RAEB-2,* refractory anemia with excess of blasts type 2; *WHO,* World Health Organization.
ᵃRisk groups were determined as follows: very low (total score = 0), low (1), intermediate (2), high (3 to 4), and very high (5 to 6).
ᵇKaryotype was as follows: good: normal, –Y, del(5q), del(20q); poor: complex (≥3 abnormalities), chromosome 7 anomalies; and intermediate: other abnormalities.
ᶜRed blood cell (RBC) transfusion dependency was defined as having at least one RBC transfusion every 8 weeks over a period of 4 months.

TABLE 46.7 International Prognostic Scoring System for Myelodysplastic Disorders (IPSS)

Score	Blasts	Karyotype	Cytopeniasᵃ	Overall Score	Median Survival (Yr)
0	<5%	Normal, –Y, 5q–, 20q–	0-1 cytopenias	0	5.7
0.5	5-10%	All other abnormalities	2-3 cytopenias	0.5-1.0	3.5
1.0		Abnormal 7, >3 abnormalities		1.5-2.0	1.2
1.5	11-20%			2.5 or higher	0.4
2.0	21-30%				

ᵃCytopenias are defined as hemoglobin <10 g/dL, neutrophils <1500/μL, platelets <100,000/μL.

mutations. Although more than 40 genes are recurrently mutated in MDS, most are altered in less than 5% of MDS patients, reflecting the enormous biologic heterogeneity of this disorder. Genes implicated in MDS are involved in cell signaling, DNA methylation, chromatin regulation, and most importantly, RNA splicing. Several studies have shown that several individual gene mutations, including *EZH2, DNMT3A, SF3B1, TET2, NRAS, TP53, RUNX1,* and *ASXL1,* predict MDS outcomes independent of IPSS classification and can improve on prognostication based on clinical features alone. However, none of the current prognostic models for MDS, such as the revised IPSS,

TABLE 46.8   Revised International Prognostic Scoring System for Myelodysplastic Syndromes (R-IPSS)

Prognostic Subgroups (% of Patients)	Cytogenetic Abnormalities	Median Survival (Yr)[a]	Median Evolution to AML, 25%[b] (Yr)[a]	Hazard Ratios OS/AML[a]	Hazard Ratios OS/AML[c]
Very good (3-4%[c])	−Y, del(11q)	5.4	NR	0.7/0.4	0.5/0.5
Good (66-72%)	Normal, del(5q), del(12p), del(20q), double including del(5q)	4.8	9.4	1/1	1/1
Intermediate (13-19%[c])	del(7q), +8, +19, i(17q), any other single or double independent clones	2.7	2.5	1.5/1.8	1.6/2.2
Poor (4-5%[c])	−7, inv(3)/t(3q)/del(3q), double including −7/del(7q), complex: 3 abnormalities	1.5	1.7	2.3/2.3	2.6/3.4
Very poor (7%[c])	Complex: >3 abnormalities	0.7	0.7	3.8/3.6	4.2/4.9

Data from Schanz J, Tüchler H, Solé F, et al: New comprehensive cytogenetic scoring system for primary myelodysplastic syndromes and oligoblastic AML following MDS derived from an international database merge, J Clin Oncol 30:820-829, 2012.

AML, Acute myeloid leukemia; *NR,* not reached; *OS,* overall survival.

[a]Multivariate analysis, *N* = 7012; data from patients in the International Working Group for Prognosis in MDS (IWG-PM) database.

[b]*AML,* 25% indicates time for 25% of patients to develop AML.

[c]*N* = 2754.

currently consider somatic mutations. The development of novel prognostic models incorporating mutational signatures is eagerly awaited in order to further refine prognosis and treatment of MDS patients in the near future.

Treatment

Insights into the pathophysiology of ineffective hematopoiesis characterizing MDS has led to several therapeutic options that ideally should be individualized based on patient preference, performance status, disease biology, and importantly, prognostic risk category.

Low to intermediate-low risk patients

Transfusions, iron chelation, and growth factors. Because most patients with MDS are elderly individuals who may not tolerate or desire aggressive intervention without hope of cure, those patients with asymptomatic low-risk disease who remain transfusion independent are typically observed expectantly. Those with symptomatic anemia and thrombocytopenia can receive supportive red blood cell and platelet transfusions to maintain quality of life. Special care should be taken to initiate iron chelators (deferoxamine or oral deferiprone) to prevent complications of iron overload caused by the delivery of between 200 and 250 mg of iron with each unit of transfused red blood cells. Accumulation of excess iron initially in macrophages and eventually in the hepatic parenchyma, myocardium, skin, and pancreas can lead to secondary hemochromatosis or transfusional iron overload with clinical symptoms of liver and heart failure, hyperpigmentation, and diabetes mellitus. To mitigate this, transfusion-dependent patients with low endogenous serum EPO levels often receive recombinant EPO growth factor to reduce transfusion needs. Similarly, chronic neutropenic individuals with recurrent or refractory infections may benefit from G-CSF or GM-CSF treatment given alone or in addition to EPO and antibiotic regimens to prevent life-threatening infections.

Luspatercept is a first-in-class recombinant fusion protein derived from human activin receptor linked to a protein derived from immunoglobulin G. This agent works by binding to select TGF-β superfamily ligands to reduce aberrant signaling and enhance late-stage erythropoiesis. By interfering with the signals that suppress RBC production, this drug improves patients' ability to manufacture their own RBCs, therefore reducing the need for transfusions. In a randomized clinical trial, luspatercept safely and effectively reduced transfusion burden in over half of patients with lower risk MDS (defined as very low, low, and intermediate risk) with ring sideroblasts who had not previously responded to or were ineligible for erythropoiesis-stimulating agents.

Immunosuppressive therapy. Certain MDS disease subgroups exhibit significant overlap with AA and PNH because hematopoietic failure in all of these conditions is mediated in part by autoimmune cells selectively targeting the destruction of normal HSCs. Young patients with low-risk MDS disease and exhibiting an HLA-DR15 haplotype have demonstrated a 30% to 50% improvement in counts after T-cell immunosuppressive therapy with ATG or cyclosporine. MDS patients with isolated trisomy 8 with and without demonstrated PNH clones have also been reported to respond to treatment with immunosuppression with or without eculizumab therapy.

5q minus syndrome. Patients with lower-risk MDS characterized by deletions in the long arm of chromosome 5 (5q− aberration) typically have anemia with preserved platelet counts. Many have a disease subtype that is extraordinarily sensitive to therapy with lenalidomide, an immunomodulatory agent that exerts antigrowth effects on MDS cells and their surrounding marrow microenvironment. Complete and durable responses after lenalidomide therapy occur in up to 66% of 5q− syndrome MDS patients and are accompanied by disappearance of the abnormal cytogenetic clone in the marrow in some patients. Defects in ribosomal protein function, specifically the ribosomal subunit protein RPS14, have been identified as the cause of 5q− syndrome MDS, paralleling findings implicating a different ribosomal subunit (RPS19) in the congenital bone marrow syndrome Diamond-Blackfan anemia. Studies have demonstrated that lenalidomide targets aberrant signaling pathways caused by haploinsufficiency of specific genes in a commonly deleted region on chromosome 5 (i.e., *SPARC,*

TABLE 46.9 Suggested Therapies for Bone Marrow Failure Syndromes

Patient Population	Recommended Treatment
Low-risk MDS (LR-MDS)	Transfusions (first line), growth factors, iron chelation, clinical trials (hypomethylating agents)
Low-risk MDS with ringed sideroblasts	Luspatercept (with ringed sideroblasts) (not yet commercially available), transfusions, iron chelation
Del(5q) MDS	Lenalidomide
Hypoplastic MDS	Immunosuppressive therapy (ATG)
Intermediate- to high-risk MDS (HR-MDS)	Hypomethylating agents (azacitidine, decitabine) or intensive AML-based induction chemotherapy (see Chapter 47) ± allogeneic stem cell transplantation, transfusion support, iron chelation, clinical trials
TP53 mutant MDS	Decitabine (10-day regimen)
Therapy-related MDS	Treatment for therapy-related AML (see Chapter 47), hypomethylating agents, allogeneic stem cell transplantation
IDH1/IDH2 mutant MDS	Clinical trials (ivosidenib, enasidenib, venetoclax-based therapy)
Paroxysmal nocturnal hemoglobinuria (PNH)	Eculizimab, anticoagulation (prior thromboses)
Severe aplastic anemia	Immunosuppressive therapy (ATG, CSA, eltrombopag), Danazol (telomere abnormalities), allogeneic stem cell transplant
Clonal hematopoiesis of indeterminate potential (CHIP)/clonal cytopenia of unknown significance (CCUS)	Close monitoring of complete blood cell counts with consideration of marrow biopsy and repeat mutational profiling if progressive cytopenia develop, modification of cardiovascular risk factors

RPS14, *CDC25C*, and *PPP2CA*). The agent specifically targets del(5q) clones while also promoting erythropoiesis and repopulation of the bone marrow in normal cells. Lenalidomide induces responses in up to one third of non-5q− MDS patients who demonstrate a specific defect in erythroid differentiation on gene expression profiling.

Intermediate to high risk MDS patients

Epigenetic therapy. The recognition that epigenetic modifications of the abnormal HSC clones in MDS affect cell growth and apoptosis and are central to disease pathogenesis has led to the successful therapeutic application of two DNA methyltransferase inhibitors (i.e., azacitidine and decitabine) for this disease. These two agents, termed *hypomethylating agents (HMA)*, are hypothesized to reverse the abnormal hypermethylation and gene silencing in abnormal HSCs. Although not curative, HMA are a cornerstone of therapy for higher-risk MDS patients ineligible for and/or unwilling to pursue alloSCT. In a phase III clinical trial of intermediate-2 to high-risk MDS patients, azacitidine significantly prolonged overall survival as compared with cytotoxic chemotherapy or supportive care only. Azacitidine delayed the time to leukemic transformation in two thirds of patients with transfusion-dependent MDS, reduced transfusion requirements, and improved quality of life compared with transfusion support alone. These results were the first to demonstrate that any therapy could alter the natural history of MDS and established azacitidine as the gold standard for treatment. Decitabine, a related compound to azacytidine, is an alternative hypomethylating agent approved for high-risk MDS patients based on the results of multiple studies showing that this agent induced higher remission rates and reduced transfusion needs as compared with supportive care and historical controls. Although decitabine has not yet resulted in an overall survival benefit in MDS patients, the shorter duration of administration (5 days for decitabine vs. 7 days for azacytidine) and the more myelosuppressive nature of this agent has led it to be preferred for some patients with higher-risk MDS with increased white blood cell count and/or blasts.

Hypomethylating therapy resulting in chronic (epigenetic) modification of MDS cells differs from cytotoxic chemotherapy in several ways. Prolonged administration of HMA is needed to induce and maintain efficacy. Therapeutic responses are often not seen until at least 4 to 6 months after treatment initiation and, once achieved, require ongoing monthly administration to maintain response and transfusion-independence. Moreover, marrow responses are not required as MDS patients receiving azacitidine who did not achieve a defined complete remission still survived significantly longer than patients treated with supportive care alone. Whether outcomes of hypomethylating therapy differ based on mutational status of MDS patients is not clear. One study reported more favorable outcomes in poor prognosis MDS patients characterized by TP53 mutations who received a 10-day decitabine regimen. Despite the positive results of HMA therapy in many individuals with MDS, no patients are ultimately cured of their disease, and durable remissions are infrequent. Patients whose disease has progressed on HMA therapy have short overall survival and therefore ideally should be referred for investigational agents and/or allogeneic stem cell transplantation.

Stem cell transplantation. As in other hematologic stem cell disorders, the only curative therapy for MDS patients remains alloSCT, ideally performed at complete remission. All MDS patients younger than 40 years with an available HLA-matched sibling donor are typically offered transplantation at diagnosis. Long-term disease-free survival rates for patients with low-risk disease are greater than 50%; however, the high transplantation-related mortality, morbidity, and relapse rates associated with mismatched or unrelated donor transplants or with transplantation in older MDS patients have usually limited the use of these transplants to patients with high-risk disease. In the past, patients with intermediate-2 or high-risk MDS (i.e., MDS with cytogenetic abnormalities predisposing to leukemic transformation or high levels of blasts or intermediate-2 or higher scores on IPSS classification systems) (see Tables 46.5, 46.6, 46.7, 46.8, and 46.9) have been offered acute leukemia-based chemotherapy regimens (see Chapter 47) designed to eradicate rapidly proliferating blast cells, not dysfunctional MDS cells. Because such therapy for MDS patients is associated with a high relapse rate within 12 to 18 months and no significant prolongation of overall survival, even for patients who achieve remission, such patients are now increasingly being offered hypomethylating agents. Regardless, subsequent alloSCT offers the best long-term outcome in the majority of MDS patients.

Outcomes following alloSCT can be predicted based on molecular biology of the MDS disease. Over 90% of MDS patients proceeding to alloSCT will have at least one somatic mutation with certain mutations such as *TP53*, *RAS*, and *JAK2V617F* associated with shorter survival and increased risk of disease recurrence following transplant. Persistence or clearance of any pretransplant MDS-associated gene mutation is also important. Detection of a mutation with a variant allele frequency of at least 0.5% at 30 days after transplant correlated with disease progression. These findings point to the importance of enhancing treatment options for MDS prior to alloSCT for optimal outcomes.

PROSPECTUS FOR THE FUTURE

Modern genomic sequencing technologies have revolutionized research in stem cell biology and marrow failure syndromes by allowing parallel assessment of hundreds of genes, pathways, and biologic processes. The study of HSC function in marrow failure syndromes provides hints of specific molecular pathways disturbed in many diseases of hematopoietic and nonhematopoietic stem cells. These observations are furthering our knowledge about the complex interplay among AA, PNH, and MDS. Understanding stem cells' plasticity and regulatory roles promises new therapeutic avenues for a wide array of diseases.

Characterization of the complex genomic landscape of MDS has revealed that almost 80% of cases are characterized by at least one oncogenic mutation, and more than 40 unique genes are recurrently mutated. Much research remains to be done to determine how best to incorporate this vast amount of information into the prognosis of MDS patients. In addition, it is estimated that up to 10% to 15% of patients with MDS, particularly younger individuals, have disease arising from inherited familial genetic predisposition syndromes with germline mutations in genes such as *DDX1* and *RUNX1* that promote aberrant myeloid cell development. Careful acquisition of personal and family history is therefore key for any individual with marrow failure disorders. Routine referral of MDS patients younger than 50 years of age and/or with appropriate family history or specific gene mutations detected on molecular testing is strongly recommended.

Multiple agents targeting the unique biologic features of ineffective hematopoiesis in marrow failure syndromes have moved into the forefront of treatment for these diseases over the last few years. These include eculizumab in PNH, immunosuppressive drugs and eltrombopag in AA and MDS subsets, azacitidine and decitabine in higher-risk MDS, and lenalidomide in 5q− MDS. Advances in allogeneic stem cell transplantation, specifically the now widespread use of reduced intensity and haploidentical transplantation protocols, has made this option a reality for many individuals who would not have been eligible for this life-extending procedure in the past.

Current clinical trials are actively investigating a new wave of tailored therapies for specific MDS biologic signatures. Examples of this include a p53 reactivating agent (APR-246) for p53 mutant MDS, a telomerase inhibitor (imetelstat) for lower-intermediate-risk MDS, a CD123-directed antibody-toxin conjugate (tagraxofusp) for MPN/MDS, and multiple immune checkpoint inhibitors added to hypomethylating therapy for higher-risk MDS. Ongoing clinical trials are also exploring the potential translation of multiple agents recently approved for acute myeloid leukemia to high-risk MDS patients, given the significant clinical and biological overlap of these two disease states. These included enasidenib for *IDH2* mutant MDS, ivosidenib for *IDH1* mutant MDS, and most importantly, venetoclax plus

azacytidine or decitabine or low-dose cytarabine for MDS independent of mutation status (see Chapter 47).

Finally, the contribution of hematopoietic stem cells to global health issues is increasingly being recognized and explored. Genomic sequencing has allowed us to discern that many healthy individuals without overt hematologic abnormalities in fact have clonal somatic gene mutations in hematopoietic stem and progenitor cells (termed *clonal hematopoiesis of indeterminate potential* or *CHIP*). The incidence of CHIP appears to increase with age of the individual, likely due to mutational events over time and other yet to be determined genetic and environmental predisposing factors. Over time, individuals with CHIP have an increased risk of developing overt hematologic cancers, particularly therapy-related MDS/AML following exposure to myelosuppressive agents (chemotherapy or radiation) and depending on the specific mutation identified. In many individuals, identification of new cytopenias in these patients (termed *clonal cytopenias of unknown significance* or *CCUS*) may represent the next step in the continuum to development of MDS. CHIP has been associated with other health problems. In one study, presence of CHIP was linked to almost twice the risk of developing coronary heart disease in individuals without other risk factors. Preclinical models of CHIP in mice have demonstrated that CHIP is linked to accelerated atherosclerosis potentially due to higher baseline underlying inflammatory processes. Studies exploring how best to utilize this information for preventive and/or therapeutic purposes are ongoing.

For a deeper discussion of these topics, please see Chapter 147, "Hematopoiesis and Hematopoietic Growth Factors," in *Goldman-Cecil Medicine*, 26th Edition.

SUGGESTED READINGS

Bejar R, Stevenson KE, Caughey BA, et al: Validation of a prognostic model and the impact of mutations in patients with lower-risk myelodysplastic syndromes, J Clin Oncol 30:3376–3382, 2012.

Duncavage EJ, Jacoby MA, Chang GS, et al: Mutation clearance after transplantation for myelodysplastic syndrome, N Engl J Med 379(11):1028–1041, 2018.

Fenaux P, Mufti GJ, Hellstrom-Lindberg E, et al: Efficacy of azacitidine compared with that of conventional care regimens in the treatment of higher-risk myelodysplastic syndromes: a randomised, open-label, phase III study, Lancet Oncol 10(3):223–232, 2009.

Fenaux P, Platzbecker U, Mufti GJ, et al. The MEDALIST trial: results of a phase 3, randomized, double-blind, placebo-controlled study of Luspatercept to treat anemia in patients with very low-, low-, or intermediate-risk myelodysplastic syndromes (MDS) with ring sideroblasts (RS) who require red blood cell (RBC) transfusions. Abstract #1. Presented at the 2018 ASH Annual Meeting, December 2, 2018, San Diego, CA.

Germing U, Schroeder T, Kaivers J, et al: Novel therapies in low- and high-risk myelodysplastic syndromes, Expert Rev Hematol 12(10):893–908, 2019.

Hillmen P, Muus P, Roth A, et al.: Long-term safety and efficacy of sustained eculizumab treatment in patients with paroxysmal nocturnal haemoglobinuria, Br J Haematol 162:2–73, 2013.

Jaiswal S, Natarajan P, Silver AJ, et al: N Engl J Med 377(2):111–121, 2017.

Krönke J, Fink EC, Hollenbach PW, et al.: Lenalidomide induces ubiquination and degradation of CK1alpha in del(5q) MDS, Nature 523(7559):183–188, 2015.

Lindsley RC, Saber W, Mar BG, et al: Prognostic mutations in myelodysplastic syndrome after stem cell transplantation, N Engl J Med 376(6):536–547, 2017.

Olnes MJ, Scheinberg P, Calvo KR, et al: Eltrombopag and improved hematopoiesis in refractory aplastic anemia, N Engl J Med 367:11–19, 2012.

Papaemmanuil E, Gerstung M, Malcovati L, et al: Clinical and biological implications of driver mutations in myelodysplastic syndromes, Blood 122:3616–3627, 2013.

Platzbecker U: Treatment of MDS, Blood 133(10):1096–1107, 2019.

Risitano AM: Paroxysmal nocturnal hemoglobinuria and the complement system: recent insights and novel anticomplement strategies, Adv Exp Med Biol 735:155–172, 2013.

Steensma DP, Bejar R, Jaiswal S, et al: Clonal hematopoiesis of indeterminate potential and its distinction from myelodysplastic syndrome, Blood 126(1):9–16, 2015.

Townsley DM, Scheinberg P, Winkler T, et al: Eltrombopag for treatment of thrombocytopenia-associated disorders, N Engl J Med 376(16):1540–1550, 2017.

Welch JS, Petti AA, Miller CA, et al: TP53 and decitabine in acute myeloid leukemia and myelodysplastic syndrome, N Engl J Med 375(21):2023–2036, 2016.

47

Clonal Disorders of the Hematopoietic Stem Cell

Eunice S. Wang, Nancy Berliner

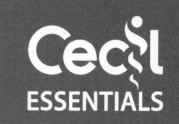

INTRODUCTION

Malignant transformation involves combined defects in cellular maturation and differentiation. The multistep theory of oncogenesis suggests that these defects are often separable and contribute to a stepwise progression from a normal to a fully transformed cell. The continuous cycling of hematopoietic cells provides a milieu for the development of clonal genetic abnormalities that supports the multistep model. Clonal defects of the hematopoietic stem cell give rise to an array of premalignant and malignant disorders. Primary defects of maturation give rise to the myelodysplastic disorders (see Chapter 46), whereas loss of normal control of proliferation results in myeloproliferative disease encompassing chronic and acute leukemias.

MYELOPROLIFERATIVE NEOPLASMS

Definition and Etiology

Myeloproliferative neoplasms (MPN), previously known as chronic myeloproliferative diseases, are clonal stem cell disorders characterized by leukocytosis, thrombocytosis, erythrocytosis, splenomegaly, and bone marrow hypercellularity. The hallmark of MPN is the failure of a transformed multipotent stem cell to respond to normal feedback mechanisms regulating hematopoietic cell mass. Stem cells from patients with MPN demonstrate clonal colony growth in vitro when they are grown in serum without the addition of exogenous cytokines, and this technique historically was used as a diagnostic test for MPN. MPN have traditionally been divided into four classic disorders based on the predominant hyperproliferative cell type: polycythemia vera (PV), essential thrombocytosis (ET), primary myelofibrosis (PMF; i.e., idiopathic myelofibrosis or agnogenic myeloid metaplasia), and chronic myelogenous leukemia (CML). Hypereosinophilic syndrome, mast cell disease, and other less common diseases characterized by profuse myeloid cell proliferation are also considered MPN but are not traditionally included among these "classic" disease subsets (Table 47.1).

The pathogenesis of MPN arises from mutational and biologic processes resulting in dysfunctional kinases that promote unabated myeloid growth and expansion. This is often accompanied by aberrant cytokine production affecting the marrow microenvironment, a gradual shift in hematopoietic cell production from the bone marrow to extramedullary sites in the liver and spleen, and altered coagulation. In CML, a well-described reciprocal translocation between chromosomes 9 and 22 termed the "Philadelphia chromosome" results in an Abelson (ABL) leukemia virus–breakpoint cluster region (BCR) fusion protein (BCR/ABL) with constitutive kinase activity. In PV, PMF, and ET, a mutation involving the substitution of a valine for phenylalanine at position 617 (V617F) in the *Janus kinase 2 (JAK2)* has been identified

in most patients and accounts for the abnormal growth properties that characterize these stem cell disorders. In those patients with MPN lacking an actual *JAK2V617F* mutation, upregulation of JAK-STAT signaling pathways has been demonstrated due to other etiologies, supporting common mechanisms of action in all MPN. Other mutations commonly identified in MPN cells include *CALR, ASXL1,* and *RUNX1.*

Clinical complications of MPN arise from the overproduction of one or more lineages in the blood. Over time, all MPN can undergo clonal evolution with acquisition of additional cytogenetic and molecular events leading to blastic transformation and eventually acute leukemia. With the exception of CML, this is an infrequent and late complication. Although all MPN are mechanistically related, significant differences still exist in each clinical disease presentation warranting specific therapeutic considerations for each type as will be discussed.

POLYCYTHEMIA VERA

Definition and Epidemiology

PV, literally meaning "increased numbers of red blood cells in the blood," is a syndrome characterized by significantly increased red blood cell mass in the peripheral blood resulting from a clonal multipotent hematopoietic stem cell (HSC) defect. PV is relatively uncommon with an incidence of 1 to 3 of 100,000 people and a median age at diagnosis of 65 years.

Clinical Presentation

PV is a primary clonal stem cell disorder of unknown origin that is characterized by predominant erythrocytosis associated with other hematopoietic abnormalities. Although one half of patients have concurrent leukocytosis or thrombocytosis, erythrocytosis is the hallmark and the cause of the most serious clinical complications of this disease. Typically, patients complain of headache, visual problems, mental clouding, and pruritus after bathing. Occlusive vascular events such as stroke, transient ischemic attacks, myocardial ischemia, and digital pain, paresthesias, or gangrene are common. Pulmonary, deep vein, hepatic, and portal vein thromboses may occur. Paradoxically, patients are also predisposed to hemorrhagic events such as gastrointestinal and mucosal bleeding caused by abnormal platelet function and also ischemic necrosis downstream from vascular occlusion. Physical examination may show retinal vein occlusion, ruddy cyanosis, digital ischemia, and splenomegaly.

Diagnosis and Differential Diagnosis

When patients are first diagnosed with an elevated hemoglobin concentration per unit volume (i.e., erythrocytosis), the initial evaluation

TABLE 47.1 World Health Organization 2016 Classification of Myeloid Neoplasms

1. Acute myeloid leukemia
2. MDS
3. MPNs
   a. Chronic myelogenous leukemia
   b. Polycythemia vera
   c. Essential thrombocythemia
   d. Primary myelofibrosis
   e. Chronic neutrophilic leukemia
   f. Chronic eosinophilic leukemia, not otherwise categorized
   g. Hypereosinophilic syndrome
   h. Mast cell disease
   i. MPNs, unclassifiable
4. MDS, MPN
5. Myeloid neoplasms associated with eosinophilia and abnormalities of PDGF-RA, PDGF-RB, or FGF-R1

From Swerdlow SH, Campo E, Harris NL, Jaffe ES, Pileri SA, Stein H, Thiele J. WHO Classification of Tumours of Haematopoietic and Lymphoid Tissues (Revised Fourth Edition), IARC, 2016.
FGF-R1, Fibroblast growth factor receptor 1; *MDS,* myelodysplastic syndrome; *MPN,* myeloproliferative neoplasm; *PDGF-RA,* platelet-derived growth factor receptor-α polypeptide; *PDGF-RB,* platelet-derived growth factor receptor-β polypeptide.

TABLE 47.2 Causes of Erythrocytosis

I. Relative or spurious erythrocytosis (normal red cell mass)
   A. Hemoconcentration due to dehydration (e.g., diarrhea, diaphoresis, diuretics, water deprivation, emesis, ethanol, hypertension, pre-eclampsia, pheochromocytoma, carbon monoxide intoxication)
II. True or absolute erythrocytosis
   A. Polycythemia vera
   B. Primary congenital polycythemia
   C. Secondary erythrocytosis due to
      1. Congenital causes (e.g., activating mutation of erythropoietin receptor)
      2. Hypoxia caused by carbon monoxide poisoning, high oxygen affinity hemoglobin, high-altitude residence, chronic pulmonary disease, hypoventilation syndromes such as sleep apnea, right-to-left cardiac shunt, neurologic defects involving the respiratory center
      3. Nonhypoxic causes with pathologic erythropoietin production
         a. Renal disease (e.g., cysts, hydronephrosis, renal artery stenosis, focal glomerulonephritis, renal transplantation)
         b. Tumors (e.g., renal cell cancer, hepatocellular carcinoma, cerebellar hemangioblastoma, uterine fibromyoma, adrenal tumors, meningioma, pheochromocytoma)
      4. Drug-associated causes
         a. Androgen therapy
         b. Exogenous erythropoietin growth factor therapy

Modified from Hoffman R, Benz EJ, Shattil SJ, et al, editors: Hematology: basic principles and practice, ed 2, New York, 1995, Churchill Livingstone.

TABLE 47.3 World Health Organization 2016 Diagnostic Criteria for Polycythemia Vera

Major criteria[a,b]
1. Hemoglobin (Hgb) >16.5 g/dL (men), >16.0 (women); *or* hematocrit (Hct) >49% (men), >48% (women) *or* increased red cell mass (RCM) (more than 25% above mean normal predicted value)
2. Bone marrow biopsy showing hypercellularity for age with trilineage growth (panmyelosis) including prominent erythroid, granulocytic, and megakaryocytic proliferation with pleomorphic, mature megakaryocytes (differences in size)
3. Presence of *JAK2* or JAK2 exon 12 mutation
Minor criteria
1. Subnormal serum erythropoietin level

From Swerdlow SH, Campo E, Harris NL, Jaffe ES, Pileri SA, Stein H, Thiele J. WHO Classification of Tumours of Haematopoietic and Lymphoid Tissues (Revised Fourth Edition), IARC, 2016.
[a]PV diagnosis requires meeting either all three major criteria or the first two major criteria and one minor criterion.
[b]Criterion number 2 (bone marrow biopsy) may not be required in cases with sustained absolute erythrocytosis: hemoglobin levels 18.5 g/dL in men (hematocrit 55.5%) or 16.5 g/dL in women (hematocrit 49.5%) if major criterion 3 and the minor criterion are present. However, initial myelofibrosis (present in up to 20% of patients) can only be detected by performing a bone marrow biopsy; this finding may predict a more rapid progression to overt myelofibrosis (post-PV MF).

absolute erythrocytosis is an absolute increase in red cell mass caused by increased red blood cell production. Under normal conditions, the body's ability to increase red blood cell production in states of hypoxemia, anemia, hemolysis, and acute blood loss ensures continuous oxygen delivery to tissues. In response to physiologic stimuli, pluripotent stem cell precursors are activated by erythropoietin (EPO) to differentiate into erythroid progenitor cells and eventually into hemoglobin-carrying erythrocytes. When numbers of mature red blood cells are adequate, a negative feedback mechanism suppresses further EPO production, and the serum hemoglobin level remains normal.

Diagnosis of PV was formerly one of exclusion based on an elevated red cell mass, splenomegaly, thrombocytosis, leukocytosis, lack of hypoxemia and other secondary causes of polycythemia, and elevated levels of leukocyte alkaline phosphatase and serum vitamin B_{12}–binding protein levels. Red blood cells in the peripheral blood often appear microcytic, with or without iron deficiency. Bone marrow examination shows a hypercellular marrow with pronounced hyperplasia of erythroid lineage cells. Cytogenetic features at the time of diagnosis are usually normal. The development of clonal cytogenetic abnormalities heralds transformation in the later stages of disease. The discovery of *JAK2* gene mutations in 97% of patients with PV as well as other mutations (such as *CALR* and *ASXL1*) and findings elucidating the underlying disease pathophysiology led to new diagnostic criteria (Table 47.3). A suspected diagnosis of PV can now be confirmed in individuals with elevated hemoglobin and/or hematocrit levels by testing for a *JAK2* mutation, bone marrow demonstrating trilineage proliferation, and documentation of subnormal serum EPO levels.

Treatment and Prognosis

Early recognition and treatment of PV are important because untreated patients with PV suffer significant morbidity and mortality from thromboembolic complications involving the cerebral, coronary, and mesenteric circulations. Twenty percent of patients show symptoms of arterial and venous thrombosis, and thrombosis remains the most common cause of death. Without treatment, up to one half of patients

should focus on whether this increase reflects an enhanced red cell mass (i.e., absolute erythrocytosis or polycythemia) or a normal red cell mass in the setting of a decreased plasma volume (i.e., relative erythrocytosis caused by reduced intravascular volume or other causes). The latter condition is not true polycythemia (Table 47.2). Polycythemia or with PV may die of thrombotic complications within 18 months of diagnosis. Realization of an individual patient's risk for life-limiting thrombotic complications dictates whether therapy is required to render PV into a chronic, progressive disease.

Low-dose aspirin and treatment of asymptomatic thrombocytosis decrease thromboembolic events in low- and high-risk PV patients and are especially important in older patients with significant cardiovascular risk factors. In younger patients, nonsteroidal anti-inflammatory drugs and antiplatelet agents should be used judiciously because of the risk of gastrointestinal hemorrhage. Patients with advanced age (>60 years), prior history of thrombosis, leukocytosis, high hematocrit values, and clinical cardiovascular factors are at high risk for subsequent vascular events. Although possible, the risk of transformation of PV to acute myeloid leukemia remains relatively low with rates of 2.3% at 10 years and 5.5% at 15 years.

Therapy varies based on risk criteria. For younger patients with lower cardiovascular risk factors, intermittent phlebotomy and aspirin prophylaxis remain the mainstays of treatment and usually result in iron deficiency anemia, which further reduces the rate of red blood cell production.

Cytoreductive therapy is indicated for patients who cannot tolerate and/or fail phlebotomy, older patients with a prior history of and/or coexisting risk factors for cardiovascular events, and those with symptomatic splenomegaly. Commonly used therapies include hydroxyurea (i.e., a low-dose oral cytotoxic agent that does not appear to increase leukemic risk), pegylated interferon-α (i.e., for young patients and women during pregnancy), and anagrelide (i.e., an oral megakaryotoxic agent for treating refractory thrombocytosis). Choice of therapy is often individualized to the patient to best meet their lifestyle requirements given the chronicity of this disease. The main goal of therapy in higher-risk individuals with PV is long-term reduction of red blood cell mass as reflected in maintenance of hematocrit values less than 45% in men (and commonly less than 42% in women). In a multicenter, prospective clinical trial, adult PV patients (largely men) randomized to maintaining a therapeutic hematocrit target of less than 45% using hydroxyurea, phlebotomy, or both had a significantly lower rate of cardiovascular death (2.7% vs. 9.8%) and major thrombosis than those with a hematocrit target maintained at a higher level between 45% and 50%. As with all myeloproliferative disorders, initiation of cytoreductive therapy may precipitate hyperuricemia that results in secondary gout and uric acid stones, warranting treatment with allopurinol.

Although low-dose chemotherapeutic agents (e.g., chlorambucil, busulfan) have historically been used to treat leukocytosis and thrombocytosis not responding to hydroxyurea, these agents have fallen out of favor due to increased toxicity and risk of secondary acute myeloid or myelogenous leukemia (AML). A randomized clinical trial of ruxolitinib, a receptor tyrosine kinase inhibitor targeting constitutively active JAK1/2 signaling pathways, in patients with PV failing prior hydroxyurea therapy, confirmed that this agent is effective in reducing phlebotomy frequency and splenomegaly in refractory patients. Reductions in white blood cell and platelet counts following ruxolitinib therapy were also reported. With effective therapy, the long-term survival of PV patients remains excellent.

ESSENTIAL THROMBOCYTHEMIA

Definition and Epidemiology

ET (also known as primary thrombocythemia) is a pluripotent stem cell disorder predominantly resulting in elevated levels of platelets and white blood cells. Platelet function and length of survival remain normal. ET is an uncommon disorder, with an increasing number of cases found on routine laboratory testing of asymptomatic patients. Although the median age at diagnosis is 60 to 65 years, 10% to 25% of patients are younger than 40 years.

TABLE 47.4　World Health Organization 2016 Diagnostic Criteria for Essential Thrombocythemia

Major criteria[a]
1. Platelet count ≥450 × 10⁹/L
2. Bone marrow biopsy showing proliferation mainly of the megakaryocyte lineage with increased numbers of enlarged mature megakaryocytes with hyperlobulated nuclei. No significant left-shift of neutrophil granulopoiesis or erythropoiesis and very rarely minor (grade 1) increase in reticulin fibers
3. Not meeting WHO criteria for *BCR-ABL1*+ CML, PV, PMF, MDS, or other myeloid neoplasms
4. Presence of JAK2, CALR, or MPL mutation

Minor criteria
1. Presence of a clonal marker (e.g., abnormal karyotype) or absence of evidence for reactive thrombocytosis

From Swerdlow SH, Campo E, Harris NL, Jaffe ES, Pileri SA, Stein H, Thiele J. WHO Classification of Tumours of Haematopoietic and Lymphoid Tissues (Revised Fourth Edition), IARC, 2016.
CML, Chronic myelogenous leukemia; *MDS,* myelodysplastic syndrome; *PMF,* primary myelofibrosis; *PV,* polycythemia vera; *WHO,* World Health Organization.
[a]ET diagnosis requires meeting all four major criteria or first three major criteria and one minor criterion.

Clinical Presentation

Up to two thirds of patients are symptomatic. Vasomotor symptoms include headache, dizziness, visual changes, and erythromelalgia (i.e., burning pain and erythema of feet and hands). Serious arterial thrombotic complications such as transient ischemic attacks, strokes, seizures, angina, and myocardial infarctions may occur. Patients may rarely have purpuric skin lesions or hematomas. The risk for gastrointestinal bleeding is less than 5%.

Diagnosis and Differential Diagnosis

Elevated platelet counts (thrombocytosis) can result as a reactive process arising from other causes (e.g., bacterial infections, sepsis, iron deficiency, autoimmune diseases, malignant diseases), which must be excluded before a diagnosis of ET is considered. The diagnosis requires a platelet count exceeding 450,000 × 10⁹/L with mutations in *JAK2, CALR,* or *MPL* genes and no evidence of reactive thrombocytosis. Bone marrow histology typically displays predominant proliferation involving the megakaryocytic lineage and little or no granulocytic or erythroid proliferation or reticulin fibrosis. Marrow immunohistochemical and cytogenetic studies are essential to exclude myelodysplasia, myelofibrosis, or the Philadelphia chromosome, which are diagnostic of CML (Table 47.4). Unlike PV, the *JAK2 V617F* mutation is only found in one half of samples from patients with ET but the presence of other clonal markers such as an abnormal karyotype can aid in making the diagnosis.

Treatment and Prognosis

Patients with ET have the most favorable outcomes of all patients with MPN with typical long-term survival rates similar to those of age-matched healthy control patients. Similar to PV, shortened overall survival is associated with high-risk features including advanced age (>60 years), prior history of thrombosis, and leukocytosis. The risk of leukemic transformation is extremely low (3% to 4%) compared with other MPNs. However, morbidity from recurrent hemorrhagic and thrombotic complications is high and cannot be reliably predicted from the platelet count or platelet function abnormalities. Because treatment requires lifelong administration for disease control, assessment of risk factors and a history of clinical signs and symptoms dictate therapeutic choices. All patients benefit from aggressive management of cardiovascular risk factors including smoking, hypertension, obesity, and hypercholesterolemia.

Although low-dose enteric coated aspirin may be used in all patients to relieve neurologic symptoms and carries a minimal risk for bleeding, excessive thrombocytosis (platelet count >1000×10^9/L) can be associated with excessive bleeding due to an acquired von Willebrand syndrome.

Although young and pregnant patients are often not treated until they become symptomatic, older patients (>60 years) and those with a history of thrombosis, long disease duration, or significant cardiovascular risk factors are most likely to benefit from the addition of platelet-lowering agents. Hydroxyurea, an oral cytotoxic and myelosuppressive agent, is the most common first-line agent and is usually well tolerated with low long-term leukemogenic risks. Anagrelide, an oral antiplatelet agent that inhibits platelet aggregation and megakaryocyte maturation, is also used, primarily as a second-line agent after hydroxyurea failure. This agent is associated with acute side effects such as fluid retention, palpitations, hemorrhage with concomitant aspirin use, and an increased risk of transformation to myelofibrosis. Both agents are known teratogens and therefore cannot be used in the significant fraction of patients with ET who are young women of childbearing age. Because patients with ET have a high incidence of fetal wastage, interferon-α (a cytokine that alters the biologic mechanisms of the malignant clone but does not cross the placenta) with low-dose heparin or aspirin prophylaxis is recommended to improve pregnancy outcomes in these patients.

PRIMARY (IDIOPATHIC) MYELOFIBROSIS

Definition and Epidemiology

PMF, also known as idiopathic myelofibrosis or previously as agnogenic myeloid metaplasia, is a clonal stem cell disorder characterized by abnormal excessive marrow fibrosis leading to marrow failure and organomegaly. PMF is a rare chronic disease that usually is seen in elderly persons. The annual incidence of PMF is 0.5 cases per 100,000 people.

Etiology

An abnormal myeloid precursor is thought to give rise to dysplastic megakaryocytes that produce increased levels of angiogenic and fibroblast growth factors. These cytokines act on normal fibroblasts and other stromal cells, a process that stimulates excessive proliferation and collagen deposition (E-Fig. 47.1A-C). Over time, increasing fibrosis of the bone marrow leads to premature release of multipotent hematopoietic precursors into the periphery (see E-Fig. 47.1D-E). These cells then migrate and reestablish themselves in other sites, thereby shifting hematopoiesis out of the bone marrow and into other tissues, specifically the spleen and liver. This process is called extramedullary hematopoiesis. Approximately 5% to 10% of cases of MF arise in individuals with prior diagnoses of PV or ET whose disease evolves over time to MF. These cases are referred to as secondary or post-PV/ET MF and are characterized by the same disease biology and clinical symptoms.

Diagnosis and Differential Diagnosis

Early in the disease, patients may be asymptomatic, with incidental findings of abnormal blood counts on routine laboratory tests. Although low blood counts may occur, overall platelet and red blood cell numbers at diagnosis may be increased or normal depending on the degree of compensatory extramedullary hematopoiesis. Review of the peripheral blood profile commonly reveals leukoerythroblastic changes characterized by teardrop-shaped erythrocytes, giant platelets, and nonleukemic immature myeloid, erythroid, and leukocyte cells.

TABLE 47.5	Causes of Bone Marrow Fibrosis

I. Neoplastic causes
  a. Chronic myeloproliferative disorders: chronic idiopathic myelofibrosis, chronic myelogenous leukemia, polycythemia vera
  b. Acute megakaryoblastic leukemia
  c. Myelodysplasia with myelofibrosis
  d. Hairy cell leukemia
  e. Acute lymphoblastic leukemia
  f. Multiple myeloma
  g. Metastatic carcinoma
  h. Systemic mastocytosis
II. Non-neoplastic causes
  a. Granulomatous diseases: mycobacterial infections, fungal infections, sarcoidosis
  b. Paget's disease of bone
  c. Hypoparathyroidism or hyperparathyroidism
  d. Renal osteodystrophy
  e. Osteoporosis
  f. Vitamin D deficiency
  g. Autoimmune diseases: systemic lupus erythematosus, systemic sclerosis

Diagnosis of PMF is made by demonstration of bone marrow fibrosis with markedly increased reticulin or collagen fibers or increased marrow cellularity. Other underlying causes of neoplastic and non-neoplastic bone marrow fibrosis (Table 47.5) should be ruled out. Testing for *JAK2*, *BCR/ABL*, or other diagnostic mutations and cytogenetic markers should be performed before a diagnosis of PMF is made (Table 47.6). In some cases, early prefibrotic changes in the marrow have been noted that signify an early phase of MF development.

Clinical Presentation

Although many patients are asymptomatic at diagnosis, most complain over time of progressive fatigue and dyspnea related to anemia or early satiety and left upper quadrant pain associated with splenomegaly and splenic infarction. More than one half of these patients develop massive hepatosplenomegaly due to extramedullary hematopoiesis. Patients with more advanced disease typically have constitutional symptoms such as fever, weight loss, night sweats, cachexia, pruritus, and bone pain, which may be debilitating. As the bone marrow failure evolves, complications of neutropenia, thrombocytopenia, and anemia develop as a result of ineffective hematopoiesis due to fibrotic changes and loss of marrow cellularity. Bleeding from occult disseminated intravascular coagulation is a risk as are infections arising from neutropenia. Extramedullary hematopoiesis in the peritoneal and pleural cavities and in the central nervous system (CNS) may also cause symptoms.

Treatment and Prognosis

Median survival of patients with PMF is poor, ranging from 2 to 5 years after diagnosis. The most commonly accepted adverse prognostic factors at onset include age greater than 65 years, hemoglobin concentration of less than 10 g/dL, leukocyte count of more than 25×10^9/L, a high percentage of circulating blasts (≥1%), and constitutional symptoms. Other important clinical factors are leukopenia, thrombocytopenia (platelets <100×10^9/L), massive hepatosplenomegaly, red cell transfusion needs, and unfavorable cytogenetic abnormalities. Over time, the disease may progress from a chronic phase to an accelerated phase, with acute leukemic transformation in 8% to 20% of patients. Treatment of PMF-related AML

TABLE 47.6 **World Health Organization 2016 Diagnostic Criteria for Primary Myelofibrosis**

Primary Myelofibrosis (PMF): Prefibrotic/Early PMF (pre-PMF)

Major criteria[a]

1. Megakaryocyte proliferation and atypia **without reticulin fibrosis > grade 1**, accompanied by increased age-adjusted bone marrow cellularity, granulocytic proliferation, and often decreased erythropoiesis
2. Not meeting WHO criteria for *BCR-ABL1+* CML, PV, MDS, or other myeloid neoplasm
3. Presence of *JAK2, CALR, or MPL* mutation or in the absence of minor reactive bone marrow reticulin fibrosis

Minor criteria

1. Presence of one or more of the following, confirmed in two consecutive determinations
   a. Anemia not attributed to a comorbid condition
   b. Leukocytosis ≥11 × 10^9/L
   c. Palpable splenomegaly
   d. LDH level above the upper limit of the institutional reference range

Primary Myelofibrosis (PMF)

Major criteria[a]

1. Megakaryocyte proliferation and atypia accompanied by either reticulin and/or collagen fibrosis (grade 2 to 3)
2. Not meeting WHO criteria for *BCR-ABL1+* CML, PV, MDS, or other myeloid neoplasm
3. Presence of *JAK2, CALR, or MPL* mutation or in the absence, the presence of another clonal marker[b] or absence of evidence for reactive bone marrow fibrosis

Minor criteria

1. Presence of one or more of the following, confirmed in two consecutive determinations
   a. Anemia not attributed to a comorbid condition
   b. Leukocytosis ≥11 × 10^9/L
   c. Palpable splenomegaly
   d. LDH level above the upper limit of the institutional reference range
   e. Leukoerythroblastosis

From Swerdlow SH, Campo E, Harris NL, Jaffe ES, Pileri SA, Stein H, Thiele J. WHO Classification of Tumours of Haematopoietic and Lymphoid Tissues (Revised Fourth Edition), IARC, 2016.
[a]Diagnosis of prefibrotic/early PMF requires all three major criteria and at least one minor criterion. Diagnosis of overt PMF requires meeting all three major criteria and at least one minor criterion.
[b]In the absence of any of the three major clonal mutations, the search for the most frequent accompanying mutations *(ASXL1, EZH2, TET2, IDH1/IDH2, SRFS2, SF3B1)* are of help in determining the clonal nature of the disease.

is usually ineffective. Other causes of nonleukemic death include heart failure, infection, intracranial hemorrhage, and pulmonary embolism.

Medical therapy for PMF is predicated on the risk category of patients. Low-risk, asymptomatic patients may be treated expectantly. All patients with symptomatic anemia benefit from palliative transfusions and administration of recombinant EPO, androgens (e.g., danazol), or low-dose thalidomide or thalidomide derivatives (i.e., lenalidomide) with or without steroids to maintain adequate red blood cell levels. Symptoms caused by excess thrombocytosis and leukocytosis or progressive extramedullary hematopoiesis may be managed with hydroxyurea as a first-line agent or pegylated interferon-α in younger or pregnant patients. Enlarging splenomegaly is best managed with medical therapy because open splenectomy is associated with significant operative morbidity and mortality, and splenic irradiation is poorly tolerated except as a palliative approach. Young patients with intermediate- to high-risk PMF and possible HLA-matched donors should be considered for potentially curative allogeneic stem cell transplantation (SCT) at academic medical centers.

Although not all patients with PMF have the *JAK2 V617F* mutation, almost all have constitutive activation of the JAK1 and JAK2 signaling pathways, rendering them potentially responsive to treatment with novel JAK1/2 inhibitors. Ruxolitinib is the first oral JAK inhibitor approved for the treatment of patients with intermediate- or high-risk myelofibrosis independent of *JAK2* mutational status, including PMF and myelofibrosis arising from prior PV or ET. In two prospective, randomized, phase III clinical trials, ruxolitinib therapy for myelofibrosis patients was compared with placebo (COMFORT-I trial) and

with best available therapy (COMFORT-II trial), respectively. Patients receiving ruxolitinib had significantly greater spleen volume reduction and overall symptom improvement in abdominal pain, early satiety, night sweats, and muscle pain, all of which correlated with overall improvement in quality of life. Updates from both trials have demonstrated significantly prolonged overall survival in the ruxolitinib-treated patients compared with control arms although neither study was designed with this as an end point. Side effects of ruxolitinib include cytopenias, specifically anemia, occurring in the first 6 to 8 weeks of therapy as well as headache, dizziness, and increased risk of herpes simplex virus (HSV) reactivation. Recently a second JAK2 inhibitor, fedratinib, was approved for the treatment of intermediate and high-risk MF as an alternative to and/or failing prior ruxolitinib therapy. Other JAK2 inhibitors are in active clinical development as single agents. Combination therapies evaluating the safety and efficacy of novel mechanistic agents alone and in addition to JAK2 inhibitors are also underway with preliminary results suggesting that even more effective therapies for PMF may be on the horizon.

CHRONIC MYELOGENOUS LEUKEMIA

Definition, Epidemiology, and Pathology

CML is the most common MPN, accounting for 15% to 20% of all leukemias and occurring in 1 of 100,000 people. The median age at diagnosis is 53 years, but patients of any age may be affected. CML is characterized by a predominant increase in the granulocytic cell line associated with concurrent erythroid and platelet hyperplasia. It is

TABLE 47.7   Definition of Phases of Chronic Myeloid Leukemia

Phase	Definition	Goal of Therapy
Chronic phase (CP)	<10% blasts <20% peripheral blood basophils	Prevent progression to AP/BP, eradicate molecular *BCR-ABL*
Accelerated phase (AP)	Peripheral blood myeloblasts ≥10% and <20% Peripheral blood myeloblasts and promyelocytes combined ≥30% Peripheral blood basophils ≥20% Platelet count ≤100 × 109/L unrelated to therapy Additional clonal cytogenetic abnormalities in Ph+ cells	Control CBC, bring back to CP and avoid progression to BP
Blast phase (BP)	≥20% blasts (myeloid or lymphoid) in peripheral blood, marrow, or both Extramedullary infiltrates of leukemic cells	Acute leukemia therapy, bridge to allogeneic stem cell transplant

unique among the MPNs in its etiology and natural history, including an inevitable transformation to acute leukemia if untreated. CML was the first malignant hematologic disease shown to be associated with a specific chromosomal abnormality. More than 95% of patients with CML have a clonal expansion of a stem cell that has acquired the Philadelphia chromosome, a balanced translocation between chromosomes 9 and 22 designated as t(9;22) (q34;q11). This translocation juxtaposes the *ABL* gene from chromosome 9 (region q34) to the *BCR* gene on chromosome 22 (region q11) and generates an oncogenic *BCR/ABL* fusion gene. The gene product, the BCR/ABL protein, is a deregulated, constitutively active cytoplasmic receptor tyrosine kinase that induces a leukemic phenotype in hematopoietic stem cells. Expression of the BCR/ABL fusion protein activates multiple downstream signal transduction pathways which permits proliferation independent of cytokine and stromal regulation and renders cells resistant to chemotherapy and normal programmed cell death.

Diagnosis and Differential Diagnosis

Laboratory tests for CML patients typically demonstrate a markedly elevated white blood cell count (median, 170×10^9/L), with low leukocyte alkaline phosphatase levels, high uric acid and lactate dehydrogenase levels, and thrombocytosis. Review of the peripheral blood smear in chronic phase CML demonstrates a full complement of myeloid cells in all stages of granulocytic development, including immature myeloblasts (usually <5%), myelocytes, metamyelocytes, basophils, eosinophils, bands, and neutrophils. In contrast, the peripheral blood smear in reactive granulocytic hyperplastic states (i.e., leukemoid reaction) caused by acute infection or sepsis consists predominantly of mature neutrophils and bands with few myelocytes, basophils, or eosinophils. The bone marrow in CML is densely hypercellular, with an overwhelming predominance of myeloid cells at all developmental stages (E-Fig. 47.2). The differential diagnosis of CML includes reactive leukocytosis (e.g., in active infection or sepsis with a profound neutrophilic response) and other MPNs (e.g., myelofibrosis).

Detection of the Philadelphia chromosome on standard cytogenetic studies and/or abnormal BCR/ABL transcripts using reverse transcription–polymerase chain reaction (RT-PCR) or fluorescent in situ hybridization (FISH) analysis is required for the diagnosis of CML. Assessment of the *BCR/ABL* fusion gene by the same methods is used to monitor disease and response to therapy. Exquisitely sensitive and quantitative RT-PCR procedures allow detection of up to a single BCR/ABL-positive cell in 10^5 to 10^6 peripheral cells and permit measurement of disease status in peripheral blood and marrow samples. A subset of patients with CML lacking a detectable Philadelphia chromosome was found to possess detectable BCR/ABL fusion products by RT-PCR, indicating a subchromosomal translocation resulting in the same pathologic gene product.

Clinical Presentation

Up to 40% of newly diagnosed CML patients are initially asymptomatic with diagnoses made on incidental laboratory results. Other patients exhibit fatigue, lethargy, shortness of breath, weight loss, easy bruising, and early satiety. Physical examination usually detects splenomegaly.

The natural history of CML is divided into three phases: chronic, accelerated, and blast phases (Table 47.7). The majority of patients are typically diagnosed during the *chronic phase of CML*, an indolent stage lasting 3 to 7 years. Peripheral white blood cell counts are elevated, with eosinophilia and basophilia (>20%) but few peripheral or marrow blasts (<5%). With control of peripheral blood cell counts, patients are essentially asymptomatic during this period.

Eventually, the disease enters the *accelerated phase*, which is characterized by fever, weight loss, worsening splenomegaly, and bone pain related to rapid marrow cell turnover. The white blood cell count rises with increased numbers of circulating or marrow blasts ranging from 10% to 19%. The increased percentage of peripheral blood basophils (>20%) results in histamine production, with symptoms of pruritus, diarrhea, and flushing. During this phase, patients may develop increasing splenomegaly, persistent thrombocytopenia, or thrombocytosis and leukocytosis, with new clonal cytogenetic abnormalities found in marrow cells.

CML blast crisis phase marks the evolution to acute leukemia, in which marrow is replaced by 20% or more immature myeloid or lymphoid blasts, with accompanying loss of normal mature cellular elements in the marrow and periphery and extramedullary blast proliferation. Untreated patients typically die in a few weeks to months. Of note, two thirds of patients develop acute myeloid leukemia, whereas the others develop acute lymphoblastic leukemia, a finding confirming that the initial neoplastic cell is an early stem cell capable of multilineage differentiation.

Treatment
Chronic Phase CML

Historically, oral cytotoxic agents such as hydroxyurea and busulfan effectively reduced myeloid cell numbers in patients with chronic phase CML but did not alter the long-term prognosis or prevent progression to blast crises.

Oral receptor tyrosine inhibitors of BCR-ABL are the mainstay of current therapy for CML. The first identified inhibitor, imatinib mesylate (formerly known as STI-571), was heralded as the first successful targeted therapy for cancer and ushered in a new era of cancer therapy. Imatinib is a rationally designed competitive oral inhibitor of multiple tyrosine kinases, including ABL, BCR/ABL, platelet-derived growth-factor receptor (PDGFR), and KIT. Inhibition of phosphorylation of BCR/ABL results in blockade of downstream signaling and growth pathways and induces apoptosis of *BCR-ABL*-positive cells. Preclinical studies demonstrated that imatinib potently inhibited the

---

TABLE 47.8   Criteria for Hematologic, Cytogenetic, and Molecular Response and Relapse in Chronic Myeloid Leukemia

Complete hematologic response
- Complete normalization of peripheral blood counts with leukocyte count $<10 \times 10^9$/L
- Platelet count $<450 \times 10^9$/L
- No immature cells, such as myelocytes, promyelocytes, or blasts in peripheral blood
- No signs and symptoms of disease with resolution of palpable splenomegaly

Cytogenetic response
- Complete cytogenetic response (CCyR): No Ph-positive metaphases
- Major cytogenetic response (MCyR): 0-35% Ph-positive metaphases
- Partial cytogenetic response (PCyR): 1-35% Ph-positive metaphases
- Minor cytogenetic response: >35-65% Ph-positive metaphases

Molecular response
- Early molecular response (EMR): *BCR-ABL1* (IS) ≤10% at 3 and 6 months
- Major molecular response (MMR): *BCR-ABL1* (IS) ≤0.1% or ≥3-log reduction in *BCR-ABL1* mRNA from the standardized baseline, if qPCR (IS) is not available
- Complete molecular response (CMR) is variably described and is best defined by the assay's level of sensitivity (e.g., MR4.5)

Relapse
- Any sign of loss of response (defined as hematologic or cytogenetic relapse)
- 1-log increase in *BCR-ABL1* transcript levels with loss of MMR should prompt bone marrow evaluation for loss of CCyR but is not itself defined as relapse (e.g., hematologic or cytogenetic relapse)

TABLE 47.9   Oral BCR-ABL1 Inhibitors for CML Therapy

Drug Name	Drug Dose	Toxicity Profile
Imatinib mesylate	400 mg po daily	Nausea, vomiting, diarrhea, peripheral and periorbital edema, myalgias, myelosuppression, increased liver function tests, rash, pleural and pericardial effusion
Dasatinib	100 mg po daily	Pulmonary arterial hypertension, pleural and pericardial effusions, headache, myelosuppression, cerebral hemorrhage (rare), ascites, peripheral or pulmonary edema
Nilotinib	400 mg po twice a day (avoid food 2 hrs before and 1 hr after drug)	Peripheral arterial occlusive disease, QTC prolongation, pancreatitis, hepatotoxicity, myelosuppression, hyperglycemia, sudden death, rash
Bosutinib	500 mg po daily	Diarrhea, myelosuppression, liver function abnormalities, fluid retention (pulmonary or peripheral edema, pleural and pericardial effusion), GI upset, rash
Ponatinib	15-45 mg po daily (45 mg daily until remission, then 15-30 mg)	Arterial and venous thrombosis and occlusions including fatal myocardial infarction and stroke (up to 35% of patients), heart failure, hepatotoxicity, cardiovascular risk, severe skin rash, pancreatitis, hepatotoxicity, hemorrhage (cerebral, gastrointestinal), cardiac arrhythmias, fluid retention, hypertension, rash, myelosuppression
Ascimimab (phase 1 trial)	Not yet determined	Pancreatitis, increased lipase levels, fatigue, headache, arthralgias, hypertension, thrombocytopenia

---

growth of BCR/ABL-expressing CML cell lines and progenitor cells in vitro and prolonged survival in animal tumor models.

Responses to BCR-ABL1 inhibitor treatment for CML are defined as hematologic (i.e., restoration of normal peripheral blood cell counts), cytogenetic (i.e., loss of the Philadelphia chromosome determined by normal karyotypic or FISH analysis), and molecular (i.e., a three log or greater reduction of detectable *BCR/ABL* transcripts below a standard baseline by RT-PCR) remissions (Table 47.8). After diagnosis, patients are typically started on tyrosine kinase inhibitor (TKI) therapy with careful interim monitoring for toxicities and clinical response. Standardized RT-PCR assays for *BCR/ABL* are used to measure disease response on a molecular level at 3, 6, and 12 months after therapy initiation. Initial clinical trials of imatinib in 1998 were notable for a hematologic remission rate of 96% in patients receiving a dose greater than 300 mg per day for 4 weeks. One third of individuals obtained cytogenetic remission after 8 weeks. Imatinib was shown to be superior to these prior therapies in individuals with newly diagnosed chronic phase CML with complete cytogenetic responses in almost 90% of patients and an overall survival of 89%. The fact that patients achieving remission could have stable disease for years, even

decades, demonstrated conclusively that this agent could effectively alter the natural history of this disease.

Despite these results, most patients achieving cytogenetic responses on imatinib demonstrate persistence of *BCR/ABL*-positive leukemic CML stem cells by sensitive molecular testing. Lifelong imatinib therapy may be required to control disease, and even patients with excellent control of chronic phase CML on imatinib therapy remain at risk for eventual disease progression and therapy failure due to development of imatinib-resistant CML cells and/or non-compliance. It is estimated that up to one third of chronic phase CML patients initiated on imatinib therapy will eventually discontinue the drug due to long-term intolerance of drug-induced side effects (e.g., nausea, vomiting, gastrointestinal issues, peripheral and periorbital edema) or development of imatinib resistance.

To address these issues, four new generation TKIs of BCR/ABL have been developed for the treatment of CML: dasatinib, nilotinib, bosutinib, and ponatinib (Table 47.9). All display increased in vitro potency against the BCR/ABL kinase compared with imatinib. At present, four (imatinib, dasatinib, nilotinib, bosutinib) are indicated for initial therapy of chronic phase CML. Multiple randomized clinical

TABLE 47.10   Scoring Systems for Risk Calculation in Newly Diagnosed Chronic Myeloid Leukemia

Risk Score	Calculation	Risk Category
Sokal score1	Exp 0.0116 × (age – 43.4) + 0.0345 × (spleen – 7.51) + 0.188 × [(platelet count ÷ 700)2 – 0.563] + 0.0887 × (blasts – 2.10)	Low <0.8 Intermediate 0.8 – 1.2 High >1.2
Hasford (EURO) score2	(0.6666 × age [0 when age <50 years; 1, otherwise] + 0.042 × spleen size [cm below costal margin] + 0.0584 × percent blasts + 0.0413 × percent eosinophils + 0.2039 × basophils [0 when basophils <3%; 1, otherwise] + 1.0956 × platelet count [0 when platelets <1500 × 109/L; 1, otherwise]) × 1000	Low ≤780 Intermediate >780-≤1480 High >1480
EUTOS long-term 3 survival (ELTS) score	0.0025 × (age/10)3 + 0.0615 × spleen size cm below costal margin + 0.1052 × blasts in peripheral blood + 0.4104 × (platelet count/1000) – 0.5	Low ≤1.5680 Intermediate >1.5680 but ≤2.2185 High >2.2185

Online calculator for the ELTS score can be found at: https://www.leukemia-net.org/content/leukemias/cml/elts_score/index_eng.html.
Calculation of relative risk based on Sokal or Hasford (EURO) score can be found at: https://www.leukemia-net.org/content/leukemias/cml/euro__and_sokal_score/index_eng.html.

trials comparing imatinib versus dasatinib or nilotinib or bosutinib in patients with newly diagnosed chronic phase CML confirmed that these newer generation TKIs outperformed imatinib as reflected by significantly higher numbers of patients achieving complete cytogenetic and molecular responses at specific time points as compared with imatinib-treated individuals. To date, however, none of these newer TKIs have significantly improved long-term overall or transformation-free survival over imatinib. Moreover, while each of these new generation TKIs have been compared in a randomized fashion with imatinib, none have been compared with any TKI other than imatinib. For this reason, recently available generic imatinib formulations continue to be recommended as the mainstay of upfront therapy for chronic phase CML.

Different scoring systems (Table 47.10) have been developed to predict the outcomes of newly diagnosed chronic phase CML patients. These scores use patient age, spleen size, platelet number, and percentage of myeloblasts as well as peripheral basophilia and eosinophilia to divide patients into low-, intermediate-, and high-risk disease. In the current era of TKI therapy, achievement of cytogenetic and molecular milestones within the first year of therapy has proven to be much more predictive of clinical outcome than these scoring systems. However, calculation of these scores has proven useful to guide selection of upfront therapy at initial presentation. Patients with low and intermediate risk scores may be assigned to standard dose imatinib while higher-risk, particularly younger patients, presenting with very high white blood cell counts and/or massive splenomegaly, may be considered for second-generation TKIs (dasatinib, nilotinib, bosutinib). Alternatively, if imatinib is used in higher-risk patients, closer monitoring for need to switch to another TKI may be warranted. Lastly, given the myriad of TKI agents available for upfront therapy, the excellent overall response (>90% for all TKIs), and the possibility that patients may need to remain on therapy for years if not the rest of their lives, consideration of other factors impacting long-term tolerability and compliance are now given increased importance in drug selection. These include patient preference (i.e., for once a day vs. twice a day administration, with food vs. empty stomach), other medical comorbidities (i.e., cardiovascular vs. pulmonary vs. gastrointestinal) that may be exacerbated by specific TKI associated toxicities, and drug-drug interactions (i.e., proton pump inhibitors and dasatinib) (see Table 47.9).

Perhaps the best indicator of the clinical success of BCR-ABL inhibitor therapy for CML is the fact that it is now possible (with careful monitoring) to permanently discontinue TKI therapy in a proportion of patients with chronic phase disease who have achieved optimal durable molecular responses on therapy. Candidates for "TKI discontinuation therapy" are individuals with chronic phase CML treated with an approved TKI agent for at least 3 years and who have obtained major molecular responses lasting for at least 2 years. Importantly, patients should have no history of accelerated or blast phase CML or demonstrated clinical or mutational resistance to prior TKI therapy. They must also be willing to undergo monthly to bimonthly visits for at least 2 years after drug discontinuation for frequent molecular testing. Although nilotinib is the only TKI with a regulatory indication for drug discontinuation, results of multiple clinical trials suggest that stopping any TKI in patients meeting these criteria results in 40% to 50% success rate (i.e., patients able to eventually permanently stop therapy). The remaining 50% to 60% will experience recurrence of disease as reflected by reemergence of molecular detectable disease by qPCR. If detected early, almost all (detected by reemergent BCR-ABL transcripts off therapy) can resume TKI therapy with re-achievement of major molecular remission. Some patients develop mild to severe musculoskeletal symptoms after discontinuing TKI (termed "TKI withdrawal syndrome"), which is managed with symptomatic medications.

The most common therapeutic strategy for chronic phase CML patients intolerant of or resistant to first-line TKI therapy based on lack of achievement of molecular and cytogenetic milestones is to switch to another TKI. Mutational analysis at the time of relapse (see Table 47.9) is essential because up to one half of CML patients who develop resistance to imatinib have cancer cells carrying single-nucleotide mutations in the BCR/ABL gene. These mutations result in conformational changes of the BCR/ABL kinase, altering drug binding and inhibitory effects. For this reason, it is recommended that patients requiring second-line therapy or beyond undergo testing for identification of mutations as a potential guide to therapy. CML patients with disease associated with a mutation at T315I are known to be resistant to imatinib, nilotinib, dasatinib, and bosutinib, but not to ponatinib, a third-generation BCR/ABL inhibitor. Use of ponatinib, a highly potent third-generation BCR-ABL inhibitor, is restricted to individuals with chronic, accelerated or blast phase CML who have failed and/or been intolerant to at least two prior TKI therapies or whose mutational testing demonstrates a BCR-ABL T315I tyrosine kinase domain mutation conferring resistance to all other TKIs. Ponatinib is not recommended for the treatment of patients with newly diagnosed chronic phase CML due to adverse events of arterial occlusion (including fatal myocardial infarction, stroke, and severe peripheral vascular disease occurring in up to 35% of patients), venous thromboembolism, heart failure, and hepatotoxicity. In patients with CML that has failed three or more TKIs, treatment with asciminib, a novel allosteric inhibitor of BCR-ABL, has shown promising activity. This agent binds a myristoyl site of BCR-ABL1 protein and thereby locks BCR-ABL1 into an inactive conformation through a mechanism distinct from all other ABL kinase inhibitors. Because asciminib targets both native and mutated BCR-ABL1, it is also effective against CML cells harboring the gatekeeper *T315I* mutation. In a phase 1 trial, almost half (48%) of patients achieved a major molecular response in 12 months, including 8 of 14 patients with prior intolerance or resistance to ponatinib.

Patients whose disease does not respond and/or who are intolerant of multiple TKIs also may receive treatment with omacetaxine mepesuccinate, a natural alkaloid product with proven antitumor activity and efficacy in CML. Its mechanisms of action are distinct from the TKIs and involve inhibition of protein synthesis and induction of apoptosis in tumor cells. Several clinical trials have confirmed the activity of this agent in patients with CML failing multiple TKIs and/or carrying the T315I mutation. A major drawback is the need for subcutaneous injections administered twice daily for 7 to 14 days of every 28 days per month and treatment-associated myelosuppression that may warrant dose reduction or interruption.

Accelerated and Blast Phase CML

Unfortunately, the majority of patients with accelerated or blast phase CML treated with new-generation TKI therapies experience only transient hematologic and cytogenetic responses. For these patients, the optimal treatment modality remains TKI therapy with newer-generation agents with or without additional chemotherapy or clinical trials followed by allogeneic stem cell transplantation (alloSCT). The novel allosteric BCR-ABL inhibitor, asciminib, reportedly induced hematologic responses in seven of eight patients with accelerated phase CML with a median duration of response of greater than 11 months. Blast phase CML patients often undergo induction chemotherapy with acute leukemia regimens with concomitant BCR/ABL inhibition. Transplantation, however, remains the only known curative therapy for these patients. Prior to the advent of targeted BCR/ABL kinase inhibitor therapy, young patients with an HLA-matched donor were routinely offered potentially curative alloSCT at the time of diagnosis of chronic phase CML. Evidence indicated that the excellent response (50% to 75%) of CML patients to SCT was partly related to the active suppression of the disease by the newly transplanted graft, called the *graft-versus-leukemia effect*. At present, in the face of the excellent control and low overall toxicity of long-term BCR/ABL inhibitors for chronic phase CML, together with the known 20% to 30% mortality and morbidity rates after alloSCT, transplantation is now viewed as an option only for patients with accelerated or blast phase disease or chronic phase CML failing multiple lines of prior therapy. Following alloSCT, it is now considered standard of care to resume TKI maintenance therapy for at least 12 months in the post-transplant setting to prevent disease relapse.

Prognosis

Overall, the transformation of CML from a progressively fatal cancer to one in which almost 90% of patients are alive with stable disease on oral kinase therapy and 10% can permanently discontinue therapy after 5 years remains one of the crowning achievements in cancer therapy in the past decade. The median overall survival for chronic phase CML patients has risen dramatically from a few months to a few years in the first half of the 20th century to 6 years for interferon-treated patients. In the era of BCR/ABL inhibition therapy, overall lifespan is expected to be almost normal for most patients on long-term TKI therapy with multiple studies demonstrating that the risk of death in these

individuals occurs not due to CML-related complications but rather to increased cardiac and vascular causes. For this reason, a focus of current CML practice is determining how best to balance the long-term toxicities of TKI therapy with its benefits. Although standard of care for CML patients who are responding optimally to treatment remains indefinite continuation of TKI therapy, selected individuals with sustained excellent molecular responses to TKI therapy for at least 3 years are now eligible to discontinue therapy with a 40% to 50% long-term success rate. Despite this therapeutic advance, a true cure for CML disease remains elusive for the majority of patients. Ongoing clinical studies are focused on strategies to further enhance this percentage by targeting CML stem cells and via combinatorial TKI approaches.

ACUTE LEUKEMIAS

Definition and Epidemiology

The acute leukemias are clinically aggressive clonal hematopoietic diseases arising from the malignant transformation of an early hematopoietic stem cell. In adults, acute leukemias are relatively uncommon and occur in 8 to 10 of 100,000 people (compared with 42 of 100,000 for prostate cancer and 62 of 100,000 for breast cancer). Acute leukemias are classified by cell lineage as AML or acute lymphocytic or lymphoblastic leukemia (ALL) based on morphology, cytogenetics, cell surface and cytoplasmic markers, and molecular studies. Between 80% and 90% of leukemia diagnoses in adults are AML. In contrast, 80% to 90% of leukemias in infants and children are ALL, and they constitute the most common cancer diagnosed in this age group.

Pathology

The pathogenesis of acute leukemia is complex and characterized by a high degree of biologic heterogeneity. Many patients with acute leukemia have detectable characteristic clonal chromosomal abnormalities and mutations that drive malignant transformation of normal hematopoietic stem cells bearing myeloid or lymphoid lineage markers. The resultant unchecked proliferation of these immature cells incapable of further differentiation (i.e., blasts) results in marrow replacement by malignant cells, peripheral leukocytosis, with and without severe cytopenias, and rapid hematopoietic failure. Known risk factors for leukemia include high-dose radiation exposure and occupational exposure to chemicals including benzene. Up to 10% of patients with prior malignancies treated with myelosuppressive chemotherapy and/or radiation develop "therapy-related" AML (t-AML). Individuals with t-AML with previous chemotherapy have usually received alkylating agents (e.g., chlorambucil, melphalan, nitrogen mustard) or topoisomerase II inhibitors (e.g., epipodophyllotoxins). Patients with chromosomal instability disorders such as Down syndrome, Bloom syndrome, Fanconi anemia, and ataxia telangiectasia also have an increased incidence of leukemia.

Diagnosis and Differential Diagnosis

To make the distinction between AML and ALL is crucial diagnostically, therapeutically, and prognostically. AML can be distinguished from ALL by cell morphology and the finding of Auer rods (sometimes multiple ones in acute promyelocytic leukemia cells), which are formed by the aggregation of myeloid granules (E-Fig. 47.3C). Further immunophenotyping of blast cells using cell surface antigens, cytochemistry, and immunohistochemistry confirms cells as having a myeloid or lymphoid origin. Morphologic subgroups of ALL and AML were originally defined by the French-American-British (FAB) classification and most recently by the 2016 World Health Organization (WHO) classification, which incorporates newer biologic information, specifically mutations and recurrent cytogenetic aberrations (Table 47.11).

TABLE 47.11   Classification of Acute Leukemias

FAB Classification of Acute Myeloid Leukemia (AML)

M0: Acute myelocytic leukemia with minimal differentiation

M1: Acute myelocytic leukemia without maturation

M2: Acute myelocytic leukemia with maturation (predominantly myeloblasts and promyelocytes)

M3: Acute promyelocytic leukemia

M4: Acute myelomonocytic leukemia

M5: Acute monocytic leukemia

M6: Erythroleukemia

M7: Megakaryocytic leukemia

FAB Classification of Acute Lymphoblastic Leukemia (ALL)

L1: Predominantly small cells (twice the size of normal lymphocyte), homogeneous population; childhood variant

L2: Larger than L1, more heterogenous population; adult variant

L3: Burkitt-like large cells, vacuolated abundant cytoplasm

WHO 2016 Classification of Acute Leukemia

I. Acute myeloid leukemia (AML)

  A. AML with recurrent genetic abnormalities

    • AML with t(8;21)(q22;q22); *RUNX1-RUNX1T1*

    • AML with inv(16)(p13;q22) or t(16;16)(p13;q22); *CBFB/MYH11*

    • Acute promyelocytic leukemia (AML with t[15;17][q22;q12]; *PML/RARA*

    • AML with t(9;11)(p21.3;q23.3); *MLLT3-KMT2A*

    • AML with t(6;9)(p23;q34.1); *DEK-NUP214*

    • AML with inv(3)(q21.3 q26.2) or t(3;3)(q21.3;q26.2); *GATA2,MECOM*

    • AML (megakaryoblastic) with t(1;22)(p13.3; q13.3); *RBM15-MKL1*

    • AML with *BCR-ABL1*

    • AML with mutant *NPM1*

    • AML with biallelic mutations of *CEBPA*

    • AML with mutated *RUNX1*

  B. AML with myelodysplasia-related changes

  C. Therapy related myeloid neoplasms

  D. AML not otherwise specified

    • AML with minimal differentiation

    • AML without maturation

    • AML with maturation

    • Acute myelomonocytic leukemia

    • Acute monoblastic/monocytic leukemia

    • Pure erythroid leukemia

    • Acute megakaryoblastic leukemia

    • Acute basophilic leukemia

    • Acute panmyelosis with myelofibrosis

  E. Myeloid sarcoma

  F. Myeloid proliferations associated with Down syndrome

  G. Blastic plasmacytoid dendritic cell neoplasm

  H. Acute leukemias of ambiguous lineage

II. Precursor lymphoid neoplasms

  A. B-lymphoblastic leukemia/lymphoblastic lymphoma, not otherwise specified

  B. B-lymphoblastic leukemia/lymphoma with recurrent genetic abnormalities

    • B-lymphoblastic leukemia/lymphoma with t(9;22)(q34.1,q11.2); *BCR-ABL1*

    • B-lymphoblastic leukemia/lymphoma with t(v;11q23.3); *KMT2A*-rearranged

    • B-lymphoblastic leukemia/lymphoma with t(12;21)(p13.2;q22.1); *ETV6-RUNX1*

    • B-lymphoblastic leukemia/lymphoma with hyperdiploidy

    • B-lymphoblastic leukemia/lymphoma with hypodiploidy

    • B-lymphoblastic leukemia/lymphoma with t95;14)(q31.1,q32.1); *IGH/IL3*

    • B-lymphoblastic leukemia/lymphoma with t(;19)(q23,p13.3); *TCF3-PBX1*

    • B-lymphoblastic leukemia/lymphoma, *BCR-ABL1*-like

    • B-lymphoblastic leukemia/lymphoma with iAMP21

  C. T-lymphoblastic leukemia/lymphoblastic lymphoma

    • Early T-cell precursor lymphoblastic leukemia

  D. NK lymphoblastic leukemia/lymphoma

From Swerdlow SH, Campo E, Harris NL, Jaffe ES, Pileri SA, Stein H, Thiele J. WHO Classification of Tumours of Haematopoietic and Lymphoid Tissues (Revised Fourth Edition), IARC, 2016.

CBF, Core binding factor; *ETO,* eight twenty-one; *FAB,* French-American-British; *MDS,* primary myelodysplastic syndrome; *MLL,* mixed-lineage leukemia; *MYH11,* myosin heavy chain gene; *PML,* promyelocytic leukemia; *RARA,* retinoic acid receptor-α; *WHO,* World Health Organization.

Clinical Presentation

Patients exhibit clinical evidence of bone marrow failure similar to other hematopoietic disorders. Complications of disease include anemia, infection, and bleeding from peripheral cytopenias. Proliferating blasts infiltrating the bone marrow may cause bone pain. Blasts may also invade other organs and lead to peripheral, mediastinal, and abdominal lymphadenopathy, hepatosplenomegaly, skin infiltration, and meningeal involvement.

Treatment

Therapy for acute leukemias is divided into several stages. *Induction therapy* is directed at reducing the number of leukemic blasts to an undetectable level and restoring normal hematopoiesis (i.e., complete remission). At complete remission, however, significant subclinical disease persists, requiring further therapy. Subsequent *consolidation therapy* involves continuing chemotherapy with the same agents to induce elimination of additional leukemic cells. With development of a wider range of effective agents, *intensification therapy* has been introduced. It involves the use of high-dose therapy with different non–cross-reactive drugs to eliminate cells with potential primary resistance to the induction regimen. *Maintenance therapy* employs low-dose, intermittent chemotherapy given over a prolonged period to prevent subsequent disease relapse. The goal of therapy is to induce remission (>5% blasts in the bone marrow and recovery of normal peripheral blood counts).

Prognosis

Adverse clinical prognostic factors for AML and ALL are similar despite widely different treatment approaches. In both leukemias, cytogenetic and molecular abnormalities represent the best independent predictors of overall survival (Tables 47.11, 47.12, and 47.13). Clinical factors that predict a poor outcome differ by specific leukemia type but generally include older age (>35 years in ALL, >60 years for AML), secondary or therapy-related disease, antecedent hematologic disorder, high initial leukocyte count (50 to 100 × 10^9/L), poor performance status and comorbidities, extramedullary disease, prolonged time (>4 weeks) or lack of response to initial treatment, and presence of detectable minimal residual disease (MRD) despite morphologic remission.

Acute Myeloid Leukemia
Definition and Epidemiology

AML represents a biologically heterogeneous group of neoplasms with widely divergent clinical outcomes. Long-term cure rates (survival >5 years) range from 5% to 60% after chemotherapy alone, with an overall cure rate of 20% to 30%. AML occurs primarily in older adults, with a median age at diagnosis of 65 years.

Clinical Presentation

Patients most often have complications related to progressively severe cytopenia, such as infection due to leukopenia, shortness of breath or fatigue due to anemia, or bleeding due to thrombocytopenia. AML patients may also have unique acute clinical emergencies requiring immediate stabilization. Leukostasis (i.e., hyperleukocytosis syndrome) caused by high levels of circulating blasts (>80,000 to 100,000) leads to diffuse pulmonary infiltrates and acute respiratory distress. Blast cells may also injure surrounding vasculature, causing life-threatening CNS bleeding and thromboses. High blast cell numbers result in the release of cellular breakdown products (i.e., tumor lysis syndrome), leading to hypokalemia, acidosis, and hyperuricemia with resultant renal failure.

Treatment of leukostasis should be instituted as soon as possible for all patients with white blood cell counts in excess of 100 to 200 ×

10^9/L. Treatment consists of leukapheresis, hydroxyurea, and initiation of induction chemotherapy to inhibit further production of circulating tumor cells. Hydration, urine alkalinization to reduce uric acid crystallization, allopurinol, or rasburicase, or a combination, should be initiated as indicated. Red blood cell transfusions are often contraindicated in patients with high numbers of circulating blast cells because of the risk of further increases in blood viscosity. CNS complications such as intracranial bleeding, cranial nerve invasion, and leukemic meningitis are treated with emergency whole brain irradiation or radiation directed to affected sites.

Laboratory evaluation of patients with AML typically shows white blood cell counts ranging from neutropenic levels (<1 × 10^9/L) to extreme leukocytosis (>100,000 × 10^9/L). Severe thrombocytopenia, normocytic anemia, and circulating peripheral blasts are common. Bone marrow aspirate and biopsy typically show a profusion of myeloblasts (20% to 100%) and depressed production of normal mature cells.

Diagnosis

Diagnostic marrow aspirates and/or peripheral blood samples require evaluation by morphology (see E-Fig. 47.3), flow cytometry, cytogenetic, and molecular analyses to distinguish between AML and ALL and to determine biologic subsets of AML disease for prognostic and therapeutic purposes.

In the past, AML subsets were classified based largely on morphologic criteria and immunohistochemical staining as FAB subtypes M0 through M7, largely defined by the stage of cellular differentiation of the abnormal cells (see Table 47.11). Some FAB subsets correlate with specific clinical syndromes, which helps to determine treatment approaches and prognosis. The most common FAB subtype of adult AML is M2. Patients with AML M3 (i.e., acute promyelocytic leukemia) often exhibit spontaneous bleeding from disseminated intravascular coagulation (discussed later). Patients with AML M4 or M5 disease (i.e., acute monocytic-myelomonocytic leukemias) have high levels of circulating white blood cells and may have swollen gums resulting from tissue infiltration with leukemic blasts. Patients with megakaryoblastic leukemia (AML M7) have significant marrow fibrosis and usually exhibit organomegaly and pancytopenia similar to those seen in patients with myelofibrosis and myeloid metaplasia.

Large-scale genomic analyses of AML samples have revealed the vast molecular complexity of this disease and identified myriad gene mutations capable of further refining AML prognosis in conjunction with karyotype. For instance, up to one third of patients with normal-karyotype AML have constitutive activation of the FMS-like tyrosine kinase 3 (FLT3) receptor as a result of point mutations or internal tandem duplications (ITDs) not seen on routine karyotypic testing. *FLT3 ITD* mutations in AML patients predict for lower remission rates, high relapse rates, and shorter overall survival compared with *FLT3*-negative AML patients. Patients with higher *FLT3 ITD* tumor burden (reflected by the ratio of mutant to wild-type *FLT3* or the allelic ratio) have particularly poor prognoses, whereas individuals with low *FLT3 ITD* allelic ratio may have outcomes similar to *FLT3* wild-type patients. Mutations that predict improved overall survival after chemotherapy include biallelic mutations in the transcription factor CCAAT/enhancer binding protein-α (*CEBPA*) and nucleophosmin 1 (*NPM1*) in the absence of *FLT3 ITDs* (see Tables 47.11 and 47.12).

The classification and prognostication of AML was refined in 2016 by the WHO to recognize biologic subtypes with unique genetic abnormalities such as t(8;21), inv(16), t(15;17), and t(9;11) as well as *BCR-ABL1*, biallelic *CEBPA*, and *RUNX1* mutations. Other categories include AML with myelodysplastic-related changes (defined by

TABLE 47.12 European Leukemia Net (ELN) Classification of Acute Myeloid Leukemia (2017)

Risk Category	Genetic Abnormality
Favorable	t(8;21)(q22;q22.1); *RUNX1-RUNX1T1*
	inv(16)(p13.1q22) or t(16;16)(p13.1;q22): *CBFB-MYH11*
	Mutated *NPM1* without *FLT3-ITD* or with *FLT3-ITD*low
	Biallelic mutated *CEBPA*
Intermediate	Mutated *NPM1* and *FLT-ITD*high
	Wild-type NPM1 without *FLT3-ITD* or with *FLT3* ITDlow (without adverse genetic lesions) t(9;11)(p21.3;q23.3): *MLLT3-KMT2A*
	Cytogenetic abnormalities not classified as favorable or adverse)
Adverse	t(6;9)(p23;q34.1); *DEK-NUP214*
	t(v;11q23.3): *KMT2A* rearranged
	t(9;22)(q34.1:q11.2): *BCR-ABL1*
	inv(3)(q21.3q26.2) or t(3;3)(q21.3;q26.2);*GATA2, MECOM (EV11)*
	−5 or del(5q); −7; −17/abn(17p)
	Complex karyotype, monosomal karyotype
	Wild-type *NPM1* and *FLT3-ITD*high
	Mutated *RUNX1*
	Mutated *ASXL1*
	Mutated *TP53*

From Dohner H, Estey EH, Grimwade D, et al. Diagnosis and management of AML in adults: 2017 ELM recommendations from an international expert panel. Blood 129(4): 424-447, 2017.
ITDs, Internal tandem duplications.

TABLE 47.13 Prognostic Factors in Acute Lymphoblastic Leukemia

Factor	Favorable	Unfavorable
Age	2-10 yr	<2 yr or >10 yr
White blood cell count at diagnosis	<30,000/μL	>50,000/μL
Phenotype	Precursor B	Precursor T
Chromosome number	Hyperdiploidy	Pseudo/hypodiploidy, near tetraploidy
Chromosome abnormality	t(12;21)	*MYC* alterations: t(8;14), t(2;8), t(8;22) mixed-lineage leukemia alterations (11q23)
		Philadelphia chromosome: t(9;22), creating *BCR-ABL*
Central nervous system disease at diagnosis	No	Yes
Sex	Women	Men
Ethnicity	White	African American, Hispanic
Time to remission	Short (7-14 days)	Prolonged time to remission or failure to achieve remission

the presence of multilineage dysplasia, prior clinical and pathologic results, and/or characteristic karyotypic aberrations) and therapy-related AML (based on clinical history of prior chemotherapy, irradiation, or other myeloablative therapy preceding AML diagnosis). In the latter case, any marrow dysplasia together with cytopenias is now considered therapy-related AML rather than MDS regardless of blast count (see Table 47.11).

Treatment and Prognosis

Upfront chemotherapy for AML has changed drastically over the last few years due to the advent of multiple new drugs for specific clinical and biological subsets of disease. For decades, it has been known that the clinical factors predictive of poor outcome include advanced age (>60 years old), therapy-related or with antecedent hematologic disorder (termed secondary AML), poor performance status, elevated initial white blood cell counts (>20-30K to >100K), and presence of disease outside the bone marrow. Extramedullary disease includes leukemic involvement in the central nervous system, skin and soft tissues (myeloid or granulocytic sarcoma), and any other organ involvement outside of the bone marrow and peripheral blood. Although these clinical factors are still considered, in this era the most important factors impacting treatment decisions for newly diagnosed patients are (1) overall functionality/comorbidities and (2) AML risk category.

AML is known to be a biologically heterogeneous disease with vast differences in outcomes based on underlying disease. Early AML risk prognostication was based primarily on karyotypic aberrations that have stood the test of time as the most robust independent predictors of response to intensive (cytarabine and anthracycline based) chemotherapy approaches. However, recent advances in genomic and molecular technologies have shed much light on the role of diverse gene mutations to AML pathogenesis. Genes involved in at least eight different biologic processes have been identified in primary AML samples. The most recent AML risk classification proposed by the European Leukemia Net delineates three risk categories (favorable, intermediate, and poor risk) incorporating diagnostic cytogenetic and molecular information (see Table 47.12). Because the presence of certain "actionable" mutations (specifically *CBF, FLT3, NPM1, IDH1,* and *IDH2*) can significantly alter upfront therapy selection, it is recommended that molecular tests evaluating these aberrations be performed in an expedited manner (turnaround time of 3-5 days) in all suspected AML cases (see Table 47.12).

Treatment based on disease subsets

Patients who are younger than 60 years and/or fit for intensive chemotherapy. The "traditional" induction regimens administered in the inpatient setting consist of 7 days of cytosine arabinoside (i.e., cytarabine) and 3 days of high-dose anthracycline (i.e., daunorubicin or idarubicin) and is commonly referred to as "7+3." Once morphologic remission (marrow blasts <5%) and count recovery (WBC >1000, platelets >100,000/mcL) have occurred, an additional two to four cycles of consolidation chemotherapy with high-dose cytarabine with or without anthracycline are administered over 4 to 6 months. Standard 7+3 induction regimens lead to complete remission in 60% to 80% of younger adults with de novo AML. Lower remission rates are achieved for older adults (>60 years) and in patients with antecedent hematologic diseases evolving into AML. After achieving complete remission after induction, patients may be offered additional consolidation chemotherapy or treatment with allogeneic or autologous SCT (see Chapter 46). Decisions about the best time to perform SCT in patients are most often guided by clinical risk factors and prognostic risk category. Although clinical outcomes are improved when patients undergo SCT after initial induction chemotherapy (i.e., during the first complete remission) rather than after disease relapse, chemotherapeutic regimens are also more effective in the first remission than they are after transplantation, and they may be better tolerated than SCT, which carries an overall mortality rate of

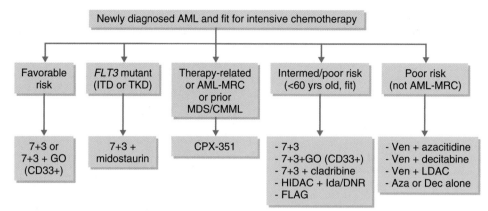

Fig. 47.1 Treatment of patients with newly diagnosed acute myeloid leukemia AML and considered fit for intensive chemotherapy. *7+3*, 7 days of continuous infusional cytarabine 100-200 mg/m²/day plus 3 days of anthracycline (daunorubicin 45-90 mg/m²/day or idarubicin 12 mg/m²/day); *AML*, acute myeloid leukemia; *AML-MRC*, acute myeloid leukemia with myelodysplastic related changes; *CD33+*, expressing CD33 surface antigen; *CMML*, chronic myelomonocytic leukemia (a subtype of MDS); *CPX-351*, liposomal formulation of cytarabine and daunorubicin; *Dec*, decitabine; *DNR*, daunorubicin; *FLAG*, intensive chemotherapy regimen consisting of fludarabine, intermediate-dose cytarabine, and G-CSF; *FLT3*, fms-like tyrosine kinase 3; *GO*, gemtuzumab ozogamicin; *HIDAC*, high-dose cytarabine; *Ida*, idarubicin; *ITD*, internal tandem duplication mutation; *LDAC*, low-dose cytarabine; *MDS*, myelodysplastic syndrome; *TKD*, tyrosine kinase domain mutation; *Ven*, venetoclax.

25% to 30%. Patients whose AML fails to respond to initial induction therapy have a grim overall prognosis and are eligible for treatment with high-dose cytarabine–containing regimens or low-dose therapy incorporating hypomethylating agents (azacitidine, decitabine) and/or experimental agents in order to obtain remission.

Treatment of younger (<60 years old) individuals with AML should be tailored based on specific AML risk classification (Fig. 47.1). Patients with favorable risk AML characterized by t(8;21), inv(16) or del(16q) aberrations are unusually responsive to induction chemotherapy followed by two to four cycles of high-dose cytosine arabinoside consolidation. Long-term 5-year survival rates of 55% to 60% can be obtained. Further improvement in outcomes has been demonstrated with the addition of gemtuzumab ozogamicin (GO), an antibody drug conjugate directed against the CD33+ surface antigen expressed on the majority of myeloid blasts. In a meta-analysis of five randomized controlled clinical trials, the addition of GO to 7+3-based induction and consolidation therapy improved overall survival by 20% over chemotherapy alone. AML patients with favorable disease features potentially responsive to high-dose cytarabine chemotherapy are encouraged to delay SCT until the time of relapse.

Some cytogenetic aberrations confer poor prognosis and are associated with resistance to and/or early relapse following standard chemotherapy regimens. These "poor-risk" cytogenetics include deletions in chromosome 5 or 7, inv(3q), t(3;3), t(6;9), t(9;22) (also known as the Philadelphia chromosome), monosomal karyotype, and three or more karyotypic abnormalities (i.e., complex karyotype). Mutations associated with poor prognosis are *FLT3-ITD*, *RUNX1*, *ASXL1*, and *TP53*. Remission rates for these poor-risk cytogenetic and molecular subtypes of AML are low; if remission is achieved, patients remain at high risk for AML relapse within the first 12 months due to presence of chemotherapy-refractory disease. Overall survival rates for poor-prognosis AML are 5% to 15%. AlloSCT is recommended for and represents the best chance for long-term cure of patients with poor-risk AML such as disease associated with unfavorable cytogenetic and molecular features, antecedent hematologic disease, or therapy-related or primary refractory disease. Poor-risk AML patients younger than 60 years undergoing allogeneic bone marrow transplantation from a

matched donor have long-term overall survival rates of 40% to 60%, compared with cure rates after conventional chemotherapy of only 5% to 20%. For younger individuals with poor-risk AML appropriate for intensive chemotherapy, the preferred approach is 7+3-based induction (without GO) followed by alloSCT in first remission.

Outcomes of standard cytarabine- and anthracycline-based intensive chemotherapy in patients with therapy-related AML (tAML) or secondary AML (sAML) arising out of antecedent myelodysplastic syndrome (MDS) or with MDS-related changes (AML-MRC) remains dismal. Long-term survival ranges from 10% to 20% regardless of age, and alloSCT is universally considered the only curative approach. Patients 60 years or older with these difficult-to-treat AML subtypes (tAML, sAML, AML, with MRC) achieve improved remission rates and prolonged overall survival, particularly in the context of subsequent alloSCT, following treatment with a liposomal cytarabine and daunorubicin formulation (formerly known as CPX-351) as compared with standard infusion cytarabine and daunorubicin. It has been speculated that the improved drug pharmacokinetics, specifically enhanced marrow drug delivery and retention, may lead to improved eradication of AML blasts in these specific subsets.

FLT3 mutations are the most common gene mutations in AML and constitute an "actionable" mutation because patients with *FLT3*-mutant AML benefit from treatment with oral TKI of mutant FLT3 signaling pathways, similar to BCR/ABL inhibitors in CML. In newly diagnosed patients with *FLT3*-mutant disease, the addition of midostaurin, a first-generation FLT3 TKI, to upfront cytarabine and anthracycline induction and consolidation chemotherapy improved overall survival (but not remission rate) as compared to chemotherapy alone. Of note, these improved outcomes were dependent in part on the majority of patients with *FLT3*-mutant AML undergoing alloSCT at time of remission.

The remaining half of AML patients have intermediate-risk cytogenetics, which is defined as a normal karyotype, trisomy 8, t(9;11), or other cytogenetic abnormalities not included in the other groups. These patients have a 30% to 45% long-term survival rate with standard 7+3 chemotherapy (see Table 47.12). Actionable mutations in *FLT3*, *NPM-1*, *IDH1*, and *IDH2* genes occur most frequently in intermediate-risk disease and carry significant therapeutic and prognostic implications. Multiple alternative

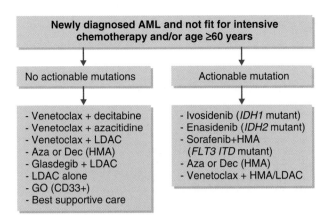

Fig. 47.2 Treatment of patients with newly diagnosed acute myeloid leukemia and considered not fit for intensive chemotherapy and/or age 60 years old or older. *AML,* Acute myeloid leukemia; *Aza,* azacytidine; *CD33+,* expressing CD33 surface antigen; *Dec,* decitabine; *FLT3,* fms-like tyrosine kinase 3; *GO,* gemtuzumab ozogamicin; *HMA,* hypomethylating agents consisting of azacytidine and decitabine; *IDH1,* isocitrate dehydrogenase isoform 1; *IDH2,* isocitrate dehydrogenase isoform 2; *LDAC,* low-dose cytarabine.

induction regimens other than 7+3 have been explored to improve prognosis for intermediate- and poor-risk AML patients. These include substitution of higher-dose intermittent-dosed cytarabine instead of 7-day infusional cytarabine and the addition of other agents (such as cladribine or fludarabine) to cytarabine and anthracycline in attempts to enhance responses. The addition of GO to 7+3 has been shown to improve overall survival in intermediate-risk AML, albeit to a much lesser degree (5.7%) than in favorable-risk patients. Risks of GO include prolonged myelosuppression with associated hemorrhagic complications and increased risk of fatal veno-occlusive disease (VOD), particularly in patients undergoing subsequent alloSCT. Recently, the rate of VOD appears to have been significantly mitigated (4%) by the use of fractionated (i.e., 3 mg/m² on days 1, 4, and 7) GO dosing. Intermediate-risk AML patients with unfavorable prognosis (based on clinical or molecular data) ideally should be offered alloSCT, particularly younger individuals with few comorbidities and related family donors. Those patients who are ineligible for allogeneic transplantation because of advanced age, other medical issues, or lack of HLA-compatible donors may be offered chemotherapy or autologous SCT instead. Whether autologous transplantation improves AML outcomes compared with chemotherapy alone is a matter of debate. However, the long-term survival rates after autologous transplantation range from 20% to 40% and are at least equivalent to consolidation chemotherapy regimens for these patients.

Patients 60 years or older and/or not fit for aggressive therapy now have a number of therapeutic options (Fig. 47.2). Because the median age at diagnosis of AML is 65 years, a sizable proportion of AML patients are elderly individuals with major comorbidities or antecedent hematologic or malignant diseases, rendering them poor candidates for intensive induction chemotherapeutic regimens or myeloablative SCT. Infectious complications remain the major cause of morbidity and mortality during intensive inpatient chemotherapy despite advances in prophylactic growth factor support, antibiotics, and antifungal agents. The low expected remission rates (30% to 50%) and high mortality and morbidity rates associated with induction are additional reasons for many patients to decline aggressive therapy. Fortunately, multiple therapeutic options are now available specifically for treatment of these older adults who in the recent past would have been offered only supportive therapy with hydroxyurea, transfusion support alone, and hospice.

Patients older than 75 years old and/or those unfit for and who choose not to receive intensive therapy now have a panoply of

low-dose chemotherapy options. Historically, chemotherapy regimens for older patients consisted of either low-dose cytarabine (LDAC) or hypomethylating therapy (HMA) (azacytidine, decitabine). These regimens have been well tolerated, but both are associated with disappointing response rates and median survival duration of less than 6 to 7 months. Low-dose subcutaneous cytarabine resulted in remission rates of about 18%, whereas HMA induced remissions ranging from 20% to 47%. Some individuals treated with HMA also experience hematologic improvement, disease stabilization, and prolonged overall survival, even in absence of complete remission.

Combination regimens adding therapeutic agents to HMA or LDAC backbones now constitute the new standard of care for individuals unable to receive intensive chemotherapy. Venetoclax is a highly potent oral inhibitor of BCL-2, upon which AML cells are dependent for viability. The addition of venetoclax to HMA therapy in older unfit patients resulted in remissions in 67% of patients with a median overall survival of 17.5 months. Of note, almost two thirds of patients with traditionally unfavorable prognostic factors including poor-risk cytogenetics, age 75 years old or older, and secondary AML attained complete remission or complete remission with incomplete count recovery. Venetoclax combined with LDAC resulted in slightly lower overall response rates (54%) and in specific subsets including poor-risk cytogenetics (42%) and secondary AML (35%). Patients who had previously received HMA therapy for MDS prior to venetoclax and LDAC therapy also had lower remission rates (33%) as compared to no prior HMA exposure (62%). Adverse events included significant myelosuppression with risk of infection, sepsis, and pneumonia leading to early death in a proportion of patients. Glasdegib is an oral inhibitor of sonic hedgehog signaling important for leukemia stem cell survival and expansion with minimal single agent activity but improved efficacy when combined with LDAC. Addition of glasdegib to LDAC significantly improved remission rate to 19% and extended overall survival to 8.8 months as compared to LDAC alone (4.9 months). Treatment was well tolerated with relatively little myelosuppression or cytopenia. The excellent tolerability of this regimen with relatively little myelosuppression and the ability to treat patients completely in the outpatient setting makes it an option for select individuals. Gemtuzumab ozogamicin monotherapy represents yet another option for these patients with CD33+ AML with survival duration of less than 6 months.

Treatment decisions may also be altered by the presence of actionable mutations in *FLT3, IDH1,* and *IDH2* genes. Patients with *IDH1*- or *IDH2*-mutant disease are eligible to receive therapy with oral inhibitors of IDH1 (ivosidenib) and IDH2 (enasidenib), respectively. These agents, originally evaluated in the relapsed/refractory setting, result in overall response rates of approximately 40% and are well tolerated without myelosuppression. One unusual toxicity of IDH inhibitors is development of differentiation syndrome, similar to that seen with treatment of acute promyelocytic leukemia (APL), and characterized by elevated white count, fever, edema, and pulmonary infiltrates. Of note, *IDH1/2*-mutant AML patients also experienced very high response rates (80% to 90%) following venetoclax plus HMA/LDAC, making this the preferred regimen over targeted IDH inhibitors for upfront therapy if tolerable in specific patients.

Addition of a first-generation FLT3 TKI (sorafenib) to HMA therapy is recommended for upfront therapy of *FLT3-ITD*–mutant AML in unfit patients. Use of newer-generation TKIs for this indication is currently under investigation. Venetoclax plus HMA or LDAC is also effective in *FLT3*-mutant AML, raising the question of whether FLT3 TKI or venetoclax is the better therapeutic partner to combine with HMA in *FLT3*-mutant AML. However, recent clinical and preclinical data have suggested that *FLT3* mutations may constitute an overall mechanism of resistance to venetoclax based therapy.

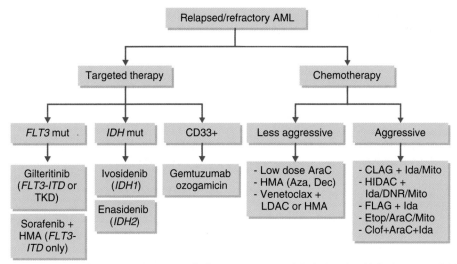

Fig. 47.3 Treatment of patients with relapsed/refractory acute myeloid leukemia. *AML,* Acute myeloid leukemia; *AraC,* cytarabine; *Aza,* azacytidine; *CD33+,* expressing CD33 surface antigen; *CLAG,* intensive chemotherapy regimen including cladribine, intermediate-dose cytarabine, and G-CSF; *Clof,* clofarabine; *Dec,* decitabine; *DNR,* daunorubicin; *Etop/AraC/Mito,* intensive chemotherapy regimen consisting of etoposide, intermediate dose cytarabine, and mitoxantrone; *FLAG,* intensive chemotherapy regimen consisting of fludarabine, intermediate-dose cytarabine, and G-CSF; *FLT3,* fms-like tyrosine kinase 3; *HIDAC,* high-dose cytarabine; *HMA,* hypomethylating agents consisting of azacytidine and decitabine; *Ida,* idarubicin; *IDH,* isocitrate dehydrogenase; *IDH1,* isocitrate dehydrogenase isoform 1; *IDH2,* isocitrate dehydrogenase isoform 2; *ITD,* internal tandem duplication mutation; *LDAC,* low-dose cytarabine; *Mito,* mitoxantrone; *TKD,* tyrosine kinase domain mutation.

Relapsed or refractory disease. Similar to newly diagnosed patients, individuals with AML relapsing following or refractory to standard upfront therapy should be assessed for their overall ability to tolerate aggressive versus less-aggressive therapy and for the presence of actionable mutations (Fig. 47.3).

Next-generation and single cell sequencing technology has demonstrated the importance of repeat molecular testing at the time of AML recurrence. Clonal evolution or emergence as a consequence of prior therapy can lead to a significantly different mutational profile at relapse than at initial AML presentation with significant therapeutic implications. For instance, patients with relapsed/refractory *FLT3*-mutant AML (both ITD and TKD mutations) benefit more from single-agent therapy with a potent next-generation FLT3 TKI, gilteritinib, than from therapy with either intensive or low-dose chemotherapy. Complete remission rate (37% vs. 17%) and overall survival (9.3 vs. 5.6 months) are both improved with FLT3 TKI monotherapy over any non-FLT3 TKI–containing regimen. Patients with relapsed/refractory *IDH1* or *IDH2*-mutant disease can be treated with ivosidenib (IDH1 inhibitor) or enasidenib (IDH2 inhibitor) with complete remission rates of 20% and overall response rates of 40%.

Patients with recurrent AML not characterized by actionable mutations may be treated with aggressive intensive salvage chemotherapy regimens (i.e., cladribine or fludarabine containing programs) or low-dose chemotherapy (i.e., venetoclax plus HMA or LDAC, HMA or LDAC or GO alone). If possible, all patients with relapsed/refractory AML should be considered for alloSCT and clinical trials. Experimental therapies for AML including nontraditional alloSCT have resulted in durable long-term remissions in a proportion of older AML patients and should be pursued based on patient preference, overall health status, and availability of an appropriate HLA-matched donor.

Acute Promyelocytic Leukemia
Definition, Epidemiology, and Pathology
APL, formerly known as the FAB M3 subtype of AML (see Table 47.11), is a rare malignancy that represents 10% to 15% of adult AML.

The incidence is increased among younger patients (median age, 40 years). The annual incidence in the United States ranges from 600 to 800 cases. APL is different from other acute leukemias because of its unique disease biology. Morphologically, APL blasts are distinctive immature promyelocytic cells containing large granules and typically high numbers of Auer rods diagnostic of AML. APL is characterized by a chromosomal translocation—t(15;17)(q22;q12)—involving the promyelocytic leukemia gene *(PML)* on chromosome 15 and the retinoic acid receptor-α gene *(RARA)* on chromosome 17. Sequestration of the resulting PML/RARA fusion protein with other proteins produces a complex that represses the gene transcription essential for granulocytic differentiation, effectively arresting differentiation of leukemia cells at the promyelocyte stage.

Clinical Presentation
Clinically, patients with APL often exhibit life-threatening bleeding caused by disseminated intravascular coagulation related to high levels of procoagulant factors released from APL granules. Bleeding complications in the CNS and other sites can be rapidly fatal if the disease is not recognized and treated as a medical emergency. All patients suspected of having APL should be started empirically with all-*trans*-retinoic acid (ATRA) therapy (discussed later) and treated aggressively with transfusions of fresh-frozen plasma, fibrinogen, and platelets until resolution of coagulopathy and disease confirmation. Unlike patients with other AML subsets, APL patients typically have cytopenias rather than leukocytosis. High-risk APL patients are defined as those with white blood cell counts greater than 10×10^9/L.

Treatment and Prognosis
Treated appropriately, APL is the most curable acute leukemia in adults. The centerpiece of APL treatment is the use of agents that induce the terminal differentiation of leukemic promyelocytes followed by senescence and spontaneous apoptosis. ATRA is an oral derivative of vitamin A shown to overcome growth arrest and permit

differentiation of immature APL blast cells into neutrophils by altering the configuration of *PML/RARA* to allow normal gene transcription.

Patients initiated on ATRA must be closely observed for development of retinoic acid or APL differentiation syndrome, which is life-threatening acute cardiopulmonary distress characterized by bilateral pulmonary effusions and infiltrates. This serositis-like disorder is attributed to adhesion of differentiating neoplastic cells to the pulmonary vasculature and carries a 5% to 10% mortality rate. Treatment consists of early initiation of corticosteroids and aggressive diuresis. In severe cases, ATRA should be temporarily withheld.

Although ATRA alone induces clinical remissions in up to 90% of patients with APL, high relapse rates observed after monotherapy led to the practice of combining ATRA with anthracycline with or without cytarabine chemotherapy in initial induction regimens. Using this approach, complete remission rates for APL rose to between 90% and 95%, and more than two thirds of patients with APL treated with standard ATRA-containing induction, consolidation, and maintenance chemotherapy regimens achieved long-term remission.

Relapsed APL patients were treated with arsenic trioxide, a naturally occurring compound used both as a poison and a drug in many countries. Low-dose arsenic therapy promotes APL cell differentiation and apoptosis and induces remission rates in up to 90% of relapsed APL cases. APL differentiation syndrome and prolongation of the QT interval are common side effects of arsenic therapy. Based on its tolerability and non-overlapping cytotoxicities with conventional cytotoxic drugs, arsenic was successfully used for consolidation therapy in APL patients and improved clinical outcomes.

Although highly effective, combination ATRA and chemotherapy regimens for newly diagnosed APL patients are associated with an overall mortality rate of 10% to 20% during the first month of treatment. Most deaths result from uncontrolled hemorrhage, differentiation syndrome, and complications of prolonged myelosuppression after cytotoxic therapy, particularly in older individuals. To address these concerns, a phase III trial randomized lower-risk APL patients to dual-differentiation therapy with ATRA and arsenic only (without cytotoxic chemotherapy) or to standard ATRA and chemotherapy during induction and consolidation. The trial demonstrated that ATRA plus arsenic treatment was not inferior to ATRA plus chemotherapy and was not associated with increased toxicity. Importantly, the trial results led to establishment of differentiation therapy alone without any cytotoxic agents as the standard of care for lower-risk APL patients. Patients with residual *PML/RARA*-positive cells after standard induction and consolidation therapy containing ATRA and arsenic should be considered for autologous or allogeneic SCT. Patients with high-risk APL should continue to receive cytarabine with or without anthracycline drugs in addition to ATRA and arsenic induction, consolidation, and maintenance for curative intent. Given the high cure rates, autologous or allogeneic stem cell transplant is not indicated for APL except for relapsed disease (which often is associated with CNS disease). Newer oral formulations of arsenic are being developed.

Acute Lymphoblastic Leukemia
Definition, Epidemiology, and Pathology

ALL is a neoplasm of immature lymphoblasts expressing markers of B-cell or T-cell lineage. ALL is predominantly a pediatric malignancy, with most cases occurring in children younger than 6 years. In the United States, 5960 new cases were diagnosed in 2018 with 1470 deaths. The median age of onset was 15 years with 27% diagnosed in individuals older than 45 years.

The prior FAB classification system divided ALL into three subtypes (i.e., L1, L2, and L3) based on the morphology of malignant cells (see E-Fig. 47.3). The WHO system reclassified the disease as precursor B-cell or T-cell ALL based on the lineage of specific cell surface

antigens found on these cells during normal maturation (see Table 47.11). T-cell ALL represents 15% to 25% of ALL diagnoses. More than 50% of T-cell ALL cases have activating mutations in *NOTCH1*, a key regulator of T-cell fate. One third of adult and 20% of pediatric B-cell ALL cases are associated with detection of the Philadelphia chromosome, t(9;22).

Clinical Presentation

Patients often present with life-threatening cytopenias, or complications of leukostasis. On examination, enlarged lymph nodes, liver, spleen, or testicles are common. Neurologic symptoms including headaches, cranial nerve deficits, or new neuropathies may be indicative of CNS involvement. Several clinical and biologic features at diagnosis have traditionally been identified as poor prognostic factors for survival (see Table 47.13). These include age (in pediatrics <2 years or >10 years, in adults >35 years), elevated white blood cell count at presentation (>100,000/mcL), precursor T phenotype, chromosome number (pseudo/hypodiploidy or near tetraploidy) and specific chromosome abnormalities (such as complex karyotype or Philadelphia chromosome).

Treatment

Newly diagnosed ALL. Progress in the understanding and treatment of this disease over the last few decades has led to cure rates of greater than 90% for children with ALL. Despite this success, only 20% to 40% of adult patients with ALL achieve cure with elderly individuals demonstrating a five-year survival of less than 20%. The poorer outcomes for adults are attributed to differences in the biologic mechanisms of disease in the different age groups and the inability of older patients to tolerate the intensive chemotherapy or transplantation procedures required to achieve long-term responses.

Standard treatment of ALL is lengthy and involves multiple chemotherapeutic agents given over 2 to 3 years. Induction chemotherapy typically includes vincristine, corticosteroids, and L-asparaginase with the addition of an anthracycline, cytarabine, or cyclophosphamide (or a combination) for adult patients. Given the propensity of ALL cells to reside in the CNS and testes (so-called sanctuaries for leukemia cells because standard systemic chemotherapy does not penetrate into these sites), routine administration of intrathecal chemotherapy at the time of diagnosis, followed by multiple additional treatments to prevent leukemia seeding in the CNS is considered a necessary adjunct to systemic chemotherapy for all patients. Younger patients with CD20+, Ph-negative ALL have been shown to have worse outcomes than those with CD20-negative B-ALL. Addition of anti-CD20 antibody (rituximab) directed against B-cell antigens on abnormal lymphoblasts has been shown to enhance outcomes of chemotherapy for these individuals. The benefit of CD20 antibodies in older patients is less certain.

Current complete remission rates following induction chemotherapy range from 97% to 99% for children and 75% to 90% for adults. After normal hematopoiesis returns, patients typically undergo consolidation and intensification therapy with the same drugs, including high-dose methotrexate, cytarabine, and asparaginase to eradicate disease. Thereafter, maintenance chemotherapy given for up to 2 to 3 years after initial remission achievement is usually recommended for all patients. Prolonged treatment is intended to eliminate slow-growing leukemic clones, prevent further transformation, or destroy occult disease in other sites, particularly the CNS.

Although clinical factors (i.e., older age, Philadelphia chromosome–positive disease, high white blood cell count at presentation, or prolonged time to first remission) are important, current ALL therapeutic approaches in both children and adults are primarily guided by measurable (or minimal) residual disease (MRD) status. MRD is defined as the detection of malignant lymphoblasts by highly sensitive

PCR or multi-parameter flow cytometry following induction and consolidation therapy at the time of morphologic marrow remission. MRD has been established as an independent predictor of disease relapse and shorter survival with or without subsequent alloSCT. Patients with MRD positive CD19+ B-cell ALL are usually treated with blinatumomab (BiTE), a bispecific single-chain antibody that binds the T-cell receptor CD3 on T cells and the B-cell antigen CD19 expressed by malignant lymphoblasts. Dual binding of CD3 and CD19 by BiTE brings reactive T cells close to tumor cells, redirects T cell lysis, and eliminates disease. Administration of BiTE to ALL patients in clinical remission but with evidence of MRD after standard chemotherapy has been shown to eradicate detectable disease in 76% of patients.

In ALL, as in AML, the worse the prognosis, the earlier transplantation should be offered. Patients with MRD+ disease are considered to have chemoresistant disease, and studies have shown that high-risk ALL patients clearly benefit from alloSCT, preferably from an HLA-matched sibling, during the first remission. Unfortunately, outcomes for high-risk ALL patients without an available HLA-matched donor are poor, and these individuals should pursue alternative transplant options or experimental therapies. No significant benefit has been seen with autologous transplantation over standard chemotherapy for these patients. In contrast, low- and standard-risk ALL patients, particularly pediatric patients, with high rates of long-term remission and survival after conventional chemotherapy and maintenance are recommended to avoid allogeneic SCT unless disease recurs.

In the modern era, ALL therapy is increasingly being tailored for specific patient populations (Table 47.14), including adolescent and young adult (AYA) patients as well as elderly individuals and those with Philadelphia chromosome–positive (Ph+) ALL, Ph-like ALL, and T-cell ALL (T-ALL) subtypes.

Age remains an important determinant of ALL therapy. Historically, adult patients diagnosed with ALL receive treatment regimens with attenuated doses or even omissions (i.e., asparaginase) of the same chemotherapy agents routinely used so successfully in pediatric patients. This is due to significantly higher rates of treatment-related toxicities and death in older individuals with medical comorbidities and decreased tolerance of prolonged chemotherapy. In contrast, multiple retrospective and prospective trials have now demonstrated that AYA patients aged 15 to 39 years of age can benefit from "pediatric-inspired" chemotherapy regimens with dose intensification of corticosteroids, vincristine, asparaginase, and intrathecal chemotherapy. This is reflected in improved overall survival rates of over 70%. In contrast, elderly patients (>60 years old) are increasingly being offered low-intensity regimens designed to preserve outcomes while minimizing toxicity. To further improve responses, recent trials have explored the addition of BiTE and anti-CD20 antibodies to chemotherapy with promising results.

Philadelphia chromosome–expressing (Ph+) ALL is a previously notoriously chemoresistant ALL subtype that occurs much more commonly in adults than children. Treatment has been dramatically altered by the incorporation of newer-generation BCR-ABL1 TKIs into conventional chemotherapy regimens (see Table 47.9). Dasatinib is a second-generation TKI with known CNS penetration that results in superior outcomes over imatinib plus chemotherapy. Ponatinib is a third-generation TKI with activity against ALL cells bearing *BCR-ABL1* tyrosine kinase mutations conferring resistance to other TKIs. Although associated with increased cardiovascular and thrombotic complications, ponatinib and chemotherapy results in very high response rates and 3-year remission rates of over 80%, Five-year overall survival for Ph+ ALL now ranges between 60% and 70%, raising the question of whether alloSCT should be performed for all patients or solely for individuals with persistent MRD+ disease following frontline therapy. Upfront TKI therapy in combination with corticosteroids now leads to almost universal remission rates without requiring cytotoxic agents. Older patients with Ph+ALL are now able to receive much less chemotherapy than previously and continue therapy with sustained responses for months if not years.

Genomic analyses have revealed a biologic subset of ALL with similar gene expression patterns as Ph+ ALL but no evidence of BCR-ABL protein or t(9;22). This so-called "Ph-like" ALL subtype occurs in up to 30% of AYA patients and is associated with Hispanic ethnicity and poor outcomes. Discovery of specific kinase mutations in these patients, such as *JAK1, JAK2, ABL2, CRLF2*, has led to clinical trials incorporating specific TKIs (i.e., ruxolitinib, dasatinib) into treatment regimen to enhance antileukemic efficacy.

T-cell ALL occurs far less frequently than B-cell disease and until recently was believed to confer worse prognosis following treatment with standard ALL chemotherapy regimens. Nelarabine is a purine analogue that is incorporated into malignant lymphoblasts, leading to inhibition of DNA synthesis and apoptosis. This single agent resulted in overall response rates of 20% to 30% in patients with relapsed/refractory T-ALL. This agent is being incorporated into upfront treatment regimens, particularly for high risk patients with ALL, with encouraging results to date.

TABLE 47.14   Treatment of Acute Lymphoblastic Leukemia

Treatment	Patient Population	Clinical Notes
Intensive induction chemotherapy	Newly diagnosed pediatric patients	High remission rates of >90%; long-term survival in pediatric patients >90% vs. 30-40% in adults
Pediatric inspired regimens	Newly diagnosed AYA	Improved 3-year survival of 73%; Dose intensification of steroids, IT chemotherapy, asparaginase and vincristine
Low-intensity chemo regimens	Newly diagnosed older adults	Lower-dose chemotherapy with omission of anthracycline
Rituximab (anti-CD20 ab)	Younger patients with CD20+ disease	Added to standard chemotherapy; not indicated for older patients or CD20-negative disease
BCR-ABL1 inhibitors	Ph-positive ALL	Combined with steroids and standard chemotherapy
Blinatumomab (CD19-CD3 bispecific antibody)	MRD+ and Relapsed refractory CD19+ ALL	Toxicities of cytokine release syndrome and CNS effects. Eliminates MRD+ disease in >70%. Overall survival of 7.7 months in relapsed disease.
Inotuzumab ozogamicin	Relapsed/refractory CD22+ ALL	Risk of veno-occlusive disease (15%) and hepatotoxicity, particularly with prior allogeneic stem cell transplant
Tisagenlecleucel (CD19 chimeric antigen receptor T cells)	Relapsed/refractory CD19+ ALL aged 25 and younger	Response rates of 80%. Toxicities of cytokine release and neurologic symptoms require treatment with steroid and anti-IL-6 antibody

Relapsed or refractory disease. Although late recurrences can emerge at any time, most ALL relapses arise within 2 years of the initial diagnosis, with recurrence of chemoresistant leukemia cells in the bone marrow, CNS, or testes. All patients with relapsed ALL should be considered for additional therapy followed by alloSCT, which represents the only known cure for disease. Autologous SCT is not routinely recommended. Overall response rates to multiagent salvage chemotherapy incorporating the same agents used in frontline therapy range from 20% to 50% with duration of second remissions lasting less than 6 months. Other chemotherapy agents specifically indicated for relapsed disease include nelarabine for T-ALL, clofarabine for patients younger than 21 years old, and a liposomal formulation of vincristine in patients receiving at least two prior lines of therapy. Each drug induces clinical responses in up to a third of heavily pretreated patients as a single agent with tolerable toxicities.

Perhaps the most exciting strategies for ALL therapy involve technologies specifically exploiting patient host immune responses to induce responses. Numerous immunotherapies targeting the leukemia cell antigens CD19 and CD22 have entered mainstream therapy for ALL as well as other lymphoid malignancies. BiTE results in significantly improved overall survival (7.7 months) as compared with standard chemotherapy (4 months). Patients with lower marrow disease burden and receiving treatment in first relapse benefit most, with 30% of patients proceeding on to alloSCT. Unique side effects of therapy include neurologic symptoms (ranging from change in mental status to seizures to encephalopathy) and cytokine release syndrome characterized by fever, hemodynamic instability, and life-threatening organ damage. Severity of complications is related to extent of tumor burden and is higher than experienced in BiTE therapy of MRD-positive ALL.

Inotuzumab is a CD22-directed antibody conjugated to a DNA damaging agent (calicheamicin). Binding of this antibody drug conjugate to surface CD22 expressed on the ALL surface leads to its internalization, induction of DNA strand breakage, and cell death. In a randomized controlled trial, inotuzumab induced higher overall responses (88%) in patients with first relapsed ALL than standard chemotherapy (32%). Forty percent of patients receiving inotuzumab underwent subsequent alloSCT. However 15% of patients developed VOD, which was largely fatal and occurred primarily in individuals with prior alloSCT who had received multiple doses of therapy.

Cellular immunotherapies that have revolutionized the treatment of all B-cell malignancies were first validated for the treatment of relapsed B-ALL. Chimeric antigen receptor T (CART) cells are autologous T cells collected from patients with relapsed ALL and genetically modified ex vivo to express CD19 chimeric antigen receptors. This effectively reprograms them to recognize and destroy CD19-expressing tumor cells. Infusion of a single dose of CART cells (tisagenlecleucel) following lymphodepleting chemotherapy in individuals (both children and young adults) with multiple relapsed/refractory ALL resulted in the complete eradication of disease in 80% to 90%. Although CART-mediated cytokine release and neurotoxicity can be life-threatening, strategies to mitigate these adverse events with early administration of steroids and the anti-IL-6 antibody (tocilizumab) have allowed CART to be successfully administered at numerous academic centers across the world.

PROSPECTUS FOR THE FUTURE

Insights into the molecular and biologic underpinnings of MPNs and acute leukemia have led to an explosion of novel therapeutic approaches that have transformed the clinical approach to each of these diseases in the past few years.

Myeloproliferative Disease

The importance of the spectacular success of imatinib as targeted therapy for CML cannot be overstated. As the first successful therapy based on an understanding of pathogenesis, imatinib has become emblematic of the translation of an understanding of disease pathogenesis into tangible innovations in clinical care. At present, there are four additional new-generation TKIs for CML therapy in addition to imatinib. The best indicator of how these agents have altered the natural history of disease is the fact that certain patients with sustained undetectable disease for 2 to 3 years are now able to permanently discontinue TKI therapy without disease recurrence.

Similarly, the discovery of *JAK2* mutations in non-CML myeloproliferative diseases opened new avenues for targeted intervention in diseases for which previous therapy was largely supportive. JAK2 inhibition now constitutes standard-of-care therapy for PV and MF independent of *JAK2* mutation status. Newer agents are actively being investigated for MPN therapy including hypomethylating agents, *MDM2* inhibitors, antibody-drug conjugates, and anti-fibrosis agents.

Acute Leukemia

Acute leukemias are clinically aggressive malignancies with survival rates of weeks to a few months if untreated. The availability of multiple targeted and nontargeted agents for distinct biological subsets has changed the therapeutic landscape for these diseases. The first acute leukemia exemplifying this was APL. The discovery of the link between the retinoic acid receptor and the origins of APL provided important insights into the unique sensitivity of this disease to ATRA therapy and paved the road for successful implementation of dual differentiation therapy with ATRA and arsenic. This regimen marks the first time that any acute leukemia was cured without cytotoxic chemotherapy or SCT.

At present, pediatric ALL is now considered a highly curable cancer with long-term remission and survival rates of over 90%. Patients with relapsed disease are eligible to receive the latest advances in novel immunotherapeutic approaches. CART therapy has revolutionized therapy not only for ALL but for all B-cell malignancies such as lymphoma and myeloma. However, durability of response and disease relapse remain major issues. It is uncertain whether patients undergoing CART should also pursue subsequent alloSCT. Antibodies including anti-CD20 antibody (rituximab), the CD19-CD3 bispecific agent (blinatumomab), and the CD22 antibody drug conjugate (inotuzumab) have expanded the armamentarium of strategies for ALL. Incorporation of new-generation oral BCR/ABL kinase inhibitors to routine chemotherapy for Philadelphia chromosome–positive ALL has altered expectations for this subtype.

Tailoring of therapy to disease subtype as well as different age groups (pediatric, AYA, and elderly) has led to true personalized therapy. Future directions include moving agents known to be effective in the relapsed/refractory setting to earlier in the treatment course during induction and/or consolidation. Examples include upfront therapy with BiTe and dasatinib for Ph+ disease or inotuzumab plus mini-hyper CVD or CART cells with MRD testing.

In AML, the "gold standard" (7+3) for induction chemotherapy since the 1970s has finally been replaced, at least in older unfit individuals, by venetoclax-based therapy. The latter results in overall response rates of 60% to 70% and provides a new backbone regimen on which to potentially add novel experimental agents. Single-agent inhibitors of mutant *FLT3*, *IDH1*, and *IDH2* have been shown to be superior to conventional chemotherapy in patients with appropriately mutant disease. Newer clinical trials are exploring combinations of targeted agents (FLT3 and IDH inhibitors) with different chemotherapy backbones (i.e., venetoclax plus HMA) or with each other (i.e., venetoclax and gilteritinib). Development of reduced intensity and haploidentical alloSCT strategies has permitted specific older AML patients the opportunity to be cured of their disease. Similar approaches may soon provide therapeutic entry points into the treatment of other acute leukemias associated with pathognomonic chromosomal translocations and genetic and molecular aberrations.

SUGGESTED READINGS

Arber DA, Orazi A, Hasserjian R, et al: The 2016 revision to the World Health Organization classification of myeloid neoplasms and acute leukemia, Blood 127(20):2391–2405, 2016.

Baxter EJ, Scott LM, Campbell PJ, et al: Acquired mutation of the tyrosine kinase JAK2 in human myeloproliferative disorders, Lancet 365(9464):1054–1061, 2005.

Byrd J, Mrozek K, Dodge R, et al: Pretreatment cytogenetic abnormalities are predictive of induction success, cumulative incidence of relapse, and overall survival in adult patients with de novo acute myeloid leukemia, Blood 100(13):4325–4336, 2002.

Cortes JE, Heidel JH, Hellman A, et al: Randomized comparison of low dose cytarabine with or without glasdegib in patients with newly diagnosed acute myeloid leukemia or high-risk myelodysplastic syndrome, Leukemia 33(2):379–389, 2019.

DiNardo CD, Pratz K, Pullarkat V, et al: Venetoclax combined with decitabine or azacitidine in treatment-naive, elderly patients with acute myeloid leukemia, Blood 133(1):7–17, 2019.

DiNardo CD, Stein EM, de Botton S, et al: Durable remissions with ivosidenib in IDH1-mutated relapsed or refractory AML, N Engl J Med 378(25):2386–2398, 2018.

Dohner H, Estey EH, Grimwade D, et al: Diagnosis and management of AML in adults: 2017 ELM recommendations from an international expert panel, Blood 129(4):424–447, 2017.

Döhner H, Estey EH, Amadori S, et al: Diagnosis and management of acute myeloid leukemia in adults: recommendations from an international expert panel, on behalf of the European LeukemiaNet, Blood 115(3):453–474, 2010.

Harrison CN, Campbell PJ, Buck G, et al: Hydroxyurea compared with anagrelide in high-risk essential thrombocythemia, N Engl J Med 353(1):33–45, 2005.

Harrison CN, Vannucchi AM, Kiladjian JJ, et al: Long-term findings from COMFORT-II, a phase 3 trial of ruxolitinib versus best available therapy for myelofibrosis, Leukemia 30(8):1701–1707, 2016.

Hasford J, Pfirrmann M, Hehlmann R, et al: A new prognostic score for survival of patients with chronic myeloid leukemia treated with interferon alfa. Writing Committee 3 for the Collaborative CML Prognostic Factors Project Group, J Natl Cancer Inst 90(11):850–858, 1998.

Hughes TP, Mauro MJ, Cortes JE, et al: Asciminib in chronic myeloid leukemia after ABL kinase inhibitor failure, N Engl J Med 381(24):2315–2326, 2019.

Kantarjian HM, DeAngelo DJ, Stelljes M, et al: Inotuzumab ozogamicin versus standard therapy for acute lymphoblastic leukemia, N Engl J Med 375(8):740–753, 2016.

Kantarjian H, Stein A, Gokbuget N, et al: Blinatumomab versus chemotherapy for advanced acute lymphoblastic leukemia, N Engl J Med 376(9):836–847, 2017.

Lambert J, Pautas C, Terre C, et al: Gemtuzumab ozogamicin for de novo acute myeloid leukemia: final efficacy and safety updates from the open-label, phase III ALFA-0701 trial, Haematologica 104(1):113–119, 2019.

Landolfi R, Marchioli R, Kutti J, et al: Efficacy and safety of low-dose aspirin in polycythemia vera, N Engl J Med 350(2):114–124, 2004.

Maude SL, Laetsch TW, Buechner J, et al: Chimeric antigen receptor T cells for sustained remissions in leukemia, N Engl J Med 378(5):439–448, 2018.

Perl S, Martinelli G, Cortes JE, et al: Gilteritinib or chemotherapy for relapsed or refractory FLT3-mutated AML, N Engl J Med 381(18):1728–1740, 2019.

Pfirrman M, Baccarani M, Saussele S, et al: Prognosis of long-term survival considering disease-specific death in patients with chronic myeloid leukemia, Leukemia 30(1):48–56, 2016.

Pullarkat V, Slovak ML, Kopecky KJ, et al: Impact of cytogenetics on the outcome of adult acute lymphocytic leukemia: results of the Southwest Oncology Group 9400 study, Blood 111(5):2563–2572, 2008.

Sokal J, Cox EB, Baccarani M, et al: Prognostic discrimination in "good-risk" chronic granulocytic leukemia, Blood 63(4):789–799, 1984.

Stein EM, DiNardo CD, Pollyea DA, et al: Enasidenib in mutant IDH2 relapsed or refractory acute myeloid leukemia, Blood 130(6):722–731, 2017.

Stock W, Luger SM, Advani AS, et al: A pediatric regimen for older adolescents and young adults with acute lymphoblastic leukemia: results of CALGB 10403, Blood 133(14):1548–1559, 2019.

Stone RM, Mandrekar SJ, Sanford BL, et al: Midostaurin plus chemotherapy for acute myeloid leukemia with a FLT3 mutation, N Engl J Med 377(5):454–464, 2017.

Vannucchi AM, Kiladjian JJ, Greisshammer M, et al: Ruxolitinib versus standard therapy for treatment of polycythemia vera, N Engl J Med 372(5):426–435, 2015.

Wei AH, Strickland SA, Hou JZ, et al: Venetoclax combined with low-Dose cytarabine for previously untreated patients with acute myeloid leukemia: results from a phase Ib/II study, J Clin Oncol 37(15):1277–1284, 2019.

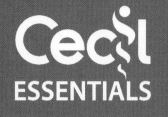

48

Disorders of Red Blood Cells

Ellice Wong, Michal G. Rose, Nancy Berliner

NORMAL RED BLOOD CELL STRUCTURE AND FUNCTION

Erythrocytes, or red blood cells (RBCs), deliver oxygen to all the tissues in the body and carry carbon dioxide back to the lungs for excretion. The erythrocyte is uniquely adapted to these functions. It has a biconcave disk shape that maximizes the membrane surface area for gas exchange, and it has a cytoskeleton and membrane structure that allow it to deform sufficiently to pass through the microvasculature. Passage through capillaries whose diameter may be one fourth the resting diameter of the erythrocyte is made possible by interactions between proteins in the membrane (band 3 and glycophorin) and underlying cytoplasmic proteins that make up the erythrocyte cytoskeleton (spectrin, ankyrin, and protein 4.1).

The mature RBC contains no nucleus and is dependent throughout its life span on proteins synthesized before extrusion of the nucleus and release of the cell from the bone marrow into the peripheral circulation. About 98% of the cytoplasmic protein of the mature erythrocyte is hemoglobin. The remainder is mainly enzymatic proteins, such as those required for anaerobic metabolism and the hexose monophosphate shunt.

Defects in any of the intrinsic structural features of the erythrocyte can result in hemolytic anemia. Abnormalities of the membrane or cytoskeletal proteins are the causes of alterations in erythrocyte shape and flexibility. Inborn defects in the enzymatic pathways for glucose metabolism decrease the resistance to oxidant stress, and inherited abnormalities of hemoglobin structure and synthesis lead to polymerization of abnormal hemoglobin (sickle cell disease) or to the precipitation of unbalanced hemoglobin chains (thalassemia). All of these changes result in decreased erythrocyte survival.

Oxygen is transported by hemoglobin, a tetramer composed of two α chains, two β-like (β, γ, or δ) chains, and four heme molecules, each of which is composed of a protoporphyrin molecule complexed with iron. In fetal life, the main hemoglobin is fetal hemoglobin (HbF: α_2, γ_2); the switch from HbF to adult hemoglobin (HbA: $\alpha_2\beta_2$) occurs in the perinatal period. By 4 to 6 months of age, the level of HbF has fallen to about 1% of total hemoglobin. HbA_2 ($\alpha_2\delta_2$) is a minor adult hemoglobin, representing about 1% of adult hemoglobin (Table 48.1).

CLINICAL PRESENTATION

Anemia, defined as a reduction in RBC mass, is an important sign of disease. It may be caused by decreased production of erythrocytes from nutritional deficiencies, primary hematologic disease, or a response to systemic illness. Alternatively, anemia may be caused by increased blood loss or cellular destruction from hemolysis. Hemolysis may occur as a result of intrinsic abnormalities of the RBC, immune-mediated RBC destruction, or a systemic vascular process. The investigation of anemia is a critical component of the evaluation of the patient and commonly provides valuable insight into systemic illness. Fig. 48.1 provides an overview of the differential diagnosis of anemia.

The symptoms of anemia reflect both the severity and the rapidity with which the reduction in erythrocyte mass has occurred. Patients with acute hemorrhage may exhibit symptoms of hypovolemic shock. Massive hemolysis may result in neurologic impairment or cardiovascular collapse. However, most patients develop anemia more slowly and have few symptoms. Usual complaints are fatigue, decreased exercise tolerance, dyspnea, and palpitations. In patients with coronary artery disease, anemia may precipitate angina. On physical examination, the major sign of anemia is pallor. Patients may be tachycardic and often have significant flow murmurs. Patients with hemolysis often exhibit jaundice and splenomegaly. Patients with iron deficiency may occasionally exhibit signs of pica (i.e., craving for ice or nonfood items such as dirt).

LABORATORY EVALUATION

The key components of the laboratory evaluation of anemia are the reticulocyte count, the peripheral blood smear, erythrocyte indices, nutritional studies, and in some cases the bone marrow aspirate and biopsy.

The *reticulocyte count* allows the critical distinction between anemia arising from a primary failure of RBC production and anemia resulting from increased RBC destruction or bleeding. Erythrocytes newly released from the marrow still contain small amounts of RNA; these cells, termed *reticulocytes,* can be detected with the use of automated counters and fluorescent nucleic acid–binding dyes or manually by staining of the peripheral blood smear with new methylene blue or other supravital stains. In response to anemia, erythropoietin (EPO) production increases, promoting the production and release of increased numbers of reticulocytes. The number of reticulocytes in the peripheral blood therefore reflects the response of the bone marrow to anemia.

The reticulocyte count can be expressed either as a percentage of the total number of RBCs or as an absolute number. In patients without anemia, the normal reticulocyte count is 0.5% to 1.5% of RBCs or 20,000 to 75,000/μL. When the anemia is caused by decreased RBC survival, the appropriate marrow response results in a reticulocyte count greater than 2%, with an absolute count of more than 100,000/μL. If the reticulocyte count is not elevated, a cause of failure of RBC production should be sought. Reticulocyte counts that are expressed as a percentage of total RBCs must be corrected for anemia because decreasing the number of circulating cells increases the reticulocyte percentage without any increase in release from the marrow.

The *corrected reticulocyte count* is calculated by multiplying the reticulocyte count by the ratio of the patient's hematocrit to a normal hematocrit. An additional calculation, the reticulocyte index or reticulocyte production index (RPI), determines whether the reticulocyte count is appropriate for the degree of anemia. The RPI corrects for both the degree of anemia and release of reticulocytes from the marrow by multiplying the ratio of the patient's hematocrit to a normal hematocrit by the reticulocyte percentage divided by a maturation term. The maturation term signifies the time in days for RBCs to mature (ranging from 1 for a hematocrit ≥40% to 2.5 for a hematocrit <20%). An RPI greater than 3 is considered an appropriate marrow response (e.g., from increased RBC destruction or bleeding) and an RPI less than 2 is an inappropriate marrow response (e.g., a RBC production problem).

Evaluation of the *peripheral blood smear* may provide important clues to the cause of anemia. Erythrocyte morphologic examination is especially critical in the evaluation of anemia associated with

reticulocytosis, wherein an examination of the smear is essential to distinguish between immune hemolysis (which results in spherocytes) and microangiopathic hemolysis (which causes schistocytes or erythrocyte fragmentation). Changes associated with other causes of anemia include sickle and target cells that are characteristic of hemoglobinopathies, teardrop cells and nucleated RBCs associated with myelofibrosis and marrow infiltration, intracorpuscular parasites in malaria and babesiosis, and pencil-shaped deformities associated with severe iron deficiency. Examination of myeloid cells and platelets may also be helpful. Hypersegmented neutrophils and large platelets support the diagnosis of megaloblastic anemia, and the presence of immature blast forms may be diagnostic of leukemia. Fig. 48.2 presents some common peripheral blood smear findings in patients with anemia.

In patients with anemia and an elevated reticulocyte count, the vigorous production of new erythroid cells suggests that marrow function is normal and is responding appropriately to the stress of the anemia. Bone marrow examination in this situation is rarely indicated because the marrow will simply show erythroid hyperplasia, usually without revealing any primary pathologic anomaly of the marrow. Evaluation in these cases should be focused on determining whether the cause of RBC consumption is bleeding or hemolysis. In contrast, bone marrow examination is more often required for the evaluation of hypoproliferative anemia. After common abnormalities such as iron deficiency and other nutritional deficiencies have been ruled out, marrow aspiration and biopsy are indicated to search for abnormalities such as marrow infiltration, marrow involvement with granulomatous disease, marrow aplasia, or myelodysplasia.

The *mean corpuscular volume* (MCV) is an extremely helpful tool in the diagnosis of anemia with a low reticulocyte count (hypoproliferative

TABLE 48.1   Structure and Distribution of Human Hemoglobins

Name of Hemoglobin (Hb)	Distribution	Structure
A	95-98% of adult Hb	$\alpha_2\beta_2$
A_2	1.5-3.5% of adult Hb	$\alpha_2\delta_2$
F	Fetal, 0.5-1.0% of adult Hb	$\alpha_2\gamma_2$
Gower 1	Embryonic	$\zeta_2\varepsilon_2$
Gower 2	Embryonic	$\alpha_2\varepsilon_2$
Portland	Embryonic	$\zeta_2\gamma_2$

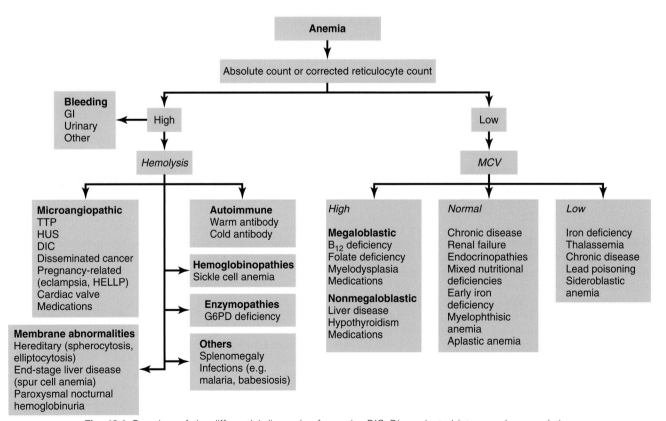

Fig. 48.1 Overview of the differential diagnosis of anemia. *DIC,* Disseminated intravascular coagulation; *G6PD,* glucose-6-phosphate dehydrogenase; *GI,* gastrointestinal; *HELLP,* hemolysis, elevated liver enzyme levels, and low platelet count; *HUS,* hemolytic-uremic syndrome; *MCV,* mean corpuscular volume; *TTP,* thrombotic thrombocytopenic purpura.

anemia). The size of the RBCs (measured in femtoliters per cell) is used to characterize the anemia as microcytic (MCV <80), normocytic (MCV 80 to 96), or macrocytic (MCV >96).

EVALUATION OF HYPOPROLIFERATIVE ANEMIAS

Microcytic Anemias

The differential diagnosis of microcytic anemia is outlined in Table 48.2. Microcytosis and hypochromia are the hallmarks of anemias caused by defects in hemoglobin synthesis, which can reflect either failure of heme synthesis or abnormalities in globin production. The leading cause of microcytic anemia is iron deficiency, in which lack of heme synthesis results from the absence of iron to incorporate into the porphyrin ring (see later discussion). Up to 30% of patients with anemia of chronic inflammation have microcytosis. Lead poisoning blocks the incorporation of iron into heme, also resulting in a microcytic anemia.

Sideroblastic anemias arise from failure to synthesize the porphyrin ring, usually as a result of inhibition of the heme synthetic pathway enzymes. Congenital sideroblastic anemia may respond to pyridoxine, a cofactor for several of the heme synthetic pathway enzymes. A more common cause of acquired sideroblastic anemia is alcohol use; ethanol inhibits most of the enzymes in the heme synthetic pathway. Failure of globin synthesis occurs in thalassemic syndromes (see "Hemoglobinopathies"). All these disorders lead to decreased mean corpuscular hemoglobin concentration, resulting in hypochromia and a decrease in RBC size (i.e., low MCV).

Iron Deficiency Anemia

Iron deficiency is the leading cause of anemia worldwide. Although the presentation of classic iron deficiency anemia is linked with a microcytic anemia, early iron deficiency is associated with a normocytic anemia. Consequently, iron deficiency should be considered in all patients with anemia, and iron indices should be a part of the evaluation of any patient with hypoproductive anemia, regardless of the MCV.

Iron is acquired in the diet from heme sources (i.e., meat) and from nonheme sources (e.g., vegetables such as spinach). Iron from heme is better absorbed than nonheme iron. Iron absorption is increased in iron deficiency, hypoxia, ineffective erythropoiesis, and hereditary hemochromatosis (most commonly caused by mutations in the *HFE* gene). Iron is absorbed from the proximal small intestine; it is transported in the cell bound to ferroportin and through the plasma bound to transferrin. Its uptake into the RBC precursors is mediated through the transferrin receptor. Iron absorption from the intestine is further regulated by hepcidin (see "Anemia of Inflammation"). Iron outside hemoglobin-producing cells is stored in ferritin. Men and women have

TABLE 48.2 Differential Diagnosis of Anemia With Low Reticulocyte Count

Microcytic Anemia (MCV <80 fL/cell)
Iron deficiency
Thalassemia minor
Anemia of chronic inflammation
Sideroblastic anemia
Lead poisoning

Macrocytic Anemia (MCV >100 fL/cell)
Megaloblastic anemias
Folate deficiency
Vitamin B$_{12}$ deficiency
Drug-induced megaloblastic anemia
Myelodysplasia
Nonmegaloblastic macrocytosis
Liver disease
Hypothyroidism
Reticulocytosis

Normocytic Anemia (MCV 80-100 fL/cell)
Early iron deficiency
Aplastic anemia
Myelophthisic disorders
Endocrinopathies
Anemia of chronic inflammation
Anemia of renal failure
Mixed nutritional deficiency

MCV, Mean corpuscular volume.

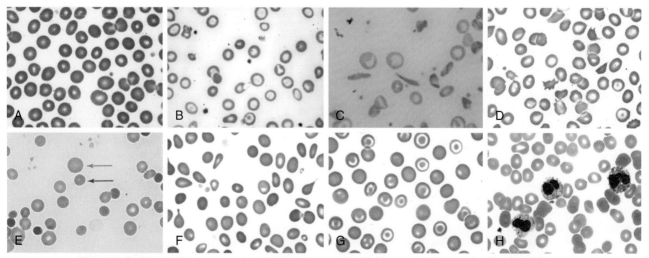

Fig. 48.2 Peripheral blood smears in patients with anemia. (A) Normal red blood cells. (B) Iron deficiency anemia. (C) Sickle cell anemia. (D) Microangiopathic hemolytic anemia. (E) Spherocytosis *(blue arrow)* and reticulocytosis *(red arrow)* in autoimmune hemolytic anemia. (F) Teardrops in myelofibrosis. (G) Target cells. (H) Pseudo-Pelger-Huet anomaly in myelodysplasia.

total-body iron concentrations of 50 mg/kg and 40 mg/kg, respectively. Between 60% and 75% of the iron is found in hemoglobin. A small amount (2 mg/kg) is found in heme and nonheme enzymes, and 5 mg/kg is found in myoglobin. The remainder is stored in ferritin, which resides primarily in liver, bone marrow, spleen, and muscle. The capacity for excreting iron is limited, and iron overload occurs in patients with excessive absorption from the gastrointestinal tract (as a result of ineffective erythropoiesis or congenital hemochromatosis) and in those receiving chronic transfusions. Iron overload leads to increased iron deposition in these tissues and secondary deposition in endocrine and other organs, resulting in liver dysfunction, heart failure, diabetes, and other endocrine abnormalities.

The most frequent cause of iron deficiency is occult blood loss. All men and postmenopausal women who are found to be iron deficient should have an evaluation for a source of gastrointestinal blood loss and malignancy, regardless of the detection of occult blood. In premenopausal women, iron deficiency is most frequently related to loss of iron with menstruation (about 15 mg per month) and during pregnancy (about 900 mg per pregnancy). *Helicobacter pylori* infection can cause iron deficiency even in the absence of intestinal bleeding. Dietary deficiency of iron is most commonly seen in multiparous women of childbearing age, in young children whose growth outstrips their intake of iron, and in babies who drink mostly milk at the expense of an intake of iron-containing foods.

Laboratory evaluation. As previously stated, early iron deficiency does not exhibit the hallmark microcytosis and hypochromia that characterize classic iron deficiency. Evaluation of the blood smear in advanced iron deficiency often demonstrates hypochromic RBCs, target cells, and pencil-shaped elongated cells. Iron deficiency is frequently associated with reactive thrombocytosis.

The mainstay of the diagnosis of iron deficiency is the peripheral blood iron indices. These include iron concentration, total iron-binding capacity (TIBC), transferrin saturation, and ferritin concentration. The transferrin saturation is the ratio of serum iron to transferrin concentration; it is normally at least 20%. Iron deficiency results in a decrease in serum iron and an increase in iron-binding capacity, decreasing this ratio to less than 10%. Chronic inflammatory conditions (e.g., infection, inflammation, malignancy) often decrease both iron and TIBC, but the transferrin saturation usually remains above 20%. The ferritin level is a reflection of total-body iron stores. The liver synthesizes ferritin in proportion to total-body iron, and a level of less than 12 ng/mL strongly supports a diagnosis of iron deficiency. Unfortunately, ferritin is an acute phase reactant, and levels rise in the setting of fever, inflammatory disease, infection, or other stresses. However, ferritin levels in response to stress do not often rise above 100 ng/mL, and levels higher than 100 ng/mL usually rule out iron deficiency.

If the indirect measurement of iron indices does not definitively confirm or refute a diagnosis of iron deficiency, a therapeutic trial of iron supplementation may be considered. Alternatively, a bone marrow examination can be performed to provide a direct assessment of marrow iron stores. Presence of iron in the marrow excludes iron deficiency anemia because marrow iron stores will be depleted before there is any fall in RBC production resulting from iron deficiency; conversely, complete absence of marrow iron confirms the diagnosis of iron deficiency.

Treatment. Oral iron supplementation (e.g., ferrous sulfate or ferrous gluconate two or three times daily) has been the standard treatment for uncomplicated iron deficiency, but patient compliance is often limited by gastrointestinal side effects, notably dose-dependent constipation or diarrhea. However, emerging data suggest that standard iron dosing may be counterproductive. A recent study demonstrated that a large oral dose of iron stimulates an increase in hepcidin (regulator of iron balance), which in turn suppresses further iron absorption up to 48 hours later, supporting an every-other-day dosing strategy. In iron-deficient women without anemia, cumulative iron absorption was superior in those receiving an alternate-day dosing over daily dosing and better tolerated. Larger prospective studies in patients with iron deficiency anemia are needed to confirm these findings. Overall, iron should be administered for several months after resolution of anemia to allow for the reconstitution of iron stores.

In patients with malabsorption, a complete inability to tolerate oral iron, or iron demands that outstrip replacement with oral supplements, parenteral iron may be administered. Historically, intravenous iron, specifically high-molecular-weight iron dextran, has been associated with anaphylaxis and was subsequently removed from markets globally. The newer parenteral iron formulations are safe and effective, including low-molecular-weight iron dextran, ferric gluconate, iron sucrose, ferumoxytol, iron isomaltoside, and ferric carboxymaltose. As previously stated, all male patients and postmenopausal women with iron deficiency require evaluation for a source of gastrointestinal bleeding.

Macrocytic Anemias

Two categories of hypoproductive macrocytic anemias exist: megaloblastic anemias and nonmegaloblastic macrocytic anemias. Megaloblastic anemias arise from a failure of DNA synthesis and result in lack of synchrony between the maturation of the nucleus and the cytoplasm of hematopoietic cells. Nonmegaloblastic macrocytic anemias usually reflect membrane abnormalities resulting from defects in cholesterol metabolism and are most commonly found in patients with advanced liver disease or severe hypothyroidism. Reticulocytosis greater than 10% causes an elevated MCV on automated blood counts because reticulocytes are larger than mature RBCs.

Megaloblastic Anemias

Megaloblastic anemias result from a block in the synthesis of critical nucleotide precursors of DNA, which leads to a cell cycle arrest in S phase. Cytoplasmic maturation occurs, but maturation of the nucleus is arrested. Cells take on a bizarre appearance, with large immature nuclei surrounded by more mature-appearing cytoplasm. Interference with DNA synthesis affects all rapidly dividing cells, so patients with megaloblastic syndromes often have pancytopenia and gastrointestinal symptoms such as diarrhea and malabsorption. In women, megaloblastic changes of the cervical mucosa occur and may cause abnormal results on Papanicolaou smears. The most common causes of megaloblastic anemia are deficiencies of vitamin B_{12} or folate, medications that inhibit DNA synthesis or that block folate metabolism, and myelodysplasia.

Cobalamin deficiency. Cobalamin (vitamin B_{12}) is absorbed from animal protein in the diet. The process of cobalamin absorption and metabolism is complex because cobalamin is always bound to other proteins. In the stomach, protein-bound vitamins are released by digestion with pepsin and are bound to haptocorrin (transcobalamin I). Within the proximal duodenum, pancreatic proteases digest cobalamin away from haptocorrin, and cobalamin binds to intrinsic factor (IF), also known as transcobalamin III. IF is secreted by the parietal cells of the stomach and mediates absorption of cobalamin through the cubam receptor in the distal ileum. Within the ileal mucosal cell, the IF-cobalamin complex is again digested, and cobalamin is released into the plasma bound to haptocorrin and transcobalamin II.

Within the cell, cobalamin is a cofactor for two intracellular enzymes, L-methylmalonyl–coenzyme A (CoA) mutase and homocysteine-methionine methyltransferase (Fig. 48.3). Methylmalonyl-CoA

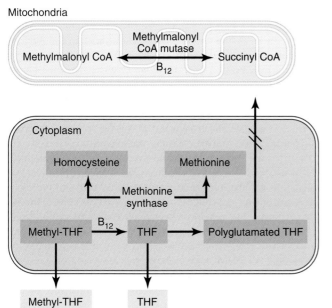

Mitochondria

Cytoplasm

Fig. 48.3 Metabolic pathways of folic acid and cobalamin. *CoA,* Coenzyme A; *THF,* tetrahydrofolate.

TABLE 48.3 Causes of Cobalamin Deficiency

Malabsorption of vitamin B$_{12}$
Pernicious anemia
Partial or total gastrectomy
Pancreatic insufficiency
Bacterial overgrowth
Diseases of the terminal ileum
Tapeworm infection
Nutritional (vegans)
Congenital deficiency of intrinsic factor or haptocorrin

TABLE 48.4 Causes of Folate Deficiency

Dietary Insufficiency
Increased Folate Requirements
Pregnancy
Lactation
Hemolysis
Exfoliative dermatitis
Malignancy

Malabsorption
Sprue
Crohn's disease
Short bowel syndrome

Antifolate Medications
Chemotherapy agents (e.g., methotrexate, pemetrexed)
Sulfa drugs

mutase is a mitochondrial enzyme that functions in the citric acid cycle to convert methylmalonyl-CoA to succinyl-CoA. The cytoplasmic enzyme homocysteine-methionine methyltransferase is necessary for the transfer of methyl groups from *N*-methyltetrahydrofolate to homocysteine to form methionine. Demethylated tetrahydrofolate is necessary as a carbon donor in the conversion of deoxyuridine to deoxythymidine. Absence of cobalamin results in a *trapping* of tetrahydrofolate in its methylated form, which blocks the synthesis of thymidine 5′-triphosphate for incorporation into DNA. The megaloblastic changes induced by cobalamin deficiency are mediated through this functional folate deficiency, which explains the similarity in the hematologic abnormalities induced by cobalamin and folate deficiency.

Causes of cobalamin deficiency. The most common cause of cobalamin deficiency is pernicious anemia, an autoimmune disease associated with gastric parietal cell atrophy, defective gastric acid secretion, and absence of IF. Anti–parietal cell and anti-IF antibodies are frequently found in patients with pernicious anemia and other autoimmune conditions such as type 1 diabetes, vitiligo, Graves' disease, Addison's disease, and hypoparathyroidism. Many other lesions in the gastrointestinal tract can interfere with absorption of cobalamin (Table 48.3). Gastrectomy causes loss of parietal cell function and IF secretion. Pancreatic insufficiency interferes with

digestion of the haptocorrin-cobalamin complex, thus hindering the binding of cobalamin to IF and ileal absorption. Resection of the terminal ileum prevents vitamin B$_{12}$ absorption, as do diseases that affect ileal mucosal function, such as Crohn's disease, sprue, intestinal tuberculosis, and lymphoma. Because the body stores of cobalamin are large and daily loss of cobalamin is low, the stores of cobalamin are adequate for 3 to 4 years if intake stops abruptly; signs of cobalamin deficiency do not develop until defective absorption has occurred for several years. Nutritional cobalamin deficiency is rare and is seen only in individuals who have been on strict vegan diets that exclude all animal products for many years. Infants born to vegan mothers who are breastfed are also at risk for development of cobalamin deficiency.

Folate deficiency. Folate is widely present in foods such as leafy vegetables, fruits, and animal protein. However, because it is destroyed by prolonged cooking, fresh fruits and vegetables are the most reliable sources of folate. Consequently, nutritional folate deficiency is common in malnourished individuals who eat very little fresh fruits and vegetables. Folate deficiency can also be caused by increased demand, as occurs with pregnancy, hemolysis, or exfoliative dermatitis, and by increased losses, which occur with dialysis (Table 48.4). Folate is absorbed in the proximal small intestine, and malabsorption of folate can also lead to folate deficiency.

Other causes of megaloblastic anemia. Drugs and toxins are common causes of megaloblastic anemia. Some drugs, such as methotrexate and sulfa drugs, act as direct folate antagonists and mimic folate deficiency. Purine and pyrimidine analogue chemotherapeutic agents (e.g., azathioprine, 5-fluorouracil) are direct DNA-synthesis inhibitors. Antiviral agents cause megaloblastic changes by unclear mechanisms. Alcohol interferes with folate metabolism, increasing the effect of frequent concomitant nutritional folate deficiency. Myelodysplastic syndrome commonly appears as a macrocytic anemia, with megaloblastic changes primarily in the erythroid series.

Clinical manifestations of megaloblastic anemia. The development of megaloblastic anemia is usually gradual, allowing adequate time for concomitant plasma expansion to prevent hypovolemia. Consequently, patients are frequently severely anemic at presentation. They may have yellowish skin as the result of a combination of pallor from reduced red cell mass and jaundice from ineffective erythropoiesis and intramedullary hemolysis. Some patients have glossitis and cheilosis. With severe anemia, patients usually have an MCV greater than 110 fL/cell, although concomitant iron deficiency, caused by malabsorption secondary to megaloblastic changes in the intestinal tract, may decrease the macrocytosis. Patients frequently have pancytopenia.

A peripheral blood smear demonstrates large, oval cells (macro-ovalocytes), hypersegmented neutrophils, and large platelets. The bone marrow is hypercellular, with megaloblastic changes and abnormally large erythroid series precursors. In addition, intramedullary destruction of erythrocytes (ineffective hematopoiesis) causes elevated concentrations of bilirubin (hence the jaundice described earlier) and lactate dehydrogenase.

Cobalamin deficiency is associated with neurologic abnormalities that are not seen with other causes of megaloblastic anemia. The neurologic signs may range widely, from a subtle loss of vibratory sensation and position sense caused by demyelination of the dorsal columns to frank dementia and neuropsychiatric disease. The neurologic changes may be present without anemia, especially if a patient with cobalamin deficiency is treated with folate, which may correct the hematologic manifestations of megaloblastic anemia but does not treat the neurologic abnormalities. The neurologic manifestations of cobalamin deficiency are thought to be secondary to loss of function of the mitochondrial enzyme methylmalonyl-CoA mutase. One proposed explanation is that the failure to metabolize odd-chain fatty acids, which results in their improper incorporation into myelin, causes the neurologic dysfunction. This explains why these findings are uniquely seen in patients with cobalamin deficiency and are not seen in those with the megaloblastic anemias caused by abnormalities in the folate pathway.

Serum levels of both cobalamin and folate should be measured in patients with megaloblastic anemia because megaloblastic changes in the gut mucosa can cause concomitant malabsorption of folate in the presence of cobalamin deficiency and vice versa. RBC folate levels better reflect the body folate stores and should be measured if a deficiency is clinically suggested but the serum folate levels are normal. Recent studies have shown, however, that many patients with pernicious anemia may have normal serum cobalamin levels. Homocysteine levels are elevated in cobalamin and folate deficiency, and methylmalonic acid levels are elevated in cobalamin deficiency. These levels should be measured if cobalamin deficiency is suggested but serum cobalamin levels are in the normal range. Anti-IF and anti–parietal cell antibodies may help determine the cause of cobalamin deficiency.

Treatment of megaloblastic anemia. For patients with cobalamin deficiency, both high-dose oral and parenteral cobalamin administration have been shown to be effective. The oral dose should be at least 1000 µg daily. Patients with neurologic abnormalities or medication noncompliance and those who have not responded to oral therapy should receive parenteral therapy with 1000 µg subcutaneously or intramuscularly several times per week for four to eight doses. Maintenance therapy should then be instituted with 1000 µg parenterally monthly. Therapy with cobalamin should be accompanied by folate therapy because concomitant secondary folate deficiency may develop when RBC production increases with the availability of cobalamin. Treatment of pernicious anemia should be continued for life.

Patients with folate deficiency should receive replacement with 1 to 5 mg per day of oral folate. As previously stated, it is critical to be certain that patients are not cobalamin deficient: Replacement of folate may correct the hematologic parameters in patients with cobalamin deficiency, but it will not improve the neurologic sequelae.

After treatment of megaloblastic anemia, a rapid response usually occurs. Reticulocytosis is seen as early as 2 days after therapy and peaks within 7 to 10 days. Despite rapid resolution of neutropenia, hypersegmentation of neutrophils may persist for several days. During this period, rapid cellular proliferation and turnover occur, which may precipitate hypokalemia, hyperuricemia, or hypophosphatemia. Patients should also be monitored for the development of iron deficiency, which may occur in the face of increased hematopoiesis. Anemia and other cytopenias should respond completely within 1 to 2 months, but the neurologic manifestations of cobalamin deficiency improve slowly and may be irreversible.

Normocytic Anemias

The differential diagnosis of a normocytic hypoproductive anemia is extensive. Most nutritional anemias that cause microcytosis or macrocytosis begin as a normocytic anemia. Patients with combined nutritional deficiencies may also have a normal MCV. The measurement of EPO levels may be helpful in the diagnosis of anemia resulting from renal failure, and many of the anemias associated with chronic inflammation and endocrinopathies exhibit a depressed EPO level. However, interpretation of EPO levels can be difficult in patients with mild anemia because the levels do not usually rise above the normal range until the hematocrit is depressed below 30%. Even with a hematocrit level of 30%, the EPO level is often in the normal range, but such levels are inappropriately low in the setting of anemia. An elevated EPO level suggests an inadequate marrow response to anemia and increases the likelihood of myelophthisis or primary bone marrow failure. In patients for whom the diagnosis is not clear after routine nutritional and endocrine studies, a bone marrow examination is indicated to rule out primary pathologic conditions of the marrow.

Anemia of Inflammation

The anemia of inflammation (previously called anemia of chronic disease) occurs in patients with chronic inflammatory, infectious, malignant, or autoimmune disorders. Patients have low-serum iron levels, but in contrast to the iron indices in iron deficiency anemia, the iron-binding capacity is also reduced, and the transferrin saturation is usually greater than 10%. Ferritin levels are often elevated, both as an acute phase reactant and as a reflection of decreased iron incorporation. These patients have inappropriately high levels of hepcidin, an acute phase reactant that facilitates the metabolism of ferroportin and reduces both intestinal iron absorption and iron mobilization from macrophages. Cytokines, including tumor necrosis factor, the interleukins, and interferon, also play a role in the anemia of inflammation, both by inducing hepcidin and by directly increasing EPO resistance in erythroid progenitors. Patients have an absolute or relative EPO deficiency, poor iron incorporation into developing erythrocytes, and shortened erythrocyte survival time. The prevalence of anemia of inflammation increases with age; most likely, this is related to age-related comorbidities and mediated through an increase in inflammatory cytokines and a relative EPO resistance.

Treatment of normocytic anemias. The mainstay of therapy for the anemia of chronic inflammation is treatment of the underlying condition and correction of nutritional deficiencies. Iron supplementation should be offered to all patients with a ferritin level lower than 100 ng/mL. Erythroid-stimulating agents (ESAs) have been shown to reduce transfusion needs in many of these patients. However, randomized studies and meta-analyses have shown that their use is associated with an increased incidence of arterial and venous thromboembolic events, an increased risk of mortality from cancer, and a reduced survival time. ESA should be avoided in cancer patients if they are being treated with curative intent, and in all other patients with cancer they should be offered only after a careful discussion of the risks and benefits (grade 1B recommendation).

Anemia of Chronic Kidney Disease

Most patients who have a glomerular filtration rate of less than 30 mL/min have anemia primarily reflecting low EPO levels. ESAs can

TABLE 48.5 Differential Diagnosis of Hemolytic Anemia

Immune Hemolytic Anemia
Immunoglobulin G (warm antibody)–mediated hemolysis
Immunoglobulin M (cold antibody)–mediated hemolysis

Hemolysis From Causes Extrinsic to the Erythrocyte
Microangiopathic hemolysis
Disseminated intravascular coagulation
Thrombotic thrombocytopenic purpura
Preeclampsia, eclampsia, HELLP syndrome
Drugs (mitomycin, cyclosporine, gemcitabine)
Valvular hemolysis
Splenomegaly
Infection (e.g., malaria, babesiosis)

Hemolytic Anemia Caused by Disorders of the Erythrocyte Membrane
Inherited membrane abnormalities
Hereditary spherocytosis
Hereditary elliptocytosis
Hereditary pyropoikilocytosis
Hereditary stomatocytosis

Acquired Membrane Abnormalities
Paroxysmal nocturnal hemoglobinuria
Spur cell anemia

Hemolysis Caused by Erythrocyte Enzymopathies
Glucose-6-phosphate dehydrogenase deficiency
Other enzyme deficiencies

Hemoglobinopathies
Sickle cell disease
Other sickle syndromes
Thalassemia

HELLP, Hemolysis, elevated liver enzymes, and low-platelet count in association with preeclampsia.

help prevent transfusions in this population; however, their use has been associated with an increased risk of stroke, access thrombosis, hypertension, and even mortality in some studies, especially when the hemoglobin levels were normalized. Therefore, most guidelines recommend a target hemoglobin concentration of 10 to 11.5 g/dL when using ESA in patients with chronic kidney disease (grade IB). As in the management of anemia of chronic inflammation, nutritional deficiencies should be corrected before the use of ESAs. The evaluation and treatment of primary marrow failure syndromes and hematologic malignancies are discussed in Chapters 46 and 47 respectively.

EVALUATION OF ANEMIA WITH RETICULOCYTOSIS

An elevated reticulocyte count in the setting of anemia signals a compensatory response by a normal marrow to premature loss of erythrocytes. Hemolysis is the premature destruction of RBCs in the reticuloendothelial system (extrinsic hemolysis) or in blood vessels (intrinsic or intravascular hemolysis). The only other condition that causes anemia with reticulocytosis is acute bleeding. The differential diagnosis of hemolytic anemia is outlined in Table 48.5.

Whereas examination of the peripheral blood smear is helpful in characterizing any anemia, it is absolutely critical in the evaluation of

hemolytic anemia. Morphologic examination of the erythrocytes is helpful in distinguishing immune hemolysis from microangiopathic hemolytic anemia. In addition, other RBC morphologic abnormalities are characteristic for specific diseases such as sickle cell disease (sickled cells), enzyme defects (*bite* cells), and erythrocyte membrane abnormalities (spherocytes, elliptocytes, stomatocytes).

Immune Hemolytic Anemia

Immune-mediated hemolysis results from coating of the erythrocyte membrane with antibodies or complement, or both. It may be mediated by immunoglobulin G (IgG) antibodies (*warm* antibody) or by IgM antibodies (*cold* antibody). The designations *warm* and *cold* denote the temperature at which maximal antibody binding takes place and the clinical syndromes caused by the two types of antibodies are distinct.

The diagnosis of hemolytic anemia is based on the direct and indirect antiglobulin (Coombs) tests. To perform a direct Coombs test, the patient's erythrocytes are mixed with antisera or monoclonal antibodies directed against human immunoglobulins and human complement. The cells are then monitored for agglutination, the presence of which confirms the presence of antibody or complement on the patient's RBCs. The indirect Coombs test is performed by mixing the patient's serum with ABO-compatible erythrocytes and then combining this mixture with antisera against IgG; the indirect Coombs tests allows for the evaluation of antibody in the patient's serum.

IgG-Mediated (Warm) Hemolytic Anemia

Classic autoimmune hemolytic anemia (AIHA) is caused by IgG antibody directed against erythrocyte antigens. Warm type hemolysis may be primary (idiopathic) or associated with autoimmune disease, lymphoproliferative disorders, or drugs. Patients exhibit acute anemia, jaundice, and an elevated reticulocyte count. Some patients have splenomegaly. The peripheral blood smear demonstrates spherocytes (see Fig. 48.2E). Laboratory analysis confirms the presence of IgG on the erythrocyte membrane, as demonstrated by a positive Coombs test; in some patients, the erythrocytes are also coated with complement. Some patients do not have reticulocytosis; in them, the antibody may be destroying both reticulocytes and mature erythrocytes.

The mainstay of therapy for AIHA is corticosteroids. Patients are usually treated with 1 to 2 mg/kg of prednisone, and in responding patients, doses are tapered slowly over several months. Patients who fail to respond to prednisone or cannot be tapered off the prednisone can be treated with other immunosuppressive agents, such as cyclophosphamide, azathioprine, chlorambucil, or rituximab. Some patients respond to intravenous immunoglobulin. Splenectomy is effective in many patients who are corticosteroid refractory or corticosteroid resistant, and it is associated with greater sustained response rates than other immunosuppressive therapies in corticosteroid-resistant patients. However, patients who do not respond and who have ongoing hemolysis after splenectomy are at high risk for secondary thromboembolic events.

Warm antibodies mediate *drug-induced hemolysis.* Several mechanisms exist through which drugs may induce AIHA (Table 48.6). Penicillin produces hemolysis by binding to erythrocytes and acting as a hapten; the antibody is directed against the drug, and hemolysis occurs only in the presence of the drug. Type 2 hemolysis is caused by the formation of an antibody-drug complex that binds to the erythrocyte membrane and activates complement. Drugs associated with this type of hemolysis include quinidine, quinine, and rifampin. Still other drugs, including methyldopa and procainamide, cause hemolysis by inducing the production of *true* antierythrocyte antibodies

TABLE 48.6 **Drug-Induced Autoimmune Hemolytic Anemia**

Type	Mechanism	Common Drugs Implicated	Direct Coombs Test	Indirect Coombs Test
1	Hapten mediated	Penicillin Cephalothin	IgG positive Complement positive or negative	Positive only in the presence of drug
2	Immune complex mediated	Quinine Quinidine Phenacetin Rifampin Isoniazid Tetracycline Chlorpromazine	IgG negative Complement positive	Positive only in the presence of drug
3	True anti-RBC antibody	Methyldopa Levodopa Procainamide Ibuprofen Interferon-α	IgG positive Complement negative	Positive also in absence of drug

IgG, Immunoglobulin G; *RBC,* red blood cell.

directed against Rh and other RBC antigens. Antibody may persist in the absence of the drug, but not all patients with a positive Coombs test have evidence of hemolysis.

IgM-Mediated (Cold) Hemolytic Anemia

Cold-type immune hemolysis is usually postinfectious. The most common associated infectious agents are *Mycoplasma pneumoniae* and Epstein-Barr virus (EBV). IgM antibodies are produced that are directed against the RBC antigen I *(Mycoplasma)* or i (EBV). The antibodies bind at lower temperatures, present in fingers and toes, and bind complement. During the return to the central circulation, the IgM falls off the RBC, leaving complement bound. The Coombs test is negative for IgG and IgM but positive for complement. Hemolysis is self-limited, is rarely severe, and resolves with supportive therapy. In cases of severe hemolysis requiring transfusion, the patient should be kept warm, and blood should be administered through a blood warmer to minimize further hemolysis.

Cold agglutinin disease is a chronic IgM antibody–mediated hemolysis that is usually seen in association with lymphoproliferative diseases. Hemolysis is usually low grade; if severe, it responds poorly to steroids and splenectomy. Acute severe IgM-mediated hemolysis may respond to plasmapheresis, rituximab, and treatment directed against the lymphoproliferative disorder when present. Supportive therapy includes avoidance of exposure to the cold.

Hemolysis From Causes Extrinsic to the Erythrocyte
Microangiopathic Hemolysis

Microangiopathic hemolytic anemia (MAHA) is caused by traumatic destruction of RBCs as they pass through small vessels. The leading causes of MAHA include thrombotic thrombocytopenic purpura and hemolytic-uremic syndrome (TTP/HUS) (see Table 48.5 and Fig. 48.1). Other causes include pregnancy-related syndromes such as preeclampsia, eclampsia, and the HELLP syndrome (*h*emolysis, *e*levated *l*iver enzyme levels, and *l*ow *p*latelet count); drugs; and metastatic cancers. A similar hemolytic picture can be seen in traumatic hemolysis on a damaged cardiac valve (native or prosthetic).

The finding of schistocytes (fragmented erythrocytes) on the peripheral blood smear confirms the diagnosis of MAHA (see Fig. 48.2D). The presence of normal prothrombin and partial thromboplastin times supports a diagnosis of TTP/HUS over that of disseminated

TABLE 48.7 **Congenital Red Blood Cell Membrane Abnormalities**

Condition	Abnormal Membrane Proteins	Inheritance
Spherocytosis	Spectrin, ankyrin, band 3, protein 4.2	Autosomal dominant Recessive (rare)
Elliptocytosis	Spectrin, protein 4.1	Autosomal dominant Recessive (rare)
Pyropoikilocytosis	Spectrin	Recessive
Stomatocytosis	Sodium channel permeability defect	Autosomal dominant

intravascular coagulation. Diagnosis and management are described further in Chapter 52.

Infection

Hemolysis can be caused by direct infection of RBCs by parasites, as seen in malaria, babesiosis, and bartonellosis. Severe, overwhelming hemolysis can be seen in clostridial sepsis, in which bacterial toxins directly damage the membrane.

Hemolytic Anemias Caused by Disorders of the Erythrocyte Membrane
Inherited Membrane Abnormalities

Hereditary spherocytosis (HS) is caused by heterogeneous congenital abnormalities in proteins of the erythrocyte cytoskeleton (Table 48.7). Most patients with HS have dominantly inherited mutations in spectrin or ankyrin. HS is characterized by hemolytic anemia, splenomegaly, and the presence of prominent spherocytes in the peripheral blood. Spherocytes are the result of *conditioning* of the erythrocytes in the spleen, during which venous sinus endothelial cells and reticuloendothelial cells remove portions of the abnormal membrane that are caused by the disordered cytoskeleton. Spherocytes reflect membrane loss that decreases the membrane-to-cytoplasm ratio. Because a high membrane-to-cytoplasm ratio is responsible for the flexible, biconcave shape of the normal erythrocyte, the erythrocyte loses its biconcave morphologic characteristics and assumes a spherocytic shape with loss of membrane. Spherocytes are less flexible and may be destroyed in the microvasculature. The laboratory finding characteristic of HS is increased osmotic fragility, which is caused by the loss of distensibility associated with a decrease in surface membrane. HS is usually a mild disorder with well-compensated hemolysis. Patients typically have exacerbations during infections or when given marrow-suppressing medication. Patients with significant hemolysis should receive folate supplementation. Many patients require cholecystectomy for pigment stones. Severe, symptomatic anemia is treated with partial or total splenectomy.

Hereditary elliptocytosis (HE) is caused by dominantly inherited mutations affecting the interactions between membrane proteins and underlying cytoplasmic proteins. The most common abnormalities affect the interactions with spectrin and protein 4.1, which causes the RBCs to assume an elliptical shape. As in HS, patients usually have mild hemolysis and splenomegaly.

Hereditary pyropoikilocytosis (HPP) is a rare recessive disorder that is frequently caused by the inheritance of two different membrane disorders (e.g., one allele for HS and one for HE). Patients have severe hemolysis with microspherocytes and elliptocytes on the peripheral blood smear. As with HS, treatment for symptomatic anemia in HE and HPP is splenectomy.

Hereditary stomatocytosis is caused by autosomal dominant mutations leading to abnormalities in RBC permeability and volume, either in an overhydrated form (OHS), dehydrated form (DHS) or near normal form. These rare membranopathies are heterogeneous in presentation with syndromic and nonsyndromic forms with varying degrees of hemolytic anemia and are confirmed with genetic testing. Treatment is supportive but splenectomy should be avoided due to increased risk of thrombosis in certain types and care should be made to distinguish from hereditary spherocytosis for which splenectomy is the indicated therapy.

More information on hemolytic anemias caused by inherited membrane disorders can be found in Chapter 152, "Hemolytic Anemias: Red Cell Membrane and Metabolic Defects," in *Goldman-Cecil Medicine*, 26th Edition.

Acquired Membrane Abnormalities

Paroxysmal nocturnal hemoglobinuria. Paroxysmal nocturnal hemoglobinuria (PNH) is an acquired clonal disease that is associated with an abnormality of complement regulation. Normal erythrocytes are protected from complement-mediated cell lysis by the presence of membrane proteins, including delay-accelerating factor (DAF or CD55) and membrane inhibitor of reactive lysis (MIRL or CD59). Both these proteins are members of a family of proteins that are anchored to the membrane by a glycosyl phosphatidylinositol (GPI) anchor. Patients with PNH have clonal mutations in phosphatidyl inositol glycan A (PIG-A), the enzyme required for synthesis of GPI. These mutations arise in the hematopoietic stem cell, and subsequently all hematopoietic cells lack GPI-anchored proteins. Absence of GPI-anchored proteins from erythrocytes renders them susceptible to complement-mediated lysis. The diagnosis can be made by flow cytometric documentation of the absence of CD55 or CD59 on the surface of RBCs or leukocytes.

PNH is a clonal stem cell disorder with several unique characteristics. Patients suffer from episodic acute intravascular hemolysis with a release of free hemoglobin that results in the hemoglobinuria for which the disease is named. The dark, hemoglobin-pigmented urine is most prominent in the morning after concentrating overnight during sleep. Patients are also susceptible to venous thrombotic complications, including Budd-Chiari syndrome, portal vein thrombosis, cerebro-vascular thrombosis, and peripheral veins. The disease is associated with a risk for development of myelodysplasia, myelofibrosis, acute

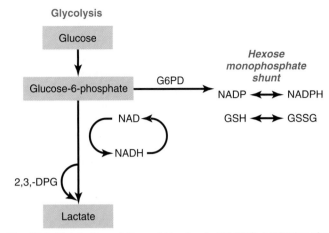

Fig. 48.4 Metabolism of the red blood cell. *2,3-DPG,* 2,3-Diphosphoglycerate; *G6PD,* glucose-6-phosphate dehydrogenase; *GSH,* reduced glutathione; *GSSG,* reduced and oxidized glutathione; *NAD,* nicotinamide adenine dinucleotide; *NADH,* reduced form of NAD; *NADP,* nicotinamide adenine dinucleotide phosphate; *NADPH,* reduced form of NADP.

leukemia, or aplastic anemia. Furthermore, patients with aplastic anemia who respond to immunosuppressive therapy frequently develop PNH-like clones. In the past, treatment has been largely supportive. However, treatment with eculizumab and ravulizumab, monoclonal antibodies that bind to the C5 component of complement, have been shown to reduce hemolysis and transfusion requirements in this disease. Eculizumab also reduces thromboembolic events; this end point has not yet been addressed in the more recently approved ravulizumab. Young patients should be considered for allogeneic stem cell transplantation.

Spur cell anemia. Spur cells (acanthocytes) are cells with abnormal membrane morphology found in patients with advanced liver disease, severe malnutrition, malabsorption, or asplenia. The membrane acquires protrusions as a result of the presence of abnormal lipids. The changes may be associated with mild hemolysis, although in patients with advanced liver disease, it is difficult to distinguish hemolysis from hypersplenism. Similar changes may be observed in patients with abetalipoproteinemia.

Hemolytic Anemias Caused by Disorders of Erythrocyte Enzymes
Glucose-6 Phosphate Dehydrogenase Deficiency

Glucose-6-phosphate dehydrogenase (G6PD) is a critical enzyme in the hexose monophosphate shunt pathway. By maintaining intracellular stores of reduced glutathione, it protects erythrocytes from membrane and hemoglobin oxidation (Fig. 48.4). The gene for G6PD resides on the X chromosome, and therefore almost all patients with G6PD deficiency are male. Most G6PD mutations are found in African and Mediterranean populations, most likely because they confer resistance to malaria. The African form of G6PD deficiency is relatively mild, whereas the Mediterranean form is severe.

Absence of G6PD renders erythrocytes sensitive to oxidative stress. In the setting of infection, inflammation acidosis, or oxidant drugs, hemoglobin may precipitate within the cells, causing hemolysis. Many drugs are associated with hemolysis in the setting of G6PD deficiency, including sulfonamides, antimalarials, dapsone, aspirin, and phenacetin. The diagnosis should be considered in male patients of African or Mediterranean extraction who have evidence of hemolysis in the setting of acute infection or recent exposure to oxidant drugs. Patients with the Mediterranean variant of G6PD deficiency may develop hemolysis on exposure to fava beans (favism). Cells with precipitated hemoglobin contain Heinz bodies that can be visualized with crystal violet staining of the peripheral blood smear. These inclusions are removed in the spleen, resulting in the additional finding of bite cells in the blood smear. The diagnosis can be confirmed with measurement of G6PD levels in the peripheral blood. However, reticulocytes and young RBCs in patients with G6PD deficiency have a higher enzyme level; consequently, if the diagnosis is probable, the patients with a normal G6PD level should be retested at a time removed from the acute episode, when the percentage of young RBCs is high. The mainstay of preventing hemolysis in these patients is avoidance of oxidative stress, especially drugs implicated in causing hemolysis. Splenectomy is recommended only for patients with severe episodic or chronic hemolysis.

Other Enzyme Deficiencies

Enzyme deficiencies as rare causes of hemolytic anemia have been reported involving almost all of the enzymes of the glycolytic pathway. The most common of these is pyruvate kinase deficiency. Autosomal genes encode these enzymes, and the pattern of inheritance is therefore autosomal recessive.

More information on hemolytic anemias caused by inherited enzyme deficiencies can be found in Chapter 152, "Hemolytic Anemias: Red Cell Membrane and Metabolic Defects," in *Goldman-Cecil Medicine*, 26th Edition.

Hemoglobinopathies

Hemoglobinopathies are disorders caused by mutations that result in the synthesis of quantitatively or qualitatively abnormal hemoglobins. The most common of these are the sickle syndromes and the thalassemias, which, like G6PD deficiency, arose in areas of the world with endemic malaria.

Sickle Cell Disease

Sickle cell disease, the most common of the sickle syndromes, arises from a point mutation that causes a substitution of valine for glutamic acid in the sixth amino acid of the β-globin gene. It has arisen as an independent mutation in diverse populations in Africa, India, the Mediterranean, and the Middle East. The substitution of a hydrophobic for a hydrophilic residue renders the deoxygenated sickle hemoglobin (HbS) less soluble and therefore susceptible to polymerization and precipitation. The rate of precipitation of HbS is exquisitely sensitive to the intracorpuscular concentration of deoxygenated hemoglobin. Sickling is therefore increased in settings in which that concentration is increased, either by changes in cellular hydration (dehydration) or by changes in the oxygen dissociation curve (e.g., hypoxia, acidosis, high altitude).

Acute manifestations. Most of the acute complications of sickle cell disease are related to vaso-occlusion (Table 48.8). Painful crises, secondary to occlusions of the microvasculature and ischemia of organs and tissues, can occur anywhere, with pain most commonly experienced in the extremities, chest, abdomen, and back. Painful crises are commonly precipitated by infections, dehydration, rapid changes in temperature, and pregnancy. Often, however, no obvious precipitating cause is found for an acute painful crisis.

Vaso-occlusion in the pulmonary circulation can be a particularly ominous complication of sickle cell disease. It results in the *acute chest syndrome*, which is characterized by chest pain, hypoxemia, and pulmonary infiltrates. The roles of infection, infarction, and in situ thrombosis in the acute chest syndrome are indistinguishable, but all patients should receive antibiotics for presumed pneumonia. Because hypoxemia predisposes to further sickling and increasing respiratory

TABLE 48.8 Clinical Manifestations of Sickle Cell Disease

Acute Manifestations	Chronic Manifestations
Vaso-occlusive crisis	Chronic renal disease
Painful crisis	Isosthenuria
Acute chest syndrome	Chronic renal failure
Priapism	Chronic pulmonary disease
Cerebrovascular events	Sickle hepatopathy
Thrombotic stroke	Proliferative retinopathy
Hemorrhagic stroke	Avascular necrosis
Aplastic crisis	Skin ulcers
Splenic sequestration	
Osteomyelitis	

compromise, the acute chest syndrome is life-threatening and is an indication for emergent exchange transfusion.

Neurologic events are a major cause of morbidity in patients with sickle cell disease. Acute large-vessel occlusions occur in children, with a recurrence rate of 70% if untreated; such strokes are an indication for long-term exchange transfusion, which has been shown to decrease the rate of repeated occlusions. For reasons that are poorly understood, such large-vessel occlusions rarely occur in adults. Adults may suffer hemorrhagic strokes as a result of aneurysmal dilation of proliferative vessels that form in response to repeated micro-occlusions in the cerebral vessels.

Any toxic or infectious insult that transiently suppresses bone marrow activity can cause an *aplastic crisis*. The shortened survival time of the RBC in sickle cell disease renders patients highly dependent on vigorous ongoing marrow activity, and short intervals of decreased reticulocyte formation can cause profound anemia. Most dramatic are infections associated with parvovirus B19, which directly infects erythroid precursors. Supportive care is usually all that is required. However, some patients go on to develop bone marrow necrosis, with a leukoerythroblastic picture; this development may be further complicated by bone marrow embolization to the lungs.

Certain vascular beds are especially prone to complications of sickle cell disease. The renal medulla is highly susceptible to damage by vaso-occlusion because its high tonicity and low oxygen tension both significantly increase the concentration of HbS. All patients with sickle cell disease develop defects in the ability to concentrate urine, and by adulthood, they are uniformly isosthenuric. Acute episodes of hematuria secondary to papillary necrosis are common.

The spleen is another site in which recurrent sickling uniformly occurs. Although in childhood the spleen can sequester blood cells, by adulthood all patients have become functionally asplenic from repeated infarctions of the microvasculature. This contributing factor increases the susceptibility of patients with sickle cell disease to infections with encapsulated organisms. Acute infection remains a significant cause of death. For unclear reasons, patients with sickle cell disease are particularly prone to osteomyelitis, and there is an unusually high incidence of *Salmonella* as the responsible organism.

Chronic manifestations. Sickle cell disease used to be a disease of childhood. As more patients survive to adulthood, it has become clear that repeated episodes of vaso-occlusion lead to damage to almost every end organ (see Table 48.8). Renal failure and pulmonary failure are leading causes of death in adult patients with sickle cell disease. Other long-term complications include chronic skin ulcers, retinopathy, and liver dysfunction. In addition, most patients require cholecystectomy for pigment stones.

TABLE 48.9 Thalassemic Syndromes		
Disorder	**Genotypic Abnormality**	**Clinical Phenotype**
β-Thalassemia		
Thalassemia major (Cooley's anemia)	Homozygous β^0-thalassemia	Severe hemolysis, ineffective erythropoiesis, transfusion dependency, iron overload
Thalassemia intermedia	Compound heterozygous β^0- and β^+-thalassemia	Moderate hemolysis, severe anemia, but not transfusion dependent; iron overload
Thalassemia minor	Heterozygous β^0- or β^+-thalassemia	Microcytosis, mild anemia
α-Thalassemia		
Hydrops fetalis	--/--	Severe anemia, intrauterine anasarca from congestive heart failure; death in utero or at birth
Hemoglobin H	α-/--	Microcytic anemia and mild hemolysis; not transfusion dependent
α-Thalassemia trait	$\alpha\alpha$/-- (α-thalassemia 1) or -α/-α (α-thalassemia 2)	Mild microcytic anemia
Silent carrier	-α/$\alpha\alpha$	Normal complete blood count

Treatment. Treatment of sickle cell disease remains largely supportive. Painful crises are treated with fluid, oxygen supplementation, and analgesics. Patients with any indication of infection should receive antibiotics. Patients with symptomatic anemia should be transfused. Exchange transfusion is indicated for chest syndrome, stroke, bone marrow necrosis, and priapism. More controversial indications for exchange transfusion include intractable pain and slow response to other supportive measures. The goal of exchange transfusion is to achieve a level of 30% to 40% HbS. As previously mentioned, patients who have sustained a thrombotic large-vessel stroke should undergo chronic exchange transfusion.

Hydroxyurea has been the main disease-modifying agent for patients with sickle cell disease. Treatment with hydroxyurea, an agent that increases the concentration of HbF in patients with sickle cell disease, reduces the incidence of vaso-occlusive crises. The efficacy of hydroxyurea in patients with recurrent crises has been demonstrated in a randomized study, and follow-up studies have revealed a survival advantage for patients treated with hydroxyurea. More recently, three additional agents have been approved; two further reduced sickle cell crises (L-glutamine and crizanlizumab) and the last increased hemoglobin levels (voxelotor). In a randomized study, L-glutamine therapy demonstrated significantly fewer sickle cell crises with most patients on both arms already receiving hydroxyurea. L-glutamine is hypothesized to reduce oxidative stress and potential pain crises by increasing reduced nicotinamide adenine dinucleotide in sickle cells. In another randomized trial, crizanlizumab, a P-selectin inhibitor, also significantly reduced sickle cell crises. P-selectin initiates the process of leukocyte adhesion to vascular endothelium during inflammation that leads to vaso-occlusion. Most recently, voxelotor, an agent that inhibits HbS polymerization by stabilizing the oxygenated hemoglobin state, has led to decreased hemolysis and improved anemia and is now an approved therapy.

The only curative treatment for sickle cell disease is allogeneic stem cell transplant although lack of donor matches remains a barrier.

Other Sickle Syndromes

Hemoglobin C. Hemoglobin C (HbC) is caused by another substitution, glutamic acid to lysine, in the sixth position of the β-globin chain. Homozygous HbC causes very mild symptoms of anemia and is usually clinically silent. Patients with hemoglobin S-C (HbSC) are compound heterozygotes for HbS and HbC. These patients are symptomatic, although the clinical manifestations are milder than in patients with homozygous HbS (HbSS). They have a higher hematocrit, but the higher viscosity increases the degree of retinopathy. They do not sustain splenic infarctions; unlike patients with HbSS, they usually have splenomegaly. Consequently, they occasionally have episodes of acute splenomegaly associated with profound decreases in hemoglobin concentration and hematocrit (splenic sequestration crisis). Although such crises also occur in children with HbSS, functional asplenia prevents this complication in adults with HbSS.

Sickle cell β-thalassemia. Patients who are double heterozygotes for HbS and β-thalassemia have a spectrum of disease dependent on the level of β-globin that they produce. Sickle cell β^+-thalassemia is a milder disease than HbSS, probably because of the decreased intracorpuscular concentration of HbS. Patients with sickle cell β^0-thalassemia (see discussion that follows) produce no normal β chains and have essentially the same phenotype as patients with HbSS.

Thalassemia

The thalassemic syndromes (Table 48.9) are a heterogeneous group of disorders associated with decreased or absent synthesis of either α- or β-globin chains. Severe thalassemic syndromes are associated with severe hemolytic anemia and are diagnosed in early childhood. However, mild forms of thalassemia minor frequently cause mild microcytic anemia with little or no evidence of hemolysis. These syndromes are often confused with iron deficiency because of the decreased MCV.

β-Thalassemia. Over 100 mutations have been described that lead to β-thalassemia, causing a decrease or absence of expression from the β-globin locus. The decreased expression of β-globin can be caused by structural mutations in the coding region of the gene, which result in nonsense mutations, truncated messenger RNA (mRNA), and no expression of intact globin from the affected allele (β^0-thalassemia). However, a large number of mutations that result in decreased transcription or translation or altered splicing of the β-globin mRNA result in reduction but not elimination of globin-chain expression from the affected allele (β^+-thalassemia).

Defective globin-chain synthesis in β-thalassemia causes both decreased normal hemoglobin production and the production of a relative excess of α chains. The decrease in normal hemoglobin synthesis results in a hypochromic anemia, and the excess α chains form insoluble α-chain complexes and cause hemolysis. In mild thalassemic syndromes, the excess α chains are insufficient to cause significant hemolysis, and the primary finding is a microcytic anemia. In severe forms of thalassemia, hemolysis occurs both in the peripheral blood and in the marrow, with intense secondary expansion of the marrow production of RBCs. The expansion of the marrow space causes severe skeletal abnormalities, and the ineffective erythropoiesis also provides a powerful stimulus to absorb iron from the intestine.

The clinical spectrum of β-thalassemia reflects the heterogeneity of the molecular lesions causing the disease (see Table 48.9). β-Thalassemia major results from homozygous β^0-thalassemia, leading to severe hemolytic anemia; such patients are diagnosed in infancy and are transfusion dependent from birth. Patients with β-thalassemia intermedia also have two β-thalassemia alleles, but at least one of them is a mild β^+ mutation. These patients have severe chronic hemolytic anemia but do not require transfusions. Because of ineffective erythropoiesis, the patients chronically hyperabsorb iron and may develop iron overload in the absence of transfusions. β-Thalassemia minor is usually caused by heterozygous β-thalassemia, although it may reflect the inheritance of two mild thalassemic mutations. These are the patients in whom iron deficiency is often misdiagnosed. Iron studies show normal to increased iron with normal iron saturation. Documentation of a compensatory increase in HbA_2 and HbF on hemoglobin electrophoresis confirms the diagnosis.

α-Thalassemia. α-Thalassemia is almost always caused by mutations that delete one or more of the α-chain loci on chromosome 16. Four α-chain loci exist with two, almost identical, copies of the α-globin gene on each chromosome. The spectrum of α-thalassemia therefore reflects the lack of one, two, three, or all four α-globin genes (see Table 48.9). In general, the clinical manifestations of α-thalassemia are milder than those of β-thalassemia for two reasons. First, the presence of four α-chain genes allows for adequate α-chain synthesis unless three or four loci are deleted. Second, β-chain tetramers are more soluble than their α-chain counterparts and do not cause hemolysis. Patients with the loss of a single α-chain gene are silent carriers and have a normal hematocrit and MCV. Patients with deletion of two α chains, either on the same chromosome (−−/αα, called α-thal 1) or on different chromosomes (−α/−α; α-thal 2), are microcytic and mildly anemic. Patients who inherit one α-thal 1 allele and one α-thal 2 allele (−−/−α) have hemoglobin H disease. Hemoglobin H is the product of excess β-chain production, specifically β_4; it causes mild hemolytic anemia and minimal or no intramedullary erythrocyte destruction. Inheritance of the homozygous α-thal 2 allele results in no functional α-chain loci and is incompatible with life. The fetus is unable to make any functional hemoglobin beyond embryonic development because HbF also requires α chains. Free γ chains form tetramers, termed *hemoglobin Barts.* Hemoglobin Barts have an extremely high oxygen affinity, and failure to release oxygen in peripheral tissues results in severe congestive heart failure and anasarca, a clinical picture termed *hydrops fetalis.* Affected fetuses are stillborn or die soon after birth.

Treatment. Though management of patients with thalassemia is mainly supportive (transfusion therapy, folic acid supplementation, iron chelation as needed), a disease-modifying erythroid maturation agent, luspatercept, has recently been approved. Luspatercept binds to specific TGFβ ligands that inhibit aberrant Smad2/3 signaling and results in improved erythropoiesis. A randomized trial of luspatercept demonstrated lowered transfusion burden in adults primarily with β-thalassemia.

More information on the thalassemias, sickle cell disease, and other hemoglobinopathies can be found in Chapter 153, "The Thalassemias," and Chapter 154, "Sickle Cell Disease and Other Hemoglobinopathies," in *Goldman-Cecil Medicine,* 26th Edition.

PROSPECTUS FOR THE FUTURE

Anemia is increasingly recognized as a marker of increased morbidity and mortality in adults with a wide range of medical conditions, including renal failure, malignancy, cardiac disease, inflammatory conditions, and other chronic diseases. Advances in understanding the pathophysiology of anemia of chronic inflammation are contributing to knowledge of iron metabolism and the roles cytokines play in hematopoiesis. These developments are paving the way for the development of new therapies for patients with anemia and iron overload. Ongoing progress in stem cell transplantation will contribute to the ability to treat and potentially cure various hemoglobinopathies, and gene therapy approaches are also being piloted.

SUGGESTED READINGS

Andrews NC: Forging a field: the golden age of iron biology, Blood 112:219–230, 2008.

Auerbach M, Macdougall I: The available intravenous iron formulations: History, efficacy, and toxicology, Hemodial Int 21:S83–S92, 2017.

Bain BJ: Diagnosis from the blood smear, N Engl J Med 353:498–507, 2005.

Bennett CL, Silver SM, Djulbegovic B, et al: Venous thromboembolism and mortality associated with recombinant erythropoietin and darbepoetin administration for the treatment of cancer-associated anemia, J Am Med Assoc 299:914–924, 2008.

Cappellini MD, et al: The Believe trial: results of a phase 3, randomized, double-blind, placebo-controlled study of luspatercept in adult beta-thalassemia patients who require regular red blood cell (RBC) transfusions. Abstract #164, ASH Annual Meeting, December 1, 2018; San Diego, CA.

Finberg KE: Unraveling mechanisms regulating systemic iron homeostasis, Hematology Am Soc Hematol Educ Program 2011:532–537, 2011.

Ganz T: Anemia of inflammation, N Engl J Med 381:1148–1157, 2019.

Kenneth AI, Kutlar A, Kanter J, et al: Crizanlizumab for the prevention of pain crises in sickle cell disease, N Engl J Med 376:429–439, 2017.

Kidney Disease: Improving Global Outcomes (KDIGO): Anemia Work Group: KDIGO clinical practice guidelines for anemia in chronic kidney disease, Kidney Int Suppl 2:279–335, 2012.

Lee JW, Sicre de Fontbrune F, Wong Lee Lee L, et al: Ravulizumab (ALXN1210) vs eculizumab in adult patients with PNH naïve to complete inhibitors: the 301 study, Blood 133:530–539, 2019.

Lin JC: Approach to anemia in the adult and child. In Hoffman R, Benz EJ, Silberstein LE, et al, editors: Hoffman: hematology—basic principles and practice, ed 7, Philadelphia, 2018, Elsevier, pp 458–467.

Moretti D, Goede JS, Zeder C, et al: Oral iron supplements increase hepcidin and decrease iron absorption from daily or twice-daily doses in iron-depleted young women, Blood 126:1981–1989, 2015.

Niihara Y, et al: A phase 3 trial of L-glutamine in sickle cell disease, N Engl J Med 379:226–235, 2018.

Stabler SP: Vitamin B12 deficiency, N Engl J Med 368:149–160, 2013.

Stoffel NU, Cercamondi CI, Brittenham G, et al: Iron absorption from oral iron supplements given on consecutive versus alternative days and as single morning doses versus twice-daily split in iron-depleted women: two open-label, randomized controlled trials, Lancet Haematol 4:PE524–E533, 2017.

Thompson A, Walters MC, Kwiatkowski J, et al: Gene therapy in patients with transfusion-dependent β-thalassemia, N Engl J Med 378:1479–1493, 2018.

Vichinsky E, Hoppe CC, Ataga KI, et al: A phase 3 randomized trial of voxelotor in sickle cell disease, N Engl J Med 381:509–519, 2019.

Yutaka N, Miller ST, Kanter J, et al: A phase 3 trial of L-glutamine in sickle cell disease, N Engl J Med 379:226–235, 2018.

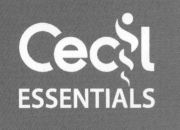

49

Clinical Disorders of Granulocytes and Monocytes

Ellice Wong, Michal G. Rose, Nancy Berliner

INTRODUCTION

Leukocytes, or white blood cells (WBCs), provide the main defense against bacterial infection. Granulocytes (primarily neutrophils) and monocytes are phagocytic cells that can kill ingested bacteria through the generation of reactive intermediates. Monocytes also release inflammatory mediators that increase the activity of lymphocytes. Lymphocyte function is discussed in Chapter 50.

NORMAL GRANULOCYTE DEVELOPMENT, STRUCTURE, AND FUNCTION

Neutrophils

Neutrophils (i.e., polymorphonuclear leukocytes) are the predominant WBC in the peripheral blood. They are morphologically recognizable by their characteristic segmented nucleus and cytoplasmic granules that are functionally important (Fig. 49.1).

Neutrophils achieve intracellular killing of bacteria through chemotaxis, margination, adhesion, and phagocytosis (Fig. 49.2). *Chemotaxis* is the ordered movement of the cell toward an attracting stimulus, such as bacterial formyl peptides or complement fragments (i.e., C3b and C5a). In *margination,* neutrophils move toward endothelial cells lining the blood vessel walls. Neutrophils attach to endothelial cells by interaction of neutrophil surface glycoproteins (i.e., CD11b/CD18) with endothelial adhesion molecules (i.e., intercellular adhesion molecule 1 and endothelial leukocyte adhesion molecule 1) in a process called *adhesion.* In response to a chemotactic stimulus, the adherent neutrophils move toward the target along the endothelial surface.

The leukocyte adhesion deficiency (LAD) syndromes are associated with impaired migration of leukocytes (particularly neutrophils) from the vasculature into tissues resulting in neutrophilia, inability to form pus, impaired wound healing, and recurrent bacterial infections. This rare group of congenital diseases is characterized by beta integrin defects, selectin receptor abnormalities, as well as loss of the C3b receptor (which mediates opsonin-induced phagocytosis). Disease therefore results both from failure of adhesion and from failure to phagocytose opsonized bacteria.

Phagocytosis requires recognition of target bacteria or debris by the neutrophil. Targets are opsonized by the surface binding of immunoglobulin or complement factor C3b. The neutrophil has surface receptors for C3b and the Fc portion of immunoglobulin G, which allows recognition and binding to the opsonized target. The target then becomes engulfed in a phagocytic vacuole, which fuses with neutrophil granules inside the cell.

Intracellular killing occurs by oxygen-dependent and oxygen-independent mechanisms. Contents of the primary granules, including cathepsin G, defensins, and lysozyme, break down the bacterial cell wall and kill the target organism. However, the major mechanism of bacterial killing is the *respiratory burst.* Stimulation of the neutrophil activates a membrane-bound oxidase complex, which generates superoxide through the transfer of an electron from reduced nicotinamide-adenine dinucleotide phosphate (NADPH). The interaction of superoxide with water generates hydroxyl ions. Myeloperoxidase catalyzes the formation of hypochlorite ion from hydrogen peroxide and chloride. The NADPH oxidase is a multisubunit enzyme. Absence or decreased activity of any one subunit impairs bacterial killing and results in chronic granulomatous disease, a congenital illness in which patients are predisposed to life-threatening bacterial infections.

More recently, *neutrophil extracellular traps (NETS)* have been proposed as an extracellular mechanism for neutrophil-induced antimicrobial activity. Activated neutrophils have been shown to release nucleic acids with histones and granule proteins extracellularly to trap and kill bacteria.

Neutrophil granules give neutrophils their characteristic appearance and have important functions in neutrophil-mediated activation and killing. *Primary granules* arise early in myeloid differentiation and are found in neutrophils and monocytes. They contain a large number of proteins, including myeloperoxidase, acid hydrolases, and neutral proteases. These granules fuse with the phagocytic vacuole and aid in the digestion of ingested bacteria. *Secondary granules* arise later in the differentiation pathway and give the neutrophil its characteristic granular (electron-dense) appearance. These granules contain lactoferrin, transcobalamin, and the matrix-modifying enzymes collagenase and gelatinase. On neutrophil stimulation, the granules are released into the extracellular space. Lactoferrin and transcobalamin act as antibacterial proteins by sequestering iron and vitamin B_{12} away from bacteria, and collagenase and gelatinase break down connective tissue at the site of inflammation.

Abnormalities in neutrophil granules have been described in rare clinical syndromes. Absence of myeloperoxidase produces surprisingly mild symptoms and may be associated with defects in control of fungal infections. Secondary granule deficiency is rare and is associated with a slight increase in the risk of bacterial infections.

Eosinophils and Basophils

In addition to neutrophils, eosinophils and basophils are granulocytes that arise from myeloid precursors in the bone marrow. They transit rapidly from the marrow to the blood and into the peripheral tissues, where they play a role in allergic and inflammatory reactions. Like neutrophils, they have secondary granules that give them a characteristic appearance and are functionally important. Both cell types occur in small numbers under normal conditions.

Although eosinophils are capable of phagocytosis, most of the activity of these cells is mediated through the release of granule

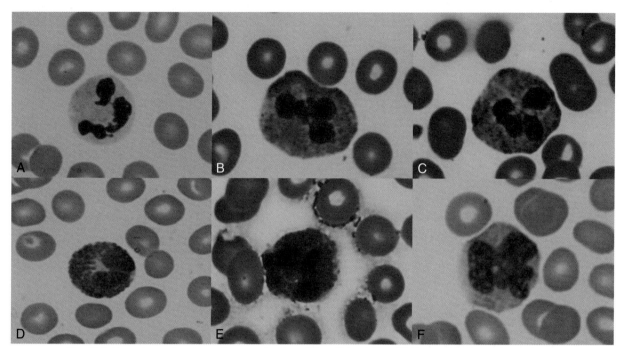

Fig. 49.1 Normal granulocytes and monocytes in peripheral blood. (A to C) Neutrophils (i.e., polymorphonuclear cells). (D) Eosinophils. (E) Basophils. (F) Monocytes. (Courtesy Robert J. Homer, MD, PhD, Yale School of Medicine, New Haven, Conn.)

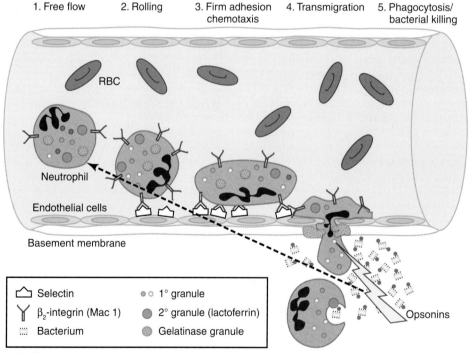

Fig. 49.2 Sequence of neutrophil activation shows the process of rolling, engagement with the vessel wall, attachment, diapedesis, and phagocytosis. *Mac 1,* Macrophage antigen 1 (CDI lb/CD18); *RBC,* red blood cell.

contents. The eosinophil numbers are elevated in parasitic and helminthic infections, in which these cells are thought to play a role in the allergic response to those organisms. Cell numbers are also elevated in allergic reactions and in collagen vascular diseases, linking their function to immunomodulation. Hypereosinophilic syndromes, in which extremely high levels of eosinophils can be seen, are rare, and hypereosinophilia can be associated with

damage to the lung, peripheral nervous system, and endocardial tissues. The differential diagnosis of eosinophilia is outlined in Table 49.1.

Basophils play a role in immediate hypersensitivity reactions and chronic inflammatory conditions including tuberculosis, ulcerative colitis, and rheumatoid arthritis. Their numbers are also notably increased in chronic myeloid leukemia.

TABLE 49.1 Differential Diagnosis of Eosinophilia

Causes	Comments
Infection[a]	Especially parasites; less commonly mycobacteria
Allergic diseases[a]	Drugs, asthma, allergic rhinitis, atopy, urticaria
Pulmonary diseases[a]	Churg-Strauss disease, Löffler's pneumonia, pulmonary infiltrates with eosinophilia
Drug reactions[a]	Usually disappears when drug discontinued
Malignancy[a]	Paraneoplastic, angioimmunoblastic T-cell lymphoma, Hodgkin's and non-Hodgkin's lymphoma
Connective tissue diseases[a]	Rheumatoid arthritis, eosinophilic fasciitis, vasculitis
Primary hypereosinophilic syndrome	More than 6 months of >1500 eosinophils/μL with no other apparent cause

[a]Reactive forms.

Monocytes

Monocytes arise from a common myeloid precursor along with granulocytes under the influence of granulocyte-macrophage colony-stimulating factor (GM-CSF) and macrophage colony-stimulating factor (M-CSF). Most circulating monocytes are marginated along the walls of blood vessels. They migrate from the vessels into tissues, where they develop into macrophages.

The monocyte-macrophage lineage has many diverse functions. These phagocytic cells perform chemotaxis, phagocytosis, and intracellular killing in much the same manner as neutrophils. They are especially important in killing infectious mycobacterial, fungal, and protozoal species.

Monocytes interact with other components of the immune system. They are antigen-presenting cells for T lymphocytes, they are capable of cellular cytotoxicity, and they secrete cytokines. The macrophages (i.e., differentiated monocytes) that process antigens and present them to T lymphocytes take on different forms in different tissues such as Langerhans cells in the skin, interdigitating cells in the thymus, and dendritic cells in the lymph nodes. Antigen-presenting cells are nonphagocytic, and the process by which they internalize antigen is not fully understood. Protein antigens are partially digested and expressed on the cell surface in association with major histocompatibility complex class II (Ia) antigens. This feature permits interaction with and activation of helper T cells. Other macrophages, such as Kupffer cells of the liver and alveolar macrophages of the lung, play an important role in removing particulate and cellular debris and senescent erythrocytes from the circulation.

Monocytes are capable of antibody-dependent and antibody-independent cytotoxicity against tumor cells. Cytotoxicity is increased by tumor necrosis factor, interleukin-1, and interferon, which are secreted by monocytes. Monocytes secrete large numbers of immunomodulatory proteins (e.g., tumor necrosis factor, interleukin-1, interferon), cytokines (e.g., granulocyte colony-stimulating factor [G-CSF], GM-CSF), coagulation proteins, cell adhesion proteins, and proteases.

Monocytosis can be present in inflammatory as well as primary hematologic conditions. Infections such as tuberculosis, endocarditis, and syphilis are commonly associated with a reactive monocytosis. Hematologic malignancies such as chronic myelomonocytic leukemia, juvenile myelomonocytic leukemia, and some types of acute myeloid leukemia have clonal monocytosis as a hallmark feature. A reactive monocytosis has also been observed in some lymphomas.

Monocytopenia is observed in stress states including severe sepsis and as a result of myelosuppressive chemotherapy. Low monocyte counts can also be found in acquired bone marrow failure states including aplastic anemia and myelodysplastic syndrome (MDS) and in hairy cell leukemia. Monocytopenia associated with natural killer cell deficiency and B-cell lymphoma have been linked to disorders involving GATA2 or SAMD9L mutations.

DETERMINANTS OF PERIPHERAL NEUTROPHIL NUMBERS

Most granulocyte precursors are in the bone marrow, where maturation occurs over 6 to 10 days. Marrow precursors represent 20% of the granulocyte mass, and the storage pool represents 75% of the granulocyte mass. Peripheral neutrophils represent only 5% of the total granulocyte mass.

Neutrophils circulate in transit between the marrow and peripheral tissues. More than one half of the circulating neutrophils adhere to the vascular endothelium (margination). The half-life of a neutrophil in the circulation was thought to be 6 to 12 hours, but more recent studies suggest it may be as long as 3 to 4 days. After neutrophils migrate into tissues, they survive another 1 to 4 days. The peripheral neutrophil count therefore represents a sampling of less than 5% of the total granulocyte pool and is taken during a very short interval of the total neutrophil lifespan.

The peripheral white cell count is a poor reflection of granulocyte kinetics. Abnormalities in neutrophil number can occur rapidly and may reflect a change in marrow granulocyte production or a shift among various cellular compartments. An elevated peripheral white cell count may result from increased marrow production, or it may reflect mobilization of neutrophils from the marginated pool or release from the marrow storage pool. Similarly, a low granulocyte count may reflect decreased marrow production, increased margination or sequestration in the spleen, or increased destruction of peripheral cells.

The *total peripheral white cell count* represents the sum of lymphocytes, monocytes, and granulocytes. The significance of an elevated or depressed leukocyte count depends on the nature of the cellular elements that are increased or decreased. *Leukocytosis* is a nonspecific term that may denote an increase in lymphocytes (i.e., lymphocytosis) or neutrophils (i.e., neutrophilia). In rare cases, increases may reflect excessive numbers of monocytes, eosinophils, or basophils.

Extreme elevation of the white blood cell count to more than 50,000 cells/μL of blood with the premature release of early myeloid precursors is called a *leukemoid reaction,* which may be associated with inflammation and infection. It requires consideration of a diagnosis of myeloproliferative disease, especially chronic myelogenous leukemia (CML). Evaluation of the peripheral blood smear may reveal characteristic changes that provide clues to the underlying disorder. A leukoerythroblastic smear shows immature granulocytes, teardrop-shaped erythrocytes, nucleated erythrocytes, and increased platelets. These changes reflect marrow infiltration (i.e., myelophthisis) by fibrous tissue, granulomas, or neoplasm. As with leukocytosis, leukopenia may reflect lymphopenia or neutropenia. Neutropenia is generally defined by an absolute neutrophil count of less than 1500 cells/μL, although institutional laboratory reference ranges may vary slightly.

NEUTROPHILIA

Neutrophilia usually results from other processes, and it rarely indicates a primary hematologic disorder (Table 49.2). However, patients with a persistently elevated neutrophil count, especially when associated with an elevated hematocrit or platelet count, should be evaluated to rule out a primary myeloproliferative neoplasm. Peripheral blood evaluation for

TABLE 49.2 Differential Diagnosis of Neutrophilia

Primary Hematologic Disease
Congenital neutrophilia
Leukocyte adhesion deficiency
Myeloproliferative disorders

Due to Other Disease Processes
Infection (acute or chronic)
Acute stress
Drugs (e.g., steroids, lithium)
Cytokine stimulation (e.g., granulocyte colony-stimulating factor)
Chronic inflammation
Malignancy
Myelophthisis
Marrow hyperstimulation
Chronic hemolysis, immune thrombocytopenia
Recovery from marrow suppression
Asplenia
Smoking
Metabolic and endocrine disorders (e.g., pregnancy, eclampsia, thyroid storm, Cushing disease)

TABLE 49.3 Differential Diagnosis of Neutropenia

Decreased Production of Neutrophils	Increased Peripheral Destruction
Congenital and/or constitutional cause	Sepsis
Constitutional neutropenia	Immune destruction
Benign chronic neutropenia	Drug related
Kostmann syndrome	Associated with collagen vascular disease
Cyclic neutropenia	Isoimmune (in newborns)
Postinfectious cause	Large granular lymphocyte leukemia
Nutritional deficiency (B$_{12}$, folate, copper)	Hypersplenism and/or sequestration
Drug-induced cause	
Primary marrow failure	
Aplastic anemia	
Myelodysplastic syndromes	
Acute leukemias	

the BCR/ABL fusion product can be performed to consider CML, and assays for JAK2 V617F, JAK2 exon 12, calreticulin, and MPL mutations can help to consider non-CML myeloproliferative neoplasms.

Neutrophilia related to acute infection, stress, toxic exposures like smoking, or corticosteroid administration primarily reflects demargination and is usually transient. Persistent neutrophilia usually reflects chronic bone marrow stimulation. Nevertheless, a bone marrow aspirate and biopsy are rarely indicated in the work-up of neutrophilia. The exception is for patients who demonstrate leukoerythroblastic changes, for which a bone marrow examination and culture may be indicated to consider tuberculosis or fungal infection, marrow infiltration with tumor, or marrow fibrosis. Cytogenetic and molecular studies should be performed to help eliminate the diagnosis of marrow malignancies, and the marrow should be cultured for mycobacteria and fungi.

NEUTROPENIA

Differential Diagnosis

Neutropenia may reflect decreased production, increased sequestration, or peripheral destruction of neutrophils (Table 49.3). Patients should first be evaluated for splenomegaly to consider the possibility of sequestration.

For patients who are asymptomatic and for whom previous studies are unavailable, the possibility of constitutional or cyclic neutropenia should be entertained and can be evaluated by serial peripheral blood counts. The normal neutrophil count varies among ethnic groups and is most commonly lower in individuals with African ancestry as compared to white individuals (i.e., constitutional or benign ethnic neutropenia [BEN]). The absence of the red blood cell Duffy antigen has been demonstrated to be associated with BEN. As the Duffy antigen is utilized by the parasite *Plasmodium vivax* to enter the red blood cell, it is believed that positive selection for the null allele enabled individuals in West Africa to be protected against malaria and have a survival advantage. Cyclic neutropenia is a relatively benign disorder, in which cyclical changes occur in all hematopoietic cell lines but are most dramatic in the neutrophil lineage. At the nadir of the neutrophil counts, patients may have infections, but the condition is often clinically silent.

In contrast, patients with congenital agranulocytosis or severe congenital neutropenia (SCN) exhibit profound neutropenia and infections in the perinatal period. Kostmann syndrome is a subset of SCN that was described more than 50 years ago as an autosomal recessive disorder; later studies demonstrated that SCN can reflect autosomal dominant, autosomal recessive, X-linked, or sporadic mutations.

About 50% of autosomal dominant SCN and almost 100% of cyclic neutropenia cases are associated with inherited mutations in the neutrophil elastase gene. The mutations are thought to produce a misfolded neutrophil elastase protein, which accumulates in the endoplasmic reticulum and activates the unfolded protein response. This complex cellular stress response coordinates the degradation of misfolded protein in the endoplasmic reticulum and can trigger cellular apoptosis if the stress is severe. Later studies have established that autosomal recessive SCN (i.e., Kostmann syndrome) is caused by mutations in the *HAX1* gene, which encodes a mitochondrial protein that is required for stabilization of the mitochondrial membrane. Absence of HAX1 results in loss of the mitochondrial membrane potential and induction of apoptosis.

Until G-CSF became available, most patients with SCN died in early childhood, but the availability of cytokine therapy has prolonged survival. However, SCN is also associated with a significantly increased incidence of acute leukemia, a complication that has become apparent as patients survive longer. Up to 30% of patients with SCN develop acute myelogenous leukemia over 10 years. Acute myelogenous leukemia in these patients is often associated with truncation mutations in the G-CSF receptor. These acquired somatic mutations may contribute to the pathogenesis of leukemia but do not contribute to the congenital neutropenia. The role of the G-CSF receptor mutations in the pathogenesis of leukemic transformation is controversial, as is the relationship between G-CSF therapy and the acquisition of these mutations.

Neutropenia may occur during or after viral, bacterial, or mycobacterial infections. Postviral neutropenia is especially common in children and probably reflects increased neutrophil consumption and a viral suppression of marrow neutrophil production. Neutropenia may be seen as a complication of overwhelming sepsis and is associated with a poor prognosis.

Drug-induced neutropenia may reflect dose-dependent marrow suppression or an idiosyncratic immune response. The former is one of the most common complications of chemotherapeutic drugs and is also common with antibiotics such as sulfamethoxazole-trimethoprim.

Chloramphenicol causes dose-dependent marrow suppression, although its more ominous complication is the rare idiosyncratic reaction that gives rise to marrow aplasia. Drugs that are most commonly associated with neutropenia include clozapine, sulfasalazine, ticlopidine, and the thionamide antithyroid agents. Most drug-induced neutropenias respond rapidly to discontinuation of the offending agent. The administration of G-CSF may speed recovery.

Autoimmune neutropenia may be seen as a primary disease or as a secondary manifestation of systemic autoimmune disease or lymphoproliferative disease. Primary autoimmune neutropenia is a disorder of infants and young children that resolves spontaneously in more than 90% of patients within 2 years. Secondary autoimmune neutropenia is a common accompaniment to systemic lupus erythematosus. Although not usually clinically severe, neutropenia is often a marker of disease activity.

Neutropenia in rheumatoid arthritis may be associated with splenomegaly (i.e., Felty syndrome) and is part of the spectrum of large granular lymphocyte (LGL) leukemia. LGL leukemia is a clonal expansion of suppressor T cells. Patients who develop LGL leukemia in association with rheumatoid arthritis share a common HLA-DR4 haplotype with patients with Felty syndrome, suggesting that they are in a common spectrum of disease. LGL leukemia is also a relatively common cause of acquired neutropenia in elderly patients in the absence of rheumatoid arthritis. Recent data have linked LGL leukemia to mutations in the *STAT3* gene.

Laboratory Evaluation

Unless the diagnosis of benign ethnic or cyclic neutropenia is likely, the evaluation of the patient with neutropenia should include stopping all potentially offending drugs and performing serologic studies to rule out collagen vascular disease. Unlike the evaluation of patients with leukocytosis, bone marrow examination is indicated early for those with neutropenia and is frequently diagnostic. Neutropenia often reflects primary hematologic disease, and bone marrow examination enables the physician to diagnose marrow failure syndromes, leukemia, and MDS. In the absence of bone marrow failure, other causes of neutropenia may give a characteristic bone marrow picture. All patients undergoing bone marrow examination should have cytogenetic and molecular studies performed to aid in the diagnosis of MDS.

Sudden onset of agranulocytosis that does not affect platelets or erythrocytes typically is attributable to drug or toxin exposure. Bone marrow examination is rarely necessary. If performed, drug-induced neutropenia produces a characteristic maturation arrest of myeloid cells. Rather than actual inhibition of neutrophil maturation, this feature reflects the immune destruction of myeloid precursors that leaves only the earliest cells behind.

Treatment

The therapeutic approach to patients with neutropenia depends on the degree of depression of the neutrophil count. Neutrophil counts between 1000 and 1500 cells/μL are not usually associated with significant impairment of the host response to bacterial infection and require no intervention beyond that demanded for diagnosis and treatment of the underlying cause. Patients with neutrophil counts between 500 and 1000 cells/μL should be alerted to their slightly increased risk of infection, although serious problems are rarely encountered in patients with functional neutrophils and counts higher than 500 cells/μL.

Patients with neutrophil counts lower than 500 cells/μL are at significant risk for infection, although this is especially true of patients with acute or chemotherapy-induced neutropenia. In contrast, patients with chronic idiopathic neutropenia may be asymptomatic with absolute neutrophil counts below 100. All patients with neutrophil counts below 500 cells/μL should be instructed to notify the physician at the

first sign of infection or fever, and they must be managed aggressively with intravenous antibiotics regardless of the documentation of a source or infecting organism. Patients with a significantly depressed neutrophil count may exhibit few signs of infection because much of the inflammatory response at the site of infection is generated by the neutrophils themselves.

In patients with severe immune-mediated neutropenia, corticosteroids and intravenous immunoglobulin may be helpful in elevating the neutrophil count and in preventing infectious complications. G-CSF may increase the peripheral white cell count and may help resolve infections in neutropenia induced by drugs, including chemotherapy. It has been efficacious for some patients with immune-mediated neutropenia and those with MDS.

For a deeper discussion of these topics, please see Chapter 158, ❖ "Leukocytosis and Leukopenia" in *Goldman-Cecil Medicine*, 26th Edition.

PROSPECTUS FOR THE FUTURE

Significant progress has been made in elucidating the molecular pathogenesis of severe congenital neutropenia and cyclic neutropenia. Compounds that modulate the unfolded protein response may play a role in the treatment of these disorders. Other studies of the molecular basis of myeloid differentiation are establishing the importance of transcription factor function in neutrophil maturation and are providing insights into the pathogenesis of leukemia and myelodysplasia. Their findings may delineate pathways with entry points for therapeutic intervention in myeloid malignancies.

SUGGESTED READINGS

Aktari M, Curtis B, Waller EK: Autoimmune neutropenia in adults, Autoimmun Rev 9:62–68, 2009.

Andres E, Maloisel F: Idiosyncratic drug-induced agranulocytosis and acute neutropenia, Curr Opin Hematol 15:15–21, 2008.

Beekman R: Touw IP: G-CSF and its receptor in myeloid malignancy, Blood 115:5131–5136, 2010.

Berliner N: Lessons from congenital neutropenia: 50 years of progress in understanding myelopoiesis, Blood 111:5427–5432, 2008.

Berliner N: Leukocytosis and leukopenia. In Goldman L, Schafer AI, editors: Goldman-Cecil Medicine, ed 26, Philadelphia, 2019, Elsevier Saunders.

Brinkmann V, Reichard U, Goosmann C, et al: Neutrophil extracellular traps kill bacteria, Science 303:1532–1535, 2004.

Dinauer MC, Coates TD: Disorders of phagocyte function. In Hoffman R, Benz EJ, Heslop H, Weitz J, editors: Hematology: basic principles and practice, ed 7, Philadelphia, 2018, Elsevier, pp 691–709.

Glogauer M: Disorders of phagocyte function. In Goldman L, Schafer AI, editors: Goldman-Cecil Medicine, Philadelphia, 2011, Elsevier Saunders, p 24.

Mortaz E, Alipoor SD, Adcock IM, Mumby S, Koenderman L: Update on Neutrophil Function in Severe Inflammation, Front Immunol 9:1–14, 2018.

Nauseef WM, Borregaard N: Neutrophils at work, Nature Immunology 15:602–611, 2014.

Pillay J, den Braber I, Vrisekoop N, et al: In vivo labeling with 2H₂O reveals a human neutrophil lifespan of 5.4 days, Blood 116:625–627, 2010.

Rappoport N, Simon AJ, Amariglio N, Rechavi G: The Duffy antigen receptor for chemokines, ACKR1,- 'Jeanne DARC' of benign neutropenia, Br J Haematol 184:497–507, 2019.

Xia J, Link DC: Severe congenital neutropenia and the unfolded protein response, Curr Opin Hematol 15:1–7, 2008.

Yipp BG, Paul K: NETosis: how vital is it? Blood 122:2784–2794, 2013.

Zhang R, Shah MV, Loughran Jr TP: The root of many evils: indolent large granular lymphocyte leukaemia and associated disorders, Hematol Oncol 28:105–117, 2010.

50

Disorders of Lymphocytes

Iris Isufi, Stuart Seropian

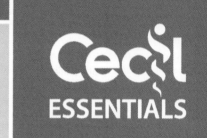

INTRODUCTION

The central cell of the immune system is the lymphocyte. Lymphocytes mediate the adaptive immune response, providing specificity to the immune system by responding to specific pathogens and conferring long-lasting immunity to reinfection. Lymphocytes are derived from hematopoietic stem cells that reside in the bone marrow and give rise to all of the cellular elements of the blood. The two major functional classes of lymphocytes—B lymphocytes (B cells) and T lymphocytes (T cells)—are distinguished by their site of development, antigenic receptors, and function.

The major disorders of lymphocytes include neoplastic transformations of specific subsets of lymphocytes that result in an array of lymphomas or leukemias, congenital or acquired defects in lymphocyte development or function with resultant immunodeficiency, and physiologic responses to infection or antigenic stimulation that lead to lymphadenopathy, lymphocytosis, or lymphocytopenia.

LYMPHOCYTE DEVELOPMENT, FUNCTION, AND LOCALIZATION

B Cells

B cells are characterized by surface immunoglobulins (i.e., antibodies). Their major function is to mount a humoral immune response to antigens by producing antigen-specific antibodies.

B cells develop in the bone marrow in a series of highly coordinated steps that involve sequential rearrangement of the heavy- and light-chain immunoglobulin genes and expression of B-cell–specific cell surface proteins (Fig. 50.1). Rearrangement of the immunoglobulin genes results in generation of a large repertoire of B cells that are each characterized by an immunoglobulin molecule with unique antigenic specificity. Mature B cells migrate from the bone marrow to lymphoid tissue throughout the body and are readily identified by cell surface immunoglobulin and antigens that are B cell specific, including CD19, CD20, and CD21.

In response to antigen binding to cell surface immunoglobulin, mature B cells are activated to proliferate and undergo differentiation to end-stage plasma cells, which lose most of their B-cell surface markers and produce large quantities of soluble antibodies. Neoplastic disorders of B cells arise from B cells at different stages of development, and B-cell lymphomas can have highly varied morphology and cell surface expression of B-cell antigens (i.e., immunophenotype).

T Cells

T cells perform an array of functions in the immune response, including those that are regarded as classic cellular immune responses. T-cell precursors migrate from the bone marrow to the thymus, where they differentiate into mature T-cell subsets and undergo selection to eliminate autoreactive T cells that respond to self-peptides. In the thymus, T-cell precursors undergo a coordinated process of differentiation that involves rearrangement and expression of the T-cell receptor (TCR) genes and acquisition of cell surface proteins that are unique to T cells, including CD3, CD4, and CD8.

As T cells mature in the thymus, they ultimately lose the CD4 or CD8 protein. Mature T cells are composed of two major groups: CD4$^+$ and CD8$^+$ cells. After T-cell maturation and selection in the thymus, mature CD4$^+$ and CD8$^+$ T cells migrate to lymph nodes, spleen, and other sites in the peripheral immune system. Mature T cells constitute about 80% of peripheral blood lymphocytes, 40% of lymph node cells, and 25% of splenic lymphoid cells.

Mature CD4$^+$ and CD8$^+$ T-cell subsets mediate distinct immune functions. CD8$^+$ cells *(cytotoxic T cells)* kill virus-infected or foreign cells and suppress immune functions. CD4$^+$ cells *(helper T cells)* activate other immune cells such as B cells and macrophages by producing cytokines and through direct cell contact.

Similar to B cells, T cells express unique TCR molecules that recognize specific peptide antigens. In contrast to B cells, T cells respond only to peptides that are processed intracellularly and bound to (or presented by) specialized cell surface antigen-presenting proteins, designated major histocompatibility complex (MHC) molecules. CD4$^+$ and CD8$^+$ T cells are MHC class restricted in their response to peptide-MHC complexes. CD4$^+$ cells recognize antigenic peptide fragments when they are presented by MHC class II molecules, and CD8$^+$ cells recognize antigenic peptide fragments when they are presented by MHC class I molecules. Binding of the TCR by a specific peptide-MHC complex triggers activation signals that lead to the expression of gene products that mediate the wide diversity of helper functions of CD4$^+$ cells or cytotoxic effector functions of CD8$^+$ cells.

Lymphoid System

Lymphocytes localize to peripheral lymphoid tissue, which is the site of antigen-lymphocyte interaction and lymphocyte activation. The peripheral lymphoid tissue is composed of lymph nodes, the spleen, and mucosal lymphoid tissue. Lymphocytes circulate continuously through these tissues through the vascular and lymphatic systems.

Lymph nodes are highly organized lymphoid tissues that are sites of convergence of the lymphatic drainage system, which carries antigens from draining lymph to the nodes, where they are trapped. A lymph node consists of an outer cortex and an inner medulla (Fig. 50.2). The cortex is organized into lymphoid follicles composed predominantly of B cells. Some of the follicles contain central areas or germinal centers, where activated B cells proliferate after encountering a specific antigen, that are surrounded by a mantle zone. The T cells are distributed more diffusely in paracortical areas surrounding follicles.

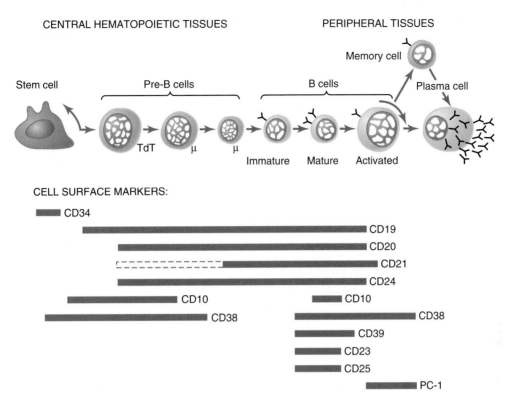

Fig. 50.1 The maturation of B lymphocytes. *Top,* The changes in immunoglobulin production and maturation. *Bottom,* The appearance and disappearance of surface markers. *TdT,* Terminal deoxynucleotidyl transferase. (Modified from Ferrarini M, Grossi CE, Cooper MD: Cellular and molecular biology of lymphoid cells. In Handin RI, Lux SE, Stossel TP, editors: *Blood: Principles and Practice of Hematology,* Philadelphia, 1995, JB Lippincott, p 643.)

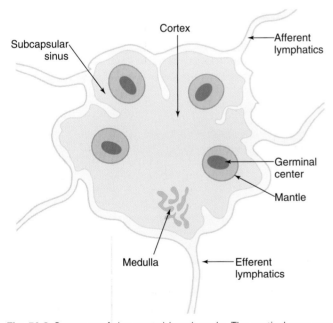

Fig. 50.2 Structure of the normal lymph node. The cortical area contains the follicles, which consist of a germinal center and a mantle zone. The medulla contains a complex of channels that lead to the efferent lymphatics.

The spleen traps antigens from blood rather than from the lymphatic system and is the site of disposal of senescent red cells. Lymphocytes in the spleen reside in the areas described as white pulp, which surround the arterioles entering the organ. As in lymph nodes, the B and T cells are segregated into a periarteriolar lymphoid sheath that is composed of T cells and flanking follicles composed of B cells.

The mucosa-associated lymphoid tissues (MALTs) collect antigen from epithelial surfaces and include the gut-associated lymphoid tissue (i.e., tonsils, adenoids, appendix, and Peyer patches of the small intestine) and more diffusely organized aggregates of lymphocytes at other mucosal sites.

Lymphocytes circulate in the blood and represent 20% to 40% of peripheral blood leukocytes in adults; the proportion is higher in newborns and children. The majority of peripheral blood lymphocytes are T cells, and the remaining lymphocytes are largely B cells. A small percentage of peripheral blood lymphoid cells represents a third category of lymphoid cells referred to as natural killer (NK) cells. These cells do not bear the characteristic cell surface molecules of B or T cells, and their immunoglobulin or TCR genes have not undergone rearrangement. Morphologically, the cells are large, with abundant cytoplasm containing azurophilic granules, and they are often called *large granular lymphocytes.* Functionally, they are part of the innate immune system, responding nonspecifically to a wide range of pathogens without requiring prior antigenic exposure.

NEOPLASIA OF LYMPHOID ORIGIN

Malignant transformation of lymphocytes leads to a diverse array of lymphoid cancers, including tumors that arise from T cells, B cells, or NK cells. Lymphoid malignancies usually involve lymphoid tissues, but they can arise in or spread to any site. The major clinical groupings of lymphoid malignancies include non-Hodgkin's lymphomas (NHLs), Hodgkin's lymphoma, lymphoid leukemias, and plasma cell dyscrasias.

Non-Hodgkin's Lymphomas
Definition and Epidemiology
The NHLs comprise a heterogeneous group of lymphoid malignancies that have different histologic appearances, cells of origin and

TABLE 50.1   2016 WHO Classification of Mature Lymphoid, Histiocytic, and Dendritic Neoplasms

Mature B-Cell Neoplasms
Chronic lymphocytic leukemia/small lymphocytic lymphoma
Monoclonal B-cell lymphocytosis[a]
B-cell prolymphocytic leukemia
Splenic marginal zone lymphoma
Hairy cell leukemia
Lymphoplasmacytic lymphoma
    Waldenström's macroglobulinemia
Monoclonal gammopathy of undetermined significance (MGUS), IgM[a]
μ Heavy-chain disease
γ Heavy-chain disease
α Heavy-chain disease
Monoclonal gammopathy of undetermined significance (MGUS), IgG/A[a]
Plasma cell myeloma
Solitary plasmacytoma of bone
Extraosseous plasmacytoma
Monoclonal immunoglobulin deposition diseases[a]
Extranodal marginal zone lymphoma of mucosa-associated lymphoid tissue
    (MALT lymphoma)
Nodal marginal zone lymphoma
Follicular lymphoma
    In situ follicular neoplasia[a]
    Duodenal-type follicular lymphoma[a]
Pediatric-type follicular lymphoma[a]
Primary cutaneous follicle center lymphoma
Mantle cell lymphoma
    In situ mantle cell neoplasia[a]
Diffuse large B-cell lymphoma (DLBCL), NOS
    Germinal center B-cell type[a]
    Activated B-cell type[a]
T-cell/histiocyte-rich large B-cell lymphoma
Primary DLBCL of the central nervous system (CNS)
Primary cutaneous DLBCL, leg type
EBV+ DLBCL, NOS[a]
DLBCL associated with chronic inflammation
Lymphomatoid granulomatosis
Primary mediastinal (thymic) large B-cell lymphoma
Intravascular large B-cell lymphoma
ALK+ large B-cell lymphoma
Plasmablastic lymphoma
Primary effusion lymphoma
Burkitt lymphoma
High-grade B-cell lymphoma, with MYC and BCL2 and/or BCL6
    rearrangements[a]
High-grade B-cell lymphoma, NOS[a]
B-cell lymphoma, unclassifiable, with features intermediate between DLBCL
    and classical Hodgkin lymphoma

Mature T and NK Neoplasms
T-cell prolymphocytic leukemia
T-cell large granular lymphocytic leukemia
Aggressive NK-cell leukemia
Systemic EBV+ T-cell lymphoma of childhood[a]
Hydroa vacciniforme–like lymphoproliferative disorder[a]
Adult T-cell leukemia/lymphoma
Extranodal NK-/T-cell lymphoma, nasal type
Enteropathy-associated T-cell lymphoma
Monomorphic epitheliotropic intestinal T-cell lymphoma[a]
Hepatosplenic T-cell lymphoma
Subcutaneous panniculitis-like T-cell lymphoma
Mycosis fungoides
Sézary syndrome
Primary cutaneous CD30+ T-cell lymphoproliferative disorders
    Lymphomatoid papulosis
    Primary cutaneous anaplastic large cell lymphoma
Primary cutaneous γδ T-cell lymphoma
Peripheral T-cell lymphoma, NOS
Angioimmunoblastic T-cell lymphoma
Anaplastic large-cell lymphoma, ALK+
Anaplastic large-cell lymphoma, ALK−[a]

Hodgkin's Lymphoma
Nodular lymphocyte predominant Hodgkin's lymphoma
Classical Hodgkin's lymphoma
    Nodular sclerosis classical Hodgkin's lymphoma
    Lymphocyte-rich classical Hodgkin's lymphoma
    Mixed cellularity classical Hodgkin's lymphoma
    Lymphocyte-depleted classical Hodgkin's lymphoma

Posttransplant Lymphoproliferative Disorders (PTLD)
Plasmacytic hyperplasia PTLD
Infectious mononucleosis PTLD
Florid follicular hyperplasia PTLD[a]
Polymorphic PTLD
Monomorphic PTLD (B- and T-/NK-cell types)
Classical Hodgkin's lymphoma PTLD

Provisional entities, histiocytic and dendritic cell entities are not included.
[a]Denotes new entities.

immunophenotypes, molecular biologic factors, clinical features, prognoses, and outcomes with therapy. According to the Surveillance, Epidemiology, and End Results (SEER) database, the NHLs are the seventh most common cancer type, with an estimated 74,200 cases occurring in 2019 and 19,970 patients succumbing to these diseases. The NHLs occur at a median age of 67 and are more common in men and in white individuals. The rate of NHLs increased slowly between 2000 and 2010 but has been decreasing slowly since that time. The annual death rate has fallen an average of 2.2% from 2007 to 2016.

Pathology

In view of the heterogeneity of NHLs, classification systems have been devised to identify specific pathologic subtypes that correlate with distinct clinical entities. These systems have evolved steadily over the past 50 years as correlations between histopathologic and biologic behavior have emerged. Pathologic classification schemes have attempted to correlate malignant NHL subtypes with normal cellular counterparts. The World Health Organization (WHO) classification (Table 50.1) is the most current and incorporates morphologic features, immunophenotype, genetic features, and molecular features, with an emphasis on biologic

TABLE 50.2 Causes of Lymphadenopathy

Infectious Diseases
Viral: infectious mononucleosis syndromes (cytomegalovirus, Epstein-Barr virus), acquired immunodeficiency syndrome, rubella, herpes simplex, infectious hepatitis
Bacterial: localized infection with regional adenopathy (streptococci, staphylococci), cat-scratch disease (*Bartonella henselae*), brucellosis, tularemia, listeriosis, bubonic plague (*Yersinia pestis*), chancroid (*Haemophilus ducreyi*)
Fungal: coccidioidomycosis, histoplasmosis
Chlamydial: lymphogranuloma venereum, trachoma
Mycobacterial: scrofula, tuberculosis, leprosy
Protozoan: toxoplasmosis, trypanosomiasis
Spirochetal: Lyme disease, syphilis, leptospirosis

Immunologic Diseases
Rheumatoid arthritis
Systemic lupus erythematosus
Mixed connective tissue disease
Sjögren's syndrome
Dermatomyositis
Serum sickness
Drug reactions: phenytoin, hydralazine, allopurinol

Malignant Diseases
Lymphomas
Solid tumors metastatic to lymph nodes: melanoma, lung, breast, head and neck, gastrointestinal tract, Kaposi's sarcoma, unknown primary tumor, renal, prostate

Atypical Lymphoid Proliferations
Giant follicular lymph node hyperplasia
Transformation of germinal centers
Castleman disease

Miscellaneous Diseases and Diseases of Unknown Cause
Dermatopathic lymphadenitis
Sarcoidosis
Immunoglobulin G4 (IgG4) lymphadenopathy
Amyloidosis
Mucocutaneous lymph node syndrome (Kawasaki disease)
Sinus histiocytosis (Rosai-Dorfman syndrome)
Multifocal Langerhans cell (eosinophilic) granulomatosis
Lipid storage diseases: Gaucher's and Niemann-Pick diseases

Epstein-Barr virus (EBV) is associated with several biologically aggressive NHLs, including acquired immunodeficiency syndrome (AIDS)–related diffuse, aggressive lymphomas, the lymphoproliferative disorders that arise in immunosuppressed patients after organ transplantation, and the form of Burkitt lymphoma that is endemic in Africa. Human T-cell lymphotropic virus type 1 (HTLV-1) is causally linked with adult T-cell leukemia/lymphoma, which is endemic in areas of Japan and the Caribbean basin. The human herpesvirus 8 (HHV-8) of Kaposi's sarcoma has been implicated in a variant of diffuse, aggressive NHL that arises in serosal cavities and is encountered almost exclusively in patients infected with human immunodeficiency virus (HIV).

Several indolent lymphomas have been linked to infectious agents that appear to indirectly promote lymphomagenesis through chronic antigen stimulation, resulting in B-lymphocyte proliferation. *Helicobacter pylori* infection is linked to gastric MALT lymphomas in this manner; eradication of infection with antibiotics is often associated with regression of the lymphoma.

Clinical Presentation

Although numerous subtypes of NHL are recognized, most disease entities may be viewed conceptually as clinically indolent (i.e., low grade) or aggressive (i.e., high grade). Indolent lymphomas typically grow slowly, do not always require therapy, and have a long natural history. A clinical history of recurring and regressing adenopathy may be elicited. Constitutional symptoms such as fever, weight loss, or night sweats occur in about 20% of patients with NHL at the time of onset. These symptoms are more common in patients with aggressive subtypes of NHL. Aggressive lymphomas are associated with limited survival in the absence of therapy.

Most patients with NHL exhibit painless lymphadenopathy involving one or more peripheral nodal sites. NHL can involve extranodal sites, and patients can exhibit a variety of symptoms that reflect the site of involvement. Common sites of extranodal disease include the gastrointestinal tract, bone marrow or focal bone lesions, liver, skin, and Waldeyer ring in the nasopharynx and oropharynx, although virtually any site can be involved. Aggressive subtypes of NHL are more likely than indolent lymphomas to involve extranodal sites.

Central nervous system involvement, including leptomeningeal spread, rarely occurs with the indolent subtypes but does occur with the aggressive variants. The most aggressive NHLs (i.e., Burkitt and lymphoblastic lymphomas) have a particular propensity to spread to the leptomeninges.

Diagnosis and Differential Diagnosis

Many causes of lymphadenopathy exist in addition to lymphoid malignancies (Table 50.2). A thorough history and careful physical examination are important before performing a lymph node biopsy. The investigation of lymphadenopathy can be organized according to the location of the enlarged nodes (i.e., localized or generalized) and clinical symptoms.

Cervical lymphadenopathy is most often caused by infections of the upper respiratory tract, including infectious mononucleosis syndromes, viral syndromes, and bacterial pharyngitis. Unilateral axillary, inguinal, or femoral adenopathy may be caused by skin infections involving the extremity, including cat-scratch fever. Generalized lymphadenopathy may be caused by systemic infections (e.g., HIV, cytomegalovirus), drug reactions, autoimmune diseases, or one of the systemic lymphadenopathy syndromes. If the cause of persistent lymphadenopathy is not apparent after a thorough evaluation, an excisional lymph node biopsy should be undertaken. An enlarged supraclavicular lymph node strongly suggests malignancy and should always be sampled.

The accurate diagnosis of lymphoma requires excisional biopsy of a lymph node or generous biopsy of involved lymph tissue. Fine-needle aspiration or needle biopsy is rarely sufficient. Analysis of the

and therapeutic implications. The most common NHLs encountered in the United States are diffuse large B-cell lymphoma (DLBCL), follicular lymphoma, small lymphocytic lymphoma or leukemia (i.e., chronic lymphocytic leukemia [CLL]), and mantle cell lymphoma.

Etiology

The cause of most NHLs is unknown. In most patients no apparent genetic predisposition or epidemiologic or environmental factor can be identified. Many of the NHL subtypes carry pathognomonic chromosomal translocations that often involve an immunoglobulin locus (or TCR locus in T-cell NHLs) and an oncogene or growth regulatory gene. The cause of these aberrant chromosomal rearrangements is unknown.

Patients with congenital immunodeficiency syndromes or autoimmune disorders are at increased risk for NHL. Oncogenic human viruses play a causal role in some of the less common NHL variants.

TABLE 50.3 Staging Evaluation for Lymphomas

Required Evaluation Procedures

Biopsy of lesion with review by an experienced hematopathologist

History with attention to the presence or absence of B symptoms

Physical examination with attention to node-bearing areas (including Waldeyer ring) and size of liver and spleen

Standard blood work:
Complete blood count
Lactate dehydrogenase and β_2-microglobulin
Evaluation of renal function
Liver function tests
Calcium, uric acid

Bone marrow aspirate and biopsy

Radiologic studies, including:
Chest radiograph (posteroanterior and lateral)
Chest, abdomen, and pelvic CT scans
PET scan (in Hodgkin's and aggressive lymphomas)

Procedures Required Under Certain Circumstances

Plain bone radiographs of symptomatic sites or abnormal areas on bone scan

Brain or spinal CT or MRI if neurologic signs or symptoms

Serum and urine protein electrophoresis

Lumbar puncture with cerebrospinal fluid cytology (Burkitt and lymphoblastic lymphoma)

B symptoms, Fever, sweats, and weight loss >10% of body weight; *CT,* computed tomography; *MRI,* magnetic resonance imaging; *PET,* positron emission tomography.

TABLE 50.4 Staging System for Hodgkin and Non-Hodgkin's Lymphoma

Stage[a]	Involvement	Extranodal E Status
I	One node or a group of adjacent nodes	Single extranodal lesions without nodal involvement
II	Two or more nodal groups on the same side of the diaphragm	Stage I or II by nodal extent with limited contiguous extranodal involvement
II bulky	As above with bulky disease[b]	
III	Nodes on both sides of the diaphragm; nodes above the diaphragm with spleen involvement	
IV	Additional noncontiguous extralymphatic involvement	

[a]Staging systems for Hodgkin's and non-Hodgkin's lymphomas are similar. For Hodgkin's lymphoma, the presence or absence of symptoms should be documented with each stage designation: A (asymptomatic) or B (fever, sweats, and weight loss >10% of body weight).

[b]For Hodgkin's lymphoma bulky disease includes nodal mass >10 cm or >1/3 of the transthoracic diameter

pathologic specimen should include routine histologic examination and immunophenotyping, immunohistochemistry, chromosome analysis, fluorescence in situ hybridization (FISH) testing, and molecular studies. Immunophenotyping can determine the cell of origin (i.e., B cell, T cell, NK cell, or nonlymphoid cell), and the pattern of cell surface antigens aids subclassification. In the case of B-cell NHLs, immunophenotyping can also reveal whether the process is monoclonal in origin (i.e., neoplastic) by determining if surface immunoglobulin is restricted to κ or λ light chain. Immunohistochemistry utilizing stains to assess expression levels of proteins such as MYC and BCL-2 provides prognostic information. In some cases, cytogenetic analysis or molecular studies of immunoglobulin or TCR gene rearrangement may be required to determine the pathologic subtype of lymphoma or to establish a monoclonal process. Chromosome analysis may reveal a complex karyotype often associated with worse prognosis, or deletion of chromosome 17p where the tumor suppressor gene p53 locus is found. FISH probes can identify translocations such as t(8;14) leading to high MYC expression in Burkitt lymphoma, t(14;18) leading to deregulated expression of the BCL-2 gene in follicular B-cell lymphoma, or t(11;14) leading to cyclin D1 (a regulator of the G1-S transition) overexpression in mantle cell lymphoma, among other abnormalities. If a lymph node biopsy is nondiagnostic and unexplained lymph node enlargement persists, biopsy should be repeated.

For patients with bone marrow and peripheral blood involvement, such as in small lymphocytic lymphoma or CLL, the diagnosis may be made based on immunophenotyping of peripheral blood lymphocytes by flow cytometry. Care must be taken to exclude the possibility of aggressive lymphoma with involved lymph nodes or extranodal sites in a patient harboring a low-grade or indolent lymphoma such as small lymphocytic lymphoma that is confined to the blood or bone marrow.

Treatment

After a lymphoma has been diagnosed, patients should undergo complete staging evaluation (Table 50.3). Staging determines the extent of involvement, provides prognostic information, and may influence the choice of therapy. The Lugano modification of the Ann Arbor staging classification is used to stage patients with NHL and Hodgkin's lymphoma (Table 50.4).

A variety of ancillary tests may be performed in specific situations. For example, a test for HTLV-1 and HIV should be performed if adult T-cell leukemia/lymphoma is suspected. Patients with a clinical history suggesting immunodeficiency or behavioral risk factors should be tested for HIV. A gastrointestinal series or endoscopy may be warranted for patients with gastrointestinal symptoms or patients at risk for gastrointestinal involvement (i.e., mantle cell and other lymphomas involving the Waldeyer ring). The choice of therapy is guided by stage, specific subtype, and clinical considerations such as age and the medical condition of the patient. Multiple novel agents are available for therapy of lymphoid neoplasms (Table 50.5). Such agents may be combined or used with traditional chemotherapy.

Lymphoma Subtypes

Indolent non-Hodgkin's lymphomas. The common low-grade or indolent conditions include follicular lymphoma, small lymphocytic lymphoma (which is identical to CLL), and marginal zone lymphomas.

Follicular lymphoma (FL) accounts for 20% of adult lymphomas and is the most common indolent lymphoma. It is a mature clonal B-cell neoplasm that histologically retains nodular architecture in the lymph node, which is infiltrated by small, mature-appearing lymphocytes. The immunophenotype is positive for surface markers (CD10, CD19, CD20, CD21) and negative for CD5. Follicular lymphomas are characterized by the t(14;18) translocation that juxtaposes the immunoglobulin heavy chain *(IGH)* locus with the antiapoptotic B-cell CLL/lymphoma 2 gene *(BCL2)*; the BCL2 protein is uniformly overexpressed in follicular lymphomas, immortalizing affected cells. Additional gain of function mutations and altered T-cell function in the malignant microenvironment are thought to play a role in pathogenesis.

TABLE 50.5   New Therapeutic Agents in Use for Lymphoma and Plasmacytic Disorders

Class	Agents	Target	Mechanism of Action	Indications
Monoclonal Antibodies	Rituximab Obinutuzumab	CD20	Complement-mediated and anti- body-dependent cytotoxicity. Apopto- sis of tumor cells	Most B-cell lymphomas
	Daratumumab	CD 38		Multiple myeloma
Antibody-Drug Conjugates	Brentuximab	CD 30	Antibody bound tubulin inhibitor deliv- ered to tumor cell	Hodgkin's lymphoma and CD30+ lymphomas
	Polatuzumab	CD79a		DLBCL
Imids	Thalidomide Lenalidomide	Cereblon, immune-modulation	Bind cereblon, activating E3 ubiquitin ligase complex	Multiple myeloma
	Pomalidomide			NHL subtypes (lenalidomide)
Kinase Inhibitors				
BTK Inhibitors	Ibrutinib Acalabrutinib Zanubrutinib	Bruton tyrosine kinase	Blocks B-cell receptor signaling	CLL, MCL, MZL, WM
Pi3k Inhibitors				CLL, FL
	Idelalisib Copanlisib	Phosphatidylinositol-3-kinase	Blocks B-cell receptor signaling	
BCL-2 Inhibitor	Venetoclax	BCL-2	Blocks antiapoptotic protein BCL-2 leading to programmed cell death	CLL
Proteosome Inhibitors	Bortezomib Carfilzomib Ixazomib	Proteasome	Inhibition of toxic protein degradation in malignant cells	Multiple myeloma MCL
CAR-T Cells	Axicabtagene ciloleucel Tisagenlecleucel	CD19	Direct binding of genetically engineered T cell to malignant B cells	DLBCL ALL

ALL, Acute lymphocytic leukemia; *BTK,* Bruton tyrosine kinase; *CLL,* chronic lymphocytic leukemia; *DLBCL,* diffuse large B-cell lymphoma; *FL,* follicular lymphoma; *IMIDS,* Immunomodulatory agents; *MCL,* mantle cell lymphoma; *MZL,* marginal aone lymphoma; *WM,* Waldenström's macroglobulinemia.

Follicular lymphoma is a low-grade, indolent neoplasm with a long natural history (median survival approaches 10 years), but 70% of patients have advanced-stage (III/IV) disease at diagnosis, often with bone marrow involvement, and cure is not considered feasible with standard treatment modalities for most patients. Follicular NHL may eventually transform to a more aggressive lymphoma, characterized pathologically by diffuse large cell infiltrates and clinically by rapidly expanding lymph nodes or tumor masses, rising lactate dehydrogenase (LDH) levels, and the onset of disease-related symptoms.

Management of follicular lymphomas is influenced by the stage. For the rare patient with early-stage (I/some non-bulky II) disease after clinical staging, the appropriate treatment is radiation therapy. With the use of locoregional lymphoid irradiation, more than one half of patients with early-stage disease achieve a durable remission or cure.

For patients with advanced-stage disease, management is more controversial. Although advanced-stage indolent NHL is responsive to a variety of treatments, incurability and long natural history have led to the practice of deferring treatment until symptoms develop. This strategy is referred to as the *watch and wait approach.* A prospective study of early intervention compared observation to the anti-CD20 monoclonal antibody rituximab alone and to rituximab followed by maintenance but found no difference in overall survival or histologic transformation rates. Indications for treatment include cosmetic or mechanical problems caused by enlarging lymph nodes, high tumor burden, constitutional symptoms, and evidence of marrow compromise.

Multiple treatment options are available, including monoclonal antibody therapies, targeted agents, immunomodulatory agents, chemotherapeutic agents, and radiolabeled antibodies. For most patients appropriate treatment includes the chimeric anti–B-cell monoclonal antibody rituximab, with or without systemic chemotherapy. The addition of rituximab to chemotherapy has increased response rates, duration of remission, and in some studies, overall survival (level I evidence obtained from at least one properly designed, randomized controlled trial).

The choice of chemotherapy to employ in combination with rituximab may be influenced by patient age and medical condition. Multiple options are available, and no regimen has proved superior with regard to overall survival. The combination of bendamustine, a unique agent with properties similar to alkylating agents and purine analogues, plus rituximab appeared advantageous compared with the CHOP regimen (i.e., cyclophosphamide, hydroxydaunorubicin [doxorubicin], Oncovin [vincristine], and prednisone) plus rituximab in a randomized trial with regard to toxicity, response rate, and progression-free survival (level I evidence).

Most patients respond to treatment, and at least one third achieve a clinical complete remission. The combination of bendamustine-rituximab results in median time to progression of 5 to 6 years. Treatment with cytotoxic agents is typically discontinued when the maximum response has been achieved, but rituximab may be continued on an intermittent schedule to maintain remission. It has been shown to prolong remission times in randomized studies (level 1 evidence). Risk of recurrence and cost considerations may influence the use of this therapy because rituximab may also be used at the time of recurrence with similar outcomes.

After a patient relapses, subsequent remissions may be achieved but are often less durable compared to first remission. Therapeutic options for patients who relapse include retreatment with chemotherapy, often with a different drug or combination than that used initially. Patients in relapse can also be treated with rituximab as a single agent. For patients who are refractory to rituximab, several humanized anti-CD20 antibodies have been developed. Obinutuzumab is a humanized glycoengineered anti-CD20 antibody with enhanced antibody-dependent cellular cytotoxicity function. It has single agent activity in relapsed FL and has shown high response rates in combination with chemotherapy. Immunomodulators such as lenalidomide also have strong activity in combination with anti-CD20 antibodies in the relapsed setting. PI3 kinase inhibitors idelalisib and copanlisib have an overall response rate of 56% with median response duration of 12 months. Radioactively labeled anti-CD20 antibodies such as ibritumomab tiuxetan (yttrium labeled) have also been used for patients with relapsed or refractory follicular lymphoma and have been associated with high response rates. Administration of radiolabelled antibodies requires treatment in a specialized center with nuclear medicine expertise and has limited the use of these agents. For patients who have clinical or pathologic evidence of transformation to a higher grade of lymphoma, treatment that is appropriate for a diffuse, aggressive histology should be offered (discussed later).

High-dose chemotherapy with autologous or allogeneic stem cell transplantation for follicular NHLs may be appropriate for selected patients with recurrent or refractory disease. Long-term follow-up of patients undergoing allogeneic transplantation suggests that some patients are cured with this modality, but the morbidity associated with allogeneic transplantation has limited its widespread use for indolent lymphomas.

In addition to the follicular NHLs, the MALT lymphomas and closely related marginal zone lymphomas are considered low-grade, indolent subtypes. Given the excellent prognosis, localized nature, and long natural history of the MALT lymphomas, they are usually managed conservatively with local treatment modalities (i.e., radiation or surgery) and avoidance of systemic chemotherapy. The monoclonal antibody rituximab has activity against MALT lymphomas and may be used when systemic therapy is desired. The gastric MALT lymphomas are highly associated with *H. pylori* infection, and remissions may be achieved with eradication of the infection. Antibiotic therapy is therefore first-line treatment for early *H. pylori*–positive gastric MALT lymphoma.

Aggressive non-Hodgkin's lymphomas. Aggressive NHLs include DLBCL, high-grade lymphoma with C-MYC and BCL-2 and/or BCL-6 rearrangements, B-cell lymphoma unclassifiable with features intermediate between DLBCL and classical Hodgkin's lymphoma, Burkitt lymphoma, lymphoblastic lymphoma, anaplastic large cell lymphoma, and peripheral T-cell lymphomas. Most of the aggressive lymphomas are B cell in origin; aggressive T-cell lymphomas are managed similarly but have an overall worse prognosis compared with their B-cell counterparts.

DLBCL is the most common subtype of NHL, constituting up to 30% of adult NHL in Western countries. Patients present with rapidly enlarged nodal masses; about 30% will have fevers, night sweats or weight loss, and 40% may have involvement of organs outside of lymph nodes. In contrast to patients with low-grade NHLs, all patients with aggressive histology should be offered immediate therapy because these lymphomas are life-threatening and potentially curable. The standard initial therapy for all patients with diffuse, aggressive NHL, regardless of stage, is a multidrug chemotherapy regimen that includes an anthracycline in combination with rituximab.

For DLBCL, CHOP plus rituximab (R-CHOP) is the most widely used treatment regimen. Patients with early-stage disease (I/nonbulky II) may be treated with local radiation therapy after a minimum of three cycles of R-CHOP if there is a need to limit exposure to chemotherapy. Patients with advanced-stage disease require six cycles of R-CHOP; the role of local radiation to sites of bulky disease in the setting of advanced-stage disease is not well established. Complete remissions can be achieved with R-CHOP or similar regimens, and more than 50% of patients are cured. Identifying prognostic biomarkers for the subset of patients who respond less well or who suffer early disease relapse is a priority.

In the early 2000s, gene expression profiling (GEP) using microarrays shed significant light into the biologic heterogeneity of DLBCL. Three distinct signatures were identified corresponding to potential cells of origin (COO): germinal center B-cell–like (GCB), activated B-cell–like (ABC), and primary mediastinal large B-cell lymphoma (PMBL), with approximately 15% of cases remaining unclassifiable. The GCB subtype arises from centroblasts, whereas the ABC subtype arises from a plasmablastic cell just prior to germinal center exit. These gene signatures have prognostic implications, with GCB-DLBCLs having a more favorable overall survival than ABC cases. PMBL displays a GEP profile that resembles that of Hodgkin's lymphoma and has a more favorable prognosis than either DLBCL subtype.

In addition to the COO, molecular subtypes of DLBCL have prognostic impact. Up to 15% of DLBCL cases contain translocations involving the MYC gene on chromosome 8q24 in combination with BCL-2 and/or BCL-6 translocations (referred to as "double or triple hit" NHL). C-MYC is a pro-oncogene that encodes a transcription factor that when dysregulated leads to uncontrolled cellular proliferation and survival. BCL-2 is an oncogene on chromosome 8q21 that when translocated leads to dysregulation of the antiapoptotic protein BCL-2. BCL-6 is a master regulator of the germinal center reaction and a transcriptional repressor. Double or triple hit NHL has the worst clinical outcome and is insufficiently treated with R-CHOP. Most patients have advanced stage disease, elevated LDH, bone marrow and CNS involvement. In general, more intensive regimens such as dose-adjusted EPOCH-R (etoposide, prednisone vincristine [Oncovin], cyclophosphamide, hydroxydaunorubicin [doxorubicin]-rituximab) or HyperCVAD-R (hyperfractionated doses of cyclophosphamide, vincristine, doxorubicin [Adriamycin], dexamethasone-rituximab) are used.

MYC and BCL-2 proteins can be overexpressed in DLBCL in the absence of gene translocation. Such "double-expressor" lymphomas have an intermediate prognosis. Most cases of double-hit lymphoma are of GCB origin whereas most cases of double-expresser lymphomas are of ABC origin.

Many studies have examined alternatives to R-CHOP therapy, including study of more intensive chemotherapy combinations or with addition of new agents such as ibrutinib or lenalidomide. To date, these approaches have largely failed to show improvements in disease control and survival for standard-risk patients and, therefore, R-CHOP remains the default standard of care for initial treatment of most patients.

Published studies of consolidation with high-dose chemotherapy and autologous stem cell transplantation (ASCT) following R-CHOP induction have also been largely negative. In particular, ASCT does not abrogate the negative prognostic impact of C-MYC translocations. In retrospective study, no difference in relapse-free and overall survival with ASCT has been identified in double hit patients who received intensified upfront treatment regimens such as DA-EPOCH-R (dose adjusted EPOCH-R) or HyperCVAD-R. However, a survival benefit for ASCT has been noted in double hit patients treated with R-CHOP, emphasizing the inferior outcomes with R-CHOP in this specific patient population.

Patients who relapse after achieving a remission may be cured with high-dose chemotherapy and ASCT, which is standard therapy if relapsed disease remains responsive to regular doses of chemotherapy. In the pre-rituximab era, cure rates with salvage chemotherapy and ASCT approached 50%. However, the large lymphoma CORAL study showed that patients who received rituximab with CHOP as part of upfront therapy had poor PFS (progression-free survival) of 21%. Patients who relapsed within a year of treatment with R-CHOP had very poor outcomes as well.

This high-risk relapsed patient population is now the target of clinical trials with chimeric antigen receptor T-cell (CAR-T) therapy. In this type of cellular immunotherapy, patients' autologous T cells are collected and genetically modified to express a chimeric T-cell receptor that recognizes one or more surface antigens, such as CD19, on the lymphoma cell. There are two FDA-approved CAR-T products for patients whose disease does not respond adequately to salvage chemotherapy, tisagenlecleucel and axicabtagene ciloleucel. Complete remission rates are in the order of 40% for a group of patients with otherwise poor outcomes. These therapies are being compared to ASCT in randomized trials. Despite promising efficacy, CAR-T cell therapy can result in considerable toxicities, including cytokine release syndrome, neurotoxicity, cytopenias, hypogammaglobulinemia, and infections. Patients are carefully monitored by a multidisciplinary team of physicians with experience in delivering cellular therapies.

Mantle cell lymphoma. Mantle cell lymphoma (MCL) accounts for 3% to 10% of adult NHL in Western countries and is most common in older male patients. Caucasians have a higher incidence compared to other ethnicities. The median age at presentation is 68. Mantle cell lymphomas are mature B-cell neoplasms that appear to arise in the mantle zone of the lymphoid follicle and display a highly characteristic immunophenotype, expressing the CD5 antigen and other B-cell markers, but CD23 expression is absent, in contrast to CLL. Mantle cell lymphomas are characterized by a pathognomonic t(11;14) chromosomal translocation that juxtaposes the immunoglobulin heavy chain gene (14q32 locus) with the *BCL1* gene, which encodes the growth-promoting protein cyclin D1. Demonstration of the translocation or expression of cyclin D1 protein by immunohistochemistry allows a definitive diagnosis in most cases. Pathologic classification as a blastoid or pleomorphic subtype and a high proliferation rate are features associated with more aggressive behavior and a poor outcome. TP53, Notch-1, and Notch-2 mutations are also associated with an aggressive clinical course. Two MCL subtypes are recognized in the WHO 2016 classification with different clinical manifestations and molecular pathways: Nodal MCL, the most common variant with an aggressive clinical course and multiple oncogenic mutations, and a leukemic, non-nodal subtype of MCL seen in 10% to 20% of patients, who have an indolent clinical course. These latter patients present with lymphocytosis, splenomegaly, and bone marrow involvement.

Patients are usually treated with systemic chemotherapy combined with rituximab, but durable remissions are difficult to achieve. High-dose chemotherapy with autologous stem cell transplantation is often applied during first remission for younger patients and has been associated with more durable remissions (level II-1 evidence, which is evidence obtained from well-designed controlled trials without randomization). Patients with TP53 mutations do not benefit from high-dose chemotherapy and are preferentially enrolled in clinical trials of new agents. Multiple agents and regimens are available for those who are not candidates for transplantation and patients with recurrent disease.

The Bruton tyrosine kinase (BTK) inhibitors ibrutinib and acalabrutinib and the BCL-2 inhibitor venetoclax have shown remarkable activity in relapsed MCL in combination with anti-CD20 antibodies. They are also being investigated as frontline treatment in combination with immunochemotherapy or in chemotherapy-free combinations. CAR-T cell therapy trials are ongoing in MCL and provide hope for patients who have progressed on the BTK inhibitors. Allogeneic SCT can provide a cure in 30% of patients with MCL and is a considered in relapsed patients and those with TP53 mutations.

High-grade non-Hodgkin's lymphomas. The two high-grade subtypes, Burkitt lymphoma (BL) and lymphoblastic lymphoma, are rare in the adult population. Nonetheless, these subtypes are important because they are potentially curable with appropriate therapy and often require urgent, inpatient treatment at the time of diagnosis due to their highly aggressive nature, rapid growth, and tendency to develop tumor lysis on initiation of therapy.

Lymphoblastic lymphoma in adults is an aggressive lymphoma that is considered the lymphomatous counterpart of acute T-cell lymphocytic leukemia. B-cell lymphoblastic lymphoma is less common. Lymphoblastic lymphoma usually afflicts young adult men and involves the mediastinum and bone marrow, with a propensity to relapse in the leptomeninges.

Burkitt lymphoma is a rare B-cell lymphoma in adults that is highly aggressive with a propensity to involve the bone marrow and central nervous system. Burkitt lymphoma is characterized cytogenetically by the pathognomonic t(8;14) translocation that moves the *MYC* oncogene from chromosome 8 to a location close to the enhancers of the antibody heavy-chain genes (*IGH* locus) on chromosome 14. In central Africa, where Burkitt lymphoma is endemic in children, it is usually associated with EBV. However, in the United States, it is uncommon for sporadic Burkitt lymphoma to be EBV positive. Recently, Burkitt-like lymphoma with 11q aberrations has been included in the WHO classification as a provisional entry. The 11q aberrations are particularly frequent in immunocompromised hosts, such as patients after organ transplantation. Recurrent ID3 mutations are found in about 30% of cases of BL, and ID3 has been recently implicated as a tumor suppressor gene with a role in pathogenesis.

Burkitt lymphoma and lymphoblastic lymphomas require treatment with intensive multiagent chemotherapy, including intrathecal chemotherapy to prevent leptomeningeal relapse. These lymphomas undergo rapid tumor lysis on initiation of chemotherapy, and all patients must receive prophylaxis against tumor lysis syndrome before and during their first course of chemotherapy. Prophylaxis includes hydration, alkalinization of the urine, allopurinol, and consideration of rasburicase therapy for rapid lowering of elevated uric acid levels.

Prognosis

A variety of prognostic variables have been identified for NHL, and specific prognostic schemes have been devised for common diseases, including DLBCL, follicular NHL, and mantle cell lymphomas. The predictors for poor survival for most subtypes include advanced stage (III/IV) at onset, involvement of multiple extranodal sites of disease, elevated LDH, B symptoms (e.g., fever, night sweats, weight loss), and poor performance status.

The International Prognostic Index (IPI) stratifies patients based on age, performance status, stage, and number of extranodal sites. The likelihood of cure and long-term, disease-free survival ranges from more than 75% for patients with one or no adverse factors to less than 50% for patients with four or more adverse factors.

Factors associated with shortened survival in follicular NHL include older age, advanced stage, anemia, multiple lymph node sites (more than four), and elevated LDH levels. Patients with three or more of these factors have a median survival of 5 years, roughly one half of that of patients with zero or one risk factor. Cytogenetic and molecular abnormalities that result in increased lymphoma cell proliferation and survival are taking center stage as prognostic variables, with some incremental improvement in outcomes with aggressive upfront treatment strategies and cellular therapies.

Aggressive T-cell lymphomas usually fare more poorly than B-cell NHL, and patients are typically considered candidates for investigational studies and upfront transplantation. Anaplastic large cell lymphoma (ALCL) ALK+, however, has a favorable outcome with chemotherapy alone. The anti-CD30 antibody-drug conjugate brentuximab vedotin has strong activity in ALCL and other types of T-cell lymphomas that express CD30.

❖ For a deeper discussion of these topics, please see Chapter 176, "Non-Hodgkin's Lymphomas," in *Goldman-Cecil Medicine*, 26th Edition.

Hodgkin Lymphoma

Hodgkin's lymphoma (HL) is a node-based lymphoid malignancy characterized by the neoplastic Reed-Sternberg (RS) cell in an inflammatory background. Hodgkin's lymphoma accounts for 10% of lymphomas, with about 8110 new cases diagnosed in the United States in 2019, and it is the most common lymphoma among young adults. The peak incidence of HL occurs between the ages of 20 and 35. The incidence of HL and death rate have declined in the past decade.

The cause of Hodgkin's lymphoma remains enigmatic. Risk factors include a history of infectious mononucleosis, high socioeconomic status, immunosuppression (e.g., HIV infection, allograft transplantation, immunosuppressive drugs), and autoimmune disorders. Although EBV is frequently detected in patients, a direct causal role has not been established.

Pathology

Hodgkin's lymphoma is diagnosed by identifying the malignant RS cell in involved lymphoid tissue. The classic RS cell is large and binucleate, with each nucleus containing a prominent nucleolus, suggesting the appearance of owl eyes. Although the cellular origin of the RS cell was debated for decades, molecular studies have confirmed that RS cells are B cells with clonal rearrangement of the germline *IG* locus. Unlike NHL, the bulk of the infiltrate in lymph nodes in HL is usually composed of benign reactive inflammatory cells, and the RS cells can be difficult to find. Immunophenotyping of RS cells shows CD30 (Ki-1) and CD15 positivity and negative CD20, CD45, and cytoplasmic or surface immunoglobulin. EBV is identified in the RS cells in about 50% of cases.

The pathologic subtypes of classic HL include four variants—nodular sclerosing (NS), mixed cellularity (MC), lymphocyte depleted (LD), and lymphocyte rich (LR)—plus the non-classic variant, nodular lymphocyte-predominant (NLP). The NS form is the most common variant (60% to 80%) and is characterized by fibrous bands separating the node into nodules and by the lacunar type of RS cells. It is the predominant type encountered in adolescents and young adults and typically involves the mediastinum and supradiaphragmatic nodal sites. In the MC type (15%), band-forming sclerosis is absent, and RS cells are easily identified in a diffuse inflammatory infiltrate that is more heterogeneous than that seen in the NS variant. The LR variant (5%) is characterized by classic RS cells in a background of small lymphocytes. LD is a rare variant (<1%) that is associated with advanced age, HIV infection, and low socioeconomic status. The pathologic hallmarks of LD HL include a notable paucity of inflammatory cells and sheets of RS cells.

The NLP variant is a distinct entity that is more closely related to indolent NHL than to classic HL. The NLP form is characterized by a nodular growth pattern with variants of RS cells that have polylobated nuclei (i.e., popcorn cells); classic RS cells are usually absent. The immunophenotype of these variant cells is distinct from classic RS cells, with expression of B-cell antigens (CD19 and CD20) and CD45 and absence of CD15 and CD30. The existence of CD20 allows the therapeutic use of rituximab, an agent not typically employed in classic Hodgkin's lymphoma. The NLP variant accounts for 5% of Hodgkin's lymphoma cases, has a strong male preponderance, and tends to involve peripheral nodes but spare the mediastinum. The prognosis is excellent, although late relapses are more common than in classic HL.

Clinical Presentation

Hodgkin's lymphoma arises in lymph nodes, most commonly in the mediastinum or neck, and spreads to adjacent contiguous or noncontiguous nodal sites, including retroperitoneal nodes and the spleen. As the disease progresses, it may spread hematogenously to involve extranodal sites, including bone marrow, liver, and lung. Unlike NHL, Hodgkin's lymphoma rarely arises in extranodal sites, although it can involve extranodal sites by contiguous spread from an adjacent lymph node (e.g., vertebrae from retroperitoneal lymph nodes, pulmonary parenchyma from hilar nodes).

Hodgkin's lymphoma usually produces painless enlargement of lymph nodes, most often in the neck. Mediastinal adenopathy may be found incidentally in an asymptomatic patient on routine chest radiography. Massive mediastinal or hilar adenopathy, with or without adjacent pulmonary involvement, may cause cough, shortness of breath, wheezing, or stridor. At clinical presentation, about one third of patients have constitutional symptoms of fever, night sweats, or weight loss (i.e., B symptoms). Generalized pruritus is associated with the NS subtype, and patients may give a history of troubling pruritus for months to years before the diagnosis. Rarely, patients may also complain of prompt marked chest discomfort induced by alcohol, the etiology of which is uncertain, but has been observed in patients with HL and carcinoid syndromes.

If left untreated, the natural history is one of inexorable, albeit often slow, progression to involve multiple nodal sites, followed by hematogenous spread to the bone marrow, liver, and other viscera. As the disease advances, patients experience B symptoms, malaise, cachexia, and infectious complications. Patients with progressive disease ultimately die of complications of bone marrow failure or infection.

Accurate staging of newly diagnosed HL is important for treatment planning, prognosis, and assessing response to therapy. A modification of the Ann Arbor classification is used (see Table 50.4), and the suffix A or B is appended to denote the absence or presence, respectively, of B symptoms. The staging work-up of a newly diagnosed patient is similar to that for patients with NHL (see Table 50.3) and includes a history and physical examination; complete blood work, including erythrocyte sedimentation rate (ESR) and HIV serology; computed tomography (CT) scan of the chest, abdomen, and pelvis; positron emission tomography (PET) scan; and in selected cases, a bone marrow aspirate and biopsy. Additional radiographic tests (e.g., bone films, spinal magnetic resonance imaging [MRI]) should be obtained only if symptoms suggest involvement of these structures. Patients also require evaluation of cardiac and pulmonary function before administration of chemotherapy and testing for hepatitis B due to the risk of reactivation during chemotherapy. The information derived from this noninvasive work-up defines the clinical stage of a patient with HL.

Diagnosis and Differential Diagnosis

The diagnosis requires an adequate biopsy of the involved nodal tissue. Immunophenotyping is routinely performed to confirm the diagnosis made on routine light microscopy and to differentiate HL from morphologically similar NHLs (e.g., T-cell–rich large B-cell lymphoma, anaplastic large cell lymphoma).

Treatment

Hodgkin's lymphoma is highly curable; the cure rate exceeds 80% with the use of current treatment modalities. The optimal treatment, including the duration of chemotherapy and the use and dose of radiation therapy, is determined by the stage (i.e., early stage [I/II] vs. advanced stage [III/IV]) and additional prognostic features. Because most patients are young adults and experience long-term, disease-free survival, the goal of therapy has shifted to minimizing treatment-related morbidity and mortality without sacrificing curative potential. Primary radiation therapy is rarely used because of delayed toxicities, which include a substantial risk of secondary solid tumors within the radiation field a decade or more after treatment, including a high risk of breast cancer in young patients. Historically noted long-term sequelae of standard doses of chest irradiation include thyroid dysfunction (usually hypothyroidism) and accelerated coronary artery disease.

Most patients with early-stage (I/II) Hodgkin's lymphoma are treated with the ABVD chemotherapy regimen (i.e., doxorubicin [Adriamycin], bleomycin, vinblastine, and dacarbazine) that may be followed by a course of low-dose radiation (<30 Gy) to involved lymph node sites, which has not been associated with an increased risk of secondary solid tumors. The duration of chemotherapy and the dose of radiation depend on whether the patient has favorable or unfavorable early-stage disease. The definition of favorable disease usually incorporates the absence of a large mediastinal mass, a limited number of involved nodal sites, absence of B symptoms, younger age, and a low ESR. Patients with favorable early-stage disease typically receive two to four cycles of ABVD followed by 20 Gy of radiation, whereas four to six cycles of ABVD and 30 Gy of radiation are required for patients with unfavorable disease (level I evidence). The option for limited course chemotherapy without radiotherapy has also been confirmed as feasible in randomized study. The choice of treatment in early-stage disease requires a detailed conversation with the patient regarding the side effects and potential risks of treatment options.

Patients with advanced-stage (III/IV) Hodgkin's lymphoma are treated primarily with chemotherapy. The ABVD regimen is the most widely used initial treatment in the United States. ABVD is more effective and less toxic than the older MOPP regimen (i.e., nitrogen mustard, vincristine, [Oncovin], procarbazine, and prednisone) and does not cause the long-term sequelae of sterility, infertility, or treatment-induced leukemias associated with MOPP (level I evidence). Long-term toxicity concerns with the ABVD regimen include potential for cardiomyopathy (Adriamycin), pulmonary toxicity (bleomycin), and neuropathy (vincristine). Roughly 60% of patients with stage III or IV disease are cured with six cycles of ABVD. A recent randomized trial confirmed the efficacy of ABVD with elimination of bleomycin after two full cycles of treatment in patients with evidence of early response to treatment.

The intensive regimen of BEACOPP (i.e., bleomycin, etoposide, Adriamycin, cyclophosphamide, vincristine, prednisolone, and procarbazine) has been associated with higher rates of complete response and freedom from treatment failure compared with ABVD-based regimens in patients with advanced disease, although overall survival has not been increased in all studies (level I evidence). BEACOPP is used increasingly in selected patients with high-risk features. Gonadal toxicity with permanent infertility may occur after BEACOPP, and an increased risk of secondary leukemia has been reported. Late sequelae and acute toxicities must be considered when choosing this regimen.

Radiation therapy in combination with chemotherapy is typically not used to treat advanced-stage disease. However, in patients with bulky mediastinal disease, consolidative radiation to the mediastinum after completion of chemotherapy has decreased the rate of relapse.

Evaluating the response to therapy involves repetition of the staging evaluation (i.e., physical examination, CT, and PET) during and at the completion of treatment. A mid-treatment PET scan after two full cycles of ABVD for advanced disease is prognostically informative because persistent metabolic activity in tumor sites correlates with resistance or subsequent relapse of disease. Conversely, patients may be cured despite the common finding of a residual abnormality on CT (e.g., enlarged nodes, residual mediastinal mass) when residual disease is not seen on PET imaging. A persistently positive PET scan during or after treatment with residual radiographic abnormalities is associated with a high rate of subsequent relapse, and these patients should be considered for immediate repeat biopsy or salvage therapy. The

more intensive BEACOPP regimen may increase the primary cure rate in such cases. Most patients destined to relapse do so within 2 years; relapses after 5 years are rare except for patients with the NLP variant.

Patients who relapse or fail to respond after initial therapy have several options for secondary therapy which may still prove curative. Second-line therapy is often employed with a plan to pursue high-dose chemotherapy and autologous hematopoietic cell transplantation, which may be associated with cure in patients with chemosensitive disease (level I evidence).

Effective novel agents to treat recurrent HL include brentuximab vedotin, an immunotoxin composed of a CD30-directed antibody linked to an antitubulin agent, and the checkpoint inhibitors pembrolizumab and nivolumab. Brentuximab is associated with high response rates, including complete responses in more than 30% of patients with relapsed disease after autologous transplantation (level II-1 evidence). A randomized study of brentuximab versus placebo after transplantation for high-risk HL patients showed a significant prolongation of progression-free survival. The checkpoint inhibitors are also highly active agents in HL patients with recurrent or refractory disease. Roughly two thirds of patients are expected to respond to therapy, although complete responses occur in a minority of patients. Allogeneic transplantation may also be considered for medically fit patients and has curative potential. Novel transplant therapy from haploidentical (half-matched) donors incorporating post-transplant cyclophosphamide has shown encouraging results with lower transplant-related morbidity and is an area of active investigation.

Prognosis

Most patients with Hodgkin's lymphoma are cured. Prognostic factors that influence risk of relapse or survival include MC or LD histology, male sex, large numbers of involved nodal sites, age older than 40 years, B symptoms, high ESR, and bulky disease (i.e., mediastinum widening by more than one third or a mass larger than 10 cm). The International Prognostic Score, based on seven variables at diagnosis, is a validated predictor of outcome in advanced disease.

Lymphoid Leukemias
Acute Lymphocytic Leukemias
The acute lymphocytic leukemias that arise from precursor B or T cells are described in detail in Chapter 47.

Chronic Lymphocytic Leukemia and Small Lymphocytic Lymphoma
Definition and epidemiology. B-cell CLL is a malignant disorder of lymphocytes characterized by expansion and accumulation of small lymphocytes of B-cell origin. CLL is essentially identical to B-cell small lymphocytic lymphoma but represents the leukemic form of the disease. CLL is the most common form of leukemia in the United States and affects twice as many men as women. There were 20,720 estimated new cases in 2019 and 3,930 deaths. Although it can occur at any stage of life, the incidence increases with age, and more than 90% of cases are diagnosed in adults older than 50 years of age.

The cause of CLL is unknown. Familial clustering of CLL suggests a genetic basis in some cases. First-degree relatives of CLL patients have an 8.5-fold increased risk of developing CLL and a 2.6-fold increased risk of developing another indolent lymphoma. The risk of developing CLL is increased by exposure to organic solvents, Agent Orange, and insecticides. Dietary and lifestyle factors have not been associated with an increased risk of CLL.

CLL is preceded by a clinically asymptomatic stage involving a proliferation of clonal B cells. This condition is referred to as a monoclonal B lymphocytosis (MBL). MBL is detectable in more than 5% of people aged over 60. The risk of transformation into CLL requiring treatment is approximately 1% per year. Such patients are observed.

Pathology. The common form of CLL is a clonal proliferation of mature B cells expressing characteristic mature B-cell markers and low levels of surface immunoglobulin M (IgM) that is light chain restricted, reflecting the clonal origin of this malignancy.

The diagnostic immunophenotype of CLL is unique, with expression of CD5 and CD23 along with the mature B-cell markers CD19, CD20 (dim expression), and CD21. Although a pathognomonic chromosomal abnormality has not been identified, 30% to 50% of patients have cytogenetic abnormalities, more so if sensitive assays such as FISH are employed. The most frequent abnormalities involve chromosomes 12 (often trisomy 12), 13, and 14. Cytogenetic abnormalities of chromosomes 17 and 11 are associated with an adverse prognosis.

Mutations that contribute to the development of CLL may occur at any stage of B-cell development. CLL cells originating from B cells that have not passed through and experienced the lymph node germinal center reaction have unmutated immunoglobulin heavy-chain variable-region (IgVH) genes and are defined as unmutated CLL (U-CLL). CLL cells that have incurred immunoglobulin (Ig) somatic mutation express mutated IgVH genes and are defined as mutated CLL (M-CLL). Unmutated IgVH genes are associated with a more aggressive form of CLL.

The B-cell receptor pathway has been recognized as the most prominent pathway activated in CLL cells. The B-cell receptor in CLL is activated via recognition and binding of autoantigens and antigens that are present in the microenvironment. Multiple kinases including BTK, spleen tyrosine kinase (SYK), and phosphatidylinositol 3-kinase (PI3K) are activated. This triggers a signaling cascade that activates downstream pathways, including $NF\kappa\beta$ pathway, ultimately promoting malignant B-cell survival and proliferation.

Diagnosis and differential diagnosis. The diagnosis of CLL is often made incidentally on a routine blood cell count that shows a leukocytosis with a predominance of small lymphocytes. Flow cytometric analysis of peripheral blood or bone marrow aspirate reveals the characteristic clonal B-cell population that is CD5 and CD23 positive. There is monoclonal expression of either Ig kappa or lambda and weak or absent expression of CD20, CD79b, FMC7. Smears of the bone marrow or peripheral blood reveal a predominance of small lymphocytes with inconspicuous nucleoli; ruptured cells (i.e., smudge cells) are often observed. Examination of involved lymph nodes reveals a diffuse infiltrate of small lymphocytes effacing the normal architecture.

CLL must be distinguished from reactive causes of lymphocytosis and other forms of lymphoma or leukemia. Mantle cell lymphoma may appear similar morphologically and with a similar immunophenotype, although CD23 is typically absent and cyclin D1 expression is detected. An absolute lymphocytosis of more than 5000 cells/μL is required for the diagnosis of CLL.

Clinical presentation. CLL cells accumulate in bone marrow, peripheral blood, lymph nodes, and spleen, resulting in lymphocytosis, lymphadenopathy, splenomegaly, and ultimately decreased bone marrow function. CLL is also frequently associated with immune dysregulation, exhibited as hypogammaglobulinemia with an increased risk of bacterial infections and autoimmune phenomena such as Coombs-positive hemolytic anemia or immune thrombocytopenia. Some patients exhibit lymphadenopathy, symptoms related to cytopenias, or recurrent infections. As the disease progresses, patients develop generalized lymphadenopathy, hepatosplenomegaly, and bone marrow failure. Death may occur from infectious complications or bone marrow failure after patients have become refractory to

treatment. In about 5% of cases, CLL transforms to a highly malignant diffuse large cell lymphoma, which may prove rapidly fatal. This transformation is commonly referred to as Richter syndrome.

Treatment. CLL is a low-grade disease typically characterized by a long natural history with slow progression over years or decades. Median survival is in excess of 6 years. The extent of disease (stage) at onset is the best predictor of survival. Genomic aberrations such as 17p or 11q deletions and unmutated IgVH status predict for significantly shorter median survival in patients with otherwise early stage disease.

Because standard therapy is not curative and CLL may have an asymptomatic phase lasting years, specific treatment is often withheld until signs of disease progression or development of symptoms (e.g., bulky lymphadenopathy, constitutional symptoms such as fevers, cytopenias caused by bone marrow infiltration). The rate of rise of the white blood cell count may also be used to predict development of symptoms and the need for therapy.

When treatment is required, multiple options for therapy are available. The patient's age, medical condition, and cytogenetic abnormalities may influence the choice of therapy. Active chemotherapeutic agents include several alkylating agents (e.g., chlorambucil, cyclophosphamide), the nucleoside analogue fludarabine, or the novel agent bendamustine. The fludarabine/cyclophosphamide (FC) regimen became a standard of care in 2005 combined with rituximab (FCR), achieving high complete remission rates. The FCR regimen was shown to improve overall survival in patients with CLL in a randomized phase 3 trial. This came at the expense of higher infection risks, particularly in older patients who tolerate bendamustine and rituximab (BR) better. There is also a risk of marrow stem cell injury. Patients with del(17p) did not respond to fludarabine-based regimens, however, and had a median survival of only 16 months after first-line treatment. FCR has been shown to provide the greatest benefit to young and fit patients with IgVH mutated CLL. Some of these patients have not relapsed with over 10 years of follow-up and may have been cured. For this subgroup of patients, the potential for cure needs to be balanced against the risks associated with FCR, including secondary malignancies.

The monoclonal anti-CD20 antibody rituximab has activity against CLL, but it is most effectively employed in combination with chemotherapeutic agents.

Most patients respond to therapy with significant reductions in tumor burden. Patients with recurrent or refractory disease may respond to a growing list of monoclonal antibodies. Alemtuzumab, a humanized monoclonal antibody to the CD52 molecule that occurs on most lymphocytes, is efficacious, including in patients with a 17p deletion, though the median response duration for this subset of patients is only 8 months. Additional agents include the anti-CD20 antibodies ofatumumab and obinutuzumab, which were shown to improve remission duration in previously untreated patients when administered in combination with chlorambucil (level I evidence).

Improved understanding of the mechanisms of CLL cell proliferation, mediated through BCR and $NF\kappa\beta$ signaling, has led to the development of a number of targeted inhibitors with favorable efficacy/toxicity profiles in recent years. In 2013 and 2014, respectively, the BTK inhibitor ibrutinib and the PI3K inhibitor idelalisib were shown to be highly active in patients with refractory and high-risk CLL [del(17p), del(11q) and IgHV unmutated]. At 3 years of follow-up an unprecedented 50% of del(17p) patients taking ibrutinib were alive without progression of disease. In 2016, the BCL-2 inhibitor venetoclax was shown to be active in patients with refractory and high-risk CLL. A randomized phase 3 trial comparing venetoclax-rituximab to bendamustine-rituximab showed a major advantage in 2-year PFS (84.9% vs. 26.3%) in the venetoclax-rituximab group. This was true among patients with del (17p) as well, with 2-year PFS of 81.5% versus 27.8%.

Randomized comparisons of ibrutinib with or without rituximab to BR or FCR in untreated patients with CLL also favor ibrutinib-based therapy with improvements in PFS.

With continued use of ibrutinib, resistance mutations may develop and next-generation BTK inhibitors are in development. Combination strategies with BCL-2 inhibitors to circumvent resistance are in phase 3 studies. CAR-T cell therapy has also shown activity in ibrutinib-resistant CLL. While allogeneic transplantation may provide a cure through a graft versus leukemia immune phenomenon, it bears with it potential for significant morbidity and mortality and has been deferred in most CLL treatment algorithms to make room for the promising new targeted therapies.

Patients who develop autoimmune phenomena require treatment with corticosteroids, and intravenous gamma globulin may be used to reduce the frequency of infections in patients who have developed hypogammaglobulinemia. The development of a rapidly enlarging mediastinal mass, constitutional symptoms, and high serum LDH level suggests transformation of the disease to a diffuse large cell lymphoma (i.e., Richter syndrome), which is associated with a poor prognosis.

Plasma Cell Disorders

The plasma cell disorders, or dyscrasias, are a group of clonal B-cell diseases that are related to each other by virtue of their production and secretion of monoclonal immunoglobulin, called the *M protein*. The laboratory hallmark of plasma cell dyscrasias is a homogeneous immunoglobulin molecule (whole or part) that can be detected in the serum or urine by protein electrophoresis. Clinically, these disorders may be characterized by the systemic effects of the M protein and by the direct effects of bone and bone marrow infiltration. Primary amyloidosis, for instance, results in tissue injury through deposition of light chains produced by a clonal population of plasma cells in the absence of an observable proliferation of the plasma cell clone. Waldenström's macroglobulinemia is a disorder with features of NHL and plasma cell disorders. It is discussed in this section because of the distinct clinical effects of the IgM paraprotein produced in this disease.

The most common plasma cell dyscrasia is *monoclonal gammopathy of uncertain significance* (MGUS), followed by multiple myeloma and the closely related plasmacytoma, which is a solitary tumor comprised of clonal plasma cells of bone or extramedullary soft tissue. Less common plasma cell dyscrasias include POEMS (polyneuropathy, organomegaly, endocrinopathy, monoclonal gammopathy and skin abnormalities) syndrome (see later in the chapter), also known as osteosclerotic myeloma, heavy-chain disease, and primary amyloidosis.

When an M protein is found on serum protein electrophoresis from an individual with no apparent associated disease and in the absence of any other laboratory or clinical evidence of a plasma cell disorder, it is designated as MGUS. MGUS is defined by low serum levels of M protein (<3 g/dL), no urinary Bence Jones protein, less than 10% clonal bone marrow plasma cells, and absence of anemia, hypercalcemia, renal failure, and lytic bone lesions. MGUS is more common than myeloma and increases in frequency with aging, occurring in 3% of the population older than 50 years. MGUS is considered a premalignant condition, and patients are at increased risk (7-fold) for overt myeloma or related malignant plasma cell dyscrasias compared with the general population. Nonetheless, progression of MGUS to a frank plasma cell neoplasm occurs only in about 1% of patients per year.

Distinguishing patients with stable, nonprogressive MGUS from patients in whom multiple myeloma will eventually develop is difficult. The risk of progression is greater among patients with IgA or IgM-type M proteins, in patients with initial concentrations of M protein in excess of 1.5 g/dL, and in patients with an abnormal free κ-to-λ light-chain ratio. Although no definitive evidence has been found that monitoring patients with the diagnosis of MGUS improves survival, it is recommended that patients undergo annual evaluation, including serum electrophoresis, to detect progression to multiple myeloma before the onset of overt symptoms or complications.

M proteins can be found in benign and malignant conditions other than the plasma cell dyscrasias (Table 50.6). About 10% of patients with CLL have detectable levels of monoclonal IgG or IgM in their sera. M proteins can also be detected in a variety of autoreactive or infectious disorders.

Multiple Myeloma

Definition and epidemiology. Multiple myeloma is a malignant plasma cell disorder characterized by neoplastic infiltration of the bone marrow and bone and by monoclonal immunoglobulin or light chains in the serum or urine. The cause of myeloma is uncertain.

The disease is more common in men than women and in African Americans than white individuals. Myeloma risk increases with age, with a median age of 69 years at diagnosis (SEER data). There were an estimated 32,110 new cases in the United States in 2019. Myeloma risk is increased for patients with first-degree relatives with a plasma cell dyscrasia. Associations have been described with occupational exposures to organic solvents, pesticides, petroleum products, and ionizing radiation; however, most patients with myeloma have no history of exposure to such agents.

Pathology. The tumor cell exhibits features of a differentiated plasma cell that is adapted to synthesize and secrete immunoglobulin at a high rate. Biopsies of bone marrow or targeted bone biopsies of tumor sites reveal infiltration by plasma cells with light-chain restriction, defining clonality. Cell surface markers useful in identifying and enumerating plasma cells include CD38, CD 138, and immunoglobulin light chains; the B-cell marker CD20 is typically absent and aids in distinguishing other lymphoproliferative disorders from myeloma.

Genetic aberrations are detectable in most patients with myeloma if adequately sensitive tests are applied. Standard karyotyping and FISH are performed routinely on marrow samples to determine abnormalities of prognostic significance, including translocations involving the immunoglobulin heavy-chain locus on chromosome 14, hyperploidy, or abnormalities of chromosomes 1, 13, or 17.

Diagnosis and differential diagnosis. Myeloma must be distinguished from related disorders, including MGUS and plasmacytoma. The diagnosis of multiple myeloma is made by identifying some combination of an increase (>10%) in the number of plasma cells in the bone marrow, a serum M protein other than IgM exceeding 3 g/dL, or a clonal protein in the urine. Asymptomatic myeloma (i.e., stage I myeloma or "smoldering myeloma") is diagnosed when clonal plasma cells are found in 10% to 59% of the bone marrow or monoclonal protein occurs in an amount greater than 3 g/dL in the absence of end organ–related injury, significant elevation in clonal free light chains or evidence of bone disease on advanced imaging (whole body MRI or PET-CT scan).

Patients with disease-related organ dysfunction (e.g., anemia, lytic bone lesions, hypercalcemia, renal dysfunction) are considered to have symptomatic myeloma, for which therapy is indicated. Recurrent infection with hypogammaglobulinemia is also considered a criterion for symptomatic myeloma. Solitary plasmacytoma is diagnosed when a single clonal plasma cell tumor is identified in bone or soft tissue in the absence of bone marrow involvement or other end organ–related injury.

Evaluation of the patient with suspected myeloma includes bone marrow biopsy; measurement of hemoglobin, calcium, renal function, and the serum free κ-to-λ light-chain ratio; serum and urine protein electrophoresis; immunoelectrophoresis; and a skeletal survey. PET

TABLE 50.6 **Classification of Disorders Associated With Monoclonal Immunoglobulin (M Protein) Secretion**

Disorder	M Protein Pattern
Plasma Cell Neoplasms	
Multiple myeloma	IgG > IgA > IgD; ± free light chain or light chain alone (κ > λ)
Solitary myeloma of bone	IgG > IgA > IgD; ± free light chain or light chain alone (κ > λ)
Extramedullary plasmacytoma	IgA > IgG > IgD; ± free light chain or light chain alone (κ > λ)
Waldenström's macroglobulinemia	IgM ± free light chain (κ > λ)
Heavy-chain disease	γ, α, μ heavy chain or fragment
Primary amyloidosis	Free light chain (λ > κ)
Monoclonal gammopathy of unknown significance	IgG > IgM > IgA, usually without urinary light-chain secretion
Other B-Cell Neoplasms	
Chronic lymphocytic leukemia	M protein occasionally secreted; IgM > IgG
B-cell non-Hodgkin's lymphomas; Hodgkin's disease	M protein occasionally secreted; IgM > IgG
Nonlymphoid Neoplasms	
Chronic myelogenous leukemia	No consistent patterns
Carcinomas (e.g., colon, breast, prostate)	No consistent patterns
Autoimmune or Autoreactive Disorders	
Cold agglutinin disease	IgM κ most common
Mixed cryoglobulinemia	IgM or IgA
Sjögren's syndrome	IgM
Miscellaneous Inflammatory, Storage, or Infectious Disorders	
Lichen myxedematosus	IgG λ
Gaucher's disease	IgG
Cirrhosis, sarcoid, parasitic diseases, renal acidosis	No consistent pattern

Ig, Immunoglobulin.
Modified from Salmon SE: Plasma cell disorders. In Wyngaarden JB, Smith LH Jr, editors: *Cecil Textbook of Medicine,* ed 18, Philadelphia, 1988, WB Saunders, p 1026.

and MRI are considered to further evaluate bone disease and may be necessary for patients with oligosecretory or nonsecretory disease to define disease and evaluate after therapy. Conventional bone scans are less useful due to the osteolytic nature of myeloma.

About 20% of patients with multiple myeloma do not have detectable serum M protein by standard electrophoresis but have circulating free light chains that may be detectable by serum free light-chain assays. Free light chains may appear in the urine (i.e., Bence Jones protein) and can also be detected in a 24-hour urine collection by urine protein electrophoresis. Free light-chain assays are quite sensitive and may provide measurement of clonal protein in patients thought to have non-secretory disease by other methods. Free light chains have a relatively short half-life (2 to 6 hours) in the circulation compared with a half-life of weeks for intact immunoglobulin molecules and may therefore be used to obtain a more rapid assessment of disease response once therapy is initiated. In rare cases, patients may have true non-secretory myeloma with no detectable serum or urine M protein by any assay.

Clinical presentation. The clinical manifestations of multiple myeloma are the direct effects of bone marrow and bone infiltration by malignant plasma cells, the systemic effects of the M protein, and the effects of the concomitant deficiency in humoral immunity that occurs in this disease. The most common symptom is bone pain. Bone radiographs typically show pure osteolytic punched-out lesions, often in association with generalized osteopenia and pathologic fractures. Bony lesions can show as expansile masses associated with spinal cord compression. Hypercalcemia caused by extensive bony involvement

is common in myeloma and may dominate the clinical picture. Anemia occurs in most patients as a result of marrow infiltration and suppression of hematopoiesis and causes fatigue; granulocytopenia and thrombocytopenia are less common.

Patients with myeloma are susceptible to bacterial infections because of impaired production and increased catabolism of normal immunoglobulins. Gram-negative urinary tract infections are common, as are respiratory tract infections caused by *Streptococcus pneumoniae, Staphylococcus aureus, Haemophilus influenzae,* and *Klebsiella pneumoniae.*

Renal insufficiency occurs in about 25% of patients with myeloma. The cause of renal failure is often multifactorial; hypercalcemia, hyperuricemia, infection, and amyloid deposition can contribute. Direct tubular damage from light-chain excretion also occurs. Because of their physicochemical properties, M proteins can cause a host of diverse effects, including cryoglobulinemia, hyperviscosity, amyloidosis, and clotting abnormalities resulting from interaction of the M protein with platelets or clotting factors.

Several staging or classification systems exist for myeloma. The Revised International Staging System (R-ISS) for myeloma identifies three stages with distinct prognoses based on β_2-microglobulin and albumin levels, LDH, and cytogenetic/FISH abnormalities (Table 50.7).

Treatment. Most patients with myeloma exhibit symptomatic, advanced-stage disease and require therapy. Patients with asymptomatic myeloma may have an indolent course and do not always require immediate therapy. Disease progression occurs at a rate of 5% to 10% per year, and patients should be monitored for disease progression

TABLE 50.7 Revised International Staging System for Multiple Myeloma

Stage	Criteria	Survival Rate at 5 Years (Months)
I	B2M <3.5 mg/L	82
	Albumin ≥3.5 g/dL	
	LDH ≤ ULN	
	Standard-risk chromosomal abnormalities by FISH	
II	Not stage I or III	62
III	B2M >5.5 mg/L	40
	High-risk chromosomal abnormalities or elevated LDH	

Palumbo A et al. Revised international staging system for multiple myeloma: a report from International Myeloma Working Group. *J Clin Oncol*, 2015;33:2863.
High-risk chromosomal abnormalities include deletion 17p and/or translocation t(4;14) and/or t(14;16).
B2M, β2-Microglobulin.

by serial quantification of M protein and serum free light chains and evaluation for disease-related signs or symptoms. For patients with solitary bone or extramedullary plasmacytomas, particularly in the head and neck region, local radiation therapy can induce long-term remissions and is the treatment of choice. Patients with a solitary plasmacytoma of bone are often found on routine MRI of the spine to have asymptomatic bone disease at other sites and should be treated as symptomatic myeloma.

Patients with symptomatic myeloma require systemic therapy and meticulous supportive care. Although myeloma is not a curable malignancy, systemic therapy prolongs survival and dramatically improves quality of life. Options for treatment have expanded in the past two decades to include multiple novel compounds in three broad classes of agents, the immunomodulatory drugs (IMIDs), proteasome inhibitors, and monoclonal antibodies. These agents may be used as single agents or in combinations for more intensive therapy. The novel agents are typically administered in combination with high doses of dexamethasone, which is a potent antimyeloma therapy. The IMIDS include thalidomide, lenalidomide, and pomalidomide. Proteasome inhibitors include bortezomib, carfilzomib, and ixazomib. The anti-CD38 monoclonal antibody daratumumab was approved for use in the United States in 2015. These agents have largely supplanted traditional chemotherapeutic agents as the cornerstone of initial and secondary therapies because they are efficacious and well tolerated. Multiple combination regimens have been devised that also incorporate chemotherapeutic agents in modest doses.

Thalidomide is the first-in-class IMID and was initially used as a sedative in the United Kingdom in the 1960s, but it was found to cause birth defects (phocomelia) when used to combat nausea during pregnancy. The antiangiogenic properties of thalidomide subsequently led to its development as an anticancer agent. The molecular target of the IMID class was recently elucidated as cereblon, an E3 ligase protein crucial to the activity of B cell–specific transcription factors that influence myeloma cell viability. The IMIDs are typically used in combination with dexamethasone, and when used as initial therapy, they have good tolerability and result in high response rates.

Toxicity related to thalidomide includes peripheral neuropathy, constipation, somnolence, and rash. Later-generation IMIDs have a more favorable side effect profile. Myelosuppression is more likely, but neuropathy and constitutional symptoms occur less frequently.

The second-generation IMID lenalidomide is more commonly used in North America due to its favorable tolerability. A troublesome and unique side effect of the IMID-steroid combination programs is development of deep vein thrombosis in up to 25% of patients, and some form of preventative therapy is required.

Bortezomib is the first-in-class proteasome inhibitor and is an important therapy for patients with adverse cytogenetic risk factors. Bortezomib is typically administered subcutaneously and may cause thrombocytopenia, asthenia, and neuropathy.

Most patients respond to initial therapy with a reduction in bone pain, hypercalcemia, and anemia in association with a decline in the M protein level. The selection of initial therapy depends on stage, cytogenetic risk, and candidacy for high-dose chemotherapy and autologous stem cell transplantation. The use of high-dose chemotherapy with alkylating agents followed by autologous peripheral stem cell infusion during first or second remission improves progression-free survival and quality of life compared with conventional therapy. Although this approach is not curative, it does represent an important treatment option for some patients and has an acceptable toxicity profile, even in older patients. Allogenic stem cell or bone marrow transplantation may be associated with durable remission in selected patients, but it carries a high near-term risk of morbidity and mortality. Patients who experience relapse after standard therapy or transplantation may be treated with alternative chemotherapy regimens or with novel combination therapies, including newer agents and chemotherapy drugs. The first-in-class *selective inhibitor of nuclear export*, selinexor was recently added to the antimyeloma armamentarium for patients with relapsed or refractory disease as a fifth-line therapy. CAR-T cell therapy has shown high response rates in clinic trials and is expected to become available as a standard therapy soon.

Supportive care directed toward anticipated complications of myeloma is an important aspect of management. Bone resorption can be reduced with regular injections of the diphosphonates zoledronic acid or pamidronate, reducing pain and pathologic fractures. The monoclonal antibody denosumab targets RANKL, inhibiting osteoclast activity, and may also be used to treat bone disease. Bony lesions, particularly those involving weight-bearing bones, may require palliative irradiation for controlling pain and preventing pathologic fractures. Vertebral bony lesions may lead to spinal cord compression, with increasing back pain and neurologic symptoms. Symptoms suggesting cord compression require prompt evaluation with spinal MRI and, if necessary, local irradiation of involved areas.

Avoidance of nephrotoxins, including intravenous contrast media, is important to prevent renal failure. All patients should receive pneumococcal and *H. influenzae* vaccines, and intravenous gamma globulin may be useful in preventing recurrent infections in patients with profound hypogammaglobulinemia. Use of erythropoietin may alleviate anemia and decrease the need for blood transfusions in patients with treatment-related anemia or concomitant renal insufficiency.

Prognosis. Multiple myeloma is considered incurable, but the overall survival of these patients has improved considerably with the use of newer agents and autologous stem cell transplantation. The five-year survival as reported by the SEER database is 52.2%.

Prognosis depends on stage of disease and cytogenetic profile. Patients with an adverse karyotype, including t(14;16), t(4;14), and 17p deletion, have a less favorable prognosis and are considered for more intensive therapies or clinical investigation. Adverse factors also include advanced stage, impaired renal function, elevated LDH levels, depressed serum albumin levels, and elevated β2-microglobulin levels.

Waldenström's Macroglobulinemia

Waldenström's macroglobulinemia (WM) is a malignancy of plasmacytoid lymphocytes that secrete large quantities of IgM. It is a chronic disorder affecting elderly patients (median age 64 years) that shares features of the low-grade lymphomas and myeloma. Unlike myeloma, Waldenström's macroglobulinemia is associated with lymphadenopathy and hepatosplenomegaly, and although bone marrow involvement invariably occurs, lytic lesions and hypercalcemia are rare. Diagnostic work-up for WM should include polymerase chain reaction analysis for mutation in the MYD88 gene, which is present in most patients and carries diagnostic and therapeutic relevance.

The major clinical manifestations of WM include symptomatic anemia and the hyperviscosity syndrome caused by the physical properties of IgM. In contrast to IgG, IgM remains largely confined to the intravascular space, and as IgM levels rise, plasma viscosity increases. Epistaxis, retinal hemorrhages, dizziness, confusion, and congestive heart failure may occur as a result of the hyperviscosity syndrome. About 10% of IgM proteins have properties of cryoglobulins, and patients show symptoms of cryoglobulinemia or cold agglutinin syndrome demonstrated as acrocyanosis, Raynaud's phenomenon, and vascular symptoms or hemolytic anemia precipitated by exposure to cold. Some patients with WM may develop a peripheral neuropathy that may antedate the appearance of the neoplastic process.

The approach to and treatment of WM is similar to those of other low-grade B-cell lymphomas. The use of fludarabine or an alkylating agent, typically employed in combination with prednisone and rituximab, is effective in decreasing adenopathy and splenomegaly and controlling the M spike but is not curative. Rituximab has activity against WM, as has the proteasome inhibitor bortezomib. The use of rituximab as a single agent may be complicated by initial worsening of hyperviscosity in patients with high IgM burdens. The novel agent ibrutinib, an inhibitor of Bruton tyrosine kinase, is an effective oral therapy for Waldenström's and may be combined with rituximab. Although complete remissions are rare, patients who respond to therapy have median survivals of 4 years, and some patients survive more than a decade.

Rare Plasma Cell Disorders

Heavy-chain disease is a rare lymphoplasmacytoid neoplasm characterized by production of a defective heavy chain of the γ, α, or μ type. The clinical manifestations vary with the type of heavy chain secreted. The γ-type heavy-chain disease is associated with lymphadenopathy, Waldeyer ring involvement with palatal edema, and constitutional symptoms. The α-type heavy-chain disease, also known as Mediterranean lymphoma, is characterized by lymphoid infiltration of the small intestine with associated diarrhea and malabsorption. The μ-type heavy-chain disease is associated with CLL.

Primary amyloidosis. Primary AL amyloidosis is a systemic illness characterized by deposition of immunoglobulin light chains in organs and tissue, resulting in an array of symptoms caused by organ dysfunction. Congestive heart failure, bleeding diathesis, nephrotic syndrome, and peripheral neuropathy are common complications. Patients with primary amyloidosis may respond to selected treatments similar to therapy for myeloma. The combination of bortezomib, cyclophosphamide, and dexamethasone is effective in some patients. Selected patients may respond well to high-dose chemotherapy and autologous stem cell support, but there are increased risks of morbidity and mortality if significant end-organ dysfunction such as cardiomyopathy occurs. It is important to note that not all amyloidosis is AL (light chain), and documentation of the source and type of amyloid protein is vital to appropriate management.

POEMS syndrome. POEMS syndrome is a rare disorder characterized by polyneuropathy, sclerotic bone lesions, endocrinopathy, monoclonal gammopathy, and skin lesions. The cause of POEMS syndrome is unknown, but the disease may be progressive, causing severe disability, third spacing of fluid, and elevated vascular endothelial growth factor (VEGF) levels. Monoclonal λ light chains are typically elevated. Limited bone disease may be treated with radiotherapy. High-dose therapy and autologous stem cell transplantation is effective in patients with extensive disease.

For a deeper discussion of these topics, please see Chapter 178, "Plasma Cell Disorders," and Chapter 179, "Amyloidosis," in *Goldman-Cecil Medicine*, 26th Edition.

CONGENITAL AND ACQUIRED DISORDERS OF LYMPHOCYTE FUNCTION

Several congenital disorders affect lymphocyte maturation or function, resulting in immunodeficiency disorders. Acquired disorders of lymphocyte function are far more common than congenital disorders. HIV infection is the most important infectious cause of acquired immunodeficiency (see Chapter 103). Patients with HIV infection are at increased risk for NHL. NHLs that occur in the setting of HIV have diffuse, aggressive B-cell histology and include DLBCL and Burkitt lymphoma. They are frequently associated with EBV infection and are often advanced stage (III or IV) at diagnosis, with extranodal sites of involvement.

Patients with HIV-associated NHL are potentially curable with the multidrug chemotherapy regimens used for treating NHL found in the general population. Treatment of the underlying HIV infection with highly active antiretroviral therapy (ART) has improved the outcome and prognosis of patients with HIV-associated NHL.

Patients who have undergone allogeneic organ transplantation require potent immunosuppressive drugs (e.g., cyclosporine, tacrolimus, mycophenolate, corticosteroids, methotrexate) to prevent graft-versus-host disease in the case of bone marrow transplantation or allograft rejection in the case of solid organ transplantation. These medications cause defects in T-cell function with an associated immunodeficiency state, which increases risk for a post-transplant lymphoproliferative disorder (PTLD). PTLD is an EBV-associated lymphoproliferative disorder characterized by a polymorphous or monomorphous population of B cells that can be monoclonal or polyclonal. Patients are treated by reducing doses of immunosuppressive drugs whenever possible. Patients with polymorphous disease early after organ transplantation may respond well to this approach. Patients who are not candidates for withdrawal of immunosuppression because of allograft rejection or who develop late monophorphic disease may respond better to treatment with rituximab alone or in combination with chemotherapy.

SUGGESTED READINGS

Canellos GP, Anderson JR, Propert KJ, et al: Chemotherapy of advanced Hodgkin's disease with MOPP, ABVD, or MOPP alternating with ABVD, N Engl J Med 327:1478–1484, 1992.

Cheson B, Fisher R, Barrington S, et al: Recommendations for initial evaluation, staging, and response assessment of Hodgkin and non-Hodgkin lymphoma: the Lugano classification, J Clin Oncol 32:3059–3068, 2014.

Coiffier B, Lepage E, Briere J, et al: CHOP chemotherapy plus rituximab compared with CHOP alone in elderly patients with diffuse large-B-cell lymphoma, N Engl J Med 346:235–242, 2002.

Dispenzieri A: POEMS Syndrome: 2019 Update on diagnosis, risk-stratification, and management, Am J Hematol 94(7):812–827, 2019.

Engert A, Plütschow A, Eich HT, et al: Reduced treatment intensity in patients with early-stage Hodgkin's lymphoma, N Engl J Med 363:640–652, 2010.

Fisher RI, Gaynor ER, Dahlberg S, et al: Comparison of a standard regimen (CHOP) with three intensive chemotherapy regimens for advanced non-Hodgkin's lymphoma, N Engl J Med 328:1002–1006, 1993.

Geisler CH, Kolstad A, Laurell A, et al: Long-term progression-free survival of mantle cell lymphoma after intensive front-line immunochemotherapy with in vivo purged stem cell rescue: a nonrandomized phase 2 multicenter study by the Nordic Lymphoma Group, Blood 112:2687–2693, 2008.

Hasenclever D, Diehl V: A prognostic score for advanced Hodgkin's disease. International prognostic factors project on advanced Hodgkin's disease, N Engl J Med 339:1506–1514, 1998.

Howlader N, Noone AM, Krapcho M, et al (eds): SEER Cancer Statistics Review, Bethesda, MD, 1975-2016, National Cancer Institute, based on November 2018 SEER data submission, posted to the SEER web site. https://seer.cancer.gov/csr/1975_2016/. Accessed April 2019.

Kyle RA, Therneau TM, Rajkumar SV, et al: A long-term study of prognosis in monoclonal gammopathy of undetermined significance, N Engl J Med 346:564–569, 2002.

Maloney DG, Grillo-Lopez AJ, White CA, et al: IDEC-C2B8 (rituximab) anti-CD20 monoclonal antibody therapy in patients with relapsed low-grade non-Hodgkin's lymphoma, Blood 90:2188–2195, 1997.

McSweeney PA, Niederwieser D, Shizuru JA, et al: Hematopoietic cell transplantation in older patients with hematologic malignancies: replacing high-dose cytotoxic therapy with graft-versus-tumor effects, Blood 97:3390–3400, 2001.

Philip T, Guglielmi C, Hagenbeek A, et al: Autologous bone marrow transplantation as compared with salvage chemotherapy in relapses of chemotherapy-sensitive non-Hodgkin's lymphoma, N Engl J Med 33:1540–1545, 1995.

Rummel MJ, Niederle N, Maschmeyer G, et al: Bendamustine plus rituximab versus CHOP plus rituximab as first-line treatment for patients with indolent and mantle-cell lymphomas: an open-label, multicentre, randomised, phase 3 non-inferiority trial, Lancet 381:1203–1210, 2013.

Singhal S, Mehta J, Desikan R, et al: Antitumor activity of thalidomide in refractory multiple myeloma, N Engl J Med 341:1565–1571, 1999.

Swerdlow SH, Harris NL, Jaffe ES, et al: World Health Organization classification of tumours of hematopoietic and lymphoid tissues, revised ed 4, Lyon, 2017, IARC Press.

Wang ML, Rule S, Martin P: Targeting BTK with ibrutinib in relapsed or refractory mantle-cell lymphoma, N Engl J Med 369:507–516, 2013.

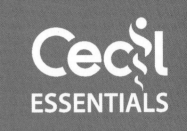

51

Normal Hemostasis

Lauren Shevell, Alfred I. Lee

INTRODUCTION

Hemostasis is the physiologic balance of procoagulant and anticoagulant forces that provide structural integrity of vasculature while maintaining circulating blood flow. Vascular damage initiates clotting, which results in a localized platelet-fibrin plug at the site of injury to prevent blood loss. This is followed by clot containment, wound healing, eventual clot dissolution, and tissue regeneration. In healthy individuals, procoagulant and anticoagulant reactions occur continuously and in a balanced fashion so that bleeding is contained while blood vessels simultaneously remain patent to deliver adequate organ blood flow. If any of these processes is disrupted, either from inherited defects or acquired abnormalities, disordered hemostasis may result in either bleeding diatheses or thromboembolic disease.

Traditionally, hemostasis has been conceptualized in two parts: *primary hemostasis*, resulting in adhesion and activation of platelets, and *secondary hemostasis*, resulting in activation and regulation of the coagulation cascade. More recent studies, however, demonstrate a considerable amount of interplay between primary and secondary hemostatic components.

This chapter briefly details the physiologic and interdependent mechanisms of vascular hemostasis, including the normal balance of procoagulant and anticoagulant functions of the blood vessel wall and platelets, receptor-ligand interactions that are critical for hemostasis, as well as the highly complex, interwoven pathways that represent the coagulation cascade.

VASCULATURE PHYSIOLOGY

Blood flow in the arterial system differs from that in the venous system and imposes different coagulation requirements. In the pressurized arteries, relatively minor vascular damage can rapidly result in massive exsanguination; therefore, the procoagulant response in the arteries must rapidly arrest bleeding. Platelets are critical to the arterial response; they initially contain the blood loss and then provide an active surface for soluble coagulation factors to both localize and accelerate formation of fibrin for a strong fibrin clot. In contrast, the slower flow rates in the venous circulation produce slower bleeding, a feature that makes platelets less critical; instead, the balance of venous hemostasis is most dependent on the rate of thrombin generation. These differences are underscored clinically by the antithrombotic agents used in these distinct clinical settings: antiplatelet agents such as aspirin and clopidogrel are used to prevent coronary and cerebral artery thrombosis, whereas anticoagulants such as heparins, warfarin, and direct oral anticoagulants (e.g., direct thrombin inhibitors like dabigatran, or Xa inhibitors like rivaroxaban or apixaban) are used for the treatment and prophylaxis of venous disease.

Vascular endothelial cells (ECs) that line the luminal surfaces of blood vessels contribute both procoagulant and anticoagulant forces depending on circumstances. When the vasculature is intact, healthy ECs exert anticoagulant activity to maintain blood fluidity. This is done through several mechanisms. First, ECs act as a barrier, separating blood from subendothelial procoagulants such as tissue factor (TF) and collagen (Fig. 51.1A). ECs also contribute to hemostatic balance by secreting several products including prostacyclin, nitric oxide, adenosine diphosphatase, and tissue factor pathway inhibitor (TFPI). Prostacyclin and nitric oxide release by ECs leads to vascular smooth muscle relaxation, reducing shear injury. These chemicals also promote the generation of cyclic adenosine monophosphate (cAMP), thus inhibiting platelet activation and aggregation. Adenosine diphosphatase degrades extracellular platelet-released ADP, inhibiting platelet recruitment into the growing platelet clot. TFPI acts by blunting the initiation of the coagulation cascade (described in more detail in the "Termination of Clotting" section).

When ECs are physically damaged or activated, their balance of coagulant properties is shifted to favor a procoagulant state. This is mediated by both the ECs themselves and subendothelial matrix that is exposed when the vascular wall is disrupted. Activated ECs express ligands on their surfaces allowing for platelet adhesion and increased inflammatory responses. These include E-selectin and P-selectin, β_1 and β_2 integrins, platelet EC adhesion molecule-1 (PECAM-1), and von Willebrand factor (VWF) multimers (Table 51.1). On the activated EC surface, VWF multimers localize and promote platelet adhesion, whereas integrins mediate adhesion and subsequent transendothelial migration of leukocytes into the tissues. After EC damage, the exposed subendothelial matrix also binds VWF multimers to further enhance platelet adhesion. Subendothelial procoagulant proteins such as thrombospondin, fibronectin, and especially collagen function both as ligands to capture platelets and as activators of adherent platelets. Collagen, in particular, is both a platelet ligand and a strong platelet agonist and causes platelets to undergo alpha and dense granule release and to express conformationally active ligands such as glycoprotein IIb/IIIa (GPIIb/IIIa, also known as integrin $\alpha_{IIb}\beta_3$) (described in detail later). Another critical procoagulant mediator exposed by EC damage is TF, which is constitutively expressed by subendothelial smooth muscle cells and fibroblasts. As outlined further later, TF is the major initiator of the soluble coagulation system that, along with activated platelets, results in the formation of a definitive platelet-fibrin clot.

VON WILLEBRAND FACTOR

VWF is an essential component of coagulation. Produced by ECs and megakaryocytes, the VWF protein is stored within platelets in alpha granules and within ECs in rodlike granules known as Weibel-Palade

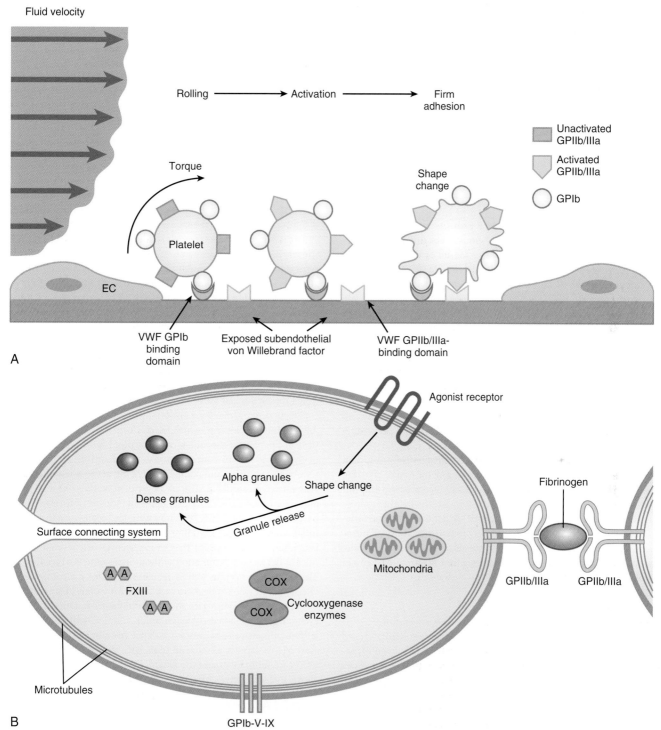

Fig. 51.1 (A) The adhesive interactions that produce stable platelet attachment to subendothelial von Willebrand factor (VWF). The initial attachment between platelet glycoprotein Ib (GPIb) and its binding domain on VWF is rapid but has a short half-life, and the result is a rolling movement caused by torque generated by flowing blood. The VWF-GPIb interaction produces transmembrane signaling that activates the platelet to change shape and simultaneously transforms GPIIb/IIIa into an activated conformation capable of binding to a distinct arginine-glycine-aspartate domain on VWF. This secondary adhesion causes the platelet to firmly adhere to the exposed subendothelial VWF. (B) The internal and external anatomy of a platelet. The platelet consists of several important external, transmembrane, and internal components that help to promote platelet activation, adhesion, aggregation/agglutination, and general coagulation factor–based hemostasis. The most important and most clinically relevant aspects of platelet anatomy are shown. Details regarding the steps leading to platelet activation and release of granules and cytosolic contents are discussed in the text. *A,* A subunits of factor XIII; *COX,* cyclooxygenase; *EC,* endothelial cell; *FXIII,* factor XIII; *GP,* glycoprotein complex.

TABLE 51.1	**Properties of Endothelial Cell Coagulants**	
Procoagulant	**Anticoagulant**
Collagen	Vasodilation
Factor VIII	Adenosine diphosphatase
Fibronectin	Heparan sulfates
Integrins	Nitric oxide
Platelet-endothelial cell adhesion molecule-1 (PECAM-1)	Prostacyclin
Selectins (E and P)	Thrombomodulin
Vasoconstriction	Tissue factor pathway inhibitor
von Willebrand factor	Tissue plasminogen activator

bodies. In both platelets and ECs, VWF proteins multimerize in the Golgi apparatus; about 95% of VWF multimers are constitutively released into the plasma and can be detected on electrophoretic gels as high-, intermediate-, and low-molecular-weight VWF forms. The remaining 5% of VWF multimers are stored either in platelet alpha granules or in EC Weibel-Palade bodies in the form of ultra-large VWF multimers. Following platelet stimulation or EC damage, ultra-large VWF multimers are released into the plasma and have high affinity for platelets and subendothelial collagen, forming string-like structures that must then be cleaved into smaller VWF proteins for proper function. Cleavage of ultra-large VWF multimers is performed by a metalloproteinase, ADAMTS13 (a disintegrin and metalloproteinase with a thrombospondin type 1 motif, member 13). In addition to platelet and subendothelial collagen binding, VWF in the plasma serves as a second role in binding and stabilizing coagulation factor VIII and preventing its degradation.

The importance of VWF is underscored clinically by von Willebrand disease (VWD), the most common inherited bleeding condition in the world, characterized by defects in either the amount or the activity of VWF protein; and alternatively by thrombotic thrombocytopenic purpura, an inherited or acquired disease arising from defects in ADAMT13 that lead to accumulation of ultra-large VWF multimers, causing microvascular thrombosis, platelet consumption, shearing of red blood cells and multiple end-organ complications.

PLATELET PHYSIOLOGY

Platelets are anucleated cells measuring 2 to 4 μm in diameter and are derived from megakaryocyte cytoplasm (Fig. 51.1B). Each megakaryocyte contributes 1000 to 3000 platelets in its lifetime. After platelets are released into the circulation, they survive 7 to 10 days. The normal platelet count ranges between 150,000 to 450,000/μL; only approximately 7100 platelets/μL are required for hemostasis per day if vascular structures are intact (i.e., in the absence of any recent surgeries or trauma) and if there is no increase in normal platelet consumption (e.g., as might occur in sepsis or disseminated intravascular coagulation).

The bleeding time, an in vivo measure of hemostasis, is usually less than 8 minutes if the platelet count is within the normal limit. It is used as a screening test for platelet function defects, VWD, and sometimes other bleeding disorders. The bleeding time is dependent on the platelet count and will naturally be prolonged if the platelet count falls to less than 100,000/μL. Therefore, in the setting of thrombocytopenia, a prolonged bleeding time cannot be used to determine whether bleeding is caused by abnormal platelet function, VWD, another bleeding problem, or thrombocytopenia. Because the bleeding time is an

operator-dependent, highly variable in vivo assay that causes trauma to patients, most laboratories now use the Platelet Function Analyzer-100 (PFA-100) (Fig. 52.2), which uses anticoagulated blood to examine the amount of time required for platelets to form a plug in response to either collagen and ADP or collagen and epinephrine (i.e., the "closure time"). The PFA-100 is similar to the bleeding time test in that both may be used to assess platelet function and to screen for VWD but are unable to distinguish between thrombocytopenia and abnormal platelet function when the platelet count is lower than 100,000/μL.

Platelet Activation

In the setting of vascular injury, platelets are recruited to the area by exposure to local agonists (collagen, epinephrine and thrombin) and by release of agonists within platelets into the local microenvironment (ADP, thromboxane). The most potent platelet activators, collagen and thrombin, interact with their specific platelet receptors to strongly activate platelets. Epinephrine alone is not a powerful platelet agonist, but stimulation of the α-adrenergic receptor on platelets primes them for synergistic activation by relatively weak agonists such as ADP. Platelets also release activating compounds, including thromboxane A2 (TXA_2), which is formed in the platelet cytosol after cyclooxygenase 1 (COX1)-mediated cleavage of arachidonic acid, which is then released into the clot milieu. TXA_2 is both a platelet agonist and vasoconstrictor and is rapidly degraded to its inert by-product, thromboxane B2. Notably, the exact roles of different platelet agonists depend on a spatial hierarchy within the platelet plug. Thrombin activates platelets within the core of the hemostatic plug, whereas ADP and TXA_2 activate platelets in the loosely packed shell surrounding the core.

Of particular clinical importance, platelet COX1 activity is irreversibly inhibited by aspirin, which blocks formation of TXA_2 for the lifetime of the platelet through a covalent bond causing steric hindrance of the active site. In contrast, nonsteroidal anti-inflammatory drugs (NSAIDs) reversibly and competitively bind at the active site; thus, the antiplatelet effects of NSAIDs are dependent on the continual presence of plasma levels of the NSAID. COX2 is an induced isoform of the cyclooxygenase enzyme that is present within leukocytes and that mediates inflammation and pain. Mature platelets do not possess COX2 activity, providing the rationale for the development of selective COX2 inhibitors to decrease inflammation without increasing the bleeding risk of platelet dysfunction (as well as decreasing risk for gastrointestinal side effects, which will not be addressed here). However, ECs are reliant on COX2 activity to synthesize the antithrombogenic compound prostacyclin. Downregulation of prostacyclin, coupled with preserved platelet function, tips the hemostatic balance in favor of clot formation. In view of this, large-scale clinical trials have shown that highly selective COX2 inhibitors increase the likelihood of hypertension and vascular events including myocardial infarction and stroke.

Platelet Adhesion

Platelet activation leads to a functional shape change of the platelet from a disk to an irregular sphere with pseudopod extensions, as well as exposure of platelet binding domains. This enhances platelet adhesion capabilities and maximizes the interaction of coagulation factors with the platelet surface. Initial platelet adhesion is primarily mediated by the glycoprotein 1b-IX-V (GP1b-IX-V) complex on the platelet surface binding to multimeric VWF, which is immobilized by adherence to exposed subendothelial collagen. The weak binding of GP1b-IX-V to VWF contributes to transmembrane signaling with downstream effects that include a change in platelet shape (see Fig. 51.1A) and a change in GPIIb/IIIa (integrin $\alpha_{IIb}\beta_3$) from a low-affinity to a high-affinity state, facilitating binding of the latter to fibrinogen and VWF (see Fig. 51.1B). A deficiency of the GP1b-IX-V complex leads to

Bernard-Soulier syndrome, a congenital bleeding disorder characterized by giant platelets that are dysfunctional.

GPIIb/IIIa (integrin $\alpha_{IIb}\beta_3$) is a member of the integrin superfamily and the most abundant receptor on the platelet surface. Prior to platelet activation, the GPIIb/IIIa ($\alpha_{IIb}\beta_3$) receptor sits on the platelet surface and has low affinity for binding. However, upon platelet activation and its consequent conformational changes, the GPIIb/IIIa receptor adopts a high-affinity conformation that facilitates binding both to VWF, securing platelets strongly on the subendothelial surface, and to fibrinogen, linking platelets together and reinforcing the platelet plug. Further, after binding to VWF, the cytosolic side of the GPIIb/IIIa ($\alpha_{IIb}\beta_3$) receptor binds to the cytoskeleton of the platelet, fostering further changes to platelet shape change and spreading via cytoskeletal reorganization. These roles of GPIIb/IIIa ($\alpha_{IIb}\beta_3$) in platelet adhesion and platelet plug formation provide the rationale for use of GPIIb/IIIa ($\alpha_{IIb}\beta_3$) antagonists in treatment of coronary artery disease. Of note, mutations in the gene encoding GPIIb/IIIa ($\alpha_{IIb}\beta_3$) lead to Glanzmann thrombocythemia, another congenital bleeding disorder leading to platelet dysfunction.

Platelet Secretion

After activation, dense granules and alpha granules within platelets fuse with the canalicular membrane and liberate their procoagulant contents into the extracellular fluid. Dense granules contain serotonin, ADP, ATP, ionized calcium, and histamine. Serotonin and ADP both activate and recruit platelets to sites of vascular injury. Additionally, serotonin, similarly to TXA_2, acts as a vasoconstrictor. ADP acts purely as a platelet agonist through the G protein–linked P2RY12 receptor and has no vasoactive properties. The importance of dense-granule release is illustrated by the severe bleeding seen in patients with congenital dense-granule deficiencies such as Hermansky-Pudlak syndrome or Chediak-Higashi syndrome.

Alpha granules contain numerous proteins including many adhesive molecules (fibrinogen, VWF, thrombospondin), cellular mitogens (platelet-derived growth factor, transforming growth factor beta), coagulation factors (factor V), and physiologically important receptors (P-selectin, $\alpha_{IIb}\beta_3$). The importance of platelet alpha granules is illustrated in patients with gray platelet syndrome, an inherited deficiency of alpha granules leading to bleeding. Other components within platelets, including factor XIII, are also released upon platelet activation and act as clot stabilizers (see Fig. 51.1B).

COAGULATION

Coagulation Cascade Model

The classical coagulation cascade (Fig. 51.2A), first described over 50 years ago, features two starting points, the intrinsic and extrinsic pathways, that flow in a step-wise waterfall of proteolytic reactions and converge in a common pathway. The common pathway culminates with the generation of thrombin, which converts fibrinogen to fibrin. Fibrin then cross-links platelets and strengthens the platelet plug.

In the classical model, coagulation begins with the extrinsic pathway, which is initiated by the exposure of TF and activated factor VIIa, leading to activation of factor X in the common pathway.

The intrinsic pathway is initiated by the activation of proteins circulating in plasma—namely, factor XII (Hageman factor), high-molecular-weight kininogen (HMWK, also known as Fitzgerald factor), and prekallikrein (PPK, also known as Fletcher factor). This pathway is also referred to as the contact activation pathway because these proteins are activated by contact with negatively charged surfaces. Factor XIIa and HMWK activate factor XI, leading to the activation of factor IX, which in conjunction with factor VIII activates factor X to initiate the common pathway (see Fig. 51.2AB). The importance of the intrinsic coagulation

cascade is demonstrated in patients with hemophilias, which are congenital bleeding disorders due to deficiencies in factor VIII (hemophilia A), factor IX (hemophilia B), or factor X (hemophilia C).

Notably, all procoagulants are produced almost exclusively in the liver aside from factor VIII, which is produced in both liver sinusoidal cells and ECs, and VWF, which is produced in ECs and megakaryocytes. The procoagulant factors II, VII, IX, and X, and the anticoagulant proteins C and S, all undergo post-translational modification in the form of vitamin K–dependent g-carboxylation of the amino terminal domains, which is critical for calcium binding and determining the three-dimensional structure of proteins. The importance of vitamin K–dependent g-carboxylation is demonstrated by the anticoagulant warfarin, which acts by blocking vitamin K epoxide reductase, thereby reducing the generation of these specific proteins.

In the classical coagulation model, the prothrombin time (PT) serves as a measure of extrinsic pathway activity while the activated partial thrombin time (aPTT) measures activity of the intrinsic pathway. Therapeutically, the PT and aPTT are used to guide warfarin and heparin dosing, respectively. Although the classical model of coagulation is workable for some clinical scenarios, more recent models have made strides to more accurately elucidate and depict the physiology and complex interplay of different components of coagulation.

Cell-Based Model of Coagulation

The cell-based coagulation model (see Fig. 51.2B) has largely been established as the most physiologically accurate in vivo model of coagulation. This model proposes that coagulation takes place on the surfaces of different cells in a three-step fashion: initiation, amplification, and propagation.

The *initiation phase* begins as exposed TF on the EC surface binds to picomolar amounts of factor VIIa, present in the circulation at all times. The VIIa-TF complex (termed the extrinsic Xase) activates factors IX and X. The conversion of a small amount of X to Xa produces a tiny amount of thrombin. The nearly trivial amount of thrombin sparks feedback to activate factor XI, leading to *amplification* of thrombin generation. Factor VIII, conveniently brought to the bleeding site by its carrier VWF, is also activated by thrombin, a step that causes release of VWF. Factor VIIIa then complexes with the picomolar amounts of factor IXa generated by the TF-VIIa complex during the initiation phase to create the VIIIa-IXa complex, known as the intrinsic Xase complex. Notably, IXa generation by the TF-VIIa complex is limited by TFPI, so factor IX is secondarily activated by platelet-bound factor XIa (catalyzed by factor XIIa in conjunction with high molecular weight kininogen), providing sufficient amounts of factor IXa in the intrinsic Xase complex. The formation of this complex on the platelet surface heralds the *propagation phase*, and the switch of the primary path of Xa generation from the TF-VIIa complex, the extrinsic Xase complex, to the intrinsic Xase. This switch is of significant kinetic advantage, with the intrinsic Xase complex exhibiting a 50-fold higher efficiency than the extrinsic Xase. More than 96% of the total thrombin that is generated during clotting occurs during the propagation phase. The bleeding diathesis associated with hemophilia is a testament to the physiologic importance of the exuberant thrombin generation engendered by the switch from extrinsic to intrinsic Xase. The aPTT, which measures the initiation phase of clotting begun by an artificial in vitro stimulant, is prolonged by severe deficiencies of either VIII or IX, but it is thrombin generation during the propagation phase, a function not evaluated by the aPTT, that is more impaired in hemophilia.

Thrombin generated during the initiation phase is a potent platelet activator. The activated platelet expresses receptors for VIIIa and IXa, and binding of these active proteases in complex with membrane phosphatidylserine enhances the binding of the enzyme's substrate,

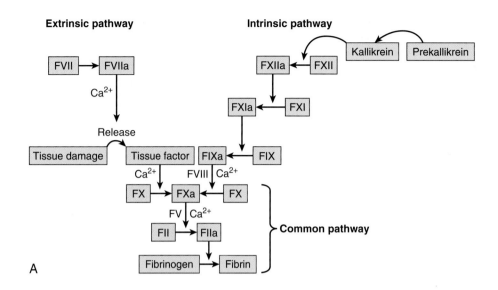

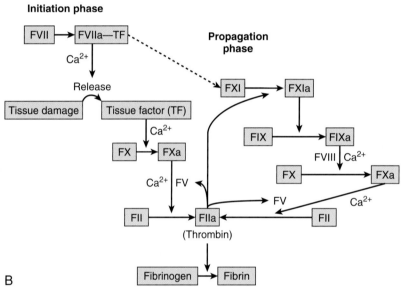

Fig. 51.2 (A) The classic view of the coagulation cascade. The laboratory-defined *extrinsic* and *intrinsic* pathways allow monitoring of anticoagulation by serial measurements of the prothrombin time (PT) and partial thromboplastin time (PTT), respectively. The PT primarily monitors factor VII activity, whereas the PTT is the best measure of XI and the hemophilic factors IX and VIII; both assays will detect deficiency of the common pathway factors (X, V, and II). (B) In the more modern view of the coagulation cascade, initiation of clotting begins with exposure to tissue factor (TF), which combines with small amounts of circulating factor (F) VIIa to form the extrinsic tenase (Xase) complex and generate FXa. FXa forms the prothrombinase complex with FVa and FII, generating small amounts of thrombin (FIIa), which begins to cleave fibrinogen into weak fibrin monomers in the initiation phase of coagulation. Thrombin's ability to activate factors, especially on the activated platelet surface, is responsible for propagation of the coagulant response. Thrombin generates FXIa, which in turn activates FIX; the TF-VIIa complex (before it is shut down by TFPI) also generates FIXa. Thrombin-activated FVIIIa then combines with IXa to form the intrinsic Xase complex, generating large amounts of FXa and prothrombinase complex on the platelet surface to further amplify thrombin generation. The large amounts of thrombin now generate enough fibrin monomers to form stable polymers and fibrin clot. *HMWK,* High-molecular-weight kininogen; *PK,* prekallikrein; *TFPI,* tissue factor pathway inhibitor.

factor X, increasing the kinetic efficiency of the intrinsic Xase complex. The activated platelet (Table 51.2) also enhances coagulation by supplying the developing clot with an activated platelet surface membrane (i.e., anionic lipids, primarily phosphatidylserine) and abundant factor V, stored in platelet granules. Factor V is then promptly activated to Va by the trace amount of thrombin produced by TF-VIIa complex. In combination with membrane phospholipids and calcium, activated Xa and its cofactor Va form the prothrombinase complex, which cleaves prothrombin to thrombin. The prothrombinase complex is several hundred thousand times more efficient at converting prothrombin to thrombin than free factor Xa acting on prothrombin alone. The role of the procoagulant effects of activated platelets on thrombosis is highlighted by Scott syndrome, a condition in which the platelet phospholipid membrane does not change in response to activation, and thus phosphatidylserine is not rearranged from the inner membrane surface to the outer membrane surface, leading to decreased thrombin generation and prolonged bleeding as a result of platelet dysfunction.

TABLE 51.2 Procoagulant Properties of Platelets

Receptor-Ligand Interactions Promoting Adhesion
[a]GPIb-IX-V-VWF
[b]GPIIb/IIIa-fibrinogen and GPIIb/IIIa-VWF
[c]GPIa/IIa-collagen
[d]P-selectin–P-selectin glycoprotein ligand-1

Receptor-Ligand Interactions Mediating Activation
GPV-thrombin
GPVI-collagen

Secreted Alpha-Granule Proteins
Ligands (fibrinogen, fibronectin, thrombospondin, vitronectin, von Willebrand factor)
Enzymes (α_2-antiplasmin; factors V, VIII, and XI)
Antiheparin (platelet factor 4)

Secreted Dense-Granule Agonists
Adenosine diphosphate, serotonin

Components and Functions of Platelets That Promote Coagulation
Thromboxane A_2 formation, phosphatidylserine expression

GP, Glycoprotein.
[a]GPIb-IX-V complex is also known as CD42.
[b]GPIIb/IIIa (integrin $\alpha_{IIb}\beta_3$) complex is also known as CD41.
[c]GPIIa is also known as CD29.
[d]P-selectin is also known as CD62P and P-selectin glycoprotein ligand-1 as CD162.

Of note, polyphosphate has been shown to have a critical role in coagulation and acts as a procoagulant, initiating clotting through several mechanisms. First, polyphosphate contains numerous negatively anionic charged surfaces leading to activation of plasma factor XII, HMWK, and PPK that set off the intrinsic pathway. Polyphosphate also mitigates the inhibitory effects of TFPI, enhances the activation of factor V and factor IX, and leads to thickened fibrin fibrils by increasing fibrin polymerization.

Termination of Clotting

The rapid production of thrombin at a localized site of vascular injury could quickly lead to extensive clotting if left unchecked; thus, there are several mechanisms in place to ensure proper modulation. This includes endogenous inhibitors of the coagulation pathway (Fig. 51.3) that limit coagulation initiation, dilution of procoagulants at the site of injury by flowing blood, and removal and inactivation of activated factors.

Endogenous anticoagulants can either prevent thrombin generation or inactivate formed thrombin. Among endogenous anticoagulants that target thrombin generation, the earliest in the coagulation process is TFPI. TFPI acts by both inactivating factor Xa and the TF-VIIa complex. TFPI is constitutively released by ECs into the microvasculature. Nascent TFPI has direct activity only against Xa, but after exposure to Xa, TFPI acquires activity against the TF-VIIa complex. Notably, C1 esterase inhibitor also inhibits factors early in the coagulation cascade, including factor XIIa and PK, although a deficiency of C1 esterase inhibitor, which causes angioedema, does not result in a hypercoagulable state.

The most important natural anticoagulant is antithrombin (AT), which inactivates several activated factors in the clotting cascade including factors IIa (thrombin), IXa, Xa, XIa and XIIa. AT is physiologically present at more than twice the concentration of the highest local thrombin concentration that can be reached during clotting. AT activity against thrombin is potentiated 1000-fold by endogenous EC-associated heparin sulfate proteoglycans. This is also the mechanism of anticoagulation employed by the anticoagulant medications

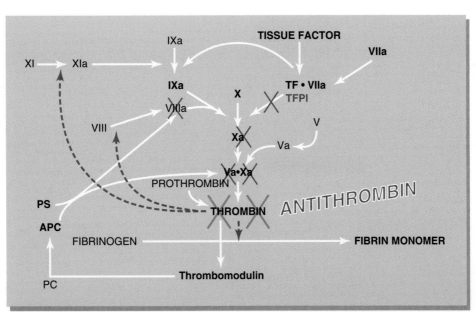

Fig. 51.3 Endogenous anticoagulant pathways. Tissue factor pathway inhibitor (TFPI) shuts off tissue factor (TF) stimulation and blocks the TF-VIIa-X complex; in addition, the clotting cascade is further downregulated by the natural anticoagulants. This inhibition is partly generated by thrombin, which activates thrombomodulin. Circulating antithrombin inhibits thrombin activity and Xa generation of thrombin. The complex of thrombin and thrombomodulin activates protein C (PC) to become activated protein C (APC), which combines with protein S (PS) to cleave and inactivate VIIIa and Va, further blocking thrombin generation.

heparin, low-molecular-weight heparin, and fondaparinux. Platelet surface membranes and platelet factor 4 protect thrombin from inactivation at the clot. However, any thrombin that escapes into the circulation is immediately inhibited by AT, and free thrombin is neutralized instantaneously. Therefore, early thrombin generation is critically dependent on protection by the activated platelet membrane to allow sufficient time to make the transition from initiation to propagation phase. Notably, during the initiation phase, platelet-bound factor Xa is protected from inactivation by both TFPI and AT.

Activated protein C (APC) has anticoagulant, anti-inflammatory, and profibrinolytic properties that make it an important regulator of both thrombosis and inflammation. Like TFPI, protein C becomes activated only after coagulation is underway. Formed thrombin binds to thrombomodulin, a proteoglycan associated with endothelial and monocyte cell surfaces. Thrombomodulin-bound thrombin loses its procoagulant abilities such as activating platelets and fibrin clot formation and instead activates protein C. On the EC surface, nascent protein C binds to EC protein C receptor (EPCR), which positions it for activation by the adjacent thrombomodulin-bound thrombin. In a reaction that is enhanced by EPCR and protein S, APC inactivates factors VIIIa and Va (components of the Xase and prothrombinase complexes, respectively), thereby limiting procoagulant self-amplification. Notably, a common mutation in factor V known as factor V Leiden results in the arginine at position 506 being replaced by glutamine, rendering the mutated factor V resistant to cleavage by APC and resulting in a hypercoagulable state. As with other coagulation factors, the activated platelet membrane protects VIIIa and Va from APC inactivation. In addition to its effects on thrombin generation, APC neutralizes plasminogen activator inhibitor-1 (PAI-1, described further in the fibrinolysis section) to enhance clot remodeling. APC has anti-inflammatory properties as well; recombinant APC reduces production of tumor necrosis factor-α after endotoxin challenge, and protein C–deficient mice exhibit higher levels of proinflammatory cytokines.

Several other molecules have been identified as contributing to antithrombotic effects. As discussed previously, prostacyclin and nitric oxide, both released from ECs, exert antithrombotic properties through vasodilation and inhibition of platelet aggregation and adhesion. Poly(adenosine 5′-diphosphate [ADP]-ribose) polymerase (PARP) protein regulates TF mRNA levels. Activated macrophages and monocytes express TF on their surfaces, and modulating TF mRNA may prevent some degree of thrombosis in the setting of inflammation. Thrombospondin 5 (also known as cartilage oligomeric matrix protein), an extracellular matrix protein, has been shown to inhibit thrombin and thrombin-dependent platelet aggregation in mouse models.

Fibrin Clot Architecture

The architecture of the fibrin clot is surprisingly variable. Although genetic factors unquestionably play a role in determining clot structure, two dominant factors are the local concentrations of thrombin and fibrinogen, whose reactions yield the fibrin strands. A thrombin-rich microenvironment typically results in thinner, more tightly cross-linked fibers, making the overall fibrin clot virtually impermeable to lytic enzymes. In thrombin-poor locations, the fibrin strands are thicker and the structure more porous, making the clot vulnerable to thrombolysis. Similarly, high fibrinogen concentrations are associated with larger thrombi whose tight, rigid meshwork makes them less deformable and more resistant to lysis. Low fibrinogen concentrations produce a less compact clot that is highly lysis prone. As mentioned previously, one of the major roles of polyphosphate on thrombosis is contributing to thicker fibrin fibrils.

Factor XIII plays a critical role in stabilization of the forming clot. Factor XIII circulates in the plasma and is also stored within platelets (see Fig. 51.1B). Notably, 50% of the total fibrin-stabilizing activity in blood resides in the platelet and is released by activation. Thrombin-activated factor XIIIa binds to fibrin and cross-links the fibrin units, thereby rendering them less permeable and more resistant to lysis. Furthermore, factor XIIIa cross-links the major plasmin inhibitor, α2-antiplasmin, directly to fibrin, positioning it for neutralization of any invading plasmin.

Fibrinolysis

The fibrinolytic system (Fig. 51.4) operates to restore patency and prevent fibrin from occluding healthy vessels. During clot formation, factor Xa and thrombin stimulate healthy ECs to release tissue-type plasminogen activator (t-PA) and urokinase-type plasminogen activator (u-PA), both of which activate plasminogen to plasmin. Plasmin then cleaves the fibrin strands of the platelet plug, producing fibrin degradation products, including D-dimer. Additionally, factor XIIIa is also cleaved by plasmin, further destabilizes the platelet plug by reducing fibrin cross-linking.

The vast excess of plasminogen in the plasma dictates that under normal circumstances, the concentrations of t-PA and u-PA comprise the rate-limiting step for plasmin formation. The kinetic efficiency of

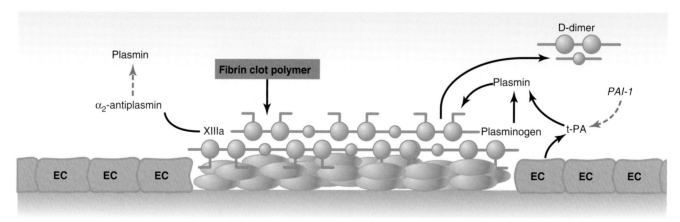

Fig. 51.4 Balanced fibrinolysis limits the platelet-fibrin clot. The platelet plug and fibrin matrices are strengthened by incorporation of factor XIIIa into the fibrin clot. Factor XIIIa also binds α2-antiplasmin to the clot to protect it from plasmin-mediated fibrinolysis. At the same time, nearby intact endothelial cells (ECs) secrete tissue plasminogen activator (t-PA). t-PA that evades plasminogen activator inhibitor-1 (PAI-1) converts clot-bound plasminogen to plasmin and leads to fibrin clot degradation and release of soluble fibrin peptides and D-dimer. Therefore, detection of circulating D-dimer usually indicates active fibrinolysis.

t-PA is improved by at least an order of magnitude in the presence of fibrin. This helps to keep t-PA most active in the microenvironment of the clot. By contrast, u-PA appears to require binding to activated platelets for its ability to liberate plasmin.

Acting to contain fibrinolysis are plasma mediators that either inactivate formed plasmin (e.g., α_2-antiplasmin and possibly α_2-macroglobulin) or block plasmin formation (e.g., PAI-1). α_2-Antiplasmin rapidly inactivates plasmin in plasma but is present in lower concentrations than plasminogen and thus can become depleted while plasmin continues to be formed. Additionally, the α_2-antiplasmin protein cross-links to the fibrin clot providing resistance to cleavage by plasmin. PAI-1 is present in several-fold molar excess in the plasma and is also released by both ECs and activated platelets, thereby protecting clots from premature lysis. Plasma levels of PAI-1 are highly variable due to a circadian pattern of secretion; polymorphisms of the *PAI-1* gene leading to higher PAI-1 levels are associated with a higher risk for thromboembolic disease, whereas rare congenital deficiencies in PAI-1 protein are associated with increased bleeding tendencies.

Another mediator that limits fibrinolysis in the vicinity of the clot is thrombin activator fibrinolysis inhibitor (TAFI). TAFI is synthesized in an inactive form by the liver and circulates in the plasma, possibly in a complex with plasminogen. TAFI cleaves specific fibrin lysine residues that would otherwise promote binding of fibrinolytic enzymes (e.g., plasmin). TAFI requires either plasmin or thrombin for activation; however, thrombin activation of TAFI requires extraordinarily large amounts of free thrombin. By contrast, EC-associated thrombomodulin increases thrombin-induced TAFI activation 1250-fold, making this an essential cofactor and one that is predominantly available only at the interface between the blood and the vessel wall.

In addition to the EC surface, macrophages are also critical to fibrinolysis. Macrophages degrade the fibrin clot through lysosomal proteolysis by a plasmin-independent mechanism. The macrophage binds to fibrin and fibrinogen through its surface integrin receptor, CD11b/18; this binding is followed by internalization of the complex into the lysosome, where fibrin and fibrinogen are degraded.

Tissue repair and regeneration are the physiologic end points of clotting, and they eventually lead to dissolution of the fibrin-based clot. Besides t-PA and u-PA, the intrinsic pathway activators kallikrein, factor XIIa, and factor XIa also generate active plasmin from plasminogen. Plasminogen binding to cell surface receptors promotes its own activation to plasmin by placing it in proximity to t-PA and the fibrin clot and protects plasmin from inactivation by circulating α_2-antiplasmin. Plasmin eventually dissolves the fibrin matrix to produce soluble fibrin peptides and D-dimer and also activates metalloproteinases that further degrade damaged tissue. Fibroblasts and leukocytes migrate into the wound, the latter mediated by selectin binding, and these inflammatory cells act in concert with growth factors secreted by leukocytes and activated platelets to enhance vascular repair and tissue regeneration.

Laboratory Testing of Coagulation

As described previously, for purposes of laboratory testing, the extrinsic pathway of the classical coagulation cascade is measured by the PT, while the intrinsic pathway is measured by the aPTT. The PT is assessed by measuring the interaction of circulating factor VIIa with exogenously added TF (also known as thromboplastin). The PT is highly sensitive to deficiencies in factors II, V, VII, and X, all of which may be associated with bleeding, but is unaffected by deficiencies in intrinsic pathway factors (i.e., factors XII, XI, IX, or VIII).

Because factors II, VII, and X are also vitamin K–dependent factors, with factor VII having the shortest half-life, the PT is also the main lab test used for monitoring warfarin therapy. The degree of prolongation of the PT by warfarin depends on the strength of the particular thromboplastin agent and the specific coagulation instrument used for the assay. A blood test known as the international normalized ratio (INR), calculated by dividing the patient's PT by a mean control PT, takes these factors into account in order to standardize variations among laboratories in PT measurements and is the preferred test for warfarin monitoring.

The aPTT measurement is based on in vitro contact activation (e.g., plasma stimulation with a negatively charged compound such as kaolin). The aPTT is sensitive to deficiencies of factors in the contact (i.e., PK, HMWK, and factor XII), intrinsic (factors XI, IX, and X), and common (factors II, V, and X) pathways but not in the extrinsic pathway (factor VII). As detailed previously, deficiencies of factors VIII, IX, or XI comprise the basis of the congenital hemophilias A, B, and C, respectively, all of which are characterized by bleeding. By contrast, deficiencies of PK, HMWK, and factor XII, while all prolonging the aPTT, do not result in significant bleeding.

The aPTT is also highly sensitive to unfractionated heparin and is used to monitor heparin activity although the therapeutic index of the aPTT in patients on heparin is rather wide owing to natural fluctuations in aPTT measurements. Alternatively, heparin, low-molecular-weight heparin, and fondaparinux activity may be measured via an anti-Xa activity, which assesses the level of inhibition of factor Xa.

In surgical settings, trauma units, and intensive care units, there may be a need for immediate turnaround in coagulation testing. One specific point-of-care test used for real-time coagulation testing is thromboelastography (TEG), a global test of hemostasis. TEG uses whole blood to monitor all components of hemostasis, including the initiation and termination phases of the coagulation cascade, fibrinolysis, and platelet function. TEG has been demonstrated to improve outcomes in trauma by guiding transfusion therapy and may have roles in surgery and in assessing coagulation status in patients with advanced liver disease, although its utility outside of these indications is uncertain.

SUGGESTED READINGS

Büller HR, Bethune C, Bhanot S, et al: Factor XI antisense oligonucleotide for prevention of venous thrombosis, N Engl J Med 372(3):232–240, 2015.

Esmon CT: The protein c pathway, Chest 124(26s), 2003.

Ho K, Pavey W: Applying the cell-based coagulation model in the management of critical bleeding, Anaesth Intensive Care 45(2):166–176, 2017.

Hoffman M, Monroe 3rd DM: A cell-based model of hemostasis, Thromb Haemost 85(6):958–965, 2001.

Manly DA, Boles J, Mackman N: Role of tissue factor in venous thrombosis, Annu Rev Physiol 73:515–525, 2011.

Morrissey JH, Choi SH, Smith SA: Polyphosphate: an ancient molecule that links platelets, coagulation, and inflammation, Blood 119(25):5972–5979, 2012.

Shen J, Sampietro S, Wu J, et al: Coordination of platelet agonist signaling during the hemostatic response in vivo, Blood Adv 1(27):2767–2775, 2017.

52

Disorders of Hemostasis: Bleeding

Aric Parnes

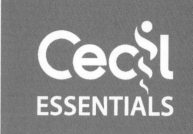

INTRODUCTION

The complex network maintaining a balance between bleeding and clotting functions in fine equilibrium. However, each component of this network can falter. This chapter describes the imbalances that result in bleeding. It covers platelet disorders, vascular abnormalities, and clotting factor deficiencies. In addition to reviewing the pathophysiology and clinical manifestations of these disorders, it covers a general approach to the evaluation of a bleeding patient and how to treat each disease. How the equilibrium shifts to favor coagulation is covered in a separate chapter.

HEMOSTASIS

Hemostasis, the ability to stop bleeding, can be simplified into two phases called primary and secondary hemostasis. However, the reality is more complex than this because primary and secondary hemostasis frequently interact and blend together. Primary hemostasis reflects an initial phase of platelet activation, adhesion, and aggregation with help from von Willebrand factor. Secondary hemostasis involves the coagulation factors activating in a cascade to augment and stabilize clotting. The clotting cascade is explained in more detail in Chapter 51. To initiate bleeding, the integrity of the endothelium is disrupted most commonly by trauma or surgery but sometimes through a vascular defect. Regardless of the inciting event, collagen and other platelet activators are released from endothelial tissue triggering primary hemostasis, whereas the release of tissue factor activates the clotting cascade.

CLINICAL EVALUATION OF BLEEDING

The evaluation of bleeding requires a careful history and physical examination. The history includes the details of the current bleeding event as well as past bleeding events. Spontaneous bleeding without a traumatic event points to a severe defect in hemostasis. Lifelong recurring bleeding events and a family history of such suggest congenital disease whereas new bleeding despite previous "hemostatic stress tests" such as surgery or dental extraction without bleeding favor an acquired disorder or a medication effect. Disorders of primary hemostasis including causes of thrombocytopenia or platelet dysfunction or diseases of von Willebrand factor lead to mucocutaneous superficial bleeding, but disorders of secondary hemostasis with missing coagulation factors cause deeper bleeding, for example muscle hematomas, hemarthroses, and intracranial hemorrhages. Superficial bleeding can be easy bruising, gum bleeding when brushing teeth, frequent epistaxis, and heavy menstrual bleeding. When uncovering family history, distinguishing between X-linked genetic disease (e.g., hemophilia A and B) and autosomal disease, such as most von Willebrand disease cases, can be vital. The X-linked inheritance pattern for hemophilia A and B

means that more severe disease manifests in males than in females and subsequently may appear to skip generations.

Similar distinctions appear in the physical examination. Hemarthroses result in joint swelling, tenderness, and moderate warmth, and multiple joint hemorrhages cause arthritis and deformity. Without imaging or laboratory tests, hemarthrosis can be indistinguishable from septic arthritis or other causes of joint pain. Platelet disorders classically result in petechiae, small subcutaneous hemorrhages that typically appear on the legs, a result of gravity dependence. Sometimes vascular anomalies can be seen on physical examination. For example, small ectatic vessels, prone to bleeding, can be seen on oral mucosa in hereditary hemorrhagic telangiectasia.

Liver disease can cause bleeding through a decline in production of coagulation factors and a decline in platelet count, due to hypersplenism and decreased thrombopoietin production by the liver. Hallmark features of liver disease can be obvious on examination, such as jaundice and abdominal distension from ascites, but can be overlooked if not searched for. This includes spider angioma, gynecomastia, Dupuytren contracture, and asterixis.

Rare causes of aplastic anemia can be determined by physical examination. Fanconi anemia patients have short stature, café au lait spots, hypoplastic thenar eminences, and absent radii. Dyskeratosis congenita, a disease of short telomeres, leads to leukoplakia, nail dystrophy, and hyperpigmented macules.

Importantly, the timing of a thorough examination and subsequent laboratory testing must be tempered in order to control rapid bleeding and hemodynamic instability. Airway, breathing, and circulation, the A-B-C's, take precedence in emergency situations, and recognizing that bleeding can evolve quickly is critical. Life-threatening hemorrhage requires immediate treatment while simultaneously pursuing diagnostic testing. Life-threatening blood loss is not limited to trauma or gastrointestinal sites but also includes small bleeds near the airway or neck and hemorrhages around other vital organs. Heart rate and blood pressure are first steps in assessing volume of blood loss.

LABORATORY EVALUATION OF BLEEDING

The initial laboratory assessment of the bleeding patient (Table 52.1) should include complete blood cell counts (CBC), prothrombin time (PT), activated partial thromboplastin time (aPTT), and fibrinogen (Fig. 52.1). The CBC marks a critical first step in this evaluation because it includes the platelet count as well as hemoglobin and hematocrit, which are essential for monitoring the rate of blood loss (as are vital signs). The CBC also contains the mean corpuscular volume (MCV), measuring the size of the red blood cell. A low MCV can suggest a slower chronic blood loss resulting in iron deficiency. A peripheral blood smear should be examined to confirm thrombocytopenia. Pseudothrombocytopenia occurs when platelets clump from EDTA

TABLE 52.1 Screening Assays for Hemostasis

Laboratory Test	Aspect of Hemostasis Tested	Causes of Abnormalities
Blood counts (CBC) and peripheral blood smear	Platelet count and morphologic features	Thrombocytopenia, thrombocytosis, gray platelet and giant platelet syndromes
Prothrombin time (PT)	Factor VII–dependent pathways	Vitamin K deficiency and warfarin, liver disease, DIC, factor deficiency (VII, V, X, II), factor inhibitor
Partial thromboplastin time (aPTT)	Factor XI–, IX–, and VIII–dependent pathways	Heparin, DIC, lupus anticoagulant[a], VWD, factor deficiency (XII[a], XI, IX, VIII, V, X, II), factor inhibitor
Thrombin time	Fibrinogen	Heparin, hypofibrinogenemia, dysfibrinogenemia, DIC
Platelet aggregation and platelet function analysis	Platelet and VWF function	Aspirin, VWD, storage pool disease
Mixing study	Factor inhibitors or deficiencies	Abnormal clotting time corrects for a factor deficiency; does not correct for an inhibitor

DIC, Disseminated intravascular coagulation; VWD, von Willebrand disease; VWF, von Willebrand factor.
[a]Lupus anticoagulant and factor XII deficiency are not associated with bleeding.

antibodies and are then read as white blood cells instead of platelets by automated counters. Other helpful findings on a peripheral blood smear include schistocytes, suggesting microangiopathic hemolytic anemia. Teardrop cells with immature white and red blood cells characterize the myelophthisic blood smear, indicative of marrow replacement by solid tumor, lymphoma, granuloma, or fibrosis.

PT and aPTT are two commonly used broad measures of the coagulation cascade. PT assesses the extrinsic and common pathways, that is clotting factors, in order of activation: VII, X, V, II, and fibrinogen. aPTT covers the intrinsic and common pathways: Clotting factors XII, XI, IX, VIII, X, V, II, and fibrinogen. Both PT and aPTT become abnormal with deficiencies of the common pathway (X, V, II, and fibrinogen) or multiple clotting factor deficiencies involving both the intrinsic and extrinsic pathways. The International Normalized Ratio (INR) represents a standardized correlate of PT so that measurements of vitamin K–dependent anticoagulation can be compared despite interlaboratory variation. Abnormal PT and aPTT should be repeated to verify the elevation was not in error. Specific factor deficiencies may be suspected based on elevations in PT or aPTT and these factor activities can be tested to confirm the diagnosis and monitor effects of treatment.

Factor deficiencies can be congenital (e.g., hemophilia A) or acquired (e.g., acquired hemophilia, liver disease, disseminated intravascular coagulopathy [DIC]). A mixing study can distinguish a factor deficiency resulting from a decline in production from a decline due to inhibition from an autoantibody. Mixing studies combine patient plasma with control plasma so that missing factors are replaced and the abnormal clotting times correct (i.e., prolonged PT or PTT becomes normal). A positive mixing study does not correct because of the presence of an inhibitor, blocking the factor from the normal control plasma. Mixing studies can also be useful in finding a lupus anticoagulant, which is important for the diagnosis of antiphospholipid syndrome (see Chapter 53), but a lupus anticoagulant does not affect bleeding and should not be in the differential diagnosis of the bleeding patient.

Fibrinogen can be decreased through a decline in production or consumption, as in DIC. The assay is an easy, rapid, and cheap test to run and should be run early in the evaluation of the bleeding patient. Many fibrinogen assays incorporate function into the quantitative measurement, but since this information may not be readily available, thrombin time is able to measure the function of fibrinogen by adding thrombin to plasma and then measuring the conversion of fibrinogen to fibrin.

Similarly, platelet function may be helpful if a defect in primary hemostasis is suspected, but platelet count and von Willebrand factor testing are normal. Platelet dysfunction disorders can be induced by

many different medications, although they are often not clinically significant and rarely are congenital. Platelet function can be assessed by platelet aggregation studies or Platelet Function Analyzer-100 (PFA-100; Fig. 52.2), which both use platelet activators to trigger platelet activation and aggregation. Different platelet activators such as adenosine diphosphate (ADP), collagen, epinephrine, and ristocetin may detect subtle differences in platelet function. These tests, not surprisingly, fail to work when platelets are absent or low. Bleeding time, a test measuring the time it takes to stop bleeding after making a small incision in the forearm as a gauge of platelet function, should no longer be performed because numerous studies have shown poor sensitivity, specificity, and reproducibility with significant technician variability.

Testing for von Willebrand disease (VWD) is as complicated as the disease, which has multiple subtypes, each with different means of diagnosing. A typical von Willebrand factor (VWF) panel includes VWF activity (a functional test measured by ristocetin-mediated binding of VWF to platelets, VWF antigen (the quantitative level), and clotting factor VIII, which declines without the presence of its stabilizer, VWF. Other tests that may be required to determine the subtype of VWD include VWF multimer analysis, VWF-factor VIII binding assay, and a measure of platelet aggregation as induced by ristocetin (RIPA). As with any congenital disorder, gene sequencing may be the only way to confirm the diagnosis, but it adds time and expense and is frequently normal in mild cases of VWD.

Additional laboratory tests useful in evaluating bleeding include factor Xa activity for measurement of low-molecular-weight heparin effect, heparin neutralization (with heparinase, hexadimethrine bromide [Polybrene], or protamine), and euglobulin clot lysis time as a measure of fibrinolysis, the time to dissolve a fibrin clot. Currently, the new class of anticoagulants, direct oral anticoagulants (DOACs), do not have readily available methods for measurement of plasma concentrations or activity. Because vitamin C deficiency (scurvy) can cause bleeding, measuring ascorbic acid can be helpful when nutrient deficiency is suspected. Thromboelastography (TEG) and rotational thromboelastometry (ROTEM) use torque to measure clotting of whole blood. These methods have many proponents but remain investigational. A rapid approach to identifying possible causes of bleeding (Fig. 52.3) considers several major disease categories: (1) VWD, thrombocytopenia, or abnormal platelet function; (2) low levels of multiple coagulation factors resulting from vitamin K deficiency, liver disease, or DIC; (3) single-factor deficiency (usually inherited); and, more rarely, (4) an acquired inhibitor to a coagulation factor such as factor VIII. The laboratory evaluation is most efficient when it is performed in this context.

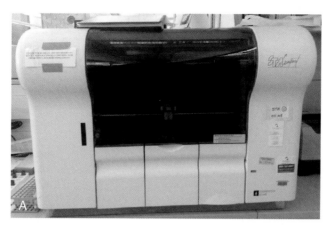

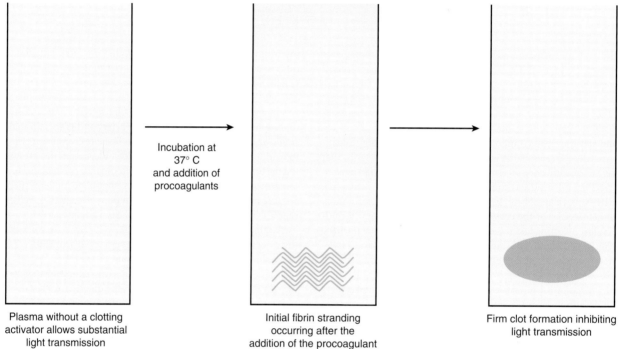

Incubation at
37° C
and addition of
procoagulants

Plasma without a clotting
activator allows substantial
light transmission

Initial fibrin stranding
occurring after the
addition of the procoagulant

Firm clot formation inhibiting
light transmission

B

Fig. 52.1 Basic methodology underlying measurement of prothrombin (PT) and activated partial thrombo-plastin time (aPTT). (A) Typical laboratory instrument used to perform basic and complex coagulation assays. (B) Plasma specimens are incubated at 37° C and then mixed with tissue factor and phospholipid (PT) or a surface activator and phospholipid (aPTT). The time it takes for clot formation to block light passage through the specimen is measured and compared with a reference range. Prolongation of the PT or aPTT clotting time can be associated with many congenital or acquired coagulation factor defects. Abnormal PT or aPTT values are typically followed by more specific coagulation factor assays, depending on the type of prolongation and the suspected underlying clinical disease.

BLEEDING CAUSED BY VASCULAR DISORDERS

Vascular purpura (i.e., bruising) is defined as bleeding caused by intrinsic structural abnormalities of blood vessels or by inflammatory infiltration of blood vessels (i.e., vasculitis). Although vascular purpura usually causes bleeding in the setting of normal platelet counts and normal coagulation tests, vasculitis and vessel damage may be severe enough to cause secondary consumption of platelets and coagulation factors.

Collagen breakdown and thinning of the subcutaneous tissue that overlies blood vessels is often observed in older patients (i.e., senile purpura), and similar atrophic skin changes are a common effect of steroid therapy. Another acquired cause of vascular purpura is scurvy (i.e.,

deficiency of vitamin C [ascorbic acid]). Patients with scurvy have bleeding around individual hair fibers (i.e., perifollicular hemorrhage) and corkscrew-shaped hair. Bruising occurs in a classic saddle pattern over the upper thighs. The bleeding gums are caused by gingivitis and not by the subcutaneous tissue defect. Edentulous patients with scurvy do not have bleeding gums, and scurvy should not be excluded on this basis.

Congenital defects of the vessel wall can cause bruising. These rare syndromes include pseudoxanthoma elasticum, a defect of the elastic fibers of the vasculature associated with severe gastrointestinal (GI) and genitourinary bleeding, and Ehlers-Danlos syndrome, which is characterized by abnormal collagen in blood vessels and subcutaneous tissue. Both syndromes cause bruising in the skin, but only patients with pseudoxanthoma elasticum develop significant GI bleeding.

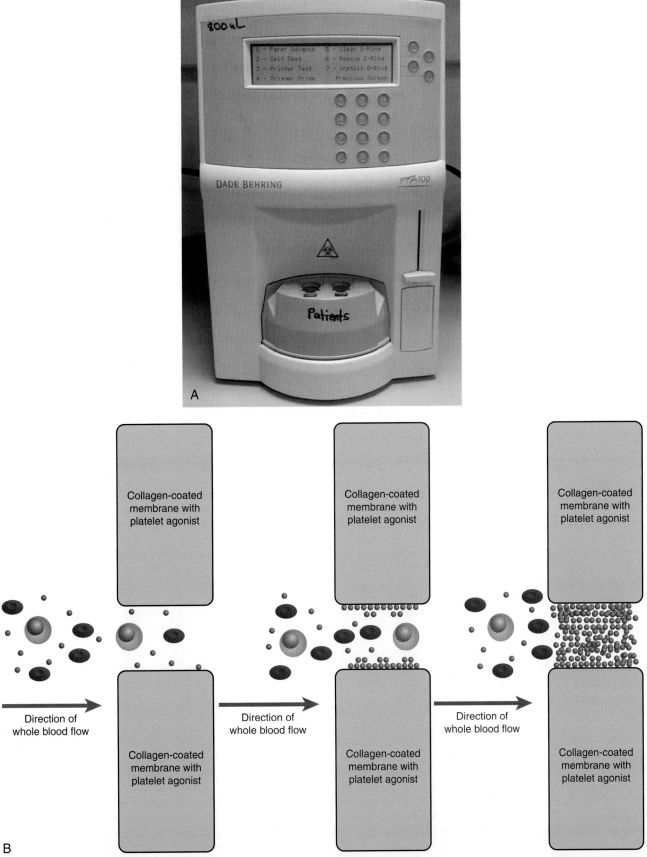

Fig. 52.2 Methodology underlying the Platelet Function Analyzer-100 (PFA-100). (A) Whole blood platelets are streamed toward a collagen-based aperture. The membrane is infused with a potent platelet agonist (i.e., adenosine diphosphate or epinephrine). (B) Streaming the platelets through the instrument channels induces shear-based activation, which in conjunction with the agonists should yield an initial wave of platelet adhesion and aggregation. Over time, activated platelets continue to aggregate, closing off the aperture to whole blood flow. The time it takes for aperture closing is measured in seconds and compared with a reference range. Abnormally prolonged closure times can be associated with von Willebrand disease due to the reliance on adhesion in this assay or with a platelet functional defect due to the reliance on aggregation for complete aperture closure.

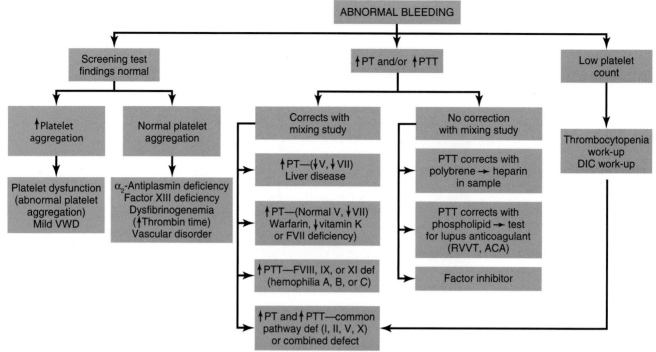

Fig. 52.3 Algorithm for the evaluation of bleeding. Screening laboratory tests for platelet and factor deficiencies are used to narrow the work-up for bleeding, followed by specific factor and other coagulation studies (e.g., mixing studies, D-dimer) to confirm the diagnosis. *ACA*, Anticardiolipin antibody; *DIC*, disseminated intravascular coagulation; *FVIII*, factor VIII; *PFA-100*, Platelet Function Analyzer-100; *PT*, prothrombin time; *PTT*, partial thromboplastin time; *RVVT*, Russell viper venom time; *VWD*, von Willebrand disease; *↑*, increased; *↓*, decreased.

Another inherited vessel wall defect associated with GI bleeding is hereditary hemorrhagic telangiectasia (Osler-Weber-Rendu syndrome). This disorder is characterized by degeneration of the blood vessel wall that results in angiomatous lesions resembling blood blisters on mucous membranes, including the lips and GI tract. The frequency of bleeding caused by breakdown of these lesions increases with age, and GI lesions commonly cause significant chronic bleeding, resulting in iron deficiency anemia.

The sudden onset of palpable purpura (i.e., localized, raised hemorrhages in the skin) associated with rash and fever may be caused by aseptic or septic vasculitis. Septic vasculitis can be caused by meningococcemia and other bacterial infections and is often accompanied by thrombocytopenia and prolongation of clotting times. One cause of aseptic vasculitis in young children and adolescents is Henoch-Schönlein purpura, a vasculitis of the skin, GI tract, and kidneys that is usually accompanied by abdominal pain from bleeding into the bowel wall. This syndrome may occur after a viral prodrome and appears to be caused by an immunoglobulin A (IgA) hypersensitivity reaction, as evidenced by serum IgA immune complexes and renal histopathologic features resembling IgA nephropathy.

The therapy for bleeding from vascular disorders depends upon the diagnosis. Senile purpura and steroid-induced purpura do not usually require treatment. Scurvy is corrected by vitamin C supplementation. In congenital disorders, including Ehlers-Danlos syndrome, hereditary hemorrhagic telangiectasia, and pseudoxanthoma elasticum, patients should avoid medications (e.g., aspirin) that may aggravate their bleeding tendencies, and they should receive supportive therapy (e.g., iron supplementation, red blood cell transfusion). Systemic administration of estrogen to patients with hereditary hemorrhagic telangiectasia may

help to decrease epistaxis by inducing squamous metaplasia of the nasal mucosa, which protects lesions from trauma.

Treatment of septic vasculitis focuses on appropriate antibiotic therapy. In the case of aseptic vasculitis, steroids and immunosuppressive agents are most effective. When vasculitis is severe enough to cause consumption of platelets and coagulation factors (see section on disseminated intravascular coagulation), transfusions of platelets, cryoprecipitate, and fresh-frozen plasma (FFP) may be indicated.

BLEEDING CAUSED BY THROMBOCYTOPENIA

With thrombocytopenia, bleeding does not occur until platelets are less than 20,000/μL unless platelet dysfunction accompanies the thrombocytopenia as it frequently does in myelodysplastic syndromes or when aspirin or nonsteroidal anti-inflammatory drugs have been used (Fig. 52.4). Platelets less than 100,000/μL can be problematic after trauma or during surgery. Since most patients do not bleed from mild thrombocytopenia (50,000 to 150,000/μL), treatment is often not required, but thrombocytopenia should be investigated to determine the cause, expected trajectory, and a plan for when treatment is needed. Broadly, thrombocytopenia results from a decline in platelet production, hypersplenism/sequestration, or destruction/consumption. However, determining which category to focus attention on can be challenging. Bone marrow biopsy can help because megakaryocyte hyperplasia implies increased production, a means of compensating for peripheral platelet destruction, whereas megakaryocyte hypoplasia suggests decreased platelet production. Still, bone marrow biopsy is often unnecessary in the evaluation. Hypersplenism is usually associated with an enlarged spleen, but splenic overactivity can be seen when the spleen is normal

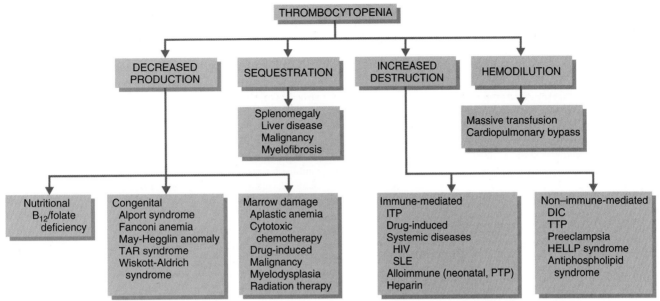

Fig. 52.4 Differential diagnosis of thrombocytopenia. Disorders resulting in a decreased circulating platelet number can be classified by four main pathophysiologic mechanisms: hypoproduction, sequestration, peripheral destruction, and hemodilution. The history, physical examination, and bone marrow evaluation usually narrow the range of possible causes. *DIC,* Disseminated intravascular coagulation; *HELLP,* hemolysis, elevated liver enzymes, and low-platelet count in association with pregnancy; *HIV,* human immunodeficiency virus; *ITP,* immune thrombocytopenic purpura; *PTP,* post-transfusion purpura; *SLE,* systemic lupus erythematosus; *TAR,* thrombocytopenia-absent radius syndrome; *TTP,* thrombotic thrombocytopenic purpura.

in size, as it is in immune thrombocytopenic purpura. Conversely, not all enlarged spleens are associated with hypersplenism (see Fig. 52.4).

Decreased Marrow Production of Platelets

Decreased production of platelets in the bone marrow is characterized by decreased or absent megakaryocytes on the bone marrow aspirate and biopsy. Suppression of normal megakaryopoiesis occurs after marrow damage and destruction of stem cells (such as occurs with cytotoxic chemotherapy); destruction of the normal marrow micro-environment and replacement of normal stem cells by invasive malignant disease, aplasia, infection (e.g., miliary tuberculosis), or myelofibrosis; specific but rare intrinsic defects of the megakaryocytic stem cells; and metabolic abnormalities affecting megakaryocyte maturation.

Drug-Associated Thrombocytopenia

Many drugs cause immune-mediated thrombocytopenia. However, some can have a direct cytotoxic effect on stem cells and megakaryocytes, causing a decline in platelet production. The classic example of this is cytotoxic chemotherapy used to treat malignancies. These medications are used to stop malignant cells from dividing, but they have the same effect on nonmalignant proliferating cells such as in the bone marrow. This myelosuppression frequently results in thrombocytopenia as well as neutropenia and anemia. Other drugs including thiazide diuretics and alcohol can have similar effects. Diagnostic confirmation comes from recovery of platelets after withdrawal of the medication. Recovery usually occurs within 7 days but can take several weeks. After repeated injury, stem cells may not recover, resulting in chronic thrombocytopenia.

Nutrition-Associated Thrombocytopenia

Deficiencies in copper, folate, and vitamin B12 can cause thrombocytopenia. However, they typically will cause other cytopenias prior to

affecting platelet production. Megaloblastic anemia refers to the effects of impaired DNA synthesis on bone marrow causing dyssynchrony between slowed maturation of the nucleus and continued maturation of cytoplasm with unimpaired protein synthesis. This process results in large erythroid precursors called megaloblasts and mature large red blood cells (macrocytes). Certain medications can have this effect: azathioprine, 5-fluorouracil, methotrexate, and others. Folate and vitamin B12 deficiencies are classic causes of megaloblastic anemia and when severe can cause pancytopenia. These deficiencies are most commonly caused by poor absorption either from autoimmune interference of intrinsic factor (pernicious anemia), other causes of atrophic gastritis, celiac disease, or previous gastrointestinal surgery. Less commonly, folate and vitamin B12 deficiency arise from a poor diet (e.g., strict vegans and alcoholics), an inherited defect in transcobalamin, or competition for vitamin B12 absorption from *Diphyllobothrium latum* parasitic infection.

Copper deficiency causes leukopenia and anemia before affecting platelet production. It occurs in two settings, first through malabsorption from celiac disease and past bowel surgeries, and second, through copper transport blockage from zinc excess. Zinc levels should be tested when copper is found to be low. Zinc excess occurs from zinc-containing denture cream and improper use of zinc supplements.

Bone Marrow Invasion

When the bone marrow is replaced by non-marrow elements, space for hematopoiesis becomes limited. In addition, the microenvironment necessary to supply proper nutrients, growth factors, and neuroendocrine stimulation is damaged. The prototypic disease of marrow invasion is myelofibrosis, either primary (a chronic myeloproliferative disease) or secondary, from other myeloproliferative disease (polycythemia vera, essential thrombocythemia), hematologic malignancy, autoimmune disease, or infection. Rarely, myelofibrosis is associated with systemic mastocytosis and osteogenesis imperfecta. In myelofibrosis, the marrow is replaced by fibrotic strands causing immature erythroid (nucleated red blood cells) and myeloid cells ("left-shift") to enter the peripheral blood stream. In addition, red blood cells become deformed (teardrop cells) as they squeeze between narrow spaces. This combination of teardrop cells and immature blood cells is called the myelophthisic blood smear. It can be seen when bone marrow is replaced by fibrotic tissue, malignant cells, or granuloma from sarcoidosis or tuberculosis. Confirmation of marrow invasion requires a bone marrow biopsy.

Myelodysplastic Syndrome

Myelodysplastic syndrome (MDS) (see also Chapter 47) is a clonal stem cell disorder resulting in ineffective hematopoiesis and cytopenias, either unilineage or multilineage. The diagnosis requires a bone marrow biopsy. Dysplasia (abnormal appearing cells) in the bone marrow and cytopenias fulfill the criteria for diagnosis. Subtypes depend on the number of blasts present in the bone marrow (must be <20%), the number of involved lineages, and the presence or absence of ringed sideroblasts, a nucleated erythroid cell with iron-laden mitochondria surrounding the nucleus (requires iron stain to see). The cytopenias tend to progress slowly, over months to years. MDS causes infection through neutropenia, symptoms of anemia, and easy bleeding/bruising from thrombocytopenia. It is also a precursor to acute myelogenous leukemia (AML).

Prior to the advent of next-generation sequencing (NGS), proving clonality in MDS was challenging because about one third of cases have normal cytogenetics. Now, NGS has become a routine part of the diagnostic evaluation and provides prognostic information as well as occasionally targetable mutations for treatment. RUNX1 is a transcription factor that leads to upregulation of the thrombopoietin receptor. When RUNX1 has a pathologic mutation as part of MDS or leukemia, patients become thrombocytopenic.

Recent studies have found MDS-associated mutations in people with normal blood counts. These mutations, for example DNMT3A, TET2, and ASXL1 among others, confer an increased risk for MDS/AML (and cardiac disease). The state of having MDS-associated mutations but normal blood counts is called clonal hematopoiesis of indeterminate potential (CHIP). Gene sequencing data are rapidly being incorporated into the pathogenesis, diagnosis, and treatment of MDS and other hematologic malignancies.

Other Hematologic Malignancies

Any hematologic malignancy can cause thrombocytopenia through marrow invasion, particularly common in acute leukemias and aggressive lymphomas. Chronic lymphocytic leukemia (CLL) progresses slowly, eventually causing thrombocytopenia from marrow invasion (defined as Rai stage IV). Additionally, CLL at any stage can cause thrombocytopenia through immune-mediated platelet destruction.

Aplastic Anemia

Aplastic anemia can cause severe pancytopenia and occurs when the bone marrow hematopoietic elements are replaced by adipose cells. The diagnosis requires a bone marrow biopsy to show decreased cellularity (hypoplasia). Once the diagnosis is established, the cause for marrow failure must be explored. Aplastic anemia can be caused by congenital or acquired diseases. Congenital causes include Fanconi anemia (mutations in the *FANC* gene leading to chromosomal instability), dyskeratosis congenital (mutations in the telomerase complex leading to short telomeres), Shwachman-Diamond syndrome

(mutation on the *SBDS* gene leading to ribosomal dysfunction), and amegakaryocytic thrombocytopenia (mutations in the thrombopoietin or thrombopoietin receptor c-mpl genes).

Acquired causes of aplastic anemia include medication effects such as chloramphenicol, sulfa, antithyroid medications, gold, allopurinol, and chemotherapy; infections such as hepatitis, HIV, and Epstein-Barr virus (EBV); and paroxysmal nocturnal hemoglobinuria (PNH). PNH is due to an acquired mutation in the gene *PIG-A*, which provides a protective coating around red blood cells (CD55 and CD59). CD55 and CD59 prevent complement from binding and hemolyzing red blood cells. When they are absent as in PNH, patients develop chronic hemolysis, causing the dark urine that accumulates overnight, thus the name nocturnal hemoglobinuria. PNH patients frequently develop aplastic anemia (see Chapter 46).

Aplastic anemia is treated with supportive transfusions of red blood cells and platelets as needed, immunosuppression (anti thymocyte globulin and cyclosporine), platelet growth factors (eltrombopag), and sometimes stem cell transplant. Interestingly, the platelet growth factor eltrombopag increases white blood cells and red blood cells as well as platelets, because thrombopoietin receptors are also on stem cells.

Other congenital diseases causing thrombocytopenia will be discussed in the later sections on platelet dysfunction.

Platelet Sequestration

Up to 30% of circulating platelets are normally sequestered within the spleen at any time. Thrombocytopenia due to sequestration is common when the spleen is enlarged as in advanced liver disease. Platelets continue to decline the larger the spleen becomes. Rarely are platelets less than 50,000/μL. Besides chronic liver disease, splenic lymphomas, chronic myelogenous leukemia and other myeloproliferative diseases, hemoglobinopathies, and Gaucher's disease, an inherited glycolipid storage disease, can cause splenomegaly with cytopenias.

The diagnosis of platelet sequestration may be suspected by physical examination findings or imaging studies demonstrating splenomegaly. Bone marrow studies typically reveal normal megakaryocyte numbers and morphology. Given the lack of specific tests for platelet sequestration, the diagnosis often is one of exclusion of other causes of thrombocytopenia.

Treatment of thrombocytopenia due to splenomegaly frequently depends on the underlying cause of increased spleen size. Splenectomy immediately resolves the thrombocytopenia when the thrombocytopenia is caused by hypersplenism. However, this must be weighed against the potential complications of surgery, an increased risk of thrombosis, and a lifelong increased risk of infection.

Platelet Destruction

Platelets can be removed from circulation by various means. One common process is through an immune mechanism, where antibodies target platelets, either from autoimmune disease (e.g., immune thrombocytopenic purpura [ITP]) or a drug effect. Another manner of platelet destruction is by consumption, for instance the rapid dissipation of platelets in DIC or hemophagocytic lymphohistiocytosis (HLH).

Immune-Mediated Platelet Destruction

Immune platelet destruction typically refers to antibody-mediated clearance. Platelet destruction can be further divided into autoimmune forms (i.e., antibody against self-antigens) and alloimmune forms (i.e., antibody against nonself-antigens). Autoimmune thrombocytopenia is the most commonly encountered form of immune-mediated platelet destruction. It may be a primary disorder directed only at platelets or a secondary complication of another autoimmune disease, such as systemic lupus erythematosus (SLE). Alloimmune-mediated platelet destruction is rare and encountered in neonates as a result of maternal antibodies formed against fetal platelet antigens or in chronically transfused individuals, who form alloantibodies against foreign platelet antigens.

In autoimmune and alloimmune thrombocytopenia, immune platelet destruction is caused by increased levels of polyclonal antiplatelet antibodies directed against platelet membrane glycoprotein receptors, most often cryptic neoepitopes of glycoprotein IIb/IIIa (GPIIb/IIIa) and less commonly glycoprotein Ib (GPIb) or human leukocyte antigens (HLAs). Coating of the platelet with these antibodies leads to opsonization of platelets by Fc receptors on macrophages in the reticuloendothelial system (RES). Antibody-coated platelets are cleared by the spleen and, to a lesser extent, by the liver.

These disorders involve a dramatic increase in marrow platelet production reflected by increased numbers of marrow megakaryocytes. The younger platelets produced have relatively high granule contents, providing increased hemostatic function. Bone marrow examination for increased or normal megakaryocyte numbers can help distinguish platelet destruction from decreased production.

Thrombocytopenia resulting from immune clearance may be severe, and platelet survival is often reduced from the normal 7 to 10 days to less than 1 day. Despite severe thrombocytopenia, serious bleeding or hemorrhagic death is uncommon, partly because the function of young platelets is increased and partly because the number of circulating platelets required to maintain vascular integrity is relatively low, estimated at 7100/µL per day.

Immune thrombocytopenic purpura. Autoimmune destruction of platelets is referred to as ITP. This can be primary or secondary to other autoimmune diseases (e.g., SLE), hematologic malignancy (especially CLL), or infections, mostly viral. ITP in children is self-limiting in more than 80% of cases and they often recover without treatment. In adults, however, it frequently remains a chronic relapsing and remitting disease. Presentations in children and adults are the same with petechiae on examination and mucocutaneous bleeding. Platelet count is varied but can be extremely low, frequently less than 10,000/µL and occasionally below the limit of detection. Blood blisters in the mouth (wet purpura) may carry a higher risk for life-threatening hemorrhage such as in the central nervous system and warrant rapid intervention. Hemorrhagic deaths are rare in children (<2%), but mortality is higher if the ITP is chronic. Fatal hemorrhage in adults is approximately 5%.

A characteristic feature of ITP is that the other cell lines are intact, so that only the platelets are affected. There are two caveats to this rule. First, bleeding patients can become anemic, and second, ITP can overlap with warm autoimmune hemolytic anemia (AIHA). When ITP occurs in conjunction with AIHA, the disease is called Evans syndrome and tends to be more resistant to treatment. The confirmatory test for the warm autoimmune hemolytic component is a direct antiglobulin Coombs test, which adds anti-IgG and anti-C3 sera to the patient's serum. The added antibodies bind to the autoantibodies, which are bound to the red blood cells, causing the red blood cells to agglutinate. The agglutination, the mark of a positive test, can be visualized in a test tube.

Besides the Coombs test for Evans syndrome, there is no confirmatory test for ITP, making it a diagnosis of exclusion. Antiplatelet antibody testing has poor sensitivity and specificity and should not factor into treatment decision making, so its diagnostic role is doubtful. Similarly, mean platelet volume (MPV) tends to be increased in ITP because younger platelets are larger, but MPV lacks sensitivity and specificity and cannot be relied upon. Revealing increased megakaryocytes as the bone marrow tries to compensate for the peripheral platelet destruction, bone marrow biopsy can be helpful, particularly

in unclear cases, but is not usually necessary. More often, confirmation of the diagnosis of ITP stands in its response to treatment.

ITP can be associated with HIV and hepatitis. It can also be the presenting manifestation of SLE. Patients should be screened for these diseases and treated if any are present because treating the underlying disease will also help control the ITP.

Therapy for ITP starts with corticosteroids, although treatment is not necessary if platelets are stable above 20 to 50,000/µL. A recent randomized control trial found faster time to response and more complete responses when using pulse dexamethasone 40 mg daily for 4 days repeated in monthly cycles compared to a prolonged taper of prednisone. An added benefit was decreasing the total long-term exposure to steroids, which comes with many complications including weight gain, infection, and osteoporosis. Response rates were high, but so were relapses. In patients who relapse, repeating cycles of dexamethasone may help, but additional therapeutic options are often necessary. Intravenous immunoglobulins (IVIG) 1 g/kg daily for 1 to 2 days or 400 mg/kg daily for 5 days are two common regimens used as first-line therapy with or without corticosteroids. Its response rates are similar to corticosteroids and it works by mopping up the autoantibody as well as blocking the Fc receptors on splenic macrophages. The order of second-line therapy for ITP is unclear and controversial. Splenectomy, with response rates of approximately 50%, offers a potential cure, but patients frequently opt for noninvasive approaches. Relapses after splenectomy warrant a search for an accessory spleen missed during surgery.

Rituximab is a chimeric monoclonal antibody that targets CD20, a B-cell antigen, thus working by decreasing the autoantibody production. It is given by intravenous infusion, weekly for 4 weeks. Response rates are around 60% but can take weeks to work and relapses often occur after 1 year. Hypersensitivity infusion reactions are common with rituximab. Infection, though rare, is also a concern. Thrombomimetics are a newer class with high efficacy. They work as thrombopoietin agonists and come as a subcutaneous injectable called romiplostim, given in weekly doses, or an oral agent called eltrombopag, mentioned previously as a treatment for aplastic anemia. The newest therapeutic option in ITP is fostamatinib, a small molecule Syk inhibitor, preventing macrophage binding to opsonized platelets, thus decreasing platelet consumption without affecting autoantibody production, similar to one of the mechanisms of IVIG. All of these newer targeted therapies are expensive, so patients need to be intolerant to or have failed steroids before using them.

There are many other treatment options that have been used with moderate success. Anti-Rh(D) immunoglobulin can be used to saturate Fc receptors on splenic macrophages, preventing these cells from consuming platelets. There is probably competitive inhibition and blockade of the mononuclear phagocytic system/RES by sensitized red blood cells in the spleen. However, this only works if patients are blood type Rh(D)+, still have their spleen, and do not have concomitant hemolytic anemia. Danazol, azathioprine, mycophenolate, cyclosporine, and cyclophosphamide can regulate autoimmunity. Platelet transfusions are necessary in bleeding patients even though the transfused platelets will be destroyed along with the endogenous platelets. Platelet transfusions should be continued until bleeding stops.

Drug-induced platelet destruction. Immune-mediated platelet destruction associated with specific drugs is an often overlooked cause of thrombocytopenia. Unlike some of the drugs mentioned earlier (e.g., chemotherapeutic agents) that act by directly suppressing megakaryocyte production, drugs in this category of thrombocytopenia induce an immune response against platelet antigens.

Drugs may induce an autoimmune response by several mechanisms. One is the development of an antibody response against soluble drug molecules. When soluble drugs bind to the platelet membrane, drug-induced antibodies act to destroy circulating platelets through the RES. Other mechanisms of drug-induced thrombocytopenia include formation of an immunogenic neoantigen through drug-platelet interactions (hapten response) with autoantibodies against drugs cross-reacting with platelet antigens. Occasionally, immune complexes that include the drug and circulating platelets are formed.

Historically, quinidine or quinine-based formulations were among the first class of drugs to be associated with platelet antibodies. The antibodies can be detected by tests using a drug coupled to a carrier protein. As awareness of drug-induced thrombocytopenia has grown, scores of drugs, including antibiotics, anticonvulsants, psychotropic drugs, and antiplatelet agents, have been reported to mediate platelet destruction (Table 52.2).

Heparin also induces thrombocytopenia, but unlike other drugs, this reaction paradoxically leads to a prothrombotic state referred to as heparin-induced thrombocytopenia (HIT) syndrome. The mechanism of heparin-induced thrombocytopenia and its prothrombotic effects are discussed in greater detail in Chapter 53.

When eliciting the medical history from patients with acute-onset thrombocytopenia, a careful review of all medications, particularly those initiated just before the development of low platelet counts, may help to deduce the cause and reverse the platelet count decline. Regardless of the mechanism of induction, development of thrombocytopenia is temporally related to exposure to the drug and is usually rapid. Discontinuation of the offending drug results in an increase in platelet count over days to weeks. For some patients with prolonged thrombocytopenia after drug removal, immunosuppression with steroids or IVIG (2 g/kg in two to three divided doses) may restore baseline platelet counts.

Although confirmation of drug-induced thrombocytopenia can often be made by testing for antibodies with drug specificities, these tests are not routinely available, are performed only by specialty reference laboratories, and take weeks to complete, by which time the offending drug has already been identified by stopping it and recovering the platelet count. When drug-induced thrombocytopenia is suspected, clinicians should not wait for results of drug-specific antibody tests before discontinuing potential offending agents.

Platelet alloimmunization. Patients who receive multiple platelet transfusions such as those with MDS may develop alloantibodies to platelets rendering future platelet transfusions less beneficial. Some do not respond to platelet transfusion at all. Alloimmunization can be assessed by measuring serial platelet counts after receiving a platelet transfusion to confirm the expected rise. Panel reactive antibody testing can also help. This test provides a percentage of HLA antigens that react with the patient's antibodies, giving the likelihood that the patient will consume a random platelet transfusion. In order to overcome this platelet destruction for those who are alloimmunized, HLA-matched platelets can be transfused, but this can take the blood bank days to find the right matched units (see "Platelet Transfusion Failure and Platelet Refractoriness" section).

Fetal and neonatal alloimmune thrombocytopenia. Fetal and neonatal alloimmune thrombocytopenia (FNAIT) occurs when a mother is homozygous for an uncommon platelet alloantigen, most often human platelet antigen 1b (HPA-1b) on the platelet GPIIIa receptor, and a fetus expresses the HPA-1a haplotype inherited from the father. The pathogenesis of alloimmune thrombocytopenia is analogous to the mechanism by which Rh(D) sensitization induces hemolytic disease of the newborn. The mother is exposed to the HPA-1a antigen during a first pregnancy, and during that or subsequent pregnancies, she produces high-titer IgG antibody against HPA-1a.

TABLE 52.2	**Commonly Used Drugs Associated With Immune Thrombocytopenia**
Drug Class	**Examples**
Antibiotics	Penicillins
	Cephalosporins (cephalothin, ceftazidime)
	Vancomycin
	Sulfonamides (sulfisoxazole)
	Rifampin
	Linezolid
	Quinine
Antiepileptics, antipsychotics, and sedative-hypnotics	Benzodiazepines (diazepam)
	Haloperidol
	Carbamazepine
	Lithium
	Phenytoin
Antihypertensives	Diuretics (chlorothiazide)
	Angiotensin-converting enzyme inhibitors (ramipril)
	Methyldopa
Analgesics and anti-inflammatories	Acetaminophen
	Ibuprofen
	Naproxen
Antiplatelet agents	Abciximab
	Tirofiban
Anticoagulants	Heparin
	Low-molecular-weight heparin

These antibodies cross the placenta, react with HPA-1a–positive fetal platelets, and cause peripheral platelet destruction through the RES.

A diagnosis of FNAIT is frequently suspected when in utero fetal bleeding is observed by imaging studies or when an otherwise healthy newborn has unexpected bleeding or bruising associated with thrombocytopenia (typically with platelet counts of 50,000 to 75,000/µL or lower). A maternal history of FNAIT is a strong predictor of its occurrence during future pregnancies.

After a diagnosis of FNAIT is suspected, it may be confirmed by examining maternal sera for anti-HPA alloantibodies and through platelet typing of the mother and father. Although bleeding may be severe in cases of FNAIT, the antibody does not necessarily predict whether bleeding will occur in utero, at delivery, or in the first days of life, and it is used primarily for confirmatory purposes.

Transfusion of washed maternal platelets (washed to remove the mother's anti-HPA-1a antibodies) or random platelets lacking the HPA-1a antigen and IVIG are useful for treating bleeding and restoring the platelet count. For newborns who recover from bleeding, there are few long-lasting deficits from FNAIT after circulating maternal antibodies are cleared from the circulation. For future pregnancies, IVIG with or without corticosteroids is given weekly throughout the second and third trimesters to prevent FNAIT.

Post-transfusion purpura. Alloimmune thrombocytopenia can occur in adults after transfusion, known as post-transfusion purpura (PTP). As in neonates, this condition is based on exposure to a common platelet alloantigen that is not present on the patient's native platelets. For instance, PTP can occur after transfusion of a blood product in an individual who lacks HPA-1a and who has been previously alloimmunized to this antigen during a prior pregnancy or transfusion. Because more than 95% of blood donors express HPA-1a and the antigen is shed by platelets, any blood product

TABLE 52.3   Molecular Basis for Alloimmune Thrombocytopenia

Glycoprotein	Alleles (Alloantigens)	Phenotype/Frequency	Amino Acid and Location
IIIa	HPA-1a/1b	0.98/0.25	Leucine/proline; 33
Ib	HPA-2a/2b	0.99/0.14	Threonine/methionine; 145
IIb	HPA-3a/3b	0.91/0.70	Isoleucine/serine; 843
IIIa	HPA-4a/4b	0.99/0.01	Arginine/glutamine; 143
Ia	HPA-5a/5b	0.99/0.21	Glutamic acid/lysine; 505
IIIa	HPA-6a/6b	NA	Proline/glutamic acid; 407
IIIa	HPA-7a/7b	NA	Proline/glutamic acid; 407
IIIa	HPA-8a/8b	NA	Arginine/cystine; 636

HPA, Human platelet antigen; *NA,* data not available.

TABLE 52.4   Causes of Disseminated Intravascular Coagulation

Sepsis or Endotoxin
Gram-negative bacteremia

Tissue Damage
Trauma
Closed-head injury
Burns
Hypoperfusion or hypotension

Malignant Disease
Adenocarcinoma
Acute promyelocytic leukemia

Primary Vascular Disorders
Vasculitis
Giant hemangioma (Kasabach-Merritt syndrome)
Aortic aneurysm
Cardiac mural thrombus

Exogenous Causes
Snake venom
Activated-factor infusions (prothrombin-complex concentrate)

can contain HPA-1a. Although not clearly understood, some investigators have speculated that soluble HPA antigens are deposited onto endogenous platelets, resulting in their rapid clearance by anti-HPA alloantibodies.

The diagnosis of PTP can be confirmed by demonstrating anti-HPA antibodies in the serum of an affected individual. Patients are typically treated with IVIG, and additional transfusions must be derived from donors lacking the implicated HPA. Although HPA-1a is the most common cause of alloimmune thrombocytopenia, other platelet alloantigens can cause this clinical syndrome (Table 52.3).

Non–Immune-Mediated Platelet Destruction

Disseminated intravascular coagulation. One of the most common and potentially life-threatening causes of nonimmune platelet destruction is DIC, which is associated with sepsis, malignancy, advanced liver disease, and other disorders that trigger endotoxin release or cause severe tissue damage (Table 52.4). In DIC caused by bacterial sepsis, circulating endotoxin induces expression of tissue factor on circulating monocytes and endothelial cells, a process leading to overwhelming thrombin and fibrin generation. Deposition of fibrin occurs throughout the vasculature, with relatively inadequate concurrent fibrinolysis, leading to a thrombotic microangiopathic vasculopathy and subsequent organ damage. Thrombin activation of platelets and circulating factors eventually overwhelms the bone marrow and liver synthetic capability, respectively, resulting in thrombocytopenia and prolongation of the PT and aPTT.

Although the primary lesion of DIC is thrombin and clot generation, the clinical end point is usually a consumptive coagulopathy with depletion of platelets and coagulation factors. Mucosal bleeding, especially in the GI tract and oozing from intravenous puncture sites are signs of DIC.

Fibrinogen levels decrease in DIC but may be normal in earlier compensated stages and from the acute phase reaction to the underlying disorder, which increases fibrinogen production and secretion. DIC should not be ruled out because fibrinogen is in the normal range. Fibrinolysis in DIC is triggered by fibrin clot formation and the action of tissue-type plasminogen activator. Laboratory testing shows increased levels of fibrin split products (i.e. cleavage of fibrin monomers) and D-dimer (i.e., cleavage of fibrin-fibrin bonds), although these findings are nonspecific. The peripheral blood smear often contains schistocytes. Schistocytes are seen in other microangiopathic hemolytic anemias such as thrombotic thrombocytopenic purpura and hemolytic uremic syndrome (TTP/HUS), but these lead to excessive clotting, not bleeding (see Chapter 53).

Chronic DIC may be triggered by consumption of platelets and factors in large blood clots associated with aneurysms, hemangiomas, and mural thrombi. Another cause of chronic DIC is malignant disease, often adenocarcinoma or acute promyelocytic leukemia. Malignant cells in these disorders promote thrombin formation through secretion of tissue factor, cysteine proteases that activate factor X, induction of platelet-ligand binding, and upregulation of endothelial cell plasminogen activator inhibitor-1 (PAI-1) or cyclooxygenase 2 (COX2). Chronic DIC associated with malignancy usually causes enough factor consumption that the PT and aPTT are prolonged. Clinically, patients exhibit migratory thrombophlebitis (i.e., Trousseau syndrome) or nonbacterial thrombotic (marantic) endocarditis.

Therapy for DIC should be aimed at (1) treatment of the underlying disorder, such as antibiotics for sepsis or chemotherapy for malignant disease; (2) supportive hemostatic therapy, including platelets, cryoprecipitate (for fibrinogen), and FFP (for clotting factors); and (3) disruption of the activation of coagulation factors and platelets. For the last approach, anticoagulation is usually not indicated unless the balance of procoagulant and anticoagulant activity actively favors clotting, such as arterial thromboemboli with mural thrombus or migratory thrombophlebitis. These thrombotic complications of chronic DIC are often resistant to warfarin therapy and usually require more intensive anti-Xa therapy with unfractionated or low-molecular-weight heparin.

TABLE 52.5	Disorders Causing Abnormal Platelet Aggregation				
	RESPONSE TO AGONIST				
Disorder	**Epinephrine**	**Adp**	**Collagen**	**Arachidonic Acid**	**Ristocetin**
Aspirin and NSAIDs	PW	PW	NL, ↓[a]	↓	NL
Glanzmann disease	Absent	Absent	Absent	Absent	PW
Bernard-Soulier syndrome	NL	NL	NL	NL	Absent
Storage pool disease	↓	PW	↓	NL, ↓	PW
Hermansky-Pudlak syndrome	↓	PW	↓	NL	PW
Gray platelet syndrome	↓	↓	↓	NL	NL
von Willebrand disease	NL	NL	NL	NL	↓, NL[b]

ADP, Adenosine diphosphate; *NL,* normal; *NSAIDs,* nonsteroidal anti-inflammatory drugs; *PW,* primary wave aggregation only; *↓,* decreased.
[a]Aspirin results in decreased aggregation with most collagen doses.
[b]In von Willebrand disease type 2B, patients have increased aggregation with low-dose ristocetin and decreased or normal aggregation with standard doses of ristocetin.

Thrombocytopenia with pregnancy-induced hypertension. Mild thrombocytopenia in pregnant women called gestational thrombocytopenia represents an effect of hemodilution as plasma volume increases through pregnancy, a normal physiologic response that can bring platelet counts into the range of 100,000 to 150,000/µL; these counts are not associated with maternal or fetal bleeding. However, pregnancy-induced hypertension can result in platelet counts of less than 100,000/µL, and these conditions can be associated with complications.

The spectrum of pregnancy-induced hypertension includes hypertension progressing to proteinuria and renal dysfunction (i.e., pre-eclampsia) and then to cerebral edema and seizures (i.e., eclampsia). Thrombocytopenia may appear as a late finding accompanying pregnancy-induced hypertension, often occurring at the time of delivery or late in the third trimester. HELLP syndrome in pregnancy (characterized by *h*emolysis, *e*levated *l*iver enzymes, and *l*ow *p*latelet counts) is occasionally associated with hypertension. The thrombocytopenia associated with pregnancy-induced hypertension or HELLP may result from abnormal vascular prostaglandin metabolism or placental dysfunction that leads to platelet consumption, vasculopathy, and microvascular occlusions. Both disorders are usually reversed by delivery of the fetus and placenta. Occasionally, IVIG or plasmapheresis is required when the disorder does not resolve after delivery.

Hemophagocytic lymphohistiocytosis. HLH is a deadly disease of T-cell and NK-cell dysregulation causing macrophage activation and extreme cytokine inflammatory responses. Histiocytes ingest blood in bone marrow and other organs. Cytopenias, fever, splenomegaly, liver function abnormalities, coagulopathy, and high levels of ferritin (typically >1000) ensue. In children, congenital causes can be found in perforin or granule fusion defects. In adults, an underlying malignancy (usually lymphoma) catalyzes the syndrome and is fatal without a stem cell transplant. Treatment otherwise entails chemotherapy with etoposide, steroids, and other immunosuppression. When associated with a rheumatologic disease, the name macrophage activation syndrome is used.

Consumption and dilutional thrombocytopenia. In addition to sequestration, hypoproductive, and destructive causes of thrombocytopenia, low platelet counts occasionally result from consumption and hemodilution. The pathophysiology of thrombocytopenia in these cases is directly attributable to the underlying cause of the bleeding, frequently large-scale trauma.

Overwhelming hemorrhage causes the consumption of endogenous platelets in an attempt to curb bleeding, and platelets are consumed faster than they can be released by the spleen or generated in the bone marrow. Resuscitative efforts after trauma, including infusion of massive volumes of intravenous fluids, red blood cells, and FFP, result in the dilution of circulating platelet numbers. The combination of platelet consumption and dilution during trauma can have catastrophic consequences and historically has been a leading cause of death in this setting. In addition to identifying the source of a large bleed, aggressive platelet transfusions in the setting of trauma may provide the greatest benefit in overcoming the effects of consumption and dilution (discussed in the "Standard Platelet Therapy" section).

BLEEDING CAUSED BY PLATELET FUNCTION DEFECTS

The ability of platelets to adhere to damaged vasculature and to recruit additional platelets into the clot is essential for primary hemostasis, especially when patients are challenged by trauma or surgery. Unlike bleeding caused by thrombocytopenia, individuals with platelet function defects bleed because their platelets cannot adhere or aggregate appropriately in response to in vivo stimuli.

These qualitative platelet disorders are most frequently encountered in individuals with normal or near-normal platelet counts. Evaluation often relies on tests that assess the function (rather than the number) of circulating platelets. From an epidemiologic standpoint, acquired qualitative platelet defects are much more frequently encountered than their congenital counterparts.

Acquired Causes of Platelet Dysfunction
Antiplatelet Therapy
The patient's history and preoperative screening should assess whether patients are taking medications that interfere with platelet function, such as aspirin and nonsteroidal anti-inflammatory drugs (NSAIDs). Aspirin irreversibly blocks arachidonic acid metabolism, and all exposed platelets are irreversibly affected so that affected platelets do not respond to stimulation even after aspirin is discontinued. The characteristic aspirin-induced platelet aggregation pattern is shown in Table 52.5 and Fig. 52.5.

Nonsteroidal anti-inflammatory drugs (NSAIDs) (e.g., indomethacin) reversibly inhibit cyclooxygenase (COX), and platelet function is restored within 48 hours after discontinuing the drug. Bleeding after most surgical procedures that is associated with aspirin or NSAIDs is

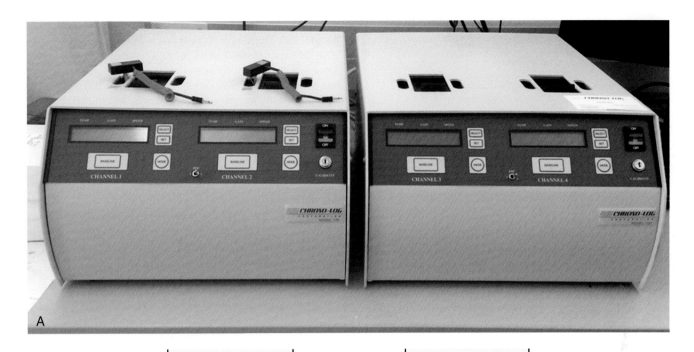

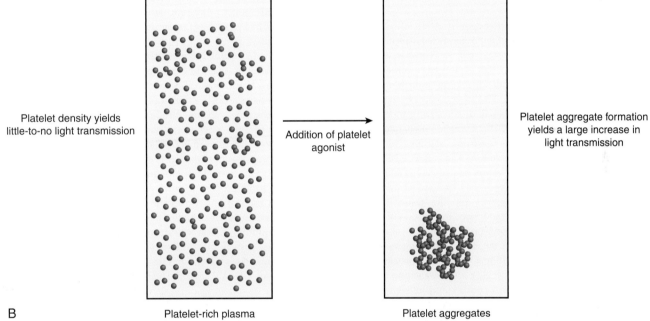

Platelet density yields little-to-no light transmission

Addition of platelet agonist

Platelet aggregate formation yields a large increase in light transmission

Platelet-rich plasma

Platelet aggregates

Fig. 52.5 Methodology underlying light transmission aggregometry. (A) Typical laboratory light transmission aggregometer. (B) Platelet function is directly proportional to light transmission in this assay. Platelet-rich plasma, which prevents light transmission, is exposed to various agonists (i.e., adenosine diphosphate, epinephrine, collagen, arachidonic acid, and ristocetin). As platelets begin to aggregate or agglutinate, light transmission increases over time and is typically reflected as a primary or secondary wave of aggregation for most agonists. Low or no increase in light transmission typically correlates with diminished platelet function.

usually mild, so aspirin may not need to be discontinued before surgery, especially considering aspirin-induced platelet dysfunction is desirable in patients at risk for stroke or myocardial infarction.

The aspirin effect is restricted to COX1, and various NSAIDs have different relative affinities for COX1 and COX2. COX2 is an inducible enzyme that is synthesized in endothelial cells in response to inflammatory cytokines. Suppression of COX2 reduces synthesis of endothelial cell prostaglandin I_2 (i.e., prostacyclin), a molecule that exhibits antithrombotic effects through inhibition of platelet aggregation. The net effect of nonselective NSAIDs on the prothrombotic

or antithrombotic balance favors bleeding because NSAID-induced COX1 inhibition means that thromboxane A_2 production in platelets is blocked. In contrast, the increased cardiovascular risk with administration of more selective COX2 inhibitors is probably attributable to the COX2-induced lack of endothelial cell prostacyclin production, coupled with intact platelet function (i.e., no inhibition of thromboxane A_2 by COX2 blockade).

Another category of antiplatelet agents acts independently of the COX1/2 pathways. These drugs are P2Y12 receptor antagonists (e.g., clopidogrel, prasugrel). They disrupt function by irreversibly binding

TABLE 52.6   Drugs Affecting Platelet Function

Strong Inhibitors
Abciximab (and other anti-GPIIb/IIIa or anti-RGD compounds)
Aspirin (often contained in over-the-counter medications)
Clopidogrel, ticlopidine (ADP-receptor blockers)
Nonsteroidal anti-inflammatory drugs

Moderate Inhibitors
Antibiotics (penicillins, cephalosporins, nitrofurantoin)
Dextran
Fibrinolytics
Heparin
Hetastarch

Weak Inhibitors
Alcohol
Nitroglycerin
Nitroprusside

ADP, Adenosine diphosphate; *GP,* glycoprotein; *RGD,* arginine-glycine-aspartate.

to the surface receptor for the platelet agonist, ADP. P2Y12 receptor antagonists are primarily used as adjunctive anticoagulant therapy for individuals at risk for thrombosis associated with coronary artery disease and stroke. These drugs can inhibit platelet activation at the site of injury, not unlike the effect in an individual taking aspirin, and further potentiate bleeding.

Regardless of the type of agent used, discontinuing an antiplatelet drug is a reasonable first step for a patient who has moderate to severe bleeding while on the therapy. Discontinuation of aspirin will not help the affected platelets because its inhibition is irreversible, but this will allow newly produced platelets to be free of drug effect and function appropriately at the site of an injury.

Beyond stopping the offending drug, bleeding caused by aspirin or other antiplatelet agents may be addressed by infusion of 1-deamino-(8-D-arginine)-vasopressin (DDAVP, desmopressin), although the results of small clinical trials have been mixed regarding its benefit to platelet function and bleeding cessation. Occasionally, platelet transfusion is necessary. In most cases, a single platelet transfusion of 4 to 6 random donor units (or one apheresis unit) contributes enough normal platelets (>10% of total circulating number) to restore primary hemostasis. Platelet dysfunction and bleeding caused by other drugs is similarly treated by discontinuing the drug and providing platelet transfusions when needed (Table 52.6).

Uremic Platelet Dysfunction

Renal insufficiency can be associated with the accumulation of toxic proteins, which induce high levels of nitric oxide formation by vascular endothelial cells and inhibit platelet function. The uremic state can also suppress platelet secretory pathways and platelet adhesion to exposed endothelium through mechanisms that are not well understood. Nonetheless, the uremic state does put an individual at risk for platelet dysfunction–related bleeding. Because no formal tests are available, the diagnosis should be suspected in individuals with acute or chronic renal failure who demonstrate bleeding.

Short-term treatment of uremic platelet dysfunction includes administration of DDAVP. This increases circulating von Willebrand factor, which can help to overcome some of the uremia-associated platelet deficits. Transfusion of red blood cells also seems to help by

increasing volume, thereby pushing platelets to the margins of the blood vessel, where they become easily activated and more likely to plug the gaps between endothelial cells. Conjugated estrogens are of some benefit for long-term treatment. Platelet transfusions may be marginally useful in patients with life-threatening bleeding and acute renal failure, but the effect of this treatment is short lived because the transfused platelets rapidly acquire the uremic defect. Platelet transfusion should not be considered as a first-line therapy for most forms of uremic bleeding. Ultimately, renal replacement therapy, including dialysis or renal transplantation, may be necessary.

Congenital Causes of Platelet Dysfunction
Platelet Glycoprotein Defects

Inherited qualitative platelet defects include abnormalities of platelet receptors and granules. Two rare but well-characterized platelet receptor disorders are Bernard-Soulier syndrome and Glanzmann thrombasthenia.

Bernard-Soulier syndrome is caused by decreased surface expression of platelet GPIb, a key receptor for von Willebrand factor and less commonly by diminished GPIb function. The syndrome is characterized by mild thrombocytopenia, large platelets, and mild to moderate bleeding symptoms. The diagnosis is usually made in childhood, but some patients may be discovered in adulthood. Laboratory testing for Bernard-Soulier syndrome shows an absent platelet aggregation response to ristocetin (see Table 52.5 and Fig. 52.5) despite adequate VWF activity.

Glanzmann thrombasthenia is characterized by an increased bleeding time and abnormally low levels of expression of platelet GPIIb/IIIa (receptor for VWF and fibrinogen) or, less commonly, normal expression but absent GPIIb/IIIa function, while platelet count remains normal. Patients usually exhibit bleeding in childhood. Whereas patients with Bernard-Soulier syndrome have an elevated mean platelet volume (MPV), MPV is normal in Glanzmann thrombasthenia. In cases of Glanzmann thrombasthenia, platelet aggregation testing confirms an absent or diminished response to all agonists except ristocetin (see Table 52.5 and Fig. 52.5).

Platelet transfusions correct the bleeding in Bernard-Soulier syndrome and Glanzmann thrombasthenia. However, because of the high risk for alloimmunization with frequent platelet transfusions (particularly because patients lack GPIb or GPIIb/IIIa), this therapy should be used sparingly. Instead, factor VIIa can be used with high efficacy for both diseases. DDAVP has some benefit in Bernard-Soulier syndrome.

Platelet Granule or Secretory Defects

Inherited platelet granule disorders are defined by the type of granule that is absent or defective. Storage pool disease is characterized by a relative decrease or absence of dense granules and correspondingly moderate to severe mucosal bleeding. Release of dense granule contents that recruit and activate platelets is impaired. Storage pool disease has a diminished or absent secondary wave of aggregation in response to most agonists (see Table 52.5 and Fig. 52.5).

Hermansky-Pudlak syndrome is a dense granule deficiency associated with oculocutaneous albinism, nystagmus, and pulmonary fibrosis. Multiple gene defects have been attributed to Hermansky-Pudlak syndrome and cause lysosome dysfunction. Patients may have spontaneous bleeding, but bleeding more often occurs with surgical procedures or trauma. This can be particularly problematic for the patients who undergo lung transplant for pulmonary fibrosis.

Chédiak-Higashi syndrome is a rare dense granule disorder characterized by mild bleeding, partial albinism, and recurrent pyogenic infections. It is caused by a mutation in the *LYST* gene leading to lysosome dysregulation. Large, irregular, gray-blue inclusions (granules) are seen in neutrophils and other white blood cells. Many patients with Chédiak-Higashi syndrome develop an accelerated phase with HLH.

Gray platelet syndrome is characterized by colorless or gray platelets that lack normal staining on the peripheral smear. Electron microscopy confirms the loss of α-granules or their contents. A mutation in the gene *NBEAL* disrupts vesicle trafficking, leading to a deficiency of the α-granules. Patients with gray platelet syndrome have a history of mild bleeding, and aggregation testing detects diminished responses to epinephrine, ADP, and collagen.

Thrombocytopenia with small platelets is characteristic of Wiskott-Aldrich syndrome, an X-linked recessive disorder with eczema and immunodeficiency that can be diagnosed by the lack of CD43 expression on T lymphocytes. A *WAS* gene mutation results in a defect in the actin cytoskeleton followed by a deficiency in platelet dense granules. Most patients with Wiskott-Aldrich syndrome will not survive without a stem cell transplant.

May-Hegglin anomaly and related myosin heavy-chain 9 gene (*MYH9*) diseases are characterized by giant platelets and Döhle bodies (i.e., basophilic inclusions in leukocytes). Platelet count is low and a family history of bleeding is common because the inheritance pattern is autosomal dominant. Unlike the other diseases in this section, *MYH9* diseases have normal granules and normal platelet aggregation, but the *MYH9* mutation impairs the platelet cytoskeleton, which affects clot retraction. With thrombopoietin agonists, the additional platelets produced are also dysfunctional, but the quantitative increase in platelets may be enough to stop bleeding.

All the platelet dysfunction disorders are treated by avoiding antiplatelet drugs, using hormonal control of menses in women, and transfusing platelets when bleeding occurs.

Platelet Transfusion Therapy
Standard Platelet Therapy
Platelet transfusions derived from the whole blood of healthy donors can be used to stop or prevent bleeding. The two broad categories of platelet transfusion support are based on the conditions previously discussed: prophylactic platelet transfusions for thrombocytopenia in nonbleeding patients and platelet transfusion for acute bleeding.

For the nonbleeding thrombocytopenic patient, several triggers can prompt platelet transfusion in the absence of frank hemorrhage. Patients receiving chemotherapy may be severely thrombocytopenic and should be transfused when their platelet counts are less than 10,000/μL to prevent spontaneous bleeding. This is a safe and appropriate threshold for patients with relatively uncomplicated clinical pictures without fever, sepsis, or bleeding. The threshold of 10,000/μL, which was rigorously established through several prospective, randomized, controlled trials, significantly decreases the frequency of platelet transfusion and thereby reduces risks associated with multiple blood product exposures. If the patient has complicating circumstances, prophylactic transfusions may be given when platelet counts are lower than 20,000/μL, although this threshold is not rigorously based on clinical trial evidence.

For patients undergoing invasive procedures or who suffer trauma, it is reasonable to transfuse platelets when counts are lower than 50,000/μL. Higher platelet counts (>100,000/μL) are recommended for patients undergoing neurologic surgery. The thresholds of 50,000/μL and 100,000/μL are based primarily on experience and published guidelines. Clinical trials are lacking in these settings.

For the acutely bleeding patient, the decision to transfuse platelets depends on several factors, of which thrombocytopenia is the most straightforward and useful criterion. Platelet counts higher than 50,000/μL are a reasonable goal for most cases of acute bleeding,

whereas counts higher than 100,000/μL may be necessary for neurologic bleeding.

Congenital or acquired platelet dysfunction must be considered for acutely bleeding patients. Those with significant bleeding who have taken an antiplatelet drug such as aspirin may benefit from platelet transfusion regardless of baseline counts. Another consideration is the volume of blood products and fluids received. Trauma patients may receive more than 10 units of transfused red blood cells in addition to plasma, volume expanders, and saline solutions. Resuscitation with large fluid volumes (≥10 units transfused) reduces the platelet count to less than 50% of baseline, resulting in a significant dilutional coagulopathy. In these scenarios, repeated platelet counts must be obtained and platelets liberally transfused to maintain adequate hemostasis. Similarly, clotting factors need repletion during massive transfusion (see "Dilutional Coagulopathy" section).

Blood banks provide random-donor pooled platelets and apheresis platelets (E-Fig. 52.1). Random-donor pooled platelets consist of platelet concentrates from four to six donors combined (pooled) into one large dose. For the adult patient with uncomplicated thrombocytopenia, a single random-donor platelet concentrate unit typically raises the platelet count by about 8000 to 10,000/μL. Between 4 and 6 units pooled together can be expected to raise counts by 30,000 to 60,000 platelets/μL. Apheresis platelets are collected from one donor using automated apheresis instruments. The dose of these *single-donor platelets* is almost equivalent to that of a 6-unit platelet pool and is estimated to increase platelet count by up to 50,000/μL in an uncomplicated patient.

Based on the expected increments and typical transfusion goals outlined previously, one random-donor platelet pool (6 units pooled together) or one apheresis platelet product should sufficiently raise platelet counts to improve thrombocytopenia and prevent spontaneous bleeding. These doses should also be sufficient to stop or prevent bleeding associated with thrombocytopenia in the setting of invasive procedures, mild to moderate trauma, or bleeding associated with platelet dysfunction. For the complicated patient (e.g., thrombocytopenia with intracranial hemorrhage, massive trauma), additional platelet doses may be necessary to achieve adequate hemostasis.

Platelet Transfusion Failure and Platelet Refractoriness
Platelet transfusions in thrombocytopenic patients are not successful in all cases. Uremia causes an acquired dysfunction of transfused platelets, limiting their hemostatic capabilities in vivo. Patients who are thrombocytopenic due to conditions such as ITP usually do not show increased platelet counts after transfusion because circulating autoantibodies cause rapid destruction of both endogenous and infused (exogenous) platelets. This phenomenon, known as platelet transfusion refractoriness, can be caused by many other recipient problems, including fever, sepsis, splenomegaly, and DIC. Although the pathophysiology of refractoriness is well understood for conditions such as ITP or DIC (in which platelets are cleared from the circulation), few data are available to suggest why individuals with conditions such as fever or infection have an inappropriate response to platelet transfusion.

When approaching a patient with platelet transfusion refractoriness, the physician should consider whether it is mediated by nonimmune or immune factors. Immune refractoriness indicates antibody-mediated clearance. For nonimmune-mediated refractoriness, as in fever or DIC, the underlying conditions usually decrease transfused platelet survival over time but do not affect immediate platelet recovery.

A standard diagnostic approach to platelet refractoriness involves measuring the platelet count 10 minutes to 1 hour after completion of the platelet transfusion. The patient with non–immune-mediated refractoriness typically shows an initial increase at 10 minutes but then a blunted increase in the platelet count 1 hour after transfusion, with a subsequent decline at a steeper rate than expected because of the underlying disorder. For patients with this type of platelet refractoriness, addressing the underlying illness often increases the effectiveness of platelet transfusions.

For patients with immune-mediated platelet refractoriness, there is virtually no increase in the platelet count, even minutes after completion of a transfusion. The antiplatelet antibodies are most frequently encountered in individuals who have been recurrently transfused. Repeated exposures to transfused products can induce alloantibodies, most commonly to HLA antigens. Over time and with multiple transfusion exposures, the titer of alloantibodies can increase sharply and cause rapid clearance of incompatible platelets after infusion.

For the alloimmunized patient, immunosuppression fails to decrease platelet alloantibodies, and efforts to improve platelet recovery after transfusion are focused on finding compatible platelet units. The first step in managing transfusion of the alloimmunized patient is to provide ABO antigen–matched platelets to minimize clearance caused by naturally occurring ABO antibodies; this is often helpful because platelets express A and B antigens on their surface. If this step fails to yield increases in platelet counts, donor platelets that lack target antigens for the detected alloantibodies should be pursued. One strategy is to use the patient's serum to crossmatch platelet donor units, with selection of those units demonstrating compatibility for subsequent transfusion.

If crossmatch-compatible platelets fail to induce adequate platelet recovery, blood banks should provide platelets that are matched to the recipient's HLA system in the hope of evading HLA-based antibodies. HLA-matched platelets are collected from compatible donors using apheresis at frequent intervals until the patient's platelet count recovers and they are no longer transfusion dependent. Many blood banks and transfusion services have attempted to address the problem of platelet HLA alloimmunization through prevention. They provide blood products that have undergone filtration to reduce their white blood cell content, a process called *leukoreduction*. Because contaminating leukocytes are the primary sources of exposure to HLAs, their removal can be quite effective in preventing subsequent alloimmunization, even in chronically transfused patients.

BLEEDING CAUSED BY VON WILLEBRAND DISEASE

Von Willebrand disease is caused by either a deficiency or dysfunction of von Willebrand factor. Because VWF is a key component to primary hemostasis, its deficiency results in easy bleeding, typically superficial (bruising, mucosal). However, VWF is a stabilizer of factor VIII and when VWF is low, factor VIII is rapidly cleared, resulting in declining factor VIII levels and an elevated aPTT. If factor VIII levels are low enough, patients can have deeper bleeding as in hemophilia A and B with muscle hematomas, hemarthroses, and bleeding into the central nervous system. VWF is synthesized in endothelial cells and megakaryocytes and functions in plasma to mediate platelet adhesion to the damaged site. VWF is a large, multimeric protein; the largest multimers contain the greatest number of adhesive sites and confer greater hemostatic ability than smaller VWF molecules. In patients with low VWF levels, platelet adhesion to damaged vessels is delayed.

VWD is grouped into three main subtypes (E-Table 52.1). Type 1 VWD results from a decline in VWF antigen. Decline in VWF antigen parallels a decline in VWF activity. Type 2 VWD represents a dysfunctional VWF, leading to a more significant decline in VWF activity than VWF antigen. Type 3 VWD is the most severe type. Patients with type 3 VWD do not make any VWF.

Type 1 von Willebrand Disease

Type 1 VWD is the most common type. Although severity can vary significantly, it tends to be mild. The cause is not always clear because many cases of type 1 VWD have a normal VWF gene sequence. Therefore, other factors must be in play such as the rate of VWF secretion, storage, and clearance. Blood type O is associated with a 25% decline in VWF levels. However, this decline does not affect bleeding rates, possibly due to enhanced secretion and decreased clearance of VWF with age. Inheritance of type 1 VWD tends to be autosomal dominant. VWF antigen levels decline in parallel with VWF activity, reported as VWF:ristocetin (RCo), and increasing severity. VWF:RCo measures the ability of the patient's VWF (plasma) to agglutinate normal platelets in the presence of ristocetin. VWF:RCo 30% to 49% is referred to as "low VWF" but not true VWD. Diagnostic criterion for VWD is VWF:RCo less than 30%. Repeating VWF testing is wise because significant variability occurs within individuals and between labs.

VWF levels also increase with age, inflammation, liver disease, and estrogen such as while on oral contraception or during pregnancy. Patients with mild and moderate VWD rarely have bleeding during pregnancy as the baseline VWF levels increase. However, days to weeks after delivery, bleeding becomes more common as levels fall back to the original baseline. Pregnant women should be alerted to this possibility so they contact a provider if postpartum bleeding occurs. Postpartum bleeding should be carefully assessed so it is not dismissed as expected lochia.

Treatment for VWD focuses on modalities to increase VWF. DDAVP increases production of VWF and its release from stores in the Weibel-Palade bodies in endothelial cells. It also increases factor VIII levels. Increased VWF levels can be detected within minutes of DDAVP administration, either intravenous or intranasal. Prior to relying on DDAVP for prevention of bleeding with surgeries or treatment of acute bleeds, a DDAVP challenge should be undertaken, where VWF and factor VIII levels are measured at baseline and then at specified timed intervals (e.g., 1 hour, 2 hours, and 6 hours) after administration of DDAVP to confirm an adequate response. Once this is done, intravenous DDAVP 0.3 μg/kg (capped at 20 μg max dose) can be given 30 to 60 minutes prior to surgeries, and intranasal DDAVP can be prescribed so patients can self-treat at home for bleeds or heavy menstrual periods.

The drawbacks to DDAVP include common side effects such as flushing, headache, malaise, and nausea, but also importantly hyponatremia, which becomes more severe with every dose. This can be circumvented by instructing patients to incorporate a 1-week drug holiday after every three doses and to limit free water intake during DDAVP days. A drug holiday is also important because tachyphylaxis develops, meaning that subsequent doses have diminishing returns on their ability to raise VWF levels (i.e., the third dose does not work as well as the first dose) as VWF stores become depleted. When DDAVP responses are inadequate or when patients do not tolerate DDAVP, VWF concentrates must be used. VWF concentrates come as plasma-derived or recombinant. Recombinant VWF contains no factor VIII, while plasma-derived VWF has factor VIII attached. This is important for treatment decisions because many patients with VWD also have low factor VIII levels. In that situation, both VWF and factor VIII need to be replaced to effectively treat acute bleeding. Thus, if recombinant VWF is used, a separate infusion of factor VIII concentrate also needs to be infused if factor VIII is low. For severely affected patients who need prophylaxis (regularly infused VWF to prevent spontaneous bleeding), either type of product is adequate because factor VIII levels become normal several hours after VWF is infused since the VWF stabilizes endogenous factor VIII. If baseline VWF levels of zero are assumed, VWF concentrates of 50 U/kg intravenous will bring

VWF to 100%. The half-life of these products is about 12 hours, so doses need to be repeated every 12 to 24 hours.

Type 2 von Willebrand Disease

Type 2 VWD is characterized by heterozygous mutations that produce a qualitative defect in the VWF molecule. Because the defect causes a dysfunction in VWF, DDAVP, which will increase the dysfunctional endogenous VWF levels, may not work as well as it does for type 1 VWD.

A variety of VWF mutations can cause VWD type 2A, which result in decreased VWF secretion or increased clearance through ADAMTS-13 (a disintegrin and metalloprotease with thrombospondin-1-like-domains-13). These patients show disproportionately low VWF:RCo activity compared with the VWF antigen level (VWF RCo:Ag < 0.6) and large or high-molecular-weight VWF multimers are absent (see E-Table 52.1). Platelet aggregation is decreased in response to ristocetin. Patients with type 2A VWD respond to VWF concentrate and less commonly to DDAVP.

Type 2B VWD represents a gain-of-function mutation in exon 28 of VWF that augments VWF binding to the platelet GP1b receptor. This leads to mild thrombocytopenia that worsens with exposure to DDAVP. Therefore, DDAVP is contraindicated in type 2B VWD. High-molecular-weight multimers are absent and platelet aggregation is increased by ristocetin (see E-Table 52.1). Patients are treated with VWF concentrate.

The same scenario can be found with platelet-type VWD (previously called pseudo-VWD), where the mutation is not on VWF but instead on the GP1b receptor, and this also augments the interaction of VWF with GP1b. GP1b can be sequenced to verify the diagnosis. These patients are treated with platelet transfusions, not VWF, because the VWF is normal.

Type 2M VWD has a VWF mutation causing decreased binding to GP1b, the opposite of type 2B VWD. These patients have normal platelet counts and normal VWF multimers. Gastrointestinal bleeding is more common in type 2M VWD than in other types. Some patients with type 2M VWD respond to DDAVP, but most require VWF concentrate. The platelet version of type 2M VWD is called Bernard-Soulier syndrome, which is caused by a mutation in GP1b leading to decreased VWF binding (see "Congenital Causes of Platelet Dysfunction").

In type 2N VWD, the abnormal VWF molecule has decreased binding affinity for factor VIII, which decreases factor VIII survival and produces a bleeding phenotype similar to hemophilia A (e.g., hemarthroses) except that it affects males and females equally because it has an autosomal recessive inheritance pattern, unlike the X-linked hemophilia A and B. The diagnosis of type 2N VWD should be considered in females who have hemophilia A. VWF levels are normal because the mutated region is isolated to the factor VIII binding site and not affecting the other functions of VWF. To confirm the diagnosis, tests for VWF binding to factor VIII are available in reference laboratories. The low factor VIII levels respond poorly to factor VIII infusions because the infused factor is rapidly cleared without functioning VWF to stabilize it. Instead, type 2N VWD is treated with VWF concentrates with or without factor VIII concentrates.

Type 3 von Willebrand Disease

Patients with type 3 VWD have a complete deficiency of VWF, often as a result of the inheritance of two abnormal VWF alleles (i.e., compound heterozygous). This VWD type is the most severe and can mimic hemophilia because factor VIII levels are also severely decreased without VWF protection. It does not respond to DDAVP and requires VWF with factor VIII concentrates to treat bleeding. Many patients with type 3 VWD require regular prophylaxis of VWF concentrates infused every 2 to 3 days to prevent spontaneous bleeding.

Acquired von Willebrand Disease

The acquired form of VWD usually appears as a severe, type 2A–like defect without larger VWF multimers in a patient with no history of bleeding. Acquired VWD is caused by abnormal clearance of the larger VWF multimers and is associated with essential thrombocythemia, monoclonal gammopathies, multiple myeloma, lymphoproliferative disorders, and other malignancies. For some patients, no etiology is apparent. Unlike ITP, acquired VWD is not associated with pregnancy. Acquired VWD has been successfully treated with IVIG and treatment for the underlying disorder. Another cause of abnormal VWF multimer clearance resulting in acquired VWD is critical aortic stenosis (Heyde syndrome). It is corrected with successful surgical repair.

BLEEDING CAUSED BY COAGULATION FACTOR DISORDERS

Unlike disorders of platelets and von Willebrand factor, which favor mucocutaneous bleeding, coagulation factor defects generally cause deeper hemorrhages, such as bleeding into muscle and joints. Because the initial platelet plug is not solidified by secondary hemostasis, the effects are clot breakdown and at times delayed bleeding.

Most patients with significant factor deficiencies have abnormal screening laboratory test results (E-Table 52.2, Table 52.1, and Fig. 52.1), although patients with mild deficiencies can have bleeding and only borderline-abnormal coagulation factor values. Like other hemostasis abnormalities previously discussed, coagulation factor problems can be classified as congenital deficiencies or acquired.

Congenital Factor Deficiencies

Hemophilia A and B

After VWD, hemophilia A and B are the two most common factor deficiencies, corresponding to factor VIII and factor IX deficiency, respectively. Hemophilia A, with an incidence of 1:10,000 live male births, is approximately four times more common than hemophilia B. They are both X-linked and clinically indistinguishable from each other. Although more prominent in males, females can also have hemophilia as symptomatic carriers and by skewing of X chromosomal inactivation (i.e., favoring one chromosome over the other).

More than 2000 different mutations have been reported to cause hemophilia A and more than 1000 to cause hemophilia B. About 50% of severe hemophilia A patients have an inversion of a major portion of the gene at intron 22 (inversion 22) that results in complete loss of activity. Smaller missense mutations tend to result in mild or moderate disease. One third of cases are de novo, therefore there is no family history.

Hemophilia A and B are stratified by severity: Severe hemophilia is defined as a factor activity of less than 1%, moderate hemophilia as a factor activity of 1% to 5%, and mild hemophilia as a factor activity of 6% to 40%. These distinctions appear small, but are not. Severely affected patients bleed often and spontaneously. Moderately affected patients occasionally bleed spontaneously, whereas mildly affected patients typically bleed only after trauma or surgery. The most common locations for hemorrhages are joints and muscles, but bleeding can occur anywhere. They can be life-threatening, particularly when intracranial. Hemarthroses cause intra-articular inflammation and synovial hyperplasia. Subsequent cartilage and bone damage worsens with repeated hemorrhages. Hemophilic arthropathy results in chronic pain and limitations in joint function. Prior to the advent of prophylaxis, patients often needed joint replacement surgery early in life.

Currently, patients who bleed frequently take factor prophylaxis by self-infusing factor intravenously every few days to maintain detectable baseline factor levels so that spontaneous bleeding does not occur. When acute hemorrhages occur, patients are instructed to infuse factor as early as possible. Most severely affected patients know how to self-infuse intravenously at home. DDAVP, given intravenously or intranasally, can rapidly raise factor VIII levels in mild hemophilia A patients but not in patients who are severely affected. It does not raise factor IX levels in hemophilia B patients either.

A newly approved therapy for prophylaxis is emicizumab, a bispecific antibody that mimics the function of factor VIII by binding to factors IXa and X. This has several advantages over traditional factor products. First, administration is subcutaneous, not intravenous like all other previous factor products. Second, the half-life is substantially longer. Traditional factor's half-life was roughly 12 hours, some extended to nearly 24 hours by the addition of extra moieties such as polyethylene glycol, albumin, or the Fc receptor domain of immunoglobulin, all slowing the metabolism of factor VIII. Emicizumab's half-life is 30 days. The third advantage of emicizumab is that it is not a clotting factor and, therefore, factor VIII inhibitors do not interfere with its efficacy. The disadvantages of emicizumab are that clotting assays (PTT, factor VIII, and others) no longer provide accurate results and that emicizumab is only used for prophylaxis, so acute bleeds are still treated by infusing factor VIII, although acute bleeds are significantly less common with emicizumab versus traditional factor VIII prophylaxis. Emicizumab works only for factor VIII deficiency, not in hemophilia B.

Inhibitors remain the largest problem for hemophilia patients. In up to one third of hemophilia A patients (much less common in hemophilia B), an alloantibody against factor VIII or IX forms, blocking the utility of factor infusions. In this situation, a bypass to work around the inhibitor in the clotting cascade is required to treat hemorrhage. There are two types of bypass agents: activated factor VII and activated 4-factor prothrombin complex concentrates (aPCC), which contain activated factors II, VII, IX, and X. Inhibitor titers can be measured in Bethesda units (BU); 1 BU is defined as the amount of inhibitor that neutralizes 50% of factor activity. High-titer inhibitors (>5 BU) completely neutralize the activity of infused factor concentrates, while low-titer inhibitors can be out-competed by using higher doses of factor, but at the risk of subsequently increasing the titer level. Inhibitors are sometimes transient, sometimes permanent, and sometimes able to be eradicated by immune tolerance induction, by giving frequent high doses of factor infusions to desensitize patients to the factor. Patients with inhibitors have more severe disease and poorly respond to available treatments. Inhibitors make an already costly disease much more expensive.

Not just a footnote in history, many hemophilia patients continue to struggle with the sequelae of human immunodeficiency virus (HIV) and viral hepatitis after contracting them from contaminated blood and factor products in the 1980s and 1990s. In fact, a large percentage of hemophilia patients died from complications of these infections. Recombinant factor was developed in the 1990s and most patients switched even though plasma-derived factor products became safe again through viral testing and inactivation procedures. In addition, a large randomized control trial has shown that plasma-derived factor leads to fewer inhibitors than recombinant, yet most patients remain on recombinant products.

The future has taken a rapid upward swing for hemophilia patients, with curative therapies for hepatitis C, emicizumab, other novel agents coming soon from development and the imminent arrival of gene therapy through coagulation factor DNA deployed into the liver by a viral vector. Multiple studies for gene therapy have shown early success and are already in phase III trials with approval for wider use expected in the coming years.

Hemophilia C

Hemophilia C refers to factor XI deficiency. Although one step prior to factor IX in the clotting cascade, factor XI deficiency is very different than hemophilia A and B. First of all, bleeding tends to be mucocutaneous, similar to platelet and VWF disorders. Second, bleeding risk does not parallel factor activity level and tends to be mild. For example, some patients with zero factor XI activity rarely bleed. Bleeding risk is best determined by a patient's bleeding history; therefore, the need for presurgical factor replacement depends on whether or not a patient tends to bleed. Factor XI replacement is done with fresh-frozen plasma (FFP) in the United States. Some countries have an available factor XI concentrate. Hemophilia C is inherited autosomal recessively and is common in Ashkenazi Jewish people.

Other Congenital Factor Deficiencies

Factor deficiencies can occur in any clotting factor (see E-Table 52.2). Patients with factor V deficiency usually lack plasma factor V and platelet factor V and have joint and muscle bleeding similar to patients with hemophilia. Some patients who are plasma factor V deficient are asymptomatic until they are challenged with the stress of surgery or trauma, and these patients are thought to have normal platelet factor V levels. Rarely, patients inherit combinations of factor deficiencies, such as combined factors V and VIII deficiencies. Some factor deficiencies have specific factor concentrations available for treatment such as factor VIIa, factor X, and factor XIII. However, others do not have specific concentrates available; those would be treated with FFP.

In neonates, factor XIII deficiency manifests with late umbilical stump bleeding or intracranial hemorrhage. Bleeding is delayed, but severe. Factor XIII deficiency does not affect PT or aPTT. It is diagnosed by screening for increased clot solubility in urea; if the clot dissolves abnormally quickly, an enzyme-linked immunosorbent assay for the precise factor XIII level should be performed. Factor XIII deficiency is treated with factor XIII concentrate or cryoprecipitate. Because of the long half-life of factor XIII, prophylactic therapy for severe deficiency is provided only in single doses on a 3- to 4-week recurring schedule.

Fibrinogen (factor I) functions as a bridging ligand for the platelet receptor GPIIb/IIIa in the platelet-platelet matrix at sites of vascular damage. It also functions in the final steps of the coagulation cascade to form the fibrin clot after activation from thrombin (factor IIa). This dual role leads to a varied phenotype of bleeding with superficial and deeper bleeding when defects in fibrinogen exist. Congenital abnormalities of fibrinogen include low levels (hypofibrinogenemia), absent fibrinogen (afibrinogenemia), and abnormally functioning fibrinogen (dysfibrinogenemia). The diagnosis can be established by screening assays (see E-Table 52.2), laboratory assays to measure fibrinogen levels, and tests such as thrombin time that are designed to measure fibrinogen function. Reptilase time can also confirm dysfibrinogenemia; heparin does not interfere with this assay like it does with thrombin time. PT and aPTT are prolonged in disorders of fibrinogen. Fibrinogen concentrates can be used for replacement, but if not available, cryoprecipitate offers high concentrations of fibrinogen compared to FFP.

Acquired Factor Inhibitors

Acquired inhibitors can occur in congenital hemophilia as described above (see "Hemophilia A and B" section), but they can also occur in those born with a normal coagulation system. Acquired factor VIII inhibitors are the most common and are associated with pregnancy, autoimmune disease, and malignancy, especially lymphoproliferative disorders. Some are idiopathic. The mechanisms underlying acquired factor inhibitors remain poorly understood.

The diagnosis of an acquired inhibitor can be made by laboratory techniques similar to those detailed for patients with congenital hemophilia. A mixing study can be a critical piece to the evaluation. It mixes control plasma with patient plasma, correcting any deficiencies unless an inhibitor is present since the inhibitor will also block the factor in the control plasma. For the treatment of bleeding, patients with acquired inhibitors to factors VIII or IX are administered factor VIIa or aPCC to promote hemostasis by bypassing the inhibitor. Rituximab, an anti-CD20 agent, has become the mainstay for successful treatment along with steroids and should be started as soon as possible to eradicate the inhibitor.

Acquired factor X deficiency can occur in patients with amyloidosis, a condition in which the abnormal circulating light chains adsorb and clear factor X, producing low levels and severe bleeding.

Vitamin K Deficiency

Bleeding in inpatients and outpatients who are severely ill may be caused by acquired coagulation factor deficiencies from vitamin K deficiency. Because vitamin K is fat-soluble, biliary tract disease can interfere with its absorption. Antibiotics can sterilize the gut and reduce bacterial sources of vitamin K. Other drugs such as cholestyramine directly block vitamin K absorption. Vitamin K deficiency also may reflect poor nutritional status due to malabsorption, chronic disease, or reduced oral intake in patients who are acutely or chronically ill.

Factors II, VII, IX, and X are vitamin K–dependent procoagulant factors and proteins C and S are the natural vitamin K-dependent anticoagulants. In addition to disease-associated vitamin K deficiency, the anticoagulant warfarin blocks vitamin K–dependent γ-carboxylation of factors II, VII, IX, and X and causes an acute decrease in functional factor VII levels because factor VII has the shortest half-life (4-6 hours) of all vitamin K–dependent factors in vivo. Individuals who experience bleeding while on warfarin may be treated with vitamin K or, for life-threatening bleeding, a 4-factor PCC or FFP infusion.

Dilutional Coagulopathy

As with platelets, coagulation factors can be depleted through the dilutional effects of a pure red blood cell transfusion or with the administration of massive amounts of volume expanders or saline solutions. For every 10 units of red cells acutely transfused, there is a concomitant increase in the international normalized ratio (INR) to greater than 2. Acute bleeding and trauma can also lead to consumption of circulating coagulation factors.

In the setting of trauma, it is important to maintain adequate coagulation factor activity through plasma transfusions. Evidence from the trauma literature suggests that transfusion ratios of red cells to plasma should approach 1:1 to optimize hemostasis. However, even this may not fully restore depleted coagulation factors. The effects of dilutional coagulopathy should be monitored by repeated testing of PT and aPTT and supported with a liberal plasma transfusion strategy. As described above (see "Standard Platelet Therapy" section), caregivers must also be vigilant about repletion of platelets.

Liver Disease

Unlike patients with vitamin K deficiency or those receiving warfarin, patients with liver disease have low levels of most factors, not just the vitamin K–dependent factors. The exception is factor VIII. Factor VIII levels are usually normal with liver disease because factor VIII is produced in endothelial cells and megakaryocytes. Seemingly in contrast to this, factor VIII levels in hemophilia A patients normalize after liver transplant because factor VIII is synthesized in endothelial cells within the transplanted liver. If factor VIII levels are decreased in patients with liver disease, consideration should be given to superimposed DIC.

Evaluating a prolonged PT, measurement of factor VII and a non–vitamin K–dependent factor, such as factor V, is useful. In vitamin K deficiency, the level of factor VII is low, and that of factor V is normal; levels of both factors are low in patients with generalized liver disease. The PT is a sensitive measure of liver function and becomes prolonged in patients with even mild liver disorders; elevation precedes a significant decrease in the albumin or prealbumin levels and is usually coincident with transaminase changes. In patients with mild to moderate liver disease, the PT is prolonged, but the aPTT usually remains within the normal range. In severe liver disease, the PT becomes even more prolonged, and the aPTT also becomes abnormal.

Other causes of bleeding in liver disease include associated DIC, inhibition of platelet function and production, removal of platelets from hypersplenism, and increased levels of tissue plasminogen activator. Treatment of bleeding associated with liver disease is based primarily on replacement of coagulation factors by plasma transfusions, although they only temporarily correct abnormalities. Liver transplantation is the only definitive treatment for these synthetic defects.

Acquired Fibrinogen Loss or Defects

Congenital fibrinogen disorders were described earlier, but more common are acquired causes such as DIC, causing a consumption of fibrinogen, and liver disease, where defects in post-translational modification of fibrinogen lead to dysfunction or dysfibrinogenemia. The abnormal fibrinogen molecules cannot undergo normal cross-linking or polymerization, resulting in bleeding.

BLEEDING IN PATIENTS WITH NORMAL LABORATORY VALUES

Sometimes confirmatory testing of a bleeding disorder can be elusive. Bleeding diathesis from connective tissue disease and vascular causes may have normal coagulation tests. Vitamin C deficiency can lead to bleeding through an acquired connective tissue disease (scurvy). Low VWF and mild deficiencies of clotting factors may not prolong PT and aPTT. Factor XIII deficiency does not affect PT, aPTT, and other tests. Tests of fibrinolysis (plasminogen activator inhibitor-1, alpha-2 antiplasmin, plasminogen, and tissue plasminogen activator) may find rare causes of bleeding. Often cases with significant bleeding histories remain unsolved.

Plasma and Coagulation Factor Transfusion Therapy

For patients with one or multiple defects in coagulation proteins, there are several options for replacement therapy. The most widely used product for replacement of coagulation factors is FFP (E-Fig. 52.2). It is collected from the whole blood of healthy donors and is frozen within 8 hours of collection. It contains normal (i.e., therapeutic) levels of all coagulation factors necessary to maintain hemostasis. FFP is an excellent choice for replacement of coagulation factors for many conditions, including liver failure and deficiencies of factors II, V, X, and XI.

FFP is commonly used with vitamin K therapy for the reversal of warfarin before invasive procedures or for the onset of bleeding. The appropriate dose of FFP is weight based and does not depend on the extent of prolongation in coagulation studies alone. Administration of FFP at 10 to 15 mL/kg should be sufficient to replace deficient coagulation factors and correct abnormal coagulation values. Assuming a volume of about 200 mL per unit of FFP, a reasonable dose for a 70-kg individual is 4 units of FFP. Administration is time sensitive because coagulation factors degrade at standard half-lives on infusion.

FFP should be provided immediately before an intended procedure to ensure adequate hemostasis.

In some cases, patients may not be able to tolerate the infusion of the large volume of FFP required to reverse coagulopathic states. Prothrombin complex concentrate (PCC) offers quick reversal of prolonged PT and aPTT without the need for large volumes of FFP. Four-factor PCC is a concentrated, lyophilized, human-derived concentrate containing factors II, VII, IX, and X that can be reconstituted in small volumes and provided by intravenous bolus injection. A 4-factor PCC was approved for clinical use in 2013 by the U.S. Food and Drug Administration (FDA). A variant PCC (FEIBA) containing activated factors II, VII, IX, and X is used as a bypass agent to treat bleeding in the setting of an inhibitor and is administered in doses of 50 to 100 U/kg every 8 to 12 hours.

Vitamin K can be given in addition to plasma infusion or factor concentrates. Oral or parenteral replacement of vitamin K (1 to 10 mg/day for 1 to 3 days) restores coagulation factor synthesis in patients with normal liver function and vitamin K deficiency.

For patients with hemophilia A or B, multiple virally inactivated, human-derived or recombinant factor VIII and IX concentrates are available (see "Hemophilia A and B"). Patients with severe hemophilia often infuse themselves with prophylactic factor on a regular basis (25-50 U/kg three times per week for hemophilia A; 50-100 U/kg twice per week for hemophilia B) and boost their dose or frequency of infusion when they sense internal bleeding, sustain trauma, or undergo dental procedures (see E-Table 52.3). Patients with mild hemophilia A may not need factor infusions for minor surgery. Their disease is often managed with DDAVP (0.3 μg/kg) or antifibrinolytic agents such as tranexamic acid 1300 mg three times a day or ε-aminocaproic acid 4 g every 4 to 6 hours.

Most patients with hemophilia require factor infusions prophylactically or at times of surgery or trauma. Factor VIII products are infused every 8 to 12 hours, and 1 U/kg of factor VIII concentrate raises plasma factor VIII activity by 2%; 50 U/kg of factor VIII theoretically yields 100% factor VIII activity in a patient with severe hemophilia A. Factor IX has a longer half-life and is infused every 18 to 24 hours; factor IX requires 1 U/kg for a 1% increase in factor IX activity (i.e., 100 U/kg for 100% activity). Major surgery in patients with hemophilia requires intensive factor therapy to achieve normal factor levels (>80%) in the intraoperative period and the early postoperative period to prevent wound hematoma formation. The dose of factors (see E-Table 52.3) is adjusted downward from this intensity, depending on the severity of the insult, the patient's response to previous factor infusions, and whether factor inhibitors have developed.

Hemophilia patients with inhibitors need bypass agents, allowing activation of the extrinsic and common pathways of the clotting cascade. Activated 4-factor PCC is given at doses of 50 to 100 U/kg every 6 to 12 hours.

Another widely used bypass agent is activated factor VII (factor VIIa), a recombinant factor protein administered at 90 μg/kg every 2 hours until the bleeding is controlled. This agent is used to control bleeding in patients with hemophilia inhibitors, acquired hemophilia, congenital factor VII deficiency, and Glanzmann thrombasthenia. It has also been used successfully in Bernard-Soulier syndrome.

Several virally inactivated plasma-derived VWF concentrate products and one recombinant VWF are available. The plasma-derived VWF products also contain factor VIII and are particularly useful for bleeding or prophylaxis in moderate to severe VWD when factor VIII levels are low. Recombinant VWF has no factor VIII, so it would need additional factor VIII infused if factor VIII levels were low, as can happen in VWD.

Cryoprecipitate Transfusion Therapy

Cryoprecipitate is an often overlooked but important blood product for the treatment of a variety of bleeding disorders. It is prepared by thawing frozen plasma and removing the precipitated portion. It contains a narrow array of coagulation factors, but fibrinogen, factor VIII, VWF, and factor XIII occur in high concentrations. A major advantage of cryoprecipitate is that the average single unit is only 10 to 20 mL (E-Fig. 52.3).

Based on its contents and small volume, cryoprecipitate is useful for the replacement of fibrinogen in DIC or in patients with hypofibrinogenemia or dysfibrinogenemia. The product may be helpful for isolated factor XIII deficiency or factor XIII consumption in DIC. Mounting evidence suggests that the VWF and factor VIII in cryoprecipitate can be used to overcome bleeding in uremia by enhancing the adhesive properties of circulating platelets.

Cryoprecipitate is most frequently administered for hypofibrinogenemia, and appropriate dosing should take into account a patient's total plasma volume, baseline fibrinogen levels, and goal fibrinogen levels. For most bleeding associated with hypofibrinogenemia, a goal fibrinogen of more than 100 mg/dL is reasonable. For a 70-kg adult with a fibrinogen level less than 100 mg/dL, a 10-unit pool (total volume of about 150 to 200 mL) should be sufficient to provide adequate fibrinogen. For more complex dosage protocols, such as for children, obese patients, or those with extreme hypofibrinogenemia, consultation with the blood bank is strongly recommended for specific calculations.

PROSPECTUS FOR THE FUTURE

Novel modalities continue to be developed for the diagnosis of patients with bleeding disorders. For instance, assays measuring thrombin generation, thromboelastography (TEG), and rotational thromboelastometry (ROTEM) offer a quantitative view of coagulation that may provide greater insight into the source of abnormal bleeding than current tests. Alternatives and improvements in transfusion are also being developed, including cells harvested from induced progenitor cells that can be customized for specific needs. Progress continues to be made in the development and application of novel therapies for hemophilia. Finally, gene therapy and gene editing portend an exciting shift in hematology and medical care, in general.

SUGGESTED READINGS

Altomare I, Wasser J, Pullarkat V: Bleeding and mortality outcomes in ITP clinical trials: a review of thrombopoietin mimetics data, Am J Hematol 87:984–987, 2012.

Hayward CP, Moffat KA, Liu Y: Laboratory investigations for bleeding disorders, Semin Thromb Hemost 38:742–752, 2012.

Hod E, Schwartz J: Platelet transfusion refractoriness, Br J Haematol 142:348–360, 2008.

Kearon C, Akl EA, Ornelas J, et al: Antithrombotic therapy for VTE disease, ed 10, American College of Chest Physicians Guideline and Expert Panel Report, Chest 149:315–352, 2016.

Levy JH, Greenberg C: Biology of factor XIII and clinical manifestations of factor XIII deficiency, Transfusion 53:1120–1131, 2013.

Mahlangu J, Oldenburg J, Paz-Priel I, et al: Emicizumab prophylaxis in patients who have hemophilia A without inhibitors, N Engl J Med 379:811–822, 2018.

Mannucci PM: New therapies for von Willebrand disease, Hematology Am Soc Hematol Educ Program 590–595, 2019.

Menegatti M, Biguzzi E, Peyvandi F: Management of rare acquired bleeding disorders, Hematology Am Soc Hematol Educ Program 80–87, 2019.

Roback JD, Caldwell S, Carson J, et al: Evidence-based practice guidelines for plasma transfusion, Transfusion 50:1227–1239, 2010.

Rydz N, James PD: Why is my patient bleeding or bruising?, Hematol Oncol Clin North Am 26:321–344, viii, 2012.

Seligsohn U: Treatment of inherited platelet disorders, Haemophilia 18(Suppl 4):161–165, 2012.

Sharma R, Haberichter SL: New advances in the diagnosis of von Willebrand disease, Hematology Am Soc Hematol Educ Program 596–600, 2019.

Wada H, Matsumoto T, Hatada T: Diagnostic criteria and laboratory tests for disseminated intravascular coagulation, Expert Rev Hematol 5:643–652, 2012.

Weyand AC, Pipe SW: New therapies in hemophilia, Blood 133:389–398, 2019.

Winkelhorst D, Murphy MF, Greinacher A, et al.: Antenatal management in fetal and neonatal alloimmune thrombocytopenia: a systematic review, Blood 129:1538–1547, 2017.

53

Disorders of Hemostasis: Thrombosis

Rebecca Zon, Nathan T. Connell

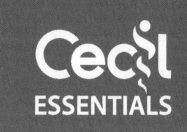

PATHOLOGY OF THROMBOSIS

The Virchow triad defines the pathologic mechanisms underlying thrombosis: diminished blood flow, damage to the vascular wall, and an imbalance favoring procoagulant over anticoagulant factors. The first two factors are clearly localized to specific vascular beds; although the last element of the triad may be systemic, data show at least partial regulation of the hemostatic balance by anatomic region. For example, congenital deficiency of antithrombin, protein C, or protein S typically leads to venous thromboembolism (VTE) of the lower extremities. In contrast, the inherited hypercoagulable disorders associated with the factor V Leiden and prothrombin G20210A mutations not only produce lower extremity VTE but also are associated with thrombosis of the cerebral veins and sinuses.

This hemostatic regulation in vascular tissues is mediated by multiple factors that include (1) microenvironmental signals, such as shear stress resulting from turbulence in the disrupted flow of damaged vessels, that affect endothelial cell (EC) expression of thrombomodulin, tissue factor, and nitric oxide synthase as well as platelet activation; (2) EC subtype–specific signaling (e.g., shear stress upregulates aortic, but not pulmonary artery, nitric oxide synthase); (3) differences in EC transcriptional regulation of proteins such as von Willebrand factor (VWF) and its cleaving protease, ADAMTS13; and (4) the increasingly appreciated important link between inflammation and thrombosis that is mediated in both physiologies by selectin and integrin ligands.

Atherothrombosis

This section briefly discusses hematologic factors that predispose to thrombosis in the setting of atherosclerotic plaque (atherothrombosis); the pathophysiologic mechanisms of atherogenesis are discussed in Chapter 8.

Atherothrombosis and Fibrinolysis

In addition to EC-directed regulation of hemostasis, the interaction of EC with the fibrinolytic system is important in the development of atherothrombotic disease because it affects the degree of clot propagation. The breakdown of stable fibrin polymers into fibrin split products, including the D-dimer segments that are routinely measured in the laboratory to detect recent thrombosis, is mediated by plasmin. Plasmin is converted from its inactive form, plasminogen, by tissue-type plasminogen activator (t-PA), the activity of which is regulated by plasminogen activator inhibitor-1 (PAI-1). Abnormal levels of both t-PA and PAI-1 are epidemiologically associated with an increased risk for arterial thrombosis, but the degree to which absolute levels contribute to arterial thrombosis remains controversial. For this reason, the current clinical utility of t-PA and PAI-1 measurements is limited.

There is a correlation between higher PAI-1 levels and atherosclerotic disease, which is possibly due to the fact that PAI-1 is markedly increased in generalized inflammation and there is known thrombosis-inflammation interplay. This is especially prominent in patients with type 2 diabetes with acute myocardial infarction and stroke. Elevated PAI-1 levels systemically may prevent thrombi removal from vessels, whereas locally it contributes to increased fibrin deposition in the lumen of the vessels. Currently there are agents that indirectly decrease PAI-1 levels, including angiotensin-converting enzyme (ACE) inhibitors and diabetes medications (including thiazolidinediones and metformin). The first PAI-1 antagonist, tiplaxtinin, has been studied in experimental models and was found to decrease VTE and atherosclerosis, although the clinical trial was discontinued given unfavorable risk-benefit outcomes. Also, meta-analyses have demonstrated PAI-1 4G/5G polymorphisms represent a risk candidate locus for higher VTE risk, which is even further heightened in patients with genetic thrombophilic disorders.

Hyperhomocysteinemia in Arterial Disease

Increased levels of plasma homocysteine (HCY) are linked to atherothrombosis. The rare congenital syndromes (e.g., cystathionine β-synthase deficiency) that are characterized by homocystinuria and hyperhomocysteinemia are associated with both VTE and premature atherosclerosis. Elevated HCY induces EC dysfunction and apoptosis, triggering normal coagulation pathways designed to respond to EC damage but without the corresponding upregulation of EC-dependent anticoagulant function (e.g., activated protein C [APC]). Even moderate elevations in HCY may thus contribute to coronary, peripheral, and cerebral arterial disease. Mildly elevated HCY levels are associated with the thermolabile form of the methylene tetrahydrofolate reductase (MTHFR) enzyme, which results from a polymorphism (C677T) in the coding region of the MTHFR binding site. This isoform occurs in 30% to 40% of the general population and introduces a higher set point for regulation of HCY concentration (the substrate for MTHFR), particularly when a relative folate deficiency exists. In fact, deficiency of any of the vitamin cofactors of HCY metabolism (folate, vitamin B_6, and vitamin B_{12}) may lead to mild hyperhomocysteinemia.

Reduction in HCY levels by supplementation with vitamin B_6, vitamin B_{12}, and folate is probably the most effective means of reducing modest HCY elevations, but such supplementation and ultimately lower HCY levels does not decrease atherothrombotic risk, regardless of the cause of hyperhomocysteinemia or the presence of the MTHFR polymorphism. Therefore, the origin of the connection between high HCY and thrombosis remains incomplete, and the search for associated factors that link HCY and hypercoagulability continues.

TABLE 53.1 Antiplatelet Therapies

Inhibitors of Cyclooxygenase
Aspirin
Nonaspirin NSAIDs (not COX2 selective)

P2Y12 Antagonists
Prasugrel
Ticagrelor
Clopidogrel

Phosphodiesterase Inhibitors
Dipyridamole
Prostacyclin

GPIIB/IIIA Blockers
Abciximab
Integrilin
Tirofiban

COX2, Cyclooxygenase 2; *GPIIb/IIIa*, glycoprotein IIb/IIIa complex; *NSAIDs*, nonsteroidal anti-inflammatory drugs.

Role of Platelets in Atherothrombosis

Although EC-associated abnormalities clearly influence hemostasis, platelet activation and adhesion are also critical to the development of atherothrombosis, especially in patients with acute coronary syndrome or ischemic stroke. Antiplatelet therapies are the primary modalities for maintaining short- and long-term patency in arteries, especially after coronary revascularization. Antiplatelet therapy can be targeted against specific platelet functions, including cyclooxygenase-mediated formation of thromboxane A_2, interaction of adenosine diphosphate (ADP) with its platelet receptor, and binding of the glycoprotein IIb/IIIa complex (GPIIb/IIIa) to fibrinogen for aggregation (Table 53.1).

Aspirin has long been a mainstay in the treatment of myocardial infarction, angina, and stroke because of its irreversible inhibition of platelet cyclooxygenase, a process that blocks the release of thromboxane A_2. Aspirin effectively prevents platelet aggregation over the lifetime of a platelet (7 to 10 days); however, aspirin is usually unable to inhibit platelet activation, secretion, and aggregation by thrombin or other strong agonists such as collagen. Therefore, blockade of other platelet activation pathways is important for patients who are at risk for arterial thrombosis.

Some drugs used to treat stroke or coronary disease (i.e., clopidogrel and prasugrel) specifically block platelet P2Y12, the ADP receptor, from interaction with ADP in the clot milieu, thereby decreasing platelet recruitment by preventing locally released ADP from activating additional platelets.

The CHANCE Trial (2013) and POINT Trial (2018) have shown reduced 90-day stroke risk with the combination of ASA/clopidogrel compared with ASA alone, although results are conflicting between the trials about increased bleeding risk with dual antiplatelet therapy (DAPT). In symptomatic peripheral arterial disease (PAD), where there is poor flow in the extremities due to atherosclerotic plaque, there are benefits with using clopidogrel compared to aspirin (demonstrated by the CAPRIE Trial 1996) but no additional benefit to using both clopidogrel and aspirin together as compared to clopidogrel monotherapy (demonstrated by the MATCH Trial 2004).

Antiplatelet therapy with aspirin and a P2Y12 inhibitor (clopidogrel, prasugrel, or ticagrelor) also reduces the risk of stent thrombosis and subsequent cardiovascular events after percutaneous coronary intervention and should be administered for at least 12 months unless the patient is at high risk for bleeding. The PLATO Trial (2009) showed, in acute coronary syndrome, prasugrel and ticagrelor further reduce cardiovascular ischemic events compared with clopidogrel, although they are associated with higher bleeding risk. This effect occurs because drug interactions and variant cytochrome genotypes do not significantly affect production of the active metabolites of prasugrel and ticagrelor; the result is greater and more rapid inhibition of P2Y12 receptor–mediated platelet aggregation in most patients. The EUCLID Trial showed that in PAD, there was no improvement with ticagrelor compared to clopidogrel in terms of cardiovascular death, myocardial infarction, or stroke.

Despite its wide use, a significant proportion (up to one third) of patients demonstrate functional platelet resistance to clopidogrel. Under such circumstances, clopidogrel is poorly metabolized to its active form because of the presence of polymorphisms in the cytochrome P-450 gene, *CYP2C19*, that cause loss of function. The more potent inhibitor, prasugrel, is not affected by cytochrome P-450 genotypes, although nongenetic factors such as platelet turnover, absorption, and compliance also play important roles in response variability.

A third avenue for blocking platelet activation targets GPIIb/IIIa, the primary platelet receptor for binding to fibrinogen and VWF. Abciximab, a modified monoclonal antibody, prevents GPIIb/IIIa from binding to fibrinogen and blocks platelet aggregation after angioplasty, stent placement, or pharmacologic thrombolysis. Abciximab has been shown to reduce the incidence of recurrent acute ischemic events after percutaneous coronary revascularization in patients with myocardial infarction or unstable angina, mainly by decreasing the incidence of platelet-mediated thrombosis within the infarct-related vessel during and after the procedure. Other GPIIb/IIIa blockers, including eptifibatide (Integrilin) and tirofiban (Aggrastat), interfere with the GPIIb/IIIa arginine-glycine-aspartate (RGD) binding sites; they are used acutely for parenteral administration in patients with acute coronary syndrome or to maintain coronary patency after percutaneous coronary intervention. Thrombocytopenia is an uncommon (<2%) complication of all the GPIIb/IIIa inhibitors; it is most likely related to exposure of neoepitopes on the receptor and immune-mediated platelet destruction. Clearance of the drug typically resolves the thrombocytopenia within 1 week. Platelet transfusion should be considered only if there is significant thrombocytopenic bleeding because of the higher incidence of stent thrombosis after stent implantation with platelet transfusion.

Additional novel strategies for mediating platelet activity include inhibition of cyclic nucleotide phosphodiesterases (e.g., dipyridamole, cilostazol) and blockade of proteinase-activated receptor 1 (PAR-1). Phosphodiesterase inhibitors most likely have multiple mechanisms of action. They result in decreased signal transduction within platelets, which impairs their responsiveness. PAR-1 is one of two principal recognized targets for thrombin stimulation of platelets, the other being PAR-4. The potential benefit of adding phosphodiesterase or PAR-1 inhibitors to aspirin and/or clopidogrel (e.g., prevention of restenosis in atherothrombosis) is being evaluated. As shown in ESPS-2 (1996) and ESPRIT (2006), aspirin/dipyridamole outperformed aspirin alone in secondary prevention of ischemic strokes—current guidelines recommended either aspirin monotherapy or aspirin/dipyridamole as secondary prevention for ischemic stroke. Additionally, for recent stroke, there appears to be no difference in recurrence rates of ischemic stroke when comparing aspirin/dipyridamole to clopidogrel, as shown in the PRoFESS Trial (2008). Currently, either of these options or aspirin monotherapy is recommended after noncardioembolic ischemic stroke; aspirin in combination with clopidogrel is not recommended given increased bleeding risk (POINT Trial 2018).

TABLE 53.2 Prevalence and Thrombotic Relative Risk Associations of Laboratory Findings[a]

Prevalence in General Population	Venous RR	Arterial RR
Hyperhomocysteinemia (25%)	1-2	1.16
Activated protein C resistance (5%)		
Heterozygous FVL	7	1
Homozygous FVL	20-80	
Prothrombin G20210A mutation (1-2%)		
Heterozygous	2-5	1
Homozygous	>5	1
Platelet GPIIb/IIIa HPA-Ib homozygosity (2-3%)		4 (MI in men)
Protein C deficiency (0.2-0.5%)	7	1
Protein S deficiency (0.1%)	8.5	1
AT deficiency (0.02-0.05%)	8	1
Dysfibrinogenemia (rare)	≈1	1.5

AT, Antithrombin; *FVL*, factor V Leiden; *GPIIb/IIIa*, glycoprotein IIb/IIIa complex; *HPA-1b*, human platelet antigen-1b; *MI*, myocardial infarction; *RR*, relative risk.

[a]Data on prevalence and relative risk vary widely, often with conflicting results. This information represents an interpretation of data collected from various sources, mainly meta-analyses.

When using platelet inhibitors, physicians and patients must also consider the risk of bleeding if they are on anticoagulation therapy. RE-DUAL (2017) and WOEST (2013) concluded that in patients on anticoagulation prior to percutaneous coronary intervention (PCI) it is recommended to use additionally only clopidogrel rather than ASA/clopidogrel after PCI given the increased bleeding risk with triple therapy.

Venous Thromboembolism: Inherited Risk Factors

The balance between thrombin formation and anticoagulant pathways has been extensively studied in patients with inherited deficiencies of naturally occurring anticoagulants (Table 53.2). These patients are predisposed to VTE, which includes deep vein thrombosis (DVT) and pulmonary embolism (PE).

Factor V Leiden

The most common inherited disorder leading to VTE is the factor V Leiden (FVL) mutation although it remains a fairly weak risk factor for VTE overall. About 5% of individuals of European ancestry are heterozygous for FVL. The FVL mutation increases VTE risk by decreasing the susceptibility of factor Va to APC-mediated inactivation and by impairing the APC-cofactor activity of factor V in factor VIIIa inactivation, all of which lead to increased thrombin generation. APC resistance can be demonstrated by specialized clotting tests in which the addition of APC fails to inhibit thrombin generation. About one fourth of patients with their first VTE are heterozygous for FVL, and this percentage increases to almost 60% among those with recurrent VTE or a strong family history of VTE.

Heterozygous FVL mutation conveys a 7-fold increased risk for VTE. However, at 50 years of age, only 25% of persons with heterozygous FVL mutation have had VTE, compared with much higher percentages in other inherited thrombophilias. It is with concomitant *acquired* risk factors such as immobilization, pregnancy, or oral contraceptive use that the risk for VTE in persons with FVL mutation becomes more significant. The prothrombin G20210A mutation demonstrates a synergistic effect with FVL mutation, but the MTHFR

mutation does not. Homozygous FVL mutation individuals have a 20- to 80-fold increased risk for VTE. APC resistance *without* the FVL mutation occurs rarely. Factor V Cambridge mutation, although much less common than FVL mutation, has a similar mutation at an APC cleavage site (Arg306) and is associated with APC resistance and thrombosis. Other minor alleles of factor V, including the 6755 A/G (D2194G) R2 haplotype, may enhance APC resistance. When this haplotype is on a different chromosome than the FVL mutation, it diminishes normal factor V transcription and increases the ratio of FVL to normal factor V.

Prothrombin G20210A

Another mutation associated with inherited thrombophilia is the prothrombin G20210A mutation, which occurs in the 3′-untranslated region of the prothrombin gene. This mutation leads to higher than normal prothrombin levels and a 2-fold increased risk for VTE. The heterozygous mutation is present in about 3% of European-derived populations but is identified in about 15% of patients with VTE. Patients homozygous for prothrombin G20210A are rare, but their relative risk for VTE is thought to be about 10-fold. Exactly how the prothrombin mutation affects thrombus development has not been fully defined, but changes in polyadenylation of the prothrombin messenger RNA (mRNA) during transcription appear to be involved. The distribution of circulating prothrombin levels overlaps significantly between those with and without the mutation, so Factor II levels are not helpful in diagnosing the condition. Diagnosis of the G20210A genotype is made by examination of the patient's DNA for this specific mutation; no screening or functional assays are available.

Inherited Deficiency of Natural Anticoagulants

Deficiencies in the natural anticoagulant proteins (antithrombin, protein C, and protein S) are less common than FVL or prothrombin G20210A, but they are more likely to produce symptomatic VTE at an earlier age. Only about one half of the cases of VTE occurring in patients with these deficiencies are associated with acquired risk factors such as pregnancy, surgery, or immobilization. Deficiencies of antithrombin, protein C, or protein S are detected by functional or antigenic assays because some mutations cause a quantitative decrease in the factor, whereas others produce a dysfunctional protein. Many gene mutations have been associated with these deficiencies, but none is predominant. Deficiencies of antithrombin (AT), protein C, and protein S in the aggregate account for fewer than 5% to 10% of all patients with VTE.

Antithrombin is a naturally occurring anticoagulant that complexes with endogenous heparin sulfates to inhibit both formed thrombin and factor Xa. Heterozygous antithrombin deficiency leads to antithrombin activity levels less than 70% of normal and a 20-fold increase in the risk for VTE; VTE usually occurs by the age of 25 years in 50% of such patients. More than 200 associated mutations are known. Homozygous mutations are very rare, likely because of lethality *in utero*.

Acquired causes of antithrombin deficiency are more common. Because antithrombin has a low molecular weight, it is lost in the proteinuria of nephrotic syndrome. Acquired antithrombin deficiency is common in patients receiving asparaginase therapy for acute lymphocytic leukemia and may also be associated with severe hepatic veno-occlusive disease after stem cell transplantation; antithrombin and protein C may be excessively consumed in the damaged hepatic microvasculature. Low levels of antithrombin are also associated with poorer outcomes in severely ill patients. Successful treatment of symptomatic patients with heterozygous antithrombin deficiency has included short-term replacement with fresh-frozen plasma or recombinant AT protein, usually coupled with unfractionated heparin (UFH) anticoagulation; long-term therapy for congenitally deficient patients has consisted primarily of warfarin although the direct oral anticoagulants have become increasingly popular due to their lack of requiring functional antithrombin activity in order to cause an anticoagulant effect.

The complex of thrombin and thrombomodulin on the EC surface activates protein C; APC coupled with its cofactor, protein S, cleaves and inactivates factors Va and VIIIa. These actions downregulate the prothrombinase and tenase complexes, respectively, to slow the rate of thrombin generation. Like antithrombin deficiency, heterozygous protein C and protein S deficiencies are observed with venous, and occasionally arterial, thrombosis in younger patients (median age at occurrence, 20 to 40 years).

The rare homozygous protein C deficiency manifests in the neonate as *purpura fulminans* with widespread VTE and skin necrosis. A similar clinical presentation has been reported in heterozygous protein C–deficient adults after institution of warfarin therapy without simultaneous heparinization; this is called *warfarin-induced skin necrosis*. About one third of these patients are deficient in protein C on a hereditary basis, whereas the rest appear to have acquired protein C deficiency, possibly associated with vitamin K deficiency. Warfarin is a vitamin K antagonist that inhibits production of vitamin K–dependent protein C synthesis; and because of its short half-life, protein C levels rapidly fall before a decline in the levels of the procoagulant factors II, IX, and X. This imbalance shortly after starting warfarin favors a procoagulant state and may result in widespread microvascular thrombosis. Therefore, patients with active VTE should be fully anticoagulated with UFH or low-molecular-weight heparin (LMWH) before concurrent warfarin therapy is begun. UFH/LMWH should be continued for at least 48 hours, warfarin has a full therapeutic effect.

Inherited deficiency of protein S has similarly been implicated in warfarin-induced skin necrosis. Protein S deficiency is commonly acquired in acute illness. Protein S circulates in a free form and is bound by complement 4b (C4b)-binding protein; only free protein S is active as a cofactor for protein C. Because C4b-binding protein is an acute phase reactant, its increase with severe illness can decrease the level of free protein S. A similar effect is seen in normal pregnancy.

Short-term therapy for homozygous protein C deficiency or for doubly heterozygous protein C or S deficiency, especially in the setting of neonatal purpura fulminans, has included plasma or protein C concentrate with full-dose UFH anticoagulation. Functional and antigenic levels of antithrombin, protein S, and protein C can be assessed to define whether functional deficiency is caused by a dysfunctional protein or by diminished synthesis. As with AT deficiency, initial heparin therapy followed by long-term treatment with warfarin has been successful in heterozygous protein C or S deficiency. As expected, both protein C and protein S levels are decreased during warfarin therapy; therefore, for adequate evaluation of protein C and S, the patient must not be taking warfarin when tested.

Venous Thrombosis: Acquired Risk Factors
Surgery and Medical Hospitalization

Medical and surgical illnesses convey increased thrombotic risk; these *acquired* risk factors are well accepted, even though the pathophysiologic features favoring thrombosis may be uncertain (Table 53.3). Stasis of blood flow is a clear risk factor for thrombus formation (e.g., VTE in immobilized inpatients). Other high-risk situations, including surgery (especially orthopedic) and trauma, are similarly associated with immobilization and stasis of lower extremity blood flow. When evidence of thrombosis is thoroughly sought, both surgery and trauma can be shown to be associated with extremely high (>50%) incidences

TABLE 53.3	Acquired Risk Factors for Thrombosis

Medical and Surgical Illnesses
Antiphospholipid antibody, lupus anticoagulant
Artificial heart valves
Atrial fibrillation (nonvalvular)
Congestive heart failure
Hemolytic anemias (autoimmune hemolysis, sickle cell, thrombotic thrombocytopenic purpura, paroxysmal nocturnal hemoglobinuria)
Hyperlipidemia
Immobilization
Malignancy
Myeloproliferative disorders with thrombocytosis
Nephrotic syndrome
Orthopedic procedures
Pregnancy
Trauma, fat embolism

Medications
Heparin-induced thrombocytopenia
Oral contraceptives, hormone replacement therapy
Prothrombin complex concentrates

of VTE. Fat embolism and tissue damage may also contribute to the risk for VTE with surgery and trauma, particularly in closed head injuries that result in massive tissue factor release. Prophylactic inferior vena cava (IVC) filters are often placed in trauma patients to protect against PE, especially in high-risk patients for whom anticoagulation is contraindicated because of the increased risk for bleeding, but there remains a high risk for thrombus formation proximal to the filter with subsequent pulmonary embolism. IVC filters should be removed as soon as patients may be safely anticoagulated.

All hospitalized medical patients should be considered for venous thromboprophylaxis with UFH or LMWH. Factors that increase bleeding risk that argue against anticoagulation include thrombocytopenia (typically a platelet count <50,000), coagulopathy (with or without liver disease), and recent hemorrhage. Risk factors that warrant aggressive prophylaxis include malignancy, prior VTE, immobilization, and thrombophilic conditions.

Pregnancy and Fetal Loss

Pregnancy is a hypercoagulable state associated with venous stasis; the risk for VTE during pregnancy and in the postpartum period for women with identified thrombophilia is about 5-fold higher than it is for nonpregnant women. Pregnancy increases procoagulant proteins, including fibrinogen, VWF, and factors VII, VIII, and X, and decreases natural anticoagulants such as protein S and antithrombin as well as fibrinolytic inhibitors such as PAI-1 and thrombin activator fibrinolysis inhibitor (TAFI). VTE can occur at any time during pregnancy or the puerperium. The risk of postpartum VTE is significantly higher in women with any of the following conditions: stillbirth, pre-term delivery, obstetric hemorrhage, caesarean procedure, medical comorbidities, or a pre-pregnancy body mass index greater than 30 kg/m^2.

Inherited maternal thrombophilia can compound the procoagulant state of pregnancy and predispose to both fetal loss and VTE in the mother. The principal inherited associated risk factors for fetal loss are FVL mutation, the G20210A prothrombin mutation, antithrombin deficiency, and protein C or protein S deficiency. The relative risk for fetal loss is markedly higher in those mothers with a history of prior

VTE, although this particular risk appears to be restricted to the period after 9 weeks' gestation. In fact, inherited thrombophilia may be protective against fetal loss during the first 9 weeks, possibly by limiting oxygen toxicity to the early embryo. Therefore, recommended indications for evaluating the inherited thrombophilia risk in women seeking to become pregnant are a history of VTE or recurrent fetal loss after 9 weeks of gestation when no other specific cause (e.g., antiphospholipid syndrome) can be identified. Both antithrombin deficiency and hyperhomocysteinemia have also been associated with placental abruption.

In the absence of an identified inherited thrombophilia or a diagnosis of antiphospholipid syndrome (discussed later), no role has been identified for prophylactic anticoagulant therapy with recurrent pregnancy loss although prophylactic aspirin is increasingly used in many women with high-risk pregnancy.

Oral Contraceptives and Hormone Replacement

Estrogen-containing oral contraceptive use conveys an increased risk for VTE, and a similar increased risk is seen early after institution of hormone replacement therapy in postmenopausal women. Concomitant heterozygosity for FVL mutation synergistically increases the risk for VTE in women who take estrogen-based oral contraceptives or hormone replacement therapy. Cigarette use in women using oral contraceptives also increases the risk of thrombosis, possibly through increased platelet reactivity mediated by increased thromboxane synthesis. On the arterial side, epidemiologic evidence clearly points to smoking as the main cardiovascular risk factor. Paradoxically, most data suggest a protective role for hormone replacement therapy in cardiovascular disease. As discussed previously, acquired APC resistance and decreases in the levels of both free and functional protein S occur with oral contraceptive use.

VTE in Malignancy

VTE is the second leading cause of death in malignancy. VTE occurs in a wide spectrum of malignancies, including mucin-producing malignancies (i.e., pancreatic, gastric, ovarian), gastrointestinal, lung, breast, lymphoma, and more. Interestingly, the part of the Virchow triad that is most affected can vary; for example, adenocarcinoma is known to increase hypercoagulability, whereas lymphoma can lead to VTE through compression of blood vessels and thus blood flow stasis.

When idiopathic VTE occurs in a cancer-free individual, an intensive work-up to find an occult malignancy is not necessarily warranted and has not been shown to improve subsequent cancer-related morbidity or mortality, as shown in the SOME Trial (2015). However, once a cancer diagnosis is established in patients with prior VTE, they are at increased risk for subsequent VTE events, especially if the FVL or G20210A prothrombin mutation is present. LMWH prophylaxis after malignancy-associated VTE achieves superior prevention compared to warfarin, possibly because of better maintenance of an anticoagulated state. Direct oral anticoagulants (DOACs) are being increasingly used given numerous recent clinical trials (see section "Therapy for VTE in Malignancy").

In the special case of myeloproliferative disorders (e.g., essential thrombocythemia), abnormal platelet physiologic mechanisms causing hyperaggregation are often present and require platelet-specific inhibition (see "Hypercoagulability and Platelet Disorders").

Other Prothrombotic Disease States

As described earlier, thrombosis in nephrotic syndrome is associated with loss of antithrombin through the kidneys. Hemolysis is a general prothrombotic state that appears to be mediated through blood cell destruction, perhaps through increased exposure to procoagulant membrane phospholipids; hemolysis with thromboembolic

complications has been observed in patients who have artificial heart valves, sickle cell disease, and other hemolytic anemias, including Coombs-positive autoimmune hemolytic anemia. In the case of paroxysmal nocturnal hemoglobinuria (PNH), complement activation may directly mediate platelet activation, and therapy with the complement inhibitor eculizumab has significantly decreased the rate of thromboembolic disease in PNH.

Platelet activation and clearance appear to be the primary prothrombotic manifestations of heparin-induced thrombocytopenia (HIT) and thrombotic thrombocytopenic purpura (TTP).

Additionally, chronic disseminated intravascular coagulation (DIC) is classically associated with certain malignancies such as mucinous adenocarcinoma and promyelocytic leukemia. In that setting, known as Trousseau syndrome, there is an increased risk in malignancy for VTE that is not related to DIC.

Antiphospholipid Antibody Syndrome

Another acquired prothrombotic disorder is the antiphospholipid antibody syndrome (APS). APS is a primary disorder, unlike the occasional association of lupus anticoagulant or antiphospholipid antibodies with other autoimmune diseases such as systemic lupus erythematosus (SLE). The etiologic connection with SLE has not been fully defined, but replacement of the host immune system after hematopoietic stem cell transplantation for refractory SLE has the potential to eradicate the lupus anticoagulant and thromboembolic risk. All of the manifestations of APS are related to hypercoagulability, including recurrent venous or arterial thrombosis, thrombocytopenia caused by microcirculatory platelet clearance, and recurrent fetal loss resulting from placental vascular insufficiency. Serologic markers of APS include *anticardiolipin antibodies, anti-β_2-glycoprotein I antibodies*, and *lupus anticoagulants*. The Sydney Consensus Criteria for Antiphospholipid Syndrome (also known as the revised Sapporo criteria) are the current standard for diagnosis of APS. Diagnosis requires both the clinical criterion of radiologically or pathologically confirmed thrombosis or thrombosis-related fetal loss and the laboratory criterion of positive tests on two or more occasions at least 12 weeks apart. Anticardiolipin and anti-glycoprotein antibodies are detected by enzyme-linked immunosorbent assay (ELISA), whereas lupus anticoagulants are defined by correction of prolonged phospholipid-dependent clotting tests (most commonly hexagonal phase partial thromboplastin time [PTT] or Russell viper venom clotting time), with addition of excess phospholipid. Therefore, *lupus anticoagulant* is a misnomer; its presence predisposes the patient to clotting rather than to bleeding, and the risk for thrombosis is highest when a lupus anticoagulant is detectable. Another misleading aspect of this nomenclature is that phospholipid-reactive antibodies are actually directed against phospholipid-binding proteins in plasma (e.g., $\beta2$-glycoprotein I antibody, annexin V, prothrombin). Anti–$\beta2$-glycoprotein I antibody is detected by immunoassay, and high titers of this marker are also correlated with thromboembolic risk.

In patients with recurrent pregnancy loss in the context of APS, LMWH during pregnancy can help reduce further miscarriages.

Hypercoagulability and Platelet Disorders

Essential thrombocythemia and polycythemia vera are clonal myeloproliferative disorders commonly associated with somatic mutations in the *JAK2* gene. In essential thrombocythemia, mutations are also found in CALR and MPL in those negative for *JAK2* mutations. They are wholly (essential thrombocythemia) or partially (polycythemia vera) characterized by thrombocytosis, and patients with these disorders are at increased risk for thrombosis. Platelet aggregometry in these disorders often shows abnormal responses, especially to epinephrine and ADP; however, the abnormal aggregation does not correspond to either bleeding or thrombosis risk. Patients with polycythemia vera in particular have a high incidence of thrombosis in the mesenteric, portal, and hepatic venous circulation.

Thrombotic complications, both arterial and venous, occur in essential thrombocythemia, even in young patients. The risk of arterial thrombosis in essential thrombocythemia (and probably also in primary myelofibrosis and polycythemia vera) is most increased by a history of previous thrombosis or the presence of the *JAK2* V617F mutation. Therefore, prophylaxis with low-dose aspirin is probably justified in patients with high-risk essential thrombocythemia and other myeloproliferative disorders.

Increased platelet turnover in thrombocytosis is also associated with thromboembolic complications, but this does not necessarily involve high platelet counts, as has been demonstrated by radioactive platelet survival studies and an increase in reticulated (young) platelets in thrombotic essential thrombocytopenia. Moreover, successful treatment of symptomatic patients with aspirin increases platelet survival by decreasing platelet clearance. Concomitant therapy to prevent thrombotic complications of thrombocytosis includes lowering the platelet count with hydroxyurea, pegylated alpha interferon or anagrelide. Evidence suggests that patients with essential thrombocythemia who are at high risk for thrombosis (prior thrombosis or over age 60) are most effectively treated with the combination of hydroxyurea and low-dose aspirin. Patients with reactive (secondary) thrombocytosis resulting from iron deficiency anemia, chronic infection, or rheumatoid arthritis do not generally have increased thrombotic risk and do not require aspirin prophylaxis.

Heparin-Induced Thrombocytopenia

HIT must be distinguished from other drug-induced forms of immune thrombocytopenia because of its potentially catastrophic *thrombotic* complications and its unique pathophysiologic features. Almost 25% of patients who are exposed to UFH develop antibodies (detected by ELISA) that recognize the complex of heparin and platelet factor 4 (PF4), the latter being released from activated platelets, although most will not develop the clinical syndrome of HIT. When such patients receive heparin again, between 5% and 10% develop HIT, most with platelet counts between 50,000 and 100,000/μL. HIT rarely occurs in patients who have not been previously exposed to heparin (0.3% incidence).

Surgery is a specific risk factor for HIT; the incidence of HIT in surgical patients is about 2.6%, compared with 1.7% in medical patients. HIT antibodies occur with high frequency in patients undergoing either cardiac surgery with cardiopulmonary bypass or an orthopedic procedure such as hip replacement. The incidence of HIT in patients who have received only LMWH is far lower, only about one tenth the rate seen with UFH. However, the mechanism of thrombocytopenia for both UFH and LMWH appears to be similar: Platelet Fc-receptor binding of the heparin-PF4 antibody complex causes signal transduction and platelet activation with enhanced thrombin generation on the platelet surface.

The diagnosis is predominantly clinical (e.g., using the 4Ts algorithm for scoring HIT—magnitude of *t*hrombocytopenia, *t*iming of platelet fall, *t*hrombotic sequelae, and ruling out o*t*her causes of thrombocytopenia), but the rapid ELISA test will detect heparin-PF4 antibodies in serum. The main drawback of ELISA is that it does not indicate whether the antibody complex is a functional activator of platelets; therefore, it is sensitive but not specific for HIT. The serotonin release assay is the functional test for HIT; it detects platelet activation after exposure to serum antibody in the presence of a therapeutic heparin level. However, a low probability for HIT based on the 4Ts score can be used to exclude the HIT diagnosis.

The thrombin-based procoagulant response in HIT incorporates platelets into microcirculatory clots, leading to thrombocytopenia; about 30% of HIT patients have overt thromboembolic complications, which can be severe or life-threatening. Thromboembolic events can occur before, concurrent with, and after development of thrombocytopenia in HIT, with about equal frequency. Although thrombosis is more frequent in patients with both HIT and concomitant cardiovascular disease and in those receiving full-dose heparin, any heparin dose (even intravenous catheter heparin flushes) can result in thrombosis in HIT. Arterial and venous thromboembolic disease can occur even weeks after heparin has been discontinued, an effect perhaps mediated by EC glycosaminoglycan binding to PF4, which serves as a target for circulating HIT antibodies.

Discontinuation of all heparin is critical; moreover, although the antibody may have been induced by treatment with UFH, more than 80% of these antibodies cross-react with LMWH. Therefore, the preferred therapy for short-term anticoagulation in patients with HIT is a direct thrombin inhibitor (DTI), such as argatroban or bivalirudin, which is not a target for the heparin-PF4 antibodies. Indeed, because the event rate for subsequent thrombosis, limb amputation, and death is increased in patients with HIT even if they do not have thrombosis at presentation, DTI therapy is mandated after discontinuation of heparin. The choice of DTI may be dictated by other clinical conditions; for example, renal insufficiency slows bivalirudin clearance, increasing bleeding risk, whereas argatroban is cleared by hepatic metabolism. For patients who develop HIT after warfarin has already been started, in addition to substituting a DTI, one should administer vitamin K to correct protein C levels. Although it has not been approved by the US Food and Drug Administration (FDA) for this clinical scenario, the synthetic pentasaccharide indirect Xa inhibitor fondaparinux has the advantages of once-daily subcutaneous administration without need for laboratory monitoring and of having no effect on the International Normalized Ratio (INR). DOACs are also an attractive option for treatment with clinical trials ongoing to determine safety and efficacy.

DTI therapy should be continued until the platelet count is higher than 100,000 to 150,000/μL. Warfarin can then be added, and the two therapies should overlap for at least 5 days with the INR at a therapeutic level for at least 48 hours. Because DTIs prolong the INR, a therapeutic warfarin level after 5 days may result in a supratherapeutic INR (usually >4); gradual downward titration of the DTI as the INR increases is a logical management strategy. Once DTIs are stopped, it is essential to repeat the INR measurement after 4 to 6 hours to confirm that it remains within the therapeutic range.

If there is no thrombosis with HIT, the total duration of anticoagulation should be at least 4 weeks; if thrombosis is present, anticoagulation should be continued for 3 to 6 months. Warfarin should never be used as initial therapy to treat HIT, and it should not later be instituted without simultaneous DTI coverage because it may induce acquired protein C deficiency leading to venous limb gangrene. One hallmark of protein C depletion in HIT is a sudden rise in the INR (to >3.5) after a single warfarin dose; in that circumstance, warfarin should be discontinued and the patient repleted with vitamin K. Patients with a history of HIT who need surgery requiring cardiopulmonary bypass can be safely reexposed to brief systemic UFH if ELISA testing is negative for the antibody at least 100 days after the previous UFH exposure.

Thrombotic Thrombocytopenic Purpura

Another cause of thrombocytopenia resulting from platelet activation and clearance is TTP. In patients with congenital or familial TTP, mutations in the VWF-cleaving protease, ADAMTS13 (*a* *d*isintegrin *a*nd *m*etalloproteinase with *t*hrombo*s*pondin type 1 motif, member 13), abrogate its activity. Patients with acquired TTP usually have an antibody that blocks the normal function of VWF-cleaving protease to less than 10% of normal. Ultralarge VWF multimers released by EC normally anchor to EC through P-selectin and form long strings that adhere and aggregate platelets in the microcirculation. ADAMTS13 downregulates the size of these multimers by docking to the A1/A3 VWF domains and cleaving within the A2 site. Deficient cleaving protease function in TTP leads to an increase in the larger, highest-molecular-weight VWF multimers, which are most effective in anchoring and activating platelets. These, in turn, cause increased platelet adhesion and clearance *without* activating the coagulation cascade. Therefore, both the prothrombin time (PT) and the PTT are normal in TTP, unlike the case in DIC.

TTP after chemotherapy (mitomycin C) or in association with pregnancy, stem cell transplantation, lupus, or HIV infection appears to have a similar pathogenic mechanism of thrombosis. Thrombocytopenia (often severe) is accompanied by microangiopathy with schistocytes on smear and increased serum lactate dehydrogenase. Microvascular occlusions in multiple organs cause symptoms, especially in the kidney and brain. The classic pentad (fever, thrombocytopenia, microangiopathic hemolysis, neurologic symptoms, and renal insufficiency) is present in fewer than 5% of patients with TTP. The diagnosis is typically made based on the clinical assessment of thrombocytopenia and microangiopathic hemolytic anemia; assays for ADAMTS13 activity and inhibitor do not have a rapid turnaround time in most laboratories. Clinical prediction scores (e.g., the PLAMIC score) are helpful as an additional piece of clinical information in the decision to initiate treatment for TTP but cannot be used on their own to exclude TTP. In validation studies, some patients ultimately found to have an ADAMTS13 activity level, less than 10% were noted to have low PLASMIC scores.

Treatment of familial TTP is based on replenishment of cleaving protease activity with plasma transfusion; acquired TTP additionally requires removal of the antibody. The latter is accomplished by therapeutic plasma exchange, whereby patient plasma is removed (plasmapheresis) and replaced with fresh-frozen plasma, which often has been made "cryo-poor" to reduce ultralarge VWF multimers in transfused plasma. Corticosteroids are often administered simultaneously, but any added benefit to plasma exchange remains unclear. Platelet transfusions are relatively contraindicated in TTP because of the risk of thrombosis, and they should not be given for thrombocytopenia in the absence of significant bleeding. When plasma exchange fails to remit acquired TTP or when early relapse occurs, immunosuppressive therapy with anti-CD20 may be successful and data suggest that early rituximab will reduce the risk of relapse. The mortality rate associated with severe TTP (defined as undetectable ADAMTS-13 activity) is still significant, almost 10% at 18 months after therapy with plasma exchange. Replacement of ADAMTS-13, which is present in fresh-frozen plasma and in cryoprecipitate, is a potential treatment. Clinical trials have shown the anti-VWF therapy caplacizumab to have benefit in reducing the number of days of plasma exchange needed to achieve a normal platelet count and also reductions in mortality, although with increasing bleeding risk. The ideal subset of patients to receive caplacizumab in conjunction with other therapies for TTP remains to be defined. Caplacizumab does not address the underlying autoantibody causing ADAMTS13

deficiency and use of rituximab for inhibitor eradication is most likely to be beneficial in patients receiving caplacizumab therapy.

The *hemolytic-uremic syndrome* (HUS) is part of the TTP spectrum of disease and also is associated with microvascular platelet thrombi. However, the hemolytic anemia and renal failure of HUS are not usually accompanied by neurologic impairment, and HUS usually does not produce the same degree of thrombocytopenia or microangiopathy as TTP. Moreover, fewer than 3% of HUS cases are associated with any decrease in VWF-cleaving protease activity. Unlike TTP, HUS is usually diagnosed in children (and less commonly in adults) who have hemorrhagic colitis caused by Shiga-like, toxin-producing bacteria, especially the *Escherichia coli* O157:H7 serotype. Atypical HUS (i.e., without diarrhea or Shiga-like toxin) is rarely associated with other bacterial infections or with complement dysregulation due to mutations or polymorphisms in factors H, I, and B. These mutations increase platelet activation through complement (C3) deposition on the platelet surface. Atypical HUS cases are those that are clinically consistent with HUS but are not associated with toxin-producing bacteria. Some HUS cases, particularly atypical forms, may temporarily respond to plasma exchange along with maintenance hemodialysis until renal function recovers. Data support use of the anti-C5a complement therapy eculizumab to prevent the complement-mediated damage associated with this disease. More recently, a modified form of eculizumab with a longer half-life, ravulizumab, has been approved to treat atypical HUS, allowing patients longer intervals between therapeutic infusions.

CLINICAL EVALUATION OF THROMBOSIS

The approach to patients with thromboembolism is defined by the clinical history, results of laboratory studies, and even physical findings. Events that trigger VTE disease include immobilization, orthopedic and other surgical procedures, use of oral contraceptives, and pregnancy. VTE that is recurrent (thrombophilia) may manifest at an early age or at unusual thrombotic sites (e.g., cerebral vessels) and may be accompanied by a family history of VTE, suggesting an inherited disorder. Acquired VTE risk may be associated with systemic disorders such as hemolysis (e.g., PNH, autoimmune hemolytic anemia), collagen vascular disorders (e.g., lupus), or various malignant diseases (e.g., adenocarcinoma). In contrast, arterial thromboembolic disease is more commonly superimposed on ruptured atherosclerotic plaque (e.g., coronary artery disease) or on atheroembolic disorders (e.g., ischemic stroke, peripheral arterial disease). Arterial vascular disease is mainly associated with metabolic risk factors including hypertension, hypercholesterolemia, and diabetes. The clinical approach to thrombotic disease is tailored to the location of the disease (arterial vs. venous and the specific vascular bed) and whether there are abnormalities of the vascular endothelium, platelets, or soluble coagulation factors that predispose the patient to thromboembolic risk.

Laboratory Diagnostics

Recurrent VTE is a strong indication for laboratory testing for causes of thrombophilia, especially in patients younger than 50 years of age, in those with unexplained VTE, and in those with a first-degree family history of VTE. Any risk factors that may predispose these individuals to recurrence must be defined, as well as any inherited disorders that may necessitate family counseling or avoidance of additional environmental risks. The current work-up for VTE thrombophilia includes the following: (1) APC resistance, (2) genotyping for prothrombin G20210A, (3) lupus anticoagulant assay and anticardiolipin and anti–β_2-glycoprotein I antibody serologies, (4) functional AT and protein C levels, and (5) free protein S (Table 53.4).

TABLE 53.4 Laboratory Evaluation of Venous Thrombosis

Activated protein C resistance, factor V Leiden
Lupus anticoagulant
Anticardiolipin, anti-β_2-glycoprotein I antibody serology
Homocysteine level: fasting or after methionine load
Prothrombin G20210A mutation
Antithrombin activity
Protein C activity
Free protein S level
Paroxysmal nocturnal hemoglobinuria (select patients)
Myeloproliferative disorders (in select patients)

Genotyping for the FVL mutation can substitute for APC resistance and also determines whether the patient is heterozygous or homozygous, although it may miss rare variants of APC resistance. Patients need to be off of warfarin during these tests and they should not be performed during the acute episode, given the changes in protein levels during these instances.

The utility of laboratory testing in the setting of atherothrombosis and arterial thromboembolism is unclear. In the setting of a myeloproliferative disorder, the use of hydroxyurea and/or aspirin therapy may be justified by platelet count and platelet function testing, but typically risk prediction models based on age and prior thrombosis are used to guide management decisions. In patients with unusual or recurrent arterial disease, other assays can be justified, including testing for t-PA and PAI-1 levels and for dysfibrinogenemia (thrombin time and antigen activity ratio), all of which should be performed in consultation with specialists in hemostasis.

THERAPY FOR VENOUS THROMBOEMBOLISM

Once VTE has been diagnosed, immediate therapy is required. In most patients, anticoagulation options include heparin, LMWH, or the newer direct oral anticoagulants (DOACs) (i.e., apixaban, rivaroxaban) initially and then warfarin or DOACs thereafter. The DOACs edoxaban and dabigatran require initial parenteral anticoagulation prior to use of the DOAC, but apixaban and rivaroxaban may be started as initial therapy with higher doses. Thrombolytic therapy is indicated for patients with extensive proximal venous clots or PE. IVC filters are used in patients with contraindications to anticoagulation, complications of anticoagulation (usually active bleeding), or failure of anticoagulation (recurrent PE). IVC filters clearly decrease the incidence of early PE, but their use is also associated with thrombosis at the insertion site and late complications of IVC thrombosis as well as a 10% to 20% incidence of postphlebitic syndrome. In patients who may be safely anticoagulated, IVC filters do not reduce the risk of pulmonary embolism and appear to be associated with a higher risk of PE. Temporary IVC filters are often used in trauma patients and appear to be most efficacious when they are placed for fewer than 7 to 10 days.

UFH is often the anticoagulation therapy of choice for many inpatients because of its short half-life and reversibility, but LMWH is increasingly used for this indication. UFH is begun as a bolus intravenous infusion of 80 U/kg, followed by a continuous infusion of 18 U/kg/hour; UFH doses in excess of 30,000 U/day have been shown to be most efficacious at preventing recurrent VTE. UFH is monitored by the PTT, and the therapeutic PTT range determined by each hospital corresponds to anti-Xa levels of 0.3 to 0.7 U/mL. Many hospitals have established protocols for adjustment of UFH infusion based on the patient's weight and PTT monitoring.

UFH should be continued for at least 5 days (longer in patients with extensive clots) and may be discontinued after the patient has been fully anticoagulated with warfarin (INR ≥2 for 2 consecutive days). Some patients receiving large doses of heparin (usually >40,000 U/day) do not develop a therapeutic PTT. This heparin resistance can be caused by a variety of mechanisms, including increased heparin-binding proteins, counteracting medications (e.g., protamine), and decreased antithrombin. An *apparent* heparin resistance is often seen in patients with coexistent inflammatory disease with high plasma levels of factor VIII and fibrinogen; direct monitoring of anti-Xa levels is indicated. It is important to remember that the anti-Xa level is a measurement of anticoagulant level in the blood but is not a direct measure of the anticoagulant effect present. Some patients may require a higher anti-Xa level in order to achieve therapeutic anticoagulation.

LMWH is an excellent alternative to UFH in the treatment of thromboembolism and acute coronary events. The small controlled-size elements of LMWH stimulate antithrombin activity that is more restricted to factor Xa compared with UFH, which has effects on thrombin, factor IX, and factor XI, in addition to others. The practical advantages of LMWH over UFH include increased plasma half-life, more predictable dose response allowing for intermittent fixed dosing, a lower *de novo* incidence of HIT (10% to 20% of the rate for UFH), and significantly reduced monitoring requirements. LMWH levels are prolonged in renal failure and in those circumstances may need to be monitored and adjusted based on anti-Xa levels. Peak anti-Xa levels (0.5 to 1 U/mL for twice-daily dosing and 1 to 2 U/mL for once-daily dosing) typically occur between 3 and 5 hours after subcutaneous LMWH injection. As with UFH, switching from LMWH to warfarin for long-term management can be accomplished after therapeutic INR values have been present for at least 2 days.

Supratherapeutic INR levels commonly occur with warfarin therapy, with or without bleeding. In patients with moderately elevated INR values (>5) and little or no bleeding, temporary discontinuation of warfarin and reinstitution of the drug at a lower maintenance dose may be sufficient. Patients with higher INR values (5 to 9) who are without serious bleeding should have warfarin withheld and should receive low doses (1 to 2.5 mg/day) of oral vitamin K to reach therapeutic INR levels; parenteral vitamin K may be given if gastrointestinal function is problematic. If serious active bleeding occurs with high INR values, especially if surgery is required to correct the bleeding, a combination of vitamin K and transfusion of plasma (see Chapter 52) will rapidly correct the INR. The INR can become elevated as a result of concurrent use of drugs that increase free warfarin levels (Table 53.5). Whenever bleeding occurs as a complication of anticoagulation, serious consideration must be given to future bleeding risks and to whether the patient requires placement of a filter for prophylaxis.

Recently, DOACs have been used with increased frequency because their efficacy and safety have now been evaluated in many circumstances. For patients with acute DVT, the initial anticoagulation (within the first week or two) options include: oral factor Xa inhibitors rivaroxaban or apixaban (in addition to the previously mentioned LMWH, subcutaneous fondaparinux, or unfractionated heparin). The decision of which agent to use is based on risk of bleeding, clinician comfort, patient comorbidities, and cost. The doses are: rivaroxaban 15 mg twice daily for 21 days then 20 mg daily; apixaban 10 mg twice daily for 7 days then 5 mg twice daily. For long-term, maintenance therapy, the DOACs approved are: direct factor Xa inhibitors (rivaroxaban, apixaban, edoxaban), thrombin inhibitors (dabigatran); as mentioned, warfarin, LMWH and fondaparinux can also be used for

TABLE 53.5 Guidelines for Duration of Prophylactic Anticoagulation After VTE

Condition	Duration of Therapy
Distal or superficial vein thrombus	3-12 wk
First Proximal VTE	
No risk factors	3-6 mo[a]
Correctable risk factor (e.g., surgery, trauma)	3-6 mo
Malignancy	Long-term[b]
Antiphospholipid syndrome	Long-term
Inherited risk factor[c]	>6 mo
Recurrent VTE/PE	Lifelong

PE, Pulmonary embolism; *VTE,* venous thromboembolism (includes deep vein thrombosis, pulmonary embolism, and sinus or cerebral thrombosis).

[a]Evaluation of D-dimer after 3-6 mo may assist in the decision to stop prophylaxis.

[b]Long-term therapy must be adjusted individually according to presence of other diseases, risks for bleeding, presence of transient risk factors, and ease of compliance.

[c]Inherited risk factors include factor V Leiden; prothrombin 20210A; deficiencies of antithrombin, protein C, or protein S.

long-term therapy. Dosing is as follows: dabigatran 150 mg BID (needs renal dose adjustment 75 mg BID if CrCl 15-30), edoxaban (after acute phase parenteral anticoagulation). DOACs are not recommended with severe renal impairment. However, apixaban can be dose adjusted for renal impairment and other variables. If creatinine is greater than 1.5, age older than 80, or weight 60 kg or less, decrease apixaban dosing to 2.5 mg orally twice daily. RE-COVER (2009) demonstrated, in patients with acute VTE, the oral direct thrombin inhibitor, dabigatran, was found to be as effective as warfarin for reducing recurrence risk and is associated with less bleeding. The benefit is that the DOACs have less variability in therapeutic range compared with warfarin and patients do not need to have blood drawn for INR checks when on the DOACs, as they have to do on warfarin.

In summary, based on the most recent American College of Client Physicians (ACCP) Antithrombotic Therapy for VTE Disease Guidelines (2016), DVT of the leg or PE without cancer, dabigatran, rivaroxaban, apixaban, or edoxaban is preferred over vitamin K antagonist therapies as treatment for the 3 months of maintenance therapy.

The treatment duration varies based on unprovoked or provoked DVT, location of clot, and initial or recurrent DVT. For most patients with a first episode of DVT (provoked and unprovoked, proximal and distal), treatment should be for 3 months. If proximal DVT or PE and low/moderate bleeding risk, this should be extended beyond 3 months. In patients with recurrent VTE, regardless of bleeding risk, the duration should be greater than 3 months and depending on risk factors of bleeding and patient comorbidities, indefinite anticoagulation may be recommended. The duration of therapy greater than 3 months has not been fully specified and will vary on a case-to-case basis. For patients who have received at least 6 to 12 months of anticoagulant therapy and have clinical equipoise to continue anticoagulation, low-dose rivaroxaban (10 mg once daily) or apixaban (2.5 mg twice daily) is safe and effective to reduce VTE risk with little to no increased bleeding risk as shown in the EINSTEIN Choice and AMPLIFY-EXT trials, respectively.

After stopping anticoagulation for unprovoked proximal DVT or PE, guidelines suggest aspirin over no aspirin to prevent recurrent DVT in patients with no contraindication to aspirin but in whom anticoagulant is not continued.

Therapy for VTE in Malignancy

In patents with malignancy, LMWH is preferred to warfarin. Based on the CLOT trial in 2003, dalteparin (LMWH) had a lower recurrent VTE risk without increasing bleeding risks or deaths compared to warfarin. These were confirmed in the 2006 LITE and ONCENOX trials. The Hokusai VTE Cancer Trial (2018) demonstrated that in patients with VTE and malignancy edoxaban was noninferior to dalteparin for recurrent VTE in an open label study but had higher bleeding risk. For specific malignancies, such as gastrointestinal cancer, LMWH is preferred to edoxaban for long-term anticoagulation (see Raskob 2017). Additionally, some studies recommend not using edoxaban if the CrCl is greater than 95, although the data for avoiding this medication in VTE are not clear. The SELECT-D pilot trial compared rivaroxaban todalteparin in cancer-associated VTE and showed a decreased rate of recurrent VTE in the rivaroxaban group compared to dalteparin but an increased rate of non-major bleeding. There are multiple current trials studying apixaban versus dalteparin for patients with malignancy-associated VTE: the Caravaggio Trial is ongoing, and preliminary results for ADAM-VTE suggest low bleeding risk and low VTE recurrence rates.

In summary, based on the most recent ACCP Antithrombotic Therapy for VTE Guidelines (2016), for patients with cancer-associated VTE, as therapy for the first 3 months, LMWH is recommended over other agents whereas ASCO guidelines suggest DOACs may be used as first-line therapy. As mentioned previously, duration of therapy for VTE depends on cancer type (clotting and bleeding risks) and treatment plan for the malignancy.

Given known interactions and lack of safety data, DOACs should not be prescribed for patients on dual P-glycoprotein and strong CYP3A inhibitors, including medications such as carbamazepine, phenytoin, ketoconazole, ritonavir, rifampin, and more. Certain antibiotics (i.e., erythromycin or clarithromycin) may increase levels of DOACs, especially in individuals with renal dysfunction.

Prophylaxis of VTE

Even with the advent of the DOACs, both warfarin and LMWH are often used for treatment of VTE. Warfarin should be begun during the first 24 hours after presentation with VTE, concurrent with heparin treatment. The PT is prolonged within hours by warfarin because of a rapid decrease in factor VII levels; however, therapeutic warfarin anticoagulation does not occur until other vitamin K–dependent factors (II, IX, and X) also decrease. Therapeutic warfarin anticoagulation is usually achieved within 4 to 5 days with adequate warfarin dosing; UFH or LMWH may be discontinued after the INR has been greater than 2 for at least 2 consecutive days. One long-standing problem with warfarin anticoagulation is the interindividual variability in INR response; at least 50% of this variability in sensitivity to warfarin may be explained by polymorphisms in the *CYP2C9* and *VKORC1* genes. Although these have been incorporated into models for predicting safe and therapeutic warfarin dosing, most clinicians simply begin dosing and adjust therapy as needed based on periodic monitoring.

The therapeutic INR range depends on the condition predisposing the patient to thromboembolism. Prophylaxis after uncomplicated VTE in a patient without known risk factors requires an INR between 2 and 3; in contrast, warfarin prophylaxis for patients with APS and recurrent VTE may require INR values as high as 3 to 4 (Table 53.6).

The duration of warfarin or LMWH prophylaxis varies depending on the circumstances of the VTE, the risk for bleeding, and the potential for recurrence. In general, the longer the period of anticoagulation with warfarin, the less the chance of recurrence. Short-term warfarin (6 weeks) is less effective at preventing recurrence than longer courses (6 months). Patients with definite transient risk factors such

TABLE 53.6 Drugs That Affect Warfarin Levels

Increased Warfarin Levels: Prolonged INR
↓ Warfarin clearance
Disulfiram
Metronidazole
Trimethoprim-sulfamethoxazole
↓ Warfarin-protein binding
Phenylbutazone
↑ Vitamin K turnover
Clofibrate

Decreased Warfarin Levels: Subtherapeutic INR
↑ Hepatic metabolism of warfarin
Barbiturates
Rifampin
↓ Warfarin absorption
Cholestyramine

↑, Increased; *↓*, decreased; *INR*, international normalized ratio.

TABLE 53.7 Therapeutic International Normalized Ratio (INR) Ranges for Warfarin

Patient Subgroup	INR Range
Venous Thrombosis	
Treatment	2.0-3.0
Prophylaxis	1.5-2.5
Artificial Heart Valves	
Tissue	2.0-2.5
Mechanical	3.0-4.0
Atrial Fibrillation (Nonvalvular)	
Prophylaxis	1.5-2.5
Lupus Anticoagulant	
Treatment, prophylaxis	2.0-3.0
Refractory thromboembolism	3.0-4.0

as orthopedic surgery have low recurrence rates, even with short-term therapy; still, prolonged thromboprophylaxis (>21 days) after total hip replacement is more efficacious than shorter therapy (7 to 10 days). It is not clear that oral Xa inhibitors and dabigatran provide any additional benefit over LMWH for thromboprophylaxis after total hip or knee replacement (Table 53.7).

Additionally, DOACs have been studied as thromboprophylaxis in specific patient settings. The MARINER trial evaluated patients who were discharged after medical illness with increased risk of VTE and showed that rivaroxaban 10 mg by mouth daily for 45 days after discharge did not reduce VTE or VTE mortality compared with placebo.

In contrast, patients with "unprovoked" VTE (i.e., outside the setting of trauma, surgery, immobilization, pregnancy, or cancer) have significant recurrence rates, even after 3 to 6 months of warfarin therapy. Because the risk for recurrence in patients with unprovoked proximal VTE or PE is relatively low when D-dimer levels are normal 3 weeks after cessation of anticoagulation, this measure may help providers decide whether anticoagulation past 3 to 6 months is necessary.

Given increased risk of recurrence in patients without reversible risk factors for VTE, extended-duration anticoagulation is sometimes warranted. Two studies evaluated using aspirin 100 mg versus placebo after anticoagulation therapy for unprovoked VTE. ASPIRE 2012 found a nonsignificant trend towards fewer recurrent VTE events and a nonsignificant trend towards higher bleeding risk, whereas WARFASA 2012 found statistically significant demonstration of fewer VTE recurrences without differences in major bleeding. There is thought that the trials differ in outcomes due to ASPIRE's lack of enrollment for prespecified power, differences in inclusion criteria, and that only two thirds of ASPIRE patients had received 6 or more months of anticoagulation prior to initiation of aspirin.

Furthermore, the EINSTEIN-CHOICE Trial demonstrated that, in patients with VTE who have completed 6 to 12 months of anticoagulation, there was reduced risk of recurrent VTE without significant bleeding when using both 10 or 20 mg/day of rivaroxaban compared to aspirin 100 mg/day. In AMPLIFY-EXT, another oral factor Xa inhibitor, apixaban, was studied for extended anticoagulation at doses of 5 mg (treatment) or 2.5 mg (prophylactic) and was found to have statistically decreased number of recurrent VTE and no increased bleeding risk compared to placebo.

Thus, current management for an unprovoked acute VTE includes use of either rivaroxaban or apixaban for the initial 6 months of therapy followed by a dose reduction in either agent. For patients with a provoked VTE, initial anticoagulation practice is the same, but anticoagulation may be stopped 3 months after the provoking risk factor has resolved.

Evidence also indicates that inherited hypercoagulable disorders (e.g., FVL mutation) probably confer a lifelong increased risk for VTE or PE, but whether the index VTE was provoked or unprovoked determines length of therapy. Some studies have shown that the bleeding risks incurred by long-term, low-intensity warfarin use are favorably balanced by the decreased incidence of recurrent thrombosis. Therefore, the presence of inherited thrombophilia may warrant continuation of anticoagulation for a longer period, depending on the patient's other medical illnesses and whether transient circumstances may have predisposed the patient to VTE. Patients who develop recurrent VTE after discontinuation of anticoagulation should receive long-term anticoagulation regardless of whether they have a defined cause of thrombophilia. Patients with APS and a first episode of VTE are at very high risk for recurrent VTE (up to 50% per year) after anticoagulation is discontinued, clearly supporting the rationale of testing for antiphospholipid. Table 53.8 suggests broad guidelines for the duration of warfarin therapy in specific patient subgroups. Because warfarin is a teratogen, effective contraception should be used concurrently in women of childbearing age.

Prophylaxis for VTE in Orthopedic Surgeries

RECORD1 and RECORD3 (both published 2008) demonstrated improved efficacy of short-course rivaroxaban over short-course enoxaparin in prevention of VTE after hip and knee replacements, respectively, without increased bleeding risk. RECORD2 (2008) demonstrated that extended-course rivaroxaban was more effective in preventing VTE than short-course enoxaparin without increasing bleeding rates following hip replacement.

Prophylactic Anticoagulation in Hospitalized Medically Ill Patients

MEDENOX, PREVENT, and ARTEMIS demonstrated promise of in-hospital thromboprophylaxis with LMWH with a relative risk reduction of 45% to 63% compared to placebo. In acutely medically ill hospitalized patients, MAGELLAN (2013) demonstrated short-course rivaroxaban (10 mg daily for 10 days) is noninferior to short-course

TABLE 53.8 Direct Oral Anticoagulants (DOAC) and Their Indications

DOAC	Indications
Dabigatran	Direct thrombin inhibitor for nonvalvular atrial fibrillation (to prevent stroke and non-CNS embolism); VTE as maintenance therapy (after initial therapy); VTE prophylaxis of VTE after hip replacement
Rivaroxaban	Anti-Xa for nonvalvular atrial fibrillation (to prevent stroke and non-CNS embolism); treatment of VTE and subsequent prophylaxis; and VTE prophylaxis of VTE after hip or knee replacement
Apixaban	Anti-Xa for nonvalvular atrial fibrillation (to prevent stroke and non-CNS embolism); VTE as initial therapy or maintenance therapy; VTE prophylaxis of VTE after hip or knee replacement
Edoxaban	Anti-Xa for prevention of VTE as maintenance therapy (after initial therapy); prevention of embolism in atrial fibrillation; has been studied for treatment of VTE in patients with malignancy and is noninferior to dalteparin (a LMWH) with an increased bleeding risk

CNS, Central nervous system; *VTE,* venous thromboembolism; *Xa,* activated factor X.

enoxaparin (40 mg daily for 10 days) in preventing VTE, although it increases risk of bleeding. Extended rivaroxaban (10 mg daily for 35 ± 4 days) was also found to be superior to short-course enoxaparin for prevention of VTE and its complications but also had increased bleeding risk.

The APEX trial studied acutely ill medical patients and showed that extended-duration betrixaban for 35 to 42 days did not reduce the primary end point of asymptomatic proximal clot or symptomatic VTE compared to standard enoxaparin for 6 to 14 days.

Prophylactic Anticoagulation in High-Risk Patients With Malignancy in the Ambulatory Setting

The CASSINI trial evaluated ambulatory cancer patients at high risk for thromboembolism (Khorana score ≥2) and whether low-dose rivaroxaban (10 mg daily) is more effective than placebo in reducing incidence of venous thromboembolism. Rivaroxaban did not result in statistically significant reduction in incident thromboembolism at 180 days when compared to placebo and had a small, not statistically significant increase in bleeding risk; however, when only time on the drug was considered, there was an absolute reduction in VTE with rivaroxaban compared to placebo. On the other hand, the AVERT trial studied apixaban 2.5 mg twice daily versus placebo in ambulatory cancer patients at intermediate-to-high risk for venous thromboembolism (Khorana score ≥2). Prophylactic apixaban reduced the risk of VTE in these patients but increased the risk of major bleeding episodes. Major bleeding was most common in those with GI or GU malignancy. Of note, the trial populations were different, with AVERT having a significant proportion of patients with lymphoma and CASSINI having a higher proportion of pancreatic cancer.

Antithrombotic Therapy During Pregnancy

Heparins, both UFH and LMWH, are the safest therapy for venous thrombosis treatment and prevention during pregnancy. Heparin does not cross the placenta, unlike warfarin, which causes a characteristic fetal embryopathy. Warfarin also causes fetal hemorrhage and placental abruption and should be avoided during pregnancy. VTE or PE during pregnancy should be treated with intravenous UFH for 5 to 10 days, followed by an adjusted-dose regimen of subcutaneous UFH, starting with 20,000 U every 12 hours and adjusted to achieve a PTT higher than 1.5 times baseline at 6 hours after injection. An attractive alternative to UFH during pregnancy is LMWH, which can be given subcutaneously once or twice daily and does not require monitoring. Suprarenal IVC filters have also been used successfully during pregnancy without significant morbidity. In women with APS who become pregnant, therapy is critical to prevent fetal loss; aspirin is combined with prophylactic doses of either subcutaneous UFH (10,000 to 15,000 U/day in divided doses) or LMWH (to achieve an anti-Xa level of 0.1 to 0.3 U/mL). When such women have a history of thromboembolic disease, therapeutic doses of LMWH or UFH plus aspirin are employed.

Heparin should be discontinued at the time of labor and delivery, although the risk for hemorrhage is not high during delivery, especially if anti-Xa levels are less than 0.7 U/mL. One concern with residual anticoagulation at delivery is the risk for spinal hematoma with epidural anesthesia; this concern has been reported with both UFH and LMWH. The anti-Xa level that is safe for an epidural procedure is not known. Protamine sulfate can be used to neutralize UFH if the PTT is prolonged during labor and delivery; however, LMWH is only partially (10%) reversed by protamine.

Anticoagulation during the postpartum period can be carried out with heparin (either UFH or LMWH) or warfarin; neither drug is contraindicated during breast-feeding. Women receiving long-term warfarin therapy (e.g., for valvular heart disease) who wish to become pregnant need to be switched to a fully anticoagulating dose of UFH or LMWH; warfarin treatment may be restarted after delivery.

There is limited evidence to support use of DOACs in pregnancy. There are concerns about a higher incidence of miscarriages and fetal anomalies with DOACs. There is currently not enough data to show safety and suggest use of the DOACs during pregnancy, so they are not recommended.

Perioperative Anticoagulation

A common clinical problem is the management of anticoagulation in patients who require surgery. The principles of care in this situation reflect the need for adequate hemostasis during and immediately after surgical procedures as well as the critical importance of restarting anticoagulation as soon as possible postoperatively, especially because surgery itself represents a relative hypercoagulable state. The perceived risk for thromboembolism in patients with atrial fibrillation clearly affects the management of perioperative anticoagulation; in this clinical situation, the CHADS-2 score (cardiac failure, *h*ypertension, *a*ge, *d*iabetes, and *s*troke) may estimate postoperative stroke risk and thus dictate the need for bridging anticoagulation with UFH/LMWH when stopping vitamin K antagonist. For patients with VTE who are anticoagulated on a short-term basis (<1 month), elective surgical procedures should be postponed; if such patients must undergo urgent surgery, discontinuation of anticoagulation and placement of a temporary IVC filter may be the best option. In most patients receiving long-term anticoagulation for VTE, preoperative heparin is not typically used; vitamin K antagonist should be discontinued for at least 4 days preoperatively to allow the INR to decrease gradually to less than 1.5, a level that is safe for surgery. Postoperatively, intravenous heparin (or subcutaneous LMWH) can be safely used for anticoagulation until therapeutic INR levels are reached after warfarin has been restarted. Increasingly, restarting a DOAC postoperatively at pre-surgery therapeutic dosing is safe and effective to avoid the need for bridging with parenteral therapy. As with all guidelines, individual patient circumstances may dictate changes. For example, institution of heparin immediately after a major surgical procedure may be contraindicated because of the high risk for hemorrhage, and reinstitution of anticoagulation may need to be delayed for 12 to 24 hours postoperatively.

Risk of postoperative VTE in patients undergoing hip or knee arthroplasty without postoperative anticoagulation is estimated at 6% by Caprini score. Thus, VTE prophylaxis is standard of care. EPCAT II 2018 showed extended thromboprophylaxis with aspirin 81 mg was noninferior to rivaroxaban 10 mg daily for 5 days in preventing symptomatic VTE in low-risk patients after total hip or knee arthroplasty.

❖ For a deeper discussion on this topic, please see Chapter 162, "Approach to the Patient with Bleeding and Thrombosis," in *Goldman-Cecil Medicine*, 26th Edition.

SUGGESTED READINGS

Adam SS, McDuffie JR, Lachiewicz PF, et al: Comparative effectiveness of new oral anticoagulants and standard thromboprophylaxis in patients having total hip or knee replacement, Ann Intern Med 159:275–284, 2013.

Barbui T, Finazzi G, Carobbio A, et al: Development and validation of an international prognostic score of thrombosis in World Health Organization-essential thrombocythemia (IPSET-thrombosis), Blood 120:5128–5133, 2012.

Basurto L, Sánchez L, Díaz A, et al: Differences between metabolically healthy and unhealthy obesity in PAI-1 level: Fibrinolysis, body size phenotypes and metabolism, Thrombosis Research vol 180:110–114, 2019.

Beer PA, Erber WN, Campbell PJ, et al: How I treat essential thrombocythemia, Blood 117:1472–1482, 2011.

Brilakis ES, Patel VG, Banerjee S: Medical management after coronary stent implantation, JAMA 310:189–198, 2013.

Carrier M, Abou-Nassar K, Mallick R, et al: AVERT Investigators. Apixaban to prevent venous thromboembolism in patients with cancer, N Engl J Med 380(8):711–719, 2019.

Cattaneo M: The platelet P2Y12 receptor for adenosine diphosphate: congenital and drug-induced defects, Blood 117:2102–2112, 2011.

Connors JM: Thrombophilia testing and venous thrombosis, N Engl J Med 377(12):1177–1187, 2017.

Cuker A, Gimotty PA, Crowtheer MA, et al: Predictive value of the 4Ts scoring system for heparin-induced thrombocytopenia, Blood 120:4160–4167, 2012.

Dobromirski M, Cohen AT: How I manage venous thromboembolism risk in hospitalized patients, Blood 120:1562–1569, 2012.

Douketis JD: Perioperative management of patients who are receiving warfarin therapy: an evidence-based and practical approach, Blood 117:5044–5049, 2011.

Khorana AA, Soff GA, Kakkar AK, et al: CASSINI Investigators. Rivaroxaban for thromboprophylaxis in high-risk ambulatory patients with cancer, N Engl J Med 380(8):720–728, 2019.

Lameijer H, Aalberts J, van Veldhuisen D, et al: Efficacy and safety of direct oral anticoagulants during pregnancy; a systematic literature review, Thrombosis Research 169:123–127, 2018.

Raskob GE, van Es N, Verhamme P, et al: Hokusai VTE Cancer Investigators. Edoxaban for the treatment of cancer-associated venous thromboembolism, N Engl J Med 378(7):615–624, 2018.

Scully M, Cataland SR, Peyvandi F, et al: HERCULES Investigators. Caplacizumab treatment for acquired thrombotic thrombocytopenic purpura, N Engl J Med 380(4):335–346, 2019.

Sobieraj DM, Lee S, Coleman CI, et al: Prolonged versus standard-duration venous thromboprophylaxis in major orthopedic surgery, Ann Intern Med 156:720–727, 2012.

Sultan AA, Tata LJ, West J, et al: Risk factors for first venous thromboembolism around pregnancy: a population-based cohort study from the United Kingdom, Blood 121:3953–3961, 2013.

Tosetto A, Iorio A, Marcucci M, et al: Predicting disease recurrence in patients with previous unprovoked venous thromboembolism: a proposed prediction score (DASH), J Thromb Haemost 366:1019–1025, 2012.

SECTION IX

Oncologic Disease

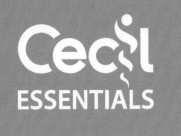

54

Cancer Biology

Andre De Souza, Wafik S. El-Deiry

INTRODUCTION

Cancer is a complex genetic disease that is defined by the transition of a normal cell, governed by processes that control its replication, into a cancer cell that is typified by unrestrained proliferation and dissemination. The underlying landscape of cancer genetics is now fully defined for many cancers, aided by the evolving technologies in gene sequencing. Many therapeutic advances of the last decade have successfully focused on targets identified by the study of genetic mutations. This chapter reviews the essential elements of cancer biology and key underlying genetic alterations driving this biology.

THE GENETICS OF CANCER

Cancer is a genetic disease. Carcinogens are chemical mutagens or physical insults that result in DNA alterations. Each of these insults produce different alterations with distinct outcomes for a cancer cell. These alterations can also be derived from random mutations enabled by failure of DNA repair mechanisms.

The most common gene alterations in cancer are nonsynonymous point mutations. A synonymous point mutation is a single nucleotide exchange (also called single nucleotide polymorphism [SNP] or single nucleotide variant [SNV]) that does not affect the final resultant amino acid and therefore does not affect the function of a protein. By contrast, a nonsynonymous mutation will result in an amino acid change that may be beneficial for the survival of a cancer cell. Dr. Bert Volgelstein described the stepwise acquisition of mutations as drivers of cancer progression. Using the progressive histopathological stages of colorectal cancer as a model, he depicted carcinogenesis as a sequence of alterations in genes such as APC, KRAS, TP53, and SMAD4 (small mothers against decapentaplegic 4). In recognizing TP53 as a tumor suppressor gene and determining its central role in the transformation of a preneoplastic adenoma to colorectal cancer, Dr. Volgelstein linked the most common tumor suppressor gene to one of the most prevalent human malignancies. He further unraveled the role of mutations as "drivers" and "passengers" in the pathogenesis of cancer and its heterogeneity. The genetic changes associated with cancer paved the way for screening tests that could be used for early detection and prevention of cancer development.

Copy number variation or gene amplification denotes the loss or gain of a whole copy of a gene. When a cell has extra copies of genes, it can produce twice or more the amount of proteins. On the other hand, when just parts of a gene are lost (deletions) or anomalous sequences are inserted amid the full gene sequence (insertions), these events are called indels (insertions and deletions). Indels have a knack for activating the immune system. Why? When proteins transcribed from genes with indels are presented in the regular health cellular checkup we call antigen presentation, they look more foreign to immune cells than point mutations. Lastly, mitosis malfunction may be conducive to fusion of distinct segments of

chromosomes. Natural selection can then favor gene fusions from translocational events that stimulate cell survival. Much progress has been made in the past several decades to unravel oncogenic fusions in various leukemias and solid tumors (Fig. 54.1). The classical Philadelphia chromosome in chronic myelogenous leukemia creates a fusion of the *BCR-ABL* genes. Tyrosine kinase inhibitors such as Imatinib block the transforming ability of *BCR-ABL* and have led to prolonged patient survival. The *BCL-2* gene translocated in follicular lymphoma can be therapeutically inhibited by venetoclax, while various NRTK fusions driving cancer can be treated with larotrectinib or entrectinib. Other common translocations in Burkitt's lymphoma, Ewing's sarcoma, or prostate cancer are well-known but not yet therapeutically targeted.

THE TUMOR MICROENVIROMENT

Tissues are made of a myriad of cells, each contributing to a state of homeostasis that controls unchecked growth of individual cells. Our understanding of cancer is evolving from a cellular disease to an infirmity of tissues.

There is a growing body of evidence that bone marrow–derived and stromal–derived cells contribute to the evolution of cancer. Myeloid-derived suppressor cells (MDSCs) have been shown to suppress NK and cytotoxic T cells (CD8⁺) in the tumor microenvironment, whereas cancer-associated fibroblasts (CAFs) synthesize the thick extracellular matrix (desmoplasia) that serves as a scaffold and a shield for drugs targeting stroma-rich tumors such as pancreatic cancer (Fig. 54.2). The tumor microenvironment (TME) is complex and includes multiple immune, stromal, endothelial cells, altered extracellular matrix, proinflammatory, immunosuppressive, and chemoattracting cytokines, and physical changes such as hypoxia, altered tumor metabolism leading to low pH, a dysregulated metabolome. The TME promotes cancer progression and resistance to therapy.

HALLMARKS OF CANCER

The hallmarks of cancer were established by Hanahan and Weinberg and updated in 2011. These hallmarks are products of driver mutations that incapacitate selective pressures restricting tumor growth. The hallmarks include acquisition of immortality, genomic instability, hyperactive proliferative signaling pathways, growth checkpoint disruption, angiogenesis, metabolism reprogramming, invasion and metastasis, and immune escape.

Immortality: Apoptosis Suppression, and Telomerase Activation

Apoptosis or programmed cell death occurs in adult cells when DNA damage or other forms of cellular stress elicit a suicidal program to

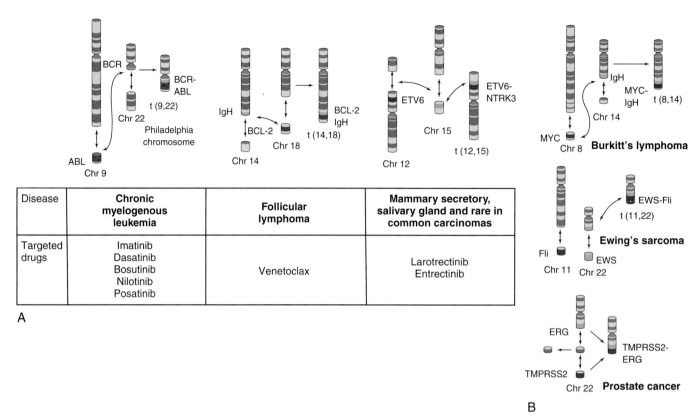

The table within figure A:

Disease	Chronic myelogenous leukemia	Follicular lymphoma	Mammary secretory, salivary gland and rare in common carcinomas
Targeted drugs	Imatinib Dasatinib Bosutinib Nilotinib Posatinib	Venetoclax	Larotrectinib Entrectinib

A

B

Fig. 54.1 Chromosomal translocations and oncogene activation in human cancer. (A) Depicted are several classical translocations associated with different types of cancer and the FDA-approved drugs used to treat them. These include chronic myelogenous leukemia t(9,22)(BCR-ABL), follicular lymphoma t(14,18) *(IgH/ BCL2)*, and *NTRK* gene fusions that occur in various solid tumors (e.g., *ETV-6/NTRK3*). (B) Major chromosomal translocations associated with Burkitt's lymphoma t(8,14) *(MYC/IgH)*, Ewing's and other sarcomas *(EWS/FLI)*, and prostate cancer *(TMPRSS2/ERG)*. Other translocations are being recognized as they contribute to therapy resistance including *ESR1* whose translocation (not shown) confers resistance to hormonal therapy in breast cancer. Not shown are common translocations in mantle cell lymphoma t(11,14) (Cyclin D, IgH) or other *NTRK* genes such as *NTRK1* and *NTRK2*.

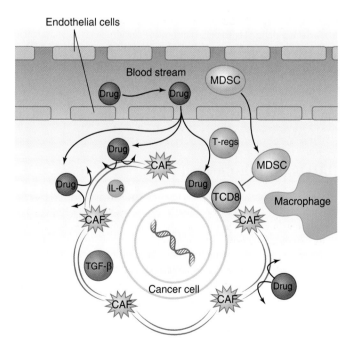

Fig. 54.2 The tumor microenvironment promotes cancer progression and impedes cancer therapy. The tumor microenvironment (TME) is composed of different cell types in addition to cancer cells. The TME of a growing tumor typically has hypoxic regions, low pH due to altered metabolism, and low levels of nutrients. Cancer associated fibroblasts (CAF) create a thick connective tissue mesh which acts as a mechanical barrier to drug delivery to cancer cells. This connective tissue shell is also known as desmoplasia, here stylized as *blue concentric curves*. A small molecule or biologic drug is represented as *red circles* crossing through the endothelial lining of a blood vessel. Although some drug does make it to the tumor cell, some bounces off the desmoplastic shell. Once cancer evolves, the body tries to fight it off with an adaptative immune response, which ultimately delivers cytotoxic T cells (TCD8) to kill cancer cells, enabled by chemical mediators such as Interleukin-6 (IL-6) and attenuated by immunosuppressive factors such as transforming growth factor β (TGF-β). Immunosuppressive cells include macrophages and T regulatory cells (T-regs). The cytotoxic T cells are characterized by specific transmembrane receptors, the cluster of differentiation (CD) 8 proteins, and are regulated in part by myeloid-derived suppressor cells (MDSCs), which dampen an overstimulated immune response that otherwise would result in autoimmune disease. MDSCs are generated in the bone marrow and also cross endothelial cell gaps to render TCD8 cells anergic. MDSCs are hijacked by tumors to serve as one of the mechanisms of immune evasion. Some of these concepts have been recently summarized in a review of the physical hallmarks of cancer (Nia HT, Munn LL, Jain RK: *Science* October 2020; 370[546]: 1–11).

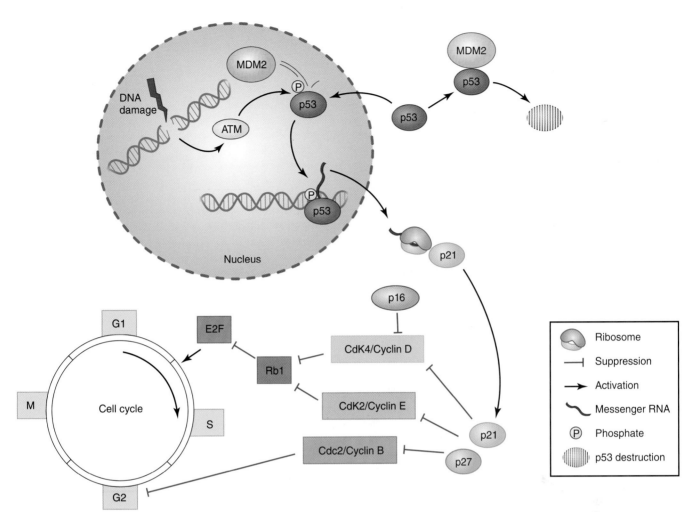

Fig. 54.3 DNA damage stalls the cell cycle. DNA damage, for example after exposure to ionizing radiation, triggers ATM phosphorylation of the p53 protein. Other kinases induced by DNA damage include ATR, Chk1, and Chk2 (not shown). The p53 protein is constitutively tagged to proteasomal destruction by the E3 ligase MDM2; p53 phosphorylation stabilizes the protein by blocking its binding to MDM2. The p53 protein transcriptionally activates the expression of the p21 gene *(CDKN1A, WAF1)*. The p21 protein is the cell checkpoint of all three CDK and cyclin complexes (CDK4/Cyclin D, CDK2/Cyclin E, CDC2/Cyclin B). Therefore, p53, through p21, arrests the cell cycle to allow repair after DNA damage and thereby prevent cancer. *TP53* is the most commonly mutated gene in human cancer. The p27 protein is another universal inhibitor of CDK complexes. By contrast, the p16 protein, encoded by the *CDKN2A* gene, inhibits CDK4/Cyclin D. Inhibition of CDK4 and CDK2 complexes allows unphosphorylated RB to bind E2F proteins and inhibit entry of cells into S-phase where the DNA is replicated. CDK4 and 6 inhibitors are approved for therapy of estrogen receptor positive breast cancer. MDM2, ATR, ATM, Chk1, and Chk2 inhibitors are currently in clinical trials for cancer therapy. The *"p"* denotes protein, followed by molecular weight in Kilodaltons, as in p21 and p53. *Arrows* indicate activation processes in a pathway. *Red "T"* symbols indicate suppression of a pathway. *ATM*, Ataxia telangiectasia mutated; *CDK*, cyclin-dependent kinase; *E2F*, a family of transcription factors which activate genes required for S-phase; *MDM2*, mouse double minute 2; *RB*, retinoblastoma.

save the organism as a whole. This program is actioned by extracellular ligands (extrinsic pathway) or intracellular mediators (intrinsic pathway). The extracellular ligand FASL or TRAIL (in immune cells) or soluble ligands (in the extracellular space) bind to FAS and TRAIL receptors in the cell that undergoes apoptosis. The intrinsic pathway culminates in release of cytochrome c to the cytosol. Caspase activation in response to either the extrinsic or intrinsic cell death pathways results in proteolytic cleavage of thousands of cellular proteins that result in cell detachment, shrinkage, nuclear fragmentation and engulfment by macrophages. Several pro- and anti-apoptotic regulator proteins, such as Bcl-2, are deregulated in cancer (Figs. 54.3–54.5). Telomere shortening is the prime cellular timekeeper process

only avoided by the enzyme telomerase, dormant in most tissues. Telomerase reactivation induces cancer cell immortality and is a key early event in carcinogenesis. However, the telomerase target is yet to be meaningfully exploited in cancer therapy.

Genomic Instability: Impairing DNA Repair Genes

Alterations in DNA repair genes increase tumor mutation burden. It was also observed that some cancer cells had frail chromosomes, prone to breakage. While some tumor cells have chromosomal instability, others have microsatellite instability characterized by mutations including frequently at repetitive DNA sequences. This microsatellite instability (MSI) is a result of mutations in DNA repair

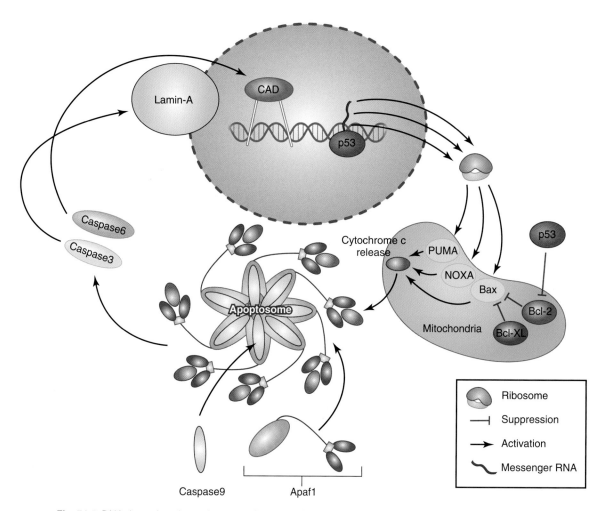

Fig. 54.4 DNA damaging chemotherapy activates p53 leading to tumor cell death through the intrinsic apoptosis pathway. This figure shows the central role of the p53 protein in the intrinsic apoptosis pathway, which culminates in apoptosome activation. Oncogene activation or cytotoxic DNA damaging chemotherapies stabilize and activate the p53 protein. If the damage is repaired, cells survive and do not become transformed. If there is too much damage, cells undergo p53-dependent cell death. When p53 is mutated in cancer, its tumor suppressor function is lost. As part of its normal function after DNA damage, the p53 protein modulates the intrinsic apoptosis pathway by regulating the balance of the proapoptotic proteins PUMA, NOXA, and BAX and the antiapoptotic proteins BCL-XL and BCL-2, resulting in the release of cytochrome c from the mitochondria. When cytochrome c binds to the apoptosome, a multimer of caspase 9 and APAF1, it activates caspases 3 and 6, which promote nuclear membrane destruction by Lamin-A and DNA fragmentation by CAD. The *"p"* denotes protein, followed by molecular weight in Kilodaltons, as in p53. *Arrows* indicate activation processes in a pathway. *Red "T" symbols* indicate suppression of a pathway. *APAF1,* Apoptosis protease activating factor 1; *BAX,* BCL-associated X; *BCL-2,* B-cell lymphoma 2; *BCL-XL,* BCL-extra-large; *CAD,* caspase-activated deoxyribonuclease; *NOXA,* Latin for damage; *PUMA,* p53 upregulated mediator of apoptosis. For a more detailed review of the apoptosis pathway and its exploitation in cancer therapy, see Carneiro BA, El-Deiry WS, *Nat. Rev. Clin. Oncol.* 2020 Jul;17(7):395–417.

genes. When the repair system is defective, the number of mutations increases. The total number of mutations in a cancer cell is called tumor mutation burden. MSI correlates with tumor mutation burden. The processing of the mutant proteins from MSI-high tumor cells in the endoplasmic reticulum and their presentation by the main histocompatibility complex-I (MHC-I) as neo-antigens predicts response to immunotherapy. Furthermore, mutations in components of the FANC complex (including BRCA genes) affect DNA double-strand break repair, resulting in homologous recombination deficiency (HRD) observed in subsets of ovarian, breast, prostate, and pancreatic cancer patients. Some of these cancers use a rescue DNA repair system, the poly-ADP ribose polymerase (PARP) system,

which can be targeted with inhibitors, a concept often named synthetic lethality (specifically in the BRCA-mutated cells). PARP inhibitors are oral medications available in the oncology clinic for patients with HRD. Both MSI and HRD may be acquired through germline (inherited from parents) or somatic (originated in the tumor) mutations.

Oncogenes Unleash Proliferation

Oncogene mutations convert a normal cell into a cancerous cell (Fig 54.6). Oncogenes often activate pathways that are important for cancer. For example, chronic myelogenous leukemia (CML) occurs when the proto-oncogene ABL from chromosome 9 translocates to

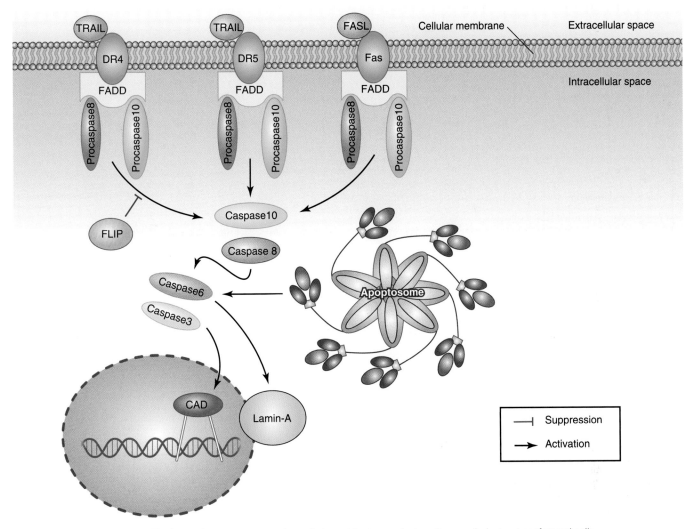

Fig. 54.5 The innate immune system, through the extrinsic apoptosis pathway, eliminates transformed cells. Extracellular molecules (TRAIL and FASL) bind to transmembrane receptors (DR4, DR5, and FAS), anchoring the intracellular adaptor protein FADD to the cellular membrane. Then, FADD recruits initiators Pro-caspase 8 and Pro-caspase 10, which are then cleaved to their active forms, caspase 8 and caspase 10. This activation reaction is tightly regulated by c-FLIP. The apoptosome, a multimer of caspase 9 and APAF1, leads to activation of executioner caspases 3 and 6, promoting nuclear membrane destruction by Lamin-A and DNA fragmentation by CAD, respectively. The *TRAIL, DR5,* and *FAS* genes are regulated by p53. The *"p"* denotes protein, followed by molecular weight in Kilodaltons, as in p53. *Arrows* indicate activation processes in the pathway. *"T" symbols* indicate suppression of a pathway. *DR,* Death receptor; *FADD,* FAS-associated protein with death domain; *FAS,* FS-7 (a cell line)-associated surface antigen; *FASL,* FAS ligand; *FLIP,* FADD-like interleukin 1 beta-converting enzyme inhibitory protein; *TRAIL,* tumor necrosis factor-related apoptosis inducing ligand. For a more detailed review of the apoptosis pathway and its exploitation in cancer therapy, see Carneiro BA, El-Deiry WS, *Nat. Rev. Clin. Oncol.* 2020 Jul;17(7):395–417.

the *BCR* gene on chromosome 22. The new protein formed by expression of the combined gene *BCR-ABL* sends unchecked growth-promoting signals to the nucleus. An activating mutation in one allele of an oncogene is usually sufficient to promote tumorigenesis (e.g., *KRAS*).

Because oncogenes activate pathways that drive cancer growth, their discovery has led to specifically designed drugs that target the products of these genes and the pathways they control. For example, among patients with breast cancer, HER2 amplification serves as a biomarker that identifies those who will benefit from treatment with the anti-HER2 monoclonal antibody trastuzumab. Similarly, activating mutations in EGFR serve to identify patients with non–small cell lung cancer who will improve with the use of drugs (erlotinib, gefitinib, afatinib, dacomitinib, osimertinib) that specifically inhibit the mutated form of EGFR. Another example is BRAF mutations in melanoma, which are inhibited by the FDA-approved drugs dabrafenib, vemurafenib, and encorafenib. This paradigm—identify a mutated oncogene, find a specific drug that inhibits the activated mutant protein, and treat patients who have the specific mutation with a drug that affects the mutated protein—has

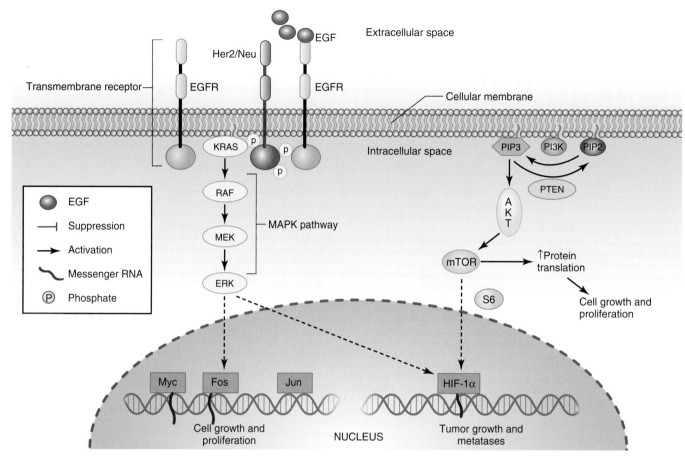

Fig. 54.6 Principles of intracellular cancer signaling and targeted therapeutics. Ligands are extracellular molecules such as the epidermal growth factor (EGF) which binds to a transmembrane receptor known as the EGF receptor (EGFR), to activate intracellular cancer pathways. Illustrated here are the MAPK (mitogen-activated protein kinase) and the phosphatidyl inositol-3 kinase/mammalian target of rapamycin (PI3K/mTOR) pathways. These pathways converge into proliferative genetic programs mediated by transcription factors including myelocytomatosis (Myc), Fos, Jun, hypoxia-inducing factor-1α (HIF-1α), and others. These transcription factors turn on genes that promote cell growth and proliferation as well as tumor growth and metastases. The major effect of mTOR signaling is to stimulate protein translation that is required for cell growth and proliferation. Modern cancer therapy has evolved to include therapeutic agents targeting most of these tumor promoting proteins. Examples include trastuzumab (Her2/neu), cetuximab (EGFR), dabrafenib (RAF), trametinib (MEK), copanlisib (PI3K), mTOR (everolimus), and many others. *Yellow "p"* denotes phosphate. *Arrows* indicate activation processes in the pathway. *Red "T" symbols* indicate suppression of a pathway. Activation of Myc, Fos, and Jun by the MAPK pathway and HIF-1α by mTOR and S6 kinase is indirect. *AKT,* AK mouse strain transforming retrovirus (AKT is also known as PKB [protein kinase B]); *ERK,* extracellular signal regulated kinase; *Her2/neu,* human EGF receptor 2/neural; *KRAS,* Kirsten rat sarcoma; *MEK,* MAP (mitogen-activated protein)/ERK kinase; *PIP3,* phosphatidylinositol (3,4,5)-trisphosphate; *PTEN,* phosphatase and tensin homolog; *RAF,* rapidly accelerating fibrosarcoma.

repeatedly been proven to be a successful approach. Recently, targeting of a specific KRAS G12C driver mutation has been achieved through a small molecule that covalently attaches to the cysteine, and this appears efficacious in some patients with non-small cell lung cancer and colon cancer. Other significant advances involved the development and FDA-approval of Ret inhibitors selpercatinib and pralsetinib for multiple tumor types including non-small cell lung cancer. Capmatinib inhibits Met exon-skipping mutant non-small cell lung cancers and sonic hedgehog pathway inhibitors vismodegib and sonidegib are used for the treatment of advanced basal cell carcinoma. Ongoing research aims to target additional oncogenic cancer pathways such as the Wnt/Beta-catenin and Notch pathways (Fig. 54.7).

Tumor Suppressor Genes Disrupt Growth Checkpoints

The inactivation of both alleles of a tumor suppressor gene (e.g., retinoblastoma, *RB1*) results in cancer, most commonly by an inherited mutation in an allele followed by loss of heterozygosity due to epigenetic events or aneuploidy (loss or gain of part of chromosomes). The tumor suppressor gene *TP53* is the most commonly mutated gene in human cancer. The p53 protein is a transcription factor that activates various genes such as p21 (WAF1) and multiple genes that induce cell death (Figs. 54.3–54.5). Mutation of this *TP53* gene can be inherited (Li-Fraumeni syndrome) in families that have higher rates of a variety of leukemia, sarcoma, breast, and brain tumors, or most commonly is acquired during cancer growth. Loss of two copies of a tumor suppressor gene leading

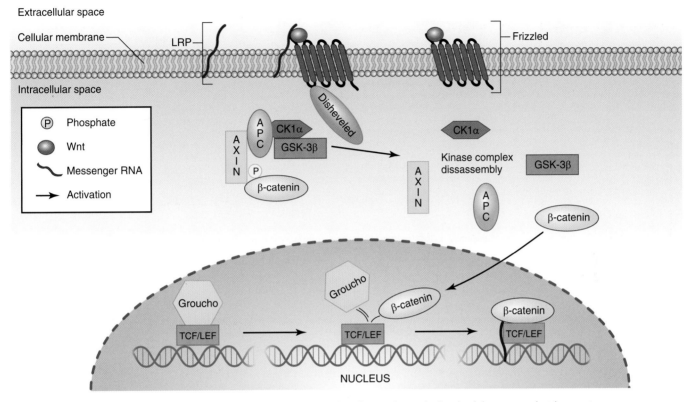

Fig. 54.7 The beta-catenin intracellular cancer signaling pathway is involved in cancer development. The extracellular molecule Wnt engages the transmembrane proteins LDL receptor related protein (LRP) and Frizzled, which activate the intracellular adaptor protein Disheveled. Then, Disheveled disassembles the kinase complex composed of the proteins Adenomatous Polyposis Coli (APC), Axin, Glycogen Synthase Kinase-3β (GSK-3β), and Casein Kinase-1α (CK-1α). This kinase complex usually breaks down beta-catenin by tagging it for destruction through phosphorylation. However, the activation of Disheveled by Frizzled bound to Wnt promotes kinase complex disassembly, stabilizing beta-catenin. Finally, beta-catenin crosses the nuclear membrane displacing the transcription repressor Groucho, which enables TCF/LEF transcriptional activity that activates target genes such as *MYC* and the Cyclin D gene (*CCND1*). This pathway is deregulated in most colon cancers through *APC* mutation (both sporadic and inherited forms of colon cancer such as Familial Adenomatous Polyposis). In other tumors, β-catenin mutations are more commonly observed. This pathway remains largely untapped for cancer therapeutic development. Inhibitors of GSK-3β, Wnt, and β-catenin are currently under development. *Arrows* indicate activation processes in a cellular pathway. *TCF/LEF*, T-cell factor/lymphoid enhancer-binding factor; *Wnt*, wingless/integrated.

to cancer was predicted by Knudson's two-hit hypothesis. Tumor suppressor genes can be inactivated by viral genes including Human Papilloma Virus (HPV) E6 and E7 that target p53 and Rb. HPV types 16 and 18 can cause cervical cancer and head and neck cancer, and there is a preventative vaccine.

Hypoxia, Angiogenesis, Invasion, and Metastases

Under hypoxic pressure from the tumor microenvironment, cancer cells shift their metabolism towards aerobic glycolysis. This so-called Warburg effect diverts Krebs cycle intermediate metabolites towards nucleic acid and amino acid production, favoring cell growth. Although mutations affecting enzymes from the Krebs cycle are uncommon in cancer (i.e., fumarate hydratase in certain kidney tumors and succinate dehydrogenase in pheochromocytomas), isocitrate dehydrogenase (IDH) 1 or 2 are commonly mutated in certain brain, bile duct, and acute myelogenous

leukemia and are targeted by the FDA-approved drugs ivosidenib (mutant IDH1 inhibitor) and enasidenib (mutant IDH2 inhibitor). Also, the upregulation of a transcription factor known as hypoxia-inducing factor induces overexpression of the vascular endothelial growth factors (VEGF). VEGF then co-opts endothelial cells to form new aberrant vessels (angiogenesis), allowing the growing mass to survive hypoxia. These ill-walled vessels allow elopement of cancer cells to the bloodstream, priming distant organ colonization (metastasis). The angiogenesis inhibitors include the biologic agents bevacizumab, ramucirumab, and ziv-aflibercept and some small molecules such as sunitinib, sorafenib, regorafenib, lenvatinib, cabozantinib among others. Finally, hypoxia upregulates a series of transcription factors (Snail, Slug, TWIST, ZEB 1 and 2) that coordinate cell-to-cell adhesion dysregulation promoting phenotypic changes (epithelial-mesenchymal transition) that enable cell migration and metastasis. Such is the importance of the hypoxia

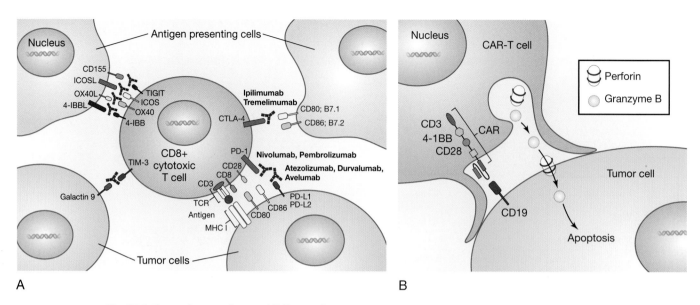

Fig. 54.8 Cancer immunotherapy. (A) Targets for cancer immune checkpoint therapy. Depicted here is a CD8+ cytotoxic T cell, an antigen presenting cell, and a tumor cell. These cell-cell interactions may take place within a primary tumor, draining lymph nodes, or metastatic sites. On the right of the T cell are immune checkpoints that have been successfully targeted in cancer therapy with now FDA-approved antibodies. Examples include ipilimumab and tremelimumab that target CTLA-4, nivolumab and pembrolizumab that target PD-1, and atezolizumab, avelumab, and durvalumab that target PD-L1. These therapeutics are currently being combined with chemotherapy or targeted therapy in the clinic. To the left of the T-cell are a number of checkpoints for which therapeutics are being tested in clinical trials. They include the T cell targets TIGIT, ICOS, OX40, TIM-3, and 4-1BB. (B) Cellular chimeric antigen receptor-T cell (CAR-T) therapy has been developed and is now FDA-approved in the treatment of acute lymphocytic leukemia and diffuse large B cell lymphoma. Shown is an engineered CAR-T cell with an immune synapse, with binding of different receptors, release of granzyme B and perforin, leading to apoptosis of a target tumor cell.

pathways in cancer that the Physiology or Medicine Nobel prize of 2019 was bestowed on William G. Kaelin, Gregg L. Semenza, and Peter J. Ratcliffe.

Immune Escape

The immune system is constantly killing cancer cells. Under pressure of this constant immune vigilance, cancer cells with random mutations that allow re-expression of useful genes that are usually dormant survive. Among the genes involved in this "immune escape," one of the best studied is *PD-L1* (programmed-death ligand 1). *PD-L1* usually is expressed in the placenta, preventing a mother's immune system from attacking her fetus, ultimately a foreign body. When tumors express *PD-L1* it binds its receptor PD-1 in cytotoxic T CD8+ cells, rendering them ineffective. One of the most revolutionary therapies in oncology is use of monoclonal antibodies to *PD-L1* and other so-called immune checkpoints (Fig. 54.8). They have been so successful that the scientists James Allison and Tasuku Honjo who were responsible to bring them to the clinic were awarded the Nobel Prize in Physiology or Medicine in 2018.

Dr. Steven Rosenberg observed that T cells fighting cancer could be removed from patients, cultured ex-vivo, and used as cancer therapies. This adoptive cell therapy acquired an iteration when Carl June selected patient-derived (autologous) cells through special magnetic beads, introduced genetically engineered antibodies linked to immune checkpoint receptors through viral vectors, and infused it back to the same patients who donated the cells. Chimeric antigenic receptor (CAR)-T cell therapy has been developed to target surface proteins in various tumors, such as CD19 in acute lymphocytic leukemia, which was approved by the FDA in 2017. The first patient treated in a clinical trial in 2012 is cancer free by 2020. Off-the-shelf CAR-T cells, extracted from allogeneic donors and engineered to avoid rejection by the recipient, are in development. Umbilical cord-derived CAR-natural killer (CAR-NK) cells are also under development.

SUGGESTED READINGS

Chae YK, Anker JF, Carneiro BA, et al: Genomic landscape of DNA repair genes in cancer, Oncotarget 7(17):23312–23321, 2016.

Classon M, Harlow E: The retinoblastoma tumour suppressor in development and cancer, Nat Rev Cancer 2(12):910–917, 2002.

El-Deiry WS: p21(WAF1) Mediates cell-cycle inhibition, relevant to cancer suppression and therapy, Cancer Res 76(18):5189–5191, 2016.

Hanahan D, Weinberg RA: Hallmarks of cancer: the next generation, Cell 144(5):646–674, 2011.

Kamps R, Brandão RD, Bosch BJ, et al: Next-Generation sequencing in oncology: genetic Diagnosis, Risk prediction and cancer classification, Int J Mol Sci (2)18, 2017.

Koike T, Kimura N, Miyazaki K, et al: Hypoxia induces adhesion molecules on cancer cells: a missing link between Warburg effect and induction of selectin-ligand carbohydrates, Proc Natl Acad Sci U S A 101(21):8132–8137, 2004.

Shay JW: Role of Telomeres and telomerase in Aging and cancer, Cancer Discov 6(6):584–593, 2016.

Vogelstein B, Lane D, Levine AJ: Surfing the p53 network, Nature 408(6810):307–310, 2000.

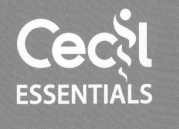

55

Cancer Epidemiology

Gary H. Lyman, Nicole M. Kuderer

INTRODUCTION

Globally, more than 18 million individuals are diagnosed with cancer and nearly 10 million die annually from the disease. At the same time, the number of cancer survivors worldwide is increasing dramatically each year. In the United States in 2020, it is estimated that more than 1.8 million individuals will be diagnosed with cancer, for an age-adjusted incidence rate of 448 per 100,000 population. At the same time, more than 600,000 individuals will die from cancer, for an age-adjusted death rate of 158 per 100,000. Cancer has become the leading cause of mortality among both women and men between the ages of 40 and 80 and the second leading cause of death for most other age groups, including children between 1 and 14 years of age.

The leading types of new invasive cancer cases and cancer-specific deaths are shown in Table 55.1. While breast cancer and prostate cancer are the most common noncutaneous forms of cancer in men and women, respectively, lung cancer is the leading cause of cancer-specific mortality accounting for nearly 30% of cancer deaths in both genders. While mortality rates for gastric and cervical cancers have decreased steadily for decades, overall cancer death rates have decreased some 20% since their height in the early 1990s, with the greatest declines for colorectal, prostate, and lung cancers in men and colorectal and breast cancer in women (Fig. 55.1). Disparities in cancer occurrence and mortality persist despite a reduction in the overall age-adjusted mortality from cancer. Cancer incidence remains highest in the United States among white individuals, likely due to their high rates of lung and female breast cancer. However, black men continue to have the highest gender-specific cancer incidence among men and the highest mortality rates despite considerable reductions in cancer mortality for all genders and races. While white women have the highest cancer incidence among women, black women have the highest gender-specific cancer mortality rate despite gradually falling rates for all races. Cancer mortality rates in developed countries are consistently higher among those from racial and ethnic minority groups, especially African Americans, and among those from lower socioeconomic strata. Greater mortality rates among racial and ethnic minorities are not fully explained by differences in the stage at diagnosis. Socioeconomic factors, access to appropriate treatment, and comorbidities represent additional determinants of greater cancer mortality.

CANCER EPIDEMIOLOGY METHODS

Epidemiologists study disease variation among populations and the factors that influence such variation. The proportion of individuals with disease in the population at a given point in time is the *prevalence* whereas *incidence and mortality rates* represent the number of events in a population over a defined period of time (e.g., cancers per

100,000 per year). To facilitate comparisons of rates between populations, rates are often adjusted for age, sex, race, or other demographic characteristics. The association between a characteristic or exposure with cancer risk is generally assessed in either cohort or case-control studies. *Cohort studies* are generally prospective and evaluate disease experience in exposed and unexposed individuals whereas *case-control studies* assess the exposure experience in individuals with and without disease. The *relative risk (RR)* is a measure of association between exposure and disease with estimates above 1.0 representing an increase in risk. In case-control studies, RR is estimated by the odds ratio because the sizes of the exposed and unexposed populations are often not known. The larger the study population, the more precise the estimate of association is between exposure and disease. However, proper interpretation of the results must explore whether any systematic error or bias has been introduced during the study design or analysis. Confounding factors may obscure or weaken a true association or create a false association because of an association between the factor and both the exposure and disease. Confounding can be evaluated and adjusted for in stratified or multivariate analysis if the potential confounder is recognized and has been properly measured in the data. It is generally not safe to assume that all possible confounding factors have been considered. Therefore, causal inference is seldom justified on the basis of a single study but evolves gradually with study repetition and consideration of other information including animal and other laboratory results, the strength of the association, and a careful consideration of likely confounding factors. Interventions for cancer prevention and screening are generally studied in randomized controlled trials requiring large numbers of participants, close monitoring for adherence in the intervention, long-term follow-up, and appropriate ascertainment of disease and disease-free status.

RISK FACTORS

Genetic

Risk factors for developing cancer can be grouped as either genetic (inherited) or acquired. While important for our understanding of carcinogenesis, only a small proportion of cancers are inherited in a mendelian fashion. Neoplasms inherited in an autosomal dominant manner include retinoblastomas, multiple endocrine neoplasia syndromes, and polyposis coli. Several additional pre-neoplastic conditions demonstrate mendelian inheritance with variable penetrance. Several common malignancies demonstrate familial risk patterns with low penetrance, including breast cancer and colorectal cancer. Genetic testing and potential preventative measures are available for several inherited cancer syndromes (Table 55.2). Although genetic testing is available for several identified cancer susceptibility genes, care must be

TABLE 55.1   US 2020 Cancer Statistics

ESTIMATED NEW CANCER CASES[a]

Females (912,930)		Males (893,660)	
Breast	30%	Prostate	21%
Lung and bronchus	12%	Lung and bronchus	13%
Colon and rectum	8%	Colon and rectum	9%
Uterine corpus	7%	Urinary bladder	7%
Thyroid	4%	Melanoma of the skin	7%
Melanoma of the skin	4%	Kidney and renal pelvis	5%
Non-Hodgkin lymphoma	4%	Non-Hodgkin lymphoma	5%
Kidney and renal pelvis	3%	Oral cavity and pharynx	4%
Pancreas	3%	Leukemia	4%
Leukemia	3%	Pancreas	3%
All other sites	22%	All other sites	22%

ESTIMATED CANCER DEATHS

Females (285,360)		Males (321,160)	
Lung and bronchus	22%	Lung and bronchus	23%
Breast	15%	Prostate	10%
Colon and rectum	9%	Colon and rectum	9%
Pancreas	8%	Pancreas	8%
Ovary	5%	Liver and intrahepatic bile duct	6%
Uterine corpus	4%	Leukemia	4%
Liver and intrahepatic bile duct	4%	Esophagus	4%
Leukemia	3%	Urinary bladder	4%
Non-Hodgkin lymphoma	3%	Non-Hodgkin lymphoma	4%
Brain and other nervous system	3%	Brain and other nervous system	3%
All other sites	24%	All other sites	25%

Data from Siegel RL, Miller KD, Jemal A: Cancer statistics, 2020. CA: A Cancer Journal for Clinicians. (70)1:7-30, 2020.
[a]Excludes basal cell and squamous cell skin cancers and in situ carcinoma except urinary bladder.

utilized in selecting individuals for such testing. Such testing requires a reasonable understanding of cancer genetics as well as the target population along with relevant ethical, economic, and societal issues.

At the same time, acquired somatic mutations are universally identified in malignant cells with some clearly driving the development and progression of cancer. While random genetic mutations occur frequently, proto-oncogenes involved in cell growth and proliferation, tumor suppressor genes involved in regulation of cellular proliferation, and mismatch repair genes associated with chromosomal instability play critical roles in carcinogenesis, tumor growth, progression, invasion, and metastasis. Fortunately, the spontaneous mutation rate is relatively low, and more than one mutational event is usually necessary for complete carcinogenic transformation resulting in a malignancy.

Lifestyle

Acquired risk factors for cancer include lifestyle factors as well as occupational and other environmental exposure to carcinogenic substances. Major lifestyle risk factors include tobacco, alcohol and other dietary factors, as well as lack of physical activity (Table 55.3).

Tobacco

Tobacco products are, by far, the single greatest contributor to cancer incidence and mortality worldwide. Cigarette smokers have a 20-fold or greater risk for developing cancer compared with nonsmokers, with smoking being the single largest cause of lung cancer. Tobacco accounts for one third of all cancers in the United States, contributing to the more than 1 million people annually who are estimated

to die from tobacco-induced cancers globally. The vast majority of lung cancers are attributable to cigarette smoking while exposure to secondhand smoke increases the risk for lung cancer in nonsmokers. Cigarette and cigar smoking and chewing tobacco are major risk factors for head, neck, mouth, and esophageal cancers and are associated with development of stomach, pancreas, kidney, bladder, and cervical cancer as well. While tobacco use has declined in the United States over the past two decades, it continues to be unacceptably high, especially among younger women, and continues to increase in many parts of the developing world.

Nutrition

Diet and body weight appear to play an important role in cancer causation. Excess alcohol use is clearly a significant risk factor for cancers of the liver, head and neck, esophagus, and breast. Obesity and dietary fat intake are associated with colon and breast cancers, but the exact nature of the relationship is still under investigation. Central or visceral adiposity in both men and women is associated with increased incidence and mortality from a number of cancers, including endometrium, breast in postmenopausal women, kidney, gallbladder, pancreas, esophagus, colon, and prostate.

Infection

Several chronic infections, including bacterial, viral, and parasitic, have been associated with an increased risk of different types of cancer. In certain parts of the developing world, infection with *Schistosoma haematobium* is a major cause of squamous cell carcinoma of the bladder.

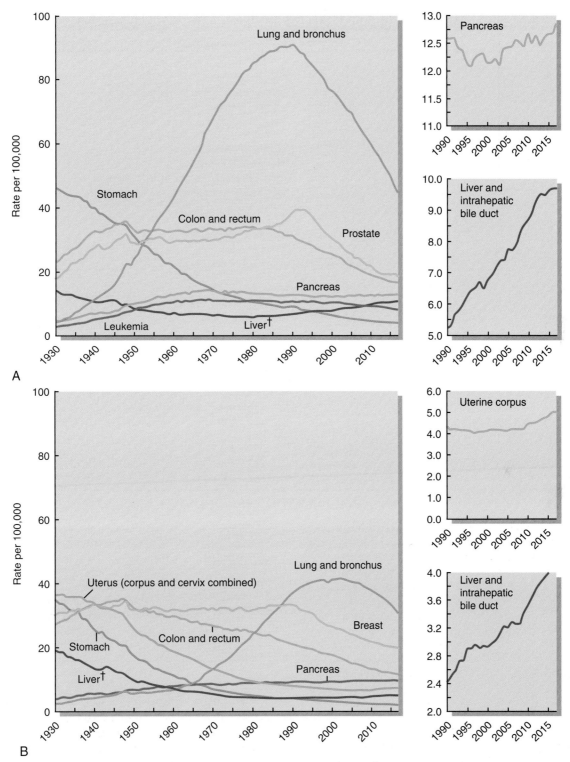

Fig. 55.1 US cancer mortality rates, 1930-2017. (A) Males. (B) Females. †Includes intrahepatic bile duct, gall bladder, and other biliary. (From Siegel RL, Miller KD, Jemal A: Cancer statistics, 2020, CA: A Cancer Journal for Clinicians [70]1:7-30, 2020.)

Both DNA and RNA viruses have been associated with human cancers. Viruses associated with human malignancies include the Epstein-Barr virus (EBV) (nasopharyngeal cancer and Burkitt lymphoma) and human T-cell leukemia virus type I (HTLV-1). Patients with the acquired immunodeficiency syndrome (AIDS) associated with the human immunodeficiency virus (HIV) are at increased risk of Kaposi's sarcoma, non-Hodgkin lymphoma, and anogenital squamous cell carcinoma. Chronic hepatitis B and C viral infections have been linked with the development of hepatocellular carcinoma. Human papillomaviruses 16 and 18 have been linked with cervical cancer, with vaccines against these virus strains and those causing genital warts, both on the market.

TABLE 55.2 **Genetic Testing for Selected Hereditary Cancer Syndromes**

Cancer: Involved Genes	Prevention Measures
Breast	
BRCA-1, BRCA-2	Prophylactic mastectomy
PTEN, STK-11, TP53	Selective estrogen receptor modulators
	Lifestyle measures
	Increased intensity of screening, including breast MRI
Lobular Breast Cancer and Gastric Cancer	Prophylactic mastectomy
	Prophylactic gastrectomy
CDH-1 (E-cadherin)	Increased intensity of screening, including breast MRI
	Selective estrogen receptor modulators
Ovarian	
BRCA-1, BRCA-2	Prophylactic oophorectomy
	Oral contraceptives
Colon	
Familial adenomatous	Prophylactic colectomy
Polyposis (FAP)	Nonsteroidal anti-inflammatory drugs
APC	Lifestyle measures
Hereditary nonpolyposis	Lifestyle measures
Colon cancer (HNPCC)	Nonsteroidal anti-inflammatory drugs
MLH-1, MSH-2	Increased surveillance
MSH-6, PMS-2	Prophylactic total abdominal hysterectomy and oophorectomy
MYH-associated polyposis	Lifestyle measures
MYH	Nonsteroidal anti-inflammatory drugs
	Prophylactic colectomy
Uterine	
PTEN, MLH-1, MSH-2, MSH-6, PMS-2	Prophylactic hysterectomy
	Increased surveillance

FAP, Familial adenomatous polyposis; HNPCC, hereditary nonpolyposis colorectal cancer; MRI, magnetic resonance imaging; MYH, mutY homologue.

TABLE 55.3 **Cancer Risk Factors**

Lifestyle Factor	Associated Cancers
Tobacco	Lung, bronchus, esophagus, head and neck, stomach, pancreas, kidney, bladder, cervix
High alcohol consumption	Liver, rectum, breast, oral cavity, pharynx, larynx, esophagus
Obesity, high dietary fat	Colon, breast, endometrium, kidney, pancreas, esophagus, prostate
Low dietary fiber	Colon
Sedentary lifestyle	Colon, breast
Environmental Exposures	**Associated Cancers**
Human papillomavirus:16,18	Cervical
Hepatitis B and C viruses	Liver and hepatocellular cancers
Asbestos	Mesothelioma and other types of lung cancer
Radon	Lung
Ultraviolet radiation	Melanoma, basal and squamous cell carcinomas
Ionizing radiation	Leukemia, thyroid, lung, breast

Cancer and the Severe Acute Respiratory Syndrome Coronavirus 2 (SARS-Cov-2)

The 2020 pandemic from SARS-Cov-2 has placed patients with cancer at disproportionately greater risk of contracting COVID-19, as well as greater risk of serious medical complications including hospitalization, need for intensive care and ventilator support, and a greater risk for mortality. The reason for this impact is multifactorial and includes greater exposure to the health care system and infected patients and staff as well as greater risk from the immunosuppression resulting from disease and cancer therapies. Other factors that lead to greater

risk include older age, one or more serious medical comorbidities, and concurrent complications from other infectious agents and a range of demographic and geographic disparities.

Given the sudden and urgent crisis of this global pandemic, much of the epidemiologic information currently available has risen out of crowd-sourcing efforts to rapidly and broadly gather as much information as possible on the impact of COVID-19 on patients with cancer and their management. The major driving force has been the need to gather and disseminate this information as quickly as possible for both clinical and public heath purposes or containment and mitigation. While the resulting case experience and cohort studies have provided much important and timely information from across the globe, it has come with analytic challenges and interpretation. Confounding by indication has complicated the rush to evaluate both preventive and therapeutic interventions in these largely uncontrolled and non-randomized studies. In the meantime, large-scale conventional epidemiologic studies are under development that should provide longer-term and more reliable information about the risk of COVID-19 in patients with cancer. Such studies may also provide data about the concurrent factors that impact the most on the risk of infection in the critically ill patient and disease and treatment-related predictors of serious and even fatal outcomes, while we are awaiting the development of effect treatments and vaccines. Nevertheless, the essentially exponential spread of SARS-Cov-2 both globally and in multiple specific sites, and the apparent, albeit limited, success of mitigation measures such as social distancing and masking, have reminded us of epidemiologic and public health measures of the past, which are equally if not more relevant today and critically important for patients with cancer.

Radiation

Non-ionizing radiation. Excess to ultraviolet (UV) radiation is unquestionably associated with an increased risk of skin cancers including basal and squamous cell carcinomas as well as cutaneous melanoma, with observed rates increasing directly with the amount of daily sunlight exposure. Most of the harmful effects from sun exposure are thought to be related to direct DNA damage associated with exposure to intermediate wavelength UV-B. The use of tanning beds and other frequent exposures to sunlight are of particular concern given the rapid increase in rates of melanoma among younger individuals.

Ionizing radiation. Ionizing radiation is arguably the most extensively studied carcinogen and has been unequivocally associated with an increased risk of both hematologic malignancies and various solid tumors in humans. Radiation-induced malignancies including leukemia and solid tumors are most extensively studied in the occupational settings among radiation workers and miners, among survivors of the atomic weapons used in Hiroshima and Nagasaki in World War II, and among those exposed to radiation for various medical indications. Excess cancer risk from radiation exposure can be seen with a latency period ranging from a few years (leukemia) to decades (solid tumors) and correlates with the cumulative exposure dose. As the survivors of the atomic bombing of Japan age, estimates of the associated risk of cancer have continued to increase.

Natural sources account for at least 80% of human exposure to radiation, most notably from radon. It has been estimated that radon exposure is the second leading cause of lung cancer due to widespread low-level exposure in the residential setting. In the occupational setting, there is a strong interaction between smoking and radon such that most radon-induced lung cancers are among smokers. Medical exposure accounts for most of the remaining average annual radiation exposure in the United States. There is increasing evidence that repeated exposure to radiation from multiple imaging studies such as CT scans, especially at a young age, is associated with an increased risk of cancer later in life.

Chemicals

Various pharmacologic agents have been associated with an increased risk for specific cancers. As with radiation, these agents may be used in the occupational setting, for diagnostic or therapeutic medical use, as well as for various purposes in the home setting. Organic and inorganic chemical compounds linked to human cancers including benzene (leukemia), benzidine (bladder), arsenic, soot and coal tars (lung and skin), and wood dusts (nasal). Arguably, asbestos is probably the most common cause of occupational cancer because of its link with the development of mesothelioma and other types of lung cancer. Nearly all mesotheliomas diagnosed in the United States are associated with prior asbestos exposure. A strong interaction exists between asbestos exposure and cigarette smoking for lung cancer.

A range of medications are associated with an increased risk of cancer, including the alkylating agents, anthracyclines, and other classes of cancer chemotherapy and immunosuppressants. Estrogen use in postmenopausal women increases the risk of endometrial cancer, while the rates drop when combined with progesterone. Synthetic estrogens, such as diethylstilbestrol (DES), administered to mothers during pregnancy increase the risk of vaginal cancer in offspring. Lifestyle exposures to carcinogenic chemicals covered previously include multiple carcinogens in tobacco products and dietary factors including aflatoxins in many part of the world.

CANCER PREVENTION

Cancer prevention strategies can be thought of as primary or secondary based on whether they reduce risk of exposure or detect cancer at an early stage when intervention can change the natural history of the disease. Reasonable primary prevention strategies include reductions in lifestyle risks (smoking cessation; use of sunscreen; adherence to a low-fat, high-fiber diet), avoidance of occupational or environmental risks, and chemoprevention (see Table 55.3).

Lifestyle Changes

Smoking cessation is unquestionably the most direct and effective cancer prevention strategy available. More than 1 million people die from tobacco-induced cancers globally each year, and tobacco accounts for one third of all cancer diagnoses in the United States. Although tobacco prevention and control programs have resulted in a decline in smoking prevalence in the United States, tobacco use continues to be high and has been increasing in a number of countries. There is also evidence from epidemiologic studies that other lifestyle changes including regular exercise and dietary modification may also reduce the risk of cancer. Central adiposity is associated with increased incidence and mortality from a number of cancers, including breast and endometrium. Sufficient dietary intake of fruits and vegetables appears to reduce the risk for gastric and esophageal cancers. Avoidance of excessive sun exposure and the use of artificial tanning devices also is important to reversing recent upward trends in cutaneous malignancies. Reduction in exposures to known carcinogenic agents is an important goal in both the occupational and domestic setting. Evidence for an association between air pollution and lung cancer incidence illustrates how difficult that may be. However, prudent use of potentially carcinogenic chemicals and radiation in the medical setting will hopefully minimize exposures to settings where the benefit clearly outweighs the potential harms.

Chemoprevention

Chemopreventive agents are drugs, vaccines, or micronutrients (e.g., minerals, vitamins) used to prevent the development of cancer. Both randomized trials and epidemiologic studies have suggested that a number of strategies may be capable of reducing the risk of some common types of cancer. Recent data from multiple studies have provided suggestive evidence that daily aspirin use may reduce the risk of several types of cancer, including colon and melanoma. Evidence suggests that hepatitis B vaccination can reduce the incidence of hepatocellular cancer. The vaccine directed against specific strains of the human papillomavirus (HPV) offers the strong promise of preventing cervical cancer.

CANCER SCREENING

Cancer screening programs should be able to detect premalignant states or early-stage cancer before the onset of symptoms with relatively high sensitivity. Likewise, for cancer screening to be useful there must be a treatment available that improves the outcome of patients with premalignant or early-stage disease. Such cancer screening programs should also, ideally, be noninvasive, inexpensive, and associated with high specificity (low false-positive rate). Identification of high-risk individuals can be of value to the effective and cost-effective application of genetic counseling and testing as well as cancer screening efforts.

Proper interpretation of the results of cancer screening studies must consider both *lead-time bias* and *length-time bias*. Lead time is the time between detection of disease by screening and the actual appearance of symptomatic disease. Diagnosing the disease earlier with screening may make it appear that the patient lived longer even when the survival of the patient from the onset of disease has not been altered. Length-time bias occurs when subsets of the cancer under study have different growth rates. Screening is more likely to detect cancers that grow slowly because of the greater prevalence of asymptomatic people with slow-growing tumors than with fast-growing tumors. Thus patients with cancer that is detected with screening appear to have longer survival as a result of screening, when in fact the longer course of their disease results from the behavior of the tumor itself. While randomized controlled trials of cancer screening programs require large numbers of participants and take years to complete, such trials are needed to accurately estimate screening performance and to address both lead-time and length-time bias.

It is important to note that screening tests may also be associated with false-negative and false-positive results. *False-negative results* fail to obtain a proper diagnosis and patients, therefore, are not provided the opportunity for effective early treatment. *False-positive results* may also cause harm by leading to unnecessary testing and treatment as well as contributing to patient costs and emotional stress.

A number of cancer screening tests are currently recommended, including clinical examination and mammography to detect breast cancer, Papanicolaou smears and HPV DNA tests to detect cervical dysplasia or cancer, colonoscopy to detect polyps or colon cancer, and digital rectal examination and serum PSA to detect prostate cancer. Low-dose CT scanning for screening appropriate high-risk individuals for lung cancer has recently been recommended based on several large randomized controlled trials.

SUGGESTED READINGS

Colditz GA, Sellers TA, Trapido E: Epidemiology-Identifying the causes and preventability of cancer, Nat Rev Cancer 6:75–83, 2006.

Dai M, Liu D, Liu M, Zhou F, Li G, Chen Z, et al: Patients with cancer appear more vulnerable to SARS-COV-2: a multicenter study during the COVID-19 Outbreak, Cancer Discov 10(6):783–791, 2020.

Desai A, Warner J, Kuderer N, Thompson M, Pinter C, Lyman G, Lopes G: Crowdsourcing a crisis response for COVID-19 in oncology, Nat Cancer Apr 21:1–4, 2020.

Detterbeck FC, Mazzone PJ, Naidich DP, et al: Screening for lung cancer: diagnosis and management of lung cancer, 3rd ed: American College of Chest Physicians evidence-based clinical practice guidelines, Chest 143:e78S–e92S, 2013.

Kuderer NM, Choureiri TK, Shah DP, et al: Clinical impact of COVID-19 on patients with cancer (CCC19): a cohort study, Lancet 395:1907–1918, 2020.

Kushi LH, Doyle C, McCullough M, et al: American Cancer Society Guidelines on nutrition and physical activity for cancer prevention: reducing the risk of cancer with healthy food choices and physical activity, CA Cancer J Clin 62:30–67, 2012.

Lyman GH, Dale DC, Wolff DA, et al: Acute myeloid leukemia or myelodysplastic syndrome in randomized controlled clinical trials of cancer chemotherapy with granulocyte colony-stimulating factor: a systematic review, J Clin Oncol 28:2914–2924, 2010.

Raaschou-Nielsen O, Andersen ZJ, Beelen R, et al: Air pollution and lung cancer incidence in 17 European cohorts: prospective analyses from the European Study of Cohorts for Air Pollution Effects (ESCAPE), Lancet Oncol 14:813–822, 2013.

Rivera DR, Peters S, Panagiotou OA, et al: Utilization of COVID-19 treatments and clinical outcomes among patients with cancer: a COVID-19 and Cancer Consortium (CCC19) cohort study, Cancer Discovery, 2020 (epub ahead of print July 22 2020).

Schottenfeld D, Beebe-Dimmer JL: Advances in cancer epidemiology: understanding causal mechanisms and the evidence for implementing interventions, Annu Rev Public Health 26:37–60, 2005.

Schottenfeld D, Beebe-Dimmer J: Alleviating the burden of cancer: a perspective on advances, challenges and future directions, Cancer Epidemiol Biomarkers Prev 15:2049–2055, 2006.

Siegel RL, Miller KD, Jemal AJ: Cancer statistics, CA Cancer J Clin 70:7–30, 2020, 2020.

Smith RA, Brooks D, Cokkinides V, et al: Cancer screening in the United States, 2013: a review of current American Cancer Society guidelines, current issues in cancer screening, and new guidance on cervical cancer screening and lung cancer screening, CA Cancer J Clin 63:88–105, 2013.

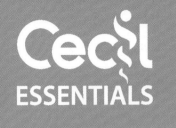

56

Principles of Cancer Therapy

Davendra P.S. Sohal, Alok A. Khorana

INTRODUCTION

The treatment of cancer includes a rapidly growing portfolio of modalities and agents: locoregional therapies (surgery, radiation), systemic therapies (chemotherapy, targeted therapies, immunotherapies), and supportive care agents. Surgery and radiation therapy are safe and effective treatments for localized cancers, and techniques continue to be refined. In most settings (particularly advanced stages), however, cancer is a systemic disease and requires systemic treatment. Chemotherapy—the "first generation" of cancer drugs—is the current mainstay of systemic treatment. The explosive increase in our knowledge of cancer biology and genomics has allowed the development of both specific targeted agents and drugs harnessing the immune system to fight cancer. Many new drugs have been approved, and many more are in clinical trials—more than for any other class of medicine. Moreover, cancer treatment incurs many side effects. Symptom control, therefore, is a very important component of cancer therapy. All these modalities make it imperative that patients with cancer be treated by multidisciplinary teams at dedicated cancer centers. This chapter reviews the principles of the various components of cancer therapy.

DIAGNOSIS AND STAGING

Definitive treatment for cancer usually requires histologic diagnosis. This typically involves an invasive biopsy to obtain sufficient material to evaluate the morphology and invasiveness of the tumor and the expression of various molecular markers. Noninvasive tests such as radiologic imaging are seldom substitutes for tissue diagnosis. (There are occasional exceptions, such as an elevated α-fetoprotein level along with imaging evidence in a patient with cirrhosis, which can be used to make a diagnosis of hepatocellular carcinoma.)

Once the diagnosis of cancer has been made, for most solid-organ tumors, the next step is to systematically determine the extent of tumor spread, a process called *staging*. Tumor staging can be clinical or pathologic. *Clinical staging* involves physical examination and imaging studies, including targeted ultrasound (percutaneous or using invasive endoscopy devices), computed tomography scans, magnetic resonance imaging, whole-body positron-emission tomography scans, and radionuclide scans, usually in some combination, depending on the propensity of particular tumors to spread to particular organs. *Pathologic staging* is more definitive and follows the tumor-node-metastasis (TNM) method developed by the American Joint Committee on Cancer and the International Union against Cancer. This system requires a careful evaluation of the primary resection specimen for three measurements: (1) the size and extent of invasion of the primary tumor (the T score), (2) the number and location of histologically involved regional lymph nodes (the N score), and (3) the presence or absence of distant metastases (the M score). The M score is based on information derived from both clinical and pathologic staging. TNM scores are then grouped into a pathologic stage, typically from I through IV, reflecting an increasing burden of disease. The final TNM stage has both prognostic and therapeutic implications. For instance, a resected colon cancer that invades the muscularis propria, involves 2 of 16 lymph nodes, but shows no evidence of distant metastases is staged as a T2 N1 M0 (stage III) colon cancer. The likelihood of tumor recurrence is 40% to 50%; and patients are recommended 3 to 6 months of chemotherapy after surgery. On the other hand, if no lymph nodes are involved (T2 N0 M0, stage I), the likelihood of recurrence is less than 10%, and chemotherapy is usually not recommended.

Biomarkers provide additional prognostic information, such as the absence of hormone receptors or expression of HER2 in breast cancer, which are indicative of a poor prognosis. Such markers can also be predictive; for instance, overexpression of HER2 in breast cancer predicts response to trastuzumab. Similarly, *KRAS* mutations in colorectal cancer predict lack of response to antibodies (e.g., cetuximab, panitumumab) that are directed against the epidermal growth factor receptor (EGFR) (Fig. 56.1). Both prognostic and predictive biomarkers provide important information in addition to the formal TNM stage. With an increasing array of biomarkers being identified, a panel of them are now usually tested, using next-generation sequencing (NGS) platforms that can sequence hundreds of relevant genes to identify point mutations, translocations, copy number alterations, and expression level changes. All of this information is compiled into a final assessment of whether the cancer is curable or not.

The next step is to evaluate the patient's overall clinical condition with respect to comorbidities affecting major organ function and the patient's functional ability, termed *performance status*. Performance status is assessed with the use of various history-based methods, such as the Eastern Cooperative Oncology Group (ECOG) or Karnofsky performance score. Patients with poor performance status or major comorbid conditions may not derive a benefit from cancer-directed therapy and are at greater risk for adverse events. This comprehensive assessment—diagnosis, stage, prognostic and predictive markers, and patient condition—dictates the management plan: either curative or palliative.

PRINCIPLES OF CANCER SURGERY

Surgery can prevent cancer by removal of precancerous lesions or organs that are at high risk for cancer (e.g., bilateral mastectomy in those with hereditary defects that can lead to breast cancer). Surgery can also make the diagnosis of cancer by biopsy; assist in staging by sampling lymph nodes; provide definitive treatment by removing the primary tumor; reconstruct the limb or organ sacrificed; and provide palliative treatment of cancer (e.g., intestinal bypass for obstruction, spinal cord decompression, or orthopedic procedures to prevent or

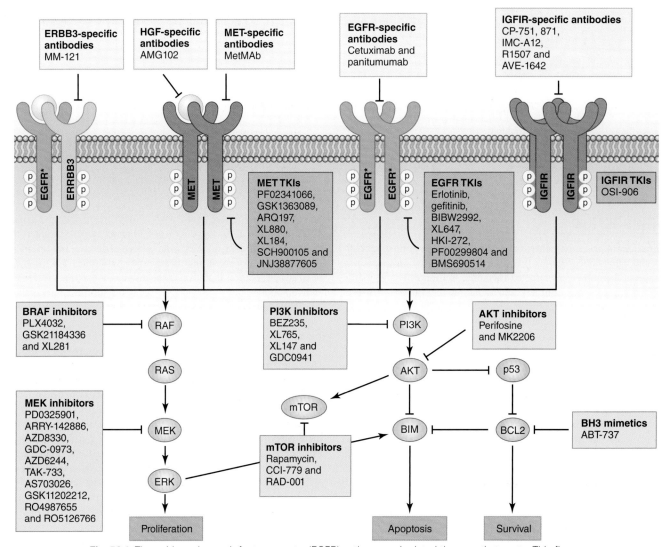

Fig. 56.1 The epidermal growth factor receptor (EGFR) pathway and related therapeutic targets. This figure depicts the transmembrane receptors of the EGFR family and the molecules involved in downstream signal transduction that ultimately lead to control of key proteins affecting cell survival, growth, and proliferation.

treat pathologic fractures). Invasive procedures, such as biopsies and the insertion of various access devices, tubes, stents, catheters, and drains, are also performed by interventional specialists, such as radiologists, gastroenterologists, and pulmonologists.

When a solid organ cancer is localized, surgery is the most effective curative treatment available. The intent is to completely remove the tumor, regional lymph nodes, and adjacent involved tissue, along with a safe margin of normal tissue. At surgery, the tumor is isolated and is almost never opened during the procedure. Refinements in cancer surgery include increasing use of minimally invasive methods in selected cancers and the identification of a sentinel lymph node by injection of a dye during surgery, which avoids a full lymph node dissection if the sentinel node is uninvolved by cancer.

PRINCIPLES OF RADIATION THERAPY

Radiation therapy can sometimes be used as definitive treatment, either alone or in combination with systemic therapy. Unlike surgery, local or regional treatment with radiation can preserve organ structure and function, improving quality of life for patients. For example, use of radiation with chemotherapy for treatment of localized laryngeal cancer has outcomes similar to those of surgery but allows preservation of the larynx. Radiation therapy is also effective in the palliative setting, where it is used to control various cancer-related problems such as pain, mechanical obstruction of a luminal organ, and bleeding.

Ionizing radiation damages cellular DNA directly or indirectly through free radical intermediates. Cells are most susceptible to radiation during the M and G_2 phases of the cell cycle. The aim of radiation therapy is to deliver the highest dose possible to the tumor with minimal toxicity to adjacent normal tissues. Dividing the total planned radiation dose into small daily fractions takes advantage of the difference in repair capability between normal and malignant tissue and improves the tolerance of normal tissue. The biologic effects of radiation can be modified by numerous factors, including the amount of oxygen in the irradiated tissue and the use of chemotherapy for sensitizing tissue to radiation.

The goal of treatment planning for radiation therapy is to precisely define the dose and volume to be irradiated. The dose of radiation is measured in units of absorbed dose, Gray (Gy), which has replaced the older unit, rad (1 Gy = 100 rad). Conventional radiation treatments deliver 1.8 to 2 Gy/day on 5 days per week, over a period of 5 to 6 weeks. For palliative treatment, higher doses per fraction may be used to deliver an effective dose over a shorter period.

TABLE 56.1 Commonly Used Chemotherapy Agents

Drug	Cancers Treated	Specific Class or Mechanism of Action	Common Side Effects
Cell Cycle–Specific			
5-Fluorouracil	Gastrointestinal, head and neck, breast	Antimetabolite, inhibits thymidylate synthase	Myelosuppression, mucositis, diarrhea
Gemcitabine	Pancreas, lung, breast, bladder	Antimetabolite, deoxycytidine analogue	Myelosuppression, nausea, emesis
Methotrexate	ALL, choriocarcinoma, bladder, lymphoma	Antimetabolite, folic acid antagonist	Myelosuppression, mucositis, acute renal failure
Doxorubicin	Breast, lung, NHL	Anthracycline, intercalates into DNA	Myelosuppression, nausea, emesis, cardiomyopathy
Irinotecan	Colorectal, lung	Camptothecin, topoisomerase I inhibitor	Myelosuppression, diarrhea
Paclitaxel	Breast, lung, Kaposi's sarcoma, ovarian	Plant alkaloid, inhibits microtubule formation	Myelosuppression, hypersensitivity reaction, neuropathy
Vincristine	ALL, lymphomas, myeloma, sarcoma	Plant alkaloid, disrupts microtubule assembly	Peripheral neuropathy, constipation
Cell Cycle–Nonspecific			
Cyclophosphamide	Breast, NHL, CLL, sarcoma	Alkylating agent, cross-links DNA	Myelosuppression, hemorrhagic cystitis, nausea, emesis
Cisplatin	Lung, bladder, ovarian, testicular, head and neck	Alkylating agent, cross-links DNA	Nephrotoxicity, nausea, emesis, ototoxicity, sensory neuropathy

ALL, Acute lymphoblastic leukemia; *CLL,* chronic lymphocytic leukemia; *NHL,* non-Hodgkin's lymphoma.

Ionizing radiation can be administered as external-beam therapy with the use of a linear accelerator to generate electrons or high-energy radiographs. Electrons have a limited depth of penetration and are useful for superficial tumors. High-energy radiographs deliver the radiation deep into the body while reducing the dose to the skin as they enter. Brachytherapy uses radioactive sources to deliver ionizing radiation (gamma rays) directly to the tumor. An example is the implantation of iodine-125 seeds into the prostate as definitive therapy for early prostate cancer. Current approaches to improving radiation therapy include the use of advanced technology that allows delivery of a higher dose of radiation to specific areas of the tumor and sparing of normal tissue (conformal and intensity-modulated radiation therapy).

Injury to normal tissue from radiation therapy can be either acute or late. Acute effects occur within days to weeks after irradiation and are seen primarily in rapidly proliferating tissues such as skin and gastrointestinal mucosa. The severity depends on the total dose, but the damage can usually be repaired. Late effects, such as necrosis, fibrosis, or organ failure, appear months or years after irradiation and are dependent on fraction size. Another late complication of radiation therapy is the development of secondary malignancies of organs in the radiation field, sometimes decades after radiation.

PRINCIPLES OF MEDICAL THERAPY

The term *chemotherapy* refers to the use of cytotoxic agents, singly or in combination, for the systemic treatment of cancer. Most such agents are general antiproliferative agents that are more effective against rapidly growing tumors and have significant adverse effects on normal tissues that also divide rapidly, such as bone marrow and digestive tract mucosa. Newer agents, including monoclonal antibodies and signal transduction inhibitors, are directed against targets that are relatively specific to tumor cells and therefore may have less toxicity. These drugs are classified separately from chemotherapy as *targeted therapy* agents. The newest class of anticancer drugs is *immunotherapy*. These drugs stimulate the T cell cytotoxic machinery to allow cancer cell kill by native immunologic mechanisms. Related to these immunotherapy drugs is the use of the T-cell arsenal from a donor (stem cell transplantation) or self (chimeric antigen receptor–T cells).

Mechanisms of Chemotherapy

Chemotherapeutic agents can be cell cycle–specific or cell cycle–nonspecific. Cell cycle–nonspecific agents have a greater effect on cells traversing the cell cycle but also affect noncycling cells; cell cycle–specific agents affect only cycling cells. Chemotherapy agents are further classified according to their mechanism of action into alkylating agents, antimetabolites, antitumor antibiotics, and mitotic spindle inhibitors (Table 56.1). Most chemotherapy agents suppress the bone marrow, increasing the risk of neutropenic infections, anemia, and exacerbated bleeding. For most drugs, treatment schedules involve successive doses every 2 to 4 weeks. This interval between successive doses, the *cycle* of chemotherapy, allows recovery of blood counts and other side effects before administration of the next dose. The concept of *dose intensity* is also important. Cellular killing with chemotherapy follows first-order kinetics: A given dose of drug kills only a fraction of tumor cells. The dose-response curve for chemotherapy drugs is steep. Therefore, the greater the dose administered, the greater the kill: A 2-fold increase in dose can lead to a 10-fold increase in tumor cell kill. This also means that dose reductions may adversely affect the eventual cure rate. Shortening of the duration of cycles of chemotherapy using growth factor support—a "dose-dense" approach—has been shown to improve survival in selected patients when compared with traditional chemotherapy for breast cancer.

Single chemotherapy agents seldom cure cancer. Combination chemotherapy regimens have therefore been developed for a variety of cancers. Combination therapy provides maximal cell kill and broader coverage of resistant cells; it may also prevent or slow the development of resistant cells. Drugs used in a combination are chosen because they have known efficacy as single agents but have differing mechanisms of action and non-overlapping toxicity profiles. These regimens are commonly referred to by acronyms, such as CHOP (cyclophosphamide, doxorubicin, vincristine, and prednisone) for lymphoma or FOLFOX (5-fluorouracil, leucovorin, and oxaliplatin) for colorectal cancer.

Indications for Chemotherapy

Chemotherapy outcomes in general for localized or advanced cancers are summarized in Table 56.2. *Adjuvant* chemotherapy refers to its use after the primary tumor has been resected. Here, chemotherapy is

TABLE 56.2   Efficacy of Medical Therapy in Selected Cancers

Cure Possible Even in Advanced Disease
Testicular cancer
Acute leukemia: lymphocytic, promyelocytic, selected myelocytic
Lymphomas: Hodgkin's lymphoma, selected non-Hodgkin's lymphomas
Childhood solid tumors: rhabdomyosarcoma, Ewing sarcoma, Wilms tumor
Choriocarcinoma
Small cell lung cancer

Cure Likely in Locoregional Disease
Breast cancer
Colorectal cancer
Prostate cancer
Renal cancer
Head and neck cancer

Long-Term Control Possible in Advanced Disease
Melanoma
Non-small cell lung cancer
Chronic myeloid leukemia

directed against presumed systemic micrometastases in patients who are at high risk for recurrence. In the example of stage III colon cancer (described earlier), 3 to 6 months of adjuvant chemotherapy after primary tumor resection can reduce the patient's likelihood of developing recurrent cancer from 50% to 25%. Adjuvant chemotherapy has been shown to increase cure rates in many other cancers.

Neoadjuvant or *preoperative* chemotherapy refers to the use of chemotherapy before surgery, sometimes in combination with radiation therapy. If successful, neoadjuvant therapy can reduce the size of the tumor and consequently permit less removal of normal tissue, such as a lumpectomy instead of a mastectomy in breast cancer or limb-sparing surgery instead of amputation in extremity sarcoma.

Chemotherapy can be curative on its own in cancers such as germ cell tumors, lymphomas, and leukemias. Most often, chemotherapy is employed in the treatment of metastatic disease for which surgery or radiation therapy is ineffective. Even when it is not curative, chemotherapy often extends survival and improves cancer-related symptoms and quality of life.

Limitations of Chemotherapy

Chemotherapy is curative only under certain circumstances, because it is inherently limited by side effects (i.e., the dose ceiling). There are several reasons for the inability of standard doses of chemotherapy to cure cancer. First, tumor cell kinetics naturally protect against chemotherapy. When chemotherapy was initially developed, it was believed that tumors contained a percentage of cells traversing the cell cycle. However, most human tumors display Gompertzian growth kinetics—that is, the rate of tumor cell doubling *slows* progressively as tumor size increases. Therefore, the growth fraction of tumors is greatest when a tumor is clinically undetectable. By the time the patient is symptomatic and has clinically evident disease, the growth fraction of tumors can be less than 5%. Chemotherapy can be successful in the adjuvant setting (when the burden of disease is minimal), but it rarely results in cure in the metastatic setting.

Second, cancer cells can become resistant to chemotherapy. One of the most important forms of resistance is intrinsic and is mediated by an evolutionarily conserved cell membrane efflux pump called *P-glycoprotein.* Resistance can also be acquired after a period

of exposure to chemotherapy agents by a variety of mechanisms; for example, tumor cells can decrease the uptake of methotrexate by decreasing the expression of the folate transporter, or they can amplify expression of the target enzyme thymidylate synthase when treated with 5-fluorouracil.

Third, mutations in the *TP53* gene are common in various cancers. The TP53 protein causes cell-cycle arrest and mediates apoptosis when DNA damage occurs. In the absence of a functioning TP53, cancer cells are protected from chemotherapy-induced apoptosis.

Targeted Therapy

The limitations of chemotherapy, coupled with a greater understanding of cancer cell biology, has led to the development of a new class of drugs directed against targets that are relatively specific to cancer cells: growth factors and signaling molecules that are essential for proliferation of tumor cells; cell-cycle proteins; regulators of apoptosis; and molecules mediating host-tumor interactions such as angiogenesis and tumor immunity. These agents include monoclonal antibodies directed against cell surface antigens or growth factors, specific or multitargeted receptor tyrosine kinase inhibitors, specific pathway signal transduction inhibitors, antisense oligonucleotides, and gene therapies. Additional agents are under development. The usual side effects of chemotherapy, such as myelosuppression, nausea, emesis, diarrhea, and alopecia, are not necessarily observed with these drugs. However, other target-specific toxicities require careful monitoring and management (Table 56.3).

The best-known targeted therapy agent is imatinib, which inhibits both BCR-ABL, the constitutively active fusion product arising from the Philadelphia chromosome of CML, and KIT (c-kit, CD117), which is overexpressed in gastrointestinal stromal tumors (GIST). The daily oral administration of imatinib results in complete hematologic responses in more than 90% of patients in chronic-phase CML and partial responses in more than 50% of patients with metastatic GIST. Ibrutinib is another novel agent, targeting Bruton tyrosine kinase, with excellent efficacy in CLL and Waldenström's macroglobulinemia.

In many other malignancies, there are multiple redundant signaling pathways that are dysregulated. Increasingly, tyrosine kinase inhibitors with multiple (as opposed to specific) targets have been developed to treat such cancers. Sorafenib and sunitinib are two examples of such agents that inhibit various pathways, including vascular endothelial growth factor (VEGF), platelet-derived growth factor (PDGF), and KIT. Studies have shown these drugs to be effective in renal and liver cancers.

Targeted therapy drugs can also increase the efficacy of chemotherapy, through various mechanisms. For instance, the EGFR antagonists cetuximab and panitumumab increase the efficacy of irinotecan-based chemotherapy in colorectal cancer and that of definitive radiation therapy in oropharyngeal cancers. The availability of these agents has increased the number of drug combinations that can be used in particular cancers. As multiple combinations of chemotherapy and targeted therapy have become available for the treatment of advanced colon cancer the median survival time of patients with this disease has more than doubled. Targeted therapy agents are also increasingly being used in the adjuvant setting—imatinib in patients with resected GIST or trastuzumab in patients with resected HER2-positive breast cancer have substantially improved outcomes for these malignancies.

Endocrine Therapy

Cancers originating from organs that are regulated by hormones, such as breast and prostate, may be susceptible to hormonal control mechanisms even when metastatic. Endocrine therapy includes the use of both hormonal and antihormonal agents that work as antagonists or partial agonists.

TABLE 56.3 Examples of Targeted Therapy Agents

Drug	Cancers Treated	Targets	Common Side Effects
Monoclonal Antibodies			
Alemtuzumab	CLL	CD52	Myelosuppression, fever, rash
Bevacizumab	Colorectal, renal, lung	VEGF	Hypertension, proteinuria, bleeding, thromboembolism
Cetuximab	Colorectal	EGFR	Rash
Ipilimumab	Metastatic melanoma	CTLA4	Cytokine release storm
Ofatumumab	CLL	CD20	Rash, diarrhea, respiratory tract infections
Panitumumab	Colorectal	EGFR	Rash
Pertuzumab	Breast	HER2	Rash, diarrhea
Rituximab	NHL	CD20	Infusional reaction, skin reactions
Trastuzumab	Breast	HER2/Neu	Infusional reaction, congestive heart failure
Signal Transduction Inhibitors			
Axitinib	Renal	VEGF, PDGF, KIT	Hypertension, hand-foot syndrome, diarrhea
Crizotinib	Lung	EML4-ALK	Edema, diarrhea
Dasatinib	CML	BCR-ABL	Myelosuppression, pleural effusions
Imatinib	CML, GIST	BCR-ABL	Diarrhea, fluid retention, myelosuppression
Erlotinib	Lung, pancreas	EGFR tyrosine kinase	Rash, diarrhea
Gefitinib	Lung	EGFR tyrosine kinase	Rash, hypertension
Ibrutinib	CLL, Waldenström's macroglobulinemia	Bruton tyrosine kinase	Bacterial infections
Imatinib	CML, GIST	BCR-ABL	Diarrhea, fluid retention, myelosuppression
Lapatinib	Breast	HER2, EGFR	Rash, diarrhea
Regorafenib	GIST, colorectal	VEGF	Hypertension, hepatotoxicity, dysphonia
Sunitinib	Renal, GIST	VEGF, PDGF, KIT	Rash, diarrhea, fatigue
Sorafenib	Liver, renal	VEGF, PDGF, KIT	Hypertension, fatigue, diarrhea, hand-foot syndrome
Vandetanib	Medullary thyroid	VEGF, EGFR, RET	Rash, abdominal pain, diarrhea
Vemurafenib	Melanoma	BRAF	Rash, skin lesions, arthralgia
Others			
All-trans-retinoic-acid	Acute promyelocytic leukemia	Differentiating agent	Vitamin A toxicity, retinoic acid syndrome, hyperlipidemia
Azacitidine	Myelodysplasia	Hypomethylating agent	Myelosuppression, injection site reactions
Bortezomib	Lymphoma, myeloma	Proteasome inhibitor	Rash, nausea, emesis, neuropathy
Everolimus	Renal, breast, neuroendocrine	mTOR inhibitor	Hyperglycemia, diarrhea, fatigue

CLL, Chronic lymphocytic leukemia; *CML,* chronic myelogenous leukemia; *CTLA4,* cytotoxic T lymphocyte–associated protein 4; *EGFR,* epidermal growth factor receptor; *GIST,* gastrointestinal stromal tumor; *mTOR,* mammalian target of rifampin; *NHL,* non-Hodgkin's lymphoma; *VEGF,* vascular endothelial growth factor.

Many patients with metastatic breast cancer express hormone receptors (estrogen or progesterone) in tumor cells. Most of these patients respond either to tamoxifen, an estrogen receptor modulator, or to aromatase inhibitors (letrozole, anastrozole, or exemestane), which inhibit adrenal steroid production. Similar responses are observed in men with metastatic prostate cancer treated with the luteinizing hormone–releasing hormone agonists leuprolide or goserelin, which decrease testosterone to castrate levels.

In selected breast and prostate cancer patients, metastatic disease can be controlled for years with only endocrine therapy. Tamoxifen and the aromatase inhibitors are also highly effective adjuvant treatments after breast cancer resection. Furthermore, tamoxifen has been shown to reduce the incidence of breast cancer by 50% in healthy women who are at high risk for developing breast cancer.

Personalized Medicine

These targeted therapies—kinase inhibitors, antibodies, hormones—work only when their specific targets are present in the cancer cells. The paradigm of evaluation of tissue specimens for such targets to allow the use of drugs impinging on those targets is referred to as *precision* or *personalized medicine/oncology.* The time and costs involved in analyzing genomic alterations from a patient's tumor are now much reduced. In addition to DNA, transcriptomic (RNA), epigenomic (DNA methylation), and single-nucleotide polymorphism (SNP array) analyses can also be performed. Several cancers have already been sequenced completely. Such work creates "reference libraries" against which a patient's tumor can be tested. Based on findings from such analyses, specific drugs or regimens can be recommended for individual patients. Most of the targeted therapies, and even immunotherapies, have predictive molecular markers: microsatellite instability, tumor mutation burden, *NTRK* and *FGFR* fusions, *KRAS* and *BRAF* mutations, HER2 and cMET overexpression being prominent examples. A prominent success story has been lung cancer, where therapies targeting EGFR mutations, ALK fusions, MET alterations, and others are now front-line treatments with much greater clinical benefit than traditional cytotoxic agents.

Immunotherapy

Immunotherapy agents act by altering the host immune response to the tumor. They either stimulate the cytotoxic T-cell machinery directly or counter the inhibitory mechanisms keeping these cells quiescent, the result being that T cells get primed to recognize and kill cancer cells. Cancer vaccines, such as the dendritic cell vaccine sipuleucel-T for prostate cancer, exploit the presence of specific tumor antigens that can serve as targets of the stimulated T cells. Their use is so far limited to a handful of scenarios.

More recently, antibodies targeting CTLA4 and PD1, which are inhibitory receptors on the surface of cytotoxic T-cells (or PD-L1, the ligand on tumor cells that corresponds to PD1), have achieved great success in the treatment of various malignancies. These checkpoint inhibitors—so called because they block the molecular "checkpoints" that normally inhibit cytotoxic T-cells—unleash the body's immune response to recognize cancer cells as "foreign" and kill them. This is akin to the graft-versus-tumor response used in allogeneic hematopoietic stem cell transplantation; only here, the body's native immune system is primed to achieve the desired effect, with much less toxicity. A major toxicity observed with this approach is the possibility of "autoimmune" reaction whereby uncontrolled T-cell cytotoxicity damages normal cells and tissues. These drugs are now routinely used to treat melanoma, kidney cancer, and lung cancer, and achieve remarkably durable clinical responses.

The ability of these checkpoint inhibitors to work is dependent largely on their ability to see the cancer cells as "different" from the normal cells. Because cancer cells frequently have mutations that lead to the production of abnormal proteins, these neopeptides serve as neoantigens for the T cells, allowing differential identification and targeting of cancer cells. Therefore, the higher the tumor mutation burden, the more likely the efficacy of these drugs. This is clearly evident in high mutational load tumors such as ultraviolet light–associated melanoma, smoking-associated lung cancer, and cancers with high microsatellite instability, which respond very well to these drugs.

Stem Cell Transplantation

The traditional model of using T-cell immunity to counter cancer has been allogeneic stem cell transplantation. By using harvested stem cells (typically from the bone marrow of an HLA-matched donor), the immunologic response mounted by the donor cells, termed *graft-versus-tumor* effect, can lead to durable cures in various leukemias. However, allogeneic transplantations can be offered only to a minority of patients because of the limited availability of matched donors (particularly in ethnic minority populations) and the inability of older patients and those with comorbid illnesses to tolerate this procedure. To increase the availability of donors, umbilical cord blood is being studied as a source of stem cells.

The complications of stem cell transplantation are primarily related to the toxicity of chemotherapy and radiation therapy to vital organs, including lungs and liver. Long-term morbidity and mortality after allogeneic transplantation can result from *graft-versus-host disease* and from complications of immunosuppressive agents used to treat it.

CAR-T Cell Therapy

The newest advance in the field of using T cell cytotoxicity to kill cancer cells is chimeric antigen receptor–T (CAR-T) cells. This involves extracting a cancer patient's T cells and then modifying them using retroviral, lentiviral, or CRISPR/Cas9 gene editing methods. This editing process attaches a chimeric receptor on the surface of these T cells: the chimeric receptor combines a cancer cell–specific antigen binding site and a T cell activating site. These primed T cells are then infused back into the patient after depleting native T cells using chemotherapy. Extensive cytotoxic T cell activity leads to a "cytokine storm" that requires aggressive supportive care, but eventually, durable clinical responses in leukemias and lymphomas have been achieved. The efficacy of this approach in patients with solid organ malignancies is currently being tested.

EVALUATION OF RESPONSE

The efficacy of cancer-directed therapies is gauged by various methods and has been granted its own vocabulary. In patients with metastatic disease, all known sites of disease are monitored by physical examinations and serial radiologic imaging. Responses are judged according to the internationally accepted Response Evaluation Criteria in Solid Tumors (RECIST) rules. Disappearance of all known lesions is called a *complete response*, whereas a 30% or greater reduction in size is called a *partial response*. Appearance of new lesions or an increase in the size of known lesions by 20% is termed *progression of disease* and implies failure of treatment. A tumor that is neither responding nor progressing is termed *stable disease.*

The percentage of patients who experience a response is called the *response rate* to the agent or agents being administered. New drugs are often evaluated on the basis of response rates. However, a response does not imply cure. Even a drug with a 100% response rate is not curative if all patients relapse. Therefore, the "gold standard" for measuring the efficacy of a drug is considered to be an improvement in *overall survival*, or its surrogate, *disease-free survival*—the time interval during which the patient is alive without disease. The use of effective second-line therapies may minimize the survival differences between two treatments prescribed as initial therapy, and in this context, disease-free survival can serve as an important end point in evaluating new regimens. Increasingly, quality-of-life end points such as use of pain medications or patient-reported outcomes are also being used to assess the efficacy of drugs in palliation.

SUPPORTIVE CARE

Supportive care interventions can improve the safety and tolerability of cancer treatments. Many drugs can mitigate chemotherapy-related side effects. Serotonin receptor antagonists and neurokinin-1 receptor antagonists, in combination with older antiemetic drugs, may control chemotherapy-induced nausea and vomiting. Granulocyte colony-stimulating factor (filgrastim) and granulocyte-macrophage colony-stimulating factor (sargramostim) stimulate the proliferation and differentiation of myeloid progenitor cells and can prevent or minimize the duration of chemotherapy-induced neutropenia and reduce the likelihood of neutropenic fever. These agents are also used to mobilize and collect stem cells for transplantation.

Supportive care is an integral part of the treatment of cancer, particularly in noncurative settings. Palliative aspects of treating cancer address not only physical symptoms in particular pain syndromes but also psychosocial and spiritual concerns. Chemotherapy and radiation therapy are often used with palliative intent and can improve quality of life.

Acknowledgments

Dr. Khorana would like to acknowledge support from the Sondra and Stephen Hardis Endowed Chair in Oncology Research and the National Institutes of Health (U01-HL143402).

SUGGESTED READINGS

DeVita VT, Rosenberg SA: Two hundred years of cancer research, N Engl J Med 366:2207–2214, 2012.

Khalil DN, Smith EL, Brentjens RJ, Wolchok JD: The future of cancer treatment: immunomodulation, CARs and combination immunotherapy, Nat Rev Clin Oncol 13:273–290, 2016.

Mardis ER: The impact of next-generation sequencing on cancer genomics: from discovery to clinic, Cold Spring Harb Perspect Med 3:a036269, 2019.

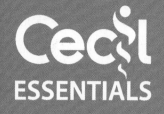

57

Lung Cancer

Zoe G.S. Vazquez, Jason M. Aliotta, Christopher G. Azzoli

DEFINITION AND EPIDEMIOLOGY

Lung cancer is the second most common cancer in the United States and the leading cause of cancer death. Worldwide, an estimated 1 million people die of lung cancer each year. Despite recent advances in understanding of the biology and genetics of lung cancer and the advent of novel therapeutic agents for its treatment, the 5-year survival rate for patients with lung cancer is below 20%. The relatively poor long-term survival partly stems from the fact that most patients with lung cancer have an advanced stage of the disease at the time of diagnosis.

Historically, lung cancer has been divided into two major types: *small cell lung carcinoma* (SCLC) (E-Fig. 57.1) and *non–small cell lung carcinoma* (NSCLC). It is increasingly important to recognize the subtypes of NSCLC (based on histologic, or genetic differences), and it is essential to do so when selecting drug therapy for stage IV (metastatic) NSCLC. Histologic subtypes of NSCLC include adenocarcinoma (40% of lung cancers) (E-Fig. 57.2), squamous cell carcinoma (30% of lung cancers) (E-Fig. 57.3), large cell carcinoma (10% of lung cancers) (E-Fig. 57.4), and some more poorly differentiated histologic subtypes not otherwise specified (NOS).

A current or prior history of cigarette smoking remains the leading known risk factor for the development of lung cancer. SCLC, in particular, is so causally linked to tobacco smoking that its prevalence (currently <15% of all lung cancers) is falling as smoking prevalence falls. Still, up to 15% of newly diagnosed NSCLCs (usually adenocarcinoma) are seen in never-smokers. In recent years, it has been recognized that lung cancer in smokers is a different disease from lung cancer in never-smokers and impacts prognosis, genetic underpinnings, and response to immune therapy.

The risk for lung cancer is generally proportional to the number of cigarette pack-years smoked (packs per day × years smoked), and the incidence peaks in the sixth and seventh decades of life. Former-smokers have a persistent risk for lung cancer throughout life. Second-hand smoking is also a risk factor for lung cancer in a portion of nonsmokers who develop the disease. Nonsmokers who live with smokers have a more than 30% increased risk of developing lung cancer than those who live with nonsmokers. Other risk factors for lung cancer include environmental hazards such as asbestos and petroleum exposure. Smoking is considered an important cofactor of lung cancer in the setting of asbestos exposure. Radon exposure also increases the risk for developing lung cancer (see Chapter 55).

An ever-growing list of genetic alterations have been identified in terms of both proto-oncogenes and tumor suppressor genes. Unique molecular-genomic subgroups of lung cancer have been recognized, including those harboring (1) mutated epidermal growth factor receptor *(EGFR/ERBB1)*, (2) mutated Kirsten rat sarcoma viral oncogene homolog *(KRAS)*, and (3) anaplastic lymphoma kinase *(ALK)* 2p23

chromosomal rearrangement, more commonly known as *EML4-ALK*, a fusion with echinoderm microtubule-associated protein-like 4 *(EML4)*. Importantly, these oncogenic alterations inform gene-targeted drug selection in that the cancer is dependent upon a single oncogenic pathway for sustained proliferation and/or survival (oncogene addiction).

Several targeted therapies have been approved by the US Food and Drug Administration (FDA) for the treatment of advanced NSCLCs containing mutated *EGFR* (gefitinib, erlotinib, afatinib, osimertinib) or the *ALK* 2p23 rearrangement (crizotinib, ceritinib, alectinib, brigatinib, lorlatinib). Lung cancers with *EGFR* mutations are more frequently identified in never-smokers or in those with a light smoking history. They are more often of the adenocarcinoma subtype and more commonly found in women and in patients of East Asian descent. *KRAS*-mutated lung cancers are found primarily in patients with a more extensive smoking history. Lung cancers with mutated *EGFR* and those with the *ALK* 2p23 rearrangement are typically seen in younger patient populations, with a median age at diagnosis of approximately 55 years.

PATHOLOGY

Histologic Subgroups
Non–Small Cell Lung Carcinomas
Most lung cancers fall under the major histologic subgroup of NSCLC. Of these, *adenocarcinomas* and *squamous cell carcinomas* are the most common.

Adenocarcinomas. Adenocarcinoma is the most commonly diagnosed subtype of lung cancer, accounting for approximately 40% of lung cancer diagnoses and 65,000 deaths each year in the United States. It is the histologic subtype most commonly diagnosed in never-smokers. Primary lung adenocarcinomas are usually found in the periphery of the lung (75%) (E-Fig. 57.5), in contrast to squamous cell carcinomas that may arise in central airways.

Histologically, adenocarcinomas typically form glandular structures and produce mucin. *EGFR* mutations are more commonly associated with nonmucinous lung adenocarcinoma, whereas the mucinous subtype is more commonly associated with mutated *KRAS*. The tumor cells typically stain positive for cytokeratin 7 (CK7) and thyroid transcription factor 1 (TTF-1) and stain negative for cytokeratin 20 (CK20). *Lepidic adenocarcinomas* (previously known as bronchioloalveolar carcinomas) grow along alveolar spaces and allow air to enter the tumor. These adenocarcinomas manifest as translucent *ground-glass* lung infiltrates on computed tomography (CT) scan. Mucinous adenocarcinomas can cause dense lung consolidation and can be accompanied by copious sputum production, known as *bronchorrhea*.

Squamous cell carcinomas. Squamous cell carcinomas arise from the epithelial layer of the bronchial wall. Normal columnar epithelial cells undergo metaplasia, dysplasia, and then localized carcinoma formation *(carcinoma in situ)*, which can then further extend and invade beyond the bronchial mucosa as it acquires a full malignant invasive phenotype. Most squamous cell carcinomas arise within central airways (E-Fig. 57.6). Therefore, the airway lumen may become obstructed, leading to collapse of the lung or postobstructive pneumonia. Although necrosis and cavity formation can occur in any lung tumor, this feature is more common in squamous cell carcinomas. Squamous lung cancers have a lower potential for metastatic spread compared to invasive adenocarcinomas. Histologically, squamous cell carcinomas can be distinguished from other NSCLCs by the presence of keratinization, pearl formation, intercellular bridging, and staining positive for p40 and/or p63.

Adenosquamous carcinomas. Adenosquamous carcinomas constitute between 0.4% and 4% of all lung cancers and have a worse prognosis. They have components of both adenocarcinoma and squamous cell carcinoma, each comprising at least 10% of the tumor. It is important to recognize intratumor heterogeneity and mixed histology NSCLCs, especially when the diagnosis is based on a single needle biopsy. Most molecular pathology guidelines recommend genetic analysis of small biopsy specimens so as not to miss the druggable gene mutations that are more common to adenocarcinoma.

Sarcomatoid carcinomas. Sarcomatoid carcinomas, also known as *giant cell* or *pleiotropic carcinomas*, are high-grade lung cancers with a poor prognosis but that may harbor druggable oncogene drivers (especially MET exon 14 skipping) or may be particularly susceptible to immune checkpoint inhibitors.

NSCLC not otherwise specified. These NSCLCs are poorly differentiated tumors that defy specific classification based on their histology and immunophenotyping profile, but they may still be subtyped based on gene mutation analyses.

Small Cell Lung Carcinoma

SCLC cells are of pulmonary neuroendocrine cell origin and are often associated with paraneoplastic syndromes (Table 57.1). SCLCs typically are perihilar in location. They often originate from the main bronchi and have associated malignant adenopathy (E-Fig. 57.7). These tumors have a high propensity for metastasis, most commonly to the thoracic lymph nodes, bones, liver, adrenal glands, and brain. Most patients are already affected with metastatic disease at the time of presentation. SCLC is an aggressive lung tumor. In fact, without treatment, the median survival time of patients with SCLC is less than 5 months. The overall survival for all patients is 5% at 5 years and has not improved over the past several decades.

Molecular-Genomic Subtypes

Lung cancer is now increasingly regarded as a disease with distinct genetic subgroups (Table 57.2). Many of these molecular-genomic alterations can inform the use of targeted therapeutics and predict responses.

Mutant *EGFR*

EGFR mutation testing and targeted therapy are essential to the care of patients with stage IV (metastatic) NSCLC. Specific somatic *EGFR* activating-sensitizing mutations predict clinical response to *EGFR* tyrosine kinase inhibitors (gefitinib, erlotinib, afatinib, osimertinib). These mutations are usually found in never-smokers with adenocarcinoma. *EGFR* mutations are more prevalent in women and patients of Asian race (30%, compared with 7% to 10% in Caucasians).

ALK 2p23 Rearrangement

The *EML4-ALK* fusion is an oncogenic driver that occurs in 3% to 7% of NSCLCs and is often found in light smokers (<10 pack-years) or never-smokers. In most cases, *EML4-ALK* fusions do not overlap with other oncogenic mutations of *EGFR* or *KRAS*. Patients with *ALK* rearrangements can be treated with *ALK* inhibitors (crizotinib, ceritinib, alectinib, brigatinib, lorlatinib).

ROS-1 Rearrangement

ROS-1 is a receptor tyrosine kinase of the insulin receptor family. *ROS-1* gene rearrangements are found in approximately 2% of NSCLCs. There is protein homology between the *ALK* and *ROS-1* kinase domain, such that the lists of active drugs overlap. FDA-approved drugs for *ROS-1* include crizotinib and entrectinib. Other *ALK*-inhibitors (ceritinib, lorlatinib) are effective against both *ALK* and *ROS-1*.

Mutant *KRAS*

KRAS gene mutations are uncommon in squamous cell carcinomas but are present in 15% to 25% of lung adenocarcinomas. *KRAS* mutations are more commonly seen in former or current cigarette smokers than in never-smokers or light smokers. There is currently no FDA-approved treatment for mutated *KRAS*, but covalent modifiers of the *KRAS G12C* oncoprotein show promise and have moved into phase 2 clinical testing.

TABLE 57.1   Paraneoplastic Syndromes Associated With Lung Cancer

Syndrome	Cell Type	Mechanism
Hypertrophic pulmonary osteoarthropathy and clubbing	All except small cell	Unknown
Hyponatremia	Small cell most common; may be any type	SIADH, ectopic antidiuretic hormone production by tumor
Hypercalcemia	Usually squamous cell	Bone metastases, osteoclast-activating factor, parathyroid hormone–like hormone, prostaglandins
Cushing syndrome	Usually small cell	Ectopic ACTH production
Eaton-Lambert myasthenic syndrome	Usually small cell	Voltage-sensitive calcium-channel antibodies in >75%; affects presynaptic neuronal calcium channel activity
Other neuromyopathic disorders	Small cell most common; may be any type	Antineuronal nuclear antibodies, also known as anti-Hu; others unknown
Thrombophlebitis	All types	Unknown

ACTH, Adrenocorticotropic hormone; *SIADH,* syndrome of inappropriate secretion of antidiuretic hormone.

TABLE 57.2 Selected Molecular-Genomic Subtypes of NSCLC

Oncogene	Class of Molecular-Genomic Alterations	Characteristics
EGFR-mutant	Somatic missense mutations (most common with L858R in exon 21) and exon 19 deletions	More frequent in Asians, females, never-smokers or light smokers; most frequently adenocarcinoma subtype Sensitizing to EGFR inhibitors gefitinib, erlotinib, afatinib, osimertinib T790M mutation in EGFR is resistant to gefitinib, erlotinib, afatinib
EML4-ALK	ALK 2p23 chromosomal translocation	3-7% of NSCLCs More common in light smokers (<10 pack-years) or never-smokers Sensitizing to ALK inhibitors crizotinib, ceritinib, alectinib, brigatinib, lorlatinib
KRAS-mutant	Somatic mutations	Found in 15-25% lung adenocarcinomas More commonly seen in former or current cigarette smokers No effective targeted treatment at present but covalent inhibitors of G12C are in phase 2 development
BRAF-mutant	Somatic mutations	Belong to a family of serine-threonine protein kinases Identified in 1-3% of cases Only BRAF V600E is sensitive to trametinib, dabrafenib
HER2-mutant	Exon 20 insertion	HER2 alterations were identified in ≈2-4% of NSCLCs In the selected population of EGFR/KRAS/ALK-mutation–negative patients, HER2 mutations can reach up to 6% Predominantly found in females, nonsmokers; predominantly adenocarcinoma subtype May be associated with sensitivity to HER2-targeting drugs (trastuzumab, lapatinib, pertuzumab, and T-DM1)
STK11/LKB1	Inactivating mutations, deletion	A tumor suppressor gene Mutational frequency about 17-35% of NSCLCs, associated with resistance to immune checkpoint inhibition
RET-fusion	Chromosomal translocations	Occur in lung adenocarcinomas (1-2%). Respond to vandetanib, cabozantinib with off-target toxicity. On-target TKIs with fewer side effects are in late-phase development.
ROS-1-fusion	Chromosomal translocations	ROS-1 is a receptor tyrosine kinase of the insulin receptor family ROS-1-fusions were identified in ≈2% of NSCLCs More commonly found in younger people, more likely in never-smokers, and Asian patients are overrepresented Similar protein structure to other RTKs leads to overlapping active drug list (crizotinib, entrectinib, ceritinib, lorlatinib)
MET	Alternative spliced variant, mutations, amplification, receptor overexpression	The MET proto-oncogene is a receptor tyrosine kinase that binds to hepatocyte growth factor MET gene amplification can be found in 2-4% of NSCLCs, whereas overexpression of its receptor protein is much more common. May respond to crizotinib. MET exon 14 skipping results in lung cancers that respond to crizotinib. Several more potent MET inhibitors are in late-phase development.
NTRK	Chromosomal translocations	Rare, <1%. The NTRK genes encode the tropomyosin receptor kinases, which are receptors for nerve growth factors. When detected in lung cancer, patients respond to TKIs larotrectinib, entrectinib.

EGFR, Epithelial growth factor receptor; FDA, US Food and Drug Administration; NSCLC, non–small cell lung cancer; RTK, receptor tyrosine kinase.

The Lung Cancer Genome

In the last decade, The Cancer Genome Atlas (TCGA) project has provided a more comprehensive understanding of lung cancer by defining many of its nuances on a genomic level. The TCGA analysis of lung adenocarcinoma identified a relatively high exonic somatic mutation rate (mean, 12.0 events per megabase), similar to the rate found in squamous cell lung carcinoma. Three distinct expression subtypes of lung adenocarcinoma were identified from RNA-sequencing data: bronchioid, magnoid and squamoid. In addition, multiple gene fusions were found to be expressed in lung adenocarcinomas and multiple mechanisms for inactivation of the tumor suppressor gene CDKN2A were discovered.

For squamous cell NSCLCs, a most unexpected finding in the TCGA study was the identification of loss-of-function mutations in the HLA-A gene, which plays an important role in tumor cell surface antigen presentation and immune recognition. This is regarded as the first evidence of somatic cancer genome alterations evading the immune system by changing their surface antigens. Potential therapeutic targets were identified in most tumors, offering new therapeutic avenues of investigation for targeted therapy in lung cancer.

CLINICAL PRESENTATION

Initial symptoms of lung cancer are usually nonspecific (cough, dyspnea, sputum production, chest pain, weight loss) and are often attributed to bronchitis or pneumonia. The cancer has often invaded adjacent structures or metastasized when first recognized, causing symptoms that reflect the site of involvement. For example, destruction of blood vessels can cause hemoptysis, and tumor invasion of the pleura or chest wall can cause pleuritic chest pain. Involvement of the left recurrent laryngeal nerve or esophagus can cause hoarseness or dysphagia, respectively. Pleural effusions can develop either due to direct tumor involvement of the pleura or obstruction of lymph flow from the mediastinal nodes (E-Fig. 57.8). By a similar mechanism, malignant pericardial effusions can form, which can progress to *cardiac tamponade*. Patients might develop focal neurologic deficits due to spinal cord compression or brain metastasis. Superior vena cava obstruction may result in the *superior vena cava syndrome,* with edema of the face and upper extremities due to impaired venous return. Tumors in the apex of the lung (called *Pancoast tumors* or *superior sulcus tumors* [E-Fig. 57.9]) can invade adjacent chest wall structures and compress the brachial plexus, resulting in ipsilateral upper extremity weakness and/or pain. Tumor erosion into the cervical sympathetic chain causes *Horner syndrome,* with ptosis, miosis, and anhidrosis over the face and forehead.

Physical examination can be normal but may reveal changes in the lungs that reflect the impact of the tumor, such as crackles (e.g., postobstructive pneumonia [E-Fig. 57.10]); inspiratory wheezes, suggestive of airway obstruction; dullness to percussion at the lung bases from underlying pleural effusion; and lymph node enlargement in the supraclavicular (E-Fig. 57.11) or cervical and axillary areas. The most common sites of metastases are the lymph nodes, liver (E-Fig. 57.12), brain, adrenal glands, kidneys, and lungs.

DIAGNOSIS AND DIFFERENTIAL DIAGNOSIS

Prevention and Screening

The most effective lung cancer prevention strategy is smoking cessation. In addition, the United States Preventive Services Task Force (USPSTF) recommends lung cancer screening by yearly, low-dose, noncontrast CT scan in patients between the ages of 55 and 80 years who are either current smokers or former smokers who quit less than 15 years ago, with a smoking history of 1 pack per day for 30 years (or 30 pack-year equivalent). This recommendation is based on a prospective clinical trial showing a 20% reduction in lung cancer–specific mortality in a CT-screened population of heavy smokers.

Diagnostic and Staging Work-Up

Early diagnosis of lung cancer is essential and can potentially lead to cure in the case of a malignant tumor. Diagnostic evaluation should consider the patient's age, sex, smoking history, family history of lung and other types of cancer, and other relevant risk factors.

When lung cancer is suspected, either incidentally or because of symptoms, a tissue diagnosis is essential unless the patient is not eligible for treatment because of comorbidity. After assessment for metastases, the site of biopsy should be chosen to determine the highest stage of the tumor, if this is feasible. If the apparent tumor is confined to the chest, bronchoscopy is appropriate for central masses and transthoracic needle aspiration for peripheral lesions. Pleural effusion should be sampled to assess for malignant cells, which would indicate stage IV (metastatic) disease.

Contrast-enhanced chest CT, including images of the abdomen, is useful to delineate the location and size of the primary tumor and to examine for mediastinal lymph nodes, pleural disease, and adrenal or liver metastases. CT has limited ability to distinguish benign from malignant lymphadenopathy in the mediastinum. Positron emission tomography (PET) using 18-fluorodeoxyglucose (FDG) is more sensitive and more specific than CT in the detection of mediastinal lymph node metastases and may also detect unexpected metastases elsewhere. In principle, any suspected mediastinal or extrathoracic metastases identified by imaging alone should be confirmed with

tissue sampling before the patient is excluded from being considered an operative candidate. Techniques for invasive staging of the mediastinal lymph nodes include endobronchial ultrasound (EBUS)–guided needle aspiration and/or mediastinoscopy. EBUS is best for ruling in lymph node metastases. Mediastinoscopy can assess mediastinal spread of disease in patients without definite imaging evidence of lymph node involvement and is used to rule out lymph node metastases prior to surgery. PET scanning is limited in its ability to detect brain lesions, and magnetic resonance imaging (MRI) of the brain with intravenous contrast (or CT scanning if MRI cannot be done) should be performed if brain metastases are suspected or prior to surgery for stage IB or higher. Bone scans are useful for suspected symptomatic bony metastases.

Once a diagnosis of lung cancer is established, staging is necessary for prognostication and treatment. Staging of NSCLC determines whether surgical resection for cure, radiation, and/or chemotherapy is indicated. The tumor-node-metastasis (TNM) system is used to stage NSCLCs (Table 57.3). Using the TNM staging system, patients are classified as having stage I to IV disease (Table 57.4). For staging of SCLC, the Veterans Administration Lung Study Group designations of limited-stage (confined to one hemithorax) and extensive-stage (beyond one hemithorax) are used. Combined chemoradiation therapy with curative intent is considered for limited-stage SCLC, whereas extensive-stage SCLC is treated with palliative chemotherapy.

Metastatic NSCLC is subdivided into disease that is confined to the chest (M1a)—malignant pleural/pericardial effusion or separate tumor nodule(s) in the contralateral lung—which has a better prognosis compared to patients with disseminated disease in liver, bone, brain, or adrenal gland (M1b/M1c). Of patients with widely disseminated disease, there is a better prognosis in patients with a single site of metastasis in a single organ (M1b) compared to multiple metastases (M1c).

Solitary Pulmonary Nodule

A *solitary pulmonary nodule* (SPN) is a single, rounded lesion in the lung that is 3 cm in diameter or smaller. Although these lesions are commonly lung cancers in certain patient populations, the differential diagnosis of SPN includes many other malignant and benign processes. In addition to primary lung cancer (adenocarcinoma; see E-Fig. 57.5), other possible causes include bronchial carcinoid tumors and metastases from extrapulmonary malignancies (e.g., malignant melanoma, sarcoma, colon, kidney, breast, and testicular cancers). Benign etiologies include benign tumors of the lung (hamartomas) (E-Fig. 57.13), infectious granulomas (from fungal diseases, including histoplasmosis and coccidioidomycosis, and mycobacterial disease), lung abscess, vascular abnormalities (arteriovenous malformation), rounded atelectasis (E-Fig. 57.14), and pseudotumor (pleural fluid trapped within a fissure).

Radiographic features of an SPN can be helpful diagnostically. Larger lesions are more likely to be malignant. Lesions 4 to 7 mm in diameter in patients without a history of cancer have a 0.9% chance of being malignant; this probability rises to 18% for lesions 8 mm to 2 cm in diameter and 50% for those larger than 2 cm. Benign tumors are more likely to have smooth, discrete borders, whereas malignant tumors often have irregular or spiculated borders. Central, popcorn, diffuse and laminated (onion-skin) calcification patterns are associated with benign tumors. Conversely, lesions with eccentric (asymmetrical) or stippled calcifications are more likely to be malignant (E-Fig. 57.15). It is important to assess the rate of progression of an SPN or its stability by comparing imaging studies with previous scans whenever available. An SPN that has not changed in size for more than 2 years is unlikely to be malignant, with the exception of ground-glass nodules that might represent slowly growing adenocarcinoma in situ.

TABLE 57.3 TNM Staging System for Lung Cancer (2018)

T (Primary Tumor)

TX	Primary tumor cannot be assessed
	Or tumor proven by the presence of malignant cells in sputum or bronchial washings but not visualized by imaging or bronchoscopy
T0	No evidence of primary tumor
Tis	Carcinoma in situ
T1	Tumor ≤3 cm in greatest dimension, surrounded by lung or visceral pleura, without bronchoscopic evidence of invasion more proximal than the lobar bronchus (i.e., not in the main bronchus)
T1a	Tumor ≤1 cm in greatest dimension
T1b	Tumor >1 cm but ≤2 cm in greatest dimension
T1c	Tumor >2 cm but ≤3 cm in greatest dimension
T2	Tumor >3 cm but ≤5 cm or tumor with any of the following features (T2 tumors with these features are classified T2a if ≤4 cm):

- Involves main bronchus
- Locally invades visceral pleura
- Locally invades the diaphragm
- Associated with obstructive atelectasis (either partial or whole lung)

T2a	Tumor >3 cm but ≤4 cm in greatest dimension
T2b	Tumor >4 cm but ≤5 cm in greatest dimension
T3	Tumor >5 cm or tumor with local invasion to any of the following structures:

- Chest wall (including superior sulcus tumors)
- Phrenic nerve
- Parietal pericardium

OR

If tumor is associated with a satellite nodule in the same lobe

T4	Tumor of any size that invades any of the following:

- Mediastinum
- Heart or great vessels
- Trachea
- Recurrent laryngeal nerve
- Esophagus
- Vertebrae
- Carina

OR

If tumor is associated with an ipsilateral satellite nodule in a different lobe

N (Regional Lymph Nodes)

NX	Regional lymph nodes cannot be assessed
N0	No regional lymph node metastases
N1	Metastasis in ipsilateral peribronchial and/or ipsilateral hilar lymph nodes and intrapulmonary nodes, including involvement by direct extension
N2	Metastasis in ipsilateral mediastinal and/or subcarinal lymph node(s)
N3	Metastasis in contralateral mediastinal, contralateral hilar, ipsilateral or contralateral scalene, or supraclavicular lymph node(s)

M (Distant Metastasis)

MX	Distant metastasis cannot be assessed
M0	No distant metastasis
M1	Distant metastasis
M1a	Separate tumor nodule(s) in a contralateral lobe; tumor with pleural nodules or malignant pleural (or pericardial) effusion
M1b	Single extrathoracic metastasis or involvement of single distant lymph node
M1c	Multiple extrathoracic metastases

TABLE 57.4 Staging Using TNM Score (AJCC 8th Edition)

	N0	N1	N2	N3
T1a	Early (Stage I-II)		Locally Advanced (Stage IIIa)	
T1b				
T1c				
T2a				
T2b				
T3			Locally Advanced (Stage IIIb)	
T4				
M1a/b/c	Metastatic (Stage IV)			

TREATMENT

Small Cell Lung Cancer

SCLCs can occasionally be resected if no evidence of metastasis is found, but most SCLCs are treated with chemotherapy for systemic disease. Limited-stage SCLC is treated with combination chemoradiation with curative intent. Extensive-stage SCLC is treated with chemotherapy alone with palliative intent. Carboplatin plus etoposide has the lowest rate of side effects and best survival, making it the chemotherapy of choice for extensive-stage disease. Recent phase 3 data demonstrate an improvement in overall survival with the addition of the immune checkpoint inhibitor (ICPI), atezolizumab, to first-line carboplatin plus etoposide. Previously treated patients can benefit from re-treatment with carboplatin plus etoposide if they achieve at least 6 months of disease control with initial therapy. Second-line therapies include topotecan or alternative immune checkpoint inhibitors (nivolumab or pembrolizumab) for patients who did not receive first-line atezolizumab. Durable responses to both chemotherapy and radiation therapy and long-term survival are possible. However, relapse with progressive therapeutic resistance is usual despite initial treatment response. Prophylactic cranial irradiation (PCI) improves overall survival in limited-stage disease after completion of chemoradiation. PCI is also favored for patients with extensive-stage disease following good response to primary chemotherapy, but recent evidence allows for active surveillance as a reasonable alternative.

Non–Small Cell Lung Cancer
Early-Stage Disease (Stages I and II)

Surgery is potentially curative for early-stage NSCLC and is indicated for patients with stage I or II disease who are eligible as operative candidates. Anatomic resection (lobectomy or pneumonectomy) is favored to remove the primary tumor as well as its draining lymph nodes (N1 disease). Lesser resections (wedge resections or segmentectomies) are favored to spare lung for clinically N0 peripheral tumors that are 2 cm or smaller, radiographically noninvasive cancers (ground glass), in patients with limited pulmonary function, or for multiple primary lung cancers. Stereotactic body radiation therapy (SBRT) or needle-directed thermal ablation may be used to cure stage I NSCLCs that are not amenable to surgery due to medical comorbidities. Once spread to lymph nodes is suspected, patients unable to tolerate anatomic resection are best treated as locally advanced.

Locally Advanced Disease (Stages IIIA and IIIB)

Stage III NSCLC is a heterogeneous disease and the optimal treatment strategy is unclear. For stage IIIA/N2 disease, "tri-modality" therapy with neoadjuvant chemotherapy or chemoradiation followed by surgery may be offered. Most patients with stage III NSCLC are not surgical candidates and are treated with chemoradiation followed by immune checkpoint blockade.

Advanced Metastatic Disease (Stage IV)

Molecular testing of diagnostic biopsy material is essential for optimal palliative drug selection for patients with stage IV NSCLC. Tumors that do not have any targetable mutations ("wild-type" patients) should be treated with immune checkpoint inhibitor therapy, either alone or in combination with chemotherapy. Prospective, randomized (phase 3) trials have shown that gene-targeted therapy is superior to chemotherapy for stage IV NSCLC with *EGFR* activating-sensitizing mutations or *ALK* gene rearrangement. In addition, single-arm (phase 2) studies have shown durable responses to targeted therapy for patients with *BRAF V600E*, rare *EGFR*, *HER2* mutations, or *ROS-1*, *RET*, *MET* or *NTRK* gene rearrangements with outcomes superior to chemotherapy (E-Fig. 57.16).

These targeted drugs provide durable disease control but do not cure patients. Acquired drug resistance inevitably leads to disease progression and death. A repeat biopsy can be used to determine the molecular mechanism of acquired resistance to targeted therapy, which can be used to inform subsequent drug selection. Patterns of resistance have been used to refine first-line drug selection. For example, the predominant mechanism of gefitinib/erlotinib/afatinib resistance is the emergence of the *EGFR T790M* mutation (located on exon 20), which accounts for about half of all resistant cases. Patients who have progression of disease despite gefitinib/erlotinib/afatinib therapy are routinely tested for *T790M* mutation, and, if present, are candidates for osimertinib therapy. First-line osimertinib proved to be superior to gefitinib/erlotinib in a randomized phase 3 trial.

Acquired genetic changes may occur in "off target" genes, shifting oncogenic signal to so-called "bypass tracts." These include druggable targets such as *BRAF*, or *HER2* mutations, *RET* rearrangements, and *MET* amplification. Adenocarcinomas may undergo histologic transformation to squamous histology or SCLC. Patterns of primary sensitivity and acquired resistance may guide multiple lines of therapy in patients with *EGFR*, *ALK*, and *ROS-1* genetic changes, keeping their management pathway distinct compared to wild-type patients.

In wild-type patients, the decision whether or not to use chemotherapy is based on measurement of programmed death-ligand 1 (PD-L1) expression. PD-L1 expressed on cancer cells or nearby immune cells binds with the PD-1 receptor on T cells and blocks anticancer immunity. Patients with PD-L1 expression on more than 50% of cancer cells are candidates for single-agent pembrolizumab, an ICPI that is a monoclonal IgG antibody against PD-L1. In a phase 3 trial, pembrolizumab was associated with improved survival and fewer adverse events than chemotherapy in patients with metastatic NSCLC without *EGFR* or *ALK* mutations and high PD-L1 expression.

Cytotoxic chemotherapy plus pembrolizumab is used for wild-type patients with low PD-L1 expression. Cytotoxic drugs include platinum (carboplatin or cisplatin), which cause DNA double-strand breaks, combined with drugs that block DNA synthesis (pemetrexed, gemcitabine) or cellular mitosis (paclitaxel, docetaxel, *nab*-paclitaxel, vinorelbine). Cytotoxic chemotherapy lowers the neutrophil count, which can lead to septicemia. ICPIs cause autoimmune side effects, most commonly dermatitis, colitis, or thyroiditis, but also vital organ inflammation (pneumonitis, hepatitis, nephritis), which requires stopping the ICPI and consideration of corticosteroids. Targeted drug therapy is not without difficult or dangerous side effects, including skin rash, diarrhea, gastrointestinal side effects, and rarely cardiac or lung toxicity.

PROGNOSIS

The most important prognostic factor in lung cancer is the TNM stage of the disease at the time of initial diagnosis. Poor performance status and weight loss are negative prognostic factors for survival of patients with lung cancer.

For a deeper discussion on this topic, please see Chapter 182, "Lung Cancer and Other Pulmonary Neoplasms," in *Goldman-Cecil Medicine*, 26th Edition.

SUGGESTED READINGS

Gandhi L, Rodriguez-Abreau D, Gadgeel S, et al: Pembrolizumab plus chemotherapy in metastatic non-small-cell lung cancer, N Engl J Med 378(22):2078–2092, 2018.

Hirsch FR, Jänne PA, Eberhardt WE, et al: Epidermal growth factor receptor inhibition in lung cancer: status 2012, J Thorac Oncol 8:373–384, 2013.

Imielinski M, Berger AH, Hammerman PS, et al: Mapping the hallmarks of lung adenocarcinoma with massively parallel sequencing, Cell 150:1107–1120, 2012.

National Lung Screening Trial Research Team, Aberle DR, Adams AM, et al: Reduced lung-cancer mortality with low-dose computed tomographic screening, N Engl J Med 365:395–409, 2011.

Reck M, Rodriguez-Abreu D, Robinson AG, et al: Pembrolizumab versus chemotherapy for PD-L1-positive non-small-cell lung cancer, N Engl J Med 375(19):1823–1833, 2016.

Rosell R, Bivona TG, Karachaliou N: Genetics and biomarkers in personalization of lung cancer treatment, Lancet 382:720–731, 2013.

Sequist LV, Waltman BA, Dias-Santagata D, et al: Genotypic and histological evolution of lung cancers acquiring resistance to EGFR inhibitors, Sci Transl Med 3(75):75ra26, 2011.

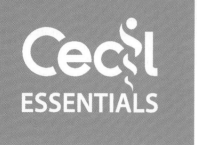

Gastrointestinal Cancers

Khaldoun Almhanna

INTRODUCTION

Gastrointestinal (GI) cancers are among the most common cancers worldwide. In the United States, approximately 300,000 new cases of GI cancer were expected in 2018 with an estimated 150,000 deaths. Gastrointestinal cancers are typically epithelial malignancies—carcinomas—with well-defined pathologic patterns of neoplastic transformation. The incidence of GI malignancies is increasing. Screening and early detection have been established for colon cancer and hepatocellular cancer. Asian populations should be screened for gastric and esophageal cancer. Risk factors, presentations, and management of GI malignancies are site specific. Management usually involves advanced diagnostic procedures and multidisciplinary treatment including advanced endoscopy, chemotherapy, radiation, and surgical intervention. Complications of advanced disease including bowel and biliary obstruction, liver failure, bleeding, and impaired nutrition play a significant role in the prognosis and mortality of these diseases. Recent advances in immunotherapy and checkpoint inhibitors, although promising, have not yet significantly improved the overall outcome of these diseases.

ESOPHAGEAL CANCER

Epidemiology

The incidence rates of esophageal cancer vary by geographic region with the highest incidence in Asia and Eastern Africa and the lowest in Western countries. The incidence of squamous cell carcinoma in the United States is decreasing while the incidence of adenocarcinoma, mostly in the gastroesophageal junction, is increasing in part due to obesity, reflux disease, and Barrett esophagus.

Pathology

Squamous cell carcinoma (SCC) is commonly seen in the upper esophagus and is associated with smoking, alcohol use, and dietary intake. Consuming hot beverages in certain areas is thought to be responsible for a higher incidence of SCC (e.g., China, Iran). On the other hand, most adenocarcinomas arise in background of Barrett esophagus. Interestingly, only 50% of patients with Barrett esophagus report a history of chronic reflux. The risk of developing esophageal cancer is increased at least 30-fold in patients with Barrett esophagus and is higher in the presence of high-grade dysplasia.

Clinical Presentation

Progressive dysphagia and weight loss are the most common presenting symptoms in patients with esophageal cancer. Chronic blood loss leading to iron deficiency anemia is not an uncommon presentation as well. History of longstanding reflux disease is not as common as expected. Early stage tumors are usually asymptomatic and are diagnosed as part of GI bleeding work-up or Barrett esophagus follow-up.

Diagnosis and Staging

Upper endoscopy remains the preferred diagnostic test for esophageal cancer. The diagnosis of cancer will require a histologic examination of the primary tumor or, in case of advanced disease, of metastatic lesions. Endoscopic ultrasound (EUS) provides detailed images of the depth of invasion into the esophagus wall (T stage) and peri-esophageal lymphadenopathy (N stage). EUS also visualizes the left lobe of the liver and can identify metastatic lesions (M stage). Bronchoscopy is recommended in patients with tumors located at or above the carina. Contrast-enhanced computed tomography (CT) and 18-fluorodeoxy-glucose positron emission tomography (FDG-PET) scans are helpful in detecting occult metastatic disease.

Treatment

Early stage esophageal cancer with negative lymph nodes (T1a: invasion into the mucosa) can be treated with endoscopic mucosal resection. T1b tumors (tumor invades the submucosa) should be treated with upfront surgery. For locally advanced disease, multimodality therapy is recommended. Neoadjuvant concurrent chemotherapy and radiation followed by surgical resection is the standard of care, at least in the United States. Definitive chemotherapy and radiation is an acceptable alternative for patients who are not surgical candidates. The combination of carboplatin and paclitaxel with radiation is currently the most commonly used neoadjuvant (chemotherapy administered before surgery) or definitive therapy. Esophagectomy can be performed with a transthoracic (Ivor-Lewis) or a transhiatal technique, with comparable clinical outcomes.

Advanced (stage IV) esophageal cancer is a highly lethal disease with poor outcome. The goals of treatment are to improve survival and quality of life. Several chemotherapeutic agents have shown benefits in patients with advanced esophageal cancer as a single agent or in combination including 5-fluorouracil (5-FU), platinum agents, irinotecan, and taxanes.

Two targeted agents, trastuzumab, a monoclonal antibody directed against human epidermal growth factor receptor 2 (HER2), and ramucirumab, a monoclonal antibody against vascular endothelial growth factor receptor 2 (VEGFR 2), have shown activity in metastatic esophageal cancer when combined with chemotherapy. Trastuzumab is indicated in patients who overexpress Her-2 neu. The recently developed PD-1/PDL-1 antibodies are showing some promising activity in this setting for patients with metastatic disease who progressed on first-line therapy. Ongoing studies are currently evaluating these agents alone and in combination with chemotherapy and radiation. Supportive care and localized therapy to the primary tumor might be indicated to help with pain, obstruction, bleeding, and other localized symptoms. Nutritional support in this patient population is always challenging and might require parenteral administration of nutrients.

589

GASTRIC CANCER

Epidemiology

Gastric adenocarcinoma is one of the most common malignancies worldwide. The disease has shown a remarkable decline in incidence and mortality worldwide secondary in part to refrigeration and the decreased use of food preservatives as well as the recognition of *Helicobacter pylori* infection as a risk factor. However, this disease remains common in Asian countries (China, Japan, and Korea), in the Middle East, and in Eastern Europe, placing it among the five most common cancers worldwide.

Pathology

There are two main histologic subtypes of gastric adenocarcinoma: diffuse and intestinal. The diffuse type (undifferentiated) is increasing in incidence and is associated with younger age, signet ring cells, early metastasis, and worse prognosis. The intestinal type (differentiated) is seen in older patients, is differentiated with a background of intestinal metaplasia, and has a declining incidence and a somewhat better prognosis. The main carcinogenic event in diffuse carcinomas is loss of expression of E-cadherin, the protein responsible for intercellular connections and the organization of epithelial tissues.

Clinical Presentation

Weight loss, nausea, and epigastric abdominal pain are the most common symptoms of gastric cancer at initial diagnosis. Early satiety (with the linitis plastica subtype), dysphagia (gastroesophageal junction or cardia tumors), and gastrointestinal bleeding are also commonly seen. Symptoms of distant metastatic disease might be seen at diagnosis. The most common metastatic sites are the liver, peritoneal surfaces (causing ascites), distant lymph nodes, and less commonly, the ovaries (Krukenberg tumor) and lungs.

Diagnosis

Upper gastrointestinal endoscopy is the standard diagnostic test to obtain tissue and localize the tumor. Endoscopic ultrasound will help with the TNM staging in combination with CT scans of the chest, abdomen, and pelvis. The role of PET scans is still evolving. The diagnosis of the linitis plastica subtype can be challenging because overt mucosal lesions are often not evident. Radiologic and endoscopic features can guide the diagnosis as well as deep biopsies. Staging laparoscopy can upstage 20% to 30% of patients with gastric cancer with otherwise negative work-up and will spare the patient unnecessary laparotomy. Screening endoscopy is recommended in high-incidence countries as well as high-risk patients.

Treatment

Surgery remains the cornerstone of treatment for nonmetastatic disease. The most controversial areas in the surgical management of gastric cancer are whether to perform total gastrectomy for tumors in the upper third of the stomach versus partial gastrectomy for tumors in the lower two thirds. Also controversial is the extent of lymph node dissection. Extended D2 dissection to remove the stomach, all surrounding lymph nodes, and the spleen is superior and recommended compared to D1 dissection (refers to a limited dissection of only the perigastric lymph nodes), but it is associated with excess morbidity and mortality and should be performed by an experienced surgeon. For locally advanced disease, in addition to surgery, either perioperative chemotherapy with a platinum-based regimen or postoperative chemoradiation with 5-FU is an acceptable approach. For metastatic disease, first- and second-line palliative chemotherapy can improve outcomes, including survival. Similar to esophageal cancer (mentioned previously), trastuzumab and ramucirumab have shown activities in metastatic disease when combined with chemotherapy. The role of immune checkpoint inhibitors in gastric cancer is still evolving as with esophageal cancer.

Prognosis

Clinical outcomes depend on the stage at diagnosis. Five-year survival rates are 65%, 40%, 15%, and 5% for stages I, II, III, and IV, respectively. Survival outcomes in Japan and Korea are better than in most Western countries; this disparity may be attributable to routine screening endoscopies or to differences in disease biology.

PANCREATIC CANCER

Epidemiology

Pancreatic cancer is the eighth leading cause of cancer deaths worldwide and is more common in the Western part of the world (see also Chapter 39). Smoking, obesity and chronic pancreatitis are established clinical risk factors. Pancreatic cancer risk increases with inherited mutations in *BRCA1*, *BRCA2*, and *PALB2* and with familial syndromes. Intraductal papillary mucinous neoplasms of the pancreas (IPMN) are at risk for malignant degeneration and are commonly managed with surveillance.

Pathology

Pancreatic ductal adenocarcinoma is the main histologic type of pancreatic cancer (85% of cases). Adenocarcinoma develops with an accumulation of mutations in the pancreatic duct epithelium. Histologic progression occurs in various stages of pancreatic intraepithelial neoplasia, leading to invasive adenocarcinoma with desmoplastic reaction. Neuroendocrine neoplasms of the pancreas are composed of epithelial neoplastic cells with phenotypic neuroendocrine differentiation. Pancreatic neuroendocrine tumors are uncommon malignancies that originate from the endocrine cells in the pancreas. They may be nonfunctional, or they may secrete hormones such as insulin (insulinoma), gastrin (gastrinoma), glucagon (glucagonoma), or vasoactive intestinal peptide (VIPoma).

Clinical Presentation

Pain, jaundice, and weight loss are the most common presenting symptoms in patients with pancreatic ductal adenocarcinoma. New-onset type 2 diabetes mellitus in an adult older than 50 years of age without overt obesity-related risk factors should raise suspicion for pancreatic cancer. Venous thromboembolism is commonly associated with pancreatic cancer and can rarely be a presenting feature. Pancreatic neuroendocrine tumors are usually diagnosed incidentally or can cause symptoms related to excess hormone production including hypoglycemia (insulinoma), Zollinger-Ellison syndrome (gastrinoma), hyperglycemia (glucagonoma), and diarrhea with electrolyte disturbances (VIPoma).

Diagnosis

Imaging of the abdomen using ultrasound can be utilized as an initial screening test if pancreatic cancer is suspected. CT or magnetic resonance imaging (MRI) can further identify the lesions and their relation to the surrounding vessels as well as metastatic disease. Endoscopic ultrasound and endoscopic retrograde cholangiopancreatography help visualize the lesions better, relieve any obstruction by stent placement, and obtain histologic confirmation by biopsies with fine-needle aspirations or bile duct brushings. Somatostatin-receptor scintigraphy can be helpful in localizing occult neuroendocrine tumors.

Treatment

Pancreatic adenocarcinomas are some of the most difficult cancers to treat. Their anatomic locations make them poor candidates for resection. Only 15% to 20% of patients are candidates for surgical resection at the time of diagnosis because the tumor frequently involves the celiac arterial axis and superior mesenteric artery and vein and even the portal vein. Whipple procedure (pancreatoduodenectomy) and distal pancreatectomy are the standard surgeries; however, the 5-year overall survival rate after pancreatic adenocarcinoma resection is less than 20%.

The role of adjuvant therapy following resection is not well established. Recent studies with multiagent regimens such as a combination of 5-FU, irinotecan, and oxaliplatin (FOLFIRINOX) or combined gemcitabine and nab-paclitaxel have demonstrated improved overall survival for metastatic pancreatic cancer and following resection as well. Observation only or somatostatin analogues are both acceptable first-line treatment for unresectable pancreatic neuroendocrine tumors. Recent studies in neuroendocrine tumors have also shown improvement in outcomes with targeted agents such as everolimus and sunitinib. Palliation of symptoms is a large component of care. Early referral to palliative care should be considered, especially in symptomatic patients with adenocarcinoma. Referrals to nutrition consultants, opioids, celiac nerve plexus block, biliary drainage, as well palliative surgeries can help improve patients' quality of life.

Prognosis

Pancreatic adenocarcinoma carries a very poor prognosis; the 5-year overall survival rate remains less than 10%. Survival has not improved significantly over the last few decades, in contrast to several other cancers. Neuroendocrine tumor carries a better prognosis, depending on the stage and the grade of the tumor, with survival measured in years.

CHOLANGIOCARCINOMA (BILE DUCT CANCERS)

Epidemiology

Cholangiocarcinomas (bile duct cancers) arise from the intrahepatic and extrahepatic biliary epithelium of the bile ducts. Cancer of the gallbladder or the ampulla of Vater are sometimes included with cholangiocarcinomas but have different risk factors and clinical behavior. Although uncommon in the United States, the incidence of cholangiocarcinomas has been on the rise for unclear reasons. Established risk factors include sclerosing cholangitis, cholelithiasis, cholecystitis, chronic liver disease, toxin exposure, metabolic syndrome, and infections. Gallbladder cancer is particularly prevalent in South American countries—especially Chile—as well as southeastern Asian countries.

Pathology

The majority of cholangiocarcinomas are adenocarcinoma. Immunohistochemistry staining might appear similar to other malignancies, in particular pancreatic cancer and upper gastrointestinal malignancies. Imaging and clinical correlation might aid in the differential diagnosis.

Clinical Presentation

Painless jaundice, pruritus, dark urine, and light color stool are usually the presenting symptoms of extrahepatic cholangiocarcinoma and are caused by biliary obstruction. Intrahepatic cholangiocarcinoma usually presents with vague right upper quadrant pain or is found incidentally on imaging. Gallbladder cancer can sometimes be an incidental finding during histologic evaluation after cholecystectomy, which is commonly performed for presumed cholelithiasis or cholecystitis.

Diagnosis

Transabdominal ultrasonography can be used to confirm biliary dilation, but to confirm the diagnosis of cholangiocarcinoma, computed tomography scanning or magnetic resonance imaging with magnetic resonance cholangiopancreatography MRCP should be performed. In some patients, an endoscopic retrograde cholangiopancreatography (ERCP) is used as the first test because it allows direct visualization of the suspected area, helps obtain a tissue diagnosis, and allows for therapeutic intervention to alleviate the obstruction. Endoscopic ultrasound can aid in identifying tumor location and extension as well.

Treatment

A negative margin surgical resection is the only curative treatment for intrahepatic and extrahepatic cholangiocarcinoma. Distal cholangiocarcinomas have the highest rate of complete resection (R0), compared to proximal and intrahepatic cholangiocarcinoma. Adjuvant chemotherapy (with or without radiation), following curative resection, is recommended in general, and based upon meta-analysis. Gemcitabine, platinum and 5-fluouracil based treatments are usually recommended in the adjuvant setting.

Surgical resection with lymph node dissection is the standard treatment for gallbladder cancer and ampullary cancer as well. The role of adjuvant therapy is less clear in this setting. Gallbladder cancer is treated in a similar fashion to cholangiocarcinoma, while recommendations following ampullary cancer resection are less clear. Many clinicians recommend surveillance-only, given the more favorable prognosis of ampullary cancer as compared with other biliary tract cancers and the lack of data supporting a survival advantage with further therapy. However, some oncologists tend to treat these patients as they would resected pancreatic cancer, even for those with the intestinal histology. Enrollment in clinical trials in always preferred.

Treatment with gemcitabine and cisplatin is the standard treatment for stage IV cholangiocarcinoma and gallbladder cancer. Stage IV ampullary carcinoma is treated like pancreatic cancer. Tumor profiling and the role of targeted therapy is evolving. The overall prognosis is still poor for all of these stage IV malignancies, with median overall survival less than 12 months.

Prognosis

Even following curative resection, cholangiocarcinoma still carries a poor prognosis. Five-year overall survival rate ranges from 30% in patients with negative lymph nodes to 2% in patients with metastatic disease. Enrollment in clinical trials is always recommended. Several new agents and pathways are being evaluated in this patient population.

HEPATOCELLULAR CARCINOMA

Epidemiology

Hepatocellular carcinoma (HCC), or primary liver cancer, is a common disease around the world. It is the second most common cause of cancer-related death in men worldwide.

Pathology

Most HCCs arise in the setting of underlying cirrhosis, with alcohol use, hepatitis B, and hepatitis C being the most common causes of cirrhosis. Other diseases causing cirrhosis such as hemochromatosis, primary biliary cirrhosis, and α_1-antitrypsin deficiency are also contributory. Cirrhosis involves chronic hepatocyte injury and ensuing cell regeneration, which provides the substrate for cancer development: inflammatory cytokine stress, constant cell cycling, and aberrant cell development and differentiation.

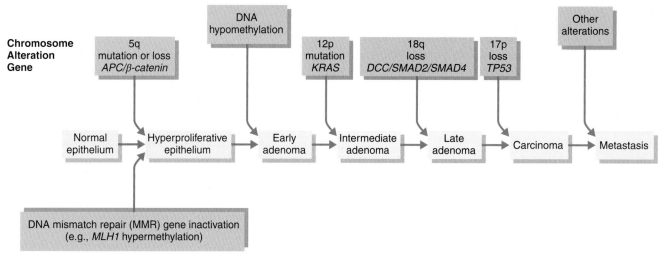

Fig. 58.1 Model of colorectal carcinogenesis. Several genes are involved in the stepwise progression from normal colonic epithelium to adenocarcinoma.

Clinical Presentation

HCC is frequently masked by the underlying liver disease. Abdominal distention from ascites, fatigue, muscle wasting, anorexia, and encephalopathy are features of cirrhosis. Acute hepatic decompensation or right upper quadrant pain may herald the development of HCC. HCC can also be an incidental finding during routine surveillance by screening ultrasound for patients with cirrhosis.

Diagnosis

HCC is one of those rare malignancies for which a diagnosis can be made without histologic confirmation. Nonhistologic criteria for diagnosis include underlying cirrhosis, elevated α-fetoprotein level (>400 ng/mL), and a characteristic appearance on contrast-enhanced CT or MRI (arterial enhancement and rapid washout). In the absence of underlying cirrhosis, however, a tissue diagnosis must be obtained. For patients with cirrhosis, a surveillance program incorporating regular measurements of α-fetoprotein and ultrasound imaging can detect early lesions.

Treatment

For small lesions, surgical resection can be curative. Preoperative assessment of liver function to ensure that the patient is an appropriate candidate for partial liver resection is critical. Liver transplantation is an option that will address HCC as well as the underlying cirrhosis. Strict criteria, such as the Milan criteria (i.e., single tumor ≤5 cm, or up to three tumors each <3 cm, and no vascular invasion), are used to determine which patients are eligible for transplantation. For those who are ineligible for surgical approaches, radiofrequency ablation, transarterial chemoembolization, yttrium-90 embolization, and percutaneous ethanol injection can provide local control. Until recently, Sorafenib, a multikinase inhibitor, was the only proven treatment for metastatic HCC. In the last 2 years, two other kinase inhibitors, lenvatinib and cabozantinib, have been approved for the treatment of HCC. Immune check point inhibitors including pembrolizumab and nivolumab are both approved for the second line treatment of HCC after failure of tyrosine kinase inhibitors.

Prognosis

The prognosis in HCC is often determined by the severity of the underlying liver disease. The 5-year survival rate approaches 50% with complete surgical resection or liver transplantation. For advanced HCC, the median overall survival time with therapy is approximately 1 year.

COLORECTAL CANCER

Epidemiology

Colorectal cancer is the third most common cancer as well as the third most common cause of cancer-related death in the United States, with approximately 150,000 new cases diagnosed each year. Worldwide, it is a growing problem and one of the most common cancers. There appears to be an increased association between colon cancer and high dietary fat, red meat consumption, low dietary fiber, obesity, and alcohol use. Conversely, increased physical activity and use of supplemental estrogen, folate, vitamin, aspirin, and nonsteroidal anti-inflammatory drugs appear to be protective. A history of inflammatory bowel disease is a risk factor for colorectal cancer.

Pathology

Adenocarcinoma of the colon progresses from normal epithelium to frank cancer in a stepwise fashion, as illustrated in Fig. 58.1. Most colon cancers arise in polyps. Hamartomatous polyps usually are non-neoplastic but can be part of juvenile polyposis or Peutz-Jeghers polyposis where they can undergo malignant transformation. Serrated polyps 10 mm or greater with dysplasia should be managed as high-risk adenoma. Adenomatous polyps are the most common neoplastic polyps in the colon and can progress to cancer.

Several inherited abnormalities lead to a genetic predisposition to colon cancer. Such syndromes are responsible for 3% to 5% of all colon cancers. They can be divided into syndromes associated with underlying polyps and those without polyps. Classic familial adenomatous polyposis (FAP) is caused by an autosomal dominant mutation in the APC gene. The colon is full of polyps—hundreds to thousands—that start forming during adolescence, leading to development of cancer in early adulthood. Patients with attenuated FAP have fewer polyps and later development of malignancy. MYH-associated polyposis is caused by an autosomal recessive mutation in the *MYH* gene, and the phenotype mimics that of attenuated FAP. Peutz-Jeghers syndrome, juvenile polyposis, and Cowden syndrome are other uncommon conditions that are associated with an inherited predisposition to colorectal polyps leading to cancer.

The classic nonpolyposis syndrome is hereditary nonpolyposis colorectal cancer, also called Lynch syndrome. Germline recessive mutations in genes involved in the mismatch repair pathway *(MSH2, MSH3, MSH6, MLH1, MLH3, PMS1, PMS2)* lead to adenocarcinoma. These cases are indistinguishable from sporadic cases associated with defective mismatch repair, except for the family history of colon and other associated cancers in the inherited syndrome (e.g., endometrial, ovarian, gastric, and small bowel cancer).

Clinical Presentation

Hematochezia and altered bowel habits are the classic symptoms of colon cancer. Early cases are essentially asymptomatic and are typically identified by screening. Advanced cases can manifest with bowel obstruction or perforation, frank rectal bleeding, weight loss, abdominal pain, and ascites due to hepatic or peritoneal metastases. Cancers associated with the mismatch repair pathway have certain typical features: They are right-sided, more common in women, and occur in younger patients. They are usually poorly differentiated and locally advanced without significant lymph node involvement.

Diagnosis

Screening for colorectal cancer is an important public health tool. Screening methods include fecal occult blood testing, imaging (barium enema, CT-guided colonography), and endoscopy (flexible sigmoidoscopy, colonoscopy). Colonoscopy is the "gold standard" for visual confirmation and histologic diagnosis of colon cancer. Once a cancer diagnosis is established, CT scans of the chest, abdomen, and pelvis are indicated to evaluate for distant disease. MRI of the pelvis or endoscopic ultrasound are used in rectal cancer to determine the exact tumor location and its extent prior to neoadjuvant therapy.

Treatment

For patients with resectable disease, surgical resection is the treatment of choice. Removal of the involved segment of the colon, along with the associated mesentery containing all draining lymph nodes, is recommended. Such procedures are being increasingly performed with the use of laparoscopic techniques, resulting in decreased perioperative morbidity. Decisions regarding chemotherapy after surgery (i.e., adjuvant chemotherapy) are based on the pathologic findings. For stage I disease (T1 or T2, N0), no chemotherapy is recommended. For stage III disease (any T, N+), chemotherapy is strongly recommended. A combination of a fluoropyrimidine (5-FU, capecitabine) with oxaliplatin, administered for 6 months, is the standard of care. For stage II disease (T3 or T4, N0), data are controversial. A careful risk-benefit evaluation for each patient is recommended to determine whether adjuvant chemotherapy is appropriate. Rectal cancer is associated with a high rate of local recurrence that can lead to significant morbidity. To improve outcomes, preoperative chemotherapy and radiation therapy are used, and surgery should include total mesorectal excision.

For metastatic colorectal cancer, treatment options include chemotherapy agents such as fluoropyrimidines, oxaliplatin, and irinotecan. The advent of targeted therapies has improved clinical outcomes. These therapies include anti-angiogenic agents (bevacizumab, ziv-aflibercept, ramucirumab), anti–epidermal growth factor receptor antibodies (cetuximab, panitumumab). The multikinase inhibitors (regorafenib) and trifluridine-tipiracil (Lonsurf) are both approved for patients who progress after first- and second-line chemotherapy but efficacy is only modest. Another option for patients with metastatic colorectal cancer who have MSI-H/dMMR tumors is immunotherapy. The immune checkpoint inhibitor nivolumab, both as a single agent or in combination with ipilimumab, are approved by the FDA for patients who progressed after standard of therapy. Colon cancer is one of the few malignancies in which some cases of metastatic disease can also be cured with aggressive systemic therapy and surgery. Therefore, close surveillance after treatment of the initial cancer is recommended to detect early recurrences. Surveillance should include regular physical evaluation, CT scanning, and measurement of serum levels of carcinoembryonic antigen (CEA), a protein synthesized disproportionately by malignant epithelial cells. Increased physical activity and dietary modifications (reduced red meat and fat; increased fruits, vegetables, and fiber) following treatment have been associated with improved outcomes. Another important component of colorectal cancer care is family risk assessment, because this is a common disease, with up to 7500 cases each year in the United States being attributable to heritable syndromes. Referral for genetic counseling should be made if such a syndrome is suspected.

Prognosis

Among gastrointestinal cancers, colorectal cancer has the best overall prognosis. For nonmetastatic disease, the 5-year survival rate ranges from 50% to 95%, depending on the extent of lymph node involvement. For metastatic disease, newer therapies, given in succession, can achieve a median overall survival time of more than 2 years. The key remains early detection by screening, which can improve outcomes.

ANAL CANCER

Epidemiology

Anal cancer is an uncommon malignancy, with about 7000 cases reported annually in the United States. It is strongly associated with human papillomavirus (HPV) infection. It is also more common in patients with human immunodeficiency virus (HIV) infection and in those who engage in anal-receptive sexual intercourse, most likely because of poor host immunity and increased transmission of HPV, respectively. Condyloma acuminata are precursor lesions for this cancer.

Pathology

The histology is typical of a squamous cell carcinoma, with sheets of hyperproliferative keratinized cells. HPV, especially types 16 and 18, causes inactivation of the tumor suppressor genes *TP53* and *RB1* via the viral proteins E6 and E7, predisposing to eventual development of carcinoma. Chronic local inflammation due to inflammatory bowel disease or recurrent anal fissures and fistulas can also lead to anal cancer.

Clinical Presentation

Local symptoms, such as perianal pruritus or pain, bleeding, discharge, and a masslike sensation, are common presentations. In cases of chronic underlying disease such as Crohn's disease, the presence of a nonhealing anal or perianal lesion despite good disease control elsewhere should raise suspicion for malignancy.

Diagnosis

Physical examination is adequate to identify suspicious lesions. A biopsy should be obtained to confirm the diagnosis. Evaluation for distant spread should include CT scans of the chest, abdomen, and pelvis. Special attention should be paid to examination of inguinal lymph nodes, because they are common sites of early spread.

Treatment

Anal cancer is one of the few solid tumor malignancies that are curable without surgical resection. For very small, early lesions, complete excision may suffice. However, for most cases, combined chemotherapy with 5-FU and mitomycin, together with radiation therapy, is the standard curative modality. This regimen has significant short-term toxicities that should be managed aggressively. This treatment can obviate the need for a large operation that would result in a permanent colostomy.

Prognosis

More than 70% of cases can be cured with chemoradiation. Relapsed disease is usually treated with surgical excision (if local) or systemic chemotherapy (if distant). Widespread vaccination against HPV, anal Pap smears in high-risk populations, and better prevention and treatment of HIV infection should lower the incidence of anal cancer.

SUGGESTED READINGS

Bang YJ, Van Cutsem E, Feyereislova A, et al: Trastuzumab in combination with chemotherapy versus chemotherapy alone for treatment of HER2-positive advanced gastric or gastro-oesophageal junction cancer (ToGA): a phase 3, open-label, randomised controlled trial, Lancet 376:687–697, 2010.

Conroy T, Desseigne F, Ychou M, et al: FOLFIRINOX versus gemcitabine for metastatic pancreatic cancer, N Engl J Med 364:1817–1825, 2011.

Grothey A, Van Cutsem E, Sobrero A, et al: Regorafenib monotherapy for previously treated metastatic colorectal cancer (CORRECT): an international, multicentre, randomised, placebo-controlled, phase 3 trial, Lancet 381:303–312, 2013.

Hvid-Jensen F, Pedersen L, Drewes AM, et al: Incidence of adenocarcinoma among patients with Barrett's esophagus, N Engl J Med 365:1375–1383, 2011.

Valle J, Wasan H, Palmer DH, et al: Cisplatin plus gemcitabine versus gemcitabine for biliary tract cancer, N Engl J Med 362:1273–1281, 2010.

van Hagen P, Hulshof MC, van Lanschot JJ, et al: Preoperative chemoradiotherapy for esophageal or junctional cancer, N Engl J Med 366:2074–2084, 2012.

Von Hoff DD, Ervin T, Arena FP, Chiorean EG, et al: Increased survival in pancreatic cancer with nab-paclitaxel plus gemcitabine, N Engl J Med 369(18):1691–1703, 2013.

Yao JC, Shah MH, Ito T, et al: Everolimus for advanced pancreatic neuroendocrine tumors, N Engl J Med 364:514–523, 2011.

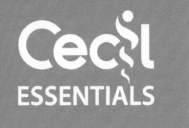

59

Genitourinary Cancers

Andre De Souza, Benedito A. Carneiro, Anthony Mega, Timothy Gilligan

RENAL CELL CARCINOMA

Definition and Epidemiology

Renal cell carcinoma (RCC) represents approximately 3% to 5% of all malignancies and 85% of kidney tumors. It is the sixth most common cancer in men and the eighth most common cancer in women, with approximately 74,000 new cases diagnosed in the United States in 2019 that will contribute to 14,770 deaths. Aside from age and male sex, most patients do not have an identifiable risk factor. The median age of diagnosis is about 65 years and the incidence is twice as high in men as in women. Smoking, obesity, and hypertension are well-established risk factors for RCC. Smokers have a relative risk 2-fold greater than that of nonsmokers whereas hypertension is associated with a 70% increased risk. RCC is also more common in patients with end-stage renal failure. A small number (3%) of cases of RCC are inherited. Approximately 65% of cases of RCC are diagnosed as localized disease with an estimated 5-year survival of 92%. The 5-year survival for advanced disease is 12%.

The most recognized inherited RCC is Von Hippel–Lindau (VHL) syndrome, an autosomal dominant disorder that is characterized by the development of multiple vascular tumors including clear cell RCC. The genetic events underlying VHL syndrome (loss of function truncating mutations or deletions of the *VHL* gene) also occur in sporadic (noninherited) clear cell tumors, leading to the remarkable RCC reliance on blood vessels for growth. Research into this syndrome has led to modified treatment options for advanced disease (see later discussion).

Pathology

The histologic subtypes of RCC are characterized by distinct genetic characteristics, histologic features, and clinical phenotypes. Clear cell RCC (75% of all RCCs) is the most common subtype and is characterized by *VHL* gene inactivation. Less common are the papillary, chromophobe, unclassified subtypes, and medullary RCC, which occurs almost exclusively in patients with sickle cell trait. Although these RCC subtypes are biologically distinct, the current surgical approaches are most frequently uninfluenced by subtype. However, the histologic subtype impacts the medical treatment of advanced disease.

Diagnosis and Differential Diagnosis

Masses in the kidney may be benign or malignant, with an increasing likelihood of malignancy with increasing size. Most clear cell RCC tumors are distinguishable based on their contrast enhancement. Other considerations for renal masses include benign tumors (e.g., oncocytoma), metastatic disease from another primary site (rare), angiomyolipoma, a lipid-containing benign tumor (most commonly occurring in young females), and infectious processes. The diagnosis is made on the basis of a biopsy or at the time of nephrectomy, although the radiographic appearance of each of the differential diagnoses is often characteristic.

Clinical Presentation

RCC is more common in males (2:1), and the median age at presentation is approximately 65 years. Patients diagnosed with RCC below 46 years of age and those presenting with multifocal or bilateral renal masses should be considered for genetic counseling because these features can be associated with hereditary RCC. In the United States, most RCCs are diagnosed as incidental findings on imaging studies (70% of the cases). Classic signs and symptoms include hematuria, flank pain, and a palpable abdominal mass. Systemic symptoms can include pain caused by bone metastases or adenopathy, respiratory symptoms related to involvement of lung parenchyma, or neurologic symptoms when presenting with brain metastases. Symptoms also occur with paraneoplastic syndromes. A renal mass is discovered, usually on computed tomography (CT) scanning, and has an appearance that is characteristic of RCC (i.e., highly vascular). Subsequently, a full staging work-up is performed, including CT scanning of the chest; CT or MRI of the brain is performed if signs or symptoms suggest brain metastases; bone scan is recommended in the presence of bone pain or elevation of alkaline phosphatase. Diagnosis is usually made at the time of nephrectomy, although a biopsy of the renal mass may be indicated, such as in a patient with distant metastases in whom nephrectomy is not pursued or in a patient with a small renal mass that may be initially observed.

Treatment
Renal Masses

Some renal masses (approximately 20%) are not cancerous, and the likelihood of malignancy increases with size, so a diagnostic biopsy should be considered for lesions smaller than 4 cm to confirm diagnosis and guide local treatment or surveillance strategies. If the mass has a radiographic appearance suggestive of RCC, biopsy is often not necessary before surgery, and larger masses are more likely to have such features. The differential diagnosis for enhancing renal masses includes non-RCC malignancies (e.g., upper tract urothelial carcinoma), metastases, and benign tumors. One option for small renal masses, even if proven to be RCC, is initial observation. Retrospective series have defined this approach for renal masses smaller than 4 cm in a select group of patients with significant comorbidities or limited life expectancy. The growth rate is approximately 3 mm/year, and the reported incidence of development of metastases is very low. If surgery is pursued, then removal of either part of the kidney (partial nephrectomy or nephron-sparing surgery) or the entire kidney (radical nephrectomy) is the standard of care, depending on factors such as the extent and anatomy of the tumor, native renal function, and surgical skill. Cancer outcomes are equivalent, although renal

TABLE 59.1   Therapeutic Approaches in Metastatic RCC

Agent	Objective Response Rate	PFS (mo)	Comments
Hormonal therapy	2%	N/A	Limited, palliative role in the treatment of metastatic RCC
Chemotherapy	5-6%	N/A	Not generally used
Interleukin-2	≈20-25% (high dose)	3.1	Durable complete response rate of 7-8%
Interferon-α	10-15%	4.7	Modest improvement in overall survival compared with inactive therapy
VEGF inhibitors[a]	≈30%	9-11	Common toxicity includes fatigue, mucositis, hand-foot syndrome, diarrhea, hypertension, and hypothyroidism
Checkpoint inhibitors[b]	25-42%	4.6-11	Adverse effects include fatigue, pruritus and immune-related hypothyroidism, colitis, adrenal insufficiency. Complete response rates of 9% were observed with the combination of nivolumab (anti-PD-1) and ipilimumab (anti-CTLA4).
mTOR inhibitors[c]	2% (treatment refractory) to 9% (treatment naive)	4	Increased overall survival of temsirolimus monotherapy vs. IFN monotherapy in poor-risk patients Toxicity includes fatigue, mucositis, rash, and hypertriglyceridemia/hyperglycemia/hypercholesterolemia
mTOR inhibitor (everolimus) + lenvatinib	41%	14.6	Combination of everolimus with lenvatinib improved the outcomes compared to everolimus monotherapy

IFN, Interferon; mTOR, mammalian target of rapamycin; N/A, not applicable; PFS, progression-free survival; RCC, renal cell carcinoma; VEGF, vascular endothelial growth factor.

[a]VEGF inhibitors: sorafenib, sunitinib, pazopanib, axitinib.

[b]Anti-PD-1 agents such as pembrolizumab and avelumab have also been combined with axitinib.

[c]mTOR inhibitors: temsirolimus, everolimus.

function is better preserved with partial nephrectomy. Another management option for renal masses is exposure to temperature extremes: freezing (cryotherapy) or burning (radiofrequency ablation). This approach is usually pursued in patients with contraindications to surgery, significant comorbidities, and/or small tumors (<3 cm). Although metastasis-free survival and cancer-specific survival rates for partial nephrectomy and ablation techniques are comparable, local recurrence rates can be higher with ablation. Biopsy of kidney mass is recommended prior to ablation to confirm diagnosis and guide subsequent surveillance strategies.

Surgery in Metastatic RCC

Removal of the primary renal tumor in the face of metastatic disease (i.e., debulking or cytoreductive nephrectomy) has been pursued in patients with good performance status, limited extrarenal disease, and low comorbidities based on results from patients receiving systemic treatment with interferon-α (INF-α) in the 1990s. However, results of a randomized clinical trial showed that systemic treatment alone with contemporary tyrosine kinase inhibitor (TKI) sunitinib had comparable overall survival to nephrectomy followed by sunitinib in patients with intermediate- or poor-risk disease, but the study did not address cytoreductive nephrectomy in patients with good-risk disease. In addition, surgical removal of solitary metastatic sites is associated with disease control in up to 30% of highly selected patients.

One randomized clinical trial demonstrated that 1 year of treatment with sunitinib administered following nephrectomy (i.e., adjuvant treatment) improved the disease-free survival of patients at high risk for recurrence, but no difference in overall survival or quality of life was reported. Patient selection and shared decision making are critical in light of treatment toxicities, lack of demonstrated overall survival benefit, and negative results of other clinical trials. To date, no clinical trial evidence has demonstrated improvement in patient outcome with systemic therapy administered before nephrectomy (i.e., neoadjuvant treatment).

Systemic Therapy for Metastatic RCC

The initial treatments for metastatic RCC—hormone therapy and chemotherapy—produced only minimal benefits (Table 59.1). Immunotherapy with cytokines interleukin-2 (IL-2) and INF-α has yielded modest benefits, the majority of benefit realized in highly selected patients who have a durable complete response to high-dose IL-2. The discovery of clear cell RCC reliance on stimulation of the vascular endothelial growth factor (VEGF) pathway, which results from VHL gene inactivation, led to the clinical development of several VEGF pathway inhibitors that include TKIs and monoclonal antibodies against VEGF (see Table 59.1). In general, 70% to 75% of patients who receive these drugs have some reduction or stabilization of tumor burden. Periods of disease control typically last for months, although they can extend to several years in a small minority of patients. The incorporation of immune checkpoint inhibitors, such as antibodies against cytotoxic T lymphocyte–associated protein 4 (CTLA-4) and programmed death receptor-1 (PD-1) or its ligand (PD-L1), represents another relevant advancement in the treatment of metastatic RCC. These agents promote antitumor immune response by blocking stimulation of PD-1 or CTLA-4 receptors that suppress T cell immune function. These agents have significant antitumor activity both as anti-PD-1 monotherapy (e.g., nivolumab) or in combination with ipilimumab (anti-CTLA4). Anti-PD-1 and PD-L1 antibodies (pembrolizumab and avelumab, respectively) have also shown strong antitumor activity in combination with the multikinase inhibitor axitinib. Inhibitors of mammalian target of rapamycin (mTOR) represent treatment alternatives as monotherapy or in combination with the multikinase inhibitor lenvatinib. The data supporting the use of TKIs and checkpoint inhibitors for RCC are strongest for clear cell RCC; the optimal treatment of non–clear cell RCC is much less well defined. In the context of growing treatment options, advances in biomarkers of treatment response as well as molecular drivers of prognosis will guide optimal sequencing of agents.

Prognosis

The prognosis of localized kidney cancer is determined largely by the stage and grade of the primary tumor. In metastatic disease, established schemas divide patients into prognostic groups based on performance status, time from diagnosis to metastatic disease, and laboratory values (lactate dehydrogenase [LDH], hemoglobin, calcium, neutrophils, and platelets). Good-, intermediate- and poor-risk groups have median survivals of about 43, 22, and 8 months, respectively.

BLADDER CANCER

Definition and Epidemiology

Urothelial carcinoma of the bladder (UCB) represents 4% of all malignancies and about 3% of cancer-related deaths in the United States. It is more common in developed countries and is the fourth most common cancer among men and ninth among women in the Western world. Smoking is an established risk factor for bladder cancer; the incidence rate is four times higher for smokers than for nonsmokers. Occupational exposures from a range of agents that contain aromatic amines, as chlorinated hydrocarbons and polycyclic aromatic hydrocarbons are believed to account for up to 20% of all bladder cancers. Genetic susceptibility is increasingly recognized as an important risk factor. The risk of bladder cancer is doubled in first-degree relatives of patients with bladder cancer. Inherited genetic factors, such as the slow acetylator N-acetyltransferase 2 (NAT2) variants and the glutathione S-transferase Mu 1 (GSTM1)–null genotypes, are established risk factors.

Pathology

Urothelial carcinoma is the predominant histologic subtype in the United States and Europe, where it accounts for 90% of all bladder cancers. Adenocarcinoma, squamous cell carcinoma, and small cell cancers account for most of the remaining 10%, although there are parts of the world where nonurothelial carcinomas are more common. The bladder wall consists of four layers: urothelium (the innermost epithelial lining), lamina propria, muscularis propria (detrusor muscle), and adventitia (serosa).

Clinical Presentation

UCB is more common in males (3:1), and the median age at presentation is 73 years. Approximately 75% of newly diagnosed cases of UCB are not muscle invasive; the remaining 25% exhibit de novo invasion of the muscle wall of the bladder at presentation.

Patients with bladder cancer typically have painless hematuria at presentation, although irritative voiding symptoms (frequency, urgency, and dysuria) can be the initial manifestation. Patients with more advanced disease may have progressive flank or pelvic pain from direct extension of disease or as a consequence of ureteral obstruction.

Diagnosis and Differential Diagnosis

The initial evaluation typically involves an office-based cystoscopic evaluation, with the collection of urine for cytology. Upper urinary tract evaluation with either a CT urogram or retrograde pyelogram is also important. When a bladder tumor is found, patients undergo a transurethral resection of bladder tumor (TURBT) under anesthesia to obtain tissue for histologic diagnosis. Inclusion of muscle in the pathologic specimen is necessary to exclude muscle invasion. For patients with muscle-invasive disease, CT imaging of the chest is indicated, and bone scintigraphy in patients with bone pain. Most new cases of UCB are staged as Ta (involvement of epithelial lining), T1 (invasion of lamina propria), or carcinoma in situ (CIS) (Fig. 59.1); these are

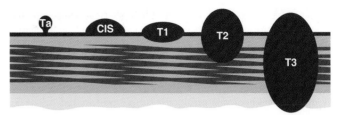

Fig. 59.1 Bladder cancer presentations by depth of invasion.

typically grouped and considered as non–muscle-invasive bladder cancer (NMIBC).

Patients with low-grade, low-stage urothelial carcinoma of the bladder remain at high risk for non–muscle-invasive recurrence but low risk for progression to more advanced stage disease. In contrast, patients with intermediate- or high-grade disease are at increased risk for both recurrence and progression to muscle-invasive and metastatic disease. Secondary involvement of the bladder with other cancers (e.g., lymphoma, sarcoma) is uncommon.

Treatment

Organ-Confined Disease

Low-grade non–muscle-invasive UCBs are typically managed with TURBT and intravesically administered cytotoxic agents. Multifocal, low-grade recurrent disease is managed with intravesically administered bacillus Calmette-Guérin (BCG). High-grade NMIBC (including CIS) is managed with BCG or cystectomy.

Muscle-invasive bladder cancer is optimally managed with radical cystectomy and bilateral pelvic lymphadenectomy. For patients who are deemed poor surgical candidates or who refuse cystectomy, external beam radiotherapy or chemoradiation and TURBT are alternative management options.

Cisplatin-based multiagent chemotherapy administered before cystectomy (i.e., neoadjuvant chemotherapy) has been shown by level I evidence to improve survival. Although it has not been prospectively evaluated in the neoadjuvant setting, the regimen of gemcitabine plus cisplatin (GC) is widely substituted for the older combination of methotrexate, vinblastine, doxorubicin, and cisplatin (M-VAC). Ongoing clinical trials are evaluating the role of perioperative immunotherapy.

Metastatic Disease

Level I evidence from a series of phase III trials provides evidence that cisplatin-based chemotherapy (i.e., M-VAC or GC) in patients with de novo metastatic disease leads to median survival times in the range of 14 to 15 months, with 5% to 15% of patients likely to be cured. The latter group is made up primarily of patients with nodal metastatic disease.

Although there have been no completed randomized phase III trials comparing cisplatin-based chemotherapy with carboplatin-based therapy in patients with advanced UCB, multiple randomized phase II trials have reported superior activity with cisplatin-based regimens. However, between 30% and 50% of patients with advanced UCB are ineligible for cisplatin because of concomitant renal insufficiency, typically as a consequence of age-related renal comorbidity or disease-related extrinsic obstruction. Immunotherapy with checkpoint inhibitors, such as pembrolizumab (anti-PD-1) and atezolizumab (anti-PD-L1), is approved for cisplatin-ineligible patients whose tumors have high expression of PD-L1 (the specific PD-L1 expression cutoff is specific to the immune checkpoint inhibitor used) as well as for patients who have already received or who are ineligible for carboplatin.

The management of advanced disease after front-line therapy has evolved with various options beyond single-agent chemotherapy. Novel treatments include PD1 and PD-L1 checkpoint inhibitors and the TKI erdafitinib targeting of fibroblast growth factor receptor 3 (FGFR3) in tumors displaying FGFR3 activating mutations or gene fusions. The best sequencing of agents beyond the front-line treatment remains to be defined. Antibodies targeting cell surface protein and delivering cytotoxic payloads (antibody drug conjugates), such as the Nectin-4 antibody enfortumab that delivers the cytotoxic drug vedotin and the trophoblast cell surface 2 antibody sacituzumab with its topoisomerase inhibitor SN-38 payload, have shown promising antitumor activity in advanced bladder cancer, and ongoing trials are comparing these drugs to standard of care treatments. Enfortumab vedotin was granted accelerated approval in the United States for patients previously treated with or ineligible for platinum-based chemotherapy and an immune checkpoint inhibitor.

Prognosis

Patients with low-grade, low-stage NMIBC typically do not progress to muscle-invasive disease. Their disease does not alter life expectancy but is associated with morbidity and use of health care resources and requires long-term follow-up. Patients with muscle-invasive disease who undergo cystectomy are at risk for systemic failure based on the T stage and extent of nodal involvement. Patients with organ-confined disease without nodal involvement have cure rates greater than 50%. Patients with metastatic disease have median survival times in the range of 14 to 16 months with systemic therapy, and only a small subset (5% to 15%) are long-term survivors, although immune checkpoint blockers and new targeted therapies may change these metrics in the near future.

PROSTATE CANCER

Definition, Epidemiology, and Screening

Prostate cancer is the most common malignancy among men in the United States; more than 174,000 cases were expected to be diagnosed in 2019 with 31,000 deaths. The lifetime risk of diagnosis and death is roughly 12% and 2.4%, respectively. The incidence has declined since the United States Preventative Service Task Force (USPSTF) recommended against prostate-specific antigen (PSA)-based screening in 2012 (D recommendation). In 2018, the USPSTF revised the recommendation to shared decision making with men age 55 to 69 years (C Recommendation). Evidence from randomized clinical trials reveals that PSA-based screening programs in men aged 55 to 69 years may prevent 1.3 prostate cancer deaths and three cases of metastatic prostate cancer per 1000 men screened. The USPSTF recommends against PSA-based screening in men 70 years and older (D recommendation).

Multiple risk factors, including age, race, dietary factors, and genetic factors, have been linked to prostate cancer. The median age at diagnosis is 65 years, and younger men (<40 years) rarely develop prostate cancer. African American men have a greater risk of developing prostate cancer compared with white men (16% vs. 11% lifetime risk of diagnosis). Although it is possible that screening may offer greater benefit for African American men, there is no conclusive evidence to support race-based screening recommendations. A man with first-degree relatives affected by prostate cancer has a 5-fold to 10-fold increased risk of prostate cancer. Whereas high animal fat intake has been linked to an increased risk of prostate cancer, no foods, vitamins or dietary supplements have been shown to reduce the likelihood of being diagnosed with the disease.

A large chemoprevention trial (SELECT) demonstrated that intake of selenium and vitamin E does not reduce the risk of prostate cancer. Two studies evaluating the 5α-reductase inhibitors finasteride and dutasteride demonstrated a 23% to 25% reduction in relative risk of prostate cancer. Despite these benefits, the use of these agents remains low. Adverse effects such as erectile dysfunction, loss of libido, and gynecomastia along with concern of a small increase in high-grade tumors have resulted in low acceptance and adoption.

Clinical Presentation

Because prostate cancer can be detected in small subsets even with very low PSA levels (i.e., <1 ng/mL) there is no "normal" PSA value below which there is no risk of prostate cancer. PSA values can be affected by rectal examination, ejaculation, infection, bicycle riding, and urinary obstruction.

Most men with early disease have no symptoms; however, urinary frequency, urgency, nocturia, and hesitancy do occur. The presence of hematuria or hematospermia should prompt consideration of prostate cancer. An abnormal rectal examination result (asymmetric mass/nodule) is also suggestive of cancer.

Men with advanced, metastatic prostate cancer are more frequently symptomatic. Given the proclivity for bone metastasis, skeletal pain is common. Because of the frequency of spine metastases, malignant spinal cord compression and resulting neurologic injury is part of the natural history of prostate cancer. Adenopathy in the abdomen and pelvis is also common, as are deep venous thromboses, and men may thus present with lower extremity edema. Men can also experience urinary obstruction with hydronephrosis due to ureteral obstruction or bladder outlet obstruction. Constitutional symptoms such as weight loss and night sweats have also been described, especially with visceral metastasis.

Diagnosis and Staging

Most patients with prostate cancer are diagnosed with local disease with the use of extended core biopsies (12 cores). Multiparametric magnetic resonance imaging (MRI) is increasingly being utilized in initial assessment of a man with an abnormal PSA. MRI is interpreted using the Prostate Imaging-Reporting and Data System (PI-RADS), a 1-5 scale, with higher numbers indicating a greater likelihood of clinically significant cancer (Gleason score 7-10). In patients with MRI PI-RADS 3 to 5, biopsies can be done with MRI guidance to improve diagnostic accuracy.

After diagnosis, risk stratification based on PSA level, Gleason score, and clinical stage becomes crucial to define management. Bone scans and CT scans are not indicated for men with a new diagnosis of prostate cancer unless they have certain intermediate-risk or high-risk features. In addition to stage, grade, and PSA level, important features determining treatment include age, comorbidities, patient preferences, and life expectancy.

Pathology, Prognosis, and Genetic Mutations

Adenocarcinoma accounts for more than 95% of all prostate cancers. The remaining histologic subtypes include neuroendocrine (small cell carcinoma), squamous, and basal cell neoplasms.

The Gleason scoring system is pivotal in the management of prostate cancer, but its interpretation requires expertise in pathology. The score is based on growth pattern and degree of differentiation and ranges from 3 to 5 (5 being the least differentiated). The composite Gleason score is derived by adding together the numerical values for the two most prevalent differentiation patterns. For instance, if a specimen comprises primarily a grade 3 pattern and secondarily a grade 4 pattern, the score is reported as 7 (3 + 4). In 2016 the World

TABLE 59.2	**WHO/ISUP Prostate Cancer Histologic Grading System**
Grade Group 1	Gleason 3 + 3 = 6
Grade Group 2	Gleason 3 + 4 = 7
Grade Group 3	Gleason 4 + 3 = 7
Grade Group 4	Gleason 4 + 4 = 8, 3 + 5 = 8, 5 + 3 = 8
Grade Group 5	Gleason 4 + 5 = 9, 5 + 4 = 9, 5 + 5 = 10

Health Organization (WHO) defined a new prostate grading system to improve prognostic strata. The WHO histologic grading system includes five grade groups as defined in Table 59.2.

Prognosis and primary management of localized prostate cancer depends on tumor (T) stage, PSA level, tumor grade, and number of positive biopsies. Risk stratification includes very low, low, favorable intermediate, unfavorable intermediate, high, and very high risk prostate cancer.

Genes in the DNA repair pathway, such as *BRCA1/2*, *ATM*, and *CHEK2*, have been found to be pathologically mutated in approximately 20% of metastatic castrate-resistant prostate cancer (mCRPC) and 8% to 12% of localized prostate cancer. *BRCA2* mutations have been associated with more aggressive prostate cancers with higher recurrence and mortality. Recommendations for genetic counseling in men with prostate cancer include presenting with de novo metastatic prostate cancer, significant family history of prostate, breast, pancreatic cancer, and Gleason 8 to 10 disease, and Ashkenazi Jewish heritage.

Treatment

Available treatment options for localized prostate cancer include radical prostatectomy, radiation therapy (either external beam radiation or brachytherapy), and active surveillance. Consensus recommendation favors active surveillance over primary treatment for very-low-risk and low-risk prostate cancer (Gleason score 6, PSA <10 ng/mL, low tumor burden). The selection between radical prostatectomy and radiation therapy is based on risk stratification and patient preferences. Surgery carries risks of urinary incontinence and erectile dysfunction. Radiation therapy has lower rates of urinary incontinence but also causes erectile dysfunction. Late complications from radiation therapy include radiation cystitis and proctitis. There is a small increased risk of second malignancies after radiation therapy, especially bladder cancer in smokers. Primary radiation therapy for intermediate- and high-risk patients is often given in combination with androgen deprivation therapy leading to additional adverse effects.

Once patients have developed advanced disease, androgen deprivation therapy (chemical or surgical castration) is widely used. Intermittent androgen deprivation therapy is an effective alternative for patients whose only sign of recurrence is a rising PSA level. In men with metastatic disease, continuous therapy with luteinizing hormone releasing hormone (LHRH) agonist or antagonist is used. Androgen deprivation therapy also has major side effects, including night sweats, hot flashes, erectile dysfunction, weight gain, loss of muscle mass, fatigue, bone loss, and metabolic syndrome. In men with metastatic prostate cancer, randomized controlled trials have reported longer overall survival when androgen deprivation therapy was combined with any of the four following medications: abiraterone (a novel CYP17A1 inhibitor), docetaxel chemotherapy, or the androgen receptor antagonists enzalutamide and apalutamide.

Bone health is a significant problem in men with prostate cancer. Osteoporosis due to androgen deprivation therapy and skeletal-related events from metastases are both common. Two agents are available to prevent these complications: zoledronic acid, a bisphosphonate, and denosumab, a RANK-ligand inhibitor. Their benefit is primarily in men with mCRPC and skeletal metastasis. All men on ADT should be counseled on osteoporosis screening and prevention and lower-dose bisphosphonate or denosumab can be used if significant bone loss develops.

All patients with metastatic prostate cancer eventually develop castrate-resistant prostate cancer (CRPC), defined by serologic, clinical, or objective progression in the setting of a castrate testosterone level. Although the mechanism of CRPC is not well understood, several treatment options are now available. Sipuleucel-T, an autologous antigen-presenting cell product shown to prolong survival in a randomized trial, is sometimes used in the prechemotherapy setting, but its use has been limited by the fact that it is not associated with a reduction in PSA, and there is thus no way to measure whether it is controlling the cancer. If not used in the castrate-sensitive setting, either abiraterone or one of the new androgen receptor antagonists (enzalutamide, apalutamide, or darolutamide) can be prescribed. Radium 223 improves survival outcomes and reduces skeletal events in men with symptomatic skeletal metastasis and without visceral or bulky, soft tissue metastasis. Two chemotherapy agents, docetaxel and cabazitaxel, are therapeutic options. Finally, the poly ADP-ribose polymerase (PARP) inhibitors are beneficial in men with mCRPC and a documented DNA repair defect.

TESTICULAR CANCER

Definition and Epidemiology

It is estimated that 9,610 new cases of testicular cancer will be diagnosed in men in the United States in 2020 and 440 men are predicted to die from the disease. It accounts for 1% of all cancers in men. The incidence of testis cancer varies widely among racial groups and geographic regions. In the United States, it is the most common cancer diagnosed in men aged 20 to 40 years of age, but it is rarely diagnosed before age 15 or after age 55. It is four times more common in white than in Black individuals. The incidence has increased by more than 50% since 1975. Risk factors include cryptorchidism, a personal or family history of testis cancer, gonadal dysgenesis, and Klinefelter's syndrome. Cryptorchidism increases risk in the undescended testicle and the normally descended contralateral testicle. Orchiopexy for cryptorchidism before puberty reduces the risk of testis cancer.

Pathology

Approximately 98% of testis cancers are germ cell tumors; the others are lymphomas, sex-cord stromal tumors, and adenocarcinomas of the rete testis. Germ cell tumors are divided into two broad categories: seminomas and nonseminomas (i.e., nonseminomatous germ cell tumors, or NSGCTs). Seminomas by definition are 100% seminoma, whereas most NSGCTs are a mixture of two or more of the five types of germ cell tumors: seminoma, embryonal carcinoma, teratoma, yolk sac tumor, and choriocarcinoma. A tumor that contains any elements of embryonal carcinoma, teratoma, yolk sac tumor, or choriocarcinoma is considered to be an NSGCT even if most of the tumor is seminoma. Because seminomas do not produce α-fetoprotein (AFP), patients who have a significantly elevated AFP level have an NSGCT regardless of the histopathology.

Diagnosis and Differential Diagnosis

Whenever a testis tumor is suspected, transscrotal ultrasound should be performed; if a mass suspicious for cancer is seen, the standard diagnostic procedure is an inguinal orchiectomy. Transscrotal orchiectomy or biopsy is contraindicated because of the risk of seeding the tumor in the scrotum and altering the pattern of spread. Differential diagnosis includes testicular lymphoma, torsion, epididymitis, orchitis, and other benign scrotal lesions.

Clinical Presentation

Testis cancer most often manifests as testicular enlargement, mass, or induration. It may or may not be painful or tender, and the presence of pain does not exclude a diagnosis of cancer. Testicular atrophy, gynecomastia, back pain, and thromboembolic disease can also occur.

Staging the cancer requires measuring postorchiectomy levels of serum AFP, human chorionic gonadotropin (β-HCG), and LDH as well as assessing for nodal and organ metastases, which should be done with a CT scan of the abdomen and pelvis and either chest CT or a chest radiography. The testes drain to the retroperitoneal lymph nodes, and retroperitoneal nodal spread constitutes stage II disease. In practice, testis cancer is divided into three categories: stage I (localized), with no evidence of spread to lymph nodes or beyond; stage II (regional), with enlarged retroperitoneal lymph nodes but no distant metastases; and disseminated disease. Disseminated disease includes stage I or II disease in which serum AFP and/or β-HCG levels are persistently elevated after orchiectomy, bulky stage II disease, and all stage III disease. Metastases to other organs or to pelvic or other non-retroperitoneal lymph nodes represent stage III disease, as does spread to retroperitoneal nodes in the setting of highly elevated serum tumor markers. Disseminated disease is divided into three categories: good-risk, intermediate-risk, and poor-risk disease; treatment differs for the different risk groups.

Treatment

Stage I seminomas and NSGCTs are usually managed with surveillance after surgery. The risk of relapse is about 18% for seminomas and 30% for NSGCTs. For pure seminomas, larger tumor size and lymphovascular invasion are each associated with a higher risk of recurrence. For nonseminomas, lymphovascular invasion has been most strongly associated with risk of relapse and tumors that are pure or predominantly embryonal carcinoma are also at higher risk. Alternatives to surveillance are single-agent carboplatin chemotherapy or radiation therapy for seminomas and bleomycin and etoposide and cisplatin (BEP) chemotherapy or retroperitoneal lymph node dissection (RPLND) for NSGCTs. Long-term disease-specific survival for stage I disease is 99% regardless of which of these approaches is used.

Stage II seminomas are usually treated with radiation therapy or chemotherapy (with BEP or etoposide plus cisplatin [EP]). Chemotherapy is preferred when the disease bulk is greater than 5 cm and sometimes for less bulky tumors. Management of stage II NSGCTs depends on the disease bulk and the levels of serum AFP and β-HCG. If either marker is elevated, then chemotherapy is preferred regardless of disease bulk. If no nodes are bigger than 2 cm and there are fewer than six enlarged nodes, then RPLND or chemotherapy can be considered. For bulkier disease, chemotherapy is preferred.

Treatment of stage III disease depends on the sites of metastases and the levels of serum tumor markers. For good-risk disease, the treatment is three cycles of BEP or four cycles of EP chemotherapy. For intermediate- and poor-risk disease, the treatment is four cycles of BEP chemotherapy (or etoposide, ifosfamide, and cisplatin [VIP] chemotherapy). In NSGCT, all residual masses should be resected after chemotherapy if feasible. In cases of seminoma, residual masses are typically observed unless they grow. Sometimes, post-chemotherapy residual masses greater than 3 cm in patients with pure seminoma are evaluated with an FDG-PET/CT, but the value of that approach is limited by the incidence of false-positive results. Patients with pure seminomas and residual masses after chemotherapy are the only testis cancer patients who should be considered for PET scans.

Relapsed disease after chemotherapy is treated with salvage chemotherapy given either at standard doses or at high doses with hematopoietic stem cell support.

Prognosis

Overall, the long-term disease-specific survival rate for testis cancer is 96%. By stage, the survival rates are 99% for stage I, 96% for stage II, and 73% for stage III. By disseminated disease risk category, survival is about 90% for good-risk disease, about 80% for intermediate-risk disease, and about 50% for poor-risk disease.

SUGGESTED READINGS

Burger M, Oosterlinck W, Konety B, et al: ICUD-EAU international consultation on bladder cancer 2012: non–muscle-invasive urothelial carcinoma of the bladder, Eur Urol 63:36–44, 2012.

Calabrò F, Albers P, Bokemeyer C, et al: The contemporary role of chemotherapy for advanced testis cancer: a systematic review of the literature, Eur Urol 61:1212–1220, 2012.

Capitanio U, Bensalah K, Bex A, et al: Epidemiology of renal cell carcinoma, Eur Urol 75(1):74–84, 2019.

Choueiri TK, Motzer RJ: Systemic therapy for metastatic renal-cell carcinoma, N Engl J Med 376(4):354–366, 2017.

Cooperberg MR, Carroll PR, Klotz L, et al: Active surveillance for prostate cancer: progress and promise, J Clin Oncol 29:3669–3676, 2011.

Eulitt P, Bjurlin M, Milowsky M: Perioperative systemic therapy for bladder cancer, Curr Opin Urol 29(3):220–226, 2019.

Gakis G, Efstathiou J, Lerner S, et al: ICUD-EAU international consultation on bladder cancer 2012: radical cystectomy and bladder preservation for muscle-invasive urothelial carcinoma of the bladder, Eur Urol 63:45–57, 2013.

Gourdin T: Optimization of therapies for men with advanced prostate cancer, Curr Opin Oncol 31(3):188–193, 2019.

Honecker F, Aparicio J, Berney D, et al: ESMO consensus conference on testicular germ cell cancer: diagnosis, treatment and follow-up, Ann Oncol 29(8):1658–1686, 2018.

Inamura K: Prostate cancer: understanding their molecular pathology and the 2016 WHO Classification, Oncotarget 9(18):14723–14737, 2018.

James N, Hussain S, Hall E, et al: Radiotherapy with or without chemotherapy in muscle-invasive bladder cancer, N Engl J Med 366:1477–1478, 2012.

James ND, Sydes MR, Clarke NW, et al: STAMPEDE investigators addition of docetaxel, zoledronic acid, or both to first-line long-term hormone therapy in prostate cancer (STAMPEDE): survival results from an adaptive, multiarm, multistage, platform randomised controlled trial, Lancet 387:1163–1177, 2016.

Kasivisvanathan V, Ranikko A, Borghi M, et al: MRI-Targeted or standard biopsy for prostate cancer diagnosis, N Engl J Med 378:1767–1777, 2018.

Motzer RJ, Escudier B, McDermott DF, et al: Nivolumab versus everolimus in advanced renal-cell Carcinoma, N Engl J Med 373(19):1803–1813, 2015.

Motzer RJ, Penkov K, Haanen J, et al: Avelumab plus axitinib versus sunitinib for advanced renal-cell carcinoma, N Engl J Med 380(12):1103–1115, 2019.

Motzer RJ, Tannir NM, McDermott DF, et al: Nivolumab plus ipilimumab versus sunitinib in advanced renal-cell carcinoma, N Engl J Med 378(14):1277–1290, 2018.

Nadal R, Bellmunt J: Management of metastatic bladder cancer, Cancer Treat Rev 76:10–21, 2019.

Ravaud A, Motzer RJ, Pandha HS, et al: Adjuvant sunitinib in high-risk renal-cell carcinoma after nephrectomy, N Engl J Med 375(23):2246–2254, 2016.

Rini BI, Plimack ER, Stus V, et al: Pembrolizumab plus axitinib versus sunitinib for advanced renal-cell carcinoma, N Engl J Med 380(12):1116–1127, 2019.

Siegel R, Miller K, Ahmedin J: Cancer statistics 2019, CA Cancer J Clin 69:7–34, 2019.

United States Preventative Service Task Force recommendation Statement. JAMA 319(18): 1901–1913, 2018.

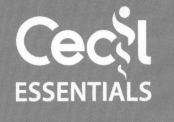

60

Breast Cancer

Mary Anne Fenton, Rochelle Strenger

EPIDEMIOLOGY

Worldwide and in the United States, breast cancer is the number one malignancy in women. In 2019 in the United States approximately 271,270 new cases were diagnosed including 268,600 in females and 2670 in males. Breast cancer is the second leading cause of female cancer deaths in the United States. Projected 2019 breast cancer mortality is estimated to be 42,260 (41,760 female, 500 male breast cancer patients). A woman has a 12.4% lifetime risk of breast cancer, and her risk increases with age (Table 60.1). The mortality risk from breast cancer in the United States declined by 39% between 1989 and 2015 due to early detection and more effective treatment; the current 5-year survival rate is 90%. For most solid tumors 5-year survival is predictive of a cure. Unfortunately, however, for the ER+ breast cancer subtype systemic recurrences continue to occur beyond 20 years.

Not all women share equally in improved breast cancer outcomes. Socioeconomic barriers may limit access to early detection and effective therapies. In addition, there are significant ethnic differences in breast cancer incidence and outcome. While breast cancer is less common in African American women, they are more likely to present at a later stage, have a higher incidence of the more aggressive triple-negative subtype and have a higher breast cancer specific mortality rate. The difference in mortality rate is in part related to tumor biology comorbidities, access and adherence to care.

RISK FACTORS

A women's risk of breast cancer increases with age (see Table 60.1) with a lifetime risk of 12%. To put it another way, 1 in 8 women in the United States will develop breast cancer during the course of their lifetime. Reproductive factors such as early onset of menses, late onset of menopause, first live birth after age 35 or nulliparity correlate with a mild increased risk of breast cancer. A positive personal history of dense breasts, findings on a breast biopsy of atypical ductal hyperplasia (ADH) or lobular carcinoma in situ (LCIS) increase breast cancer risk 4-fold.

The risk of breast cancer is increased when there is family history of breast cancer and other cancers such as ovarian, high-risk pancreatic, and prostate. When there is one family member with breast cancer the risk is increased 2-fold. The presence of a familial breast cancer predisposition to gene mutation BRCA1/2 increases breast cancer risk over 4 fold (Table 60.2).

Breast Cancer Genetics

Approximately 10% of breast cancers are associated with inheritable genetic mutations. The first high-penetrance genes, *BRCA1* and *BRCA2,* were identified by screening families with early-onset breast cancer. Mutations in the tumor suppressor genes *BRCA1/2* are also associated with ovarian cancer and other malignancies. Screening recommendations and guidelines for genetic testing and counseling from organizations such as Medicare and the National Comprehensive Cancer Network (NCCN) Guidelines focus on individuals with first-, second-, and third-generation maternal and paternal family histories of cancer, including age of onset.

NCCN guidelines from 2019 recommend referral for genetic counseling for patients diagnosed with breast cancer below the age of 50, or triple-negative (ER/PR, HER2-negative) disease below the age of 60, two breast primaries in an individual, family member with diagnosis of breast cancer below age of 50, family member with ovarian cancer, patient or relative with male breast cancer, and individuals of Eastern European Jewish ancestry who may be at risk for founder mutations. Unfortunately, many individuals are unaware of their family history of cancer including site of cancer and age of onset (Table 60.3).

The identification of a high-penetrant mutation in a family member without breast cancer will afford them the opportunity to consider preventative and early detection strategies. Prior to 2012, breast cancer genetic testing focused on *BRCA1/2* testing and was performed by the Sanger method of sequencing a single DNA fragment at a time, a sequencing technique known to miss large deletions. Next-generation sequencing (NGS) allows for testing of multiple genes, and the number of "clinically actionable mutations" has increased beyond *BRCA1/2*. Patients with *BRCA1/2* testing with negative results prior to 2012 should be referred for genetic counseling and updated testing. In the metastatic setting, patients with germline *BRCA1/2* (gBRCA1/2) mutations may be candidates for PARP inhibitor therapy (see metastatic breast cancer section).

CLINICAL PRESENTATION AND DIAGNOSIS

In the United States, over 50% of breast cancers are detected on a screening mammogram, and 33% of cases will present with a self-detected or clinically detected breast mass. In the majority of mammogram and ultrasound detected masses, calcifications and clinically palpable lesions are amenable to core needle biopsy in order to establish a diagnosis, determine breast cancer histology, assess tumor grade, and assess ER, PR, and HER2 expression by immunohistochemistry. The presence or absence of estrogen receptor (ER), progesterone receptor (PR), and human epidermal growth factor receptor 2/neu (HER2) are prognostic for survival and predict response to systemic therapies for breast cancer. Patients presenting with a palpable mass should be referred for diagnostic mammogram and ultrasound and biopsy. If imaging and biopsy are not concordant with the patient's presentation and clinical examination the patient should be referred to a breast surgeon.

TABLE 60.1 Age-Specific Probabilities of Developing Invasive Breast Cancer for US Women

Age	10-Year Probability	Or 1 in
20	0.1%	1567
30	0.5%	220
40	1.5%	68
50	2.3%	43
60	3.4%	29
70	3.9%	25
Lifetime	12.4%	8

Note: Probability is among those free of cancer at the beginning of each age interval based on cases diagnosed 2012-2014 American Cancer Society, Inc. Surveillance Report 2017.
From Desantis C, Ma J, Goding Sauer A, et al. Breast Cancer Statistics, 2017, Racial Disparity and Mortality by State, CA Cancer J Clin 67;439-448, 2017.

TABLE 60.2 Risk Factors for Breast Cancer

		Relative Risk
Family history of breast cancer	First-degree relative	2
	More than one first degree relative	3-4
	BRCA1/2 mutation carrier	>4
Age over 65		>4.0
Early menses	age < 12	1.1-2
Nulliparous		1.1-2
First birth	>35 years	1.1-2
Late menopause	>55 years	1.1-2
Never breast fed		1.1-2
Postmenopausal obesity (BMI greater than or equal to 30)		1.1-2
Mammographically dense breasts		4
Proliferative breast lesions	Atypical ductal hyperplasia	4
	Lobular carcinoma in situ	
High-dose radiation to the chest	Hodgkin's lymphoma age 10-30	2.1-4

Data from American Cancer Society. Breast Cancer Facts and Figures 2017-2018 Atlanta, GA; American Cancer Society, 2017.

Traditionally, breast cancer histology and anatomic stage have driven patient stage, prognosis, and decision making for surgery, radiation, and medical oncology care. In current practice, and as delineated in the latest American Joint Commission (AJCC) 8th edition *Staging Manual*, ER, PR, HER2 status, tumor grade, and genomics impact breast cancer prognosis in the prognostic breast cancer stage.

Histology

Breast cancer arises from the epidermal cells of the terminal ductal lobular unit and progresses in a continuum from intraductal hyperplasia, atypia, ductal carcinoma in situ, to invasion through the basement membrane of the duct.

Ductal Carcinoma in Situ

Ductal carcinoma in situ (DCIS) is a clonal disorder of cancer cells contained within the milk duct basement membrane with the potential to

TABLE 60.3 NCCN Guideline on Referral for Genetic Counseling 2019

No history of breast cancer	Personal history of ovarian cancer
	Family history of pancreatic cancer
	Family history of metastatic prostate cancer
	Eastern European Jewish ancestry and personal history of breast cancer or high-grade Gleason 7 or greater prostate cancer in family member
Patient with breast cancer	Age under 50
	Triple-negative breast cancer under the age of 60
	Ovarian cancer
	Two breast primaries
	Male breast cancer
	Pancreatic cancer
	Greater than or equal to two family members with breast cancer
	Family member with ovarian cancer Gleason 7 or greater or metastatic prostate cancer

Data from National Comprehensive Cancer Network Genetic/familial high-risk assessment: breast/ovarian version 3.2019 http://www.nccn.org/professionals/physician_gls/pdf/breast.pdf. Accessed September 25, 2019.

progress to invasive ductal carcinoma (Fig. 60.1). Twenty-five percent of breast cancers diagnosed each year in the United States are classified as DCIS (Tis, Stage 0). Fifteen to fifty percent of DCIS will progress to invasive cancer. Treatment for DCIS is excision to 2-mm negative margins and local breast radiation. Low-grade DCIS less than 2.5 mm considered "low risk" DCIS may be treated with excision alone. The option of "watchful waiting" is being investigated in ongoing studies on molecular features of DCIS. Patients with DCIS are not at risk for systemic spread unless it progresses or recurs as invasive disease.

DCIS treated with mastectomy has a local regional recurrence rate less than 1%. Lumpectomy and radiation recurrence rate is 6% to 16%, of which 50% of recurrences are invasive. There is no difference in survival for mastectomy versus lumpectomy/radiation therapy. For ER-positive DCIS, tamoxifen or anastrozole (reserved for postmenopausal patients) reduces local recurrence by 32% and contralateral breast cancer by 50%.

Lobular Carcinoma in Situ

LCIS is a spectrum of lobular cells with varying potential for invasion. A patient with LCIS and/or atypical ductal hyperplasia has an increased risk of bilateral breast cancer. Patients with DCIS, LCIS, and atypical hyperplasia are candidates for risk reduction with selective estrogen receptor modulators (SERMS) such as tamoxifen and raloxifene or aromatase inhibitors.

Invasive Breast Cancer

Breast cancer is classified histologically by morphology and grade based on nuclear pleomorphism, gland formation, and mitotic index. The most commonly used grading system is Bloom Richardson or Nottingham, with grade 1 less aggressive and grade 3 more aggressive and with higher invasion potential.

Infiltrating ductal carcinoma (IDC) (49% to 75%), is the most common histology, seen as a density on mammography and gross pathology assessment. The clinical behavior of IDC is dependent on grade and ER, PR and HER2 expression. **Invasive lobular carcinoma (ILC)** comprises 5% to 15% of invasive breast cancer, has a slight increased risk of bilateral

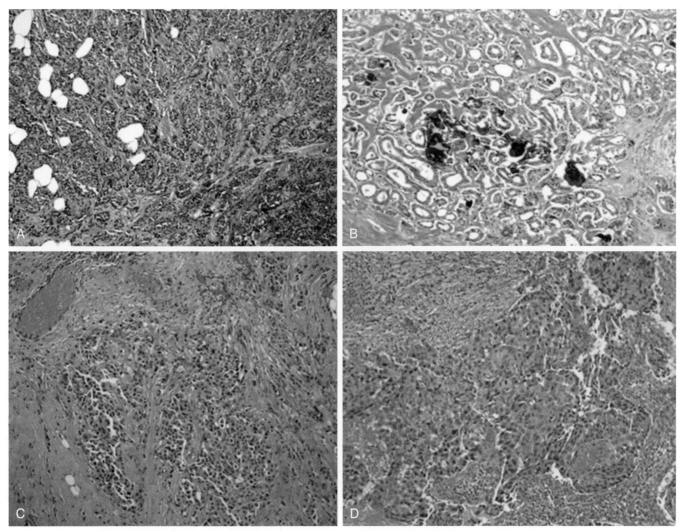

Fig. 60.1 (A-D) Four cases of invasive ductal carcinoma. (Korourian S: Infiltrating carcinomas of the breast: not one disease. In: Bland K, editor. The Breast: Comprehensive Management of Benign and Malignant Diseases, 145-155.e4, 64, 2018, Elsevier Press.).

breast cancer and slight propensity for abdominal mesenteric dissemination. ILC is characterized by single cell tissue infiltration, loss of heterozygosity or 16q chromosome, and absence of epithelial e-cadherin. **Medullary carcinoma** (3% to 9%) is associated with *BRCA1* germline mutations and higher grade. The histologic appearance is described as "pushing borders" rather than single cell invasion. **Mucinous and tubular breast cancer** subtypes, 1% to 2% and 1% to 3% respectively, are less common and present a lower risk for systemic metastasis.

BREAST CANCER STAGING

Approximately 90% of breast cancer at presentation is confined to the breast and axilla. Clinical evaluation includes history, including careful review of systems; screening for signs or symptoms of metastasis such as headache, weight loss, and bone pain; clinical examination; and laboratory evaluation including CBC, liver tests, and alkaline phosphatase. Clinical breast cancer staging is based on clinical breast exam including breast inspection for nipple discharge or retraction, skin dimpling, ulceration, erythema, edema, and palpable masses, and palpation of supraclavicular, axillary, and cervical lymph nodes.

Inflammatory breast cancer (Fig. 60.2) is an aggressive subtype of breast cancer with tumor invasion of the dermal lymphatics presenting with rapid skin changes of edema, erythema, and *peau d'orange* change,

involving greater than one third of the breast. Patients with breast cancer considered clinical stage III or signs or symptoms concerning for distant metastasis should be referred for systemic staging with bone scan and CT scan and in select cases PET scan. If a suspicious site is noted on staging, biopsy should be performed to confirm distant spread of breast cancer.

Breast cancer staging is based on the AJCC of anatomic cancer staging using tumor size (T in centimeters), regional node metastasis (N), and distant metastasis (M). The TNM system has prognostic significance. In the AJCC 8th edition *Staging Manual*, released in 2019, clinical stage (c) and pathologic stage (p) are supplemented with an additional pathologic prognostic stage incorporating grade and ER, PR, and HER2 gene overexpression. As an example, patients with T2 (2 to 5 cm) node-negative (N0) ER-positive HER2-negative tumors with gene expression profiles such as an Oncotype® Recurrence Score less than 11 have an excellent 5-year prognosis. This is reflected in the patient's AJCC 8th edition pathological prognostic stage of 1A (previously, by the AJCC 7th edition system, the patient would have been staged as IIA).

TREATMENT

Breast cancer is a story of the old and the new. Tamoxifen, the first cancer targeted therapy, was approved for ER-positive metastatic breast

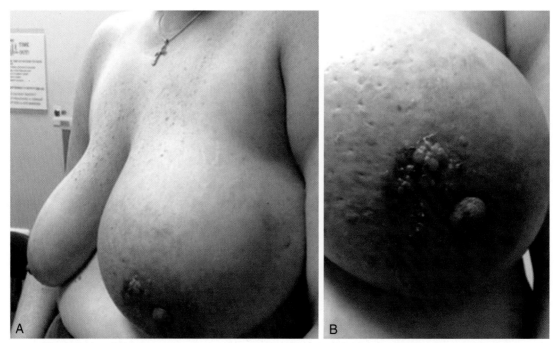

Fig. 60.2 (A and B) Inflammatory breast cancer with erythema and edema occupying the majority of the breast. (Somlo G, Jones V: Inflammatory breast cancer. In: Bland K, editor. The Breast: Comprehensive Management of Benign and Malignant Diseases, 2018, Elsevier Press.).

cancer in 1977. In the adjuvant setting for the most common type of breast cancer, tamoxifen has proven to reduce systemic recurrence by 50%. Scientific discoveries of pathways of tamoxifen resistance have led to additional therapeutic strategies for ER-positive breast cancer including aromatase inhibition to decrease estrogen production in postmenopausal patients, ovarian suppression of estrogen production in the premenopausal setting, and estrogen receptor downregulation with fulvestrant. Recent discoveries have led to FDA approval of cell cycle inhibitors of cyclin D 4/6 in combination with endocrine therapy with improved overall survival of ER-positive metastatic breast cancer.

By gene expression profiling, ER-positive breast cancer is further subdivided into luminal A, with a low cell proliferation signature and high endocrine therapy response, and luminal B, with a high cell proliferation signature and higher recurrence rate indicating relative endocrine insensitivity and relatively higher chemotherapy sensitivity. In the current era of personalized medicine, gene expression profiles such as Oncotype Recurrence Score testing of ER-positive node-negative breast cancer can identify patients who can forgo chemotherapy.

Other applications of personalized medicine for metastatic breast cancer include screening tumor samples with genomic sequencing for actionable mutations with specific targeted agents. PIK3CA-mutant ER-positive stage IV breast cancer patients have improved progression-free survival (PFS) with the PIK3CA inhibitor alpelisib. Approximately 10% of patients with breast cancer harbor somatic mutations in specific tumor suppressor genes such as BRCA1 and BRCA2. These patients are at higher risk of breast cancer and other malignancies with early age of onset. Some patients who harbor these genes are candidates for more intense screening and prevention strategies. Patients with stage IV disease who are BRCA1/2 mutation carriers may benefit from PARP inhibitor therapy.

Early-Stage Breast Cancer
Local Therapy
Stage I and II breast cancer clinical trials demonstrate equivalent outcomes of overall survival with breast preservation surgery with lumpectomy or segmental mastectomy to achieve negative surgical margins and breast external beam radiation compared to modified radical

mastectomy and axillary dissection. Patients age 70 and older with ER+ stage 1 disease willing to take 5 years of endocrine therapy have an equivalent overall survival with or without radiation and can safely omit radiation.

Unfortunately, not all breast cancer patients are candidates for breast preservation. Patients with multicentric disease (more than one breast quadrant), extensive malignant appearing calcifications, surgical inability to achieve negative margins, prior breast radiation, connective tissue disorder or who are unable to access a radiation facility treatment center are candidates for mastectomy. Patients with inflammatory breast cancer need neoadjuvant chemotherapy, prior to surgery, to eradicate dermal lymphatic cancer metastasis from the skin. In addition, patients with large unresectable tumors or large tumor-to-breast ratio may be candidates for neoadjuvant chemotherapy or endocrine therapy to downstage the tumor and allow for breast preservation.

For patients with no palpable lymph nodes on clinical exam, sentinel lymph node staging with removal and examination of the first draining lymph node accurately reflects the status of axillary metastases. Based on the ACOSZ-0011 trial of patients with clinically negative axillary lymph nodes staged with sentinel lymph nodes (with up to two positive lymph nodes), radiation and systemic therapy provide adequate local control.

Systemic Therapy
Prognosis estimation of systemic recurrence. The indication for breast cancer staging is to estimate the risk of systemic metastasis and help direct therapy. Historically, the most accurate indicators are tumor size, axillary metastasis, tumor grade, and ER, PR, and HER2 neu expression. ER, PR, and HER2 gene expression are detected by immunohistochemistry (IHC). Equivocal HER2 IHC testing is further evaluated by HER2 gene duplication detected by invitro hybridization (ISH).

Another chapter in breast cancer care is systemic therapy to reduce the risk of recurrence by elimination of micro-metastatic disease. Effective systemic therapy for breast cancer is the result of patient participation in well-designed randomized sequential clinical trials and identification of effective systemic therapies to decrease recurrence. The use of genomic signatures for personalized medicine allows us to move beyond "chemo for all" to an understanding of which breast cancers are chemotherapy sensitive or require chemotherapy. Tools such as PREDICT.NHS.UK calculate risk of mortality based on a patient's age, anatomic stage, and prognostic factors and assist clinicians and patients in estimating risk of recurrence and mortality reduction from chemotherapy, endocrine therapy, and validated genomic assays.

Therapy for HR+ Breast Cancer

Hormone receptor positive (HR+) breast cancer is the most common form of breast cancer and HR positivity is prognostic for a better 5-year disease-free survival compared to HR-negative breast tumors. HR+ also predicts those who will respond to antiestrogen directed therapies, although the risk of local and systemic recurrence extends past 10 years and is estimated to occur at a rate of 2% per year.

Tamoxifen was the first "targeted therapy" and ER expression the first biomarker for response to therapy. The Early Breast Cancer Trialists Group (EBCTCG) published series of breast cancer trial meta-analyses. EBCTCG trials of tamoxifen for HR+ breast cancer showed decreases in systemic recurrence by 50% and mortality by 25%; reduction in recurrence continues after 5 years. Further incremental improvement for subsets of patients include ovarian suppression for high-risk HR+ premenopausal patients and addition of aromatase inhibitors for postmenopausal patients. Based on the persistent risk of late recurrences in HR+ disease, trials of extended endocrine therapy with tamoxifen or aromatase inhibitors have shown further decrease in disease recurrence. Extended therapies and ovarian suppression come at a cost of increase in side effects and symptoms including hot flashes, decreased bone density, and for tamoxifen, increase in vaginal bleeding and risk of endometrial cancer.

A subset of HR+ patients is less responsive to endocrine therapy. In the current era of personalized medicine, gene expression profiles such as Oncotype Recurrence Score for HR+ node-negative breast cancer evaluates 16 genes including ER, proliferation, and invasion genes and predicts for risk of recurrence with endocrine therapy as well as a response to chemotherapy. Luminal A patients have low Oncotype Recurrence Scores and can forgo chemotherapy, and luminal B patients may derive benefit from addition of chemotherapy to endocrine therapy. Results of these assays can be used by clinicians for risk-benefit discussions with patients.

Approximately 20% of breast cancers are HER2 positive. *HER2* gene overexpression is a marker of a more aggressive phenotype. Targeted therapy with trastuzumab, a humanized monoclonal antibody to HER2 in combination with chemotherapy reduces systemic recurrence by 40%. Since the identification of trastuzumab, additional HER2-directed monoclonal antibodies have been developed and documented to have clinical utility. Pertuzumab, a monoclonal antibody directed to HER2 that prevents HER2 heterodimerization and cell activation added to trastuzumab and chemotherapy clinically improves the pathologic response rate. Future directions with HER2-directed therapies may be the ability to tailor therapy based on response and potentially to deescalate chemotherapy for HER2-positive patients.

Triple-negative breast cancer, defined as the absence of ER, PR and HER2 expression, is an aggressive breast cancer phenotype and comprises 10% to 15% of all breast cancers. Gene array analysis has identified six subtypes. Triple-negative breast cancer has a high systemic recurrence rate that typically occurs within the first 5 years of diagnosis. Due to high recurrence rates and shortened life expectancy after triple-negative breast cancer recurrence, systemic chemotherapy should be considered for a triple-negative breast cancer greater than 0.5 cm. Neoadjuvant chemotherapy may be considered if tumor size is over 2 centimeters.

Metastatic Breast Cancer

Metastatic breast cancer is "treatable not curable," and while the goal of therapy is palliative, many patients will live months to years on systemic therapy. The most frequent sites of breast cancer systemic recurrence are bone, lung, liver, and for lobular cancer, abdominal recurrences including ovaries and mesentery. Patients presenting with clinical or radiographic evidence of systemic recurrence should have a biopsy to confirm diagnosis including evaluation of ER, PR, and HER2 expression of metastatic cells. Results from a small series indicate receptor status on metastasis may change from the original breast cancer approximately 10% of the time. Next-generation sequencing of tumor metastasis screening for actionable mutations may direct cancer therapies in patients demonstrating PIK3CA-mutant ER-positive stage IV, to include alpelisib and fulvestrant. For triple-negative breast cancers, testing for programmed death ligand 1 (PD-L1) expression predicts response to checkpoint inhibitor therapy with atezolizumab. Single-agent chemotherapy for stage IV breast cancer is as effective as combination chemotherapy. Combination chemotherapy is reserved for patients at risk for a visceral crisis.

ER-Positive HER2-Negative Metastatic Breast Cancer

Bone only metastatic disease may have a long disease-free interval and patients may live many months to years with treatment as a chronic disease. Recurrence of ER-positive breast cancer within 6 months of initiation of antiestrogen therapy may indicate primary endocrine therapy resistance. Although chemotherapy response rate is more rapid, in the absence of impending visceral crisis there is no advantage in survival to chemotherapy over initial endocrine therapy.

Triple-Negative Breast Cancer

Unfortunately, systemic recurrence of triple-negative breast cancer (TNBC) frequently occurs in first 2 years after diagnosis. Chemotherapy options for stage IV ER-positive breast cancer resistant to endocrine therapy or TNBC include anthracyclines, taxanes, eribulin, carboplatin, and other single agents.

Targeted therapies for TNBC subtypes have expanded therapeutic options for selected patients. Patients with *BRCA1/2* germline mutations may benefit from disease control with an oral polyadenosine diphosphate-ribose polymerase (PARP) inhibitor. Olaparib and talazoparib are FDA approved for *BRCA*-associated *HER2*-negative breast cancer based on improved progression free survival. Immune checkpoint inhibition is one of many pathways for cancer to evade the immune system. Tumors expressing PD-L1 may activate PD-1 on tumor infiltrating immune cells resulting in immune cell apoptosis. In the Impassion130 trial of checkpoint inhibitor therapy, tumor-infiltrating immune cells with expression of 1% or greater PD-L1 expression derive increase in progression free survival with nab-paclitaxel and atezolizumab.

Special Circumstances
Bone Metastasis

Osteoclast inhibitors zoledronic acid bisphosphonates or denosumab, a RANK ligand inhibitor, prolong the time to skeletal related events such as pathologic fractures or need for surgery or radiation for bone metastases. Risks include renal dysfunction, hypocalcemia, and osteonecrosis.

Survivorship

A cancer patient becomes a cancer survivor on the day of diagnosis, regardless of whether they are currently without evidence of disease or are living with advanced or metastatic breast cancer. There are 15 million cancer survivors in the United States. Forty-four percent are breast cancer survivors. The Institute of Medicine report on cancer survivorship notes the transition of patients from active treatment to cancer survivor. The concern for patients "lost in transition" led the American College of Surgeons Commission on Cancer and the American Society of Clinical Oncology (ASCO) to recommend the creation of a survivorship plan for patient and primary care practitioner and follow-up care as quality standards.

Endocrine Therapy Compliance

It is estimated that 50% of ER-positive breast cancer patients do not complete adjuvant endocrine therapy due to side effects or barriers such as cost. Side effects that may affect quality of life and compliance include hot flashes from chemotherapy-induced menopause, tamoxifen or aromatase inhibitors. A recent study showed improvement in hot flashes and sleep quality with the use of cognitive behavioral therapy. Arthralgias from aromatase inhibitors may be attenuated by rotation through drug regimens and/or acupuncture, duloxetine or yoga.

Sexual Dysfunction

Unfortunately, sexual dysfunction is a common side effect following a breast cancer diagnosis secondary to surgery, radiation, chemotherapy, and adjuvant endocrine therapy. Practitioners should use open-ended questions about intimacy issues to normalize patients' concerns. Patients note change in self-image, decrease in sexual drive, vaginal dryness, and dyspareunia. Effective interventions can include use of vaginal moisturizers and lubricants, gabapentin and venlafaxine for hot flashes, topical lidocaine for tender vestibule, and referral to a sexual health expert.

Fertility Preservation

Pregnancy following a breast cancer diagnosis does not appear to increase risk for breast cancer recurrence, based on case control studies. Fertility may be compromised by chemotherapy, and fertility preservation options include egg retrieval and invitro fertilization. A general rule is to avoid pregnancy for 2 years after diagnosis, because this time period is a high-risk time for cancer recurrence. The PROMISE trial will follow a cohort of women following breast cancer diagnosis and treatment for breast cancer outcomes who chose to stop adjuvant endocrine therapy for pregnancy.

Lymphedema

Breast and arm lymphedema can be a complication from surgery and may be exacerbated by radiation. Physical therapy, manual massage, and compression bras and sleeves may attenuate this side effect.

Male Breast Cancer

Male breast cancer represents 1% of all breast cancers in the United States. Approximately 2500 men are diagnosed with breast cancer yearly and 500 men will die each year from male breast cancer. Risk factors for male breast cancer include *gBRCA2* mutations, Klinefelter's syndrome, undescended testes or testicular injury, and environmental radiation exposure, as documented in atomic bomb survivors. Male breast cancer patients are not represented in clinical trials. Available data on male breast cancer are primarily from small cohort studies. Mirroring women, incidence increases with age, but unlike women it is slightly higher in black men than in non-Hispanic white men. Presentation is with a palpable breast mass. Initial evaluation includes diagnostic mammogram, ultrasound, and core needle biopsy. On histologic diagnosis, 90% are ER-positive, HER2-positive. Surgical options and systemic therapy are similar to those of female counterparts. Tamoxifen reduces the risk of systemic disease in male breast cancer, with similar side effects as seen in women. The utility of aromatase inhibitor therapy is unknown in the adjuvant or metastatic setting.

Breast Cancer in Older Women

Breast cancer risk increases with age (see Table 60.1). In the United States a woman has a 1 in 8 risk of breast cancer diagnosis. The majority of patients diagnosed with breast cancer are ER-positive and over 65 years old. Patients age 70 and older with ER-positive stage 1 disease willing to take 5 years of endocrine therapy have an equivalent overall survival with or without radiation therapy and can therefore safely omit radiation. For women over 70 years of age with more aggressive or higher stage breast cancer, estimation of risk of recurrence, life expectancy, comorbidities, and toxicities of therapies are necessary to tailor therapy. Tools such as "ePrognosis" can be used for life-expectancy estimates based on comorbidities and PREDICT.NHS.UK for estimation of mortality based on tumor stage and prognostic features.

SCREENING

One outcome of advances in breast imaging techniques has been earlier detection of invasive and noninvasive breast cancers. Multiple guidelines have attempted to address screening of women without symptoms of breast cancer. In 2019, The American College of Physicians issued an updated guidance statement that addresses the use of screening mammography in women aged 50 to 74.

These guidelines do not address high-risk patients such as those with a personal history of breast cancer, prior abnormal mammogram or who carry a genetic mutation known to predispose to an increased risk of breast cancer.

CONCLUSION AND FUTURE DIRECTIONS

Breast cancer 5-year survival overall is 90% due to early detection and effective therapies such as chemotherapy and endocrine therapy. Unfortunately, chemotherapy and endocrine therapy have short- and long-term side effects of fatigue, cardiac toxicity, neuropathy, hot flashes, and sexual dysfunction. In an era of personalized medicine, ER-positive, node-negative breast cancer gene expression profile has identified a large proportion of patients who do not benefit from chemotherapy. Ongoing prospective trials will aid in decision making for ER-positive node-positive patients. For stage IV ER-positive patients, CDK 4/6 inhibitors and PIK3CA inhibitors appear to prolong time to progression. Triple-negative breast cancer continues to have a high proportion of patients who relapse and die within a few years of diagnosis; novel therapies are currently in phase 3 trials.

SUGGESTED READINGS

Bland KI, Copeland III EM, Klimberg VS, Gradishar WJ: The breast: comprehensive management of benign and malignant diseases, ed 5, Elsevier Inc, 2018.

DeSantis CE, etal: Breast cancer statistics, 2017, racial disparity in mortality by state, CA Cancer J Clin 67:439–448, 2017.

Giordano S: Breast cancer in men, N Engl J Med 378:2311–2320, 2018.

National Comprehensive Cancer Network Breast Cancer Version 3.2019. http://www.nccn.org/professionals/physician_gls/pdf/breast.pdf. Accessed September 25, 2019.

National Comprehensive Cancer Network Genetic/Familial High-Risk Assessment: Breast/Ovarian Version 3.2019. http://www.nccn.org/ professionals/physician_gls/pdf/breast.pdf. Accessed September 25, 2019.

Runowicz C, Leach CR, Henry NL, et al: ACS/ASCO breast cancer survivorship guidelines, J Clin Oncol 34:611–635, 2015.

Screening for Breast Cancer in Average-risk Women: A guidance statement from the American College of Physicians, Ann Intern Med 170(8):547–560, 2019. https://doi.org/10.7326/M18-2147.

Siegel R, Miller KD, Jemal A: Cancer statistics, 2019 CA Cancer J Clin 69:7–34, 2019.

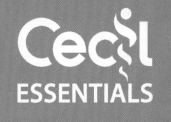

61

Gynecological Cancer

Christina Bandera, Tarra B. Evans, Don Dizon

OVARIAN CANCER

Epidemiology

Ovarian cancer is the most difficult gynecologic cancer to cure, because over 70% of cases present with metastatic disease, and over 80% of cases will recur despite treatment. Ovarian cancer is the seventh most common cancer affecting women worldwide. In North America, Europe, Australia, and New Zealand it is the most common cause of death from a gynecologic malignancy.

A woman's lifetime risk of developing ovarian cancer is 1.4%. Most ovarian cancers are sporadic; however, a family history of ovarian cancer is the strongest risk factor for developing disease due to inherited genetic mutations. For example, inherited BRCA1 and BRCA2 mutations carry a 40% to 60% and a 15% to 20% risk of developing ovarian cancer, respectively. Lynch syndrome, the result of inherited mutations in mismatch repair genes, portends a 12% risk of ovarian cancer.

Currently, guidelines recommend that all women with ovarian carcinoma receive genetic counseling. Multigene panel testing is available to detect mutations that may confer a greater risk of developing the disease and can help guide targeted treatment recommendations. Furthermore, genetic screening enables identification of family members at risk who may benefit from prophylactic removal of the ovaries and fallopian tubes, as well as specialized screening programs for other cancers. (Please see Chapter 55.)

Other significant risk factors for ovarian cancer include reproductive factors associated with increased ovulation such as early menarche, late menopause, and nulliparity. Protective factors against ovarian cancer include pregnancy, breast-feeding, and use of oral contraceptives. Talcum powder has been associated with asbestos contamination, and its use on the perineum has been studied for a potential link to ovarian cancer, with conflicting results.

Pathology

Ovarian carcinoma refers to a family of tumors arising from the epithelial lining of the ovary, fallopian tube, and peritoneum. More recently, it is thought that the majority of ovarian cancers originate in the fallopian tube due to the frequent concurrent finding of premalignant serous tubal intraepithelial carcinoma (STIC). The most common cell type is serous carcinoma. Other histologies include endometrioid, mucinous, and clear cell patterns.

Borderline ovarian neoplasms are an unusual category of ovarian neoplasm with a favorable prognosis that can spread and recur but do not exhibit invasion of tissue. Treatment is surgical because these tumors do not respond to chemotherapy.

Nonepithelial ovarian cancers account for less than 5% of ovarian cancers and originate from sex-cord cells, stromal cells, and germ cells of the ovary. These rare tumors often occur in adolescent females, and pathologic classification determines treatment and prognosis.

Clinical Presentation

Ovarian cancer is often called the cancer that "whispers" because symptoms are subtle and nonspecific. Bloating, abdominal pain, gastrointestinal disturbance, and bladder symptoms may present once diffuse carcinomatosis develops with nodules of cancer and ascites throughout the abdomen and pelvis. Cancer is often detected during imaging for work-up of sudden GI or GU symptoms. Common sites of metastasis include the omentum, peritoneal surfaces, lymph nodes in the pelvis and abdomen, and pleural effusions. Distant metastases to the lungs, liver, bone and brain are less common. Over 70% of patients are diagnosed with disease beyond the pelvis considered stage IIIC or IV.

Diagnosis and Staging

Ovarian cancer is diagnosed with histologic confirmation of a pelvic mass or abnormal tissue typically identified on ultrasound, computed tomography (CT), or magnetic resonance imaging (MRI). Advanced ovarian cancer is suspected on imaging with the presence of an adnexal mass accompanied by ascites, peritoneal carcinomatosis or enlarged pelvic and para-aortic lymph nodes. Patients with an enlarged complex ovarian mass and no evidence of metastatic disease should have surgery for resection of the mass with effort made to avoid disrupting the integrity of the neoplasm, because rupture may spread cancer if present. If widespread disease is seen on imaging, a clinician may recommend an image-guided biopsy of solid tumor, drainage of ascites or surgical resection to obtain tumor for tissue diagnosis.

The tumor biomarker carbohydrate antigen 125 (CA 125) is a mucin-type glycoprotein secreted into the bloodstream by cancer cells and can be useful in the initial work-up and for monitoring response to treatment, but the test should not be used for diagnostic purposes alone as the marker is nonspecific. CA 125 may be elevated in noncancer conditions such as menstruation, benign ovarian tumors, endometriosis, fibroids, pelvic infection, congestive heart failure, and pleural effusions.

Ovarian cancer stage is assigned by review of clinical, pathologic, and radiologic evaluation. Early disease is isolated to the ovaries or fallopian tubes (FIGO [International Federation of Gynecology and Obstetrics] stage I) or to the true pelvis (stage II). Diffuse carcinomatosis or abdominal/pelvic adenopathy (FIGO stage III) and distant metastases to sites including liver parenchyma, lungs, bone and brain (FIGO stage IV) comprise advanced stage disease.

Treatment

The treatment for presumed early stage ovarian carcinoma is surgical resection and staging to evaluate for metastatic disease. Because

TABLE 61.1   Addition of Maintenance Bevacizumab to Front-Line Therapy for Ovarian Cancer Shows Improved Progression-Free Survival (PFS) in Two Studies

Study	Randomization	N	Median PFS	Hazard Ratio	*P*-value	Survival Advantage
GOG-218	C/P + placebo	625	10.3 mo	0.91	0.16	No
	C/P + bev	625	11.2 mo	0.72	<0.001	
	C/P + bev →7 bev-M	623	14.1 mo			
ICON7	C/P	764	17.3	0.81	0.004	Yes (for those at high risk for PD)
	C/P + bev →7 bev-M	764	19.0			

Data from Burger RA, et al. NEJM 2011; 365:2473-83; Perren TJ, et al. NEJM 2011; 365:2484-96; Tewari, et al. J Clin Oncol. 2019;37:2317-2328.
bev, Bevacizumab; *bev-M,* bev maintenance; *C/P,* cisplatin + paclitaxel; *PD,* progression of disease.

ovarian cancer may spread through peritoneal shedding of cells, lymphatically or through the bloodstream, staging includes removing the ovaries, fallopian tubes, uterus, omentum, lymph nodes, and peritoneal biopsies. High-grade cancers isolated to the ovary, or cancer with any sign of spread beyond the ovary, is treated with adjuvant chemotherapy. The standard of care calls for the administration of intravenous carboplatin and paclitaxel every 3 weeks. For early stage ovarian carcinoma, there is no consensus on whether three or six cycles should be administered; one study that looked at the impact of histology on outcomes following chemotherapy suggested that compared to three cycles, six cycles was associated with a significantly lower risk of recurrence for women with serous cancers (HR 0.33, 95% CI 0.14-0.77) but not for those with nonserous cancers (HR 0.94, 95% CI 0.60-1.49). We continue to recommend six cycles for women with early stage ovarian cancer, though have a lower threshold to discontinue treatment after three cycles for women with nonserous cancers, if they opt to stop or if side effects intervene.

In advanced stage disease, the care team must decide whether to begin treatment with a primary "debulking" surgery or neoadjuvant chemotherapy (NACT). Debulking is favored when imaging suggests all visible tumor may be resected at the time of surgery. NACT is favored with a low likelihood of achieving cytoreduction to no visible disease or in patients with major perioperative risk factors related to comorbidities and frailty, which is consistent with the ASCO/SGO Clinical Guidelines in this population. After three to four cycles of NACT, patients are assessed for an interval debulking surgery (IDS) followed by additional chemotherapy. One randomized trial showed a survival advantage in favor of heated intraperitoneal chemotherapy for patients undergoing an IDS; confirmatory trials are underway. In either case, adjuvant therapy is indicated, and we suggest patients receive up to three cycles following surgery to complete at least six cycles total of chemotherapy. Finally, data show that bevacizumab confers a progression-free survival advantage, though this did not translate into an overall survival benefit in the American trial, GOG 218 (Table 61.1).

Following first-line chemotherapy, women with newly diagnosed ovarian cancer should be offered maintenance treatment using a poly-ADP-ribose polymerase (PARP) inhibitor. Multiple trials have shown that treatment is associated with significant improvement in disease-free survival, particularly in those with a mutation in BRCA (mBRCA, germline or somatic), with one trial also supporting its use in combination with bevacizumab in those without a mutation but with evidence of homologous recombination deficiency (HRD). While niraparib was associated with a survival advantage in women without mBRCA or HRD, the benefit was much smaller than in other groups. As such, while we offer PARP inhibition as maintenance treatment to all patients after completion of adjuvant therapy, we strongly recommend it for women with mBRCA or evidence of HRD.

Recurrent ovarian cancer can be treated with additional chemotherapy and surgery can be considered if there are resectable sites of limited disease. If the recurrence occurs more than 6 months after completing primary platinum-based treatment, the tumor is considered "platinum sensitive" and retreatment with a platinum combination is preferred. In these patients, evidence supports the use of PARP inhibitors in the maintenance setting, regardless of whether patients have mBRCA or HRD. When recurrence occurs in less than 6 months, the cancer is considered "platinum resistant," and an alternative agent is chosen. Patients with recurrent ovarian cancer do not have curable disease; therefore, clinical trials should be offered whenever possible.

Prognosis

Early ovarian cancer is often curable with surgery and chemotherapy. Stage I disease has an 80% to 90% 5-year survival, and stage II disease portends a 60% to 70% 5-year survival. Unfortunately, patients with advanced stage disease usually recur and develop treatment resistance. Eventually treatment turns to best supportive care. Bowel obstruction from massive carcinomatosis is a common terminal event for women with ovarian cancer. Five-year survival for women with stage III to IV disease ranges from 18% to 50% depending on the pattern of disease.

UTERINE CANCER

Epidemiology

Endometrial cancer is the most common gynecologic cancer in North America and in Northern and Eastern Europe. Worldwide, it is the sixth most common malignancy affecting women, and it ranks as the fourteenth cause of cancer death.

Increased circulating estrogen without progesterone to balance stimulation of the endometrial lining is associated with endometrial cancer development. Obesity is a strong risk factor due to high levels of circulating estrogen via conversion of androgens to estrogen by aromatase within adipose cells. Other increased estrogen-related risk factors include anovulatory menstrual cycles, nulliparity, early menarche, late menopause, estrogen producing ovarian neoplasms (benign thecomas and malignant dysgerminomas), and estrogen replacement without the use of protective progesterone. Breast cancer treatment with tamoxifen blocks estrogen action in the breast but has pro-estrogen effects on the endometrium resulting in a 2- to 5-fold increased risk of endometrial cancer after 5 years of use.

Women with hereditary Lynch syndrome (see section on epidemiology of ovarian cancer) have a 60% lifetime risk of developing endometrial cancer and require screening with annual endometrial biopsy, and when childbearing is complete, a hysterectomy with bilateral salpingo-oophorectomy is recommended. Diabetes and hypertension are associated with increased risk of endometrial cancer. Smoking is associated with a decreased rate of endometrial cancer, likely due to the association with low circulating estrogen.

Pathology

Endometrial cancer traditionally has been divided into two categories: type 1 and type 2. Type 1 endometrial cancers are hormone-induced, arising from the hyperplastic precursor endometrioid intraepithelial neoplasia (EIN). These low-grade endometrioid type cancers are usually limited to the uterus and have a good prognosis. Type 2 endometrial cancer is the more aggressive form of cancer, more likely to metastasize, and carries a worse prognosis. Type 2 histologies include high-grade endometrioid, serous, clear cell, and carcinosarcoma. More recently, genomic analysis has been used to stratify endometrial cancer into four groups: (1) *POLE* gene ultramutated; (2) tumors with microsatellite instability hypermutated; (3) copy number low; and (4) copy number high (serous tumors and one quarter of high-grade endometrioid tumors). Data suggest that the groups confer prognostic information in terms of progression-free survival with POLE-type tumors having the best prognosis and those with high copy number having the worst prognosis.

Mesenchymal cancers of the uterus are rare and include cancers, such as sarcoma, arising from the myometrial wall of the uterus and cancers arising from the endometrial stromal cells.

Clinical Presentation

Studies show that 70% to 90% of women with endometrial cancer present with postmenopausal bleeding. In premenopausal women, irregular or heavy vaginal bleeding is the most common symptom. An abnormal Papanicolaou (Pap) smear, or abnormal imaging of the uterus, may also lead to a diagnosis of endometrial cancer. Mesenchymal cancers may present with abnormal uterine bleeding or pain.

Diagnosis and Staging

Postmenopausal women with any uterine bleeding, even spotting, should be evaluated for endometrial cancer. The work-up includes a full gynecologic exam with endometrial sampling and imaging to evaluate the appearance of the endometrium (normal endometrial thickness measures ≤4 mm after menopause). Endometrial biopsy may be performed as an office procedure and has a high sensitivity when the endometrial lining measures 11 mm or less. A thicker lining may require further evaluation with a dilatation and curettage of the uterus to definitively rule out malignancy. Premenopausal women with persistent bleeding between menses should also be evaluated with endometrial sampling and radiographic imaging, especially those presenting with known risk factors for endometrial cancer.

If a high-grade cancer is identified on endometrial sampling, then CT of the abdomen and pelvis is recommended to assess for the presence of metastatic disease.

Staging of endometrial cancer is surgical. FIGO stage I disease is cancer limited to the uterus, whereas stage II involves the cervical stroma. Stage III includes disease involving the ovaries, tubes, and regional lymph nodes. Stage IV is defined as peritoneal carcinomatosis, liver metastases, or other metastases beyond the abdomen and pelvis.

Treatment

Unless widespread metastatic disease is identified on preoperative imaging, standard treatment for endometrial cancer is a simple hysterectomy (Fig. 61.1) with bilateral salpingo-oophorectomy and assessment for lymph node metastases. If the uterus is small, this procedure may be performed with a laparoscopic or robot-assisted laparoscopic technique. Laparotomy may be indicated for a large uterus that cannot be extracted vaginally. Sentinel nodal evaluation has largely replaced complete pelvic and para-aortic lymphadenectomy. This procedure

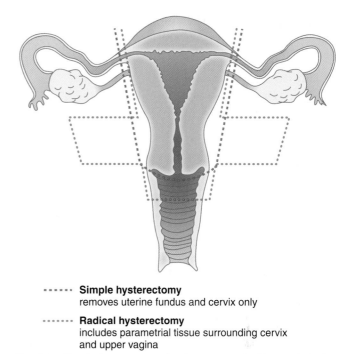

- - - - - **Simple hysterectomy**
removes uterine fundus and cervix only

- - - - - **Radical hysterectomy**
includes parametrial tissue surrounding cervix and upper vagina

Fig. 61.1 Simple hysterectomy involves removal of uterus including fundus and cervix. Radical hysterectomy extends the surgical margin with removal of surrounding parametrial tissue and upper vagina.

involves injecting the cervix with dye and removing lymph nodes that collect the dye. The advantages of sentinel node dissection include a limited, more targeted surgery, with less risk of surgical complications including lower extremity lymphedema.

Early stage endometrial cancer with low grade histology that invades less than 50% of the myometrium has an excellent prognosis for cure with surgery alone. The protocols for administering adjuvant therapy for endometrial cancer after surgical staging are complex. A careful review of pathologic risk factors by a multidisciplinary team that considers the patient's comorbidites is important in the treatment planning process. Recommendations may include vaginal cuff brachytherapy, pelvic radiation, and/or chemotherapy. Stage 1 tumors that invade more than 50% of the myometrium are typically treated with vaginal radiation to prevent local recurrence of cancer. Tumors with cervical stromal involvement are treated with additional whole pelvic radiation. If lymph node metastases or other disease beyond the uterus is identified, then chemotherapy with intravenous carboplatin and paclitaxel with or without radiation is typically recommended. Some patients with high grade cancer such as the serous subtype may also benefit from chemotherapy even if cancer is isolated to the uterus.

Treatment for recurrent endometrial cancer is tailored to the site of recurrence. A vaginal recurrence is typically treated with localized radiation. Distant recurrences often require platinum-based chemotherapy; however, a low-grade metastatic endometrial cancer may respond to antiestrogen hormonal therapy alone. For those who progress on first-line chemotherapy, clinical trials should be pursued. To date, there are no FDA-approved agents in the second- or later-line setting for these patients.

A subset of women with early endometrial cancer may opt to forego standard hysterectomy. This includes young women wishing to preserve fertility and elderly, or frail women, who have a high surgical risk. These women may be treated with high-dose progesterone therapy using a progesterone secreting intrauterine device or oral tablets. Success rates greater than 80% are reported for women with low-grade cancers without evidence of myometrial invasion on pretreatment

MRI imaging. Ongoing surveillance or hysterectomy when childbearing is complete is recommended for young patients. For frail patients, progesterone therapy is continued indefinitely.

Prognosis

Endometrial cancer isolated to the uterus is curable in 80% to 90% of cases. Rates of cure for more advanced disease are lower, while advanced stage IV disease remains incurable. Sadly, for women with endometrial cancer presenting with carcinomatosis, the 5-year survival rate is less than 25%.

CERVICAL CANCER

Epidemiology

Cervical cancer is the most preventable gynecologic cancer. Unfortunately, it remains the most common malignancy of the female reproductive tract worldwide and is a leading cause of cancer-related death in developing countries. In the United States, it is the third most common gynecologic cancer. The primary risk factor for developing cervical cancer is infection with a high-risk subtype of the human papillomavirus (HPV). As nearly all cancers of the cervix are the result of HPV-associated cytopathologic changes, infection with the virus is considered a necessary cause in disease development. The incidence and mortality of cervical cancer are influenced by access to screening programs. Thus, resource poor settings with limited access to Pap screening have higher rates of cervical cancer morbidity and mortality. Other risk factors for cervical cancer include smoking, immunosuppression, and diethylstilbestrol (DES) exposure.

HPV infects the female genital tract via sexual transmission. Subtypes are termed high-risk (HR) when they are associated with preinvasive and invasive cervical disease. There are 15 primary HRHPV subtypes associated with the development of cervical cancer; however, HPV-16 and -18 are responsible for 50% and 20% of cervical cancer cases, respectively. While many individuals will clear the HPV virus, persistence of HPV infection is associated with an increased risk for developing preinvasive neoplasia or invasive cervical cancer. Due to the causal relationship of HPV and cervical cancer, vaccines have been developed targeting HRHPV subtypes to prevent the development of HPV associated cervical pathology. In 2006, the FDA approved use of the Gardasil quadrivalent vaccine for the prevention of anogenital lesions, which covered six HRHPV subtypes for females aged 9 to 26 years old. Currently, the only FDA-approved vaccine in the US is Gardasil 9, covering HPV types 6, 11, 16, 18, 31, 33, 45, 52, and 58 for females and males ages 9 to 45 years old.

Pathology

The outer cellular layer of the cervix that lies within the vagina is comprised of squamous epithelium. The endocervical canal is comprised of columnar epithelium. The region where endocervical columnar epithelium is replaced by squamous epithelium—the transformation zone—serves as the primary site of HPV-related preinvasive and invasive lesions of the cervix. The majority of cervical cancers are squamous carcinomas (75%) and adenocarcinomas (25%). Other extremely rare types of cervical cancer include neuroendocrine, adenosquamous, clear cell, and undifferentiated carcinoma.

Clinical Presentation

In early stage disease, patients do not typically experience symptoms. If symptoms are present, they often include abnormal vaginal bleeding, bleeding with intercourse, discharge, or pelvic discomfort.

Cervical cancer spreads by local extension to surrounding tissues, followed by nodal metastasis and then hematologic dissemination.

Patients with advanced stage disease may have symptoms related to involvement of surrounding structures. Local tumor infiltration may result in significant vaginal bleeding and pelvic pain or urinary or bowel complaints. These patients are often noted to have a large cervical mass on physical examination or imaging.

Diagnosis and Staging

The majority of cervical cancers are diagnosed through cervical biopsies performed as a result of a screening Pap that identifies abnormal cervical cytology or persistent HRHPV. In patients who have not undergone routine Pap screening, cervical cancer is diagnosed through biopsies of grossly abnormal appearing cervical tissue or masses. Regardless of PAP smear cytology, patients with persistent HRHPV subtypes should have a diagnostic biopsy for the presence of cervical pathology.

Cervical cancer is clinically and radiographically staged FIGO I through IV. Subcategories within each stage are based on the extent of disease. Cervical cancer is categorized into early stage disease (stages IA-IB1), locally advanced disease (stages IB2-IVA), and metastatic disease (stage IVB). Early stage cancers are small tumors limited to the cervix. Locally advanced disease refers to larger tumors and tumors that have invaded beyond the uterus and extend into nearby pelvic structures, including the bladder and rectum. Metastatic disease refers to cancer that has spread beyond the pelvic organs to distant sites. A complete physical examination and thorough pelvic examination is important in evaluating both localized and distant spread of disease.

Helpful imaging modalities in assessing the extent of disease in cervical cancer include CT of the chest, abdomen, and pelvis; positron emission tomography–computed tomography (PET/CT), which is often helpful in evaluation of nodal involvement or smaller metastasis; and MRI, which can aid in assessment of local spread to soft tissues and adjacent pelvic structures. If imaging identifies sites of metastatic disease, image-guided biopsy should be performed for confirmation of stage.

Treatment

Treatment for cervical cancer is dependent on whether the disease is early, locally advanced or has distant metastases. Both early stage tumors and locally advanced tumors are treated with curative intent. Early stage disease is managed surgically with simple hysterectomy or radical hysterectomy (see Fig. 61.1). Pelvic lymph node dissection is performed as part of the procedure, with the exception of smaller tumors (<3 mm depth of invasion) and no evidence for lymphovascular space invasion. In reproductive age patients with early stage disease who would like to maintain fertility, options include cone excisional procedures or trachelectomy (surgical removal of only the cervix), and the uterus is left intact for future childbearing.

For larger cervical tumors (>4 cm) and locally advanced disease, concurrent chemotherapy and radiation are the mainstays of treatment. The addition of chemotherapy (cisplatin or cisplatin and 5-fluorouracil) to radiation is utilized as a radiosensitizer to increase the effectiveness of radiation. Chemoradiation in locally advanced disease is associated with improved survival and reduction in recurrence rates. Surgical management is not favored for larger cervical tumors and locally advanced disease, because the goal of surgery is to obtain negative margins. With surgery, large tumors and locally advanced disease have higher rates of recurrence, decreased survival, and a high likelihood for requiring postoperative radiation, which is associated with increased complication rates when compared with radiation without prior surgery.

Unfortunately, widely metastatic cervical cancer is not considered curable and treatment is aimed at controlling the spread of disease and palliating bothersome symptoms. Treatment involves combination platinum-based chemotherapy with the addition of bevacizumab to improve survival outcomes. Pelvic radiation in these patients is reserved for palliative treatment intended to decrease symptomatic pelvic disease burden or to control vaginal bleeding. For those who experience recurrence despite first-line chemotherapy, testing for PD-L1 is recommended because the FDA has approved the immune checkpoint inhibitor pembrolizumab for use in these patients if their tumors are positive.

For patients with recurrent disease localized to the central pelvis and no evidence of distant metastatic spread, pelvic exenterative procedures that remove remaining pelvic structures with urinary and stool diversion may be curative but are associated with high rates of perioperative morbidity. For patients with recurrent disease who are not candidates for operative management or radiation therapy, chemotherapy such as cisplatin with paclitaxel or gemcitabine can help control disease.

New advances in the treatment of cervical cancer are now examining the role of HPV vaccination for active disease, as well as the utilization of immunotherapy as part of systemic treatment.

Prognosis

Outcomes in cervical cancer depend on stage at diagnosis. Patients with nodal disease have higher rates of relapse and poorer prognosis. Five-year survival rates are roughly 92%, 56%, and 17% for localized, regional, and distant disease, respectively.

VULVAR CANCER

Epidemiology

Vulvar cancer is the most frequently overlooked gynecologic cancer and is the fourth most common gynecologic cancer in the United States. A woman's lifetime risk of developing vulvar cancer is roughly 0.3%. Most vulvar cancers arise from either oncogenic HPV-associated preinvasive vulvar intraepithelial neoplasia (VIN) or through autoimmune or inflammatory related changes, such as lichen sclerosus, leading to differentiated VIN (dVIN). While vulvar cancer most commonly occurs in women over the age of 60, HPV-related vulvar cancer occurs more commonly in younger women. Atypical moles of vulva are associated with an increased risk for the development of vulvar melanomas. Other risk factors for developing vulvar cancer include advanced age, smoking, HIV, and a personal history of cervical cancer or preinvasive cervical lesions.

Pathology

The vulva includes the clitoris, mons, labia majora and minora, vestibule, and the perineal body. Squamous cell carcinoma (SCC) accounts for more than 80% of all vulvar cancers. Melanomas are the second most common type accounting for 10%, followed by basal cell carcinomas (2% to 4%), verrucous carcinomas—an indolent variant of SCC—and sarcomas (1% to 2%). Paget's disease of the vulva is a glandular-like intraepithelial neoplasm that can develop into or harbor underlying adenocarcinoma. Bartholin gland carcinomas account for 0.1% to 5% of vulvar cancers and are typically adenocarcinomas. Other rarer types of vulvar cancers include germ cell tumors, urothelial/transitional cell carcinoma, and neuroendocrine tumors.

Clinical Presentation

Vulvar cancers typically present as an irritated or pruritic solitary vulvar lesion that may be flat, raised, indurated, cauliform, ulcerated or discolored. Occasionally the lesions can be multifocal or may be associated with vulvar bleeding or dysuria. Vulvar cancers metastasize by local extension, lymphatic drainage to the inguinofemoral nodes, and hematogenous spread to distant sites. Patients with more advanced stage disease may present with evidence of a large ulcerated or verrucous (wartlike) mass extending to surrounding tissues or involving large areas of the vulva, vagina, or the anal verge. Often, enlarged groin lymph nodes can be palpated. Other signs related to local extension may include profound vulvar pain, urinary outlet obstruction or dysuria. As the development of vulvar cancer generally has an indolent growth rate, most patients presenting with locally advanced or advanced stage disease are elderly women who are disconnected from routine gynecologic care, or women with limited access to gynecologic care.

Diagnosis and Staging

Vulvar cancer is pathologically diagnosed and staged. Both patients and providers frequently ignore symptoms of perineal itching and discomfort that are typical for the cancer. Patients who present with a suspicious or bothersome lesion on the vulva should undergo a biopsy to evaluate for the presence of vulvar cancer. In addition to biopsy of the gross lesion for histologic confirmation, a complete pelvic examination should be performed including visual inspection of the entire vulva, vagina, cervix, and anus. The groin nodes are palpated to assess for inguinofemoral adenopathy. Enlarged lymph nodes should be biopsied to confirm the presence of disease versus reactive nodes.

After histologic confirmation, the next step is determining the extent of disease. Vulvar cancer is staged with a combination of clinical examination, pathologic confirmation, and radiographic findings. Helpful imaging modalities include CT of the chest, abdomen, and pelvis, or PET/CT. MRI can often be helpful in ambiguous cases to better characterize local extension of disease into surrounding soft tissues and can aid in operative decision making.

Vulvar cancers spread by local extension, and by lymphatic channels to inguinofemoral nodes then pelvic nodes. FIGO stage I disease defines tumor confined to the vulva. Stage II disease involves cancer extending to the adjacent perineal structures including the urethra, anus, and lower one third of the vagina. Stage III disease is comprised of tumor involving the inguinofemoral lymph nodes and stage IV tumor involves the upper two thirds of the urethra and vagina or any distant structures. Roughly 60% of vulvar cancers are localized to the primary site at diagnosis, approximately one third are diagnosed with regional spread, and roughly 6% present with distant metastasis.

Treatment

Treatment of vulvar cancer depends on the histologic subtype and stage of the disease. Treatment courses for vulvar cancer should be individualized because many affected patients are elderly or medically frail.

For patients with apparent early stage disease, treatment includes a radical wide local excision of the lesion with at least a 2-cm lateral margin. Because inguinofemoral node status is the most important prognostic factor, groin nodal evaluation should be assessed for tumors having more than 1 mm depth of invasion. Sentinel lymph node dissection to diagnose nodal involvement has largely replaced full groin nodal dissection because it is associated with less perioperative morbidity. Bilateral groin nodes are evaluated for midline tumors and tumors larger than 4 cm. Postoperative radiation therapy is typically recommended if two or more lymph nodes are involved or nodal extracapsular spread is present and is associated with improved survival outcomes.

For vulvar cancers that have spread beyond the vulva, treatment is highly individualized with careful consideration of goals of care and patient functional status. These tumors are typically not amenable to surgical management and treatment options include primary chemoradiation, radiation alone, palliative radiation to burdensome disease sites or systemic chemotherapy. Chemoradiation with sensitizing cisplatin chemotherapy is considered superior to radiation alone for locally advanced disease. Radiation fields typically include the primary tumor site, inguinofemoral nodes, and pelvic lymph nodes. If there is residual primary tumor after radiation, resection, if technically feasible, may improve survival or alleviate symptoms. A palliative care approach to provide supportive care is important for patients with advanced stage disease because they often have a high symptom burden pre- and postradiation.

Patients who present with distant metastasis are treated with systemic chemotherapy such as carboplatin and paclitaxel, and radiation can be offered in palliative doses to highly symptomatic disease sites. Recurrent vulvar cancer is treated with surgical excision if localized to the vulva. Systemic carboplatin/paclitaxel is administered for recurrent vulvar cancer at distant sites.

Prognosis

The most important prognostic factor in vulvar cancer is inguinofemoral nodal involvement. Estimated 5-year survival rates for localized, regional, and distant disease are 86%, 53%, and 19%, respectively. Risk factors for recurrent disease include inguinofemoral nodal involvement, close postoperative surgical margins (<5 mm), and higher stage of disease at diagnosis. Patients with HPV-associated vulvar cancers have improved outcomes with radiation treatment relative to non-HPV-associated vulvar cancers.

VAGINAL CANCER

Epidemiology

Primary vaginal cancer is the rarest gynecologic cancer, accounting for only 1% to 2% of gynecologic malignancies. Extension of primary cancers of the uterus, cervix, and vulva, or metastasis from another primary site, should be ruled out to confirm vaginal origin. Vaginal cancer is typically diagnosed in patients older than 60 years. Risk factors include HRHPV, in utero DES exposure, HIV, history of pre-cancers or cancers of the cervix, and the presence of high-grade vaginal intraepithelial neoplasia.

Pathology

The main histopathologic subtype of vaginal cancer is squamous cell carcinoma (90%). Less common types include adenocarcinomas such as clear cells (8% to 14%), melanomas, sarcomas, lymphomas, neuroendocrine, and yolk sac tumors.

Clinical Presentation

Most patients with vaginal cancer present with vaginal bleeding or abnormal vaginal discharge. Alternatively, asymptomatic patients are diagnosed via biopsy of a grossly abnormal appearing lesion at time of routine annual pelvic examination or colposcopic directed biopsy after abnormal cervical or vaginal cytology is detected. Lesions have a variety of appearances and can be soft, friable, nodular, raised, papillary, flat, erythematous, hyper- or hypopigmented. Lesions are most commonly found in the upper one third of the vagina, but distal lesions can be seen as well. Primary vaginal cancers spread by direct extension, the lymphatics, and hematologically to distant sites. The lymphatic drainage of the upper vagina involves the internal iliac lymph nodes and the lower vagina drains to the inguinal lymph nodes. Patients with more advanced disease may present with symptoms related to local extension such as painful urination or defecation; pelvic, vulvar or vaginal pain; hematochezia or hematuria.

Diagnosis and Staging

The diagnosis of vaginal cancer is made by histologic confirmation via biopsy of visible tumor. Because most vaginal cancers are the result of

metastasis from another primary site, it is important to rule out other primary gynecologic cancers of the cervix, uterus, ovaries, or vulva as well as nongynecologic cancers that may have vaginal extension such as colorectal or urethral/bladder cancers.

FIGO stage I vaginal cancer includes small tumors limited to the vagina. Stage II disease has extended through the vaginal walls. Stage III tumors invade into the pelvic wall or lower one third of the vagina and may obstruct urinary outflow or cause hydronephrosis. Stage IV tumors include nodal metastasis and spread to the rectum, bladder or distant sites.

Vaginal cancer is the only gynecologic cancer that remains clinically staged (physical examination, cystoscopy, proctoscopy, chest radiograph); however, more advanced imaging modalities such as pelvic MRI, PET/CT or CT chest, abdomen, and pelvis can be used to help assess the full extent of disease not detected by clinical examination alone. While these studies help to guide treatment, they are not currently used to assign the stage of disease.

Treatment

Treatment for vaginal cancer is based on location of tumor and stage of the disease. Aside from stage I disease confined to the mucosa, vaginal cancer is typically treated with a combination of primary chemotherapy and radiation.

An important consideration for surgical resection in vaginal cancer is location (upper vagina or lower vagina) and size of the lesion, as the goal is to achieve negative resection margins. Candidates for primary operative management of vaginal cancers include stage I disease limited to the upper or lower vagina. These lesions are best treated surgically when superficial and smaller than 2 cm. Surgery has become the mainstay of treatment for such lesions, with survival rates ranging from 75% to 100%. If the vaginal tumor includes the upper vagina, a radical hysterectomy with a radical upper vaginectomy and pelvic lymph node dissection may be performed. For stage I disease in the lower vagina, a radical vaginectomy and potentially a vulvovaginectomy may be performed with an inguinofemoral nodal dissection.

For stage II to IV tumors, primary chemoradiation is the mainstay of treatment because it is associated with improved disease control and reduction in locoregional recurrence rates. Due to the rarity of vaginal cancer, studies are few and treatment approaches are often derived from favorable outcomes demonstrated in cervical cancers utilizing a combination of chemotherapy and radiation. For a central pelvic recurrence of vaginal cancer after radiation treatment, total pelvic exenteration may be curative in approximately 50% of correctly selected cases.

Prognosis

Outcomes in vaginal cancer vary by stage at diagnosis, reflecting the size of the tumor and spread of disease. Stage I disease has the most favorable prognosis with survival rates ranging from 70% to 90%, and treatment at this early stage can be curative. Overall, 5-year relative survival rates in vaginal cancer are 67%, 52%, and 19% for localized, regional, and distant disease, respectively. Vaginal melanoma has an extremely poor prognosis with 5-year survival of 15%.

GESTATIONAL TROPHOBLASTIC DISEASE AND GESTATIONAL TROPHOBLASTIC NEOPLASIA

Epidemiology

Gestational trophoblastic disease (GTD) and gestational trophoblastic neoplasia (GTN) are unusual gynecologic conditions as they arise from fetal tissue. GTD is a benign growth of placental tissue arising from an

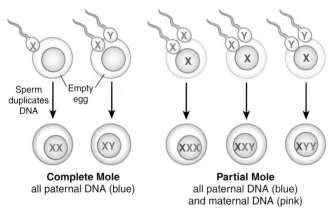

Fig. 61.2 Complete molar pregnancy versus partial molar pregnancy. (Adapted from Ning F, et al. F1000Research 2019;8:428.)

abnormal pregnancy. The frequency is 1:1000 to 1:1500 pregnancies in the United States and 1:125 pregnancies in Asia. Proposed reasons for the regional variation include heredity and dietary differences such as low vitamin A and low animal fat diet in the East. While GTD is considered benign, it may be a precursor to GTN, which is a neoplastic process associated with pregnancy. GTN includes invasive molar pregnancy, choriocarcinoma, placental site trophoblastic tumor (PSTT), and epithelioid trophoblastic tumors (ETT).

Pathology

The term "complete mole" refers to an abnormal pregnancy that contains only paternal DNA. For example, an egg devoid of maternal DNA may be fertilized by one sperm that duplicates or two sperm (most commonly XX or XY, with all paternal DNA). A "partial" mole refers to an egg with maternal DNA that has been fertilized by two sperm (69 XXX, 69 XXY or 69XYY) (Fig. 61.2). An invasive mole is a molar pregnancy that has grown into myometrial tissue. Choriocarcinoma is an aggressive form of cancer that can occur following a normal pregnancy, abortion, or complete molar pregnancy, and is comprised of cytotrophoblast and syncytiotrophoblast. It may be associated with local extension beyond the uterus and metastatic disease. PSTT arises in the placental bed of an antecedent pregnancy and has the pathologic appearance of sheets of intermediate trophoblast invading the myometrial wall of the uterus. ETT is composed of neoplastic chorionic-type intermediate trophoblast. Choriocarcinoma, PSTT, and ETT may occur after molar and nonmolar pregnancies.

Clinical Presentation

The majority of molar pregnancies present with symptoms of bleeding, pain, hyperemesis, and uterine size too large for suspected dates. The pregnancy hormone, human chorionic gonadotropin (hCG), is abnormally elevated in cases of complete molar pregnancy. Pelvic ultrasound usually shows globular vesicles that are pathognomonic for the disease (Fig. 61.3). Other rarer symptoms may include ovarian theca lutein cysts and hyperthyroidism caused by the alpha subunit of hCG mimicking the effects of thyroid stimulating hormone.

Invasive moles typically present with bleeding due to uterine or vaginal disease. GTN may also present with symptoms of hemoptysis (lung disease), abdominal complaints (abdominal disease), or neurologic symptoms (brain disease). Choriocarcinoma often presents with high hCG levels and bleeding metastatic sites. PSTT and ETT can present years after a prior pregnancy and typically have low elevations in hCG levels and a uterine mass on imaging.

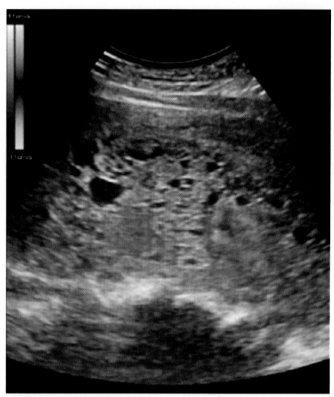

Fig. 61.3 Ultrasound showing classic snowstorm pattern of a complete mole at 24 weeks' gestation. (From J Ultrasound Med 2020;39:597-613.)

Diagnosis and Staging

When clinical presentation and imaging suggest a molar pregnancy, pathologic evaluation of products of conception obtained at time of D&C confirm the diagnosis. Although most patients with molar pregnancy are cured with D&C alone, 20% of patients will have a plateau, increase, or persistence of hCG over time not explained by other causes, which confirms the diagnosis of GTN. When this occurs, a metastatic work-up should be performed including physical exam for vaginal metastasis, chest radiograph, CT imaging of abdomen and pelvis or chest, and consideration of head CT or MRI. Biopsy of GTN is hazardous because these lesions are prone to excessive bleeding; therefore, tissue sampling is not required for diagnosis.

The most commonly used staging systems for GTN are the FIGO staging system, which reflects sites of metastases, and the WHO prognostic scoring system, which takes into account a number of prognostic factors including the patient's age, type and timing of antecedent pregnancy, pretreatment hCG level, tumor size, sites and number of metastases, and chemotherapy treatment. Low-risk metastases include disease in lungs and vagina, while high-risk metastases involve other organs including the brain and liver.

Treatment

The primary treatment of a molar pregnancy is a D&C, followed by weekly monitoring of hCG levels until undetectable. For an invasive mole isolated to the uterus, hysterectomy can be a curative treatment for women who do not wish to preserve fertility. Otherwise GTN is treated with chemotherapy, and regimens are determined by stratifying patients into low-risk and high-risk categories. If no evidence of metastatic disease is identified (low risk), then single agent chemotherapy is administered using methotrexate or dactinomycin. If high-risk metastatic disease is identified, or if disease persists despite single agent treatment, then patients are treated with an aggressive regimen such as the combination of etoposide, methotrexate, dactinomycin, calcium leucovorin, cyclophosphamide, and vincristine (EMA-CO). PSTT and ETT differ in that they are less chemoresponsive and thus are typically treated with hysterectomy and surgical removal of metastatic sites. The use of chemotherapy for PSTT and ETT is controversial.

Prognosis

For patients with low-risk GTN, the cure rate with single agent chemotherapy is nearly 100%. Cure rates with metastatic disease depend on the site of disease. Survival rates for lung, brain, and liver metastases are greater than 90%, 70% to 90%, and 40% to 50%, respectively. Prognosis is poor if metastatic PSTT or ETT is identified.

SUGGESTED READINGS

Brown J, Naumann RW, Seckl MJ, Schink J: 15 years of progress in gestational trophoblastic disease: scoring, standardization, and salvage, Gynecol Oncol 144(1):200–207, 2017.

Harkenrider MM, Markham MJ, Dizon DS, et al: Moving forward in cervical cancer—enhancing susceptibility to DNA repair inhibition and damage: NCI clinical trials planning meeting report, J Natl Cancer Inst djaa041, 2020. https://doi.org/10.1093/jnci/djaa041.

Konstantinopoulos PA, Lheureux S, Moore KNL: PARP inhibitors for ovarian cancer: current indications, future combinations, and novel assets in development to target DNA damage repair. American Society of Clinical Oncology Educational Book 40 (April 30, 2020):e116-e131. https://doi.org/10.1200/EDBK_288015.

Liontos M, Kyriazoglou A, Dimitriadis I, et al: Systemic therapy in cervical cancer: 30 years in review, Crit Rev Oncol Hematol 137:9–17, 2019.

McAlpine J, Leon-Castillo A, Bosse T: The rise of a novel classification system for endometrial carcinoma; integration of molecular subclasses, J Pathol 244(5):538–549, 2018.

Wright AA, Bohlke K, Armstrong DK, et al: Neoadjuvant chemotherapy for newly diagnosed, advanced ovarian cancer: society of gynecologic oncology and American society of clinical oncology clinical practice guideline, J Clin Oncol 34(28):3460–3473, 2016.

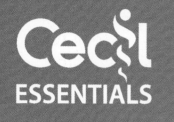

62

Other Solid Tumors (Head and Neck, Sarcomas, Melanoma, Unknown Primary)

Christopher G. Azzoli, Ariel E. Birnbaum, Maria Constantinou, Thomas A. Ollila

INTRODUCTION

Head and neck cancer, melanoma, sarcoma, and carcinoma of unknown primary site (CUP) are distinct malignancies each with its own epidemiology, pathology, treatment, and prognosis. Head and neck cancers and melanoma are more common, and sarcomas and CUP are relatively rare. Recent advances in understanding of the molecular biology of cancer and immune therapies have refined diagnosis and improved treatment for each of these diseases.

HEAD AND NECK CANCER

Definition and Epidemiology

Head and neck cancers are squamous cell carcinomas that arise from the mucosal lining of the oral cavity, oropharynx, hypopharynx, and larynx. Other cancers arising from the head and neck include salivary gland cancers and thyroid cancers. These differ in regard to biology, presentation, natural history, pathology, and therapy.

Head and neck cancer accounts for 4% of new cancer diagnoses in the United States. In 2019, it was estimated that 53,000 patients would be diagnosed with, and 10,860 Americans would die of, head and neck cancer. Historically, tobacco and alcohol have been the strongest risk factors for developing this disease. Over the last 20 years, human papilloma virus (HPV) has been responsible for an increase in the incidence of oropharyngeal squamous cell carcinoma. Patients with HPV-associated oropharyngeal cancer are typically younger than patients with HPV-negative disease, and often have minimal tobacco or alcohol use. Nasopharyngeal squamous cell carcinoma is uncommon in the United States and is distinct from other head and neck cancers given its association with Epstein-Barr virus (EBV).

Pathology

Approximately 95% of all cancers arising from the squamous epithelium of the head and neck are squamous cell carcinomas. Other cancers include mucosal melanoma, adenocarcinomas, and neuroendocrine cancers. Poorly differentiated cancers have a worse prognosis.

The increasingly common HPV-associated oropharyngeal cancers differ in molecular profile from HPV-negative cancers. HPV-negative cancers are associated with mutations in the tumor suppressor gene TP53 and decreased expression of the cell cycle regulatory protein p16-INK4a. HPV-positive cancers display a wild-type TP53 with increased expression of p16-INK4a. P16 expression by immunohistochemistry staining of greater than 70% establishes the diagnosis of HPV-positive disease. Most but not all nasopharyngeal carcinomas are non-keratinizing and associated with EBV infection, which is detected by immunohistochemistry for Epstein-Barr–encoding RNAs (EBER).

Clinical Presentation

The presenting symptoms of head and neck cancer depend on the location of the primary cancer and extent of local disease. Tumors of the nasopharynx can present with a blocked eustachian tube or epistaxis. Oral cavity cancers present with a painful ulcerative lesion. HPV-associated oropharyngeal cancers present with enlarged cervical lymph nodes, often larger than the primary lesion. Laryngeal and hypopharyngeal cancers present with dysphagia and hoarseness.

Diagnosis and Staging

The diagnosis of a squamous cell carcinoma requires a biopsy. A direct laryngoscopy and biopsy is recommended to find the site of origin. Patients who have cervical lymphadenopathy and no apparent primary site require random biopsies of the tongue base and the surrounding tissues and often a tonsillectomy. CT scan, MRI, and positron emission tomography (PET) are used to detect nodal involvement and metastatic disease.

Treatment and Prognosis

Prognosis of head and neck cancer depends on tumor stage. The American Joint Committee of Cancer (AJCC) TNM, 8th edition, incorporates HPV status into its staging system, specifically for the base of tongue and tonsil. Patients with early-stage disease (no cervical lymphadenopathy) have an excellent prognosis. The majority of cancers are diagnosed at the locally advanced stage that has spread to the cervical lymph nodes. Average 5-year survival for all patients is approximately 50%.

Prognosis for HPV-associated disease is usually better. Both biology of disease and comorbidities impact prognosis. HPV-negative patients are at higher risk for developing second primary cancers of the lung and esophagus.

Surgery and radiation therapy are potentially curative treatments for head and neck cancer. Stage IV head and neck cancer may still be cured if all disease can be encompassed by treatment. Chemotherapy by itself is not curative. The combination of chemotherapy and radiation therapy improves rates of cure. The combination is also more toxic than radiation by itself. Choice of treatment is determined by location of the cancer and extent of disease. Locally advanced cancers usually require a combination of surgery, radiation therapy, and chemotherapy. Radiation treatment may be used instead of surgery to preserve organ function. In laryngeal cancer, chemoradiation therapy can be used without the need to remove the larynx. Chemoradiation therapy may permit organ preservation, but it has both acute and chronic toxicity.

Disease that has spread through the blood to distant sites is not curable. Chemotherapy may be used to control the disease and extend life.

A major advance in medical therapy for metastatic head and neck cancer are anti-PD1 immune checkpoint inhibitors (pembrolizumab and nivolumab) that can provide immune-mediated and durable control for a subset of patients. As with other metastatic cancers, enrollment in clinical trials and early integration of palliative care consultants is recommend for optimal patient care.

MELANOMA

Definition and Epidemiology

Melanoma is an aggressive form of skin cancer that originates from melanocytes, a pigment-producing cell found in the basal layer of the epidermis. Melanoma accounts for 1% of all skin cancers but it represents the fifth most common cancer in men and women.

The incidence of melanoma has been rising rapidly over the past five decades. An estimated 96,480 cases of melanoma were diagnosed in the United States in 2019 with approximately 7230 deaths. Melanoma is more common among people aged 65 to 74. Ultraviolet (UV) sun exposure is the main risk factor for development of melanoma.

Individuals with high recreational/intermittent sun exposure, history of blistering sunburns in childhood or adolescence, and exposure to artificial UV radiation from use of tanning beds have a higher risk for developing melanoma. In addition, family history of melanoma and certain phenotypic traits such as fair skin, red/blonde hair, light eyes, the presence of multiple nevi, and atypical or congenital nevi appear to also increase the risk.

Pathology

Melanoma can be classified based on four major histopathologic subtypes: superficial spreading melanoma (SSM), nodular melanoma (NM), lentigo maligna melanoma (LMM), and acral lentiginous melanoma (ALM).

SSM is the most common subtype, representing 70% of all melanomas. It typically affects individuals between the ages of 30 and 50 years. These melanomas spread in a radial growth pattern and develop in intermittently sun-exposed skin, often in a preexisting nevus. It commonly appears on the trunk in males and legs in females. It clinically presents as a flat lesion with irregular borders.

NM accounts for 10% to 15% of all melanomas. It has a vertical growth phase and is usually associated with dermal invasion at the time of diagnosis, hence a worse prognosis. It clinically presents as a deeply pigmented nodule, typically blue-black or polypoid, but 5% of nodular melanomas may be amelanotic (no pigment). It usually develops de novo on the trunk, head, and neck of middle-aged individuals.

LMM accounts for 5% of all melanomas. It affects older individuals with peak incidence in the seventh to eighth decade of life. It originates from a large brown patch on chronically sun-damaged skin (lentigo). Lentigo maligna is associated with slow progression and may evolve for decades before invading into the dermis.

ALM is uncommon and represents less than 5% of all melanomas. It is the most common type seen among Asians and African Americans. The median age of diagnosis is 65. ALM arises on palmar, plantar, and subungual surfaces, the nail matrix being the most common site, and it is not associated with sun exposure. Clinically, it appears as a dark brown to black patch on the palms, soles or under the nails.

Pathologic features that have prognostic relevance include the depth of invasion (Breslow thickness) and the presence of ulceration. Breslow thickness represents the depth of melanoma invasion from the upper epidermal layer. It is measured in mm and it defines the T stage. It is one of the most important prognostic and predictive factors for lymph node involvement. The risk of nodal spread increases with the depth of invasion. The presence of lymph node metastases in melanomas with Breslow thickness less than 0.8 mm is less than 5% and increases to 40% in patients with primary melanomas with Breslow thickness greater than 4 mm.

Another adverse predictor for the development of melanoma metastasis is the presence of microscopic ulceration within the primary site. Patients with ulcerated localized melanoma have a significant decrease in 5 year survival, from 80 to 55%.

Clinical Presentation

Most patients with cutaneous melanoma present with disease confined to the primary site.

Approximately 10% of patients have disease spread to regional lymph nodes, and 4% have distant metastasis at the time of diagnosis. A number of benign lesions share morphologic features with melanoma, making the diagnosis challenging. A lesion that is changing in shape, size, or color should be considered suspicious. Melanomas commonly arise within a preexisting nevus in sun-exposed areas such as the face, upper back, and extremities.

The ABCDE criteria encompass several features that increase the accuracy of skin examination for detection of melanoma: asymmetry (A), border irregularity (B), color change (C), diameter greater than 6 mm (D), and evolution or change (E).

Melanoma can metastasize to regional sites such as the nearby skin, subcutaneous tissue, and lymph nodes or distant sites such as skin, lung, liver, brain, and bone. Regional skin and nodal examination should be performed regularly. Symptoms of advanced disease are highly variable.

Diagnosis and Differential Diagnosis

Pathologic examination with an excisional biopsy is the "gold standard" for diagnosis of melanoma. Such approach allows sufficient depth assessment to ensure that the lesion is not transected at the base of the biopsy. The depth of invasion guides surgical decision making regarding the need for a sentinel lymph node biopsy (sampling the first lymph node that cancer cells are likely to spread to) and the optimal size of resection margin with subsequent excision. If an excisional biopsy cannot be performed, a full-thickness punch biopsy is recommended. Shave biopsies may lead to inadequate sampling and underestimation of the depth of the lesion. The histologic diagnosis is based on characteristic morphology and on immunohistochemical staining for markers such as S100, HMB45, and MART1/Melan A.

In general, imaging investigations for staging purposes are not required for patients with thin (<1 mm) or intermediate-thickness melanoma (1-4 mm). The likelihood of demonstrating metastatic disease is low. Patients with thick melanomas (>4 mm) or lymph node metastasis detected on clinical examination or by sentinel lymph node biopsy are at high risk for disease dissemination and need radiographic staging by CT of the chest, abdomen, and pelvis. Metastasis to the brain is observed in 10% to 40% of melanoma patients and imaging with a brain MRI is warranted for any patient with neurologic symptoms.

Treatment and Prognosis

The prognosis of melanoma can be accurately estimated using the AJCC TNM staging system. Overall survival depends on the thickness of the primary tumor and the presence and number of regional lymph node metastases. Tumor ulceration and high mitotic rate are associated with a poor prognosis. Metastatic disease is incurable, and the clinical course depends on the pattern and extent of dissemination. An elevated serum lactate dehydrogenase (LDH) level is an independent poor prognostic factor for patients with metastases.

Surgery with wide margins is the cornerstone of curative therapy for nonmetastatic disease. The optimal margin depends on the depth of invasion and the location of the primary lesion but is typically between 1 and 2 cm. Biopsy of the sentinel lymph node (first lymph node to which cancer cells are likely to spread) is recommended for all patients with intermediate-thickness melanoma (1-4 mm) and should also be considered in patients with T1b melanomas 0.8 to 1.0 mm or less than 0.8 mm with ulceration. Despite adequate surgical resection of the primary melanoma, 15% to 36% of patients with early-stage melanoma with no lymph node involvement will develop disease recurrence or metastasis.

Patients who are found to have micrometastatic disease to the sentinel node may choose careful observation with routine nodal ultrasonography or immediate complete lymph node dissection. However, studies have shown that immediate completion of lymph node dissection has not shown to improve melanoma-specific survival in this group of patients. All patients with enlarged lymph nodes that test positive for melanoma, in the absence of distant metastasis, should undergo complete lymph node dissection.

Anti–programmed death (PD-1) agents nivolumab and pembrolizumab have recently gained regulatory approval for treating patients with a high risk of recurrence after complete resection—that is, those with lymph node involvement. These monoclonal antibodies are immune checkpoint inhibitors that block negative regulators of T cell immune function, leading to immune system activation. A year of therapy is associated with significantly longer relapse-free survival.

Approximately 50% of cutaneous melanomas have activating mutations of the proto-oncogene *BRAF*, a component of the mitogen-activated protein kinase (MAPK) signaling pathway. The MAPK pathway plays an important role in cell proliferation, differentiation, and apoptosis. BRAF-MEK inhibition with combination dabrafenib plus trametinib therapy is associated with improved clinical benefit and is an alternative adjuvant option for patients whose tumor contains a *BRAF* V600 mutation.

Immunotherapy and kinase inhibitors are the backbone of systemic therapy for patients with metastatic melanoma. Anti-PD1 antibodies and anti-CTLA4 antibodies (ipilimumab) have shown durable responses with improvement in survival. In *BRAF* V600–mutant melanoma, the use of BRAF inhibitors with MEK inhibitors has led to high response rates (70%) and a rapid response to induction and symptom control, with a progression-free survival of approximately 12 months.

Cytotoxic chemotherapy is generally not effective for treatment of metastatic melanoma. Radiation therapy is often used for management of brain metastases or central nervous system symptoms, pain associated with bone metastases, spinal cord compression, and superficial skin and subcutaneous metastases.

SARCOMA

Definition and Epidemiology

Sarcomas are heterogeneous solid tumors of mesenchymal origin, with over 70 different clinicopathologic subtypes. These tumors are broadly categorized as sarcomas of bone or sarcomas of soft tissue. There were expected to be 12,750 new diagnoses of soft tissue sarcoma and 3500 new diagnoses of bone sarcoma in the United States in 2019, causing nearly 7000 deaths. Overall, sarcomas account for fewer than 1% of all new cancer diagnoses in adults; however, they are relatively common in children and represent 15% of all pediatric malignancies.

Most sarcomas are sporadic, but risk factors include prior radiation exposure, chemical carcinogens, and genetic predisposition (familial adenomatous polyposis [FAP] and Li-Fraumeni syndrome). Human herpesvirus 8 (HHV-8) infection is associated with the development of Kaposi's sarcoma. Most genetic abnormalities that define sarcomas are sporadic and not inherited.

Soft tissue sarcomas can be classified by their anatomic site of origin: head and neck, visceral, retroperitoneal, intra-abdominal, and extremity. This categorization is useful for staging, assessing prognosis, and establishing a therapeutic approach. The most common soft tissue sarcomas are gastrointestinal stromal tumors (GISTs), pleomorphic sarcoma, liposarcoma, leiomyosarcoma, and synovial sarcoma. The most commonly encountered sarcomas of bone are the Ewing family of sarcomas, chondrosarcomas, and osteosarcomas.

Clinical Presentation

Given the heterogeneity of this group of diseases, including differences in tumor biology and in anatomic site of origin, the clinical presentation is highly variable. Soft tissue sarcomas of the extremities and of the head and neck usually manifest as a progressively enlarging, often painless, mass. Visceral and intra-abdominal sarcomas including GISTs are often found incidentally and are not symptomatic until they are locally advanced. Symptoms are often nonspecific but may include early satiety, abdominal fullness, bloating, or discomfort. Bone sarcomas, such as Ewing sarcoma and osteosarcoma, typically manifest with pain. The most frequently involved locations are the femur, tibia, and humerus. The physical examination may reveal a palpable mass, which is often tender to palpation. Symptoms may be present for several months before diagnosis. Most patients have locally confined disease at diagnosis. The lungs and bone are the most common sites of metastatic spread.

Diagnosis and Differential Diagnosis

The diagnosis of sarcoma can only be established by histologic confirmation, which requires a tissue biopsy. Large biopsy specimens are often necessary to accurately identify and subclassify sarcoma. Sarcoma must be distinguished from more common malignancies such as lymphoma, melanoma, and poorly differentiated carcinoma. The diagnosis of sarcoma is based on characteristic morphology but may be aided by the use of immunohistochemical and molecular studies.

For example, Ewing sarcoma is often associated with a characteristic reciprocal translocation between chromosomes 11 and 22, t(11:22), resulting in gene rearrangements between the EWS and ETS family of genes. Synovial sarcoma is characterized by a reciprocal t(X;18) translocation resulting in a chimeric SS18-SSX fusion protein. Dozens of other gene rearrangements have been identified such that routine molecular pathology testing is often required to establish a specific diagnosis.

For bone sarcomas, plain films often demonstrate a mixture of lytic and blastic components with associated soft tissue edema. For osteosarcoma, the periosteal reaction produces a "sunburst" appearance as new bone forms at right angles to the tumor, as opposed to the "onion peel" appearance caused by layering of reactive bone, which is more commonly associated with Ewing sarcoma.

Treatment and Prognosis

Surgery is the primary therapy for locally confined disease. Radiotherapy before or after surgery may decrease the likelihood of local recurrence. Chemotherapy may be used in resectable sarcoma for certain histologic subtypes (primarily Ewing sarcoma and osteosarcoma) to improve local control and decrease the risk of distant recurrences; however, whether drugs improve overall survival in resectable sarcoma remains uncertain.

Patients with metastatic sarcoma may occasionally benefit from surgical removal of their disease. However, once metastatic dissemination has been detected, the intent of therapy is primarily to control the disease and not to cure. Chemotherapy can reduce the overall tumor burden and minimize cancer-related symptoms.

Historically, the most active drugs for sarcoma were cytotoxic drugs like doxorubicin, ifosfamide, and gemcitabine. These drugs damage or block production of DNA and inhibit cell division. Newer drugs also block cell division. Trabectedin is a DNA damaging agent used as salvage treatment of metastatic liposarcoma, or leiomyosarcoma. Eribulin is a nontaxane inhibitor of microtubules, which blocks cell division and is used for previously treated liposarcoma.

Other new drugs have diverse mechanisms of action and reflect the diverse biology of sarcoma. Imatinib is a small-molecule tyrosine kinase inhibitor (TKI) that blocks the activity of KIT and is highly active in patients with GISTs, which are commonly driven by KIT mutations. Imatinib is used to control metastatic GIST and also improves survival when combined with surgery in patients with resectable GIST. Pazopanib and regorafenib are multitargeted TKIs that have been tested in patients with soft tissue sarcomas (excluding GIST and liposarcoma). The activity of these drugs is limited, and they provide only a few more months of disease control compared to placebo. Other multitargeted TKIs have limited activity against chondrosarcoma, chordoma, osteosarcoma, and desmoid tumors. A small percentage of sarcomas (less than 1%) have a mutation in the neurotrophic receptor tyrosine kinase (NTRK) gene that responds to TRK inhibitors (larotrectinib, entrectinib).

Currently available immune therapies have only limited activity in the treatment of sarcoma. Single-agent anti-PD1 therapy is rarely effective, except in the 1% of sarcomas that are microsatellite instability-high (MSI-H) or mismatch repair deficient (dMMR). A combination of anti-PD1 and anti-CTLA4 drugs is being developed for unselected patients. There is activity of chimeric antigen receptor (CAR) T cells for the treatment of synovial sarcoma on research protocols, making it one of the first solid tumors to be targeted with cellular immune therapy.

CANCER OF UNKNOWN PRIMARY SITE

Definition and Epidemiology

CUPs occur when a malignancy is identified, but no primary site can be identified following pathology review, complete diagnostic imaging or invasive procedures. Once accounting for 5% to 10% of malignancies, improvements in histopathologic techniques have lessened the frequency of CUPs to 3% to 5% of all malignancies. Patients with CUP tend to be older, with median age 65 to 90 years. CUPs are heterogeneous, with adenocarcinoma, squamous cell carcinoma, neuroendocrine tumors, and poorly differentiated carcinoma all fulfilling criteria. Debate exists as to whether CUPs are simply malignancies where the primary is not found, or if they are truly a separate entity.

Treatment typically includes platinum-based chemotherapy unless a high clinical suspicion for a primary site provides a more specific guide. Molecular profiling suggests that CUP is frequently a result of occult lung, kidney, bladder, or pancreaticobiliary cancer.

Clinical Presentation

Many patients with CUP present with advanced disease. Symptoms can be based upon location of metastatic disease or general nonspecific complaints including fatigue, fevers, anorexia or weight loss. Examples of presenting signs and symptoms can include neurologic deficit from brain or spinal cord metastatic disease, ascites, or general malignancy-associated symptoms such as increased risk for thrombotic events, hypercalcemia, paraneoplastic syndrome or pain. Some patients with CUP present earlier with only mild symptoms, such as an enlarged lymph node or skin lesion. Also, some are found incidentally on imaging performed for another indication.

Diagnosis and Pathology

When considering the origin of a metastatic cancer, it is important to do a thorough history and physical exam, including breast, GU/pelvic, and rectal exam; review of prior malignancies; and available imaging (CT scan of the chest/abdomen/pelvis, which should include neck if there is disease in axillary or supraclavicular lymph nodes). Careful pathologic review of biopsy material is essential. The first step in pathologic evaluation is through immunohistochemistry. Adenocarcinoma constitutes around 70% of CUPs, followed by poorly differentiated carcinoma at 20%, squamous cell carcinoma around 5%, and neuroendocrine carcinoma and other rare subtypes at under 1%. Caution must be used in evaluation of the poorly differentiated carcinomas, because choice of treatment for a specific disease could be radically different. For example, melanoma is typically treated with targeted or immune-based therapy rather than chemotherapy as would be the case for a CUP.

Immunohistochemistry may disclose the site of origin. For example, in the case of poorly differentiated tumors, the presence of S100 and HMB45 supports a diagnosis of melanoma, whereas CD45 supports a diagnosis of lymphoma. Chromogranin and synaptophysin suggest neuroendocrine differentiation. Cytokeratin 5 (CK5) and CK6 are strongly expressed by squamous cell carcinomas, whereas the expression pattern of CK7 and CK20 can limit the differential diagnosis of adenocarcinomas.

Multiple groups have attempted to define genetic and molecular features of CUPs. The success of gene expression profiling to determine the origin of CUP varies widely in published reports, from 33% to nearly 100%, depending on the technique and patient population studied. Gene expression profiling points to biliary tract, urothelial, colorectal, and lung as common sites.

Treatment and Prognosis

Outcomes in CUP remain poor with a median survival of 8 to 12 months. Despite advances in many cancers, survival of CUP patients has not improved in greater than 30 years. Because CUP is typically widespread at time of presentation, treatment is usually palliative rather than curative in intent. There are situations where the histology suggests a favorable type, for example a germ cell tumor and lymphoma, and cure might still be possible. Occasionally CUPs are identified as localized disease, in which case an attempt should be made at definitive treatment.

For example, a woman presenting with adenocarcinoma isolated to unilateral axillary lymph nodes should be evaluated and treated as for a locally advanced breast cancer, even if imaging does not demonstrate a primary breast malignancy. Likewise, a patient with squamous cell carcinoma isolated to cervical lymph nodes at presentation should receive therapy for locally advanced head and neck cancer, again even if a primary lesion is not identified. In both of these circumstances, therapy may prove curative. Another clinical scenario for which specific therapy is beneficial is that of a young man with a poorly differentiated midline chest tumor, in which case a favorable response to a chemotherapy regimen for germ cell cancers may lead to long-term survival.

Whether or not gene expression profiling and next-generation sequencing can improve outcomes remains to be seen. A multicenter phase II trial of 130 patients with gene expression–guided treatment versus empiric carboplatin and paclitaxel in CUP found non–statistically significant inferior outcomes with 1-year survival at 44% in the guided group versus 55% for the empiric group. Despite these results, hope exists that with further study gene expression profiling can offer guidance to improve outcomes.

SUGGESTED READINGS

D'Angelo SP, Melchiori L, Merchant MS, et al: Antitumor activity associated with prolonged persistence of adoptively transferred NY-ESO-1 c259T cells in synovial sarcoma, Cancer Discov 8(8):944–957, 2018.

Drilon A, Laetsch TW, Kummar S, et al: Efficacy of larotrectinib in TRK fusion-positive cancers in adults and children, N Engl J Med 378(8):731–739, 2018.

El Rassy E, Pavlidis N: The current evidence for a biomarker-based approach in cancer of unknown primary, Cancer Treat Rev 67:21–28, 2018.

Hainsworth JD, Rubin MS, Spigel DR, et al: Molecular gene expression profiling to predict the tissue of origin and direct site-specific therapy in patients with carcinoma of unknown primary site: a prospective trial of the Sarah Cannon Research Institute, J Clin Oncol 31(2):217–223, 2013.

Hayashi H, Kurata T, Takiguchi Y, et al: Randomized phase II trial comparing site-specific treatment based on gene expression profiling with carboplatin and paclitaxel for patients with cancer of unknown primary site, J Clin Oncol 37(7):570–579, 2019.

Pollack SM, Ingham M, Spraker MB, Schwartz GK: Emerging targeted and immune-based therapies in sarcoma, J Clin Oncol 36(2):125–135, 2018.

Siegel RL, Miller KD, Jemal A: Cancer statistics, 2019, CA Cancer J Clin 69(1):7–34, 2019.

Tawbi HA, Burgess M, Bolejack V, et al: Pembrolizumab in advanced soft-tissue sarcoma and bone sarcoma (SARC028): a multicentre, two-cohort, single-arm, open-label, phase 2 trial, Lancet Oncol 18(11):1493–1501, 2017.

Wisco OJ, Sober AJ: Prognostic factors for melanoma, Dermatol Clin 30:469–485, 2012.

Zandberg DP, Bhargava R, Badin S, et al: The role of human papillomavirus in nongenital cancers, CA Cancer J Clin 63:57–81, 2013.

63

Complications of Cancer and Cancer Treatment

Pamela Egan, Ari Pelcovits, John Reagan

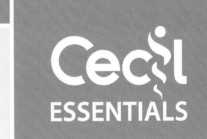

INTRODUCTION

The complications of cancer and its associated treatments are myriad. Although many of these complications require the expert management of hematologists and oncologists, all physicians who may encounter these patients should be prepared to recognize their manifestations and understand both their basic management and indications for specialist referral.

Cancer complications can be localized or systemic (Table 63.1). Cancer treatments, which can include radiation, chemotherapy, and hormonal therapy, have potentially significant side effects and complications. Most are temporary, but some, such as peripheral neuropathy, can become permanent (Table 63.2). Complications from cancer-directed therapy can affect not just quality of life for cancer patients, but can also result in treatment delays or discontinuation, hospitalization, and even death. The management of cancer- and treatment-related complications often requires a multidisciplinary approach. This chapter highlights some important complications of cancer and its treatment.

CANCER-ASSOCIATED THROMBOSIS

Epidemiology

Venous thromboembolism (VTE) is a common complication of cancer and is often its initial presenting event. Approximately 15% of patients with cancer develop VTEs during their illness, and it is a major cause of mortality among cancer patients.

Pathology

The primary drivers of the hypercoagulable state in cancer patients are the procoagulant factors associated with the tumor cells. Other contributing factors include immobilization due to illness, venous compression from tumor and resultant vascular stasis, chemotherapies such as platinum compounds and vascular endothelial growth factor (VEGF) inhibitors, hormonal therapies, and central venous catheters placed for treatment or in the setting of critical illness. Gastric, brain, and pancreas cancers pose the highest risk for development of VTE, but any tumor type can trigger a hypercoagulable state, including blood cancers.

Clinical Presentation

Symptoms and signs that should prompt a work-up for VTE include dyspnea, chest pain, tachycardia, unexplained low-grade fever, calf pain, and swelling of either the upper or lower extremities. Patients may present in either the inpatient or outpatient setting, and even those who are already anticoagulated may still thrombose. VTE may be discovered incidentally on staging scans; these should typically be treated even if asymptomatic.

The Khorana score is a widely used validated risk assessment tool that calculates the risk of developing VTE in cancer patients and may be used to guide consideration of prophylactic anticoagulation in these patients.

Treatment

Treatment of cancer-associated VTE with low-molecular-weight heparin (LMWH) has long been the "gold standard." In a pivotal trial, LMWH was shown to reduce VTE recurrence rate in cancer patients when compared with warfarin. More recently, the direct oral anticoagulants (DOACs) apixaban, edoxaban, and rivaroxaban have been studied in comparison with LMWH in cancer patients. Edoxaban was demonstrated to be noninferior to LMWH in reducing VTE recurrence risk, while apixaban and rivaroxaban were demonstrated to be superior with respect to this outcome. Some DOACs may have more bleeding complications in certain subsets of cancer patients, and the decision to use these agents should be made in consultation with a hematologist. Drug-drug interactions, including certain chemotherapeutic agents, may also preclude the use of DOACs. The duration of anticoagulation depends on the clinical scenario and requires a more nuanced approach than can be detailed here. In general, inferior vena cava (IVC) filters should only be placed if patients have a strong indication for anticoagulation that is contemporaneous with a strong contraindication.

SPINAL CORD COMPRESSION

Epidemiology

Approximately 3% of cancer patients will develop spinal cord compression as a result of their disease. Spinal cord compression is most prevalent in patients with lung and prostate cancers, as well as multiple myeloma.

Pathology

Most cases occur at the level of the thoracic spine, followed by the lumbar, then cervical spine. Spinal cord compression commonly develops when tumor extends from the bone into the epidural space, or as the result of a pathologic fracture. Compression of the spinal cord obstructs venous flow and results in vasogenic edema. When epidural disease occurs below the level of L1-L2 (where the conus medullaris terminates), cauda equina syndrome develops.

Clinical Presentation

The first symptom of spinal cord compression is typically pain. Patients will describe pain that is aggravated in the supine position or during a Valsalva maneuver, and may interfere with sleep. Motor weakness

TABLE 63.1   Complications of Cancer

Localized	Systemic
Brain metastases	Anorexia/cachexia
Cancer-related pain	Cancer-associated thrombosis
Cord compression/cauda equina syndrome	Cancer-related anemia
Malignant effusions	Cancer-related fatigue
Pathologic fractures	Hypercalcemia
Superior vena cava syndrome	Paraneoplastic syndromes
Visceral obstruction	Tumor lysis syndrome

TABLE 63.2   Complications of Cancer Treatment

Alopecia
Central line thrombosis/infections
Cytopenias
Febrile neutropenia
Hot flashes
Hypertension
Nausea and vomiting
Peripheral neuropathy
Secondary malignancies
Skin toxicity
Stomatitis
Tumor lysis syndrome

and sensory deficits, specifically saddle anesthesia, can be present at diagnosis. These symptoms, however, typically herald advanced cord compression and are associated with a lower likelihood of functional recovery. Patients may also present with urinary retention (early) or bowel and bladder incontinence (later).

Diagnosis

A high clinical suspicion for spinal cord compression should develop when patients with known cancer present with any new back pain, and rapidly investigated with spinal imaging. Though plain radiographs of the vertebrae can certainly reveal abnormalities such as lytic lesions or vertebral fractures, time should not be wasted obtaining these studies because negative results in the setting of high clinical suspicion will not rule out spinal cord compression. Magnetic resonance imaging (MRI) is the preferred diagnostic imaging modality and should be obtained unless there is a contraindication to MRI, in which case computed tomography myelography should be performed. Imaging of the full spine is recommended even with localized symptoms because frequently multiple vertebral levels are affected.

Treatment

Dexamethasone and narcotic analgesia are the cornerstones of immediate treatment for cord compression. The optimal dose of corticosteroid is controversial. The most widely accepted dosing of dexamethasone is 10 mg IV followed by 4 to 6 mg IV every 6 hours, although some providers advocate an initial dose as high as 96 mg. This large dose, however, has been demonstrated to result in significant toxicity with questionable benefit.

Surgery and radiation therapy (RT) are the cornerstones of definitive therapy for spinal cord compression. Large randomized studies have demonstrated conflicting evidence about the benefits of surgery followed by RT versus RT alone. Though the presence of neurologic deficits is typically considered to be a clear indication for surgical intervention, goals

of care, patient and tumor characteristics, and other comorbidities factor in to decision making regarding the most appropriate course of therapy.

SUPERIOR VENA CAVA SYNDROME

Definition

Superior vena cava (SVC) syndrome in malignancy is the result of flow obstruction by either external compression or intravascular thrombosis. The superior vena cava is thin walled and therefore easily compressed. The most common malignant causes are lung cancer and lymphoma.

Clinical Presentation

The presenting symptoms and signs of SVC syndrome depend on the rate of vessel obstruction. Slow compression allows for the development of collaterals from the azygos, internal mammary, paraspinous, lateral thoracic, and esophageal venous systems. Of these collateral tributaries the azygos vein is the most important because obstruction below its level is not well tolerated. Symptoms can be sudden or insidious. Most patients experience dyspnea (60% to 70%) and facial or neck swelling (50%). Cough, pain, arm swelling, and dysphagia are less common. Symptoms are frequently positional and exacerbated by leaning forward or lying down. Physical findings may include venous distention of neck and chest wall, facial edema, plethora, cyanosis, and upper extremity edema.

Diagnosis

Plain chest radiographs are usually abnormal; mediastinal widening (64%) and pleural effusion (26%) are the most common findings. The diagnosis is best established with contrast-enhanced computed tomographic scanning of the chest. It demonstrates the location and size of masses, the presence of intravascular thrombosis, and collateral venous drainage. When SVC syndrome is the initial manifestation of malignancy, pathologic diagnosis is the first step in establishing the proper initial treatment modality.

Treatment

The goals of treatment are to alleviate symptoms urgently and to treat the underlying malignancy. General supportive measures include head elevation and administration of glucocorticoids and diuretics. It is essential not to start radiation or glucocorticoids before obtaining a biopsy because these therapies can cloud the pathologic diagnosis. Specific management depends on the underlying pathology. Chemotherapy is the preferred first line of therapy for chemosensitive malignancies such as lymphoma, small cell lung cancer, or germ cell tumors. For non–small cell lung cancers and other less chemosensitive tumors, initial radiation therapy may be preferred.

Symptomatic relief can occur within 2 weeks but is often temporary; therefore, systemic management should be initiated as soon as possible with either chemotherapy, chemoradiation, or surgical resection. Persistent symptoms not relieved by chemotherapy or irradiation and those severe enough to warrant intervention before diagnosis can be successfully managed with endovascular stent placement with or without balloon angioplasty. The treatment of catheter-related SVC syndrome from thrombosis is anticoagulation. The decision regarding catheter removal is case dependent. Typically, catheters may remain in place provided they continue to function without evidence for clot propagation.

HYPERCALCEMIA

Epidemiology

Hypercalcemia complicates cancer in up to 10% of cases, occurring in both hematologic and solid malignancies. The most common etiologies are multiple myeloma, breast cancer, and squamous cell carcinoma.

Pathology

Mechanisms leading to hypercalcemia include osteolysis due to bony involvement or tumor production of parathyroid hormone–related protein (PTHrP), calcitriol, or cytokines. Primary hyperparathyroidism should always be ruled out even in cancer patients. Because most cancer patients also have hypoalbuminemia, calcium levels should either be corrected or ionized calcium levels should be obtained.

Clinical Presentation

Early symptoms of hypercalcemia include altered mental status, constipation, polydipsia, polyuria, nausea, vomiting, and bradycardia. Many patients also have hypovolemia because of the polyuria. The severity of symptoms depends on the time course over which hypercalcemia has developed rather than the absolute calcium level.

Treatment

First and foremost, all calcium supplements, vitamin D, and diuretics should be stopped. Initial aggressive fluid resuscitation with normal saline at 200 to 300 mL/hour should be started to maintain a high urine output. This should be done carefully in patients with compromised cardiac or renal function while loop diuretics can be considered to maintain urine output in all patients who show signs of volume overload.

More definitive treatment for almost all cases of hypercalcemia in cancer patients is centered on bisphosphonates, which inhibit osteoclast activity and bone resorption. Intravenous pamidronate and zoledronic acid are the two most commonly used bisphosphonates. In a pooled analysis, zoledronic acid was associated with a higher rate of calcium normalization and longer control. Calcium response to bisphosphonates can take a few days, so if a rapid reduction in calcium is required then subcutaneous calcitonin (4 units/kg) can be given two to four times daily. Tachyphylaxis occurs with calcitonin so its use should be limited to 48 hours. Calcitonin works by increasing calcium renal excretion and reducing bone resorption. Ultimately, management should eventually include control of the underlying disease, which in the case of myeloma and lymphoma, includes glucocorticoids. Frequently new or recurring hypercalcemia indicates disease progression or treatment resistance and should be addressed with systemic therapy.

FEBRILE NEUTROPENIA

Definition

Febrile neutropenia is another common complication of chemotherapy and is defined as a temperature of 100.4° F sustained over 1 hour, or a one-time reading of 101.0° F in the setting of a neutrophil count lower than 1000/μL. The risk of febrile neutropenia increases with the intensity of the chemotherapy regimen and the severity and duration of neutropenia. It can lead to treatment delays or interruptions, prolonged hospitalizations, decreased quality of life, and increased morbidity and mortality. Febrile neutropenia is a medical emergency and delays in assessment and treatment should be avoided.

Treatment

Although most cases are managed in the hospital, low-risk patients may occasionally be successfully managed as outpatients. The American Society of Clinical Oncology (ASCO) has published guidelines for outpatient management that are based on a risk-stratified scoring system, including the Multinational Association for Supportive Care in Cancer (MASCC) and Clinical Index of Stable Febrile Neutropenia (CISNE) scores. All patients should have a history and physical examination to identify possible focal sources of infection. Attention should be given to the presence of mucositis and to swelling or induration and

erythema around indwelling catheters as possible sources of infection. The initial work-up should include a full chemistry profile, complete blood count with differential, two sets of blood cultures, urinalysis, and chest radiography. ASCO guidelines allow for institutional variation in whether one set of blood cultures should be drawn from central venous access devices.

Prompt initiation of broad-spectrum antibiotics as soon as febrile neutropenia is identified is critical. Empirical antimicrobial therapy should consist of an antipseudomonal β-lactam such as cefepime or piperacillin-tazobactam for patients who require inpatient treatment and a fluoroquinolone for those whose risk profile allows for outpatient therapy. Patients with risk factors for antimicrobial resistance should have their regimens tailored accordingly; for example, vancomycin should be added if the clinical picture is consistent with pneumonia or there is hemodynamic instability. Often, no source is identified; in this case, antibiotics are continued until the neutrophil count exceeds 500 (provided that the fever resolves). When a source has been identified, antibiotic duration is dictated by the standard course for that particular type of infection. Certain high-risk chemotherapeutic regimens include the use of prophylactic myeloid growth factors such as filgrastim or pegfilgrastim to shorten the duration of neutropenia, and with that, the risk of developing febrile neutropenia. Routine use of growth factor support is not recommended in the management of febrile neutropenia in the absence of critical illness because there is little evidence to support its use in this clinical scenario.

CHEMOTHERAPY-INDUCED NAUSEA AND VOMITING

Definition

Nausea and vomiting are common adverse effects of chemotherapy, but prevention and management of this toxicity has evolved significantly in the last 2 decades. Nausea and emesis are typically categorized as acute, delayed, or anticipatory. Acute nausea and vomiting occur during the first 24 hours of treatment, whereas delayed nausea occurs 2 to 5 days after treatment initiation. Patients with high levels of anxiety or prior poor control of nausea may also suffer symptoms in anticipation of starting treatment. The risk of chemotherapy-induced nausea and vomiting is greater in younger patients, women, and those with a history of motion sickness.

Pathology

The mechanism by which chemotherapy induces nausea is complex. Proposed mechanisms involve the transmission of signals from neurotransmitter receptors in the gut to the nucleus tract solitarius, the area postrema, and the central pattern generator (in the brainstem) and involve the neurotransmitters dopamine, serotonin, and substance P.

Treatment

The best approach for treatment is prevention. The prophylactic antiemetic protocol depends on the chemotherapy regimen and emetic risk (Table 63.3). Randomized clinical trials have established that the combination of a neurokinin 1 (NK1) receptor antagonist (aprepitant or fosaprepitant), a 5HT3 serotonin receptor antagonist (ondansetron), olanzapine, and dexamethasone is the regimen of choice for highly emetogenic chemotherapy. For moderately emetogenic chemotherapy, a three-drug regimen of an NK1 receptor antagonist, 5HT3 antagonist with dexamethasone is recommended, although for some regimens just a 5HT3 receptor antagonist and dexamethasone alone may be adequate. All patients should be given a dopamine receptor antagonist such as prochlorperazine or a 5HT3 receptor antagonist

TABLE 63.3 Nausea and Vomiting Risk With Cancer Therapy

Emetic Risk	Percentage of Patients Affected	Representative Agents	Recommended Preventive Antiemetic
High	>90	Cisplatin, high-dose cyclophosphamide	NK1 antagonist + 5HT3 antagonist + olanzapine + dexamethasone
Moderate	30-90	Oxaliplatin, doxorubicin, irinotecan	NK1 antagonist + 5HT3 antagonist + dexamethasone
Low	10-30	Paclitaxel, etoposide, gemcitabine	5HT3 antagonist OR dexamethasone
Minimal	<10	Vincristine, bleomycin	No routine prophylaxis

5HT3, Serotonin receptor; *NK1*, neurokinin 1.

such as ondansetron as rescue therapy for intermittent nausea, and the addition of olanzapine for breakthrough nausea and vomiting is appropriate in some circumstances.

Dexamethasone is the preferred treatment for delayed nausea and vomiting in highly and moderately emetogenic chemotherapy. Anticipatory nausea or vomiting is best treated with proper control of symptoms in the initial cycles. When it occurs, it is best treated with behavioral therapy, and benzodiazepines can be useful as adjunctive therapy.

DERMATOLOGIC TOXICITY

Many chemotherapeutic and targeted agents are associated with dermatologic toxicity, which can lead to patient morbidity, alter quality of life, and affect therapeutic dosing.

Clinical Presentation

Acneiform eruptions are observed with agents targeted against epidermal growth factor receptor (EGFR) in 70% to 80% of patients. The rash is usually erythematous with pustulopapular eruptions over the face, scalp, and upper trunk.

Palmar-plantar erythema, or so-called hand-foot syndrome, is seen with chemotherapeutic agents such as 5-fluorouracil and capecitabine or with tyrosine kinase inhibitors such as sorafenib, sunitinib, and regorafenib. Manifestations can differ slightly between classes of drugs, but they usually involve symmetrical redness of the palms or soles. Tingling and pain may accompany erythema. With progression, painful blistering or skin peeling may occur. Symptoms are frequently observed at pressure areas, such as on the soles of the feet after prolonged standing or running.

Treatment

Treatment of skin rash associated with anti-EGFR therapies is tailored to the severity of the rash and may include topical steroids, oral antibiotics (minocycline or doxycycline), and dose modification or cessation. Sunscreens, reduced sun exposure, and lotions for dry skin should be used for prevention. For hand-foot syndrome, preventive measures such as sunscreens and routine application of lotion to hands and feet are helpful. The most effective treatment is a brief treatment break (typically for several days, until complete resolution occurs), followed by resumption but with a reduced dose of the inciting agent.

TUMOR LYSIS SYNDROME

Definition

Tumor lysis syndrome (TLS) occurs when tumor cells break up and release toxic contents into the blood stream. It most commonly occurs in hematologic malignancies such as acute leukemias and non-Hodgkin's lymphoma, but can occur in almost any malignancy.

It is typically triggered by the initiation of therapy in aggressive malignancies but can occur spontaneously, especially when there is a high tumor burden.

Pathology

Lysis of tumor cells causes the release of intracellular contents, including nucleic acids, potassium, and phosphate, into the bloodstream. The breakdown of nucleic acids results in high levels of uric acid, which can precipitate in the renal tubules and cause acute kidney injury (AKI). High levels of phosphate result in precipitation of calcium phosphate, which can cause symptomatic hypocalcemia, renal tubular injury and cardiac arrhythmias. High levels of potassium can also result in life-threatening cardiac arrhythmias.

Diagnosis

The recognition of patients who are at high risk for TLS should begin before therapy, and most patients in this category are given prophylactic allopurinol before initiation of treatment. The formal diagnosis of TLS is guided by the Cairo-Bishop criteria, which involves identifying both laboratory abnormalities suggestive of TLS (hyperkalemia, hypocalcemia, hyperphosphatemia, and hyperuricemia) and clinical criteria (AKI, cardiac arrhythmia, and seizure). The prompt diagnosis of TLS is critical to treatment and prevention of life-threatening electrolyte disturbances.

Treatment

Treatment involves aggressive hydration and meticulous management of electrolyte abnormalities. Patients are given 2 to 3 L of normal saline over 24 hours, which is sometimes augmented with loop diuretics to increase urine output. Allopurinol, if not given as a preventative measure, is given at a dose of 300 mg daily. If uric acid rises above 8, or is rapidly rising, rasburicase is given for a reduction in serum uric acid levels, although the magnitude of benefit with respect to preservation of renal function has not been solidly established. Most patients with a diagnosis of TLS require close monitoring, with laboratory checks three to four times a day and telemetry monitoring for cardiac arrhythmias, and sometimes require ICU level of care.

IMMUNE CHECKPOINT INHIBITOR TOXICITY

Definition

The use of recently discovered checkpoint inhibitors (e.g., pembrolizumab, nivolumab) is radically changing prognosis and treatment for several malignancies. With these new drugs, however, has also come new immunotherapy-induced toxicity. These are almost all related to an autoimmune-like response induced by these medications, resulting in inflammation of various organ systems. These include colitis, hepatitis, pneumonitis, dermatitis, encephalitis, and hypophysitis (panhypopituitarism).

Pathophysiology

Immune checkpoint inhibitors work by "releasing the brakes" on the immune system imposed by cancer cells. Co-stimulatory cell surface antigens such as PD-1/PDL-1 and CTLA-4, needed for activation of the immune system, are often downregulated by tumor cell surface markers. Immunotherapy reactivates the immune system, removing the tumor blockades and allowing the body's own immune system to attack the tumor cells. In doing so, the immune system may be mobilized indiscriminately, resulting in its activation not only against the cancer but also against the patient's own healthy tissue.

Diagnosis

Immune-mediated toxicity should be considered in all patients on immunotherapy presenting with symptoms consistent with immune-mediated phenomena. These include diarrhea (colitis), shortness of breath or cough (pneumonitis), rash (dermatitis), or altered mentation (encephalitis). In addition, patients are also monitored for laboratory evidence of hepatitis and hypophysitis (most specifically hypothyroidism). These signs and symptoms can be mild and treated symptomatically, but on rare occasions can be life-threatening.

Treatment

Patients with mild signs and symptoms can often be treated symptomatically while remaining on the medication, or with a brief interruption in treatment, which can be restarted once signs and symptoms have resolved. Patients with findings of hypothyroidism can be started on thyroid hormone replacement without need for immune checkpoint discontinuation. In more severe cases, such as with new oxygen requirement, severe diarrhea, or significant elevations in liver function tests (LFTs), the immunotherapy needs to be discontinued and patients should be started on corticosteroids to try to decrease the inflammatory response, typically at doses of 1 to 2 mg/kg of methylprednisolone (or its equivalent) per day. In rare cases of severe toxicity, immunomodulatory medication such as mycophenolate mofetil or infliximab is utilized in addition to corticosteroids. In most cases, expert consultation should be obtained to guide the management of these toxicities.

For a deeper discussion on this topic, please see Chapter 73, ❖ "Thrombotic Disorders: Hypercoagulable States," Chapter 232, "The Parathyroid Glands, Hypercalcemia, and Hypocalcemia," and Chapter 372, "Mechanical and Other Lesions of the Spine, Nerve Roots, and Spinal Cord," in *Goldman-Cecil Medicine*, 26th Edition.

SUGGESTED READINGS

Hesketh P, Kris MG, Basch E, et al: Antiemetics: american society of clinical oncology clinical practice guideline update, J Clin Oncol 35(28):3240–3261, 2017.

Howard SC, Jones DP, Pui CH: The tumor lysis syndrome, N Engl J Med 364:1844–1854, 2011.

Kraaijpoel N, Carrier M: How I treat cancer-associated venous thromboembolism, Blood 133:291–298, 2019.

Lawton AJ, Lee KA, Cheville AL, et al: Assessment and management of patients with metastatic spinal cord compression: a multidisciplinary review, J Clin Oncol 37(1):61–71, 2019.

Postow MA, Sidlow R, Hellmann MD: Immune-related adverse events associated with immune checkpoint blockade, N Eng J Med 378:158, 2018.

Taplitz R, Kennedy EB, Bow EJ, et al: Outpatient management of fever and neutropenia in adults treated for malignancy: American Society of Clinical Oncology and Infectious Diseases Society of America Clinical Practice Guideline Update, J Clin Oncol 36(14):1443–1453, 2018.

Endocrine Disease and Metabolic Disease

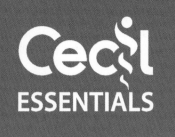

64

Hypothalamic-Pituitary Axis

Diana Maas, Jenna Sarvaideo

ANATOMY AND PHYSIOLOGY

The pituitary gland sits in the skull base in a bony structure called the sella turcica. It weighs approximately 600 mg and is composed of three lobes, the adenohypophysis (anterior lobe), the neurohypophysis (posterior lobe), and the intermediate lobe. The intermediate lobe regresses in humans at about 15 weeks' gestation and is absent in the adult normal pituitary gland. The infundibular stalk, which contains the portal plexus circulation, connects the hypothalamus to the pituitary gland. The pituitary gland is surrounded by important structures that can be compromised by its enlargement, including the optic chiasm, located superior to the gland, and the cavernous sinuses, located on both sides of the gland. The cavernous sinuses each contain the internal carotid artery and cranial nerves III, IV, V1, V2, and VI (Fig. 64.1).

The anterior pituitary gland produces six hormones that are produced by specific cell types within the gland: adrenocorticotropic hormone (ACTH), follicle-stimulating hormone (FSH), luteinizing hormone (LH), growth hormone (GH), prolactin (PRL), and thyroid-stimulating hormone (TSH or thyrotropin). These hormones are regulated by stimulatory and inhibitory peptides produced within the hypothalamus and are transported to the anterior pituitary gland by the infundibular portal system. The posterior pituitary gland makes up about 20% of the total pituitary mass and stores and secretes two major peptide hormones: vasopressin (AVP or antidiuretic hormone) and oxytocin. These neurohypophyseal hormones are synthesized by the supraoptic and paraventricular nuclei of the hypothalamus and transported to the posterior lobe in neurosecretory granules along the supraopticohypophyseal tract (Table 64.1).

On imaging studies, the normal adult pituitary gland has a flat superior border and a vertical height of approximately 8 to 10 mm. The anterior pituitary is homogeneous in signal on magnetic resonance imaging (MRI), the preferred imaging method, and enhances homogeneously after intravenous administration of a contrast agent (see Fig. 64.1). The posterior pituitary lobe is distinguished from the anterior lobe on T1-weighted MRI as a bright spot in the posterior aspect of the gland, best seen on a sagittal view. The bright appearance is thought to result from the presence of AVP and/or phospholipid vesicles within the normal neurohypophysis.

PITUITARY TUMORS

Pituitary tumors account for approximately 10% to 15% of intracranial tumors. They are the most common tumors in the sella, accounting for more than 90% of masses that develop in that area, and they are usually benign. Their true incidence is difficult to determine because they are often asymptomatic, but the prevalence is about 10% to 20% in radiologic studies. Most pituitary tumors are slow growing, but some have higher growth rates and can be invasive. Pituitary carcinomas are very

rare and are defined by the presence of a metastasis that is noncontiguous with the original tumor, or cerebrospinal fluid dissemination.

Pituitary tumors are classified by size and secretory capacity. Tumors that are smaller than 10 mm in diameter are called *microadenomas*, whereas lesions 10 mm or larger are called *macroadenomas*. Hormone-producing tumors are called *secretory adenomas,* and those that do not secrete a hormone are known as *nonsecretory adenomas*. Pituitary tumors may be composed of any of the anterior pituitary cell types, with multiple cell types forming plurihormonal tumors. Prolactin-secreting pituitary tumors are the most common type. Table 64.2 reviews the prevalence of the various pituitary tumors, and Table 64.3 describes the screening tests used to determine the secretory status of a new pituitary tumor.

The clinical manifestations of pituitary tumors are usually signs and symptoms caused by hormone overproduction or underproduction or mass effect. Common clinical features of pituitary mass effect include headaches, visual field defects, and cranial nerve palsies. Superior extension of a tumor compresses the optic chiasm, causing bitemporal hemianopsia; lateral extension into the cavernous sinuses results in ophthalmoplegia, diplopia, or ptosis due to compression of cranial nerves III, IV, or VI or facial pain due to compression of V1 or V2. Compromise of normal pituitary tissue by a tumor can cause hormone loss or hypopituitarism. Screening tests for and causes of pituitary hormone deficiency are shown in Tables 64.3 and 64.4, respectively.

DISORDERS OF ANTERIOR PITUITARY HORMONES

Prolactin
Definition and Epidemiology

The mature prolactin polypeptide contains 199 amino acids and is formed after a 28-amino-acid signal peptide is proteolytically cleaved from the prolactin prohormone (pre-prolactin). Prolactin synthesis and secretion by pituitary lactotrophs is under tonic inhibitory control by hypothalamic-derived dopamine, which keeps prolactin at its basal levels. Factors stimulating prolactin synthesis and secretion, in addition to reduced dopamine availability to the lactotrophs, include thyrotropin-releasing hormone (TRH), estrogen, vasoactive intestinal polypeptide (VIP), AVP, oxytocin, and epidermal growth factor.

Prolactin levels physiologically increase during pregnancy. After delivery, prolactin induces and maintains lactation of the breast. Hyperprolactinemia, regardless of the etiology, can cause hypogonadism through its inhibitory effect on gonadotropin release, infertility, galactorrhea, and/or bone loss from the hypogonadism.

Prolactinomas and hyperprolactinemia are more common in women, with a peak prevalence between 25 and 35 years of age. The mean prevalence of patients medically treated for hyperprolactinemia is approximately 20 per 100,000 in men and approximately 90 per 100,000 in women. Prolactinomas are rare in childhood or adolescence.

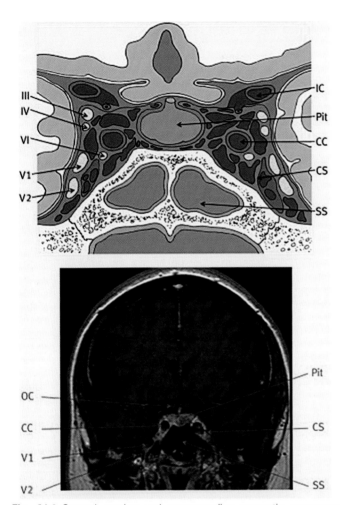

Fig. 64.1 Coronal section and corresponding magnetic resonance imaging scan of the pituitary gland and surrounding structures, including cranial nerves III (oculomotor), IV (trochlear), V1 (trigeminal, ophthalmic branch), V2 (trigeminal, maxillary branch), and VI (abducens). *CC,* Carotid artery (intracavernous); *CS,* cavernous sinus (left); *IC,* internal carotid artery; *OC,* optic chiasm; *Pit,* pituitary gland; *SS,* sphenoid sinus. (From Jesurasa A, Kailaya-Vasan A, Sinha S: Surgery for pituitary tumors, Surgery 29:428-433, 2011, Figure 1.)

Clinical Presentation

The clinical presentation of a prolactinoma varies with the age and gender of the patient. Typically, the patient is a young woman with menstrual irregularities, galactorrhea, and infertility. Galactorrhea occurs in 50% to 80% of affected women. Men may report a decrease in libido and erectile dysfunction as a result of hypogonadism caused by reduced secretion of LH and FSH. Typically, however, their tumors are diagnosed after symptoms of tumor compression appear, including headache, neurologic deficits, and vision changes. Galactorrhea and gynecomastia are rare in men. Because of the early presentation of menstrual irregularities in women, microprolactinomas are more common in women; macroprolactinomas are more frequent in men and in postmenopausal women.

Diagnosis and Differential Diagnosis

Hyperprolactinemia is diagnosed by a serum prolactin above the upper limit of normal. This can be drawn at any time of day. For prolactinomas, serum prolactin levels typically parallel tumor size. A prolactin level greater than 250 ng/mL is usually diagnostic of a prolactinoma,

but smaller prolactinomas may have lower levels. Dynamic testing is not needed to diagnose hyperprolactinemia.

Two types of artifacts can occur during the standard measurement of prolactin: the presence of macroprolactin and the hook effect. When a patient with mild hyperprolactinemia does not have the expected clinical features of hyperprolactinemia (e.g., galactorrhea, menstrual disturbance, infertility), one should consider the presence of macroprolactin. Macroprolactin is a polymeric form of prolactin that is biologically inactive. Most commercially available prolactin assays do not detect macroprolactin, but it can be detected inexpensively in the serum by polyethylene glycol precipitation. The estimated incidence of macroprolactin accounting for a significant proportion of hyperprolactinemia is 10% to 20%. The hook effect should be considered in a patient who has a very large pituitary mass and only a mild elevation in prolactin. The hook effect is an assay artifact that occurs when very high serum prolactin concentrations saturate antibodies in the standard two-site immunoradiometric assay, resulting in falsely low levels. This artifact can be overcome by repeating the prolactin measurement on a 1:100 serum sample dilution.

Physiologic increases in prolactin occur with pregnancy, physical or emotional stress, exercise, and chest wall stimulation. Mild to moderate hyperprolactinemia (25 to 200 ng/mL) in the presence of a larger pituitary mass is more likely to be caused by a non–prolactin-secreting tumor with infundibular stalk compression and inhibition of dopamine transport to the lactotroph. Other common causes for hyperprolactinemia are shown in Table 64.5. Some drugs such as metoclopramide and risperidone can increase prolactin to greater than 200 ng/mL.

Treatment and Prognosis

Medical management with a dopamine agonist—bromocriptine or cabergoline—is the recommended treatment. The dopamine agonists normalize prolactin, decrease tumor size, and restore gonadal function in more than 80% of patients with prolactinomas. Because of the rapidity and efficacy of the dopamine agonists in treating these tumors, they are also the initial treatment for macroprolactinomas that have caused compromise in vision, neurologic deficits, or pituitary dysfunction.

Cabergoline, the newer agent, is preferred to other dopamine agonists because it has higher efficacy in normalizing prolactin levels and shrinking tumor size and has fewer side effects. The most common side effects seen with dopamine agonists are nausea, vomiting, orthostatic lightheadedness, dizziness, and nasal congestion. Because of the concern for cabergoline-related cardiac valvulopathy that was reported in patients who had Parkinson's disease treated with higher doses of cabergoline than used in prolactinomas, baseline echocardiogram and regular cardiac auscultation is recommended in patients taking greater than 2 mg weekly. Transsphenoidal resection of the tumor is indicated for patients who cannot tolerate the dopamine agonists or who do not respond to medical treatment. No treatment is required for patients who have microprolactinomas that are asymptomatic.

Studies have shown that dopamine agonists may be safely withdrawn in patients who have maintained normal prolactin levels for 2 years and who have no visible tumor on low doses of dopamine agonist. Once the dopamine agonist is discontinued, prolactin levels should be checked every 3 months for 1 year and then annually. An MRI should be obtained only if the prolactin level becomes elevated again. Recurrence risk after drug withdrawal ranges from 26% to 69% and is predicted by the initial prolactin level and tumor size.

TABLE 64.1 Pituitary–Target Organ Hormone Axis

Hypothalamic Hormone	Pituitary Target Cell	Pituitary Hormone Affected	Peripheral Target Gland	Peripheral Hormone Affected
Stimulatory				
Anterior Lobe of Pituitary Gland				
Thyrotropin-releasing hormone (TRH)	Thyrotroph	Thyroid-stimulating hormone (TSH)	Thyroid gland	Thyroxine (T_4) Triiodothyronine (T_3)
Growth hormone-releasing hormone (GHRH)	Somatotroph	Growth hormone (GH)	Liver	Insulin-like growth factor-I (IGF-I)
Gonadotropin-releasing hormone (GnRH)	Gonadotroph	Luteinizing hormone (LH)	Ovary Testis	Progesterone Testosterone
		Follicle-stimulating hormone (FSH)	Ovary Testis	Estradiol Inhibin
Corticotropin-releasing hormone	Corticotroph	Adrenocorticotrophic hormone (ACTH)	Adrenal gland	Cortisol
Posterior Lobe of Pituitary Gland				
Vasopressin (AVP)			Kidney	
Oxytocin			Uterus Breast	
Inhibitory				
Somatostatin	Somatotroph Thyrotroph	Growth hormone (GH) Thyroid stimulating hormone (TSH)	Liver Thyroid	IGF-I T_4 and T_3
Dopamine	Lactotroph	Prolactin (PRL)	Breast	

TABLE 64.2 Prevalence of Pituitary Tumors

Tumor	Prevalence (%)
Prolactin-secreting adenomas	40-45
Gonadotropin-secreting adenomas	20
Growth hormone–secreting adenomas	10-15
Adrenocorticotrophic hormone–secreting adenomas	10-15
Null cell adenomas	5-10
Thyroid-stimulating hormone–secreting adenomas	1-2

TABLE 64.3 Biochemical Tests for Pituitary Disorders

Disorder	Tests
Pituitary Tumor	
GH-secreting adenomas	IGF-I
	OGTT: measure blood sugar and GH (0, 60, 120 min)
PRL-secreting adenomas	Basal serum prolactin
ACTH-secreting adenomas	24-hr urine-free cortisol and creatinine level
	1-mg overnight dexamethasone suppression test
	11 PM salivary cortisol
	Serum ACTH
TSH-secreting adenomas	Serum TSH, Free T_4, Free T_3, alpha subunit
Gonadotropin-secreting adenomas	FSH, LH, alpha subunit estradiol (women), testosterone (men)
Hypopituitarism	
GH deficiency	IGF-I
	Glucagon stimulation test
	Arginine-GHRH (GHRH not available in the United States)
	Arginine-L-DOPA
	ITT
Gonadotropin deficiency	Women: basal estradiol, LH, FSH
	Men: 8 AM fasting testosterone (total; free), LH, FSH
TSH deficiency	Serum TSH, free T_4
ACTH deficiency	8 AM fasting ACTH and cortisol
	Cosyntropin-stimulation test (1 μg and 250 μg)

ACTH, Adrenocorticotropic hormone; *CRH,* corticotropin-releasing hormone; *FSH,* follicle-stimulating hormone; *GH,* growth hormone; *GHRH,* growth hormone-releasing hormone; *IGF-I,* insulin-like growth factor-I; *ITT,* insulin tolerance test; *LH,* luteinizing hormone; *OGTT,* oral glucose tolerance test; *PRL,* prolactin; T_4, thyroxine; *TFT,* thyroid function test; *TSH,* thyroid-stimulating hormone.

Growth Hormone

Definition

GH is a single-chain polypeptide hormone consisting of 191 amino acids that is synthesized, stored, and secreted by the anterior pituitary somatotrophs. GH secretion is regulated by two factors derived from the hypothalamus: growth hormone–releasing hormone (GHRH) and somatostatin. GHRH stimulates somatotroph GH release, and somatostatin inhibits it. GH stimulates secretion of insulin-like growth factor-I (IGF-I) by the liver. IGF-I circulates in the blood attached to binding proteins; although there are six binding proteins in serum, more than 80% of IGF-I is bound to a protein called IGFBP3. Postnatally and through puberty, GH and IGF-I are critical in determining longitudinal skeletal growth, skeletal maturation, and bone mass. In adulthood, they are instrumental in the maintenance of skeletal architecture and bone mass. GH also has effects on the metabolism of carbohydrates, lipids, and proteins by antagonizing insulin action, increasing lipolysis and free fatty acid production, and increasing protein synthesis.

Growth Hormone Deficiency

Epidemiology. Childhood-onset GH deficiency is most commonly idiopathic, but it may be genetic or associated with congenital anatomic malformations in the brain or sellar region. The most common cause of GH deficiency in adults is a pituitary macroadenoma and its treatment;

TABLE 64.4 Causes of Pituitary Hormone Deficiency

Causes	Examples
Sellar masses	Pituitary macroadenomas, craniopharyngiomas
Treatment of sellar, parasellar, and hypothalamic tumors	Pituitary/hypothalamic surgery, radiotherapy, radiosurgery (gamma knife)
Infiltrative diseases	Lymphocytic hypophysitis, hemochromatosis, sarcoidosis
Trauma	Head injury, perinatal trauma
Vascular	Sheehan syndrome, pituitary apoplexy
Medications	Opiates, glucocorticoids
Infections	Fungal, tuberculosis
Genetic	Combined or isolated pituitary hormone deficiencies
Developmental	Pituitary hypoplasia or aplasia, midline cerebral and cranial malformations
Empty sella	

TABLE 64.5 Causes of Hyperprolactinemia

Causes	Examples
Medications	Methyldopa, estrogens, metoclopramide, domperidone, neuroleptics and antipsychotics
Hypothalamic-infundibular stalk damage	Infiltrative disorders (sarcoidosis), brain irradiation, trauma, surgery, tumors
Pituitary	Prolactinomas, non-PRL-secreting pituitary macroadenomas with stalk compression
Medical	Renal failure, primary hypothyroidism

deficiency of one or more pituitary hormones occurs in 30% to 60% of such cases. The incidence of hypopituitarism 10 years after irradiation of the sellar region is approximately 50%.

Clinical presentation. Children with GH deficiency exhibit growth retardation, short stature, and fasting hypoglycemia. Manifestations of adult GH deficiency include reduced bone density, decreased muscle strength and exercise performance, decreased lean body mass with increase in fat mass and abdominal adiposity, glucose intolerance and insulin resistance, abnormal lipid profile including elevated low-density lipoprotein (LDL) and triglyceride levels with decreased high-density lipoprotein (HDL), depressed mood, and impaired psychosocial well-being.

Diagnosis and differential diagnosis. Because of the pulsatile nature of pituitary GH secretion, a single random measurement of serum GH is not helpful to diagnose GH deficiency. In adults with GH deficiency due to a pituitary tumor and concomitant hypopituitarism involving any three other pituitary hormones, a low IGF-I level is sufficient to diagnose GH deficiency, and provocative testing is not warranted. Falsely low IGF-I levels are seen in malnutrition, acute illness, celiac disease, poorly controlled diabetes mellitus, and liver disease. In children, there tends to be greater variation in IGF-I levels that do not correspond to the true GH status, so provocative testing is required.

The historical "gold standard" stimulatory test is insulin-induced hypoglycemia (insulin tolerance test or ITT). Symptomatic hypoglycemia with a serum glucose level lower than 45 mg/dL is a potent stimulus for GH secretion; the normal GH response is greater than 10 ng/mL in children and greater than 5 ng/mL in adults. Because of the unavailability in the United States of GHRH, which is as sensitive and specific as the ITT in stimulating GH secretion, glucagon stimulation is being used, especially in adults with ischemic heart disease or seizures. A normal adult response with the glucagon stimulation test is defined

as a GH peak greater than 3 ng/mL for those with normal weight, but in obese patients, a cutoff of 1 ng/mL is used.

Treatment and prognosis. The US Food and Drug Administration (FDA) has approved recombinant human growth hormone (hGH) in both the adult and pediatric populations. It is used in conditions involving complete absence of GH associated with severe growth retardation or partial GH deficiency resulting in short stature. Short stature is defined as height more than 2.5 standard deviations below the mean for age-matched normal children, growth velocity less than the 25th percentile, delayed bone age, and predicted adult height less than the mean parental height. Other conditions approved by the FDA to use hGH include Turner syndrome, Prader-Willi syndrome, chronic kidney disease, AIDS-associated muscle wasting, *SHOX* gene deficiency, Noonan syndrome, and children born small for gestational age. Combined clinical evaluations, along with an inadequate pituitary GH response to provocative testing, are used in the assessment of childhood GH deficiency. Higher doses of GH are recommended for children without GH deficiency disorders or with partial GH deficiency.

In adults, hGH is administered as a daily subcutaneous injection starting at 0.1 to 0.3 mg, with dose increases at 6-week intervals based on clinical response, side effects, and IGF-I levels. Absolute contraindications to hGH therapy in adults include active neoplasm, intracranial hypertension, and proliferative diabetic retinopathy; uncontrolled diabetes and untreated thyroid disease are relative contraindications. Side effects of hGH therapy are usually transient and include arthralgias, fluid retention, carpal tunnel syndrome, and glucose intolerance. Additional side effects in children include slipped capital femoral epiphysis and hydrocephalus.

Acromegaly or Growth Hormone Hypersecretion

Definition and epidemiology. Acromegaly is literally translated as abnormal enlargement of the extremities of the skeleton. It is caused by hypersecretion of GH in adulthood. In children, excessive GH secretion before closure of the epiphyseal growth plate leads to gigantism. In both cases, the cause is almost always a GH-secreting pituitary tumor. Approximately 30% of GH-secreting pituitary adenomas are bihormonal and also secrete prolactin. The incidence of acromegaly is about 2 to 4 per million population, and the mean age at diagnosis is 40 to 50 years. GH-secreting tumors are caused by a clonal expansion of pure somatotrophs or mixed somatomammotrophs. A variety of genetic abnormalities can be found in GH-secreting pituitary adenomas including McCune-Albright syndrome, multiple endocrine neoplasia type 1 and 4, Carney complex, and familial isolated pituitary adenoma.

TABLE 64.6 Clinical Features of Acromegaly

Change	Manifestations
Somatic Changes	
Acral changes	Enlarged hands and feet
Musculoskeletal changes	Arthralgias
	Prognathism
	Malocclusion
	Carpal tunnel syndrome
Skin changes	Sweating
	Skin tags
	Nevi
Colon changes	Polyps
	Carcinoma
Cardiovascular symptoms	Cardiomegaly
	Hypertension
Visceromegaly	Tongue
	Thyroid
	Liver
Endocrine-Metabolic Changes	
Reproduction	Menstrual abnormalities
	Galactorrhea
	Decreased libido
Carbohydrate metabolism	Impaired glucose tolerance
	Diabetes mellitus
	Insulin resistance
Lipids	Hypertriglyceridemia

Clinical presentation. Acromegaly is a rare disease, and the rate of change of symptoms and signs is slow and insidious. The usual period from earliest onset of symptoms and signs to diagnosis is 8 to 10 years, during which time many patients undergo medical and surgical treatments for many of the metabolic abnormalities and morbidities caused by GH excess. Characteristic clinical findings of this disease include physical changes of the bone and soft tissue and multiple endocrine and metabolic abnormalities (Table 64.6).

Diagnosis and differential diagnosis. Measurement of serum IGF-I can be used to diagnose excess GH in most patients with acromegaly. An alternative is an oral glucose tolerance test using a 75 g glucose load. Normally, glucose suppresses GH levels to less than 1 ng/mL after 2 hours; in patients with acromegaly, GH levels may paradoxically increase, remain unchanged, or decrease but not below 1 ng/mL. Most acromegalic patients have GH-secreting pituitary tumors, and approximately 70% of cases of acromegaly present with pituitary macroadenomas. Rarely, GH hypersecretion is caused by ectopic GHRH-secreting tumors, including hypothalamic hamartomas and gangliocytomas, pancreatic islet cell tumors, small cell carcinoma of the lung, carcinoid, adrenal adenomas, and pheochromocytomas. Ectopic GH secretion has also been reported in pancreatic, lung, and breast cancers.

Treatment and prognosis. Treatment of acromegaly requires both treatment of the tumor and normalization of GH and IGF-I levels, along with management of the comorbidities and metabolic abnormalities caused by the excess GH. Treatment often requires the use of multiple modalities to achieve adequate control of the disease. Primary therapy is almost always transsphenoidal surgery, with the cure rate being directly proportional to tumor size. Patients with intrasellar microadenomas have a 75% to 95% cure rate with surgery.

In patients with noninvasive macroadenomas, surgical removal results in normalization of GH and IGF-I in 40% to 68% of patients.

Approximately 40% to 60% of tumors are not controlled with surgery alone because of cavernous sinus invasion or intracapsular intra-arachnoid invasion. Additional treatment options include primary medical therapy or primary surgical debulking of the tumor followed by medical therapy for hormonal control and/or radiation therapy for treatment of residual tumor. Conventional radiotherapy can normalize GH and IGF-I levels in more than 60% of patients, but the maximum response takes 10 to 15 years to achieve. Focused single-dose gamma knife radiotherapy has a 5-year remission rate of 29% to 60%. Hypopituitarism is seen in more than 50% of patients within 5 to 10 years after radiotherapy.

Currently, three drug classes are used to treat acromegaly: dopamine agonists, somatostatin receptor ligands (SRLs) such as octreotide, lanreotide, and pasireotide, and GH receptor antagonists. SRLs work mainly through the somatostatin receptor subtypes 2 and 5 (except pasireotide works through receptor subtypes 1, 2, 3, and 5), causing a decrease in tumor GH secretion. In acromegaly, SRLs are indicated for first-line treatment when there is low probability of surgical cure, after a failed surgical cure of GH hypersecretion, and to provide GH and IGF-I control while waiting for radiotherapy to achieve its maximum effect. SRLs reduce GH and IGF-I levels to normal in 40% to 65% of patients and shrink tumor size in approximately 50% of cases. Side effects of SRLs include diarrhea, abdominal cramping, flatulence, and cholelithiasis (15%).

Pegvisomant is the only GH receptor antagonist available. It works by blocking the peripheral action of GH through blockade of the GH receptors located on the liver. Pegvisomant is indicated for patients who have persistent elevation in IGF-I even with maximum doses of SRLs. This drug is highly effective in the treatment of acromegaly and normalizes IGF-I levels in 97% of patients; transient elevation in liver function enzymes is seen in 25% of those treated and tumor growth in fewer than 2%. After starting pegvisomant, GH levels are often elevated and are no longer helpful in guiding treatment.

Cabergoline is the most efficacious of the dopamine agonists for treatment of acromegaly, but it is effective in fewer than 10% of patients, working best in bihormonal PRL and GH-secreting tumors.

Thyroid-Stimulating Hormone

Definition

TSH is a glycoprotein secreted from the thyrotroph cells of the anterior pituitary. It is composed of alpha and beta subunits with the beta subunit giving its specific biological activity. Its release is regulated by TRH (stimulatory) and somatostatin (inhibitory). In addition, it is subject to the negative feedback of thyroid hormones released from the thyroid gland. Assessment of the pituitary-thyroid axis requires checking levels of TSH as well as thyroid hormones released by the thyroid gland (i.e., thyroxine [T_4] and triiodothyronine [T_3]).

Deficiency of TSH

Definition and epidemiology. Deficiency of TSH leads to secondary hypothyroidism. The diminished secretion of TSH from the pituitary provides inadequate stimulation to the thyroid gland for thyroid hormone release. The estimated prevalence of TSH deficiency is about 1 in 80,000 to 120,000 individuals. The more common causes of TSH deficiency are found in Table 64.4, listing causes of hypopituitarism.

Clinical presentation. The usual signs and symptoms of hypothyroidism are weight gain, fatigue, cold intolerance, and constipation. If the condition is caused by an underlying sellar tumor, symptoms of mass effect may also be present, depending on the size of the tumor.

Diagnosis and differential diagnosis. Secondary hypothyroidism is characterized by low levels of free T_4 along with low or inappropriately normal TSH. The differential diagnosis includes euthyroid sick syndrome, which is often seen in the setting of an acute illness. This syndrome does not require any intervention, and the laboratory results normalize on repeat testing after resolution of the acute illness.

Treatment and prognosis. Management focuses on replacement of the thyroid hormones, as in primary hypothyroidism. However, measurement of free T_4, rather than TSH, is used as a guide to adjust therapy. Underlying adrenal insufficiency should always be excluded and treated before treatment of secondary hypothyroidism to avoid precipitating an adrenal crisis.

TSH-Secreting Pituitary Tumors

Definition and epidemiology. TSH-secreting pituitary tumors are rare and are characterized by inappropriate release of TSH that is refractory to the negative feedback mechanism of the thyroid hormones released by the thyroid gland. The prevalence of TSH-secreting pituitary adenomas is 1 to 2 cases per million in the general population. The pathogenesis of TSH-secreting pituitary tumors is unknown.

Clinical presentation. The most common age of presentation is in the early fifth decade, and there is no gender predilection. Presenting symptoms can be the result of a mass effect of the tumor or, most commonly, there are symptoms and signs of hyperthyroidism, including weight loss, tremors, heat intolerance, and diarrhea. Diffuse goiter is observed in up to 80% of patients. Many times, these tumors are initially misdiagnosed as primary hyperthyroidism and patients are mistakenly treated with radioactive iodine. Sometimes, the TSH produced by these tumors is biologically inactive and the tumors are diagnosed as an incidental finding on imaging studies.

Diagnosis and differential diagnosis. The diagnosis is made in the setting of elevated or inappropriately normal TSH and alpha subunit along with elevated levels of thyroid hormones (free and total T_4 and T_3). The differential diagnosis includes genetic resistance to thyroid hormone and euthyroid hyperthyroxinemia, which is characterized by normal TSH, high total T_4, normal free T_4, and elevated thyroxine-binding globulin levels. Imaging studies (MRI) should be done only after biochemical confirmation because of the high incidence of incidental pituitary tumors.

Treatment and prognosis. Surgery (transsphenoidal resection) is the first-line treatment. Radiotherapy can be used if surgery is declined or contraindicated, but normalization of thyroid hormones can take years. Medical therapy with somatostatin analogues (e.g., octreotide, lanreotide) is used for first-line drug treatment for persistent hyperthyroidism after surgery. Most patients on SRLs achieve control of symptoms of thyrotoxicosis through normalization of thyroid function as well as reduction in tumor burden.

Adrenocorticotropic Hormone

ACTH is a 39-amino-acid peptide hormone that is formed from a precursor molecule, pro-opiomelanocortin (POMC) and is synthesized and secreted by corticotrophs in the anterior pituitary. It is stimulated by hypothalamic corticotropin-releasing hormone (CRH). ACTH, in turn, stimulates release of glucocorticoids and androgens from the adrenal cortex.

ACTH Deficiency

Definition. ACTH deficiency causes secondary adrenal insufficiency leading to decreased cortisol and adrenal androgens. Aldosterone secretion from the adrenal glands is not impaired because it is maintained via the renin-angiotensin axis. Causes of ACTH deficiency can be found in Table 64.4. Central (secondary and tertiary) adrenal insufficiency is most commonly iatrogenic, caused by the use of steroids for other disease processes.

Clinical presentation. Both primary and central adrenal insufficiency are characterized by weight loss, fatigue, muscle weakness, orthostatic symptoms, nausea, vomiting, diarrhea, and abdominal pain. Biochemical abnormalities include hyponatremia, hypoglycemia, eosinophilia, and anemia. Importantly, hyperpigmentation of the skin and hyperkalemia are seen only with primary adrenal insufficiency, not with ACTH deficiency.

Diagnosis and differential diagnosis. Typically, an 8 AM fasting serum cortisol greater than 10 mcg/dL suggests against adrenal insufficiency whereas a value less than 3 mcg/dL is strongly suggestive of adrenal insufficiency. An inappropriately low morning cortisol and ACTH likely suggests secondary adrenal insufficiency. Many times, it is appropriate to perform an ACTH stimulation test. This test measures the cortisol response to synthetic ACTH or cosyntropin. ACTH and cortisol levels are measured at baseline, followed by cortisol levels at 30 and 60 minutes. A peak plasma cortisol level higher than 14 mcg/dL by liquid chromatography tandem mass spectrometry (LC-MS/MS) is considered a normal response. It is important to keep in mind that if secondary adrenal insufficiency is recent, the adrenal glands may initially respond appropriately to cosyntropin because they have not had time to atrophy.

Treatment. Glucocorticoid therapy in the form of hydrocortisone (10 mg in AM and 5 mg in PM) or prednisone (5 to 7.5 mg/day) should be initiated for replacement. Patient education regarding stress dosing of steroids is important. Mineralocorticoids are usually not needed in patients with central secondary adrenal insufficiency.

ACTH-Secreting Pituitary Tumors (Cushing's Disease)

Definition and epidemiology. ACTH-secreting pituitary tumors (by definition, Cushing's disease) account for about 80% of the cases of Cushing's syndrome; they are usually microadenomas. Cushing's syndrome includes any condition of hypercortisolism regardless of the cause. There is a female preponderance (female-to-male ratio, about 3:1). The chronic stimulation by excessive ACTH causes simple diffuse hyperplasia of the bilateral adrenal glands or sometimes multinodular hyperplasia, both leading to excessive cortisol production.

Clinical presentation. Signs and symptoms of Cushing's disease are related to the hypercortisolism and include central obesity, hirsutism, facial plethora, violaceous striae, supraclavicular and dorsocervical fat pads, and proximal muscle weakness (Fig. 64.2). Additional manifestations of Cushing's disease are type 2 diabetes mellitus, hypertension, dyslipidemia, premature coronary artery disease, osteoporosis, and hypogonadism.

Diagnosis and differential diagnosis. Three different tests are performed in combination to assess for endogenous hypercortisolism. A 24-hour urine collection may show an elevated cortisol level, but this test is not reliable in patients with renal dysfunction. A second test, the 1-mg dexamethasone suppression test, measures an 8 AM fasting cortisol level after a dose of 1 mg dexamethasone given at 11 PM the night before. Cortisol suppression to less than 1.8 µg/dL is considered a normal response. Another diagnostic test is the late-night salivary cortisol measurement, using saliva collected at 11 PM on two consecutive nights. The test relies on a normal sleep cycle. Individuals who are using inhaled or topical steroids are not good candidates because of a high rate of false-positive results. A single positive finding is not sufficient to make this diagnosis and must be repeated and confirmed by doing additional tests. Because of the potential of cyclic ACTH overproduction by these tumors, repeat testing is recommended for individuals with high clinical suspicion but negative initial testing.

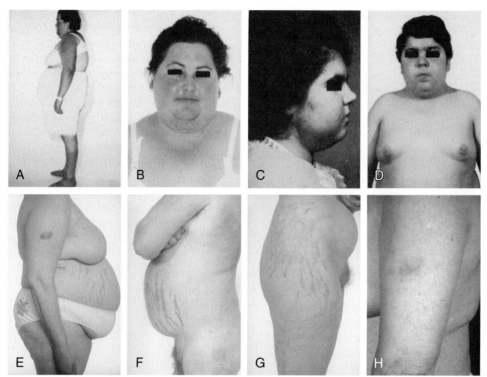

Fig. 64.2 Clinical features of Cushing's syndrome. (A) Centripetal and some generalized obesity and dorsal kyphosis in a 30-year-old woman with Cushing's disease. (B) Moon facies, plethora, hirsutism, and enlarged supraclavicular fat pads in the same woman as in A. (C) Facial rounding, hirsutism, and acne in a 14-year-old girl with Cushing's disease. (D) Central and generalized obesity and moon facies in a 14-year-old boy with Cushing's disease. Typical centripetal obesity with livid abdominal striae in a 41-year-old woman (E) and a 40-year-old man (F) with Cushing's disease. (G) Striae in a 24-year-old patient with congenital adrenal hyperplasia treated with excessive doses of dexamethasone as replacement therapy. (H) Typical bruising and thin skin of a patient with Cushing's disease. In this case, the bruising has occurred without obvious injury. (From Larsen PR, Kronenberg H, Melmed S, et al: Williams Textbook of Endocrinology, ed 10, Philadelphia, 2003, Saunders.)

Pathologic hypercortisolism should be differentiated from physiologic activation of the hypothalamic-pituitary-adrenal axis or pseudo-Cushing's syndrome, which can be observed in conditions such as critical illness, eating disorders, alcoholism, pregnancy, severe neuropsychiatric illness, and poorly controlled diabetes. The desmopressin (DDAVP) stimulation test may be useful to distinguish patients with Cushing's disease from those with pseudo-Cushing's syndrome. Further, pathologic hypercortisolism can be ACTH dependent or independent. Once the diagnosis of ACTH-dependent hypercortisolism is established, a pituitary MRI should be performed looking for a corticotroph adenoma; however, 40% to 45% of ACTH-secreting pituitary tumors are not seen on MRI. In those cases with no or small pituitary tumors and ACTH-dependent Cushing's syndrome, inferior petrosal sinus sampling (IPSS) for ACTH with CRH stimulation differentiates between pituitary and ectopic ACTH overproduction by demonstrating a pituitary-to-peripheral ACTH gradient.

Treatment and prognosis. The treatment involves removal of the pituitary tumor by an experienced neurosurgeon. Options after a failed resection include reoperation, bilateral adrenalectomy, radiotherapy, or pharmacotherapy. Pharmacotherapeutic agents include ketoconazole, metyrapone, mitotane, cabergoline, pasireotide, and mifepristone. In severe cases, intravenous etomidate may be used to stabilize patients for surgery. Long-term remission after resection of a pituitary microadenoma ranges from 69% to 98%, with a recurrence rate of 3% to 19%.

Gonadotropins
Definition
The two gonadotropins, LH and FSH, are glycoprotein hormones that are synthesized and secreted by gonadotrophs in the anterior pituitary. They are both composed of an alpha and a beta subunit, the latter of which gives each its specific biologic function. These hormones bind to the receptors in the gonads (ovaries and testes) and modulate gonadal function. Secretion is regulated both by gonadotropin-releasing hormone (GnRH) from the hypothalamus and by feedback from circulating sex steroids (estrogen and testosterone).

Gonadotropin Deficiency (Hypogonadotropic Hypogonadism)

Definition. Hypogonadotropic hypogonadism is characterized by low levels of sex steroids (estrogen or testosterone) along with low or inappropriately normal FSH and LH.

Clinical presentation. Signs and symptoms depend on the time of onset and the extent of gonadotropin deficiency. If deficiency occurs during fetal life, it can cause ambiguous genitalia. If deficiency occurs after birth but before puberty, it can cause delayed or absent sexual development. Onset after puberty causes menstrual disturbances in women and sexual dysfunction and gynecomastia in men. Osteoporosis and infertility can be present in both sexes.

Diagnosis and differential diagnosis. The diagnosis is made by the presence of low or inappropriately normal FSH and LH levels along with low sex steroids (estrogen or testosterone). Causes of gonadotropin deficiency can be congenital (Kallman syndrome,

Prader-Willi syndrome, septo-optic dysplasia) or acquired, as in hemochromatosis, hyperprolactinemia, sellar tumors, cranial irradiation, and inflammatory and infiltrative disorders.

Treatment and prognosis. For women, replacement therapy in the form of oral or transdermal estrogen should be continued until the age of natural menopause. Progesterone is essential in women with an intact uterus to prevent endometrial hyperplasia. For men, testosterone replacement is available in multiple forms, including injections, implantable pellets, several gels, and a patch. Exogenous testosterone does not restore fertility and in fact inhibits spermatogenesis. For both men and women, fertility treatment requires the use of gonadotropin therapy.

Gonadotropin-Secreting Pituitary Tumors

Definition and epidemiology. Gonadotropin-secreting pituitary tumors are considered nonfunctional. They are usually large and known as the most common macroadenoma. These tumors can secrete FSH, LH, and/or alpha subunit. Nonfunctioning pituitary adenomas are the second most common pituitary adenoma after prolactinomas. They have a prevalence of 7 to 22 per 100,000 population.

Diagnosis and differential diagnosis. Gonadotropin-secreting pituitary tumors typically manifest with signs and symptoms of mass effect. Patients can also have symptoms of pituitary hormone deficiencies. Hormonal evaluation reveals elevated FSH, LH, and/or alpha subunit in the absence of low estrogen or testosterone. Immunoperoxidase staining on tumor tissue is also needed to establish the diagnosis, especially as seen in postmenopausal women when gonadotropins are appropriately elevated.

Treatment and prognosis. Primary treatment is transsphenoidal surgical removal, which is generally successful. Radiation therapy may be used as an adjunct treatment because of the larger size of these tumors at diagnosis. Medical therapy is not used because no effective therapy exists.

DISORDERS OF POSTERIOR PITUITARY HORMONES

AVP and oxytocin are the two hormones that are produced in the hypothalamus and stored in and released from the posterior pituitary.

Diabetes Insipidus

Definition

Diabetes insipidus (DI) is characterized by AVP deficiency and excretion of large volumes of dilute urine. Central DI (posterior pituitary in origin) can be familial due to an autosomal dominant mutation in the vasopressin gene that affects the functioning of the AVP-producing neurons. It can also be acquired secondary to intrasellar and suprasellar tumors, infiltration of the hypothalamus and posterior pituitary, infection, trauma or surgery, or as part of an autoimmune condition. Table 64.7 gives a more extensive list of causes of diabetes insipidus.

Clinical Presentation

Polyuria (defined as excretion of more than 3 L of urine per day) and polydipsia are the clinical hallmarks of DI.

Diagnosis and Differential Diagnosis

DI can be central, caused by AVP deficiency, or nephrogenic, caused by resistance to AVP. As long as access to free water is maintained and the thirst mechanism is intact, patients with DI are usually able to maintain normal serum sodium levels and osmolality. The water deprivation test is the primary test used to make the

TABLE 64.7 Causes of Diabetes Insipidus
Central Diabetes Insipidus
Idiopathic
Familial
Hypophysectomy
Infiltration of hypothalamus and posterior pituitary
Langerhans cell histiocytosis
Granulomas
Infection
Tumors (intrasellar and suprasellar)
Autoimmune
Nephrogenic Diabetes Insipidus
Idiopathic
Familial
V_2 receptor gene mutation
Aquaporin-2 gene mutation
Chronic renal disease (e.g., chronic pyelonephritis, polycystic kidney disease, or medullary cystic disease)
Hypokalemia
Hypercalcemia
Sickle cell anemia
Drugs
Lithium
Fluoride
Demeclocycline
Colchicine

diagnosis and to differentiate the cause of DI. In patients with DI, the serum sodium level and osmolality increase in response to water deprivation. The response to a synthetic analogue of vasopressin is analyzed if the normal rise in urine osmolality and decrease in urine volume are not seen. Patients with central DI respond to the synthetic analogue by increasing urine osmolality and decreasing urine volume. In contrast, patients with nephrogenic DI do not respond to the synthetic vasopressin. Patients with partial central DI may have a limited response. Primary polydipsia is characterized by increased water intake without a deficiency or resistance to AVP. Patients with primary polydipsia concentrate their urine without the need for synthetic vasopressin. Copeptin, also derived from arginine vasopressin prohormone, is recently being studied as an arginine vasopressin surrogate to differentiate central and nephrogenic DI and primary polydipsia, using a direct measurement of hypertonic saline-stimulated plasma copeptin rather than the indirect water deprivation test.

Treatment

Replacement therapy with DDAVP, an analogue of AVP, is available in oral (desmopressin), parenteral, and intranasal forms. Aqueous vasopressin is a shorter-acting analogue of AVP that can be given subcutaneously in the immediate postoperative period. Because of the transient nature of DI and a possible shift to a transient syndrome of inappropriate secretion of antidiuretic hormone (SIADH) phase in the patient who has undergone pituitary surgery, AVP is given cautiously and not as a scheduled medication in order to avoid hyponatremia.

Syndrome of Inappropriate Secretion of Antidiuretic Hormone

SIADH is covered in the discussion of hyponatremia in Chapter 25.

SUGGESTED READINGS

Biller BM, Grossman AB, Stewart PM, et al: Treatment of adrenocorticotropin-dependent Cushing's syndrome: a consensus statement, J Clin Endocrinol Metab 93:2454–2462, 2008.

Dichtel LE, Yuen KCJ, Bredella MA, et al: Overweight/obese adults with pituitary disorders require lower peak growth hormone cutoff values on glucagon stimulation testing to avoid overdiagnosis of growth hormone deficiency, J Clin Endocrinol Metab 99(12):4712–4719, 2014.

Fenske W, Refardt J, Chifu I, et al: A copeptin-based approach in the diagnosis of diabetes insipidus, N Engl J Med 379(5):428–439, 2018.

Fleseriu M, Petersenn S: Medical management of Cushing's disease: what is the future? Pituitary 15:330–341, 2012.

Freda P, Beckers A, Katznelson L, et al: Pituitary incidentaloma: an Endocrine Society clinical practice guideline, J Clin Endocrinol Metab 96:894–904, 2011.

Melmed S, Casanueva F, Hoffman A, et al: Diagnosis and treatment of hyperprolactinemia: an Endocrine Society clinical practice guideline, J Clin Endocrinol Metab 96:273–288, 2011.

Melmed S, Colao A, Barkan A, et al: Guidelines for acromegaly management: an update, J Clin Endocrinol Metab 94:1509–1517, 2009.

Melmed S: Medical progress: acromegaly, N Engl J Med 355:2558–2573, 2006.

Melmed S: The pituitary, ed 4, 2017, Elsevier.

Nieman L, Biller B, Findling J, et al: The diagnosis of Cushing's syndrome: an Endocrine Society clinical practice guideline, J Clin Endocrinol Metab 93:1526–1540, 2008.

Swearingen B, Biller B: Diagnosis and management of pituitary disorders, New York, 2008, Humana Press.

Ueland GÅ, Methlie P, Øksnes M, et al: The short cosyntropin test revisited: new normal reference range using LC-MS/MS, J Clin Endocrinol Metab 103(4):1696–1703, 2018.

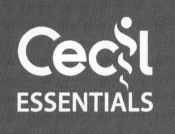

65

Thyroid Gland

Theodore C. Friedman

INTRODUCTION

The thyroid gland secretes thyroxine (T_4) and triiodothyronine (T_3), both of which modulate energy utilization and heat production and facilitate growth. The gland consists of two lateral lobes joined by an isthmus (E-Fig. 65.1). The weight of the adult gland is 10 to 20 g. Microscopically, the thyroid is composed of several follicles that contain colloid surrounded by a single layer of thyroid epithelium. The follicular cells synthesize thyroglobulin, which is stored as colloid. Biosynthesis of T_4 and T_3 occurs by iodination of tyrosine molecules in thyroglobulin.

THYROID HORMONE PHYSIOLOGY

Thyroid Hormone Synthesis

Dietary iodine is essential for the synthesis of thyroid hormones. Iodine, after conversion to iodide in the stomach, is rapidly absorbed from the gastrointestinal tract. After active transport from the bloodstream across the follicular cell basement membrane, iodide is enzymatically oxidized by thyroid peroxidase, which also mediates the iodination of the tyrosine residues in thyroglobulin, to form monoiodotyrosine and diiodotyrosine. The iodotyrosine molecules couple to form T_4 (3,5,3′,5′-tetraiodothyronine) or T_3 (3,5,3′-triiodothyronine). Once iodinated, thyroglobulin containing newly formed T_4 and T_3 is stored in the follicles. Secretion of free T_4 and T_3 into the circulation occurs after proteolytic digestion of thyroglobulin, which is stimulated by thyroid-stimulating hormone (TSH). Deiodination of monoiodotyrosine and diiodotyrosine by iodotyrosine deiodinase releases iodine, which then reenters the thyroid iodine pool (E-Fig. 65.2).

Thyroid Hormone Transport

T_4 and T_3 are tightly bound to the serum carrier proteins thyroxine-binding globulin (TBG), thyroxine-binding prealbumin, and albumin. The unbound or free fractions are the biologically active fractions; they represent only 0.04% of the total T_4 and 0.4% of the total T_3.

Peripheral Metabolism of Thyroid Hormones

The normal thyroid gland secretes T_4, T_3, and reverse T_3, a biologically inactive form of T_3. Most of the circulating T_3 is derived from deiodination of circulating T_4 in the peripheral tissues. Deiodination of T_4 can occur at the outer ring (5′-deiodination), producing T_3 (3,5,3′-triiodothyronine), or at the inner ring (5-deiodination), producing reverse T_3 (3,3,5′-triiodothyronine).

Control of Thyroid Function

Hypothalamic thyrotropin-releasing hormone (TRH) is transported through the hypothalamic-hypophyseal portal system to the thyrotrophs of the anterior pituitary gland, stimulating synthesis and release

of TSH (Fig. 65.1). TSH, in turn, increases thyroidal iodide uptake and iodination of thyroglobulin, releases T_3 and T_4 from the thyroid gland by increasing hydrolysis of thyroglobulin, and stimulates thyroid cell growth. Hypersecretion of TSH results in thyroid enlargement (goiter). Circulating T_3 exerts negative feedback inhibition of TRH and TSH release.

Physiologic Effects of Thyroid Hormones

Thyroid hormones increase the basal metabolic rate by increasing oxygen consumption and heat production in several body tissues. Thyroid hormones also have specific effects on several organ systems (Table 65.1). These effects are exaggerated in hyperthyroidism and reduced in hypothyroidism, accounting for the well-recognized signs and symptoms of these two disorders.

THYROID EVALUATION

A careful thyroid examination is essential in evaluating a patient with thyroid disease (Video 65.1). Thyroid gland function and structure can be evaluated by (1) determining serum thyroid hormone levels, (2) imaging thyroid gland size and architecture, (3) measuring thyroid autoantibodies, and (4) performing a thyroid gland biopsy by fine-needle aspiration (FNA).

Tests of Serum Thyroid Hormone Levels

Measurements of total serum T_4 and total T_3 indicate the total amount of hormone bound to thyroid-binding proteins by radioimmunoassay. Total T_4 and T_3 levels are elevated in hyperthyroidism and low in hypothyroidism. Increased production of TBG (as with pregnancy or estrogen

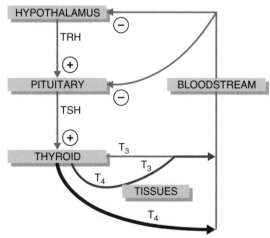

Fig. 65.1 Hypothalamic-pituitary-thyroid axis. T_4 is converted to T_3 in peripheral tissues. *T_3,* Triiodothyronine; *T_4,* thyroxine; *TRH,* thyrotropin-releasing hormone; *TSH,* thyroid-stimulating hormone.

therapy) increases the total T_4 and T_3 levels without actual hyperthyroidism. Similarly, total T_4 and T_3 are low despite euthyroidism in conditions associated with low levels of thyroid-binding proteins (e.g., congenital decrease, protein-losing enteropathy, cirrhosis, nephrotic syndrome). Therefore, further tests to assess the free hormone levels, which reflect biologic activity, must be performed. Free T_4 and free T_3 levels can be measured directly or by dialysis or ultrafiltration and have, at most institutions, replaced measuring total T_4 and T_3 levels.

Serum TSH is measured by a third-generation immunometric assay that accurately discriminates between normal TSH levels and levels below the normal range. Thus, the TSH assay can diagnose clinical hyperthyroidism (elevated free T_4 and free T_3 and suppressed TSH) and subclinical hyperthyroidism (normal free T_4 and free T_3 and suppressed TSH). In hyperthyroidism, the free T_3 may be elevated in the presence of a normal free T_4. In primary (thyroidal) hypothyroidism, serum TSH is supranormal because of diminished feedback inhibition. The TSH is usually low but may be normal in secondary (pituitary) or tertiary (hypothalamic) hypothyroidism.

Serum thyroglobulin measurements are useful in the follow-up of patients with papillary or follicular carcinoma. After thyroidectomy and iodine-131 (^{131}I) ablation therapy, thyroglobulin levels should be less than 0.5 ng/mL while the patient is on suppressive levothyroxine treatment. Levels in excess of this value indicate the possibility of persistent or metastatic disease.

Calcitonin is produced by the C cells of the thyroid and has a minor role in calcium homeostasis. Calcitonin measurements are invaluable in the diagnosis of medullary carcinoma of the thyroid and for monitoring the effects of therapy for this entity.

Thyroid Imaging

Technetium-99m (^{99m}Tc) pertechnetate is concentrated in the thyroid gland and can be scanned with a gamma camera, yielding information about the size and shape of the gland and the location of the functional activity in the gland (thyroid scan). The thyroid scan is often performed in conjunction with a quantitative assessment of radioactive iodine (^{123}I) uptake by the thyroid. Functioning thyroid nodules are called *warm* or *hot* nodules; *cold* nodules are nonfunctioning.

Malignancy is usually associated with a cold nodule; 16% of surgically removed cold nodules are malignant.

Thyroid ultrasound evaluation is useful in the differentiation of solid nodules from cystic nodules and to determine which patients should undergo an FNA. The use of thyroid ultrasounds in patients with thyroid nodules is discussed later.

Thyroid Antibodies

Autoantibodies to several different antigenic components in the thyroid gland, including thyroglobulin (TgAb), thyroid peroxidase (TPO Ab, formerly called *antimicrosomal antibodies*), and the TSH receptor, can be measured in the serum. A strongly positive test for TPO Ab indicates autoimmune thyroid disease. Elevated TSH receptor antibody occurs in Graves' disease (see later discussion).

Thyroid Biopsy

FNA of a nodule (E-Fig. 65.3) to obtain thyroid cells for cytologic evaluation is the best way to differentiate benign from malignant disease. FNA requires adequate tissue samples and interpretation by an experienced cytologist.

HYPERTHYROIDISM

Thyrotoxicosis is the clinical syndrome that results from elevated levels of circulating thyroid hormones. Clinical manifestations of thyrotoxicosis result from the direct physiologic effects of the thyroid hormones as well as the increased sensitivity to catecholamines. Tachycardia, tremor, stare, sweating, and lid lag are all caused by catecholamine hypersensitivity.

Signs and Symptoms

Table 65.2 lists the signs and symptoms of hyperthyroidism. Thyrotoxic crisis, or *thyroid storm*, is a life-threatening complication of hyperthyroidism that can be precipitated by surgery, radioactive iodine therapy, or severe stress (e.g., uncontrolled diabetes mellitus, myocardial infarction, acute infection). Patients develop fever, flushing, sweating, significant tachycardia, atrial fibrillation, and cardiac failure. Significant agitation, restlessness, delirium, and coma frequently

TABLE 65.1 Physiologic Effects of Thyroid Hormone	
System	**Effects**
Cardiovascular	Increased heart rate and cardiac output
Gastrointestinal	Increased gut motility
Skeletal	Increased bone turnover and resorption
Pulmonary	Maintenance of normal hypoxic and hypercapnic drive in the respiratory center
Neuromuscular	Increased muscle protein turnover and increased speed of muscle contraction and relaxation
Metabolism of lipids and carbohydrates	Increased hepatic gluconeogenesis and glycogenolysis, as well as intestinal glucose absorption
	Increased cholesterol synthesis and degradation
	Increased lipolysis
Sympathetic nervous system	Increased numbers of β-adrenergic receptors in the heart, skeletal muscle, lymphocytes, and adipose cells
	Decreased cardiac α-adrenergic receptors
	Increased catecholamine sensitivity
Hematopoietic	Increased red blood cell 2,3-diphosphoglycerate, facilitating oxygen dissociation from hemoglobin with increased oxygen available to tissues

TABLE 65.2 Signs and Symptoms of Hyperthyroidism
Symptoms
Palpitations
Nervousness
Shortness of breath
Heat intolerance
Fatigue and weakness
Increased appetite
Weight loss
Oligomenorrhea
Signs
Tachycardia
Atrial fibrillation
Wide pulse pressure
Brisk reflexes
Fine tremor
Proximal limb-girdle myopathy
Chemosis (swelling of conjunctiva)
Thyroid bruit (Graves' disease)

occur. Gastrointestinal manifestations may include nausea, vomiting, and diarrhea. Hyperpyrexia out of proportion to other clinical findings is the hallmark of thyroid storm.

Differential Diagnosis

Thyrotoxicosis usually reflects excess secretion of thyroid hormones resulting from Graves' disease, toxic adenoma, multinodular goiter, or thyroiditis (Table 65.3 and Fig. 65.2). However, it may be the result of excessive ingestion of thyroid hormone or, rarely, thyroid hormone production from an ectopic site (as in struma ovarii).

Graves' Disease

Graves' disease, the most common cause of thyrotoxicosis, is an autoimmune disease that is more common in women, with a peak incidence between 20 and 50 years of age. One or more of the following features are present: (1) goiter; (2) thyrotoxicosis; (3) eye disease ranging from tearing to proptosis, extraocular muscle paralysis, and loss of sight as a result of optic nerve involvement; and (4) thyroid dermopathy, usually observed as significant skin thickening without pitting in a pretibial distribution (*pretibial myxedema*). (Do not confuse this use of myxedema with that described below under the discussion of the clinical features of *hypothyroidism*.)

Pathogenesis. Thyrotoxicosis in Graves' disease is caused by overproduction of an antibody that binds to the TSH receptor. These thyroid-stimulating immunoglobulins increase thyroid cell growth and thyroid hormone secretion. Ophthalmopathy results from inflammatory infiltration of the extraocular eye muscles by lymphocytes with mucopolysaccharide deposition. The inflammatory reaction that contributes to the eye signs in Graves' disease may be caused by sensitization of lymphocytes to antigens that are common to the orbital muscles and the thyroid.

Clinical presentation. The common manifestations of thyrotoxicosis (see Table 65.2) are characteristic features of younger patients with Graves' disease. In addition, patients may exhibit a diffuse goiter or the eye signs characteristic of Graves' disease. Older patients often do not have the florid clinical features of thyrotoxicosis, and the condition termed *apathetic hyperthyroidism* is exhibited as flat affect, emotional lability, weight loss, muscle weakness, congestive heart failure, and atrial fibrillation resistant to standard therapy.

Eye signs associated with Graves' disease may also occur as a nonspecific manifestation of hyperthyroidism from any cause (e.g., thyroid stare). In Graves' disease, a specific inflammatory infiltrate of the orbital tissues leads to periorbital edema, conjunctival congestion and swelling, proptosis, extraocular muscle weakness, or optic nerve damage with visual impairment (E-Fig. 65.4).

Pretibial myxedema (thyroid dermopathy) (E-Fig. 65.5) occurs in 2% to 3% of patients with Graves' disease and results in a thickening of the skin over the lower tibia without pitting. Onycholysis, characterized by separation of the fingernails from their beds, often occurs in patients with Graves' disease. Thyroid acropachy, or clubbing, may also occur.

Diagnosis. Elevated total or free T_4 or T_3 (or both) and a suppressed TSH confirm the clinical diagnosis of thyrotoxicosis. TSH receptor antibody is usually elevated, and its measurement may be useful in patients with eye signs who do not have other characteristic clinical features. Increased uptake of ^{123}I differentiates Graves' disease from early subacute or Hashimoto thyroiditis, in which uptake is low in the presence of hyperthyroidism. Magnetic resonance imaging or ultrasonography of the orbit usually shows orbital muscle enlargement, whether or not clinical signs of ophthalmopathy are observed.

Treatment. Three treatment modalities are used to control the hyperthyroidism of Graves' disease: antithyroid drugs, radioactive iodine therapy, and surgery. In Europe, Latin America, and Japan, antithyroid drugs are the favored therapy while in the United States, radioactive iodine is the main therapy. However, more recently antithyroid drugs are becoming the mainstay of treatment for Graves' disease worldwide.

Antithyroid drugs. The thiocarbamide drugs propylthiouracil, methimazole, and carbimazole block thyroid hormone synthesis

TABLE 65.3	Causes of Thyrotoxicosis

Common Causes
Graves' disease
Toxic adenoma (solitary)
Toxic multinodular goiter

Less Common Causes
Subacute thyroiditis (de Quervain or granulomatous thyroiditis)
Hashimoto thyroiditis with transient hyperthyroid phase
Thyrotoxicosis factitia
Postpartum thyroiditis (probably variant of silent thyroiditis)

Rare Causes
Struma ovarii
Metastatic thyroid carcinoma
Hydatidiform mole
TSH-secreting pituitary tumor

TSH, Thyroid-stimulating hormone.

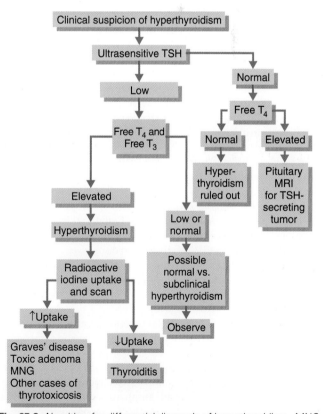

Fig. 65.2 Algorithm for differential diagnosis of hyperthyroidism. *MNG*, Multinodular goiter; *MRI*, magnetic resonance imaging; *RIA*, radioimmunoassay; T_3, triiodothyronine; T_4, thyroxine; *TSH*, thyroid-stimulating hormone.

by inhibiting thyroid peroxidase. Propylthiouracil also partially inhibits peripheral conversion of T_4 to T_3. Medical therapy is usually administered for a prolonged period (1 to 3 years), with the dose gradually reduced until spontaneous remission occurs. Many patients can remain on low doses of thiocarbamide drugs for long periods of time without significant side effects. One approach is to gradually decrease the dose while maintaining T_4 and T_3 in the normal range, leaving patients on low doses of thiocarbamide drugs if T_4 and T_3 remain high after a gradual taper. After cessation of medication, 40% to 60% of patients remain in remission. Those who experience relapse can either resume therapy with thiocarbamide drugs or undergo definitive surgery or radioactive iodine treatment. Side effects of the thiocarbamide regimen include pruritus and rash (in about 5% of patients), elevated liver function enzymes, cholestatic jaundice, acute arthralgias, and, rarely, agranulocytosis (<0.5% of patients).

Methimazole was found to be more effective at normalizing thyroid hormone levels and led to a lower rate of transaminase elevation and leukopenia than propylthiouracil; it has now become the preferred medical treatment for hyperthyroidism. Methimazole can be given once a day as long as the total dose is 30 mg or less, leading to better compliance, whereas PTU is usually given two to three times a day. At the onset of treatment during the acute phase of thyrotoxicosis, β-adrenergic receptor blockers can be used to help alleviate tachycardia, hypertension, and atrial fibrillation in symptomatic patients. As the thyroid hormone levels return to normal, the treatment with β-blockers is tapered off.

Radioactive iodine. Radioactive iodine (^{131}I) can be used for treating adults with Graves' disease. However, 80% to 90% of patients become hypothyroid after radiotherapy and require lifelong thyroid hormone replacement. As discussed later, a percentage of patients treated with levothyroxine for hypothyroidism continue to have hypothyroid symptoms despite normalization of TSH; this has caused a shift in the paradigm that radioactive iodine is the preferred treatment of hyperthyroidism, with a greater emphasis on using thiocarbamide drugs. ^{131}I has been found to increase the incidence of cancer mortality. ^{131}I is contraindicated in women who are pregnant, but it does not increase the risk of birth defects in offspring conceived after ^{131}I therapy. Patients with severe thyrotoxicosis, very large glands, or underlying heart disease should be rendered euthyroid with antithyroid medication before receiving radioactive iodine, because ^{131}I treatment can cause a release of preformed thyroid hormone from the thyroid gland that could precipitate cardiac arrhythmias and exacerbate symptoms of thyrotoxicosis.

After administration of radioactive iodine, the thyroid gland shrinks; patients become euthyroid and later hypothyroid over a period of 6 weeks to 3 months. Serum free T_4 and TSH levels should be monitored, and replacement with levothyroxine should be instituted when hypothyroidism occurs. Hypothyroidism always occurs after surgical total thyroidectomy, frequently after subtotal thyroidectomy or administration of radioactive iodine, and in a smaller percentage of patients after antithyroid medication; therefore, lifelong monitoring of all patients with Graves' disease is mandated.

Surgery. Either subtotal or total thyroidectomy is the treatment of choice for patients with very large glands and obstructive symptoms, those with multinodular glands, and sometimes in those who desire pregnancy within the next year. It is essential that the surgeon be experienced in thyroid surgery. Preoperatively, patients receive 6 weeks of treatment with antithyroid drugs to ensure that they are euthyroid at the time of surgery. Two weeks before surgery, oral saturated solution of potassium iodide is administered daily to decrease the vascularity of the gland. Permanent hypoparathyroidism and recurrent laryngeal nerve paralysis occur postoperatively in fewer than 2% of patients, although the rate of transient postoperative hypocalcemia is higher.

Graves' orbitopathy can be treated with glucocorticoids, orbital radiotherapy, or surgery. It was recently found that selenium is effective for Graves' orbitopathy.

Toxic Adenoma

Solitary toxic nodules, which are usually benign, occur more frequently in older patients. The clinical manifestations are those of thyrotoxicosis. Physical examination shows a distinct solitary nodule. Laboratory investigation shows suppressed TSH and significantly elevated T_3 levels, often with only moderately elevated T_4. Thyroid scan shows a hot nodule in the affected lobe with partial or complete suppression of the unaffected lobe. Solitary toxic nodules are usually treated with radioactive iodine. Euthyroidism results if the unaffected lobe has suppressed uptake on a thyroid scan, and often hypothyroidism occurs if the unaffected lobe does not have suppressed uptake. For large nodules, unilateral lobectomy after the administration of antithyroid drugs to render the patient euthyroid may be required.

Toxic Multinodular Goiter

Toxic multinodular goiter occurs in older patients with long-standing multinodular goiter, especially in patients from iodine-deficient regions when they are exposed to increased dietary iodine or iodine-containing radiocontrast dyes. The presenting clinical features are frequently tachycardia, heart failure, and arrhythmias. Physical examination shows a multinodular goiter. The diagnosis is confirmed by laboratory features of suppressed TSH, elevated T_3 and T_4, and a thyroid scan showing multiple functioning nodules. The treatment of choice is often ^{131}I ablation. It is especially effective in patients with small glands and a high degree of radioactive uptake. Larger glands may require surgery.

Subclinical Hyperthyroidism

In subclinical hyperthyroidism, total or free T_4 and T_3 levels are normal and TSH is suppressed. The causes of this condition include early presentation of any form of hyperthyroidism (e.g., Graves' disease, toxic adenoma, toxic multinodular goiter). Because these patients, especially those who are older, are at an increased risk for cardiac dysrhythmias, many patients with a persistently suppressed TSH should be treated with thiocarbamide drugs, β-blockers or, less commonly, radioactive iodine. A decreased bone mineral density is another indication for treatment.

Thyroiditis

Thyroiditis may be classified as acute, subacute, or chronic. Although thyroiditis may eventually result in clinical hypothyroidism, the initial presentation is often that of hyperthyroidism as a result of acute release of T_4 and T_3. Hyperthyroidism caused by thyroiditis can be readily differentiated from other causes of hyperthyroidism by suppressed uptake of radioactive iodine in the thyroid gland, reflecting decreased hormone production by damaged cells.

A rare disorder, acute suppurative thyroiditis, is caused by an infection, usually bacterial. Patients exhibit high fever, redness of the overlying skin, and thyroid gland tenderness; the condition may be confused with subacute thyroiditis. If blood cultures are negative, FNA should identify the organism. Intensive antibiotic treatment and, occasionally, incision and drainage are required.

Subacute Thyroiditis

Subacute thyroiditis (also known as de Quervain thyroiditis or granulomatous thyroiditis) is an acute inflammatory disorder of the thyroid gland that is probably caused by a viral infection and resolves completely in 90% of cases. Patients with subacute thyroiditis complain of fever and anterior neck pain. The patient may have symptoms and signs of hyperthyroidism. The classic feature on physical examination is an exquisitely tender thyroid gland. Laboratory findings vary with the course of the disease. Initially, the patient may be symptomatically thyrotoxic with elevated serum T_4, depressed serum TSH and low radioactive iodine uptake on the thyroid scan. Subsequently, the thyroid status fluctuates through euthyroid and hypothyroid phases and may return to euthyroidism. An increase in radioactive iodine uptake on the scan reflects recovery of the gland. Treatment usually includes high-dose aspirin or other nonsteroidal anti-inflammatory drugs, but a short course of prednisone may be required if pain and fever are severe. During the hypothyroid phase, replacement therapy with levothyroxine may be indicated.

Postpartum thyroiditis resembles subacute thyroiditis in its clinical course. It usually occurs within the first 6 months after delivery and goes through the triphasic course of hyperthyroidism, hypothyroidism, and then euthyroidism, though it may develop with only hypothyroidism. Some patients have underlying chronic thyroiditis.

Chronic Thyroiditis

Chronic thyroiditis (Hashimoto or lymphocytic thyroiditis), caused by destruction of the normal thyroidal architecture by lymphocytic infiltration, results in hypothyroidism and goiter. Riedel struma is probably a variant of Hashimoto thyroiditis; it is characterized by extensive thyroid fibrosis resulting in a rock-hard thyroid mass. Hashimoto thyroiditis is more common in women and is the most common cause of goiter and hypothyroidism in the United States. Occasionally, patients with Hashimoto thyroiditis have transient hyperthyroidism with low radioactive iodine uptake owing to the release of T_4 and T_3 into the circulation. Chronic thyroiditis can be differentiated from subacute thyroiditis in that in the former, the gland is nontender to palpation and antithyroid antibodies are present in high titer. TPO Ab is usually present early and typically remains present for years. The presence of TgAb does not reflect Hashimoto thyroiditis and does not provide additional information beyond the TPO Ab finding. Serum T_3 and T_4 levels are either normal or low; when they are low, the TSH is elevated. FNA of the thyroid shows lymphocytes and Hürthle cells (enlarged basophilic follicular cells). Hypothyroidism and significant glandular enlargement (goiter) are indications for levothyroxine therapy. Adequate doses of levothyroxine are administered to normalize TSH levels and shrink the goiter. Recent evidence that symptoms of profound fatigue, poor sleep quality, and muscle joint pain persist despite levothyroxine supplementation leading to euthyroidism suggests that symptoms may be related to the autoimmune disease per se rather than hypothyroidism.

Thyrotoxicosis Factitia

Patients with thyrotoxicosis factitia ingest excessive amounts of thyroxine, often in an attempt to lose weight, and exhibit typical features of thyrotoxicosis. Serum T_3 and T_4 levels are elevated and TSH is suppressed, as is the serum thyroglobulin concentration. Radioactive iodine uptake is absent. Patients may require psychotherapy.

Rare Causes of Thyrotoxicosis

Struma ovarii occurs when an ovarian teratoma contains thyroid tissue that secretes thyroid hormone. A body scan confirms the diagnosis by demonstrating uptake of radioactive iodine in the pelvis.

Hydatidiform mole is caused by proliferation and swelling of the trophoblast during pregnancy, with excess production of chorionic gonadotropin, which has intrinsic TSH-like activity. The hyperthyroidism remits with surgical and medical treatment of the molar pregnancy.

HYPOTHYROIDISM

Hypothyroidism is a clinical syndrome caused by deficiency of thyroid hormones. In infants and children, hypothyroidism causes retardation of growth and development and may result in permanent motor and mental retardation. Congenital causes of hypothyroidism include agenesis (complete absence of thyroid tissue), dysgenesis (ectopic or lingual thyroid gland), hypoplastic thyroid, thyroid dyshormonogenesis, and congenital pituitary diseases. Adult-onset hypothyroidism results in a slowing of metabolic processes and is reversible with treatment. Hypothyroidism is usually primary (thyroid failure), but it may be secondary (hypothalamic or pituitary deficiency) or rarely the result of resistance at the thyroid hormone receptor (Table 65.4).

In adults, autoimmune thyroiditis (Hashimoto thyroiditis) is the most common cause of hypothyroidism. This condition may be

TABLE 65.4 Causes of Hypothyroidism
Primary Hypothyroidism
Autoimmune
Hashimoto thyroiditis
Part of polyglandular failure syndrome, type II
Iatrogenic
^{131}I therapy
Thyroidectomy
Drug-Induced
Iodine deficiency
Iodine excess
Lithium
Amiodarone
Antithyroid drugs
Opioids
Glucocorticoids
CTLA-4 inhibitors
PD-1 inhibitors
Congenital
Thyroid agenesis
Thyroid dysgenesis
Hypoplastic thyroid
Biosynthetic defects
Secondary Hypothyroidism
Hypothalamic Dysfunction
Neoplasms
Tuberculosis
Sarcoidosis
Langerhans cell histiocytosis
Hemochromatosis
Radiation treatment
Pituitary Dysfunction
Neoplasms
Pituitary surgery
Postpartum pituitary necrosis
Idiopathic hypopituitarism
Glucocorticoid excess (Cushing's syndrome)
Radiation treatment to the pituitary

isolated, or it may be part of polyglandular failure syndrome type II (Schmidt syndrome), which also includes insulin-dependent diabetes mellitus, adrenal insufficiency, pernicious anemia, vitiligo, gonadal failure, hypophysitis, celiac disease, myasthenia gravis, and primary biliary cirrhosis. Iatrogenic causes of hypothyroidism include ^{131}I therapy, thyroidectomy, and treatment with lithium, amiodarone, opioids, and glucocorticoids, as well as CTLA-4 and PD-1 inhibitors (cancer immunotherapy agents), with the last two drug classes causing painless thyroiditis and transient hyperthyroidism followed by hypothyroidism. Iodine deficiency or excess can also cause hypothyroidism.

Clinical Presentation

The clinical presentation of hypothyroidism (Table 65.5) depends on the age at onset and the severity of the thyroid deficiency. Infants with congenital hypothyroidism (also called *cretinism*) may exhibit feeding problems, hypotonia, inactivity, an open posterior fontanelle, and edematous face and hands. Mental retardation, short stature, and delayed puberty occur if treatment is delayed.

Hypothyroidism in adults usually develops insidiously. Patients often complain of fatigue, lethargy, and gradual weight gain for years before the diagnosis is established. A delayed relaxation phase of deep tendon reflexes (*hung-up* reflexes) is a valuable clinical sign that is characteristic of severe hypothyroidism. Subcutaneous infiltration by mucopolysaccharides, which bind water, causes the edema; this condition, termed *myxedema*, is responsible for the thickened features and puffy appearance of patients with severe hypothyroidism.

Severe untreated hypothyroidism can result in *myxedema coma*, which is characterized by hypothermia, extreme weakness, stupor, hypoventilation, hypoglycemia, and hyponatremia and is often precipitated by cold exposure, infection, or psychoactive drugs. (Do not confuse the uses of myxedema here with *pretibial myxedema* seen in Graves' disease, where it refers to thyroid dermopathy—skin thickening without pitting.)

Diagnosis

Because the initial manifestations of hypothyroidism are subtle, early diagnosis demands a high index of suspicion in patients with one or more of the signs and symptoms (see Table 65.5), though hypothyroidism is often picked up in patients who have a TSH measured as part of routine laboratories. Early symptoms that are often overlooked include menstrual irregularities (usually menorrhagia), arthralgias, and myalgias.

Laboratory abnormalities in patients with primary hypothyroidism include elevated serum TSH and low total and free T_4. A low or low-normal morning serum TSH level in the setting of hypothalamic or pituitary dysfunction characterizes secondary hypothyroidism. Often, the serum total and free T_4 levels are at the lower limits of normal.

Hypothyroidism is often associated with hypercholesterolemia and elevated creatine phosphokinase skeletal muscle (MM) fraction (the fraction representative of skeletal muscle). Anemia is usually normocytic and normochromic but may be macrocytic (with vitamin B_{12} deficiency resulting from associated pernicious anemia) or microcytic (caused by nutritional deficiencies or menstrual blood loss in women). Because TPO Ab is usually positive in Hashimoto thyroiditis, the major cause of hypothyroidism in adults, its measurement is helpful in deciding whether levothyroxine treatment is appropriate in patients with subclinical hypothyroidism (discussed later).

Treatment

Hypothyroidism should be treated initially with synthetic levothyroxine (T_4). Administration of levothyroxine results in physiologic levels of bioavailable T_3 and T_4. Levothyroxine has a half-life of 8 days; consequently, it needs to be given only once a day. The average replacement dose of levothyroxine for adults is 75 to 150 µg/day. In healthy adults, 1.6 µg/kg/day is an appropriate starting dose. In some older patients and patients with cardiac disease, levothyroxine should be increased gradually, starting at 25 µg/day and increasing the dose by 25 µg every 2 weeks; however, most patients can safely be started on a full replacement dose. The therapeutic response to levothyroxine therapy should be monitored clinically and with measurement of serum TSH levels 6 to 8 weeks after a dose adjustment. TSH levels between 0.5 and 2 mU/L are considered optimal. Because TSH measurements are not a useful guide in patients with secondary hypothyroidism (pituitary or hypothalamic dysfunction), these patients should be given levothyroxine until their free T_4 is in the mid- to upper-normal range.

Recent studies have suggested that a percentage of patients treated with levothyroxine for hypothyroidism continue to have hypothyroid symptoms despite normalization of TSH. Furthermore, a large study found that more than 20% of athyreotic patients (those who have absence or functional deficiency of the thyroid gland) treated with levothyroxine replacement did not maintain free T_3 or free T_4 values in the normal range despite normal TSH levels. This reflects the inadequacy of peripheral deiodination to compensate for the absent T_3 secretion. Because of these studies, there is renewed interest (accompanied by a large amount of controversy) in treating hypothyroid patients who have not had an adequate clinical response to levothyroxine replacement with a combination of levothyroxine and liothyronine (a manufactured form of T_3) or with desiccated thyroid preparations that contain levothyroxine and liothyronine.

In patients with myxedema coma, 500 to 800 µg of levothyroxine is administered intravenously as a loading dose, followed by 100 µg/day of levothyroxine, hydrocortisone (100 mg IV intravenously three times daily), and intravenous fluids. Corticosteroids should be given before thyroxine in autoimmune conditions. The underlying precipitating event should be corrected. Respiratory assistance and treatment of hypothermia with warming blankets may be required. Although myxedema coma carries a high mortality rate despite appropriate treatment, many patients improve in 1 to 3 days.

TABLE 65.5 Clinical Features of Hypothyroidism

Children
Learning disabilities
Mental retardation
Short stature
Delayed bone age
Delayed puberty

Adults
Fatigue
Cold intolerance
Weight gain
Constipation
Menstrual irregularities
Dry, coarse, cold skin
Periorbital and peripheral edema
Delayed reflexes
Bradycardia
Arthralgias, myalgias

Subclinical Hypothyroidism

In subclinical hypothyroidism, free or total T_4 and T_3 levels are normal or low-normal, and TSH is mildly elevated. Some of these patients develop overt hypothyroidism. The decision as to when to treat patients who have a mildly elevated TSH level is controversial. It is frequently recommended that patients should be treated with levothyroxine if they have a TSH level greater than 5 mU/L on two occasions and either positive anti–TPO Ab test results or a goiter. If the patient does not have an appreciable goiter and has negative anti–TPO Ab test results, many experts suggest that levothyroxine should be given only if the TSH level is greater than 10 mU/L on two occasions. Other experts suggest treatment at lower TSH levels depending on the presence of TPO antibody.

GOITER

Enlargement of the thyroid gland is called a *goiter*. Patients with goiters may be euthyroid (simple goiter), hyperthyroid (toxic nodular goiter or Graves' disease), or hypothyroid (nontoxic goiter or Hashimoto thyroiditis). Thyroid enlargement (often focal) may also be the result of a thyroid adenoma or carcinoma. In nontoxic goiter, inadequate thyroid hormone synthesis leads to TSH stimulation with resultant enlargement of the thyroid gland. Iodine deficiency (endemic goiter) was once the most common cause of nontoxic goiter. Since the widespread availability of iodized salt, endemic goiter is less common in North America.

Goitrogens are agents that can cause a goiter, and iodine and lithium are the two chemicals or drugs that frequently cause a goiter. Natural goitrogens include thioglucosides found in vegetables such as cabbage, broccoli, Brussels sprouts, turnips, cauliflower, kale, and other greens. Other foods that are goitrogens include soybeans and soybean products, peanuts, spinach, sweet potatoes, and some fruits (e.g., strawberries, pears, and peaches). Thyroid hormone biosynthetic defects can cause goiter associated with hypothyroidism (or, with adequate compensation, euthyroidism).

A careful thyroid examination coupled with thyroid hormone tests can reveal the cause of the goiter. A smooth, symmetrical gland, often with a bruit, and hyperthyroidism are suggestive of Graves' disease. A nodular thyroid gland with hypothyroidism and positive antithyroid antibodies is consistent with Hashimoto thyroiditis. A diffuse, smooth goiter with hypothyroidism and negative antithyroid antibodies may be indicative of iodine deficiency or a biosynthetic defect. Goiters can become very large, extending substernally and causing dysphagia, respiratory distress, or hoarseness. An ultrasound evaluation or radioactive iodine scan delineates the thyroid gland, and measurement of the TSH level determines the functional activity of the goiter.

Hypothyroid goiters are treated with thyroid hormone at a dose that normalizes TSH. Previously, euthyroid goiters were treated with levothyroxine therapy; however, regression with levothyroxine therapy is unlikely and is no longer recommended. Surgery is indicated for nontoxic goiter only if obstructive symptoms develop or substantial substernal extension is present.

SOLITARY THYROID NODULES

Thyroid nodules are common. They can be detected clinically in about 4% of the population and are found in about 50% of the population at autopsy. Benign thyroid nodules are usually follicular adenomas, colloid nodules, benign cysts, or nodular thyroiditis. Patients may have one prominent nodule on clinical examination, but thyroid ultrasound evaluation may reveal multiple nodules. Although most nodules are benign, a small percentage are malignant. Fortunately, most thyroid cancers are low-grade malignancies.

The major etiologic factor for thyroid cancer is childhood or adolescent exposure to head and neck radiation. Previously, radiation was used to treat an enlarged thymus, tonsillar disease, hemangioma, or acne. Exposure to radiation from nuclear plants (e.g., Chernobyl, Ukraine; Fukushima Daiichi, Japan) contributes to an increased incidence of thyroid cancer. Patients with a history of irradiation should have a baseline thyroid ultrasound study, then a repeat study every 5 years.

All patients with a thyroid nodule noticed by the patient or during physical examination by a clinician should undergo a thyroid ultrasound. Patients who are found to have asymptomatic, incidental, non-suspicious thyroid nodules on imaging performed for other reasons should be referred for diagnostic thyroid ultrasound only if they meet the following criteria: (1) younger than 35 years of age with normal life expectancy and nodule 1 cm or greater, or (2) 35 years of age or older with normal life expectancy and nodule 1.5 cm or greater. Radiologists have a standard report and score on thyroid ultrasounds called TI-RADS that ranges from 1 (looks very benign) to 5 (looks like it might be malignant) (Fig. 65.3). Thus, the TI-RADS helps to distinguish which patient with a thyroid nodule should get a biopsy. If the TI-RADS score is 3 and the nodule is larger than 2.5 cm, if the score is 4 and the nodule is larger than 1.5 cm, or if the score is 5 and the nodule is larger than 1 cm, then an FNA is recommended. If the TI-RADS score is lower and the nodule is smaller, a repeat ultrasound in 1 year is recommended, and for even smaller, more benign looking nodules, no follow-up is needed. FNA should be done under ultrasound guidance if possible.

The Bethesda system for reporting thyroid cytopathology (Table 65.6) is used to report FNA results. Molecular testing can now be performed on FNA specimens to help determine whether follicular lesions have molecular characteristics of malignancy and should be removed.

Although in the past benign thyroid nodules were treated with levothyroxine suppression, this is no longer recommended because it is uncommon for thyroid nodules to shrink substantially with levothyroxine.

THYROID CARCINOMA

The types and characteristics of thyroid carcinomas are presented in Table 65.7. Papillary carcinoma is associated with local invasion and lymph node spread. Indicators of poor prognosis include thyroid capsule invasion, size greater than 2.5 cm, age at onset older than 45 years, tall cell or Hürthle cell variant, and lymph node involvement. Follicular carcinoma is slightly more aggressive than papillary carcinoma and can spread by local invasion of lymph nodes or hematogenously to bone, brain, or lung. Many tumors show both papillary and follicular cell types. Patients may exhibit metastases before diagnosis of the primary thyroid lesion. Anaplastic carcinoma tends to occur in older individuals, is very aggressive, and rapidly causes pain, dysphagia, and hoarseness.

Medullary thyroid carcinoma is derived from calcitonin-producing parafollicular cells and is more malignant than papillary or follicular carcinoma. It is multifocal and spreads both locally and distally. It may be either sporadic or familial. When familial, it is inherited in an autosomal dominant pattern and is part of multiple endocrine neoplasia type IIA (medullary carcinoma of the thyroid, pheochromocytoma, and hyperparathyroidism) or multiple endocrine neoplasia type IIB (medullary carcinoma of the thyroid, mucosal neuromas, intestinal ganglioneuromas, marfanoid habitus, and pheochromocytoma). Elevated basal serum calcitonin levels confirm the diagnosis. Evaluation for *RET* proto-oncogene mutations should be performed

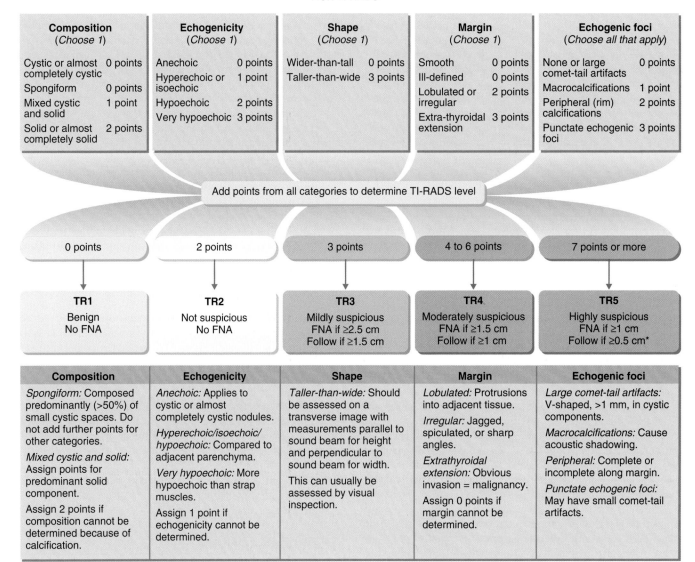

Fig. 65.3 Chart showing five categories on the basis of the ACR Thyroid Imaging, Reporting and Data System (TI-RADS) lexicon, TR levels, and criteria for fine-needle aspiration or follow-up ultrasound. Explanatory notes appear at the bottom.

in patients with medullary carcinoma; if mutations are present, all first-degree relatives should be examined.

Treatment

Lobectomy may be performed for low-risk patients. This includes papillary nodules less than 2.5 cm, TI-RADS score less than 4, absence of neck lymph nodes seen on neck ultrasound, and most follicular tumors. Nodules less than 1 cm with papillary carcinoma can be observed. However, higher risk patients with larger tumors (>3 cm) and/or positive lymph nodes should have a total thyroidectomy. Routine central neck dissection is not needed unless lymph nodes are seen on preoperative imaging or if the surgeon discovers nodes during examination during surgery.

Patients with a lobectomy usually do not need thyroid hormone replacement but should have their TSH monitored. If the TSH goes above range, the patient should be started on levothyroxine. They should have thyroglobulin measured and a thyroid ultrasound every 6 months for the first 2 years and then yearly. A thyroglobulin greater than 30 ng/mL and/or enlarging nodule on the contralateral lobe or lymph nodes draw concern for recurrent disease and should be evaluated for completion of the thyroidectomy.

After total thyroidectomy, patients with low-risk, small carcinomas may be administered doses of levothyroxine sufficient to keep the TSH level in the low-normal or slightly suppressed range and monitored with serum thyroglobulin determinations and yearly neck ultrasound examinations. In the presence of a stable serum TSH level, one should follow the trend in thyroglobulin values with a rising value being concerning. Ideally the thyroglobulin should be less than 0.5 ng/mL, although values less than 2.5 ng/mL may not require an intervention if the thyroid ultrasound does not show detectable thyroid tissue. Patients with large lesions and those at high risk for persistence or metastatic disease should be treated with radioactive iodine with sufficient levothyroxine administration to suppress serum TSH to subnormal levels for about 5 years after thyroidectomy; after that, normal TSH levels can be targeted if no sign of tumor recurrence is seen.

TABLE 65.6 Bethesda System for Reporting Thyroid Cytopathology

Bethesda Category	Diagnosis	Disposition	Notes
I	Nondiagnostic/Unsatisfactory	Repeat FNA (under ultrasound guidance)	
II	Benign	Clinical follow-up and a repeat ultrasound and a possible repeat biopsy needed if the patient or provider notices the nodule is growing.	
III	Atypia of Undetermined Significance (AUS) or Follicular Lesion of Undetermined Significance (FLUS)	If pathologist determines a FLUS/AUS reading, one additional biopsy should be performed 3-6 months after the initial biopsy. The repeat FNA should include a sample for molecular testing and if the pathology still shows FLUS/AUS, then the sample should be sent out for molecular testing with the results guiding further treatment. If it is still unclear if surgery is needed, ultrasound should be performed to determine if the nodule grows or changes characteristics (higher TI-RADS score). If it does not grow or change characteristics, the nodule could be watched.	A TPO antibody should also be obtained because FLUS/AUS may occur in the context of a Hashimoto gland and its measurement may assist the pathologist. Molecular testing can be used to determine likelihood of malignancy.
IV	Follicular Neoplasm (FN) or Suspicious for a Follicular Neoplasm (SFN)	If initial biopsy shows FN/SFN, a repeat biopsy should be performed 3-6 months later and include a sample for molecular testing with the results guiding further treatment.	Follicular carcinomas cannot be diagnosed on FNA because definitive diagnosis requires identification of capsular/vascular invasion. Molecular testing can be used to determine likelihood of malignancy.
V	Suspicious for Malignancy	As for malignant	
VI	Malignant	Referral to surgery if nodule is >1 cm. Nodules with papillary carcinoma less than 1 cm may not need to be removed and the option of serial ultrasounds (every 6-12 months) should be discussed with the patient. If the patient feels more comfortable with surgery, that can also be an option.	The most common malignancies of the thyroid are well-differentiated malignancies with a favorable prognosis. Of these, the most common is papillary thyroid carcinoma. Other malignancies include medullary thyroid carcinoma, poorly differentiated thyroid carcinoma, undifferentiated (anaplastic) thyroid carcinoma, squamous cell carcinoma, and malignant lymphoma. Metastases to the thyroid from other malignancies can occur as well

TABLE 65.7 Characteristics of Thyroid Cancers

Type of Cancer	Percentage of Thyroid Cancers	Age at Onset (Yr)	Treatment	Prognosis
Papillary	85	40-80	Lobectomy or thyroidectomy, aggressive cases should receive radioactive iodine ablation	Good
Follicular	10	45-80	Lobectomy or thyroidectomy in aggressive cases	Fair to good
Medullary	3	20-50	Thyroidectomy and central compartment lymph node dissection	Fair
Anaplastic	1	50-80	Isthmusectomy followed by palliative radiograph treatment	Poor
Lymphoma	1	25-70	Radiograph therapy or chemotherapy or both	Fair

A rise in serum thyroglobulin levels suggests recurrence of thyroid cancer and should prompt testing for recurrence and/or metastases. These are evaluated by ^{131}I whole body scans carried out under conditions of TSH stimulation, which increases ^{131}I uptake by the thyroid tissue. Elevated TSH levels can be achieved by withdrawal of thyroxine supplementation for 6 weeks or by treatment with recombinant human TSH administered while the patient maintains therapy with thyroid hormone replacement. The latter avoids symptomatic hypothyroidism. Local or metastatic lesions that take up ^{131}I on whole body scanning can be treated with radioactive iodine after the patient has stopped thyroid hormone replacement, whereas those that do not take up ^{131}I can be treated with surgical excision or local radiograph therapy. Conventional chemotherapy has limited efficacy in the treatment of differentiated thyroid cancer, but newer biologic agents targeting the molecular pathogenesis of these tumors appear promising.

Medullary carcinoma of the thyroid requires total thyroidectomy with removal of the central lymph nodes in the neck. Completeness of the procedure and monitoring for recurrence are determined by measurements of serum calcitonin.

Anaplastic carcinoma is treated with isthmusectomy to confirm the diagnosis and to prevent tracheal compression, followed by palliative radiograph treatment. Thyroid lymphomas are also treated with radiograph therapy, chemotherapy, or both.

The prognosis for well-differentiated thyroid carcinomas is good. The patient's age at the time of diagnosis and sex are the most important prognostic factors. Men older than 40 years of age and women older than 50 years of age have higher recurrence and death rates than do younger patients. The 5-year survival rate for invasive medullary carcinoma is 50%, whereas the mean survival time for anaplastic carcinoma is 6 months.

For a deeper discussion on this topic, please see Chapter 213, ❖ "Thyroid," in *Goldman-Cecil Medicine*, 26th Edition.

SUGGESTED READINGS

Burch HB: Drug effects on the thyroid, N Engl J Med 381(8):749–761, 2019.

Cibas ES, Ali SZ: The 2017 Bethesda system for reporting thyroid cytopathology, Thyroid 27:1341–1346, 2017.

Gullo D, Latina A, Frasca F, et al: Levothyroxine monotherapy cannot guarantee euthyroidism in all athyreotic patients, PloS One 6:e22552, 2011.

Haugen BR, Alexander EK, Bible KC, et al: 2015 American thyroid association management guidelines for adult patients with thyroid nodules and differentiated thyroid cancer: the American Thyroid Association Guidelines Task Force on Thyroid Nodules and Differentiated Thyroid Cancer, Thyroid 26:1–133, 2016.

Ross DS, Burch HB, Cooper DS, et al: 2016 American Thyroid Association Guidelines for Diagnosis and Management of Hyperthyroidism and Other Causes of Thyrotoxicosis, Thyroid 26(10):1343–1421, 2016.

Welch HG, Doherty GM: Saving thyroids—overtreatment of small papillary cancers, N Engl J Med 379:310–312, 2018.

Wiersinga WM: Do we need still more trials on T4 and T3 combination therapy in hypothyroidism? Eur J Endocrinol 161:955–959, 2009.

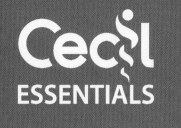

66

Adrenal Gland

Theodore C. Friedman

PHYSIOLOGY

The adrenal glands (Fig. 66.1) lie at the superior pole of each kidney and are composed of two distinct regions: the cortex and the medulla. The adrenal cortex comprises three anatomic zones: the outer *zona glomerulosa*, which secretes the mineralocorticoid aldosterone; the intermediate *zona fasciculata*, which secretes cortisol; and the inner *zona reticularis*, which secretes adrenal androgens. The adrenal medulla, lying in the center of the adrenal gland, is functionally related to the sympathetic nervous system and secretes the catecholamines epinephrine and norepinephrine in response to stress.

The synthesis of all steroid hormones begins with cholesterol and is catalyzed by a series of regulated, enzyme-mediated reactions (Fig. 66.2). Glucocorticoids affect metabolism, cardiovascular function, behavior, and the inflammatory and immune responses (Table 66.1). Cortisol, the natural human glucocorticoid, is secreted by the adrenal glands in response to adrenocorticotropic hormone (ACTH), a 39-amino-acid neuropeptide that is regulated by corticotropin-releasing hormone (CRH) and vasopressin (AVP) produced in the hypothalamus (see Chapter 64). Glucocorticoids exert negative feedback on CRH and ACTH secretion. The brain hypothalamic-pituitary-adrenal (HPA) axis (Fig. 66.3) interacts with and influences the functions of the reproductive, growth, and thyroid axes at many levels, with major participation of glucocorticoids at all levels.

The renin-angiotensin-aldosterone system (Fig. 66.4) is the major regulator of aldosterone secretion. Renal juxtaglomerular cells secrete renin in response to a decrease in circulating volume, a reduction in renal perfusion pressure or both. Renin is the rate-limiting enzyme that cleaves the 60-kD angiotensinogen molecule, synthesized by the liver, to produce the bioactive decapeptide angiotensin I. Angiotensin I is rapidly converted to the octapeptide angiotensin II by angiotensin-converting enzyme in the lungs and other tissues. Angiotensin II is a potent vasopressor; it stimulates aldosterone production but does not stimulate cortisol production. Angiotensin II is the predominant regulator of aldosterone secretion, but plasma potassium concentration, plasma volume, and ACTH level also influence aldosterone secretion. ACTH also mediates the circadian rhythm of aldosterone, and as a result, the plasma concentration of aldosterone is highest in the morning. Aldosterone binds to the type I mineralocorticoid receptor. In contrast, cortisol binds to both the type I mineralocorticoid and type II glucocorticoid receptors. The intracellular enzyme 11β-hydroxysteroid dehydrogenase (11β-HSD) type II, which catabolizes cortisol to inactive cortisone, limits the functional binding to the former receptor. The availability of cortisol to bind to the glucocorticoid receptor is modulated by 11β-HSD type I, which interconverts cortisol and cortisone. Binding of aldosterone to the cytosol mineralocorticoid receptor leads to sodium (Na^+) absorption and potassium (K^+) and hydrogen (H^+) secretion by the renal tubules. The resultant increase in plasma Na^+ and decrease in plasma K^+ provide a feedback mechanism for suppressing renin and, subsequently, aldosterone secretion.

Adrenal androgen precursors include dehydroepiandrosterone (DHEA) and its sulfate and androstenedione. These are synthesized in the zona reticularis under the influence of ACTH and other adrenal androgen-stimulating factors. Although they have minimal intrinsic androgenic activity, they contribute to androgenicity by their peripheral conversion to testosterone and dihydrotestosterone. In adult men, excessive levels of adrenal androgens have negligible clinical consequences, but in women they result in acne, hirsutism, and virilization. Because of gonadal production of androgens and estrogens and the secretion of norepinephrine by sympathetic ganglia, deficiencies of adrenal androgens and catecholamines are not clinically recognized.

SYNDROMES OF ADRENOCORTICAL HYPOFUNCTION

Adrenal Insufficiency

Glucocorticoid insufficiency can be primary, resulting from destruction or dysfunction of the adrenal cortex, or secondary, resulting from ACTH hyposecretion (Table 66.2). Medications and supplements affecting cortisol levels are shown in Table 66.3. Autoimmune destruction of the adrenal glands (Addison's disease) is the most common cause of primary adrenal insufficiency in the industrialized world, accounting for about 65% of cases. Usually, both glucocorticoid and mineralocorticoid secretions are diminished in this condition that, if left untreated, can be fatal. Isolated glucocorticoid or mineralocorticoid deficiency may also occur, and it is becoming apparent that mild adrenal insufficiency (similar to subclinical hypothyroidism, discussed in Chapter 65) should also be diagnosed and, in some cases, treated. Adrenal medulla function is usually spared. About 80% of patients with Addison's disease have antiadrenal antibodies directed at 21α-hydroxylase (CYP21A2), though in clinical practice this may be lower due to poor quality of commercial autoantibody testing.

Tuberculosis used to be the most common cause of adrenal insufficiency. However, its incidence in the industrialized world has decreased since the 1960s, and it now accounts for only 15% to 20% of patients with adrenal insufficiency; calcified adrenal glands can be observed in 50% of these patients. Rare causes of adrenal insufficiency are listed in Table 66.2. Many patients with human immunodeficiency virus (HIV) infection have decreased adrenal reserve without overt adrenal insufficiency.

Addison's disease may be part of two distinct autoimmune polyglandular syndromes. The triad of hypoparathyroidism, adrenal insufficiency, and mucocutaneous candidiasis characterizes *type I polyglandular autoimmune syndrome*, also called autoimmune polyendocrinopathy 1 (APECED), which usually manifests in childhood. Other, less common manifestations include hypothyroidism, gonadal failure,

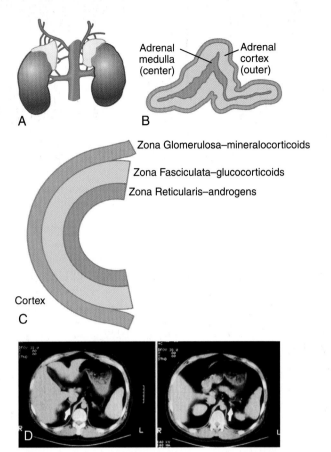

Fig. 66.1 (A) Anatomic location of the adrenal glands. (B) Distribution of adrenal cortex and medulla. (C) Zones of the adrenal cortex. (D) Magnetic resonance images of the abdomen showing the position and relative size of the normal adrenal glands *(arrows)*. (D, From Nieman LK: Adrenal cortex. In Goldman L, Schafer AI, editors: Goldman-Cecil medicine, ed 24, Philadelphia, 2012, Saunders, Figure 234-1.)

gastrointestinal malabsorption, insulin-dependent diabetes mellitus, alopecia areata and totalis, pernicious anemia, vitiligo, chronic active hepatitis, keratopathy, hypoplasia of dental enamel and nails, hypophysitis, asplenism, and cholelithiasis. *Type II polyglandular autoimmune syndrome*, also called *Schmidt syndrome*, is characterized by Addison's disease, autoimmune thyroid disease (Graves' disease or Hashimoto thyroiditis), and insulin-dependent diabetes mellitus. Other associated diseases include pernicious anemia, vitiligo, gonadal failure, hypophysitis, celiac disease, myasthenia gravis, primary biliary cirrhosis, Sjögren's syndrome, lupus erythematosus, and Parkinson's disease. This syndrome usually develops in adults.

Common manifestations of adrenal insufficiency are anorexia, weight loss, increasing fatigue, occasional vomiting, diarrhea, and salt craving. Muscle and joint pain, abdominal pain, and postural dizziness may also occur. Signs of increased pigmentation (initially most significant on the extensor surfaces, palmar creases, and buccal mucosa) often occur secondary to the increased production of ACTH and other related peptides by the pituitary gland (E-Fig. 66.1). Laboratory abnormalities may include hyponatremia, hyperkalemia, mild metabolic acidosis, azotemia, hypercalcemia, anemia, lymphocytosis, and eosinophilia. Hypoglycemia may also occur, especially in children.

Acute adrenal insufficiency is a medical emergency, and treatment should not be delayed pending laboratory results. In a critically ill patient with hypovolemia, a plasma sample for cortisol, ACTH, aldosterone, and renin should be obtained, and then treatment with

hydrocortisone (100 mg IV bolus) and parenteral saline administration should be initiated. Sepsis-induced adrenal insufficiency is recognized by a basal cortisol level lower than 10 μg/dL or a change in cortisol of less than 9 μg/dL after administration of 0.25 mg ACTH (1-24) (cosyntropin). In severe illness, albumin and cortisol-binding globulin (CBG) are low, resulting in a low level of total cortisol but not free cortisol; therefore, a low total cortisol level may not be diagnostic of adrenal insufficiency in this setting.

In a patient with chronic symptoms suggestive of adrenal insufficiency described previously, a basal early morning plasma cortisol measurement, a 1-hour cosyntropin test, or both, should be performed. These tests are not recommended in patients without symptoms of adrenal insufficiency. In the latter test, 0.25 mg of cosyntropin is given intravenously or intramuscularly, and plasma cortisol is measured after 0, 30, and 60 minutes. A normal response is a plasma cortisol concentration higher than 18 μg/dL at any time during the test. A patient with a basal morning plasma cortisol concentration lower than 5 μg/dL and a stimulated cortisol concentration lower than 18 μg/dL probably has adrenal insufficiency and should receive treatment. A basal plasma morning cortisol concentration between 10 and 18 μg/dL in association with a stimulated cortisol concentration lower than 18 μg/dL probably indicates impaired adrenal reserve and a requirement for receiving cortisol replacement under stress conditions (see later discussion). Birth control pills and oral estrogens increase CBG levels; therefore, a patient on those agents may have a normal basal or cosyntropin-stimulated cortisol level and have a low free cortisol level, making interpretation of the test difficult for these patients.

Once the diagnosis of adrenal insufficiency is made, the distinction between primary and secondary adrenal insufficiency needs to be established. Secondary adrenal insufficiency results from inadequate stimulation of the adrenal cortex by ACTH (see Chapter 64). Hyperpigmentation does not occur. In addition, because mineralocorticoid levels are normal in secondary adrenal insufficiency, symptoms of salt craving, as well as the laboratory abnormalities of hyperkalemia and metabolic acidosis, are not present, although hyponatremia may be observed. Hypothyroidism, hypogonadism, and growth hormone deficiency may also be present. To distinguish primary from secondary adrenal insufficiency, a basal morning plasma ACTH value should be obtained, along with a serum aldosterone level and a measurement of plasma renin activity (PRA). A plasma ACTH value greater than 20 pg/mL (normal, 5 to 30 pg/mL) is consistent with primary adrenal insufficiency, whereas a value lower than 20 pg/mL probably represents secondary adrenal insufficiency. A PRA value greater than 3 ng/mL/hour in the setting of a suppressed aldosterone level is consistent with primary adrenal insufficiency, whereas a value lower than 3 ng/mL/hour probably represents secondary adrenal insufficiency. The 1-hour cosyntropin test is suppressed in both primary and secondary chronic adrenal insufficiency.

Secondary adrenal insufficiency occurs commonly after the discontinuation of exogenous glucocorticoids. Alternate-day glucocorticoid treatment, if feasible, results in less suppression of the HPA axis than does daily glucocorticoid therapy. Complete recovery of the HPA axis can take 1 year or more, and the rate-limiting step appears to be recovery of the CRH-producing neurons.

Under stress, cortisol secretion is increased. Therefore, the concept of adrenal fatigue, proposed by some alternative providers, has no biologic validity.

After stabilization of acute adrenal insufficiency, patients with Addison's disease require lifelong replacement therapy with both glucocorticoids and mineralocorticoids. Many patients are overtreated with glucocorticoids and undertreated with mineralocorticoids. Because overtreatment with glucocorticoids results in insidious weight

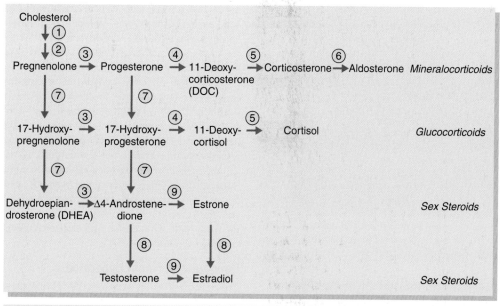

Enzyme Number	Enzyme (Current and Trivial Name)
1	StAR; Steroidogenic acute regulatory protein
2	CYP11A1; Cholesterol side-chain cleavage enzyme/desmolase
3	3β-HSD II; 3β-Hydroxylase dehydrogenase
4	CYP21A2; 21α-Hydroxylase
5	CYP11B1; 11β-Hydroxylase
6	CYP11B2; Corticosterone methyloxidase
7	CYP17; 17α-Hydroxylase/17, 20 lyase
8	17β-HSD; 17β-Hydroxysteroid dehydrogenase
9	CYP19; Aromatase

Fig. 66.2 Pathways of steroid biosynthesis.

TABLE 66.1   Actions of Glucocorticoids

Metabolic Homeostasis
Regulate blood glucose level (permissive effects on gluconeogenesis)
Increase glycogen synthesis
Raise insulin levels (permissive effects on lipolytic hormones)
Increase catabolism, decrease anabolism (except fat), inhibit growth hormone axis
Inhibit reproductive axis
Stimulate mineralocorticoid receptor by cortisol

Connective Tissues
Cause loss of collagen and connective tissue

Calcium Homeostasis
Stimulate osteoclasts, inhibit osteoblasts
Reduce intestinal calcium absorption, stimulate parathyroid hormone release, increase urinary calcium excretion, decrease reabsorption of phosphate

Cardiovascular Function
Increase cardiac output
Increase vascular tone (permissive effects on pressor hormones)
Increase sodium retention

Behavior and Cognitive Function
Daytime fatigue
Nocturnal hyperarousal
Decreased short-term memory
Decreased cognition

Euphoria or Depression
Immune System
Increase intravascular leukocyte concentration
Decrease migration of inflammatory cells to sites of injury
Suppress immune system (thymolysis; suppression of cytokines, prostanoids, kinins, serotonin, histamine, collagenase, and plasminogen activator)

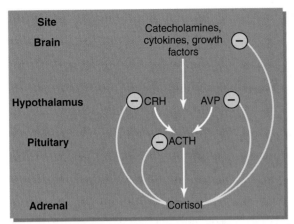

Fig. 66.3 Brain hypothalamic-pituitary-adrenal axis. Minus signs indicate negative feedback. *ACTH*, Adrenocorticotropic hormone; *AVP*, arginine vasopressin; *CRH*, corticotropin-releasing hormone.

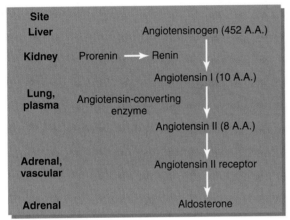

Fig. 66.4 Renin-angiotensin-aldosterone axis. *A.A.*, Amino acids.

gain and osteoporosis, the minimal cortisol dose that can be tolerated without symptoms of glucocorticoid insufficiency (usually joint pain, abdominal pain, or diarrhea) is recommended. An initial regimen of 10 to 15 mg hydrocortisone first thing in the morning plus 5 mg hydrocortisone at about 3:00 PM mimics the physiologic dose and is recommended; a third dose is occasionally needed. Whereas glucocorticoid replacement is fairly uniform in most patients, the requirement for mineralocorticoid replacement varies greatly. The initial dose of the synthetic mineralocorticoid fludrocortisone should be 100 µg/day (often in divided doses), and the dosage should be adjusted to keep the standing PRA value between 1 and 3 ng/mL/hr.

Under the stress of a minor illness (e.g., nausea, vomiting, fever >100.5° F), the hydrocortisone dose should be doubled for as short a period as possible. An inability to ingest hydrocortisone pills may necessitate parenteral hydrocortisone administration. Patients undergoing a major stressful event (e.g., surgery necessitating general anesthesia, major trauma) should receive 150 to 300 mg parenteral hydrocortisone daily (in divided doses) with a rapid taper to normal replacement during recovery. All patients should wear a medical information bracelet and should be instructed in the use of intramuscular emergency hydrocortisone injections or alternatively hydrocortisone suppositories as another option.

Hyporeninemic Hypoaldosteronism

Mineralocorticoid deficiency can result from decreased renin secretion by the kidneys. Resultant hypoangiotensinemia leads to hypoaldosteronism with hyperkalemia and hyperchloremic metabolic acidosis. The plasma sodium concentration is usually normal, but total plasma volume is often deficient. PRA and aldosterone levels are low and unresponsive to stimuli, including hypokalemia. Diabetes mellitus and chronic tubulointerstitial diseases of the kidney are the most common underlying conditions leading to impairment of the juxtaglomerular apparatus. A subset of hyporeninemic hypoaldosteronism is caused by autonomic insufficiency and is a frequent cause of orthostatic hypotension. Stimuli such as upright posture or volume depletion, mediated by baroreceptors, do not cause a normal renin response. Administration of pharmacologic agents such as nonsteroidal anti-inflammatory agents, angiotensin-converting enzyme inhibitors, and β-adrenergic antagonists can also produce conditions of hypoaldosteronism. Salt administration often with fludrocortisone and the α1-receptor agonist midodrine are effective in correcting the orthostatic hypotension and electrolyte abnormalities caused by hypoaldosteronism.

Congenital Adrenal Hyperplasia

Congenital adrenal hyperplasia (CAH) refers to autosomal recessive disorders of adrenal steroid biosynthesis that result in glucocorticoid and mineralocorticoid deficiencies and compensatory increase in ACTH secretion (see Fig. 66.2). Five major types of CAH exist, and the clinical manifestations of each type depend on which steroids are in excess and which are deficient. CYP21A2 deficiency is the most common of these disorders and accounts for about 95% of patients with CAH. In this condition, there is a failure of 21-hydroxylation of 17-hydroxyprogesterone and progesterone to 11-deoxycortisol and 11-deoxycorticosterone, respectively, with deficient cortisol and aldosterone production. Cortisol deficiency leads to increased ACTH release, resulting in adrenal hyperplasia and overproduction of 17-hydroxyprogesterone and progesterone. Increased ACTH production also leads to increased biosynthesis of androstenedione and DHEA, which can be converted to testosterone. Patients with CYP21A2 deficiencies can be divided into two clinical phenotypes: classic 21-hydroxylase deficiency, which usually is diagnosed at birth or during childhood, and late-onset 21-hydroxylase deficiency, which develops during or after puberty. Two thirds of patients with classic CYP21A2 deficiency have various degrees of mineralocorticoid deficiency (salt-losing form); the remaining one third have the non–salt-losing type (simple virilizing form). Both decreased aldosterone production and increased concentrations of precursors that are mineralocorticoid antagonists (progesterone and 17-hydroxyprogesterone) contribute to salt loss.

Late-onset 21-hydroxylase deficiency represents an allelic variant of classic 21-hydroxylase deficiency and is characterized by a mild enzymatic defect. This deficiency is the most common autosomal recessive disorder in humans and is present at high frequency in Ashkenazi Jews. The syndrome usually develops at the time of puberty with signs of virilization (hirsutism and acne) and amenorrhea or oligomenorrhea. This diagnosis should be considered in women who have unexplained hirsutism and menstrual abnormalities or infertility.

The most useful initial measurement for the diagnosis of classic 21-hydroxylase deficiency is that of plasma 17-hydroxyprogesterone. A value greater than 200 ng/dL is consistent with the diagnosis. The diagnosis of late-onset 21-hydroxylase deficiency is based on the finding of an elevated level of plasma 17-hydroxyprogesterone (>1500 ng/dL) 30 minutes after administration of 0.25 mg of synthetic ACTH (1-24).

The aim of treatment for classic 21-hydroxylase deficiency is to replace glucocorticoids and mineralocorticoids, suppress ACTH and androgen overproduction, and allow for normal growth and

TABLE 66.2   Syndromes of Adrenocortical Hypofunction

Primary Adrenal Disorders
Combined Glucocorticoid and Mineralocorticoid Deficiency
Autoimmune
   Isolated autoimmune disease (Addison's disease)
   Polyglandular autoimmune syndrome, type I
   Polyglandular autoimmune syndrome, type II
Infectious
   Tuberculosis
   Fungal
   Cytomegalovirus
   Human immunodeficiency virus
Vascular
   Bilateral adrenal hemorrhage
   Sepsis
   Coagulopathy
   Thrombosis, embolism
   Adrenal infarction
Infiltration
   Metastatic carcinoma and lymphoma
   Sarcoidosis
   Amyloidosis
   Hemochromatosis
Congenital
   Congenital adrenal hyperplasia
   21-Hydroxylase deficiency
   3β-ol Dehydrogenase deficiency
   20,22-Desmolase deficiency
   Adrenal unresponsiveness to ACTH
   Congenital adrenal hypoplasia
   Adrenoleukodystrophy
   Adrenomyeloneuropathy
Iatrogenic
   Bilateral adrenalectomy
   Drugs and supplements: See Table 66.3
Mineralocorticoid Deficiency Without Glucocorticoid Deficiency
   Corticosterone methyl oxidase deficiency
   Isolated zona glomerulosa defect
   Heparin therapy
   Critical illness
   Angiotensin-converting enzyme inhibitors

Secondary Adrenal Disorders
Secondary Adrenal Insufficiency
Hypothalamic-pituitary dysfunction
Exogenous glucocorticoids
After removal of an ACTH-secreting tumor
Hyporeninemic Hypoaldosteronism
Diabetic nephropathy
Tubulointerstitial diseases
Obstructive uropathy
Autonomic neuropathy
Nonsteroidal anti-inflammatory drugs
β-Adrenergic drugs

ACTH, Adrenocorticotropic hormone.

sexual maturation in children. A proposed approach to treating classic 21-hydroxylase deficiency recommends physiologic replacement with hydrocortisone and fludrocortisone in all affected patients. Virilizing effects can be prevented by the use of an antiandrogen (spironolactone or flutamide). Although the traditional treatment for late-onset 21-hydroxylase deficiency is dexamethasone (0.5 mg/day), the use of an antiandrogen such as spironolactone (100 to 200 mg/day) or flutamide (125 mg/day) is probably equally effective and has fewer side effects. Mineralocorticoid replacement is not needed in late-onset 21-hydroxylase deficiency.

11β-Hydroxylase (CYP11B1) deficiency accounts for about 5% of patients with CAH. In this condition, the conversions of 11-deoxycortisol to cortisol and 11-deoxycorticosterone to corticosterone (the precursor to aldosterone) are blocked. Affected patients usually have hypertension and hypokalemia because of increased amounts of precursors with mineralocorticoid activity. Virilization occurs, as with 21-hydroxylase deficiency, and a late-onset form manifesting as androgen excess also occurs. The diagnosis is made from the finding of elevated plasma 11-deoxycortisol levels, either basally or after ACTH stimulation.

Rare forms of CAH are 3β-HSD type II deficiency, 17α-hydroxylase (CYP17) deficiency, and steroidogenic acute regulatory protein (StAR) deficiency. Patients previously diagnosed with 3β-HSD type II deficiency most likely had polycystic ovarian syndrome (PCOS), which is associated with high DHEAS levels.

SYNDROMES OF ADRENOCORTICAL HYPERFUNCTION

Hypersecretion of the glucocorticoid hormone cortisol results in Cushing's syndrome, a metabolic disorder that affects carbohydrate, protein, and lipid metabolism (see Table 66.1). Hypersecretion of mineralocorticoids such as aldosterone results in a syndrome of hypertension and electrolyte disturbances.

Cushing's Syndrome
Pathophysiology
Cushing's syndrome refers to any condition of endogenous glucocorticoid excess, while Cushing's disease refers to an ACTH-secreting pituitary tumor leading to glucocorticoid excess. Increased production of cortisol is seen in both physiologic and pathologic states (Table 66.4). Physiologic hypercortisolism occurs with stress, during the last trimester of pregnancy, and in persons who regularly perform strenuous exercise. Pathologic conditions of elevated cortisol levels include exogenous or endogenous Cushing's syndrome and several psychiatric states, such as depression, alcoholism, anorexia nervosa, panic disorder, and alcohol or narcotic withdrawal.

Cushing's syndrome may be caused by exogenous administration of ACTH or glucocorticoid or by endogenous overproduction of these hormones. Endogenous Cushing's syndrome is either ACTH dependent or ACTH independent. ACTH dependency accounts for 85% of patients and includes pituitary sources of ACTH (Cushing's disease) and ectopic sources of ACTH. Pituitary Cushing's disease accounts for 90% of patients with ACTH-dependent Cushing's syndrome. Ectopic secretion of ACTH occurs most commonly in patients with small cell lung carcinoma. These patients are older, usually have a history of smoking, and primarily exhibit signs and symptoms of lung cancer rather than those of Cushing's syndrome. Patients with the clinically apparent ectopic ACTH syndrome, in contrast, have mostly lung, thymic or pancreatic carcinoid tumors. ACTH-independent causes account for 15% of patients with Cushing's syndrome and include adrenal adenomas, adrenal carcinomas, micronodular adrenal disease, and autonomous macronodular adrenal disease. The female-to-male ratio for noncancerous forms of Cushing's syndrome is 4:1.

TABLE 66.3 Medications and Supplements Affecting Cortisol Levels

Type of Drugs	Generic Name	Brand Name	Effect on Cortisol	Comments
Cushing's drugs	**Ketoconazole**	**Nizoral**	↓	Decreases cortisol biosynthesis
	Mifepristone	**Korlym**	↑	Blocks cortisol at the receptor
	Somatostatin analogues (octreotide, lanreotide, pasireotide)	**Sandostatin, Somatuline, Signifor**	↓	Lowers cortisol mildly
	Metyrapone	**Metopirone**	↓	High rate of adrenal insufficiency
	Etomidate	**Amidate**	↓	Can be given IV
	Mitotane	**Lysodren**	↓	Adrenolytic
Antidepressant	**Citalopram**	**Celexa**	↑	
	Sertraline	**Zoloft**	↑	
	Fluoxetine	Prozac	–	
	Imipramine	Tofranil	↓	
	Desipramine	Norpramin	↓	
	Trazodone	Desyrel	↓	
	Mirtazapine	Remeron	↓	
Antipsychotic	Olanzapine	Zyprexa	↓	
	Quetiapine	Seroquel	↓	
Anti-anxiety	Temazepam	Restoril	↓	
	Alprazolam	**Xanax**	↓	
	Lorazepam	Ativan	↓/–	Anecdotal-lowers cortisol, literature no effect
Dopamine agents	Cabergoline	Dostinex	↓	Variable effect
	Bromocriptine	Parlodel	↓	Variable effect
	Metoclopramide	Reglan	↑	
	Methylphenidate	Ritalin	↑	Found in one study but not another study
Antihypertensives	**Clonidine**	**Catapres**	↓	
Opioids/anti-opioids	Loperamide	Imodium	↓	
	Morphine, Methadone, Codeine	**Various**	↓	
	Buprenorphine	Buprenex	↓	
	Naloxone	**Narcan**	↑	
	Naltrexone	**Revia**	↑	Unclear if low-dose naltrexone (LDN) has the same effect
Drugs of abuse	**Heroin**		↓	
	Cocaine		↑	
	Alcohol		↑	
	Tobacco/nicotine		↑	
Hormones	Progesterone	Provera, Prometrium	↓	Binds to the cortisol receptor, so Cushingoid features could occur, even though cortisol levels are decreased
	Megestrol	**Megace**	↓	Used for weight gain
	Growth hormone	Various	↓	Increase catabolism of cortisol
	Thyroid hormone	Synthroid, Levoxyl, Cytomel Armour, etc.	↓	Increase catabolism of cortisol
	Raloxifene	Evista	↓	Used for osteoporosis
	Estrogens, birth control pills		–	Raises cortisol-binding protein and raises total cortisol, does not affect free cortisol
	DHEA		↓	
	Desmopressin	DDAVP	↑	
	Oxytocin		↓	Anecdotal reports of lowering cortisol

TABLE 66.3	Medications and Supplements Affecting Cortisol Levels—cont'd			
Type of Drugs	**Generic Name**	**Brand Name**	**Effect on Cortisol**	**Comments**
Diabetes medications	Rosiglitazone	Avandia	↓/–	Initial studies found a reduction in cortisol, not confirmed by additional studies
	Pioglitazone	Actos	↓/–	
Supplements	**Phosphatidyl serine**	**Seriphos**	↓	Effective at night, Seriphos and phosphatidyl serine are slightly different
	Gingko biloba		↓	
	St. John's wort		↑	
	Rhodiola		↓	

Bold indicates substantial effect.

Clinical Presentation

The clinical signs, symptoms, and common laboratory findings of hypercortisolism observed in patients with Cushing's syndrome are listed in Table 66.5. Patients with Cushing's syndrome often have some, but not all, of the signs and symptoms discussed here. Typically, the obesity is centripetal, with a wasting of the arms and legs, which is distinct from the generalized weight gain observed in idiopathic obesity. Rounding of the face (called *moon facies*) and a dorsocervical fat pad *(buffalo hump)* may occur in obesity not related to Cushing's syndrome, whereas facial plethora and supraclavicular filling are more specific for Cushing's syndrome. Patients with Cushing's syndrome may have proximal muscle weakness; consequently, the inability to stand up from a squat or to comb their own hair can be revealing. Sleep disturbances and insomnia, hyperarousal in the evening and night, mood swings, and other psychological abnormalities are frequently seen. Cognitive dysfunction and severe fatigue are often present. Menstrual irregularities often precede other Cushingoid symptoms in affected women. Patients of both sexes complain of a loss of libido, and affected men frequently complain of erectile dysfunction. Adult-onset acne or hirsutism in women could also suggest Cushing's syndrome. The skin striae observed in patients with Cushing's syndrome are often violaceous (i.e., purple or dark red, from hemorrhage into the striae) depending on the level of hypercortisolism. Thinning of the skin on the top of the hands is a specific sign in younger adults with Cushing's syndrome. Old pictures of patients are extremely helpful for evaluating the progression of the physical stigmata of Cushing's syndrome.

Associated laboratory findings in Cushing's syndrome include elevated plasma alkaline phosphatase levels, granulocytosis, thrombocytosis, hypercholesterolemia, hypertriglyceridemia, and glucose intolerance, and/or diabetes mellitus. Hypokalemia or alkalosis usually occurs in patients with severe hypercortisolism as a result of the ectopic ACTH syndrome.

Diagnosis

If the history and physical examination findings are suggestive of hypercortisolism, then the diagnosis of Cushing's syndrome can usually be established by collecting urine for 24 hours and measuring the urinary free cortisol (UFC). This test is extremely sensitive for diagnosis of Cushing's syndrome because in 90% of affected patients the initial UFC level is greater than 50 μg/24 hours (Fig. 66.5).

Cortisol is normally secreted in a diurnal manner: The plasma concentration is highest in the early morning (between 6:00 and 8:00 AM) and lowest around midnight. Most patients with Cushing's syndrome have blunted diurnal variation. Nighttime plasma cortisol values greater than 50% of the morning values are considered to be consistent with Cushing's syndrome. Because of the difficulty of obtaining nighttime plasma cortisol levels, measurement of late-night salivary cortisol has been developed to assess hypercortisolism. This test has a high degree of sensitivity and specificity for the diagnosis of Cushing's syndrome and is convenient for patients. Multiple measurements of UFC or salivary cortisol may be needed to either diagnose or exclude Cushing's syndrome, especially in subjects with convincing and progressive signs and symptoms of hypercortisolism.

The overnight dexamethasone suppression test has been widely used as a screening tool to evaluate patients who may have hypercortisolism. Dexamethasone, 1 mg, is given orally at 11:00 PM or midnight, and plasma cortisol is measured the following morning at 8:00 AM. A morning plasma cortisol level greater than 1.8 μg/dL suggests hypercortisolism. This test produces a significant number of both false-positive and false-negative results, but it is recommended in the 2008 Endocrine Society consensus guidelines.

Differential Diagnosis

Once the diagnosis of Cushing's syndrome is established, the cause of the hypercortisolism needs to be ascertained by biochemical studies that evaluate the HPA axis; this should be accompanied by imaging procedures and at times, venous sampling. The initial approach is to measure basal ACTH levels, which are normal or elevated in Cushing's disease and the ectopic ACTH syndrome but are suppressed in primary adrenal Cushing's syndrome. Patients with a suppressed ACTH level can proceed to adrenal imaging studies. To distinguish between Cushing's disease and the ectopic ACTH syndrome, the 2-day dexamethasone suppression test or 8-mg overnight dexamethasone suppression test and bilateral simultaneous inferior petrosal sinus sampling (IPSS) may be used.

In the dexamethasone suppression test (Liddle test), 0.5 mg of dexamethasone is given orally every 6 hours for 2 days (low dose), followed by 2 mg of dexamethasone every 6 hours for another 2 days (high dose). On the second day of high-dose dexamethasone, the UFC level will be suppressed to less than 10% of the baseline collection value in patients with pituitary adenomas but not in patients with the ectopic ACTH syndrome or adrenal cortisol-secreting tumors. The Liddle test has some methodologic drawbacks, and results should be interpreted cautiously; other confirmatory tests should be performed before surgery is recommended.

An overnight high-dose dexamethasone suppression test can be helpful in establishing the cause of Cushing's syndrome. In this test, a baseline cortisol level is measured at 8:00 AM, and then 8 mg of dexamethasone is given orally at 11:00 PM. At 8:00 AM the following morning, a plasma cortisol measurement is obtained. Suppression, which occurs in patients with pituitary Cushing's disease, is defined as a decrease in plasma cortisol to less than 50% of the baseline level.

TABLE 66.4   Syndromes of Adrenocortical Hyperfunction

States of Glucocorticoid Excess
Physiologic States
Stress
Strenuous exercise
Last trimester of pregnancy
Pathologic States
Psychiatric conditions (pseudo-Cushing's disorders)
Depression
Alcoholism
Anorexia nervosa
Panic disorders
Alcohol and drug withdrawal
ACTH-dependent states
  Pituitary adenoma (Cushing's disease)
  Ectopic ACTH syndrome
  Bronchial carcinoid
  Thymic carcinoid
  Islet cell tumor
  Small cell lung carcinoma
  Ectopic CRH secretion
ACTH-independent states
  Adrenal adenoma
  Adrenal carcinoma
  Micronodular adrenal disease
Exogenous Sources
Glucocorticoid intake
ACTH intake

States of Mineralocorticoid Excess
Primary Aldosteronism
Aldosterone-secreting adenoma
Bilateral adrenal hyperplasia
Aldosterone-secreting carcinoma
Glucocorticoid-suppressible hyperaldosteronism
Adrenal Enzyme Deficiencies
11β-Hydroxylase deficiency
17α-Hydroxylase deficiency
11β-Hydroxysteroid dehydrogenase type II deficiency
Exogenous Mineralocorticoids
Licorice
Carbenoxolone
Fludrocortisone
Secondary Hyperaldosteronism
Associated with hypertension
  Accelerated hypertension
  Renovascular hypertension
  Estrogen administration
  Renin-secreting tumors
Without hypertension
  Bartter syndrome
  Sodium-wasting nephropathy
  Renal tubular acidosis
  Diuretic and laxative abuse
  Edematous states (cirrhosis, nephrosis, congestive heart failure)

ACTH, Adrenocorticotropin hormone; *CRH*, corticotropin-releasing hormone.

Bilateral IPSS is an accurate and safe procedure for distinguishing pituitary Cushing's disease from the ectopic ACTH syndrome.

Venous blood from the anterior lobe of the pituitary gland empties into the cavernous sinuses and then into the superior and inferior petrosal sinuses. Venous plasma samples for ACTH determination are obtained from both inferior petrosal sinuses, along with a simultaneous peripheral sample, both before and after intravenous bolus administration of ovine corticotropin-releasing hormone (oCRH). Significant gradients at baseline and after oCRH stimulation between petrosal sinus and peripheral samples suggest pituitary Cushing's disease. In baseline measurements, an ACTH concentration gradient of 1.6 or more between a sample from either of the petrosal sinuses and the peripheral sample is strongly suggestive of pituitary Cushing's disease, whereas patients with the ectopic ACTH syndrome or adrenal adenomas have no ACTH gradient between their petrosal and peripheral samples. After oCRH administration, a central-to-peripheral gradient of more than 3.2 is consistent with pituitary Cushing's disease. An ACTH gradient ipsilateral to the side of the tumor is found in 70% to 80% of pituitary Cushing's disease patients sampled. Although this procedure requires a radiologist who is experienced in IPSS, it is available at many tertiary care facilities. The test cannot be done to distinguish patients with Cushing's syndrome from those without the condition, and the test needs to be done when the patient is hypercortisolemic, making it less helpful in those with episodic cortisol secretion.

Magnetic resonance imaging (MRI) with gadolinium is the preferred procedure for localizing a pituitary adenoma. In many centers, a *dynamic* MRI is performed; the pituitary is visualized as the gadolinium enters and leaves the gland. Because about 10% of normal individuals are found to have a nonfunctioning pituitary adenoma on pituitary MRI, pituitary imaging should not be the sole criterion for the diagnosis of pituitary Cushing's disease.

Treatment

The preferred treatment for all forms of Cushing's syndrome is appropriate surgery or, in some cases, radiation therapy (see Chapter 64). A more appealing option for many patients with Cushing's disease who remain hypercortisolemic after pituitary surgery is bilateral adrenalectomy followed by lifelong glucocorticoid and mineralocorticoid replacement therapy.

In patients with the ectopic ACTH syndrome, the goal is to localize the tumor by appropriate scans so it can be removed surgically. A unilateral adrenalectomy is the treatment of choice in patients with a cortisol-secreting adrenal adenoma. Cortisol-secreting adrenal carcinomas initially should also be managed surgically; however, the prognosis is poor, with only 20% of patients surviving more than 1 year after diagnosis.

Medical treatment for hypercortisolism may be needed to prepare patients who are undergoing or have undergone pituitary irradiation and are awaiting its effects before surgery; it may also be needed for those who are not surgical candidates or elect not to have surgery. Ketoconazole, *o,p′*-DDD (mitotane), metyrapone, aminoglutethimide, mifepristone (FDA approved for Cushing's syndrome if accompanied by hypertension or glucose intolerance/diabetes), and trilostane are the most commonly used agents for adrenal blockade and can be used alone or in combination. The somatostatin analogue, pasireotide, which decreases ACTH and may decrease tumor size, is an FDA-approved drug for treating Cushing's disease.

Primary Mineralocorticoid Excess
Pathophysiology

The causes of primary aldosteronism (see Table 66.4) are aldosterone-producing adenoma (75%), bilateral adrenal hyperplasia (25%), adrenal carcinoma (1%), and glucocorticoid-remediable hyperaldosteronism (<1%). Adrenal enzyme defects (11β-HSD type II,

TABLE 66.5   Signs, Symptoms, and Laboratory Abnormalities of Hypercortisolism

Feature	Percentage of Patients
Fat redistribution (dorsocervical and supraclavicular fat pads, temporal wasting, centripetal obesity, weight gain)	95
Menstrual irregularities	80 (of affected women)
Thin skin and plethora	80
Moon facies	75
Increased appetite	75
Sleep disturbances	75
Nocturnal hyperarousal	75
Hypertension	75
Hypercholesterolemia and hypertriglyceridemia	70
Altered mentation (poor concentration, decreased memory, euphoria)	70
Diabetes mellitus and glucose intolerance	65
Striae	65
Hirsutism	65 (of affected women)
Proximal muscle weakness	60
Psychological disturbances (emotional lability, depression, mania, psychosis)	50
Decreased libido and erectile dysfunction	50 (of affected men)
Acne	45
Osteoporosis and pathologic fractures	40
Easy bruisability	40
Poor wound healing	40
Virilization	20 (of affected women)
Edema	20
Increased infections	10
Cataracts	5

11β-hydroxylase, and 17α-hydroxylase deficiencies) and apparent mineralocorticoid excess (from ingestion of licorice or carbenoxolone, which inhibit 11β-HSD type II, or from a congenital defect in this enzyme) are also states of functional mineralocorticoid overactivity. Secondary aldosteronism (see Table 66.4) results from an overactive renin-angiotensin system.

Primary aldosteronism is usually recognized during evaluation of hypertension or hypokalemia and represents a potentially curable form of hypertension. Up to 5% of patients with hypertension have primary aldosteronism. These patients are usually between the ages of 30 and 50 years, and the female-to-male ratio is 2:1.

Clinical Presentation

Hypertension, hypokalemia, and metabolic alkalosis are the main clinical manifestations of hyperaldosteronism; most of the presenting symptoms are related to hypokalemia. Symptoms in patients with mild hypokalemia are fatigue, muscle weakness, nocturia, lassitude, and headaches. If more severe hypokalemia exists, polydipsia, polyuria, paresthesias, and even intermittent paralysis and tetany can occur. Blood pressure can range from minimally elevated to very high. A positive Trousseau or Chvostek sign may occur as a result of metabolic alkalosis.

Diagnosis and Treatment

Initially, hypokalemia in the presence of hypertension should be documented (Fig. 66.6), although mild cases of hyperaldosteronism without hypokalemia exist. The patient must have adequate salt intake and discontinue diuretics before potassium measurement. A morning plasma aldosterone level (measured in ng/dL) and a PRA value (in ng/mL/hour) should be obtained. A ratio of serum aldosterone to PRA greater than 20 with a serum aldosterone level greater than 15 ng/dL suggests the diagnosis of hyperaldosteronism.

Confirmatory tests for hyperaldosteronism should be performed, such as oral sodium loading, saline infusion, fludrocortisone suppression, or captopril challenge.

Once the diagnosis of primary aldosteronism has been demonstrated, it is important to distinguish between an aldosterone-producing adenoma and bilateral hyperplasia, because the former is treated with surgery and the latter is treated medically. A computed tomography (CT) scan of the adrenal glands should be performed to localize the tumor. Prior to surgery, imaging should be confirmed with adrenal venous sampling for cortisol due to the high degree of adrenal incidentalomas. The patient should undergo unilateral adrenalectomy if a discrete adenoma is observed in one adrenal gland, the contralateral gland is normal, and the adrenal venous sampling lateralizes to the side of the adenoma. Patients in whom biochemical and localization study findings are consistent with bilateral hyperplasia should be treated medically with a potassium-sparing diuretic, usually eplerenone or spironolactone. Hyperaldosteronism and hypertension secondary to activation of the renin-angiotensin system can occur in patients with accelerated hypertension, in those with renovascular hypertension, in those receiving estrogen therapies, and, rarely, in patients with renin-secreting tumors. Hyperaldosteronism without hypertension occurs in patients with Bartter syndrome, sodium-wasting nephropathy, or renal tubular acidosis, as well as those who abuse diuretics or laxatives.

ADRENAL MEDULLARY HYPERFUNCTION

The adrenal medulla synthesizes the catecholamines norepinephrine, epinephrine, and dopamine from the amino acid tyrosine. Norepinephrine, the major catecholamine produced by the adrenal medulla, has predominantly α-agonist actions, causing vasoconstriction. Epinephrine acts primarily on the β-receptors, having positive

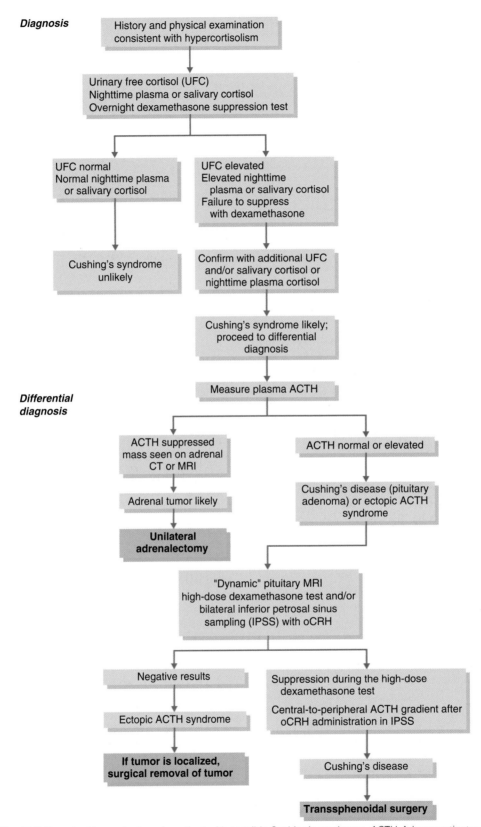

Fig. 66.5 Flowchart for evaluation of a patient with possible Cushing's syndrome. *ACTH,* Adrenocorticotropic hormone; *CT,* computed tomography; *MRI,* magnetic resonance imaging.

inotropic and chronotropic effects on the heart causing peripheral vasodilation and increasing plasma glucose concentrations in response to hypoglycemia. The action of circulating dopamine is unclear. Whereas norepinephrine is synthesized in the central nervous system and sympathetic postganglionic neurons, epinephrine is synthesized almost entirely in the adrenal medulla. The adrenal medullary contribution to total body norepinephrine secretion is relatively small. Hypofunction of the adrenal medulla has little physiologic effect, whereas hypersecretion of catecholamines produces the clinical syndrome of pheochromocytoma.

Pheochromocytoma

Pathophysiology

Although pheochromocytomas can occur in any sympathetic ganglion in the body, more than 90% arise from the adrenal medulla. Most extra-adrenal tumors occur in the mediastinum or abdomen. Bilateral adrenal pheochromocytomas are present in about 5% of the cases and may occur as part of familial syndromes. Pheochromocytoma occurs as part of multiple endocrine neoplasia type IIA or IIB. The former, type IIA, is also called Sipple syndrome and is marked by medullary carcinoma of the thyroid, hyperparathyroidism, and pheochromocytoma; the latter, type IIB, is characterized by medullary carcinoma of the thyroid, mucosal neuromas, intestinal ganglioneuromas, marfanoid habitus, and pheochromocytoma. Pheochromocytomas are also associated with neurofibromatosis, cerebelloretinal hemangioblastoma (von Hippel–Lindau disease), and tuberous sclerosis.

Clinical Presentation

Because most pheochromocytomas secrete norepinephrine as the principal catecholamine, hypertension (often paroxysmal) is the most common finding. Other symptoms include the triad of headache, palpitations, and sweating as well as skin blanching, diarrhea, anxiety, nausea, fatigue, weight loss, and abdominal and chest pain. Emotional stress, exercise, anesthesia, abdominal pressure, or intake of tyramine-containing foods may precipitate these symptoms. Orthostatic hypotension can also occur. Wide fluctuations in blood pressure are characteristic, and the hypertension associated with pheochromocytoma usually does not respond to standard antihypertensive medicines. Cardiac abnormalities, as well as idiosyncratic reactions to medications, may also occur.

Diagnosis and Treatment

Although measurements of fractionated catecholamine and metanephrine levels in the urine are often used as screening tests, plasma free metanephrine and normetanephrine levels are the best tests for confirming or excluding pheochromocytoma. A plasma free metanephrine level greater than 0.61 nmol/L and a plasma free normetanephrine level greater than 0.31 nmol/L are consistent with the diagnosis of a pheochromocytoma. If these levels are only mildly elevated, a clonidine suppression test can be performed. In patients with pheochromocytoma, levels are unchanged or increased. Once the diagnosis of pheochromocytoma is made, a CT scan of the adrenal glands should be performed. Most intra-adrenal pheochromocytomas are readily visible on this scan and enhance with contrast. If the CT scan is negative, then extra-adrenal pheochromocytomas can often be localized by iodine 131–labeled metaiodobenzylguanidine (^{131}I-MIBG), positron emission tomography, octreotide scan, or abdominal MRI. Pheochromocytomas show high signal intensity on MRI T2-weighted images.

The treatment of pheochromocytoma is surgical if the lesion can be localized. Patients should undergo preoperative α-blockade with phenoxybenzamine 1 to 2 weeks before surgery. About 5% to 10% of pheochromocytomas are malignant. ^{131}I-MIBG or chemotherapy may be useful, but the prognosis is poor. α-Methyl-*p*-tyrosine, an inhibitor of tyrosine hydroxylase, the rate-limiting enzyme in catecholamine biosynthesis, may be used to decrease catecholamine secretion from the tumor.

Incidental Adrenal Mass

Clinically inapparent adrenal masses may be discovered inadvertently in the course of diagnostic testing or treatment for other clinical conditions not related to the signs and symptoms of adrenal disease; they are commonly known as *incidentalomas* (E-Fig. 66.2). Some of these

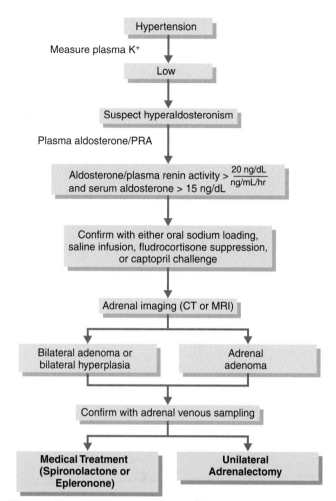

Fig. 66.6 Flowchart for evaluation of a patient with probable primary hyperaldosteronism. Plasma aldosterone is measured in ng/dL, and plasma renin activity (PRA) is measured in ng/mL/hour. *CT,* Computed tomography; *MRI,* magnetic resonance imaging.

tumors secrete a small amount of excess cortisol, leading to a condition that used to be called subclinical Cushing's syndrome and is now called *mild autonomous cortisol excess (MACE)* or *autonomous cortisol secretion,* a condition associated with comorbidities including hypertension, glucose intolerance/diabetes, obesity, dyslipidemia, osteoporosis, and increased cardiovascular events. This condition does not progress to overt Cushing's syndrome. An overnight 1-mg dexamethasone test is recommended for all patients with an adrenal mass seen on imaging. A morning cortisol post-dexamethasone of between 1.8 and 5 μg/dL suggests possible autonomous cortisol secretion that usually does not need surgery, whereas values greater than 5 μg/dL should be worked up for Cushing's syndrome as described previously. Under certain circumstances, surgical removal should be performed. Patients with hypertension should also undergo measurement of serum potassium, plasma aldosterone concentration, PRA, and plasma free metanephrines (only if the unenhanced CT attenuation value is greater than 10 Hounsfield units). Surgery should be considered for all patients with functional adrenal cortical tumors that are hormonally active or larger than 4 cm. Tumors not associated with hormonal secretion that are smaller than 4 cm and have benign imaging characteristics do not need follow-up.

Primary Adrenal Cancer

Primary adrenal carcinomas are rare, with an incidence of 1 to 5 per 1 million persons. The female-to-male ratio is 2.5:1, and the mean age at onset is 40 to 50 years. About 25% of patients have symptoms, including abdominal pain, weight loss, anorexia, and fever. Eighty percent of primary adrenal carcinomas are functional, with secretion of glucocorticoid alone (45%) or glucocorticoid plus androgens (45%) being most common.

At presentation, metastatic spread is evident in 75% of cases. An incidentally discovered adrenal mass that is large is more likely to be malignant. Resection is recommended for tumors larger than 6 cm and often for those larger than 4 cm. In patients who do not have a known cancer, most adrenal masses that turn out to be malignant are primary adrenocortical carcinomas, whereas in patients with a known malignancy, an adrenal mass is likely to be a metastasis in about 75% of cases.

The treatment of adrenocortical carcinomas is surgery. These cancers are usually resistant to radiation and chemotherapy, but the adrenolytic compound mitotane has been shown to improve survival. Adrenocortical carcinomas carry a poor prognosis, with overall 5-year survival rates of less than 20%.

❖ For a deeper discussion on this topic, please see Chapter 214, "Adrenal Cortex," in *Goldman-Cecil Medicine*, 26th Edition.

SUGGESTED READINGS

Annane D, Pastores SM, Rochwerg B, et al: Guidelines for the diagnosis and management of critical illness-related corticosteroid insufficiency (CIRCI) in critically ill patients (Part I): Society of Critical Care Medicine (SCCM) and European Society of Intensive Care Medicine (ESICM) 2017, Intensive Care Med 43:1751–1763, 2017.

Bornstein SR, Allolio B, Arlt W, et al: Diagnosis and treatment of primary adrenal insufficiency: an Endocrine Society clinical practice guideline, J Clin Endocrinol Metab 101:364–389, 2016.

Fassnacht M, Arlt W, Bancos I, et al: Management of adrenal incidentalomas: European Society of Endocrinology clinical practice guideline in collaboration with the European Network for the Study of Adrenal Tumors, Eur J Endocrinol 175:G1–G34, 2016.

Nieman LK, Biller BM, Findling JW, et al: The diagnosis of Cushing's syndrome: an Endocrine Society clinical practice guideline, J Clin Endocrinol Metab 93:1526–1540, 2008.

Rushworth RL, Torpy DJ, Falhammar H: Adrenal crisis, N Engl J Med 381:852–861, 2019.

Speiser PW, Arlt W, Auchus RJ, et al: Congenital adrenal hyperplasia due to steroid 21-hydroxylase deficiency: an Endocrine Society clinical practice guideline, J Clin Endocrinol Metab 103:4043–4088, 2018.

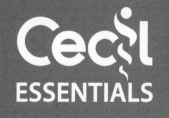

67

Male Reproductive Endocrinology

Glenn D. Braunstein

INTRODUCTION

The testes are composed of Leydig (interstitial) cells, which secrete testosterone and estradiol, and the seminiferous tubules, which produce sperm. They are regulated by the luteinizing hormone (LH) and follicle-stimulating hormone (FSH), which are secreted by the anterior pituitary under the influence of the hypothalamic decapeptide gonadotropin-releasing hormone (GnRH) (Fig. 67.1). LH stimulates the Leydig cells to secrete testosterone, which feeds back in a negative fashion at the level of the pituitary and hypothalamus to inhibit further LH production. FSH stimulates sperm production through interaction with the Sertoli cells in the seminiferous tubules. Feedback inhibition of FSH is through gonadal steroids, as well as through inhibin, a glycoprotein produced by Sertoli cells.

Biochemical evaluation of the hypothalamic-pituitary-Leydig axis is carried out by measurement of serum LH and testosterone concentrations, whereas a semen analysis and serum FSH determination provide an assessment of the hypothalamic-pituitary-seminiferous tubular axis. The ability of the pituitary to release gonadotropins can be tested dynamically through GnRH stimulation, and the ability of the testes to secrete testosterone can be evaluated through injections of human chorionic gonadotropin (HCG), a glycoprotein hormone that has biologic activity similar to that of LH.

HYPOGONADISM

Either testosterone deficiency or defective spermatogenesis constitutes *hypogonadism*. Often both disorders coexist. The clinical manifestations of androgen deficiency depend on the time of onset and the degree of deficiency. Testosterone is required for development of the Wolffian duct into the epididymis, vas deferens, seminal vesicles, and ejaculatory ducts, as well as for virilization of the external genitalia through the major intracellular testosterone metabolite, dihydrotestosterone (DHT). Consequently, early prenatal androgen deficiency leads to the formation of ambiguous genitalia and to male pseudohermaphroditism. Androgen deficiency occurring later during gestation may result in micropenis or *cryptorchidism*, the unilateral or bilateral absence of testes in the scrotum resulting from the failure of normal testicular descent.

During puberty, androgens are responsible for male sexual differentiation, which includes growth of the scrotum, epididymis, vas deferens, seminal vesicles, prostate, penis, skeletal muscle, and larynx. Additionally, androgens stimulate the growth of axillary, pubic, facial, and body hair and increase sebaceous gland activity. They are also responsible through conversion to estrogens for the growth and fusion of the epiphyseal cartilaginous plates, clinically seen as the *pubertal growth spurt*. Prepubertal androgen deficiency leads to poor muscle development, decreased strength and endurance, a

high-pitched voice, sparse axillary and pubic hair, and the absence of facial and body hair. The long bones of the lower extremities and arms may continue to grow under the influence of growth hormone; this condition leads to eunuchoid proportions (i.e., arm span exceeding total height by ≥5 cm) and greater growth of the lower extremities relative to total height. Postpubertal androgen deficiency may result in a decrease in libido, impotence, low energy, fine wrinkling around the corners of the eyes and mouth, and diminished facial and body hair.

Male hypogonadism may be classified into three categories according to the level of the defect (Table 67.1). Diseases directly affecting the testes result in *primary* or *hypergonadotropic hypogonadism*, which is characterized by oligospermia or azoospermia and low testosterone levels but exhibits elevations of LH and FSH because of a decrease in the negative feedback regulation on the pituitary and hypothalamus by androgens, estrogens, and inhibin. In contrast, hypogonadism from lesions in the hypothalamus or pituitary gives rise to *secondary* or *hypogonadotropic hypogonadism*; the low testosterone level or ineffective spermatogenesis results from inadequate concentrations of the gonadotropins. The third category of hypogonadism is the result of defects in androgen action.

Hypothalamic-Pituitary Disorders

Panhypopituitarism occurs congenitally from structural defects or from inadequate production or release of the hypothalamic-releasing factors. The condition may also be acquired through replacement by tumors, infarction from vascular insufficiency, infiltrative disorders, autoimmune diseases, trauma, and infections.

Kallmann syndrome is a form of hypogonadotropic hypogonadism that is associated with problems in the ability to discriminate odors, either incompletely *(hyposmia)* or completely *(anosmia)*. This syndrome results from a defect in the migration of the GnRH neurons from the olfactory placode into the hypothalamus. Therefore, it represents a GnRH deficiency. Patients remain prepubertal, with small, rubbery testes, and they develop eunuchoidism (E-Fig. 67.1).

Hyperprolactinemia may result in hypogonadotropic hypogonadism because prolactin elevation inhibits normal release of GnRH, decreases the effectiveness of LH at the Leydig cell level, and also inhibits some of the actions of testosterone at the level of the target organ. Normalization of prolactin levels through withdrawal of an offending drug, by surgical removal of the pituitary adenoma, or with the use of dopamine agonists reverses this form of hypogonadism.

Weight loss or systemic illness in male patients can cause another form of secondary hypogonadism, *hypothalamic dysfunction*. Weight loss or illness induces a defect in the hypothalamic release of GnRH and results in low levels of gonadotropin and testosterone. This condition is commonly observed in patients with cancer, AIDS, or chronic

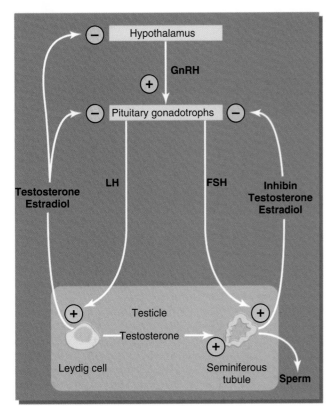

Fig. 67.1 Regulation of the hypothalamic-pituitary-testicular axis. The *plus (+)* and *minus (−)* symbols indicate positive and negative feedback, respectively. *FSH,* Follicle-stimulating hormone; *GnRH,* gonadotropin-releasing hormone; *LH,* luteinizing hormone.

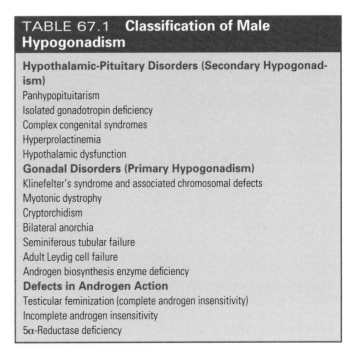

TABLE 67.1   **Classification of Male Hypogonadism**
Hypothalamic-Pituitary Disorders (Secondary Hypogonadism)
Panhypopituitarism
Isolated gonadotropin deficiency
Complex congenital syndromes
Hyperprolactinemia
Hypothalamic dysfunction
Gonadal Disorders (Primary Hypogonadism)
Klinefelter's syndrome and associated chromosomal defects
Myotonic dystrophy
Cryptorchidism
Bilateral anorchia
Seminiferous tubular failure
Adult Leydig cell failure
Androgen biosynthesis enzyme deficiency
Defects in Androgen Action
Testicular feminization (complete androgen insensitivity)
Incomplete androgen insensitivity
5α-Reductase deficiency

inflammatory processes. Prolonged use of opioids and therapeutic doses of glucocorticoids may suppress gonadotropin production and cause secondary hypogonadism.

Primary Gonadal Abnormalities

The most common congenital cause of primary testicular failure is *Klinefelter's syndrome,* which occurs in about 1 of every 600 live male births and is usually caused by a maternal meiotic chromosomal nondisjunction that results in an XXY genotype. At puberty, clinical findings include the following: a variable degree of hypogonadism; gynecomastia; small, firm testes measuring less than 2 cm in the longest axis (normal testes, 3.5 cm or greater); azoospermia; eunuchoid skeletal proportions; and elevations of FSH and LH (E-Fig. 67.2). Primary gonadal failure is also found in patients with another congenital condition, *myotonic dystrophy,* which is characterized by progressive weakness; atrophy of the facial, neck, hand, and lower extremity muscles; frontal baldness; and myotonia.

About 3% of full-term male infants have *cryptorchidism,* which spontaneously corrects during the first year of life in most cases; consequently, by 1 year of age, the incidence of this condition is about 0.8%. When the testes are maintained in the intra-abdominal position, the increased temperature leads to defective spermatogenesis and oligospermia. Leydig cell function usually remains normal, resulting in normal levels of adult testosterone.

Bilateral anorchia, also known as the vanishing testicle syndrome, is a rare condition in which the external genitalia are fully formed, indicating that ample quantities of testosterone and DHT were produced during early embryogenesis. However, the testicular tissue disappears before or shortly after birth, and the result is an empty scrotum. This condition is differentiated from cryptorchidism by an HCG stimulation test. Patients with cryptorchidism have an increase in serum testosterone level after an injection of HCG, whereas patients with bilateral anorchia do not.

Acquired gonadal failure has numerous causes. The adult seminiferous tubules are susceptible to a variety of injuries, and seminiferous tubular failure is found after infections such as mumps, gonococcal or lepromatous orchitis, irradiation, vascular injury, trauma, alcohol ingestion, and use of chemotherapeutic drugs, especially alkylating agents. The serum FSH concentration may be normal or elevated, depending on the degree of damage to the seminiferous tubules. The Leydig cell compartment may also be damaged by these same conditions. In addition, some men experience a gradual decline in testicular function as they age, possibly because of microvascular insufficiency. Patients with decreased testosterone production may clinically exhibit lowered libido and potency, emotional lability, fatigue, and vasomotor symptoms such as hot flashes. The serum LH concentration is usually elevated in this situation.

Defects in Androgen Action

When either testosterone or its metabolite, DHT, binds to the androgen receptor in target cells, the receptor is activated and binds DNA; the resulting stimulation of transcription, protein synthesis, and cell growth collectively constitutes androgen action. An absence of androgen receptors causes the syndrome of *testicular feminization,* a form of male pseudohermaphroditism. These genetic males have cryptorchid testes but appear to be phenotypic females. Because androgens are inactive during embryogenesis, the labial-scrotal folds fail to fuse, and a short vagina results. The fallopian tubes, uterus, and upper portion of the vagina are absent because the fetal testicular Sertoli cells secrete Anti-Müllerian duct hormone (Müllerian duct inhibitory factor) during early fetal development. At puberty, these patients have breast enlargement because the testes secrete a small amount of estradiol and the peripheral tissues convert testosterone and adrenal androgens to estrogens. Axillary and pubic hair does not grow because androgen action is required for their development. The serum testosterone concentrations are elevated as a result of continuous stimulation by elevated concentrations of LH. LH is high because of the inability of the testosterone to act in a negative feedback fashion at

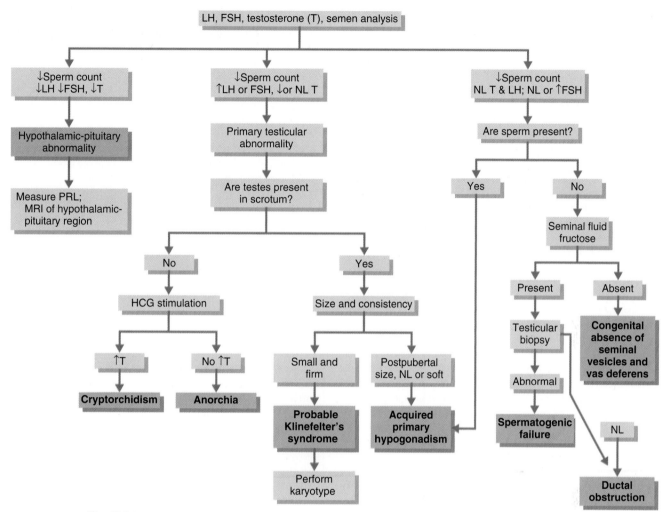

Fig. 67.2 Laboratory evaluation of hypogonadism. *↑*, Elevated; *↓*, decreased or low; *FSH*, follicle-stimulating hormone; *HCG*, human chorionic gonadotropin; *LH*, luteinizing hormone; *MRI*, magnetic resonance imaging; *NL*, normal; *PRL*, prolactin.

the hypothalamus. Patients may have incomplete forms of androgen insensitivity caused by point mutations affecting the androgen receptor gene, and clinically these patients show varying degrees of male pseudohermaphroditism.

Patients who lack the 5α-reductase enzyme that is required to convert testosterone to DHT are born with a *bifid scrotum*, which reflects abnormal fusion of the labial-scrotal folds, and *hypospadias*, in which the urethral opening is in the perineal area or in the shaft of the penis. At puberty, androgen production is sufficient to partially overcome the defect; the scrotum, phallus, and muscle mass enlarge, and these patients appear to develop into physiologically normal men.

Diagnosis

Fig. 67.2 illustrates an algorithm for the laboratory evaluation of hypogonadism in a phenotypic man. Serum concentrations of LH, FSH, and testosterone should be obtained, and a semen analysis should be performed. A low testosterone level with low concentrations of gonadotropins indicates a hypothalamic-pituitary abnormality, which needs to be evaluated with serum prolactin determination and radiographic examination. Elevated concentrations of gonadotropins with a normal or low testosterone level reflect a primary testicular abnormality. If no testes are palpable in the scrotum and careful *milking* of the patient's

lower abdomen does not bring retractile testes into the scrotum, an HCG stimulation test should be performed. A rise in serum testosterone concentrations indicates the presence of functional testicular tissue, and a diagnosis of cryptorchidism can be made. Absence of a rise in testosterone suggests bilateral anorchia. Small, firm testes in the scrotum are highly suggestive of Klinefelter's syndrome; this diagnosis needs to be confirmed with a chromosomal karyotype. Testes that are more than 3.5 cm in longest diameter and that are either of normal consistency or are soft indicate postpubertal acquired primary hypogonadism.

If the major abnormality is a deficient sperm count with or without an elevation of FSH, differentiation between a ductal problem and acquired primary hypogonadism must be made. If spermatozoa are present, at least the ducts emanating from one testicle are patent; this condition indicates an acquired testicular defect. If the patient has no sperm in the ejaculate, a primary testicular or ductal problem may be responsible. The seminal vesicles secrete fructose into the seminal fluid. Therefore, the presence of fructose in the ejaculate should be followed by a testicular biopsy to determine whether the defect results from spermatogenic failure or from an obstruction of the ducts leading from the testes to the seminal vesicles. Absence of seminal fluid fructose indicates a congenital absence of the seminal vesicles and vas deferens.

Male Infertility

The inability to conceive after 1 year of unprotected sexual intercourse affects about 15% of couples, and male factors appear to be responsible in about 20% of cases. Female factors account for close to 40%, and a couple factor is present in about 25% of cases with about 15% being undefined. In addition to the defects in spermatogenesis that occur in patients with hypothalamic, pituitary, testicular, or androgen action disorders, hyperthyroidism, hypothyroidism, adrenal abnormalities, and systemic illnesses can result in defective spermatogenesis, as can microdeletions of genetic material on the Y chromosome. Disorders of the vas deferens, seminal vesicles, and prostate may also lead to infertility, as may diseases affecting the bladder sphincter that result in *retrograde ejaculation*, in which the sperm passes into the bladder rather than through the penis. Anatomic defects of the penis (as observed in patients with hypospadias), poor coital technique, and the presence of antisperm antibodies in the male or female genital tract also are associated with infertility.

Therapy for Hypogonadism and Infertility

Treatment of androgen deficiency in patients who have hypothalamic-pituitary or primary testicular abnormalities is best accomplished with exogenous testosterone administration—either intramuscular injection of intermediate (1-3 weeks)- or long (3 months)-acting testosterone esters or transdermal testosterone patches or gel. Buccal, nasal, and subcutaneous testosterone pellets are also available but are less often used. Testosterone therapy increases libido, potency, muscle mass, strength, athletic endurance, hair growth on the face and body, and bone density. The most common side effect is erythrocytosis. Other side effects include acne, fluid retention, benign prostate hyperplasia, and, rarely, sleep apnea. This therapy is contraindicated in patients with cancer of the prostate.

If fertility is desired, patients with hypothalamic abnormalities may develop virilization and spermatogenesis with the use of GnRH delivered in a pulsatile fashion subcutaneously by an external pump. Direct stimulation of the testes in patients with hypothalamic or pituitary abnormalities may be accomplished with the use of exogenous gonadotropins, which increase testosterone and sperm production. If primary testicular failure is present and the patient has oligospermia, an attempt can be made to concentrate the sperm for intrauterine insemination or in vitro fertilization. If the azoospermia is caused by ductal obstruction, repair of the obstruction may be undertaken or aspiration of sperm from the epididymis may be accomplished for in vitro fertilization.

GYNECOMASTIA

Gynecomastia refers to a benign enlargement of the male breast that results from proliferation of the glandular component. This common condition is found in close to 70% of pubertal boys and in about one third of adults 50 to 80 years old. Estrogens stimulate and androgens inhibit breast glandular development; gynecomastia results from an imbalance between estrogen and androgen actions at the breast tissue level. This condition may result from an absolute increase in free estrogens, a decrease in endogenous free androgens, androgen insensitivity of the tissues, or enhanced sensitivity of the breast tissue to estrogens. Table 67.2 lists the common conditions associated with gynecomastia.

Gynecomastia must be differentiated from fatty enlargement of the breasts without glandular proliferation and from other disorders of the breasts, especially breast carcinoma. *Male breast cancer* usually manifests as a unilateral, eccentric, hard or firm mass that is fixed to the underlying tissues. It may be associated with skin dimpling or

TABLE 67.2 **Conditions Associated With Gynecomastia**
Physiologic Conditions
Neonatal
Pubertal
Involutional
Pathologic Conditions
Neoplasms
Testicular
Adrenal
Ectopic production of human chorionic gonadotropin
Primary gonadal failure
Secondary hypogonadism
Enzyme defects in testosterone production
Androgen insensitivity syndromes
Liver disease
Malnutrition with refeeding
Dialysis
Hyperthyroidism
Excessive extraglandular aromatase activity
Drugs
Estrogens and estrogen agonists
Gonadotropins
Antiandrogens or inhibitors of androgen synthesis
Cytotoxic agents
Highly active antiretroviral therapy (ART)
Spironolactone
Cimetidine
Growth hormone
Alcohol
Human immunodeficiency virus infection
Idiopathic

retraction or with crusting of the nipple or nipple discharge. In contrast, gynecomastia occurs concentrically around the nipple and is not fixed to the underlying structures. Although physical examination is usually sufficient to differentiate gynecomastia from breast carcinoma, mammography or ultrasonography may be required.

Painful and tender gynecomastia in a pubertal adolescent should be monitored with periodic examinations because, in most patients, pubertal gynecomastia disappears within 1 year. Incidentally discovered, asymptomatic gynecomastia in an adult requires a careful assessment for alcohol, drug, or medication use; liver, lung, or kidney dysfunction; and signs and symptoms of hypogonadism or hyperthyroidism. If these conditions are not present, only follow-up is required. In contrast, in an adult with recent onset of progressive painful gynecomastia, thyroid, liver, and renal function should be determined. If test results are normal, serum concentrations of HCG, LH, testosterone, and estradiol should be measured. Further evaluation should be carried out according to the schema outlined in Fig. 67.3.

Removal of the offending drug or correction of the underlying condition causing the gynecomastia may result in regression of the breast glandular tissue. If the gynecomastia persists, an off-label trial of antiestrogens (e.g., tamoxifen) may be given for 3 months to see whether regression occurs. Gynecomastia that has been present for longer than 1 year usually contains a fibrotic component that does not respond to medications. In these cases, correction usually requires surgical removal of the tissue.

For a deeper discussion on this topic, please see Chapter 223, "Reproductive Endocrinology and Infertility," in *Goldman-Cecil Medicine*, 26th Edition.

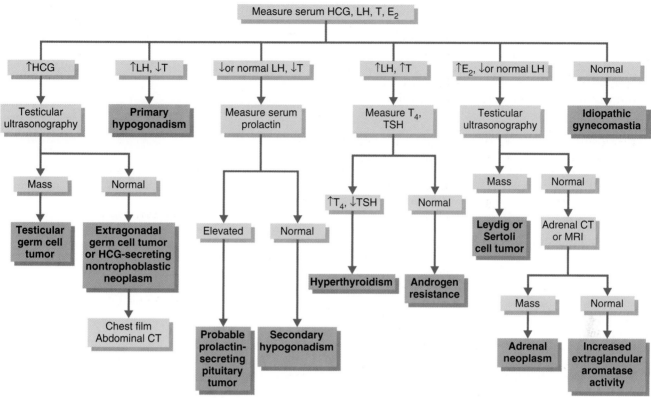

Fig. 67.3 Diagnostic evaluation for causes of gynecomastia based on measurements of serum human chorionic gonadotropin (HCG), luteinizing hormone (LH), testosterone (T), and estradiol (E$_2$). *↑*, Increased; *↓*, decreased; *CT*, computed tomography; *MRI*, magnetic resonance imaging; *T$_4$*, thyroxine; *TSH*, thyroid-stimulating hormone. (From Braunstein GD: Gynecomastia, N Engl J Med 328:490-495, 1993.)

SUGGESTED READINGS

Bhasin S, Brito J, Cunningham GR, et al: Testosterone therapy in men with hypogonadism: an Endocrine Society clinical practice guideline, J Clin Endocrinol Metab 103:1715–1744, 2018.

Gravholt CH, Chang S, Wallentin M, Fedder J, Moore P, Skakkebaek A: Klinefelter syndrome: integrating genetics, neuropsychology, and endocrinology, Endocr Rev 39:389–423, 2018.

Irwin GM: Erectile dysfunction, Clinics in Office Practice 46:249–255, 2019.

Pan MM, HGockenberry MS, Kirby EW, Lipshultz LI: Male infertility diagnosis and treatment in the era of in vitro fertilization and intracytoplasmic sperm injection, Med Clin N Amer 102:337–347, 2018.

Practice Committee of the American Society for Reproductive Medicine in collaboration with the Society for Male Reproduction and Urology: Evaluation of the azoospermic male: a committee opinion, Fertil Steril 109:777–782, 2018.

Sansone A, Romanelli F, Sansone M, Lenzi A, Luigi LD: Gynecomastia and hormones, Endocrine 55:37–44, 2017.

Shepard CL, Kraft KH: The nonpalpable testis: a narrative review, J Urol 198:1410–1417, 2017.

68

Diabetes Mellitus, Hypoglycemia

Robert J. Smith

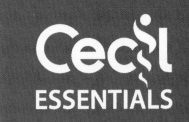

DIABETES MELLITUS

Definition and Diagnostic Criteria

Diabetes mellitus is not a single disease but a group of disorders that develop as a consequence of absolute or relative deficiency of the hormone insulin. Inadequate actions of insulin in stimulating the uptake of glucose by body tissues and regulating the metabolism of carbohydrate, fat, and protein result in *hyperglycemia*. Other metabolic disturbances in addition to hyperglycemia typically occur in uncontrolled diabetes, including altered lipoprotein dynamics and elevated free fatty acid levels. These abnormalities contribute to the acute and chronic clinical consequences of diabetes.

The criteria used to diagnose diabetes mellitus in nonpregnant individuals are summarized in Table 68.1. The diagnosis can be made on the basis of a fasting blood glucose level of 126 mg/dL or higher, a random blood glucose concentration (i.e., determined at any time in association with meals or fasting) of 200 mg/dL or higher, or a 2-hour glucose level of 200 mg/dL or higher as part of a 75-g oral glucose tolerance test. Alternatively, diabetes can be diagnosed if the hemoglobin A_{1c} (HbA_{1c}) level is 6.5% or higher. HbA_{1c}, a measure of the percentage of hemoglobin in circulating erythrocytes that is glycosylated, correlates with mean circulating glucose levels. HbA_{1c} provides an index of the average blood glucose level over the preceding 2 to 3 months. Because HbA_{1c} accumulates progressively throughout the lifespan of an erythrocyte, spurious values may occur in states of altered erythrocyte turnover (e.g., with various anemias) or with certain hemoglobinopathies that increase or decrease the susceptibility of hemoglobin to glycosylation. In patients with marked elevations in blood glucose or HbA_{1c} and coincident symptoms typical for hyperglycemia (e.g., polyuria and polydipsia), the diagnosis can be made based on a single test result. With less marked glucose elevations in the absence of symptoms, the diagnosis should be confirmed by repeat testing on a separate day.

Patients who have mild elevations in plasma glucose levels that do not reach the threshold for diagnosis of diabetes (e.g., HbA_{1c} levels between 5.7% and 6.4%) are at increased risk for progression to diabetes and therefore are considered to have *prediabetes*. Prediabetes patients with fasting blood glucose levels between 100 and 125 mg/dL are more specifically labeled as having *impaired fasting glucose*, and those with 2-hour postprandial plasma glucose levels between 140 and 199 mg/dL (most reliably measured after a standardized 75-g oral glucose load) have *impaired glucose tolerance* (see Table 68.1). Although not all individuals with prediabetes will become diabetic, the mean progression rate to overt diabetes is approximately 6% per year. There also is evidence from observational studies that the prediabetic state is associated with an increased risk of cardiovascular disease.

Gestational diabetes mellitus (GDM) is a term applied to diabetes first recognized during pregnancy. The most widely accepted thresholds for diagnosis of GDM are a fasting plasma glucose level of 92 mg/dL or higher at any gestational stage and values on a 75-g oral glucose tolerance test at 24 to 28 weeks' gestation of 92 mg/dL or higher fasting, 180 mg/dL or higher at 1 hour, or 153 mg/dL or higher at 2 hours after glucose loading (Table 68.2). Untreated diabetes in pregnancy is associated with increased fetal malformations, problems in delivery, and possibly more frequent diabetes complications in the mother.

Etiologic Classification

Once the diagnosis is made based on elevated blood glucose or HbA_{1c} values, it is important to establish the specific subtype of diabetes based on a combination of clinical and molecular pathophysiologic features Table 68.3.

Type 1 diabetes (T1DM) is characterized by extensive destruction of the insulin-producing beta cells within the islets of Langerhans in the pancreas and dependence on insulin therapy for survival. In previous medical literature, the terms *juvenile-onset diabetes* or *insulin-dependent diabetes* were used for T1DM. This terminology is no longer used, because T1DM not uncommonly has its onset in adulthood, and multiple other forms of diabetes often require treatment with insulin. T1DM accounts for 5% to 10% of all diabetes in the United States. In most patients, it involves autoimmune mechanisms leading to beta cell destruction (the *type 1A* form). Rare individuals have no markers for autoimmunity and are classified as having *type 1B (idiopathic) diabetes*. Most patients with T1DM progress to marked insulin deficiency over a period of several weeks to months after initial presentation. A smaller number of individuals with evidence of beta-cell autoimmunity but much slower disease progression have a variant form of T1DM that has been designated *latent autoimmune diabetes of adulthood* (LADA).

In patients with marked elevations in glucose and accompanying ketoacidosis, particularly if they are young and nonobese, the diagnosis of T1DM is highly probable. This can be confirmed by measuring autoantibodies against glutamic acid decarboxylase (GAD65), insulin, tyrosine phosphatases (IA-2 and IA2-beta), and zinc transporter 8 (ZnT8), with several of these often obtained as a panel, and also by a clinical course demonstrating an ongoing need for insulin to control hyperglycemia. A fasting C-peptide level can be measured later in the disease to confirm marked deficiency in insulin secretion. C-peptide is a fragment of the insulin precursor proinsulin, which is cleaved during the synthesis of insulin. It is secreted and circulates in proportion to endogenous insulin production but is absent from injected exogenous insulin preparations.

Type 2 diabetes (T2DM) is a heterogeneous, clinically defined subtype that accounts for more than 90% of all diabetes in the United States. It typically has a gradual onset with progression over multiple years or even decades. There is often prolonged preservation of at least partial insulin secretory capacity together with evidence

TABLE 68.1 Criteria for the Diagnosis of Diabetes Mellitus

Measurement	Normal	Prediabetes	Diabetes Mellitus
Plasma glucose (mg/dL)			
Fasting[a]	<100	100-125[b]	≥126
2-hr Postload[c]	<140	140-199[d]	≥200
Random[e]			≥200
Hemoglobin A$_{1c}$ (%)	≤5.6	5.7-6.4	≥6.5

[a]Fasting: no caloric intake for ≥8 hr.
[b]Impaired fasting glucose.
[c]Postload: Following a standardized 75-g oral glucose load or after a meal.
[d]Impaired glucose tolerance.
[e]Random: any time of day, unrelated to meals.
Data from the American Diabetes Association Standards of Medical Care in Diabetes 2019, Diabetes Care 42(Suppl 1):S13-S28, 2019.

TABLE 68.2 Criteria for the Diagnosis of Gestational Diabetes Mellitus

Measurement	Diagnostic Threshold (mg/dL)
Plasma glucose	
Fasting[a]	≥92
After 75-g oral glucose load	
1 hr	≥180
2 hr	<153

[a]Fasting: no caloric intake for ≥8 hr.
Data from the American Diabetes Association Standards of Medical Care in Diabetes 2019, Diabetes Care 42(Suppl 1):S13-S28, 2019.

of insulin resistance. Most patients have associated obesity (80% to 90%), although a subset of patients with a clinical picture otherwise typical for T2DM are nonobese. T2DM usually can be presumptively distinguished from T1DM by its indolent course in the presence of risk factors such as obesity and by the milder hyperglycemia and absence of ketoacidosis due to residual insulin secretion. If there is clinical suspicion of T1DM based on earlier age at onset, degree of hyperglycemia, absence of obesity, or presence of ketoacidosis, an autoantibody panel (which should be negative) and a C-peptide level (which should be positive) can be measured.

An expanding number of diabetes etiologies distinct from T1DM and T2DM are classified under a broad category designated *other specific types*. Although these forms of diabetes are uncommon (<5% of all diabetes), it is important to recognize them in clinical practice. They include a group of inherited, monogenic, autosomal dominant disorders that previously were designated *maturity-onset diabetes of the young (MODY)*; many of these patients have clinical features similar to those of T2DM but onset typically before 25 years of age. Patients with hepatocyte nuclear factor-1alpha mutations (MODY3) are particularly sensitive to sulfonylureas, whereas those with glucokinase mutations (MODY2) have mild, nonprogressive blood glucose elevations and often require no treatment except during pregnancy. Because the genetic diagnosis can direct the treatment plan for these individuals, patients with early-onset diabetes, lack of autoimmune markers, and family histories suggestive of autosomal dominant inheritance should be considered for MODY gene sequencing.

TABLE 68.3 Etiologic Classification of Diabetes Mellitus

Type 1 Diabetes Mellitus
Immune-mediated (type 1A)
Idiopathic (type 1B)

Type 2 Diabetes Mellitus
Other Specific Types
Genetic defects of beta-cell function
    Maturity-onset diabetes of the young (MODY) and other disorders
Genetic defects in insulin action
    Insulin receptor mutations and other disorders
Diseases of the exocrine pancreas
Endocrinopathies
    Cushing's syndrome, acromegaly, and other disorders
Drug- or chemical-induced
    Glucocorticoids most common
Infections
Uncommon forms of immune-mediated diabetes
    Insulin receptor–blocking antibodies and other disorders
Other genetic syndromes sometimes associated with diabetes

Gestational Diabetes Mellitus

Classification consistent with the American Diabetes Association Standards of Medical Care in Diabetes 2019, Diabetes Care 42 (Suppl 1):S13-S28, 2019.

Much less common monogenic causes include mutations in insulin receptors or various other genes involved in insulin action. Exocrine pancreatic disease from disorders such as chronic pancreatitis or surgery results in loss of the glucagon-producing islet alpha cells as well as the insulin-producing beta cells. These patients often exhibit greater sensitivity to insulin and more of a propensity for hypoglycemia than T1DM patients because of the absent insulin counter-regulatory effects of glucagon. Endocrine disorders with excess production of hormones that counteract insulin, such as growth hormone in acromegaly or cortisol in Cushing's syndrome, are important to recognize as causes of diabetes because removal of the source of excess hormone can lead to resolution of the diabetic state. Many drugs have been associated with diabetes, most notably glucocorticoids.

The category GDM includes any woman in whom diabetes is first recognized during pregnancy and usually represents T2DM.

Type 1 Diabetes
Epidemiology and Pathology
The principal features of T1DM, contrasted with T2DM, are summarized in Table 68.4. The peak incidence occurs between the ages of 6 and 14 years, but onset in approximately half of patients with T1DM occurs after the age of 20. The role of genetic factors in T1DM risk is supported by an observed increased incidence of T1DM among family members of affected patients: approximately 5% in siblings, 6% in offspring of a diabetic father, and 2% in offspring of a diabetic mother. It is hypothesized that the immune destruction of beta cells is predisposed by genetic risk factors and precipitated by environmental factors, the latter possibly including microbial, chemical, or dietary triggers (Fig. 68.1). The operation of a combination of genetic and environmental factors is thought to explain the high but not absolute concordance observed in monozygotic twins (30% to 50%).

The prevalence of T1DM varies substantially in different populations; for example, it is relatively high in northwestern Europe and much lower in parts of Asia. The overall prevalence in the United

TABLE 68.4	General Comparison of the Two Most Common Types of Diabetes Mellitus	
	Type 1	**Type 2**
Previous terminology	Insulin-dependent diabetes mellitus, type I; juvenile-onset diabetes	Non–insulin-dependent diabetes mellitus, type II; adult-onset diabetes
Age at onset	Usually <30 yr, particularly childhood and adolescence, but any age	Usually >40 yr, but increasingly at younger ages
Genetic predisposition	Moderate; environmental factors required for expression; 35-50% concordance in monozygotic twins; multiple candidate genes proposed	Strong; 60-90% concordance in monozygotic twins; many candidate genes proposed
Human leukocyte antigen associations	Linkage to DQA and DQB, influenced by DRB3 and DRB4 (DR2 protective)	None known
Other associations	Autoimmune; Graves' disease, Hashimoto thyroiditis, vitiligo, Addison's disease, pernicious anemia	Heterogeneous, ongoing subclassification based on identification of specific pathogenic processes and genetic defects
Precipitating and risk factors	Largely unknown; microbial, chemical, dietary, other	Age, obesity (central), sedentary lifestyle, previous gestational diabetes
Findings at diagnosis	85-90% of patients have one and usually more autoantibodies to GAD_{65}, insulin, IA-2, IA-2β, ZnT8	Possibly complications (microvascular and macrovascular) caused by significant hyperglycemia in the preceding asymptomatic period
Endogenous insulin levels	Low or absent	Usually present (relative deficiency), early hyperinsulinemia
Insulin resistance	Only with hyperglycemia or coincident obesity	Mostly present
Prolonged fast	Hyperglycemia, ketoacidosis	Euglycemia
Stress, withdrawal of insulin	Ketoacidosis	Nonketotic hyperglycemia, occasionally ketoacidosis

GAD, Glutamic acid decarboxylase; *IA-2,* IA-2β, insuloma-associated protein 2 and 2β (tyrosine phosphatases); *ZnT8,* zinc transporter 8.

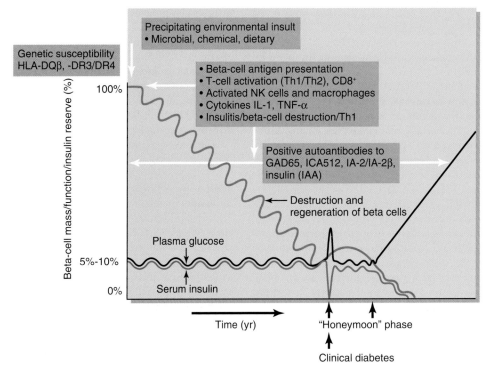

Fig. 68.1 Natural history of type 1 diabetes mellitus. The honeymoon period with temporary improvement in beta-cell function occurs with the initiation of insulin therapy at the time of clinical diagnosis. *GAD,* Glutamic acid decarboxylase; *HLA,* human leukocyte antigen; *IA-2,* IA-2β, tyrosine phosphatases; *ICA,* islet cell antibody; *ICA512,* islet cell autoantigen 512 (fragment of IA-2); *IL-1,* interleukin-1; *NK,* natural killer; *Th1,* subset of CD4+ helper T cells responsible for cell-mediated immunity; *Th2,* subset of CD4+ helper T cells responsible for humoral immunity; *TNF-α,* tumor necrosis factor-α.

States is approximately 2.4 cases per 1000 individuals. The frequent onset before age 20 makes T1DM one of the most common chronic, serious childhood diseases. It is the most common subtype of diabetes in childhood, accounting for approximately 70% of all cases, with T2DM accounting for most of the remainder. LADA, an uncommon variant form of autoimmune T1DM, is characterized by onset in adulthood and a more prolonged waxing and waning course than is typical for T1DM.

The onset of overt T1DM follows a preclinical phase of variable duration (typically extending from months to years) during which there is destruction of beta cells resulting predominantly from cell-mediated immune mechanisms (mononuclear cells; mainly CD8$^+$ T lymphocytes). It is believed that the autoantibodies (against glutamic acid decarboxylase, insulin, tyrosine phosphatases, and zinc transporter 8) are generated for the most part in response to exposure of beta-cell and islet antigens and do not function as primary mediators of the destructive process. Nevertheless, demonstration of one or more autoantibodies represents the most sensitive and useful way to establish preclinical disease in patients at risk (e.g., first-degree relatives of patients with T1DM).

The complement of beta cells in a healthy individual normally provides enough excess insulin secretory capacity to maintain blood glucose levels until 80% to 90% of beta cells have been lost. In some patients, the subclinical loss of beta cells may be unmasked, resulting in hyperglycemia and possibly diabetic ketoacidosis (DKA) during the course of an intercurrent illness such as an incidental upper respiratory tract infection. This reflects a lack of adequate insulin reserve to compensate for stress-induced insulin resistance. After institution of insulin and other therapy, stress-induced insulin resistance resolves, and there may be an improvement in beta-cell function. Some patients then revert to a state in which no insulin is required. This phenomenon, designated the *honeymoon* period, can last for several weeks to as long as 1 year. Patients generally should continue insulin administration at doses low enough to be tolerated during this interval, because progressive beta-cell function can be expected eventually to result in recurrent hyperglycemia and, potentially, DKA.

Screening for T1DM is not a part of standard medical care. Autoantibody determinations in individuals with a family history of T1DM can help to define risk but do not reliably predict time of onset or otherwise guide clinical care. Screening for thyroid, adrenal, or other associated autoimmune disorders should be considered in patients with T1DM on an individual basis.

Clinical Presentation

T1DM most often manifests clinically with symptoms resulting from hyperglycemia and consequent osmotic diuresis. Patients typically have a history extending over days to weeks of worsening polyuria, plus polydipsia (as a compensatory response to hypovolemia and increased serum osmolality). The polyuria may be evident as bed wetting or daytime incontinence in children and as nocturia in adults. There typically also is weight loss, and patients often describe low energy and lethargy. Approximately 25% of patients with T1DM have progressed to DKA by the time of clinical presentation.

Treatment

The management of T1DM involves immediate treatment at the outset to correct hyperglycemia, fluid deficits, and DKA, if present, plus attention to possible precipitating or complicating factors such as infection. The initial treatment of T1DM should be coupled with education of patients and their family members (appropriate to the patient's age) concerning the needed skills to manage insulin administration, blood glucose testing, nutrition, and exercise. This often is best accomplished

by a team involving the physician, educators (typically specially trained nurses or pharmacists), and a dietician. Medical advice, patient education, and psychological support should be provided on an ongoing, long-term, individualized basis. The primary goal of glucose management is to minimize the degree of hyperglycemia and its attendant risks of long-term complications of diabetes, while avoiding the acute and chronic risks of hypoglycemia. Medical care should include attention to control of lipid levels, blood pressure, and other factors that affect the risks of long-term diabetes complications. Routine assessments of foot care, peripheral nerve function, retinal status, and renal function should be used to detect incipient diabetes complications and enable early treatment interventions. Other sources should be consulted for information on specific issues related to T1DM management in children and adolescents.

Blood glucose control. Patients with T1DM have an absolute requirement for exogenous insulin. The Diabetes Control and Complications Trial (DCCT) and other studies have established that improved glycemic control in patients with T1DM decreases long-term microvascular complications (retinopathy, nephropathy, and neuropathy). A follow-up study of the same patients (the Epidemiology of Diabetes Interventions and Complications [EDIC] study) further demonstrated lower cardiovascular morbidity and mortality with intensive insulin management. Based on these and other studies, the most generally accepted target goal for HbA$_{1c}$ in T1DM is 7.0%, although selected individuals may safely target HbA$_{1c}$ of 6.5%. For patients who have difficulty sensing hypoglycemia or who have other factors complicating blood glucose management (e.g., renal failure), it is appropriate to set an individualized HbA$_{1c}$ goal of 8.0% or even higher.

Many preparations of insulin are available. They differ in rapidity of absorption, degree of peaking of blood levels, and duration of action after subcutaneous injection (Table 68.5). The different kinetics of recombinant human insulin preparations derive from their specific complexing with proteins and zinc. Additionally, multiple analogues of human insulin are available that have rapid or slow kinetics as a consequence of altered solubility at subcutaneous injection sites. Most insulin preparations are provided at a concentration of 100 U/mL (U-100), with some available at higher concentrations (200 or 500 U/mL). Self-monitoring of blood glucose (SMBG) by patients using glucose meters is critical to the implementation of an effective insulin regimen. Ideally, SMBG should be performed as frequently as practicable: fasting, preprandial, 2 hours postprandial, at bedtime, and occasionally at 2:00 to 3:00 AM. Values and times are saved in most meters for subsequent review. It is helpful for patients to manually record these data on a flowchart, and it is also possible to download meter data to a computer. SMBG records are most useful when annotated with relevant details on food intake, exercise, or the occurrence of symptoms. HbA$_{1c}$ determinations generally should be obtained every 3 months.

Most cases of T1DM should be managed with an *intensive insulin therapy regimen* involving multiple (three or more) daily subcutaneous injections or continuous subcutaneous insulin infusion (CSII) using an insulin pump. Multiple-injection regimens, also termed *basal-bolus therapy*, typically involve injections of a long-acting insulin analogue (glargine, detemir, or degludec) once or twice daily to establish a stable basal insulin level. Regular insulin or a rapid-acting insulin analogue is additionally injected three or more times daily (before each meal and sometimes before snacks) to provide appropriate post-meal peaks in insulin levels. Usually, once glucose levels are stabilized on a regimen, the doses of long-acting insulin are kept constant from day to day. The rapid-acting insulin doses can be kept constant with efforts to ingest a fixed amount of carbohydrate and total calories at each meal. Alternatively, better control and greater flexibility can be achieved if

TABLE 68.5 Types of Insulin[a]

Insulin Type	Generic Name	Preprandial Injection Timing (hr)	Onset (hr)	Peak (hr)	Duration (hr)	Bg Nadir (hr)
Rapid-acting	Lispro[b]	0-0.2	0.1-0.5	0.5-2	<5	2-4
	Aspart[c]	0-0.2	0.1-0.3	0.6-3	3-5	1-3
	Glulisine[d]	0-0.25 (15 min before a meal or within 20 min after starting a meal)	0.15-0.3	0.5-1.5	1-5.3	2-4
Short-acting	Regular	0.5-1	0.3-1	2-6	4-8	3-7
Intermediate-acting	NPH	0.5-1	1-3	6-15	16-26	6-13
Long-acting	Glargine[e,f]	Once daily[g] or twice daily (approx 12 hourly)	1-4	Little or no peak	10.8->24	Before next dose
	Detemir[f]	Once daily[g] or twice daily (approx 12 hourly)	1-4	Little or no peak	12-24	Before next dose
	Degludec	Once daily	0.5-1.5	Little or no peak	42	Before next dose
Human Premixed						
NPH/regular	70/30	0.5-1	0.5-1	2-12	14-24	3-12
NPH/regular	50/50	0.5-1	0.5-1	2-5	14-24	3-12
Insulin Analogue Premixed						
NPL/lispro	75/25	0.25	0.15-0.25	1	14-24	—
NPA/aspart	70/30	0.25	0.15-0.3	2-4	24	—
NPL/lispro	50/50	0.25	0.15-0.25	1	14-24	—

BG, Blood glucose; *NPA*, neutral protamine aspart; *NPH*, neutral protamine Hagedorn; *NPL*, neutral protamine lispro.

[a]Time profiles depend on several factors, including dose, anatomic site of injection, method (profiles in this table are for subcutaneous injections), duration of diabetes, type of diabetes, degree of insulin resistance, level of physical activity, presence of obesity, and body temperature. Preprandial injection timing depends on premeal BG values and insulin type.

[b]Insulin analogue with reversal of lysine and proline at positions 28 and 29 on the B chain of the insulin molecule.

[c]Insulin analogue with substitution of aspartic acid for proline at position 28 on the B chain of the insulin molecule.

[d]Insulin analogue with substitution of lysine for asparagine at position 3 on the B chain and glutamic acid for lysine at position 29 on the B chain of the insulin molecule.

[e]Insulin analogue with substitution of glycine for asparagine at position 21 on the A chain and addition of two arginines to the carboxyl terminus of the B chain of the insulin molecule.

[f]Do not mix glargine or detemir in the same syringe with other insulins.

[g]Administer at same time each day, unrelated to meals. Morning administration may result in greater glucose lowering and less nocturnal hypoglycemia.

rapid-acting insulin doses are adjusted according to the blood glucose level (measured before each meal) and the carbohydrate calories ingested with the meal. The long-acting insulin glargine and detemir analogues cannot be mixed in a single syringe with other insulins; for this reason, basal-bolus regimens often require four or more daily injections.

For patients newly diagnosed with T1DM, a typical starting dose of insulin is a total of 0.2 to 0.4 U/kg/day, with the expectation that this will be increased to 0.6 to 0.7 U/kg/day over time. Approximately half of the total dose should be given as basal insulin. Basal glargine or detemir insulin may be administered as a single daily dose (in the morning or at bedtime), or two equally divided doses may be required, depending on individual patient blood glucose responses. Degludec normally requires only once daily injection. For a basal regimen using intermediate acting insulin (NPH), two thirds of the dose typically is given in the morning and one third at bedtime. This decreases the risk of nocturnal hypoglycemia and times the maximum NPH peak to approximately match the midday meal. The rapid-acting component of the daily insulin dose is distributed before meals according to meal size and content.

An insulin pump (continuous subcutaneous insulin infusion, CSII) represents the preferred method of insulin administration for many T1DM patients. These small, wearable devices contain a reservoir of

rapid-acting insulin that is infused via an easily placed subcutaneous catheter. A microprocessor-controlled pump provides the basal insulin infusion and can be programmed to adjust basal rates at multiple points during the day according to predetermined patient needs. The patient further instructs the pump to make bolus insulin injections to cover meals, snacks, or needed corrections in hyperglycemia. Controlled studies have shown that modestly better blood glucose control can be achieved with CSII, compared to basal-bolus regimens with multiple daily injections. When used appropriately, CSII represents the most flexible means of managing insulin doses, with options for dose adjustments and supplementation that do not require separate injections. Limitations include need for greater patient involvement, lack of a protective, long-acting subcutaneous insulin reservoir, and pump failure. Newly diagnosed T1DM should be managed for a period of time (at least 6 to 12 months) with intermittently injected insulin before transition to a pump is considered. During the transition from intermittent insulin injections to CSII in a patient with well-controlled blood glucose levels (HbA$_{1c}$ ≤7.0%), the total daily insulin dose typically is decreased by 10% to 20% initially.

Many CSII patients require a slightly higher basal infusion rate in the early morning hours to accommodate the *dawn phenomenon*, a period of decreased insulin sensitivity secondary to circadian changes in secretion of insulin counter-regulatory hormones such as growth hormone and cortisol. Adjustments in the basal rate may also be needed at other times of day because of changes in insulin sensitivity (e.g., in response to exercise). Premeal insulin boluses are calculated to include a correction dose if needed, based on the premeal blood glucose level, plus a meal coverage dose calculated from the patient's predetermined individual carbohydrate/insulin ratio. It often is most effective for a patient to be seen in a specialty setting during transition to CSII, so that an experienced educator (often a specially trained RN) can assist with needed patient education. Devices are available that provide continuous glucose monitoring (CGM), either as a separate device or integrated into a sensor-augmented insulin pump. Some of the latter devices have the capacity to automatically interrupt insulin delivery for a proscribed period in response to low blood glucose levels as a protection against hypoglycemia (especially useful for nocturnal hypoglycemia). One approved sensor-augmented insulin pump can adjust the basal insulin infusion rate based on the CGM data but still requires manual control of premeal insulin boluses and periodic confirmation of blood glucose levels by fingerstick testing.

Intensive insulin therapy is not appropriate for all T1DM patients. Some patients are unwilling or unable to manage the required frequent glucose monitoring, diet adherence, and multiple insulin boluses. In other patients, the tight blood glucose control and low HbA_{1c} targets that are the goals of intensive insulin therapy may not be feasible. For example, there may be an increased risk of hypoglycemia because of autonomic neuropathy and inability to sense hypoglycemia, or gastrointestinal neuropathy may cause gastroparesis resulting in unpredictable variations in nutrient digestion and absorption. Under such circumstances, simpler approaches to insulin therapy and blood glucose management, previously termed *conventional insulin therapy*, may be appropriate. Such a regimen may be based, for example, on two injections per day of intermediate-acting insulin with or without short- or rapid-acting insulin. As one example, a *split-mixed regimen* uses NPH/regular or NPH/lispro (or aspart or glulisine) formulations twice daily. Initially, two thirds of the estimated total daily dose is given before breakfast and one third before dinner; at each of these times, two thirds of the insulin is given as NPH and one third as regular or rapid-acting insulin. The amount of each insulin type at each of the injection times is then adjusted according to measured blood glucose levels, with the expectation that the peak of the morning NPH will cover lunch, the rapid-acting insulins will cover the other meals, and the NPH will otherwise ensure adequate basal blood glucose control. Two daily injections are made possible by mixing the intermediate- and rapid-acting insulins in a single syringe. Premixed insulin preparations, such as 70% NPH plus 30% rapid-acting insulin or 50% NPH plus 50% regular insulin, also are available for injection with syringes or with preloaded insulin pens. Premixed insulins provide greater ease of use but are less likely to achieve good glycemic control.

Hypoglycemia management. Irrespective of the specific treatment regimen, patients with T1DM need to learn how to manage hypoglycemia. Patients usually experience adrenergic symptoms (e.g., sweating, anxiety, tremulousness) as blood glucose levels decrease below the normal range (<50 to 70 mg/dL). If a patient is taking β-blockers, symptoms such as tachycardia and tremulousness might be blunted or absent. If glucose levels decrease markedly enough, patients may experience central nervous system (CNS) symptoms ranging from difficulty thinking clearly to confusion, obtundation, and loss of consciousness. If low blood glucose is confirmed (e.g., <70 mg/dL), 10 to 15 g of rapidly absorbed carbohydrate should be ingested. For a glucose level lower than 50 mg/dL, 20 to 30 g of carbohydrate is advisable. This can be provided as orange juice or crackers, or patients can carry glucose tablets or squeeze tubes of glucose solution (obtainable over the counter from pharmacies) for use in treating hypoglycemia.

The blood glucose level should be retested after 15 minutes, and the treatment should be repeated as needed until hypoglycemia is resolved. An alternative is to inject glucagon. For patients who have a history of hypoglycemia severe enough (including loss of consciousness) to require assistance from others, it often is helpful for a family member to be trained in glucagon injection. With severe hypoglycemia, there is a risk of injury, such as from a fall or automobile accident, as well as neurologic damage if hypoglycemia is sustained.

Nutritional management. Appropriate nutritional management is an essential component of an effective T1DM treatment program, both to facilitate blood glucose control and reduce risks of long-term diabetes complications. Patients should work with a medical professional who is trained in diabetes care to establish nutritional goals. Rather than target specific percentages or sources of dietary carbohydrate, protein, and fat, the diet should be individualized to the patient's lifestyle, exercise regimen, eating habits, culture, and financial resources.

Most diets focus on measuring and controlling the amounts rather than the sources of carbohydrates. Patients can learn how to estimate the grams of carbohydrate in a meal *(carbohydrate counting)* as a means of ensuring that a consistent amount of carbohydrate is ingested. Alternatively, they can use carbohydrate counting with each meal as part of a strategy that enables day-to-day variations in consumption with adjustments of mealtime insulin doses according to a predetermined, patient-specific *insulin/carbohydrate ratio*.

Because of the contribution of excess body weight to increased cardiovascular risk, a fundamental goal of nutritional management should be to maintain normal body weight or to achieve weight reduction in overweight or obese patients. Eating disorders including binge eating, anorexia nervosa, and bulimia are relatively common in T1DM, especially among younger female patients.

Exercise. Regular physical exercise should be encouraged for its beneficial effects on weight control, risks of long-term complications, and overall quality of life. The general recommendation of several expert panels is 30 minutes or more of moderate-intensity physical exercise on at least 5 days per week. Physical exercise burns calories in proportion to its duration and intensity and also may result in increased insulin sensitivity after exercise (sometimes lasting for many hours). It often is most effective for patients to schedule exercise periods with a consistent temporal relationship to meals and insulin injections. Blood glucose should be tested before and after exercise, and exercise should not be undertaken if the initial blood glucose level is low (because of increased risk of hypoglycemia) or if it is higher than 250 mg/dL (because of risk of inducing further blood glucose elevation and development of ketosis). Patients with T1DM should be encouraged to pursue age- and overall health-appropriate athletic interests, including competitive sports, but this should be done only with careful attention to blood glucose monitoring and appropriate adjustments in insulin regimen and diet.

Type 2 Diabetes
Epidemiology and Pathology

T2DM is an extraordinarily common disorder, affecting nearly 10% of the population in the United States and with a similar prevalence in most other developed or developing countries. Many additional individuals (approximately 8% of the US population) have a prediabetic state. T2DM is characterized by varying degrees of insulin resistance and insulin deficiency, which are believed to result from the impact of environmental factors on a background of genetic risk. The principal features of T2DM, contrasted with T1DM, are summarized in Table 68.4. The prevalence of T2DM has increased more than 10-fold over the past 50 years, driven primarily by population-wide increased

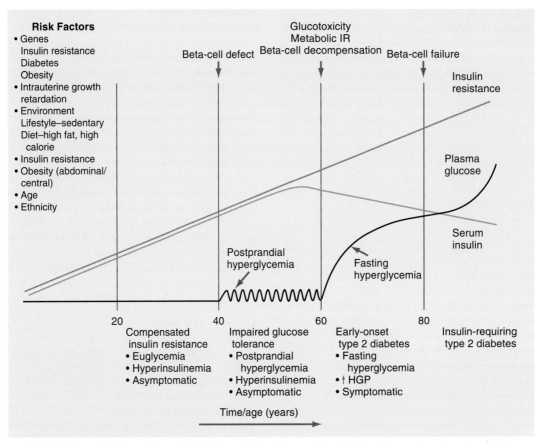

Fig. 68.2 Natural history of type 2 diabetes mellitus. The numbers for time/age markers in years for the different phases of beta-cell decompensation toward overt diabetes and an insulin-requiring state are approximate guides. Certain groups are more insulin sensitive and require a greater loss of beta-cell function to precipitate diabetes, compared with obese insulin-resistant people, who develop diabetes after small declines in beta-cell function. Use of insulin in patients with type 2 diabetes varies considerably and is not age dependent. *HGP,* Hepatic glucose production; *IR,* insulin resistance.

calorie intake, decreased exercise, and resulting obesity. More than 80% of patients with T2DM are obese. The peak incidence of T2DM occurs in the fifth and sixth decades; however, T2DM now accounts for up to 30% of childhood diabetes in some populations. The lifetime risk of developing T2DM is approximately 40% among the offspring of a single affected parent, and approximately 70% if both parents are affected. The incidence of T2DM in the United States is higher in Hispanic/Latino populations, among African Americans, and in some east Asian populations, compared to populations of northern and western European ancestry. This is thought to result in part from effects of socioeconomic and cultural factors (e.g., differences in consumption of low-cost, calorie-dense foods) and also from genetic differences among these populations. The genetic predisposition is thought to reflect the combined influence of more than 100 genes. No single gene or small group of genes with dominant influence on diabetes risk in any population has been identified.

T2DM is typically preceded by a prolonged preclinical or prediabetic phase during which there is a gradual deterioration in glucose tolerance (Fig. 68.2). This process occurs over a decade or more on average, with marked individual variation in the rate of progression. Most patients are insulin resistant during the preclinical phase but are able to compensate by producing enough insulin to maintain euglycemia. With time, there is progressive deterioration in the capacity to compensate for the insulin resistance. This is associated with a decrease in beta cell-mass during the preclinical phase of T2DM, but substantial

residual beta cells (typically 40% to 50% of the normal complement) are still present at the time that overt hyperglycemia develops. Therefore, there is compromised function as well as a reduced number of beta cells in T2DM. As blood glucose levels rise, the hyperglycemia itself may contribute to progression of the diabetic state by further decreasing insulin secretion and insulin resistance through mechanisms that are not well understood (referred to as *glucotoxicity*).

Screening of certain high-risk populations for T2DM and prediabetes by determination of a fasting or random plasma glucose measurement is considered cost-effective. Approximately 25% of people with T2DM and an even higher percentage of those with prediabetes are undiagnosed. Expert panel recommendations from the ADA for screening based on age, lifestyle factors, family history, and ethnicity are summarized in Table 68.6. Because of the insidious nature of T2DM, patients have a high risk for development of complications by the time of clinical diagnosis (see later discussion).

Clinical Presentation

Many patients are asymptomatic and are diagnosed on routine blood glucose testing. Blood glucose levels that rise high enough to exceed the renal threshold for glucose reabsorption (>170 mg/dL) induce an osmotic diuresis, resulting in the typical presenting symptoms of polyuria and polydipsia, as well as blurred vision secondary to osmotic shifts in the lens. Patients may also have weight loss or bacterial urinary tract or cutaneous fungal infections at presentation. Osmotic diuresis

TABLE 68.6   Screening Criteria for Diabetes in Asymptomatic Adults

1. Testing for diabetes should be considered in all persons ≥45 yr of age; if normal, the test should be repeated at 3-yr intervals.
2. Testing should be considered at a younger age (<30 yr) or performed more frequently in individuals who
   a. Have BMI ≥ 25 kg/m² (≥ 23 kg/m² in Asian Americans)
   b. Have a sedentary lifestyle
   c. Have a first-degree relative with diabetes (i.e., parent or sibling)
   d. Are members of a high-risk ethnic population (e.g., African American, Latino/Hispanic American, Native American, Asian American, Pacific Islander)
   e. Have been diagnosed with gestational diabetes
   f. Are hypertensive (≥140/90 mm Hg)
   g. Have an HDL cholesterol level <35 mg/dL (0.9 mmol/L) and/or a triglyceride level >250 mg/dL (2.82 mmol/L)
   h. Have other clinical conditions associated with insulin resistance (e.g., PCOS, acanthosis nigricans)
   i. Have a history of cardiovascular disease
   j. Had prediabetes on previous testing (see criteria in Table 68.1); should be tested annually

BMI, Body mass index (weight [kg]/height [m²]); *HbA₁c,* glycosylated hemoglobin; *HDL,* high-density lipoprotein; *PCOS,* polycystic ovary syndrome; *T1DM,* type 1 diabetes mellitus; *T2DM,* type 2 diabetes mellitus. Modified from the American Diabetes Association Clinical Practice Recommendations 2013, Diabetes Care 36(Suppl 1):S11-S66, 2013.

secondary to hyperglycemia may lead to electrolyte abnormalities and even occasionally to a severe hyperosmolar state associated with clinical symptoms and signs including fatigue, weakness, and ultimately compromised mental status that can range from confusion to coma (see later discussion). This most frequently occurs in elderly patients who may have compromised baseline renal function. In contrast to patients with T1DM, those with T2DM usually have enough residual insulin activity to partially suppress lipolysis, and this protects them from developing DKA. In a subset of T2DM patients, DKA can develop, possibly reflecting individual variations in the degree of suppression of insulin secretion by glucotoxicity.

As a consequence of prolonged exposure to hyperglycemia and associated metabolic disturbances, patients with T2DM may already have developed long-term microvascular or macrovascular complications of diabetes by the time of diagnosis. Therefore, patients may experience a cardiovascular event, such as acute myocardial infarction, and then incidentally be found to have T2DM.

The metabolic syndrome. Susceptibility to cardiovascular disease is further increased by the frequent association of insulin resistance, prediabetes, and T2DM with other cardiovascular risk factors, including abdominal or visceral obesity, dyslipidemia, and hypertension. The term *metabolic syndrome* has been applied to patients who have a combination of these risk factors. Different but overlapping diagnostic criteria for the metabolic syndrome have been proposed by various expert panels. The National Cholesterol Education Program Adult Treatment Panel III (ATP III) defines this syndrome as the presence of any three of the following five characteristics:

1. Fasting blood glucose level ≥100 mg/dL or drug treatment for elevated blood glucose
2. High-density lipoprotein (HDL)-cholesterol <40 mg/dL in men or <50 mg/dL in women or drug treatment for low HDL-cholesterol
3. Plasma triglycerides ≥150 mg/dL or drug treatment for elevated triglycerides

4. Abdominal obesity (waist ≥102 cm in men or ≥88 cm in women
5. Blood pressure ≥130/85 mm Hg or drug treatment for hypertension.

There is debate about whether the metabolic syndrome represents a discrete pathologic entity, but its recognition does draw attention to the frequent clustering of cardiovascular risk factors.

Treatment

Patients with T2DM should receive nutrition counseling starting at the time of diagnosis. This should include efforts at weight loss in overweight or obese patients. Adjustments in diet, especially reductions in calorie intake, can rapidly improve blood glucose levels in many patients independent of other interventions. Weight reduction by as little as 10% to 20% of body weight can have marked beneficial effects on insulin resistance and glycemia in some patients.

Depending on initial blood glucose levels, the presence or absence of symptoms related to hyperglycemia, and the presence of other complicating medical conditions, a decision can be made on whether to treat the patient initially with diet alone or to also start medication. Patients with marked hyperglycemia, fluid deficits, altered mental status related to hyperosmolar state, and DKA should be hospitalized for acute treatment (see later discussion).

For most patients, treatment of T2DM can be conducted on an outpatient basis. Useful guidelines are available online from the American Diabetes Association (ADA) and the European Association for the Study of Diabetes. Most expert panels recommend starting with one or two oral glucose-lowering medications (depending on the degree of hyperglycemia) with progression to a third oral agent or insulin if this proves ineffective. In patients with marked hyperglycemia (≥300 mg/dL or HbA₁c >10%), consideration should be given to starting insulin from the outset. There typically is gradually progressive loss of beta-cell function in T2DM, extending sometimes over many years, and this results in a need over time for increased doses or additional glucose-lowering agents and often, ultimately, the use of insulin. As for T1DM, the overall management of T2DM should include not only the treatment of hyperglycemia but also interventions that assess, decrease the risks for, and treat long-term microvascular and macrovascular complications.

Blood glucose control. The United Kingdom Prevention of Diabetes Study (UKPDS) and other randomized, controlled trials have established that improved blood glucose control lowers the risk of microvascular long-term complications (retinopathy, nephropathy, and neuropathy) in T2DM. The risk appears to increase progressively, starting with any increment above normoglycemia. Randomized clinical trial data have not convincingly demonstrated improved macrovascular (i.e., cardiovascular disease) outcomes in response to improved blood glucose control in T2DM. T2DM patients, particularly those who are older or have complicating comorbid conditions, may have limited capacity to manage a tight blood glucose control regimen and also increased susceptibility to adverse effects of hypoglycemia. HbA₁c goals therefore should be developed on an individualized basis, such that the benefits of improving microvascular complications are balanced against the risks of hypoglycemia. Whereas HbA₁c of 7% or less is an appropriate target for younger T2DM patients, 8% or less may be an acceptable and safer target for older patients with complicating medical conditions and limited life expectancy. HbA₁c should be measured every 6 months, or at intervals of 3 months if glucose control is unstable or the treatment regimen is being adjusted. SMBG should be performed on a regular basis if patients are being treated with agents that can cause hypoglycemia (sulfonylureas, meglitinides, and insulin). Regular SMBG is not generally needed for patients on agents that do not cause hypoglycemia, although testing during intercurrent

TABLE 68.7	Non-Insulin Antidiabetic Agents by Drug Class[a]		
Drug Class	**Available Agents (Generic Name)**	**Route of Administration**	**Mode of Action**
Biguanide	Metformin	Oral	Insulin sensitizer
SGLT2 inhibitors	Canagliflozin, dapagliflozin, empagliflozin, ertugliflozin	Oral	Increase urinary glucose excretion
GLP-1 receptor agonists	Dulaglutide, exenatide, liraglutide, lixisenatide, semaglutide	Subcutaneous injection, semaglutide oral	Incretin mimetic
DPP-4 inhibitors	Alogliptin, linagliptin, saxagliptin, sitagliptin	Oral	Incretin amplifier
Thiazolidinediones	Pioglitazone, rosiglitazone	Oral	Insulin sensitizer
Sulfonylureas	Glipizide, glyburide, glimepiride, gliclazide, chlorpropamide, tolazamide	Oral	Insulin secretagogue
Meglitinides	Repaglinide, nateglinide	Oral	Insulin secretagogue
α-Glucosidase inhibitors	Acarbose, miglitol	Oral	Delay carbohydrate digestion/absorption
Amylin mimetics	Pramlintide	Subcutaneous injection	Delay gastric emptying, suppress glucagon

DPP-4, Dipeptidyl peptidase-4; *GLP-1*, glucagon-like peptide-1; *SGLT2*, sodium glucose co-transporter 2.
[a]Consult current manufacturer information for details on available combinations, prescribing, and safety.

illnesses or with occurrence of symptoms suggestive of hyperglycemia is advisable.

Non-insulin pharmacologic (antidiabetic) agents in T2DM. Non-insulin pharmacologic agents from many different drug classes are available for treatment of T2DM, some taken orally and others by injection (Table 68.7). When non-insulin pharmacologic agents are appropriate, metformin is generally preferred as first-line therapy because of its glucose-lowering efficacy, absence of weight gain and hypoglycemia, favorable safety and tolerability profile based on many years of clinical experience, and low cost. For patients who are unable to tolerate metformin, the choice of an alternative drug may be influenced by considerations such as glucose-lowering efficacy, patient preference for an oral versus an injectable agent, potential adverse effects (e.g., hypoglycemia, weight gain, or fluid retention), the presence of comorbidities (cardiovascular disease, heart failure, or chronic renal insufficiency), and cost. For patients with established atherosclerotic cardiovascular disease or chronic kidney disease (CKD), a sodium glucose cotransporter (SGLT2) inhibitor or glucagon-like peptide-1 (GLP-1) receptor agonist with established cardiovascular disease or CKD benefit should be considered. For patients with atherosclerotic heart disease and heart failure or high risk of heart failure, an SGLT2 inhibitor might be most appropriate. Dipeptidyl peptidase-4 (DPP-4) inhibitors represent another reasonable option as well-tolerated agents with established cardiovascular safety. When drug cost is a critical issue, a sulfonylurea is a reasonable choice, although these drugs have the disadvantages of inducing modest weight gain and causing hypoglycemia. Pioglitazone is another low-cost agent that is effective in lowering blood glucose, but it is associated with increased risk of fluid retention and heart failure.

If a single drug is tolerated but does not adequately control blood glucose levels, the usual practice is to continue that drug and add a second from a distinct drug class with choice of agent influenced by the factors stated previously. In patients with marked hyperglycemia (e.g., with HbA$_{1c}$ ≥1.5% above target) that is not judged severe enough to merit insulin treatment, two agents may be started from the outset. This has the potential advantage of more rapidly achieving blood glucose control but the disadvantage of exposing patients to the potential side effects of taking two drugs simultaneously. Many combination preparations are available for administration of more than one drug; these are more convenient for patients and sometimes less expensive than taking the multiple drugs separately.

Available non-insulin antidiabetic agents are summarized here and in Table 68.7. Current manufacturer information should be consulted before prescribing these drugs to ensure updated and adequately detailed information on available single and combination agents and their effective and safe use.

Metformin. Metformin is an oral agent in the biguanide class that produces its most prominent effects by decreasing gluconeogenesis and thus reducing hepatic glucose production. This insulin-sensitizing effect is associated with a low risk of hypoglycemia. It has been in use for more than 30 years and is available in inexpensive generic form. The usual starting dose is 500 mg once or twice daily with incremental advancement at several-week intervals to a usual maximum of 2000 mg daily in two or three divided doses. Metformin typically decreases HbA$_{1c}$ by up to 1.5%. Further benefits include modest weight loss (approximately 3 kg on average) and a small improvement in plasma lipid profile (decrease in low-density lipoprotein [LDL]-cholesterol and triglycerides and increase in HDL). Adverse reactions include gastrointestinal effects and, rarely, lactic acidosis. The drug should be avoided in patients with an estimated glomerular filtration rate (eGFR) of <30 mL/min/1.73m^2 and used at decreased dosage with an eGFR of 30 to 45 mL/min/1.73m^2.

SGLT2 inhibitors. Canagliflozin, dapagliflozin, empagliflozin, and ertugliflozin function by inhibiting SGLT2. SGLT2 mediates more than 90% of glucose reabsorption in the proximal renal tubule, and the drug lowers blood glucose levels by promoting excretion of glucose in the urine. This typically results in a decrease in HbA$_{1c}$ in the range of 0.5% to 1.0%, plus modest weight loss (2-3 kg on average) and decrease in blood pressure. The mechanism of action is independent of insulin, and this class of drugs does not cause hypoglycemia. Large-scale, prospective, randomized clinical trials have shown decreased major cardiovascular events in T2DM patients with established cardiovascular disease with canagliflozin and empagliflozin. These studies, plus a similar trial with dapagliflozin in T2DM patients with milder cardiovascular disease history, have shown decreases in hospitalization for heart failure and progression of diabetic nephropathy. As a result, drugs in this class appear to be a favorable choice in patients with established cardiovascular disease or diabetic nephropathy. Concerns about potential side effects include urinary and genital infections, hypotension, acute renal injury, fractures in the context of low bone mineral density, increased lower extremity amputations, and DKA. Further studies will be needed to validate the benefits and potential adverse effects of these drugs and determine whether some of these responses are specific to individual members of the drug class. They are taken orally once daily, with dosage specific to each drug.

Glucagon-like peptide-1 receptor agonists. GLP-1 is one of several hormones produced in the small intestine (designated *incretins*) that modify gastrointestinal motility and insulin secretion. The GLP-1 receptor agonists, dulaglutide, exenatide, liraglutide, lixisenatide, and semaglutide, bind to GLP-1 receptors and improve blood glucose control by enhancing glucose-dependent insulin secretion, slowing gastric emptying, suppressing postprandial glucagon production, and decreasing food intake through enhanced satiety. This results in decreases in HbA$_{1c}$ by 0.5% to 1.5% and modest weight loss (in the range of 3 kg). There is evidence for improved cardiovascular outcomes for several of these agents in patients with established cardiovascular disease and possibly an improvement in CKD outcomes. They may be a favorable choice as a second-line drug for glycemia management if weight loss is a goal and in patients with established cardiovascular disease, with attention to the data available for specific agents. Because of their relatively high efficacy, GLP-1 receptor agonists are a reasonable option to consider before starting insulin in patients not adequately controlled on other agents. Most members of this drug class are administered via injection with prefilled pens, twice daily, once daily, or once weekly depending on the specific drug, and semaglutide also is available in an orally administered form. The most common side effects are nausea and sometimes diarrhea, likely related to effects on gastrointestinal motility, and these agents should not be used in patients with a history of pancreatitis or in combination with DPP-4 inhibitors.

Dipeptidyl peptidase-4 inhibitors. DPP-4 inhibitors (alogliptin, linagliptin, saxagliptin, and sitagliptin) block the deactivation of GLP-1 (described in the previous section) and glucose-dependent insulinotropic peptide (GIP), peptide hormones that are important in the regulation of glucose homeostasis. DPP-4 inhibitors are taken orally and result in decreased HbA$_{1c}$ in the range of 0.5% to 1.0%. They have a low risk of causing hypoglycemia, have neutral effects on cardiovascular disease outcomes and body weight, and can be used in the context of CKD with agent-specific dose reductions. They have generally favorable side effect profiles, although there is concern that some members of the class may increase heart failure risk. They should not be used in combination with GLP-1 receptor agonists.

Pioglitazone. The thiazolidinedione, pioglitazone, activates the nuclear peroxisome proliferator-activated receptor-γ, which leads to changes in transcription rates of multiple genes. The net effect is reduced insulin resistance, resulting in increased glucose uptake in peripheral tissues and reduced hepatic glucose production. Pioglitazone typically lowers HbA$_{1c}$ by 0.5% to 1.4% and is available as a low-cost drug. It carries a low risk of hypoglycemia, but potential side effects include weight gain, fluid retention and heart failure, hepatoxicity, concerns about increased fracture risk in the setting of low bone density, and a potential link to bladder cancer. Another member of this drug class, rosiglitazone, is little used because of its potential link to increased cardiovascular events.

Sulfonylureas. Sulfonylureas stimulate endogenous insulin secretion by binding and activating potassium channels in beta cells. In patients with adequate residual beta-cell function, they can lower HbA$_{1c}$ levels by 1% to 2%. Drugs in this class have been in clinical use for more than 40 years, and many inexpensive, generic sulfonylureas are available that differ in duration of action, metabolism, and mode of clearance. Because they can increase insulin secretion even in the absence of hyperglycemia, they have significant potential to cause hypoglycemia. Patients need to be instructed how to recognize and treat hypoglycemia before starting a sulfonylurea. Factors that increase the risk for hypoglycemia with sulfonylureas include advanced age, poor nutrition, alcohol ingestion, and hepatic and renal insufficiency. Other disadvantages of this drug class are a tendency to cause weight gain and a yet unresolved concern about increased risk for cardiovascular events.

Meglitinides. Repaglinide and nateglinide activate beta cell potassium channels and thus stimulate endogenous insulin secretion

through a mechanism similar to that of sulfonylureas, although they generally result in less reduction in blood glucose than sulfonylureas. They have rapid action and have less tendency to cause hypoglycemia than sulfonylureas. Their use has been limited by high cost and lack of advantage over the sulfonylureas.

α-Glucosidase inhibitors. The α-glucosidase inhibitors, acarbose and miglitol, are oral agents that improve glycemia by inhibiting the enzymatic breakdown of complex carbohydrates within the lumen of the small intestine. They have modest glucose-lowering effects, decreasing HbA$_{1c}$ in the range of 0.5% to 0.8%. Their use is limited by the frequent occurrence of flatulence and diarrhea as a consequence of undigested carbohydrates reaching lower intestinal regions.

Pramlintide. Pramlintide is a stable analogue of the beta-cell peptide, amylin, which has actions that include slowing of gastric emptying, satiety effects that decrease food intake, and decrease in postmeal glucagon. It is not widely used because of required multiple injections and limited efficacy in lowering HbA1c.

Insulin treatment in T2DM. For patients who have inadequate glycemic control with oral agents, insulin may be started as a basal supplement to the oral regimen. Frequently used choices include glargine or detemir (once or twice daily), degludec (once daily), or NPH (once daily at bedtime) (see later discussion and Table 68.5 for more details on different types of insulin). Starting doses are typically in the range of 10 U (or can be more specifically calculated as 0.2 U/kg), with increases of 2 to 4 U at intervals of 3 days or longer based on blood glucose response. Oral agent regimens commonly are simplified at the time of starting insulin (e.g., shifting from multiple agents to a single oral agent). For patients who do not achieve adequate control with basal insulin, mealtime coverage is provided by a rapid-acting insulin. Often, under this circumstance, all oral agents are discontinued, and blood glucose control is achieved with the use of exogenous insulin alone. Compared to patients with T1DM, those with T2DM may not require as tight a match of carbohydrate to insulin doses at meals, perhaps because of some residual insulin secretion. For this reason, insulin pumps are less frequently used in T2DM.

Nutritional and weight management. Patients should receive counseling from a dietician and be assisted in developing a nutritional plan that is individualized to their lifestyle, exercise, culture, and financial resources. Guidelines from many current expert panels allow flexibility in the relative amounts of carbohydrate, fat, and protein. Nutritional management in T2DM often has a major focus on achieving reductions in calorie intake and weight loss. Achieving weight loss may be made more difficult by a tendency of some oral antidiabetic agents and also insulin to induce a degree of weight gain.

An important goal of nutritional management should be to balance the timing and quantities of ingested macronutrients with medications and exercise to help achieve targets for blood glucose control without periods of hypoglycemia.

For overweight or obese patients, it often is practical to set an initial goal of losing 5% to 10% of body weight. This may significantly improve diabetes control and increase the patient's motivation to then set goals for further weight loss (see Chapter 69).

Bariatric surgical procedures represent a method for achieving weight loss and potentially dramatic improvements in glycemia and risk factors for long-term complications in T2DM. Patients typically have improvements in glycemic control and lower requirements for antidiabetic medications within days after undergoing the Roux-en-Y gastric bypass procedure. This is thought to reflect changes in gut hormones and metabolic factors independent of weight loss. Beneficial effects on glucose control develop more gradually after the placement of an adjustable gastric band, sleeve gastrectomy, or other device.

Randomized trials comparing bariatric surgery with medical nutrition therapy alone for weight loss have shown greater efficacy in achieving HbA$_{1c}$ goals with surgery, and some studies have shown dramatic rates of remission, with 75% of patients or more becoming normoglycemic off all antidiabetic agents (see Chapter 69).

Exercise. Physical exercise should be encouraged in T2DM as an important component of weight loss regimens and also for its beneficial effects in decreasing the risks of long-term complications. The general recommendation of several expert panels is 30 minutes or more of moderate-intensity physical exercise on at least 5 days per week, but the regimen needs to be highly individualized according to a patient's capabilities and limitations imposed by other medical conditions such as cardiovascular disease. Patients who are unwilling or unable to undertake significant aerobic exercise should be encouraged to do daily walking or other physical activities within their limitations.

Standards of Care in T1DM and T2DM in Addition to Blood Glucose Control

A number of assessments and interventions should be performed at intervals in patients with T1DM or T2DM. These include blood pressure measurement and examination of the feet at each physician visit. Patients who smoke should receive counseling at each visit about the importance of and strategies for discontinuing. A dilated eye examination should be performed annually, or more often in patients with diabetic eye disease. A dental examination also should be performed at least annually. Starting 5 years after disease onset in T1DM and at the time of diagnosis in T2DM, patients should have annual measurement of their urinary albumin/creatinine ratio with confirmation if elevated (>30 mg albumin per gram of creatinine). A fasting lipid profile should be obtained annually. Aspirin (75 to 162 mg daily) is usually recommended for secondary prevention of cardiovascular disease (supported by clinical trial evidence) or for primary prevention in patients with a 10-year cardiovascular risk greater than 10% (based on expert opinion). Influenza vaccination should be provided yearly; pneumococcal immunization should be given once and then repeated after age 65 (see latest CDC recommendations).

Management of Diabetes During Intercurrent Illness

Diabetes often requires changes in the blood glucose management regimen during an intercurrent illness to accommodate potential decreases in nutrient intake and increases in insulin resistance secondary to disease-related release of stress hormones. Patients with T1DM require exogenous insulin administration at all times to prevent marked hyperglycemia and DKA, even if they are unable to consume nutrients during an illness (e.g., with gastroenteritis). Depending on the degree and duration of interruption of food intake, they may require a transient, partial reduction in insulin dosage as well as more frequent glucose monitoring. Alternatively, if they are consuming a normal diet, they may require a modest increase in insulin dose because of insulin resistance related to the stress of illness. T2DM patients taking oral agents who are undergoing surgical procedures or are hospitalized for serious illness often require discontinuation of the oral agents and use of insulin to control blood glucose until normal eating patterns are resumed.

For hospitalized patients, blood glucose target goals are adjusted to prevent marked hyperglycemia and at the same time protect against hypoglycemia. For noncritical illness, typical blood glucose targets include lowest levels of 90 to 100 mg/dL, premeal levels lower than 140 mg/dL, and random levels lower than 180 mg/dL. For critically ill patients, intravenous insulin infusion may be needed to allow for rapid

adjustments in dosage, and the blood glucose range recommended by most expert panels is 140 to 180 mg/dL.

Gestational Diabetes Mellitus

The hormonal environment of pregnancy results in insulin resistance and therefore predisposes to the development or unmasking of diabetes during pregnancy. GDM occurs in 2% to 5% of all pregnancies and is associated with consequences for both mother and fetus if untreated. For this reason, screening for GDM is routinely performed between 24 and 28 weeks of gestation in women older than 25 years of age and in younger women who fulfill one or more of the risk criteria in Table 68.6 (2a through 2d and 2g). Women who are at high risk (i.e., those who are obese, have a personal history of GDM, glycosuria, or have a first-degree relative with diabetes) should be screened at their initial obstetric or prenatal visit. A broadly accepted approach to screening is a 2-hour 75-g oral glucose tolerance test with cutoff values as specified in Table 68.2.

A detailed discussion of the approach to managing GDM and also preexisting diabetes during pregnancy is beyond the scope of this chapter. The fundamental principles include diet, exercise, and glucose-lowering oral agents or insulin as needed. Blood glucose goals are set lower than in nonpregnant individuals because of the importance of minimizing exposure of the fetus to hyperglycemia: fasting, 95 mg/dL (5.3 mmol/L) or lower; 1-hour postprandial, 140 mg/dL (7.8 mmol/L) or lower; and 2-hours postprandial, 120 mg/dL (6.7 mmol/L) or lower. HbA$_{1c}$ levels may be useful in establishing the presence of hyperglycemia before its discovery during pregnancy, but they have limited value in managing GDM. Women with GDM should be reevaluated with a 75-g glucose tolerance test 6 to 12 weeks after delivery, at which point approximately 10% will still have overt diabetes. Up to 40% of women with GDM go on to develop diabetes in the subsequent 20 years, with this risk varying substantially depending on ethnic background and obesity. Pregnancy serves as a provocative test and not as a risk factor for the future development of diabetes.

Management of Severe Metabolic Decompensation in Diabetes
Diabetic Ketoacidosis

DKA develops most commonly in patients with T1DM (approximately 2.5 cases per 100 T1DM patients per year). It also can occur in those with T2DM, especially during acute illness (severe infection, medical illness, or trauma), and in a subset of *ketosis-prone* T2DM patients. DKA is present in approximately 25% of T1DM patients at diagnosis and otherwise most often develops when patients with known T1DM stop taking prescribed insulin. It is a potentially life-threatening condition that has an overall mortality rate of approximately 1% to 2%, with most deaths resulting from complicating or precipitating medical conditions rather than the metabolic disturbances of DKA itself.

The pathophysiology of DKA results from the combined effects of insulin deficiency and increased levels of *insulin counter-regulatory (stress) hormones*. With insulin deficiency, glucose levels rise as a consequence of decreased uptake and metabolism by body tissues, the breakdown of hepatic glycogen stores (*glycogenolysis*), and net glucose production by the liver and kidney (*gluconeogenesis*). Catabolism of muscle proteins as a result of low insulin levels leads to the release of amino acids, which provide substrate that further drives gluconeogenesis. Because glucose is being synthesized endogenously, blood glucose levels rise markedly, even in the fasted state. Blood glucose levels greater than 170 mg/dL result in glycosuria. Excretion of glucose in the urine necessitates the co-excretion of large amounts of water and electrolytes (Na$^+$ and K$^+$). Patients experience polyuria but cannot compensate adequately and become progressively more fluid and electrolyte depleted. The osmotic diuresis is characterized by greater losses of water than electrolytes, and this leads to progressively increasing hyperosmolality. Because of insulin deficiency, there is decreased *lipogenesis* and accelerated *lipolysis* leading to increased levels of circulating free fatty acids, which serve as a substrate for the hepatic synthesis of ketone bodies (β-hydroxybutyrate, acetoacetate, and acetone). β-Hydroxybutyrate and acetoacetate are acids, and their rising plasma levels contribute to the development of a metabolic acidosis.

These processes can result from simple insulin deficiency, but often they are exacerbated by an underlying or precipitating illness, such as an infection. Infection results in insulin resistance secondary to increased levels of *stress hormones* (cortisol, catecholamines, glucagon, and growth hormone). A series of positive feedback loops are thus generated and lead to ever-accelerating hyperglycemia, fluid and electrolyte depletion, ketosis, and metabolic acidosis. More than simple restoration of insulin dosing is required, and patients usually need hospital admission and multicomponent interventions.

Common presenting symptoms in DKA include polyuria, thirst and polydipsia, recent weight loss (especially in new-onset diabetes), blurred vision, weakness, anorexia, nausea and vomiting, abdominal pain (which can mimic acute abdomen), and mental status changes varying from somnolence to coma. DKA and these associated symptoms usually evolve over 2 to 4 days but can have an onset of less than 12 hours in patients using insulin pumps. On physical examination, patients typically have evidence of dehydration, especially intravascular volume depletion, including decreased skin turgor, hypotension, and tachycardia (best assessed in skin overlying the sternum and forehead). The skin may be warm and dry from the vasodilating effects of acidosis, and marked hypotension should generate concern for impending vascular collapse. Patients often have deep, rapid respirations (Kussmaul breathing) as respiratory compensation for the metabolic acidosis, together with a characteristic fruity odor on their breath from exhaled acetone. The diagnosis is made in patients who have (1) a high blood glucose concentration (>250 mg/dL), (2) moderate to severe ketonemia (β-hydroxybutyrate >5 mmol/L or positive ketone levels by Ketostix at a serum dilution of 1:2 or higher), and (3) acidosis (pH <7.3 or plasma bicarbonate ≤15 mEq/L). Measurements of urine ketones may be misleading, because urinary ketones can be positive during fasting in the absence of DKA.

Additional evaluation besides the diagnostic tests already mentioned should include electrolytes, blood urea nitrogen, creatinine, phosphate, liver function tests, and amylase; arterial or mixed venous blood gases (including pH); complete blood count; urinalysis; electrocardiogram; and chest radiographs. The serum anion gap, which is usually greater than 12 mEq/L in DKA, should be calculated (anion gap = $[Na^+] - [Cl^- + HCO_3^-]$). Serum osmolality should be measured directly or calculated: estimated osmolality = $(2 \times [Na^+]) + ([glucose\ in\ mg/dL]/18)$.

Precipitating causes of DKA include infection (most common), myocardial infarction (including silent infarction), inflammatory processes (appendicitis, pancreatitis), and medications (especially glucocorticoids).

Treatment of DKA should start promptly with institution of measures to correct life-threatening abnormalities, including insulin deficiency, fluid and electrolyte depletion, potassium (K^+) depletion, and metabolic acidosis. In a typical regimen, regular insulin or a rapid-acting insulin analog is administered as a bolus (0.1 U/kg) followed by a continuous intravenous infusion at 0.1 U/kg/hour. Plasma glucose is monitored hourly until it is less than 250 mg/dL, and the rate of insulin infusion is adjusted as needed to target a rate of blood glucose

decline of 75 to 100 mg/dL/hour to avoid potential complications of rapid shifts in osmolality.

At the time of starting insulin, it is essential to begin fluid and electrolyte replacement. The initial fluid deficit should be estimated based on the magnitude of weight loss (if known), mucous membrane dryness, skin turgor, and whether or not there is postural hypotension, with the knowledge that losses in DKA usually range from 3 to 8 L. A typical program for intravenous fluid replacement starts with 1 L of normal saline in the first hour. Normal saline may then be continued at 15 mL/minute for a second hour depending on the estimated severity of initial fluid depletion. This then may be changed to 0.45% (half-normal) saline at 7.5 mL/minute for the next 2 hours and gradually tapered thereafter to achieve full replacement of the estimated fluid deficit in approximately 8 hours. During that time, there should be frequent monitoring for jugular venous distention and chest auscultation to ensure early detection of fluid overload. Central venous pressure should be monitored in patients who are at risk for congestive heart failure.

Potassium repletion is needed in all patients, and there should be careful monitoring and replacement to ensure that patients do not develop potentially harmful hypokalemia or hyperkalemia. Urine output should be verified with the use of a Foley catheter if necessary before K^+ replacement is started. Unless patients are anuric, K^+ replacement should be initiated within 1 to 2 hours after starting insulin. A key goal is to maintain serum K^+ at all times higher than 3.5 mEq/L, and it is especially important to administer K^+ early in the course of treatment if there is initial hypokalemia or if bicarbonate is administered to correct acidosis, because the latter action promotes a shift of extracellular K^+ into cells. Potassium typically is withheld if the serum K^+ is 5 mEq/L or higher; otherwise, it is administered as part of the intravenous fluid regimen at 10 to 40 mEq/hour depending on the measured serum level. Serum K^+ should be monitored every 2 hours if it is less than 4 or greater than 5 mEq/L.

Bicarbonate infusion in general should be avoided but needs to be considered for patients who have a pH lower than 7, a serum bicarbonate level lower than 5.0 mEq/L, a K^+ concentration greater than 6.5 mEq/L, hypotension unresponsive to fluid replacement, severe left ventricular failure, or respiratory depression. Under these circumstances, 50 to 100 mEq (1 to 2 ampules) of bicarbonate may be infused intravenously over 2 hours. Serum phosphate should be measured, and phosphate repletion should be considered if the level falls below 1 mg/dL, especially if there is coincident heart failure, respiratory depression, or hemolytic anemia. Under these circumstances, 20 to 30/L potassium or sodium phosphate can be added to IV fluids. Phosphate repletion is not recommended with less marked decreases in serum levels, because this has not been shown to improve outcomes in DKA and may lead to hypocalcemia or hypomagnesemia.

As DKA resolves, it is important to continue providing adequate insulin to effectively resolve the ketosis, which may correct more slowly than the other abnormalities. This can be accomplished by adding glucose to the intravenous regimen (e.g., 5% glucose in half-normal saline) when blood glucose levels decrease to less than 200 to 250 mg/dL and continuing insulin infusion at 1 to 2 U/hour.

In patients with resolved DKA, transition to subcutaneous insulin can be made when the patient is clinically stable with normal vital signs, the acidosis is fully corrected, the patient is able take fluids orally without nausea or vomiting, and any precipitating conditions (e.g., infection) are controlled.

Hyperglycemic Hyperosmolar State

A hyperglycemic hyperosmolar state (HHS) occurs almost exclusively in patients with T2DM, one third of whom have not been previously diagnosed. Patients often are elderly and frequently have compromised renal function. Insulin deficiency, often exacerbated by insulin resistance resulting from the stress of an intercurrent illness, leads to hyperglycemia, glucosuria, and an osmotic diuresis. However, the presence of some endogenous insulin secretion suppresses lipolysis and ketogenesis enough to prevent ketoacidosis. Patients with HHS typically develop more marked hyperglycemia, fluid and electrolyte deficits, and hyperosmolality compared to those with DKA. HHS usually develops insidiously over days to weeks, and patients may be vulnerable to development of more severe hyperglycemia and volume deficits over this extended period.

HHS is associated with infections (40%), diuretic use (35% to 40%), and residency in nursing homes (25% to 30%). Other precipitating and complicating factors may include intestinal obstruction, mesenteric thrombosis, pulmonary embolism, peritoneal dialysis, subdural hematoma, and an extensive list of medications. The overall mortality rate exceeds that of DKA (10% to 40%), with higher mortality rates associated with age older than 70 years, nursing home residency, and higher osmolality or serum Na^+ concentration. Clinically, patients have evidence of the marked fluid and electrolyte deficits and tend to have more prominent neurologic abnormalities than those with DKA, including confusion, obtundation, and coma.

Therapy for HHS follows the same general principles as that for DKA, with a greater volume replacement required (typically 8 to 12 L in fully developed HHS). Restoration of the fluid and electrolyte deficits should proceed more slowly than in DKA (e.g., over 36 to 72 hours). Insulin therapy should be started only after rehydration is in progress. There is a need for K^+ replacement, but less than in DKA. Patients with HHS may be more sensitive to insulin than those with DKA and may require lower insulin doses. In view of the severe dehydration and predisposition to vascular thrombosis, heparin prophylaxis usually should be provided. Despite the very marked hyperglycemia of HHS, patients may be able to ultimately return to oral medications.

Chronic Complications of Diabetes

Chronic complications of T1DM and T2DM are similar and include microvascular complications (nephropathy, retinopathy, and neuropathy) and macrovascular or cardiovascular complications (coronary artery disease, peripheral vascular disease, and cerebrovascular disease). The long-term complications of diabetes result in substantial morbidity and shorten average lifespan by approximately 10 years. Candidate mechanisms for microvascular and macrovascular complications include activation of the polyol pathway (with accumulation of sorbitol), formation of glycated proteins and advanced glycation end products (cross-linked glycated proteins), abnormalities in lipid metabolism, increased oxidative damage, hyperinsulinemia, hyperperfusion of certain tissues, hyperviscosity, platelet dysfunction (increased aggregation), endothelial dysfunction, and activation of various growth factors.

Microvascular Complications

Retinopathy. Diabetic retinopathy affects almost all patients with T1DM and 60% to 80% of those with T2DM by 20 years after the diagnosis of diabetes. It is the most common cause of blindness in persons between the ages of 20 and 74 years in the developed world. The incidence and progression of diabetic retinopathy increase with duration of diabetes, poor glycemic control, the type of diabetes (T1DM more than T2DM), and the presence of hypertension, smoking, dyslipidemia, nephropathy, and pregnancy.

Early interventions often are beneficial in slowing or sometimes reversing diabetic retinopathy, but most patients have no symptoms until the lesions are advanced. Therefore, annual ophthalmologic screening is recommended starting at 5 years after diagnosis in T1DM and at the time of diagnosis in T2DM.

In nonproliferative retinopathy, the progression to visual loss in patients with clinically significant macular edema is improved by focal laser photocoagulation. Panretinal photocoagulation improves outcomes in patients with proliferative retinopathy and also in the subset of T2DM patients with severe nonproliferative diabetic retinopathy. Patients who have had vitreous hemorrhage and resulting visual loss may have significant restoration of vision with vitrectomy. Patients with macular edema also may benefit from intravitreous anti–vascular endothelial factor (VEGF) pharmacotherapy. In addition to diabetic retinopathy, patients with diabetes are at increased risk for development of cataracts.

Nephropathy. Diabetic nephropathy is the most common cause of end-stage renal disease (ESRD) in developed countries (about 30% of cases). However, the risk of progression to ESRD has been markedly decreasing over the last several decades. ESRD now appears to affect fewer than 10% of patients. The risk of developing advanced renal disease in diabetes is increased by poor glycemic control, hypertension, smoking, and possibly use of oral contraceptives, obesity, dyslipidemia, and more advanced age.

Diabetic nephropathy is primarily a glomerulopathy, with pathologic features that include mesangial expansion, glomerular basement membrane thickening, and glomerular sclerosis. Many but not all patients develop albuminuria early in the course, and the level of albumin correlates with the rate of progression and the degree of renal injury. For this reason, patients should be monitored annually for albuminuria starting 5 years after diagnosis in T1DM and at the time of diagnosis in T2DM. Measurement of the ratio of microalbumin to creatinine in a random urine sample is adequate, because this ratio correlates well with results from 24-hour collections. Albumin excretion of 30 to 300 mg per gram of creatinine (designated *moderately increased albuminuria*) indicates probable diabetic nephropathy. Albumin excretion of greater than 300 mg per gram of creatinine (designated *severely increased albuminuria*) indicates high risk for progression to nephrotic-range proteinuria and ESRD.

Efforts to achieve blood glucose targets and rigorously control blood pressure (appropriate to age and overall risk profile) should be part of the strategy for primary prevention of nephropathy in all patients with diabetes. For patients with greater than 300 mg protein per gram creatinine and an eGFR greater than 30 mL/min/1.73m², canagliflozin should be considered for blood glucose management, since it has been shown to delay progression to ESRD. Blood pressure should be maintained lower than 140/90 mm Hg unless otherwise contraindicated. In patients with high risk for adverse cardiovascular events, a target of 130/80 mm Hg should be considered. Angiotensin-converting enzyme (ACE) inhibitors or angiotensin receptor blockers (ARBs) are preferable first-line agents. The calcium-channel blockers diltiazem and verapamil can be used as alternatives in patients who are unable to tolerate ACE inhibitors or ARBs, or as additive therapy in patients who need multiple drugs to control blood pressure. Diuretics and moderate Na^+ restriction also frequently are needed to reach blood pressure goals.

Neuropathy. The likelihood of development of diabetic neuropathy increases with duration of disease and is influenced by the degree of glycemic control (occurring overall in up to 70% of people with diabetes). Any part of the peripheral or autonomic nervous system may be affected. *Peripheral polyneuropathy* occurs most commonly, usually manifesting as a bilaterally symmetrical, distal, primarily sensory polyneuropathy (with or without motor involvement) in a *glove-and-stocking* distribution. Pain, numbness, hyperesthesias, and paresthesias progress to sensory loss. This condition, together with loss of proprioception, can lead to an abnormal gait with repeated trauma and potential for fractures of the tarsal bones, sometimes resulting in the development of Charcot joints. These changes lead to abnormal pressures in the feet that, together with the soft tissue atrophy related to peripheral arterial insufficiency, result in foot ulcers that may progress to osteomyelitis and gangrene. Detailed, regular neurologic examination of all patients is essential to elicit the early loss of light touch (using a size 5.07/10-g monofilament), reflexes, and vibratory sensation.

A second common form of diabetic neuropathy is autonomic neuropathy, which may develop in concert with or separate from distal polyneuropathy. Resulting symptoms can be debilitating, including postural hypotension leading to falls or syncope, gastroparesis, enteropathy with constipation or diarrhea, and bladder outflow obstruction with urinary retention. Diabetic autonomic neuropathy together with vascular disease is a contributor to erectile dysfunction in males. Gastrointestinal dysfunction with autonomic neuropathy can complicate efforts to achieve blood glucose control by causing variable absorption of food. A suspected diagnosis of autonomic neuropathy can be strengthened by demonstrating loss of normal variability in heart rate with deep respirations or the Valsalva maneuver.

Other, less common manifestations of diabetic neuropathy include thoracic and lumbar nerve root *polyradiculopathies*, individual peripheral and cranial nerve *mononeuropathies*, and asymmetrical neuropathies of multiple peripheral nerves (mononeuropathy multiplex). Diabetic amyotrophy causing muscle atrophy and weakness most often involving the anterior thigh muscles and pelvic girdle is an uncommon form of diabetic neuropathy that often resolves after several months.

The primary approach to all diabetic neuropathies consists of efforts to improve blood glucose control. Clinical trials have shown decreased development of distal polyneuropathy with improved glycemia in T1DM. It also is particularly important for patients with neuropathies to receive regular foot care, including daily self-inspection of the feet, regular physician examinations, and early interventions for developing calluses, infections, or other foot lesions. Painful polyneuropathies cause substantial morbidity and are difficult to treat. First-line drugs include amitriptyline, venlafaxine, duloxetine, and pregabalin. For patients who do not respond adequately to one drug, combination therapy with two drugs of different classes can be tested. Alternative treatments that may be effective in some patients include topical capsaicin cream, lidocaine patch, α-lipoic acid, isosorbide dinitrate topical spray, and transcutaneous electrical nerve stimulation (TENS). *Gastroparesis* secondary to autonomic neuropathy may improve symptomatically with metoclopramide or domperidone (dopamine D2 antagonists), erythromycin (motilin agonist) for bacterial overgrowth, cisapride (cholinergic agonist), or mosapride (selective serotonin 5-HT4 receptor agonist). Diarrhea may respond to loperamide or diphenoxylate and atropine. Orthostatic hypotension can be treated by attention to mechanical factors such as elevation of the head of the bed, gradual rising from a lying to standing position, use of support stockings, and sometimes use of the mineralocorticoid fludrocortisone.

Macrovascular Complications

The risk of macrovascular disease including cardiovascular disease, transient ischemic attacks and strokes, and peripheral vascular disease is increased 2-fold to 4-fold and accounts for 70% to 80% of deaths in patients with diabetes. This increased risk is believed to result from the altered metabolism in diabetes and also from the frequent occurrence of associated risk factors in diabetic patients, including hypertension and dyslipidemia. Screening for macrovascular disease and predisposing factors were discussed earlier. Approaches to decreasing the risk of macrovascular disease should include optimization of blood glucose

control (including consideration of specific drugs for T2DM that may decrease cardiovascular event risk as discussed previously), weight loss for overweight and obese patients, smoking cessation, control of blood pressure, and treatment of dyslipidemia. (See Chapter 71 for details on the management of dyslipidemia.)

HYPOGLYCEMIA

Definition

Hypoglycemia most often occurs in patients with T1DM or T2DM under circumstances in which insulin or other antidiabetic therapies result in blood glucose levels decreasing below the lower limit of normal (<50 to 60 mg/dL for most laboratories). This may be caused by overtreatment with glucose-lowering agents, failure to take in anticipated calories, or the combination of increased glucose utilization and increased insulin sensitivity induced by exercise.

Hypoglycemia much less commonly occurs as a primary disorder in patients who do not have drug-treated diabetes. Under these circumstances, clinically significant hypoglycemia can be difficult to identify based on blood glucose measurements alone, because the normal lower limit of blood glucose varies in individuals and is influenced by duration of fasting and gender. Plasma glucose levels during a fast in men decrease to approximately 55 mg/dL at 24 hours and 50 mg/dL at 48 and 72 hours, whereas in premenopausal women they may be as low as 35 mg/dL at 24 hours without symptoms of hypoglycemia. In evaluating glucose determinations, it is important to recognize that plasma levels are approximately 15% higher than glucose levels in whole blood. Clinically significant hypoglycemia can be most readily established if patients manifest *Whipple triad*, which refers to the combination of: (1) symptoms suggestive of hypoglycemia, (2) documented low plasma glucose levels (<50 to 60 mg/dL), and (3) prompt resolution of symptoms when the low blood glucose is corrected.

Signs and Symptoms

Typical signs and symptoms of hypoglycemia are listed in Table 68.8. *Autonomic* symptoms result from sympathetic neural outflow that occurs as part of the counter-regulatory response to hypoglycemia. Although most patients appear to fully recover CNS function after a neuroglycopenic episode, there is a risk of irreversible brain damage or death with sustained or repeated episodes of severe neuroglycopenia.

Pathology

Hypoglycemic disorders can result when there is overproduction of hormones that lower glucose concentrations, underproduction of hormones that serve to elevate glucose levels, deficiency of substrates for endogenous glucose synthesis, or changes in cells and tissues that result in their increased consumption of glucose.

Etiologic Classification

Causes of hypoglycemia by etiologic categories are listed in Table 68.9.

Drug-Induced

The most common causes of hypoglycemia are excess insulin or insulin secretagogues (especially sulfonylureas) administered in the treatment of diabetes. Ethanol can cause hypoglycemia, most often in the context of chronic alcoholism in an individual who is nutritionally depleted after binge drinking for several days or longer. Under these circumstances, hepatic glycogen stores become depleted, and the process of alcohol metabolism blocks gluconeogenesis by depriving the liver of nicotinamide adenine dinucleotide (NAD+). Commonly used pharmacologic agents that have been associated with hypoglycemia include β-blockers (especially nonselective β$_2$-adrenergic antagonists), ACE

TABLE 68.8   Signs and Symptoms of Hypoglycemia

Autonomic

Sweating	Palpitations	Hunger
Pallor	Tachycardia	Nausea
Anxiety	Hypertension	Vomiting
Tremor	Irritability	Paresthesias

Neuroglycopenic

Difficulty thinking	Dizziness	Seizures
Fatigue, weakness	Visual blurring	Loss of consciousness
Somnolence	Confusion	Coma
Headache	Abnormal behavior	Death

TABLE 68.9   Etiologic Classification of Hypoglycemic Disorders Manifesting in Adults

Drug-Induced
Antidiabetic agents (insulin, sulfonylureas, meglitinides)
Alcohol
Other pharmacologic agents (β-blockers, ACE inhibitors, pentamidine, quinine, quinolones and many others)

Altered Gastrointestinal Function
Alimentary hypoglycemia

Beta-Cell Insulin Oversecretion
Insulinoma
Non-insulinoma pancreatogenous hypoglycemia (without or with bariatric surgery)

Non–Islet Cell Neoplasms
Tumor insulin-like growth factor-II secretion
Tumor glucose consumption

Autoimmune
Circulating insulin antibodies
Insulin receptor activating antibodies

Endocrine Deficiencies
Glucocorticoids (adrenal insufficiency), growth hormone, catecholamines, glucagon

Severe Illness
Sepsis
Hepatic failure
Renal failure

Malnutrition
Anorexia nervosa

ACE, Angiotensin-converting enzyme.

inhibitors, pentamidine (through toxic effects on beta cells), quinine, and quinolones.

Excess Endogenous Insulin or Insulin-like Hormones

Alimentary hypoglycemia is a disorder in which low blood glucose levels occur typically 90 to 180 minutes after meals in patients who have undergone gastric outlet surgery with resulting accelerated gastric emptying. This is distinct from the more common *dumping syndrome*, which results from rapid entry of an osmotic load into the small intestine and associated fluid shifts and autonomic responses and is not associated with hypoglycemia. "Reactive hypoglycemia" is a now outmoded term that previously was applied to adrenergic symptoms occurring 2 to 4 hours after a meal in patients who are not hypoglycemic; these individuals may experience decreased symptoms with frequent feedings and avoidance of high-carbohydrate meals.

Tumors of islet beta cells *(insulinomas)* can cause hypoglycemia by producing excess insulin in an unregulated manner. They are uncommon (1 in 250,000 patient-years) but important to recognize when they do occur. Insulinomas usually are small (1 to 2 cm), benign (>90%), solitary (>90%), and confined to the endocrine pancreas (99%). Some patients have an indolent course extending over many years before diagnosis, but insulinomas can produce profound hypoglycemia. There is a tendency for adrenergic symptoms to become suppressed as a consequence of repeated exposures to hypoglycemia, and neuroglycopenic symptoms may predominate, including sometimes bizarre behavioral abnormalities. Patients may eat frequently in response to the hypoglycemia and exhibit moderate weight gain.

Non-insulinoma pancreatogenous hypoglycemia is a disorder that may manifest with symptoms similar to those of insulinomas, but the pathology involves beta-cell hypertrophy and hyperplasia rather than the presence of a discrete tumor. More recently, the development of hypoglycemia with similar beta-cell hyperplasia has been described in some patients months to years after Roux-en-Y gastric bypass surgery.

Non–islet cell neoplasms are a rare cause of hypoglycemia; they produce an insulin-like growth factor (IGF), usually a partially processed form of IGF-II designated *big IGF-II*, that can have insulin-like effects. The tumors typically are large and malignant and are most often located in the retroperitoneal space, abdomen, or thoracic cavity. Tumor types include hemangiopericytomas, hepatocellular carcinomas, lymphomas, adrenocortical carcinomas, gastrointestinal carcinoids, and mesenchymal tumors. Some large tumors cause hypoglycemia in the absence of detectable insulin-like factors.

Hormone Deficiencies

Deficiencies of insulin counter-regulatory hormones, which normally function to raise glucose levels, can result in or contribute to

hypoglycemia. An example is low levels of corticosteroids caused by primary or secondary adrenocorticoid insufficiency. Deficiencies of other hormones, including catecholamines, glucagon, and growth hormone, also can cause hypoglycemia.

Severe Illness

Hypoglycemia can occur during severe illness through a number of different mechanisms in association with sepsis, hepatic insufficiency, and renal failure. Patients with severe illness appear to be particularly vulnerable to hypoglycemia when they are poorly nourished, although malnutrition alone is rarely associated with hypoglycemia.

Approach to the Diagnosis

For patients who have well-documented hypoglycemia, the diagnosis often is evident or strongly suggested by the clinical setting, history, and physical examination findings. Hypoglycemia induced by insulin or other glucose-lowering agents in diabetic patients often is immediately apparent from the medical history. Alcohol-induced hypoglycemia may be suspected in a patient with a known or suspected history of alcohol use and binge drinking. Identification of other candidate drugs as a cause of hypoglycemia requires a thorough medical history, and the condition can be expected to resolve if the suspect medication is stopped. The patient may have a known diagnosis of adrenal insufficiency, or this may be suggested by other clinical findings (e.g., orthostatic hypotension, increased skin pigmentation) or the development of markedly increased insulin sensitivity in a patient with T1DM. The patient may have a known tumor, suggesting the possibility of a non–islet cell neoplasm as a cause of hypoglycemia. There may be a history of Roux-en-Y bypass surgery, raising the possibility of beta-cell hyperplasia. The co-occurrence of sepsis, hepatic failure, renal failure, profound malnutrition, or a diagnosis of anorexia nervosa may suggest one of these potential underlying causes.

A number of algorithms have been developed to guide the evaluation of documented or potential hypoglycemia, including a recommended approach from an expert panel published by the Endocrine Society. If there is an opportunity to observe the patient during a symptomatic episode of presumed hypoglycemia, plasma should be obtained, if possible before treatment, for measurement of glucose, insulin, proinsulin, C-peptide, β-hydroxybutyrate, and screening for sulfonylureas and meglitinides. Hypoglycemia can be rapidly, provisionally confirmed with a test meter and later confirmed by laboratory analysis. After blood samples have been obtained for the tests described, glucose should be administered orally (15 to 30 g) or intravenously (25 g, or 1 ampule of 50% dextrose), and recovery of glucose levels and symptoms should be observed.

For patients with suspected or confirmed hypoglycemia developing specifically in the fasted state, it may be possible to replicate the condition by observing during several hours of daytime fasting, with or without a preceding overnight fast. The same laboratory testing panel as described earlier then can be obtained if symptoms suggestive of hypoglycemia occur. For patients who describe postprandial hypoglycemic symptoms (within 5 hours after a meal), a mixed meal (not a pure glucose load) should be provided, with blood sampling at baseline and every 30 minutes thereafter for 5 hours.

For patients who do not manifest hypoglycemia with the testing procedures described despite a strong suspicion of hypoglycemia, the most frequently utilized approach is a 72-hour fast according to a protocol developed at the Mayo Clinic. Blood is obtained every 6 hours and at test termination. The test is ended at 72 hours or at an earlier time point if the plasma glucose level decreases (by glucose meter testing) with associated symptoms to 45 mg/dL (2.5 mmol/L) or lower or to less than 55 mg/dL (3 mmol/L) in a patient with prior documentation of Whipple triad. At the end of the 72-hour test period, the patient is given 1 mg of glucagon intravenously, and blood is obtained at 10, 20, and 30 minutes, after which the patient is given a meal. The final blood sample obtained at the end of the fast (before glucagon administration) is analyzed additionally for β-hydroxybutyrate and a sulfonylurea/meglitinide panel.

For any of these test protocols, elevations of insulin, proinsulin, and C-peptide associated with hypoglycemia at the same time point are consistent with an insulinoma, beta-cell hyperplasia, the effects of an insulin secretagogue (sulfonylurea or meglitinide), or the presence of insulin antibodies. An elevation in these three hormones during a meal test in a patient who has had gastric surgery is suggestive of alimentary hypoglycemia. Plasma insulin, proinsulin, and C-peptide are not elevated in patients with hypoglycemia secondary to extrapancreatic neoplasms. This diagnosis usually can be further confirmed by evidence of a large tumor with various imaging techniques. High insulin levels, together with low proinsulin and C-peptide concentrations in the presence of hypoglycemia, are indicative of exogenous insulin administration. Factitious hypoglycemia secondary to insulin or insulin secretagogue administration is uncommon and has been observed in individuals with or without diabetes.

Treatment

The most important therapeutic step in hypoglycemia is to identify and treat the underlying causes, including drugs, alcohol, serious infection, tumors, and hypoadrenalism. The occurrence of hypoglycemia usually can be substantially improved in patients with alimentary hypoglycemia by a modified feeding regimen with frequent, small meals and avoidance of concentrated sources of rapidly digested and absorbed carbohydrate.

Non–islet cell tumor hypoglycemia is treated by tumor resection if possible. For nonresectable tumors, a debulking procedure may be effective in reducing hypoglycemia. Hypoglycemia in patients with insulinomas can be cured by resection. Persistent hypoglycemia secondary to nonresectable insulinoma can sometimes be treated effectively with diazoxide, long-acting somatostatin analogues (octreotide or lanreotide), verapamil, or phenytoin. For patients with beta-cell hyperplasia after bariatric surgery, first-line treatment includes diet modifications with more frequent, small meals and avoidance of concentrated sources of carbohydrate to decrease meal-induced insulin secretion.

For a deeper discussion of this topic, please see Chapter 216, ❖ "Diabetes Mellitus," and Chapter 217, "Hypoglycemia and Pancreatic Islet Cell Disorders," in *Goldman-Cecil Medicine*, 26th Edition.

SUGGESTED READINGS

ACOG Practice Bulletin No. 190: Gestational diabetes mellitus. Committee on practice bulletins—obstetrics, Obstet Gynecol 131:e49–e64, 2018.

American Diabetes Association Standards of Medical Care in Diabetes 2019: Diabetes Care 42(Suppl 1):S1–S193, 2019.

Cryer PE, Axelrod L, Grossman AB, et al: Evaluation and management of adult hypoglycemic disorders: an Endocrine Society clinical practice guideline, J Clin Endocrinol Metab 94:709–728, 2009.

Davies MJ, D'Alessio DA, Fradkin J, et al: Management of hyperglycemia in type 2 diabetes, 2018. A consensus report by the American Diabetes Association (ADA) and the European Association for the Study of Diabetes (EASD), Diabetes Care 41:2669–2701, 2018.

Eckel RH, Grundy SM, Zimmet PZ: The metabolic syndrome, Lancet 365:1415–1428, 2005.

Forbes JM, Cooper ME: Mechanisms of diabetic complications, Physiol Rev 93:137–188, 2013.

Nathan DM, Cleary PA, Backlund JY, et al: Intensive diabetes treatment and cardiovascular disease in patients with type 1 diabetes. Diabetes Control and Complications Trial/Epidemiology of Diabetes Interventions and Complications (DCCT/EDIC) Study Research Group, N Engl J Med 353:2643–2653, 2005.

Pathak V, Pathak NM, O'Neill CL, et al: Therapies for type 1 diabetes: current scenario and future perspectives, Clin Med Insights Endocrinol Diabetes 12:1179551419844521, 2019.

Pop-Busu R, Boulton AJM, Feldman EL, et al: Diabetic neuropathy: a position statement by the American Diabetes Association, Diabetes Care 40:136–154, 2017.

Sanyoura M, Philipson LH, Naylor R: Monogenic diabetes in children and adolescents: recognition and treatment options, Curr Diab Rep 18:58, 2018. https://doi.org/10.1007/s11892-018-1024-2.

Seaquist ER, Anderson J, Childs B, et al: Hypoglycemia and diabetes: a report of a workgroup of the American Diabetes Association and the Endocrine Society, J Clin Endocrinol Metab 98:1845–1859, 2013.

Tauschmann M, Hovorka R: Technology in the management of type 1 diabetes mellitus—current status and future prospects, Nat Rev Endocrinol 14:464–475, 2018.

Torres JM, Cox NJ, Philipson LH: Genome wide association studies for diabetes: perspective on results and challenges, Pediatr Diabetes 14:90–96, 2013.

Warren AM, Knudsen ST, Cooper ME: Diabetic nephropathy: an insight into molecular mechanisms and emerging therapies, Expert Opin Ther Targets 23:579–591, 2019.

69

Obesity

Osama Hamdy, Marwa Al-Badri

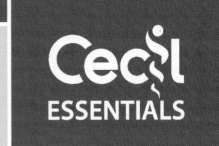

DEFINITION AND EPIDEMIOLOGY

Obesity is a disease that is usually defined as a body mass index (BMI) greater than or equal to 30 kg/m² (weight [kg]/(height [m])²). A BMI of 30 to 34.9 is considered class 1 obesity, 35 to 39.9 is class 2 obesity, and 40 or higher is class 3 or severe obesity. The term "morbid obesity" previously was applied to individuals weighing at least 45 kg (100 lb) more than, or typically about 60% more than, desirable body weight; the term also has been applied to any individual with BMI greater than or equal to 40 kg/m².

There is increasing recognition of limitations to defining obesity based on BMI resulting from the variable correlation between BMI and amount of body fat in different ethnic (genetic) populations or in individuals with different degrees of muscularity. Many investigators and clinicians are moving toward a definition that defines obesity as an excess of body fat sufficient to confer risk. According to the percentage of body fat, obesity is defined in men as percentage of body fat greater than 25%, with 21% to 25% being borderline, and in women as percentage of body fat greater than 33%, with 31% to 33% being borderline.

Linking obesity to cardiometabolic risk, body fat distribution, and waist circumference is more important than measuring percentage body fat or BMI alone. People who accumulate abdominal visceral fat and clinically have higher waist circumference (metabolic obesity) are at much higher risk for cardiovascular disease and diabetes than those with the same BMI or the same percentage of body fat but with lower waist circumference. The National Cholesterol Education Program Adult Treatment Panel III (ATP III) considered a waist circumference greater than 40 inches (102 cm) in American men or 35 inches (88 cm) in American women to be among the five criteria that define the cardiometabolic syndrome. In spite of its limitations, BMI remains a simple measurement with utility in estimating a person's health risks and comparing outcomes between trials.

During the last 30 years, there has been a dramatic increase in the percentage of both adults and children in the United States who are overweight (defined as BMI of 25 to 30) or obese. According to the 2015-2016 National Health and Nutrition Examination Survey (NHANES) conducted by the Centers for Disease Control and Prevention (CDC), 39.8% of US adults were obese, including 7.6% with severe obesity, and an additional 31.8% are overweight. This was more than double the prevalence in the 1976-1980 NHANES data (15.0%). Mexican Americans had the highest age-adjusted percentage of obesity (49.25%), followed by all Hispanic individuals (46.85%), non-Hispanic black (45.8%), and non-Hispanic white individuals (37.95%). More recently, there appears to have been a slowing in the rate of obesity increase or even a leveling off. In 2017, obesity prevalence seemed to vary significantly across states, from 20% or less in Colorado, Hawaii, and District of Columbia to 35% or more in seven states (Alabama, Arkansas, Iowa, Louisiana, Mississippi, Oklahoma, and West Virginia). In general, higher prevalence of adult obesity was found in the south (32.4%) and the midwest (32.3%) and lower prevalence in the northeast (27.7%) and the west (26.1%). The percentage of children and adolescents who are overweight or obese has almost tripled since 1980. Currently, 18.5% of children and adolescents aged 2 to 19 years are obese, including 5.6% with severe obesity, and another 16.6% are overweight. NHANES data from 1976-1980 and from 2015-2016 show that the prevalence of obesity increased from 5.0% to 13.9% for children aged 2 to 5 years and from 5.0% to 20.6% for those aged 12 to 19 years. Among low-income preschool children, the prevalence of obesity increased between 1998 and 2016 from 13.0% to 13.9% and severe obesity from 1.8% to 2.1%.

Overweight and obesity and their associated health problems have a significant economic impact on the US health care system through direct medical expenses and indirect costs (e.g., loss of work time and productivity). Medical costs of obesity and their associated health problems account for an estimated 10% of total US medical expenditures.

PATHOLOGY OF OBESITY

Obesity develops as a consequence of genetic-environmental interactions, such that genetically prone individuals who lead a sedentary lifestyle and consume larger amounts of dietary calories are at higher risk. For example, children of obese parents are 80% more likely to become obese, and it is believed that this results from a combination of genetic and environmental influences.

The genetic contributions to obesity are most commonly considered to reflect the combined effects of variations in multiple genes and only rarely appear to result from a defect in a single powerful gene. Single-gene defects identified in experimental animals have been useful to demonstrate appetite and satiety mechanisms. Mutations in some of these same genes have subsequently been identified in rare human forms of genetic obesity. For example, loss-of-function mutations in the leptin gene and in the cellular receptor for leptin were first identified as a cause of obesity in laboratory mice (*ob/ob* and *db/db* mice, respectively). Leptin is a hormone that is produced in fat cells, mostly in subcutaneous fat. It is a potent satiety factor that acts in the arcuate nucleus of the hypothalamus to reduce the production of neuropeptide Y, a stimulator of food intake. After its discovery in mice, leptin gene mutations were identified as a cause of a rare form of heritable human obesity. Affected individuals develop marked obesity in childhood as a consequence of increased food intake. Leptin secretion normally follows a circadian pattern, with higher levels during evening and night hours. Loss of leptin secretion has particularly marked effects during these hours, resulting in a phenomenon known as the night-eating syndrome, in which patients tend to consume large amounts of food during the night.

Other single-gene defects identified as rare causes of human obesity include loss-of-function mutations in genes encoding carboxypeptidase E, melanocortin-4 or melanocortin-3 receptors, and serotonin-2C or serotonin-1B receptors. Obesity is also a feature of many other genetic disorders in which the specific mechanisms of the obesity are less well understood. These different syndromes may have autosomal dominant, autosomal recessive or X-linked inheritance patterns, consistent with multiple different genetic causes. Among the best known of these disorders is the Bardet-Biedl syndrome, which is an autosomal recessive disorder characterized by obesity and other abnormalities, including hypogonadism in men, mental retardation, retinal dystrophy, polydactyly, and renal malformations. In Prader-Willi syndrome, loss of portions of the long arm of chromosome 15 (q11-13) is associated with obesity, poor muscle tone in infancy, defects in cognition, behavioral abnormalities (irritability), short stature, and hypogonadotropic hypogonadism.

Although known single-gene mutations account for only a small percentage of human obesity, there is evidence for widespread heritable influences in more common forms of human obesity. For example, in twin and adoptee studies, both members of identical twin pairs tend to become obese in concordance with the same weight pattern as their biologic parents, even when raised apart. Metabolic rate, spontaneous physical activity, and thermic response to food seem to be heritable to a variable extent, but the specific genes that contribute to prevalent forms of human obesity have not yet been identified. Genomic analyses in large populations have identified multiple genes or genetic regions in which polymorphisms are associated with obesity risk. These include polymorphisms in or near genes for the melanocortin-4 receptor (a protein involved in appetite suppression pathways in the hypothalamus), brain-derived neurotrophic factor (role in energy balance), the β_3-adrenergic receptor (role in visceral fat accumulation), and peroxisome proliferator-activated receptor-$\gamma2$ (PPAR-$\gamma2$), a transcription factor involved in adipocyte differentiation. Multiple other sites of genetic variation associated with increased obesity risk have been identified for which potential mechanistic links to obesity are not yet apparent. It is hypothesized that the heritable component of common forms of human obesity derives from the effects of variations in these and many yet unidentified genes acting both additively and synergistically.

Important environmental factors driving the recent increased prevalence of obesity include increased caloric intake (reflecting greater availability of high-calorie, low-cost foods) and decreased energy expenditure (as a consequence of decreased physical activity). Lower socioeconomic status, lower education level, cessation of smoking, and high consumption of carbohydrates with a high glycemic index have been identified as specific confounders of obesity. Additional factors that may influence obesity risk include intrauterine growth, weight gain during pregnancy, hormonal changes during menopause, history of depression, use of major antipsychotic medications, and factors that may alter the feedback between energy intake and expenditure.

Many hormones affect appetite and food intake. Ghrelin, which is secreted from the stomach fundus, is a major hunger hormone. Endocannabinoids, through their effects on endocannabinoid receptors in the brain, increase appetite, promote nutrient absorption, and promote lipogenesis. Melanocortin hormone, through its effects on various melanocortin receptors in the brain, modifies appetite. Meanwhile, several gut hormones play significant roles in influencing satiety, including glucagon-like peptide-1 (GLP-1), neuropeptide YY (PYY), and cholecystokinin. Leptin and pancreatic amylin are other potent satiety hormones. Ultimately, an increase in total body fat results from an increase in energy intake that exceeds energy expenditure.

This occurs through the operation of genetic and environmental influences, together with individual behavioral characteristics.

PATHOLOGY OF OBESITY-ASSOCIATED HEALTH RISKS

Adipose tissue is not just a passive depot for lipids. Adipocytes also function as a complex and active endocrine organ with metabolic and secretory products (hormones, prohormones, cytokines, and enzymes) that play a major role in whole-body metabolism. Relationships between obesity and both insulin resistance and endothelial dysfunction (the early stage of atherosclerosis) are mediated through the release of several hormones from adipose tissue. These hormones, designated adipocytokines or adipokines, comprise a group of pharmacologically active low- and medium-molecular-weight proteins that possess autocrine and paracrine effects and are known products of the inflammatory and immune systems. They play an important role in adipose tissue physiology and in initiating metabolic and cardiovascular abnormalities, not only in overweight and obese individuals, but also in lean persons with higher visceral fat mass. These adipokines include adiponectin, leptin, tumor necrosis factor-α (TNF-α), interleukin-6 (IL-6), resistin, plasminogen activator inhibitor-1 (PAI-1), angiotensinogen, and monocyte chemoattractant protein-1 (MCP-1). An increased amount of adipose tissue or its disproportionate distribution between central and peripheral body regions is related to altered serum levels of these factors. With the exceptions of leptin and adiponectin, the adipokines are produced both from fat cells and from adipose tissue–resident macrophages in the stromal tissues surrounding fat cells. For unknown reasons, an increase in the amount of body fat is associated with increases in the number of adipose tissue macrophages and their production of cytokines.

Human adiponectin is a relatively abundant, 244-amino-acid polypeptide in plasma, accounting for 0.01% of total plasma proteins. Adiponectin gene expression in adipose tissue is associated with obesity, insulin resistance, and type 2 diabetes (T2DM). Hypoadiponectinemia is more strongly related to the degree of insulin resistance than to the degree of adiposity or glucose intolerance. Genetic polymorphisms may influence the regulation of adiponectin and lead to variations in its levels among different individuals. Several human studies have shown that high adiponectin levels protect against development of T2DM and point to the possible future use of adiponectin as an indicator of diabetes risk. Low plasma concentrations of adiponectin are observed in patients with coronary artery disease (CAD), and lower adiponectin levels have been found in patients with diabetes and CAD than in those without CAD. In obesity, a 10% reduction in body weight leads to a significant increase in adiponectin (40% to 60%) in both patients with and without diabetes. Adiponectin is also involved in the modulation of inflammatory responses through attenuation of TNF-α–mediated inflammatory effects, regulation of endothelial function, and inhibition of growth factor–induced proliferation of vascular smooth muscle cells.

Leptin is a 167-amino-acid adipocyte-derived hormone that circulates in the plasma in free and bound forms. It affects energy balance by activating specific centers in the hypothalamus to decrease food intake, increase energy expenditure, modulate glucose and fat metabolism, and alter neuroendocrine function. Leptin plasma levels increase exponentially with increased fat mass (4-fold higher in obese compared with lean individuals in one study), and this is thought to reflect resistance to leptin in obesity. Leptin therapy in lipodystrophic patients has been shown to lower blood glucose, improve insulin-stimulated hepatic and peripheral glucose metabolism, and reduce hepatic and muscle triglyceride content, suggesting that leptin acts as a signal that contributes to regulation of total body sensitivity to insulin. It has also been found that leptin is independently associated with cardiovascular mortality. Although both adiponectin and leptin are integrally related to insulin resistance, adiponectin is more strongly related to visceral abdominal fat stores, whereas leptin is more closely related to subcutaneous fat.

Adipose tissue, especially visceral fat and intermuscular fat, serves as a major source of TNF-α and substantial amounts of IL-6. Levels of these two proinflammatory cytokines correlate with obesity and are strongly related to insulin resistance. Several studies have demonstrated a strong link between TNF-α and cardiovascular disease. Plasma levels of TNF-α are increased in individuals with premature cardiovascular disease independent of insulin sensitivity. Conversely, circulating levels of TNF-α decrease after weight reduction in parallel with the improvement in endothelial function.

Resistin is an adipocyte-derived, cysteine-rich signaling protein that is expressed predominantly in white adipose tissue and is also detectable in serum. Resistin is thought to act at sites remote from adipose tissue, similar to other adipokines, and to contribute to insulin resistance in obesity. *PAI-1* is another bioactive peptide produced by subcutaneous and visceral fat. Its circulating levels correlate better with visceral than with subcutaneous adiposity and are strong predictors of CAD. High PAI-1 levels are associated with increased blood coagulability. Improvement in insulin sensitivity by either weight reduction or medication lowers circulating levels of PAI-1. This decrease in PAI-1 correlates with the amount of weight loss and the decline in serum triglycerides.

Visceral, subcutaneous, and intermuscular fat differ in their production of specific adipokines, pointing to differences in endocrine function between these three adipose depots. Removal of a significant amount of only subcutaneous fat by liposuction in obese individuals with and without diabetes resulted in reduction in serum leptin but did not change the serum levels of other cytokines or any other metabolic parameters. It also did not improve insulin sensitivity or decrease the high serum insulin level observed initially in those individuals. In animal models, removal of subcutaneous fat resulted in an increase in mesenteric fat volume and increased production of TNF-α by visceral fat. Although surgical removal of visceral fat has not been attempted in humans, two studies of aging in rodent models showed that removal of visceral fat reduces the production of inflammatory adipokines and improves glucose tolerance and insulin sensitivity. More recently, it was shown that inflammatory adipokines are also secreted from intermuscular and subfascial fat and in excess of those secreted from abdominal visceral fat. Excess accumulation of intermuscular and subfascial fat (myosteatosis) is seen with ageing in both men and women and is strongly associated with insulin resistance.

Risks Associated With Obesity

Individuals who are overweight or obese are at increased risk for the following health conditions:

- Cardiometabolic syndrome
- T2DM
- Hypertension
- Dyslipidemia
- Coronary heart disease
- Congestive heart failure
- Atrial fibrillation
- Osteoarthritis
- Stroke
- Gallbladder disease
- Hepatic steatosis and nonalcoholic steatohepatitis (NASH)
- Obstructive sleep apnea
- Asthma
- Gastroesophageal reflux (GERD)
- Some cancers (endometrial, breast, and colon)
- Gynecologic disorders (abnormal menses, infertility, polycystic ovarian syndrome)
- Erectile dysfunction
- Depression

Weight loss of 7% to 10% is associated with reduced risk for many if not all of these disorders. Recent studies have shown that significant weight reduction (15% to 25% of initial body weight) after bariatric surgery in class 2 and class 3 obese patients with T2DM may result in partial or complete remission of diabetes, especially in patients with recent history of diabetes.

DIAGNOSIS AND ASSESSMENT OF OBESITY

The form of obesity that characteristically occurs in men—android or abdominal obesity (apple-shaped body configuration)—is closely associated with metabolic complications such as insulin resistance, hypertension, dyslipidemia, and hyperuricemia. By contrast, the typical female or gynecoid obesity (pear-shaped body configuration), in which fat accumulates in the hips and gluteal and femoral regions, has milder metabolic complications. The waist-to-hip circumference ratio (WHR) has been used to distinguish these forms of obesity. A ratio greater than 1.0 in men or greater than 0.8 in women, indicative of visceral fat deposition and abdominal obesity, correlates with increased health risks.

Standard laboratory studies in the evaluation of obesity should include the following:

- Fasting lipid panel
- Liver function tests
- Thyroid function tests
- Fasting plasma glucose
- Hemoglobin A1c (A1C)

Previously, the "gold standard" technique for measuring total body fat was *hydrodensitometry* (underwater weighing). This is based on the principle that fatty tissue is less dense than muscle. Currently, *dual-energy x-ray absorptiometry (DXA)* scanning is used to accurately measure body composition, particularly fat mass and fat-free mass. It has an additional advantage of measuring regional fat distribution. DXA is more accurate than anthropometric measures and is more cost-effective than computerized tomography (CT) or magnetic resonance imaging (MRI) scans. However, DXA cannot distinguish between subcutaneous and visceral abdominal fat depots, or between subcutaneous and intramuscular peripheral fat depots. Bioelectric impedance is a simpler and less expensive method for measuring total body fat, but it is greatly affected by the hydration state of the body and is less accurate than DXA.

BMI is widely used as a measure of obesity. It is calculated by dividing a person's body weight in kilograms by the square of the person's height in meters; alternatively, weight in pounds multiplied by 703 is divided by the square of the height in inches). A BMI between 19 and 27 has little association with cardiometabolic risk in white individuals. Adverse health consequences occur with a BMI of 27 or more and increase with increasing levels of BMI. Risks associated with increased BMI are more pronounced in older patients.

Waist circumference or *WHR* or both are often used to indirectly estimate intra-abdominal fat volume in epidemiologic studies. Although these measures show good correlation with intra-abdominal fat volume as measured by CT, they are less accurate than CT. At present, waist circumference is the easiest anthropometric measurement for routine use by health care professionals to estimate visceral adiposity and monitor changes in visceral fat volume.

The current gold standard techniques for measuring visceral fat volume are abdominal CT (at the L4-L5 vertebral level) and MRI. These methods are not widely used because of high cost. In contrast to CT, MRI requires additional definition of adipose tissue by adjusting settings on the MRI scanner. Several commercial software packages are available for calculation of visceral fat volume, and it is possible to further subdivide body fat into at least three separate and measurable compartments; subcutaneous, intramuscular, and visceral fat.

Visceral fat volume determination by abdominal ultrasonography has been investigated for use in research and clinical settings. Several studies found good correlation between intra-abdominal fat volume measured by abdominal ultrasound and that measured by abdominal CT scanning. Measurements should be performed with the patient in the supine position at the end of a quiet inspiration with compression of the transducer against the abdomen. Intra-abdominal fat is quantified based on the distance between the peritoneum and the lumbar spine. Studies have shown that intra-abdominal fat measured by ultrasound has a stronger association with metabolic risk factors for CAD than does waist circumference or WHR. Recently, visceral fat has been measured using *bioelectric impedance*, but this technique is less accurate than CT. Determinations of intrahepatic fat by ultrasonography, CT and *vibration controlled transient elastography* (VCTE) are of significant clinical value. Determination of intermuscular and subfascial fat volume by CT has been investigated for use in research but not used yet in routine clinical setting.

TREATMENT OF OBESITY

Current guidelines for treatment of obesity are summarized in Table 69.1. The preferred intervention varies with the obesity level based on five BMI categories. The major four therapeutic options are lifestyle modification (diet and exercise), behavior modification, pharmacologic intervention, and bariatric surgery. In general, better results are obtained with a combination of different interventions rather than a single modality.

Lifestyle Modification

Key components of effective lifestyle modification most often include structured dietary interventions and individualized physical activity programs. Behavior modification strategies and patient education are also critical for achievement and maintenance of target weight loss. Evidence-based dietary guidelines should be used to design individualized patient plans in consultation with a registered dietitian or qualified health care provider. First, daily caloric intake should be reduced by a modest 250 to 500 calories. Reasonable and paced reductions can help patients continue on the recommended dietary plan for a longer time. Daily calories from carbohydrate should be reduced to

approximately 40% to 45% of intake, with a total daily carbohydrate intake of no less than 130 g/day. Except in patients with renal impairment (creatinine clearance <60 mL/min) or significant microalbuminuria, protein intake should not be less than 1.2 g/kg of adjusted body weight (adjusted body weight = ideal body weight + 0.25 [current weight − ideal body weight]). This typically accounts for 20% to 30% of total calorie intake and is intended to minimize loss of lean body mass during weight reduction. The remaining 30% to 35% of calorie intake should come from fat. *Trans*-fats should be eliminated, and saturated fat, especially from meat and meat-products, should be reduced. Meal plans should also include substantial soluble fiber (e.g., from fresh fruits) and insoluble fiber (e.g., from vegetables) and consumption of healthy carbohydrates, especially foods that have a low glycemic index and high fiber content. Approximately 14 g of fiber per 1000 calories (20 to 35 g of fiber) per day is recommended.

Caloric intake should be adjusted downward over time until weight loss is achieved. Underlying all of these steps should be the goal of designing an individualized plan that can be maintained over the long term. Many patients find it helpful to receive a structured dietary intervention that includes specific suggestions for daily meals and snacks. Such structured diets may increase adherence and can be easier to follow than a list of general guidelines. Nutritionally complete meal replacement (e.g., in the form of shakes or bars) can be useful for some patients, especially at the start of a weight reduction program. If meal replacement is used, 100- to 200-calorie snacks (e.g., fruits and nuts) may be added at breakfast, lunch, or between meals. A recent study showed that a structured meal plan that includes menus, snack lists, and meal replacements in obese patients with T2DM resulted in 2.7 to 3.5 kg weight loss over 16 weeks in comparison to individualized meal plans.

Each patient should meet with an exercise physiologist to construct an individualized plan that is responsive to his or her lifestyle, capabilities, and potential cardiovascular risks. Because obese individuals frequently have difficulty exercising, this process requires careful attention. A balanced exercise plan incorporates a mix of cardiovascular, stretching, and strength exercises and should be graded to increase gradually in both duration and intensity. Patients can start with 10 to 20 minutes of daily stretching and aerobic exercise (e.g., moderate-intensity walking) with subsequent progressive increases. Any exercise should be preceded by a warm-up period to minimize injuries.

Long-term lifestyle modification trials, such as the Diabetes Prevention Program, have targeted 150 minutes of exercise per week. Newer guidelines recommend 60 to 90 minutes of daily exercise, with a minimum of 150 to 175 minutes per week needed to obtain weight loss benefit. Emphasis should be placed on moderate-intensity exercise, such as walking 20-minute miles, rather than strenuous exercise. Because patients who are not used to exercising may find it difficult

TABLE 69.1	Guide to Selecting Treatment Based on BMI Category[a]				
	BMI CATEGORY				
Treatment	25-26.9	27-29.9	30-34.9	35-39.9	≥40
Diet, physical activity, behavior therapy	Yes with comorbidities	Yes with comorbidities	Yes	Yes	Yes
Pharmacotherapy	No	Yes with comorbidities	Yes	Yes	Yes
Weight-loss surgery	No	No	Yes with comorbidities	Yes with comorbidities	Yes with comorbidities

[a]"Yes" indicates that the treatment is indicated regardless of comorbidities.
From National Institutes of Health (NIH), National Heart, Lung, and Blood Institute (NHLBI), North American Association for the Study of Obesity (NAASO): The practical guide to the identification, evaluation, and treatment of overweight and obesity in adults. NIH Publication No. 00-4084, Bethesda, Md., October 2000, NIH. http://www.nhlbi.nih.gov/files/docs/guidelines/prctgd_c.pdf. Accessed November 2014.

to incorporate physical activity into daily practice, it is also important to use a variety of exercises to maintain interest. Increasing exercise duration to 300 minutes/week was found to help in long-term maintenance of weight reduction. Frequent short bouts of exercise as brief as 10 minutes each can increase adherence to an exercise regimen and increase overall duration of exercise.

Behavior Modification and Patient Education

Cognitive-behavioral intervention and patient education are important components of successful weight loss programs. Whenever possible, cognitive-behavioral intervention should be conducted by an experienced psychologist. The fundamental principles of intervention typically include behavioral goal setting, stimulus control techniques, cognitive restructuring, assertive communication skills, stress management, and relapse prevention. Cognitive-behavioral support conducted in a group setting with weekly meetings is frequently successful. Patients should learn how to set *SMART* goals (*s*pecific, *m*easurable, *a*ction-oriented, *r*ealistic, *t*ime-limited). It can be helpful to emphasize real-life examples (e.g., success stories, logbook learning, recommitting to progress). The behavioral modification strategy should assist patients in identifying precipitants for deviations from a diet (e.g., timing, types of food or exercise, situations, feelings), overcoming challenges (planning ahead, delay and distraction, problem solving), managing automatic negative thinking ("detour thoughts"), coping with cravings through mindful strategic eating, preventing relapses using logbook learning, navigating social eating, and setting personal weight maintenance plans.

Pharmacologic Treatment of Obesity

Several anti-obesity drugs are currently approved by the US Food and Drug Administration (FDA) for use in the United States. These drugs include orlistat, phentermine, lorcaserin, a combination of phentermine and long-acting topiramate, liraglutide, and a combination of bupropion and naltrexone. Generally, all these medications are indicated for patients with a BMI of 30 kg/m^2 or more or with BMI of 27 kg/m^2 or more with other weight-related comorbidities (e.g., diabetes, hypertension, dyslipidemia, obstructive sleep apnea) in combination with caloric restriction, increased physical activity, and behavioral modifications.

Orlistat

Orlistat limits caloric intake through inhibition of the lipase-mediated breakdown of fat in the gastrointestinal tract. This mechanism results in an approximately 30% reduction of fat absorption and an increase in fecal fat content. In addition to weight loss, orlistat use has been associated with decreased incidence of diabetes, improved concentrations of total cholesterol and low-density lipoprotein (LDL)-cholesterol, and improved blood pressure and glycemic control in patients with diabetes. However, high-density lipoprotein (HDL)-cholesterol has been found to be slightly lowered. Most people develop side effects with variable degrees of diarrhea, flatulence, oily stools, fecal urgency, and, rarely, fecal incontinence. There also is an increased risk of cholelithiasis. Gastrointestinal side events are usually proportional to the amount of fat intake. Supplemental fat-soluble vitamins A, D, E, and K must be taken to prevent possible deficiencies. The usual dose of orlistat is 120 mg before each meal. A 60 mg dose formulation is currently available over the counter. The lower dose is less effective but is associated with fewer side effects.

Phentermine

Phentermine is approved for short-term treatment of obesity (up to 6 months). Because phentermine has actions similar to amphetamines, it can elevate blood pressure, increase heart rate, and stimulate the central nervous system (frequently causing insomnia), in addition to suppressing the appetite. The recommended phentermine dose is 30 mg once daily. Combining phentermine with tricyclic antidepressants or monoamine oxidase inhibitors may result in substantial increases in blood pressure and other serious reactions because of elevated serotonin levels in the blood.

Lorcaserin

Lorcaserin is a selective serotonin (5-hydroxytryptamine) receptor agonist with specificity for the 5-HT2C receptor subtype. The activation of these receptors in the hypothalamus is thought to activate production of pro-opiomelanocortin (POMC) and, consequently, to promote weight loss through satiety signals. Lorcaserin has 100-fold higher selectivity for 5-HT2C versus the closely related 5-HT2B receptor. Activation of the 5-HT2B receptor by the less selective agents like fenfluramine and dexfenfluramine was linked to serious cardiac valvulopathy, but there is no evidence for this adverse effect with lorcaserin. Clinical trials showed that 47.5% of patients treated with lorcaserin lost at least 5% of their initial body weight, and 22.6% lost at least 10%, in 1 year. Lorcaserin treatment also resulted in significantly lower A_{1C} values in patients with T2DM and improved lipid profile and decreased blood pressure in clinical studies.

Lorcaserin is approved for use as an adjunct to a reduced-calorie diet and exercise for chronic weight management in patients with initial BMI values of 30 kg/m^2 or higher and in those with BMI values of 27 kg/m^2 or higher with at least one weight-related comorbid condition. It is given in a dose of 10 mg twice daily or 20 mg of extended release (XR) form once daily. Side effects usually are mild to moderate, with the most common being headache, upper respiratory tract infection, nasopharyngitis, sinusitis, dizziness, nausea, and fatigue. The US Drug Enforcement Administration has classified lorcaserin as a schedule IV drug because it has hallucinogenic properties that could lead to psychiatric complications.

Phentermine and Long-Acting Topiramate

Phentermine is an appetite suppressant and stimulant of the amphetamine and phenethylamine class (see earlier discussion for details on the use of phentermine alone for weight reduction). Topiramate is an anticonvulsant that was found to have weight loss side effects. The combination of phentermine plus low doses of topiramate has been shown to have synergistic effects on weight loss. As with lorcaserin, this combination tablet is indicated as an adjunct to a reduced-calorie diet and exercise for chronic weight management. Clinical trials showed that average weight loss after 1 year of 10.9% for patients receiving the maximum dose (phentermine/topiramate, 15 mg/92 mg) and 5.1% for those taking the recommended starting dose (3.75 mg/23 mg). The drug is taken once daily in the morning to avoid insomnia caused by the phentermine component. The initial dose of 3.75 mg/23 mg is given for 2 weeks before titration to 7.5 mg/46 mg for another 12 weeks. If a patient has not lost at least 3% of baseline body weight on the higher dosage, the drug may be discontinued or the dose may be escalated to 11.25 mg/69 mg for an additional 2 weeks before a further increase to the maximum dose of 15 mg/92 mg. If a patient has not lost at least 5% of baseline body weight after 12 weeks, the drug is discontinued gradually. Side effects include paresthesias, dry mouth, constipation, metabolic acidosis, nasopharyngitis, upper respiratory infection, and headache.

Data indicate that fetuses exposed during the first trimester to topiramate (when used alone as an anticonvulsant) have an increased risk (9.6%) of cleft lip with or without cleft palate. Therefore, the drug should not be given to women of childbearing age unless an effective method of contraception is used and a pregnancy test is conducted monthly during use. Phentermine/topiramate may increase resting heart rate up to 20 beats/minute, so the drug should be used cautiously in patients with a history of cardiac or cerebrovascular disease. Topiramate also increases the risk of suicidal thoughts or behaviors and mood disorders including depression, anxiety, and insomnia. It can also cause cognitive dysfunction, including impairment of concentration or attention, difficulty with memory, and speech or language problems, particularly word-finding difficulties. It is contraindicated in patients with closed-angle glaucoma because it increases intraocular pressure and the risk of permanent loss of vision.

Bupropion and Naltrexone

This combination is thought to cause a reduction in appetite and an increase in energy expenditure by increasing activity of POMC neurons. Bupropion is a dopamine and norepinephrine reuptake antagonist, which increases dopamine activity in the brain and in turns leads to reduction in appetite and increase in energy expenditure by increasing activity of POMC neurons. Naltrexone blocks opioid receptors on the POMC neurons, preventing feedback inhibition of these neurons and further increasing POMC activity.

The combination tablet of 8 mg of naltrexone and 90 mg of bupropion is initially taken once daily in the morning for 1 week then increased each week by one tablet until reaching the effective dose of two tablets taken twice daily. Average weight loss after 56 weeks of full dose of 32 naltrexone/360 bupropion was 8.4% of the initial body weight (6.4% in intention to treat analysis). The major side events include nausea, constipation, headache, vomiting, dizziness, and insomnia. Bupropion also increases the risk of suicidal thoughts similar to all other antidepressant medications.

Liraglutide

Liraglutide is a GLP-1 analog. GLP-1 is a physiologic regulator of appetite and calorie intake, and the GLP-1 receptor is present in several areas of the brain involved in appetite regulation. GLP-1 analogs, including liraglutide, are used for management of T2DM, but liraglutide dose for obesity indication is much higher, up to 3 mg/day by subcutaneous injection in comparison to a maximum dose of 1.8 mg/day for treatment of T2DM. The dose is escalated gradually every week from 0.6 mg/day to 1.2, 1.8, 2.4, and finally 3 mg/day to reduce nausea. Average weight loss with liraglutide 3 mg daily for 56 weeks is around 5.9%. Side effects include nausea, vomiting, constipation, diarrhea or, rarely, acute pancreatitis. There is an FDA warning about the possibility of developing medullary-cell carcinoma of the thyroid gland, which was seen in experimental animals during preclinical studies, but this is very rare in humans.

Other Drugs for Short-term Treatment of Obesity

Besides phentermine, three other FDA-approved drugs are available in the United States for the short-term (8-12 weeks) treatment of obesity:

diethylpropion, phendimetrazine, benzphetamine. Any of these drugs can be used as an adjunct in a regimen of weight reduction based on caloric restriction in patients with an initial BMI of 30 kg/m^2 or higher who have not responded to an appropriate weight-reduction regimen alone.

Bariatric Surgery

At present, there are three broad categories of bariatric surgical procedures: (1) pure gastric restriction; (2) gastric restriction with some malabsorption, as represented by the Roux-en-Y gastric bypass (RYGB) procedure; and (3) gastric restriction with significant intestinal malabsorption. The number of bariatric procedures performed in the United States increased from an estimated 13,365 in 1998 to almost 228,000 in 2017. Bariatric surgery is considered to be indicated for adults with class 3 obesity (BMI ≤40 kg/m^2). In patients with less severe obesity (BMI 35 to 40 kg/m^2), bariatric surgery can be considered if there are one or more high-risk comorbid conditions present, such as life-threatening cardiopulmonary disease (e.g., severe obstructive sleep apnea, obesity-related cardiomyopathy) or uncontrolled T2DM. Bariatric surgery is sometimes performed for patients with diabetes or metabolic syndrome and a BMI of 30 to 35 kg/m^2, although current evidence on benefit in this weight bracket is limited. For teenagers younger than 17 years old who have attained skeletal maturity (usually by 13 years for girls and 15 years for boys), bariatric surgery has been recommended with different guidelines: BMI 35 to 40 kg/m^2 with at least one serious comorbid condition (e.g., T2DM, obstructive sleep apnea, pseudotumor cerebri) or BMI 50 kg/m^2 or higher with less serious comorbidities. Contraindications for bariatric surgery include high operative risk (e.g., congestive heart failure, unstable angina), active substance abuse, and significant psychopathology.

The three most common bariatric procedures are RYGB, sleeve gastrectomy (SLG), and laparoscopic adjustable gastric banding (LAGB). Currently, the most common bariatric procedure in the United States is sleeve gastrectomy. Other procedures such as biliopancreatic diversion (BPD), biliopancreatic diversion with duodenal switch (BPD/DS), and staged bariatric surgical procedures are less commonly performed. Different types of commonly used bariatric procedures are shown in Fig. 69.1. Gastric restriction procedures induce weight loss by producing early satiety and limiting food intake.

LAGB carries a very low operative mortality rate (0.1%). However, it is associated with significantly lower loss of excess weight at 5 years and 10 years and with higher risk of weight regain compared with RYGB and sleeve gastrectomy. LAGB has been demonstrated to be safe in patients older than 55 years of age. Complications associated with the LAGB procedure include band slippage, band erosion, balloon failure, injection port malposition, band and port infections, and esophageal dilatation. Some of these problems have been decreased by

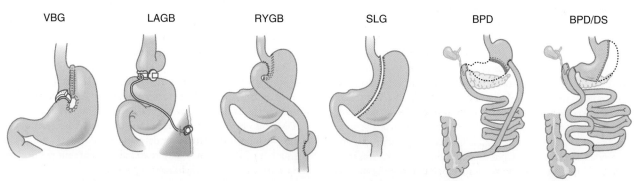

VBG   LAGB   RYGB   SLG   BPD   BPD/DS

Fig. 69.1 Common bariatric procedures. *BPD*, Biliopancreatic diversion; *BPD/DS*, BPD with duodenal switch; *LAGB*, laparoscopic adjustable gastric band; *RYGB*, Roux-en-Y gastric bypass; *SLG*, sleeve gastrectomy; *VBG*, vertical banded gastroplasty.

use of a different method of band insertion and revision of the port connection. Because the absorptive surface of the entire small intestine remains intact, nutritional deficiencies are rare.

In RYGB, the upper stomach is transected, thereby creating a very small proximal gastric pouch measuring 10 to 30 mL. The gastric pouch is anastomosed to a Roux-en-Y proximal jejunal segment, bypassing the remaining stomach, duodenum, and a small portion of jejunum. The standard Roux (alimentary) limb length is about 50 to 100 cm, and the biliopancreatic limb is 15 to 50 cm. As a result, the RYGB serves to limit food intake and induces some nutritional deficiencies such as vitamin B_{12}, vitamin B_1 (thiamine), iron, calcium, copper and vitamin D, which can be corrected by supplementation. It may also lead to protein malnutrition. Dumping syndrome is another complication that occurs as a result of mechanical and hormonal changes that are commonly seen after any gastric restrictive procedure such as RYGB. The primary management of dumping syndrome is dietary modification for prevention of symptoms.

SLG is another popular restrictive surgery in which the stomach is reduced to about 25% of its original size by surgical removal of a large portion of the stomach fundus, resulting in a tube-like structure. Although the procedure permanently reduces stomach size, some dilatation of the stomach may occur later. The procedure is frequently performed by a laparoscopic technique. Sleeve gastrostomy is a similar procedure done by gastroenterologists through gastroscopy without surgical removal of the stomach fundus. Nutritional deficiencies are less common in SLG when compared to RYGB and include vitamin D, vitamin B_{12}, vitamin B_1, folic acid, and iron. Dumping syndrome may also occur but to a lesser extent than with RYGB. This could be caused by an increase in gastric motility consequent to the increase in intraluminal pressure within the remaining stomach.

Currently, most bariatric procedures are performed laparoscopically. This approach has the advantages of fewer wound complications, less postoperative pain, a shorter hospital stay, and more rapid postoperative recovery with comparable efficacy.

The Agency for Healthcare Research and Quality (AHRQ) identified a 0.19% in-hospital mortality rate for all bariatric discharges in the United States. One meta-analysis showed that the mortality rate from bariatric surgery within 30 days was 0.08% and the mortality rate after 30 days was 0.31%. Bariatric surgery is not uniformly a "low-risk" procedure, and judicious patient selection and diligent perioperative care are mandatory. Preoperative patient selection and education as well as careful postsurgical follow-up are important for successful outcomes.

The mortality rate associated with standard bariatric surgical procedures in an experienced center should not exceed 1.5% to 2%. The surgical mortality rate is less than 0.5% at centers specializing in bariatric surgery. Mortality rates exceeding 2% suggest a risk-to-benefit ratio that probably is unacceptable.

The benefits of bariatric surgery extend beyond calorie restriction and weight loss. Foregut bypass leads to improvement in the physiologic responses of gut hormones involved in glucose regulation and appetite control, including ghrelin, GLP-1, and peptide YY[3-36] (PYY). Mechanical improvements include less weight-bearing burden on joints, improved lung compliance, and reduced fatty tissue around the neck, which can relieve obstruction to breathing and sleep apnea.

In an extensive meta-analysis of 22,000 bariatric surgeries, patients lost on average 61% of excess body weight and exhibited improvements in T2DM, hypertension, sleep apnea, and dyslipidemia. The beneficial effect of bariatric surgery on T2DM is one of the most important outcomes observed, with RYGB, SLG, and malabsorptive procedures having the greatest impact. A shorter duration of diabetes and greater weight loss are independent predictors of diabetes partial or complete remission after bariatric surgery. Improvements in fasting blood glucose levels occur before significant weight loss is achieved. Insulin-treated patients experience significant decreases in insulin requirements, and most T2DM patients are able to discontinue insulin therapy by 6 weeks after surgery. Euglycemia is maintained in some patients for up to 5 years after RYGB and SLG. Two recent randomized controlled studies compared RYGB to intensive lifestyle intervention in moderately obese patients with T2DM and found RYGB to be superior in inducing diabetes remission and reducing use of antihyperglycemic medications.

Weight loss after malabsorptive bariatric surgery usually reaches a nadir after 12 to 18 months. Over the following decade, there is weight regain of approximately 10% of body weight. In purely restrictive procedures, failure to experience optimal weight loss has been associated with increased consumption of calorically dense liquids that can pass through the stoma without producing satiety.

Other FDA-approved procedures include *gastric pacing*. Gastric pacing achieved by using implantable electrodes induces weight loss. This outcome was initially discovered with the use of gastric pacemaker devices for gastroparesis in patients with diabetes. Currently, it is an FDA-approved procedure for obesity management.

Gastric aspiration system is an obesity management technique which consists of an endoscopically placed gastrostomy tube and siphon assembly that allows patients to aspirate gastric contents 20 min after meal consumption three times daily. Aspiration takes about 10 min to perform and removes approximately 30% of ingested calories. The side effects include pain, leakage or tube displacement, and stoma site–related problems.

Intra-gastric balloons are used to occupy space in the stomach. Each inflated balloon with air occupies approximately 250 mL volume. Up to three balloons can be placed over a 6-month treatment period, then deflated and removed with an endoscopic procedure.

PROGNOSIS

Although recent clinical data show that patients on average can maintain a 4% to 6.9% weight loss for 10 years with ongoing medically supervised intensive lifestyle intervention, many patients are subjected to less intensive intervention and regain their initial weight loss over months or years. Weight regain even after bariatric surgery is not uncommon and most often occurs after 2 years of peak weight loss. Loss of 10% to 20% of the initial body weight is associated with a decrease in total and resting energy expenditure, a change that retards further weight loss. Similarly, weight gain is associated with an increase in energy expenditure, which retards further weight gain. These observations suggest that the human body adopts a biologic set point or mechanism that tends to maintain body weight, and they lend support to the theory that behavior is not the sole determinant of obesity. Although long-term intensive lifestyle intervention in obese patients with T2DM resulting in approximately 5% body weight loss can significantly decrease the risks of chronic kidney disease and depression and further improve glucose control, blood pressure, physical fitness, and some lipid parameters in patients with T2DM and obesity, it has not been shown to reduce cardiovascular events or mortality. Further understanding of genetic and hormonal regulation of obesity may help researchers create more effective and long-lasting interventional tools.

For further discussion on this topic, please see Chapter 207, "Obesity," in *Goldman-Cecil Medicine*, 26th Edition.

SUGGESTED READINGS

Aldahi W, Hamdy O: Adipokines, inflammation, and the endothelium in diabetes, Curr Diabetes Rep 3:293–298, 2003.

Angrisani L, Lorenzo M, Borrelli V: Laparoscopic adjustable gastric banding versus Roux-en-Y gastric bypass: 5-year results of a prospective randomized trial, Surg Obes Relat Dis 3:127–134, 2007.

Chang SH, Stoll CR, Song J, et al: The effectiveness and risks of bariatric surgery: an updated systematic review and meta-analysis, 2003-2012, JAMA Surg 149:275–287, 2014.

Després J-P, Moorjani S, Lupien PJ, et al: Regional distribution of body fat, plasma lipoproteins, and cardiovascular disease, Arteriosclerosis 10:497–511, 1990.

Hales CM, Carroll MD, Fryar CD: Ogden CL prevalence of obesity among adults and youth: United States, 2015–2016. NCHS data brief, no 288, Hyattsville, MD, 2017, National Center for Health Statistics.

Hamdy O: Obesity chapter. Medscape. https://emedicine.medscape.com/article/123702-overview. Updated: Mar 20, 2018.

Hamdy O: The role of adipose tissue as an endocrine gland, Curr Diabetes Rep 5:317–319, 2005.

Hamdy O, Carver C: The Why WAIT program: improving clinical outcomes through weight management in type 2 diabetes, Curr Diabetes Rep 8:413–420, 2008.

Hamdy O, Mottalib A, Morsi A, et al: Long-term effect of intensive lifestyle intervention on cardiovascular risk factors in patients with diabetes in real-world clinical practice: a 5-year longitudinal study, BMJ Open Diabetes Res Care 5(1):e000259, 2017.

Ikramuddin S, Korner J, Lee WJ, et al: Roux-en-Y gastric bypass vs intensive medical management for the control of type 2 diabetes, hypertension, and hyperlipidemia: the Diabetes Surgery Study randomized clinical trial, J Am Med Assoc 309:2240–2249, 2013.

Look AHEAD Research Group, Wing RR, Bolin P, et al: Cardiovascular effects of intensive lifestyle intervention in type 2 diabetes, N Engl J Med 369:145–154, 2013.

Maggard MA, Shugarman LR, Suttorp M, et al: Meta-analysis: surgical treatment of obesity, Ann Intern Med 142:547–559, 2005.

Mottalib A, Salsberg V, et al: Effects of nutrition therapy on HbA1c and cardiovascular disease risk factors in overweight and obese patients with type 2 diabetes, Nutr J 17(1):42, 2018.

Schauer PR, Bhatt DL, Kirwan JP, et al: Bariatric surgery versus intensive medical therapy for diabetes—5-year outcomes, N Engl J Med 376(7):641–651, 2017.

Schauer PR, Kashyap SR, Wolski K, et al: Bariatric surgery versus intensive medical therapy in obese patients with diabetes, N Engl J Med 366:1567–1576, 2012.

Sjostrom L, Lindroos AK, Peltonen M, et al: Swedish Obese Subjects Study Scientific Group. Lifestyle, diabetes, and cardiovascular risk factors 10 years after bariatric surgery, N Engl J Med 351:2683–2693, 2004.

Strauss RS, Bradley LJ, Brolin RE: Gastric bypass surgery in adolescents with morbid obesity, J Pediatr 138:499–504, 2001.

70

Malnutrition, Nutritional Assessment, and Nutritional Support in Adult Patients

Thomas R. Ziegler

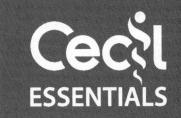

MALNUTRITION IN HOSPITALIZED PATIENTS

Numerous surveys conducted in developed countries in the 21st century continue to demonstrate the frequent rate of protein-energy malnutrition as well as depletion of specific micronutrients in hospitalized patients with chronic illnesses and those requiring elective or emergent hospital admission. Hospitalized patients commonly receive inadequate amounts of calories, protein, vitamins, and minerals during their stay, and ad libitum intake of prescribed diets is typically inadequate. Studies have shown that worsening of malnutrition during hospitalization is common. This is problematic because adequate intake of essential macronutrients (energy, carbohydrate, protein/amino acids, and fats) and micronutrients (vitamins, minerals, and electrolytes) is critical for optimal cellular and organ structure and function, muscle mass, tissue repair, immune function, ambulatory capacity, and patient recovery. Significant erosion of lean body mass (predominately derived from skeletal muscle) and deficiencies of specific vitamins and minerals are variously associated with weakness and fatigue, increased rates of infection, impaired wound healing, and delayed convalescence. This relationship is especially apparent in patients with chronic protein-energy malnutrition and body weight loss associated with illness.

Patients with acute or chronic illnesses typically have experienced several days to several months of continuous or intermittent decreased food intake due to anorexia, gastrointestinal symptoms, depression and anxiety, and other medical factors. They may also have had food intake restricted by surgical operations or diagnostic or therapeutic procedures and recovery from these. Some patients have abnormal nutrient losses due to diarrhea (e.g., with chronic malabsorptive and maldigestive disorders or infectious diarrhea), vomiting, polyuria (as in uncontrolled diabetes mellitus), wound drainage, dialysis, or other causes. Certain drugs, including corticosteroids, chemotherapeutic agents, antirejection drugs, and diuretics, are associated with skeletal muscle breakdown, gastrointestinal injury, or loss of electrolytes or water-soluble vitamins. Bedrest or markedly decreased ambulation are common in outpatient and inpatient settings and are associated with skeletal muscle wasting and impaired protein synthesis.

Catabolic and critical illnesses are associated with concomitantly increased blood concentrations of "counterregulatory" hormones derived from the adrenal glands and pancreas (e.g., cortisol, catecholamines, glucagon); release of pro-inflammatory cytokines from stimulated immune, endothelial, and epithelial cells, such as interleukins (e.g., IL-1, IL-6, IL-8) and tumor necrosis factor-α (TNF-α); and peripheral tissue resistance to anabolic hormones such as insulin and insulin-like growth factor-I (IGF-I). These hormonal and cytokine alterations increase the availability of endogenous metabolic substrates that are critical for cellular and organ function, wound healing, and host survival (e.g., glucose via glycogenolysis and gluconeogenesis, amino acids via skeletal muscle breakdown, and free fatty acids via lipolysis). This combination of decreased nutrient intake and increased tissue nutrient losses (from the actions of these hormones and cytokines), coupled with increased energy (calorie), protein, and micronutrient needs due to inflammation, infection, and cytokinemia, is responsible for the wasting and micronutrient depletion commonly observed in medical patients with acute and chronic illnesses. Common causes of protein-energy malnutrition and micronutrient depletion in medical patients are shown in Table 70.1. Obesity has become a widespread medical problem and is also a form of malnutrition; it is considered in detail in Chapter 69.

NUTRITIONAL ASSESSMENT

Serial assessment of nutritional status is a critically important component of routine medical care. The major objectives are to detect preexisting depletion of body protein, energy reserves, and micronutrients; to identify risk factors for malnutrition (see Table 70.1); and to take steps to prevent nutrient deficiencies, depletion of lean body mass, and loss of skeletal muscle. There are still no practical "gold standard" tests that can provide an index of general nutritional status. Blood concentrations of specific micronutrients (e.g., copper, zinc, thiamine, 25-hydroxyvitamin D, vitamin B_6, folate, vitamin B_{12}) and electrolytes (e.g., magnesium, potassium, phosphorus) are important to guide needs and repletion responses. Nutritional assessment involves an integration of multiple factors, including the patient's medical and surgical history, type and severity of the acute or chronic underlying illness and its anticipated medical and surgical course, fluid drainage sites and amounts, physical examination findings, history of body weight change (degree and temporal aspects), dietary intake pattern, use of nutritional supplements including prior administration of specialized enteral nutrition (EN) or parenteral nutrition (PN), evaluation of current organ function and fluid status, and determination of selected vitamin, mineral, and electrolyte concentrations in blood (E-Table 70.1). In the intensive care unit (ICU) setting, measured body weight typically reflects recent intravenous fluid administration and is typically much higher than recent "dry" or preoperative body weight, which is the best parameter to use.

Integration of the factors outlined in E-Table 70.1 provides important information on whether patients are likely to be adequately nourished; to have mild, moderate, or severe protein-energy malnutrition; or to have depletion or deficiency of specific vitamins, minerals, or electrolytes. Patients who have experienced an involuntary

TABLE 70.1 Common Causes of Protein-Energy Malnutrition and Micronutrient Depletion in Medical Patients With Acute or Chronic Illnesses

Decreased spontaneous food intake due to anorexia from chronic or acute illness, gastrointestinal symptoms (e.g., nausea, vomiting, abdominal pain), or depression and anxiety

Restricted food intake required for surgical operations or diagnostic or therapeutic procedures and gastrointestinal dysfunction after these procedures

Abnormal macronutrient and micronutrient losses from the body due to malabsorption (e.g., celiac sprue, short gut syndrome, inflammatory bowel disease, cystic fibrosis, diarrhea), maldigestion (e.g., pancreatitis), emesis, polyuria (e.g., in diabetes), wound drainage, or renal replacement therapy

Periods of increased energy expenditure (caloric needs), protein requirements, and micronutrient needs (e.g., critical illness, increased inflammation)

Catabolic effects of counterregulatory hormones (e.g., cortisol, catecholamines, glucagon), release of pro-inflammatory cytokines from stimulated immune cells and endothelial and epithelial cells such as interleukins (e.g., IL-1, IL-6, IL-8) and tumor necrosis factor-α (TNF-α), and peripheral tissue resistance to the anabolic hormones insulin and insulin-like growth factor-I (IGF-I)

Bedrest, decreased ambulation, and chemical paralysis during mechanical ventilation (skeletal muscle wasting due to impaired protein synthesis)

Administration of drugs that induce skeletal muscle breakdown, gastrointestinal injury, or loss of electrolytes and water-soluble vitamins (e.g., corticosteroids, chemotherapeutic agents, diuretics, antirejection regimens)

Socioeconomic deprivation, inadequate caregivers, ambulation difficulties in the home setting

Inadequate provision of calories, protein, and essential micronutrients (vitamins, minerals, trace elements) during hospitalization

---

body weight loss of 5% to 10% or more of their usual body weight in the previous few weeks or months, those who weigh less than 90% of their ideal body weight (IBW), and those who have a body mass index (BMI) lower than 18.5 kg/m² should be carefully evaluated, because these individuals are likely to be malnourished.

Among hospitalized patients, especially those in the ICU, circulating concentrations of proteins (e.g., albumin, prealbumin) are often quite low and not useful as protein nutritional status biomarkers given their lack of specificity. Plasma concentrations of albumin and prealbumin typically fall during active inflammation or infection, in critical illness, and after traumatic injury (due to deceased synthesis by the liver and catabolism of blood proteins). They are markedly affected by non-nutritional factors, including fluid status, capillary leak, decreased hepatic synthesis, and increased clearance from blood. Because of the long circulating half-life of albumin (18 to 21 days), concentrations in blood remain low despite adequate feeding and are slow to respond to nutritional repletion, irrespective of other confounding factors. Prealbumin has a much shorter circulating half-life (several days), and serial blood levels can be used as a general indicator of protein status in clinically stable outpatients. E-Table 70.2 illustrates physical examination findings that may be observed in associated with depletion of specific nutrients.

Energy requirements can be estimated with the use of standard equations, such as the Harris-Benedict equation, which incorporate the patient's age, gender, weight, and height to determine basal energy expenditure (BEE) (see E-Table 70.1). Recently published European and American Clinical Practice Guidelines suggest that an adequate

energy goal for most patients can be estimated at 20 to 25 kcal/kg/day (using the most recent prehospital clinic dry body weight), which is approximately equivalent to measured or estimated BEE multiplied by 1.0 to 1.3. Ongoing RCTs are designed to better define caloric dosing guidelines in hospitalized general and ICU patients.

Typically, lower amounts of calories are now given to ICU patients (as discussed later). Use of data obtained from a bedside metabolic cart machine (indirect calorimeter), which measures expired breath to determine oxygen consumption and carbon dioxide production, provides accurate actual energy expenditure in most settings and can be very useful (see E-Table 70.1).

In ICU patients, even lower caloric doses (equivalent to 15-20 kcal/kg dry weight/day) have been advocated by some, based on known complications of overfeeding (see later discussion) and limited data on clinical outcome as a function of energy dose. In clinically stable, malnourished, non-ICU patients who require nutritional repletion, higher doses of calories (up to 35 kcal/kg/day) appear to be generally well tolerated if refeeding syndrome is avoided (see later discussion). In obese subjects (defined for these calculations as patients with body weight 20% to 25% greater than ideal), an adjusted body weight value should be used for calculation of energy and protein needs, as determined by the following equation:

$$\text{Adjusted body weight} = (\text{current weight} - \text{IBW}) \times 0.25 + \text{IBW}$$

Guidelines for protein or amino acid administration are given in E-Table 70.3. Studies in nonburned ICU patients indicate that protein loads of more than 2.0 g/kg/day may not be efficiently utilized for protein synthesis, and the excess may be oxidized, contributing to azotemia. In most catabolic patients requiring specialized feeding, a recommended protein dose is 1.5 g/kg/day for individuals with normal renal function. This is about twice the recommended dietary allowance (RDA) for healthy adults of 0.8 g/kg/day. The administered protein dose should be adjusted downward as a function of the degree and tempo of azotemia (in the absence of dialysis therapy) and of hyperbilirubinemia (see E-Table 70.3). These strategies take into account the relative inability of catabolic patients to efficiently use exogenous nutrients and knowledge that most protein and lean tissue repletion occurs over a period of several weeks to months during posthospital convalescence. Adequate nonprotein energy is essential to allow amino acids to be effectively used for protein synthesis and not oxidized for production of energy (adenosine triphosphate, or ATP). The commonly recommended protein/amino acid dose range is 1.2 to 1.5 g/kg/day for most adults with normal renal and hepatic function (50% to 100% above the RDA of 0.8 g/kg/day); although some guidelines recommend higher doses (up to 2.0 to 2.5 g/kg/day) in specific conditions such as in patients requiring renal replacement therapy or burns.

NUTRITIONAL SUPPORT

Table 70.2 lists common clinical scenarios in which specialized oral/EN or PN support may be indicated. In these settings, consultation with a multidisciplinary nutrition support team, if available, has been shown to reduce complications and costs and to increase the appropriate use of EN and PN in both academic and community medical centers.

Oral Nutrition Support

Oral nutrition supplementation includes provision of balanced oral diets of usual foods supplemented with complete liquid (or solid) nutrient products, protein supplements (e.g., hydrolyzed whey or casein powder that can be mixed with dietary beverages), high-potency multivitamin-multimineral supplements, and/or specific micronutrients required to treat a diagnosed deficiency (e.g., zinc, copper, vitamin B₆, vitamin

TABLE 70.2   Some Clinical Indications for Specialized Oral/Enteral or Parenteral Nutrition Support

Patient currently exhibits moderate to severe protein or protein-energy malnutrition or has evidence of specific deficiency of one or more essential micronutrients

Patient with involuntary body weight loss of 5-10% or more of their usual body weight in the previous few weeks or months, weighs less than 90% of ideal body weight, or has a BMI lower than 18.5 kg/m²

Dietary food intake in a hospital or outpatient setting likely to be <50% of needs for more than 5-10 days due to underlying illness

Patient with severe catabolic stress (e.g., ICU care, serious infection) and adequate nutrient intake unlikely for >3-5 days

After major gastrointestinal surgery or other major operation (e.g., hip replacement, partial organ resection)

Medical illness associated with prolonged (>5-10 days) GI dysfunction (diarrhea, nausea and vomiting, GI bleeding, severe ileus, partial obstruction) and/or short bowel syndrome, chronic or severe diarrhea, or other malabsorptive disorders

Clinical settings in which adequate oral food intake may be contraindicated or otherwise significantly decreased, such as respiratory or other acute or severe organ failure, dementia, dysphagia, chemotherapy or irradiation, inflammatory bowel disease, pancreatitis, high-output enterocutaneous fistula, alcoholism, drug addiction

Chronic obstructive lung disease, chronic infection, or other chronic inflammatory or catabolic disorders with documented poor nutrient intake and/or recent weight loss

BMI, Body mass index; *GI,* gastrointestinal; *ICU,* intensive care unit; *PN,* parenteral nutrition.

B₁₂, vitamin D). Special supplements designed for patients with chronic renal failure (featuring concentrated calories and low amounts of protein and electrolytes) are available, as are a variety of formulations designed for other specific disease categories (see later discussion). Several studies have shown that convalescence after stresses such as total hip replacement or gastrointestinal surgery is enhanced with the addition of one or two containers per day of complete liquid nutrient supplements. These provide calories, carbohydrate, high-quality protein, fat, and micronutrients; are lactose and gluten free; and may contain small peptides and medium-chain triglycerides to facilitate absorption of amino acid and fat, respectively. Some formulations also contain soluble fiber or prebiotics (e.g., fructo-oligosaccharides) designed to decrease diarrhea. It is probably prudent to place outpatients who exhibit or are at risk for undernutrition (see E-Tables 70.1 and 70.2) and can tolerate oral medications on a potent oral multivitamin-multimineral preparation, at least for several months.

Administration of Enteral Tube Feeding

Patients with conditions outlined in Table 70.2 may have a functional gastrointestinal tract and yet be unable to consume adequate diet orally due to medical or surgical conditions (e.g., mechanical ventilation, pancreatitis, dementia, dysphagia, trauma, or burns). Although PN is commonly administered in these settings, this practice is not evidence based; academic guidelines strongly suggest that oral nutritional supplements or enteral tube feedings should be used if specialized nutrition support is indicated in patients with a functional gastrointestinal tract ("if the gut works, use it"). EN is more physiologic, associated with less severe infectious, mechanical, and metabolic complications, and is less costly than PN. Although not evidence based, common contraindications to EN include paralytic ileus, bowel ischemia, and hemodynamic

instability requiring mid- to high-dose vasopressors, inability to gain access to the gastrointestinal (GI) tract, intestinal obstruction, intractable vomiting, severe diarrhea, and peritonitis.

E-Table 70.4 shows major characteristics of common complete liquid tube feeding formulations and the types of patients for which these are typically prescribed. These products can be used for oral nutrient supplementation as tolerated. When delivered in appropriate amounts, the liquid diets provide complete nutrition for most patients, although some ICU patients and patients with malabsorption or other conditions may have special needs (see later discussion).

The feedings can be delivered by conventional nasogastric tubes into the stomach or by small-bore nasogastric or nasojejunal tubes, percutaneous gastrostomy or jejunostomy tubes, or percutaneous gastrojejunostomy tubes (in which the gastric port may be used for suction and the jejunal port for feeding). Gastric feedings can be administered by either continuous or bolus feeds, whereas small bowel feeds must employ a continuous slow infusion using an infusion pump to avoid diarrhea. Tube feedings should be initiated at a slow rate (e.g., 10 to 20 mL/hr) for 8 to 24 hours and slowly advanced to the goal rate in 8- to 24-hour increments to deliver the calculated caloric and protein needs over the next 24 to 48 hours, depending on clinical tolerance and clinical conditions. Recent guidelines emphasize placing tube-fed patients in the semirecumbent position (e.g., increase head of bed), advancing feedings cautiously (with serial evaluations for diarrhea, nausea, emesis, abdominal distention, and significant gastric residuals), and using prokinetic agents and/or postpyloric feedings if gastric feedings are not well tolerated. Recent data suggest that higher volumes of gastric residuals (e.g., >250 mL) are usually well tolerated in patients being tube fed.

Primarily based on results of animal studies, EN is associated with improved gut barrier function, decreased infectious complications, less hypermetabolism, and decreased morbidity and mortality in catabolic models, compared with PN. Salutary clinical outcomes have been shown in randomized clinical trials in patients with pancreatitis receiving EN into the jejunum, compared with PN. The current Society for Critical Care Medicine (SCCM) and American Society for Parenteral and Enteral Nutrition (ASPEN) guidelines recommend starting early EN (within 24-48 hours) in ICU patients who cannot achieve adequate caloric needs (e.g., >60%) with oral diet and supplements alone, especially for patients with existing malnutrition. Many studies have shown that ICU patients actually receive only 60% to 75% of the amount of tube feeding ordered by physicians. This can occur because of tube feeding intolerance (e.g., high gastric residuals, emesis, diarrhea, tube dislodgement) or discontinuation of feeding for diagnostic tests or therapeutic interventions. Although supplemental PN (see later discussion) is commonly ordered in patients who are not able to achieve tube-feeding rates adequate for their needs, this practice remains controversial because of the limited number of good clinical trials. Rigorous studies are now in progress to address the efficacy of this approach, motivated by data suggesting that an increase in net caloric deficit (i.e., the difference between daily calorie requirements and daily actual calories delivered, summed over time) is associated with worse clinical outcomes in medical and surgical ICU patients.

Most outpatients and hospitalized ICU and non-ICU patients tolerate standard, inexpensive enteral formulas delivered via gastric or intestinal routes that provide between 1.0 and 1.5 kcal/mL. A large variety of enteral tube-feeding products are available for clinical use. The specific product chosen should be based both on clinical conditions and underlying organ function, as outlined in E-Table 70.4. Because EN products can be marketed without efficacy data from randomized, controlled clinical trials, there remains a clear need for such trials to determine optimal EN formulations for different clinical conditions.

Complications of enteral feeding include diarrhea. Diarrhea is common in hospital patients receiving tube feedings but is typically caused by factors independent of the feeding, including administration of antibiotics, sorbitol-containing or hypertonic medications (e.g., acetaminophen elixir), and infections. Diarrhea caused by tube feeding itself does occur with rapid formula administration, in patients with underlying gut mucosal disease, and in those with severe hypoalbuminemia, which causes bowel wall edema. A fiber-containing enteral formula is sometimes useful to decrease diarrhea. Other complications of tube feeding include aspiration of tube feedings into the lung; mechanical problems with nasally placed feeding tubes, including discomfort, sinusitis, pharyngeal or esophageal mucosal erosion due to local tube trauma; and, with percutaneous feeding tubes, entrance site leakage, skin breakdown, cellulitis, and pain. Metabolic complications of tube feeding include fluid imbalances, hyperglycemia, electrolyte abnormalities, azotemia, and, occasionally, refeeding syndrome (discussed later). In general, if tube feedings are deemed to be required for more than 4 to 6 weeks, a percutaneous feeding tube should be placed.

In tube-fed patients who are receiving either subcutaneous or intravenous insulin to control hyperglycemia, significant hypoglycemia due to the continued actions of insulin may occur if tube feedings are discontinued inadvertently or for diagnostic or therapeutic tests. Hospitalized patients receiving tube feedings should have their blood glucose concentration monitored on a daily basis (or several times per day as indicated) and their blood electrolytes (including magnesium, potassium, and phosphorus) and renal function monitored several times each week (or daily in the ICU setting). Other blood chemistries should be determined at least weekly. This should be accompanied by close monitoring of intake and output records (including urine, stool, and drainage outputs) and gastrointestinal tolerance. When patients are able to consume oral food, tube feeding should be decreased and then discontinued (e.g., with daily calorie counts by a registered dietitian). For patients requiring home tube feeding, it is important to consult social service professionals to ensure appropriate care and follow-up.

EN administration must be individualized to each patient's specific needs. In order to determine the appropriate EN delivery method, GI tract integrity and functional capacity, presence and degree of malnutrition, underlying disease states, and patient tolerance must be assessed prior to and following the initiation of tube feeding. Gastrointestinal, mechanical, and metabolic complications, as well as pulmonary aspiration of feeds, can occur with enteral tube feeding. It is therefore essential to monitor enterally fed patients closely in order to identify complications.

A recent randomized study of 894 clinically similar, critically ill adults with medical or surgical issues at seven academic centers assigned patients to permissive enteral underfeeding (40-60% of calculated energy needs) versus standard EN (70-100% of calculated energy needs), with similar daily protein intake (approximately 60 g/day). During intervention, the permissive underfed group received 835 plus or minus 297 kcal/day versus 1299 plus or minus 467 kcal/day in the standard group; no difference in mortality or other clinical outcomes occurred.

Administration of Parenteral Nutrition

The basic principle in considering PN therapy is that the patient must be unable to achieve adequate nutrient intake via the enteral route. PN support includes administration of standard complete nutrient mixtures that contain dextrose, L-amino acids, lipid emulsion, electrolytes, vitamins, and minerals (in addition to certain medications as indicated, such as insulin or octreotide), given via a peripheral or central vein. Administration of complete PN therapy to patients with gastrointestinal tract dysfunction has become a standard of care in most hospitals and ICUs throughout the world, although use in individual institutions varies widely. PN is life-saving in patients with intestinal

failure (e.g., short bowel syndrome). Existing data indicate that PN benefits patients with preexisting moderate to severe malnutrition or critical illness by decreasing overall morbidity, and possibly mortality, compared with patients receiving inadequate EN or hydration (intravenous dextrose) therapy alone. A consensus is emerging, based on recent rigorous studies in critical illness, that PN should probably not be initiated until days 3 to 4 after ICU admission in patients who are unable to tolerate adequate EN.

Compared with PN, EN is less expensive, probably maintains intestinal mucosal structure and function to a greater extent, is safer in terms of mechanical and metabolic complications (see later discussion), and is associated with reduced rates of nosocomial infection. Therefore, the enteral route of feeding should be used and advanced whenever possible, and the amount of administered PN should be correspondingly reduced.

Generally recognized indications for PN include the following situations:
1. Patients with short bowel syndrome or other conditions causing intestinal failure (e.g., motility disorders, obstruction, severe ileus, severe inflammatory bowel disease), especially those with preexisting malnutrition.
2. Clinically stable patients in whom adequate enteral feeding (e.g., >50% of needs) is unlikely for 7 to 10 days because of an underlying illness.
3. Patients with severe catabolic stress requiring ICU care in whom adequate enteral nutrient intake is unlikely for more than 3 to 5 days.

There is no reason to withhold PN in hospitalized patients for any period of time if they exhibit preexisting moderate to severe malnutrition and are deemed to be unlikely to meet their needs by the oral or enteral route.

Generally accepted contraindications for PN include the following conditions:
1. If the GI tract is functional and access for enteral feeding is available.
2. If PN is thought to be required for 5 days or less.
3. If the patient cannot tolerate the extra intravenous fluid required for PN or has severe hyperglycemia or electrolyte abnormalities on the planned day of PN initiation.
4. If the patient has an uncontrolled bloodstream infection or severe hemodynamic instability.
5. If new placement of an intravenous line solely for PN poses undue risks based on clinical judgment.
6. On an individualized basis, if aggressive nutritional support is not desired by the competent patient or legally authorized representative, such as in premorbid patients or those with terminal illness.

PN can be delivered either as peripheral vein solutions or as central vein solutions through a percutaneous subclavian vein or internal jugular vein catheter for infusion into the superior vena cava (nontunneled in the hospital setting), through a subcutaneously tunneled central venous catheter (e.g., Hickman catheter) or central venous port (for chronic home PN therapy), or through a peripherally inserted central venous catheter (PICC). Although data are limited, it is clearly preferable to manage long-term central venous PN to be managed at home with the use of a tunneled central venous catheter rather than a PICC line because of the higher rate of local complications (e.g., phlebitis, catheter breakage) and possibly catheter-associated infections with PICC lines.

A comparison of typical fluid, macronutrient, and micronutrient content of peripheral and central vein PN solutions is shown in Table 70.3. Complete PN provides intravenous lipid emulsions (IVF) as a source of both energy and essential linoleic and linolenic fatty acids.

In the United States, historically the only commercially available lipid emulsion was soybean oil (SO)-based; now, an intravenous soybean oil/olive oil emulsion, an intravenous soybean oil/medium-chain triglyceride mixture, a fish oil/medium-chain triglyceride/olive oil/soybean oil emulsion, and a fish oil–based emulsion have been approved for use in PN. The different formulations vary in the fatty acid content and dosing. The use of SO-based emulsions has been associated with elevated serum bilirubin levels, intestinal failure–associated liver disease, and cholestasis in some patients, particularly at chronic doses exceeding 1.0 g/kg/day. Recent reviews of fish oil–containing IVF lowered inflammatory markers, improved triglyceride levels and liver enzymes, and reduced infectious complications in ICU patients. When compared with SO-based IVF, olive oil–based IVF are a safe alternative but clinical and metabolic differences between these two IVF were not statistically significant.

The maximal recommended rate of fat emulsion infusion is approximately 1.0 g/kg/day but larger doses may be given for shorter term use in hospital settings and are well tolerated. Most patients are well able to clear triglyceride from plasma after intravenous administration of fat emulsion. It is important to monitor blood triglyceride levels at baseline and then approximately weekly and as indicated to assess clearance of intravenous fat; triglyceride levels should be maintained lower than 400 mg/dL to decrease the risk of pancreatitis or diminished pulmonary diffusion capacity in patients with severe chronic obstructive lung disease.

Central venous administration of PN allows higher concentrations of dextrose (3.4 kcal/g) and amino acids (4 kcal/g) to be delivered as hypertonic solutions; thus, lower amounts of fat emulsion are needed to reach caloric goals (see Table 70.3). Requirements for potassium, magnesium, and phosphorus are typically higher with central vein PN compared to peripheral vein PN. The higher concentrations of dextrose and amino acids allow most patients to achieve caloric and amino acid goals with only 1 to 1.5 L of PN per day. In central vein PN, initial orders typically provide 60% to 70% of non–amino acid calories as dextrose and 30% to 40% of non–amino acid calories as fat emulsion. These percentages are adjusted as indicated based on levels of blood glucose and triglyceride, respectively. Based on comprehensive data associating hyperglycemia with hospital morbidity and mortality, expert panels now recommend tight blood glucose control in ICU settings (between 80 and 130 to 150 mg/dL) and close blood glucose monitoring. Separate intravenous insulin infusions should usually be administered in the ICU when patients receiving central vein PN develop hyperglycemia.

Specific requirements for intravenous trace elements and vitamins have not been rigorously defined for patient subgroups, and in most stable patients, therapy is directed at meeting published recommended doses using standardized intravenous preparations to maintain blood levels in the normal range (see Table 70.3). Several studies have shown that a significant proportion of ICU patients have low levels of zinc, selenium, vitamin C, vitamin E, and vitamin D despite receiving specialized PN (or EN). Depletion of these essential nutrients may impair antioxidant capacity, immunity, wound healing, and other important body functions, and supplementation is recommended if serum concentrations are low. For example, zinc (and other micronutrients such as copper) should probably be increased in the PN of patients with burns, large wounds, significant gastrointestinal fluid losses, and other conditions if serum concentrations indicate low levels. Recent data suggest that thiamine depletion is not uncommon in patients receiving chronic diuretic therapy, renal replacement therapy, or in those with severe malabsorption.

The most common complication of peripheral vein PN is local phlebitis resulting from use of the catheter. In such cases, a small dose of hydrocortisone and heparin is typically added to the solution.

TABLE 70.3 Composition of Typical Parenteral Nutrition Solutions

Component[a]	Peripheral PN	Central PN
Volume (L/day)	2-3	1-1.5
Dextrose (%)	5	10-25
Amino acids (%)[b]	2.5-3.5	3-8
Lipid (%)[c]	3.5-5.0	2.5-5.0
Sodium (mEq/L)	50-150	50-150
Potassium (mEq/L)	20-35	30-50
Phosphorus (mmol/L)	5-10	10-30
Magnesium (mEq/L)	8-10	10-20
Calcium (mEq/L)	2.5-5	2.5-5
Trace elements[d]		
Vitamins[e]		

[a]Electrolytes in parenteral nutrition (PN) are adjusted as indicated to maintain serially measured serum levels within the normal range. The percentage of sodium and potassium salts as chloride is increased to correct metabolic alkalosis, and the percentage of salts as acetate is increased to correct metabolic acidosis. Regular insulin is added to PN as needed to achieve blood glucose goals (separate intravenous insulin infusions are commonly required with hyperglycemia in intensive care unit settings).
[b]Provides all essential amino acids and several nonessential amino acids. The dose of amino acids is adjusted downward or upward to goal as a function of the degree of azotemia or hyperbilirubinemia in patients with renal or hepatic failure, respectively.
[c]Lipid is given as soybean oil– or olive oil/soybean oil–based fat emulsion in the United States. Intravenous fish oil, olive oil, medium-chain triglycerides, and combinations of these are also now available for use in PN. Lipid is typically mixed with dextrose and amino acids in the same PN infusion bag ("all-in-one" solution).
[d]Trace elements added on a daily basis to peripheral vein and central vein PN are mixtures of chromium, copper, manganese, selenium, and zinc. (These elements can also be supplemented individually.)
[e]Vitamins added on a daily basis to peripheral vein and central vein PN are mixtures of vitamins A, B$_1$ (thiamine), B$_2$ (riboflavin), B$_3$ (niacinamide), B$_6$ (pyridoxine), B$_{12}$, C, D, and E, biotin, folate, and pantothenic acid. Vitamin K is added on an individual basis (e.g., for patients with cirrhosis). Specific vitamins can also be supplemented individually.

Alterations in blood electrolytes can be treated with adjustment of concentrations in the peripheral PN prescription. Hypertriglyceridemia typically responds well to lowering of the total PN lipid dose. Central vein PN is associated with a much higher rate of mechanical, metabolic, and infectious complications than peripheral vein PN. Mechanical complications include those related to insertion of the central venous catheter (e.g., pneumothorax, hemothorax, malposition of the catheter, thrombosis). Infectious complications include catheter-related bloodstream infections and non–catheter-related infections. The risk for these infections appears to be increased with use of non–subclavian vein central venous access (e.g., jugular vein, femoral vein) and multiple-use catheters with non-dedicated PN infusion ports used for additional purposes such as blood drawing or medication administration. Poorly controlled blood glucose levels (>140 to 180 mg/dL) are not uncommon in patients requiring central vein PN and are associated with an increased risk of nosocomial infection. Risk factors for hyperglycemia include poorly controlled blood glucose at PN initiation; use of high dextrose concentrations (>10%) in the initial few days of PN administration or too rapid an increase in total dextrose load; insufficient exogenous insulin administration; inadequate monitoring of blood glucose responses to central vein PN administration; and administration of corticosteroids and vasopressor agents such as norepinephrine (which stimulate gluconeogenesis and cause insulin resistance).

Studies on nutrient utilization efficiency and metabolic complications in severely catabolic patients suggest that lower amounts of total energy and protein/amino acids should be administered than were routinely given in the past, particularly in unstable and ICU patients. High calorie, carbohydrate, amino acid, and fat loads ("hyperalimentation") are easily administered via central vein PN but can induce severe metabolic complications, including carbon dioxide overproduction, azotemia, hyperglycemia, electrolyte alterations, and hepatic steatosis and injury (E-Table 70.5). Dextrose and lipid doses in PN should be advanced over several days after initiation, with close monitoring of the blood glucose concentration, electrolytes, triglycerides, organ function tests, intake and output measurements, and the clinical course.

Refeeding syndrome with central vein PN administration is relatively common in patients at risk, including those with preexisting malnutrition, electrolyte depletion, alcoholism, or prolonged periods of intravenous hydration therapy (e.g., 5% dextrose) without nutritional support, all of which are common in hospital patients. Refeeding syndrome is mediated by administration of excessive intravenous dextrose (>150 to 250 g, for example in 1 L of PN containing 15% to 25% dextrose). This, in turn, markedly stimulates insulin release, which rapidly lowers blood concentrations of potassium, magnesium, and especially phosphorus as a result of intracellular shifts and utilization in carbohydrate metabolic pathways. Administration of high doses of carbohydrate also consumes thiamine, which is required as a cofactor for carbohydrate metabolism and can precipitate symptoms of thiamine deficiency (see E-Table 70.2), especially in patients with poor thiamine nutriture at baseline. Hyperinsulinemia also tends to cause sodium and fluid retention at the level of the kidney. Together, fluid and sodium retention, the drop in electrolytes (which can cause arrhythmias), and hypermetabolism due to excessive calorie provision can result in heart failure, especially in patients with preexisting heart disease and cardiac muscle atrophy due to prolonged protein-energy malnutrition. Prevention of refeeding syndrome requires vigilance to identify patients at risk; use of initially low PN dextrose concentrations; empiric provision of higher doses of potassium, magnesium, and phosphorus based on current blood levels and renal function; and supplemental thiamine (100 mg/day for 3 to 5 days).

If home PN is indicated, the primary physician should consult with social service professionals to identify appropriate home care companies and nutrition support professionals to assess intravenous line access, metabolic status, and the home PN order and to arrange for follow-up care and monitoring of PN. It is important not to arrange for rapid discharge of hospitalized patients newly started on PN. Obtaining appropriate venous access and monitoring of fluid and electrolyte status over a 2- to 3-day period is an important aspect of care for most patients started on PN, and it is imperative for those with severe malnutrition and those at risk for refeeding syndrome.

For a deeper discussion on this topic, please see Chapters 203, "Protein-Energy Malnutrition," and 204, "Malnutrition: Assessment and Support," in *Goldman-Cecil Medicine*, 26th Edition.

SUGGESTED READINGS

Arabi VM, Aldawood AS, Haddad SH, et al: Permissive underfeeding or standard enteral feeding in critically ill adults, New Engl J Med 372:2398–2408, 2015.

Blaauw R, Osland E, Sriram K, et al: Parenteral provision of micronutrients to adult patients: an expert consensus paper, JPEN J Parenter Enteral Nutr 43(Suppl 1):S5–S23, 2019.

Boullata J, Carrera A, Harvey L, et al: ASPEN safe practices for enteral nutrition therapy, JPEN J Parenter Enteral Nutr 41:36–46, 2017.

Casaer MP, Mesotten D, Hermans G, et al: Early versus late parenteral nutrition in critically ill adults, N Engl J Med 365:506–517, 2011.

Doig GS, Simpson F, Sweetman EA, et al: Early PN Investigators of the ANZICS clinical trials group: early parenteral nutrition in critically ill patients with short-term relative contraindications to early enteral nutrition: a randomized controlled trial, J Am Med Assoc 309:2130–2138, 2013.

Harvey SE, Parrott F, Harrison DA, et al: Trial of the route of early nutritional support in critically ill adults, N Eng J Med 371:1673–1684, 2014.

Honeywell S, Zelig R, Radler DR: Impact of intravenous lipid emulsions containing fish oil on clinical outcomes in critically ill surgical patients: a literature review, JPEN J Parenter Enteral Nutr 26:112–122, 2019.

Manzanares W, Langlois PL, Hardy G: Intravenous lipid emulsions in the crucially ill: an update, Curr Opin Crit Care 22:308–315, 2016.

McClave SA, Taylor BE, Martindale RG, et al: Guidelines for the provision and assessment of nutrition support therapy in the adult critically ill patient: society of critical care medicine (SCCM) and American Society for Parenteral and Enteral Nutrition (A.S.P.E.N.), JPEN J Parenter Enteral Nutr 40(2):159–211, 2016.

Singer P, Blaser AR, Berger MM, et al: ESPEN guidelines on clinical nutrition in the intensive care unit, Clin Nutr 38:48–79, 2019.

Ziegler TR: Nutrition support in critical illness: bridging the evidence gap, N Engl J Med 365:562–564, 2011.

Ziegler TR: Parenteral nutrition in the critically ill patient, N Engl J Med 361:1088–1097, 2009.

71

Disorders of Lipid Metabolism

Russell Bratman, Geetha Gopalakrishnan

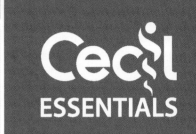

DEFINITION AND EPIDEMIOLOGY

Lipids such as free fatty acids (FFA), cholesterol, and triglycerides are hydrophobic molecules that bind proteins for transport. Nonesterified FFA travel as anions complexed to albumin. Esterified complex lipids are transported in lipoprotein particles. Lipoproteins have a hydrophobic core (cholesteryl esters and triglycerides) and an amphiphilic surface monolayer (phospholipids, unesterified cholesterol, and apolipoproteins). Ultracentrifugation separates lipoproteins into five classes based on their density (Table 71.1).

Proteins on the surface of lipoproteins (i.e., apolipoproteins) activate enzymes and receptors that guide lipid metabolism. Defects in the synthesis and catabolism of lipoproteins result in dyslipidemia. Prevalence of dyslipidemia in the United States is approximately 20% and varies with the population studied. An estimated 70% of individuals with premature coronary heart disease (CHD) have dyslipidemia. In clinical trials, treatment of dyslipidemia improved both CHD and all-cause mortality rates. Two classes of lipids, triglyceride and cholesterol, play a significant, yet modifiable, role in the pathogenesis of atherosclerosis and therefore are the focus of this chapter.

PATHOLOGY

In the intestinal lumen, dietary triglycerides and cholesterol esters are hydrolyzed by pancreatic lipase to produce glycerol, FFA, and free cholesterol. Bile acids aid in the formation of amphiphilic droplets known as micelles. Micelles enable the absorption of glycerol and FFA into the intestinal cell. The transport of free cholesterol is mediated by a cholesterol gradient that exists between the lumen and the intestinal cell. Within the cell, glycerol combines with three fatty acid chains to form triglycerides, and cholesterol is esterified to form cholesterol esters. Chylomicrons are formed from triglycerides (85% of chylomicron mass) and cholesterol esters assembled with surface lipoproteins. Chylomicrons enter the circulation and acquire more surface apolipoproteins such as apo C-II and apo E from high-density lipoprotein (HDL) particles (Fig. 71.1). Apo C-II activates lipoprotein lipase (LPL), which is located on the capillary endothelium. LPL hydrolyzes the core chylomicron triglycerides to release FFA. FFA functions as an energy source. Excess FFA are stored in adipose tissue or utilized in hepatic lipoprotein synthesis. The triglyceride-poor chylomicron remnant is then cleared from the circulation by hepatic LDL receptors. These receptors are activated by apo E located on the surface of chylomicrons.

Very-low-density lipoproteins (VLDL) are synthesized by the liver (see Fig. 71.1) using FFA and cholesterol obtained from the circulation or synthesized by the liver. Any condition that increases the flux of FFA to the liver, such as poorly controlled diabetes, will increase VLDL production. The liver assembles triglycerides (55% of VLDL mass), cholesterol (20%), and surface apolipoproteins to form VLDL particles. Apo C-II, the cofactor for LPL, hydrolyzes the triglyceride core of VLDL particles to generate VLDL remnant or intermediate-density lipoprotein (IDL). The IDL, depleted of triglycerides (25%), can be cleared from the circulation by apo E–mediated LDL receptors, or it can be hydrolyzed further to form low-density lipoprotein (LDL). LDL particles are triglyceride poor (5% of LDL mass) and consist mostly of cholesterol esters (60%) and apolipoproteins. Apo B100 on the surface of LDL binds LDL receptors and facilitates LDL clearance from the circulation. Internalized LDL-cholesterol is used to synthesize hormones, produce cell membranes, and store energy.

In the liver, LDL-cholesterol is used to synthesize bile acids (see Fig. 71.1), which are secreted into the intestinal lumen along with free cholesterol. Bile acids help transport fat. Approximately 50% of the cholesterol and 97% of the bile acid entering the lumen are reabsorbed back into the circulation. The reabsorbed cholesterol regulates cholesterol and LDL receptor synthesis.

Many cells in the body, including liver parenchymal cells, synthesize cholesterol (Fig. 71.2). Acetate is converted to 3-hydroxy-3-methylglutaryl–coenzyme A (HMG-CoA). HMG-CoA reductase converts HMG-CoA to mevalonic acid, which is then converted to cholesterol through a series of steps. HMG-CoA reductase catalyzes the rate-limiting step in the cholesterol synthesis pathway. Drugs that inhibit this enzyme decrease cholesterol biosynthesis and cellular cholesterol pools. The class of drugs that inhibit HMG-CoA inhibitors are often called "statins." Internalization of LDL particles into cells is regulated by negative feedback (see Fig. 71.2). A negative cholesterol balance increases the expression of LDL receptors and subsequent uptake of cholesterol from the circulation. A positive cell cholesterol balance suppresses LDL receptor expression and decreases uptake of LDL-cholesterol into cells. Circulating LDL then enters macrophages and other tissues via scavenger receptors. Because the scavenger receptors are not regulated, these cells accumulate excess intracellular cholesterol, resulting in the formation of foam cells and atheromatous plaques.

The anti-atherogenic effect of HDL is attributed to the removal of excess cholesterol from tissue sites and other lipoproteins. HDL is synthesized in the liver and intestine (see Fig. 71.1). Excess phospholipids, cholesterol, and apolipoproteins on remnant chylomicrons, VLDL, IDL, and LDL are transferred to HDL particles and thus increase HDL mass. Apo A-I, a surface lipoprotein on HDL particles, mobilizes cholesterol from intracellular pools and accepts cholesterol released during lipolysis of triglyceride-rich lipoproteins. It also activates lecithin-cholesterol acyltransferase (LCAT), an enzyme that esterifies cholesterol. These cholesterol esters move the hydrophilic HDL

TABLE 71.1 Properties of Lipoproteins

Lipoprotein Class	Density (g/mL)	Origin	Apolipoproteins	Lipid
Chylomicrons	<0.95	Intestine	B48, C-II, E	TG (85%), cholesterol (10%)
VLDL	<1.006	Liver	B100, C-II, E	TG (55%), cholesterol (20%)
IDL	1.006–1.019	VLDL catabolism	B100, E	TG (25%), cholesterol (35%)
LDL	1.019–1.063	IDL catabolism	B100	TG (5%), cholesterol (60%)
HDL	1.063–1.25	Liver, intestine	A-I, E	TG (5%), cholesterol (20%)

HDL, High-density lipoprotein; *IDL,* intermediate-density lipoprotein; *LDL,* low-density lipoprotein; *TG,* triglyceride; *VLDL,* very-low-density lipoprotein.

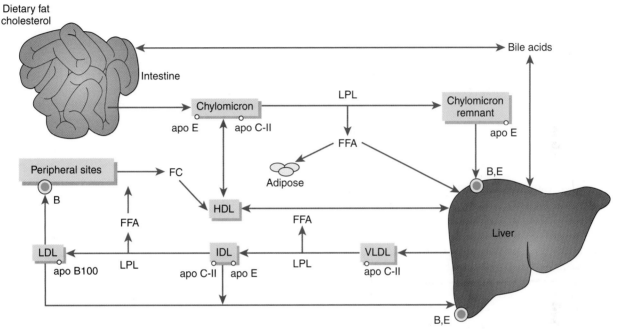

Fig. 71.1 Normal metabolism of plasma lipoproteins (see text for details). *apo,* Apolipoprotein; *B,E,* membrane receptor for lipoproteins containing apo B and apo E (synonymous with the LDL receptor); *FC,* free (unesterified) cholesterol; *FFA,* free (unesterified) fatty acids; *HDL,* high-density lipoprotein; *IDL,* intermediate-density lipoprotein; *LDL,* low-density lipoprotein; *LPL,* lipoprotein lipase; *VLDL,* very-low-density lipoprotein.

surface to the hydrophobic HDL core. Cholesterol ester transfer protein (CETP) transfers core HDL cholesterol esters to other lipoproteins such as VLDL. These lipoproteins deliver cholesterol to peripheral sites for hormone and cell membrane synthesis.

Defects in the production or removal of lipoproteins results in dyslipidemia. Both genetic and acquired conditions have been implicated in the pathogenesis of lipid disorders (Tables 71.2 and 71.3). These are discussed later in the chapter.

CLINICAL PRESENTATION

Dyslipidemia plays a significant role in the development of atherosclerosis. Increased incidence of CHD with high LDL- and low HDL-cholesterol is well documented. Excess LDL can result in the formation of cholesterol plaques that deposit in arteries (atheroma), skin and tendon (xanthomas), eyelids (xanthelasma), and iris (corneal arcus). The impact of triglycerides on vascular disease is less clear. Metabolic disorders such as diabetes and obesity are often associated with vascular disease and hypertriglyceridemia. The atherogenic impact of other elements associated with metabolic disorders is difficult to separate from the effect of hypertriglyceridemia. However, in several population-based studies, abnormal triglyceride levels correlated with

increased risk for CHD. Marked hypertriglyceridemia (>1000 mg/dL) is associated with the chylomicronemia syndrome, characterized by pancreatitis and xanthomas.

DIAGNOSIS

Dyslipidemia is defined by a total cholesterol, triglyceride, or LDL level greater than the 90th percentile or an HDL level lower than the 10th percentile for the general population. Because chylomicrons are present in plasma for up to 10 hours after a meal, fasting total cholesterol, triglyceride, and lipoprotein assessments are required for diagnosis. It is advisable to confirm dyslipidemia with two separate determinations.

Total cholesterol, triglyceride, and HDL levels can be measured directly. VLDL and LDL levels usually are calculated. If the triglyceride concentration is lower than 400 mg/dL, then VLDL is calculated by dividing the triglyceride level by 5. LDL-cholesterol is estimated by subtracting VLDL and HDL from the total cholesterol. This is known as the Friedewald equation. LDL cholesterol calculated utilizing this equation is used to set therapeutic targets in most clinical trials and treatment guidelines. However, calculated LDL cholesterol becomes progressively inaccurate with increasing triglyceride levels and should not be estimated if triglyceride levels are greater the 400 mg/dL. In

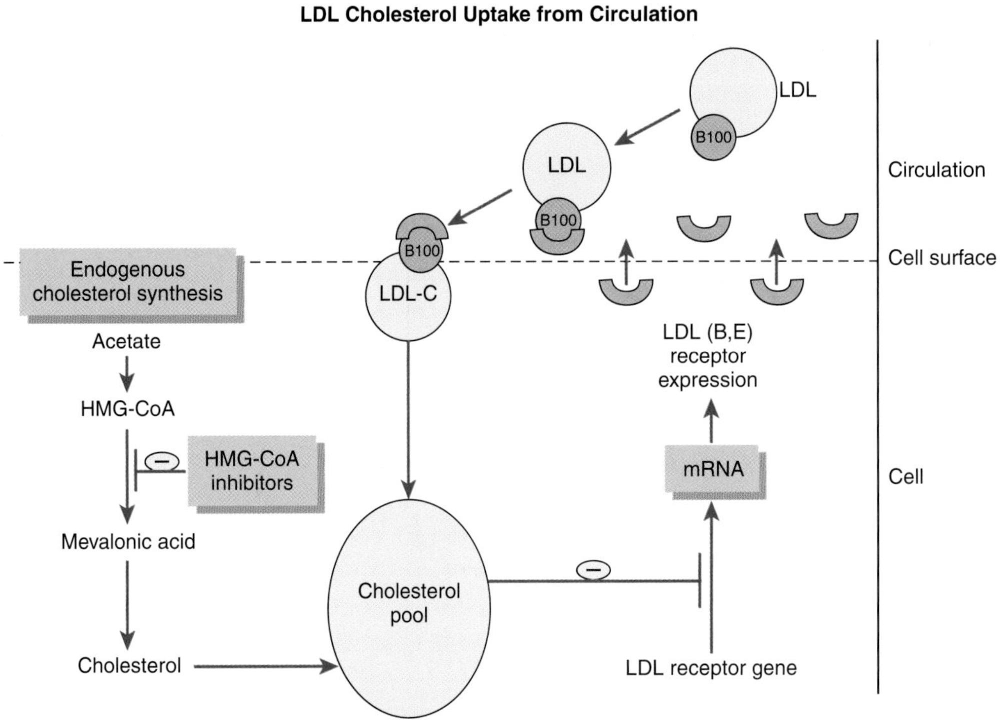

LDL Cholesterol Uptake from Circulation

Fig. 71.2 Regulation of low-density lipoprotein (LDL) receptor expression (see text for details). *B100,* Apolipoprotein B100; *B,E,* membrane receptor for lipoproteins containing apo B and apo E (synonymous with the LDL receptor); *HMG-CoA,* 3-hydroxy-3-methylglutaryl–coenzyme A; *LDL-C,* LDL-cholesterol; *mRNA,* messenger RNA.

TABLE 71.2   Genetic Disorders of Lipid Metabolism

Disorder	Genetic Defect	Dyslipidemia
Familial hypercholesterolemia	Mutation in the gene that encodes LDL receptor Gain of function mutation in *PCSK9* gene Mutation in the apolipoprotein B100 gene	Elevated TC and LDL
Elevated plasma Lp(a)	Increased binding of LDL to apolipoprotein(a)	Elevated Lp(a)
Polygenic hypercholesterolemia	Increased binding of apo E4–containing lipoprotein to LDL receptor resulting in downregulation of the LDL receptor	Elevated TC and LDL
Familial combined hyperlipoproteinemia	Polygenic disorder associated with increased hepatic VLDL production, resulting in increased LDL and decreased HDL production; some individuals have a mutation in the LPL gene that affects expression and function of LPL	Elevated TC, LDL, and TG Low HDL
Familial dysbetalipoproteinemia	Lower affinity of apo E2 for LDL receptor	Elevated TG, TC, and LDL
Lipoprotein lipase deficiency	Mutation in the *LPL* gene	Elevated TG
Apolipoprotein C-II deficiency	Decrease in activation of LPL due to a deficiency of apo CII	Elevated TG
Familial hypertriglyceridemia	Overproduction of hepatic VLDL and increased catabolism of HDL	Elevated TG Low HDL

HDL, High-density lipoprotein; *LDL,* low-density lipoprotein; *TC,* total cholesterol; *TG,* triglyceride; *VLDL,* very-low-density lipoprotein.

that case, assays are available to directly measure the concentration of LDL cholesterol. Furthermore, the lipoprotein abnormality associated with triglyceride levels greater than 400 mg/dL can be identified by inspecting the serum. When the triglyceride level exceeds 350 mg/dL, the serum is cloudy. After refrigeration, a white surface layer depicts excess chylomicrons, whereas a dispersed, opaque infranatant reflects a VLDL dysfunction.

In general, universal screening is recommended starting at 35 years of age for men and at 45 years of age for women. There is a paucity of data supporting long-term benefits from universal screening of younger individuals. Most guidelines suggest selective screening of children who have a family history of lipoprotein abnormality or premature vascular disease. Baseline lipid levels are also recommended in adults with CHD, risk factors for CHD, or CHD equivalent (i.e., symptomatic carotid artery disease, peripheral arterial disease, abdominal aortic aneurysm, or diabetes). CHD risk factors include hypertension, diabetes mellitus, cigarette smoking, and family history of premature CHD (i.e., affected male first-degree relative <55 years or female first-degree relative <65 years of age). Either a fasting or a nonfasting total cholesterol and HDL measurement can be the initial screen. Treatment initiation is based on 10-year and lifetime risk of atherosclerotic cardiovascular disease (ASCVD) (Table 71.4).

TABLE 71.3 Mechanisms of Secondary Hyperlipidemia

Clinical	Elevated Lipoprotein	Mechanism
Diabetes	Chylomicron, VLDL, LDL	Increase in VLDL production and decrease in VLDL/LDL clearance
Obesity	Chylomicron, VLDL, LDL	Increase in VLDL production and decrease in VLDL/LDL clearance
Lipodystrophy	VLDL	Increase in VLDL production
Hypothyroidism	LDL, VLDL	Decrease in LDL/LDL clearance
Estrogen	VLDL	Increase in VLDL production
Glucocorticoids	VLDL, LDL	Increase in VLDL production and conversion to LDL
Alcohol	VLDL	Increase in VLDL production
Nephrotic syndrome	VLDL, LDL	Increase in VLDL production and conversion to LDL

LDL, Low-density lipoprotein; *VLDL*, very-low-density lipoprotein.

TABLE 71.4 Cardiovascular Risk Prevention

	Primary Prevention (Age 40–75 Years)		Secondary Prevention
Risk assessment	LDL 70–190 or 10-year risk of ASCVD 7.5–20% or diabetes	LDL >190 or 10-year risk of ASCVD >20% or diabetes with risk factors	Known ASCVD
Statin dosing	Moderate intensity statin	High intensity statin	High intensity statin to lower LDL-C >50%
LDL target	<100	<100	<50–70

TABLE 71.5 Recommendations for Nutritional Intake

Nutrient	Recommended Intake
Total fat	25–35% of total calories
Saturated	<7%
Polyunsaturated	<10%
Monounsaturated	<20%
Carbohydrates	50–60% of total calories
Protein	15% of total calories
Cholesterol	<200 mg/day
Fiber	20–30 g/day

Individuals who do not meet the threshold for treatment should be screened every 3 to 5 years.

TREATMENT

Treatment of elevated total and LDL-cholesterol can slow the development and progression of CHD. Meta-analysis of primary and secondary prevention trials indicates that CHD mortality decreases by approximately 15% for every 10% reduction in serum cholesterol. LDL-cholesterol treatment strategies are based on risk indicators. There is strong evidence that dietary modifications can reduce LDL-cholesterol and triglyceride levels (Table 71.5). However, evidence that lifestyle-induced lipid modifications improve cardiovascular outcomes is limited. Ample evidence supports statin use in primary and secondary prevention of CHD (see Table 71.4 and Table 71.6). Treatment effects of statins can be assessed after 1 to 2 months. Additional agents can be considered if target goals are not achieved with maximal drug dosing (Table 71.7).

A fasting lipid panel is required to diagnose hypertriglyceridemia. Triglyceride levels higher than 200 mg/dL are classified as abnormal. Borderline triglyceride levels range from 150 to 200 mg/dL, and normal values are lower than 150 mg/dL. A diet and exercise program is recommended for all individuals with abnormal triglyceride levels. However, pharmacologic treatments to reduce triglyceride levels may be considered if fasting levels are higher than 200 mg/dL, especially if the individual is at risk for CHD or pancreatitis (see Table 71.7). Fibrates, fish oil, and nicotinic acid should be considered if the triglyceride level is higher than 500 mg/dL. However, for levels lower than 500 mg/dL, statins are first-line therapy.

Low HDL concentrations (<40 mg/dL) can also increase the risk for CHD. In the Framingham Heart Study, every decrease in HDL of 5 mg/dL increased the risk for myocardial infarction. Both lifestyle modifications (e.g., diet low in saturated fat, exercise) and pharmacologic therapy (e.g., nicotinic acid, fibrate) can improve HDL levels. However, target goals and treatment recommendations have not been established due to a lack of evidence.

Lifestyle Modification

Lifestyle modification should be the initial step in the management of hyperlipidemia (see Table 71.5). Restricting the dietary intake of fat lowers total cholesterol by approximately 15% and LDL cholesterol by 25%. Low-fat diets that limit saturated fat content promote LDL receptor expression and increase the uptake of LDL-cholesterol from the circulation. By contrast, saturated fat downregulates hepatic LDL receptors and increases circulating LDL. Because unsaturated fats (polyunsaturated and monounsaturated) generally do not have this effect, they are the preferred form of fat intake. However, polyunsaturated fats containing fatty acids with a *trans* rather than *cis* double bond configuration (*trans*-fatty acids) increase plasma cholesterol levels similarly to saturated fat.

Limiting the intake of saturated and *trans*-unsaturated fatty acids requires appropriate calorie substitutions. Increasing carbohydrate content to achieve this goal can increase the hepatic synthesis of triglyceride. Dietary substitution with soluble fibers (e.g., oat bran) has been recommended, because these fibers have a limited effect on triglyceride levels. They also bind bile acids in the gut and thereby decrease cholesterol levels. Other polyunsaturated fats, such as omega-3 fatty acids, are cardioprotective. They are abundant in fatty fish, flaxseed oil, canola oil, and nuts. They reduce VLDL production, inhibit platelet

TABLE 71.6 Statins

High-Intensity Statins: Lowers LDL-C by >50%	Moderate-Intensity Statins: Lowers LDL-C 30–50%	Low-Intensity Statins: Lowers LDL-C by 30%
Atorvastatin 40–80 mg Rosuvastatin 20–40 mg	Atorvastatin 10–20 mg Rosuvastatin 5–10 mg Simvastatin 20–40 mg Pravastatin 40–80 mg Lovastatin 40 mg Fluvastatin 80 mg Pitavastatin 2–4 mg	Simvastatin 10 mg Pravastatin 10–20 mg Lovastatin 20 mg Fluvastatin 20–40 mg Pitavastatin 1 mg

TABLE 71.7 Drugs Commonly Used for the Treatment of Hyperlipidemia

Drug Class	LDL (% Change)	HDL (% Change)	Triglycerides (% Change)	Side Effects
HMG-CoA inhibitors	↓ 20–60	↑ 5–10	↓ 10–30	Liver toxicity, myositis, rhabdomyolysis; enhanced warfarin effect
Cholesterol absorption inhibitors	↓ 17	No effect	↓ 7–8	Abnormal liver enzymes in combination with an HMG-CoA inhibitor, myalgia, hepatitis, rhabdomyolysis, pancreatitis, potential increase in cancer risk and cancer death
PCSK-9 inhibitor	↓ 38–72	↑ 4–9	↓ 2–23	Injection site reaction, hypersensitivity, drug neutralizing antibody
Bempedoic acid	↓ 15–19	No change	No change	Hyperuricemia, tendon rupture, and may potentiate statin-related myopathy
Bile acid sequestrants	↓ 15–30	Slight increase	No effect	Nausea, bloating, cramping, abnormal liver function; interferes with absorption of other drugs such as warfarin and thyroxine
Fibric acid	↓ 6–20	↑ 5–20	↓ 41–53	Nausea, cramping, myalgias, liver toxicity, enhanced warfarin effect
Nicotinic acid	↓ 10–25	↑ 15–35	↓ 25–30	Hepatotoxicity, hyperuricemia, hyperglycemia, flushing, pruritus, nausea, vomiting, diarrhea
Omega-3 fatty acids	Variable	↑ 5–9	↓ 23–45	Eructation, taste perversion, dyspepsia

HMG-CoA, Hydroxymethylglutaryl–coenzyme A reductase.

aggregation, and decrease CHD. Even two servings per week of fatty fish such as salmon can be beneficial.

Dietary restriction of fat (<10%) is essential for the treatment of marked hypertriglyceridemia. Other factors such as carbohydrate and alcohol intake can also increase the synthesis of triglyceride. Restriction of alcohol intake to one or two servings per week and adherence to a low-fat, high-fiber diet will improve hypertriglyceridemia.

Exercise has been shown to increase LPL activity. Even a single exercise session can reduce triglycerides and increase HDL. The impact of exercise on LDL is less clear. With low- to moderate-intensity exercise regimens, clearance of VLDL particles increases LDL production. However, this effect is not seen with high-intensity exercise programs. A decrease in LDL-cholesterol occurs with high-intensity exercise, and this effect is independent of weight loss.

Pharmacotherapy

In addition to diet and exercise modifications, pharmacologic agents are prescribed to reduce cardiovascular risk and to achieve therapeutic goals. The ASCVD Risk algorithm is used to calculate a 10-year risk of heart disease or stroke. This algorithm calculates risk by evaluating the following factors: history of ASCVD, LDL-cholesterol levels, age, current diagnosis of diabetes, gender, race, total cholesterol, HDL-cholesterol levels, medication controlled hypertension, and smoking history. History of the following conditions is considered as known

ASCVD: acute coronary syndrome, myocardial infarction, stable angina, coronary revascularization, stroke, transient ischemic attack, or peripheral arterial disease. Cardiovascular risk profile determines therapeutic plan including drug dosing and LDL targets in individuals 40 to 75 years of age (see Tables 71.4 and 71.6). High-risk patients may require additional agents to achieve target goals. Likely benefit of each agent needs to be balanced against potential adverse effects when determining drug therapy (see Table 71.7). In individuals younger than 40 years or with 10-year risk below 7.5%, lifestyle modification is recommended unless risk enhancers such as family history of premature ASCVD, LDL-cholesterol greater than 160 mg/dL, chronic kidney disease, and metabolic syndrome, are noted.

HMG-CoA reductase is the rate-limiting enzyme involved in cholesterol biosynthesis. Inhibition of this enzyme decreases intracellular cholesterol pools and subsequently increases uptake of LDL cholesterol from the circulation. HMG-CoA reductase inhibitors (e.g., atorvastatin and rosuvastatin) increase cholesterol utilization, decrease VLDL synthesis, and increase HDL synthesis. As a result, lower LDL and triglyceride levels and higher HDL levels are observed with treatment. Meta-analysis of primary and secondary CHD prevention trials found reductions in all-cause and cardiovascular mortality rates with statin therapy. These agents limit progression and may even cause regression of coronary atherosclerosis. Therefore, they represent first-line therapy in the management of abnormal LDL-cholesterol levels and for prevention of cardiovascular outcomes. Elevated liver enzymes and muscle toxicity are potential dose-related complications. Myositis can occur with statins alone, but the risk is higher when statins are used in combination with nicotinic acid or fibric acid derivatives.

Ezetimibe is a Niemann-Pick C1 Like 1 (NPC1L1) inhibitor. NPC1L1 is a protein that aids in the transport of cholesterol across the intestinal brush border. Ezetimibe inhibits this enzyme, decreasing cholesterol absorption and thus increasing cholesterol utilization and decreasing LDL-cholesterol levels. Ezetimibe may be used as a single agent or in combination with an HMG-CoA reductase inhibitor to lower LDL-cholesterol levels. In combination with a statin, this agent may reduce cardiovascular events in high-risk individuals.

Proprotein convertase subtilisin kexin type 9 (PCSK9) inhibitors represent an exciting new frontier in LDL-cholesterol reduction. PCSK9 is a protease whose function is the degradation of LDL receptors. Inhibition of this protease leads to increased LDL receptor survival, which in turn leads to the reduction of circulating LDL-cholesterol. The two approved agents, evolocumab and alirocumab, are both monoclonal antibodies against PCSK9 that are administered by subcutaneous injection every 2 to 4 weeks. They are indicated in patients with LDL greater than 190 mg/dL or ASCVD judged to be high risk who have not achieved desired LDL reduction on statin and ezetimibe. Cost of these therapies is significant and may be a limiting factor. Antisense therapy (injectable oligonucleotides to prevent mRNA translation) against PCSK9 mRNA is an area of active investigation.

Bempedoic acid inhibits adenosine triphosphate citrate lyase, an enzyme in the cholesterol biosynthesis pathway. This enzyme is upstream of 3-hydroxy-3methylglutarly-CoA reductase, the target of statin drugs. Bempedoic acid alone or in combination with other agents lowers LDL-cholesterol and is recommended for individuals intolerant to statins, unable to achieve target goals, and in circumstances where PCSK-9 inhibitors are not an option.

Drugs that interfere with the absorption of cholesterol from the intestinal lumen increase cholesterol utilization and decrease circulating levels of cholesterol. Bile acid sequestrants (e.g., cholestyramine, colestipol, and colesevelam) bind bile acids in the intestinal lumen and increase fecal excretion. Subsequently, more LDL-cholesterol is used by the liver to synthesis bile acids. The decrease in cellular cholesterol pools upregulates LDL receptors and decreases the amount of LDL-cholesterol in the circulation. Mild increases in HDL-cholesterol are also seen with this agent as a result of increased intestinal HDL formation. Treatment is associated with a reduction in the incidence of CHD. Bile acid sequestrants may be used alone for mild lipid dysfunction or in combination with another lipid-lowering agent such as an HMG-CoA reductase inhibitor. Abnormal liver function and gastrointestinal symptoms (e.g., nausea, bloating, cramping) are common side effects that limit the use of bile acid sequestrants. They can also interfere with the absorption of other drugs such as warfarin and thyroxine.

Fibric acid derivatives such as gemfibrozil and fenofibrate increase FFA oxidation in muscle and liver. The reduced lipogenesis in the liver decreases VLDL and subsequent LDL production. Fibric acid derivatives also enhance LPL activity and HDL synthesis. As a result, treatment is usually associated with not only lower triglyceride and LDL levels, but also higher HDL levels. Reduced cardiovascular events have been demonstrated in a subset of individuals with high triglyceride (>200 mg/dL) and low HDL (<40 mg/dL) levels, but improvements in cardiovascular or all-cause mortality otherwise have not been confirmed with these agents. Liver toxicity and myositis are potential side effects of fibric acid derivatives, and they also interfere with the metabolism of warfarin, leading to a need for its dose adjustment.

Nicotinic acid has an antilipolytic effect and therefore decreases the influx of FFA to the liver. As a result, hepatic VLDL synthesis and LDL production are reduced. Nicotinic acid also decreases HDL catabolism. Lower triglyceride and LDL levels and higher HDL levels are observed with treatment. In addition, nicotinic acid stimulates tissue plasminogen activator and prevents thrombosis. It also reduces lipoprotein(a), or Lp(a), which is an independent risk factor for developing vascular disease (discussed later). The cardioprotective effect of nicotinic acid may be linked to its effect on Lp(a) and HDL. Side effects include hepatotoxicity, hyperuricemia, hyperglycemia, and flushing.

Omega-3 fatty acids reduce VLDL production and subsequently lower triglyceride levels (by 35%). They also modestly increase HDL (3%) and LDL (5%). The impact on lipids can occur over months to years and requires treatment doses as high as 3 to 4 g of fish oil per day. Omega-3 fatty acids constitute 30% of fish oil supplements and 85% of prescribed pharmacologic preparations (i.e., Lovaza and Vascepa). In clinical trials, both Lovaza and Vascepa 4 g/day lowered triglyceride levels by 45%. Fish oil supplements seem to be a reasonable, cost-effective means to reduce triglyceride levels; side effects include eructation, taste perversion, and dyspepsia. A large clinical trial recently demonstrated that Vascepa may reduce the incidence of cardiovascular events in patients with cardiovascular disease, well-controlled LDL, and modest triglyceride elevations.

Other agents to consider are neomycin, lomitapide, and mipomersen. These agents can be considered in the management of patients with refractory LDL elevations. Neomycin complexes with bile acid and lowers LDL levels. It also inhibits production of apolipoprotein(a) in the liver and lowers Lp(a). It is recommended as adjuvant therapy for patients with familial hypercholesterolemia and Lp(a) excess. Important side effects include nephrotoxicity and ototoxicity. Lomitapide inhibits microsomal triglyceride transfer protein in the liver and decreases apo B. Significant reductions in LDL (up to 50%) are seen with treatment. Liver toxicity is a serious adverse event associated with this agent. Mipomersen is another agent approved for use in homozygous familial hypercholesterolemia. It binds apo B messenger RNA and inhibits apo B production. Apo B is a structural component of VLDL, IDL, and LDL. Treatment reduces LDL by up to 50%. Side effects include flu-like symptoms, injection site reactions, elevations in liver enzymes, and liver toxicity. The side effect profile and expense associated with both lomitapide and mipomersen limit the use of these agents to individuals with homozygous familial hypercholesterolemia.

LIPID DISORDERS

A number of specific disorders of overproduction or impaired removal of lipoproteins result in dyslipidemia (see Tables 71.2 and 71.3). These disorders are often familial, but secondary causes also need to be considered. Comorbid conditions (diabetes, hypothyroidism), medications (estrogen, glucocorticoids, β-adrenergic receptor blockers), and lifestyle factors (diet, alcohol) can increase the production and clearance of lipoproteins. Addressing these factors can often normalize lipid levels. If abnormalities persist, evaluation of genetic factors and treatment with pharmacologic therapy may need to be considered.

Familial Hypercholesterolemia

Familial hypercholesterolemia (FH) is an autosomal dominant disorder that alters LDL receptor synthesis and function. It is caused by mutations in one of three genes that decrease the clearance of LDL particles and increase circulating LDL levels. Gene mutations that result in FH exhibit an additive effect with more severe clinical presentations noted in individuals with homozygous or compound heterozygous mutations. A defect in the LDL (apo B/E) receptor gene is the most common cause of FH. Receptor defects are classified based on receptor activity: receptor-negative (<2% activity) and receptor-defective (2% to 25% activity). Defects in the PCSK9 and apolipoprotein B gene are less common. PCSK9 is a serine protease produced by the liver. It binds the LDL receptor leading to internalization and eventual destruction of the LDL receptor. Gain of function mutation in the PCSK9 gene results in decreased LDL receptor expression, decreased LDL catabolism, and increased LDL-cholesterol. Mutation in the apolipoprotein B gene results in impaired binding of LDL particles to the LDL receptors. Apo B100 protein defect has a milder presentation than LDL (apo B/E) receptor defect. This is because apo E–mediated clearance of remnant particles is still functional.

The homozygous form of the LDL receptor mutation is rare. Affected individuals present early in life with elevated levels of total cholesterol (600 to 1000 mg/dL) and LDL-cholesterol (550 to 950 mg/dL). Triglyceride and HDL-cholesterol levels are normal. These patients develop CHD, aortic stenosis due to atherosclerosis of the aortic root, and tendon xanthomas (often in the Achilles tendon). If the condition remains untreated, patients with homozygous familial hypercholesterolemia typically die of myocardial infarction before 20 years of age. The heterozygous form of FH affects 1 in every 500 individuals. Partial receptor defect results in cells that display half the normal number of fully functional LDL receptors. These individuals have lower concentrations of total cholesterol (>300 to 600 mg/dL) and LDL-cholesterol (250 to 500 mg/dL) than do those with the homozygous form. Premature CHD and tendon xanthomas are characteristic clinical findings.

Although the diagnosis of familial hypercholesterolemia can be established by genetic testing, the diagnosis is usually made based on clinical features. Elevated total cholesterol (>300 mg/dL) and LDL-cholesterol (>250 mg/dL) in an individual with a personal or family history of premature CHD and tendon xanthomas identifies patients at risk for familial hypercholesterolemia. Treatment requires a low-fat (<20% of total calories), low-cholesterol (<100 mg/day) diet in combination with drug therapy. Usually, patients with familial hypercholesterolemia require multiple agents including high-intensity statin, ezetimibe, and/or PCSK9 inhibitors to lower cholesterol levels to the target range. For patients who are unable to achieve target goals, additional intervention with liver transplantation to provide functional receptors, ileal bypass surgery to decrease gastrointestinal absorption of bile acids, LDL apheresis to remove excess LDL, and novel therapies with lomitapide and mipomersen may be considered.

Elevated Plasma Lipoprotein(a)

Lp(a) is a specialized form of LDL that is assembled extracellularly from apolipoprotein(a) and LDL. Lp(a), when present at elevated levels, interferes with fibrinolysis by competing with plasminogen. This leads to decreased thrombolysis and increased clot formation. Lp(a) also binds macrophages, promoting foam cell formation and atherosclerotic plaques. Screening should be considered in individuals who have a family or personal history of premature CHD without dyslipidemia and in those for whom cholesterol-lowering therapy has failed. The diagnosis can be made by documenting Lp(a) levels higher than 30 mg/dL in a patient with premature CHD. The primary goal of therapy is to lower LDL levels with agents such as statins, ezetimibe, and PCSK-9 inhibitors. Niacin can also reduce Lp(a); however, the effectiveness of this strategy in ASCVD prevention remains unproven.

Polygenic Hypercholesterolemia

Hypercholesterolemia in a population is mostly due to small influences of many different genes. The exact nature of these genetic defects is poorly defined, but apo E may play a role in the pathogenesis. Apo E4 on chylomicrons and VLDL remnants has a high affinity for the LDL receptor. Elevated binding of apo E4–containing lipoproteins to LDL receptors may downregulate LDL receptor synthesis and increase circulating LDL levels. Environmental factors such as diet can influence production of chylomicrons and VLDL, resulting in downregulation of the LDL receptor in conditions with high apo E4. This leads to an increased propensity for CHD, and treatment with LDL-lowering agents is recommended based on risk factors (see Table 71.7).

Familial Combined Hyperlipoproteinemia

Familial combined hyperlipoproteinemia (FCHL) is a polygenic disorder that affects 1% to 2% of the population. Factors such as diet, glucose intolerance, and medications can influence the phenotypic presentation. In FCHL, the liver synthesizes excess VLDL. VLDL is hydrolyzed by LPL to produce LDL. Mutations in the *LPL* gene affecting its expression or function can decrease the efficiency of VLDL catabolism. Dysfunction of LPL is observed in one third of patients with FCHL. Diminished LPL activity increases circulating VLDL-triglyceride; furthermore, fewer VLDL remnant particles are available for HDL synthesis. Therefore, FCHL needs to be considered in all patients whose total cholesterol level is greater than 250 mg/dL, triglycerides greater than 175 mg/dL, or HDL-cholesterol less than 35 mg/dL.

There are no definitive diagnostic tests, but family screening can help confirm the diagnosis. The phenotype of FCHL is variable, with individuals displaying high LDL-cholesterol, high VLDL-triglyceride, or both based on the genetic defect and environmental factors. Patients also typically have high apo B (>120 mg/dL) and a low ratio of LDL-cholesterol to apo B100 (<1.2). They accumulate small dense LDL particles, which are thought to be atherogenic and contribute to premature CHD. Xanthomas or xanthelasmas are not a feature of this disorder. Affected individuals require a low-fat, low-cholesterol diet plus multiple lipid-lowering drugs to achieve target goals. Statins are recommended to lower LDL-cholesterol and to reduce the risk of cardiovascular disease and mortality. Addition of ezetimibe, fibric acid derivatives, niacin, and omega-3 fatty acid are often considered to achieve LDL-cholesterol and triglyceride target goals. However, these agents have not been shown to decrease cardiovascular events or improve overall survival.

Familial Dysbetalipoproteinemia

Apo E on the surface of lipoprotein particles binds LDL receptors and facilitates clearance of remnant particles from the circulation. The apo E2 allele has a lower affinity for LDL receptors than apo E3 or apo E4. In individuals who are homozygous for apo E2, LPL hydrolyzes the triglyceride core and the resulting cholesterol-rich chylomicrons. VLDL and IDL remnant particles accumulate in the circulation. Expression of this phenotype usually requires a precipitating condition that increases lipoprotein production (e.g., diabetes, alcohol consumption) or decreases clearance (e.g., hypothyroidism). In addition to the more common autosomal recessive mutation of apo E described previously, several apo E mutations have been described that result in an autosomal dominant phenotype manifesting in childhood. Premature CHD, peripheral vascular disease, and xanthomas involving the palmar crease are characteristic clinical features. Individuals with familial dysbetalipoproteinemia have elevated levels of total cholesterol (300 to 400 mg/dL) and triglycerides (300 to 400 mg/dL). Definitive diagnosis requires genetic testing to identify apo E2 homozygosity or mutation. Treatment of coexisting conditions such as diabetes and hypothyroidism can normalize lipid levels in apo E2 homozygotes. If target levels are not achieved, dietary therapy and lipid-lowering drugs such as fibric acid derivatives and HMG-CoA reductase inhibitors should also be considered.

Familial Chylomicronemia

Mutations in the *LPL* gene resulting in deficiency of LPL synthesis or function lead to increased circulating chylomicron and VLDL particles and severe hypertriglyceridemia. Homozygous LPL deficiency is rare. It manifests in childhood with triglyceride levels higher than 1000 mg/dL. Heterozygous LPL deficiency occurs in 2% to 4% of the population and usually requires a precipitating factor, such as uncontrolled diabetes or estrogen therapy, to manifest the phenotype. These individuals have moderate hypertriglyceridemia (250 to 750 mg/dL) that can increase to levels greater than 1000 mg/dL with secondary factors. This can result in the chylomicronemia syndrome, which is characterized by marked hypertriglyceridemia (>1000 to 2000 mg/dL), pancreatitis, eruptive xanthomas, lipemia retinalis, and hepatosplenomegaly. Visual inspection demonstrates lipemic plasma. After refrigeration for 12 hours, a creamy top layer (increased chylomicrons) or turbid plasma infranatant (increased VLDL), or both, can be demonstrated. Documentation of diminished LPL activity confirms the diagnosis. A diet low in fat (<10% of total calories or 20 to 25 g/day) is the primary treatment. Secondary factors such as uncontrolled diabetes and alcohol use should be addressed, and VLDL-lowering agents (e.g., fibric acid derivatives, niacin) may be needed to prevent severe hypertriglyceridemia.

Apolipoprotein C-II Deficiency

Apo C-II is an activating cofactor for LPL. Deficiency of apo C-II is a rare autosomal recessive disorder that leads to increased chylomicrons and VLDL particles in the circulation, resulting in severe hypertriglyceridemia. Clinical manifestations are similar to those of LPL deficiency, including hypertriglyceridemia (>1000 mg/dL) and symptoms of pancreatitis, eruptive xanthomas, lipemia retinalis, and hepatosplenomegaly. Treatment recommendations include appropriate management of secondary factors such as diabetes and hypothyroidism, dietary fat restriction (<10% of calories), and drug therapy (e.g., fibric acid derivatives). For severe hypertriglyceridemia, plasma transfusion (with apo C-II) can be considered.

Familial Hypertriglyceridemia

Familial hypertriglyceridemia is an autosomal dominant disorder that is characterized by overproduction of hepatic VLDL. The exact defect or mutation is unknown. Secondary factors that increase VLDL, such as diabetes, alcohol ingestion, and estrogen therapy, appear to exacerbate this condition. Low HDL associated with familial hypertriglyceridemia is related to increased catabolism. Individuals with this condition have hypertriglyceridemia (200 to 500 mg/dL) and low HDL-cholesterol (<35 mg/dL) at presentation. This diagnosis is considered in individuals who have a family and personal history of hypertriglyceridemia, CHD, and normal LDL levels. Cloudy infranatant after overnight refrigeration of plasma identifies a disorder of VLDL metabolism. Treatment starts with management of secondary factors that may exacerbate the condition. Dietary fat restriction (<10% of calories) and drug therapy with fish oil, niacin, and fibric acid derivatives should be initiated if target goals are not achieved.

For a deeper discussion on this topic, please see Chapter 195, "Disorders of Lipid Metabolism," in *Goldman-Cecil Medicine*, 26th Edition.

SUGGESTED READINGS

Eckel RH, Jakicic JM, Ard JD, et al: 2013 AHA/ACC guideline on lifestyle management to reduce cardiovascular risk, Circulation 129:S76–S99, 2014.

Grundy SM, Stone NJ, Bailey AL, et al: 2018 AHA/ACC multisociety guideline on the management of blood cholesterol, J Am Coll Cardiol 73:e285, 2019.

Jellinger PS, Handelsman Y, Rosenblit PD, et al: American association of clinical endocrinologist and American College of Endocrinology guidelines for the management of dyslipidemia and prevention of cardiovascular disease, Endocr Pract 23:1–87, 2017.

U.S. Preventive Services Task Force: Statin use for the primary prevention of cardiovascular disease in adults: Preventive medication: U.S. Preventive Services Task Force recommendation statement, 2016, Available at: https://www.uspreventiveservicestaskforce.org/Page/Document/RecommendationStatementFinal/statin-use-in-adults-preventive-medication1. Accessed June 2020.

Women's Health

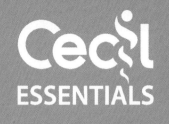

72

Women's Health Topics

Vidya Gopinath, Yael Tarshish, Kelly McGarry

INTRODUCTION

The field of women's health grew out of the recognition that certain medical conditions are unique to women. Sex- and gender-specific differences exist in disease manifestation and management. Sex differences are defined as variations between males and females due to the specific composition and expression of their chromosomes. Gender differences are derived from sociocultural origins. For instance, women are disproportionately affected by poverty, intimate partner violence (IPV), unstable housing, substance use disorders, lack of transportation, lack of insurance, and the necessity of finding child care, all of which pose barriers to care and thereby influence their health. Variations in health outcomes between men and women are related to a complex interplay among lifestyle, environmental, behavioral, molecular, and cellular differences.

Women's health as a specialty focuses on conditions unique to women, diseases that disproportionately affect women, present differently or are managed in ways that are specific to women. Diagnoses unique to women include polycystic ovarian syndrome, menstrual irregularities, and endometriosis. Conditions that disproportionately affect women include breast cancer, osteoporosis, lupus, hypothyroidism, and urinary incontinence. Women have an increased susceptibility for developing certain conditions. For example, a woman who smokes the same number of cigarettes as a man is 20% to 70% more likely to develop lung cancer. Women are also more susceptible to alcohol-induced liver disease. Among individuals who consume 28 to 41 alcoholic beverages per week, the relative risk of alcohol-induced cirrhosis is 17.0 in women and 7.0 in men. During unprotected intercourse, women are 10 times more likely to contract human immunodeficiency virus (HIV) than men. The field of women's health has become more robust and includes practitioners from a multitude of disciplines: obstetrician-gynecologists, general internists, subspecialty internists, family medicine, emergency medicine, radiologists, and surgeons. Pharmacokinetics and pharmacodynamics of numerous drugs have sex-specific differences that are being discovered and require further study. The National Institutes of Health has made significant progress in the inclusion of women in clinical trials; they were historically excluded for numerous reasons including concerns about hormonal fluctuations affecting the data and teratogenic effects in women who were or could become pregnant. In 1977, the US Food and Drug Administration (FDA) recommended excluding women with "childbearing potential" from phase 1 and early phase 2 clinical studies. There is now growing recognition of the need for research studies to fully analyze sex-specific differences and include individuals of both sexes.

The seeds of this disparity in research and representation stem in part from the fact that women have been underrepresented in the field of medicine. In 1849, Elizabeth Blackwell earned the first medical degree granted to an American woman, but the advancement of female physicians has been gradual. In 1950, only 6% of practicing physicians were female. Currently, female physicians make up 36% of the workforce. In 2017, for the first time, the number of women enrolling in US medical schools exceeded the number of men, with females representing 50.7% of the 21,338 new enrollees, compared with 49.8% in 2016. Given these statistics, women will have an expanding impact on shaping the profession and the world of health care.

In this chapter, we focus on medical issues unique to women and highlight what is known about sex and gender differences in common diseases. Although "females" and "women" are often used interchangeably, we recognize that biological sex and gender are not synonymous. We aim to be inclusive of sexual minorities and recognize that some topics may be relevant only to biological females or women who choose to have sexual relationships with males. For more detailed discussions of specific topics, please refer to the appropriate chapters in this edition of *Cecil Essentials of Medicine* and the 26th edition of *Goldman-Cecil Medicine*.

THE MENSTRUAL CYCLE

The menstrual cycle is a complex hormonal process resulting in the release of a single oocyte, an immature ovum or egg. The menstrual cycle consists of two phases, the follicular phase and the luteal phase. The follicular phase begins with the first day of menses. Several follicles grow until a single dominant follicle is selected. Meanwhile, the uterine endometrium gradually thickens. The follicular phase ends the day prior to the luteal hormone (LH) surge that marks the first day of the luteal phase. The LH surge initiates the release of the follicle from the ovary to travel down the fallopian tube to the uterine cavity. The luteal phase ends when either the oocyte becomes fertilized and implants in the endometrium or without fertilization, when levels of estradiol and progesterone decline. Without high levels of estradiol or progesterone, endometrial blood supply decreases, which then leads to sloughing of the endometrial lining and thus marks the onset of menses. The physiologic changes that define the menstrual cycle, including variations in hormones, the uterine lining, and morning basal body temperature, are graphically represented in Fig. 72.1. The average adult menstrual cycle is 28 to 35 days. Variability in length of cycle is common during adolescence; between ages 20 to 40 years old, women tend to have consistent cycle lengths.

Menstrual disorders are common and categorized as amenorrhea or abnormal uterine bleeding. Amenorrhea is defined as the lack of menses in a sexually mature female. It is further delineated as primary

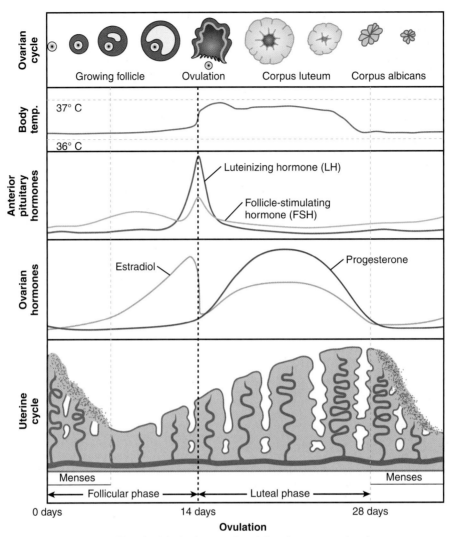

Fig. 72.1 The physiologic changes that define the menstrual cycle.

or secondary amenorrhea. These abnormalities may indicate problems related to the reproductive system or may be an early sign of an important underlying systemic illness. A pregnancy test must always be done to exclude pregnancy in cases of amenorrhea along with a thorough history and physical exam.

Primary Amenorrhea

Primary amenorrhea is most often caused by genetic or anatomic abnormalities. It is defined as the lack of menarche by age 15 or 16 despite normal sexual development or the lack of menarche by age 13 or 14 in the absence of sexual development. Breast development, the presence of a uterus, and levels of LH, follicle-stimulating hormone (FSH), thyroid-stimulating hormone (TSH), and prolactin are important factors in determining the cause of primary amenorrhea. Work-up may include karyotyping and pelvic or brain imaging. The most common cause of primary amenorrhea is gonadal dysgenesis, which is found in Turner syndrome. The second most common cause is müllerian agenesis, a congenital malformation resulting in lack of uterine development and vaginal hypoplasia. If the uterus is present, an outflow tract obstruction such as an imperforate hymen or a transverse vaginal septum may be identified. FSH and LH levels can differentiate between functional hypothalamic amenorrhea and primary ovarian insufficiency.

Secondary Amenorrhea

Secondary amenorrhea is the absence of menses for 3 months in women with regular menses or 6 months in women with irregular menses outside of the setting of pregnancy or lactation. Oligomenorrhea occurs when menses are irregular or infrequent, with a cycle length usually greater than 35 to 40 days or fewer than nine menstrual cycles in 12 months, and it is often associated with chronic anovulation or oligo-ovulation. The most common cause of secondary amenorrhea is pregnancy. Lactation causes amenorrhea for up to 6 months in women who are exclusively breast-feeding. Prolonged amenorrhea can follow cessation of some hormonal contraceptives, especially depot medroxyprogesterone acetate (DMPA). Menopause should be suspected in a woman older than 45 years of age.

Amenorrhea and oligomenorrhea may be caused by pathologic changes at any point in the endometrial-ovarian-pituitary-hypothalamic axis. The differential diagnosis for other causes of secondary amenorrhea is broad. Most cases are associated with polycystic ovary syndrome (PCOS), hypothalamic amenorrhea, hyperprolactinemia or primary ovarian insufficiency.

PCOS and hyperandrogenism are associated with hirsutism, acne, and history of irregular menses. Hypothalamic amenorrhea can be functionally caused by stress, change in weight, diet or exercise or an eating disorder. Headaches and visual field deficits are concerning for hypothalamic-pituitary disease; galactorrhea indicates hyperprolactinemia. Evidence of ovarian insufficiency includes symptoms of estrogen deficiency such as hot flashes, vaginal dryness, and decreased libido. Initial labs include FSH, TSH, prolactin, and possibly total testosterone. Pituitary MRI, progestin withdrawal test, and hysteroscopy may be a part of the work-up if initial tests are unrevealing.

Abnormal Uterine Bleeding

Abnormal uterine bleeding (AUB) affects approximately one third of women at some point in their life. Terms such as menorrhagia and metrorrhagia were updated in 2011 by the International Federation of Gynecology and Obstetrics. Instead they recommend use of the terms heavy menstrual bleeding (HMB), which is defined as ovulatory bleeding for more than 8 days or interfering with quality of life, and abnormal uterine bleeding with ovulatory dysfunction (AUB-O), which is defined as irregular bleeding.

In the PALM-COEIN classification, the etiology of HMB and AUB-O is divided into structural and nonstructural causes. The four main structural causes are *p*olyp, *a*denomyosis, *l*eiomyoma, and *m*alignancy or hyperplasia. The five nonstructural causes are *c*oagulopathy, *o*vulatory dysfunction, *e*ndometrial, *i*atrogenic, and *n*ot yet classified.

Key elements of the history include details about bleeding, including the onset, duration, pattern, and quantity of bleeding. This history and information about breast tenderness and cramping prior to onset of bleeding can establish evidence of ovulatory cycles. The evaluation should also confirm the source of bleeding as uterine and not gastrointestinal, urinary, or vulvar. Pregnancy must be ruled out in all patients including those who are using contraception or deny being sexually active.

Evaluation includes a pelvic exam with a vaginal speculum and bimanual exam to characterize the uterus. Pap smear and cervical cultures should be obtained to assess for cervical disease or infection. Laboratory testing should include a complete blood count (CBC), thyroid studies, and serum ferritin. It may also include coagulation studies because a significant fraction (5% to 32%) of women with heavy menstrual bleeding have an underlying bleeding disorder.

Endometrial sampling should be performed for women age 45 or older and for women younger than 45 years of age who are at risk for endometrial hyperplasia or endometrial cancer (i.e., women with obesity or a history of chronic anovulation, failed medical therapy or persistent symptoms). For women with suspected structural abnormalities, a transvaginal ultrasound study should be pursued.

Management of abnormal bleeding depends on the underlying pathology identified and the degree of anemia caused by the bleeding. Hemodynamically unstable women may require uterine curettage or intravenous estrogen. For hemodynamically stable women, control of bleeding is usually achieved through a combination of estrogen and progestin preparations, usually in the form of oral contraceptive pills. In women with a contraindication to estrogen, levonorgestrel-releasing intrauterine devices (IUDs) and high-dose oral progestins can be used. Irregular bleeding often continues with hormonal management but declines over time. Nonsteroidal anti-inflammatory drugs (NSAIDs) can be used by women who do not require contraception, because NSAIDs have been shown to decrease bleeding. Standard iron supplementation is recommended for patients with resultant anemia or iron deficiency. Surgical options include less-invasive treatments like endometrial ablation and uterine artery ablation as well as definitive therapy with hysterectomy. These are usually reserved for women who have failed other treatments, decline long-term medical therapy, and do not desire future pregnancy.

CONTRACEPTION

Approximately 62% of reproductive-age women in the United States are using some form of contraception and 99% of women who have

ever been sexually active with men have used a form of contraception in their lifetime. However, nearly half of pregnancies in the United States are unintended. When helping patients choose a contraceptive method, several important variables should be considered. Patient preference and likelihood of adherence to a given method are important components to consider in selecting a mode of contraception. Efficacy depends on appropriate use. Patients' past experiences with different forms of contraception and personal preferences help to predict how well they will adhere to current regimens. Observational studies have demonstrated patient-provider relationships are important in family planning care.

Obtaining a thorough personal and family medical history is important to determine what methods are appropriate for a patient. Certain medical issues can make a choice too risky for one patient but provide a health benefit for another. For example, oral contraceptives that increase the risk of thrombosis are contraindicated for a patient with a strong family history of venous thrombosis, but they could correct anemia in a patient with menorrhagia. The patient's sexual history and assessment of the risk for sexually transmitted infections (STIs) play a role in contraceptive choice and education about the use of barrier methods.

Methods of Contraception

Barrier methods include the diaphragm, cervical cap, male condom, and female condom. These methods do not disrupt fertility beyond their moment of use. The diaphragm and cervical cap need to be fitted by a medical professional and therefore require a prescription. With each sexual encounter spermicide must be applied and the device needs to be left in 6 to 8 hours after intercourse to be efficacious. The male condom can be purchased over the counter and is among the most cost-effective options. It has the added benefit of reducing the transmission of STIs. Prevention of conception and STI transmission depends on correct and consistent use: the male condom must be used during the entire sexual act. The female condom is also over the counter and protects against transmission of STIs, though there are less data on decreased STI transmission compared to male condoms.

Combination hormonal contraceptives are the most common form of hormonal birth control. They typically contain a low dose of estrogen (≤35 µg) and one of several progestins. Delivery methods include pills, patches, and intravaginal rings. These methods carry similar contraindications and have the same contraceptive mechanism: prevention of ovulation. Combined oral contraceptives (COCs) are classified as either monophasic, which release a constant hormone dose throughout the menstrual cycle, or multiphasic, which contain variable levels of hormones to be taken over the course of the month. Monophasic COCs are preferred because they have been more extensively studied, may be associated with improved mood variability compared to multiphasic formulations in susceptible women, and are simpler to use. No clear benefit has been demonstrated for multiphasic COCs. Continuous or extended cycle COCs allow for less frequent withdrawal bleeding and more control over timing of withdrawal bleeding, though this can be associated with more unpredictable bleeding. After cessation of combination hormonal contraceptives, menses typically return in 1 month. Fertility and menses are expected in all women within 90 days of stopping the medication.

The transdermal patch is applied weekly for 3 weeks per month followed by a week without the patch in order to allow for withdrawal bleeding. The patch is applied to a different site on the body each time. It delivers a higher average dose of estrogen but lower peak doses. One key difference between COCs and the patch is that the latter bypasses hepatic first pass metabolism; thus, the patch has fewer drug interactions and requires lower peak hormonal doses in order to be effective as compared to COCs. Return to fertility can occur immediately after patch discontinuation because exogenous hormones reach very low levels within 3 days.

The ring is inserted vaginally and left in place for 3 weeks and then removed for 1 week to allow for withdrawal bleeding. Extended ring regimens are possible whereby a new ring is inserted the same day as the prior one is removed. This can be done every 3 weeks for up to a year to delay withdrawal bleeding, though it is associated with spotting. The patch and the ring are reasonable options for patients concerned with taking a daily medication.

Contraindications to combination hormonal contraception are related to the estrogen component. Contraindications include a personal history of a thromboembolic event or known thrombogenic mutation, cerebrovascular accident (CVA), coronary artery disease (CAD), uncontrolled hypertension, migraine with aura, smoking after age 35, breast cancer, estrogen-dependent neoplasms, undiagnosed abnormal vaginal bleeding, liver tumors, and pregnancy. There is no evidence that COCs cause weight gain. Upon initiation, some patients report breast tenderness, nausea, and bloating. Most symptoms go away quickly with continued use. Irregular bleeding typically resolves within 3 months. If COCs are started more than 5 days since onset of menses, back-up contraception is recommended for 7 days.

Potential noncontraceptive benefits of combination oral contraceptives include regulation of menstrual flow and improvement in ovarian cyst recurrence, endometriosis, chronic pelvic pain, acne, polycystic ovarian syndrome, hyperandrogenism, and mittelschmerz (i.e., midcycle pain). Long-term use of combination oral contraceptives has been associated with a reduced lifetime risk of endometrial and ovarian cancers. Bone density is higher in perimenopausal women who used COCs compared to women who did not.

Progesterone-only contraceptives are an option for women intolerant of estrogen or at increased risk for thromboembolic events. They can be taken continuously without a hormone-free interval. Contraindications include active CAD, breast cancer, hepatic tumor, and phlebitis. They are slightly less efficacious than the combination pills, and women may experience breakthrough bleeding. They have a short duration of action and half-life so they must be taken at the same time each day. Back-up contraception is required if a dose is taken more than 3 hours late. Upon cessation, the return of fertility is rapid. Compared to COCs, ovulation is not consistently suppressed.

DMPA is a progesterone-only injection administered every 12 weeks. Major side effects include irregular bleeding (which resolves over time) and amenorrhea (50% at 1 year). Weight gain, hair changes, and acne are possible side effects. The FDA issued a black box warning that DMPA may decrease bone density, especially in adolescents and perimenopausal women. This possible association between DMPA use and fracture risk remains controversial without definitive data; however, a retrospective cohort study found no significant fracture risk difference. Return to fertility can be delayed and is dependent on body weight: women with lower body weights conceive sooner after discontinuation as compared to women with higher body weight. If conception is desired within 1 to 2 years of initiating a contraceptive method, DMPA is not recommended.

The IUD can be a great option for women who do not desire pregnancy in the next 5 to 10 years. Worldwide, it is the most widely used method of reversible contraception. Two types of IUDs are available in the United States, and both are as effective as sterilization. The copper IUD can be left in 10 years. There are four progesterone-emitting IUDs available in the United States and they can be left in from 3 to 5 years depending on the formulation. The copper IUD can be associated with heavier menstrual bleeding and cramps. The progesterone IUD may initially have breakthrough bleeding, but almost one half of users become amenorrheic. Return of fertility is rapid after removal of IUD.

The progesterone contraceptive subdermal implant was originally marketed as Implanon and is now Nexplanon. Unlike Implanon, Nexplanon is radiopaque. It is a 40-mm progesterone rod that is implanted under the skin of the upper arm and is highly effective for 3 years. It can be placed in outpatient offices and is helpful in reducing dysmenorrhea, but it is associated with irregular menses.

Postcoital emergency contraception (EC) can be achieved with one or several hormonal options or with placement of a copper IUD. EC is not considered an abortifacient. It functions to either disrupt ovulation or prevent fertilization. The copper IUD is the most effective option and can be used within 5 days of unprotected intercourse. Hormonal oral contraceptives can be used in a specifically formulated EC dose (Plan B) or off-label with a regimen of COCs. The recommendation is for use of Plan B within 72 hours of unprotected intercourse. It is available without a prescription. Efficacy of hormonal contraception decreases with increasing body mass index (BMI) above 25 kg/m^2. The only absolute contraindication to EC is pregnancy.

INFERTILITY

According to the Centers for Disease Control (CDC), 12% of US women have trouble conceiving. However, infertility is a unique medical condition in that it involves a couple rather than an individual. Infertility is a failure to conceive after 1 year of regular intercourse without contraception in women under age 35 or 6 months in women 35 years and older. The term fecundability is the probability of achieving pregnancy in one menstrual cycle. Impaired fecundity describes women who have difficulty getting pregnant or carrying a pregnancy to term. It is unclear if the prevalence of infertility has changed or if the heightened awareness of infertility is due to the combination of factors such as deferment of pregnancy to later in life, technological advances, and increase in awareness of infertility. Causes of infertility are likely varied among different demographic and socioeconomic groups.

Infertility may be caused by female factors, male factors or both. Approximately 20% to 30% of couples experience unexplained infertility. History should focus on menstrual and contraceptive history, surgeries, sexual dysfunction, medications, and family history of early menopause or reproductive issues. The physical exam should include a thyroid, breast and pelvic exam. The most common female cause is a problem involving ovulation (20% to 35%), followed by tubal disease (20% to 25%) and uterine factors (5% to 15%). Ovulatory dysfunction can be evaluated from patient report, but up to one third of women with normal menses are anovulatory; therefore, objective measures can be used to confirm ovulation with progesterone and LH levels, evaluation of cervical mucus and basal body temperature. Testing also typically includes TSH, FSH, and prolactin levels in women with irregular menses. Initial male evaluation includes semen analysis and a reproductive history. Further testing is performed by reproductive specialists and may include evaluation of ovarian reserve through a transvaginal ultrasound and hysterosalpingography to visualize the uterus and fallopian tubes and ensure tubal patency. The diagnosis of infertility is associated with significant stress for most couples and a provider's awareness can help to mitigate its effects.

PREGNANCY COMPLICATIONS AND RISK OF FUTURE DISEASES

During pregnancy, a woman is typically primarily cared for by her obstetrics provider. However, women with complex medical conditions or pregnancy complications may require a maternal fetal medicine (MFM) specialist or an obstetric medicine specialist to participate in their care. MFM is a specialty in obstetrics and gynecology that manages high-risk pregnancies as well as unexpected complications in pregnancy such as a trauma to the mother, early labor, and bleeding. Obstetric medicine is a specialty of internal medicine that manages medical problems in pregnancy such as hypertension, kidney disease, thyroid disease, diabetes mellitus, and heart disease.

Pregnancy can be associated with exacerbations of chronic illnesses, unmasking a new illness or predicting future disease. An understanding of the long-term consequences of certain complications in pregnancy can smooth the transition back to primary care.

Gestational diabetes affects 4% to 8% of pregnancies in the United States. All pregnant women receiving routine obstetric care are screened for gestational diabetes. Women with a history of gestational diabetes are at increased risk for diabetes later in life. They should be screened 6 to 12 weeks postpartum with an oral glucose tolerance test and diagnosed with nonpregnancy diagnostic criteria for diabetes. They should have lifelong screening at least every 3 years.

Women whose pregnancies were complicated by a gestational hypertensive disorder, such as preeclampsia or gestational hypertension, are at increased risk for subsequent essential hypertension. A history of preeclampsia is associated with twice the risk of heart disease and stroke and four times the risk of hypertension. Currently, there are no additional screening or preventive interventions recommended for these women.

MENOPAUSE

Menopause is defined as the absence of a menstrual period for 12 consecutive months or the cessation of the menstrual cycle due to oophorectomy. The average age at menopause in the United States is 51 years, with a range of 40 to 58 years. Natural menopause prior to the age of 40 is considered premature ovarian failure. Menopause after the age of 55 is considered late menopause. The life expectancy of women in the United States is almost 80 years; therefore, many women spend at least one third of their lifetime in the postmenopausal period. Although symptoms such as hot flashes and vaginal dryness may develop during menopause, the process itself is a normal part of aging for women.

Transition From Perimenopause to Menopause

The transition to menopause can be erratic and prolonged over a 5- to 10-year period. It is characterized by ovarian and endocrine changes that ultimately result in the depletion of primordial oocyte stores and the cessation of ovarian estrogen production. An accelerated loss of follicles begins at about 37 years of age and is correlated with a small increase in FSH and a decrease in inhibin levels. As the FSH concentration increases, the follicular phase of the cycle decreases. One of the earliest clinical signs of the menopausal transition is shortening of the menstrual cycle from a mean length of 30 days in the early reproductive years to 25 days in the early menopausal transition.

Later in the menopausal transition, the few remaining follicles respond poorly to FSH, and anovulation may occur. Menstrual cycles may become erratic with prolonged periods of oligomenorrhea. Ovulation may still occur, and women in this time period are advised to continue effective contraception until 12 months of amenorrhea have occurred. Ultimately, when ovarian follicles are depleted, the ovary no longer secretes estradiol but continues to secrete androgens due to continued stimulation by LH.

Perimenopausal Symptoms

Menstrual irregularities are experienced by almost 75% of women and are usually the first change noticed by women entering the menopausal transition. Although changes in the menstrual flow are expected and

most women can be reassured, clinicians need to be aware of bleeding patterns that may represent underlying pathology and require evaluation.

Sleep disturbances in perimenopausal women are a well-documented phenomenon. Hot flashes can disturb sleep patterns and interfere with sleep quality, resulting in fatigue, irritability, and difficulty concentrating. Vaginal dryness and dyspareunia are common symptoms that can interfere with sexual function and increase the risk of urinary tract infections. Another genitourinary symptom that increases with age is urinary incontinence, which affects approximately 25% of postmenopausal women. The etiology is multifactorial. The endothelium of the bladder and urethra become more fragile and less elastic; urethral tone decreases with age. Uterine prolapse, cystoceles, rectoceles, and increasing BMI all increase the risk of urinary incontinence.

Change in mood is a common complaint during the menopausal transition, but a causative link between hormonal fluctuations and mood disturbances has not been established. Women who experience significant depression around menopause are more likely to have experienced depression earlier in their lives, particularly at times of hormonal change (e.g., postpartum depression, premenstrual dysphoric disorder [PMDD]). Mood issues during the perimenopausal transition should be approached in the same manner as at other ages.

In addition to mood symptoms, many women in perimenopause complain of difficulties with concentration and memory. A large multisite, multiethnic cohort study, the Study of Women's Health Across the Nation (SWAN), demonstrated that women had a small, transient decline in cognitive abilities during perimenopause. However, anxiety and depression also had independent negative effects on cognition. Most epidemiologic studies do not demonstrate an increased risk of depression or a decline in cognitive skills during the menopausal transition.

Hot flashes or vasomotor symptoms are the hallmark symptom of menopause. In the United States, up to 75% of women who experience a natural menopause and 90% of women who experience surgical menopause have vasomotor symptoms. Hot flashes may occur a few times per year or several times each day; 10% to 15% of women have hot flashes that are very frequent or severe. For most women, vasomotor symptoms are self-limited, lasting on average 1 to 2 years; however, up to 25% of women may have symptoms for longer than 5 years.

The exact cause of a hot flash is not understood, although it is related to a disturbance of hypothalamic thermoregulation. A hot flash consists of a sudden onset of a warm sensation over the face and upper body that ranges from mild to markedly uncomfortable. This may be accompanied by significant perspiration and typically lasts 2 to 4 minutes. It can be followed by chills. There are racial and ethnic differences in reported hot flashes, with African American women experiencing higher rates compared with white women and Hispanic and Asian women experiencing lower rates. Frequency of hot flashes is also affected by smoking, obesity, and stress.

In the 1950s, the use of estrogen to relieve hot flashes became widespread. In 1975, a study published in the *New England Journal of Medicine* showed that women who used estrogen for more than 7 years had a 14-fold increase in uterine cancer. Subsequent research determined that the increased risk of endometrial hyperplasia and uterine cancer is reduced to essentially zero when concurrent low-dose progestin is continued for 12 to 13 days per month. Women on estrogen with an intact uterus must use progestin therapy to prevent endometrial hyperplasia and cancer.

Menopausal hormone therapy (MHT) is the use of estrogen or combined estrogen and progestin for women with an intact uterus. MHT remains the most effective treatment of menopausal vasomotor symptoms. It is also FDA approved for the treatment of urogenital atrophy and the prevention of osteoporosis. Evidence suggests that ultra-low-dose estrogen is sufficient to prevent bone loss. Although not FDA approved for treatment of osteoporosis, there is some research supporting its use in preventing fractures and increasing bone density.

Early epidemiologic studies demonstrated a decrease in coronary heart disease (CHD) events in women on MHT. However, the opposite conclusion was found in dedicated randomized trials. One large study demonstrated an overall null effect but an increased number of CHD events in the first year of treatment. Another large randomized controlled trial to evaluate MHT was stopped early because there was more harm than benefit with the treatment intervention. Therefore, menopausal hormone therapy is not recommended for primary prevention of CHD or chronic disease.

Postmenopausal Therapy

Hormone Therapy

Estrogen and estrogen-progestin therapy are appropriate and the most effective treatment for moderate to severe vasomotor symptoms. If hormone therapy is initiated, the lowest dose needed to treat the symptoms should be used and usually for short-term use. Women with a uterus require progesterone and estrogen. Combination MHT is recommended for 3 to 5 years total if initiated and limited by the increased risk of breast cancer. Estrogen-only therapy has a more favorable risk profile and can be used for 7 years in women without a uterus. Oral contraceptives can be used for management of menopausal symptoms for women who require contraception until age 51. The estrogen dose in oral contraceptives is 4 to 7 times higher than in MHT, and thus the use of COCs confers an unnecessary risk to postmenopausal women. One recommendation on determining ability to transition from oral contraception to MHT is to check FSH levels at age 50 to evaluate for menopause. Estrogen administration can be oral, transdermal, or topical. There are some minor differences in their risk profile. For example, transdermal estrogen is associated with decreases in blood pressure compared to oral administration. When administered transdermally, estrogen bypasses liver metabolism resulting in decreased angiotensin production thereby lowering blood pressure. MHT needs to be tapered when stopping because abrupt cessation could cause a recurrence of symptoms.

For women who have primarily vaginal symptoms such as vaginal dryness or urogenital atrophy, referred to as "genitourinary symptoms of menopause," estrogen can be used transvaginally. Transvaginal estrogen can be high dose, in which case it has the risk profile of systemic oral or transdermal MHT. Low-dose transvaginal estrogen does not require progesterone in women who have a uterus and does not confer the same risks as systemic estrogen. For example, the low-dose estrogen ring releases 7.5 mcg of estradiol daily compared to the high dose ring that releases 50 to 100 mcg daily and is considered systemic estrogen.

Nonhormonal Therapies

During the 1990s, newer antidepressants that affect serotonin and/ or norepinephrine (SSRIs and SNRIs) were observed to improve hot flashes. Randomized controlled trials studying the effects of SSRIs and SNRIs on vasomotor symptoms have demonstrated varied efficacy, but a large meta-analysis and systemic review found all SSRIs were more effective than placebo; escitalopram was found to be the most effective. However, the only FDA-approved nonhormonal treatment for hot flashes is paroxetine.

Gabapentin and pregabalin have also been demonstrated to decrease intensity and frequency of hot flashes. One study found the efficacy of gabapentin to be comparable to SSRIs. Clonidine is another nonhormonal option but is considered second line because it is typically poorly tolerated due to dizziness and dry mouth. In practice, the SSRIs/SNRIs and gabapentin/pregabalin are commonly used off-label given demonstrated efficacy.

Complementary Therapy

As many as 75% of menopausal women have used some form of alternative or complementary treatment to relieve menopausal symptoms. Behavioral options such as dressing in layers, regular exercise, stress reduction techniques, and avoidance of known triggers are safe and may be helpful for many women. Cognitive behavioral therapy has also been demonstrated to be modestly effective. Some of the more common herbal remedies for menopausal symptoms include isoflavones and phytoestrogens (e.g., soy, chickpeas, red clover) and black cohosh. None of these therapies has been shown to decrease hot flashes beyond placebo.

BREAST PAIN, DISCHARGE, AND MASSES

Breast pain, masses, and nipple discharge are common symptoms that providers face when taking care of female patients. Women who present with breast symptoms often fear that any abnormality indicates the presence of malignancy. Although it is essential to keep breast cancer on the differential diagnosis throughout the clinical evaluation, most breast-related complaints are not manifestations of cancer. For example, in recent studies, breast pain was a presenting symptom in close to 6% of women who had breast cancer, whereas 70% of women report breast pain over the course of their lifetime.

Mastalgia

Breast pain can originate from the breast tissue itself, which is termed "true mastalgia," or appear as referred pain from the chest wall. Chest wall pain is often isolated to the medial or lateral side of the breast. Intercostal nerves originating from T3 to T5 innervate the breast and nipple. Any irritation along their course can lead to pain experienced in the breast. Causes of nerve irritation include cervical and thoracic spondylosis, lung disease, and gallstones.

True mastalgia is often classified as cyclical or non-cyclical pain. Etiologies of non-cyclical pain include trauma, mastitis, superficial thrombophlebitis, cysts or tumors. Cyclical breast pain is the most common type of breast pain and is hormone dependent. The onset of pain occurs during the weeks before menstruation, and the start of menstruation marks resolution. A unifying etiology of cyclical breast pain remains unclear. Studies demonstrate that progesterone, prolactin, ratio of fatty acids, and type of estrogen receptors may play a role. The presence of breast pain in women on hormone replacement therapy suggests that hormones have a causative impact; however, hormone manipulation rather than concentration of estrogen appears to influence the occurrence of pain. Amount of caffeine intake has not been shown to have any impact on developing mastalgia, despite popular belief.

Evaluation of mastalgia often consists of age-appropriate breast cancer screening. Focal pain and pain that is progressively worsening may warrant further imaging. Unfortunately, obtaining a history of symptoms that follow a cyclical versus non-cyclical pattern has not proven to help differentiate between etiologies of pain.

Research shows that most women presenting with mastalgia respond well to reassurance. Adjustments in type of brassiere or additional breast support during the night can improve pain levels. Treatments with proven effectiveness for cyclical pain include danazol, tamoxifen, progestogen, and progesterone, as well as non-hormone–based therapies including selective serotonin reuptake inhibitors and the fruit extract agnus castus. Use of therapies such as danazol and tamoxifen are limited by side effects of the medications. NSAIDS and steroid injections have been effective in managing chest wall pain.

Nipple Discharge

Based on history and examination, nipple discharge can be classified into three categories to guide evaluation and management. If the discharge is serous, sanguineous, or serosanguineous, spontaneously occurring, unilateral, originating from a single duct, and found to be reproducible on examination, then a mammogram and ultrasound are recommended for women over 30. An ultrasound is recommended as initial evaluation for women under 30. If the discharge is milky and bilateral, then a pregnancy test followed by a work-up for galactorrhea should be initiated. Work-up includes measuring TSH and prolactin levels. In women over 40, if the discharge is nonspontaneous, originates from multiple ducts, and cannot be characterized as serous, sanguineous, or serosanguineous, a diagnostic mammography plus ultrasonography is recommended. For women younger than 40, observation and education around avoiding nipple manipulation is appropriate. In summary, nipple discharge suggestive of malignancy occurs without provocation, is persistent, unilateral, presents in an older patient, is of serous, sanguineous, or serosanguineous quality or is associated with a mass or lump.

Breast Masses

There are four categories of breast masses: abscesses, benign masses, benign tumors, and cancer. Benign masses are further subdivided into categories of nonproliferative (i.e., cyst), proliferative without atypia (i.e., fibroadenoma), and atypical hyperplasia, which guide further evaluation and predict risk of becoming malignant. Cancerous masses are typically painless, occur in older women, and do not vary by menstrual cycle. Although breast cancers have characteristically been described as hard and immobile with irregular borders, no self or clinical examination finding reliably distinguishes between a benign and cancerous mass.

For women over 30, any palpable mass requires a diagnostic mammogram. Further diagnostic evaluation depends on a combination of radiographic qualities (i.e., solid vs. fluid filled) classified according to the Breast Imaging Reporting Data System (BI-RADS) and level of clinical suspicion. For example, if a mass gets a BI-RADS classification of 1, then an ultrasound is recommended. If it gets a BI-RADS classification of 4, then a tissue biopsy follows. For masses rated as BI-RADS 1 to 3, ultrasound findings in combination with clinical suspicion guide further evaluation versus observation. For women under 30, if clinical suspicion for malignancy is low, then a mass can be observed for several menstrual cycles. If clinical suspicion is high, then an ultrasound is the first line of imaging. BI-RADS from the ultrasound reading guides additional testing. If biopsies prove negative for malignancy or imaging determines that the mass is a cyst, masses are surgically removed and cysts aspirated only if the patient is symptomatic.

Breast Cancer Screening

Breast cancer is the most common type of cancer in women. Despite significant prevalence, it has a high survival rate of close to 90% at 5 years, which is attributed to early detection and effective treatment. Individuals are considered high risk for breast cancer if they have a personal history of breast cancer, a previous diagnosis of a high-risk breast lesion, a genetic mutation associated with risk for developing breast cancer, or if they have received radiation therapy to the chest. Although other risk factors such as early menarche, late menopausal onset, oral contraceptive or menopausal hormone therapy, increased breast density on mammography, and family member with a history of breast cancer have been identified, they do not change an individual's

categorization as average or high risk according to most guidelines. Screening consists of a mammogram for average-risk patients and an MRI in addition to mammography for high-risk patients. Different medical societies and international health organizations offer different guidelines regarding the appropriate age to begin screening for breast cancer in average risk women. These guidelines shift based on the results of risk-benefit models and the current data available. Current recommendations from US Preventive Services Task Force (USPSTF) are for screening average-risk women at age 50 and continuing every 2 years until age 75 years. Shared decision making around starting screening between age 40 and 49 should take place between the patient and provider. The American College of Obstetrics and Gynecology, in contrast, recommends that screening should start at age 40. Harms from screening mammography include false-positive results that could lead to overdiagnosis and overtreatment. Self-exams and breast exams as part of a routine physical for the purpose of screening are no longer recommended by most medical societies.

CERVICAL CANCER SCREENING

Cervical cancer screening is an important example of success in preventative medicine over the second half of the last century: mortality rates decreased by 50% between 1975 and 2008. In women found to have cervical cancer, 50% percent of them had not undergone screening in the preceding 3 to 5 years. The success of screening rests on the fact that cervical cancer progresses slowly.

Infections with high-risk strains of HPV (16 and 18) are responsible for approximately 70% of cervical cancer cases. Peak incidence of HPV infection occurs among women younger than 25 years of age, but most of these infections are transient. Approximately 10% of women remain HPV positive 5 years after infection. Current guidelines recommend Papanicolaou (Pap) tests with cytology starting at age 21 to be repeated every 3 years if normal. At age 30, both cytology and HPV co-testing can be sent and if both are negative, then testing can be spaced to every 5 years until age 65. A Pap test obtains cervical cells that are analyzed for the presence of abnormal cells to identify squamous intraepithelial lesions (SIL). SIL identified in the cytological report mandates a cervical biopsy via colposcopy. Biopsy results are graded in terms of cervical intraepithelial lesion (CIN) 1, 2 or 3. Depending on grade, they are treated and then monitored for possible progression into cancer according to a different algorithm of surveillance than normal screening. In addition, recommendations for screening differ for women who have had diethylstilbestrol (DES) exposure in utero or for women who are immunocompromised. The CDC recommends vaccination for HPV starting at age 11 and 12 (see *CDC Vaccines and Preventable Diseases* for full recommendations).

OSTEOPOROSIS

Eighty percent of the ten million Americans with osteoporosis are women. The risk of osteoporosis increases with age. Estrogen is protective of bones and many women experience significant bone density loss in the 5 to 7 years after menopause. Approximately one in two women over the age of 50 will experience a bone fracture due to osteoporosis. These fractures are associated with significant morbidity and mortality both directly and indirectly related to the fracture, including acute myocardial infarction, pulmonary embolus, loss of independence, decreased quality of life, and multiple hospitalizations. Twenty-one percent to 30% of patients with a hip fracture die within 1 year.

The USPSTF recommends screening for osteoporosis in average risk white women age 65 and older with bone density evaluation. The most common method of bone density evaluation is dual-energy x-ray absorptiometry (DXA) of the hip and lumbar spine. Several risk assessment tools exist to evaluate a woman's risk of osteoporosis. The most commonly used is the FRAX tool. Risk factors for osteoporosis include a family history of hip fracture, smoking, long-term steroid use, and low body weight. Women younger than age 65 with at least one risk factor should have their osteoporosis risk assessed and then have bone density evaluation if their risk equals that of a 65-year-old white woman without risk factors. The recommendation is based on the risk of osteoporosis in white women because they have been historically the population studied. Ethnic background affects risk and management of osteoporosis, and racial minorities are diagnosed and treated less frequently. Women found to have osteoporosis who are treated have a moderate reduction in osteoporotic fracture. Treatment options include bisphosphonates, estrogen, and raloxifene. Individuals with osteopenia and osteoporosis are recommended to have adequate calcium and vitamin D intake through diet and/or supplements.

INTIMATE PARTNER VIOLENCE

IPV is a preventable public health problem that affects 1 in 4 American women during their lifetime. Nearly half of female homicide victims in the United States are killed by a current or former male intimate partner. IPV is any behavior that causes physical, sexual or psychological harm by a current or former intimate partner or spouse. There are numerous health consequences beyond the direct effects of IPV such as depression, anxiety disorders, chronic pain, and posttraumatic stress disorder (PTSD). Even when historical or physical examination clues are evident, IPV often remains undiagnosed by providers.

The USPSTF recommends that clinicians screen for IPV in women of childbearing age and refer women who screen positive to support services. The strongest evidence supporting screening is in women who are pregnant or postpartum, but the recommendation is to screen all women of childbearing age. There are several screening instruments to detect IPV. When screening for and discussing IPV, the clinician must be nonjudgmental, compassionate, and ensure confidentiality. Clinicians should normalize the screening interview with an explanation of IPV as an important health issue.

Identified risk factors for IPV victimization include younger age, female sex, lower SES, and a family history or personal history of violence. Suspicion for IPV should increase when there is a history of frequent emergency room visits, delay in seeking treatment, an inconsistent explanation of injuries, missed appointments, repeated abortions, late initiation of prenatal care or medication noncompliance. If a patient appears with an inappropriate affect, overly attentive or verbally abusive partner, apparent social isolation, and reluctance to undress or difficulty with examination of genitals or rectum, providers should further evaluate for IPV. Patients who are experiencing IPV present with a diverse range of complaints that include somatic and psychological symptoms as well as sexually transmitted infections. Women who screen positive for IPV should be evaluated for their risk of immediate harm. They should be provided with information about safety planning and a list of local and national resources.

OBESITY, METABOLIC SYNDROME, AND POLYCYSTIC OVARY SYNDROME

Obesity/Metabolic Syndrome

Rates of obesity (BMI >30) have increased in recent decades, yielding a rate of 40% in US adults in 2016. Overall, obesity appears to affect men and women equally, although the distribution by income varies by sex. Women in the lowest socioeconomic group have the highest rates of

obesity. Men in the highest and lowest socioeconomic groups had a higher rate of obesity compared to the middle-income group. Obesity increases the risk for many diseases. In women, central obesity (waist-hip ratio >0.9) predicts the risk of CAD. The risk of many cancers (e.g., endometrial cancer, breast cancer, kidney cancer, ovarian cancer) is increased for obese individuals. Obesity has specific implications for women during pregnancy, increasing the risk of numerous pregnancy-related complications, including gestational diabetes mellitus, fetal macrosomia, hypertension, shoulder dystocia, and cesarean delivery, and contributes to postpartum complications such as thrombosis and infection. Obesity is also associated with irregular menses and higher rates of anovulation.

The risk of cardiovascular disease related to the metabolic syndrome appears to have a stronger correlation in women. There are several definitions of the metabolic syndrome. The most commonly used defines metabolic syndrome as the presence of three or more of five risk factors that increase the chance of developing heart disease or stroke: central obesity, elevated triglyceride levels, low levels of high-density lipoprotein (HDL) cholesterol, hypertension, and impaired fasting glucose values. Women with the metabolic syndrome should be monitored and counseled about their increased risk of cardiovascular events and overt diabetes mellitus.

Polycystic Ovary Syndrome

PCOS is a complex endocrine disorder without a known etiology that affects approximately 5% to 10% of women worldwide. The key diagnostic criteria are androgen excess, ovulatory dysfunction and/or polycystic ovaries. The most commonly used diagnostic criteria is the Rotterdam 2003 criteria which requires two out of three of the above criteria. Risk factors for PCOS include first-degree relatives with PCOS, diabetes mellitus, obesity, and certain ethnic groups such as Mexican Americans. Reproductive and metabolic effects include anovulation, infertility, acne, hirsutism, obesity, nonalcoholic fatty liver disease, and metabolic syndrome. Increased insulin resistance is a significant consequence of the syndrome, increasing the risk of type 2 diabetes, particularly in obese women. Therefore, women with a diagnosis of PCOS require screening for diabetes.

Management of PCOS is primarily symptom based. For women who are overweight or obese, lifestyle modifications are recommended. COCs are the first line in PCOS to regulate menses and decrease hyperandrogenism in women not attempting to conceive. After COCs, second-line treatment for hyperandrogenism is an antiandrogen such as spironolactone or finasteride. Insulin sensitivity can be increased with metformin and thiazolidinediones. Metformin also regulates menses. These medications are contraindicated during pregnancy, and an effective form of contraception is required because these medications are teratogenic. Women with PCOS often struggle to conceive. Ovulation-inducing medications such as clomiphene citrate or letrozole are frequently required. Women with PCOS are at increased risk for endometrial and ovarian cancers. COCs decrease risk for endometrial hyperplasia and may decrease risk of endometrial cancer.

FIBROMYALGIA

The prevalence of fibromyalgia ranges from 2% to 8% depending on the diagnostic criteria used. Historically, the diagnosis of fibromyalgia has been significantly more common in women. Original diagnostic criteria involved the quantity of tender points present on exam. Either women were likely to report more tender points or the symptom manifestation between women and men differed, which led to a disproportionate number of women with the condition as compared to men. With the change in diagnostic criteria, however, the disease has a smaller female to male ratio at 2:1. Since 2011, diagnosis has been determined by a symptom survey. Because of the vague set of symptoms and lack of laboratory findings, it has been a complicated and controversial diagnosis that continues to evolve.

Fibromyalgia is characterized by persistent pain, sleep disturbance, and fatigue lasting more than 3 months. The pain state is thought to be driven by how the central nervous system interprets peripheral nociceptive input. The central nervous system magnifies a given signal based on the levels of neurotransmitters, which then intensifies the pain response. The centralized pain phenomenon can be associated with other chronic pain states that have similar pathophysiology involving a specific organ system, such as chronic headaches, dysmenorrhea, irritable bowel syndrome, interstitial cystitis, or endometriosis. In addition, 10% to 30% of rheumatologic conditions are thought to have fibromyalgia as an associated diagnosis. The etiology is likely multifactorial, involving the influence of the environment, infection, and genetic predisposition.

Physical exam without any findings other than diffuse tenderness to palpation is characteristic. Treatment recommendations involve an integrated approach including both pharmacologic and nonpharmacologic modalities. Studies show that gabapentinoids, serotonin norepinephrine reuptake inhibitors, and gamma-hydroxybutyrate have efficacy in addressing symptoms of fibromyalgia. Choice of medication should be driven by predominant symptom, but multiple agents from different classes can be used for a synergistic effect. General patient-centered education, exercise, cognitive behavioral therapy, as well as some complementary and alternative medicine therapies such as tai chi, yoga, acupuncture, and trigger point injections, have been shown to be effective in increasing functionality. Setting expectations around the fact that fibromyalgia is a chronic disease that needs to be managed is an important part of the clinical care of these patients.

INTERSTITIAL CYSTITIS/HYPERSENSITIVE BLADDER

Interstitial cystitis, bladder pain syndrome, hypersensitive bladder, or painful bladder syndrome is a diagnosis that has evolved, changed names, and included different criteria for diagnosis over time. Based on literature from the Society for Urodynamics and Female Urology (SUFU), which was adapted by the American Urological Association, the current definition of interstitial cystitis is: "an unpleasant sensation (pain, pressure, discomfort) perceived to be related to the urinary bladder, associated with lower urinary tract symptoms of more than 6 weeks' duration, in the absence of infection or other identifiable causes." Interstitial cystitis disproportionately affects women, with studies reporting ratios ranging from 2:1 to 8:1. It most often presents in the fourth decade of life. Quality-of-life scores demonstrate a significant negative impact on functioning. Diagnosis involves ruling out infection or other physiologic causes of symptoms. No lab test aids in the diagnosis of the disease; however, antinuclear antibodies are often present and can confound the diagnosis. Based on symptoms and risk factors different imaging modalities may be employed.

The exact etiology remains unknown. Possibilities include epithelial dysfunction, neurogenic inflammation on the level of the urothelium, and mast cell activation leading to a heightened pain response. Theories involving central amplification of a pain signal, similar to the pathophysiology used to explain pain in fibromyalgia, have been applied to interstitial cystitis. Hunner lesion interstitial cystitis is defined by the presence of well-circumscribed reddened mucosal areas with small vessels radiating towards a central scar visualized on cystoscopy. This form of the disease most often occurs in older patients and presents

with more severe symptoms and fewer associated other chronic pain conditions. Treatment involves an elimination diet geared towards decreasing foods with high acid and potassium content. Fulguration and electrocautery can be performed by a urologist.

Patients without identifiable lesions are more likely to have dyspareunia, vulvodynia, and bowel symptoms in addition to having more comorbid conditions. Guidelines for treatment involve starting with conservative options and progressing to more aggressive measures only in the case that initial treatments fail. Treatment often begins with diet modifications. Other nonpharmacologic approaches include pelvic floor physical therapy, cognitive behavioral therapy, and complementary therapy such as acupuncture and massage. Tricyclic antidepressants and antihistamines have led to a decrease in symptoms and an increase in functional status. Intravesical injections of BOTOX and combinations of dimethyl sulfoxide, heparin, or lidocaine, as well as nerve blocks and neuromodulators have been shown to be effective.

HUMAN IMMUNODEFICIENCY VIRUS INFECTION

HIV demands special attention in women's health care due to both epidemiologic and pathophysiologic factors. In the United States, only 7% of people with known HIV infections were women when the epidemic began; however, women now account for 25% of the population of people living with HIV, with women representing 20% of new infections in 2017. There is a higher incidence in rates of infection in African American women, which points to an inequality in education regarding HIV transmission and access to care. Heterosexual sexual encounters cause most HIV infections in women. Unprotected vaginal sex is a much higher risk for women than for men, and unprotected anal sex carries higher risk than unprotected vaginal sex.

The virus itself has a different physiologic impact on women: women typically have lower viral loads than men despite the same level of CD4 counts. Yet the rates of disease progression and opportunistic infections are similar for men and women. Awareness of gynecologic infections as initial manifestations of HIV/AIDS is important when treating women. Counseling for women of childbearing age around risk for vertical transmission and infection through breast milk are important considerations.

Although antiretroviral therapy and follow-up monitoring are similar for men and women with HIV/AIDS, general primary care for women with HIV requires special considerations. Risk for cervical abnormalities and cervical cancer is related to the degree of immunosuppression, age, and co-infection with high-risk HPV genotypes (16, 18, 52, and 58). Women with HIV infection are more likely to progress more rapidly to cervical cancer. The CDC recommends two cervical cytology screens at 6-month intervals in the first year after an HIV diagnosis and then annually. If there are three normal screens, then testing can be every 3 years. For more detail see the HIV opportunistic infection guidelines at *CDC.gov*. Vulvar and perianal intraepithelial neoplasia are more common in women with HIV than HIV-seronegative women, therefore any lesions present need careful evaluation.

EATING DISORDERS

Eating disorders are disturbances to a person's eating behaviors that result in significant health or psychosocial impairment. They often involve having a distorted body image. Common eating disorders include binge eating disorder, bulimia nervosa, and anorexia nervosa. Median age of onset is between 18 and 21 years old. The lifetime prevalence of binge eating disorder, bulimia nervosa, and anorexia nervosa are 2.8%, 1.0%, and 0.6%, respectively. Rates of eating disorders are increasing, and white females tend to be disproportionately affected. According to the National Institute of Mental Health, the prevalence of eating disorders ranges between 2 to 5 times higher in women than in men. In contrast, some studies based on clinical practice have found a 20- to 30-fold higher prevalence in women. There is a high comorbidity with other mental disorders, primarily anxiety disorders. Physicians who care for adolescents should monitor weight and BMI and screen for alterations in body image and behaviors that suggest disordered eating. A number of screening instruments are available. Somatic symptoms are common and include dyspnea, chest pain, headache, and gastrointestinal problems. Self-induced vomiting is associated with erosion of dental enamel, parotid gland swelling, scarring or calluses on the dorsum of the hand, and esophageal complications such as Mallory-Weiss syndrome. Individuals with eating disorders should be evaluated for severe medical complications that require hospitalization. Unstable vital signs, moderate to severe refeeding syndrome and dehydration are indications for hospitalization for medical stabilization. Long-term treatment of anorexia may require inpatient hospitalization if there is minimal response to outpatient treatment or weight remains under 70% to 75% of ideal body weight. Management of eating disorders often requires a multidisciplinary approach with a primary care physician, psychologist, and nutritionist. Treatment for binge eating disorder is typically CBT. Treatment for bulimia includes a combination of pharmacotherapy, of which fluoxetine is first line, and psychotherapy. Treatment for anorexia is nutritional rehab and psychotherapy. If individuals fail to respond to outpatient treatment, they may require inpatient treatment for closer monitoring and more intensive treatment.

CARDIOVASCULAR DISEASE

CAD remains the leading cause of death for both women and men; however, significant sex and gender differences in the epidemiology, pathophysiology, and clinical manifestations of cardiovascular disease exist. Women with ischemic heart disease are more likely than men to experience atypical symptoms, such as fatigue, abdominal pain, indigestion, nausea and vomiting, and shortness of breath. These non-classic symptoms may partially explain why women tend to seek health care later than men. Even when women seek health care, they have a longer time to diagnosis and a longer time to medical intervention than men. Women are also more likely to have sudden cardiac death at presentation. They are less likely to receive proven effective therapies, such as β-blockers, aspirin, thrombolytics, and statins, and they are less often referred for invasive testing and coronary artery bypass grafting (CABG). Women are also more likely to die after a myocardial infarction and CABG compared with men. Inequalities are at play in the management of heart disease along racial lines: African American women are offered reperfusion therapy and coronary angiography at lower rates, and in-hospital mortality rates are higher compared with those of white women.

Women who present with acute coronary syndrome more frequently have coronary arteries absent of thrombus, but with distal emboli. This points to pathophysiologic differences in ischemic heart disease based on sex. Vasoreactivity and endothelial dysfunction are more common in women, which is demonstrated in the phenomenon of spontaneous coronary artery dissection, an underdiagnosed cause of acute coronary syndromes (ACS) seen in women between the ages of 45 and 60 and associated with pregnancy and the postpartum period. Takotsubo syndrome (stress cardiomyopathy) represents an estimated 8% of ACS cases in women, whereas it is the cause of less than 1% of ACS cases in men. Women with ischemic heart disease tend to present with ACS an average of 7 to 10 years later than men. The predominance

of disease in women post menopause suggests the protective role of higher estrogen states. Estrogen enhances HDL cholesterol and influences atherosclerotic plaque progression and regression. Estrogen may also be beneficial due to its vasodilatory, anti-inflammatory, and antioxidative properties.

Much of the evidence used to guide the treatment of coronary disease in women is based on trials that predominantly enrolled men. The studied treatments and interventions may not induce the same benefit and may even cause harm. For example, due to the tendency for women to have smaller arteries and fewer lesions, initial noninvasive tests have a higher likelihood of producing false-positive results that lead to invasive testing for evaluation of obstructive CAD.

PRECONCEPTION COUNSELING AND PRE-PREGNANCY CARE

Preconception counseling involves a combination of taking a thorough social, family, and medical history to assess potential risks to the mother and potential fetus and offering guidance around maintaining a healthy lifestyle, nutritional supplementation, and avoidance of potential toxins. The first step of a visit involves assessing desire of the patient to become pregnant, discussing what factors are influencing her decision, and offering contraception if pregnancy is not wanted. Women with a personal or family history of genetic disorders may benefit from formal genetic counseling. During a preconception visit, blood work is assessed and immunizations can be administered.

All prescribed and over-the-counter medications and herbal supplements need review to identify potential teratogens. Medications not considered necessary for the well-being of the mother should be stopped. This is not always possible or indicated for women treated for chronic medical conditions where the risk in stopping the medication outweighs the potential harm to the fetus. All women planning pregnancy or capable of becoming pregnant should be advised to take a daily multivitamin with folic acid (400 µg) to reduce the risks of neural tube defects and other congenital anomalies, including cardiovascular defects, urinary defects, and cleft lip.

Medical conditions known to increase the risk of adverse pregnancy outcomes for women and their offspring include obesity, diabetes, thyroid disease, seizure disorders, hypertension, rheumatoid arthritis, chronic renal disease, thrombophilias, asthma, and cardiovascular disease. Preconception care of these conditions can improve pregnancy outcomes. Patients usually are referred to high-risk pregnancy care for evaluation. Addressing obesity prior to pregnancy is important because although higher BMIs lead to adverse outcomes for both the woman and baby, weight loss should not occur during pregnancy.

Approximately 1% of pregnancies in the United States are complicated by pregestational diabetes. Gestational diabetes (GDM) occurs in approximately 7% of pregnancies. GDM has a high recurrence rate (30% to 80%) in subsequent pregnancies and a significantly increased risk for future development of type 2 diabetes. In women with pregestational diabetes and GDM, adequate control of diabetes reduces the risk of congenital malformations. Goal for HbA_{1C} prior to conception is less than 6.5%.

Hyperthyroidism and overt hypothyroidism occur in approximately 0.2% and 2.5% of all pregnancies, respectively. Adequate treatment of thyroid illness improves pregnancy outcomes. Approximately 70% to 80% of women with rheumatoid arthritis experience remission of disease during pregnancy, although the remaining women have active or worsening disease in pregnancy. Women with systemic lupus erythematosus (SLE) often experience exacerbations in pregnancy. SLE increases the risk of adverse fetal outcomes, including spontaneous abortion, fetal growth restriction, and preterm birth. Maternal mortality is associated with conditions such as pulmonary hypertension (especially Eisenmenger's syndrome), congenital heart disease with hypoxia and poor functional class, and arrhythmias.

Assessing for substance use and providing support around abstinence from tobacco, alcohol, and other illicit substances is important in addressing fertility concerns, for the general well-being of the woman, and for the development of the fetus. Routine laboratory evaluation includes rubella titer, varicella titer (in women with a negative history of varicella), hepatitis B surface antigen, and a complete blood count to assess for hemoglobinopathy. Women should receive screening for HIV, chlamydia, and syphilis.

Immunity to measles, mumps, rubella, tetanus, diphtheria, poliomyelitis, and varicella should be ensured through vaccination. Women should receive influenza vaccine in pregnancy due to the increased risk of complications from influenza infection. Ideally, women should receive all indicated vaccinations at least 1 month before conception. Live vaccines (e.g., rubella) should not be given during pregnancy.

PERINATAL DEPRESSION

Depression during pregnancy and in the postpartum period is a significant and common occurrence for childbearing women. Although more efforts to understand the cause, impact, and adequate management are emerging, stigma and underdiagnosis have led to missed opportunities to provide women with appropriate care. Defining and categorizing the specific type of depression particular to this period varies, thereby making it more challenging to study, recognize, and treat. Perinatal depression as delineated by ACOG is defined as major or minor episodes of depression that occur during pregnancy or within the first 12 months after delivery. The DSM-V, however, defines postpartum depression (PPD) as the onset of depressive symptoms within the first 4 weeks of delivery. Studies show that 33% of women with PPD had symptoms during pregnancy, whereas 27% had symptoms pre-pregnancy. In 2016, USPSTF issued a recommendation for routine depression screening in the general adult population and specifically including pregnant and postpartum women, which highlights perinatal depression as a condition worthy of attention but at the same time does not clearly delineate it from other types of depression.

Changes in sleep, appetite, and libido directly caused by responsibilities associated with caring for a newborn may complicate evaluation of postpartum depression based on symptomatology. Postpartum, 50% of women experience a change in mood, called "postpartum blues," marked by intensified emotions that are transient, lasting for the first few weeks after birth. Postpartum blues can develop into PPD. Anxiety or obsessions regarding the health and safety of the baby are common in the postpartum period; the degree to which these thoughts and feelings lead to a debilitating state varies and thereby drives the diagnosis of the psychological condition of PPD. Studies of PPD have found that 20% of women with this diagnosis have suicidal thoughts. Risk factors for PPD include depression and anxiety during pregnancy, traumatic birth experience, previous history of depression, and complications in the health of the infant.

Pathophysiology is multifactorial, likely including genetic, hormonal, immune, and social influences. Although changes in hormones have been assumed to be at the center of PPD, studies have failed to demonstrate a clear association between reproductive levels in women with PPD. Management should be driven by severity of symptoms. First steps involve providing support around self-care and psychosocial needs, which includes encouraging exercise and sleep. In moderate cases, cognitive behavioral therapy and the addition of an SSRI is recommended. In severe cases, additional classes of antidepressants are added, if a switch in SSRI does not yield improvement. ECT

is recommended when suicidality and/or psychosis are present. The FDA has recently approved a treatment for severe postpartum depression that consists of an intravenous formulation of allopregnanolone, a steroid that works on GABA receptors. However, applicability only to women with severe symptoms and cost limit current use of this medication.

SEXUAL DYSFUNCTION

Sexual dysfunction is a term that describes a range of sexual health–related concerns that cause personal distress. The etiology is often multifactorial with psychological, sociocultural, biologic, and physiologic components. It is experienced by approximately 40% of women in the United States. Women around menopause, between the ages of 45 and 65, are most commonly affected. It is often underdiagnosed and undertreated. Numerous medical conditions can impact sexual function due to changes in desire, arousal, orgasm or the presence of pain. Aging itself is associated with decreased libido and sexual responsiveness. The decline in estrogen during menopause causes thinning of the vaginal epithelium, decreased vaginal elasticity, and decreased lubrication. Medications are also implicated in sexual dysfunction, most commonly SSRIs. Evaluation includes a thorough medical and sexual history and the physical exam should also include testing for STIs. Management depends on the etiology but is frequently multifactorial. Some treatment options include pelvic physical therapy, psychotherapy or sex therapy, and mindfulness-based interventions. Pharmacologic options are limited but there are two recently FDA-approved medications. Flibanserin is a daily oral medication approved for premenopausal women with low sexual desire; however, its use is limited by a black box warning, an interaction with alcohol, and significant nausea and dizziness. Bremelanotide, a subcutaneous injection administered as needed prior to sexual activity, was approved in June 2019 for premenopausal women with low sexual desire. Hormone therapies such as systemic estrogen and testosterone have been used off label. Systemic estrogen was not found to improve sexual dysfunction in postmenopausal women in the Women's Health Initiative. Testosterone has been found to improve sexual dysfunction in peri- and postmenopausal women in most studies. Testosterone is metabolized to estrogen, thus its use can be associated with abnormal uterine bleeding and breast symptoms.

PELVIC PAIN

Pelvic pain is characterized as acute or chronic, and both types are commonly encountered in primary care practice. Acute pelvic pain usually manifests over hours to days and may be gynecologic, gastrointestinal, or urologic in origin. Life-threatening conditions, including ruptured ectopic pregnancy and appendicitis, need to be ruled out. Gynecologic causes include complications of pregnancy, acute pelvic infection, and ovarian pathology, including cyst and torsion.

Chronic pelvic pain (CPP) is lower abdominal pain of at least 6 months' duration, and it is severe enough to cause functional impairment or require treatment. Approximately 10% of ambulatory gynecologic referrals are for CPP. The history obtained for evaluation of CPP should include characteristics of the pain; a thorough review of systems; prior medical, surgical, gynecologic, and obstetric history; and a thorough psychiatric and social history, including episodes of domestic violence as a child or an adult and periods of substance abuse.

The most common conditions associated with CPP are endometriosis, chronic pelvic inflammatory disease, interstitial cystitis, irritable bowel syndrome, pelvic floor myalgia, myofascial pain, and neuralgia.

Interstitial cystitis or painful bladder syndrome is a clinical diagnosis consisting of pain, pressure, or discomfort related to the bladder and associated with lower urinary tract symptoms lasting more than 6 weeks and occurring in the absence of infection or other identifiable causes. Mental health issues, including substance abuse, somatization, depression, and physical or sexual abuse, can also cause CPP and are important to identify so that women need not undergo unnecessary testing and interventions.

Physical examination should assess for focal areas of pain, scars, hernias, or masses in the abdomen, and a pelvic examination should be performed. After the most likely diagnosis has been identified, an empirical, targeted treatment may be instituted and followed for efficacy. Further work-up should be considered if the patient does not respond or symptoms change. If empirical therapy and a thorough investigation do not yield a diagnosis, laparoscopy may be considered to identify pelvic pathology.

Any identified peripheral etiology to CPP should be treated; however, CPP of unclear etiology is common and does not have definitive treatment. Depending on the underlying cause, management strategies may include heat therapy (for musculoskeletal pain), counseling and psychiatric referral, gastrointestinal referral, medications (e.g., gabapentin for neuropathic pain, NSAIDs, hormonal contraceptives), hysterectomy, and nerve transection procedures. Multidisciplinary approaches, including medications and interventions that address dietary and psychosocial factors, may be superior to medical treatment alone.

GENDER AND FEMALE SEXUAL MINORITIES

The health care needs of female sexual and gender minorities have significant overlap with the general population but require specific attention and sensitivity given significant barriers to care and differences in both sexual health concerns and certain medical issues. Females who have sex with females come from diverse racial, ethnic, and socioeconomic backgrounds and may choose to identify as lesbian, gay, or bisexual or transgender. Gender minorities, such as individuals who identify as transgender or genderqueer, identify and/or express a different gender than the gender traditionally associated with their assigned sex at birth. Gender and sexual minorities are significantly more likely than heterosexual women to experience implicit and explicit discrimination during health care visits. Many providers do not take a sexual history or inquire about sexual orientation. Health care providers may inadvertently assume heterosexuality and communicate heterosexist attitudes, making it more difficult for patients to disclose their sexual orientation. A lack of cultural competency means that providers do not understand appropriate terminology around gender identity and sexual orientation, which can create further challenges in provider-patient relationships.

Rates of STIs between females who have sex with females are not well studied; however, the assumption that there is lower risk for STIs through female-female sex as compared to heterosexual intercourse is not based in adequate research. Female-female sex allows for transmission of infection through vaginal fluids, menstrual blood, mucosal contact, and via sex toys. Dental dams, condoms, or latex sheet provide a barrier for transmission of bacterial and viral infections. Using condoms on sex toys and cleaning sex toys between use can decrease the spread of infection. Lubrication can also decrease infection transmission by preventing breakdown and bleeding of mucosal areas. Rates of bacterial vaginosis are higher in females who have sex with females, which has suggested transmissibility of bacterial vaginosis and that it should be classified as an STI.

Sexual minorities should receive the same age-appropriate preventative health care and cancer screenings as heterosexual women. For transgender individuals, the decision as to whether to screen for breast cancer or cervical cancer should be based on current anatomy and risk as opposed to gender identity of the individual. Recognition that the individual's relationship to the organ in need of cancer screening may be dysphoric for the individual should inform how screenings are introduced and discussed during a clinic visit.

Sexual and gender minority stress as a result of prejudice and systemic discrimination has direct and indirect impacts on the health of individuals. Recent studies comparing the health and health risk factors between individuals who identified as lesbian, gay or bisexual (LGB) and heterosexual individuals demonstrate LGB persons have higher rates of psychological distress, heavy alcohol and tobacco use, obesity, cardiovascular disease, type 2 diabetes, and breast and gynecological cancers compared to heterosexual women. These differences are not explained by any innate biological differences between heterosexuals/cisgendered individuals and sexual/gender minorities but are felt to be heavily influenced by minority stress and decreased access of medical care. Lifetime rates of intimate personal violence are higher for lesbian, bisexual, and transgender peoples. Although the differences in health outcomes for sexual and gender minorities do not change screening recommendations, provider awareness is important in meeting the physical and emotional health needs of all patients.

SUGGESTED READINGS

American College of Obstetricians and Gynecologists' Committee on Practice Bulletins—Gynecology: Practice bulletin No. 164: diagnosis and management of benign breast disorders, Obstet Gynecol 127(6):e141–e156, 2016.

Bots SH, Peters SAE, Woodward M: Sex differences in coronary heart disease and stroke mortality: a global assessment of the effect of ageing between 1980 and 2010, BMJ Glob Health 2(2):e000298, 2017.

Clayton AH, Margarita Valladares Juarez E: Female sexual dysfunction, Med Clin 103(4):681–698, 2019.

Eriksen EF, Díez-Pérez A, Boonen S: Update on long-term treatment with bisphosphonates for postmenopausal osteoporosis: a systematic review, Bone 58(January):126–135, 2014.

Guy J, Peters MG: Liver disease in women: the influence of gender on epidemiology, natural history, and patient outcomes, Gastroenterol Hepatol 9(10):633–639, 2013.

Han E, Nguyen L, Sirls L, Peters K: Current best practice management of interstitial cystitis/bladder pain syndrome, Ther Adv Urol 10(7):197–211, 2018.

Iddon J, Dixon JM: Mastalgia, BMJ 347(December):f3288, 2013.

Infertility Workup for the Women's Health Specialist—ACOG. n.d. https://www.acog.org/Clinical-Guidance-and-Publications/Committee-Opinions/Committee-on-Gynecologic-Practice/Infertility-Workup-for-the-Womens-Health-Specialist?IsMobileSet=false. Accessed July 3, 2019.

Kaunitz AM: Abnormal uterine bleeding in reproductive-age women, J Am Med Assoc, 2019, https://doi.org/10.1001/jama.2019.5248.

Kodner C: Common questions about the diagnosis and management of fibromyalgia, Am Fam Physician 91(7):472–478, 2015.

Mehler PS: Diagnosis and care of patients with anorexia nervosa in primary care settings, Ann Intern Med 134(11):1048–1059, 2001.

Millett ERC, Peters SAE, Woodward M: Sex differences in risk factors for myocardial infarction: cohort study of UK biobank participants, BMJ 363(November):k4247, 2018.

Nonhormonal Management of Menopause-Associated Vasomotor Symptoms: 2015 Position Statement of the North American Menopause Society. 2015. Menopause 22 (11): 1155-1172; quiz 1173-1174.

Stewart DE, Vigod SN: Postpartum depression: pathophysiology, treatment, and emerging therapeutics, Annu Rev Med 70(January):183–196, 2019.

Men's Health

73

Men's Health Topics

Niels V. Johnsen, Douglas F. Milam, Joseph A. Smith, Jr.

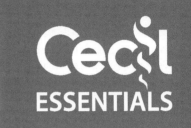

INTRODUCTION

Men's health has grown into a subspecialty field that includes primary care physicians, urologists, and endocrinologists, among others. Men's health needs and concerns are becoming more evident and often require the expertise of those with dedicated interest in men's health topics. This chapter aims to address benign disorders that are unique to men because they specifically involve the male genitalia and reproductive system. Male genitourinary malignancies and infertility are addressed in Chapters 59 and 67.

TESTOSTERONE DEFICIENCY

Definition and Epidemiology

The prescribing and use of testosterone in the United States has risen dramatically in the past decade. However, many men continue to fail to receive treatment when appropriate due to lack of provider knowledge or unsupported clinical concerns, while others continue to receive testosterone despite the lack of a clear clinical indication. Furthermore, escalations in direct-to-consumer marketing and the rise of well-publicized centers dedicated solely to the management of men's health issues have further increased patient interest in and desire to receive testosterone therapy.

Previously referred to by a number of different terms, *testosterone deficiency* is the preferred terminology adopted by the American Urological Association (AUA) to describe the condition of low serum testosterone in men in conjunction with signs or symptoms associated with low serum testosterone levels. The true prevalence of testosterone deficiency is not known. Estimates range between 2% and 77% of the US male population. This wide variability in estimates stems from inconsistencies both in definitions of testosterone deficiency applied within the literature, as well as variabilities in the assays and cut-off values used to determine low serum testosterone levels.

Testosterone deficiency does not refer to a low serum testosterone level alone, but by definition requires additional clinical signs or symptoms associated with low serum testosterone. Previous recommendations have attempted to quantify a required number of associated symptoms or signs for diagnosis of testosterone deficiency in a patient with a low total serum testosterone; however, the current AUA guidelines simply state that patients must have at least one sign or symptom in addition to low serum testosterone levels for diagnosis. These include symptoms such as fatigue, depression, erectile dysfunction, cognitive dysfunction, decreased libido, and decreased endurance; as well as signs such as loss of body hair, weight gain, or loss of lean muscle mass. Unfortunately, while some signs and symptoms are more

suggestive of testosterone deficiency, many are nonspecific and can often be manifestations of other illnesses or disease states (Table 73.1). Thus, it is vital that clinicians have a thorough understanding of testosterone deficiency in order to ensure patients are both offered appropriate care when indicated and not offered care when not indicated.

Pathophysiology

Testosterone is produced primarily by the testicles as a result of stimulation by luteinizing hormone (LH) secreted from the anterior pituitary gland, which in turn is stimulated by the hypothalamus. This hypothalamic-pituitary-gonadal (HPG) axis can often be disrupted by aging, with multiple studies showing that the prevalence of testosterone deficiency increases significantly with advancing age. Disruptions in the HPG axis can occur at multiple points and lead to differing classifications of testosterone deficiency. *Primary hypogonadism* is a condition due to testicular failure, in which the testicles fail to produce adequate amounts of testosterone (and sperm) despite adequate stimulation by LH from the anterior pituitary. *Secondary hypogonadism*, on the other hand, is a low serum testosterone level as a result of failure of the pituitary to secrete sufficient amounts of LH. In this state, the Leydig cells of the testicle are not adequately stimulated and thus do not produce testosterone. *Secondary hypogonadism* can be the result of disease processes such as pituitary tumors, hemochromatosis, or obstructive sleep apnea.

As the predominant androgen in men, testosterone circulates within the bloodstream in four distinct forms. Approximately 44% of testosterone is tightly bound to sex hormone-binding globulin (SHBG) and represents the non-bioavailable component of serum testosterone. However, 50% is loosely bound to albumin, 4% loosely bound to corticotropin-binding globulin, and 2% freely circulating within the blood stream, representing the bioavailable form of testosterone. The 2% of circulating testosterone that it is not bound to serum proteins, however, is the most biochemically active form of testosterone and referred to as free testosterone (FT).

Laboratory tests of total testosterone (TT) measure both the bound and unbound forms of testosterone. In patients with either borderline-low serum TT levels or in patients with low-normal TT levels with significant associated signs or symptoms, measurement of FT may be helpful in making a clinical diagnosis. Increased levels of SHBG in the serum can decrease the level of FT, as more testosterone becomes bound to SHBG. The level of SHBG may increase with smoking, excessive coffee consumption, age, and disease processes such as hepatitis and hyperthyroidism. Therefore, increased levels of SHBG can contribute to testosterone deficiency. Conversely, while obesity may

TABLE 73.1 Signs and Symptoms of Testosterone Deficiency

Specific Signs and Symptoms	Less Specific Signs and Symptoms
Reduced sexual desire (libido) and activity	Decreased energy and self-confidence
Decreased spontaneous erections	Feeling sad, depressed mood
Breast discomfort, gynecomastia	Poor concentration and memory
Less axillary and pubic hair and less shaving	Sleep disturbance and sleepiness
Very small or shrinking testes	Mild anemia (normochromic, normocytic)
Infertility and low sperm count	Reduced muscle bulk and strength
Height loss and low bone mineral density	Increased body fat and body mass index
Hot flashes and sweats	Diminished physical or work performance

decrease levels of SHBG, it too can contribute to testosterone deficiency through the peripheral conversion of testosterone into estrogen within adipose cells. Lastly, conditions such as extreme exercise, recreational drug use, nutritional deficiency, stress, use of certain medications, and acute illness can transiently lower serum testosterone.

Clinical Presentation

Low testosterone levels can affect a patient's general, sexual, physical, and psychological health. In Table 73.1, these symptoms are grouped according to their specific relation to testosterone deficiency. Various studies have categorized and used the symptoms of testosterone deficiency in different ways. For example, one clinical trial looking at the incidence of testosterone deficiency defined the syndrome as the presence of 3 of 12 clinical symptoms combined with a low serum FT or TT level, whereas, in a similar trial, patients were considered to be testosterone deficient if they had a low TT and exhibited three specific sexual symptoms. Current guidelines state that clinicians should use these different symptomologies as a means to determine the appropriateness and potential benefit of checking a patient's serum testosterone level, while also noting that decreased libido is the most common presenting symptom.

Diagnosis

For several reasons, the diagnosis of testosterone deficiency is not straightforward. By the very simplest of definitions, diagnosis requires a low serum testosterone level on at least two separate occasions in conjunction with at least one clinical symptom. Most clinical guidelines suggest measuring an early morning TT in any adult man who has symptoms associated with testosterone deficiency and, if low, repeating a subsequent early morning test using the same assay to confirm low testosterone. An early morning blood draw is recommended given the diurnal variation in serum testosterone levels. According to the AUA, a serum TT level of less than 300 ng/dL serves as the appropriate threshold value for identifying testosterone deficiency. However, it should be noted that there is significant variability between different testosterone assays that may alter the range of normal for each particular test, so providers should be sure to evaluate their assay-specific ranges when making determinations for therapy. In highly symptomatic patients with borderline or normal TT, FT should be assessed; however, FT tests are not recommended initially due to higher variability, increased time, and increased costs. In addition, screening of asymptomatic men for low testosterone is not medically necessary or appropriate.

In men with borderline testosterone levels, repeat measurement of a morning testosterone level is warranted because there may be significant day-to-day and diurnal variability. Ideally, levels should be checked within 4 hours of waking (usually between 7 and 11 AM), when testosterone levels are highest. It is not necessary to fast before a testosterone laboratory test; however, in a study from 2013, there was

a 25% reduction in TT levels in healthy men 60 minutes after an oral glucose tolerance test. Strength training may also transiently decrease serum testosterone levels in healthy men (but typically not outside the normal range).

Testosterone levels should not be checked during acute or subacute illness. However, physicians should have a lower threshold to check the testosterone level in patients with chronic illnesses that are known to cause a symptomatically lower testosterone concentration, such as diabetes mellitus, chronic obstructive lung disease, inflammatory arthritic disease, renal disease, human immunodeficiency virus (HIV)-related disease, obesity, metabolic syndrome, and hemochromatosis. In fact, some have argued that patients who have a pituitary mass, HIV-associated weight loss, unexplained anemia, chronic narcotic use, or chronic steroid use should have their testosterone level checked regardless of symptoms.

In patients with a confirmed low TT in the presence of symptoms, LH levels should be checked to determine the etiology of testosterone deficiency and to rule out secondary hypogonadism. Testosterone-deficient patients with a low LH likely have a defect at the level of the hypothalamus or pituitary (hypogonadotropic hypogonadism), whereas those with elevated LH levels have a primary testicular defect (hypergonadotropic hypogonadism). There are a number of conditions that may cause hypogonadotropic hypogonadism, including Kallmann syndrome, pituitary tumors, infiltrative pituitary disorders such as hemochromatosis or sarcoidosis, hyperprolactinemia, and prior head trauma. Patients with this disorder warrant further investigation to determine the source of the testosterone deficiency, such as serum prolactin measurements or possible endocrine evaluation. Hypergonadotropic hypogonadism, on the other hand, may be the result of prior infection or trauma to the testes, autoimmune damage, or possibly Klinefelter's syndrome, which would prompt karyotyping for diagnosis.

Men over the age of 40 being considered for testosterone replacement should have their prostate-specific antigen (PSA) level measured and a digital rectal examination (DRE) performed to assess the prostate. If either is abnormal, referral to a urologist should be considered. Table 73.2 provides helpful guidelines for evaluating possible testosterone deficiency. For patients with documented testosterone deficiency who are interested in future fertility, reproductive medicine evaluation should be performed because testosterone therapy markedly decreases sperm production. Return of normal spermatogenesis takes a variable amount of time, if at all.

Treatment

Testosterone therapy is recommended for men with confirmed testosterone deficiency on two separate tests who also have associated signs or symptoms of deficiency, or in the select cases mentioned above. The primary purpose of testosterone therapy is to provide symptom

TABLE 73.2 Testosterone Deficiency Diagnosis Do's and Don'ts

Do check total testosterone (TT) in every symptomatic adult male >40 yr

Do confirm low testosterone results with a second test

Do check in the morning

Do have a lower threshold to check testosterone in patients with certain chronic illnesses

Do consider measuring prolactin and LH level in patients with low testosterone

Do check hematocrit and PSA levels prior to initiating testosterone therapy

Don't check the testosterone level during acute or subacute illness

Don't start with measurement of free testosterone

Don't monitor testosterone treatment with measurements of free testosterone

Don't consider testosterone therapy in a patient trying to father a child

LH, Luteinizing hormone; *PSA,* prostate-specific antigen.

relief by returning patients to normal physiologic levels of testosterone. This, in turn, may improve symptoms such as erectile dysfunction, decreased libido, anemia, depressive mood, or low bone mineral density. However, the data are not as clear as to the benefits of testosterone therapy in improving cognitive function, fatigue, or metabolic syndrome measures. Patients should also be counseled that although the data on the cardiovascular risks or benefits of testosterone therapy are currently inconclusive, low testosterone is a known risk factor for cardiovascular disease. Clinicians should also obtain a baseline hematocrit, because polycythemia (hematocrit >52%) is known to occur significantly more frequently in men on testosterone therapy. This is especially true for men receiving intramuscular testosterone injections and those with hormone pellet implants. Polycythemia can often be addressed with dose adjustment, but it will occasionally require phlebotomy or hematology consultation.

There are numerous testosterone replacement formulations. In the United States, the most commonly used forms are testosterone enanthate or cypionate by intramuscular (IM) injection, transdermal testosterone patches, testosterone gels, and implantable timed-release pellets. The goal of therapy should be to achieve a serum TT level in the middle tertile of the reference range for the assay being used. Because of the frequency of significant skin irritation with the testosterone patch, many practitioners prefer one of the other modalities, usually based on patient preference. There is also the risk of transference with gel applications, particularly worrisome for those who come in contact with pregnant women or young children. For specifics on dosing and formulations, the AUA Guideline on Evaluation and Management of Testosterone Deficiency provides a comprehensive table with recommendations. In general though, daily gel applications mimic diurnal variation with early morning application, produce middle tertile testosterone levels, and have a relatively low rate of polycythemia. Intramuscular injection (often biweekly) does not produce diurnal variation, causes very high testosterone levels initially that often fall to subtherapeutic levels before the next injection, and is more likely to produce polycythemia than gel preparations. Pellets do not mimic diurnal variation, often produce polycythemia, but have the advantage of dosage intervals as long as 6 months.

Side Effects of Testosterone Therapy

Testosterone therapy causes decreased sperm production and usually decreased testicular volume, and it may cause acne, oily skin, and breast tenderness. Testosterone replacement is not a treatment for infertility and has, in fact, been investigated as a method of male contraception.

Patients who are interested in fathering children should not take testosterone and those with a desire for future fertility should be informed that the return of normal spermatogenesis after cessation of testosterone is variable. If necessary, human chorionic gonadotropin (HCG), selective estrogen receptor modulators (SERM), aromatase inhibitors, or a combination thereof may be administered for testosterone-deficient men wishing to preserve fertility.

In addition, as previously discussed, testosterone can increase hematocrit levels and cause life-threatening polycythemia. Generally, patients experience a rise over the first 6 months of treatment, with a plateau thereafter. If the hematocrit becomes significantly elevated, testosterone replacement should be suspended and only resumed at a modified dose after levels have normalized. Occasionally, patients require phlebotomy to avoid or treat dangerous polycythemia.

Testosterone therapy may worsen obstructive sleep apnea and congestive heart failure; therefore, patients in whom these conditions are untreated should not be started on testosterone therapy. Present data suggest that testosterone therapy does not worsen levels of high-density lipoproteins and there is no definitive evidence linking testosterone therapy to an increased risk of venothrombotic events.

Testosterone Therapy and the Prostate

It has previously been advocated that testosterone therapy should be avoided in men with a history of prostate cancer, given the known association of testosterone with prostate cancer pathophysiology. Although this topic remains controversial, a number of providers now treat patients with confirmed testosterone deficiency and a history of prostate cancer in select cases. The current AUA guidelines state that there is inadequate evidence to quantify the risk-benefit ratio of testosterone therapy in men with a history of prostate cancer. However, in patients with a history of prostatectomy with low-risk pathology, current studies show no increased risk of cancer recurrence with testosterone therapy. Similar results have been seen in low-risk prostate cancer patients treated with radiation. Patients with a history of high-risk cancer treated by radiation, however, have experienced increased rises in post-treatment PSA values and should be cautioned about the risks with testosterone therapy. These patients, as well as those with active or recurrent prostate cancer, who desire testosterone therapy should be referred to centers with experience and expertise in this clinical scenario.

Monitoring Testosterone Treatment

Patients on testosterone therapy should have regular laboratory testing to confirm that appropriate serum testosterone levels are being achieved. As stated previously, therapy should be targeted to achieving the middle tertile of normal on the particular testosterone assay being used. In general, patients using gels or patches, as well as intranasal formulations, should have levels checked within 4 weeks of initiation of treatment, and then every 6 to 12 months once on steady dosing. For patients on short-acting injectable formulations, it is generally recommended to check testosterone levels after four cycles and then every 6 to 12 months. For patients who achieve target testosterone levels for 3 to 6 months but still do not feel that their inciting symptoms have improved, testosterone therapy should likely be discontinued in all but select cases (for example, patients with prior documented bone mineral density loss).

ERECTILE DYSFUNCTION

Erectile dysfunction (ED) is defined as the inability to achieve and/or maintain an erection sufficient for satisfactory sexual performance and is known to affect some 150 million men worldwide. According to the Massachusetts Male Aging Study, 52% of men older than 40 years of age are afflicted with some degree of ED, with the prevalence of ED tripling between the ages 40 and 70 years. By age 70 years, 15% of men will experience complete ED. While age and physical health are the most important predictors of the onset of ED, smoking remains one of the most important modifiable lifestyle factors impacting one's risk for ED.

Recently, many clinics that specifically treat ED and men's sexual health have opened across America, designed to meet a growing need for treatment of this condition. However, these clinics often charge out-of-pocket fees for treatments and medications that primary care physicians can provide and that are often covered by insurance. Therefore, it is more important than ever for primary care physicians to have a thorough understanding of this disease process and its management in order to provide appropriate and medically supervised care.

Mechanism of Erection

Afferent signals capable of initiating erection can originate within the brain, as with psychogenic stimulation, or as a result of peripheral tactile stimulation. While there is no discreet center for psychogenic erections, the temporal lobe appears to be important in this process. The pelvic plexus receives input from both the sympathetic and the parasympathetic nervous system and propagates these signals into the cavernous nerves of the penis. Sympathetic fibers involved originate in the thoracolumbar spinal cord, while parasympathetic fibers originate in the second through fourth sacral spinal cord segments (S2 through S4). Afferent somatic sensory signals are carried from the penis through the pudendal nerve to the S2 through S4 nerve roots. This information is then routed both to autonomic centers of the brain and to the spinal cord. Parasympathetic innervation is largely involved in achieving an erection (tumescence), whereas sympathetic, adrenergic innervation plays a vital role in the process of ending an erection (detumescence).

Sexual stimulation and the resultant propagation of efferent signaling through the pelvic plexus causes the release of nitric oxide (NO) by the cavernous nerves into the neuromuscular junction at the level of the smooth muscle of the corpora cavernosa of the penis (Fig. 73.1). NO subsequently activates guanylyl cyclase, which converts guanosine triphosphate (GTP) into cyclic guanosine monophosphate (cGMP). Protein kinase G is activated by cGMP and in turn activates several proteins that cause a decrease in the intracellular concentration of calcium ions (Ca^{2+}). Decreased Ca^{2+} concentration in the smooth muscle results in muscular relaxation, cavernosal artery dilation, increased blood flow, and subsequent tumescence. With the resultant cavernosal expansion from increased blood flow, venous sinuses that usually drain the penis are compressed and venous outflow from the penis is reduced, allowing for a persistent increased pressure within the penis and maintenance of the erection. At the end of erection, sympathetic nerves release norepinephrine, which ultimately results in smooth muscle contraction and detumescence. Similarly, phosphodiesterase type 5 (PDE5) works within the smooth muscle cells of the cavernosal tissue to degrade cGMP, ending the propagation of the signaling cascade for erection.

Causes of Erectile Dysfunction

Although often multifactorial in etiology, ED can be generally classified into two types: psychogenic ED and organic ED. Psychogenic ED was once thought to be the most common type of ED; however, advances in understanding of the mechanics and neurophysiology of erectile function have identified other more common causes. As a result, psychogenic ED is now thought to account for fewer than 15% of patients seen by ED specialists. Patients with psychogenic ED have otherwise intact vascular and neural physiology and are often able to

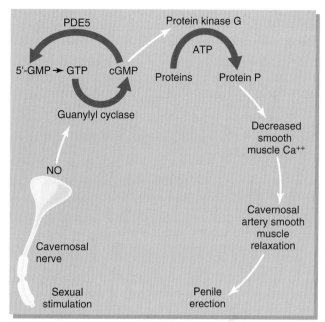

Fig. 73.1 Sexual stimulation causes the release of nitric oxide (NO) by the cavernous nerve into the neuromuscular junction. *ATP,* Adenosine triphosphate; *cGMP,* cyclic guanosine monophosphate; *GMP,* guanosine monophosphate; *GTP,* guanosine triphosphate; *PDE5,* phosphodiesterase type 5.

achieve erections either nocturnally or with self-stimulation, but continue to have difficulties with ED. This is most often related to issues such as depression, stress, anxiety or other psychiatric illness.

Organic ED represents the majority of ED seen clinically and can be classified as vasculogenic, neurogenic, endocrinologic or a combination thereof. For many patients, atherosclerotic arterial disease results in poor vascular inflow, impacting the ability to achieve an erection. Recent estimates suggest that atherosclerosis alone accounts for up to 60% of ED cases seen in men over the age of 60. Furthermore, a diagnosis of ED has been strongly associated with future cardiovascular disease in US men.

Cardiovascular Disease

In the United States, atherosclerotic vascular disease, hyperlipidemia, smoking, and hypertension are frequent causes of ED. These relationships are not surprising, as erection is achieved by a combination of relaxation of arteriolar smooth muscle and increased venous resistance of channels penetrating the wall of the corpora cavernosa. Cardiovascular disease may decrease erectile ability by decreasing blood flow to the penile arteries, mechanical obstruction of the vascular lumen, or, more commonly, due to the resultant endothelial dysfunction. Endothelial dysfunction is the most common cause of ED, in which there is an interruption of the neural control mechanism of vascular smooth muscle function due to a decreased ability of endothelial cells to release NO, leading to decreased blood flow and pressure in the corpora cavernosa. Given this close relationship between ED and cardiovascular disease, men presenting with ED should undergo appropriate cardiovascular risk factor evaluation and management. Men presenting with new onset ED in their forties are particularly at risk with an approximately 15 times increased risk of a myocardial event.

The principal blood vessels supplying the corpora cavernosa are the cavernosal arteries, which are terminal branches of the internal pudendal artery. Diseases of large and small arteries may decrease corporal blood pressure and lead to decreased penile lengthening and

TABLE 73.3   Frequency of Decreased Erectile Rigidity and Ejaculatory Dysfunction by Medication Class

Medication Class	Decreased Erectile Rigidity	Ejaculatory Dysfunction
β-Adrenergic antagonists	Common	Less common
Sympatholytics	Expected	Common
$α_1$-Agonists	Uncommon	Uncommon
$α_2$-Agonists	Common	Less common
$α_1$-Antagonists	Uncommon	Less common[a]
Angiotensin-converting enzyme inhibitors	Uncommon	Uncommon
Diuretics	Less common	Uncommon
Antidepressants	Common[b]	Uncommon[c]
Antipsychotics	Common	Common
Anticholinergics	Less common	Uncommon

[a]Patients are able to ejaculate, but retrograde ejaculation is seen in 5% to 30%.
[b]Uncommon with serotonin reuptake inhibitors.
[c]Delayed or inhibited ejaculation with serotonin reuptake inhibitors.

rigidity. Veno-occlusive disease in the penis is also a significant cause of ED. In these patients, there is often appropriate arterial inflow but an impaired ability to prevent leakage of blood through the venous system out of the penis. As such, these patients often experience normal initial rigidity but quickly lose their erection before ejaculation occurs.

Neurogenic Erectile Dysfunction

Because the nervous system plays an integral role in the physiology of erection, any disease process that affects the brain, the spinal cord, or the peripheral nerves can cause ED. For example, dementia, Parkinson's disease, and stroke are diseases of the brain associated with ED. Patients with spinal cord injury commonly have ED. Because of an intact spinal reflex pathway, most patients with spinal cord injury respond to tactile sensation, but they usually require medical therapy to maintain the erection through intercourse. Iatrogenic injury to nerves during surgery (e.g., prostatectomy, rectal surgery) is also a common cause of neurogenic ED. Neurogenic ED due to decreases in penile tactile sensation can occur with increasing age.

Endocrine Disorders

Testosterone plays a permissive role in erectile function, and many endocrine disorders can directly or indirectly decrease plasma free or bound testosterone. However, while testosterone deficiency is an uncommon primary cause of ED as erectile ability is only partially androgen dependent, the current AUA guidelines do recommend checking a morning serum testosterone in men with ED to confirm that they are not testosterone deficient. Patients with testosterone deficiency typically have decreased or absent libido in addition to loss of erectile rigidity. If testosterone deficiency is confirmed on two separate morning testosterone tests, testosterone therapy should be offered. If erectile rigidity fails to improve with 3 to 6 months of testosterone therapy, testosterone supplementation should be discontinued. Testosterone therapy is not indicated for patients with normal circulating testosterone levels and ED.

The most common endocrine disorder affecting erectile ability is diabetes mellitus. In addition to causing atherosclerosis and microvascular disease, diabetes affects both the autonomic and the somatic nervous systems, including loss of function of long autonomic nerves. The loss of function of these long cholinergic neurons results in interruptions of the efferent arm of the erectile reflex arc. Diabetes also appears to produce dysfunction of the neuromuscular junction at the level of arterial smooth muscle in the penile corpora

cavernosa. Studies have indicated markedly decreased acetylcholine and NO concentrations in the trabeculae of the corpora cavernosa in diabetic patients. These findings probably represent a combination of neural loss and neuromuscular junction dysfunction. Other endocrine disorders, such as hypothyroidism, hyperthyroidism, and adrenal dysfunction, can also cause ED. Because of the uncommon occurrence of thyroid and adrenal disorders in patients presenting for treatment of ED, testing of those axes is not a part of the routine work-up of ED.

Medication-Induced Erectile Dysfunction

Many commonly prescribed medications can cause or contribute to decreased erectile function. Table 73.3 lists the major classes of medications implicated in ED and suggests how commonly these medications interfere with erectile function. Changing medications may restore erectile function in some patients. However, proceeding directly to treatment of ED is usually a better option in all but the most straightforward cases.

Medical and Surgical Therapies

Since the introduction of sildenafil in 1998, the Process of Care Model for the evaluation and treatment of ED has been adopted. This model targets the primary care provider as the initial source of care for patients with ED. Currently available therapies for ED include oral PDE5 inhibitors, intraurethral alprostadil, intracavernosal vasoactive injection therapy, vacuum constriction devices, and penile prosthesis implantation. Although a stepwise treatment approach starting with oral agents and progressing to more invasive therapeutic interventions has generally been advocated, many men's health specialists now advocate assessing each patient individually and ensuring that all options are discussed (Fig. 73.2). All patients who are candidates for oral medications should generally try these prior to more invasive procedures given their relative high success and low risk profile; however, all patients are not required to proceed incrementally up the chain of treatment measures, as long as they are fully informed of the available options. Informed patient decision making is critical to successful progression through the Process of Care pathway. Patient referral is primarily based on the need or desire for specialized diagnostic testing and management. Most importantly, all men with comorbidities known to negatively affect erectile function should be counseled that lifestyle modifications such as improved diet and physical activity may have a significant positive impact on their erectile function.

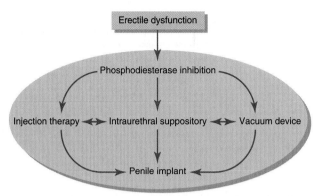

Fig. 73.2 A logical treatment algorithm for erectile dysfunction.

Oral Phosphodiesterase Type 5 Inhibitors

Current medical therapy is based on inhibition of PDE5, which degrades cGMP to inactive 5′-GMP, as shown in Fig. 73.1. Sildenafil, vardenafil, avanafil, and tadalafil all competitively inhibit PDE5 breakdown of cGMP. Use of a PDE5 inhibitor results in improved erectile rigidity even in patients with decreased NO or cGMP synthesis. However, not all patients respond to PDE5 inhibition. Adequate sexual stimulation and intact neural and vascular pathways are necessary to produce an adequate amount of NO and cGMP to increase deep penile artery blood flow. PDE5 inhibitors have been shown to be effective in men with vasculogenic, psychogenic, neurogenic, and mixed cases of ED. The overall response rate to PDE5 inhibitors is 70%.

Unless contraindicated, PDE5 inhibition should be considered first-line therapy for most men. The combination of PDE5 inhibitors and α-adrenergic receptor blockers (often used in men with lower urinary tract symptoms related to an enlarged prostate) can result in transient hypotension; however, in general it is safe to use selective α-blockers such as tamsulosin and alfluzosin with any PDE5 inhibitor, particularly once a patient is already established on therapy with the α-blocker. However, PDE5 inhibitors should not be used concurrently with nitrate medications due to the significant risk of a large (>25 mm Hg) synergistic drop in blood pressure. Periodic follow-up is necessary to determine therapeutic efficacy, assess for side effects related to PDE5 inhibition, and evaluate any changes in health status. Commonly reported side effects include headaches and flushing, while some patients have reported changes in vision due to unintended inhibition of PDE6 in the retina.

Alprostadil Intraurethral Drug Therapy

In patients for whom PDE5 inhibition is unsuccessful, one potential second-line medical treatment is intraurethral administration of prostaglandin E$_1$ (alprostadil). Alprostadil pellets are inserted directly into the urethra with the use of a pellet applicator and then diffuse into the surrounding tissue, initiating a second messenger cascade involving cAMP and inducing erection. This method of delivery assumes substantial venous communications between the corpus spongiosum surrounding the urethra and the corpus cavernosum and is effective in many patients who fail oral PDE5 inhibitor medications. A number of patients experience difficulty initiating this type of treatment due to discomfort or concerns in using the applicator, so it may be beneficial to administer the first dose in an office setting. To lubricate the urethra, patients should void prior to insertion of the pellet.

Up to one third of patients have normal, transient burning penile pain, and this should be discussed with the patient before treatment. Dizziness and presyncope are uncommon complications. Intraurethral alprostadil results in rapid onset erection after administration and has a minimal risk of priapism. It can be used with increased efficacy in combination with PDE5 inhibitors. Transient burning pain in the sexual partner can occur and is caused by leakage of the medication from the urethra into the vagina. This method of achieving erection is also contraindicated in men having intercourse with a pregnant female, due to the above risks of transference. This can be managed by wearing a condom.

Intracavernosal Injection Therapy

Pharmacologic injection therapy involves the injection of vasodilator agents into the corpora cavernosa to produce erection by stimulating dilation of the corporal artery smooth muscle. More than 90% of patients with ED respond to this type of therapy. Commonly used agents, either alone or in combination, include alprostadil, papaverine, and phentolamine. As monotherapy, alprostadil is most commonly used. Of the three, only alprostadil has been evaluated in rigorous clinical trials and has specific marketing approval from the US Food and Drug Administration for the treatment of ED. Phentolamine is often used to potentiate the action of papaverine and can be used in combination with both alprostadil and papaverine. These vasoactive drugs can be formulated with different combinations of medications and concentrations to achieve increased efficacy and decreased side effects. *Bimix* and *trimix* are terms often used to refer to a combination of two or three of these medications, respectively.

The most common side effects of this type of treatment are bruising and penile pain (50%). Penile pain is more common in young patients and is usually worse with alprostadil. Therefore, a combination using lower-dose alprostadil or formulations of papaverine and phentolamine alone might be beneficial in younger patients. Other, more serious risks of injection therapy include priapism and corporal scarring. Priapism has been reported to occur in 1% to 4% of patients but is more commonly reported in patients with neurogenic ED, especially young men with spinal cord injury. Significant acquired penile curvature due to corporal scarring (Peyronie's disease) is seen uncommonly and usually follows several years of injection therapy. Penile curvature appears to be less common with the use of alprostadil than with papaverine. The most common problem with pharmacologic injection therapy, however, is continuation of treatment, as up to 50% to 60% of patients stop using the technique within 1 year due to poor tolerance and satisfaction.

As with intraurethral alprostadil, initial treatment should be performed under the supervision of a physician. The medication can be injected using a self-contained medication-syringe kit or a 29-gauge (5/8-inch) insulin syringe with medication drawn from a refrigerated vial. It is advisable to start with a small test dose and slowly titrate the dosage for desired effect over several weeks. The patient should not use the medication more than once in a 24-hour period and should be instructed to seek medical care promptly for prolonged erections lasting longer than 4 hours. Typically, administration of the test dose should be carried out in the morning, and the patient should be expected to stay in close proximity to the medical office to monitor for priapism. Should a patient develop priapism, it usually resolves without sequelae after intracavernosal injection of phenylephrine in a setting where blood pressure and heart rate can be continuously monitored. Formal guidelines for the treatment of priapism are available on the website of the AUA.

Vacuum Constriction Devices

Vacuum constriction devices enclose the penis in a plastic tube with an airtight seal at the penile base. Air is pumped out of the cylinder, creating a vacuum and pulling blood into the corporal bodies, leading to penile erection. A constriction band is then slid from the cylinder to the base of the penis to constrict venous outflow and maintain the erection. Simultaneous use of a vacuum device and a PDE5 inhibitor is safe and has been shown to improve erectile rigidity and patient satisfaction with the vacuum device. Some of the common side effects that affect patient satisfaction with these devices are coldness, numbness, and bruising of the penis, as well as the cumbersome nature of the process.

Penile Prosthesis

A penile prosthesis is an either semirigid or inflatable device that is implanted into the penis in the operating room under general anesthesia. These devices allow for men to achieve rigid erections suitable for penetration and sexual function. In contemporary series, most patients prefer the inflatable devices over semirigid options because of the more natural erection when inflated and a fully flaccid penis when deflated. Although implantation of a penile prosthesis is more invasive than the other techniques, this device is the most effective long-term option for impotence treatment, with nearly 90% of patients and partners satisfied with the result.

Important interval improvements have been made in the design of implantable penile prostheses to make them more durable and resistant to infection. Improvements in the connections between tubing and corporal cylinders have cut the mechanical failure rate to less than 5% in 5 years. Components now also have special coatings that either contain antibiotics or absorb antibiotics applied topically at the time of implantation in order to decrease the risk of infection.

PEYRONIE'S DISEASE

Peyronie's disease (PD) is an acquired condition of the penis that involves fibrosis of the tunica albuginea, resulting in contracture and ultimately penile curvature and/or deformity. It may affect up to 6% of men in the United States. This disease can be quite debilitating to men for both psychological as well as functional reasons. Other than embarrassment related to the appearance of their penises, many men experience depression, relationship difficulties, and diminished quality of life, not to mention pain and difficulty in sexual activity, both for themselves and for their partners. There have been a number of significant advances over the past decade in the management of PD, progressing from a purely surgical disease process to one that now is often amenable to minimally invasive injection therapies.

Pathophysiology

PD is the result of fibrosis in the tunica albuginea of the penis and is believed to be secondary to repetitive microvascular trauma and buckling events over time. While some individuals will present with a clear history of a significant prior penile injury, most recall no inciting event. The natural history of PD itself is variable as well. Most men report a gradual worsening of curvature with associated penile pain for a number of months prior to presentation to a physician. For men who remain untreated for PD after presentation to a physician, approximately 12% will note improvement in their curvature over the ensuing year, while the remainder will either remain stable or worsen with time.

PD is defined temporally by *active* and *stable* phases of disease. The active phase is generally characterized by changes in the degree of curvature with time, as well as other degrees of penile modeling changes such as development of an "hourglass" appearance or induration. The prime characteristic of the active phase of disease, however, is the presence of pain, particularly with erection. The stable phase of disease is defined by at least 3 months of stable, unchanged curvature and/or other deformity. Pain with manipulation should be absent once a patient has reached the stable phase of the disease.

Differential Diagnosis

Acquired penile curvature due to PD may be difficult to differentiate from congenital penile curvature in some individuals, especially those

who become sexually active later in life. Patients with congenital curvature generally have lifelong ventral curvature and no palpable fibrotic plaque consistent with PD. Acute penile trauma may cause pain and/or induration that may be confused for the active phase of PD. Rarely, patients with acute penile fractures may develop PD later in life due to inappropriate collagen deposition following injury.

Evaluation

The most common presenting symptom for patients with PD is dorsal curvature (the penis curves up towards the abdomen) with a palpable fibrotic plaque on the dorsum of the penis. However, there is tremendous variation in the degree and extent of curvature that patients may develop, with many patients having ventral, lateral, or multiplanar, compound curvatures. Furthermore, many patients develop the previously mentioned "hourglass" appearance due to circumferential constriction of the tunica albuginea by fibrosis within the corpora cavernosa. PD has been shown to occur simultaneously in patients with Dupuytren contracture of the hands or Ledderhose disease of the plantar fascia, so patients should be appropriately evaluated for these diseases as well. While some patients will occasionally present with photographs of their erect penis for evaluation, providers should be comfortable inducing a pharmacologic erection to evaluate the degree, extent, and location of curvature in the office. Concomitant penile duplex ultrasonography may be useful to evaluate the vascular integrity of the penis, as well as for possible calcifications of the fibrotic plaque, but this is best performed by individuals specifically trained in this technique.

Measurements of penile length and specific notation on the location and size of the plaque are useful in determining treatment strategies. A thorough sexual history is similarly vital in the initial evaluation. The degree or extent of ED must be ascertained, as PD commonly coexists with ED and the presence of ED impacts potential treatment options. Treatment of penile curvature due to Peyronie's disease will not improve decreased penile rigidity. Similarly, a thorough history of the duration and stability of curvature, as well as the presence of pain with erections and/or intercourse, should be obtained in order to determine if a patient is in the active and stable phase of disease.

Treatment
Active Phase

Active phase disease represents an ongoing physiologic process in which collagen deposition is incomplete and variable. Many attempts have been made in the past to alter this process through the use of medications; however, no proven therapies have been found to be efficacious, other than simple nonsteroidal anti-inflammatory drugs (NSAIDs) for the pain associated with active disease. Surgical treatments for PD are not indicated during the active phase of the disease. Although a number of proposed oral therapies have been previously advocated with hopes of preventing or reversing curvature, there is currently insufficient evidence for their use. The most commonly used oral medication, vitamin E, has had a number of both observational and randomized control trials performed, all of which have failed to demonstrate efficacy in reducing curvature, pain or progression. The primary aim for management of patients in the active phase of disease is symptom control with NSAIDs.

Stable Phase

For patients in the stable phase of PD, in whom curvature has been stable for at least 3 months and there is no significant pain with erections, treatment is geared towards improving sexual function and quality of life. There is no urgent medical indication for intervening on PD in the absence of patient bother. Treatment decisions are based on patient wishes and tailored according to degree of erectile function, tolerance of each intervention, and ability to undergo general anesthesia.

Intralesional injection therapy. There are currently two commonly used medications for PD that are directly injected into the fibrous plaque of patients and have been shown to be effective in improving curvature. Interferon-α was the first widely successful intralesional injection therapy used in PD patients. This medication functions by decreasing the rate of fibroblast proliferation within the tissues, thus decreasing the deposition of extracellular collagen. Interferon-α has been shown to have efficacy in improving both curvature and plaque size.

More recent, however, was the FDA approval of collagenase clostridium histolyticum (CCH) in 2013 for use in PD patients. This medication contains a collagenase enzyme that, when directly injected into Peyronie's lesions, enzymatically degrades interstitial collagen, improving curvature. The IMPRESS trial, which led to the FDA approval of CCH for PD patients, consisted of up to four 6-week cycles, with each cycle including two injections of CCH 24 to 72 hours apart. The treatment group, as compared to a saline control group, was found to fare significantly better, with a mean 34% improvement in curvature (17 degrees) in the treatment group as compared to 18% (9 degrees) in the control group. While this trial excluded individuals with curvatures of less than 30 degrees, as well as those with ventral curvatures and plaques, some providers have now extrapolated these data to treat individuals not initially eligible based on these inclusion criteria. Though no head-to-head trials have been conducted, CCH appears to be more effective at decreasing penile curvature than interferon-α.

While intralesional injection therapy is generally safe and minimally invasive, there are some associated risks. Patients who receive interferon-α are at significant risk of developing sinusitis, flulike symptoms, and penile swelling. CCH, on the other hand, has been associated with rare serious adverse events such as penile fracture, while the majority of patients developed mild adverse side effects such as pain, swelling, bruising, or painful erections. Lastly, patients may require up to 24 weeks of therapy to reach maximal improvement in curvature, which may dissuade some individuals.

Surgical therapy. The goal of surgical therapy for PD is to correct the penile deformity (curvature and/or hourglass) and allow the patient to return to satisfactory intercourse. For patients with PD who are either not interested in or not candidates for intralesional injection therapies there are three primary surgical options. The primary determinant of the surgical therapy offered is the degree of ED in the patient. Improvement of penile curvature in a patient who is otherwise unable to obtain a sufficient and satisfactory erection will improve that patient's quality of life. For patients with significant ED despite pharmacotherapy, placement of a penile prosthesis may be performed (as discussed previously), often with adjunct maneuvers discussed later to obtain straightening.

The most commonly performed procedure for men with PD is tunical plication. In this procedure, the convex side of the penis is shortened with placement of sutures directly in the tunica albuginea opposite the fibrous plaque on the contralateral side of the penis. This procedure may result in perceived penile shortening and is best reserved for men with sufficient preoperative stretched penile length, as well as for those with mild to moderate degrees of curvature. Plication techniques are unable to address hourglass or other indentation deformities but are unlikely to have any significant negative impact on erectile function.

An alternative approach, particularly for men with more significant curvatures or in those in whom a plication technique may have too significant of an impact on penile length, is plaque incision (or excision) and grafting. In this procedure, the PD plaque is identified and incised (or excised if extensively calcified). Incising the plaque relieves the tension that the fibrous plaque was applying to the penis causing it to curve, allowing it to return to its normal straight position without sacrificing length. The resultant defect in the tunica albuginea is then grafted using either autologous tissues (i.e., saphenous vein) or other graft materials (allograft, xenograft, or synthetic grafts have all been utilized). Importantly, this procedure can be used to correct hourglass and other indentation deformities that other techniques cannot. Although this procedure does maintain penile length, there are increased concerns related to postoperative ED, with up to 30% of men reporting new-onset or worsening ED after the procedure. However, overall, satisfaction and straightening rates are greater than 80% for both plication and grafting techniques.

TABLE 73.4 Symptoms of Lower Urinary Tract Syndrome

Overactive Bladder	Obstructive Voiding
Frequency	Hesitancy
Nocturia	Slow stream
Urgency	Stop-and-start voiding
Urge incontinence	Sensation of incomplete emptying

BENIGN PROSTATIC HYPERPLASIA

Benign prostatic hyperplasia (BPH) is a nonmalignant enlargement of the prostate gland and is widely prevalent in the aging male patient. It is estimated that more than 90% of all men will develop histologic evidence of BPH during the course of their lifetime, with at least 50% of these men developing lower urinary tract symptoms (LUTS) that prompt them to seek medical care. Broadly speaking, LUTS can be divided into two groups: obstructive voiding symptoms and overactive bladder symptoms (Table 73.4).

Although most patients who seek medical care for BPH do so because of the associated LUTS, these same symptoms can also result from other illnesses such as diabetes mellitus, spine disease, Parkinson's disease, multiple sclerosis, and cerebrovascular disease (Fig. 73.3). It is important to evaluate all patients for these non–BPH-related conditions to ensure appropriate management is provided. It is also important to pay close attention to medication use, because a number of medications used in the elderly population can result in various urologic symptoms, including both obstructive and overactive bladder voiding symptoms. Lastly, BPH itself is a histologic diagnosis and does not in itself require intervention. Intervention is only indicated for individuals in which BPH is resulting in bothersome symptoms or complications related to impaired bladder emptying.

Pathophysiology

Prostate growth and the subsequent development of BPH occur under the influence of testosterone and the more metabolically active byproduct, dihydrotestosterone (DHT). Testosterone produced by the testes is converted to DHT by the action of the enzyme 5α-reductase within the prostate itself. DHT is the major intracellular androgen within the prostate and is believed to be responsible for the development and maintenance of the hyperplastic cell growth characteristics of BPH.

BPH develops predominantly in the periurethral prostatic tissue, referred to as the *transition zone* (Fig. 73.4). Tissue growth in this area leads to the phenomenon of bladder outlet obstruction (BOO), which causes LUTS. BOO occurs as a result of two mechanisms: first, mechanical obstruction from increased tissue volume in the periurethral zone of the prostate and, second, dynamic obstruction caused by decreased bladder neck relaxation during voiding and increased

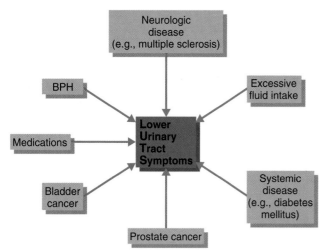

Fig. 73.3 Causes of lower urinary tract symptoms (LUTS). *BPH,* Benign prostatic hyperplasia.

smooth muscle tone in the bladder neck and prostate gland. Also important, but less well characterized, is the response of the detrusor muscle to the increase in outlet resistance provided by those two mechanisms. As bladder outlet resistance increases, the bladder responds by increasing the force of contraction. This added work results in physical and mechanical changes in bladder function over time and may contribute to the presence of overactive bladder symptomatology in patients with BOO.

Early in the course of BOO, the bladder is able to compensate to overcome the elevated outlet resistance; however, with persistent obstruction, the patient typically develops LUTS, particularly difficulty initiating the stream, weak stream, hesitancy, and intermittency. These symptoms frequently drive patients to seek medical care. Later during the course of the obstructive process, the bladder wall becomes thickened and loses compliance. The subsequent loss of compliance results in a decreased functional capacity of the bladder, which exacerbates the patient's overactive bladder symptoms such as urgency and frequency.

Diagnosis

The initial evaluation of a patient with LUTS suggestive of BPH should include a detailed medical history that focuses on the patient's urinary symptoms as well as the past medical history, including comorbid conditions and any previous surgical procedures, general health conditions, and history of alcohol and tobacco use. The assessment of symptoms can be facilitated with the use of the AUA Symptom Index (also known as the *International Prostate Symptom Score*, or IPSS). This is a self-administered, validated questionnaire consisting of seven questions related to the symptoms of BPH and BOO. The AUA Symptom Index classifies voiding symptoms as mild (0 to 7), moderate (8 to 19), or severe (20 to 35). Validated instruments such as the AUA Symptom Index are useful during the initial evaluation as an overall assessment of symptom severity and during follow-up visits to assess the effectiveness of any medical or surgical interventions.

A general physical examination should be performed that includes a DRE and a focused neurologic examination. Urinalysis, either by dipstick or by microscopic examination of urine sediment, is also mandatory to rule out hematuria and evidence of urinary tract infection. Glucosuria can be a significant finding, particularly if not previously identified, as this may indicate the presence of polyuria contributing to the patient's LUTS. The initial clinical practice guidelines for the diagnosis of BPH recommended a serum creatinine measurement to assess renal function in all patients with signs or symptoms suggestive

of BPH. However, this recommendation came under scrutiny because of its low yield for the detection of renal insufficiency secondary to obstructive uropathy. As such, serum creatinine measurement is no longer a routine part of the BPH work-up. According to the same clinical practice guidelines, PSA measurement is optional during the initial evaluation. PSA can function as a surrogate for prostate volume measurement in addition to being a screening test for prostate cancer. The Medical Therapy of Prostatic Symptoms (MTOPS) study, sponsored by the National Institutes of Health, demonstrated that PSA increases linearly with prostate volume and that a PSA level greater than 4 ng/mL conveys a 9% risk of requiring surgical therapy for benign disease over a 4.5-year period.

The following additional diagnostic tests should be considered when evaluating patients with BPH, specifically those in whom surgical therapy is being considered. Uroflowmetry is a noninvasive method of measuring urinary flow rate. The maximal urinary flow rate, Q_{max}, is considered the most useful measurement for identifying patients with BOO. However, a diminished Q_{max} alone is not diagnostic of BOO because patients with diminished flow rates may have such due to impaired bladder contraction rather than physical obstruction. Typical values range from 25 mL/second in a young man without BOO to 10 mL/second or slower in a man with significant BOO. Measurement of postvoid residual (PVR) urine may be accomplished by urethral catheterization or, preferably, by ultrasonography. Elevated PVR volumes indicate an increased risk for acute urinary retention and eventual need for surgical intervention. Elevated residuals, furthermore, put patients at risk for the formation of bladder stones, urinary tract infections, or renal deterioration with long-term retention. The MTOPS study demonstrated that 7% of men with PVR greater than 39 mL required surgical intervention over a 4.5-year period. Elevation of PVR to greater than 200 mL raises the question of functional impairment of the bladder and warrants further evaluation with urodynamic testing.

Routine evaluation of the upper urinary tracts (kidneys and ureters) with excretory urography or ultrasonography is not recommended for the average BPH patient unless there is concomitant urinary pathology (i.e., hematuria, urinary tract infection, renal insufficiency, a history of prior urologic surgery, or a history of nephrolithiasis). Likewise, transrectal ultrasonography (TRUS), CT or MRI imaging are not routinely recommended for medical therapy but should be considered in the preoperative assessment of prostate gland size prior to surgical intervention, as this may influence selection of technique.

Differential Diagnosis

A number of conditions can cause LUTS in the aging male. A DRE and PSA testing are helpful in distinguishing between BPH and prostate cancer, but neither is diagnostic. Early-stage prostate cancer is typically asymptomatic and patients can have both conditions concurrently. Although PSA testing is not sufficiently sensitive or specific to reliably differentiate BPH from prostate cancer, it is a useful tool to stratify a patient's risk for the presence of prostate cancer and assess the need for further prostate cancer evaluation. While controversy surrounding the use of PSA for prostate cancer screening persists, in general, patients between the ages of 40 and 55 at a higher risk for prostate cancer (i.e., African American men and/or those with a family history) and all men ages 55 to 69 should engage in shared decision making with their primary care providers to discuss the risks and benefits of prostate cancer screening and make an individualized decision on screening. Men with elevated PSAs or concerning DRE should be referred to a urologist for further evaluation and management.

Prostatitis is another condition that can cause LUTS. It may result from bacterial infection or from a nonbacterial inflammatory process, and the symptoms may substantially overlap those of BPH,

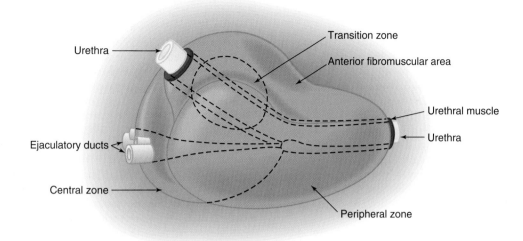

Fig. 73.4 Zonal anatomy of the prostate gland.

particularly in older men. Diabetes mellitus, neurologic diseases such as Parkinson's disease or cerebrovascular disease, and other conditions of the urinary tract, such as urethral strictures, may result in LUTS in patients with BPH. Finally, many medications, particularly those with significant anticholinergic side effects, can cause symptoms mimicking those associated with BPH.

Medical Management

Medical management is the preferred first-line treatment option for patients diagnosed with LUTS due to BPH, and most patients can be effectively managed with a minimum of side effects on medication alone. In general, medical management is initiated for patients with moderate to severe AUA symptom scores. However, in the absence of indications for surgery (refractory urinary retention, hydronephrosis with or without renal impairment, recurrent urinary tract infections, recurrent gross hematuria, or bladder calculi), the decision to embark on any course of therapy, medical or otherwise, is principally driven by the patient. Every patient has a different perception of his symptoms: nocturia twice nightly may be a minor nuisance for some but may represent a significant problem for others. There is no absolute AUA symptom score or other objective measure that dictates the need for initiation of therapy for symptomatic BPH. Each patient must be evaluated individually, and the treatment course must be tailored to the patient's individual situation.

α-Adrenergic Antagonists

α-Blockers are the most commonly prescribed medications for the treatment of LUTS associated with BPH. The bladder neck and prostate are richly innervated with α-adrenergic receptors, specifically α_{1a}-receptors, which constitute about 70% to 80% of the total number of α-receptors in these areas. α_{1b}-Receptors modulate vascular smooth muscle contraction and are located in the bladder neck and prostate to a lesser degree.

Doxazosin, terazosin, tamsulosin, and extended-release alfuzosin are long-acting α-receptor antagonists. These medications are typically administered once daily, usually at bedtime to minimize the potential side effect of orthostatic hypotension. They act through α_1-receptors and can cause vasodilation resulting in transient hypotension and lightheadedness. Blood pressure reduction is greater in patients with a history of hypertension (average reduction, 10 to 15 mm Hg)

relative to normotensive patients (average reduction, 1 to 4 mm Hg). Overall, 10% to 20% of patients experience some (often transient) side effects from these medications, including dizziness, asthenia, headaches, peripheral edema, and nasal congestion. Dose titration is recommended for doxazosin and terazosin to minimize occurrence of adverse effects and optimize the therapeutic response. Maximal response is usually seen within 1 to 2 weeks with doxazosin and within 3 to 6 weeks with terazosin. Overall, these drugs reduce symptom scores by 40% to 50% and improve urinary flow rates by 40% to 50% in about 60% to 65% of patients treated.

Tamsulosin is a selective α_{1a}-receptor antagonist with a long half-life. It has a significantly lower degree of nonspecific α-receptor binding compared with other α-receptor antagonists. Therefore, side effects such as postural hypotension and dizziness are less commonly seen. This drug does not appreciably affect blood pressure in hypertensive or normotensive patients. Maximal response is usually seen within 1 to 2 weeks after the initiation of therapy.

One notable side effect of this class of medications reported in a significant proportion of individuals is retrograde ejaculation. In this condition, the ejaculate is propelled across the bladder neck into the bladder, rather than out the urethra, as a result of the increased relaxation of the prostate and bladder neck tissues. While not medically dangerous, this can be disconcerting to many men who are unaware of this potential side effect. Tamsulosin and silodosin have been shown to have the highest rates of retrograde ejaculation of the regularly prescribed α-blockers.

5α-Reductase Inhibitors (Finasteride and Dutasteride)

Finasteride and dutasteride block the intracellular conversion of testosterone to DHT by inhibiting the action of the enzyme 5α-reductase. This results in an approximate 18% to 25% reduction in prostate gland size over 6 to 12 months. It is most effective in reducing symptoms and preventing disease progression in patients with large prostate glands (>40 g), although recent evidence suggests that symptomatic improvement and stabilization of disease progression may occur in treated men with prostates as small as 30 g. 5α-Reductase inhibition has also been shown to decrease the risk for urinary retention and subsequent surgical intervention, again predominantly in those patients with larger glands. Initial response is seen within 6 months, and maximal effect occurs 12 to 18 months after the initiation of therapy. Data from the MTOPS study demonstrated that combination therapy with an α-blocker and a 5α-reductase inhibitor was more effective than single-agent therapy alone in men with large prostates. As such, many men are placed on concomitant therapy.

It should be noted that finasteride and dutasteride have been found to reduce serum PSA by about 50%. This must be taken into consideration when interpreting PSA values for prostate cancer screening in men taking these agents. After 6 months of therapy, the effective PSA level in a patient taking finasteride or dutasteride may be calculated by doubling the measured PSA value. Free PSA (the percentage of non–protein-bound PSA) is also reduced by about 50%. Use of finasteride or dutasteride may result in sexual dysfunction, including decreased erectile rigidity, decreased libido, and decreased ejaculate volume. ED caused by 5α-reductase inhibitor therapy is reversible and returns to baseline within 2 to 6 months after discontinuation of therapy.

Phosphodiesterase Type 5 Inhibitors

Although more often thought of as medications for the treatment of ED, sildenafil, vardenafil, and tadalafil have been shown to be efficacious in the treatment of urinary symptoms related to BPH. As previously discussed, these medications work by preventing the degradation of cGMP by PDE5. This results in lower intracellular calcium levels and, consequently, smooth muscle relaxation. This process works in the vasculature of the penis as well as the smooth muscle cells of the prostate, urethra, and bladder neck. A number of randomized, double-blind, placebo-controlled trials have shown significant improvements in LUTS in men treated with a once-daily regimen of one of these medications. Although it has not been conclusively shown that PDE5 inhibitors are more efficacious than α-blockers, it does appear that the combination of the two medications works better than either one of them alone. The common side effects of these medications are headache, nasal stuffiness, and facial flushing.

Anticholinergic Medications

For most men, symptoms of overactive bladder make up a large component of LUTS associated with BPH. As previously discussed, many men with long-standing BOO have symptoms of urgency, frequency, and nocturia. One of the best ways to treat these symptoms of overactive bladder is with the daily use of anticholinergic medications such as oxybutynin, tolterodine, or solifenacin. The use of anticholinergic medications in combination with α-blockers has been shown to result in greater improvement in LUTS, quality of life, and AUA symptom scores in men with symptoms of overactive bladder due to BPH than use of either agent in monotherapy. The typical side effects of this class of medications include dry mouth, constipation, nausea, and impaired cognition. The risk of urinary retention related to the use of these medications in men appears to be minimal.

Surgical Management
Minimally Invasive Therapy

Although transurethral resection of the prostate (TURP) remains the standard for surgical treatment of BPH, substantial effort has been devoted to the development of less invasive and less morbid methods of treating patients with symptomatic BPH. This has led to a number of minimally invasive therapies, primarily using various energy platforms to cause tissue destruction within the prostate. These office-based techniques are best reserved for patients with smaller prostates and may transiently increase bladder outlet obstruction for 1 to 2 weeks due to postprocedure swelling. Maximal tissue reduction and treatment effect generally occur within 12 weeks.

Water vapor thermal therapy and transurethral microwave thermotherapy (TUMT) are the most widely used minimally invasive methods of treating symptomatic BPH. With water vapor therapy a hollow needle is placed in prostatic tissue under cystoscopic visualization which is used to inject steam. Surrounding tissue is immediately coagulated. Several puncture sites are chosen based on the prostatic anatomy. During TUMT, catheter-mounted transducers use microwave energy to heat prostatic tissue, resulting in coagulative necrosis and shrinkage of the prostate gland. The subsequent reduction in prostate transition zone volume results in an improvement in flow rates and symptom scores. Transurethral needle ablation (TUNA), which uses low-level radio frequency energy to effect similar changes within the prostate gland, is no longer recommended by the AUA guidelines. Water vapor thermal therapy and aquablation are both office-based procedures that have shown efficacy similar to TUMT in patients with prostates less than 80 g, although retreatment rates may be higher than with other interventions. Lastly, the prostatic urethral lift procedure, which involves the placement of permanent transprostatic implants to mechanically open the urethra and improve voiding, has been shown to be effective in men with small prostates and no appreciable median lobe.

The most common side effects of these treatments are temporary increases in overactive bladder symptoms, transient urinary retention, hematuria, and ejaculatory dysfunction. However, antegrade ejaculation is generally preserved in men undergoing both water vapor thermal therapy and the prostatic urethral lift procedures, so patients should be appropriately counseled. Late complications such as urethral strictures and ED have been reported but are significantly less common than with traditional surgical approaches. The major benefits of these less invasive therapies are the reduction in traditional surgical morbidities (e.g., bleeding) and risks associated with general or spinal anesthesia and decreased rates of long-term complications such as incontinence, ED, bladder neck contractures, and urethral strictures. Additionally, most of these procedures can be accomplished safely on an outpatient basis, either in the office or in an ambulatory surgical setting.

Success rates for minimally invasive therapies are intermediate between those achieved with medical management and those of traditional surgical therapy, with 65% to 75% of patients experiencing symptomatic improvement and improved flow rates. The long-term durability of these therapies appears to be good but is presently being evaluated.

Surgical Management

TURP remains the "gold standard" for the surgical management of symptomatic BPH. A TURP procedure involves removal of the transition zone of the prostate through the use of a scope passed through the urethra using a cutting electrocautery loop. The goals of the surgery are to reduce the transition zone prostate tissue to the level of the prostatic capsule and to create a smooth, open appearance of the prostatic urethra and bladder neck. Improvements in the conventional technique have included bipolar electrosurgical cutting, which allows the use of normal saline irrigation and eliminates the risks associated with the potential systemic absorption of hypotonic irrigation solutions.

Newer operating room–based therapies have evolved that produce end results similar to or better than those of TURP. Holmium laser enucleation (HoLEP) is a surgical technique performed by specially trained urologists, generally indicated for large size prostates (>80 g). In this procedure, the entirety of the prostatic adenoma is "enucleated" from the capsule of the prostate and then removed through the urethra after morcellation. Other procedures include various forms of vaporization of the transition zone tissue of the prostate. In contrast to the TURP and HoLEP, no pieces of prostate are removed with these procedures as the tissue is vaporized. The various vaporization procedures include potassium titanyl phosphate (KTP or GreenLight)

TABLE 73.5   Success in Medical Versus Surgical Management of Benign Prostatic Hyperplasia

Degree of Improvement	α_1-Blockers	Finasteride	TURP	TUIP	Open Surgery
Symptoms (%)	48	31	82	73	79
Flow rate (%)	40-50	17	120	100	185
Mean probability (%) of achieving the stated improvements	74	67	88	80	98

TUIP, Transurethral incision of the prostate; *TURP,* transurethral resection of the prostate.

laser therapy, also called photovaporization of the prostate, and bipolar plasma vaporization of the prostate (button TURP). Rates of urinary incontinence, retrograde ejaculation, and urethral stricture are all higher after operating room procedures than after office-based therapies. Perioperative morbidity, including the need for blood transfusion, although substantially decreased by technical improvements, is likewise higher after TURP and similar procedures. However, standard electrosurgical resection of the prostate (TURP) is the most effective surgical treatment for symptomatic BPH short of enucleation. Success rates, as measured by improved symptom scores and increased urinary flow rates, are 80% to 90% after TURP.

Transurethral incision of the prostate (TUIP) is a more limited surgical procedure, although still performed under anesthesia in the operating room, that consists of incising the bladder neck and proximal prostatic urethra. This procedure is generally reserved for men with smaller prostates (<30 g) who have significant LUTS. Although it is more invasive than the heat-based therapies, success rates approach those of TURP in properly selected patients. Morbidity after TUIP is significantly less than after TURP, but long-term durability of symptom relief is less than that seen with TURP.

Surgical enucleation (simple prostatectomy) is reserved for patients with very large glands. Traditionally performed via an open lower abdominal incision, this procedure involves incision into the bladder neck or the capsule of the prostate and then removal of the prostatic adenoma from within the prostatic capsule. While success rates are high, the rate of complications such as bleeding and incontinence is higher than with any of the other traditional surgical approaches (Table 73.5). With advancements in robotic technology, this surgery is now being performed with a robot-assisted laparoscopic approach that has significantly reduced the associated morbidity. For many centers, robot-assisted simple prostatectomy or HoLEP remain the mainstay for management of very large symptomatic prostates.

Conclusion

The management of LUTS resulting from BPH has undergone a dramatic shift from principally a surgical approach to more of a medical one. This evolution of care, coupled with the aging of the U.S. population, has resulted in a shift of care for these patients from the urologist to the primary care physician. In the absence of severe LUTS or indications for early surgical intervention, the primary care physician can now successfully manage most cases of mild to moderate BPH. If there is no or minimal response to therapy, a variety of minimally invasive and surgical options are now available that are all highly successful.

BENIGN SCROTAL DISEASES

Benign masses of the scrotum are some of the most common complaints of men presenting to their primary care providers. While serious concerns such as testicular cancer or an incarcerated inguinal hernia must always be considered, the majority of these masses are benign. A thorough clinical history and physical exam alone will likely lead one to the correct diagnosis; scrotal ultrasound can be used to confirm a diagnosis or aid in finding the diagnosis for those with equivocal exam findings.

Varicocele

A scrotal varicocele is an abnormal dilation of the veins of the pampiniform plexus that run along the spermatic cord and can be palpated as a "bag of worms" with or without having the patient performing the Valsalva maneuver while standing. When examining a patient for any scrotal pathology, it is important to have the patient stand. A clinical varicocele is one that can be palpated on physical examination. Because the occurrence of varicoceles increases with age, the prevalence in the literature is highly variable. The prevalence of a unilateral palpable left-sided varicocele is between 6.5% and 22%, and that of bilateral palpable varicoceles ranges from 10% to 20%. The prevalence of an isolated right-sided palpable varicocele is less than 1%. However, because of a very rare association of isolated right-sided varicocele with retroperitoneal malignancy, many clinicians perform axial imaging on patients with a unilateral right-sided varicocele. In general, a left-sided varicocele does not have clinical significance unless it can be palpated on physical examination. A varicocele that is incidentally found during ultrasonography of the scrotum and is not palpable on examination is considered a subclinical varicocele and typically does not warrant intervention.

Palpable and nonpalpable varicoceles are most commonly found incidentally and, in most cases, have no clinical significance. However, palpable varicoceles can cause ipsilateral testicular atrophy, discomfort, and/or affect semen parameters. Therefore, it is important for the clinician to compare the size of the testicles in patients who desire future fertility. If the physical examination is unclear, scrotal ultrasonography can be used to accurately measure the size of both testicles. Any patient who desires future children and has a size discrepancy greater than 20% should be monitored closely and possibly referred to a urologist. Although varicoceles are most commonly found incidentally, they may also be found during a work-up for male factor infertility, scrotal pain, or asymptomatic testicular atrophy.

The pathophysiology of varicoceles is poorly understood but involves dilation of the internal spermatic vein and transmission of increased hydrostatic pressure across dysfunctional venous valves. Stasis of blood in the venous system disturbs the countercurrent heat exchange that is responsible for maintaining testicular temperature and may result in testicular parenchymal damage and impaired spermatogenesis.

Varicoceles are the most common cause of both primary male infertility (patient has fathered no children) and secondary male infertility (patient has fathered at least one child), accounting for 33% of cases. However, most men with palpable varicoceles are able to father children without difficulty. In a man with infertility and a palpable varicocele, semen analysis commonly reveals a low sperm count and abnormal sperm morphology and motility. After surgical correction of a varicocele in a patient with infertility, semen parameters improve in 60% to 80% and subsequent pregnancy rates range from 20% to 60%.

Providers often perform scrotal ultrasonography on any patient with chronic testicular pain to determine the source. Varicoceles are commonly found during this evaluation, but usually only palpable (clinical) varicoceles are considered as a source of pain. If a nonpalpable varicocele is found on an ultrasound examination, the patient should not be told that it is the cause of his pain. However, patients with palpable varicoceles and chronic testicular pain should be referred for treatment, as more than 80% of these men will have improvement in their pain after surgical correction.

Common operative techniques for treatment of a varicocele include high retroperitoneal ligation of the internal spermatic vein, microsurgical inguinal and subinguinal varicocelectomy, laparoscopic varicocelectomy, and gonadal vein embolization. The inguinal approach using microscopic magnification has the highest success and lowest complication and recurrence rates. The most common complication is hydrocele formation, whereas a rare complication is inadvertent ligation of the testicular artery resulting in testicular atrophy and loss. Surgical intervention for subclinical (nonpalpable) varicoceles is not indicated.

Spermatocele (Epididymal Cyst)

Spermatoceles and epididymal cysts are dilations of the tubes that connect the testicle to the epididymis (ductuli efferentes). Although they are technically synonymous, many clinicians refer to small lesions as epididymal cysts and larger ones as spermatoceles. These cystic lesions are very common and are found in 29% of asymptomatic men on ultrasonography. After a vasectomy, 35% of men develop a new small spermatocele, suggesting that distal obstruction of the vasa likely contributes to their development.

On physical examination, spermatoceles are somewhat mobile, firm masses that are separate and distinguishable from the smooth border of the testicle. It may be possible to transilluminate larger lesions, but this is rarely performed in practice. Spermatoceles are filled with a clear fluid that usually contains abundant amounts of sperm. If the lesion cannot be transilluminated, it is advisable to perform an ultrasound study of the scrotum to distinguish a spermatocele from a solid mass or from other testicular lesions. Of note, should a solid mass be identified on the epididymis on imaging, the vast majority of solid masses of the epididymis are benign. However, referral to a urologist for risk evaluation is prudent. Small spermatoceles and epididymal cysts normally have no clinical significance and are typically not the source of a patient's chronic testicular pain. They can be surgically removed if they are large or are causing discomfort for the patient.

Acute Epididymitis

Acute epididymitis is a clinical syndrome that may manifest with fever, acute scrotal pain, and impressive swelling and induration of the epididymis. Epididymitis is most often caused by retrograde bacterial spread from the bladder or urethra into the vasa and then into the epididymides. In men younger than 35 years of age, the most common causative agents are those organisms associated with sexually transmitted infections—namely, *Neisseria gonococcus* and *Chlamydia trachomatis*. In older men, acute epididymitis is usually caused by a coliform bacteria such as *Escherichia coli* and often occurs in association other lower urinary tract infections or bladder outlet obstruction.

The most important consideration in diagnosing acute epididymitis is differentiating this disease from acute testicular torsion. Physical examination can be nonspecific, although focal epididymal swelling and tenderness are suggestive, and the presence of white cells and bacteria in the urine is indicative of an infectious etiology. Scrotal

ultrasonography with Doppler flow can be extremely helpful in differentiating acute epididymitis from torsion in difficult cases, as the epididymis will present with increased vascular flow (hyperemia) while torsion will show no or diminished flow within the testicle.

Patients with acute epididymitis have significant inflammation that can also involve the testicle (epididymo-orchitis). Patients with severe epididymitis involving the testicle are often systemically ill. In most instances, initial treatment should consist of antibiotics, nonsteroidal anti-inflammatory medications, and possibly oral narcotics. In some cases, broad-spectrum antibiotics or even hospital admission may be necessary. In general, patients younger than 35 years of age should be treated with ceftriaxone and doxycycline. Older patients are usually empirically treated with a fluoroquinolone for 2 to 4 weeks. Complications associated with acute epididymitis include abscess formation, reactive hydrocele formation, testicular infarction, infertility, and chronic epididymitis or orchalgia.

Hydrocele

A hydrocele is a sterile fluid collection located between the parietal and visceral layers of the tunica vaginalis of the scrotum. Noncommunicating hydroceles are commonly seen in adults and usually surround the testicle and spermatic cord. Communicating hydroceles are more common in children and actually represent indirect inguinal hernias. These communicating hydroceles contain only fluid and not bowel or fat because the opening into the peritoneal cavity is small. Communicating hydroceles can be distinguished from noncommunicating hydroceles on physical examination by gently pushing the fluid out of the scrotum and into the peritoneum, or by a history of fluctuation in size of the fluid collection throughout the day or with standing and lying down.

Patients with a noncommunicating hydrocele usually have complaints of heaviness in the scrotum, scrotal pain, or an enlarging scrotal mass. Usually the diagnosis is easily made based on the physical examination and transillumination of the scrotum. If the testis is not palpable, an ultrasound study may be performed to rule out a testicular tumor associated with a secondary or reactive hydrocele. Noncommunicating hydroceles are caused by increased secretion or decreased reabsorption of serous fluid by the tunica vaginalis. Infection, trauma, surgery, neoplastic disease, and lymphatic disease are causative in many adults, whereas the remainder of cases are idiopathic.

Asymptomatic hydroceles are benign and do not require treatment unless desired by the patient. Definitive treatment of symptomatic hydroceles requires surgical intervention. Although the recurrence rate is significantly higher with aspiration and sclerotherapy, this approach can be a good option in patients who are considered poor surgical candidates. Hydrocelectomy procedures involve drainage of the serous fluid with either excision of the redundant tunica vaginalis or plication of the sac without excision. After surgery, the rates of hydrocele recurrence and chronic pain are 9% and 1%, respectively.

Testicular Torsion

Testicular torsion is considered a true urologic emergency. The testicle receives its blood supply from the testicular artery (a branch of the aorta), the vasal artery (a branch of the inferior vesicle artery), and the cremasteric artery (a branch of the inferior epigastric artery). All three vessels are transmitted to the testicle through the spermatic cord. Torsion of the spermatic cord impairs arterial inflow as well as venous outflow. If detorsion is not performed within 6 to 8 hours, testicular infarction and hemorrhagic necrosis are likely to occur. Typically, patients are younger than 21 years of age, although testicular torsion can occur later in life. Delays in presentation and diagnosis are more common in the adult patient population and are often related to patient and physician factors.

The characteristic signs and symptoms of acute testicular torsion are the acute onset of scrotal pain, swelling, nausea, vomiting, loss of normal rugae of the scrotal skin, absent cremasteric reflex, and a high-riding, rotated, tender testicle. The diagnosis of testicular torsion remains a clinical one; however, in equivocal cases, if ultrasound equipment is readily available and obtaining an ultrasound does not negatively affect the patient promptly proceeding to the operating room, scrotal ultrasonography may be performed prior to surgery. In many cases, surgical exploration is undertaken when the index of suspicion is high but imaging is not available. Doppler ultrasonography is extremely useful in differentiating testicular torsion from other causes of acute scrotum, such as acute epididymitis, torsion of the appendix testis, and trauma, as previously discussed.

It is possible to untwist testicular torsion by manual manipulation of the testicle through the scrotum in the emergency room or in a physician's office. After giving the patient parenteral narcotics, the testicle can be untwisted by gently pulling down on it and, usually, rotating it laterally (like opening a book). If this is successful, the testicle will uncoil like a spring and fall into its normal position, with immediate relief of the patient's pain. Even if the procedure is successful, patients should still be taken to the operating room for bilateral orchiopexy to prevent future occurrences.

Important surgical principles include surgical detorsion and assessment of testicular viability in the operating room. If the testis is determined to be viable, bilateral orchiopexy is performed using the technique of three-point fixation (sutures placed medially, laterally, and inferiorly). In the presence of infarction, orchiectomy is recommended. Orchiopexy of the contralateral testicle is always performed simultaneously. When diagnosis and surgery occur in a timely fashion, testicular salvage rates approach 70%. Delayed surgical therapy significantly decreases the salvage rate to approximately 40%.

SUGGESTED READINGS

Alleman WG, Gorman B, King BF, et al: Benign and malignant epididymal masses evaluated with scrotal sonography: clinical and pathologic review of 85 patients, J Ultrasound Med 27:1195–1202, 2008.

Baillargeon J, Urban RJ, Ottenbacher KJ, et al: Trends in androgen prescribing in the United States, 2001 to 2011, JAMA Intern Med 173:1465–1466, 2013.

Bhasin S, Cunningham GR, Hayes FJ, et al: Testosterone therapy in men with androgen deficiency syndromes: an endocrine society clinical practice guideline, J Clin Endocrinol Metab 95:2536–2559, 2010.

Burnett AL, Nehra A, Breau RH, et al: Erectile dysfunction: AUA guideline, J Urol 200:633, 2018.

Capoccia E, Levine LA: Contemporary review of Peyronie's disease treatment, Curr Urol Rep 19:51, 2018.

Cappelleri JC, Rosen RC: The Sexual Health Inventory for Men (SHIM): a 5-year review of research and clinical experience, Int J Impotence Res 17:307–319, 2005.

Carson CC, Lue TF: Phosphodiesterase type 5 inhibitors for erectile dysfunction, Br J Urol Int 96:257–280, 2005.

Costa P, Potempa A-J: Intraurethral alprostadil for erectile dysfunction: a review of the literature, Drugs 72:2243–2254, 2012.

D'Amico AV, Chen MH, Roehl KA, et al: Preoperative PSA velocity and the risk of death from prostate cancer after radical prostatectomy, N Engl J Med 351:125–135, 2004.

Eggener SE, Roehl KA, Catalona WJ: Predictors of subsequent prostate cancer in men with a prostate specific antigen of 2.6 to 4.0 ng/ml and an initially negative biopsy, J Urol 174:500–504, 2005.

Feldman HA, Goldstein I, Hatzichristou DG, et al: Impotence and its medical and psychosocial correlates: results of the massachusetts male aging study, J Urol 151:54–61, 1994.

Ficarra V, Crestani A, Novara G, et al: Varicocele repair for infertility: what is the evidence? Curr Opin Urol 22:489–494, 2012.

Foster HE, Dahm P, Kohler TS, et al: Surgical management of lower urinary tract symptoms attributed to benign prostatic hyperplasia: AUA guideline amendment 2019, J Urol 202:592, 2019.

Gelbard M, Goldstein I, Hellstrom WJG, et al: Clinical efficacy, safety and tolerability of collagenase clostridium histolyticum for the treatment of Peyronie disease in 2 large double-blind, randomized, placebo controlled phase 3 studies, J Urol 190:199–207, 2013.

Kaplan SA, Roehrborn CG, Rovner ES, et al: Tolterodine and tamsulosin for treatment of men with lower urinary tract symptoms and overactive bladder: a randomized controlled trial, J Am Med Assoc 296:2319–2328, 2006.

Karmazyn B, Steinberg R, Kurareid L, et al: Clinical and radiographic criteria of the acute scrotum in children: a retrospective study in 172 boys, Pediatr Radiol 35:302–310, 2005.

Kostis JB, Jackson G, Rosen R, et al: Sexual dysfunction and cardiac risk (the second Princeton Consensus Conference), Am J Cardiol 96:313–321, 2005.

Lowe FC, McConnell JD, Hudson PB, et al: for the Finasteride Study Group, Long-term 6-year experience with finasteride in patients with benign prostatic hyperplasia, Urology 61:791-796, 2003.

Lue TF: Erectile dysfunction, N Engl J Med 342:1802, 2000.

McConnell JD, Roehrborn CG, Bautista OM, et al, for the Medical Therapy of Prostatic Symptoms (MTOPS) Research Group: The long-term effect of doxazosin, finasteride, and combination therapy on the clinical progression of benign prostatic hyperplasia, N Engl J Med 349:2387-2398, 2003.

Meriggiola MC, Bremner WJ, Costantino A, et al: Low dose of cyproterone acetate and testosterone enanthate for contraception in men, Hum Reprod 13:1225–1229, 1998.

Morgentaler A, Caliber M: Safety of testosterone therapy in men with prostate cancer, Expert Opin Drug Saf 1, 2019.

Morgentaler A, Traish A, Hackett G, et al: Diagnosis and treatment of testosterone deficiency: updated recommendations from the lisbon 2018 international consultation for sexual medicine, Sex Med Rev, 2019.

Mulhall JP, Trost LW, Brannigan RE, et al: Evaluation and management of testosterone deficiency: AUA guideline, J Urol 200:423, 2018.

Nehra A, Alterowitz R, Culkin DJ, et al: Peyronie's disease: AUA guideline, J Urol 194:745, 2015.

Neiderberger C: Microsurgical treatment of persistent or recurrent varicocele, J Urol 173:2079–2080, 2005.

Nieschlag E, Swerdloff R, Behre HM, et al: Investigation, treatment, and monitoring of late-onset hypogonadism in males: ISA, ISSAM, and EAU recommendations, J Androl 27:135–137, 2006.

Rhoden EL, Morgentaler A: Risks of testosterone-replacement therapy and recommendations for monitoring, N Engl J Med 350:482–492, 2004.

Roehrborn CG, Kaplan SA, Jones JS, et al: Tolterodine extended release with or without tamsulosin in men with lower urinary tract symptoms including overactive bladder symptoms: effects of prostate size, Eur Urol 55:472–479, 2009.

Sessions AE, Rabinowitz R, Hulbert WC, et al: Testicular torsion: direction, degree, duration and disinformation, J Urol 169:663–665, 2003.

Shridharani A, Lockwood G, Sandlow J: Varicocelectomy in the treatment of testicular pain: a review, Curr Opin Urol 22:499–506, 2012.

Stewart CA, Yafi FA, Knoedler M, et al: Intralesional injection of interferon-α2b improves penile curvature in men with Peyronie's disease independent of plaque location, J Urol 194:1704–1707, 2015.

Svartberg J, Midtby M, Bønaa KH, et al: The associations of age, lifestyle factors and chronic disease with testosterone in men: the Tromsø Study, Eur J Endocrinol 149:145–152, 2003.

Wang C: Phosphodiesterase-5 inhibitors and benign prostatic hyperplasia, Curr Opin Urol 20:49–54, 2010.

Wu FCW, Tajar A, Beynon JM, et al: Identification of late-onset hypogonadism in middle-aged and elderly men, N Engl J Med 363:123–135, 2010.

Yafi FA, Pinsky MR, Sangkum P, et al: Therapeutic advances in the treatment of Peyronie's disease, Andrology 3:650, 2015.

Diseases of Bone and Bone Mineral Metabolism

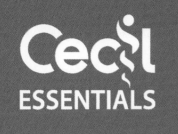

74

Normal Physiology of Bone and Mineral Homeostasis

Clemens Bergwitz, John J. Wysolmerski

CALCIUM HOMEOSTASIS

Circulating free (or ionized) calcium concentrations are maintained within a narrow normal range by an intricate series of homeostatic mechanisms. Maintaining stable calcium levels is important for at least three reasons. First, calcium along with phosphorus forms *hydroxyapatite*, the major mineral contained within the skeleton. Hydroxyapatite provides structural integrity to bones and also provides a metabolic store of calcium to maintain circulating levels if calcium is not readily available from the environment. Reductions in the mineral content of the skeleton can impair its biomechanical integrity and result in fractures. Second, the circulating ionized calcium concentration influences membrane excitability in muscle and nervous tissue. An increase in serum calcium levels produces refractoriness to the stimulation of neurons and muscle cells, which could lead to muscular weakness and even coma. Conversely, a reduction in ionized calcium levels increases neuromuscular excitability, which can translate clinically into seizures or spontaneous muscle cramps and contractions referred to as *carpopedal spasm* or *tetany*. Finally, intracellular calcium contributes to a host of cellular functions, including enzymatic reactions, intracellular signaling, vesicular trafficking, and cytoskeletal organization to name a few. Therefore, all cells require a stable source of calcium in extracellular fluid for proper function. Physicians routinely use a variety of drugs that regulate channels and intracellular calcium concentrations to manipulate cellular function for the treatment of a wide variety of human diseases.

Total circulating calcium levels, which are customarily measured for diagnostic purposes, typically fall between 8.5 to 10.5 mg/dL (4 mg/dL = 1 mmol/L). Of this total value approximately 50% of calcium circulates as free or ionized calcium, 5% circulates as insoluble complexes such as calcium sulfate, phosphate, and citrate, and the remainder (45%) is bound to serum proteins, principally albumin. It is the free, ionized calcium that is important for physiologic processes or in pathophysiologic settings. While changes in the total calcium usually reflect changes in ionized calcium levels, in some instances, total serum calcium can change without a change in the ionized calcium level. For example, if the serum albumin level declines as a result of hepatic cirrhosis or the nephrotic syndrome, the total serum calcium also declines, but the ionized serum calcium concentration remains normal. Therefore, measuring the ionized serum calcium level directly or deriving it from formula 1 and 2 can be important clinically.

Formula 1 (Payne RB, Little AJ, Williams RB, Milner JR: Interpretation of serum calcium in patients with abnormal plasma proteins, Br Med J 4:643-646, 1973) is:

$$Ca_{Ad} \text{ (mmol/L)} = Ca_T \text{ (mmol/L)} + 0.025 (40 - \text{albumin, g/L})$$

Formula 2 (Pfitzenmeyer P, Martin I, d'Athis P, et al: A new formula for correction of total calcium level into ionized serum calcium values in very elderly hospitalized patients, Arch Gerontol Geriatrics 45:151-157, 2007) is:

$$Ca^{2+} \text{ (mmol/L)} = 0.188 - 0.00469 \text{ protein (g/L)} \\ + 0.0110 \text{ albumin (g/L)} + 0.401 \, Ca_{Ad} \text{ (mmol/L)}.$$

An overview of calcium economy is represented in Fig. 74.1. As depicted, the circulating calcium level is influenced by a series of three major fluxes of calcium: (1) The net absorption of calcium from the diet in the gut, (2) the storage of calcium in and the liberation of calcium from the hydroxyapatite "warehouse" in the skeleton, and (3) the filtration and net excretion of calcium by the kidneys. Calcium homeostasis and disorders of calcium metabolism involve the hormonal regulation of fluxes between these three compartments.

Calcium Fluxes Into and Out of Extracellular Fluid
Intestinal Calcium Absorption

The average dietary calcium intake for an adult is approximately 1000 mg per day. About 300 mg of the total is absorbed (i.e., unidirectional absorption is about 30%), principally within the duodenum and proximal jejunum. However, about 150 mg of calcium per day is secreted by the liver (in bile), the pancreas (in pancreatic secretions), and the intestinal glands into the gut lumen. Thus, net absorption (called *fractional absorption*) of calcium is approximately 15% of intake and about 85% of calcium entering the gut lumen will be excreted in the feces each day.

The efficiency of calcium absorption is regulated at the level of the small intestinal epithelial cell, the enterocyte, by the active form of vitamin D, 1,25-dihydroxyvitamin D (1,25[OH]$_2$D), also called *calcitriol*. Increases in 1,25(OH)$_2$D enhance calcium absorption, and decreases in 1,25(OH)$_2$D reduce absorption of dietary calcium. Dietary calcium absorption can be increased over the short term by increasing calcium intake or by increasing plasma 1,25(OH)$_2$D concentrations, or both. Pathologic increases in serum calcium (i.e., hypercalcemia) can be caused by increases in circulating 1,25(OH)$_2$D (e.g., in sarcoidosis) or by excessive calcium intake (i.e., milk-alkali syndrome). Conversely, hypocalcemia can result from a decline in 1,25(OH)$_2$D (e.g., chronic renal failure, hypoparathyroidism, vitamin D deficiency).

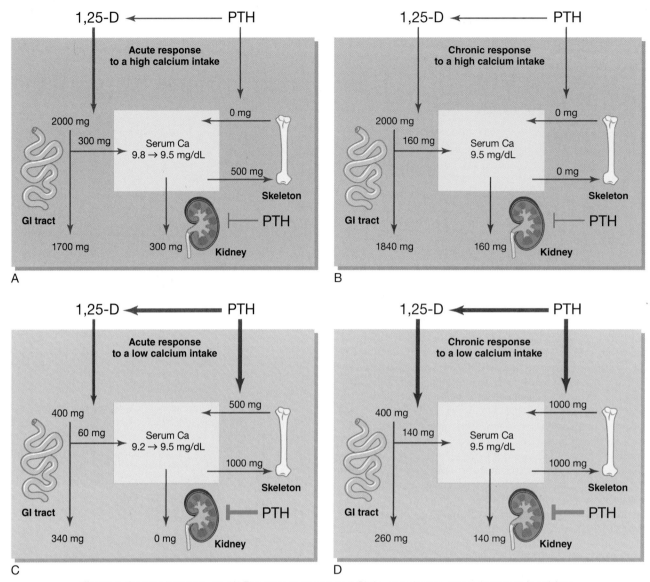

Fig. 74.1 Calcium homeostasis. (A) The acute response and (B) the chronic response to increases in calcium intake. (C) The acute response and (D) the chronic response to decreases in calcium intake. Details are provided in the text. *GI,* Gastrointestinal; *PTH,* parathyroid hormone; *1,25(OH)₂D,* 1,25-dihydroxycholecalciferol (calcitriol). SI conversion: 1 mg calcium = 0.4 mmol calcium.

Renal Calcium Handling

The filtered load of calcium by the kidneys is about 10,000 mg per day assuming a glomerular filtration rate (GFR) of 100 mL/min and serum calcium of 10 mg/dL, making the kidney the most important moment-to-moment regulator of the serum calcium concentration and, as a result, disordered renal calcium handling (e.g., thiazide diuretic use, hypoparathyroidism) can produce significant abnormalities in serum calcium homeostasis.

Of the 10,000 mg of calcium filtered at the glomerulus each day, about 9000 mg (90%) is reabsorbed *proximally* by the proximal convoluted tubule, the pars recta, and the thick ascending limb of Henle loop. This 90% is absorbed in conjunction/competition with sodium and chloride reabsorption and is not subject to regulation by parathyroid hormone (PTH). The remaining 10% (1000 mg) that arrives at the distal tubule is subject to regulation by PTH, which stimulates renal calcium reabsorption. The anticalciuric effect of PTH can be extremely efficient, and elevated PTH concentrations can essentially eliminate calcium

excretion into the urine. This action is a potent mechanism for retaining calcium under conditions of calcium deprivation (e.g., a low-calcium diet, vitamin D deficiency, intestinal malabsorption) and can contribute to hypercalcemia under pathologic conditions, as in primary hyperparathyroidism. The absence of PTH action, in turn, produces hypercalciuria and nephrolithiasis in hypoparathyroidism. Because of preserved PTH action at the distal tubules in pseudohypoparathyroidism, hypocalciuria characterizes this rare genetic condition, which is caused by end-organ resistance to PTH at the proximal tubules, leading to hypovitaminosis D and hypocalcemia despite often elevated PTH levels.

About 150 mg of calcium is excreted by the kidney in the final urine on a daily basis in a healthy individual. If the kidney filters 10,000 mg of calcium each day, and if 150 mg is excreted in the final urine, 9850 mg (98.5%) is reabsorbed at proximal and distal sites. Therefore, a healthy person is in zero calcium balance with respect to the outside world: intake (1000 mg/day) − output [(850 mg/day in feces) + (150 mg/day in urine)] = 0.

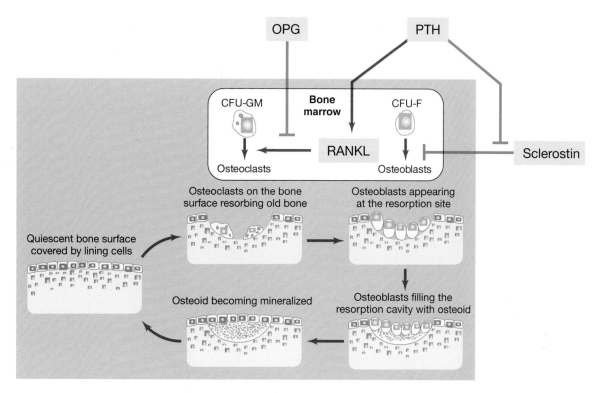

Fig. 74.2 Cellular components of bone remodeling. Bone remodeling is a continuous process that involves the activation of osteoclast precursors in the macrophage lineage (i.e., colony-forming units of granulocyte-macrophage progenitors [CFU-GM]) by RANKL that become actively resorbing osteoclasts, which tunnel into the bone surface to dig resorption lacunae. Bone resorption can be inhibited by bisphosphonates, which are toxic to osteoclasts, or by antibody drugs that inhibit RANKL, such as the decoy receptor osteoprotegerin (OPG). Osteoblast precursors in the fibroblast–bone marrow stromal cell lineage (CFU-F) then appear and become active at the sites of prior resorption, and they secrete new osteoid, which later mineralizes to fill the lacunae created by osteoclastic bone resorption. Both processes are stimulated by PTH, which inhibits the bone formation inhibitor sclerostin. PTH analogs and antibody drugs that inhibit sclerostin can be used to stimulate bone formation.

Skeletal Biology and Calcium Homeostasis

The skeleton contains about 1.2 kg of calcium in a male adult and 1.0 kg in a female adult. Most of this calcium is in the form of crystal hydroxyapatite, a calcium phosphate salt. Calcium contributes in an important way to the structural integrity of the skeleton and, in turn, the skeleton serves as a quantitatively large reservoir (i.e., a sink) for adding and removing calcium to and from the extracellular fluid (ECF) compartment at appropriate times.

The adult skeleton is composed of two types of bone: cortical (or lamellar) bone and trabecular (or cancellous) bone. Cortical bone predominates in the skull and the shafts of long bones, and trabecular bone predominates at other sites, such as the distal radius, the vertebral bodies, and the trochanters of the hip.

Bone is not an inert tissue; rather, it is continually turning over. The adult skeleton is completely remodeled every 3 to 10 years. Remodeling is perhaps best appreciated by recalling that orthopedic surgeons routinely and intentionally set fractures imperfectly, knowing that the normal processes of bone remodeling will restore the bone's original shape with the passage of time.

The cells that regulate bone turnover can be divided into those that remove old bone, those that provide new bone (Fig. 74.2) (see Chapter 76), and those that regulate these two processes. Cells that remove, or resorb, old bone are osteoclasts. These cells are large, metabolically active, multinucleated cells derived from the fusion of circulating macrophages. Following attachment to the surface of bone,

osteoclasts form a sealing zone over the bone surface into which they secrete protons (i.e., acid), proteases (e.g., collagenase), and proteoglycan-digesting enzymes (e.g., hyaluronidase). The acid solubilizes hydroxyapatite crystals, releasing calcium, and the enzymes digest bone proteins and proteoglycans (e.g., collagen, osteocalcin, osteopontin), which constitute the nonmineral, or osteoid, component of bone. Osteoclasts move along the surface of trabecular bone plates and drill tunnels in cortical bone, periodically releasing the digested contents within their sealed zones into the bone marrow space and thereby creating resorption pits, called Howship's lacunae, on the trabecular bone surface. The released calcium contributes to the ECF calcium pool, and the released proteolytic products, such as deoxypyridinoline cross-links (i.e., collagen fragments and hydroxyproline), can be used clinically as indices of bone resorption.

New bone formation is accomplished by osteoblasts, which are derived from marrow stromal cells or bone surface lining cells. Osteoblasts synthesize and secrete the components of the nonmineral phase of bone, called osteoid. The components are mostly proteins and include collagen, osteopontin, osteonectin, osteocalcin, proteoglycans, and a plethora of growth factors, including transforming growth factor-β and insulin-like growth factor-I. Osteoblasts also produce alkaline phosphatase, which inactivates the mineralization inhibitor pyrophosphate, and type 1 collagen, which forms cable-like structures in bone matrix, and they also facilitate the deposition of hydroxyapatite between these proteinaceous cables. Both the bone-specific isoform of alkaline phosphatase and procollagen can be used clinically as indices of bone formation. Maintaining the correct balance between protein and mineral in bone provides the combination of compliance and toughness needed to withstand the biomechanical forces encountered by the skeleton.

In the past decade, attention has focused on a third, previously underappreciated bone cell type, the osteocyte. These cells are descendants of osteoblasts and are embedded into the mineralized phase of bone. Osteocytes physically connect with one another and to cells at the mineral surface through long dendritic processes. The dendritic processes extensively permeate the mineralized phase of bone through an elaborate canalicular network. Osteocytes serve a critical role in sensing biomechanical strain within bone, and through their cellular extensions to the bone surface, they communicate signals that attract, activate, or repress osteoclasts and osteoblasts. In this way, they determine which areas of the skeleton require new bone formation and which need to be targets of osteoclastic bone resorption, a critical function for proper structural remodeling of bone tissue.

Bone remodeling involves the coordinated removal of old bone through osteoclastic bone resorption stimulated by receptor activator of nuclear factor κB ligand (RANKL) followed by the formation of new bone via osteoblastic bone formation. This process occurs in discrete locations called bone remodeling units, the locations of which, as described previously, are likely dictated by osteocytes. In adults, skeletal homeostasis requires the careful balancing of osteoclast and osteoblast activities so that the same amount of bone that is removed by osteoclasts is replaced by osteoblasts. This is accomplished by a complex, and only partly understood, three-way series of communications between osteoclasts, osteoblasts, and osteocytes, that are modulated by systemic hormones. Altering the relative activities of these cells can result in the net movement of calcium out of or into the skeleton on a physiologic basis but a prolonged imbalance of osteoclastic and osteoblastic activities can result in disease. For example, excessive bone remodeling leads to osteoporosis, while absent bone remodeling leads to adynamic bone disease, both conditions that can predispose to fractures. Bone remodeling is also exploited therapeutically. Anabolic agents for osteoporosis, such as sclerostin inhibitors or parathyroid hormone and parathyroid hormone-related protein analogues stimulate the activity of osteoblasts to produce new bone. In contrast, antiresorptive agents, such as estrogens, estrogen-like drugs, bisphosphonates, and RANKL inhibitors, reduce bone resorption to improve bone mass and bone mechanical properties.

Bone remodeling is important for systemic calcium homeostasis. Osteoclasts are mobilized to release calcium from the skeleton in times of need in order to maintain a normal serum calcium concentration and prevent hypocalcemia. Conversely, unmineralized osteoid produced by osteoblasts serves to deposit excess calcium to prevent hypercalcemia. Under normal circumstances, osteoclasts result in the release of about 500 mg of calcium per day from the skeleton to the ECF compartment. At the same time, osteoblasts produce osteoid that mineralizes at a rate such that about 500 mg of ECF calcium is deposited in the skeleton at new sites. From the perspective of the normal homeostatic fluxes shown in Fig. 74.1, the skeleton is in zero calcium balance with the ECF, and the whole organism is in zero calcium balance with the external environment.

Considering the complexity of this calcium homeostatic system and the importance of maintaining tight control of serum calcium levels, an obvious need exists for systemic regulation and integration of the calcium fluxes across the GI, skeletal, and renal compartments. The two key metabolic regulatory hormones that coordinate these activities are PTH and the active form of vitamin D, $1,25(OH)_2D$.

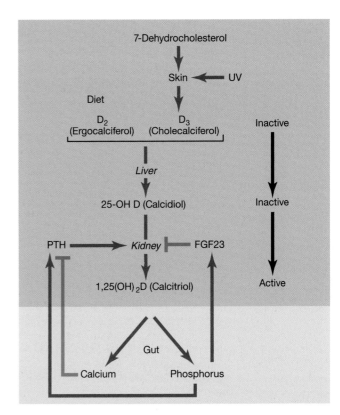

Fig. 74.3 Calcium and phosphate homeostasis are co-regulated by parathyroid hormone (PTH). PTH is secreted as an 84-amino-acid protein, which is cleaved in the liver to derivative amino-terminal and carboxyl-terminal (C-term) forms. Actions of the amino-terminally intact forms of PTH are listed in Table 74.1. It stimulates synthesis of the active form of $1,25(OH)_2D$, 1,25-dihydroxycholecalciferol, from its biologically inactive precursors, vitamin D_2 and D_3, which are either produced in the skin or absorbed from the diet in the gastrointestinal (GI) tract, and 25-hydroxylated in the liver and kidney. $1,25(OH)_2D$ stimulates absorption of calcium and phosphate from the diet in the GI tract. Different from PTH, fibroblast growth factor 23 (FGF23) stimulates renal phosphate excretion and inhibits the last step (1α hydroxylation) of vitamin D activation. Although both PTH and FGF23 lower phosphate levels, PTH primarily responds to changes in circulating calcium levels, while FGF23 responds to alterations in phosphate levels. Their different actions on vitamin D synthesis reflect their different primary functions since PTH increases 1,25 vitamin D levels to help restore low calcium levels towards normal and FGF23 suppresses 1,25 vitamin D levels to help restore elevated phosphate levels towards normal.

Regulatory Hormones
Parathyroid Hormone

PTH is a peptide hormone produced by the four parathyroid glands (Fig. 74.3 and Table 74.1). These glands are located behind the normal thyroid lobes, with two on the right and two on the left. Through the calcium sensor—a G protein–coupled receptor for calcium that is located on the surface of the parathyroid cell—the serum ionized calcium concentration is continuously monitored. In this exquisitely sensitive system, minor (e.g., 0.1 mg/dL) reductions in serum ionized calcium lead to PTH secretion, and minor increments in serum calcium lead to suppression of PTH secretion.

PTH is secreted as an 84-amino-acid peptide hormone that is rapidly (half-life of about 3 to 5 minutes) cleaved by the Kupffer cells in the liver into an active amino-terminal form and an inactive carboxyl-terminal fragment. Continuous monitoring of the serum calcium concentration by the parathyroid glands, the immediate secretion of PTH in response

TABLE 74.1 Hormone Actions

Hormone	S-CA	U-CA	P-Pi	U-Pi	S-1,25(OH)$_2$-D	S-Mg	U-Mg	Other
PTH	↑	↓	↓	↑	↑	=	=	Stimulates bone remodeling, induces hypotension
FGF23	=/↓	=/↓	↓	↑	↓	=	=	Inhibits growth plates resulting in short stature, causes left ventricular hypertrophy
1,25(OH)$_2$D	↑	↑	↑	↑	↓	=	=	Inhibits PTH secretion and stimulates FGF23 synthesis
EGF1	=/↓	=/↑	=	=	=/↓	↑	↓	

EGF1, Epidermal growth factor 1; *FGF23,* fibroblast growth factor 23; *PTH,* parathyroid hormone; *1,25(OH)$_2$D,* 1,25-dihydroxy vitamin D.

to hypocalcemia, and the rapid clearance of PTH after secretion enable the parathyroid gland and PTH to regulate serum calcium rapidly and with remarkable precision.

PTH targets three organs, two directly and one indirectly. In the kidney, PTH stimulates calcium reabsorption in the distal tubule inhibiting urinary calcium excretion. PTH also inhibits phosphate and bicarbonate reabsorption by the proximal tubules, which induces phosphaturia and hypophosphatemia and proximal renal tubular acidosis, respectively. PTH also stimulates the production of the active form of vitamin D, 1,25(OH)$_2$D by the renal tubules. These actions of PTH on the kidney are rapid and direct.

The second PTH target is the skeleton. PTH can mobilize calcium immediately from the skeleton through the activity of osteoclasts and osteocytes, without activating bone formation, which is important for the rapid delivery of calcium to the ECF. If PTH is elevated over days to weeks, it also stimulates the activity of osteoblasts directly and through inhibition of sclerostin release by osteocytes to produce new bone. This type of prolonged elevation in PTH stimulates bone resorption in excess of bone formation to maintain a net release of skeletal calcium to the ECF, enabling the skeleton to help prevent hypocalcemia in states of nutritional calcium deficiency, malabsorption or vitamin D deficiency.

The third target organ is the intestine, which PTH affects indirectly. By increasing renal synthesis of 1,25(OH)$_2$D, PTH can lead to increased intestinal calcium absorption to supply more calcium to the ECF from the diet, a response that is not immediate but occurs over several days of PTH stimulation. Seen in concert, PTH is secreted in response to hypocalcemia, and the actions of PTH combine to restore a low serum calcium concentration to normal by preventing renal calcium losses, by releasing calcium from the skeleton, and by indirectly stimulating (through 1,25[OH]$_2$D) increases in intestinal calcium absorption.

Vitamin D

Vitamin D occurs in two forms: ergocalciferol (vitamin D$_2$) and cholecalciferol (vitamin D$_3$) (Fig. 74.3 and Table 74.2). Both substances are inactive precursors. One (D$_3$) is derived principally from skin exposed to sunlight and the other (D$_2$) is derived from plant sterols in the diet. Either D$_2$, D$_3$ or both can be found in multivitamins and commercial dietary supplements.

Both precursors are constitutively converted to their respective 25-hydroxyvitamin D (25[OH]D) derivatives in the liver through the actions of the enzyme vitamin D 25-hydroxylase (CYP2R1). 25(OH)D is also called calcidiol and has 1000-fold lower affinity to the vitamin D receptor (VDR) when compared to 1,25(OH)$_2$D, but it is a helpful clinical laboratory measure of the vitamin D status (i.e., repletion or deficiency) of patients with hypocalcemia, osteomalacia or rickets, osteoporosis, intestinal malabsorption, and other similar conditions. Furthermore, severe liver disease such as cirrhosis prevents this 25-hydroxylation and leads to a vitamin D–deficiency syndrome called hepatic osteodystrophy.

25(OH)D is converted, or activated, in the renal proximal tubule by the enzyme 25-hydroxyvitamin D$_3$ 1α-hydroxylase (CYP27B1) to the active form of the vitamin, 1,25(OH)$_2$D, which is also called calcitriol.

PTH increases 1,25(OH)$_2$D levels by stimulating its formation through the activity of CYP27B1 while also inhibiting its degradation through the activity of another enzyme, CYP24A1 (24-hydroxylase), which converts 1,25(OH)$_2$D to its inactive metabolite, 24,25(OH)$_2$D. The primary action of 1,25(OH)$_2$D is to regulate intestinal calcium absorption. PTH, through 1,25(OH)$_2$D, indirectly regulates calcium absorption from the diet by the intestine. The hypocalcemia of hypoparathyroidism is a result, in part, of inadequate intestinal calcium absorption. Conversely, hyperparathyroidism is associated with hypercalciuria and nephrolithiasis, both of which directly result from increases in circulating 1,25(OH)$_2$D levels. Therefore, measurement of 1,25(OH)$_2$D can be used as an index of parathyroid function and intestinal calcium absorption.

Because of some affinity to the vitamin D receptor, high doses of calcidiol can be used to treat hypoparathyroidism. However, 1α-hydroxylated versions (i.e., hectoral), which can be 25-hydroxylated by CYP2R1 in the liver or calcitriol, have become standard of care for these disorders (see Table 74.2).

Calcitonin

Calcitonin is produced by the parafollicular or C cells of the thyroid gland in response to hypercalcemia. It was once viewed as an essential calcium-regulating hormone. Pharmacologic doses of calcitonin reduce serum calcium levels by inhibiting osteoclastic bone resorption, which is used in the emergency setting along with hydration to rapidly treat life-threatening hypercalcemia, but this effect wears off quickly due to tachyphylaxis (i.e., desensitization of osteoclasts). Little evidence exists that calcitonin has homeostatic relevance in humans, although it appears to contribute to the regulation of calcium and skeletal homeostasis during reproductive cycles in female rodents.

Integration of Calcium Homeostasis

Ingestion of a greater than normal dietary calcium load (see Fig. 74.1A) leads to a mild rise in the serum calcium level. The rise in calcium is sensed by the parathyroid glands that suppress PTH secretion causing a rapid and marked increase in renal calcium excretion by the distal tubule. It also immediately decreases osteoclastic activity, which slows continued bone resorption but allows continued calcium entry from the ECF into unmineralized osteoid. These two effects produce a rapid, short-term reduction in serum calcium to normal levels. However, if the high-calcium diet is maintained over the long term, these adaptations are insufficient. Continued renal calcium wasting leads to hypercalciuria (with nephrolithiasis and nephrocalcinosis), and unopposed osteoblastic bone formation leads to excessive skeletal mineralization (i.e., osteopetrosis).

Two additional responses (see Fig. 74.1B) are required to prevent the long-term adverse effects of a high-calcium diet. First, subacute or chronic suppression of PTH reduces circulating 1,25(OH)$_2$D. This reduces the efficiency of calcium absorption from the intestine, calcium entry into the ECF, and urinary calcium excretion. Second, a chronic decrement in PTH leads to a chronic decline in osteoblastic activity. No osteoid is formed, and the ability to deposit calcium into the skeleton is decreased.

TABLE 74.2	Phosphate and Vitamin D Metabolite Preparations			
Phosphate Preparations		**Phosphorus Content**	**Potassium (K) Content**	**Sodium (Na) Content**
Neutra-Phos powder (for mixing with liquid)		250 mg/packet	270 mg	164 mg
Neutra-Phos-K powder (for mixing with liquid)		250 mg/packet	556 mg	0 mg
K-Phos Original tablet (to mix in liquid, acidifying)		114 mg/tablet	144 mg	0 mg
K-Phos MF tablet (mixing not required, acidifying)		126 mg	45 mg	67 mg
K-Phos #2 (double strength of K-Phos MF)		250 mg	90 mg	133 mg
K-Phos Neutral tablet (nonacidifying, mixing not required)		250 mg	45 mg	298 mg
Phospho-Soda solution (small doses may be given undiluted)		127 mg/mL	0 mg/mL	152 mg/mL
Joule's solution (prepared by compounding pharmacies)		30 mg/mL	0 mg/mL	17.5–20 mg/mL
Vitamin D and Related Agents	**Available Preparations**			
Vitamin D				
Calciferol (Drisdol)	Solution: 8000 IU/mL			
	Tablets: 25,000 and 50,000 IU			
Dihydrotachysterol				
DHT (Hytakerol)	Solution: 0.2 mg/mL			
	Tablets: 0.125, 0.2, and 0.4 mg			
1,25 Dihydroxyvitamin D				
Calcitriol (Rocaltrol)	0.25 and 0.5 µg capsules and 1 µg/mL solution			
Calcijex	Ampules for IV use containing 1 or 2 µg of drug per mL			
1α-Hydroxyvitamin D				
Alfacalcidol	0.25, 0.5, and 1 µg capsules			
	Oral solution (drops): 2 µg/mL			
	Solution for IV use: 2 µg/mL			
Vitamin D Analogues				
Paricalcitol (Zemplar)	1 and 2 mcg capsules			
	2 and 5 mcg/mL injectable solution			
Doxercalciferol (Hectoral)	0.5, 1, and 2.5 µg capsules			
	2 mcg/mL injectable solution			

SI conversion: 1 mg phosphorus = 0.32 mmol phosphorus, 1 µg vitamin D = 40 IU vitamin D.
From Carpenter TO, Imel EA, Holm IA, Jan de Beur SM, Insogna KL. A clinician's guide to X-linked hypophosphatemia. J Bone Miner Res. 2011 Jul;26(7):1381-8. https://doi.org/10.1002/jbmr.340. Epub 2011 May 2.

Conversely, during brief periods of dietary calcium deficiency (see Fig. 74.1C), as occurs between meals, the serum calcium level declines almost imperceptibly and PTH levels rise, which immediately reduces renal calcium excretion. At the same time, an acute activation of osteoclasts and osteocytes delivers skeletal calcium into the ECF. The combination of reduced urinary calcium loss and increased skeletal calcium efflux rapidly returns blood calcium to normal.

Over the longer term, the initial response is inadequate and leads to skeletal demineralization. A longer-term solution is required, and the adaptation is 2-fold (see Fig. 74.1D). First, a chronic low calcium intake, as may occur in a person with lactose intolerance, leads to a chronic elevation in PTH, and over a matter of days to weeks, this leads to an increase in the 1,25(OH)$_2$D level, which increases the efficiency of calcium absorption from the intestine (i.e., increase in the fractional absorption of calcium) to compensate for the reduction in dietary intake. Second, chronically elevated PTH leads to an increase in osteoblast activity to match the increased osteoclastic activity. In this steady-state adaptation to a low-calcium diet, PTH levels are elevated, and coupled increases in osteoclastic and osteoblastic activities take place (i.e., increased bone turnover), but net skeletal calcium losses are negligible or normal. These physiologic adaptations hold for mild reductions in dietary calcium but in cases of severe calcium restriction or malabsorption, chronic and more significant elevations in PTH can

lead to an imbalance of greater bone resorption than bone formation and chronic bone loss.

From an evolutionary standpoint, as life moved from a calcium-rich marine environment to a terrestrial setting in which calcium availability was unpredictable, a complex, elegant regulatory mechanism evolved that permitted survival without requiring intentional behavioral adaptations to the vagaries of calcium supply. As discussed in Chapter 75, disorders that cause hypercalcemia or hypocalcemia are always caused by abnormalities at the interfaces of the ECF with the intestine, kidney, and skeleton. The physician needs only to recall these homeostatic premises to dissect the pathophysiologic process with precision, enabling her or him to treat the underlying disorder effectively.

PHOSPHATE HOMEOSTASIS

Phosphorus is an inorganic element, abbreviated as P in physical chemistry literature. The biologically relevant molecule is the negatively charged, divalent phosphate ion (HPO_4^{2-}), also referred to as inorganic phosphate (Pi). Phosphate is an important physiologic buffer, and at neutral pH in blood, it is apportioned between HPO_4^{2-} (divalent) and $H_2PO_4^-$ (monovalent) species. Clinical laboratories use differing methods to measure either phosphate (colorimetric assays) or phosphorus (flame photometry), but phosphate measurements are converted to phosphorus (1 mg/

dL phosphate contains 0.32 mmol/L phosphate, which is equal to 0.32 mmol/L phosphorus). Physicians need to be aware that phosphorus preparations often list the mass of the phosphate salt, which includes oxygen, sodium, and potassium (see Table 74.2). Phosphorus content varies for the specific preparation being prescribed, which should be considered in consultation with the pharmacist and hospital formulary.

Pi participates in the regulation of an enormous number of biologic processes fundamental to life. They include being an integral component of the DNA double helix, shuttling oxygen from hemoglobin to cells and vice versa using 2,3-diphosphoglycerate (2,3-DPG), intracellular signaling through kinases that attach phosphate groups to other molecules, facilitating critical intracellular messenger systems such as cyclic monophosphate (cAMP) and inositol phosphates, maintaining basic intracellular redox status through the nicotinamide adenine dinucleotide phosphate (NADP-NADPH) system, and serving as the gateway to the glucose metabolic pathway through glucose 6-phosphate.

Most phosphorus is intracellular as Pi or organophosphate. In addition to its critical intracellular roles, Pi has a key extracellular role. The anion pairs with calcium in the hydroxyapatite crystal lattice that provides structural integrity to the skeleton (discussed earlier). As with calcium, phosphate is critical to skeletal strength, and disorders of phosphorus homeostasis, such as hypophosphatemic rickets, lead to pathologic skeletal fractures. The skeleton also serves as a major storage site for phosphate that is accessed in times of severe phosphate deficiency.

The broad intracellular roles for Pi have two corollaries. First, clinically significant intracellular Pi deficiency may exist without marked hypophosphatemia. Second, life-threatening Pi deficiency is often unrecognized because its manifestations (i.e., reduced levels of consciousness, hypotension, respirator dependence, and muscular weakness) are nonspecific but common in intensive care unit settings. Astute clinicians learn to recognize general debility as a potential sign of Pi deficiency. Pi repletion in this setting may produce dramatic results.

In contrast to regulation of the serum calcium concentration, which is very tight, the regulation of the serum phosphate concentration is relatively lax. Serum phosphate levels are maintained in a range between 2.5 and 4.5 mg/dL, which is broader than the range of normal calcium concentrations. Furthermore, the normal range of infants is higher, between 3.5 and 5.5 mg/dL, and decreases to the adult range in the first few years of life. Even so, the regulation of the extracellular Pi concentrations is no less important, because hypophosphatemia and hyperphosphatemia can both cause disease. Pi is abundant in most diets, and only 33% of intestinal Pi absorption is regulated, principally by 1,25(OH)$_2$D, while 67% occurs in an unregulated fashion. Conversely, its excretion is tightly regulated in the renal proximal tubules by PTH and fibroblast growth factor 23 (FGF23).

Fig. 74.4 outlines the main fluxes of phosphate that define the circulating level as well as overall phosphate economy. The box represents the ECF, and as with calcium, it has interfaces with the GI tract, kidney, and skeleton. Because most phosphate is contained within cells, the phosphate black box has a quantitatively significant interface with the intracellular compartment.

Intestinal Phosphate Absorption

A normal diet contains about 1200 to 1600 mg of phosphorus, and about two thirds of this amount, or 800 to 1200 mg, is absorbed each day. This fixed fractional absorption of about 67% occurs in the duodenum and jejunum. In the normal world of phosphate abundance, this intake is more than ample. Under conditions of dietary phosphorus deficiency, as occurs in chronic alcoholism, intensive care units, intestinal malabsorption, or phosphate-binding antacid use, failure of adequate phosphorus absorption presents a physiologic challenge for which no physiologic remedy exists.

Skeletal Phosphate Fluxes

As with calcium, osteoclastic bone resorption and osteoblastic new bone formation (see Fig. 74.2) lead to skeletal phosphate exit or entry, respectively. Under pathophysiologic conditions, skeletal phosphate fluxes may become important. For example, skeletal destruction in multiple myeloma or severe immobilization syndromes leads to hypercalcemia and hyperphosphatemia, which can cause nephrocalcinosis and renal failure. Conversely, osteoblastic metastases in prostate and breast cancers as well as the hungry bone syndrome after parathyroidectomy can cause clinically significant hypophosphatemia. Although phosphorus has been viewed as a passive passenger with calcium in the calcium regulatory process, recent insights suggest that FGF23, whose levels are determined by phosphate concentrations, stimulates bone matrix mineralization independently of calcium by suppressing osteopontin and by stimulating alkaline phosphatase activity.

Intracellular-Extracellular Phosphate Fluxes

Phosphate shuttles from extracellular to intracellular compartments. This issue becomes important in certain clinical situations. For example, in the setting of metabolic acidosis, phosphate leaves the intracellular compartment and may lead to hyperphosphatemia, whereas under conditions of alkalosis, serum phosphate concentrations decline, and hypophosphatemia develops as phosphate enters the intracellular compartment.

The intracellular phosphate level has important clinical implications, in part, in the settings of crush injury (i.e., rhabdomyolysis) and tumor lysis syndrome. In both conditions, large intracellular loads of phosphate are delivered into the ECF and result in hypocalcemia, seizures, nephrocalcinosis, and renal failure. Conversely, glucose shifts phosphate into cells as glucose 6-phosphate, and overzealous intravenous or oral caloric restitution in the undernourished patient can result in severe hypophosphatemia and sudden death.

Renal Phosphate Handling

The most important mechanism for maintaining a normal serum phosphorus concentration is the regulation of renal phosphorus excretion. As with calcium, phosphate is filtered by the glomerulus, and 90% is reabsorbed (i.e., tubular reabsorption of filtered phosphate [TRP]). The remaining 10% is excreted (i.e., fractional excretion of phosphorus [FE$_{Pi}$]). The FE$_{Pi}$ can be calculated in a spot urine sample using formula 3:

$$FE_{Pi} = (urine\ Pi\ [mg/dL]\ /\ urine\ creatinine\ [mg/dL])$$
$$(serum\ creatinine\ [mg/dL]\ /\ serum\ phosphorus\ [mg/dL])$$

The TRP is simple to calculate using formula 4:

$$TRP = 1 - FE_{Pi}\ (expressed\ in\ \%,\ when\ multiplied\ by\ 100)$$

The renal handling of phosphorus is best considered as a tubular maximum (Tm)–regulated process. The TmP/GFR is normally identical to a normal serum phosphorus concentration in blood, 2.5 to 4.5 mg/dL. If the serum phosphate concentration rises above this level, phosphaturia occurs, and as a result the serum phosphorus returns to the normal range. If the serum phosphate concentration declines below this level, filtered phosphate is entirely reabsorbed as TRP approaches 100%. Thus, the TmP/GFR can be considered as a dam in the phosphate reservoir, over which excess phosphate spills and whose level controls the concentration of serum phosphorus. The TmP/GFR is not fixed but can be moved upward or downward, depending on metabolic needs and prevailing metabolic conditions (described later).

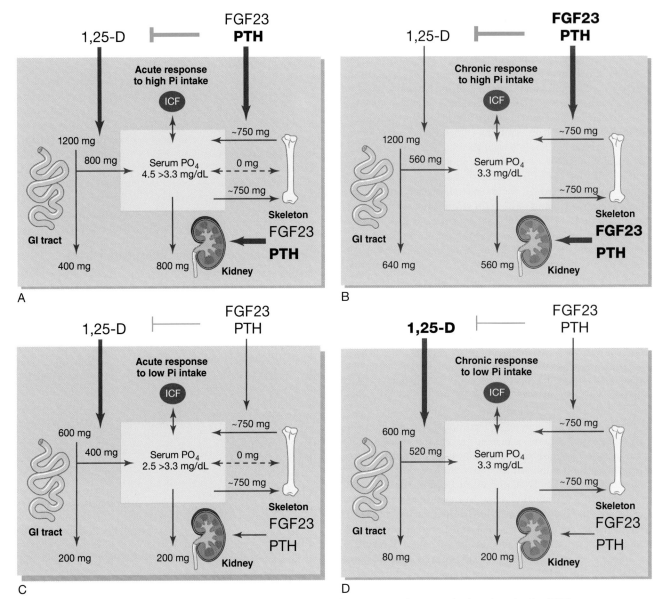

Fig. 74.4 Phosphate homeostasis. (A) The acute response and (B) the chronic response to increases in phosphate intake. (C) The acute response and (D) the chronic response to decreases in phosphate intake. Details are provided in the text. *FGF23,* Fibroblast growth factor 23; *GI,* gastrointestinal; *ICF,* intracellular fluid; *PTH,* parathyroid hormone; *1,25(OH)₂D,* 1,25-dihydroxycholecalciferol (calcitriol). SI conversion: 1 mg phosphorus = 0.32 mmol phosphorus.

The TRP can be used to derive TmP/GFR from the nomogram of Bijvoet, which is shown in Fig. 74.5. Determining renal handling of Pi by calculation of TRP and deriving TmP/GFR proves enormously useful in clinical practice because it is the central starting point for determining whether hypophosphatemia is principally renal or nonrenal in origin.

Regulatory Hormones
Fibroblast Growth Factor

In addition to PTH, which has long been appreciated to be phosphaturic, experimental dietary phosphorus deprivation in laboratory animals and humans leads to a PTH-independent increase in the TmP/GFR, and high-phosphate feeding results in a PTH-independent decline in the TmP/GFR. Over the past two decades, the principal phosphaturic hormone or phosphatonin responsible for regulating renal phosphate handling was identified as fibroblast growth factor 23 (FGF23). FGF23 also affects calcium regulatory hormones; however, the principle regulator of FGF23 is phosphate, while the principle

regulator of PTH is calcium. FGF23 together with FGF19 and FG21 define a family of evolutionarily conserved endocrine fibroblast growth factors. FGF23 elicits its phosphaturic actions in the renal proximal and distal tubules by activation of a co-receptor complex composed of FGFR1c and alpha klotho (aKL). It also acts in an aKL-independent fashion to suppress CYP27B1 and stimulate CYP24A1, leading to inactivation of 1,25(OH)₂D. This requires two different receptors, FGFR3 and FGFR4. The net effect of these actions is a decrease of serum phosphorus. FGF23 also suppresses PTH, stimulates bone mineralization, and inhibits erythropoietin-mediated synthesis of red blood cells, which are less well-understood actions.

FGF23 is produced by osteoblasts and osteocytes. Its gene expression is stimulated by a number of factors including 1,25(OH)₂D and bone matrix factors, for example phosphate-regulating neutral endopeptidase, X-linked (PHEX), the gene mutated in X-linked hypophosphatemia (XLH). Phosphate stimulates FGF23 secretion on the posttranslational level, presumably by increasing activity of the o-glycosylase, GALNT3, which prevents FGF23 inactivation. Mutations

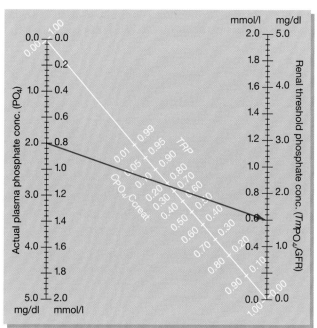

Fig. 74.5 Nomogram shows the tubular maximum for the phosphorus glomerular filtration rate (TmP-GFR). It allows conversion of the fractional excretion of phosphorus (or its inverse, the tubular reabsorption of filtered phosphate [TRP]) into the TmP-GFR. The TRP is calculated, and a line is drawn *(red arrow)* extending from the serum phosphorus level *(left vertical line)*, through the TRP *(middle diagonal line)*, to the *right vertical line*, which represents the TmP/GFR. TmP values are provided in millimolar and milligram per deciliter units. TmP values below 1.0 mmol or 2.5 mg/dL are abnormal in the setting of hypophosphatemia and indicate renal phosphate wasting. C_{creat}, Creatinine concentration; C_{PO4}, phosphate concentration.

in the o-glycosylation site of FGF23 stabilize and thereby increase its bioactivity and are responsible for autosomal dominant hypophosphatemic rickets (ADHR). FGF23 is also the factor responsible for most paraneoplastic hypophosphatemic syndromes, also referred to as tumor-induced osteomalacia (TIO).

MAGNESIUM HOMEOSTASIS

Magnesium is a divalent cation and its homeostasis parallels phosphorus homeostasis. Like Pi, magnesium is principally intracellular, with concentrations inside the cell that far exceed those outside the cell. Both substances govern key intracellular regulatory processes. In the case of magnesium, these processes include fundamental events such as DNA replication and transcription, translation of RNA, the use of adenosine triphosphate as an energy source, and regulated peptide hormone secretion.

Both substances are abundant inside all kinds of cells. Because they are well supplied in vegetarian and carnivorous diets, little evolutionary pressure exists to develop a complex regulatory network and, as with phosphate, serum magnesium concentrations are not tightly regulated. Because magnesium is principally intracellular, measurement of serum levels may provide false estimates of actual total body and intracellular magnesium status. Because magnesium is essential for fundamental processes such as gene transcription and cellular energy use, life-threatening magnesium deficiency is often unrecognized because its symptoms are nonspecific: weakness, respirator dependence, diffuse neurologic syndromes (including seizures), and cardiovascular collapse.

Magnesium has a molecular weight of 24 (1 mole = 24 g), and because it is divalent, one equivalent is 12 g. Blood magnesium

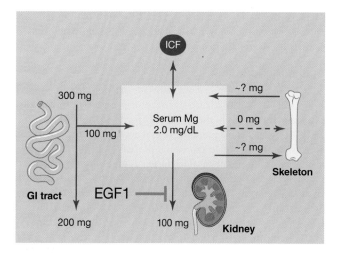

Fig. 74.6 Magnesium homeostasis. See Fig. 74.1 for nomenclature and the text for details.

measurements are often provided in milligrams per deciliter (mg/dL) or milliequivalents per liter (mEq/L); oral magnesium supplements are expressed in milligrams per tablet or milliequivalents per vial; and urinary magnesium excretion values are given in milliequivalents or milligrams per 24 hours. As with calcium and phosphate, it is helpful to examine daily magnesium fluxes. In Fig. 74.6, magnesium values are provided in milligram and milliequivalent units.

As with phosphorus, magnesium has quantitatively important interfaces with the intestine, skeleton, intracellular supplies, and kidney. At the level of the intestine, magnesium is widely available in normal diets and about one third of what is ingested is absorbed in a largely unregulated fashion. In normal circumstances, because dietary magnesium is abundant, magnesium deficiency does not occur. However, deficiency due to insufficient dietary absorption may occur with alcoholism, proton pump inhibitor or cyclosporin use, in intensive care unit settings in which adequate nutrition often is not provided, or with intestinal malabsorption.

Magnesium is incorporated into hydroxyapatite crystals in the skeleton as mineralization of osteoid occurs, and it is released by osteoclastic bone resorption (see Fig. 74.3). In quantitative terms, these fluxes are small.

Many instances of magnesium deficiency are caused by excessive renal losses. Functional examples include the magnesuria that accompanies saline infusions, aminoglycoside, diuretic, or alcohol use, and secondary hyperaldosteronism states such as cirrhosis and ascites. Genetic magnesium deficiency occurs as a result of mutations in claudin 16 and 19 (*CLCN16* and *CLCN19*), both of which encode for paracellular calcium and magnesium channels in the thick ascending limb, and transient receptor potential melastatin 6 (TRPM6) in the distal renal tubules. Gitelman-like hypomagnesemia occurs with several of the Bartter syndromes.

As with calcium and phosphorus, the fractional excretion of magnesium (FE_{Mg}) can be calculated, and it should be used as an index of whether the kidney is appropriately conserving magnesium in states of hypomagnesemia or whether renal magnesium wasting is the cause of the hypomagnesemia. The normal FE_{Mg} is 2% to 4%. Hypomagnesemic individuals have FE_{Mg} values below 1% to 2%.

Like phosphate, magnesium homeostasis can best be viewed as a renal Tm-regulated process (see "Renal Phosphate Handling"), with the renal Tm for magnesium set at a fixed level of about 2.2 mg/dL. In this scenario, abundant dietary magnesium exists, and excessive magnesium intake is managed by spillage of excess magnesium into urine when the Tm of 2.2 mg/dL is exceeded. Conversely, in settings of dietary magnesium deficiency, which equate evolutionarily with caloric deficiency, short-term deficiency is prevented when serum levels fall below the renal Tm of 2.0 mg/dL.

Regulatory Hormones

The significance of hormonal regulators for magnesium homeostasis is currently unclear. Isolated recessive hypomagnesemia is caused by loss-of-function mutations in the epidermal growth factor gene (*EGF1*; see Table 74.1). EGF1 is magnesiotropic as it acts in an autocrine or paracrine fashion to stimulate expression of TRPM6 in the distal convoluted tubules of the kidneys, which increases Mg reabsorption from the urine. Its role as magnesiotropic hormone is further supported by the hypomagnesemia in cancer patients who are treated with the chimeric human/mouse anti-EGF antibody cetuximab or with inhibitors of the EGFR tyrosine kinase (i.e., erlotinib). Magnesium deficiency can result in parathyroid failure and therefore hypocalcemia due to its important role in peptide hormone secretion.

PROSPECTUS FOR THE FUTURE

Although it may seem that calcium, PTH, vitamin D, magnesium, and phosphorus homeostasis and skeletal biology are well understood, many of the physiologic details described in this chapter have been elucidated only during the past 10 to 15 years, and new regulatory proteins (e.g., fibroblast growth factor 23, epidermal growth factor 1) and diseases continue to be identified. This area of research is dynamic, with many unanswered questions remaining.

SUGGESTED READINGS

Carpenter TO, Bergwitz C, Insogna K: Phosphorus homeostasis and related clinical disorders. In Bilezikian JP, Martin TJ, Clemens TL, Rosen CJ, editors: Principles of bone biology, ed 4, 2019, Elsevier Inc., p. 469.

Carpenter TO, Imel EA, Holm IA, Jan de Beur SM, Insogna KL: A clinician's guide to X-linked hypophosphatemia, J Bone Miner Res 26(7):1381–1388, 2011.

Chande S, Bergwitz C: Role of phosphate sensing in bone and mineral metabolism, Nat Rev Endocrinol 14(11):637–655, 2018.

Melmed S, Polonsky KS, Larsen PR, et al: In Williams textbook of endocrinology, ed 12, Philadelphia, 2012, Saunders.

Rosen CJ, editor: The American Society for Bone and Mineral Research primer on metabolic bone diseases and disorders of mineral metabolism, ed 8, Washington, D.C., 2013, American Society for Bone and Mineral Research.

Schlingmann KP, Konrad M: Magnesium homeostasis. In Bilezikian JP, Martin TJ, Clemens TL, Rosen CJ, editors: Principles of bone biology, ed 4, 2019, Elsevier Inc., p. 509.

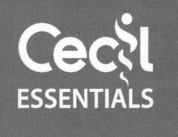

75

Disorders of Serum Minerals

Emily M. Stein, Yi Liu, Elizabeth Shane

INTRODUCTION

This chapter will provide an overview of the metabolic disorders that can impact serum calcium, phosphorus, and magnesium. We will review those disorders that manifest in both excess and deficiency. Please refer to Chapter 74 for descriptions of normal calcium, phosphorus, and magnesium metabolism. We will briefly review the pathophysiology of these disorders, the signs and symptoms, and strategies for treatment. When evaluating a patient, it is critical to consider the broad differential diagnosis for each metabolic abnormality. For all of the metabolic disturbances, the severity of presentation can vary dramatically depending not only on the magnitude of the abnormal value but also on the acuity with which it develops. Patients with chronic abnormalities may have very few symptoms, whereas those with more acute changes are more likely to be symptomatic. Even among patients who have multiple conditions that may result in metabolic disturbances, the most common diagnoses are still most likely. For example, a patient with a history of malignancy who develops hypercalcemia may have humoral hypercalcemia of malignancy, but primary hyperparathyroidism (HPT) should also be considered.

DISORDERS OF CALCIUM METABOLISM

Hypercalcemia

Pathophysiology

Serum calcium is tightly regulated by the movement of ionized calcium between the skeleton, intestines, kidney, and serum binding proteins. Hypercalcemia develops when there are abnormalities in the movement of calcium between the extracellular fluid (ECF) and one of these compartments or when there is abnormal binding of calcium to serum proteins. Hypercalcemia causes hyperpolarization of neuromuscular cell membranes, which become refractory to stimulation and can result in several symptoms, including neuropsychiatric disturbances, gastrointestinal abnormalities, renal dysfunction, musculoskeletal symptoms, and cardiovascular disease.

The physiologic black box described in Chapter 74 should be considered when diagnosing or treating patients with hypercalcemia. Causes of hypercalcemia can be grouped into factitious disorders (e.g., abnormalities in serum proteins), parathyroid mediated, non-parathyroid mediated, medication related, and miscellaneous disorders. The differential diagnosis for hypercalcemia is outlined in Table 75.1.

Symptoms and Signs

Calcium is included in the standard basic metabolic panel, and as a result asymptomatic hypercalcemia is often discovered by routine laboratory testing. Whether a patient develops symptoms depends on several factors, including the degree of hypercalcemia and the rapidity with which it develops. Typically, when absolute serum calcium is above 13 mg/dL patients are symptomatic. A gradual increase in serum calcium, even into the severe range above 15 mg/dL, may cause fewer symptoms then a rapid rise to 13 mg/dL. The overall health status and age of the person with hypercalcemia influence the severity of symptoms. Symptoms can be most severe in elderly patients.

Hypercalcemia can cause smooth muscle hypoactivity, resulting in constipation and ileus. Pancreatitis and peptic ulcer, although less commonly seen, can occur in patients with severe hypercalcemia. Hypercalcemia is also associated with neurologic dysfunction, which can range in severity from mild confusion to coma. Renal impairment can result from hypercalcemia through several mechanisms. Hypercalcemia causes afferent arteriolar vasoconstriction and activation of the calcium receptor in the distal nephron, which reduces the glomerular filtration rate (GFR). It can also cause a form of nephrogenic diabetes insipidus with associated polydipsia and polyuria. As a result, the ECF volume is reduced and the GFR further lowered. Hypercalcemia can directly cause kidney damage through deposition of calcium phosphate crystals into the renal interstitium (i.e., nephrocalcinosis or interstitial nephritis) as well as into the urine leading to nephrolithiasis and obstructive uropathy. Hypercalcemia can have severe adverse effects on the heart, including arrhythmias. Abnormalities on electrocardiogram include shortening of the QTc interval, prolonged PR interval, widened QRS complex and bradycardia. ST elevations mimicking myocardial infarctions have also been reported. Muscular weakness is also frequently seen among hypercalcemia patients.

Differential Diagnosis

Hyperproteinemia. Approximately 50% of circulating calcium is bound to serum albumin and other proteins. Increases in serum proteins lead to an artifactual increase in total, but not ionized, serum calcium concentrations. This increase is commonly observed in settings of volume depletion and dehydration. Patients with hypercalcemia as a result of hyperproteinemia do not display signs or symptoms. Treatment should be avoided in this setting as it might actually result in hypocalcemia.

Parathyroid hormone–related hypercalcemia

Hyperparathyroidism. Both primary and tertiary hyperparathyroidism are characterized by hypercalcemia. Patients who have secondary hyperparathyroidism (SHPT) in response to other abnormalities, such as vitamin D deficiency, calcium deficiency, or chronic kidney disease, will have serum calcium values that are frankly low or in the low-normal range. However, it is important to note that these disorders can coexist. Full consideration of a patient's comorbidities and laboratory test results may be necessary for making the proper diagnosis or combination of diagnoses.

Primary hyperparathyroidism. Primary hyperparathyroidism (PHPT), due to overproduction of parathyroid hormone (PTH) from

TABLE 75.1 Disorders Associated With Hypercalcemia

PTH-Related Hypercalcemia	Non-PTH Mediated Hypercalcemia
Primary hyperparathyroidism	Malignancy-associated hypercalcemia
Tertiary hyperparathyroidism	Humoral hypercalcemia of malignancy
Familial hypocalciuric hypercalcemia or familial benign hypercalcemia	Hypercalcemia caused by 1,25-dihydroxyvitamin D_3 $(1,25[OH]_2D_3)$–secreting lymphomas
	Hypercalcemia caused by direct skeletal invasion
	Granulomatous disorders
	Sarcoid
	Berylliosis
	Foreign body
	Tuberculosis
	Coccidioidomycosis
	Blastomycosis
	Histoplasmosis
	Granulomatous leprosy
	Eosinophilic granuloma
	Histiocytosis
	Inflammatory bowel disease
	Endocrine disorders other than hyperparathyroidism
	Hyperthyroidism
	Pheochromocytoma
	Addisonian crisis
	Vasoactive intestinal peptide–producing tumor (VIPoma); watery diarrhea, hypokalemia, and achlorhydria (WDHA) syndrome
	Milk-alkali syndrome
	Total parenteral nutrition (TPN)
	Calcium-containing TPN in patients with decreased glomerular filtration rate
	Chronic TPN in patients with short-bowel syndrome
	Immobilization plus high bone turnover (risk is particularly high in individuals with the following)
	Juvenile skeleton
	Paget's disease
	Myeloma and breast cancer with bone metastases
	Mild primary hyperparathyroidism
	Secondary hyperparathyroidism (e.g., from continuous ambulatory peritoneal dialysis)
	Medications
	Thiazides
	Aminophylline
	Lithium
	Estrogen/antiestrogen in breast cancer with bone metastases (estrogen flare)
	Vitamin D and derivatives (calcitriol, dihydrotachysterol)
	Vitamin A (including retinoic acid derivatives)
	Foscarnet
	Anabolic agents (teriparatide, abaloparatide)

multiple glands. Rarely, HPT may result from parathyroid carcinoma. The diagnosis of HPT is relatively straightforward in patients who have hypercalcemia in the setting of a frankly elevated serum PTH. It is important to note, however, that in a patient with normal parathyroid gland function, PTH synthesis and secretion should be suppressed by hypercalcemia. Therefore, a PTH level within the normal range should be considered inappropriately high in the setting of hypercalcemia and may indicate underlying hyperparathyroidism. Concurrent vitamin D deficiency, which predisposes to hypocalcemia, can mask elevated calcium levels in patients with HPT; in such cases, hypercalcemia may become apparent only after vitamin D is repleted. Other typical biochemical features of HPT include hypophosphatemia, increased $1,25(OH)_2D$ and chloride levels, and a reduction in serum bicarbonate.

Many patients diagnosed with PHPT are asymptomatic and have serum calcium in the mildly elevated range. Because serum calcium is typically included in chemistry panels, this diagnosis is frequently made when hypercalcemia is found during routine laboratory testing. Less frequently, patients may present with symptoms including osteoporosis, bone pain, and nephrolithiasis. Kidney stones are most often comprised of calcium oxalate and, less commonly, calcium phosphate. Osteoporosis is common among patients with HPT. In the classic densitometric pattern of HPT, bone mineral density (BMD) is relatively preserved at the spine, lower at the hip, and particularly low at the $\frac{1}{3}$ radius. This is because the $\frac{1}{3}$ radius is a predominantly cortical site, which is susceptible to the effects of excess PTH. Though rarely seen today, severe HPT can cause the classic skeletal manifestations known as *osteitis fibrosa cystica* in which there are bone cysts and "brown tumors," which are collections of osteoclasts intermixed with fibrous tissue and poorly mineralized woven bone (see Chapter 76). Some patients with HPT may develop renal disease as a result of the mechanisms described earlier.

Rarely, HPT can occur as part of one of the multiple endocrine neoplasia (MEN) syndromes. It is associated with pituitary and pancreatic neuroendocrine tumors (MEN 1) and with pheochromocytomas and medullary carcinoma of the thyroid (MEN 2).

Tertiary hyperparathyroidism. Tertiary HPT refers to HPT-associated hypercalcemia that occurs in the setting of prolonged stimulation of the parathyroid glands. Chronic hypocalcemic stimulation of the parathyroids eventually leads to hyperplasia. The abnormal glands stop responding appropriately to elevations in serum calcium, ultimately resulting in hypercalcemia. This is typically seen in patients with chronic renal failure and can be seen after renal transplantation.

Familial hypocalciuric hypercalcemia. Familial hypocalciuric hypercalcemia (FHH), or *familial benign hypercalcemia,* is an autosomal dominant genetic disorder caused by heterozygous inactivating mutations of the calcium sensing receptor. As a result of the defect, the parathyroid glands interpret normal serum calcium levels as low, increase PTH in response, and serum calcium rises. PTH in this disorder is in the high-normal to slightly high range. Hypercalcemia is typically mild, in the range of 11 to 12 mg/dL. Abnormal calcium receptors are also expressed in the kidney, leading to inappropriate renal conservation of calcium and hypocalciuria, further exacerbating hypercalcemia. With the exception of the hypocalciuria, patients with FHH have biochemical profiles similar to those with PHPT. However, affected individuals are asymptomatic and do not develop adverse sequelae from FHH. It is critical to distinguish the two disorders, particularly in patients being considered for parathyroidectomy, because patients with FHH do not require any intervention. In contrast to the mild presentation of heterozygous individuals, homozygous patients usually develop severe hypercalcemia in infancy, requiring urgent total parathyroidectomy.

abnormal parathyroid glands, is by far the most common cause of hypercalcemia among otherwise healthy outpatients. In approximately 85% of patients with HPT, a single parathyroid adenoma is responsible for excess PTH secretion, while in about 15% there is hyperplasia of

Nonparathyroid hormone–mediated hypercalcemia

Malignancy-associated hypercalcemia. The most common cause of hypercalcemia among hospitalized patients is malignancy. Cancer may lead to hypercalcemia through several mechanisms, the majority of which are PTH independent. Hypercalcemia typically occurs in patients with end-stage malignancies and progresses rapidly. Approximately 50% of patients die within 30 days of developing malignancy-associated hypercalcemia (MAHC). Hypercalcemia usually occurs in patients with large tumor burdens but can also be seen in patients who have small neuroendocrine tumors, such as islet cell tumors and bronchial carcinoids. Tumors that commonly cause hypercalcemia include breast, renal, squamous cell, ovarian carcinomas, multiple myeloma, and lymphoma.

Humoral hypercalcemia of malignancy (HHM) results from excessive secretion of parathyroid hormone–related protein (PTHrP) by tumor cells. This is the most common cause of MAHC, accounting for approximately 80% of cases. PTHrP acts on the same receptor as PTH and can induce similar systemic effects. PTHrP mimics the actions of PTH on the kidney to promote calcium retention and on the skeleton to activate osteoclasts and induce bone resorption. PTHrP is typically produced at low levels in healthy individuals; however, excess levels can cause significant hypercalcemia. Patients with HHM have elevations in PTHrP and reductions in the levels of PTH, 1,25-dihydroxyvitamin D_3 (1,25[OH]$_2$D), and serum phosphorus (see Chapter 74). Tumors classically associated with HHM include squamous cell carcinomas (i.e., larynx, lung, cervix, and esophagus), renal, ovarian, and breast carcinomas. In HHM, hypercalcemia typically occurs in the absence of skeletal metastases. If tumor resection or ablation is possible, hypercalcemia will reverse.

Another etiology of MAHC is local tumor invasion of the skeleton, a process called *local osteolytic hypercalcemia* (LOH). LOH accounts for approximately 20% of patients with MAHC. In contrast to HHM, these patients often have extensive skeletal metastases. The primary tumor is most commonly breast cancer or a hematologic neoplasm such as multiple myeloma, leukemia, or lymphoma. Local factors secreted by tumors in the bone marrow induce osteoclastic bone resorption. These include PTHrP, macrophage inflammatory protein 1α (MIP-1α), receptor-activating nuclear factor-κB ligand (RANKL), interleukin-6, and interleukin-1. Typically, patients with LOH have both hypercalcemia and hyperphosphatemia as a result of excess bone resorption. PTH, PTHrP and 1,25(OH)$_2$D levels are reduced, reflecting appropriate suppressive responses to hypercalcemia

A third, rare, form of MAHC is secretion of 1,25(OH)$_2$D by lymphomas and dysgerminomas. The increased 1,25(OH)$_2$D leads to intestinal calcium hyperabsorption as well as bone resorption. This condition is mechanistically similar to the hypercalcemia that occurs in granulomatous disease (see below).

Granulomatous diseases. Another type of PTH-independent hypercalcemia occurs in patients with granulomatous disease including sarcoidosis, tuberculosis, and fungal infections (see Table 75.1). The granulomas in these conditions contain the 1α-hydroxylase enzyme and therefore have the ability to convert inactive 25-hydroxyvitamin D to its active metabolite, 1,25(OH)$_2$D. Hypercalcemia results from intestinal calcium hyperabsorption and to a lesser extent, 1,25(OH)$_2$D-induced bone resorption. As a result of increased 1α-hydroxylase activity, patients with these disorders are susceptible to developing hypercalcemia when exposed to sunlight, ultraviolet radiation, or relatively trivial quantities of dietary vitamin D. The excess 1,25(OH)$_2$D results in an elevated serum phosphorus and suppression of endogenous PTH. The combined hypercalcemia and hyperphosphatemia can result in nephrocalcinosis and renal failure.

Other endocrine disorders. Although HPT is most common, other endocrine disorders can cause hypercalcemia as well. Hyperthyroidism can cause mild hypercalcemia through an increase in bone resorption driven by elevated thyroid hormone. This can occur in up to half of patients with this disorder. Serum calcium in these patients is usually below 11 mg/dL.

Hypercalcemia can also be seen in patients with pheochromocytoma. In patients with pheochromocytoma as part of MEN 2, hypercalcemia can result directly from PHPT, which is also part of this syndrome. In other patients, hypercalcemia is due to PTHrP secretion by the pheochromocytoma. Hypercalcemia has also been reported in patients with hypoadrenalism and those with VIPomas, a type of islet cell tumor.

Milk-Alkali syndrome. As reviewed in Chapter 74, absorption of calcium from the diet is usually well regulated. However, ingestion of very large quantities of calcium, particularly from supplements, can exceed the regulatory ability of this system and result in hypercalcemia. This can occur in patients ingesting large quantities of calcium carbonate or other calcium-containing antacids for peptic ulcer disease. This condition, known as milk-alkali syndrome, consists of the triad of hypercalcemia, metabolic alkalosis, and acute kidney injury. Severe hypercalcemia is common and may lead to renal failure. Calcium intake in patients with milk-alkali syndrome typically exceeds 4 g/day and can be in the 10- to 20-g/day range.

Parenteral nutrition. Patients receiving both enteric and parenteral nutrition can develop hypercalcemia. Hypercaloric enteric feeding regimens may contain large quantities of calcium, which can lead to a form of milk-alkali syndrome. Patients with renal impairment are at particular risk for developing hypercalcemia in this setting. Hypercalcemia has also been described in patients treated with total parenteral nutrition (TPN). In some cases, hypercalcemia results from large amounts of calcium, vitamin D, or aluminum in the TPN solution. Often patients who develop hypercalcemia have short-bowel syndrome and are on long-term TPN.

Immobilization. Hypercalcemia can occur in the setting of immobilization. Immobilization activates osteoclast mediated bone resorption and inhibits osteoblast activity, uncoupling bone turnover. As a result, there is substantial, rapid movement of calcium from the skeleton into the ECF. This condition is associated with hypercalciuria and calcium nephrolithiasis. It can result in severe skeletal demineralization if untreated. Typically, for immobilization-related hypercalcemia to occur, patients must be completely immobilized for weeks and have a concurrent underlying predisposition to hypercalcemia because of high bone turnover. This condition is most commonly seen in young adults or children, patients with HPT, Paget's disease, skeletal metastases or multiple myeloma. The most effective treatment for immobilization-related hypercalcemia is resumption of active weight bearing. Hydration and antiresorptive medications, if hypercalcemia is severe, can be used to lower serum calcium as well.

Medications. Drugs that may cause hypercalcemia include thiazide diuretics, lithium, aminophylline, theophylline, vitamins D and A, foscarnet, and osteoanabolic agents like teriparatide and abaloparatide.

Treatment of Hypercalcemia

Patients with mild, asymptomatic hypercalcemia may not require immediate treatment. For severe (Ca >14 mg/dL) or symptomatic hypercalcemia, the initial treatment includes intravenous hydration, calcitonin, and antiresorptive agents like bisphosphonates or denosumab. Volume expansion with isotonic saline is usually initiated first. Loop diuretics should be avoided unless patients have volume overload or heart failure. Subcutaneous calcitonin, which has a rapid onset of action, is usually administered in addition to fluids for the first

48 hours. However, because tachyphylaxis develops rapidly to calcitonin therapy, it should be discontinued after 24 to 48 hours. Concurrent use of intravenous bisphosphonates, preferably zoledronic acid, is often needed, particularly in patients with hypercalcemia of malignancy. Denosumab is an alternative option for patients who are refractory to bisphosphonates or have renal dysfunction that precludes bisphosphonate use. These medications have a slower onset of action, so it is important to treat concurrently with fluids and calcitonin when rapid correction of the calcium is required. Cinacalcet, a calcimimetic agent typically used in patients with secondary HPT from chronic kidney disease (CKD), can also be used to treat severe hypercalcemia from tertiary HPT or due to parathyroid carcinoma. Glucocorticoids are the preferred treatment for hypercalcemia due to overproduction of 1,25-vitamin D related to granulomatous disease or lymphomas. In cases of severe hypercalcemia that are refractory to medical treatment, or in patients with advanced CKD, dialysis against a low or zero calcium bath can be performed.

Therapy for hypercalcemia should ultimately be directed at reversing the underlying pathophysiologic abnormality. Patients with symptomatic primary HPT should undergo parathyroidectomy. For asymptomatic patients with PHPT, indications for surgery include osteoporosis, kidney stones, reduced renal function, and a serum calcium concentration greater than 1 mg/dL above normal. Other patients may be monitored conservatively. In patients who are unwilling or unable to undergo surgery, medical management of hypercalcemia may be attempted using bisphosphonates. As above, familial hypocalciuric hypercalcemia does not require treatment.

Treatment of hypercalcemia related to granulomatous diseases focuses on correcting the underlying disorder. Measures include a low dietary calcium intake, low vitamin D intake, limiting sun exposure, and hydration. If hypercalcemia is severe, glucocorticoids can be used.

Disorders associated with increased intestinal calcium absorption (e.g., sarcoid, milk-alkali syndrome, $1,25[OH]_2D_3$-secreting lymphomas) should be treated by having patients limit intake of both calcium and vitamin D. Medications that induce hypercalcemia should be discontinued.

Hypocalcemia
Pathophysiology
Hypocalcemia can be caused by several mechanisms. Apparent hypocalcemia can result from a reduction in serum proteins that bind calcium, typically albumin. In these patients, ionized calcium and calcium corrected for albumin will be normal. Increased serum phosphate can cause hypocalcemia via an increase in the calcium-phosphate solubility product. Increased renal calcium excretion or a reduction in intestinal calcium absorption can cause hypocalcemia. Hypocalcemia can also result from loss of calcium from the ECF into the skeleton, which can occur in the setting of some malignancies, after parathyroidectomy (hungry bone syndrome), or with certain medications, including bisphosphonates, denosumab, chelating agents, and foscarnet. Many disorders that cause severe hypocalcemia do so by impacting several of these processes simultaneously. In order to provide effective treatment, all of the mechanisms through which a disorder is causing hypocalcemia should be considered and addressed. Hypocalcemia leads to a reduction in the potential difference across cell membranes, producing hyperexcitability in neuromuscular cells which can spontaneously fire (see Chapter 74).

Symptoms and Signs
The seminal signs of hypocalcemia on physical exam relate to neuromuscular hyperexcitability. Hypocalcemia can cause paresthesias, seizures, and skeletal muscle contractions (i.e., carpal spasm, pedal spasm, or tetany). The *Trousseau sign* describes spontaneous contraction of the forearm muscles in response to inflation of a blood pressure cuff around the upper arm to above systolic pressure. The *Chvostek sign* describes twitching of the facial muscles that is elicited by gentle tapping of the facial nerve as it exits the parotid gland. On an electrocardiogram, hypocalcemia can manifest as a prolonged QTc interval. Patients with hypocalcemia may also have more general symptoms such as fatigue, weakness, and abdominal pain. As with hypercalcemia, the severity of symptoms will relate to both the severity and chronicity of hypocalcemia.

Differential Diagnosis
Disorders that may lead to hypocalcemia are summarized in the following sections and Table 75.2.

Hypoalbuminemia. The majority of serum calcium is bound to albumin. Low serum albumin will lead to a low measured total calcium although ionized values will be normal. This is commonly seen in patients with cirrhosis, nephrotic syndrome, malnutrition, and severe burns. The formula commonly used to correct serum calcium for low serum albumin levels is: corrected calcium = measured total calcium + $(0.8 \times [4.0 - \text{measured albumin}])$. This formula should be used to confirm the presence of hypocalcemia.

Hypoparathyroidism. In hypoparathyroidism, low levels of parathyroid hormone result in hypocalcemia through decreased intestinal calcium absorption and reduced calcium reabsorption in the distal renal tubule. Hypoparathyroidism most commonly occurs as a complication of neck surgery or as a consequence of autoimmune disease. Postoperative hypoparathyroidism typically occurs after thyroid, parathyroid, or laryngeal surgery. Autoimmune hypoparathyroidism can occur as a single entity or as part of autoimmune polyglandular syndrome, where it can be associated with primary adrenal insufficiency (Addison's disease), type 1 diabetes, autoimmune thyroid disease, vitiligo, and mucocutaneous candidiasis. Other less common causes of hypoparathyroidism include congenital hypoparathyroidism as part of DiGeorge syndrome, isolated parathyroid failure, or genetic mutations. Rarely, infiltrative conditions including sarcoidosis, hemochromatosis, HIV, and malignancy (i.e., breast cancer) can cause hypoparathyroidism.

The diagnosis of hypoparathyroidism is made by finding an inappropriately low serum PTH in a patient with hypocalcemia. The phosphorus concentration is usually high normal or frankly elevated, and plasma $1,25(OH)_2D$ concentrations are reduced. Prolonged hypoparathyroidism may be associated with asymptomatic basal ganglia calcification on computed tomography scans and plain radiographs of the skull.

Treatment for hypoparathyroidism has historically been directed at increasing intestinal calcium absorption through the use of large doses of calcium (up to 6 to 8 g of elemental calcium per day) along with active vitamin D $(1,25[OH]_2D)$ in doses of 0.25 to 1.0 μg/day. With this regimen it is possible to induce sufficient intestinal calcium hyperabsorption to overwhelm the ability of the kidney to excrete it. However, this treatment can exacerbate hypercalciuria leading to nephrocalcinosis and nephrolithiasis, making it critical to monitor 24-hour urinary calcium. Thiazide diuretics can be used as adjunctive treatment to stimulate renal calcium reabsorption, reduce hypercalciuria, and raise serum calcium. Treatment should be aimed at maintaining serum calcium concentration in the low-normal range.

The approval of recombinant PTH 1-84 by the FDA for chronic hypoparathyroidism has provided an important option for treatment that lowers the risk of some of the adverse effects of high dose calcium and calcitriol.

Pseudohypoparathyroidism. In the group of disorders known as pseudohypoparathyroidism, patients are resistant to the actions of PTH. In these disorders, resistance may result from several different inactivating mutations in the signal-transducing protein $G_{s\alpha}$. The most

TABLE 75.2 Differential Diagnosis of Hypocalcemia

Hypoparathyroidism
　Surgical
　Idiopathic and autoimmune
　Infiltrative diseases
　Wilson's disease (copper)
　Hemochromatosis
　Sarcoidosis
　Metastatic (breast) cancer
　Congenital
　Isolated, sporadic
　DiGeorge syndrome
　Infant of mother with hyperparathyroidism
Hereditary
　X-linked
　Parathyroid gland calcium receptor (Gα11 subunit)–activating mutations
　Parathyroid hormone (PTH) signal peptide mutation
　GCM2 (formerly GCMB) mutation
Pseudohypoparathyroidism
　Type Ia: multiple hormone resistance, Albright hereditary osteodystrophy
　Type Ib: PTH resistance without other abnormalities
　Type Ic: specific PTH resistance, resulting from defect in catalytic subunit of
　　PTH-receptor complex
　Type II: specific PTH resistance, postreceptor defect of adenylyl cyclase, undefined
Vitamin D disorders
　Absent ultraviolet exposure
　Vitamin D deficiency
　Fat malabsorption
　Vitamin D–dependent rickets, renal 1α-hydroxylase deficiency, 1,25-dihydroxyvitamin
　　D–receptor defects
　Chronic renal failure
　Hepatic failure

Hypoalbuminemia
Sepsis
Hypermagnesemia and hypomagnesemia
Rapid bone formation
　Hungry bone syndrome after parathyroidectomy or thyroidectomy
　Osteoblastic metastases
　Vitamin D therapy of osteomalacia, rickets
Hyperphosphatemia
　Crush injury, rhabdomyolysis
　Renal failure
　Tumor lysis
　Excessive phosphate (PO_4) administration (PO, IV, PR)
Medications
　Mithramycin, plicamycin
　Bisphosphonates
　Denosumab
　Calcitonin
　Fluoride
　Ethylenediaminetetraacetic acid (EDTA)
　Citrate
　Intravenous contrast
　Foscarnet
　Cisplatin
Pancreatitis
　Hypoalbuminemia
　Hypomagnesemia
　Calcium soap formation

common form of pseudohypoparathyroidism, Type Ia, also known as *Albright hereditary osteodystrophy,* is associated with resistance to multiple hormones and has a classic phenotype: short stature, shortened fourth and fifth metacarpals and metatarsals, obesity, mental retardation, subcutaneous calcifications, and café au lait spots. Laboratory studies in these patients demonstrate hypocalcemia and hyperphosphatemia similar to hypoparathyroidism. However, PTH levels are paradoxically elevated. Treatment involves supplementation with calcium and active vitamin D analogs.

Vitamin D deficiency. Sufficient vitamin D is necessary for maintenance of serum calcium. Active vitamin D, $1,25(OH)_2D$, is required for intestinal calcium absorption. In order to maintain sufficient vitamin D levels, individuals must have adequate intake of vitamin D from diet and supplements or sufficient sunlight exposure for cutaneous manufacture of vitamin D. As calcium and vitamin D are absorbed from the small intestine, patients with inflammatory gastrointestinal disease, including celiac disease or short-bowel syndrome, or prior upper intestinal surgery are at risk for vitamin D deficiency and hypocalcemia. Patients with hepatic disease commonly have vitamin D deficiency, due in part to impaired 25-hydroxylation. Because the majority of conversion of 25-hydroxyvitamin D to $1,25(OH)_2D$ occurs in the kidney (see Chapter 74), patients with reduced kidney function often have low $1,25(OH)_2D$, which can cause reduced intestinal absorption of vitamin D and hypocalcemia. Severe vitamin D deficiency can result in osteomalacia or rickets (see Chapter 76). Certain genetic syndromes affecting vitamin D conversion or causing vitamin D resistance can result in severe hypocalcemia.

Long-term, high-dose treatment with older antiseizure medications such as phenytoin or phenobarbital or their derivatives may lead to hypocalcemia and osteomalacia.

Sepsis. Sepsis from both gram-positive and gram-negative organisms has been associated with hypocalcemia. The mechanisms for this are poorly understood. Although hypocalcemia occurring in the setting of sepsis is typically mild, its presence is associated with a poor prognosis.

Magnesium disorders. Hypocalcemia can result from low magnesium levels. This occurs most commonly in patients with alcoholism, malnutrition, intestinal malabsorption, and cisplatin-based chemotherapy. Magnesium deficiency causes a form of functional hypoparathyroidism that is due to decreased PTH secretion and resistance to PTH at the kidney and skeleton. These abnormalities can be quickly reversed with magnesium replacement. Paradoxically, in rare instances, hypermagnesemia can cause hypocalcemia. Magnesium, like calcium, is a divalent cation. In very high concentrations, it can mimic the actions of calcium and suppress PTH, causing hypoparathyroidism and hypocalcemia.

Hyperphosphatemia. Phosphate binds calcium avidly and therefore, excess can cause hypocalcemia. This can be seen in disorders that cause severe hyperphosphatemia including rhabdomyolysis (e.g., crush injuries), renal failure, and tumor lysis syndrome. Severe hyperphosphatemia can also be caused by ingestion of large amounts of phosphate-containing purgatives in preparation for colonoscopy, inadvertent perforation of the rectum during the administration of phosphate enemas, and administration of large doses of intravenous phosphate. In these examples, the onset of hyperphosphatemia is acute, and hypocalcemia is immediate and severe. Seizures can occur as the earliest manifestation. Treatment involves reducing the serum phosphorus level. Intravenous calcium should not be given to hyperphosphatemic patients because calcium-phosphate salts can precipitate into soft tissues.

Recalcification and rapid bone formation. Increased rates of skeletal mineralization that exceed the rate of bone resorption lead to net calcium entry into the skeleton and can cause hypocalcemia. This classically occurs in patients with hyperparathyroidism following parathyroidectomy, a situation known as "hungry bone syndrome." In these patients, preoperative rates of bone turnover are very high but formation and resorption are coupled. Postoperatively, as PTH acutely drops, so do rates of osteoclastic bone resorption. However, an elevated rate of bone remineralization continues. As a result of this imbalance, there is a net influx of calcium and phosphorus into the skeleton. This disorder can persist for weeks after surgery and may require very high doses of calcium and vitamin D metabolites to treat. Hypocalcemia from rapid skeletal uptake can also occur in the setting of extensive osteoblastic bone metastases, most commonly observed in prostate or breast cancer.

Pancreatitis. In patients with pancreatitis, fatty acid soaps are formed by lipases released from the inflamed pancreas. The free lipases then autodigest omental and retroperitoneal fat into negatively charged ions that tightly bind calcium in the ECF, resulting in hypocalcemia. The hypocalcemia is reversible by calcium infusion and self-terminates when pancreatitis improves. The development of hypocalcemia in patients with pancreatitis is a poor prognostic sign.

Medications. Several medications can cause hypocalcemia, including those used to treat hypercalcemia and osteoporosis such as bisphosphonates, denosumab, and cinacalcet. Fluoride compounds (e.g., anesthetic gas), chelating agents such as ethylenediaminetetraacetic acid (EDTA) and citrate in stored blood products, radiographic intravenous contrast agents, the antiviral drug foscarnet, and chemotherapy including cisplatin, 5-fluorouracil, and leucovorin can all cause hypocalcemia. Patients with undiagnosed vitamin D deficiency may be particularly susceptible to developing hypocalcemia when they receive one of these medications.

DISORDERS OF PHOSPHATE METABOLISM

Hyperphosphatemia

Pathophysiology

Phosphate plays a key role in many ubiquitous cellular processes, including DNA synthesis and replication, energy generation and use, oxygen uptake and delivery by erythrocytes, and maintenance of the redox state (see Chapter 74). Hyperphosphatemia can develop due to one of three mechanisms: decreased renal excretion, increased phosphate load in the acute setting, and redistribution to the extracellular space. Chronic hyperphosphatemia can lead to soft tissue calcifications. Most diets naturally contain substantial quantities of phosphate, which is cleared by the kidney. However, as GFR declines below 20 to 30 mg/dL, the renal capacity to excrete phosphate diminishes. Patients with stage 4 and 5 CKD (GFR below 30 mL/min) often have some degree of hyperphosphatemia. As detailed above, excess phosphate will avidly bind calcium, and can cause hypocalcemia.

Symptoms and Signs

Hyperphosphatemia is usually identified incidentally on routine blood tests. There are no specific symptoms or signs.

Differential Diagnosis

The differential diagnosis of hyperphosphatemia is detailed in the following sections and in Table 75.3.

TABLE 75.3	Causes of Hyperphosphatemia
Artifactual
Hemolysis
Increased gastrointestinal intake
Rectal enemas
Oral Phospho-Soda purgatives
Gastrointestinal bleeding
Large phosphate loads
K-Phos
Blood transfusions
Redistribution to the extracellular space
Tumor lysis syndrome
Rhabdomyolysis (crush injury)
Hemolysis
Reduced renal clearance
Chronic or acute renal failure
Hypoparathyroidism
Acromegaly
Tumoral calcinosis

Pseudohyperphosphatemia. Hyperphosphatemia may occur artifactually as a result of hemolysis of red blood cells in blood collection tubes. This effect is also commonly seen with potassium, another ion with high intracellular concentrations. Hemolysis should be considered as a cause when unexplained hyperphosphatemia and hyperkalemia occur concurrently. In this circumstance, a new blood sample should be obtained and the levels repeated.

Reduced renal clearance. Renal clearance of phosphate is the main mechanism for maintaining phosphate homeostasis. Acute and chronic kidney disease can cause hyperphosphatemia. Parathyroid hormone promotes phosphate excretion in the proximal nephron. Therefore, patients who have hypoparathyroidism tend to have high-normal or frankly elevated serum phosphate values.

In *tumoral calcinosis*, the ability of the kidney to clear phosphate is defective, either because of genetic mutations in proteins involved in renal phosphate clearance or from advanced CKD. This reduced clearance leads to chronic hyperphosphatemia and the accumulation of calcium-phosphate salts around large joints of the appendicular skeleton. Children and adolescents have higher serum phosphate concentrations than adults and are more prone to this condition.

Increased gastrointestinal intake. Hyperphosphatemia can occur in the setting of excess oral phosphate loads. This most commonly occurs in patients using phosphate-containing purgatives as preparation for colonoscopy. Inadvertent perforation of the rectum during the administration of a Phospho-Soda enema, with delivery of large amounts of phosphate directly into the peritoneal cavity, can also cause hyperphosphatemia. Bleeding from the upper GI tract can also lead to delivery of a large GI phosphate load that is absorbed systemically, therefore leading to hyperphosphatemia.

Systemic phosphate loads. A large phosphate load delivered into the ECF through intravenous medications, or endogenous sources such as muscle or tumor necrosis, can result in hyperphosphatemia. Hyperphosphatemia is often seen in patients who receive large doses of potassium phosphate for hypokalemia (see Chapter 74).

Redistribution to the extracellular space. Hyperphosphatemia may result from the rapid destruction of large amounts of tissue. In tumor lysis syndrome, large tumors respond to chemotherapy with massive cell death and can release substantial amounts of phosphate. This is commonly seen with treatment of Burkitt lymphoma. In acute rhabdomyolysis, phosphate is released from damaged skeletal muscle.

In severe hemolysis, phosphate stored in red blood cells is released and moves to the extracellular space. In each of these conditions, renal impairment is also common and the excess phosphate combined with worsening renal dysfunction can result in progressive renal failure, severe hypocalcemia, seizures, and even death.

Hypophosphatemia
Symptoms and Signs
Because phosphate plays such a ubiquitous and critical role in cellular processes, low phosphate levels can be life threatening. Hypophosphatemia can result in generalized, nonspecific symptoms and signs ranging from generalized weakness and malaise, to hypotension, respiratory failure, congestive heart failure, and coma. Hypophosphatemia often occurs in critically ill patients. These patients are at high risk because of limited oral nutrition, as well as exposure to intravenous diuretics and saline infusions that accelerate renal phosphate losses. With correction of serum phosphate, patients can have complete recovery of mental status and respiratory capacity.

Chronic hypophosphatemia leads to defects in skeletal mineralization, a phenomenon called *rickets* in children or *osteomalacia* in adults. These syndromes produce weakness, bone pain, bowing of the long bones, and fractures or pseudofractures (see Chapter 76). Hypophosphatemia can go unnoticed if phosphate is not routinely checked because symptoms are nonspecific. Under-mineralization can cause low bone mineral density and patients with osteomalacia may be mistaken for having osteoporosis if not properly identified. This is a critical distinction because osteoporosis treatment can actually exacerbate the underlying mineralization disorder. As with acute hypophosphatemia in critically ill patients, patients with chronic hypophosphatemia will dramatically improve with correction of phosphate. Bone pain resolves and wheelchair-bound patients can regain full ambulatory ability.

Differential Diagnosis
Hypophosphatemia can result from excessive renal phosphate loss, decreased intestinal absorption, or intracellular shifts of phosphate from the ECF (Table 75.4). Once a low serum phosphate has been found, urine collection for measurement of the maximum tubular reabsorption of phosphate (TmP) can help to identify the cause (see Chapter 74). In the setting of a low serum phosphate, renal reabsorption should be high as a compensatory response. A low TmP in a patient with hypophosphatemia is therefore indicative of a renal deficit.

Excessive renal phosphate losses. Patients with hypophosphatemia resulting from renal losses will have a low TmP. Inappropriately increased renal phosphate excretion may be due to the presence of a circulating factor versus an intrinsic defect in renal phosphate reabsorption. PTH is phosphaturic, and HPT can cause hypophosphatemia in patients with normal renal function. Hypophosphatemia can be seen in patients with PHPT and in SHPT due to vitamin D deficiency and calcium malabsorption. Vitamin D deficiency can lead to decreased gastrointestinal calcium absorption and secondary HPT, resulting in increased urinary phosphate excretion. A low serum phosphate level may be the first clue to severe vitamin D deficiency. PTHrP is also phosphaturic, and as a result, patients with humoral hypercalcemia of malignancy are commonly hypophosphatemic.

Certain genetic disorders may lead to severe renal phosphate wasting (see Chapter 76). Most of these genetic disorders result in elevated levels of fibroblast growth factor 23 (FGF23), a circulating protein that both inhibits intestinal phosphate absorption and decreases renal phosphate reabsorption, resulting in hypophosphatemia. These disorders include X-linked hypophosphatemia (XLH), also called *vitamin*

TABLE 75.4 **Causes of Hypophosphatemia**
Inadequate phosphate (PO$_4$) intake
Starvation
Malabsorption
PO$_4$-binding antacid use
Alcoholism
Renal PO$_4$ losses
Primary, secondary, or tertiary hyperparathyroidism
Humoral hypercalcemia of malignancy (parathyroid hormone–related protein)
Diuretics, calcitonin
X-linked hypophosphatemic rickets
Autosomal dominant hypophosphatemic rickets
Oncogenic osteomalacia
Fanconi syndrome
Alcoholism
Excessive skeletal mineralization
Hungry bone syndrome after parathyroidectomy
Osteoblastic metastases
Healing osteomalacia, rickets
PO$_4$ shift into extracellular fluid
Recovery from metabolic acidosis
Respiratory alkalosis
Starvation refeeding, intravenous glucose

D–resistant rickets, in which there is an inactivating mutation in the enzyme PHEX that regulates FGF23. In autosomal dominant hypophosphatemic rickets (ADHR), there are mutations in FGF23 that disrupt its breakdown. Oncogenic osteomalacia or *tumor-induced osteomalacia* is an acquired renal phosphate-wasting syndrome. In this disorder, mesenchymal tumors secrete excess amounts of FGF23. Acquired or inherited diffuse proximal renal tubular disorders, such as Fanconi syndrome, may lead to hypophosphatemia as a result of renal phosphate wasting.

Thiazide and loop diuretics are potent phosphaturic agents, and their use without phosphate replacement therapy can lead to hypophosphatemia. Excessive ethanol can also have this effect. Tenofovir, an antiretroviral medication that is increasingly used for the treatment and prevention of HIV infection, can also induce renal phosphate wasting. In some cases, tenofovir can cause Fanconi syndrome, with renal loss of glucose, uric acid, amino acids, and bicarbonate in addition to phosphate. As a result of significant phosphate loss, these patients can present with bone pain, weakness, and fractures because of skeletal demineralization and osteomalacia.

Decreased intestinal absorption. Hypophosphatemia that results from inadequate phosphate intake will be associated with a high TmP. Because most foods are rich in phosphate, it is rare for an individual with a normal diet to develop phosphate deficiency. However, deficiency can occur in settings of severe caloric deprivation, such as anorexia nervosa, prisoner-of-war camps, prolonged critical illness, malabsorption syndromes, and chronic alcoholism. In the first three disorders, caloric intake is low and little phosphate is consumed. Conversely, in alcoholism, overall caloric intake may be high but is primarily derived from alcohol, which does not contain phosphate. The use of phosphate-binding antacids such as aluminum hydroxide gels may lead to severe phosphate deficiency, hypophosphatemia, and osteomalacia.

Intracellular phosphate shift. Phosphate can be shifted from serum into the intracellular compartment as a result of increased formation of phosphorylated carbohydrate compounds. Insulin increases the rate of glucose uptake into cells and its subsequent phosphorylation to glucose-6-phosphate. Patients with diabetic ketoacidosis require phosphate repletion to avoid hypophosphatemia. In the setting of significantly depleted phosphate reserves, rapid consumption of oral carbohydrates or parenteral glucose can precipitate profound hypophosphatemia and sudden death due to respiratory or circulatory failure.

Increased bone mineralization rates may result in large amounts of phosphate entering the skeleton and hypophosphatemia. One example is the hungry bone syndrome that occurs after parathyroidectomy when there is an acute drop in PTH and in bone resorption (see section on hypocalcemia). Hypophosphatemia as a result of increased skeletal uptake can also be seen in patients with osteoblastic metastases and after treatment of vitamin D–deficient rickets or osteomalacia from vitamin D deficiency.

Treatment

Oral phosphate replacement is the optimal method for correction of hypophosphatemia. Phosphate is usually provided in two to four divided doses of 2000 to 4000 mg/day. Doses greater than 1000 to 2000 mg/day can cause diarrhea and other gastrointestinal side effects, particularly at initiation. Gradual increases in doses may be helpful for minimizing GI effects. Intravenous phosphate should be given only to patients for whom oral administration is not an option. Intravenous dosages up to 500 to 800 mg/day may be required. Frequent monitoring of serum phosphate, calcium, and creatinine levels is necessary. Burosumab, a monoclonal antibody to FGF23, was recently approved by the FDA to treat XLH.

DISORDERS OF MAGNESIUM METABOLISM

Hypermagnesemia
Symptoms and Signs

Clinically significant hypermagnesemia is uncommon. The most common symptom is drowsiness. On exam, patients have hyporeflexia and if untreated, eventual neuromuscular, respiratory, and cardiovascular collapse. Hypermagnesemia can also lead to hypocalcemia through effects on PTH (see "Hypocalcemia" section).

Differential Diagnosis

Hypermagnesemia is typically encountered in two settings: patients with severe renal failure who receive magnesium-containing antacids and in women who receive large doses of intravenous magnesium sulfate for eclampsia or preeclampsia (Table 75.5). Mild hypermagnesemia is common in patients on dialysis, but severe hypermagnesemia occurs only in the settings of renal failure accompanied by parenteral or oral magnesium salt administration, such as the use of magnesium-containing antacids or phosphate binders. In women being treated for eclampsia, hypermagnesemia occurs but is rarely severe, as patients are typically closely monitored by labs and physical exam.

Hypomagnesemia
Symptoms and Signs

Hypomagnesemia is common, particularly among critically ill patients in the ICU setting. As with hypophosphatemia, it is not always detected. Magnesium is key to many biologic processes, and hypomagnesemia may cause hypocalcemia, seizures, and paresthesias as well as many neuromuscular, cardiovascular, and respiratory symptoms.

Differential Diagnosis

The differential diagnosis of hypomagnesemia is reviewed in the following sections and in Table 75.5.

Inadequate intake. Inadequate intake of magnesium is common among alcoholics and other malnourished individuals. It may occur as

TABLE 75.5 Causes of Hypermagnesemia and Hypomagnesemia

Hypermagnesemia
  Renal failure accompanied by magnesium antacid use
  Parenteral magnesium sulfate administration for eclampsia
Hypomagnesemia
  Inadequate intake
  Starvation
  Malabsorption
  Alcoholism
  Vomiting, nasogastric suction
  Excessive renal losses
  Diuretics
  Saline infusion
  Secondary aldosteronism
  Cirrhosis
  Congestive heart failure
  Osmotic diuresis, hyperglycemia
  Cisplatin, aminoglycoside antibiotics, amphotericin
  Hypokalemia
  Hypercalcemia, hypercalciuria
  Proximal tubular diseases
  Genetic defects

part of an intestinal malabsorption syndrome and in association with continuous vomiting or nasogastric suctioning.

Excessive renal losses. Excessive renal losses of magnesium are common in clinical practice. Thiazide and loop diuretics cause renal magnesium losses, and saline infusions can have a similar effect. Aldosterone can induce renal magnesium loss. This can be seen in patients with primary hyperaldosteronism and more commonly in the secondary hyperaldosteronism from cirrhosis, volume depletion, and congestive heart failure. Osmotic diuresis can cause renal magnesium loss as well, which is commonly seen in patients with poorly controlled diabetes mellitus. Certain nephrotoxic drugs such as cisplatin, aminoglycoside antibiotics, and amphotericin induce proximal renal tubular injury and severe renal magnesium wasting. Hypokalemia, hypercalcemia, and hypercalciuria can also lead to increased renal magnesium excretion. In diseases that lead to proximal tubular injury, such as Fanconi syndrome and interstitial nephritis, magnesium wasting can occur.

Treatment

Magnesium can be replaced intramuscularly or intravenously. A typical treatment regimen is 24 to 48 mEq (3 to 6 g) of magnesium sulfate given over 24 hours. Oral magnesium salts such as magnesium oxide are also available; however, oral dosing is limited to mild cases requiring low doses because of the cathartic effects of high doses of oral magnesium.

SUGGESTED READINGS

Bilezikian JP, Bandeira L, Khan A, et al: Hyperparathyroidism, Lancet 391(10116):168–178, 2018.
Bilezikian JP, editor: The American Society for Bone and Mineral Research primer on metabolic bone diseases and disorders of mineral metabolism. Regulation of calcium homeostasis, ed 9, Orlando, FL, 2019, American Society for Bone and Mineral Research, pp 165–172.
Bilezikian JP, editor: The American Society for Bone and Mineral Research primer on metabolic bone diseases and disorders of mineral metabolism.

Magnesium homeostasis, ed 9, Orlando, FL, 2019, American Society for Bone and Mineral Research, pp 173–179.

Bilezikian JP, editor: The American Society for Bone and Mineral Research primer on metabolic bone diseases and disorders of mineral metabolism. Primary Hyperparathyroidism, ed 9, Orlando, FL, 2019, American Society for Bone and Mineral Research, pp 619–628.

Bilezikian JP, editor: The American Society for Bone and Mineral Research primer on metabolic bone diseases and disorders of mineral metabolism. Non-Parathyroid hypercalcemia, ed 9, Orlando, FL, 2019, American Society for Bone and Mineral Research, pp 639–645.

Bilezikian JP, editor: The American Society for Bone and Mineral Research primer on metabolic bone diseases and disorders of mineral metabolism. Disorders of Phosphate Homeostasis, ed 9, Orlando, FL, 2019, American Society for Bone and Mineral Research, pp 674–683.

Bilezikian JP, editor: The American Society for Bone and Mineral Research primer on metabolic bone diseases and disorders of mineral metabolism.

Disorders of mineral metabolism in childhood, ed 9, Orlando, FL, 2019, American Society for Bone and Mineral Research, pp 705–712.

Christov M, Juppner H: Insights from genetic disorders of phosphate homeostasis, Semin Nephrol 33:143–157, 2013.

Kinoshita Y, Fukumoto S: X-Linked hypophosphatemia and FGF23-related hypophosphatemic diseases: prospect for new treatment, Endocr Rev 39(3):274–291, 2018.

Nazeri AS, Reilly Jr RF: Hereditary etiologies of hypomagnesemia, Nat Clin Pract Nephrol 4:80–89, 2008.

Nesbitt MA, Hanan FM, Howles SA, et al: Mutations affecting G-protein subunit alpha-11 in hypercalcemia and hypocalcemia, N Engl J Med 368:2476–2486, 2013.

Stewart AF: Translational implications of the parathyroid calcium receptor, N Engl J Med 351:324–326, 2004.

Zagzag J, Hu MI, Fisher SB, et al: Hypercalcemia and cancer: differential diagnosis and treatment, CA Cancer J Clin 68(5):377–386, 2018.

76

Metabolic Bone Diseases

Marcella D. Walker, Thomas J. Weber

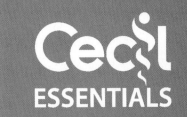

INTRODUCTION

Metabolic bone disease (MBD) is an umbrella term that describes a heterogeneous group of skeletal disorders due to focal or diffuse alterations in bone remodeling and/or mineralization, often with associated abnormalities in mineral metabolism. Bone mineral density (BMD) is usually affected, although in some cases is normal. Etiology varies by disorder but includes metabolic, pathophysiologic, nutritional, genetic, toxic, infectious, and other causes. This family of disorders encompasses common conditions such as osteoporosis (see Chapter 77), less common conditions such as osteomalacia, as well as rare disorders including osteopetrosis. This chapter provides an overview with a focus on the more common diseases (Table 76.1). Normal skeletal homeostasis and histopathology are reviewed in Chapter 74 and Fig. 76.1A.

The clinical presentation of MBD is variable, ranging from asymptomatic incidental findings on laboratory tests, or radiographs, to disabling bone pain, muscle weakness, skeletal deformity, and fractures. Common laboratory and radiologic tests are useful in the evaluation of MBD and can often be diagnostic (Table 76.2 and 76.3). The "gold standard" for assessing both static and dynamic bone metabolism, although rarely required based on clinical history, remains tetracycline-labeled undecalcified bone biopsy of the anterior iliac crest. Bone biopsy allows assessment of osteoclast and osteoblast activity as well as osteoid mineralization. Undecalcified sections (see Fig. 76.1A to F) are necessary because the acid-mediated decalcification performed during routine pathology removes calcium and cannot distinguish between mineralized mature bone and unmineralized osteoid that may be normal or pathologic. Because tetracycline is incorporated into hydroxyapatite crystals as osteoid mineralizes and fluoresces under fluorescence microscopy, administration to patients before biopsy allows evaluation of the rates and effectiveness of bone formation and mineralization (see Fig. 76.1B and F).

PAGET'S DISEASE OF BONE

Paget's disease, or *osteitis deformans,* is the second most common MBD after osteoporosis, affecting 2% to 3% of adults over age 55 years in the United States. Incidence varies geographically and by race/ethnicity (most frequent in those of European descent) and may be declining. Paget's disease is usually a focal disorder of bone remodeling, in contrast to many others, such as osteoporosis, that affect the entire skeleton. Paget's disease may be *monostotic* or *polyostotic* (affecting one vs. multiple bones). Original lesions may expand, but new lesions rarely develop. It may involve any skeletal site, but the pelvis, vertebrae, skull, femur, and tibia are most commonly affected.

Paget's disease is characterized by an increase in bone resorption by abnormal osteoclasts, followed by rapid formation of poorly organized,

structurally weak "woven" bone (see Fig. 76.1C). The markedly increased osteoblast activity accounts for the typical sclerotic lesions observed on plain radiographs (Fig. 76.2A to C), the increased uptake of radionuclide on bone scan (see Fig. 76.2D), and the concomitant increase in serum levels of alkaline phosphatase, the latter of which is a protein byproduct of bone formation and the biochemical hallmark of Paget's disease. The pathogenesis of Paget's disease is unknown, but both genetic variants and viruses may contribute. Up to 30% with Paget's have a familial history and several genes have been implicated, including *SQSTM1, ZNF687, CSF-1, RANK,* and *PML* among others. Evidence suggests Paget's disease may result from chronic paramyxovirus infection with measles, respiratory syncytial virus or canine distemper virus.

Most patients are asymptomatic and diagnosed incidentally, either by increased serum alkaline phosphatase level on routine testing or on radiographs obtained for other reasons. Depending on the location and extent of lesions, however, patients may have bone pain, skeletal deformities including long bone bowing, fractures, osteoarthritis, and signs of nerve compression (e.g., deafness, spinal stenosis). Rare sequelae include hypercalcemia (in immobilized patients) and high-output cardiac failure. Because pagetic lesions are highly vascular, the skin over affected bones may be warm. The most feared (rare) complication is development of osteosarcoma in a pagetic lesion (<1%).

Paget's disease is typically diagnosed using biochemical markers of bone turnover and radiologic studies. In most patients, elevated total serum alkaline phosphatase is an adequate and sensitive indicator of disease activity. However, the serum level of bone-specific alkaline phosphatase may be a more sensitive indicator in those with low disease activity or if hepatic-derived alkaline phosphatase levels are low. A bone scan at diagnosis defines the location and extent of pagetic lesions (see Fig. 76.2D). Radiographs of the affected areas can confirm Paget's disease and are useful for evaluating complications and local disease progression (see Fig. 76.2A to C).

Therapeutic goals include relief of symptoms and prevention of complications. Indications for treatment include alleviating symptoms (e.g., bone pain, headache, neurologic complications), decreasing blood flow preoperatively to minimize bleeding during elective surgery involving a pagetic site, managing hypercalcemia, and preventing future complications of progressive local disease (bowing of the long bones, hearing loss due to temporal bone involvement, and neurologic complications from foramen magnum or vertebral involvement). Moderate quality evidence exists only for pain reduction with bisphosphonate therapy.

Treatment of Paget's disease involves a combination of nonpharmacologic (i.e., physical therapy) and pharmacologic therapy, including antiresorptive agents and analgesics. Bisphosphonates, the mainstay of treatment, decrease bone resorption at pagetic sites by

TABLE 76.1 Conditions, Diseases, and Medications That Cause or Contribute to Metabolic Bone Disease

Osteoporosis (see also Chapter 77)
Paget's disease of the bone
Osteomalacia and rickets
  Vitamin D syndromes
  Hypophosphatemic syndromes
  Hypophosphatasia
  Medications (anticonvulsants, aluminum)
  Metabolic acidosis
Hyperparathyroid bone disease
Renal osteodystrophy/transplantation osteoporosis
Genetic diseases
  Low bone mass phenotypes
    • Osteogenesis imperfecta
    • Osteoporosis-pseudoglioma syndrome
    • X-linked osteoporosis
  High bone mass phenotypes
    • Osteopetrosis
    • Autosomal dominant (LRP-5)
    • Van Buchem disease and sclerosteosis
  Disorganized skeletal development
    • Fibrous dysplasia
Infiltrative diseases
  Multiple myeloma
  Mastocytosis
  Lymphoma, leukemia
  Sarcoid
  Malignant histiocytosis
  Gaucher's disease
  Hemolytic diseases (e.g., thalassemia, sickle cell anemia)

inhibiting osteoclasts. Intravenous zoledronic acid is the first-line treatment and leads to more rapid and sustained normalization of alkaline phosphatase than oral bisphosphonates. Surgery may be needed for an impending or complete fracture through pagetic bone, realignment of arthritic joints, and total joint arthroplasty in affected hips or knees.

OSTEOMALACIA AND RICKETS

Although common in the United States and throughout the world, osteomalacia and rickets are often underappreciated and overlooked. Osteomalacia and rickets are essentially the same disorders, but by definition, rickets occurs in children with open growth plates (i.e., epiphyses), and osteomalacia occurs in adults who are skeletally mature. The fundamental abnormality in these disorders is an inability to mineralize (i.e., form hydroxyapatite crystals) osteoid, the precursor to mineralized bone. Although osteoid is produced, there is a defect in the mineralization process. This results in the accumulation of characteristic thick osteoid seams on bone biopsy (see Fig. 76.1E and F) and a reduction in the bone mineral content that renders it mechanically inferior, leading to stress or pseudofractures, frank fractures, bowing of the long bones, and other skeletal deformities (Fig. 76.3A to C).

Mineralization disorders are due to disturbances in vitamin D, calcium, phosphorus or inhibitors of mineralization/matrix development. Vitamin D deficiency (low 25-hydroxyvitamin D level) is the most common cause of rickets and osteomalacia and is usually due to poor intake or malabsorption, but impaired hepatic production, excessive renal loss, and accelerated catabolism of vitamin D can occur in advanced liver disease, nephrotic syndrome, and with anticonvulsant use, respectively. Mutations in P450 enzymes regulating vitamin D metabolism (1α-hydroxylase and 25-hydroxylase) and the vitamin D receptor (VDR) are much rarer causes of rickets and osteomalacia.

Hypophosphatemic disorders are less frequent causes of osteomalacia, but often present with more severe symptoms. These conditions include inherited or acquired disorders, like X-linked hypophosphatemic rickets (XLH) and tumor-induced osteomalacia, respectively, due to altered metabolism or over-production of a "phosphatonin" protein, fibroblast growth factor 23 (FGF23), as well as other renal phosphate-wasting conditions such as Fanconi syndrome.

Toxins interfering with mineralization, including aluminum, fluoride, and heavy metals (e.g., cadmium), can also cause osteomalacia. In addition, because calcium salts are acid soluble, chronic metabolic acidoses can result in osteomalacia or rickets. Mutations in tissue nonspecific alkaline phosphatase (TNSALP) result in skeletal over-accumulation of the naturally occurring mineralization inhibitor, pyrophosphate, causing hypophosphatasia (HPP). HPP, which is life-threatening in neonates due to respiratory failure from lack of rib mineralization, presents less severely in adults with bone pain, lower extremity stress fractures, and dental disease/tooth loss, though it can be a source of significant morbidity. Finally, osteomalacia is rarely due to inherent defects in bone matrix, such as in type VI *osteogenesis imperfecta (OI)*.

In children, rickets presents with decreased longitudinal growth, widening of the long bone metaphyses (wrists, tibias), and bowing but may also include dental and other skeletal sequelae (i.e., rachitic rosary from enlargement of the costochondral junctions). In adults, osteomalacia presents with bone pain, proximal muscle weakness, fractures, and difficulty walking. The diagnosis of osteomalacia is suggested by the above symptoms and signs. Biochemistries, particularly serum phosphorus, vitamin D (25-hydroxyvitamin D_3 and $1,25[OH]_2D_3$), parathyroid hormone (PTH), and alkaline phosphatase reflect the underlying pathobiology. Inappropriate phosphaturia with a low tubular maximum for phosphorus or glomerular filtration rate, measured with a fasting 2-hour urine phosphorus and creatinine (see Chapter 75), typifies renal phosphate-wasting disorders.

The characteristic radiologic signs of osteomalacia are stress fractures, also known as Looser's zones or Milkman's pseudofractures, primarily in weight-bearing bones. They can be identified by plain radiographs, but computed tomography (CT), MR or whole body bone scintigraphy may be required (Fig. 76.3C).

BMD, measured by dual-energy x-ray absorptiometry or DXA, is usually low, although often is erroneously assumed to be due to osteoporosis. Given this, and that some osteoporosis treatments (i.e., bisphosphonates) can worsen osteomalacia, the physician should review the list in Table 76.1 and exclude alternative mineralization disorders prior to recommending conventional osteoporosis treatments. Finally, although the diagnosis of osteomalacia can often be made clinically, definitive diagnosis in uncertain cases relies on tetracycline-labeled undecalcified bone biopsy, which quantitates the degree of mineralization defect (see Fig. 76.1E and F).

Treatment of rickets or osteomalacia is dependent on underlying etiology. Ergocalciferol or cholecalciferol with supplemental calcium leads to fracture healing and reduced pain in severe vitamin D deficiency. Oral phosphorous salts and activated vitamin D

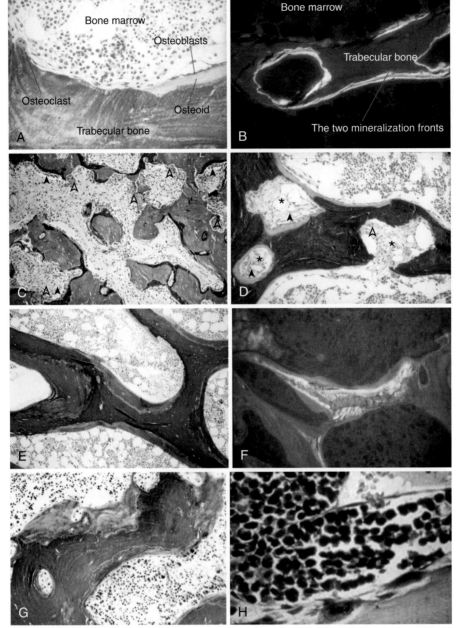

Fig. 76.1 (A) Normal bone histology, showing a normal bone-remodeling unit as seen in an undecalcified human anterior iliac crest biopsy. On the left, a multinucleated osteoclast has moved across the mineralized trabecular bone surface over the previous week or two, resorbing (removing) old bone. On the extreme right, the bone surface is covered by osteoid secreted by the overlying osteoblasts. In between the osteoclast- and osteoblast-covered surfaces of the trabecular bone are a large number of flat, fibroblastoid cells referred to as *lining cells*. No osteocytes are visible in this section. (B) Tetracycline labeling of a bone biopsy from a patient with hyperparathyroid bone disease. Notice the bright yellow parallel lines on the trabecular bone surface. These lines represent the two sets of tetracycline labeling, which occurred 14 days apart. From these sets, the mineralization rate can be described in micrometers (microns) per day, the so-called *mineral apposition rate*, and it is increased dramatically in this example, as is typical of hyperparathyroid bone disease. Contrast with example F, which has no tetracycline labeling. (C) Paget's disease. Enormous and abundant highly multinucleated osteoclasts *(open arrowheads)* are resorbing trabecular bone, and a comparably enormous number of osteoblasts *(closed arrowheads)* are making new but disorganized bone. The marrow space is replaced by fibrous cells. (D) Primary hyperparathyroidism has the classic features of osteitis fibrosa cystica. Far more osteoid and osteoblasts *(closed arrowheads)* and osteoclasts *(open arrowhead)* exist than in the normal example (A). Three large microcysts *(asterisks)* have been created by aggressive osteoclastic bone resorption. These microcysts account for the *cystica* component of osteitis fibrosa cystica. The marrow space, particularly within the microcysts, is filled with fibroblasts, which make up the *fibrosa* component of osteitis fibrosa cystica. (E) Osteomalacia or rickets. Notice the abundant quantities of partially and chaotically mineralized osteoid *(orange)*. These seams are the thick osteoid seams and represent osteoid that has been produced by osteoblasts but that cannot mineralize, which is the signature defect in osteomalacia and rickets. (F) Tetracycline labeling reveals a complete absence of mineralization, diagnostic of osteomalacia or rickets. Compare with example B. (G) Renal osteodystrophy. This photomicrograph of a biopsy from a patient on dialysis demonstrates many of the classic features of renal osteodystrophy, including evidence of aggressive osteoclastic bone resorption (i.e., numerous osteoclastic lacunae on the bone surface compared with the smooth surfaces in example A) and abundant, partially and chaotically mineralized areas of osteoid *(orange)*. (H) Infiltrative bone disease as exemplified by multiple myeloma. The bone marrow is replaced by plasma cells, and two large osteoclasts in lacunae are actively resorbing the trabecular bone surface.

analogues, such as calcitriol, improve osteomalacia in hypophos-phatemic rickets, although targeted reduction of FGF23 levels with a monoclonal antibody also improves bone pain and fracture healing in XLH. Treatment of children with HPP using recombinant TNSALP can be life-saving and markedly reduces pain and disability. Identification and withdrawal of drugs/toxins causing inhibition of mineralization generally improves osteomalacic symptoms. Treatment of these diseases is gratifying because the responses are often dramatic with restoration of normal function in patients who were severely disabled.

HYPERPARATHYROID BONE DISEASE

Hyperparathyroid bone disease can be a major cause of skeletal morbidity, though the clinical presentation varies widely, depending on the nature and severity of the underlying parathyroid disorder. Patients with primary hyperparathyroidism (PHPT), characterized by elevated serum calcium and PTH levels from a parathyroid adenoma or hyperplasia, typically have no symptoms related to accelerated bone remodeling from excess PTH. However, in many patients, osteopenia or osteoporosis can be detected by DXA, which often shows bone loss at the cortical-rich proximal one third radius and proximal femur and

sparing of the cancellous-rich lumbar spine. Fracture risk, particularly risk for vertebral fractures, is also increased in PHPT, but many vertebral fractures are clinically occult (i.e., only identified by spine imaging).

Secondary hyperparathyroidism (SHPT), which is a physiologic PTH elevation occurring in response to hypocalcemia and/or 25-hydroxyvitamin D_3 deficiency, is also associated with bone loss from cortical-rich sites. SHPT is almost always present in advanced chronic kidney disease (CKD) as a result of chronic hypocalcemia, hyperphosphatemia, and low calcitriol (1,25[OH]$_2$D$_3$) levels, as well as in malabsorptive states such as gastric bypass. Tertiary hyperparathyroidism is characterized by hypercalcemia and elevated PTH resulting from long-standing SHPT, usually from end-stage renal disease (ESRD; see Chapter 30). In tertiary hyperparathyroidism, chronic parathyroid stimulation results in hyperplasia or adenomas and autonomous gland function.

In patients with chronically, markedly elevated PTH levels, severe hyperparathyroid bone disease, known as *osteitis fibrosa cystica* (OFC), may develop. OFC was common among patients with PHPT in the United States before the onset of routine biochemical screening that began in the 1970s but occurs in fewer than 2% of patients today. OFC remains frequent in regions of the world where calcium is not routinely measured. Today, OFC is typically seen in the context of severe, prolonged, and uncontrolled secondary and tertiary hyperparathyroidism (from ESRD) and parathyroid carcinoma. OFC, a *high turnover* skeletal disease, is characterized by coupled increases in osteoclastic bone resorption and osteoblastic osteoid synthesis, accelerated rates of bone mineralization accompanied by microcysts in the cortex and trabeculae (the *cystica* of OFC), and increased numbers of fibroblasts and marrow stroma (the *fibrosa* of OFC) (see Fig. 76.1B and D). Levels of markers of bone formation (i.e., alkaline phosphatase and osteocalcin) and resorption (i.e., N-terminal and C-terminal telopeptides) are usually increased, reflecting the bone histology. The radiologic hallmarks of OFC are salt-and-pepper demineralization of the calvarium, resorption of the tufts of the terminal phalanges and distal clavicles, subperiosteal resorption of the radial aspect of the cortex of the second phalanges (Fig. 76.4), and Brown tumors (i.e., collections of osteoclasts that produce gross lytic lesions) of the pelvis and long bones. Patients with OFC may have bone pain or fractures.

The treatment involves normalizing or lowering elevated PTH concentrations. In patients with OFC, curative parathyroidectomy normalizes biochemistries and leads to resolution of the radiologic

---

TABLE 76.2   Diagnostic Studies in the Evaluation of Metabolic Bone Disease

Laboratory Evaluation
  Serum calcium, phosphate, magnesium
  Alkaline phosphatase (total and bone-specific)
  Vitamin D metabolites (25-hydroxyvitamin D and 1,25-dihydroxyvitamin D)
  Creatinine
  Parathyroid hormone
  24-hour urine calcium and creatinine
  Fasting 2-hour urine phosphorus and creatinine
  Markers of bone formation and resorption
Imaging
  Radiographs
  DXA
  Technetium-99 bone scan
Pathology
  Tetracycline-labeled bone biopsy

TABLE 76.3   Biochemical Hallmarks of Various Metabolic Bone Diseases

	Calcium	Phosphate	PTH	25-Hydroxy Vitamin D	1,25-Dihydroxyvitamin D	Alkaline Phosphatase
Vitamin D deficiency with osteomalacia	Low or low normal	Low or low normal	High	Low	High or high normal	High
Renal phosphate wasting with osteomalacia	Normal	Low	Normal or high	Normal	Low or low normal	High
Paget's disease	Normal	Normal	Normal or high	Dependent on intake; Often low	Normal	High
Primary/hyperparathyroidism	High	Low or low normal	High	Dependent on intake; Often low	High or high normal	High or high normal

signs. In hyperparathyroid patients without OFC but with osteopenia or osteoporosis, BMD typically increases robustly after parathyroidectomy, particularly in the lumbar spine. If the hypercalcemia is mild and BMD is normal, no treatment may be required. Medical therapy with cinacalcet, a *calcimimetic* (mimics the action of calcium at the calcium-sensing receptor) can be used to lower PTH levels in those with parathyroid carcinoma who have failed surgical resection and patients with severe hypercalcemia due to primary or tertiary hyperparathyroidism who are not surgical candidates. Hypocalcemia may occasionally occur after parathyroidectomy in patients with more severe disease, a condition known as *hungry bone syndrome* (see Chapter 75).

SHPT due to vitamin D deficiency is treated with oral vitamin D_3 (cholecalciferol) or D_2 (ergocalciferol). SHPT from ESRD can be treated with a combination of the active form of vitamin D $(1,25[OH]_2D_3$ [calcitriol] or analogues), calcium supplementation, phosphate binders, and cinacalcet, depending on the clinical situation.

Infrequently, parathyroidectomy is needed for severe hyperparathyroid bone disease related to SHPT.

RENAL OSTEODYSTROPHY

Renal osteodystrophy (ROD) refers to changes in bone turnover, mineralization, and morphology that occur in CKD. ROD is typically associated with abnormalities in serum calcium, phosphate, PTH, FGF23 or vitamin D metabolism and also may be accompanied by vascular and soft tissue calcification. The term *chronic kidney disease–mineral and bone disorder (CKD-MBD)* describes the systemic disorder encompassing both the mineral and bone metabolism abnormalities in CKD.

ROD may occur as early as stage 2 CKD and is prevalent among those with stage 4 to 5 CKD. Furthermore, even mild and moderate CKD confers an increased risk of fracture. The pathophysiology of ROD is complex and related to alterations in both hormonal and

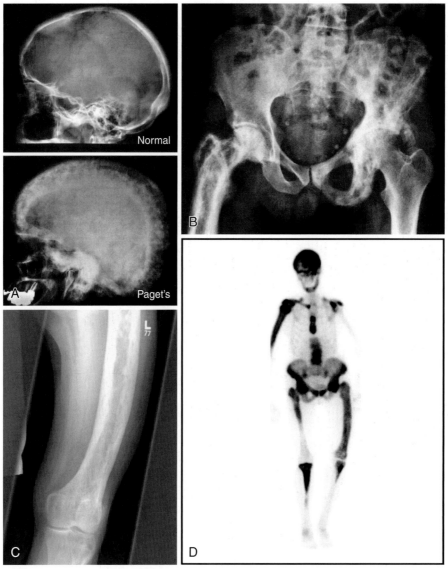

Fig. 76.2 Typical radiologic abnormalities in Paget's disease. (A) Compare the normal skull *(top)* with the skull *(bottom)* with the classic cotton-wool appearance, an expanded calvarium, and osteosclerosis of the petrous bones. (B) Classic asymmetrical involvement of the pelvis with a mixture of lytic and blastic lesions. (C) Bowing deformity of the femur with a markedly thickened cortex. (D) A whole-body radionuclide scan demonstrates polyostotic Paget's disease.

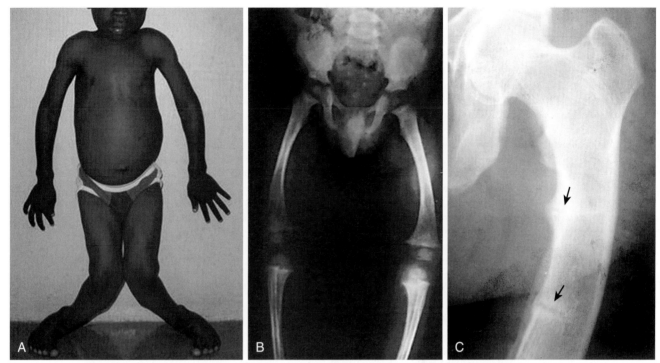

Fig. 76.3 (A) A typical example of rickets, with bowing of the femurs and tibias, wrist enlargement due to metaphyseal flaring and rachitic rosary, and enlargement of the costochondral junctions of the ribs. (From Thacher TD, Pludowski P, Shaw NJ, Mughal MZ, Munns CF, Högler W. Nutritional rickets in immigrant and refugee children. Public Health Rev. 2016 Jul 22;37:3. (B) A skeletal radiograph of a child with rickets. The weight-bearing bones of the lower extremities are bowed, and the epiphyses are open, mottled, and overgrown. (C) Looser's zones or pseudofractures *(arrows)* are characteristic of osteomalacia or rickets. The closed epiphyses indicate the patient is an adult. This radiograph is diagnostic of osteomalacia.)

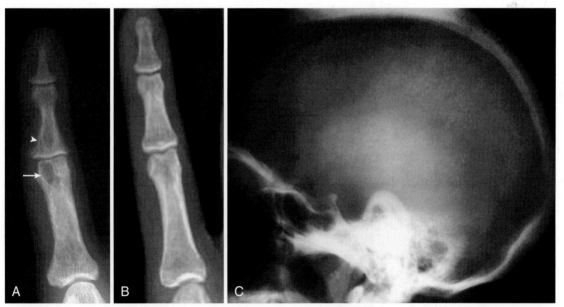

Fig. 76.4 Skeletal radiographic changes of hyperparathyroidism. (A) A hand film from a patient with primary hyperparathyroidism. The *arrow* indicates a typical giant cell tumor (brown tumor), which is a collection of osteoclasts that lead to macrocystic changes in bone. The *arrowhead* indicates the irregular radial surface of a phalanx resulting from subperiosteal bone resorption, which is typical of hyperparathyroidism. The brown tumor and the subperiosteal resorption refill and disappear when the offending parathyroid tumor or hyperplasia is resected. (B) Radiograph of a normal hand for comparison. No brown tumors are seen, and the phalangeal periosteal surfaces are smooth. (C) The classic salt-and-pepper appearance of the skull in hyperparathyroidism. The periosteal surfaces of the inner and outer cortices or tables of the calvarium are indistinct as a result of subperiosteal bone resorption. The lateral view of the calvarium is hazy and indistinct, showing micropunctations. (Courtesy J. Towers, MD, and D. Armfield, MD, University of Pittsburgh, Pittsburgh, Penn.)

mineral metabolism. In early CKD, reduced phosphorous excretion leads to increased production and circulating levels of FGF23. SHPT results from hypocalcemia due to hyperphosphatemia and its precipitation with phosphate into soft tissues as well as defective renal $1,25[OH]_2D_3$ production (see Chapters 30 and 75).

Several types of ROD can occur and are classified as high-turnover (OFC), low-turnover (adynamic bone disease or ABD), osteomalacia, or mixed ROD. Tetracycline-labeled transiliac bone biopsy is the only way to reliably distinguish which type of ROD is present, though levels of PTH and alkaline phosphatase may provide noninvasive guidance (typically high in OFC). OFC and osteomalacia were common in the past, but their prevalence has declined while that of ABD has increased. The reasons for this, and the exact mechanisms leading to development of one type of ROD versus another, are not entirely clear, but may be related to degree of PTH elevation and other pathogenic factors.

As noted previously, OFC is due to excessive PTH secretion that causes marked increases in bone turnover, demineralization, and fracture. OFC may respond dramatically to $1,25(OH)_2D_3$, cinacalcet, or both. Intravenous etelcalcetide, a newer calcimimetic, may be more effective. In contrast, ABD is characterized by little or no osteoblastic or osteoclastic activity or osteoid on bone biopsy. The condition results from excessive treatment with $1,25[OH]_2D_3$ or calcium-phosphate binders that are believed to cause "over-suppression" of PTH, although other factors may contribute as well. Patients may have bone pain, fractures, hypercalcemia, and vascular calcification. Treatment centers on reducing the dose of active vitamin D analogs, cinacalcet or other measures. Though an intuitive choice of treatment, little data confirm that osteoanabolic agents, such as PTH analogues, are beneficial in the treatment of ABD.

Severe osteomalacia, now uncommon in CKD, is characterized by bone pain, low BMD, and thickened osteoid seams with a mineralization defect on bone biopsy (see Fig. 76.1E). A major contributor to osteomalacia in the past was aluminum bone deposition from now obsolete aluminum-containing phosphate binders. More subtle defects in mineralization can be seen, however, even in early CKD from increased phosphorous and FGF23. CKD-associated osteomalacia may respond to $1,25[OH]_2D_3$ replacement. Mixed ROD is much less common and can be characterized by either high- or low-turnover bone disease along with osteomalacia (see Fig. 76.1G).

TRANSPLANTATION OSTEOPOROSIS

Patients who have undergone organ transplantation often have osteoporosis and are at high risk for fracture. Post-transplant use of immunosuppressive drugs, particularly glucocorticoids, leads to rapid bone loss. Glucocorticoids increase bone resorption, reduce bone formation, decrease gastrointestinal calcium absorption, and increase renal calcium excretion, leading to marked bone loss, and often fracture, within 6 months of initiation. Tacrolimus and cyclosporine have also been associated with bone loss.

Decreased BMD may, however, be present before transplantation as a result of organ failure and its treatment, malnutrition or malabsorption, inactivity, or hypogonadism. For example, those with primary biliary cirrhosis have reduced osteoblast function and low-turnover osteoporosis due to cholestatic toxins. Patients with cystic fibrosis have calcium and vitamin D malabsorption, malnutrition, and low weight. In those with end-stage lung or cardiac disease, physical inactivity contributes. Patients with ESRD who undergo renal transplantation often have ROD. Screening of patients at risk for transplant osteoporosis is paramount. Pretransplant DXA, measurement of vitamin D, and spine imaging is recommended. Early intervention with osteoporosis therapies in those at high risk for fracture or post-transplant bone loss may prevent post-transplant fractures.

GENETIC DISEASES

Monogenic disorders that lead to abnormal BMD (low or high) or focal skeletal disease are uncommon, but their discovery has advanced our understanding of basic skeletal biology and in turn led to the development of new therapeutic agents for osteoporosis.

The most common monogenic disorder causing low BMD is OI, the severity of which is dependent on the underlying gene involved. OI most often results from mutations in the genes for type I collagen, although defects in collagen processing and mineralization may also cause disease. Patients with OI generally have very low BMD with marked skeletal fragility and deformities but may also have involvement of collagen-containing tissues including the tendons, skin, eyes, and teeth (dentogenesis imperfecta). A much rarer but mechanistically important monogeneic form of low BMD is the osteoporosis-pseudoglioma syndrome, characterized by autosomal dominant, severe osteoporosis with blindness. This disease results from inactivating mutations in the low-density lipoprotein receptor–related protein 5 gene (LRP5), which acts in the osteoblast WNT-signaling pathway to increase bone formation. A missense mutation in WNT has also been described in a family with early-onset osteoporosis.

In contrast, activating mutations in LRP5 lead to an autosomal-dominant form of very high BMD. Mutations in the gene encoding an inhibitor of the WNT signaling pathway, sclerostin, also lead to increased bone formation and high bone mass phenotypes, such as Van Buchem disease and sclerosteosis. These latter discoveries have led to the development of a monoclonal antibody against sclerostin for the treatment of osteoporosis.

In contrast to the disorders that affect bone formation, osteopetrosis, or "marble bone disease," refers to a group of disorders resulting from mutations that impair osteoclastic bone resorption. Although osteopetrosis is associated with increased skeletal mass, fracture risk is increased, presumably due to a change in material properties or "brittleness" that results in reduced bone strength. The clinical presentation is variable depending on the underlying genetic etiology, but the features may include skeletal deformity/short stature, recurrent and poorly healing fractures, macrocephaly, dental abnormalities, overgrowth of neural foramina with nerve paralysis, and impaired hematopoiesis due to bone overgrowth crowding out the bone marrow space. Radiographic findings are diagnostic and indicate generalized sclerosis, a "bone in bone" appearance (from remaining primary spongiosa or calcified cartilage), rugger-jersey vertebrae, flaring of the long bone metaphyses (Erlenmeyer flask deformity) and calvarial and basilar thickening (Fig. 76.5A to C). There is no established treatment for osteopetrosis.

Genetic bone diseases can also present with focal skeletal lesions. Fibrous dysplasia (FD) is a rare condition characterized by fibro-osseous lesions within the skeleton and sometimes extra-skeletal manifestations. It is due to activating mutations in the GNAS gene, encoding the alpha subunit of the stimulatory G protein involved in cyclic adenosine monophosphate (cAMP) production and signaling that causes abnormal differentiation of osteoblasts and osteocytes. Mutations occur post-zygotically and are not inherited, resulting in a somatic mosaicism, with the extent of disease dependent on the timing of the mutation in development. Abnormal osteoblasts secrete a disorganized fibrotic bone matrix resulting in irregular trabeculae enmeshed within a fibrous stroma of spindle-shaped cells, as well as cytokines that result in bone resorption within lesions. Abnormal bone mineralization also

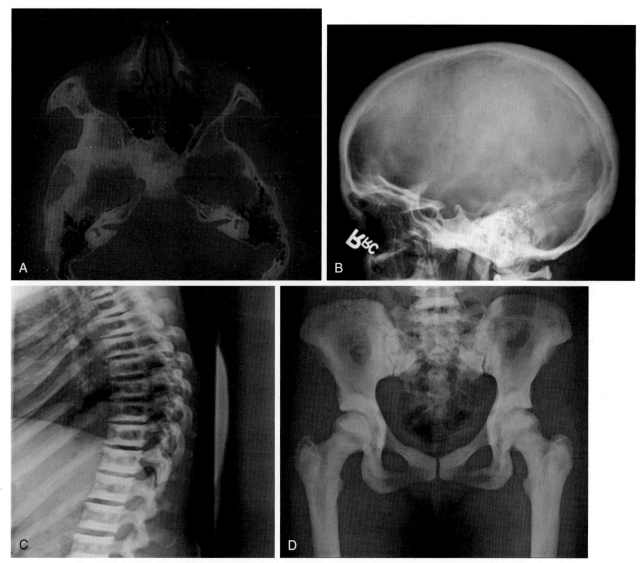

Fig. 76.5 (A) Head/face CT from a patient with fibrous dysplasia indicating expansion of the right maxilla; the cortex is intact but there are multiple lucent and sclerotic areas and some areas of ground-glass appearance; there is narrowing of the right maxillary sinus. (B–D) indicate diagnostic radiographic findings in a patient with "adult" osteopetrosis. There is generalized sclerosis. (B) The calvarium is thickened due to osteopetrosis. (C) The typical "Rugger-Jersey" spine due to bands of calcified primary spongiosa. (D) Endobones *(arrow)* or a "bone in bone" appearance can be seen in the pelvis due to calcified cartilage deposited during endochondral bone formation.

occurs locally and sometimes systemically, related to over-production of FGF23.

FD can involve one (monostotic) or multiple (polystotic) bones but can rarely affect the entire skeleton (pan ostotic). The presentation of FD varies from incidentally discovered asymptomatic radiographic findings to severe disability from fractures, pain, and skeletal deformity. FD most often affects the skull and femur, though the spine, ribs, and pelvis are commonly involved as well. Radiographically, FD lesions appear as expansile, deforming, medullary lesions with cortical thinning and overall "ground-glass" appearance (Fig. 76.5D) but can evolve over time and become sclerotic. Diagnosis is often made radiologically with plain films or CT. Bone biopsy is infrequently required. As in Paget's disease, extent of disease is best assessed with technetium-99 scan. FD also may be associated with extra-skeletal features including café au lait spots and/or hyperfunctioning endocrinopathies (McCune-Albright syndrome), resulting from mutant progeny cells within extraskeletal tissues. Skeletal malignancies are a

rare complication of FD. Depending on the extent of disease, management may include analgesia, physical therapy, orthopedic surgery for proximal femur or spine disease, monitoring for cranial nerve deficits, treatment of endocrinopathies and mineral disturbances, and bisphosphonates, though there are limited data regarding efficacy of the latter.

ISCHEMIC AND INFILTRATIVE DISEASES

Bone disease may also develop from ischemia or infiltration of the skeleton. Ischemic injury may develop due to drugs/toxins (excess glucocorticoids/alcohol), hemoglobinopathies, glycogen storage disorders (e.g. Gaucher's disease) and excess radiation, among other causes. Radiographs may show focal or diffuse changes in BMD, as well as bone collapse. In multiple myeloma, malignant infiltration of the bone marrow by plasma cells results in excessive osteoclast activation, severe osteoporosis, and commonly hypercalcemia (see Fig. 76.1H). Systemic mastocytosis, another lymphoproliferative disease that can affect multiple organs including the skin (urticaria pigmentosa), liver, spleen, and lymph nodes, may cause focal osteolytic lesions as well as diffuse osteoporosis and fractures. These and other infiltrative disorders can lead to diffuse osteopenia, bone pain, and fractures, and should be considered in unexplained osteoporosis.

SUGGESTED READINGS

Bilezikian JP: Primer on the metabolic bone diseases and disorders of mineral metabolism, ed 9, Ames Iowa, 2018, J Wiley & Sons and American Society for Bone and Mineral Research.

Christov M, Pereira R, Wesselig-Perry K: Bone biopsy in renal osteodystrophy: continued insights into a complex disease, Curr Opin Nephrol Hypertens 22:210–215, 2013.

Corral-Gudino L, Tan AJ, Del Pino-Montes J, Ralston SH: Bisphosphonates for Paget's disease of bone in adults, Cochrane Database Syst Rev 12:CD004956, 2017.

Khosla S, Westendorf JJ, Oursler MJ: Building bone to reverse osteoporosis and repair fractures, J Clin Invest 118:421–428, 2008.

Lindsay R, Cosman F, Zhao H, et al: A novel tetracycline labeling strategy for longitudinal evaluation of the short term effects of anabolic therapy with a single iliac crest bone biopsy, J Bone Miner Res 21:366–373, 2006.

Moe S, Drueke T, Cunningham J, et al: Definition, evaluation and classification of renal osteodystrophy: a position statement from Kidney Disease: Improving Global Outcomes (KIDIGO), Kidney Int 69:1945–1953, 2006.

Ralston SH: Paget's disease of bone, N Engl J Med 368:644–650, 2013.

Stewart AF: Translational implications of the parathyroid calcium receptor, N Engl J Med 351:324–326, 2004.

77

Osteoporosis

Susan L. Greenspan, Mary P. Kotlarczyk

INTRODUCTION

Osteoporosis, the most common disorder of bone and mineral metabolism, affects about 50% of women and 20% of men older than 50 years. The National Institutes of Health Consensus Development Panel on Osteoporosis Prevention defines osteoporosis as a skeletal disorder characterized by compromised bone strength, predisposing a person to an increased risk of fracture. Bone strength has two major components: bone density and bone quality. Bone density reflects the peak adult bone mass and the amount of bone lost in adulthood. Bone quality is determined by bone architecture, bone geometry, bone turnover, mineralization, and damage accumulation (i.e., microfractures) (Fig. 77.1).

DEFINITION AND EPIDEMIOLOGY

In the United States, 2 million osteoporotic fractures occur each year. There are almost 300,000 hip fractures annually, which are associated with a mortality rate of more than 20% during the first year. The mortality rate is higher in men than in women. More than 40% of patients with hip fracture are unable to return to their previous ambulatory state, and about 20% of them are placed in long-term care facilities. When defined by bone mineral densitometry, 44 million Americans have low bone mass, and 10 million have osteoporosis. Although morbidity is less with vertebral fractures, the 5-year mortality rate is similar to that for hip fractures. Only one third of radiologically diagnosed vertebral fractures receive medical attention.

PATHOLOGY AND RISK FACTORS

Peak bone mass is determined primarily by genetic factors. Men have a higher bone mass than women, and African American and Hispanic individuals have a higher bone mass than white individuals. Other factors that contribute to the development of peak bone mass include nutrition and calcium intake, physical activity, timing of puberty, chronic illness, smoking, and use of medications that harm bone such as glucocorticoids.

The causes of bone loss in adults are multifactorial. The pattern of bone loss is different in women than in men, and bone loss is greater in sites rich in trabecular bone (e.g., spine) than cortical bone (e.g., femoral neck) (Fig. 77.2). Women lose significantly more trabecular bone than men. Estrogen deficiency during menopause contributes significantly to bone loss in women, and they may lose 1% to 5% of bone mass per year in the first few years after menopause. Women continue to lose bone mass throughout the remainder of their lives, with another acceleration of bone loss occurring after age 75 years. The mechanism of this accelerated loss in old age is not clear.

Multiple causes of secondary bone loss contribute to osteoporosis and fractures. Medications that commonly cause bone loss include glucocorticoids, antiseizure medications, excess thyroid hormone, heparin, androgen deprivation therapy, aromatase inhibitors, and depo-medroxyprogesterone. Endocrine diseases resulting in female or male hypogonadism also lead to bone loss. Hyperparathyroidism, hyperthyroidism, and hypercortisolism commonly cause bone loss, as can vitamin D deficiency. Gastrointestinal problems can contribute to decreased absorption of calcium and vitamin D (Table 77.1). Risk factors for falls (e.g., age, poor vision, previous falls, immobility, orthostatic hypotension, cognitive impairment, vitamin D insufficiency, poor balance, gait problems, weak muscles, sarcopenia) also contribute to fractures.

CLINICAL PRESENTATION

Unlike many other chronic diseases with multiple signs and symptoms, osteoporosis is considered a silent disease until fractures occur. Whereas 90% of hip fractures occur after a fall, two thirds of vertebral fractures are silent and occur with minimal stress, such as lifting, sneezing, and bending. An acute vertebral fracture may result in significant back pain that decreases gradually over several weeks with analgesics and physical therapy. Patients with significant vertebral osteoporosis may have height loss, kyphosis, and severe cervical lordosis, also known as a *dowager's hump*. Prolonged bisphosphonate use (>5 years) may result in an atypical femoral fracture, which may manifest as unilateral or bilateral thigh pain and result in a femoral shaft fracture with no or minimal trauma.

Bone Mineral Density and Other Bone Mass Assessments

In 1994, the World Health Organization (WHO) developed a classification system for osteoporosis and low bone mass based on data from white, postmenopausal women (Table 77.2). Osteoporosis is defined as a bone mineral density less than or equal to 2.5 standard deviations (SDs) below young adult peak bone mass (T-score ≤ −2.5 SD). Low bone mass (i.e., osteopenia) is defined as a bone mass measurement between 1.0 and 2.5 SDs below adult peak bone mass (T-score between −1.0 and −2.5 SD). Normal bone mineral density is defined as assessments at or above 1.0 SD below adult peak bone mass (T-score ≥ −1.0 SD).

The standard for assessing bone mineral density is dual-energy x-ray absorptiometry (DXA), which has excellent precision and accuracy. Measurements are made at the hip and spine, and in about 30% of cases, discordance is found between these measurements (Fig. 77.3). Classification should be made only if two or more vertebrae are available for analysis on spine images because of the high error rate when a single vertebra is assessed. Classification is based on the lowest value (i.e., total spine, total hip, or femoral neck).

In patients with hyperparathyroidism, in which cortical bone loss is often seen, forearm DXA using the one third distal radius site should

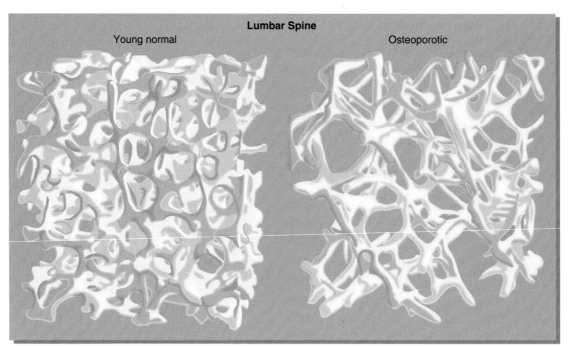

Fig. 77.1 Three-dimensional reconstruction by microcomputed tomography of a lumbar spine sample from a young adult normal woman and from a woman with postmenopausal osteoporosis. In the osteoporotic woman, bone mass is reduced and microarchitectural bone structure is deteriorated. Whereas the platelike structure in the normal case is very isotropic, the structure in the osteoporotic case shows preferential loss of horizontal struts; the plates have become rods that are thin and farther apart, and there is a concomitant loss of trabecular connectivity. These changes lead to a reduction in bone strength that is more than would be predicted by the decrease in bone mineral density. (From Riggs BL, Khosla S, Melton LJ 3rd: Sex steroids and the construction and conservation of the adult skeleton, Endocr Rev 23:279-302, 2002; Courtesy Ralph Mueller, PhD, Swiss Federal Institute of Technology [ETH] and University of Zurich, Switzerland.)

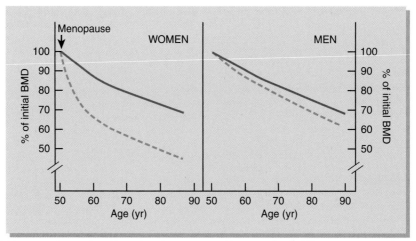

Fig. 77.2 Patterns of age-related bone loss in women and in men. *Dashed lines* represent trabecular bone, and *solid lines* represent cortical bone. The figure is based on multiple cross-sectional and longitudinal studies using dual-energy x-ray absorptiometry. *BMD,* Bone mineral density. (From Khosla S, Riggs BL: Pathophysiology of age-related bone loss and osteoporosis, Endocrinol Metab Clin North Am 34:1015-1030, 2005.)

also be assessed. Forearm assessments may be helpful in older patients who often have falsely elevated bone mineral density measurements at the spine as a result of atypical calcifications from degenerative joint disease, sclerosis, or aortic calcifications or in obese patients whose weight exceeds the table limit.

Bone mineral density can be measured by hip or spine quantitative computed tomography (QCT). However, less normative data are available for hip QCT, vertebral precision is inferior to that of DXA,

and radiation doses are significantly higher than those of DXA. Single-photon absorptiometry of the forearm and peripheral measures, such as heel ultrasound, have also been used to assess bone mass. However, the WHO classification should be used only with the central DXA measurements.

The National Osteoporosis Foundation (NOF) recommends obtaining a bone mineral density assessment in all women 65 years old or older, men aged 70 or older regardless of risk factors, and in adults

TABLE 77.1 Conditions, Diseases, and Medications That Cause or Contribute to Osteoporosis and Fractures

Lifestyle Factors
Alcohol abuse
Excessive thinness
Excess vitamin A
Falling
High salt intake
Immobilization
Inadequate physical activity
Low calcium intake
Smoking (active or passive)
Vitamin D insufficiency

Genetic Factors
Cystic fibrosis
Ehlers-Danlos syndrome
Gaucher's disease
Glycogen storage diseases
Hemochromatosis
Homocystinuria
Hypophosphatasia
Hypophosphatemia
Idiopathic hypercalciuria
Marfan syndrome
Osteogenesis imperfecta
Parental history of hip fracture or osteoporosis
Porphyria

Hypogonadal States
Anorexia nervosa and bulimia
Athletic amenorrhea
Hyperprolactinemia
Male hypogonadism
Panhypopituitarism
Premature and primary ovarian failure
Secondary gonadal failure
Turner's syndrome, Klinefelter syndrome

Endocrine Disorders
Cushing's syndrome
Diabetes mellitus (types 1 and 2)
Hyperparathyroidism
Thyrotoxicosis

Gastrointestinal Disorders
Celiac disease
Gastric bypass and bariatric surgery
Gastrointestinal surgery
Inflammatory bowel disease
Malabsorption
Pancreatic disease
Primary biliary cirrhosis

Hematologic Disorders
Hemophilia
Leukemia and lymphomas
Monoclonal gammopathies
Multiple myeloma
Sickle cell disease
Systemic mastocytosis
Thalassemia

Rheumatologic and Autoimmune Diseases
Ankylosing spondylitis
Lupus
Rheumatoid arthritis
Other rheumatic and autoimmune diseases

Neurologic Disorders
Epilepsy
Multiple sclerosis
Muscular dystrophy
Parkinson's disease
Spinal cord injury
Stroke

Miscellaneous Conditions and Diseases
Human immunodeficiency virus (HIV) infection/acquired immunodeficiency syndrome (AIDS)
Alcoholism
Amyloidosis
Chronic metabolic acidosis
Chronic obstructive lung disease
Congestive heart failure
Depression
End-stage renal disease
Hypercalciuria
Idiopathic scoliosis
Post-transplantation bone disease
Sarcoidosis
Weight loss

Medications
Aluminum (in antacids)
Anticoagulants (heparin)
Anticonvulsants
Aromatase inhibitors
Barbiturates
Cancer chemotherapeutic drugs
Cyclosporine and tacrolimus
Depo-medroxyprogesterone (premenopausal contraception)
Glucocorticoids (≥ 5 mg/day of prednisone or equivalent for ≥ 3 mo)
Gonadotropin-releasing hormone (GnRH) antagonists and agonists
Lithium
Methotrexate
Parenteral nutrition
Proton pump inhibitors
Selective serotonin reuptake inhibitors
Tamoxifen (premenopausal use)
Thiazolidinediones (e.g., Actos, Avandia)
Thyroid hormones (in excess)

Modified from National Osteoporosis Foundation: Clinician's Guide to Prevention and Treatment of Osteoporosis; 2020 (in press). Available at https://cdn.nof.org/wp-content/uploads/2016/01/995.pdf.

TABLE 77.2	World Health Organization Classification for Osteoporosis
Classification	**Criteria for Bone Mineral Density**
Normal	At or above –1.0 SD of young adult peak mean value
Low bone mass (osteopenia)	Between –1.0 and –2.5 SD of young adult peak mean value
Osteoporosis	At or below –2.5 SD of young adult peak mean value

SD, Standard deviation.

age 50 and older who have a fracture. They also suggest screening younger postmenopausal women and men age 50 to 69 with clinical risk factors for a fracture and adults with a condition or on a medication associated with low bone mass or bone loss (Table 77.3). This recommendation differs from 2018 US Preventive Services Task Force (USPSTF) guidelines that recommend screening women age 65 and older and younger women at risk (using screening tools) but did not endorse screening for men. The guidelines of the NOF concur with the Endocrine Society and International Society for Clinical Densitometry. Reference databases are available for white, African American, Asian and Hispanic men and women.

FRAX, a fracture risk assessment tool, predicts the 10-year risk for hip or any major osteoporotic fracture for women and men between 40 and 90 years of age. The FRAX for the individual patient incorporates femoral neck T-score, age, gender, height, weight, and specific risk factors, including history of adult fracture, parental hip fracture, current smoking, glucocorticoid use, rheumatoid arthritis, alcohol (three drinks or more per day), and secondary osteoporosis. The fracture risk prediction is specific for race and country and should be used for patients *not* on therapy.

Bone mineral density determined by DXA usually can be monitored after 2 years of therapy, depending on the site to be assessed and the type of therapy prescribed. For example, trabecular bone, which has greater surface area and is more metabolically active than cortical bone, is more likely to show improvements with stronger-acting antiresorptive agents. Changes in bone mass with potent antiresorptive therapy are more prominent in the spine compared with other areas. Seeing no changes in forearm bone mineral density over time is common despite good precision. Although the heel has a high percentage of trabecular bone, precision is poor, and monitoring should not be done at this site.

All patients with osteoporosis or low bone mass should have a work-up for secondary causes of bone loss. It should include a serum calcium level (corrected for albumin) to rule out hyperparathyroidism or malnutrition; a 25-hydroxyvitamin D level to assess for vitamin D deficiency or insufficiency; an alkaline phosphatase level to assess for Paget's disease, malignancy, cirrhosis, or vitamin D deficiency; liver and renal function tests to assess for abnormalities; a 24-hour urine calcium and creatinine assay to evaluate for hypercalciuria or malabsorption; a test for sprue in patients with anemia, malabsorption, or hypocalciuria; a thyrotropin level to rule out hyperthyroidism; and serum protein electrophoresis to rule out myeloma in older adults with anemia. Measurement of the parathyroid hormone (PTH) level often is needed to interpret the calcium and vitamin D levels. Total testosterone levels are recommended for men.

A more extensive work-up can be done in severe or unusual cases. A bone biopsy is rarely needed. Markers of bone turnover vary considerably in clinical practice, and these tests usually are reserved for research. However, they may be useful for assessing the rate of bone turnover after prolonged bisphosphonate use or a bisphosphonate holiday.

Radiography

Conventional radiographs and vertebral fracture assessment in adults age 50 and older can reveal a vertebral compression fracture that is diagnostic of osteoporosis (Fig. 77.4) even in the absence of a BMD. However, two thirds of vertebral compression fractures are asymptomatic. Low bone mass may not be evident on radiographs until 30% of the mass has been lost. When assessing bone mass, radiographs may be read inappropriately as a result of overpenetration or under penetration of the film. Radiographs therefore are a poor indicator of osteoporosis (with the exception of vertebral fractures), and the diagnosis is instead based on bone mineral densitometric results. A vertebral fracture assessment (VFA) can often be performed in tandem with a standard DXA and can identify vertebral compression fractures.

PREVENTION

General preventive measures for all patients include adequate calcium and vitamin D intake, exercise, and fall prevention techniques. The recommended daily allowance of calcium for adults, as reviewed by the Institute of Medicine, is 1200 mg for women 51 years or older and men 71 years or older and 1000 mg for men 50 to 70 years old. Calcium intake can be accomplished by dietary consumption, supplementation, or the combination of diet plus supplement. The supplements should be pure calcium carbonate or pure calcium citrate, taken in divided doses of approximately 500 to 600 mg twice daily. Calcium carbonate should be taken with meals for best absorption, whereas calcium citrate may be taken with or without food. Calcium supplements are available as tablets and in chewable and liquid forms. Foods such as orange juice, cereals, breads, and nutrition bars may be calcium fortified. There is no benefit to taking more than 1200 mg per day, and excess intake may increase the risk of kidney stones and cardiovascular disease (although data are controversial).

Vitamin D is important for calcium absorption and bone mineralization. Vitamin D has nonskeletal benefits and has been associated with improvement in muscle strength and prevention of falls. Vitamin D comes from two sources: diet and photosynthesis. Because dietary sources of vitamin D are limited only to certain foods (e.g., fortified milk, yogurt) and patients are often advised to avoid sun exposure for prevention of skin cancer and wrinkles, many studies have documented vitamin D deficiency and insufficiency in older adults. Older patients have a reduced ability to synthesize vitamin D in the skin. Low vitamin D levels can lead to secondary hyperparathyroidism.

Vitamin D can be taken in a multivitamin, in a calcium supplement, or in pure form and is available as cholecalciferol (D_3) or ergocalciferol (D_2). Based on data from noninstitutionalized patients without osteoporosis, the daily dose recommended by the Institute of Medicine is 600 IU per day for adults up to age 70 and 800 IU for those older than 70 years to achieve a 25-hydroxy vitamin D level of at least 20 ng/mL (50 nmol/L). However, the NOF suggests 800 to 1000 IU per day and a 25-hydroxy vitamin D level of at least 30 ng/mL for optimal calcium absorption. Elderly patients, those with malabsorption, and obese patients may need greater amounts of vitamin D. Older patients with severe vitamin D deficiency may be given 50,000 IU of vitamin D once per week for 3 months to bring serum vitamin D into the normal range to be followed by a maintenance dose of at least 1000 IU daily. The upper limit of vitamin D intake is 4000 IU/day. Activated vitamin D is rarely needed and should not be given on a regular basis for postmenopausal osteoporosis.

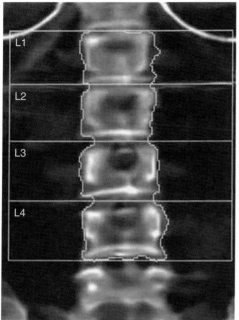

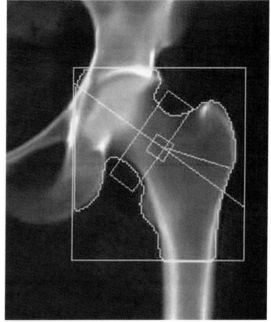

Image not for diagnostic use
k = 1.131, d0 = 47.0
116 × 117

Image not for diagnostic use
k = 1.152, d0 = 51.0
83 × 90
NECK: 49 × 15

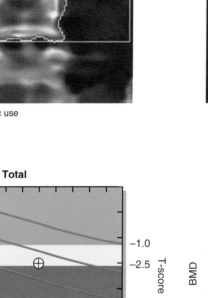

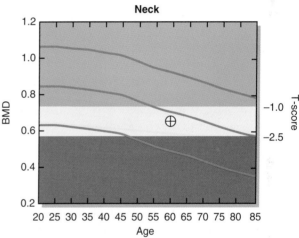

DXA results summary:

Region	Area (cm²)	BMC (g)	BMD (g/cm²)	T-score	Z-score
L1	10.29	8.63	0.839	−1.4	−0.1
L2	10.69	8.16	0.763	−2.4	−1.0
L3	11.78	9.50	0.807	−2.5	−1.1
L4	12.51	9.68	0.774	−2.6	−1.1
Total	**45.27**	**35.97**	**0.794**	**−2.3**	**−0.9**

Total BMD CV 1.0%, ACF = 1.039, BCF = 1.005, TH = 7.494
WHO classification: Osteopenia
Fracture risk: Increased

DXA results summary:

Region	Area (cm²)	BMC (g)	BMD (g/cm²)	T-score	Z-score
Neck	4.83	3.16	0.655	−1.7	−0.5
Total	**28.61**	**23.10**	**0.807**	**−1.1**	**−0.1**

Total BMD CV 1.0%, ACF = 1.039, BCF = 1.005, TH = 5.696
WHO classification: Osteopenia

Fig. 77.3 (Left) This patient has a lumbar spine (L1 through L4) bone mineral density (BMD) of 0.794 g/cm² *(white circle with cross on the graph)* as measured by dual-energy x-ray absorptiometry (DXA) and a T-score of −2.3. The reference database graph displays age- and sex-matched mean BMD levels ±2 standard deviations (SDs) derived from a normative database from the manufacturer (Hologic, Inc., Bedford, Mass.). The T-score indicates the difference in SD between the patient's BMD and that of the predicted sex-matched mean peak of a young adult; the z-value is the difference in SD between the patient's BMD and the sex-, age-, and ethnicity-matched mean BMD. (Right) This patient has a total hip BMD of 0.807 g/cm² and a femoral neck BMD of 0.655 g/cm² *(white circle with cross on the graph)* as measured by DXA, a total hip T-score of −1.1, and a femoral neck T-score of −1.7. The reference database graph displays age- and sex-matched mean BMD levels ±2 SDs derived from the third National Health and Nutrition Examination Survey. The T-score indicates the difference in SD between the patient's BMD and the predicted sex-matched mean peak young adult BMD; the z-score is the difference in SD between the patient's BMD. The 10-year fracture risk (FRAX) is 15% for a major osteoporotic fracture and 1.6% for a hip fracture (including reported risk factors: previous fracture, BMI = 24.2, using a US Caucasian database). (Bone densitometry report for the Horizon bone densitometer, Bedford, Mass., Hologic, Inc.)

TABLE 77.3 National Osteoporosis Foundation Recommendations for Bone Mineral Density Testing

- Women age ≥65 yr and men ≥70 yr, regardless of clinical risk factors
- Younger postmenopausal women, women in the menopausal transition, and men age 50–69 yr with clinical risk factors for fracture
- Adults who have a fracture after age 50 yr
- Adults who have a condition (e.g., rheumatoid arthritis) or are taking a medication (e.g., glucocorticoids in a daily dose of ≥5 mg prednisone or equivalent for ≥3 mo) associated with low bone mass or bone loss

TABLE 77.4 National Osteoporosis Foundation Guidelines for Treatment

- An adult hip or vertebral fragility fracture
- Osteoporosis by DXA T-score ≤ –2.5 SD for lumbar spine, total hip, or femoral neck after appropriate evaluation
- Low bone mass by DXA T-scores between –1.0 and –2.5 SD at the lumbar spine or femoral neck and a FRAX 10-year probability of a hip fracture ≥3% or a 10-year probability of major osteoporosis-related fractures ≥20%.

DXA, Dual-energy x-ray absorptiometry; *FRAX,* fracture risk assessment tool; *SD,* standard deviation.

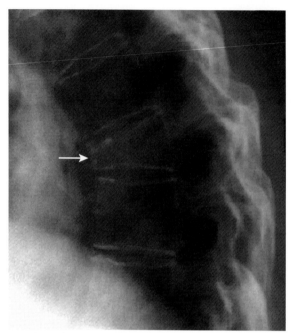

Fig. 77.4 Lateral spine radiograph demonstrates a thoracic anterior wedge compression fracture.

Weight-bearing exercise (walking, jogging, dancing, tai chi, etc.) is important for maintaining skeletal integrity. Study results are controversial concerning different types and durations of exercise by postmenopausal women and men. However, weight-bearing or resistance training exercises usually are suggested and have been shown to improve bone mass or maintain skeletal integrity. In patients with new vertebral fractures, physical therapy is important for improving posture and increasing the strength of back muscles.

Because 90% of hip fractures and a significant number of vertebral fractures occur following a fall, preventive measures are suggested for frail older patients at risk for falling. Fall-proofing the household includes installing grab bars in the bathroom and hand rails on stairways, avoiding loose throw rugs and cords, ensuring good lighting by the bedside, and moving objects within easy reach in the kitchen. Other fall prevention measures include eliminating medications that cause dizziness or postural hypotension (if possible), assessing the need for assistive devices (e.g., canes, walkers), and ensuring appropriate footwear and good vision. The benefits of hip protectors for hip fracture reduction are disappointing and controversial, and compliance with these products is often poor.

TREATMENT AND PROGNOSIS

The NOF developed treatment guidelines that incorporate a 10-year fracture risk prediction. The NOF suggests treatment for

postmenopausal women and men 50 years old or older, as shown in Table 77.4. In addition, the National Bone Health Alliance (NBHA) group of experts published an expanded version that included a fourth criterion for treatment: fracture of proximal humerus, pelvis or wrist in the setting of osteopenia (T-score between −1.0 and −2.5).

Patients taking glucocorticoids can fracture despite having normal bone density. The American College of Rheumatology suggests that patients starting glucocorticoids who will be treated for 3 months or longer have a bone density test and start antiresorptive therapy if indicated according to their guidelines.

Bisphosphonates

Bisphosphonates are the mainstay of osteoporosis prevention and treatment. They inhibit the cholesterol synthesis pathway in osteoclasts, causing early apoptosis and inhibiting osteoclast migration and attachment. Unlike other agents, bisphosphonates are incorporated into bone, the half-life is long, and the agent may be recycled.

In the United States, the bisphosphonates alendronate, risedronate, ibandronate, and zoledronic acid have been approved for the prevention and treatment of osteoporosis. Alendronate can increase bone mass by about 8% at the spine and 4% at the hip over 3 years. This increase has been associated with an approximately 50% reduction in spine, hip, and forearm fractures (Table 77.5). Alendronate is prescribed at 35 mg once weekly for osteoporosis prevention and 70 mg once weekly for the treatment of osteoporosis. Alendronate has been approved for use in men and patients with glucocorticoid-induced osteoporosis.

Risedronate is approved for the prevention and treatment of osteoporosis at a dose of 35 mg per week or 150 mg per month or as a delayed dose after breakfast of 35 mg per week. Large-scale, multicenter studies have shown improvements in bone mass of about 6% to 7% at the spine and 3% at the hip over 3 years. These studies revealed approximately 50% reduction in vertebral fractures, 40% reduction in nonvertebral fractures, and 40% reduction in hip fractures (see Table 77.5). Risedronate is approved for the treatment of osteoporosis in men and for the prevention and treatment of patients with glucocorticoid-induced osteoporosis.

Oral ibandronate is approved for the prevention and treatment of postmenopausal osteoporosis. After 3 years of treatment, ibandronate increased bone density by 6.5% at the spine and 3.4% at the hip, and it reduced new vertebral fractures by approximately 60%. No reductions in nonvertebral or hip fractures occurred. Ibandronate is approved at an oral dose of 150 mg monthly and for treatment at an intravenous dose of 3 mg every 3 months.

Zoledronic acid is approved for the prevention and treatment of postmenopausal osteoporosis, osteoporosis in men, and steroid-induced bone loss. The 3-year pivotal trial demonstrated increases of 6.9% of bone density at the spine and 6.0% at the hip, and the drug reduced spinal fractures by 70%, nonvertebral fractures by 25%, and hip fractures by 41%. Zoledronic acid is given at a dose of 5 mg intravenously once per year for treatment and 5 mg intravenously every 24 months for prevention.

There is not a simple guide for which bisphosphonate is chosen, since the order of medication selection is often determined by the cost of the medication and insurance consideration. Generally, alendronate is the most commonly used because it is usually the least expensive.

Because oral bisphosphonates are poorly absorbed, they must be taken first thing in the morning on an empty stomach with a full glass of water. Patients must wait 30 minutes (when taking alendronate and risedronate) to 60 minutes (when taking ibandronate) before eating and must not lie down. A delayed-release form of risedronate can be taken after breakfast.

Potential side effects of bisphosphonates include epigastric distress, heartburn, and esophagitis. Intravenous bisphosphonates have been associated with an influenza-like syndrome after infusion. Bisphosphonates can also cause arthralgias and myalgias. They are contraindicated in patients with renal insufficiency (i.e., estimated glomerular filtration rate of 30 to 35 mL/minute). Osteonecrosis of the jaw (ONJ) is a rare adverse event of abnormal bone growth in the jaw, which is more often associated with high-dose intravenous bisphosphonates in patients with cancer and poor oral hygiene. Atypical femoral shaft fractures (AFF) have been reported rarely after long-term use (>5 years of oral or >3 years intravenous) of bisphosphonates. These fractures may manifest with a prodrome of unilateral or bilateral thigh pain, and fractures may occur with minimal activity. These fractures are rare after osteoporosis treatment but common in cancer patients receiving frequent high doses intravenously.

Denosumab

The receptor activator of nuclear factor-κB (RANK) and its ligand (RANKL) are mediators of osteoclast activity. Compared with placebo, denosumab, an antibody to RANKL, produced a relative increase in bone mineral density at the spine of 9.2% and hip of 6.0% over 3 years, and it reduced fractures by 68% at the spine, 40% at the hip, and 20% at nonvertebral sites. Denosumab is approved for postmenopausal women and men with osteoporosis, men with prostate cancer on androgen deprivation therapy, postmenopausal women with breast cancer on aromatase inhibitors, and men and women on glucocorticoids. It is given as a 60-mg subcutaneous injection every 6 months. Denosumab may cause hypocalcemia so calcium intake by diet or supplement is encouraged. It is rarely associated with a rash or skin infection and very rarely associated with ONJ or AFF. When therapy is stopped, bone loss and vertebral compression fractures can occur, especially in patients with a previous vertebral fracture. It is suggested patients switch to an oral or intravenous bisphosphonate. Following denosumab discontinuation, teriparatide (a recombinant version of human parathyroid hormone) treatment (see later) can lead to bone loss at some sites.

Estrogen Agonists-Antagonists

Estrogen agonists-antagonists were previously called selective estrogen receptor modulators (SERMs) because they have some estrogen-like and anti-estrogen-like benefits. Raloxifene is approved for the prevention and treatment of osteoporosis in women. The Multiple Outcomes of Raloxifene Evaluation (MORE) trial found that bone mass was increased by 4% at the spine and 2.5% at the femoral neck over 3 years. This increase was associated with an approximate 50% reduction in vertebral fractures. No reduction in nonvertebral or hip fractures was seen (see Table 77.5). Treatment was associated with improved lipid status, as shown by decreased total and low-density lipoprotein cholesterol.

Raloxifene is not associated with endometrial hyperplasia, and patients should not have bleeding or spotting. They do not have breast tenderness or swelling. Raloxifene reduces the risk for invasive breast cancer in postmenopausal women with osteoporosis and in women at high risk for invasive breast cancer. Patients have the same small risk of deep vein thrombosis or pulmonary embolus that is found with hormone therapy. Raloxifene does not relieve postmenopausal symptoms and may exacerbate hot flashes. Studies have not found a significant impact on cardiovascular disease. Raloxifene can be given with or without food in a daily oral dose of 60 mg per day.

Hormone Therapy

Investigators of the Women's Health Initiative, a large, randomized, placebo-controlled, multicenter trial evaluating estrogen therapy, reported a 34% reduction in hip and vertebral fractures after 5.2 years. In addition to improvements in bone mass, benefits include an improved lipid profile, decreased colon cancer incidence, and decreased menopausal symptoms. However, because of the potential risks of hormone therapy (i.e., cardiovascular events, breast cancer, deep vein thrombosis, pulmonary embolus, and gallbladder problems), it should be used only for prevention or management of menopausal symptoms, and other agents should be used for the treatment of osteoporosis. A combination of conjugated estrogen/bazedoxifene is also approved for prevention in postmenopausal osteoporosis and other menopausal symptoms (hot flashes).

Parathyroid Hormone

Recombinant human PTH (1-34), or teriparatide, is an osteoanabolic agent that increases spinal bone mineral density by 9.7% and hip bone mineral density by 2.6% in 18 months. It is associated with a 65% reduction in vertebral fractures and a 53% reduction in nonvertebral fractures. Teriparatide is taken for up to 2 years as a subcutaneous, 20-µg daily dose for postmenopausal women and men at high risk for fracture including patients on glucocorticoids. Side effects include nausea, headache, and dizziness and may be associated with bone loss at some sites if initiated following denosumab discontinuation. After therapy, patients benefit from antiresorptive therapy to prevent bone loss. Recombinant human PTH (1-84) is approved for use in Europe.

Parathyroid Hormone-Related Peptide

Abaloparatide analog of PTHrP (1-34) is an osteoanabolic agent that increases spine bone density by 9.8% and hip bone density by 3.4% in approximately 12 months. The pivotal trial reported a reduction of vertebral fractures by 86% and nonvertebral fractures by 43%. It can be administered as a daily subcutaneous injection of 80 mg for up to 2 years for postmenopausal women. Side effects include nausea, headache, dizziness, and palpitations. A patch form is under investigation. Following therapy, an antiresorptive agent is recommended to prevent bone loss.

Romosozumab

Romosozumab is a monoclonal antibody to sclerostin that has a dual effect mechanism of action since it increases bone formation and decreases bone resorption. In pivotal trials compared to placebo, after 12 months romosozumab increased bone density by 13.7% at the spine and 6.2% at the hip and reduced vertebral fractures by 73% and hip fractures by 38%. It is approved for postmenopausal women with osteoporosis for 12 months as a subcutaneous monthly injection of 210 mg. It should be followed by an antiresorptive therapy to prevent bone loss. It is rarely associated with ONJ and AFF. In a study where romosozumab was compared to alendronate, there was an increased risk of

TABLE 77.5 US Food and Drug Administration–Approved Therapies for Prevention and Treatment of Osteoporosis

Agent	Prevention/ Treatment	Dosage	Vertebral Fracture Reduction	Hip Fracture Reduction	Women/ Men	Steroid-Induced OP
Antiresorptive Agents						
Alendronate[a]	Yes/yes	Prev: 35 mg/wk PO Treat: 70 mg/wk PO	Yes	Yes	Yes/yes	Yes
Ibandronate[a]	Yes[b]/yes	150 mg/mo PO, 3 mg q3mo IV	Yes	No	Yes/no	No
Risedronate[a]	Yes/yes	Prev/treat: 35 mg/wk PO, 35 mg/wk PO delayed release, 150 mg/mo PO	Yes	Yes	Yes/yes	Yes
Zoledronic acid[a]	Yes/yes	Prev: 5 mg q2yr IV Treat: 5 mg/yr IV	Yes	Yes	Yes/yes	Yes
Calcitonin	No/yes	200 IU/day Intranasal	Yes	No	Yes/no	No
Denosumab	No/yes	60 mg q6mo SC	Yes	Yes	Yes/yes	Yes
Hormone/Estrogen Therapy	Yes[c]/no	Various preparations available	Yes	Yes	Yes[d]/no	No
Raloxifene	Yes/yes	60 mg/day PO	Yes	No	Yes/no	No
Anabolic Agents						
Abaloparatide (PTHrP)	No/yes	80 μg/day SC	Yes	No	Yes/yes	No
Teriparatide (PTH [1-34])	No/yes	20 μg/day SC	Yes	No	Yes/yes	Yes
Dual-Action Agents						
Romosozumab	No/yes	210 mg/month SC	Yes	Yes	Yes/no	No

OP, Osteoporosis; *PO*, oral administration; *prev*, prevention; *PTH*, parathyroid hormone; *PTHtrP*, parathyroid hormone-related peptide; *SC*, subcutaneous administration; *Treat*, treatment.

[a]Alendronate, risedronate, ibandronate, and zoledronic acid are bisphosphonates.

[b]Oral only.

[c]Short-term prevention or management.

[d]For management.

cardiovascular events and strokes, so it should be avoided in patients who have had these events in the preceding year.

Calcitonin

Calcitonin is a 32-amino-acid peptide produced by the parafollicular cells of the thyroid gland. The pivotal clinical treatment trial did not show significant changes in bone mineral density after 3 years. However, the 200 IU dose of nasal calcitonin was associated with a 50% reduction in vertebral fractures (see Table 77.5). No reduction in nonvertebral or hip fractures was found. There is a possible association with development of cancer. Calcitonin may reduce pain following an acute vertebral compression fracture.

Choice of Therapy and Sequential Versus Combination Therapy

The initial choice of medication and sequence of therapy is important and under investigation. Currently, conventional therapy starts with a single agent. The choice of therapy is usually driven by the insurance provider, and often an oral antiresorptive bisphosphonate such as alendronate is the least expensive and provides fracture risk reduction at key vertebral, nonvertebral, and hip sites. If a patient has a contraindication to an oral bisphosphonate such as GERD, an intravenous bisphosphonate such as zoledronic acid is often initiated.

The concept of "treat-to-target" is based on the premise that starting *any* therapy may *not* be sufficient to achieve an acceptable level of risk. For high-risk patients with severe osteoporosis, the initial choice of therapy may be based on using the most potent therapy first

(anabolic), followed by a less potent therapy (antiresorptive) to maintain skeletal integrity. Recent studies have demonstrated greater vertebral fracture risk reduction with an anabolic therapy compared to an antiresorptive therapy.

Combination therapy with an anabolic and potent antiresorptive (denosumab) has been shown to increase bone mineral density more than monotherapy, but fracture reduction studies are needed. Combination of two antiresorptive therapies are not indicated.

Duration of Treatment

Osteoporosis is a chronic disease and requires lifelong management and follow-up. It is recommended that patients be reevaluated after 5 years of oral or 3 years of intravenous bisphosphate therapy. If they are osteopenic and without fracture risk they can begin a bisphosphate holiday, but reevaluation is suggested in 1 to 2 years. If they still have osteoporosis, have fractured on therapy, or are still at risk for fracture, therapy can be continued but a change to an alternative agent should be considered. After 2 years of an anabolic therapy with teriparatide or abaloparatide or 1 year of romosozumab, an antiresorptive therapy is suggested. There is no limit to the duration for denosumab, but following discontinuation of therapy an alternative antiresorptive therapy should be considered to prevent bone loss.

Vertebroplasty and Kyphoplasty

Vertebroplasty involves injection of cement (i.e., polymethylmethacrylate) into a compressed vertebra to prevent the vertebral body from further collapse. Kyphoplasty introduces a balloon into the vertebral body to expand it, followed by cement placement inside the vertebral body. This approach expands the vertebral body and may increase height. Some studies suggest a significant reduction in pain early on, but the long-term pain reduction may be similar to that of placebo. Ongoing studies are needed to determine whether differences in outcomes can be found between vertebroplasty and kyphoplasty. These procedures are recommended only for patients with significant pain from vertebral fractures and are not routinely performed in asymptomatic patients with vertebral osteoporosis.

SUGGESTED READINGS

Clinician's guide to prevention and treatment of osteoporosis, Washington, D.C., 2020, National Osteoporosis Foundation (in press).

Eastell R, Rosen CJ: Response to Letter to the Editor "Pharmalogical Management of Osteoporosis in Postmenopausal Women: An Endocrine Society Clinical Practice Guidelines," J Clin Endocrinol Metab 104(8):3537–3538, 2019.

Siu A, Allore H, Brown D, Charles ST, Lohman M: National Institutes of Health Pathways Workshop: Research Gaps for Long-Term Drug Therapies for Osteoporotic Fracture Prevention, Ann Intern Med 171(1):51–57, 2019.

U.S. Preventive Services Task Force: Screening for Osteoporosis to Prevent Fractures: US Preventative Services Task Force Recommendation Statement, JAMA 319(24):2521–2531, 2018.

Viswanathan M, Reddy S, Berkman N, Cullen K, Middleton JC, Nicholson WK, et al: Screening to Prevent Osteoporotic Fractures: Updated Evidence Report and Systematic Review for the US Preventative Services Task Force, JAMA 319(24):2532–2551, 2018.

Musculoskeletal and Connective Tissue Disease

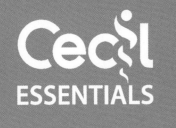

78

Approach to the Patient With Rheumatic Disease

Niveditha Mohan

INTRODUCTION

Rheumatic diseases encompass a range of musculoskeletal and systemic disorders that involve the joints and periarticular tissues in addition to other organ systems in the body. Differentiating localized from systemic processes, executing logical diagnostic procedures, and embarking on appropriate therapeutic courses demand careful clinical evaluation. The medical history and physical examination are paramount in this process. Laboratory tests are more confirmatory than diagnostic. Confirmation or exclusion of systemic connective tissue disease on the basis of laboratory results is unreliable and therefore unwise.

MUSCULOSKELETAL HISTORY

A logical approach to musculoskeletal complaints is indispensable to arriving at the correct diagnosis. Features in the medical history that are useful for distinguishing different types of arthritis are listed in Tables 78.1 and 78.2. The first step is to confirm that the complaint originates from the musculoskeletal system and is not referred pain caused by other organ system pathology (e.g., left shoulder pain due to cardiac disease). The next step is to define whether the problem is articular or extra-articular based on the history and clinical presentation.

Demographic data provide useful information. The age of the patient can point to a specific rheumatic disorder. The spondyloarthropathies are more commonly diagnosed in young men, systemic lupus erythematosus (SLE) in young women, gout in middle-aged men and postmenopausal women, and osteoarthritis in the older population. Asymmetrical pain and swelling in the knees have different connotations in a 70-year-old patient than in a 20-year-old patient.

Immune status may affect the diagnosis of rheumatic disease. Immunocompromised patients should be evaluated for infectious arthritis. Patients with human immunodeficiency virus (HIV) infection may have a severe form of Reiter syndrome or a sudden flare of psoriasis or psoriatic arthritis.

The patient's history provides the basis for differentiating inflammatory from noninflammatory arthropathies. Inflammatory arthritis is characterized by pain at rest, morning stiffness (typically greater than 60 minutes), gelling phenomenon (i.e., stiffening of joints after inactivity), and joint tenderness associated with other signs of inflammation such as swelling, erythema, and warmth. In osteoarthritis and nonarthritic musculoskeletal problems, pain usually does not occur at rest and is precipitated or worsened by activity. Some osteoarthritic joints are stiff initially but are improved with activity. The onset of

disease is abrupt in crystal-induced arthritis, less so in septic arthritis, and slow and insidious in most other disorders.

Patterns of joint involvement are typical of certain disorders: monoarthritis (one joint), as in septic or crystal-induced arthritis; pauciarthritis or oligoarthritis (two to four joints), as in Reiter syndrome or psoriatic arthritis; and polyarthritis (five or more joints), as in rheumatoid arthritis or SLE. Symmetry, migratory features, large versus small joint involvement, and axial versus appendicular locations are characteristic features of specific diseases and should be sought in the patient's history. Enthesopathy (i.e., disease at the attachment of tendons or ligaments to bone) can indicate a spondyloarthropathy.

Constitutional features such as fatigue, weight loss, and fever are seen in systemic autoimmune disease and infection but not in localized conditions. A thorough review of systems can provide clues to the primary diagnosis by defining associated systemic syndromes. Although there are many exceptions to these demographic and clinical generalizations, they provide helpful starting points when a patient is being evaluated for the first time.

PHYSICAL EXAMINATION

On physical examination, active and passive range of motion in all joints should be carefully assessed, and tenderness, swelling, warmth, erythema, deformity, and joint effusions should be evaluated (Fig. 78.1). Patients are frequently unaware of detectable joint abnormalities, including deformity and effusion, which are signs of joint disease. Reported pain may be referred from another site, which can be determined by examination. Pain in the knee is often a sign of hip disease and may be reproduced on examination of the hip. Palpable synovitis (i.e., thickening of the synovial membrane) is helpful in diagnosing inflammatory arthritides such as rheumatoid arthritis.

Different diseases have distinctive patterns of joint involvement, which provide critical diagnostic information. For example, prominent disease of distal interphalangeal joints is seen in psoriasis and inflammatory osteoarthritis. Wrist and metacarpophalangeal involvement are almost universal in rheumatoid arthritis but rare in osteoarthritis. Examination of the axial skeleton may reveal diminished lumbar flexion, decreased rotational motion of the spine, and decreased chest expansion, features of ankylosing spondylitis and other spondyloarthropathies. Patients may report symptoms in only a single joint, but finding additional affected joints on physical examination can change the entire evaluation.

Because rheumatic diseases may involve any organ system, a complete physical examination should be performed for all patients.

Alopecia and funduscopic changes (in SLE), uveitis (in spondyloarthropathy and juvenile arthritis), conjunctivitis (in reactive arthritis), sicca symptoms (in Sjögren's syndrome), oral and other mucous membrane ulcers (in reactive arthritis, SLE, and Behçet syndrome), lymphadenopathy (in SLE and Sjögren's syndrome), and cutaneous lesions (in psoriasis, dermatomyositis, scleroderma, SLE, and vasculitides) should be considered. Recurrent otorhinolaryngologic complaints, such as sinusitis, should raise suspicion for granulomatosis with polyangiitis (i.e., Wegener's granulomatosis). Lesions of psoriasis in the scalp, umbilicus, and anal crease, thickening of the skin on the fingers in scleroderma, and mucous membrane ulcers are often overlooked.

The lung examination may find evidence of interstitial fibrosis (in scleroderma, SLE, rheumatoid arthritis, and myositis), and a cardiac evaluation may reveal aortic insufficiency (in SLE and spondyloarthropathy), pulmonary hypertension (in systemic sclerosis), or evidence of cardiomyopathy (in systemic sclerosis, myositis, and amyloidosis). Pleural and pericardial rubs may be detected in SLE. Hepatosplenomegaly (in SLE and rheumatoid arthritis) and abdominal distention (in scleroderma) are also valuable clinical clues.

Muscle examination may reveal weakness from myositis, neuropathy (in vasculitis and SLE) or myopathy (in steroid myopathy). A complete neurologic examination may reveal carpal tunnel syndrome, peripheral neuropathy such as mononeuritis multiplex (i.e., asymmetrical sensory or motor neuropathy seen in many vasculitides), and central nervous system disease (in SLE and vasculitis). Recurrent miscarriages, livedo reticularis, Raynaud's phenomenon, and recurrent thrombotic events indicate antiphospholipid antibody syndrome.

The onset of systemic rheumatic diseases is usually insidious, and the clinical course is prolonged. However, presentation sometimes can be acute depending on the organ system involved. The initial evaluation must determine whether diagnosis and treatment of the patient's problem requires urgent attention. Infectious processes need immediate treatment. Acute joint inflammation, fever, and systemic signs such as chills, night sweats, and leukocytosis provide supporting evidence for infection. Gouty arthritis may share some or all of these clinical features, but its onset tends to be more abrupt. Inflammation extending beyond the margins of the joint is characteristic of septic arthritis and is otherwise seen only in crystal disease. Nonarticular processes such as cellulitis, septic bursitis, tenosynovitis, and phlebitis may mimic infectious arthritis. Analysis of synovial fluid is the key to diagnosis.

Acute nerve entrapment or spinal cord compression, tendon rupture, and fractures may occur in the absence of obvious trauma. Spinal cord compression may be the result of a herniated disk or vertebral subluxation. Tendon rupture may occur in inflammatory arthritides, particularly in the wrist of patients with rheumatoid arthritis. Pelvic and other insufficiency fractures may be seen in patients with osteoporosis or osteomalacia.

Patients with SLE or systemic vasculitis may have central or peripheral nervous system disease, including brain and peripheral nerve infarcts, glomerulonephritis, inflammatory or hemorrhagic lung disease, coronary artery involvement, intestinal infarcts, and digital infarcts. Threatened digit loss may also be seen in cases of scleroderma due to severe Raynaud's and vasculitis. Renal crisis may occur in scleroderma, with vasculopathy leading to renal infarcts, azotemia, microangiopathy, and severe hypertension. Acute blindness is a potential complication of giant cell arteritis, and the diagnosis requires urgent therapy even before confirmatory biopsy.

Acute inflammatory myositis should be promptly treated because it may progress rapidly and involve the respiratory musculature. In some cases, major organ involvement may be occult. When systemic disease is suggested, the patient's lungs and kidneys should be carefully evaluated.

TABLE 78.1 Clinical Features That Are Helpful in the Evaluation of Arthritis

Age, sex, ethnicity, family history
Pattern of joint involvement
Monoarticular, oligoarticular, polyarticular
Large versus small joints
Symmetry
Insidious versus rapid onset
Inflammatory versus noninflammatory pain (e.g., morning stiffness, gelling, night pain)
Constitutional symptoms and signs (e.g., fever, fatigue, weight loss)
Synovitis, bursitis, tendinitis
Involvement of other organ systems (e.g., rash, mucous membrane lesions, nail lesions)
Arthritis-associated diseases (e.g., psoriasis, inflammatory bowel disease)
Anemia, proteinuria, azotemia
Erosive joint disease

TABLE 78.2 Differentiating Features of Common Arthritides

Disease	Demographics	Joints Involved	Special Features	Laboratory Findings
Gout	Men, postmenopausal women	Monoarticular or oligoarticular	Podagra, rapid onset of attack, polyarticular gout, tophi	SF: Crystals, high WBC count, >80% PMNs
Septic arthritis	Any age	Usually large joints	Fever, chills	SF: High WBC count, >90% PMNs, culture
Osteoarthritis	Increases with age	Weight-bearing, hands		Noninflammatory SF
Rheumatoid arthritis	Any age, predominantly women ages 20–50 yr	Symmetrical, small joints disease	Rheumatoid nodules, extra-articular	SF: High WBC count, >70% PMNs
Reactive arthritis (Reiter syndrome)	Young males	Oligoarticular, asymmetrical	Urethritis, conjunctivitis, skin and mucous membranes	SF: Moderate WBC count, >50% PMNs
Spondyloarthropathy	Young to middle-aged men	Axial skeleton, pelvis (sacroiliac joints)	Uveitis, aortic insufficiency, enthesopathy	
Systemic lupus erythematosus	Women in childbearing years	Hands, knees	Nonerosive joint disease, autoantibodies, mostly mononuclear; multiorgan disease	SF: Low to moderate WBC count, almost 100% have antinuclear antibodies

PMNs, Neutrophils; *SF*, synovial fluid; *WBC*, white blood cell.

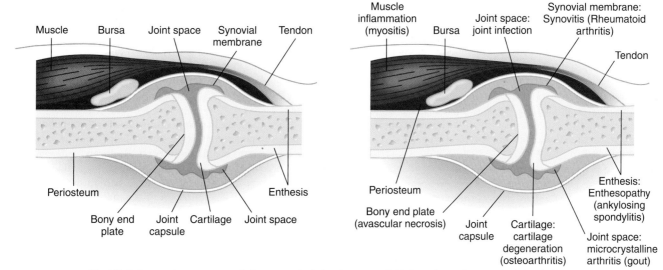

Fig. 78.1 Anatomic structures of the musculoskeletal system *(left).* Locations of musculoskeletal disease processes *(right).* (From Gordon DA: Approach to the patient with musculoskeletal disease. In Bennett JC, Plum F, editors: Cecil textbook of medicine, ed 20, Philadelphia, 1996, WB Saunders, p 1440.)

TABLE 78.3	Classification of Synovial Effusions by Synovial White Blood Cell Count			
Group	**Sample Diagnoses**	**Appearance**	**Synovial Fluid WBC Count (MM³)[a]**	**PMN Cells (%)**
Normal		Clear, pale yellow	0–200	<10
I. Noninflammatory	Osteoarthritis; trauma	Clear to slightly turbid	50–2000 (600)	<30
II. Mildly inflammatory	Systemic lupus erythematosus	Clear to slightly turbid	100–9000 (3000)	<20
III. Severely inflammatory	Gout	Turbid	2000–160,000 (21,000)	≈70
(noninfectious)	Pseudogout	Turbid	500–75,000 (14,000)	≈70
	Rheumatoid arthritis	Turbid	2000–80,000 (19,000)	≈70
IV. Severely inflammatory	Bacterial infections	Very turbid	5000–250,000 (80,000)	≈90
(infectious)	Tuberculosis	Turbid	2500–100,000 (20,000)	≈60

PMNs, Neutrophils; *WBC,* white blood cell.
[a]Range, with mean values in parentheses.

LABORATORY TESTING

Synovial fluid analysis is an important part of the evaluation of arthritis (Table 78.3). It helps to distinguish between inflammatory and noninflammatory arthritis, and results can be diagnostic of infectious arthritis or crystal disease.

Synovial fluid consists of an ultrafiltrate of plasma plus hyaluronic acid that is secreted by synovial lining cells. Evaluation of synovial fluid should include a cell count and differential, examination for sodium urate and calcium phosphate dehydrate crystals, Gram stain, and culture. Synovial fluid glucose and protein levels are not useful tests. Synovial fluid examination should be performed for all acute arthritides and all situations in which joint infection is likely. It should be performed at least once to evaluate chronic inflammatory arthritis. Aspiration and analysis of fluid before therapy are essential for appropriate decision making.

Although autoantibodies are often considered the hallmark of rheumatic diseases, their utility in diagnosing individual patients is much less than commonly assumed. Although almost 95% of patients with SLE have antinuclear antibodies (ANAs), as do most patients with scleroderma and autoimmune myositis, the proportion of patients with other rheumatic diseases who have positive test results is much lower. Conversely, 15% to 25% of healthy persons have ANAs, sometimes in high titers, when commercial test kits are used. Older persons

and patients with nonrheumatic systemic diseases such as malignancies and nonrheumatic autoimmune diseases such as thyroiditis or hypothyroidism have even higher frequencies of ANAs.

The very low specificity of a positive ANA result in the absence of clinical findings for an autoimmune disorder precludes its use as a screening test for disease in the general population. Other autoantibodies may be more useful and are discussed in subsequent chapters.

Rheumatoid factor is found in approximately 80% of patients with rheumatoid arthritis but also found in other rheumatic diseases, chronic infection, neoplasia, and almost any disease state that can cause chronic hyperglobulinemia. Neither positive nor negative test results are diagnostic, and the results should be interpreted only in the clinical context. Although the specificity of the rheumatoid factor is low, it does predict more aggressive joint disease and extra-articular joint manifestations.

Antibodies to cyclic citrullinated peptides are helpful in diagnosing rheumatoid arthritis because they have a high specificity (>90%). Their sensitivity varies from about 50% to 75%. Antibody tests should be ordered and repeated only if they can help in making the diagnosis, assessing the prognosis, or altering the treatment plan.

Tests for acute phase proteins, C-reactive protein, and the erythrocyte sedimentation rate are nonspecific, but positive results suggest an inflammatory disease. In some cases, such as in patients with giant cell arteritis and polymyalgia rheumatica, these tests may be useful for the diagnosis and monitoring the course of disease and therapy. Anemia may suggest chronic disease or hemolytic anemia. Leukopenia, especially lymphopenia, suggests SLE, and thrombocytosis indicates active inflammation. Leukocytosis may reflect inflammation or infection, and glucocorticoid therapy also elevates the neutrophil cell count by demargination. Urinalysis should always be performed in patients with systemic disease. Proteinuria, red blood cells, and casts should be considered evidence of occult renal disease. Laboratory tests should always be considered in the context of the clinical presentation.

IMAGING STUDIES

Radiographic studies often show changes characteristic of particular diseases. In patients with established rheumatoid arthritis, radiographs may demonstrate classically erosive disease of the small joints of the wrists, the ulnar styloid, the metacarpophalangeal and proximal interphalangeal joints, and the small joints in the foot. The erosions are bland and nonreactive. In contrast, erosive psoriatic arthritis causes a sclerotic reaction, and the patient may have characteristic telescoping of joints, also called *pencil-in-cup lesions.* Large erosions with overhanging sclerotic margins and even juxta-articular tophi may be seen in gout.

In ankylosing spondylitis, sacroiliitis is observed on pelvic radiograph films and has high diagnostic specificity. Syndesmophytes (i.e., calcification of the outer rim of the annulus fibrosis), bridging osteophytes, calcification of spinal ligaments, and a typical bamboo spine in the late stages are seen on lumbar and chest radiographs. Joint space narrowing, bony spurs, and sclerosis are seen in osteoarthritis. Chondrocalcinosis is a common finding. It may be asymptomatic or may lead to crystal arthritis (i.e., pseudogout). In acute arthritis, radiographs are much less helpful because bony changes take time to develop; only in septic joint disease is destruction observed in the early stages.

Imaging modalities such as magnetic resonance imaging (MRI), radionuclide scans, ultrasound, and computed tomography are often useful in assessing diseases of bones, joints, muscle, and soft tissues. Ultrasound may be used to detect synovial cysts, especially Baker cysts of the knee, and it is being used more frequently in the outpatient setting to guide procedures.

MRI is the procedure of choice for evaluating early avascular necrosis of bone, especially the hips, and for meniscal or rotator cuff disease.

MRI is preferred for evaluating intervertebral disk disease with radiculopathy and spinal stenosis, and it is useful for assessing solid lesions of bone and joints, including neoplastic lesions. The sensitivity of MRI for detecting edema (i.e., water) enables evaluation of infectious and noninfectious inflammatory muscle diseases. MRI is a sensitive but not a specific modality for evaluating osteomyelitis, properties shared with radionuclide imaging. MRI should not supplant clinical evaluation or plain radiography.

In many instances, diagnosis can be made with certainty only by pathologic examination of tissue. Muscle biopsy may be necessary to establish a diagnosis of inflammatory muscle disease, and nerve biopsy may be needed to detect vasculitis. Skin biopsy is useful in differentiating the many causes of rheumatologic skin disease. Renal biopsy is often needed for determination of the diagnosis, treatment, and prognosis.

SUMMARY

The evaluation of arthritis begins with a detailed history consisting of the location and pattern of joint involvement, differentiation of inflammatory from mechanical and other causes, and a thorough review of systems to determine the nonarticular systemic features. The patient's age and sex, family history, medication history, and coexisting medical conditions have a bearing on the diagnosis and treatment plan. Radiographic and laboratory studies, particularly synovial fluid analysis, provide confirmatory and sometimes diagnostic information.

For a deeper discussion of these topics, please see Chapter 241, ❖ "Approach to the Patient with Rheumatic Disease," in *Goldman-Cecil Medicine,* 26th Edition.

SUGGESTED READINGS

Felson DT: Epidemiology of the rheumatic diseases. In Koopman WJ, editor: Arthritis and allied conditions, ed 13, Baltimore, 1997, Williams & Wilkins, p 3.

Gordon DA: Approach to the patient with musculoskeletal disease. In Goldman L, Bennett JC, editors: Cecil textbook of medicine, ed 21, Philadelphia, 2000, WB Saunders, pp 1472–1475.

Sergent JS: Approach to the patient with pain in more than one joint. In Kelley WN, Harris Jr ED, Ruddy S, et al, editors: Textbook of rheumatology, ed 5, Philadelphia, 1997, WB Saunders, p 381.

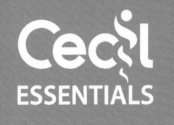

79

Rheumatoid Arthritis

Larry W. Moreland, Rayford R. June

DEFINITION

Rheumatoid arthritis (RA) is a chronic, systemic, inflammatory disorder that is characterized by symmetrical joint pain and swelling, morning stiffness, and fatigue. RA has a variable disease course, often with periods of exacerbations and, less frequently, disease quiescence. Outcomes range from rarely seen remitting disease to severe disease that produces disability and, for some patients, premature death.

Without treatment, most patients have progressive joint damage and significant disability within a few years. Since the introduction of methotrexate in 1985 and tumor necrosis factor-α (TNF-α) inhibitors in the 1990s, there has been a change in the treatment paradigm; many conventional and biologic therapies are now available to effectively treat this previously debilitating chronic disease.

EPIDEMIOLOGY

RA is a worldwide problem with a prevalence in Europe and North America of 0.5% to 1% of the adult population and an annual incidence of 25 to 50/100,000. RA is at least twice as common in women as in men and has a higher prevalence in specific patient populations such as the Pima and Chippewa Native Americans, with a respective prevalence of 5.3% and 6.8%. The disease affects individuals at any age, but most common age of onset is between 50 and 60 years. RA is uncommon among men younger than 45 years of age, but the incidence rises steeply with increasing age. Poor prognostic factors include high disease activity with many joints involved, increased inflammatory markers, high titers of rheumatoid factor (RF) and/or cyclic citrullinated peptides (CCP) antibodies, tobacco use, and erosions on radiographs. With the advent of new therapies, disease severity has decreased over time with less marked radiographic damage and fewer major orthopedic surgeries including joint replacements. However, despite these advances, work-related disability rates remain high for patients with RA. Numerous studies have demonstrated increased mortality rates for patients with RA compared with the general population, with a relative risk of 1.3. The increased mortality rate is more pronounced in males than in females with RA and is attributed to infectious complications and cardiovascular disease.

ETIOLOGY AND GENETICS

The specific underlying cause of RA (i.e., triggers in the susceptible host) is unknown. As for most autoimmune diseases, RA is thought to result from a complex interaction of genetic and environmental factors. RA may consist of multiple environmental stimuli leading to a common clinical presentation. There is not a known single mechanism of initiation or perpetuation. Various environmental triggers such as smoking, obesity, silica exposure, mineral oil, and organic solvents have been associated with the development of RA. Smoking has the most impact, particularly on CCP antibody–positive disease; CCP-positive disease has a more distinct presentation and epidemiology than CCP-negative disease.

An individual's genetic profile also plays a critical role in the susceptibility to and severity of RA. Supporting a genetic component, studies have revealed a 9% to 15% concordance in monozygotic twins that is approximately four times greater than the rate in dizygotic twins. RA is a polygenetic disease with over 100 susceptibility loci reported. The genes with the greatest impact lie in the class II major histocompatibility (MHC) locus, accounting for approximately 60% of the genetic risk for RA. A specific sequence on the HLA-DR haplotype involved in antigen recognition is called the *shared epitope*, which is strongly associated with severe RA and extra-articular manifestations. Multiple mutations in various alleles can then cause changes in the peptide binding grove leading to decreased self-tolerance. Although important, the shared epitope does not fully explain RA because it also occurs in only 25% to 35% of the white population whereas the chance of developing RA in shared-epitope carriers is only 1 in 25 (4%). Non-MHC and HLA genetic associations primarily involve pathways within CD4+ T cells and pathways affecting T- and B-cell interactions, cellular proliferation, and cytokine signaling pathways.

The interplay between environmental and genetic factors is most clearly seen with the increased risk of RA associated with smoking and the MHC class II loci. The exact association between the two is unclear, but research has shown that the bacteria in periodontal and mucosal lung disease, which are increased with smoking, can promote citrullination of bacteria leading to antibodies against multiple different citrullinated peptides. Anti-CCP antibodies are associated with aggressive disease.

For a deeper discussion of these topics, please see Chapter 248, ❖ "Rheumatoid Arthritis," in *Goldman-Cecil Medicine*, 26th Edition.

PATHOLOGY AND PATHOGENESIS

RA is a heterogeneous disease with a complex pathogenesis. RA is a clinical diagnosis presenting as a single clinical phenotype, but the underlying pathogenic immunologic genotype is more often than not unique. Instead, several signaling pathways often lead to the same clinical presentation.

Synovial membrane inflammation characterizes RA. Specific processes that lead to this inflammation and cellular proliferation are loss of tolerance, cytokine production, and autoantibody production. Several cytokine signaling pathways are involved with the predominant cytokines interleukin-1 (IL-1), IL-6, TNF-α, and granulocyte-macrophage colony-stimulating factor (GM-CSF) detected within the synovium and peripheral blood. As mentioned, in anti-CCP–positive disease, the initial site of inflammation may be in the periodontal mucosa and lung. Many advances have been made in understanding the cell-cell interactions and cytokine signaling, but little is known about the loss of tolerance and role of regulatory T cells in disease onset and propagation. Many insights into the pathogenesis of RA have resulted from analyzing the responses to cytokine inhibition (i.e., IL-1, TNF-α, and IL-6) and to specific T- and B-cell–directed therapies. For instance, TNF-α blockade therapies were initially developed for other diseases but then found to be very effective for RA.

The process of synovial inflammation and proliferation is initiated by an interaction between antigen-presenting cells (APCs) and CD4+ T cells. APCs display complexes of class II MHC molecules and peptide antigens that bind to specific receptors on the T cells. Clonal expansion of T-cell subsets occurs with an appropriate second signal, or co-stimulation, delivered by the APC to the T cell. Activated T_H1 and T_H17 T-cell subsets predominate in synovial tissues. These cell types stimulate synovial macrophages to secrete proinflammatory cytokines such as IL-1, TNF-α, GM-CSF, and IL-6 to activate inflammatory pathways.

In addition to cellular and cytokine processes, the humoral immune system is also involved in the pathogenesis of RA. The autoantibodies found most frequently in patients with RA are immunoglobulin M (IgM), RF, and anti-CCP. Positive RF and anti-CCP testing is associated with aggressive, erosive RA, and these autoantibodies are found in serum sometimes years before patients develop signs of RA. Although a causal link has not been confirmed, CCP antibodies, combined with genetic and environmental factors (e.g., smoking, periodontal disease),

are involved in the development of RA. It is not known yet how to prevent RA in people with high risk for developing it.

RA pathogenesis occurs in stages. In the induction phase, the anatomy of the synovial lining within the articular joint enables recruitment of inflammatory cells. Cigarette smoke, bacterial products, viral components, and other environmental stimuli may amplify this process and promote a dysregulated immune system. A genetic propensity for autoreactivity may initiate a then irreversible pathway to RA.

The destructive phase, which can be antigen dependent or independent, involves mesenchymal elements such as fibroblasts and synoviocytes. Bone erosions result from local differentiation and activation of osteoclasts, whereas cartilage damage appears to be caused by proteolytic enzymes produced by synoviocytes, macrophages, and synovial fluid neutrophils. Counter-regulatory mechanisms (e.g., soluble TNF-α receptors, suppressive cytokines through regulatory T cells, protease inhibitors, natural cytokine antagonists) are not produced in high enough levels, leading to a loss of tolerance.

Cytokines, which are hormone-like proteins that regulate many immune cell functions, have been implicated in synovial inflammation. The inflammatory milieu of the joint is dominated by proinflammatory factors produced by macrophages and fibroblasts, especially in the synovial intimal lining. In addition to the four cytokines mentioned previously (IL-1, IL-6, GM-CSF and TNF-alpha), many other cytokines and chemokines have been identified at the protein and mRNA level within the synovium.

Joint damage in RA results from proliferation of the synovial intimal layer forming a pannus that overgrows, invades, and destroys adjacent cartilage and bone (Fig. 79.1). Fibroblast-like synoviocytes

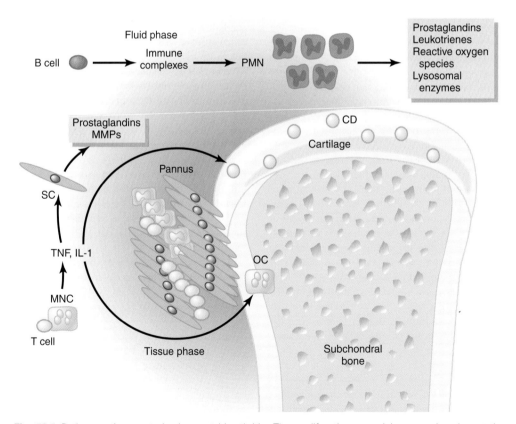

Fig. 79.1 Pathogenetic events in rheumatoid arthritis. The proliferative synovial pannus invades at the bone-cartilage interface. Interleukin-1 (IL-1) and tumor necrosis factor-α (TNF-α) activate synovial cells (SC) to produce prostaglandins and matrix metalloproteinases (MMPs). In the synovial fluid, polymorphonuclear leukocytes (PMN), activated by immune complexes and complement, produce mediators of inflammation and destruction. *CD*, Chondrocytes; *MNC*, mononuclear cell; *OC*, osteoclast.

and macrophages are the predominant cellular components of the invading pannus of the synovium. Extracellular matrix damage resulting from synovial expansion is caused by several families of enzymes, including serine proteases, cathepsins, and matrix metalloproteinases.

❖ For a deeper discussion of these topics, please see Chapter 248, "Rheumatoid Arthritis," in *Goldman-Cecil Medicine*, 26th Edition.

CLINICAL PRESENTATION

Articular Manifestations

RA manifests with a symmetrical polyarthritis that typically starts with the small joints of the hands and feet and can progress to the synovium of the wrists, elbows, shoulders, knees, and ankles. Patients have an insidious onset of inflammatory symptoms, which are fatigue, pain, and stiffness that is worse with inactivity and is improved with movement. Prolonged morning stiffness, usually lasting more than 1 hour, is a classic feature of RA (Table 79.1). Often, warm water and heat will also relieve this stiffness. Any diarthrodial (synovial) joint may be involved, including the apophyseal (spinal), temporomandibular, and cricoarytenoid joints. Involved joints are swollen, warm, and tender, and they may have effusions. The synovium, which is normally a few cell layers thick, becomes palpable on examination (i.e., synovitis).

Without treatment, RA progresses in some patients to joint destruction and deformity. Erosive lesions of bone and cartilage often are visible radiographically at the margins of bone and cartilage, the sites of synovial attachment. Not all patients with RA have erosive disease, with only 40% of patients in many present-day studies having radiographic erosions. Tenosynovitis (i.e., inflammation of tendon sheaths) leads to tendon malalignment, stretching or shortening and exacerbates joint subluxation.

Joint deformities leading to functional disability occur in RA after long-standing joint disease. Common deformities are ulnar deviation at the metacarpophalangeal joints and volar subluxation at those joints and at the wrists. Flexion and extension contractures in the proximal and distal interphalangeal (PIP and DIP) joints of the fingers lead to the characteristic swan-neck deformity (i.e., flexion contracture at the DIP joint and hyperextension at the PIP joint) or boutonnière deformity (i.e., flexion contracture at the PIP and hyperextension at the DIP joint).

Synovitis at the wrists can lead to median nerve compression and carpal tunnel syndrome. Carpal tunnel syndrome can often be the first sign of RA. Rarely, long-standing cervical spine disease may lead to C1-C2 subluxation and life-threatening spinal cord compression. Rupture of synovial fluid from the knee into the calf (i.e., Baker cyst) may mimic deep vein thrombosis or imitate cellulitis.

Extra-articular Manifestations

RA is a systemic disease in which there can be multiple extra-articular manifestations, particularly in severe uncontrolled RA (Table 79.2).

Constitutional symptoms are common with disease onset and flares; these symptoms include fatigue, low-grade fever, weight loss, and myalgia. Extra-articular manifestations are more common in RF-positive patients and some epidemiologic studies have shown a decrease in extra-articular manifestations associated with newer treatments and improved disease control.

The most common extra-articular manifestation of RA is rheumatoid nodules, which can occur in 30% to 40% of patients. These are grossly palpable nodules on the skin at pressure points along extensor surfaces, especially at the elbows. Rheumatoid nodules are associated with RF positivity and tobacco use and can also occur in the lungs, pleura, pericardium, sclerae, and other sites, including the heart in rare cases. In the eyes, RA commonly is associated with keratoconjunctivitis sicca with coexistent Sjögren's syndrome and less often with scleritis and episcleritis.

Lung involvement in RA can present as interstitial lung disease and may include pleuropericarditis, producing inflammatory exudative pleural and pericardial effusions. The cardiovascular effects of RA can range from long-term inflammation leading to accelerated coronary artery disease to pericarditis to small and medium-sized vasculitis. The vasculitis of RA can produce cutaneous lesions (e.g., ulcers, skin necrosis) and mononeuritis multiplex.

RA patients often have common hematologic manifestations such as anemia of chronic disease and thrombocytosis with uncontrolled disease and early presentation. Patients with RA also have an increased incidence of lymphoma. Larger granular lymphocyte (LGL) leukemia is a specific form of chronic leukemia associated with RA. Often LGL can present as Felty syndrome (i.e., rheumatoid arthritis, splenomegaly, and neutropenia). This rare complication can be accompanied by leg ulcers and vasculitis.

Medication side effects should also be considered as extra-articular manifestations of RA. Rheumatoid nodules can be precipitated by methotrexate with a syndrome called methotrexate nodulosis and must be differentiated from uncontrolled RA. TNF-α inhibitors, the most common biologic agent for RA, are associated with skin psoriasis and can also cause drug induced lupus.

DIAGNOSIS AND DIFFERENTIAL DIAGNOSIS

RA is a clinical diagnosis based on a thorough history and physical examination. Classic symptoms include morning stiffness associated with synovitis of small joints in a symmetrical fashion. No single diagnostic test enables a diagnosis of RA to be made with certainty. Instead, the diagnosis depends on the accumulation of characteristic symptoms, signs, laboratory data, and radiologic findings. There are no diagnostic criteria for RA but rather a pattern of clinical features and laboratory tests that aid the clinician in making the diagnosis. Classification criteria are useful in guiding the clinical diagnosis of RA and also create clear guidelines for classifying patients in research studies. The RA classification criteria were updated in 2010 to include anti-CCP testing

---

TABLE 79.1 Clinical Characteristics of Rheumatoid Arthritis

Morning stiffness or gelling

Symmetrical joint swelling

Predilection for wrists and proximal interphalangeal, metacarpophalangeal, and metatarsophalangeal joints

Erosions of bone and cartilage

Joint subluxation and ulnar deviation

Inflammatory joint fluid

Carpal tunnel syndrome

Baker cyst

TABLE 79.2 Extra-articular Features of Rheumatoid Arthritis

Rheumatoid nodules: subcutaneous, pulmonary, sclera

Interstitial lung disease

Vasculitis, especially skin and peripheral nerves

Pleuropericarditis

Scleritis and episcleritis

Leg ulcers

Felty syndrome

TABLE 79.3 2010 ACR/EULAR Classification Criteria for Rheumatoid Arthritis

For patients who have at least 1 joint with definite synovitis and for whom the synovitis is not better explained by another disease.

A. Joint involvement (0–5 points)
  1 large joint (0)
  2–10 large joints (1)
  1–3 small joints (with or without involvement of large joints) (2)
  4–10 small joints (or without involvement of large joints) (3)
  >10 joints (with involvement of at least 1 small joint) (5)
B. Serology (0–3 points)
  Negative RF and negative anti-CCP (0)
  Low-positive RF or low-positive anti-CCP (2)
  High positive RF or high positive anti-CCP (3)
C. Acute phase reactants (0–1 points)
  Normal CRP and normal ESR (0)
  Abnormal CRP or abnormal ESR (1)
D. Duration of symptoms (0–1 points)
  <6 weeks (0)
  ≥6 weeks (1)
A score of at least 6 of 10 points is needed for the classification of definite rheumatoid arthritis.

ACR, American College of Rheumatology; *CCP,* cyclic citrullinated peptide; *CRP,* C-reactive protein; *ESR,* erythrocyte sedimentation rate; *EULAR,* European League Against Rheumatism; *RF,* rheumatoid factor. Aletaha D, Neogi T, Silman AJ, et al: 2010 Rheumatoid arthritis classification criteria: an American College of Rheumatology/European League Against Rheumatism collaborative initiative, *Arthritis Rheum* 62:2569-2581, 2010.

and were designed to capture early RA (Table 79.3). Multiple studies have shown that prompt diagnosis and treatment are important to prevent disease progression, joint deformities, and disability. With the advent of specific diagnostic testing such as CCP testing and incorporation into the new classification criteria for early RA, both clinical practice and research settings have seen significant advancements with earlier treatment for patients with subsequently improved outcomes.

The differential diagnosis for RA is broad and includes viral arthritis (e.g., parvovirus, rubella, hepatitis B and C), thyroid disorders, sarcoidosis, reactive arthritis, psoriatic arthritis, Sjögren's syndrome, systemic lupus erythematosus (SLE), bacterial endocarditis, rheumatic fever, calcium pyrophosphate disease (CPPD), chronic tophaceous gout, polymyalgia rheumatica, erosive osteoarthritis, and fibromyalgia syndrome. A history and physical examination, including a thorough review of systems, persistence over time (with 6 weeks being on the most recent classification criteria; see Table 79.3), and available diagnostic testing guide the clinician in making the diagnosis. Initial laboratory tests in the evaluation should include a complete blood count, comprehensive metabolic panel, erythrocyte sedimentation rate, C-reactive protein, uric acid, RF, anti-CCP, ANA by indirect immunofluorescence, and hepatitis B and C testing. Additional tests such as viral serologies and autoantibody testing should be guided by the clinical presentation.

RF is an antibody (typically IgM but also IgG or others) that binds to the Fc fragment of IgG. RF and IgG join to form immune complexes that are detectable in the serum of 70% to 80% of patients with RA over the course of the disease. However, RF is not specific for RA and frequently occurs in patients with SLE, Sjögren's syndrome, infective endocarditis, sarcoidosis, lung and liver diseases (including infections

such as hepatitis B and C), and also in healthy individuals. In an individual patient, the RF titer does not correlate with disease activity, but high titers are associated with severe erosive arthritis and extra-articular disease. The finding of RF in serum alone does not establish a diagnosis of RA, but it can help to confirm the clinical impression. RF does not need to be repeatedly tested once the diagnosis is made.

Anti-CCP antibodies are a more specific marker for RA than RF. Anti-CCP antibodies are antibodies directed at citrullinated peptides and can be tested with one diagnostic test. Anti-CCP antibodies in the presence of at least one swollen joint have a high specificity (>95%) for RA. Compared to RF, CCP antibodies have improved specificity (96% vs. 86%), with similar sensitivity (67% vs. 70%) for RA. These antibodies can be detected several years before the development of clinical RA, and they are associated with severe RA outcomes, including radiographic joint damage and a poor prognosis. Because of their specificity for RA, anti-CCP antibodies are useful in differentiating RA from other conditions positive for RF, including Sjögren's syndrome, infection, and hepatitis.

Acute phase reactants, such as the erythrocyte sedimentation rate and C-reactive protein, are usually elevated in active inflammation but are not sensitive or specific for the diagnosis of RA. These tests are useful for differentiating RA from noninflammatory conditions such as osteoarthritis or fibromyalgia. However, even when there is clear clinical evidence of joint inflammation, the values for acute phase reactants may be normal. Inflammation in RA often leads to anemia of chronic disease and thrombocytosis.

Synovial fluid analysis is usually not necessary when there is a clear chronic inflammatory polyarthritis. Arthrocentesis should be performed to rule out infection or crystalline arthropathy in monoarthritis if only a single joint is involved. Synovial fluid analysis is nonspecific but can support the diagnosis by showing inflammatory joint fluid with cell counts between 2000 and 100,000. Radiographs, although not part of the 2010 RA classification criteria, may show characteristic periarticular osteopenia, marginal joint bone erosions, and uniform joint space narrowing in a symmetrical distribution. Often radiographs will be normal in early RA but can serve as a baseline to assess disease progression over time.

For a deeper discussion of these topics, please see Chapter 242, "Laboratory Testing in the Rheumatic Diseases," Chapter 243, "Imaging Studies in the Rheumatic Diseases," Chapter 247, "Bursitis, Tendinitis, and Other Periarticular Disorders and Sports Medicine," and Chapter 248, "Rheumatoid Arthritis," in *Goldman-Cecil Medicine,* 26th Edition.

TREATMENT

The ultimate goals for managing RA are to reduce pain and discomfort, prevent joint deformities, and maintain normal physical and social function. Although there is no cure for RA, remission can be maintained in a subset of patients. Treatment begins with effective communication between the physician and patient regarding the nature of the disease and the goals of treatment.

Nonpharmacologic therapeutic options include reduction of joint stress, often through physical and occupational therapy. Local rest of an inflamed joint can reduce joint stress, as can weight reduction, splinting, and the use of walking aids. Vigorous activity should be avoided during disease flares. Full range of motion of joints, however, should be maintained by a graded exercise program to prevent contractures and muscle atrophy. Physical therapy improves muscle strength, decreases joint stress, and maintains joint mobility. Occupational therapy can provide various appliances to protect joints and make daily activities easier.

TABLE 79.4 Conventional Disease-Modifying Antirheumatic Drugs

Conventional Agents	Toxicities
Azathioprine	Infection, nausea, bone marrow suppression, fever, pancreatitis
Baricitinib, tofacitinib (targeted synthetic oral DMARD)	Infection rate similar to biologic DMARDs; bone marrow and hepatic toxicity, hyperlipidemia, contraindicated with biologics
Hydroxychloroquine	Retinal toxicity, requires ophthalmologic monitoring
Leflunomide	Bone marrow and hepatic toxicity; cholestyramine washout if toxic; contraindicated in pregnancy
Methotrexate[a]	Oral ulcers, nausea, bone marrow suppression, pneumonitis; contraindicated in pregnancy and severe coexistent lung disease; hepatotoxicity
Sulfasalazine	Nausea, bone marrow suppression

DMARDs, Disease-modifying antirheumatic drugs.
[a]Initial recommended DMARD in moderate to severe RA.

TABLE 79.5 Biologic Disease-Modifying Antirheumatic Drugs

Biologic Agent	Targeted Mechanism
Adalimumab, certolizumab, etanercept, golimumab, infliximab	Cytokine directed, anti-TNF-α
Anakinra	Cytokine directed, anti-IL-1
Sarilumab, tocilizumab	Cytokine directed, anti-IL-6
Abatacept	T-cell directed, inhibits co-stimulation
Rituximab	B-cell directed, anti-CD20

IL, interleukin; TNF, tumor necrosis factor.

Pharmacologic Approach

Studies have revealed that disease-modifying antirheumatic drug (DMARD) therapy early in the course of RA slows disease progression more effectively than delayed therapy. Early RA is currently defined as within 6 months of diagnosis and established RA as greater than 6 months. A targeted approach at the extent of disease activity should be used to minimize joint inflammation. Effective treatment with DMARDs can improve signs, symptoms, and radiographic progression, even in long-standing disease. The inflammation of RA should be controlled as completely as possible, as soon as possible, and for as long as possible. Conventional DMARDs and biologic DMARDs prevent disease progression and disability.

Disease Activity

Establishing a diagnosis of RA enables the clinician to determine treatment and also counsel the patient regarding future disease course, need for treatment, and prognosis. Intensity of treatment is guided by the extent of disease activity. As mentioned, RA involves the diarthrodial joints but the exact pattern of joint involvement is patient specific. More joints involved means worse disease and is associated with worse outcomes of disease. Disease activity can be defined by multiple different disease activity tools that combine input from physical exam with counting the number of swollen and tender joints, patient input on their global assessment of RA disease activity, not just pain, and laboratory tests showing evidence of inflammation, most commonly by ESR and CRP. The goal of treatment should be absence of joint inflammation. When the diagnosis is made, the patient should be treated in consultation with a rheumatologist, if available, to use specialized disease activity measurements with a goal to minimize joint inflammation towards remission or low disease activity. These disease activity measures include the DAS28 (disease activity measuring involvement of 28 joints), ESR/CRP, CDAI (Clinical Disease Activity Index), SDAI (Simple Disease Activity Score), RAPID3 (Disease Activity Score developed from short and simple questionnaire), and PASDAS (PAS Disease Activity Score based on a weighted index that includes 7 components).

Conventional Disease-Modifying Antirheumatic Drugs

Many DMARDs are available for treating RA. All conventional DMARDs have a slow onset, taking 1 to 6 months to become fully effective, and they need close monitoring for toxicity (Table 79.4). Once the diagnosis of RA is made, a DMARD should be initiated.

Methotrexate is universally used as the initial DMARD in patients with early RA because of its established efficacy and known toxicity profile (evidence from multiple randomized controlled trials). It can be administered once weekly by the oral or parenteral route. Known side effects to monitor for include oral ulcers, nausea, hepatotoxicity, cytopenias, and pneumonitis. If contraindications to methotrexate exist such as chronic liver disease or alcohol use in excess of two drinks per day for males or one per females, alternative conventional DMARDs such as sulfasalazine or hydroxychloroquine should be used in monotherapy. Early in the course of disease, NSAIDs and low-dose corticosteroids can be used for rapid control of inflammation in combination with DMARDs.

In cases of methotrexate failure or inadequate response with continued moderate to high disease activity, the subsequent choice of conventional and biologic DMARDs is not standardized and is instead based on clinical factors such as route of administration, side effects and risks of adverse events, cost, and patient and physician preference. Often combination therapy of multiple DMARDs is used for RA treatment. For patients with mild RA, hydroxychloroquine or sulfasalazine, or both, may be used as first-line drugs. Triple therapy, the combination of methotrexate, hydroxychloroquine, and sulfasalazine, was shown in two randomized, controlled trials to be noninferior to biologic TNF-α inhibitors. Tofacitinib and baricitinib are a new class of synthetic DMARDS that inhibit Janus kinase (JAK)s and reduce cytokine levels. JAK inhibitors are the one class of synthetic DMARDS that should not be used in combination with biologic DMARDS due to increased risk of infections.

Biologic DMARDs

Biologic DMARDs are targeted, immune-based therapies that were introduced in the 1990s with the initiation of cytokine-directed TNF-α inhibitors. Biologics are produced by living cells using recombinant DNA technology (Table 79.5). TNF-α inhibitors were the first of 10 biologic DMARDs approved by the U.S. Food and Drug Administration (FDA) for the treatment of RA (see Table 79.3). Five TNF-α–directed therapies are available. The TNF-α inhibitors are the most widely used biologic agents because of the rapid improvement they produce in patients resistant to methotrexate therapy. They are one class of the biologics recommended in addition to methotrexate after methotrexate failure.

Most biologic DMARDs are given by intravenous or subcutaneous injection and are quite expensive but very effective treatments. Biosimilars are biologic medications with a similar molecular structure to a sister biologic medication and that have no clinically meaningful differences from FDA-approved biologic DMARDs. Multiple biosimilars are available and more are in development as cheaper alternatives to biologic DMARDs. Most biologics have an increased risk of infection, including risk of reactivation of tuberculosis. Other cytokine-directed therapies include the IL-6 receptor antagonists sarilumab and tocilizumab and the IL-1 receptor antagonist anakinra. Biologic DMARDs also include an inhibitor of T-cell co-stimulation, abatacept; and a B-cell–depleting agent, rituximab. All patients should be screened for tuberculosis within 12 months prior to starting the first biologic DMARD. Biologic DMARDs should not be used in combination with other biologics because of increased risk of atypical infections.

❖ For a deeper discussion of these topics, please see Chapter 33, "Biologic Agents and Signaling Inhibitors," in *Goldman-Cecil Medicine*, 26th Edition.

Symptomatic Control and Bridging Therapy

DMARDs often take up to 1 to 6 months to produce low disease activity or remission. Consequently, nonsteroidal anti-inflammatory drugs (NSAIDs), which are not disease modifying, are frequently used early in the disease process for symptomatic control. NSAIDs can have significant side effects, including renal toxicity and increased risk of gastrointestinal bleeding; NSAIDs should be used with caution in patients with multiple medical comorbidities but are a standby for many patients with chronic disease.

Glucocorticoids remain important in the treatment of RA, especially for acute exacerbations of disease. These agents are used for RA in low to medium doses. Glucocorticoids are useful for brief exacerbations and decrease bone erosions, but the long-term side effects of glucocorticoids can be substantial; they should be used primarily in episodes of RA flares or high disease activity as bridging therapy for further DMARD effects. Side effects include osteoporosis, avascular necrosis of bone, obesity, hypertension, and glucose intolerance. Screening, prevention, and treatment for osteoporosis should be considered for all patients who receive long-term glucocorticoid therapy for prevention of glucocorticoid-induced osteoporosis. Intra-articular glucocorticoids are extremely effective treatment for exacerbations involving only a few joints.

❖ For a deeper discussion of these topics, please see Chapter 230, "Osteoporosis," in *Goldman-Cecil Medicine*, 26th Edition.

Medical Care Specialized for Rheumatoid Arthritis

RA is a chronic disease that requires focused care for comorbidities. DMARDs themselves require frequent laboratory monitoring for toxicities, including bone marrow suppression, hepatotoxicity, and renal dysfunction.

Infection

All patients should be tested for hepatitis B and C prior to starting a DMARD or biologic. Patients should be tested for latent tuberculosis within the previous 12 months by either a purified protein derivative (PPD) or interferon-γ release assay (IGRA) before starting a biologic DMARD. Opportunistic infections can occur in patients receiving DMARDs and biologic therapies and should be considered in the clinical care if chronic cytopenias or respiratory disease. In the setting of acute infection, DMARDs and biologic therapies should be withheld.

Vaccinations

Vaccination status should be assessed by primary care and rheumatology in caring for patients with RA. Ideally, vaccinations should occur during quiescent disease and also prior to starting immunosuppressive therapy. Killed vaccines can be given to patients while on all immunosuppressive conventional and biologic therapy, but live vaccines should be avoided in patients on biologic therapy. Prophylactically, all RA patients should be vaccinated for pneumococcal, influenza, and hepatitis B infection if increased risk. Herpes zoster vaccine to prevent shingles should be given to patients greater than 50 years old. If the live vaccine is used, this should be used prior to starting or while off biologic agents.

Osteoporosis

RA itself is a risk factor for osteoporosis, and combined with glucocorticoid use, it can lead to severe osteoporosis and subsequent morbidity. In every RA patient, bone health should be addressed to prevent development of osteoporosis. Bone health can be evaluated by periodic dual-energy x-ray absorptiometry (DXA), a risk assessment tool including coexistent tobacco use, family history of fractures, and ensuring adequate vitamin D supplementation. Routine strength training and aerobic exercise in moderation is recommended to improve bone health and ensure joint stabilization.

Cardiovascular

RA is a risk factor for cardiovascular disease due to chronic inflammation and should be monitored and managed. Lipid treatment recommendations do not currently differ from the routine non-RA patient populations. Hypertension, exacerbated by both pain and coexistent medications such as NSAIDs and glucocorticoids, should be monitored and treated according to current guidelines.

Perioperative

Caution should be taken preoperatively when the RA patient is being anesthetized to avoid C1-C2 subluxation and spinal cord compression. Flexion and extension radiographs of the cervical spine should be considered preoperatively for general anesthesia to assess for atlanto-occipital joint instability. Joint replacement surgery plays an important role for patients who have had severe, destructive joint disease, particularly in the knees and hips. Medications should be evaluated preoperatively with biologic DMARDs held one treatment cycle prior to starting. Methotrexate and conventional DMARDs can be continued through joint replacement surgery with improvement in both surgical and RA outcomes.

CONCLUSION AND PROGNOSIS

Although the underlying cause of RA is unknown, advances in cell biology, immunology, and molecular biology have led to dramatic therapeutic advancements for this disease. Conventional and biologic DMARDs improve short- and long-term outcomes. Bone erosions can occur within 1 to 2 years of disease onset, and early initiation of DMARDs is essential to prevent further morbidity.

RF and/or CCP positivity and extra-articular features are characteristic of severe disease. Tobacco use is the most significant environmental risk factor for RA and smoking cessation should be recommended to patients at risk for and with RA. The incidence of lymphoma and other malignancies is increased among patients with RA, and the overall mortality rate is increased by coexisting cardiovascular disease and infection.

Although up to 15% of patients can go into drug-free remission, long-term disability is still significant for most patients. Fifty percent of patients with RA are not working in their original occupation after 10 years, approximately 10 times the rate in the normal population. Most patients fall between these disease extremes with various levels of functional impairment. Some have a waxing and waning course over a period of years, with acute episodes of single- or multiple-joint exacerbations.

Future developments in RA therapy will include guidelines about when to institute and withdraw biologic DMARDS, novel targeted biologic agents, when to use biosimilars, and personalized approaches based on an understanding of individual disease pathogenesis and disease activity.

SUGGESTED READINGS

Aletaha D, Neogi T, Silman AJ, et al: 2010 Rheumatoid arthritis classification criteria: an American College of Rheumatology/European League Against Rheumatism collaborative initiative, Arthritis Rheum 62:2569–2581, 2010.

Furer V, Rondaan C, Heijstek MW, et al: 2019 update of the ULAR recommendations for vaccination in adult patients with autoimmune inflammatory rheumatic diseases, Ann Rheum Dis 0:1–14, 2019.

Karlson EW, Ding B, Keenan BT, et al: Association of environmental and genetic factors and gene-environment interactions with risk of developing rheumatoid arthritis, Arthritis Care Res 65:1147–1156, 2013.

Kim K, Band SY, Lee HS, Bae SC: Update on the genetic architecture of rheumatoid arthritis, Nat Rev Rheumatol 13:13–24, 2017.

McInnes IB, Schett G: The pathogenesis of rheumatoid arthritis, N Engl J Med 365:22052219, 2011.

Minichiello E, Semerano L, Boissier MC: Time trends in the incidence, prevalence, and severity of rheumatoid arthritis: a systematic literature review, Joint Bone Spine 83:625–630, 2016.

Moreland LW, O'Dell JR, Paulus HE, et al: A randomized comparative effectiveness study of oral triple therapy versus etanercept plus methotrexate in early aggressive rheumatoid arthritis: the treatment of Early Aggressive Rheumatoid Arthritis Trial, Arthritis Rheum 64:2824–2835, 2012.

O'Dell JR, Mikuls TR, Taylor TH, et al: Therapies for active rheumatoid arthritis after methotrexate failure, N Engl J Med 369:307–318, 2013.

Okada Y, Wu D, Trynka G, et al: Genetics of rheumatoid arthritis contributes to biology and drug discovery, Nature 506:376–381, 2014.

Singh JA, Saag KG, Bridges Jr SL, et al: 2015 American College of Rheumatology Guideline for the Treatment of Rheumatoid Arthritis, Arthritis Care Res 68:1–26, 2016.

Smolen JS, Aletaha D, Mcinnes IB: Rheumatoid arthritis, Lancet 388:2023–2038, 2016.

Smolen JS, Landwe B, et al: EULAR recommendations for the management of rheumatoid arthritis with synthetic and biological disease-modifying antirheumatic drugs: 2016 update, Ann Rheum Dis 17:960–977, 2017.

Sparks JA: Rheumatoid arthritis, Ann Intern Med 170:ITC1–ITC16, 2019.

van der Woude D, van der Helm-van Mil HM: Update on the epidemiology, risk factors, and disease outcomes of rheumatoid arthritis, Best Pract Res Clin Rheumatol 32:174–187, 2018.

80

Spondyloarthritis

Douglas W. Lienesch

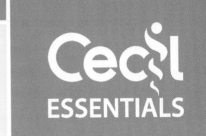

DEFINITION

Spondyloarthritis is a form of inflammatory joint disease characterized by inflammation of the axial skeleton (spine and sacroiliac joints) and/or the peripheral joints, often associated with inflammation of the eye, gastrointestinal tract, genitourinary system, and skin. *Axial spondyloarthritis* is the term used when the spine is the site of inflammation, and *peripheral spondyloarthritis* indicates inflammation of the joints and periarticular tissues in the extremities.

The cardinal clinical feature of spondyloarthritis is inflammation of the sacroiliac joints (i.e., sacroiliitis) and the spine (i.e., spondylitis). Inflammation of tendon insertion sites (i.e., enthesitis), inflammation of entire digits (i.e., dactylitis), and inflammation of one to four lower extremity joints (i.e., oligoarthritis) are extraspinal skeletal findings. A positive family history, eye inflammation (i.e., anterior uveitis or conjunctivitis), and the absence of rheumatoid factor and subcutaneous nodules are common.

Spondyloarthritis may be further subcategorized based on other clinical features. Patients with axial spondyloarthritis with typical radiographic features including sacroiliac joint erosions, spinal syndesmophytes, and ankylosis of the joints have *ankylosing spondylitis*. In the absence of these radiographic changes, *nonradiographic axial spondyloarthritis* may be present if there are typical symptoms accompanied by magnetic resonance imaging inflammatory signs at the sacroiliac joint or spine. Axial or peripheral inflammatory joint disease in the setting of psoriasis or inflammatory bowel disease (IBD) is termed *psoriatic arthritis* or *IBD-related spondyloarthritis*, respectively. *Reactive arthritis* refers to spondyloarthritis with onset within a few weeks of certain types of infection.

Spondyloarthritis is strongly associated with human leukocyte antigen B27 (HLA-27), a specific allele of the B locus of the HLA-encoding class I major histocompatibility complex genes. The frequency of HLA-B27 among white individuals is approximately 8%. However, up to 90% of white patients with ankylosing spondylitis and 80% of white patients with reactive arthritis or juvenile spondyloarthritis are HLA-B27 positive, and these percentages are even higher among patients with uveitis. The rate of HLA-B27 positivity among patients with inflammatory bowel disease or psoriasis with peripheral arthritis is not markedly increased unless they have spondylitis, in which case the frequency of HLA-B27 is 50%. The frequency of HLA-B27 varies widely among other ethnic groups and accounts for the broad variation of the prevalence of ankylosing spondylitis in different populations.

Ankylosing spondylitis is much more common among adolescent boys and young men, but this finding may reflect underdiagnosis in women, in whom disease manifestations may be milder than they are in men. Reactive arthritis is more common among men when it follows genitourinary *Chlamydia trachomatis* infection, but the sex distribution is even among patients after dysentery. Inflammatory arthritis including spondylitis affects approximately 5% to 8% of patients with psoriasis and 10% to 25% of patients with ulcerative colitis or Crohn's disease. Men and women are affected equally. The prevalence of spondyloarthritis, particularly psoriatic and reactive arthritis, is increased in populations with high human immunodeficiency virus (HIV) infection rates.

PATHOLOGY

Although the strong association of HLA-B27 with spondyloarthritis is well established, a specific role in the pathogenesis of these disorders has not been elucidated. Animal models in which rodents transgenic for HLA-B27 develop inflammatory abnormalities strikingly similar to those seen in HLA-B27–associated human diseases provide compelling indirect evidence for a pathogenic role. When raised in a germ-free environment, these animals remain disease free, suggesting a key additional environmental factor.

In addition to the strong genetic links for the risk of spondyloarthritis, important associations exist between specific bacterial agents and disease pathogenesis. Genitourinary infection with *C. trachomatis* or diarrheal illness with *Shigella*, *Salmonella*, *Campylobacter*, and *Yersinia* species can induce reactive arthritis. Several additional infectious agents are less commonly implicated. They appear to trigger an inflammatory response, possibly as a result of persistence of bacterial antigens, or cause an aberrant immunologic response to infection that results in misfolding of HLA-B27 molecules in antigen-presenting cells, generating a persistent inflammatory reaction.

No one theory of pathogenesis of spondyloarthritis explains the clinical spectrum of these disorders, and more research is clearly needed to solidify an understanding of their origin. The complex role of the immune system in spondyloarthritis is highlighted by the observation that patients infected with HIV appear more likely to have severe disease, especially psoriatic arthritis. When HIV infection is treated with antiviral agents, the incidence of spondyloarthritis declines.

Although many of the cellular and molecular mechanisms of inflammatory joint disease have been elucidated, the pathophysiology of spondyloarthritis remains incompletely understood. Inflammation of the sacroiliac joints, spine, and entheses is a unique feature of these disorders. Pathophysiologic studies show that the inflammation originates at the interface of bone and cartilage in the sacroiliac joint and bone and fibrocartilage in the enthesis. Macrophages and CD4$^+$ and CD8$^+$ T cells are present, and Th17 appears to play a critical role in the inflammatory process. Proinflammatory cytokines interleukin-17 (IL-17), interleukin-23 (IL-23), and tumor necrosis factor-α (TNF-α) and are abundant.

Synovial tissue becomes inflamed, and osteoclasts are activated, leading to bone resorption, reminiscent of rheumatoid arthritis joint

TABLE 80.1 Comparison of the Spondyloarthritis

Features	Ankylosing Spondylitis	Posturethral Reactive Arthritis	Postdysenteric Reactive Arthritis	Enteropathic Arthritis	Psoriatic Arthritis
Sacroiliitis	+++++	+++	++	+	++
Spondylitis	++++	+++	++	++	++
Peripheral arthritis	+	++++	++++	+++	++++
Articular course	Chronic	Acute or chronic	Acute or chronic	Acute or chronic	Chronic
HLA-B27	95%	60%	30%	20%	20%
Enthesopathy	++	++++	+++	++	++
Extra-articular manifestations	Eye, heart	Eye, GU, oral and/or GI, heart	GU, eye	GI, eye	Skin, eye
Other names	Bekhterev arthritis, Marie-Strümpell disease	Reactive arthritis, SARA, NGU, chlamydial arthritis	Reactive arthritis	Crohn's disease, ulcerative colitis	

GI, Gastrointestinal tract; *GU,* genitourinary tract; *HLA,* human leukocyte antigen; *NGU,* nongonococcal urethritis; *SARA,* sexually acquired reactive arthritis; *+,* relative prevalence of a specific feature.
Data from Cush JJ, Lipsky PE: The spondyloarthropathies. In Goldman L, Bennett JC, editors: *Cecil textbook of medicine,* ed 21, Philadelphia, 2000, Saunders, pp 1499-1507.

inflammation. Unlike in rheumatoid arthritis, early bone resorption is followed by a secondary phase during which osteoblast activity predominates, leading to new bone formation in periarticular bone (i.e., hyperostosis) and around joints (i.e., osteophytosis) or vertebral bodies (i.e., syndesmophytes). Ultimately, bony fusion of joints (ankylosis) occurs. The relationship between these paradoxical phases of bone resorption and proliferation is an area of active investigation.

CLINICAL PRESENTATION

Common Clinical Features of Spondyloarthritis

All forms of spondyloarthritis have considerable clinical overlap with one another and are most easily considered as a group of related disorders. Table 80.1 outlines the clinical features of these disorders. The cardinal clinical features common to all of them are inflammatory spine pain and an asymmetrical, predominantly lower extremity inflammatory joint or tendon disease. Inflammatory spine pain should be suspected in young patients (<40 years) who have an insidious onset of chronic low back pain or buttock pain associated with prolonged morning stiffness and relieved by exercise.

The characteristic peripheral joint disease involves one to four joints, usually in the lower extremities, and may be associated with tendon insertion inflammation (i.e., enthesitis) or sausage digits (i.e., dactylitis). Symmetrical polyarthropathy involving the upper extremities and clinically similar to rheumatoid arthritis is seen in some forms of psoriatic or inflammatory bowel disease–related spondyloarthritis. Anterior uveitis, enthesitis, dactylitis, psoriatic skin or nail changes, inflammatory bowel disease, a family history of spondyloarthritis, or a history of preceding gastrointestinal or genitourinary infection suggests spondyloarthritis. Subcutaneous nodules, rheumatoid factor, and antinuclear antibodies are usually absent.

In a given patient, the clinical features of these disorders may accumulate over a prolonged period. Some patients do not initially demonstrate the typical findings of a specific disorder. They are considered to have undifferentiated spondyloarthritis. Early disease can be subcategorized as predominately axial spondyloarthritis or predominately peripheral spondyloarthritis, depending on the site of the dominant symptoms. Many patients later have clinical findings consistent with a specific subtype of spondyloarthritis.

Inflammatory spine pain is the cardinal feature of axial disease and results from inflammation in the sacroiliac joints and spinal elements.

Uncontrolled disease may lead to ankylosis (i.e., bony fusion) at sacroiliac joints and throughout the vertebral column, culminating in loss of spinal and costovertebral motion, deformity, and restrictive extrapulmonary physiology.

Enthesitis can occur in many different anatomic locations. They include spinous processes, costosternal junctions, ischial tuberosities, plantar aponeuroses, and Achilles tendons.

When peripheral arthritis of spondyloarthritis occurs, it frequently begins as an episodic, asymmetrical, oligoarticular process that often involves the lower extremities. The arthritis can progress and may become chronic and disabling. A unique feature of spondyloarthritis is the appearance of fusiform swelling of an entire finger or toe, referred to as *dactylitis* or *sausage digits.*

Anterior uveitis, or inflammation of the anterior chamber of the eye, is a common extra-articular manifestation of spondyloarthritis, especially among HLA-B27–positive patients. Acute bouts of uveitis are usually monocular, painful, and accompanied by eye redness and blurred vision. Recurrent attacks are common and can lead to blindness. Scleritis, episcleritis, and conjunctivitis are less commonly associated phenomena.

Spondyloarthritis may occasionally involve other organ systems and may cause significant morbidity and mortality. Aortitis, especially occurring in the ascending segment, can result in aortic insufficiency from aortic root dilation, aortic dissection, and cardiac conduction system abnormalities. Pulmonary fibrosis of the apical regions can occur, often in an insidious fashion. Spinal cord compression can result from atlantoaxial joint subluxation, cauda equina syndrome, or vertebral fractures. In rare cases, long-standing spondyloarthritis is associated with secondary amyloidosis.

Specific Clinical Features of Spondyloarthritis
Ankylosing Spondylitis

The cardinal clinical feature of ankylosing spondylitis is inflammatory spine pain. Over time, spine involvement ascends from the sacroiliac joints to involve all levels of the spine. Progressive loss of motion results from ankylosis of the vertebral column and apophyseal joints. Costovertebral involvement leads to decreased chest expansion and restrictive lung physiology.

Loss of mobility and secondary osteoporosis of the vertebral bodies increase the risk of traumatic spine fracture. Axial involvement of the shoulders and hips is common and associated with a worse prognosis.

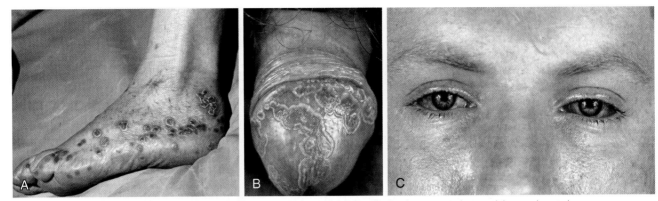

Fig. 80.1 Reactive arthritis. (A) Keratoderma blennorrhagicum. Red to brown papules, vesicles, and pustules with central erosion show characteristic crusting and peripheral scaling on the dorsolateral and plantar foot. (B) Balanitis circinata. Moist, well-demarcated erosions with a slightly raised micropustular circinate border on the glans penis. (C) Bilateral conjunctivitis associated with anterior uveitis. (From Fitzpatrick TB, Johnson RA, Wolff K, et al: *Color atlas and synopsis of clinical dermatology*, ed 3, New York, 1983, McGraw-Hill, pp 393, 395.)

Peripheral oligoarthritis, enthesitis, and dactylitis are more common in females. Diagnosis requires demonstration of radiographic sacroiliitis (i.e., sacroiliac joint erosions, sclerosis, and ankylosis). Anterior uveitis is common. Aortitis, upper lobe pulmonary fibrosis, cauda equina syndrome, and amyloidosis are less common and seen in late disease.

Reactive Arthritis (Posturethral/Postdysenteric)

Among the unique clinical features of reactive arthritis are urethritis, conjunctivitis, and certain dermatologic problems (Fig. 80.1). The urethritis may result from the chlamydial infection that triggers the disease, or it may be a sterile inflammatory discharge seen in diarrhea-associated disease. Conjunctivitis may be mild in reactive arthritis and is distinct from uveitis.

Keratoderma blennorrhagicum is a distinct papulosquamous rash usually found on the palms or soles. Circinate balanitis is a rash that may appear on the penile glans or shaft of men with reactive arthritis. Nonpitting nail thickening and oral ulcers may also occur in patients with reactive arthritis. These lesions can be confused with similar findings in patients with psoriasis and inflammatory bowel disease, respectively.

Most cases are self-limited. Chronic or relapsing arthritis and chronic spondylitis are associated with HLA-B27 and *Chlamydia* infection.

Psoriatic Arthritis

Five identifiable clinical patterns of psoriatic arthritis are recognized: distal interphalangeal joint involvement with nail pitting; asymmetrical oligoarthropathy of large and small joints; arthritis mutilans, a severe, destructive arthritis; symmetrical polyarthritis, which is identical to rheumatoid arthritis; and predominately axial disease. These patterns are not exclusive, and clinical overlap is significant.

Spondylitis or sacroiliitis may occur along with any of the other patterns. The prevalence of HLA-B27 is increased among the patients with spondylitis or sacroiliitis but not among patients with the other patterns. Psoriatic skin or nail disease predates arthritis in most cases, but both may occur concomitantly, or joint disease may precede skin involvement. Rarely, joint disease is indistinguishable from psoriatic arthritis, which can occur in patients with a family history but no personal history of psoriatic skin disease.

Enteropathic Arthritis: Inflammatory Bowel Disease

Crohn's disease and ulcerative colitis (see Chapter 38) are frequently associated with inflammatory spine disease and peripheral arthritis.

The peripheral arthritis is typically nonerosive, oligoarticular, and episodic, and the degree of joint involvement fluctuates with gut activity. A more chronic, symmetrical polyarthritis may occur in patients with Crohn's disease.

DIAGNOSIS AND DIFFERENTIAL DIAGNOSIS

The diagnosis of spondyloarthritis remains a clinical diagnosis made by identifying typical history and physical examination phenomena, analyzing selected laboratory tests, and using musculoskeletal imaging. The diagnosis is suggested by inflammatory spine pain or chronic lower extremity asymmetric inflammatory oligoarthritis in two to four joints. In this setting, features that increase the probability of spondyloarthritis include uveitis, psoriasis, enthesitis, dactylitis, inflammatory bowel disease, family history of spondylarthropathy, elevated C-reactive protein (CRP) level, HLA-B27, preceding gastrointestinal or genitourinary infection, and sacroiliitis on radiography, computed tomography (CT), or magnetic resonance imaging MRI).

Differentiating spondyloarthritis from other inflammatory or degenerative joint or spine diseases can be challenging. Crystalline arthropathies can manifest with peripheral oligoarthritis, often in the lower extremities. However, the spine is rarely involved, and intracellular crystals can be demonstrated in the synovial fluid. Rheumatoid arthritis and other systemic autoimmune diseases usually manifest with symmetrical polyarthritis of the upper and lower extremities associated with abnormal serologies such as rheumatoid factors, anti–cyclic citrullinated peptide (CCP) antibodies, or antinuclear antibodies. Predominately axial spondyloarthritis must be differentiated from indolent infections of the sacroiliac joints, vertebrae, or intravertebral disks; degenerative disease of the spine and disks (i.e., spondylosis); and diffuse idiopathic skeletal hyperostosis (DISH).

The radiographic features of the spondyloarthritis are highly specific and, in the correct clinical setting, greatly increase the certainty of the diagnosis. Sacroiliitis is usually the earliest radiographic sign of spine disease and results in sclerosis and erosions of the sacroiliac joints with eventual bony fusion (Fig. 80.2A). Many radiographic changes result from chronic spondylitis, including ossification of the annulus fibrosus, calcification of spinal ligaments, bony sclerosis and squaring of vertebral bodies, and ankylosis of apophyseal joints. These changes can lead to vertebral fusion and a bamboo spine appearance (see Fig. 80.2B).

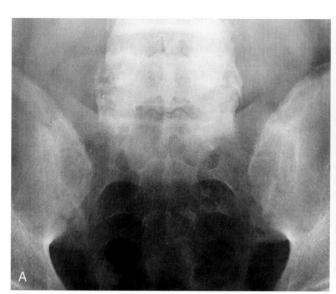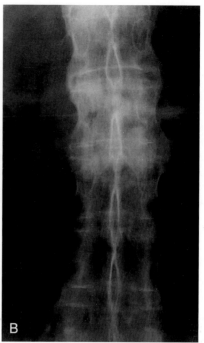

Fig. 80.2 (A) Bilaterally symmetrical sacroiliitis in ankylosing spondylitis. (B) Lumbar spondylitis in ankylosing spondylitis with symmetrical, marginal bridging syndesmophytes and calcification of the spinal ligament. (From Cush JJ, Lipsky PE: The spondyloarthropathies. In Goldman L, Bennett JC, editors: Cecil textbook of medicine, ed 21, Philadelphia, 2000, Saunders, pp 1499-1507.)

Radiographic findings progress over many years of illness and may not be apparent in early disease. However, during this preradiographic period, MRI demonstrates bone inflammation (i.e., osteitis) and erosion at the sacroiliac joints and vertebral bodies, and CT shows bony sclerosis and joint erosions.

Bone erosions, sclerosis, and new bone formation may occur at sites of enthesitis. Erosions at bone-cartilage interface (i.e., subchondral erosions), sclerosis, and bone proliferation are hallmarks of spondyloarthritis involving peripheral joints. In severe cases such as the arthritis mutilans form of psoriatic arthritis, total or subtotal bone resorption (i.e., osteolysis) of a phalange may occur.

TREATMENT

No cure has been found for any form of spondyloarthritis, but effective treatment for many of the manifestations is available. Patient education regarding the disease is essential and allows identification of affected family members and early detection of urgent clinical features such as uveitis. Physical therapy, including a daily stretching program, postural adjustments, and strengthening, helps to maintain proper bony alignment, reduce deformities, and maximize function, particularly for those with axial disease. Selective use of orthopedic surgery may be highly effective in correcting significant spinal deformities or instability.

Nonsteroidal anti-inflammatory drugs (NSAIDs) can provide significant relief of spinal pain and stiffness, and many patients take these drugs continually for years. No clear evidence indicates that systemic glucocorticoids benefit patients with spondyloarthritis, and these agents are usually avoided. Intra-articular glucocorticoid injection into the sacroiliac or other involved joints may provide temporary relief. Similarly, the role and efficacy of older immunosuppressive agents in the treatment of axial spondyloarthritis have not been established. In contrast, clinical trials have shown that the peripheral manifestations of spondylarthritis improve with sulfasalazine and methotrexate. Apremilast, a phosphodiesterase-4 inhibitor, has shown efficacy in peripheral joint inflammation in patients with psoriatic arthritis.

TNF-α blockers (i.e., infliximab, etanercept, adalimumab, certolizumab, and golimumab) represent a substantial breakthrough in the treatment of spondyloarthritis. The efficacy of these agents is well established for patients with axial inflammation who do not satisfactorily or fully respond to NSAIDs and physical therapy. TNF-α blockers can significantly reduce pain, improve function, and improve quality of life. They may also prevent or slow disease progression and structural damage. The drugs are effective in psoriatic arthritis, suppress the skin and nail disease of psoriasis, and retard radiographic progression in the peripheral joints. Infliximab and adalimumab reduce gut inflammation in ulcerative colitis and Crohn's disease, with concomitant reduction in symptoms of joint and spine inflammation. Ustekinumab, an inhibitor of IL-23, has demonstrated efficacy in psoriasis and psoriatic arthritis, as well as the intestinal manifestations of IBD. Secukinumab and ixekizumab, IL-17 inhibitors, have clinical efficacy in psoriasis, peripheral and axial spondyloarthritis.

Flares of uveitis require care by an ophthalmologist experienced in treating inflammatory eye diseases. Topical or intraocular glucocorticoids may suffice, but systemic therapy with glucocorticoids or immunosuppressive medications may be necessary to control the inflammation and prevent permanent visual loss. Methotrexate is frequently employed and the TNF-α inhibitor adalimumab has proven efficacy.

Reactive arthritis is usually self-limited, and joint symptoms are managed with NSAIDs or intra-articular corticosteroid injections. When chronic arthritis or spondylitis develops, interventions are similar to those employed for other forms of spondyloarthritis. Evaluation and treatment of C. trachomatis and associated sexually transmitted diseases in patients with reactive arthritis and their sex partners are essential. Early treatment reduces the frequency of reactive arthritis.

Long-term antibiotics are ineffective for gastroenteritis-associated reactive arthritis. Clinical trials of long-term antibiotics for reactive arthritis after *C. trachomatis* infection have had mixed results, and this practice requires further study before it can be adopted.

SUMMARY

Disability due to spondyloarthritis varies according to the subtype and severity of the specific syndrome. Historically, patients with spondyloarthritis usually experienced a lesser degree of disability compared with those with rheumatoid arthritis. Some patients with reactive arthritis experience self-limited disease with no long-term sequelae. Alternatively, those with more severe disease can have deformation and destruction of the axial and peripheral joints, leading to severe disability. Serious and potentially fatal extraskeletal manifestations can manifest.

With the advent of effective immunosuppressant medications such as methotrexate and biologic agents (i.e., TNF-α, IL-17 and IL-23 inhibitors), patients with more severe manifestations have markedly improved symptom control and quality of life.

SUGGESTED READINGS

Sieper J, Poddubnyy D: Axial spondyloarthritis, Lancet, 390:73–84, 2017.

Sieper J, Rudwaleit M, Baraliakos X, et al: The Assessment of Spondyloarthritis international Society (ASAS) handbook: a guide to assess spondyloarthritis, Ann Rheum Dis 68(Suppl lII):ii1–ii44, 2009.

Ward MW, Deodhar A, Gensler LS, et al: 2019 update of the American College of Rheumatology/Spondylitis Association of America/Spondylitis Research and Treatment Network recommendations for the treatment of ankylosing spondylitis and nonradiographic axial spondyloarthritis, Arthritis Rheumatol vol. 71(No. 10):1599–1613, 2019.

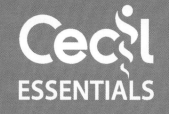

81

Systemic Lupus Erythematosus

Sonia Manocha, Tanmayee Bichile, Susan Manzi

DEFINITION AND EPIDEMIOLOGY

Systemic lupus erythematosus (SLE) is a chronic multisystem autoimmune disease characterized by autoantibody production and immune complex deposition that can lead to organ inflammation and, if left untreated, organ damage. The cause of SLE is largely unknown. Clinical manifestations are heterogeneous, ranging from milder non-organ-threatening symptoms of fatigue or oral ulcerations to life-threatening organ involvement with nephritis and neurologic disease. Diagnosing SLE is often challenging due to its varied clinical presentation, and it can take up to several years and seeing multiple health care providers to accurately come to a diagnosis.

Incidence and Prevalence

New data regarding the incidence and prevalence of SLE in the United States have been derived from several lupus registries including Michigan, Georgia, California Lupus Surveillance Project (CLSP), Manhattan Lupus Surveillance Program (MLSP), CDC funded population-based registry, Minnesota, and a large national managed-care claims database. These lupus registries allowed for a comprehensive estimation of incidence and prevalence across various ethnicities, including African American, Caucasian, Alaskan Native/American Indian, Hispanic, and Asian populations.

There remains a female predominance in both incidence and prevalence of SLE. Overall, the incidence and prevalence of SLE ranges from 5.2 to 7.4 cases per 100,000 person years and 72.8 to 178 cases per 100,000 person years, respectively. There remains ethnic diversity with a higher incidence of SLE among non-white ethnic populations, with African Americans having the highest incidence and prevalence followed by Hispanic and Asian individuals.

During childbearing years, the female-to-male ratio of SLE prevalence is 10:1 to 15:1. This gender discrepancy also exists but is less distinct (2:1) in young children and older individuals, suggesting hormonal influences.

Mortality

Mortality rates due to SLE have waxed and waned over time. Initially, there was a decrease in mortality from 1968 to 1975 followed by a steady increase from 1975 to 1999. This increase was followed by a steady decrease in mortality after 1999. However, despite this sustained decrease, SLE mortality remains high compared with those without SLE. SLE mortality has a bimodal distribution, with infection and disease activity typically increasing mortality earlier in the course of disease and cardiovascular and renal disease increasing mortality later in the course of disease. Furthermore, a study of all-cause mortality utilizing Medicaid data found ethnic variability in SLE-related mortality showing Asians and Hispanics having lower mortality as compared with African Americans, Caucasians or Native Americans.

PATHOLOGY

Although SLE pathogenesis remains poorly understood, individuals who develop SLE likely have a genetic predisposition in the setting of immune system dysregulation, environmental triggers, and altered hormonal milieu. The genetic contribution to SLE is emphasized by the high concordance rate for monozygotic twins (>20%) and a lower concordance rate among other siblings (<5%). The search for genes involved in SLE pathogenesis is an active area of research. Genes coding for certain human leukocyte antigens, complement system components, immunoglobulin receptors, and various other proteins are being considered as candidate genes for SLE.

The many immune abnormalities in SLE implicate dysregulation of the humoral and cellular immune systems in the pathogenesis of the disease. Dysregulation leads to loss of self-tolerance and autoimmune destruction of healthy tissues, hallmarked by the production of autoantibodies and immune complexes. The heterogeneity of clinical manifestations of lupus and response to treatment is likely a result of the different genetic and molecular profiles of individual patients. This has led to the notion of lupus as a spectrum disorder that includes distinct phenotypes that require customized management strategies.

Various environmental triggers, including microorganisms and ultraviolet light exposure, may influence the development of SLE and lupus activity. The striking differences in SLE prevalence between genders and the effect of pregnancy on disease activity suggest a role for hormones in SLE pathogenesis.

CLINICAL PRESENTATION

SLE can affect virtually any organ system. Typically, patients experience fluctuating periods of increased disease activity, known as flares, alternating with periods of clinical quiescence. The frequency, intensity, and duration of flares are highly variable among patients, and when left untreated, may lead to irreversible organ damage.

A challenge with establishing a diagnosis of SLE has been to accurately estimate the onset of disease. Patients with SLE often have antibody positivity for many years prior to the onset of clinical symptoms. The type and severity of chief complaint in SLE depends on underlying organ involvement at the time of presentation, varying from vague constitutional symptoms to specific organ involvement such as seizures, glomerulonephritis, serositis, and thrombosis. In one study by Cervera and colleagues, most manifestations of SLE occurred in the first 5 years. Long-term prognosis in SLE varies greatly depending on whether patients are diagnosed early or late.

Constitutional Symptoms

Constitutional symptoms of SLE include fever, lymphadenopathy, weight loss, malaise, and fatigue. These are nonspecific and can be related to other etiologies, and it is therefore imperative to be cognizant of infection in a patient with SLE presenting with fever. One way to distinguish a fever caused by infection versus a fever from SLE would be to evaluate serologic activity from lupus, especially complement levels, which are often elevated in the setting of infection because they are acute-phase reactants and decreased in the setting of active lupus.

Lymphadenopathy in lupus is often cervical and axillary and generally painful, soft, and mobile. Weight loss in SLE indicates an ongoing inflammatory state. Malaise and fatigue are among the most common but often difficult to treat presentations of SLE.

Mucocutaneous Manifestations

Skin manifestations of SLE are wide ranging and divided into categories including acute cutaneous lupus, subacute cutaneous lupus, and chronic cutaneous lupus. Acute cutaneous lupus includes a wide range of presentations. Many patients will present with a malar rash described as a butterfly rash with erythema and crusting that spares the nasolabial folds. Other presentations may include maculopapular rash, urticaria, bullous lupus and a toxic epidermal necrolysis (TEN)-like rash.

Subacute cutaneous lupus erythematosus (SCLE) typically presents as a psoriasiform or annular, polycyclic rash.

Chronic cutaneous lupus can cause disfiguration and scarring, with the most common form being discoid lupus. Other forms include lupus panniculitis (which is an inflammatory involvement of the subcutis and fat), tumid lupus, chilblains, lichen planus overlap, and mucosal lesions (oral, nasal, genital).

The majority of these rashes are photosensitive, which is an exaggerated response to ultraviolet (UV) light leading to symptoms of redness, itching or burning. Typically, skin manifestations of SLE occur within 24 to 48 hours after UV exposure.

Oral ulcerations occur in approximately 45% of SLE patients. Those involving the hard palate and buccal mucosa are more commonly associated with SLE. It is important to keep in mind that oral ulcers may also be seen in multiple other comorbid conditions such as acid reflux as well as herpetic infections.

Nonscarring alopecia involving the temporal area or diffuse thinning is another common cutaneous manifestation.

Musculoskeletal Manifestations

Arthritis is common in SLE. Usually this is an inflammatory, nonerosive arthritis. Some patients may develop deformities referred to as Jaccoud arthropathy. The hand in a patient with Jaccoud arthropathy looks similar to someone with rheumatoid arthritis except that the deformities are reducible (manually corrected) as opposed to fixed and imaging demonstrates absence of erosions.

Myalgia is another common manifestation of SLE, especially during periods of flares. Muscle weakness along with elevated CPK levels should raise suspicion of an underlying myopathy/myositis.

Hematologic Manifestations

Leukopenia (defined as white blood cell [WBC] count <4000 cells/mL), primarily lymphopenia, anemia, and thrombocytopenia, is common in SLE. Coombs positive autoimmune hemolytic anemia (AIHA) is one of the criteria for classification of SLE. Thrombocytopenia, which is an immune-mediated peripheral destruction disorder, may also be seen. Evans syndrome is rare in SLE and defined as AIHA and autoimmune thrombocytopenia. Thrombotic thrombocytopenic purpura (TTP) is also reported in SLE.

Cardiopulmonary Manifestations

Cardiac involvement in SLE is manifold. SLE can affect all parts of the cardiac system including the endocardium, myocardium, pericardium, valves, conduction pathways, and the coronary arteries. Pericarditis is the most common of cardiac manifestations in SLE. Myocarditis is rare but can be fatal. Libman-Sacks endocarditis is valvular involvement in SLE described as sterile verrucous lesions typically seen on the left-sided heart valves. Cardiovascular disease in SLE is discussed separately.

Pulmonary manifestations in SLE can involve the pleura, parenchyma, and pulmonary vessels. Pleural involvement typically occurs with pleurisy and pleural effusions. Parenchymal involvement can present as acute lupus pneumonitis, interstitial lung disease, diffuse alveolar hemorrhage, and shrinking lung syndrome. Pulmonary vessel involvement typically presents as a pulmonary embolus often in the presence of antiphospholipid antibodies and pulmonary artery hypertension.

Gastrointestinal and Hepatic Manifestations

Gastrointestinal (GI) manifestations may be seen in about 50% of patients with SLE and are often difficult to diagnose. GI manifestations are often mild but may be life-threatening. Although acute abdominal pain in SLE is more commonly attributed to non-SLE etiologies, SLE-related causes of acute abdominal pain include pancreatitis, serositis, mesenteric vasculitis, and renal vein thrombosis. Lupus hepatitis is a controversial diagnosis. This has been described in the literature in SLE patients presenting with constitutional symptoms and elevated liver enzymes five times or greater the upper limit of normal. SLE patients with persistent elevations of LFTs without other symptoms should be further evaluated for autoimmune hepatitis (AIH) because this may be seen in association.

Renal Manifestations

Nephritis, which manifests with hematuria and proteinuria, is a major cause of morbidity and mortality for SLE patients. The International Society of Nephrology/Renal Pathology Society (ISN/RPS) revisited the 1982 World Health Organization classification of lupus nephritis (classes I through VI). ISN/RPS class IV (i.e., diffuse, proliferative) lupus nephritis is the most common form and has the worst prognosis, but it is also the most amenable to aggressive immunosuppressive therapy. See Table 81.1 for more details.

Neuropsychiatric Manifestations

Neuropsychiatric manifestations of systemic lupus erythematosus (NPSLE) can vary from mild to severe and may be difficult to diagnose. NPSLE may involve any area of the nervous system with diffuse or focal involvement of the central nervous system (CNS) as well as involvement of the peripheral nervous system (PNS). Diffuse involvement may manifest as cognitive dysfunction, acute confusional state, headache, aseptic meningitis, and mood disorders. Focal involvement may present as cerebrovascular disease, myelopathy, movement disorders, demyelinating syndromes, and seizures.

Vascular Manifestations

More than 40% of SLE patients have Raynaud's phenomenon. This is typically described as cold sensitivity followed by biphasic or triphasic color changes with white discoloration followed by cyanosis and reactive hyperemia in the digits of hands and feet. Other areas affected by Raynaud's phenomenon include nose, earlobes, lips, and nipples.

Livedo reticularis is a netlike discoloration over arms or legs commonly seen in SLE. Livedo racemosa, which is a more severe form of livedo reticularis, can be seen in patients with SLE and Sneddon syndrome (ischemic cerebrovascular disease along with antiphospholipid antibodies [APLs]).

TABLE 81.1 International Society of Nephrology/Renal Pathology Society (ISN/RPS) 2003 Classification of Lupus Nephritis

Class I	**Minimal mesangial lupus nephritis**
	Normal glomeruli by light microscopy, but mesangial immune deposits by immunofluorescence
Class II	**Mesangial proliferative lupus nephritis**
	Purely mesangial hypercellularity of any degree or mesangial matrix expansion by light microscopy, with mesangial immune deposits
	May be a few isolated subepithelial or subendothelial deposits visible by immunofluorescence or electron microscopy, but not by light microscopy
Class III	**Focal lupus nephritis**[a]
	Active or inactive focal, segmental or global endo- or extracapillary glomerulonephritis involving 50% of all glomeruli, typically with focal subendothelial immune deposits, with or without mesangial alterations
Class III (A)	Active lesions: focal proliferative lupus nephritis
Class III (A/C)	Active and chronic lesions: focal proliferative and sclerosing lupus nephritis
Class III (C)	Chronic inactive lesions with glomerular scars: focal sclerosing lupus nephritis
Class IV	**Diffuse lupus nephritis**[b]
	Active or inactive diffuse, segmental or global endo- or extracapillary glomerulonephritis involving 50% of all glomeruli, typically with diffuse subendothelial immune deposits, with or without mesangial alterations. This class is divided into diffuse segmental (IV-S) lupus nephritis when 50% of the involved glomeruli have segmental lesions, and diffuse global (IV-G) lupus nephritis when 50% of the involved glomeruli have global lesions. Segmental is defined as a glomerular lesion that involves less than half of the glomerular tuft. This class includes cases with diffuse wire loop deposits but with little or no glomerular proliferation.
Class IV-S (A)	Active lesions: diffuse segmental proliferative lupus nephritis
Class IV-G (A)	Active lesions: diffuse global proliferative lupus nephritis
Class IV-S (A/C)	Active and chronic lesions: diffuse segmental proliferative and sclerosing lupus nephritis
Class IV-G (A/C)	Active and chronic lesions: diffuse global proliferative and sclerosing lupus nephritis
Class IV-S (C)	Chronic inactive lesions with scars: diffuse segmental sclerosing lupus nephritis
Class IV-G (C)	Chronic inactive lesions with scars: diffuse global sclerosing lupus nephritis
Class V	**Membranous lupus nephritis**
	Global or segmental subepithelial immune deposits or their morphologic sequelae by light microscopy and by immunofluorescence or electron microscopy, with or without mesangial alterations
	Class V lupus nephritis may occur in combination with class III or IV in which case both will be diagnosed
	Class V lupus nephritis show advanced sclerosis
Class VI	**Advanced sclerosis lupus nephritis**
	90% of glomeruli globally sclerosed without residual activity

[a]Indicate the proportion of glomeruli with active and with sclerotic lesions.
[b]Indicate the proportion of glomeruli with fibrinoid necrosis and/or cellular crescents. Indicate and grade (mild, moderate, severe) tubular atrophy, interstitial inflammation and fibrosis, severity of arteriosclerosis or other vascular lesions.
Data from Wallace D, Hahn BH: Pathogenesis of Lupus Nephritis. In Dubois' lupus erythematosus and related syndromes, ed 9, Philadelphia, 2019, Elsevier, pp 273.

Venous clots (e.g., pulmonary emboli, deep vein thrombosis) and arterial clots typically are seen in association with APLs and antiphospholipid syndrome. Leg ulcers, gangrene, thrombophlebitis, nail fold infarcts, cutaneous necrosis, and necrotizing purpura may also occur. Small vessel vasculopathy or vasculitis can be seen in lupus and may be a life-threatening manifestation.

Ocular Manifestations

Keratoconjunctivitis sicca from secondary Sjögren's syndrome is the most common ocular manifestation of SLE. Episcleritis, scleritis, uveitis, optic neuropathy, and retinal vasculitis can occur but are less frequent.

DIAGNOSIS AND DIFFERENTIAL DIAGNOSIS

SLE is a clinical diagnosis; no single test or feature is definitively diagnostic of the disease. SLE is typically suspected in patients presenting with clinical symptoms and exam findings suggesting a multisystem disease. Serologic testing is utilized to confirm the suspected diagnosis. It is important to note that many clinical manifestations and serologic tests that help to diagnose SLE can be seen in other diseases.

For example, arthralgias, myalgias, fevers, and rash are common presentations in many viral diseases that may also have a positive ANA. Anti-double-stranded DNA (anti-dsDNA) antibodies are reported in patients with hepatitis B and hepatitis C. Low complement levels could occur in patients with chronic liver disease or inherited complement deficiencies. Malignancy (lymphoma and other hematologic malignancies, solid organ cancer) is an important differential diagnosis to consider in an elderly patient with constitutional symptoms, lymphadenopathy, rash, arthralgias, myalgias and positive ANA.

Classification Criteria

Classification Criteria for SLE were designed to group similar patients for the purposes of research. There are several classification criteria currently used for SLE. The American College of Rheumatology (ACR) classification criteria for SLE were updated in 1997. Patients are considered to have SLE if they meet 4 of 11 criteria (Table 81.2).

The Systemic Lupus International Collaborating Clinics (SLICC) classification criteria were developed in 2012 to improve clinical relevance and incorporate new knowledge into the definition of SLE immunopathogenesis. Under the SLICC criteria, patients are classified to have lupus if they meet four criteria including at least one clinical and

TABLE 81.2   1997 American College of Rheumatology Criteria for Classification of Systemic Lupus Erythematosus[a]

Criteria	Definitions
Malar rash	Fixed, flat or raised erythema is observed over the malar eminences, tending to spare the nasolabial folds.
Discoid rash	Erythematous, raised patches develop with adherent keratotic scaling and follicular plugging; atrophic scarring may occur in older lesions.
Photosensitivity	Rash occurs as a result of unusual reaction to sunlight, determined by patient history or physician observation.
Oral ulcers	Oral or nasopharyngeal ulceration, usually painless, is observed by the physician.
Arthritis	Nonerosive arthritis involves two or more peripheral joints, characterized by tenderness, swelling, or effusion.
Serositis	a. Pleuritis: convincing history of pleuritic pain exists or rub is heard by a physician or pleural effusion is in evidence, *or* b. Pericarditis: documented by electrocardiogram or rub or evidence of pericardial effusion.
Renal disorder	a. Persistent proteinuria is >0.5 g/day or scored >3+ if quantitation is not performed, *or* b. Cellular casts: may be red cell, hemoglobin, granular, tubular, or mixed.
Neurologic disorder	a. Seizures: occurs in the absence of offending drugs or known metabolic derangements (e.g., uremia, ketoacidosis, or electrolyte imbalance), *or* b. Psychosis: occurs in the absence of offending drugs or known metabolic derangements (e.g., uremia, ketoacidosis, electrolyte imbalance)
Hematologic disorder	a. Hemolytic anemia: develops with reticulocytosis, *or* b. Leukopenia: <4000/mm^3 is documented on two or more occasions, *or* c. Lymphopenia: <1500/mm^3 is documented on two or more occasions, *or* d. Thrombocytopenia: <100,000/mm^3 develops in the absence of offending drugs.
Immunologic disorder	a. Anti–double-stranded DNA: antibody to native DNA in abnormal titer, *or* b. Anti-Smith: presence of antibody to Smith nuclear antigen, *or* c. Positive finding of antiphospholipid antibodies is based on (1) an abnormal serum level of IgG or IgM anticardiolipin antibodies, (2) a positive test result for lupus anticoagulant using a standard method, or (3) a false-positive serologic test for syphilis known to be positive for at least 6 months and confirmed by *Treponema pallidum* immobilization or fluorescent treponemal antibody absorption test.
ANA	An abnormal titer of antinuclear antibody is documented by immunofluorescence or an equivalent assay at any point in time and in the absence of drugs known to be associated with drug-induced lupus syndrome.

[a]This classification is based on 11 criteria. For the purpose of identifying patients in clinical studies, a patient is classified as having definite SLE if any 4 or more of the 11 criteria are present (cumulative) during any interval of observation.

one immunologic finding. SLICC criteria also allow classification of a patient with SLE with only renal-limited disease (biopsy proven) in the presence of a positive ANA (Table 81.3).

The newest criteria from 2019 are a result of collaboration between ACR and European League against Rheumatism (EULAR) (Table 81.4). There are seven clinical and three immunologic domains. Each domain has several criteria, which are weighted. Within each domain, only the highest weighted criterion is counted towards the total score. Patients are classified to have SLE if there is a positive ANA of 1:80 or greater, at least one clinical criteria and a score of 10 or greater. These classification criteria are unique in the sense that they are the first weighted criteria for SLE. These criteria are combined with a comprehensive examination to help guide a diagnosis of SLE.

The hallmark of SLE is the presence of various autoantibodies that at times may be detected before the initial clinical presentation of SLE. The prevalence of these autoantibodies varies across different SLE patient cohorts and ethnic groups; however, more than 95% of patients with SLE will have a positive ANA, often with titers 1:160 or greater. The HEP-2 indirect immunofluorescence ANA test is the preferred assay over direct ELISA testing. Indirect immunofluorescence is reported in titers and patterns, with the most common pattern reported in SLE being homogenous (diffuse). ANA is not specific for the diagnosis of SLE, particularly in the presence of low titers and can often be seen in patients with normal ageing, viral infections, malignancies, and other connective tissue diseases.

Anti-dsDNA and anti-Smith antibodies are more specific for SLE. Anti-Ro antibodies are commonly found in SLE and are associated with subacute cutaneous lupus. Anti-Ro antibodies have implications during pregnancy with increased risk of neonatal lupus. Anti-U1-RNP is associated with increased risk of pulmonary hypertension

and is discussed further in the "Overlap Syndrome" section. Antihistone antibodies are generally associated with drug-induced lupus but can be seen in patients with idiopathic lupus (Table 81.5).

The complement system plays an integral role in immune activation in SLE. Low complements (low C3, C4, CH50) are often considered hallmarks of disease activity in SLE, in particular glomerular disease, making them a valuable tool for clinicians to monitor disease activity.

Drug-Induced Lupus

Many drugs have been associated with lupus-like symptoms and development of lupus-related antibodies. Drug-induced lupus generally affects older populations, and common causative medications include procainamide, isoniazid, hydralazine, propylthiouracil, TNF inhibitors, proton-pump inhibitors, minocycline, methyldopa, levodopa, and interferon-α.

Clinical symptoms generally manifest as musculoskeletal, cutaneous, serous, and hematologic. Rarely, there may be renal or CNS involvement. The typical gender inequality in SLE is not represented in drug-induced lupus, but rather there seems to be a higher incidence in older men. Serologies often present include ANA and antihistone antibodies. The presence of anti-dsDNA antibodies is rare and is more commonly found in patients that were exposed to TNF inhibitor medications versus other medications.

In most cases, removal of the offending drug leads to improvement in symptoms. Depending on the severity of manifestations, glucocorticoids may also be helpful.

Neonatal Lupus

Neonatal lupus is a rare autoimmune disorder that develops in utero in which maternal anti-SSA/Ro and/or SSB/La antibodies cross the placenta and affect the fetus. This was first described in 1957 by G.R. Hogg

TABLE 81.3   Systemic Lupus International Collaborating Clinics (SLICC) Classification Criteria of Systemic Lupus Erythematosus

Clinical Criteria[a]	Examples
1. Acute cutaneous lupus	Bullous lupus
	Lupus malar rash (not malar discoid)
	Maculopapular lupus rash
	Photosensitive lupus rash (in the absence of dermatomyositis)
	Subacute cutaneous lupus
	Toxic epidermal necrolysis variant of SLE
2. Chronic cutaneous lupus	Classic discoid rash
	Localized (above the neck)
	Generalized (above and below the neck) Chilblains lupus
	Discoid lupus/lichen planus overlap
	Hypertrophic (verrucous) lupus
	Lupus erythematosus tumidus
	Lupus panniculitis (profundus)
	Mucosal lupus
3. Oral ulcers	Palate, buccal, tongue, *or* nasal ulcers (in the absence of other causes: vasculitis, Behçet's disease, infection, inflammatory bowel disease, reactive arthritis, and acidic foods)
4. Nonscarring alopecia	Diffuse thinning *or* hair fragility with visible broken hairs (in the absence of other causes: alopecia areata, drugs, iron deficiency, and androgenic alopecia)
5. Synovitis (≥2 joints)	Characterized by swelling or effusion *or* tenderness with ≥30 minutes of morning stiffness
6. Serositis	Typical pleurisy for >1 day *or* pleural effusions *or* pleural rub
	Typical pericardial pain for >1 day *or* pericardial effusion *or* pericardial rub *or* pericarditis by ECG (in the absence of other causes: infection, uremia, and Dressler pericarditis)
7. Renal	Urine protein/creatinine (*or* 24-hr protein) ≥500 mg of protein/24 hr *or* red blood cell casts
8. Neurologic	Acute confusional state (in the absence of other causes: toxic-metabolic, uremia, and drugs)
	Mononeuritis multiplex (in the absence of other known causes: primary vasculitis)
	Myelitis
	Peripheral or cranial neuropathy (in the absence of other known causes: primary vasculitis, infection, and diabetes mellitus)
	Psychosis
	Seizure
9. Hemolytic anemia	
10. Leukopenia	<4000 cells/mm^3 detected at least once (in the absence of other known causes: Felty syndrome, drugs, and portal hypertension)
11. or Lymphopenia	<1000 cells/mm^3 detected at least once (in the absence of other known causes: corticosteroids, drugs, and infection)
12. Thrombocytopenia	<100,000 cells/mm^3 detected at least once (in the absence of other known causes: drugs, portal hypertension, and thrombotic thrombocytopenic purpura)
Immunologic Criteria	
1. ANAs	Above laboratory reference range
2. Anti–double-stranded DNA	Above laboratory reference range, except ELISA: two times greater than laboratory reference range
3. Anti-Smith	
4. Antiphospholipid	Any of the following: lupus anticoagulant, false-positive RPR, medium- or high-titer anticardiolipin (IgA, IgG, or IgM), or anti-β_2 glycoprotein I (IgA, IgG, or IgM)
5. Low complement	Low C3
	Low C4
	Low CH50
6. Direct Coombs test	In the absence of hemolytic anemia

ANAs, Antinuclear antibodies; *ECG,* electrocardiogram; *ELISA,* enzyme-linked immunosorbent assay; *Ig,* immunoglobulin; *RPR,* rapid plasma reagin; *SLE,* systemic lupus erythematosus.

[a]Criteria are cumulative. A patient is classified as having SLE using lupus nephritis as a stand-alone criterion (in the setting of ANAs or anti-dsDNA antibodies) *or* four criteria (with at least one of the clinical criteria and one of the immunologic criteria).

Modified from Petri M, Orbai AM, Alarcon GS, et al: Derivation and validation of Systemic Lupus International Collaborating Clinics classification criteria for systemic lupus erythematosus, Arthritis Rheum 64:2677-2686, 2012.

TABLE 81.4   2019 EULAR/ACR Criteria for Classification of SLE

Entry Criterion

Antinuclear antibodies (ANA) at a titer of ≥1:80 on HEp-2 cells or an equivalent positive test (ever)

↓

If absent, do not classify as SLE
If present, apply additive criteria

↓

Additive Criteria

Do not count a criterion if there is a more likely explanation than SLE
Occurrence of a criterion on at least one occasion is sufficient
SLE classification requires at least one clinical criterion and ≥10 points
Criteria need not occur simultaneously
Within each domain, only the highest weighted criterion is counted toward the total score[a]

Clinical Domains and Criteria	Weight	Immunology Domains and Criteria	Weight
Constitutional		*Antiphospholipid antibodies*	
Fever	2	Anti-cardiolipin antibodies OR	
		Anti-β$_2$GPI antibodies OR	
		Lupus anticoagulant	2
Hematologic		*Complement proteins*	
Leukopenia	3	Low C3 OR low C4	3
Thrombocytopenia	4	Low C3 AND low C4	4
Autoimmune hemolysis	4		
Neuropsychiatric		*SLE-specific antibodies*	
Delirium	2	Anti-dsDNA antibody[b] OR	
Psychosis	3	Anti-Smith antibody	6
Seizure	5		
Mucocutaneous			
Non-scarring alopecia	2		
Oral ulcers	2		
Subacute cutaneous OR discoid lupus	4		
Acute cutaneous lupus	6		
Serosal			
Pleural or pericardial effusion	5		
Acute pericarditis	6		
Musculoskeletal			
Joint involvement	6		
Renal			
Proteinuria >0.5 g/24 h	4		
Renal biopsy Class II or V lupus nephritis	8		
Renal biopsy Class III or IV lupus nephritis	10		
Total Score:			

↓

Classify as Systemic Lupus Erythematosus with a score of ≥10 if entry criterion fulfilled.

Anti-β$_2$GPI, Anti-β$_2$-glycoprotein I; *anti-dsDNA,* anti–double-stranded DNA.
[a]Additional criteria within the same domain will not be counted.
[b]In an assay with 90% specificity against relevant disease controls.

in a full-term, 2-kg baby boy who had complete AV block and subendocardial fibrosis born to a mother with SLE. There is a 1% to 2% chance of having a child with neonatal lupus in mothers with anti-SSA/Ro or SSB/La antibodies. In women with a previous baby with neonatal lupus the risk of having a subsequent baby with cardiac involvement of neonatal lupus increases from 2% to 19%. The development of heart block is most common between 18 weeks' and 24 weeks' gestation in mothers with these antibodies; thus, screening with fetal heart tones and fetal echocardiography should begin at 16 weeks' gestation. If there are signs of heart block, the mother may be treated with fluorinated corticosteroids (i.e., dexamethasone or betamethasone). Many children with congenital heart block do not survive or have continued morbidities requiring pacemakers.

Other manifestations of neonatal SLE that are more common include rashes, cytopenias, and hepatosplenomegaly. These manifestations generally resolve after the baby begins to develop his or her own antibodies, at around 6 to 8 months. Although this is commonly a condition that is seen in children born to mothers with SLE, it may also be seen in other autoimmune conditions or in otherwise healthy mothers with SSA/Ro and/or SSB/La antibodies.

Overlap Syndrome

Some patients with clinical and laboratory features of two or more autoimmune diseases have an overlap syndrome. Mixed connective tissue disease is characterized by overlaps among SLE, scleroderma, and myositis with a high titer of anti–U1-RNP antibody levels. For

TABLE 81.5 Prevalence of Autoantibodies in Systemic Lupus Erythematosus

Target Autoantigen	Positive (%)
Nuclear antigens	>95
Double-stranded DNA	30–60
Smith	10–44
Ribonucleoprotein (U1-RNP)	25–40
SSA/Ro	30–40
SSB/La	38
Phospholipids	16–60
Ribosomal P	5–10
Histone	21–90

Data from Wallace D, Hahn BH: Other Clinical laboratory tests in SLE. In Dubois' lupus erythematosus and related syndromes, ed 8, Philadelphia, 2013, Saunders, pp 526–531.

patients who have multiple autoimmune manifestations but do not meet the criteria of a specific autoimmune disease, the term *undifferentiated connective tissue disease* is used. In some instances, these patients may be early in their disease course and eventually develop a specific autoimmune disease.

TREATMENT

There is no known cure for SLE. Management can be challenging and is aimed at treating the underlying organ manifestations. Treatment is often multipronged with patient education; one or more medications including anti-inflammatories, antimalarials, glucocorticoids and immunosuppressive drugs; and management of other aspects such as fatigue, depression, and other psychosocial factors. General goals for treatment are to achieve low disease activity or remission and prevent flares with the least amount of glucocorticoid use possible. At this time, there are only four FDA-approved treatments for SLE: aspirin, glucocorticoids, hydroxychloroquine, and belimumab.

It is essential to establish the type of SLE and the extent of organ involvement prior to initiating treatment. This is important because prognosis of SLE varies based on the severity of disease at presentation.

Every patient with SLE should be educated on sun protection techniques and smoking cessation because both are important triggers of flares and ongoing disease activity. Sunscreen with at least SPF 30 and preferably one that blocks both UVA and UVB is recommended. Avoiding sun exposure during peak hours, typically midmorning to early evening, and use of long-sleeve shirts and wide-brimmed hats are advisable. Smoking not only increases all-cause mortality but also worsens SLE activity and may decrease efficacy of certain medications such as hydroxychloroquine.

Nonsteroidal anti-inflammatory drugs (NSAIDs) are commonly used to treat certain manifestations of SLE including musculoskeletal symptoms, pericarditis, pleurisy, and fever. Typically, NSAIDs are used as short-term therapies. One should be cognizant of renal involvement prior to initiation and continuation of NSAIDs. Aspirin is often used in SLE patients with other cardiac risk factors to mitigate the increased risk of cardiovascular events. Aspirin is often used in patients with SLE who have high titer antiphospholipid antibodies without a history of thrombosis and in most pregnant women.

Glucocorticoids remain a very effective treatment modality in SLE. They are fast acting and halt ongoing inflammation in many organ systems, making them valuable during initial treatment and as bridge therapy for flares. Doses of glucocorticoids vary widely from oral low-dose

alternate-day regimen to very high doses of IV formulations. As a general rule, using the lowest effective dose for the shortest amount of time limits potential long-term side effects. Long-term use of moderate to high doses of glucocorticoids leads to a higher cumulative dose exposure over time and increased risk of toxicity. This includes obesity, diabetes mellitus, hypertension, hyperlipidemia, accelerated atherosclerosis, osteoporosis with increased risk of fracture, avascular necrosis, cataracts, glaucoma, and increased risk of infections. To avoid these toxicities, steroid-sparing immunomodulating or immunosuppressant agents are used.

Antimalarial agents are the cornerstone of therapy in SLE. Hydroxychloroquine is the most commonly used agent because it has less retinal toxicity compared to chloroquine. Quinacrine is an antimalarial agent with no retinal toxicity, but the oral formulation has to be compounded at a specialty pharmacy. Hydroxychloroquine is an immunomodulatory agent that is beneficial in treating cutaneous and musculoskeletal manifestations. It has also been shown to prevent organ flares, prevent organ damage, modulate risk factors for atherosclerosis and thrombosis, and prevent placental transfer of anti-Ro antibodies that cause congenital heart block and neonatal lupus. Newer guidelines for the screening and prevention of hydroxychloroquine retinopathy suggest use of 5 mg/kg/day or less and regular ophthalmologic monitoring. Ophthalmologic monitoring at baseline (within the first year) and then annually after 5 years (more frequent in high risk individuals) with a dilated eye exam, Humphrey visual field testing, and spectral domain optical coherence tomography (SD-OCT) is recommended to monitor for retinal toxicity. Risk for retinal toxicity is dose dependent and influenced by comorbidities.

Azathioprine (AZA), methotrexate (MTX), leflunomide (LEF), and mycophenolate mofetil (MMF) are immunosuppressive agents used in SLE. AZA is effective in treating a variety of manifestations including skin disease, musculoskeletal disease, and nephritis. It is safe during pregnancy and breast-feeding. Toxicity includes cytopenias, hepatoxicity with transaminitis, and increased risk for infections. MTX is effective in treating cutaneous, arthritis, and serositis manifestations. MTX is teratogenic and should be discontinued 3 to 6 months prior to conception. Toxicity is similar to AZA. LEF works well for cutaneous and musculoskeletal manifestations. LEF is teratogenic and contraindicated in pregnancy and lactation. MMF has been used for more than 20 years for the treatment of lupus nephritis, but it is also effective for skin disease and serositis. MMF toxicity is primarily related to gastrointestinal intolerance, cytopenias, and infectious complications. Mycophenolic acid, which is an active form of MMF, has less gastrointestinal intolerance. MMF is teratogenic and contraindicated in both pregnancy and lactation.

In organ- or life-threatening SLE, the alkylating agent cyclophosphamide (CTX) is used. Scenarios where CTX is utilized include rapidly progressive glomerulonephritis, lupus cerebritis, and diffuse alveolar hemorrhage. However, it is associated with significant toxicity, particularly bone marrow suppression, hemorrhagic cystitis, gonadal toxicity, increased risk of infections, and certain malignancies. The use of lower doses of intravenous CTX has resulted in equal efficacy and fewer side effects and has replaced many of the older regimens.

Great potential and optimism exist for biologic immunomodulating agents that focus on various aspects of the immune system, including B cells, interactions between B and T cells, and cytokines. The most promising agents are those that target B cells, which produce autoantibodies. In 2011, belimumab, a monoclonal antibody that inhibits B-lymphocyte stimulator, was the first therapeutic agent approved for the treatment of SLE in more than 50 years (Table 81.6). There are a number of other potential biologic therapies for lupus in the pipeline and currently being tested in clinical trials.

TABLE 81.6   Treatment Options in Systemic Lupus Erythematosus

Medication	Mechanism of Action	Monitoring	Pregnancy Concern
NSAIDS	Inhibits cyclooxygenase, reducing prostaglandin and thromboxane synthesis	CBC and CMP, caution with renal disease	Caution in 1st trimester, avoid use in 3rd trimester
Glucocorticoids[a]	Inhibits multiple cytokines	Electrolytes, BP, blood sugar. Caution with comorbid diabetes mellitus	May be used. Increased risk of low birth weight and premature birth.
Hydroxychloroquine[a]	Exact mechanism unknown. Inhibits TLR and various enzymes.	Ophthalmologic exam at baseline (within 6 months of starting), in 5 years then annually. If there are increased risk factors, every 6 months or annually.	Safe in pregnancy and lactation. May decrease risk of neonatal lupus in mothers with anti-Ro or anti-La antibodies
Azathioprine	Inhibits T-lymphocytes	Check TPMT[b] prior to initiation. CBC and CMP	May be used in pregnancy
Methotrexate	Inhibits dihydrofolate reductase and inhibits lymphocyte proliferation	Pregnancy test, hepatitis B and C serologies and CXR at baseline. CBC and CMP. Caution with renal disease, hepatitis or alcohol use	Teratogenic. Avoid use in both men and women considering pregnancy
Leflunomide	Inhibits pyrimidine synthesis via dihydroorotate dehydrogenase inhibition	Pregnancy test, TB test at baseline. CBC and CMP	Teratogenic
Mycophenolate mofetil	Inhibits B and T lymphocyte proliferation	Pregnancy test at baseline. CBC and CMP	Teratogenic
Belimumab[a]	Inhibits B lymphocyte stimulator (BLyS) binding to B cells which inhibits B-cell survival and decreased B-cell differentiation into immunoglobulin producing plasma cells	No routine testing	Avoid use during pregnancy and lactation. Not enough data available
Cyclophosphamide	Alkylates and cross-links DNA	Creatinine at baseline. CBC, UA and CMP. May need to adjust dose in renal impairment	May cause gonadal failure. Teratogenic. Avoid use in pregnancy as well as lactation

[a]Denotes medications that are FDA approved for the treatment of SLE.
[b]Testing for thiopurine methyltransferase deficiency.

PROGNOSIS

Prognosis in SLE has improved with early diagnosis and advances in treatment. In 1955, 5-year survival of SLE was 55%, which improved to 64% to 87% in the 1980s, and most recently, it was reported at 95%. Survival rates are influenced by geographic location and ethnicity.

With improved mortality from lupus disease activity, the focus has been on prevention and management of comorbid conditions. Premature atherosclerotic heart disease, malignancy, bone health, and psychosocial well-being may be secondary to the inflammatory state seen in lupus or as a result of treatment.

SPECIAL CONSIDERATIONS IN SYSTEMIC LUPUS ERYTHEMATOSUS

Pregnancy

Women with SLE have normal fertility but have higher rates of pregnancy loss (i.e., miscarriage and stillbirths) and preterm delivery (i.e., premature rupture of membranes, preeclampsia, and intrauterine growth restriction) than their healthy counterparts. Lupus activity preceding conception, especially nephritis, hypertension, and APS, are risk factors for pregnancy complications in SLE. Pregnancy itself may place women with SLE at a greater risk of a flare, particularly if the disease was active before conception.

With careful prenatal screening and planning, women with SLE can successfully have a healthy child. Prenatal monitoring of anti-SSA/Ro and anti-SSB/La antibodies and APLs and pre-pregnancy consultation with an obstetrician caring for high-risk pregnancies are critical. Ideally, women with SLE should have clinical quiescence for 6 months prior to a planned pregnancy.

Hormone Therapy

Contraception plays an important role in pregnancy planning for women with lupus. Often it is important to avoid unintended pregnancy during periods of severe disease activity and fetal exposure to potentially teratogenic drugs.

Because SLE is more prevalent in women of childbearing ages there has been consideration of a hormonal role in pathogenesis. There have been concerns raised that estrogen-containing compounds could induce a flare. In the past, estrogen-containing contraceptives were considered relatively contraindicated. However, randomized controlled trials evaluating the rate of disease flares in women with SLE on estrogen-containing contraceptives found no significant difference in rates of serious flares. Still, as a general rule, women with SLE who have APLs should avoid contraception with estrogen-containing compounds due to increased risk of thrombotic events. More recently, intrauterine devices are becoming a recommended alternative, given the efficacy and safety profile.

The use of postmenopausal hormone replacement therapy for treating vasomotor symptoms in SLE should be restricted to patients with negative APLs and at the lowest dose and shortest duration.

TABLE 81.7 Revised Classification Criteria of Antiphospholipid Syndrome

Classification Criteria[a]	Definition
Clinical Criteria	
1. Vascular thrombosis	One or more clinical episodes of arterial, venous, or small vessel thrombosis in any tissue or organ
	Thrombosis must be confirmed by objective validated criteria (i.e., unequivocal findings of appropriate imaging studies or histopathology). For histopathologic confirmation, thrombosis should be present without significant evidence of inflammation in the vessel wall.
2. Pregnancy morbidity	a. One or more unexplained deaths of a morphologically normal fetus at or beyond 10 weeks' gestation, with normal fetal morphology documented by ultrasound or by direct examination of the fetus
	or
	b. One or more premature births of a morphologically normal neonate before 34 weeks' gestation because of (i) eclampsia or severe preeclampsia or (ii) recognized features of placental insufficiency
	or
	c. Three or more unexplained consecutive spontaneous abortions before 10 weeks' gestation, with maternal anatomic or hormonal abnormalities and paternal and maternal chromosomal causes excluded
Laboratory Criteria	
1. Lupus anticoagulant	LAC detected in plasma on two or more occasions at least 12 weeks apart
2. Anticardiolipin antibody	The ACA antibody of IgG and/or IgM isotype in serum or plasma in medium or high titer (i.e., >40 GPL units, or >the 99th percentile) on two or more occasions at least 12 weeks apart, measured by a standardized ELISA
3. Anti-β_2 glycoprotein I antibody	β_2GPI antibody of IgG and/or IgM isotype in serum or plasma (in titer >the 99th percentile), detected on two or more occasions at least 12 weeks apart, measured by a standardized ELISA

ACA, Anticardiolipin antibody; *β_2GPI,* anti-β_2 glycoprotein I antibody; *ELISA,* enzyme-linked immunosorbent assay; *Ig,* immunoglobulin; *LAC,* lupus anticoagulant.
[a]Antiphospholipid antibody syndrome is diagnosed if at least one clinical criterion and one laboratory criterion are met.
Modified from Miyakis S, Lockshin MD, Atsumi T, et al: International consensus statement on an update of the classification criteria for definite antiphospholipid syndrome (APS), J Thromb Haemost 4:295-306, 2006.

Bone Health

Women with SLE have an increased risk for osteoporosis due to multiple factors. Some of these factors are more specific to SLE, such as chronic inflammation, renal disease, photosensitivity and avoidance of sun exposure, medication use (especially glucocorticoids), and premature ovarian failure, which may be due to SLE or the use of CTX. In addition, there are still the typical risk factors for osteoporosis such as smoking, alcohol use, family history, and low BMI. One challenging aspect in treating osteoporosis in young women with SLE is the use of bisphosphonates as these medications are not safe in pregnancy and may be present for years after discontinuation.

Cardiovascular Health

As survival and therapies for SLE have improved, and patients are living longer, cardiovascular disease (CVD) has emerged as a leading cause of morbidity and mortality. SLE patients are 5 to 10 times more likely than healthy individuals to have a coronary event. More striking, premenopausal women between 35 and 44 years of age are 50 times more likely than healthy women to have a myocardial infarction.

Autopsy series reveal atherosclerotic heart disease as the underlying mechanism of CVD in SLE. The cause of premature atherosclerosis in SLE is multifactorial and likely includes inflammatory mediators, SLE-related factors (e.g., premature menopause, corticosteroid therapy, disease activity), and traditional cardiovascular risk factors.

Although no firm cardiovascular management guidelines exist for SLE patients, the 2011 updated guidelines from the American Heart Association for prevention of CVD in women included (for the first time) autoimmune diseases (i.e., SLE and rheumatoid arthritis) in the increased-risk category. Physicians should consider premature atherosclerotic CVD and aggressively evaluate SLE patients with typical and atypical cardiac symptoms, regardless of age and sex.

Secondary Antiphospholipid Syndrome

Antiphospholipid syndrome (APS) is a condition characterized by an increased risk of thrombosis and/or pregnancy loss in the setting of APLs. The term *lupus anticoagulant* is a misnomer because the in vitro anticoagulant effect reflects the prolonged activated partial thromboplastin time (aPTT), but the term does not indicate a diagnosis of SLE or an increased risk of bleeding. In fact, lupus anticoagulant is associated with an increased risk of thrombotic events.

If APS occurs in the absence of another autoimmune disease it is considered primary APS. When it occurs in the setting of SLE or another autoimmune disease it is considered secondary APS. Both primary and secondary APS have similar clinical manifestations and the treatment is also similar. Clinical manifestations of APS typically include increased risk for venous and arterial thrombosis, pregnancy complications, cerebrovascular and cardiovascular events, pulmonary hypertension, Libman-Sacks endocarditis, and neurologic complications.

Catastrophic APS (CAPS) is the most severe manifestation of APS, which affects multiple organs with microthromboses leading to rapid organ failure and potentially death. CAPS may be difficult to discern from sepsis or TTP.

For patients with presence of APS but no thrombotic events or pregnancy loss there is no indication for anticoagulation. If there is an episode of vascular thrombosis, treatment with lifelong anticoagulation is generally recommended. Warfarin remains the drug of choice for these patients despite the development of several other novel oral anticoagulants. Unfractionated and low-molecular-weight heparin are also effective anticoagulants for APS and are used for patients who suffer recurrent events while on warfarin therapy or patients who are or plan to become pregnant (Table 81.7).

Malignancy

Patients with SLE have an increased risk of solid organ cancers as well as lymphoma. A multicenter international cohort study by SLICC of more than 16,000 SLE patients reported an increased risk of malignancy compared with the general population. Most striking was a 4-fold increased risk of non-Hodgkin's lymphoma. Other hematologic, vulvar, lung, and thyroid cancers were also increased, whereas breast and endometrial cancers were observed less often in lupus. Malignancy risk appears to be highest early in the disease course, but risk remains elevated throughout a patient's lifespan. Although lymph node enlargement is a common manifestation of SLE, physicians must consider malignancy if the lymphadenopathy does not resolve with SLE treatment, is nontender or nonmobile, or if it occurs without other lupus symptoms.

Vaccines

Patients with SLE are at an increased risk of infection due to immune dysregulation in addition to the use of immunosuppressive medications. Vaccines play a vital role in prevention of infections. As a general rule, live attenuated vaccines are contraindicated in lupus patients on biologic therapy or high-dose immunosuppressive treatments with a few exceptions. Patients with SLE should receive pneumococcal vaccines (PCV 13 and 23) and annual influenza vaccine. Patients with SLE have a higher risk of HPV-related cancers, and younger individuals should receive the HPV vaccination to mitigate this risk. There is also an increased risk of latent varicella zoster reactivation. There is now an inactivated vaccine available for the use in immunocompromised individuals such as those with SLE. The long-term safety of this vaccine is still being evaluated.

Psychosocial Effects of Systemic Lupus Erythematosus

When deciding upon management of SLE one must take into consideration other factors that influence outcomes. There is an immune response to acute stress as well as physical and emotional trauma. Although commonly reported by patients, it has been difficult to demonstrate a causal relationship between stress and increased flares in clinical studies. Regardless, anxiety, depression, and social determinants of health can impact adherence to medications and treatment plans as well as overall quality of life and should be considered when caring for patients with lupus.

Fatigue

Fatigue is extremely common in SLE, affecting up to 80% of patients. The cause is often multifactorial, and it is essential to rule out reversible etiologies that may be contributing, such as thyroid disease, depression, non-restorative sleep, obstructive sleep apnea, deconditioning, poor nutrition, celiac disease and nutritional deficiencies, fibromyalgia, and medication side effects. It is often difficult to pinpoint the exact cause of fatigue, and this makes management challenging. Treatment requires addressing the underlying causes of fatigue as well as improving nutrition, sleep, and encouraging aerobic exercise.

Depression and Anxiety

Patients with SLE are at increased risk for depression and anxiety, which have been associated with worse outcomes and medication response. Management of depression and anxiety is essential to the overall treatment of patients with SLE. Along with pharmacologic modalities such as antidepressants and anxiolytics, nonpharmacologic interventions such as psychological counseling, biofeedback, and guided imagery should be incorporated into management of lupus when appropriate.

SUMMARY

Systemic lupus erythematosus is a chronic multisystem autoimmune disease characterized by periods of disease flares and quiescence, and when left untreated it can lead to permanent organ damage and increased mortality. Diagnosis of SLE can be difficult and relies on a combination of clinical and laboratory factors. The Classification Criteria serve as a helpful reminder of common manifestations to aid in diagnosis. The heterogeneity of clinical manifestations of lupus has raised the concept of lupus as a spectrum disorder with different genetic and molecular profiles that define distinct phenotypes requiring customized management strategies.

Antimalarials remain the cornerstone of SLE treatment and have benefits beyond managing lupus disease activity. Immunosuppressive and biologic agents are available for manifestations that are not controlled by antimalarials. It is crucial to recognize the increased risk of comorbidities in lupus, including cardiovascular disease, malignancy, and bone loss. Addressing social determinants of health should be a part of the overall treatment plan in lupus. There is a pipeline of new agents currently being tested to improve management, morbidity, and mortality of patients with SLE.

SUGGESTED READINGS

Arbuckle MR, et al: Development of autoantibodies before clinical onset of systemic lupus erythematosus, N Engl J Med 314:614–619, 1986.

Aringer M, Costenbader K, Daikh D, et al: 2019 European League Against Rheumatism/American College of Rheumatology Classification Criteria for Systemic Lupus Erythematosus, Arthritis Rheumatol 71(9):1400–1412, 2019.

Bernatsky S, Ramsey-Goldman R, Labrecque J: Cancer risk in systemic lupus: an updated international multi-center cohort study, J Autoimmun 42:130–135, 2013.

Borchers AT, Keen CL, Shoenfeld Y, Gershwin ME: Surviving the butterfly and the wolf: mortality trends in systemic lupus erythematosus, Autoimmun Rev 3(6):423–453, 2004.

Buyon JP: Updates on lupus and pregnancy, Bull NYU Hosp Jt Dis 67:271–275, 2009.

Cervera R, Khamashta MA, Font J, et al: Morbidity and mortality in systemic lupus erythematosus during a 10-year period. A comparison of early and late manifestations in a cohort of 1000 patients, Medicine (Baltimore) 82(5):299–308, 2003.

Churg J, Sobin LH: Renal disease: classification and atlas of glomerular disease, Tokyo, 1982, Igaku-Shoin.

Data from Wallace D, Hahn BH: Other clinical laboratory tests in SLE. In Dubois' lupus erythematosus and related syndromes, ed 8, Philadelphia, 2013, Saunders, pp 526–531.

Data modified from Gilliam classification scheme. Gilliam JN, Sontheimer RD: Distinctive cutaneous subsets in the spectrum of lupus erythematosus, J Am Acad Dermatol 4(4):471–475, 1981.

Fanouriakis A, Kostopoulou M, Alunno A, et al: 2019 update of the EULAR recommendations on the management of systemic lupus erythematosus, Ann Rheum Dis 78:736–745, 2019.

Gomez-Puerta J, Barbhaiya M, Guan H, et al: Racial/ethnic variation in all-cause mortality among U.S. medicaid recipients with, systemic lupus erythematosus: an hispanic and asian paradox, Arthritis Rheumatol 67(3):752–760, 2015.

Hochberg MC: Updating the American College of Rheumatology revised criteria for the classification of systemic lupus erythematosus, Arthritis Rheum 40:1725, 1997.

Hull D, Binns BA, Joyce D: Congenital heart block and widespread fibrosis due to maternal lupus erythematosus, Arch Dis Child 41:688–690, 1996.

Izmirly PM, Llanos C, Lee LA, et al: Cutaneous manifestations of neonatal lupus and risk of subsequent congenital heart block, Arthritis Rheumatol 62:1153–1157, 2010.

Llanos C, Izmirly PM, Katholi M, et al: Recurrence rates of cardiac manifestations associated with neonatal lupus and maternal/fetal risk factors, Arthritis Rheumatol 60:3091–3097, 2009.

Manzi S, Meilahn EN, Rairie JE, et al: Age-specific incidence rates of MI and angina in women with SLE: comparison with Framingham study, Am J Epidemiol 145(5):408–415, 1997.

Marmor MF, Kellner U, Lai TYY, et al: Recommendations on Screening for Chloroquine and Hydroxychloroquine Retinopathy (2016 Revision), Ophthalmology 123(6):1386–1394, 2016.

Merola JF, Bermas B, Lu B, et al: Clinical manifestations and survival among adults with SLE according to age of diagnosis, Lupus 23(8):778–784, 2014.

Merrell M, Shulman LE: Determination of prognosis in chronic disease, illustrated by systemic lupus erythematosus, J Chronic Dis 1(1):12–32, 1955.

Modified from Miyakis S, Lockshin MD, Atsumi T, et al: International consensus statement on an update of the classification criteria for definite antiphospholipid syndrome (APS), J Thromb Haemost 4:295-306, 2006.

Modified from Petri M, Orbai AM, Alarcón GS, et al: Derivation and validation of Systemic Lupus International Collaborating Clinics classification criteria for systemic lupus erythematosus, Arthritis Rheum 64: 2677–2686, 2012.

Mosca L, Benjamin EJ, Berra K, et al: Circulation 123(11):1243–1262, 2011.

Petri M, Kim MY, Kalunian KC, et al: Combined oral contraceptives in women with systemic lupus erythematosus, N Engl J Med 353(24):2550–2558, 2005.

Sánchez-Guerrero J, Uribe AG, Jiménez-Santana L, et al: A trial of contraceptive methods in women with systemic lupus erythematosus, N Engl J Med 353(24):2539–2549, 2005.

Stojan G, Petri M: Epidemiology of systemic lupus erythematosus: an update, Curr Opin Rheumatol 30(2):144–150, 2018.

Tan EM, Cohen AS, Fries, et al: The 1982 revised criteria of the classification of systemic lupus erythematosus, Arthritis Rheum 25:1271, 1982.

Tench CM, McCurdie I, White PD, D'Cruz DP: The prevalence and associations of fatigue in systemic lupus erythematosus, Rheumatology 39(11):1249–1254, 2000.

Weening JJ, D'Agati VD, Schwartz MM, et al: Classification of glomerulonephritis in systemic lupus erythematosus revisited, Kidney Int 65:521–530, 2004.

82

Systemic Sclerosis

Anna Papazoglou, Robyn T. Domsic

INTRODUCTION

Systemic sclerosis (SSc) is a multisystem, autoimmune disease characterized by cutaneous and visceral fibrosis. The more common term for the disease, *scleroderma*, reflects this hallmark feature as it is derived from the Greek *scleros,* which means thick, and *derma*, which means skin. The pathology and damage from the disease reflects a complex interplay of vascular injury, immune system activation, and excessive fibrosis.

The disorder can range from a relatively benign condition to a rapidly progressive disease leading to significant morbidity or death. Although cutaneous manifestations are the most obvious features, visceral and vascular involvement can be severe and disabling. Monitoring for potential organ complications is essential in caring for SSc patients because early detection and treatment may minimize morbidity and mortality. There is ongoing research aiming to increase in-depth understanding of the complex mechanisms leading to SSc, which would facilitate the discovery of curative treatment.

EPIDEMIOLOGY

The annual US incidence of SSc is approximately 32 cases per million persons and the estimated prevalence is 254 cases per million persons. Incidence and prevalence vary somewhat throughout the world, and they typically are lower in Europe and Asia. SSc more commonly affects women, with a 3-5:1 female-to-male ratio. It occurs in individuals of all ages, from childhood to the elderly, but it most frequently affects those between the ages of 40 and 60 years. There are studies that indicate differences in the frequency and severity of SSc clinical manifestations as well as complications between men and women.

A familial pattern of inheritance is not as evident in SSc as in other connective tissue diseases, although first-degree relatives appear to be at somewhat increased risk. Twin studies have demonstrated only a 5% rate of concordance in monozygotic and dizygotic twins, implying that there are significant environmental contributions to its occurrence. Many patients with SSc, however, have family histories of other autoimmune diseases (e.g., thyroid disease, rheumatoid arthritis, systemic lupus erythematosus [SLE]). Genome-wide association studies have revealed a handful of genes associated with SSc that are shared with other diseases such as rheumatoid arthritis and SLE (e.g., major histocompatibility complex class I and II genes, *STAT4, IRF5, TNFSF4, IRF8*). These findings suggest a shared genetic predisposition to autoimmune conditions.

PATHOLOGY

The pathogenesis of SSc remains unclear. A combination of genetic and environmental factors results in complicated interaction of three clearly identified components, consisting of vascular abnormalities, immunologic abnormalities and extracellular membrane abnormalities leading to tissue fibrosis, the hallmark of SSc (Fig. 82.1).

The initial event is postulated to be tissue injury including endothelial damage with subsequent endothelial cell activation and chemokine production as well as vascular injury. Vascular damage is characterized by vascular obliteration, defective vasculogenesis, and tissue hypoxia. Vascular changes are seen in the skin and may also occur in the pulmonary, cardiac, and renal blood vessels, affecting arteries, arterioles, and capillaries. True vasculitis is conspicuously absent. Early vascular involvement consists of an imbalance between vasodilatory and vasoconstrictive factors, endothelial cell activation with resultant leukocyte migration and smooth muscle cell proliferation.

Immune system activation is evident in several respects. The secretion of multiple chemokines leads to perpetuating cycles of inflammation and autoimmunity. SSc-associated autoantibodies are detected in more than 95% of patients with SSc. All 10 of the recognized SSc-associated autoantibodies are directed against distinct nuclear antigens. They are helpful in classifying patients, but their pathogenic role has not been clarified. There is evidence of T-cell activation, with a T_H2-predominant cytokine profile. Elevated levels of interleukins (i.e., IL-1, IL-2, IL-2R, IL-4, IL-8, IL-13, and IL-17) and interferon have been reported. The role of T_H17 cells is not understood, but studies suggest that dysregulation of these proinflammatory T cells contributes to disease pathogenesis. In addition, there is increasing evidence of innate immune dysregulation in the setting of activated macrophages and altered expression and function of toll-like receptors.

The complex interplay between the chemokines produced by the inflammatory cells leads to activation of fibroblasts and presumed differentiation into myofibroblast. As such, there is overproduction of extracellular matrix, which results in progressively worsening fibrosis. Of note, fibroblasts are found in increased numbers in the skin and other tissues, and they develop an SSc phenotype when grown in vitro, producing an overabundance of collagen and living longer in tissue culture. Fibroblast persistence in culture suggests a perpetuated abnormality not requiring continued immune stimulation. Over the past decades, increasing evidence suggests that macrophages are important in the pathogenesis of systemic sclerosis through secretion of inflammatory cytokines; however, their exact role needs to be further clarified. Transforming growth factor β (TGF-β), specifically, is secreted by macrophages and has been found to have effect on the fibrotic mechanism through regulation of fibroblast function as well as various important processes in fibrosis.

CLINICAL PRESENTATION

Patients with SSc can have several clinical presentations, although Raynaud's phenomenon is the most common symptom (>95%). Distinctive phenotypes may manifest differently. SSc can have many

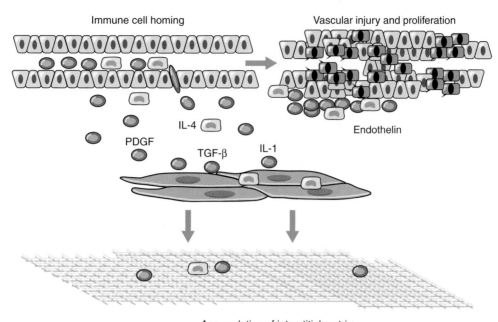

Fig. 82.1 Pathogenetic processes in systemic sclerosis. Vascular injury leads to intimal proliferation of endothelial cells *(red)* and smooth muscle cells *(blue with black nuclei)*. Immune cells consisting of T cells *(blue, small)* and monocyte/macrophages *(yellow with orange nuclei)* are activated and home to sites in the dermis. Fibroblasts are activated to deposit increased amounts of interstitial matrix. *IL,* Interleukin; *PDGF,* platelet-derived growth factor; *TGF-β,* transforming growth factor-β.

internal organ manifestations, producing various clinical presentations and requiring tailored work-up protocols.

Classification by Cutaneous Features

Historically, SSc has been separated into two major clinical subsets defined by the degree and extent of skin involvement: limited cutaneous (lc) and diffuse cutaneous (dc) disease. Patients with lcSSc experience skin thickening limited to the distal extremities (i.e., below the elbows and knees) as well as the face. The dcSSc patients have similar distal changes in addition to involvement of the upper arms, thighs, or trunk at some time during the disease course. Few patients (<1%) have no skin thickening but have one or more typical SSc visceral manifestations. The term *scleroderma sine scleroderma* has been used to describe patients with minimal or no skin involvement whose clinical course resembles that of individuals with lcSSc.

The distinct cutaneous patterns are important, because patients with dcSSc are more likely to develop internal organ complications (e.g., renal crisis, cardiac involvement) early in their illness, whereas those with lcSSc can develop internal organ involvement at any point throughout their disease, even decades after the initial symptoms. Several classification criteria have been suggested that do not particularly assist in diagnosis of SSc but are rather intended primarily to help classify SSc patients for studies (Table 82.1). These clinical characteristics are derived from a long-standing registry at the University of Pittsburgh. Some patients with lcSSc or dcSSC may have typical features of another connective tissue disease (most commonly polymyositis, SLE, or rheumatoid arthritis-like features), and they are considered to have *SSc in overlap.*

Of note, as an attempt for early identification of individuals at risk for future development of SSc, the Very Early Diagnosis of Systemic Sclerosis (VEDOSS) approach has been considered recently as a potentially useful tool for predicting SSc disease development. Its role in clinical and research work at this time still requires better understanding. This approach, which includes patients with manifestations of Raynaud's phenomenon, puffy fingers, certain positive SSc antibodies, and reported

nailfold capillaroscopy changes, may be helpful in identifying those at risk for developing established disease over shorter-term follow-up.

Serologic Classification

Serologic classification refers to SSc-associated serum autoantibodies. Patients with the same autoantibody tend to have a similar cutaneous pattern, natural history of disease, and risk of internal organ involvement.

Serologic classification can augment the clinical classification described previously. For example, 95% of patients with anticentromere antibody have lcSSc and are at increased risk for pulmonary hypertension during the course of the disease. Individuals with anti–topoisomerase I (i.e., anti-SCL70) or anti–RNA polymerase III antibody are more likely to have dcSSc. Those with anti–RNA polymerase III antibody have an increased risk of renal crisis, and those with anti-SCL70 have a higher frequency of interstitial lung disease.

The primary internal organ risks and cutaneous associations are depicted in Fig. 82.2, which illustrates the combined clinical-serologic classification of SSc. It is uncommon for patients to have more than one SSc autoantibody.

Raynaud's Phenomenon and Peripheral Vascular Involvement

Nearly all patients with SSc experience Raynaud's phenomenon during their disease course, often as the initial symptom. Raynaud's phenomenon is a triphasic vasospastic response to cold consisting of pallor (i.e., blanching) with or without cyanosis (i.e., bluish discoloration followed by reactive hyperemia manifested by erythema) with a characteristic distinct line of demarcation on the digits separating the affected from unaffected areas.

The onset of Raynaud's phenomenon can precede the development of skin changes by years in some patients. Beyond Raynaud's phenomenon, SSc patients can develop progressive peripheral vasculopathy. This may lead to loss of digital tip tissue with resulting digital pitting scars, ulcers, or gangrene (rare) that can lead to autoamputation. Digital tip ulcers occur more frequently in patients who are anticentromere or

TABLE 82.1 Manifestations of Systemic Sclerosis by Clinical Classification in the Pittsburgh Scleroderma Center Database

Manifestations	Diffuse (N = 1646)	Limited (N = 2124)
Cutaneous		
Puffy fingers	83%	80%
Skin induration, thickening	Widespread: trunk, face, extremities	Face, below the elbow and knee
Telangiectasias	62%	65%
Calcinosis	10%	13%
Peripheral Vascular		
Raynaud's phenomenon	95%	98%
Digital ulcerations	41%	37%
Pulmonary		
Interstitial lung disease	38%	34%
Pulmonary arterial hypertension	6%	18%
Cardiac		
Arrhythmias	12%	10%
Diastolic dysfunction	7%	9%
Myocarditis	3%	1%
Pericarditis	3%	2%
Renal		
Renal crisis	16%	3%
Gastrointestinal		
Esophageal hypomotility, reflux	84%	83%
Small intestine dysmotility	11%	8%
Malabsorption	5%	4%
Incontinence	3%	4%
Joint and Musculoskeletal		
Tendon friction rubs	51%	6%
Joint contractures	87%	37%
Myositis	6%	7%

Data from the University of Pittsburgh Scleroderma Databank, 1980-2018.

anti–topoisomerase I autoantibody positive. Lower extremity ulcerations in SSc patients have been increasingly reported in recent years.

Interstitial Lung Disease

Interstitial lung disease (ILD) can be one of the most serious complications of SSc and should be monitored for routinely, because it plays a major role in mortality and morbidity (see Chapter 17). The initial presentation is often a nonproductive cough and a gradual onset of dyspnea on exertion over several months to years. However, the onset can be abrupt.

High-resolution chest computed tomography (CT) typically shows bibasilar fibrotic changes, which can be progressive. Pulmonary function tests reveal reduced forced vital capacity (FVC). On pathologic examination, the most frequently seen pattern is nonspecific interstitial pneumonitis (NSIP) or fibrosing NSIP. Patients with anti-SCL70 autoantibody and U11/U12 are at the highest risk for ILD.

Pulmonary Hypertension

SSc patients can develop pulmonary hypertension of three World Health Organization (WHO) classifications (see Chapter 18 and Chapter 12). Pulmonary arterial hypertension (PAH, WHO group 1) is the most common, with an estimated 10% to 15% of patients in cohort studies developing PAH. It occurs most commonly in those with lcSSc. The clinical presentation includes rapidly progressive dyspnea occurring over several months. Pulmonary function tests reveal a reduced diffusion capacity for carbon monoxide (DLCO) out of proportion to any concomitant reduction in the FVC.

Less frequently, SSc patients develop pulmonary hypertension associated with ILD (WHO group 3) or pulmonary hypertension associated with left ventricular diastolic dysfunction from myocardial fibrosis or non–SSc-associated left ventricular disorders (WHO group 2). Screening for all types of pulmonary hypertension is performed by echocardiogram, and results should be confirmed by right heart cardiac catheterization.

Scleroderma Renal Crisis

Scleroderma renal crisis (SRC) manifests as the abrupt onset of accelerated arterial hypertension accompanied by a rise in serum creatinine levels and by microscopic hematuria and proteinuria on urinalysis. Microangiopathic hemolytic anemia and thrombocytopenia are common. Although once the major cause of mortality in SSc, SRC is now managed by aggressive blood pressure control with an angiotensin-converting enzyme (ACE) inhibitor, which should be maintained lifelong.

The typical setting for SRC is early dcSSc with a recent increase in skin thickening, palpable tendon friction rubs, and anti–RNA polymerase III antibody. During active, early dcSSc, patients should check their blood pressure once weekly and report a rise in systolic blood pressure of more than 20 mm Hg from baseline. Prednisone given at a dose of 15 mg daily or higher has been associated with the development of SRC and should be avoided in at-risk patients.

Cardiac Manifestations

In general, all cardiac structures may be affected with subsequent serious functional consequences. Underlying PAH contributes as well to cardiac manifestations of SSc. Patients with SSc have three primary types of cardiac involvement: pericarditis, myocarditis, and myocardial fibrosis. The latter can lead to congestive heart failure and arrhythmias due to fibrosis of the conduction system. These complications can be asymptomatic and underrecognized in SSc patients, but pathologic changes have been found in 70% of patients in older autopsy series. Later studies using cardiac magnetic resonance imaging (MRI) have supported the autopsy findings of subclinical cardiac involvement.

Diastolic dysfunction is becoming increasingly recognized as a complication of fibrosis and can be evaluated by echocardiogram during pulmonary hypertension screening. Many SSc deaths occur suddenly, possibly due to ventricular arrhythmias. It is prudent to obtain a resting electrocardiogram early in the disease course. Palpitations noticed by the patient should be addressed with a formal cardiac arrhythmia evaluation.

Gastrointestinal Tract Manifestations

At least one gastrointestinal manifestation will affect 80% or more of SSc patients, and all areas of the gastrointestinal tract may be affected. Gastrointestinal involvement is a significant cause of morbidity.

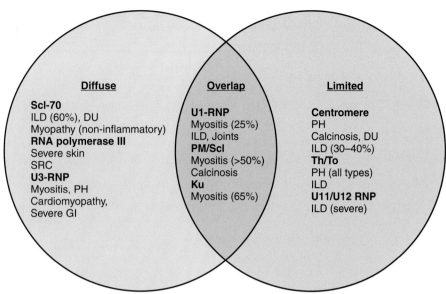

Fig. 82.2 Clinical-serologic classification of systemic sclerosis and antibody-associated internal organ manifestations. *Bold text* indicates an antibody; clinical manifestations listed below are associated with that antibody. *DU,* Digital ulcers; *ILD,* interstitial lung disease; *Ku,* 70/80-kD protein (XRCC6/XRCC5); *PH,* pulmonary hypertension; *PM,* polymyosis; *RNP,* ribonucleoprotein; *Scl,* sclerosis; *SRC,* scleroderma renal crisis.

When the esophagus is affected, patients experience heartburn and/or regurgitation due to a reduced lower esophageal sphincter pressure and distal dysphagia for solid foods due to esophageal dysmotility. The former can be determined by manometry. Less invasively, a barium swallow can reveal hypo- or aperistalsis to determine esophageal dysfunction. Neuropathic changes and fibrosis of the muscularis of the small intestine can lead to motor dysfunction and symptoms of postprandial abdominal distention. Small intestinal hypomotility may lead to bacterial overgrowth, causing bloating and diarrhea. When severe atony of the small intestine develops, patients occasionally develop a functional ileus or intestinal pseudo-obstruction. Parenteral nutrition may be necessary for severe malabsorption with accompanying weight loss and steatorrhea. Similar to the small bowel, the colon may develop impaired motor function leading to constipation and occasionally overflow diarrhea. Wide-mouthed diverticula on the antimesenteric border of the colon can be seen. The internal anal sphincter may become fibrotic, resulting in fecal incontinence.

Musculoskeletal Manifestations

Musculoskeletal manifestations are common. Tendons can become inflamed and fibrotic, particularly in early, diffuse disease. Palpable tendon or bursal friction rubs are virtually pathognomonic of SSc and often indicate progression to dcSSc before widespread skin thickening has occurred. Finger joint flexion contractures develop frequently within the first years of diffuse SSc. True arthritis with palpable synovitis should raise the question of an overlap condition or concomitant Sjögren's syndrome, because synovitis is not a typical feature of SSc.

Some patients develop a bland myopathy with nonprogressive, mild proximal muscle weakness and wasting. A few, particularly with features that overlap with other connective tissue diseases or mixed connective tissue disease, can develop true myositis, which can result in morbidity and disability.

DIAGNOSIS AND DIFFERENTIAL DIAGNOSIS

Raynaud's phenomenon is prominent in the differential diagnosis for SSc. Features that identify Raynaud's patients who have or may later develop SSc or another connective tissue disease are abnormal nail fold

capillaries (i.e., megacapillaries, hemorrhages, neovascularization, and avascular areas), tissue loss at the tips of the fingers, and a positive antinuclear antibody (ANA) test result. None of these features is found in Raynaud's disease (i.e., primary Raynaud's phenomenon).

Mixed connective tissue disease (MCTD) is also on the differential for SSc. MCTD patients have features of two or more autoimmune diseases and are U1-RNP antibody positive. This most frequently includes SSc, polymyosis, and SLE. Patients with MCTD can develop any or all of the following SSc manifestations: Raynaud's phenomenon, puffy fingers, limited or diffuse skin thickening, myositis, ILD, PAH, and esophageal dysmotility.

Scleroderma mimics are sometimes difficult to distinguish from SSc (Table 82.2). They include eosinophilic fasciitis, the localized forms of scleroderma such as linear scleroderma (more frequently seen in children), and plaque or generalized morphea.

Nephrogenic systemic fibrosis is a complication of gadolinium administration for radiographic studies that occurs in the setting of renal failure. Nephrogenic systemic fibrosis manifests as symmetrical, bilateral, fibrotic, indurated papules, plaques, or subcutaneous nodules, which can be erythematosus and occur on the lower legs or hands. The lesions are often preceded by edema and may initially be misdiagnosed as cellulitis. This diagnosis should be considered in patients being evaluated for a fibrotic disorder who have renal failure, regardless of the cause of renal disease.

Scleromyxedema and scleredema are cutaneous fibrotic disorders in which excessive mucin accumulation is found on skin biopsy. Scleromyxedema can mimic dcSSc on the physical examination or can manifest with multiple, firm, nodular skin lesions (i.e., papular mucinosis). A frequent association is a monoclonal gammopathy (i.e., immunoglobulin [IgG] paraprotein). Scleredema typically involves the nape of the neck and shoulders, sparing the distal extremities. All SSc mimics lack Raynaud's phenomenon, characteristic SSc internal organ involvement, and SSc-associated serum antibodies.

TREATMENT

No single efficacious therapy has been demonstrated in a randomized, placebo-controlled phase III study for SSc. Thus, patients must

TABLE 82.2 Scleroderma Mimics

Disorder	Distinguishing Features
Other Diseases	
Morphea	One or more discrete lesions; patchy or linear in distribution
Eosinophilic fasciitis	Finger flexures without sclerodactyly; characteristic groove sign when the arms are raised; puckering or dimpling of the upper arm and thigh skin; peripheral blood eosinophilia; fascia and deep subcutaneous fibrosis
Scleredema (Buschke disease)	Prominent involvement of neck, shoulders, and upper arms; hands spared; associated with diabetes
Scleromyxedema	Association with gammopathy; skin lichenoid and thickened but not tethered; may have Raynaud's phenomenon
Graft-versus-host disease	Skin changes similar to scleroderma; vasculopathy
Nephrogenic fibrosing dermopathy	Indurated plaques or nodules on the legs or arms, sparing the face; administration of gadolinium in the setting of renal dysfunction; often preceded by edema
Reactions to Environmental Agents and Drugs	
Bleomycin	Skin and lung fibrosis similar to scleroderma
L-Tryptophan (1980s)	Eosinophilia-myalgia syndrome from L-tryptophan contaminant or metabolite (first described in the 1980s); fever, eosinophilia, neurologic manifestations
Organic solvents (e.g., trichloroethylene)	Clinically indistinguishable from idiopathic systemic sclerosis
Pentazocine	Localized lesions at injection sites
Toxic oil syndrome	Contaminated rapeseed oil (Spanish epidemic in 1981); similar to eosinophilia myalgia syndrome
Vinyl chloride	Vascular lesions, acro-osteolysis, sclerodactyly, no visceral disease
Gadolinium	Nephrogenic fibrosing dermopathy

be appropriately monitored for visceral involvement to allow early identification and therapy targeted at specific organ complications. Consultation with a rheumatologist is helpful in this respect. Generally, patients with early diffuse or evolving diffuse scleroderma are likely to be considered for treatment with immunosuppression and treatment options specifically for those SSc patients with ILD include an anti-fibrotic agent. Given the lack of US Food and Drug Administration (FDA)- or EMA-approved therapy, SSc is an active area of therapeutic research; multiple international clinical trials are either ongoing or planned. Given this, patients should be considered for referral to a dedicated scleroderma center early in disease to have the advantage of these opportunities. Autologous stem cell transplant has been tested in the United States and Europe and has demonstrated an improvement in event-free and overall survival in patients with moderate to severe and early diffuse SSc. Treatment-related mortality must be weighed when considering stem cell therapy as an option, and we do not advise it for skin management alone.

With respect to evaluation and monitoring, all patients should undergo screening evaluation for ILD and pulmonary hypertension throughout the course of their disease. Current expert recommendations suggest that patients with early, diffuse disease should be monitored at least yearly for these complications. Patients with active dcSSc, particularly if they have tendon friction rubs, should undergo weekly blood pressure monitoring because the abrupt appearance of hypertension suggests SRC. Early dcSSc patients should also have skin thickness scores assessed for progression or regression of cutaneous disease. For dcSSc and lcSSc, initial esophageal motility studies should be considered, and further objective studies should be ordered on the basis of symptoms.

Education of patients and family members regarding the disease and an accurate prognosis based on disease subtype and stage can be helpful in management. Educational programs are available through foundations across the world. This includes the Scleroderma Foundation in the United States, Scleroderma Canada, Scleroderma and Raynaud's UK, Scleroderma Australia, and the World Scleroderma Foundation.

Raynaud's Phenomenon

Nonpharmacologic measures such as cold avoidance, warming measures, avoidance of vibratory tools, and smoking cessation are encouraged in all patients. Pharmacologic measures are recommended, because ongoing vascular injury may play a role in pathogenesis.

Calcium-channel blockers have been widely used for decades, and they are generally well tolerated by patients. Long-acting nifedipine is effective in more than one half of patients; other agents such as amlodipine are also frequently prescribed. The angiotensin-receptor blocker losartan reduced the severity and frequency of Raynaud's phenomenon attacks in a placebo-controlled trial. ACE inhibitors have not proved effective in several controlled trials. Phosphodiesterase-5 (PDE-5) inhibitors have been shown to improve Raynaud's phenomenon. Some studies have shown encouraging results with use of fluoxetine (selective serotonin reuptake inhibitor). The prostacyclin iloprost is used as a therapy for severe Raynaud's phenomenon and digital ischemia. The benefit of statin therapy for Raynaud's phenomenon has produced conflicting results, although it has benefits in endothelial dysfunction, which is a component of the vascular pathogenesis in SSc.

In patients with digital ulcerations, more aggressive therapy may be warranted. PDE-5 inhibitors have been helpful. Topical nitroglycerin as a paste, gel, or patch placed at the base of the fingers or over the dorsal wrist may be a useful adjunct. In randomized, placebo-controlled trials, bosentan, an endothelin receptor antagonist, prevented the formation of new digital ulcerations in patients with SSc and Raynaud's phenomenon, although it has not been approved by the FDA for this indication. Iloprost, an intravenous prostacyclin, has also been shown to reduce digital ulcerations and is frequently used in Europe, but it is not FDA-approved in the United States.

For patients with digital ulcers involving adjacent fingers, assessment of the ulnar and radial artery should be performed with arterial Doppler or angiography because larger arteries can become severely narrowed. Surgical interventions include sympathectomy of the digital, radial, or ulnar artery and venous bypass for ulnar or radial artery occlusion. Topical botulinum A injections are potentially helpful in selected patients who are unable to tolerate other treatments. In SSc patients with recurrent digital ulcers or other thrombotic events, evaluation for a hypercoagulable state, particularly for lupus anticoagulant, should be performed. In this circumstance, aspirin or other anticoagulants are indicated.

Cutaneous Disease

No therapeutic agent has been found to achieve a clinically significant improvement in skin thickening as measured by the modified Rodnan skin score in a randomized, placebo-controlled trial for patients with dcSSc. The Rodnan skin score was developed by Dr. Gerald Rodnan at the University of Pittsburgh. It is calculated by estimating skin thickness on a scale of 0 to 3 in 17 skin areas. Negative findings in therapeutic trials have been attributed to the type of drugs chosen, the patient populations, and trial designs. In the past, considerable attention was given to methotrexate and D-penicillamine, but no trials demonstrate a clinically significant improvement in skin score. Case series with historical controls have suggested a benefit for mycophenolate mofetil, although it has not been studied in a randomized setting. Subset analysis from the Scleroderma Lung Study 2 suggested that both mycophenolate and cyclophosphamide therapy were associated with an improvement in the skin thickness of patients with dcSSc. More recently, two studies with tocilizumab failed to demonstrate a statistically significant improvement in skin score, although there was clinical improvement during the extended open label trial. Currently, mycophenolate mofetil and methotrexate are commonly used as first-line agents in dcSSc.

Scleroderma Renal Crisis

Early diagnosis and prompt initiation of ACE inhibitors are the keys to improved survival and outcomes of SRC. ACE inhibitors should be titrated to maintain a normal blood pressure, preferably less than 125/75 mm Hg, and lifelong treatment is recommended. Second-line agents to maintain blood pressure control include calcium-channel blockers (CCB). β-Blockers are relatively contraindicated because there is concern for worsening of Raynaud's phenomenon as well as for potential vascular complications.

Even if patients with SRC become dialysis dependent initially, some may experience a slow reversal of renal vascular damage if ACE inhibitor therapy is maintained. Because up to 50% of SRC patients can spontaneously come off dialysis, transplantation evaluation should be delayed until at least 2 years after SRC onset.

Interstitial Lung Disease

Early recognition of inflammatory ILD is important if treatment is to prevent progression to distortion of lung architecture and irreversible fibrosis. Controlled clinical trials support the potential benefit of mycophenolate mofetil, particularly with early detection of underlying ILD associated with SSc and initiation of treatment. Although the choice of mycophenolate mofetil has not been proven to be more effective compared to cyclophosphamide, there is overall better tolerance of the drug and a relatively safer side-effect profile. In addition, small trials have shown hopeful results in terms of using rituximab, an anti-CD20 monoclonal antibody, for fibrotic lung complications associated with underlying scleroderma. Two randomized controlled trials of tocilizumab revealed encouraging results regarding preservation of lung function. A recent trial of nintedanib in SSc-related ILD demonstrated that the annual rate of decline in FVC was lower with nintedanib than with placebo; nearly half the patients in this trial were taking background mycophenolate therapy. Lung transplantation can be considered for end-stage ILD. In all settings, management of ILD should include management of esophageal disease.

Pulmonary Hypertension

Several agents have been approved for the treatment of PAH (see Chapter 18). Subset analyses of several placebo-controlled drug trials have shown improvement in established SSc or connective tissue disease–related PAH. They have included phosphodiesterase-5 inhibitors (e.g., sildenafil, tadalafil), endothelial receptor antagonists (e.g., bosentan, ambrisentan, macitentan), soluble guanylate cyclase inhibitors (riociguat), and prostacyclin analogues (e.g., treprostinil, epoprostenol, selexipag). There is growing interest in the potential benefit of immunosuppressive therapies for SSc-PAH in addition to vasodilators.

Theoretically, treatment of patients with early, less severe disease should improve outcomes. Because patients with SSc-related PAH have a worse prognosis than those with idiopathic PAH despite modern therapies, SSc patients with PAH should be recommended to a tertiary care facility with a dedicated pulmonary hypertension clinic.

Cardiac Manifestations

Combined corticosteroids and immunosuppression can be used for myocarditis. Conventional treatment is recommended for symptomatic pericarditis (see Chapter 10), arrhythmias (see Chapter 9), and diastolic heart failure (see Chapter 5).

Gastrointestinal Manifestations

Gastroesophageal reflux, which occurs in most SSc patients, can be treated with proton pump inhibitors and conservative measures, including elevation of the head of the bed and avoidance of alcohol and caffeine. If untreated, reflux esophagitis can progress to distal esophageal stricture formation.

Patients with severe esophageal, gastric, or small bowel dysmotility may improve with the use of prokinetic drugs such as metoclopramide, erythromycin, or octreotide. Rotating antibiotics may be of assistance for bacterial overgrowth. For advanced small bowel involvement with malabsorption, supplementation of iron, calcium, and fat-soluble vitamins may be required. Occasionally, total parental nutrition is necessary. Unexplained iron deficiency anemia in SSc patients suggests the possibility of gastric antral vascular ectasias (i.e., watermelon stomach), which are treated with laser photocoagulation as first-line therapy.

Skeletal Muscle, Joint, and Tendon Manifestations

Bland myopathy usually is nonprogressive and is treated with physical therapy. If there is evidence of myositis with elevated serum levels of muscle enzymes or abnormal electromyography or muscle biopsy, corticosteroids and immunosuppressive therapy (e.g., methotrexate, azathioprine) may be helpful.

Patients with lcSSc or dcSSc can develop contractures of the hands due to tendon involvement. Physical therapy with daily stretching exercises directed at the finger joints should be instituted as soon as possible to prevent further loss of finger motion.

For a deeper discussion of these topics, please see Chapter 251, "Systemic Sclerosis (Scleroderma)," in *Goldman-Cecil Medicine*, 26th Edition.

SPECIAL CONSIDERATIONS

Patients with SSc are at increased risk for development of cancer, particularly hematologic malignancies such as lymphoma as well as lung and breast cancer. There is ongoing research focused on understanding the exact pathogenetic mechanisms. Underlying inflammation is thought to play a major role. The existence of specific autoantibodies in addition to the use of certain immunosuppressive agents also have been implicated in playing role. Pending clarification of the pathophysiology leading to malignancy, it is important to perform age-appropriate screening in SSc patients.

SUGGESTED READINGS

Kowal-Bielecka O, Landewé R, Avouac J, et al: EULAR recommendations for the treatment of systemic sclerosis: a report from the EULAR scleroderma trials and research group (EUSTAR), Ann Rheum Dis 68:620–628, 2009.

Maurer B, Distler O: Emerging targeted therapies in scleroderma lung and skin fibrosis, Best Pract Res Clin Rheumatol 25:843–858, 2011.

Mayes MD: The scleroderma book: a guide for patients and families, New York, 1999, Oxford University Press.

Medsger TA: Natural history of systemic sclerosis and the assessment of disease activity, severity, functional status, and psychologic well-being, Rheum Dis Clin North Am 29:255–275, 2003.

83

Systemic Vasculitis

Kimberly P. Liang, Kelly V. Liang

DEFINITION AND EPIDEMIOLOGY

The primary systemic vasculitides are inflammatory disorders of blood vessels that are characterized by immune-mediated injury leading to vessel necrosis, thrombosis, stenosis, or some combination of these. Vessels in any organ may be affected, but each vasculitis is characterized by different preferential vessel size or territory and tissue targeting. Although these disorders are rare, they may be organ- or life-threatening, so prompt diagnosis and treatment are necessary. The vasculitides are defined according to the 1990 American College of Rheumatology (ACR) classification criteria and the 1994 Chapel Hill Consensus Conference (revised in 2012) (CHCC) based on generally affected vessel size (small, medium, or large). Antineutrophil cytoplasmic antibody (ANCA)–associated vasculitides (AAVs) have known associations with characteristic autoantibodies. Fig. 83.1 shows the major types of vasculitides. Although the ACR and CHCC definitions were not designed as diagnostic criteria, classification criteria such as these are important in clinical research study design, treatment, and prognosis. The ACR and the European League Against Rheumatism (EULAR) are currently in the process of refining diagnostic and classification criteria for primary vasculitides.

Determining the incidence and prevalence of each of the vasculitides is challenging given the rarity of the disorders, imperfect classification criteria and definitions for epidemiologic purposes, and some clinicopathologic overlaps that occur between certain types (e.g., AAVs).

Small Vessel Vasculitis
ANCA-Associated Vasculitides

Granulomatosis with polyangiitis (GPA; previously known as Wegener's granulomatosis), microscopic polyangiitis (MPA), eosinophilic granulomatosis with polyangiitis (EGPA; previously known as Churg-Strauss syndrome), and renal-limited vasculitis (RLV) affect small and medium-sized blood vessels and may be associated with ANCA. Various studies have shown AAVs to have an incidence of approximately 10 to 20 per million. The peak age at onset is 65 to 74 years, with a female-to-male ratio of 1.5:1. EGPA is the least common of the AAVs, with an incidence of approximately 1.0 to 3.0 per million, and it also has a weaker association with ANCA than GPA and MPA.

Henoch-Schönlein Purpura

Henoch-Schönlein purpura (HSP) is a small vessel vasculitis that occurs most frequently in young children, with a peak age at onset of 4 to 6 years, but can also occur in adults. HSP accounts for almost half of all cases of childhood vasculitis. In children younger than 17 years of age, the annual incidence of HSP is approximately 20 per 100,000. Males are more commonly affected than females (approximately 2:1), and HSP occurs more frequently during the winter and spring months.

Medium Vessel Vasculitis

Polyarteritis nodosa (PAN) is a medium vessel vasculitis that is characterized by arterial aneurysmal and stenotic lesions of muscular arteries, often located at segmental and branch points. In contrast to small vessel vasculitis, renal involvement in PAN is not characterized by glomerulonephritis but rather by aneurysms and stenoses of renal arteries that may result in hypertension or renal dysfunction or both. In addition, ANCAs are usually negative in PAN. PAN may occur either as a primary vasculitis or secondary to viral infections, mainly hepatitis B or C, or human immunodeficiency virus (HIV). Determining the incidence of this vasculitis is difficult, because PAN and MPA were not differentiated until 1994.

Kawasaki disease is a medium vessel vasculitis most often seen in boys younger than 5 years of age. It is the second most common vasculitis in childhood after HSP, accounting for about 23% of all childhood vasculitis cases. In the United States, the annual incidence in children younger than 5 years old is 20 per 100,000.

Large Vessel Vasculitis

Giant cell arteritis (GCA), also known as temporal arteritis, is the most common form of vasculitis in adults. It is a large vessel vasculitis that typically affects patients of Eastern European descent, with a mean age at onset of 70 to 75 years. It affects women more commonly than men (3:1). About 40% of patients with GCA have the related condition, polymyalgia rheumatica (PMR), which is characterized by subacute onset of aching and stiffness in the muscles of the neck, shoulder girdle, and hip girdle. However, only 10% to 25% of patients with PMR have or will develop GCA.

Takayasu's arteritis (TAK), or "pulseless disease," is a rare large vessel vasculitis that was initially identified in young women from East Asia but is now described worldwide. In adults, the female-to-male ratio is about 8:1, with an average age at diagnosis in the mid-20s.

PATHOLOGY

For most of the systemic vasculitides, the etiology and pathogenesis of disease are largely unknown. It has been proposed that a number of diverse mechanisms contribute to the development of vascular inflammation and subsequent injury on the background of genetic susceptibility (Fig. 83.2). Proposed triggers of disease include infection and environmental exposures (e.g., chemicals, pollutants). For most vasculitides, these associations remain speculative.

Humoral and cellular immune responses, cytokine release, chemokine activation, and immune complex deposition are important in disease pathogenesis. Normal protective and repair processes in the vessel can also contribute to injury and ischemia. For example, after injury, cellular migration and proliferation occurring as

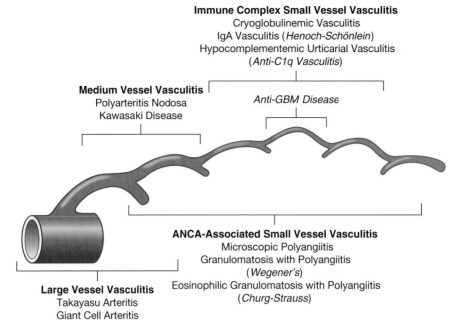

Fig. 83.1 The vascular spectrum of the vasculitides. (From Jennette JC, Falk RJ, Bacon PA, et al: 2012 revised International Chapel Hill Consensus Conference Nomenclature of Vasculitides. *Arthritis Rheum* 2013;65:1-11.)

part of vessel repair can result in intimal hyperplasia, and the procoagulant milieu that is protective against hemorrhage may lead to thrombosis and vessel occlusion. Impairment of blood flow in injured vessels results in tissue ischemia and damage. The degree of blood flow impairment varies along a broad spectrum of severity and may depend on the type of vasculitis as well as the size and location of the vessels involved.

Among the AAVs, the pathology of GPA is typically characterized by necrotizing granulomatous inflammation of small blood vessels supplying the upper and lower respiratory tract. In both GPA and MPA, renal pathology shows a pauci-immune necrotizing crescentic glomerulonephritis. In EGPA, there is a strong association with allergic and atopic disorders, including allergic rhinitis, nasal polyposis, and asthma. Approximately 70% of patients with EGPA have elevated levels of immunoglobulin E (IgE) and eosinophilia of peripheral blood and tissue. Small vessel histopathology typically reveals transmural eosinophilic infiltrates with scattered plasma cells and lymphocytes and extravascular granulomas.

The pathology of HSP is characterized by a leukocytoclastic vasculitis of small vessels with IgA deposition seen on immunofluorescence. Various infectious agents, including bacteria and viruses, have been reported as triggers for HSP.

The pathology of GCA and TAK are very similar histologically. In both, large vessels demonstrate a lymphoplasmacytic inflammatory infiltrate. Giant cells and granulomas may be seen in the media, and lumen-occlusive arteritis may occur from exuberant intimal hyperplasia. Additional pathologic features include proliferation of vascular smooth muscle cells and fragmentation of the internal elastic lamina.

CLINICAL PRESENTATION AND DIAGNOSIS

Clinical manifestations of the systemic vasculitides are diverse and differ not only among disorders but also among patients. Typical clinical manifestations associated with the size of the affected vessel are detailed in Table 83.1. Fever, weight loss, malaise, anorexia, arthralgias, and myalgias may occur with all vasculitides.

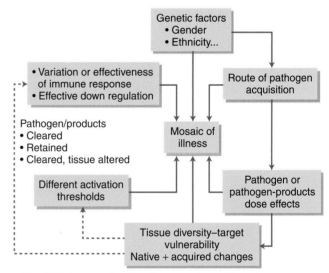

Fig. 83.2 Factors affecting disease vulnerability and expression.

Small Vessel Vasculitis
ANCA-Associated Vasculitides

GPA most commonly affects the sinuses and upper airway, the lungs, and the kidneys, although almost any organ system may be affected. Chronic refractory sinusitis, nasal crusting and ulcers, epistaxis, septal perforations, and otitis media are common presenting manifestations. Chronic nasal cartilaginous inflammation and destruction may lead to the characteristic "saddle nose" deformity. Lung involvement in GPA or MPA can include pulmonary nodules (often cavitary in GPA), infiltrates, or diffuse alveolar hemorrhage due to capillaritis. Importantly, life-threatening pulmonary hemorrhage may manifest simply as progressive acute dyspnea with hypoxia or respiratory failure, and not necessarily hemoptysis. Laryngotracheal disease may manifest as hoarseness or subglottic stenosis; orbital pseudotumors can also occur from GPA, and they may cause optic nerve compression, proptosis, and/or extraocular muscle palsies.

TABLE 83.1 Typical Clinical Features Based on Vessel Size[a]

Large	Medium	Small
Limb claudication	Cutaneous nodules	Purpura
Asymmetrical blood pressures	Ulcers	Vesiculobullous lesions
Absence of pulses	Livedo reticularis	Alveolar hemorrhage
Bruits	Digital gangrene	Glomerulonephritis
Aortic dilatation	Mononeuritis multiplex	Mononeuritis multiplex
Aortic primary branch stenoses and/or aneurysms	Microaneurysms of mesenteric and/or renal branch arteries	Cutaneous extravascular necrotizing granulomas
		Splinter hemorrhages
		Scleritis, episcleritis, uveitis

[a]Constitutional symptoms in all types are fever, weight loss, malaise, anorexia, arthralgias, and myalgias.

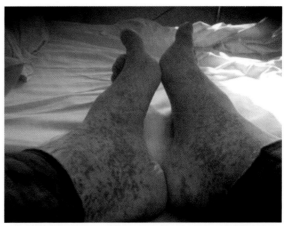

Fig. 83.3 Palpable purpura on the lower extremities of a patient with small vessel vasculitis affecting the skin. These lesions are "palpable" because they are slightly raised (i.e., palpable even with the eyes closed), and they are typically nonblanching when palpated. (Modified from Molyneux ID, Moon T, Webb AK, Morice AH: Treatment of cystic fibrosis associated cutaneous vasculitis with chloroquine, *J Cystic Fibrosis* 9:439-441, 2010. Copyright 2010 European Cystic Fibrosis Society.)

The renal manifestations in GPA, MPA, or RLV are those of nephritic syndrome, including acute renal failure, hematuria, hypertension, and subnephrotic proteinuria. Urine microscopy may reveal dysmorphic red blood cells. Renal biopsy reveals pauci-immune necrotizing crescentic glomerulonephritis. Additional organ manifestations that may occur in either GPA or MPA include neurologic, cutaneous, musculoskeletal, cardiovascular, and constitutional signs and symptoms. Patients may have subacute symptoms (weeks to months of sinusitis, arthralgias, and fatigue) or may exhibit acute "pulmonary-renal syndrome" with rapidly progressive glomerulonephritis and life-threatening alveolar hemorrhage with respiratory failure.

In EGPA, the clinical features comprise severe asthma, eosinophilia (>1500 cells/mL), and vasculitis involving two or more organs. Additional organ involvement in EGPA may include the nervous system, kidneys, skin, heart, and gastrointestinal tract. Sinus involvement in EGPA is typically not destructive as in GPA, and pulmonary infiltrates may be fleeting.

The diagnosis of any of the AAVs is most frequently established by tissue biopsy (e.g., kidney, lung, skin, sinus, nerve). ANCA testing plays an important diagnostic role in suspected small vessel vasculitis and is helpful in differentiating between GPA and MPA. Almost 90% of patients with renal disease have positive ANCA on testing. Most GPA patients have the cytoplasmic (cANCA) antiproteinase 3 (anti-PR3) type, whereas most MPA patients have the perinuclear (pANCA) antimyeloperoxidase (anti-MPO) type. The differential diagnosis for positive ANCA testing includes drug-induced effects, infections, and other autoimmune conditions. EGPA can be distinguished from other AAVs on the basis of a prior history of adult-onset asthma or allergic rhinitis and blood or tissue eosinophilia.

The differential diagnosis for any small vessel vasculitis includes infection, disorders of coagulation, drug toxicity, atherosclerotic and embolic disease, malignancy, and secondary vasculitides associated with other autoimmune diseases.

Henoch-Schönlein Purpura

Patients with HSP have lower extremity purpura, arthritis (typically of the large joints), abdominal pain, and renal disease at presentation (Fig. 83.3). In children, arthritis and abdominal pain affect about 75% of patients; the gastrointestinal manifestations may precede the purpura by up to 2 weeks and include hematochezia. The most common renal manifestation is microscopic hematuria with or without proteinuria.

The diagnosis of HSP is most often based on clinical and laboratory evidence, although skin or renal biopsy revealing IgA deposition may be helpful in solidifying the diagnosis. By classification criteria from the EULAR, patients with HSP must have purpura or petechiae with lower limb predominance and at least one of the following: arthritis or arthralgias; abdominal pain; histopathology demonstrating IgA deposition; and renal involvement. The differential for HSP includes other causes of abdominal pain, other causes of purpura in childhood, and hypersensitivity vasculitis. Hypersensitivity vasculitis is also a small vessel vasculitis that may occur in both children and adults and may be idiopathic or triggered by infections or drug exposures. It typically manifests as an isolated cutaneous leukocytoclastic (neutrophils and neutrophil debris in small vessels) vasculitis that is self-limited with treatment of the underlying cause (e.g., treatment of infection, discontinuation of drug culprit).

Medium Vessel Vasculitis
Polyarteritis Nodosa

The most common organ systems affected in PAN are the gastrointestinal, renal, and nervous systems. Mesenteric aneurysms or stenoses resulting in gut ischemia lead to symptoms of abdominal pain or "intestinal angina" (pain after eating). Renal artery aneurysms or stenoses result in hypertension or renal dysfunction, rather than glomerulonephritis as in MPA. Neurologic involvement may manifest as mononeuritis multiplex (painful asymmetrical sensory and motor peripheral neuropathy involving at least two separate nerve areas). Orchitis may be seen, manifesting as acute testicular pain. Anemia, elevated erythrocyte sedimentation rate or C-reactive protein or both, and hypertension (if renal artery involvement is present) are common. As in all vasculitides, constitutional symptoms may also be present.

The diagnosis of PAN is made based on angiographic or biopsy findings in the appropriate clinical setting. ANCAs typically are absent in PAN. A work-up for infection, including tests for hepatitis B and C and HIV, is warranted, given their known associations with PAN. The differential diagnosis includes MPA and mixed cryoglobulinemic vasculitis (defined by the presence of cryoglobulins in the blood). The latter vasculitis shares many clinical features with PAN, including peripheral neuropathy, arthralgias, myalgias, purpura, and association with hepatitis C.

Kawasaki Disease

The clinical presentation of Kawasaki disease includes fever lasting longer than 5 days, conjunctival injection, oropharyngeal changes (strawberry tongue, mucous membrane desquamation), peripheral extremity changes (cutaneous desquamation), polymorphous rash, and cervical lymphadenopathy. Arthralgias, abdominal pain, hepatitis, aseptic meningitis, and uveitis have also been reported. Coronary artery aneurysms, one of the most serious complications of this vasculitis, appear within the first 4 weeks after onset of disease and are often detectable with echocardiography. Although areas of ectasia and small aneurysms may regress, larger aneurysms often persist and can result in coronary ischemia at any time after development, even into adulthood. Kawasaki disease is a triphasic disease, consisting of an acute febrile period lasting up to 14 days, a subacute phase of 2 to 4 weeks, and a convalescent phase that can last months to years. In the acute phase, the fever is persistent and high (>38.5° C) and is minimally responsive to antipyretics.

The differential diagnosis is wide and includes viral infections, toxin-mediated illnesses (e.g., toxic shock syndrome, scarlet fever), systemic juvenile idiopathic arthritis, hypersensitivity reactions, and drug reactions (e.g., Stevens-Johnson syndrome).

Large Vessel Vasculitis
Giant Cell Arteritis or Temporal Arteritis

At presentation, patients with GCA most commonly have new continuous headache, jaw claudication, visual disturbances (e.g., amaurosis fugax, diplopia), fatigue, and arthralgias. They are usually older than 50 years of age, have tender or thickened temporal arteries, and have an elevated erythrocyte sedimentation rate (>50 mm/hr by the Westergren method). Disease onset may be insidious or acute. Blindness due to anterior ischemic optic neuropathy occurs in 10% to 15% of patients with GCA and can occur at disease onset. Given the association between GCA and PMR, patients with PMR should be educated regarding signs and symptoms of GCA, and patients with GCA should be monitored for symptoms of PMR.

The diagnosis of GCA is often made by a biopsy of the superficial temporal artery. It is important to obtain a sufficient length of tissue (2 to 3 cm) because the vasculitis can have "skip lesions."

Takayasu's Arteritis

The typical clinical manifestations of TAK include a systolic blood pressure difference of greater than 10 mm Hg between the arms, decreased brachial or radial artery pulses, bruits auscultated over the subclavian arteries or aorta, claudication of extremities, neck or jaw pain, headache, dizziness, hypertension, constitutional symptoms, arthralgias, and myalgias.

The diagnosis of TAK is often based on vascular imaging studies that demonstrate long, tapering stenotic lesions or aneurysmal lesions in the aorta and primary branches. The differential diagnosis includes syphilis, spondyloarthropathies, rheumatoid arthritis, inflammatory bowel disease, and connective tissue disorders. Vascular imaging studies including computed tomographic angiography and magnetic resonance angiography are typically performed for both diagnosis and disease surveillance.

TREATMENT AND PROGNOSIS

Small Vessel Vasculitis
ANCA-Associated Vasculitides

Glucocorticoids, often with other agents, are uniformly used to induce and maintain remission in AAV. They are typically initiated at a prednisone equivalent dose of 1 mg/kg/day with or without pulse methylprednisolone (1 g IV daily × 3 days), followed by a gradual taper over approximately 6 to 12 months. In addition, the standard of care in both GPA and MPA has traditionally been cyclophosphamide, either oral or intravenous, for 3 to 6 months. This yields remission rates varying from 30% to 93% in GPA and from 75% to 89% in MPA.

Rituximab, an anti-CD20 chimeric monoclonal antibody that depletes B cells, was shown to be noninferior to cyclophosphamide in remission induction for AAV in several randomized controlled trials (RITUXVAS and RAVE trials).

Plasmapheresis, or plasma exchange therapy (PLEX), is often used in combination with remission induction therapy in patients with life-threatening disease such as alveolar hemorrhage, or rapidly progressive glomerulonephritis (pulmonary-renal syndrome). The MEPEX study was a randomized controlled trial comparing plasmapheresis with high-dose methylprednisolone for severe renal vasculitis. PLEX was shown to be superior to methylprednisolone in reducing the number of patients remaining dependent on dialysis. The PEXIVAS trial is an ongoing multicenter randomized trial evaluating adjunctive PLEX and two oral glucocorticoid regimens in severe AAV.

For limited (early) GPA, such as disease confined to the upper respiratory tract, methotrexate may be used for remission induction, rather than cyclophosphamide; this conclusion was supported by evidence in the NORAM trial. Trimethoprim-sulfamethoxazole was shown in two randomized controlled trials to be helpful in preventing relapses after remission induction in GPA.

For EGPA, mepolizumab, an anti–interleukin-5 monoclonal antibody, has recently been shown in a multicenter double-blind placebo-controlled trial to be superior to placebo in producing a higher proportion of patients in remission and longer duration of remission in those who were relapsing or refractory to standard therapy. Only 47% of those in the mepolizumab group relapsed, compared to 81% of those in the placebo group, over 52 weeks. Hence, mepolizumab is now being used as a steroid-sparing therapy in EGPA patients who are relapsing or refractory to standard therapy.

Remission maintenance therapies in AAV include methotrexate, azathioprine, mycophenolate mofetil, and rituximab (RTX). Because there are known risks of bladder cancer, hemorrhagic cystitis, and bone marrow suppression with cumulative use of cyclophosphamide, it no longer has a role in remission maintenance in AAV. The role of RTX in remission maintenance has recently shown strong evidence of efficacy based on the MAINRITSAN Trial. In this study, patients with newly diagnosed or relapsing GPA, MPA, or renal-limited ANCA-associated vasculitis (RLV) in complete remission were recruited after a cyclophosphamide-glucocorticoid regimen. Patients were randomly assigned to receive either 500 mg of RTX on days 0 and 14 and at months 6, 12, and 18 after study entry, or daily azathioprine until month 22. At month 28, major relapse had occurred in 29% in the azathioprine group and 5% in the RTX group. RTX is now also being used to maintain remission in AAV.

Although AAVs were once considered diseases with considerable mortality (80% at 2 years if left untreated), the prognosis has improved significantly over the last 30 years because of improved treatments. Patient survival is now reported to be as high as 45% to 91% at 5 years. Among AAV patients with renal involvement at presentation, 20% develop end-stage renal disease within 5 years.

Henoch-Schönlein Purpura

In mild cases, the therapy for HSP is simply supportive care (i.e., hydration and analgesics). However, glucocorticoids are commonly used to hasten the resolution of symptoms; early use of glucocorticoids has been associated with improved outcomes, especially when there is severe gastrointestinal involvement. In life-threatening cases and in severe acute renal failure, additional immunosuppressive agents or plasmapheresis may be considered. The prognosis of HSP is generally good, with fewer than 1% of patients developing end-stage renal disease.

Medium Vessel Vasculitis
Polyarteritis Nodosa

Treatment of PAN includes glucocorticoids or nonsteroidal anti-inflammatory drugs (NSAIDs) or both. If disease is severe and persistent or relapsing, additional immunosuppressive agents are used, such as cyclophosphamide (especially for gastrointestinal or cardiac involvement), methotrexate, colchicine, or intravenous immunoglobulin (IVIG). In cases of PAN associated with hepatitis B or C, antiviral therapy is required not only for attaining control of the viral infection but also for treatment of the associated vasculitis itself. Corticosteroids and cyclophosphamide have improved patient outcomes, and the 1-year survival rate is now 85%. Prognosis is typically worse with more systemic complications such as renal or neurologic involvement.

Kawasaki Disease

Treatment of Kawasaki disease includes high-dose aspirin (30 to 100 mg/kg/day) for the first 48 hours, then 3 to 5 mg/kg/day. IVIG is standard therapy and has significantly decreased the incidence of coronary artery aneurysm complications in this disease. The initial IVIG dose is 2 g/kg within the first 10 days after presentation, with at least one repeat dose typically given if the first IVIG dose fails to improve the child's condition. The prognosis of Kawasaki disease, if promptly treated, is good; however, approximately 15% to 25% of patients develop coronary artery aneurysms that increase morbidity and mortality.

Large Vessel Vasculitis
Giant Cell Arteritis or Temporal Arteritis

Glucocorticoids are the cornerstone of therapy in GCA. To prevent vision loss, treatment should be instituted immediately (within 24 hours) if clinical suspicion for GCA is high or if visual disturbances are present. The initial dose of glucocorticoids is typically 1 mg/kg/day with a gradual taper. Most patients require a glucocorticoid treatment duration of 1 to 2 years, but it may be longer, especially in those with symptoms of PMR. In PMR without GCA, lower doses of glucocorticoids (10 to 20 mg/day of prednisone equivalent) are effective and provide prompt clinical response.

If patients experience relapse with glucocorticoid tapering, other immunosuppressive agents may be used. Methotrexate was shown in a meta-analysis of three randomized controlled trials to be a beneficial adjunctive agent in reducing risks of first and second relapses in GCA, with a significant decrease in the cumulative dose of glucocorticoids. Low-dose aspirin is an important adjunctive therapy in protecting against cranial ischemic events (level II evidence from two large retrospective studies). Recently, tocilizumab given subcutaneously weekly or every other week with a 26-week prednisone taper was found in a large 1-year randomized trial of GCA patients to result in more sustained glucocorticoid-free remission compared to either 26-week or 52-week prednisone tapering courses plus placebo. Hence, tocilizumab is now being used as an effective steroid-sparing agent to maintain remission in GCA.

Takayasu's Arteritis

Glucocorticoids are also the cornerstone of therapy for TAK; they are typically initiated at a dose of 0.5 to 1 mg/kg/day. Although most patients respond to the initial dose, relapses occur in more than 50% of patients during glucocorticoid tapering. Hence, steroid-sparing agents

are often used to aid in maintaining disease remission. The most commonly used steroid-sparing agents are methotrexate and azathioprine. In TAK, unlike in GCA and PMR, the tumor necrosis factor (TNF) inhibitors have shown promise in treating refractory disease. As in GCA, low-dose aspirin is believed to play a beneficial adjunctive role in preventing ischemic complications.

Revascularization interventions are often indicated in patients with TAK whose presenting symptoms include cerebrovascular disease, coronary artery disease, moderate to severe aortic regurgitation, renovascular hypertension, progressive limb claudication, or progressive aneurysm enlargement. Elective intervention should be performed when the disease is quiescent.

In both GCA and TAK, aortitis—a common manifestation of large vessel involvement—can lead to an increased risk of aortic aneurysm and subsequent dissection and rupture. In both GCA and TAK, disease flares occur in most patients, rendering them chronic, progressive, and relapsing conditions.

ADDITIONAL CONSIDERATIONS IN TREATMENT

Immunosuppressive therapy is associated with an increased risk of infection. Patients receiving combination therapy with moderate- to high-dose glucocorticoid (>20 mg/day of prednisone equivalents) and another immunosuppressive agent should also receive prophylaxis for *Pneumocystis jirovecii* pneumonia (previously known as PCP). Furthermore, infections can often mimic or result in flares of systemic vasculitis. Glucocorticoid therapy should never be discontinued abruptly, even in the setting of infection, because of the risk of adrenal crisis or disease relapse or both. In most cases, other immunosuppressive agents should be discontinued if infection is suspected or diagnosed.

Glucocorticoid therapy is a common cause of bone loss (osteopenia, osteoporosis). Because significant bone loss can occur even within the first 6 months of therapy, calcium and vitamin D supplementation should be initiated, and a baseline bone density study should be obtained. Consideration should be given to additional bone protection therapies (e.g., bisphosphonates). Methotrexate and cyclophosphamide are teratogenic, and cyclophosphamide may result in premature ovarian failure. These factors must be considered when choosing therapies for women of child-bearing age. Immunosuppressive agents also can be associated with bone marrow suppression and with additional long-term risks such as malignancy.

Acknowledgments

The author wishes to acknowledge the assistance of Kathleen Maksimowicz-McKinnon, DO.

For a deeper discussion on this topic, please see Chapter 254, "The Systemic Vasculitides," in *Goldman-Cecil Medicine,* 26th Edition.

SUGGESTED READINGS

Bloch DA, Michel BA, Hunder GG, et al: The American College of Rheumatology 1990 criteria for the classification of vasculitis: patients and methods, Arthritis Rheum 33:1068–1073, 1990.

Guillevin L, Pagnoux C, Karras A, et al: Rituximab versus azathioprine for maintenance in ANCA-associated vasculitis, N Engl J Med 371:1771–1780, 2014.

Hoffman GS, Cid MC, Rendt-Zagar KE, et al: Infliximab for maintenance of glucocorticosteroid-induced remission of giant cell arteritis: a randomized trial, Ann Intern Med 146:621–630, 2007.

Hunder GG, Bloch DA, Michel BA, et al: The American College of Rheumatology 1990 criteria for the classification of giant cell arteritis, Arthritis Rheum 33:1122–1128, 1990.

Jennette JC, Falk RJ, Bacon PA, et al: 2012 revised International Chapel Hill Consensus Conference Nomenclature of vasculitides, Arthritis Rheum 65:1–11, 2013.

Jones RB, Tervaert JW, Hauser T, et al: Rituximab versus cyclophosphamide in ANCA-associated renal vasculitis, N Engl J Med 363:211–220, 2010.

Specks U, Merkel PA, Seo P, et al: Efficacy of remission-induction regimens for ANCA-associated vasculitis, N Engl J Med 369:417–427, 2013.

Stone JH, Merkel PA, Spiera R, et al: Rituximab versus cyclophosphamide for ANCA-associated vasculitis, N Engl J Med 363:221–232, 2010.

Stone JH, Tuckwell K, Dimonaco S, et al: Trial of tocilizumab in giant cell arteritis, N Engl J Med 337:317–328, 2017.

Wechsler ME, Akuthota P, Jayne D, et al: Mepolizumab or placebo for eosinophilic granulomatosis with polyangiitis, N Engl J Med 376:1921–1932, 2017.

Weiss PF: Pediatric vasculitis, Pediatr Clin North Am 59:407–423, 2012.

84

Crystal Arthropathies

Pooja Bhadbhade, Ghaith Noaiseh

GOUT

Gout is a disorder resulting from deposition of monosodium urate (MSU) monohydrate crystals in and around the tissues of joints causing attacks of acute inflammatory arthritis. Gout is associated with hyperuricemia, which is defined as a serum urate level greater than 6.8 mg/dL. The risk of gout is strongly associated with the degree of hyperuricemia. However, it is not a sufficient causative factor for the development of gout.

Typically, the disease presents as an acute and episodic monoarthritis affecting the lower extremities but can become recurrent, chronic, and deforming, affecting multiple joints. Tophi are a pathognomonic feature of gout resulting from accumulation of urate crystals in soft tissues or joints.

Epidemiology

In the United States, the prevalence of gout is 3.9%, affecting 8.3 million adults. The incidence rate ranges from 0.45 to 1 cases per 1000 person-years. There is a trend towards increasing incidence and prevalence, thought to be related to the aging population, increased use of certain medications such as diuretics, and the increasing frequency of risk factors for hyperuricemia including obesity, hypertension, renal disease, cardiovascular disease, and metabolic syndrome.

Men are three to six times more likely to have gout than women, but the sex disparity decreases with age due to loss of the uricosuric effect of estrogen after menopause. This also explains why gout is less common in premenopausal women.

Pathogenesis
Pathophysiology of Hyperuricemia

Uric acid is the end product of purine metabolism in humans. Unlike many other species, humans lack the enzyme uricase, which catalyzes the conversion of uric acid into allantoin, a very soluble metabolite. Most individuals maintain uric acid levels between 4 and 6.8 mg/dL and a total body uric acid pool of approximately 1000 mg. However, uric acid levels may increase, leading to supersaturation of urate in blood. MSU crystals form in some patients with serum uric acid levels greater than 6.8 mg/dL. Only about 20% of hyperuricemic patients develop gout during their lifetime. Factors controlling crystal formation are poorly understood, but urate solubility may be affected by temperature, pH, salt concentration, and cartilage matrix components. Urate crystallization is a critical step in the progression from asymptomatic hyperuricemia to clinical gout. Unlike soluble urate molecules, MSU crystals are a potent promoter of acute inflammation.

The total body uric acid pool depends on the balance between dietary intake, synthesis, and excretion. About two thirds of the daily excretion of uric acid occurs in the kidneys; the rest is eliminated by the gut. Renal underexcretion is the cause for approximately 90% of hyperuricemia cases (Table 84.1). In the remaining 10%, hyperuricemia is caused by uric acid overproduction (>1000 mg in a 24-hour urine collection while on a standard Western diet) or by a combination of overproduction with renal underexcretion.

Fig. 84.1 summarizes the de novo biosynthesis and salvage pathways of purine metabolism. Abnormalities in the activities of key enzymes can lead to increased serum uric acid levels and development of gout. The de novo synthesis of purine is driven by the enzyme 5′-phosphoribosyl 1-pyrophosphate (PRPP) synthetase. In PRPP synthetase overactivity, overproduction of PRPP increases purine production. In salvage pathways, tissue-derived intermediate purine products (hypoxanthine, guanine, and adenine) are reutilized rather than undergoing further degradation to xanthine and uric acid. Deficiencies of hypoxanthine-guanine phosphoribosyltransferase (HGPRT) activity result in impaired purine salvage and increased substrate for uric acid generation (Lysch-Nyhan syndrome and Kelley-Seegmiller syndrome). Overall, inborn errors of metabolism account for a small fraction of uric acid overproduction.

Most cases of uric acid overproduction result from increased reutilization of purine bases through salvage pathways (see Fig. 84.1). The purine precursors come from exogenous (dietary) sources or endogenous metabolism (synthesis and cell turnover) Purine-rich foods such as red meat, organ meats (e.g., sweetbreads, liver), seafood, high-fructose corn syrup–sweetened beverages, and alcohol comprise a significant portion of the daily purine load and can worsen hyperuricemia. On the other hand, consumption of low-fat dairy products is associated with reduced serum urate levels and may decrease the risk of gout.

A very small proportion of serum urate is bound to plasma proteins; therefore, urate is almost completely filtered in the glomeruli. Subsequent reabsorption and secretion are controlled by various organic acid transporters located on the luminal side of the proximal convoluted tubule epithelium. Only 10% of the initially filtered uric acid is eventually excreted in the urine.

In addition to the bidirectional transport of uric acid, organic acid transporters are also responsible for eliminating other organic acids and certain medications. The function of these transporters is affected by certain medications, including thiazides, low-dose aspirin, and cyclosporine, leading to decreased uric acid excretion and hyperuricemia. Conversely, medications such as probenecid and losartan, when excreted in the tubular lumen, exert their uricosuric effect by displacing uric acid from the transporter and increasing uric acid excretion. Certain genetic mutations affecting these transporters may lead to uric acid underexcretion. Renal insufficiency can cause hyperuricemia though decreased uric acid filtration.

Pathophysiology of Acute Gouty Attack

In some patients with prolonged hyperuricemia, tissue deposits of MSU crystals, called microtophi, form in the synovium and on the

TABLE 84.1   Causes of Hyperuricemia

Urate Overproduction	Urate Underexcretion
Metabolic Disorders	Renal insufficiency
HGPRT deficiency (homozygous or heterozygous)	Volume depletion
PRPP synthetase hyperactivity	Metabolic acidosis (lactic acidosis and ketoacidosis)
G6PD deficiency	Obesity
Glycogen storage diseases	Ethanol
	Medications: low-dose salicylate, diuretics (thiazides, loop diuretics), cyclosporine, tacrolimus, L-dopa, ethambutol
Others	
Myeloproliferative and lymphoproliferative disorders	Familial juvenile hyperuricemic nephropathy
Erythropoietic disorders (hemolytic anemia, megaloblastic anemia, sickle cell disease, thalassemia, other hemoglobinopathies)	Medullary cystic kidney disease
	Lead nephropathy
Solid tumors	
Diffuse psoriasis	
Ethanol (particularly beer)	
Medications: cytotoxic agents, nicotinic acid	
Shellfish, organ meat, red meat	
Fructose	
Obesity	

G6PD, Glucose-6-phosphate dehydrogenase; *HGPRT,* hypoxanthine-guanine phosphoribosyltransferase; *PRPP,* 5-phosphoribosyl 1-pyrophosphate.

surface of cartilage. During an acute attack, microtophi break apart, shedding a large number of MSU crystals into the joint space and activating synovial macrophages and fibroblasts that phagocytize the crystals. This, in turn, leads to the activation of a cytosolic multiprotein complex, the NALP3 (NACHT, LRR, and PYD domains–containing protein 3) inflammasome (Fig. 84.2). There is evidence that in acute gout, MSU crystals undergo phagocytosis, which activates the NLRP3 inflammasome, leading to the release of interleukin-1β, which in turn induces further production of interleukin-1β and other inflammatory mediators and activation of synovial lining cells and phagocytes.

MSU crystals undergo clearance by inflammatory cells that then undergo apoptosis. This, along with other mechanisms, eventually leads to resolution of the acute inflammatory process, typically after 10 to 14 days. Even after complete resolution of symptoms, a low-grade level of inflammation (intercritical inflammation) can persist in the otherwise asymptomatic joint. This inflammation may become clinically apparent in long-standing gout, contributing to development of tophi, chronic synovitis, cartilage loss, and bony erosions.

Clinical Features

Gout has three stages: asymptomatic hyperuricemia, acute intermittent gout, and chronic gout.

Acute Gouty Attacks

The classic picture of acute gout is rapid development of an inflammatory arthritis involving one or occasionally two joints. Severe pain, erythema, swelling, and exquisite tenderness typically occur. This clinical picture can be easily confused with that of septic arthritis or bacterial

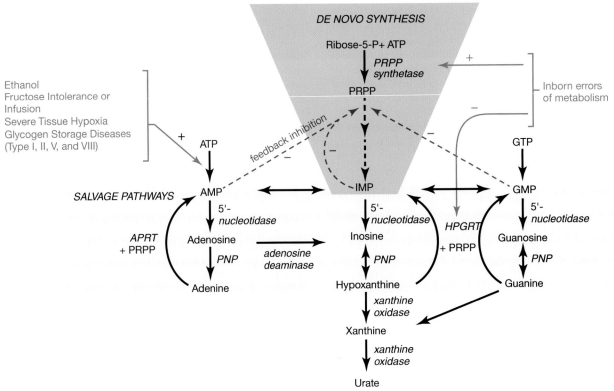

Fig. 84.1 The steps in the urate production pathways implicated in the pathogenesis of hyperuricemia and gout. *ADP,* Adenosine diphosphate; *APRT,* adenine phosphoribosyl transferase; *ATP,* adenosine triphosphate; *GMP,* guanosine monophosphate; *GTB,* guanosine triphosphate; *HPGRT,* hypoxanthine-guanine phosphoribosyl transferase; *IMP,* inosine monophosphate; *PNP,* purine nucleotide phosphorylase; *PRPP,* 5′-ribosyl 1-pyrophosphate. (From Choi HK: Epidemiology, pathology, and pathogenesis, chap 12. In Stone JH, Crofford LJ, White PH, editors: Primer on the rheumatic diseases, ed 13, New York, 2008, Springer.)

cellulitis, because many patients can mount an intense systemic inflammatory response with fever, chills, and elevated inflammatory markers. The most commonly involved joints are the first metatarsophalangeal joint (podagra), followed by the joints of the ankle, midfoot, and knee. The pain intensifies over 8 to 24 hours. Acute attacks usually resolve, even without therapy, within 5 to 14 days. The clinical resolution is complete, and the patient is asymptomatic between attacks. Subsequently, involvement of the upper extremities can occur, affecting the small joints of the hands, wrists, and elbows.

Attack-provoking factors include use of diuretics, alcohol, surgery, trauma, and consumption of foods containing high purine levels. Each of these can cause fluctuation in serum urate levels. Initiation of urate-lowering therapy can trigger attacks in the early phase by the same mechanism.

Chronic Gout

This phase, called chronic gout (also referred to as *chronic tophaceous gout* or *chronic advanced gout*), typically develops 10 or more years after the onset of acute attacks. Transition to the chronic phase occurs if hyperuricemia is inadequately treated. During this transition, the intercritical periods are no longer free of pain. The involved joints become persistently uncomfortable and swollen, although the intensity of these symptoms is significantly less pronounced compared to acute attacks. On top of this persistent background pain, acute gouty attacks continue to occur, especially in the absence of therapy. Polyarticular involvement becomes much more frequent during this time, including joints of the upper limbs.

The pathognomonic feature of chronic gout is the *tophus*, a palpable collection of MSU crystals in soft tissue or joints. It is detected in about 75% of patients who have had gout for more than 20 years. The severity and duration of hyperuricemia determine the likelihood of tophus development. While tophi most often occur over the first metatarsophalangeal

joint, fingers, wrist, olecranon bursa, and helix of the ear, they can occur anywhere in the body. Infiltration of tophi into bone is thought to be the driving mechanism for bone erosion and joint damage in gout.

Diagnosis

The typical presentation of acute gouty arthritis in a characteristic joint distribution is strongly suggestive of the diagnosis, particularly if history of similar attacks that completely resolved is reported. However, detection of MSU crystals in the synovial fluid, bursa or tophus remains the diagnostic "gold standard." Arthrocentesis is not only important to confirm clinical suspicion but also to rule out septic arthritis or other crystalline arthropathies. During acute attacks, intracellular, strongly negative birefringent, needle-shaped MSU crystals are typically identified by polarized compensated microscopy. MSU crystals can also be demonstrated in tophus aspiration (Fig. 84.3A).

Septic arthritis can coexist with urate crystals in the synovial fluid; Gram stain and culture should be performed and are necessary to exclude septic arthritis. Aspirated synovial fluid appears cloudy, and analysis shows inflammatory fluid (>2000 white blood cells per microliter), usually in the 10,000 to 100,000 white blood cells per microliter range. Serum uric acid is not a diagnostically reliable test during acute flares since serum urate level may be normal or even low. Laboratory testing may reveal leukocytosis and elevated inflammatory markers, both of which are nonspecific. Between attacks, MSU crystals can often be demonstrated in previously inflamed joints, providing support to the diagnosis.

Radiologic Features

During an acute attack, a plain radiograph may only show soft tissue swelling. In chronic advanced gout, well-defined, "punched out" juxtaarticular erosions characterized by a sclerotic rim and overhanging

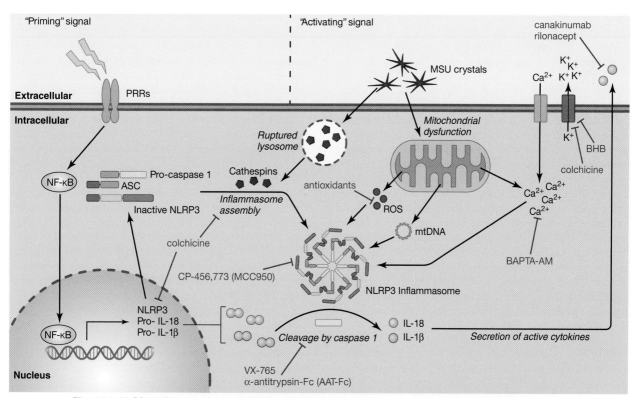

Fig. 84.2 NLRP3 inflammasome activation and potential targets in gout. *ASC,* Apoptosis-associated speck-like protein containing a CARD; *mtDNA,* mitochondrial DNA; *NF-kB,* nuclear factor kappa light-chain-enhancer of activated B cells; *PRRs,* pattern recognition receptors; *ROS,* reactive oxygen species. (From Szekanecz Z, Szamosi S, Kovács GE, et al: The NLRP3 inflammasome–interleukin 1 pathway as a therapeutic target in gout, Arch Biochem Biophys 670:82-93, 2019.)

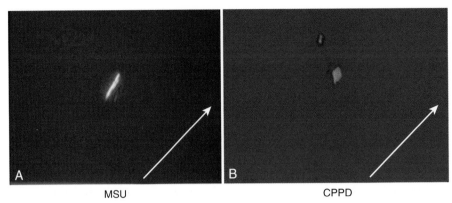

MSU   CPPD

Fig. 84.3 Polarized microscopy image of (A) strongly negative birefringent monosodium urate crystals and (B) weakly positive calcium pyrophosphate dihydrate crystals. *Arrows* indicate axis of polarization. (A, Modified from the ACR Slide Collection on the Rheumatic Diseases. Available at http://images.rheumatology.org/. Accessed January 2015; B, Modified from Saadeh C, Diamond HS: Calcium pyrophosphate deposition disease. Available at: http://emedicine.medscape.com/article/330936-overview#showall.)

edges may be seen. The joint space is preserved until late in the course of the disease. Soft tissue masses may be detected in patients with tophi.

Dual-energy CT is a useful noninvasive imaging modality that can identify and color-code urate deposits in patients with gout. Ultrasound is a promising noninvasive tool in the diagnosis and management of gout.

Gout in Transplantation Patients

Hyperuricemia occurs much more frequently in transplantation patients using cyclosporine than in the normal population. Compared to patients with classic gout, transplant patients exhibit a significantly shorter period of asymptomatic hyperuricemia (0.5 to 4 years vs. 20 to 30 years), a shorter stage of acute intermittent gout (1 to 4 years vs. 10 to 15 years), and rapid development of tophi as early as 1 year after transplantation. Gouty attacks can be atypical and less severe, in part because of the concomitant use of prednisone.

Differential Diagnosis

Acute gouty arthropathy should be distinguished from septic arthritis and other crystal-induced arthropathies such as calcium pyrophosphate dihydrate (CPPD) deposition disease. The onset of acute CPPD arthropathy is usually less abrupt, and attacks tend to last longer, up to 1 month or more. Attacks occur more often in large joints such as the knee and wrist. Forms of spondyloarthropathies including reactive arthritis, psoriatic arthritis, ankylosing spondylitis, and inflammatory bowel–related arthritis can also present with monoarticular arthritis. In these disorders, synovial fluid is inflammatory, with a leukocyte count usually in the range of 10,000 to 50,000/μL, but crystals are absent and fluid culture is negative.

The diffuse and symmetric involvement of small joints in the hands and feet seen in chronic tophaceous gout can sometimes be confused with the symmetrical polyarthritis of rheumatoid arthritis and rheumatoid nodules. Aspiration of chronically inflamed joints or a tophus can help in distinguishing the two entities.

Treatment

Management strategies should focus on treating acute attacks, long-term management of hyperuricemia, patient education, and lifestyle modification.

Management of Acute Gouty Attack

Nonsteroidal anti-inflammatory drugs (NSAIDs) (such as naproxen and indomethacin) are typically used, and all seem to be equally effective. A full dose should be immediately initiated. Therapy should be continued for 7 to 10 days to ensure complete resolution of symptoms. NSAIDs are inappropriate in patients with peptic ulcer disease, inflammatory bowel disease, or renal insufficiency, and they must be used with caution in patients at risk for cardiovascular events.

Oral colchicine can be effective if used within the first 24 to 48 hours of an acute attack. A commonly prescribed dose is 1.2 mg, followed by 0.6 mg 1 hour later in the first day, followed by dose tapering until the attack is resolved. Colchicine can cause nausea and diarrhea and therapy should be stopped if symptoms are severe. Use of intravenous colchicine is discouraged due to high risk of bone marrow suppression.

Intra-articular corticosteroid administration is a very effective therapy for patients with monoarticular or oligoarticular disease in whom other systemic therapies are contraindicated. Enteral or parenteral glucocorticosteroids are effective in patients with renal insufficiency, intolerance to NSAIDs or colchicine, or treatment resistance. This approach is usually reserved for polyarticular flares when intra-articular injection is not practical (i.e., too many involved joints). Prednisone, 30 to 50 mg daily, is commonly used.

Urate-lowering therapy (ULT) should *not* be interrupted during acute attacks. Prompt initiation of anti-inflammatory therapy at the onset of symptoms may shorten the duration of attacks.

Management of Intercritical and Chronic Gout

Urate-lowering therapy. The aim of chronic treatment is to prevent recurrent attacks and to minimize joint damage by depleting tophaceous deposits in joints and soft tissue. This is achieved by lowering uric acid level below 6 mg/dL. A target level of less than 5 mg/dL should be considered in patients with chronic tophaceous gout as this may result in a faster, more effective reduction in tophus size and flare frequency. Indications for ULT include two or more attacks in a single year, presence of tophi, chronic kidney disease CKD stage 2 or more, chronic gouty arthritis, or recurrent nephrolithiasis.

Three categories of urate-lowering therapies are available: uricostatic agents that decrease uric acid production, uricosuric agents that increase renal excretion of uric acid, and uricolytic agents that break up uric acid into other metabolites.

The optimal duration of ULT is not known, and lifelong therapy is usually recommended. ULT is typically started after resolution of an acute attack.

Uricostatic therapy. Allopurinol and febuxostat are xanthine oxidase inhibitors (XOI) that prevent urate formation. They are effective in managing gout in both overproducers and undersecretors of uric acid.

Allopurinol remains the first-line and most commonly used ULT agent, particularly in patients with chronic renal insufficiency, uric acid stones, or uric acid overproduction. If renal function is normal, a starting dose of 100 mg daily is recommended because higher doses may increase the risk of allopurinol-associated hypersensitivity, a potentially lethal complication. The risk of early flares may also be increased with higher doses. The dose should be titrated up by 100 mg increments every 2 to 5 weeks until the target uric acid level is reached. The maximal dose is 800 mg/day. Doses above 300 mg per day can be safely used in patients with renal impairment. Adverse events include rash (2%), hepatitis, vasculitis, eosinophilia, and bone marrow suppression.

Allopurinol-associated hypersensitivity is a serious side effect. Risk factors include concomitant use of thiazides and penicillin allergy. Fever, severe exfoliative dermatitis, eosinophilia, and hepatic and renal failure can occur. Febuxostat may be used in patients who do not achieve target uric acid levels despite adequate allopurinol dose titration or in patients with side effects to allopurinol.

Uricosuric therapy. Probenecid may be used as first-line ULT in uric acid undersecretors (<600 mg in a 24-hour urine collection) and in the setting of contraindication or intolerance to XOIs. Probenecid can be combined with an XOI to achieve target UA level, assuming adequate renal function. Probenecid is ineffective in patients with renal insufficiency (glomerular filtration rate <50 mL/minute) and is contraindicated in patients with nephrolithiasis. Patients should maintain high urine volume by drinking at least 1.5 L of fluid daily. Lesinurad is not used as monotherapy but can be combined with an XOI.

Uricolytic therapy. Pegloticase (pegylated recombinant uricase), administered intravenously every 2 weeks, is used in cases refractory to conventional ULT. Rasburicase, another recombinant uricase, is used to prevent tumor lysis syndrome but has no role in the management of gout.

Future directions. As previously mentioned, IL-1 is a proinflammatory cytokine that has been shown to play an important role in pathogenesis of acute gouty attacks. As a result, IL-1 antagonists have been a target for recent drug therapies (see Fig. 84.2). These include anakinra, rilonacept, and canakinumab. Anakinra has been shown to be effective at treating acute flares, whereas rilonacept may be more effective in preventing gout flares due to its longer half-life. Canakinumab may be effective for both acute flares and flare prophylaxis when used with ULT. More formal clinical trials are needed comparing these therapies with conventional gout treatment.

Non–urate-lowering prophylactic therapy. Anti-inflammatory prophylaxis using low-dose colchicine or NSAIDs is usually recommended in conjunction with ULT to decrease the risk of flares that often accompany initiation of ULT. Prophylactic treatment is usually continued for 6 months after the serum uric acid goal is achieved.

Lifestyle modifications and education. A patient newly diagnosed with gout should be evaluated for potentially modifiable risk factors and associated illnesses such as obesity, hypertension, and hyperlipidemia. Decreased consumption of high-purine food (e.g., shellfish, liver, sweetbreads) and fructose-containing beverages, as well as reduced alcohol intake, should be recommended. Diuretics should be avoided, if possible.

Treatment of hyperuricemia in patients without gout. Allopurinol and rasburicase have been used for treatment and prevention of tumor lysis syndrome–associated hyperuricemia following chemotherapy. Otherwise, there is no evidence to support their use in asymptomatic hyperuricemia.

CALCIUM PYROPHOSPHATE DIHYDRATE DEPOSITION DISEASE

CPPD deposition disease is a clinically heterogeneous disorder that is characterized by the presence of intra-articular CPPD crystals. These crystals are deposited primarily in the cartilage, in the normally unmineralized pericellular matrix of hyaline and fibrocartilage. Calcification of the cartilage is promoted by alterations in the metabolism of inorganic pyrophosphate (PPi) and extracellular matrix leading to extracellular accumulation of PPi, which is necessary to the formation of CPPD crystals. Crystals are phagocytized by resident synovial macrophages, activating the intracellular NALP3 inflammasome complex and leading to recruitment and influx of neutrophils into the joint space.

CPPD deposition disease typically affects the elderly population. Up to 50% of individuals older than 85 years of age have radiographic evidence of CPPD crystal accumulation in cartilage (chondrocalcinosis), but most are asymptomatic. The most commonly involved joints are the knee menisci and the triangular fibrocartilage of the wrist. It is uncommon for CPPD deposition disease to affect patients younger than 50 years of age, unless the disease is familial or related to a metabolic abnormality (e.g., hyperparathyroidism, hemochromatosis).

CPPD deposition disease can present with acute CPPD crystal arthritis (pseudogout), chronic arthropathy with structural changes of osteoarthritis, or may be asymptomatic, presenting as an incidental finding of chondrocalcinosis on imaging. The most common clinical manifestation, occurring in more than 50% of patients, is a peculiar type of osteoarthritis called pseudo-osteoarthritis; it is a noninflammatory arthritis involving joints not typically affected by osteoarthritis, such as the wrist, shoulder, and metacarpophalangeal joints. A chronic symmetric polyarticular arthritis pattern resembling rheumatoid arthritis and a severe destructive arthropathy that mimics neuropathic arthritis on radiographs may be seen.

Acute pseudogout attacks may be precipitated by trauma, surgery (particularly parathyroidectomy for hyperparathyroidism), or severe medical illness. Administration of intra-articular viscosupplementation may also trigger a CPPD flare. Attacks are usually monoarticular or oligoarticular, similar to an acute gouty attack; if left untreated, they may last from a few days to a few months. The vigorous inflammatory response to CPPD crystals manifests as warmth, erythema, and swelling in and around the affected joint resembling acute gouty arthritis. Fever, elevated erythrocyte sedimentation rate, and leukocytosis can occur.

The diagnosis is confirmed by assessing synovial fluid for the presence of intracellular rod- or rhomboid-shaped crystals, which exhibit weakly positive birefringence when examined by compensated polarized light microscopy (see Fig. 84.3B). CPP crystals can be difficult to detect in some patients and are frequently missed in clinical specimens.

The presence of chondrocalcinosis (radio-dense deposits on radiographs) is highly suggestive of the diagnosis in the appropriate clinical context. Joint aspiration should always be performed to rule out septic arthritis. Importantly, joint infection can cause crystal shedding, leading to a concomitant crystal-related inflammation. Synovial fluid is inflammatory (>2000 white blood cells per microliter).

Therapy for CPPD deposition disease is indicated for symptomatic patients. There is no effective treatment to remove CPPD deposits from synovium or cartilage. Intra-articular glucocorticoid administration to the affected joints is effective. NSAIDs are also effective, but their potential toxicity in elderly patients may limit their use. Severe polyarticular attacks may require short courses of systemic corticosteroids.

In patients with frequent attacks, prophylactic daily low-dose colchicine may decrease the attack frequency.

APATITE-ASSOCIATED ARTHROPATHY

Abnormal accumulation of apatite (basic calcium phosphate, or BCP) may occur in hypercalcemic states and other illnesses. Unlike MSU or CPPD crystals, individual BCP crystals are not identifiable by polarized microscopy and can only be seen using electron microscopy. The most common presentation is calcific periarteritis, which typically occurs in the shoulder.

Milwaukee shoulder is an extremely destructive BCP-associated arthropathy that tends to affect elderly women. It is characterized by a large noninflammatory effusion (i.e., <2000 white blood cells per microliter) causing destruction of the rotator cuff and marked instability of the glenohumeral joint.

Other manifestations include acute reversible inflammatory arthropathies that resemble gout, referred to as *pseudo-pseudogout*, and ossifications along the anterolateral aspect of spinal vertebrae, termed *diffuse idiopathic skeletal hyperostosis* (DISH). Acute attacks of arthritis or bursitis may be self-limited. Intra-articular or periarticular injection of corticosteroids or the use of NSAIDs may shorten the duration and intensity of symptoms.

CALCIUM OXALATE DEPOSITION DISEASE

In calcium oxalate deposition disease, or oxalosis, calcium oxalate crystals are deposited in tissue. In primary oxalosis, a hereditary metabolic disorder, this leads to nephrocalcinosis, renal failure, and early mortality. Secondary oxalosis complicates long-term hemo- and peritoneal dialysis; crystals are deposited in bone, cartilage, synovium, and periarticular tissue. Crystal shedding into the joint space may result in inflammatory arthritis of peripheral joints. Chondrocalcinosis or soft tissue calcifications can be seen on plain radiographs. The presence of strongly birefringent bipyramidal crystals in synovial fluid is characteristic. Treatment with NSAIDS, intra-articular corticosteroids, or colchicine usually results in moderate improvement.

SUGGESTED READINGS

Choi HK: Epidemiology, pathology, and pathogenesis, chap 12. In Stone JH, Crofford LJ, White PH, editors: Primer on the rheumatic diseases, ed 13, New York, 2008, Springer.

Dalbeth N, Merriman TR, Stamp LK: Gout, Lancet 388:2039–2052, 2016.

Khanna D, Fitzgerald JD, Khanna PP, et al: 2012 American College of Rheumatology guidelines for management of gout. Part 1: systematic nonpharmacologic and pharmacologic therapeutic approaches to hyperuricemia, Arthritis Care Res 64:1431–1446, 2012.

Khanna D, Khanna PP, Fitzgerald JD, et al: 2012 American College of Rheumatology guidelines for management of gout. Part 2: therapy and anti-inflammatory prophylaxis of acute gouty arthritis, Arthritis Care Res 64:1447–1461, 2012.

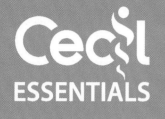

85

Osteoarthritis

Joanne S. Cunha, Zuhal Arzomand, Philip Tsoukas

DEFINITION AND EPIDEMIOLOGY

Osteoarthritis, also known as degenerative joint disease, is the most common type of arthritis and musculoskeletal disease. It is a disease of synovial joints that encompasses the pathophysiologic changes that result from alterations in joint structure due to failed repair of joint damage and the individual's experience of illness, which is most often characterized by pain.

Osteoarthritis affects more than 300 million people worldwide. The prevalence of osteoarthritis continues to rise with the aging population, obesity epidemic, and increased numbers of joint injuries. Currently, more than 30 million adult Americans have some form of osteoarthritis.

The hands, knees, and hips are commonly affected joints in osteoarthritis. Hand and knee osteoarthritis is more common among women, especially after 50 years of age. Radiographic prevalence of osteoarthritis varies by the joint involved and often predates symptomatic osteoarthritis, with higher prevalence for knee and hand osteoarthritis than hip osteoarthritis.

Osteoarthritis is associated with major morbidity, reduced quality of life, and disability. There is increasing evidence of an association between osteoarthritis and cardiovascular disease. Osteoarthritis is one of the leading causes of long-term disability in the United States. Lower extremity osteoarthritis is the most common cause of difficulty with walking or climbing stairs, preventing an estimated 100,000 elderly Americans from independently walking from their bed to the bathroom.

Osteoarthritis has a large economic impact because of direct medical costs (e.g., physician visits, laboratory tests, medications, surgery) and indirect costs (e.g., lost wages, home care). With the aging of the US population, the burden of osteoarthritis is expected to increase in the coming years.

PATHOLOGIC FACTORS

The causes of osteoarthritis are complex and heterogeneous. Osteoarthritis may be classified as primary, or idiopathic, without a specific cause. Secondary osteoarthritis has an identifiable cause and is pathologically identical to primary osteoarthritis. Causes of secondary osteoarthritis include biomechanical factors, congenital or developmental deformities of the joint that alter its shape, traumatic events, metabolic disorders, and inflammatory conditions. Genetic predisposition, age, gender, and obesity are prominent risk factors as well.

The pathophysiology of osteoarthritis is not well understood. The cardinal feature in the pathogenesis of osteoarthritis is an imbalance between the destruction and repair of the joint tissues, with failure of the repair process and progressive loss of articular cartilage with associated remodeling of subchondral bone. In normal cartilage, there is continuous extracellular matrix turnover with a balance between synthesis and degradation. In osteoarthritis, there is disproportion between these two processes, with an excess of matrix degradation that exceeds ongoing matrix synthesis. Excess degradation results from overproduction of catabolic factors such as proinflammatory cytokines and reactive oxygen species (Fig. 85.1).

Osteoarthritis is best defined as joint failure, a disease process that involves the total joint, including the subchondral bone, ligaments, joint capsule, synovial membrane, periarticular muscles, and articular cartilage. After bone trauma or repetitive injury, joint failure may result from joint instability caused by muscle weakness and ligamentous laxity, nerve injury and neuronal sensitization or hyperexcitability, or both.

Biomechanical contributors include repetitive or isolated joint trauma related to certain occupations or physical activities that involve repeated joint stress and predispose to early osteoarthritis. Altered joint shape may contribute to osteoarthritis through biomechanical factors, as may be seen with chronic patellar maltracking and the development of knee osteoarthritis and cam deformity or acetabular dysplasia in the development of hip osteoarthritis.

Obesity may contribute to osteoarthritis biomechanically or systemically through subacute or overt metabolic syndromes, both of which are associated with low-grade systemic inflammation. Age-related changes in habitus result in decreased muscle mass with a relative increase in visceral adiposity. This contributes to abnormal joint mechanics and low-grade systemic inflammation. Other age-related factors include changes in the extracellular matrix composition and structure leading to susceptibility for degeneration, mitochondrial dysfunction with increase in oxidative stress and promotion of catabolic activity, and chondrocyte dysfunction.

Inflammatory joint diseases, such as rheumatoid arthritis, may result in cartilage degradation and biomechanical effects that lead to secondary osteoarthritis. Crystal deposition diseases, osteonecrosis, Paget's disease, and metabolic disorders such as hemochromatosis, ochronosis, Wilson's disease, and Gaucher's disease are also associated with secondary osteoarthritis. High bone mineral density is associated with hip and knee involvement. Estrogen deficiency may be a risk factor for hip or knee disease, showcasing a hormonal influence. Candidate gene studies and genome-wide scans have identified several potential genetic markers. Patients often have a family history of osteoarthritis or joint replacement.

The destruction of the joint, including articular cartilage damage, osteophyte formation, and subchondral bone remodeling, is best viewed as joint failure and the final product of a variety of etiologic factors.

The earliest finding is fibrillation of the most superficial layer of the articular cartilage. Over time, disruption of the articular surface becomes deeper, with fibrillations extending to subchondral bone, fragmentation of cartilage with release into the joint, matrix degradation, and eventually, complete loss of cartilage, leaving only exposed bone.

Early in the process, the cartilage matrix demonstrates increased water and decreased proteoglycan content, unlike the dehydration of cartilage that occurs with aging. The tidemark zone, separating the calcified cartilage from the radial zone, is invaded by capillaries. Chondrocytes initially are metabolically active and release a variety of cytokines and metalloproteinases, contributing to matrix degradation. In the later stages, this results in the penetration of fissures to the

subchondral bone and the release of fibrillated cartilage into the joint space.

An imbalance between tissue inhibitors of metalloproteinases and the production of metalloproteinases may be operative in osteoarthritis. Subchondral bone remodels and increases in density. Cystlike bone cavities containing myxoid, fibrous, or cartilaginous tissue may form. Osteophytes or bony proliferations at the margin of joints at the site of the bone-cartilage interface may form at capsule insertions. Osteophytes contribute to joint motion restriction and are thought to be the result of new bone formation in response to the degeneration

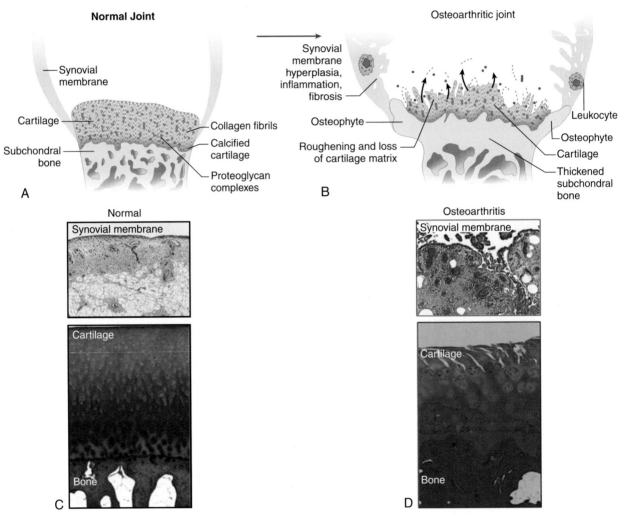

Fig. 85.1 Pathologic features of osteoarthritic joint tissues. (A) Features of a normal adult synovial joint. Healthy adult articular cartilage is characterized by a smooth surface and extracellular matrix (ECM) composed of a collagen type II fibrillar network and large proteoglycan complexes. The ECM is produced and maintained by the cellular components of cartilage, chondrocytes. The subchondral bone consists of a thin cortical layer and underlying trabecular bone. The synovial membrane lines the joint capsule and attaches at the cartilage-bone interface. In the normal state, it consists of a lining layer one or two cells thick, with underlying vascularized loose connective tissue. (B) Typical changes to tissues seen in osteoarthritis (OA). Enzymatic activities (ADAMTS4,5 and MMP-13 in particular) cleave proteoglycan and collagen components of the ECM, leading to loss of these molecules from the matrix. As the process advances, the articular cartilage thins and fibrillates, and eventually fissures down to the underlying bone are seen. Simultaneously, a remodeling response in the bone is observed. Thickening of the cortical subchondral bone layer occurs, and new bone growth at the margins appears as osteophytes. The synovial membrane changes observed in OA patients include lining layer hyperplasia, inflammation in the form of leukocyte infiltration, and fibrosis, which can be seen to varying degrees. Photomicrographs of human joint tissues showing these features are depicted in C (normal tissues) and D (OA tissues). (C and D, Courtesy Edward F. DiCarlo, MD, Hospital for Special Surgery, New York, NY.)

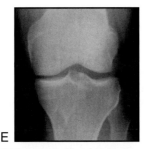

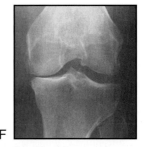

Fig. 85.1, cont'd (E and F) Radiographic features of osteoarthritic joint. Patient baseline (E) vs. 3 years later (F) showing typical features of OA progression including the development of medial joint space narrowing and osteophyte (spur outgrowth) at joint margins. The classical Kellgren and Lawrence grading system scores radiographs by five categories (scores 0–4) as follows: 0 = no osteoarthritis; 1 = small osteophyte of doubtful significance; 2 = definite osteophyte(s), possible joint space narrowing; 3 = multiple osteophytes, definite joint space narrowing, some subchondral sclerosis and possible deformity of bony ends; 4 = large osteophytes, marked narrowing of joint space, severe sclerosis of subchondral bone, and definite deformity of bone ends. (From Byers VV, Vincent TL: Osteoarthritis. In Goldman-Cecil Medicine, 26th edition, eds. Goldman L, Schafer AI, Goldman-Cecil Medicine, 1698-1703.e2, Fig. 246-3.)

of articular cartilage, but the precise mechanism for their production remains unknown.

Several crystals have been identified in synovial fluid and other tissues from osteoarthritic joints, most notably calcium pyrophosphate dehydrate and hydroxyapatite. Although these crystals have potent inflammatory potential, their role in the pathogenesis of osteoarthritis remains unclear. Frequently, the crystals are asymptomatic and do not correlate with extent or severity of disease.

The diversity of risk factors predisposing to osteoarthritis suggests that many insults to the joints, including biomechanical trauma, chronic articular inflammation, and genetic and metabolic errors, can contribute to or trigger the cascade of events that results in the characteristic pathologic features described earlier. At some point, the cartilage degradation process becomes irreversible. With progressive changes in articular cartilage, joint mechanics become altered, perpetuating the degradative process.

CLINICAL PRESENTATION

Pain is the characteristic feature of osteoarthritis and the most common presenting symptom. Pain is usually worse with activity or weight bearing and better with rest. In later stages, pain may also occur at rest. Early in the disease course, pain tends to be transient, intermittent, and unpredictable. The pain may be characterized as severe, and its unpredictable nature is an extremely bothersome feature that limits activity and affects quality of life. With disease progression, pain tends to become constant but is reported to be less severe and have an aching quality. Other prominent symptoms, such as stiffness, gelling, fatigue, and sleep disturbance, often lead to functional limitation and disability.

Pain tends to be localized to the specific joint involved, but it may be referred to a more distant site. The cause of pain is unclear but is likely to be heterogeneous. Pain may result from interactions among structural pathology; the motor, sensory, and autonomic innervation of the joint; and pain signal processing at the spinal and cortical levels. Specific individual and environmental factors also may be important. A subset of patients may have neuropathic pain.

Patient-specific factors may modify pain reception and pain reporting. Patients' affective status, such as depression, anxiety, and anger, may influence the level of pain reported. Their cognitive status, including pain beliefs, expectations, and memories of past pain, and their communication skills may determine how pain is perceived and reported. Studies have shown that demographic factors such as age,

sex, socioeconomic status, race or ethnicity, and cultural background may affect pain reporting.

Patients may have stiffness, particularly after prolonged inactivity, but it is not a major feature of osteoarthritis and usually lasts for less than 30 minutes. Patients do not report systemic features such as fever.

Examination of an involved joint may reveal tenderness and bony enlargement. Joint effusion and soft tissue swelling may occur with knee involvement, but they tend to be intermittent. Persistent inflammation with joint warmth, erythema, effusion, and soft tissue swelling is usually not seen. Crepitus with movement, limitation of joint motion, and joint deformity, malalignment, and joint laxity or instability may be detected on evaluation. Joint deformity as manifested by lateral subluxation is fixed and not reducible. Muscle weakness and gait abnormalities may be seen.

Several subtypes of osteoarthritis have been identified. The nodal form involves the distal interphalangeal joints (DIPs), also known as Heberden nodes, and the proximal interphalangeal joints (PIPs), also known as Bouchard nodes. It is most common in middle-aged women, typically those with a strong family history among first-degree relatives. Erosive, inflammatory osteoarthritis is associated with prominent destructive changes, especially in the finger joints, and it is often quite symptomatic. Generalized osteoarthritis is characterized by involvement of the DIP, PIP, and first carpal-metacarpal joints, as well as the knees, feet, and hips.

DIAGNOSIS AND DIFFERENTIAL DIAGNOSIS

The diagnosis of osteoarthritis is based on the signs and symptoms previously outlined. Although there are characteristic radiographic features, they are not necessary to make the clinical diagnosis. Imaging may be used to confirm the diagnosis and exclude other diseases, but radiographs are insensitive and may not show findings early in the disease course. Despite radiographic findings of osteoarthritis, pain may have other sources, such as bursitis, tendonitis, or referred pain. For example, hip disease may manifest as knee pain.

Osteoarthritis must be distinguished from inflammatory joint diseases such as rheumatoid arthritis and the spondyloarthropathies. This is accomplished by identifying the characteristic pattern of joint involvement and the nature of the individual joint deformity. Joints commonly involved in osteoarthritis include the DIPs, PIPs, first carpal-metacarpal, cervical and lumbar spine facet joints, hips, knees, and first metatarsophalangeal joints. Involvement of the metacarpal phalangeal joints (MCPs), wrist, elbows, shoulders, and ankles is uncommon, except in the case of trauma, congenital disease, or coexisting endocrine or metabolic disease.

The characteristic radiographic features of osteoarthritis include joint space narrowing as a surrogate for cartilage loss; osteophytes and subchondral sclerosis as an indicator of new bone formation, which is characteristic of osteoarthritis; and subchondral cysts as a manifestation of myxoid or fibrous degeneration of subchondral bone. Bone attrition and subchondral bone remodeling may result in changes in bone shape. Magnetic resonance imaging (MRI) can demonstrate additional morphologic abnormalities, such as bone marrow lesions in subchondral bone, meniscal degeneration, and synovitis. Musculoskeletal ultrasonography is an alternative imaging modality used to identify osteoarthritic pathologic changes within the joint space, soft tissue, cartilage, and bone surfaces. Ultrasound can identify osteoarthritis features such as osteophytes, morphologic degeneration in cartilage, synovitis, and synovial fluid.

The pain and swelling of erosive hand osteoarthritis may suggest rheumatoid arthritis, although systemic inflammatory signs and other typical features of rheumatoid arthritis are absent. Patients with osteoarthritis typically have a negative rheumatoid factor, normal inflammatory markers such as erythrocyte sedimentation rate and c-reactive protein, normal complete blood count, and normal antinuclear antibody tests. Synovial fluid examination is typically noninflammatory with clear viscous fluid and normal white blood cell count. The prevalence of false-positive findings of rheumatoid factor and antinuclear antibody, sometimes in significant titers, is higher with increasing age. Osteoarthritis more commonly affects the distal small joints in the hands (DIPs > PIPs > MCPs and wrists), whereas rheumatoid arthritis more commonly affects proximal small joints in the hands (MCPs and wrists > PIPs > DIPs).

TREATMENT

The natural history of osteoarthritis includes periods of relative stability interspersed with rapid deterioration. Management should be individually tailored and may include a combination of nonpharmacologic, pharmacologic, and surgical approaches. The primary goal of treatment is to improve pain and function and reduce disability.

Patients should be educated regarding the objectives of treatment and the importance of lifestyle changes, exercise, pacing of activities, and other measures to unload the damaged joints. The initial focus should be on self-help and patient-driven treatments rather than on passive therapies. Patients should be encouraged to adhere to nonpharmacologic and pharmacologic therapies. Physical therapists may be helpful in providing instruction in appropriate exercises to reduce pain and preserve functional capacity. For knee and hip osteoarthritis, assistive devices such as walking aids may be useful. In patients with first carpometacarpal joint osteoarthritis, hand orthoses are recommended. Graded regular aerobic, aquatic exercise, muscle-strengthening, and range-of-motion exercises are beneficial. Tai chi has been shown to have beneficial effects not only in the treatment of knee and hip osteoarthritis, but also in improving quality of life and depression.

Overweight patients should be encouraged to lose weight. A combination of dietary weight loss in conjunction with exercise results in improvement of both pain and function compared to either intervention alone, though long-term weight management may be challenging for patients. A knee brace can reduce pain, improve stability, and diminish the risk of falling for patients with knee osteoarthritis and mild or moderate varus or valgus instability. Advice concerning appropriate footwear is also important. Spinal orthoses may provide benefit to patients with significant cervical or lumbar involvement. Local applications of heat, ultrasound, or transcutaneous electrical nerve stimulation (TENS) may provide short-term benefit in these patients. In patients with knee and hip osteoarthritis, TENS is not recommended as there have been limited studies and lack of benefit. Acupuncture may also offer symptomatic benefit for patients with osteoarthritis, but its efficacy in knee, hip, and hand osteoarthritis is still debatable as studies have shown variable results.

Pharmacologic therapy provides symptomatic relief but does not alter the course of the disease. Pharmacologic therapy should therefore be selected based on its relative efficacy and safety. The use of concomitant medications in the setting of comorbidities should be taken into account.

Acetaminophen (up to 3 g/day with caution) may be an effective initial oral analgesic for mild to moderate pain, though it may not provide sufficient benefit on its own. In patients with symptomatic osteoarthritis, nonsteroidal anti-inflammatory drugs (NSAIDs) should be used at the lowest effective dose, although their long-term use should be avoided if possible. If patients are at risk for increased gastrointestinal toxicity, a cyclooxygenase-2 (COX2)–selective agent or a nonselective NSAID with co-prescription of a proton pump inhibitor or misoprostol for gastroprotection should be considered. All NSAIDs, including nonselective and COX2-selective agents, should be used with caution in patients with cardiovascular risk factors and chronic kidney disease. Topical NSAIDs and capsaicin may be effective alternatives to oral analgesic or anti-inflammatory agents in knee and hand osteoarthritis and may be used as adjunctive agents, particularly in elderly patients. If patients fail the aforementioned, find other therapies ineffective, and are not surgical candidates, then tramadol, a weak opioid receptor agonist, may also be used in these select cases. Non-tramadol opiates are discouraged as they pose risk for an increase of adverse effects that typically outweighs their benefits. In select patients that have exhausted other therapies and medications, non-tramadol opioids may be used for the shortest possible length of time, given the limited pain control with longer duration of these medications.

Despite the popularity of these products, meta-analyses have shown that oral glucosamine and chondroitin sulfate have limited benefit in patients with knee osteoarthritis and are currently not recommended in knee, hip or hand osteoarthritis.

Other agents, such as duloxetine, when compared to placebo, were shown to reduce pain and improve function in a meta-analysis. Duloxetine can be used in pain management and studies have shown efficacy in the treatment of osteoarthritis.

Occasional injection of intra-articular corticosteroids (usually no more than once every 4 months) may provide modest short-term symptomatic benefit with minimal toxicity, especially in the knee. Studies have shown that patients given more frequent corticosteroid injections (i.e., every 3 months) lose greater cartilage volume than those given a corticosteroid injection every 4 months, but the significance of this cartilage loss is unclear. Patients with moderate to severe pain and effusion or other local signs of inflammation may be more responsive to these injections. Intra-articular hyaluronate appears to have little or no benefit based on current evidence. Recent trials evaluated platelet-rich plasma injections and mesenchymal stem cell injections in osteoarthritis, but these are not currently recommended because there is a concern in the techniques used for these injections as well as the heterogeneity and lack of standardization of available preparations.

Surgical management includes total joint replacement, which is extremely effective in relieving pain, decreasing disability, and improving function. With improvements in surgical technique and technology, the indications for total joint replacement have expanded to include younger and older age groups. Other surgical options include osteotomy and uni-compartmental knee replacement.

Referral to an orthopedic surgeon should be considered in cases where other treatment options have been exhausted and quality of life is greatly reduced, including joint pain disrupting sleep, restriction of walking distance, and limiting participation in daily activities. Arthroscopy is not recommended for the management of knee osteoarthritis.

PROGNOSIS

Given the obesity epidemic and the marked contact loads that increased weight places on the knee, obesity is likely the most important modifiable risk factor for the development and progression of knee osteoarthritis. One kilogram of weight loss decreases the load on the knee by 4 kg. Varus and valgus malalignments have also been identified as important risk factors for the progression of knee osteoarthritis.

SUGGESTED READINGS

Blagojevic M, Jinks C, Jeffery A, et al: Risk factors for onset of osteoarthritis of the knee in older adults: a systematic review and meta-analysis, Osteoarthritis Cartilage 18:24–33, 2013.

Helmick CG, Felson DT, Kwoh CK, et al: Estimates of the prevalence of arthritis and other rheumatic conditions in the United States. Part I, Arthritis Rheum 58:15–25, 2008.

Hochberg MC, Altman RD, April KT, et al: American College of Rheumatology 2012 recommendations for the use of nonpharmacologic and pharmacologic therapies in osteoarthritis of the hand, hip, and knee, Arthritis Care Res 64:465–474, 2012.

Hunter DJ, Bierma-Zeinstra S: Osteoarthritis, Lancet 393(10182): 1745–1759, 2019.

Kolasinski SL, Neogi T, Hochberg MC, et al: 2019 American College of Rheumatology/Arthritis Foundation guidelines for the management of osteoarthritis of the hand, hip and knee, Art Rheum 72(2):220–233, 2019.

Litwic A, Edwards MH, Dennison EM, et al: Epidemiology and burden of osteoarthritis, Br Med Bull 105:185–199, 2013.

McAlindon TE, LaValley MP, Harvey WF, et al: Effect of intra-articular triamcinolone vs saline on knee cartilage volume and pain in patients with knee osteoarthritis: a randomized clinical trial, J Am Med Assoc 317:1967–1975, 2017.

Okano T, Mamoto K, Di Carlo M, et al: Clinical utility and potential of ultrasound in osteoarthritis, Radiol Med 124:1101–1111, 2019.

Wang ZY, Shi SY, Li SJ, et al: Efficacy and safety of duloxetine on osteoarthritis knee pain: a meta-analysis of randomized controlled trials, Pain Med 16(7):1373–1385, 2015.

Zhang W, Moskowitz RW, Kwoh CK, et al: OARSI recommendations for the management of hip and knee osteoarthritis, part I: critical appraisal of existing treatment guidelines and systematic review of current research evidence, Osteoarthritis Cartilage 15:981–1000, 2007.

Zhang W, Moskovitz RW, Nuki G, et al: OARSI recommendations for the management of hip and knee osteoarthritis, part II: OARSI evidence-based, expert consensus guidelines, Osteoarthritis Cartilage 16:137–162, 2008.

86

Nonarticular Soft Tissue Disorders

Niveditha Mohan

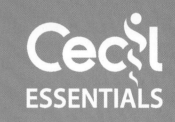

INTRODUCTION

The nonarticular soft tissue disorders account for most musculoskeletal complaints in the general population. These disorders include a large number of anatomically localized conditions (e.g., bursitis, tendinitis) and fibromyalgia syndrome, a generalized pain disorder. For most nonarticular soft tissue conditions, the etiologic factors and pathogenesis are poorly understood.

Once the location of the symptom is defined, (e.g., shoulder pain), the specific structure that is involved should be identified (e.g., supraspinatus tendon, subacromial bursa) using a careful history and physical examination. In the case of back pain, precise anatomic delineation of the structure involved (e.g., intervertebral disk, facet joint, ligament, paraspinal muscle) is more likely to require advanced imaging. When the patient complains of diffuse pain, it is imperative to evaluate for contribution of local pain that may be driving the diffuse pain, with a thorough physical examination.

EPIDEMIOLOGY

Precise data for prevalence or incidence of most nonarticular soft tissue syndromes are not available, but these conditions account for up to 30% of all outpatient visits. Fibromyalgia is considered to be the most common cause of generalized musculoskeletal pain in women between the ages of 20 and 55 years. The global mean prevalence is 2.7%.

ETIOLOGIC FACTORS AND PATHOGENESIS

The precise pathophysiology of most nonarticular soft tissue disorders remains unknown, although predisposing factors, such as trauma, overuse, repetitive activities (e.g., tennis elbow, lateral epicondylitis) or biomechanical factors (e.g., leg-length discrepancy in trochanteric bursitis), can be identified in many cases.

The term *tendinitis* implies tendon sheath inflammation, but small tendon tears, periostitis, and nerve entrapment have been proposed as potential mechanisms. Similarly, although the term *bursitis* implies bursal inflammation, demonstrable inflammation is difficult to find. In some cases (e.g., acute bursitis of the olecranon or prepatellar bursa), the mechanism is an acute inflammatory response to sodium urate crystals deposited in the soft tissue, an extra-articular manifestation of gout. The favorable response of tendinitis and bursitis to anti-inflammatory agents, including corticosteroids, supports the view that at least one component of these syndromes is the result of an inflammatory process.

Fibromyalgia is the current term for chronic widespread musculoskeletal pain for which no alternative cause can be identified. The underlying pathology is due to alterations in central nervous system (CNS) function leading to augmented nociceptive (caused by pain) processing that leads to the development of CNS-mediated somatic symptoms of fatigue, sleep, memory and mood difficulties in addition to the chronic widespread pain. There may also be alterations in the immune system leading to an enhanced inflammatory state with emerging evidence that some of the pathobiology of fibromyalgia may involve altered nociceptor sensitivity. This disorder often begins in childhood or adolescence, and individuals who eventually go on to develop FM are more likely to experience headaches, dysmenorrhea, temporomandibular joint disorder, chronic fatigue, irritable bowel syndrome and other functional gastrointestinal tract disorders, interstitial cystitis/painful bladder syndrome, endometriosis, and other regional pain syndromes (especially back and neck pain).

CLINICAL PRESENTATION

Many of the soft tissue rheumatic syndromes involve bursae, tendons, ligaments, and muscles. Bursae are closed sacs lined with mesenchymal cells that are similar to synovial cells; the sacs are strategically located to facilitate tissue gliding. Subcutaneous bursae (e.g., olecranon, prepatellar) form after birth in response to normal external friction. Deep bursae (e.g., subacromial bursa) usually form before birth in response to movement between muscles and bones and may or may not communicate with adjacent joint cavities. Adventitious bursae (e.g., over the first metatarsal head) form in response to abnormal shearing stresses and are not uniformly found. Although most forms of bursitis involve isolated, local conditions, some may be the result of systemic conditions such as gout.

Tendinitis, bursitis, and myofascial disorders should be distinguished from articular disorders. In most cases, this can be accomplished by a careful examination of the involved structure (Table 86.1). General principles of the musculoskeletal examination are as follows:

1. Observation: If deformity or soft tissue swelling is detected, is it fusiform (i.e., surrounding the entire joint in a symmetrical fashion) or is it localized? Local rather than fusiform deformity distinguishes nonarticular disorders from articular disorders.
2. Palpation: Is tenderness localized or in a fusiform distribution? Is there an effusion? Local (not fusiform or joint line) tenderness distinguishes nonarticular disorders from articular disorders. An effusion typically indicates an articular disorder.
3. Assessing range of motion: The musculoskeletal examination includes the assessment of active range of motion (i.e., patient attempts to move the symptomatic structure) and passive range of motion (i.e., examiner moves the symptomatic structure). Articular disorders usually are characterized by equal impairment in active and passive movements as a result of the mechanical limitation

TABLE 86.1   Differentiating Nonarticular Soft Tissue Disorders From Articular Disease

Manifestation	Nonarticular Soft Tissue Disorders	Articular Disease
Limitation of motion	Active > passive	Active = passive
Crepitus of articular surfaces (structural damage)	0	+/0
Tenderness		
Synovial (fusiform pattern)	0	+
Local	+	0
Swelling		
Synovial (fusiform pattern)	0	+
Local	+/0	0

+, Present; *0*, absent.

TABLE 86.2   Bursitis Syndromes

Location	Symptom	Finding
Subacromial	Shoulder pain	Tender subacromial space
Olecranon	Elbow pain	Tender olecranon swelling
Iliopectineal	Groin pain	Tender inguinal region
Trochanteric	Lateral hip pain	Tender at greater trochanter
Prepatellar	Anterior knee pain	Tender swelling over patella
Infrapatellar	Anterior knee pain	Tender swelling lateral or medial to patellar tendon
Anserine	Medial knee pain	Tender medioproximal tibia (below joint line of knee)
Ischiogluteal	Buttock pain	Tender ischial spine (at gluteal fold)
Retrocalcaneal	Heel pain	Tender swelling between Achilles tendon insertion and calcaneus
Calcaneal	Heel pain	Tender central heel pad

of joint motion resulting from proliferation of the synovial membrane, an effusion, or derangement of intra-articular structures. Impairment of active movement characterizes nonarticular disorders to a much greater degree than passive movement.

Clinical symptoms include pain, warmth, and swelling over the site of the bursa that are worse with activity and better with rest. Bursitis can be distinguished from tendinitis by the pain during active and passive range of movement; in tendinitis, pain is elicited only during active range of movement. However, for many patients there is concomitant bursitis and tendinitis.

Muscle sprains or strains are typically diagnosed based on a history of preceding activity causing the symptom along with pain and limitation of movement when the muscle is contracted against resistance. The clinical signs and symptoms of chronic myofascial pain are more nonspecific and characterized by a distribution that is frequently nonanatomic and associated with hyperalgesia in the involved area.

Fibromyalgia syndrome is characterized by widespread pain and a host of other symptoms, including insomnia, cognitive dysfunction, depression, anxiety, recurrent headaches, dizziness, fatigue, morning stiffness, extremity dysesthesia, irritable bowel syndrome, and irritable bladder syndrome.

DIAGNOSIS AND TREATMENT

Septic Bursitis

Superficial forms of bursitis, particularly olecranon bursitis and prepatellar and occasionally infrapatellar bursitis, are more frequently infected or involved with crystal deposition than are deep forms of bursitis, presumably due to direct extension of organisms through subcutaneous tissues. Most commonly, *Staphylococcus aureus* is isolated from infected superficial bursae. Septic bursitis should be suspected when there is cellulitis, erythema, fever, and peripheral leukocytosis.

Definitive diagnosis and exclusion of infection of subcutaneous bursae usually require aspiration of the distended bursa. The bursal fluid should be assessed for cell count, Gram stain, and culture and examined for crystals.

Nonseptic Bursitis

Nonseptic bursitis frequently appears as an overuse condition associated with sudden or unaccustomed repetitive activity of the associated extremity. The two most common types of bursitis are subacromial and trochanteric bursitis (Table 86.2).

Subacromial bursitis is the most common overall cause of shoulder pain over the lateral upper arm or deltoid muscle that is exacerbated with abduction of the arm. It occurs as a result of compression of the inflamed rotator cuff tendon between the acromion and humeral head. Because the rotator cuff forms the floor of the subacromial bursa, bursitis in this location often results from tendinitis of the rotator cuff. Occasionally, subacromial bursitis or rotator cuff tendinitis results from osteophyte compression of the rotator cuff tendon originating from the acromioclavicular joint. The differential diagnosis includes tears of the rotator cuff, intra-articular pathologic mechanisms of the glenohumeral joint, bicipital tendinitis, cervical radiculopathy, and referred pain from the chest.

Trochanteric bursitis is the result of inflammation at the insertion of the gluteal muscles at the greater trochanter. It produces lateral thigh pain, which is often worse when the patient lies on the affected side. Women seem to be more prone to develop this condition, perhaps because of increased traction of the gluteal muscles as a result of the relatively broader female pelvis. Other potential risk factors include weight gain, local trauma, overuse activities such as jogging, and leg-length discrepancies (primarily on the side with the longer leg). These factors are thought to lead to increased tension of the gluteus maximus on the iliotibial band, producing bursal inflammation. The differential diagnosis of trochanteric bursitis includes lumbar radiculopathy (particularly of the L1 and L2 nerve roots), meralgia paresthetica (i.e., entrapment of the lateral cutaneous nerve of the thigh as it passes under the inguinal ligament), true hip joint disease, and intra-abdominal pathologic processes. Other bursitis syndromes are less common and listed in Table 86.2.

Septic bursitis is treated with a combination of serial aspirations of the infected bursa and antibiotics, initially directed against *S. aureus* and then adjusted depending on the results of bursal fluid cultures. Recurrent septic bursitis may need surgical excision of the bursa. The approach to nonseptic bursitis should include rest, local heat, and unless contraindicated by peptic ulcer disease, renal disease, or advanced age, nonsteroidal anti-inflammatory drugs (NSAIDs).

The most effective approach usually is local injection of a corticosteroid. Superficial bursae with obvious swelling should be aspirated before the corticosteroid is injected. For deep bursae, such as the subacromial or trochanteric bursae, aspiration yields little or no fluid, and direct injection of a corticosteroid without attempted aspiration is reasonable. Caution is advised in attempted aspiration or injection of the iliopsoas bursa, the ischiogluteal bursa, and the gastrocnemius-semimembranosus bursa (i.e., Baker cyst). These bursae lie close to important neural and vascular structures, and aspiration under ultrasound guidance is recommended.

TABLE 86.3   Tendinitis Syndromes

Location	Symptom	Finding
Extensor pollicis brevis and abductor pollicis longus (de Quervain tenosynovitis)	Wrist pain	Pain on ulnar deviation of the wrist, with the thumb grasped by the remaining four fingers (i.e., Finkelstein test)
Flexor tendons of fingers	Triggering or locking of fingers in flexion	Tender nodule on flexor tendon on palm over metacarpal joint
Medial epicondyle	Elbow pain	Tenderness of medial epicondyle
Lateral epicondyle	Elbow pain	Tenderness of lateral epicondyle
Bicipital tendon	Shoulder pain	Tenderness along bicipital groove
Patella	Knee pain	Tenderness at insertion of patellar tendon
Achilles	Heel pain	Tender Achilles tendon
Tibialis posterior	Medial ankle pain	Tenderness under medial malleolus with resisted inversion of ankle
Peroneal	Lateral midfoot or ankle pain	Tenderness under lateral malleolus with passive inversion

TABLE 86.4   2011 American College of Rheumatology Fibromyalgia Diagnostic Criteria Modification

Criteria
1. 0 to 19 pain locations on the widespread pain index (WPI)
2. 6 self-reported symptoms, including difficulty sleeping, fatigue, poor cognition, headache, depression and abdominal pain. 0–3 points for fatigue, cognition, and sleep; 1 point for abdominal pain, headache, and depression
3. Symptoms are present for at least 3 months
4. Exclusion of other explanation for the pain
   Total score is calculated by adding WPI and self-reported symptom score; 12–13 is generally indicative of fibromyalgia. There has been a 2016 modification to this score to minimize misclassification of regional pain disorders.

Somatic symptoms may include muscle pain or weakness, irritable bowel syndrome, fatigue or tiredness, cognitive or memory problems, headache, numbness or tingling, dizziness, insomnia, depression, nervousness, seizures, abdominal pain or cramps (especially upper abdomen), constipation, diarrhea, nausea, vomiting, fever, dry mouth, itching, chest pain, wheezing, Raynaud's phenomenon, hives or welts, tinnitus, hearing difficulties, heartburn, oral ulcers, loss of or change in taste, dry eyes, blurred vision, shortness of breath, loss of appetite, rash, sun sensitivity, easy bruising, hair loss, frequent or painful urination, and bladder spasms.

Tendinitis

Most tendinitis syndromes are the result of inflammation in the tendon sheath. Overuse with microscopic tearing of the tendon is the most common risk factor for tendinitis. Tendon compression by an osteophyte may occur, such as in the rotator cuff tendon compressed by an osteophyte originating from the acromioclavicular joint.

A common form of tendinitis is lateral epicondylitis, also known as *tennis elbow* (Table 86.3). This is a common overuse syndrome among tennis players, but it can be seen in many other settings requiring repetitive extension of the forearm (e.g., painting overhead). The diagnosis is confirmed by exclusion of elbow joint pathology and the finding of local tenderness at the lateral epicondyle, which is typically exacerbated by forearm extension against resistance. Enthesopathies such as Achilles tendinitis and peroneal and posterior tibial tendinitis may occur in the setting of an underlying seronegative arthropathy such as Reiter disease or psoriatic arthritis. A history and clinical evaluation for these disorders should be pursued for the appropriate patient.

Therapy for tendinitis—NSAIDs, local heat, and corticosteroid injection—is similar to that for bursitis. Rest, physical therapy, occupational therapy, and occasionally ergonomic modification are useful adjuncts. The goal of corticosteroid injection in tendinitis is to infiltrate the tendon sheath rather than the tendon itself because direct injection into a tendon may result in rupture of the tendon. Corticosteroid injection of the Achilles tendon should be avoided because of the propensity of this tendon to rupture. Surgical management of tendinitis is indicated only after failure of conservative treatment. For example, chronic impingement of the supraspinatus tendon that is refractory to conservative treatment may require subacromial decompression.

Fibromyalgia Syndrome

Descriptions of fibromyalgia syndrome exist far back in the medical literature, but it remains a diagnosis of exclusion due to the lack of objective diagnostic or pathologic findings. Fibromyalgia syndrome as defined by the American College of Rheumatology (ACR) 1990 definition for use in clinical trials is a chronic, widespread pain condition with characteristic tender points on physical examination, often associated with a constellation of symptoms such as fatigue, sleep disturbance, headache, irritable bowel syndrome, and mood disorders. In 2010, the ACR developed preliminary diagnostic criteria based only on symptoms because of well-documented issues with the tender point examination (Table 86.4). These criteria do not require a tender point examination, but they provide a scale for measuring the severity of symptoms that are characteristic of fibromyalgia and show good correlation with the 1990 ACR criteria.

The clinical presentation of fibromyalgia syndrome is an insidious onset of chronic, diffuse, poorly localized musculoskeletal pain, typically accompanied by fatigue and sleep disturbance. The physical examination reveals a normal musculoskeletal system, with no deformity or synovitis. However, widespread tenderness occurs, especially at tendon insertion sites, indicating a general reduction in the pain threshold.

Approximately one third of the patients identify antecedent trauma as a precipitant for their symptoms, one third of patients describe a viral prodrome, and one third have no clear precipitant. A variety of less typical presentations has been described, including a predominantly neuropathic presentation with paresthesias (i.e., numbness and tingling) in a nondermatomal distribution, an arthralgic rather than myalgic presentation, and an axial skeletal manifestation resembling degenerative disk disease. Many patients may have undergone invasive diagnostic tests and, in some cases, inappropriate procedures such as carpal tunnel release or cervical or lumbar laminectomies.

Conditions that should be considered in the differential diagnosis of fibromyalgia syndrome include polymyalgia rheumatica (in older patients), hypothyroidism, polymyositis, and early systemic lupus erythematosus or rheumatoid arthritis. However, symptoms are exhibited for many months or years without evidence of other signs or symptoms of an underlying connective tissue disease, making other possible diagnoses unlikely.

Results of laboratory and radiographic studies are usually normal for patients with fibromyalgia syndrome. Exclusion of other conditions, such as osteoarthritis, rheumatoid arthritis, and systemic lupus erythematosus, by radiography, erythrocyte sedimentation rate, assays for rheumatoid factor or antinuclear antibody, and other tests is no longer considered necessary for the diagnosis of fibromyalgia syndrome. Fibromyalgia should be diagnosed on the basis of positive criteria.

The treatment of fibromyalgia includes reassurance that the condition is not a progressive, crippling, or life-threatening entity. A combination of treatment options, including medication and physical measures, is helpful for most patients. Medications found to be helpful in short-term, double-blind, placebo-controlled trials include amitriptyline and cyclobenzaprine. Low doses of these medications (e.g., 10 to 30 mg of amitriptyline, 10 to 30 mg of cyclobenzaprine) are moderately effective and generally well tolerated. Studies have shown that newer antidepressants of the serotonin-norepinephrine reuptake inhibitor group (e.g., duloxetine, venlafaxine, bupropion) and $\alpha_2\delta$ ligands (e.g., gabapentin, pregabalin) are also effective, particularly in combination with low doses of tricyclic agents. There is currently significant interest among patients regarding the use of cannabinoids for the management of chronic pain but very little data to support their use. However, there is evidence that chronic opioids are not indicated in these patients due to the high risk of dependence, tolerance, and possible worsening of hyperalgesia in these patients.

Patients should be encouraged to take an active role in the management of their condition. If possible, they should begin a progressive, low-level aerobic exercise program to improve muscular fitness and provide a sense of well-being. Cognitive behavioral therapy has been shown to improved function significantly. Adherence, compliance, and access to these modalities are limitations in patients. A combination approach is effective for most patients in alleviating symptoms, although a small minority of patients requires more intensive treatment strategies, such as psychiatric treatment or referral to a pain center.

SUGGESTED READINGS

Goldenberg DL, Burkhardt C, Crofford L: Management of fibromyalgia syndrome, J Am Med Assoc 292:2388–2395, 2004.

Littlejohn GO: Balanced treatments for fibromyalgia, Arthritis Rheum 50:2725–2729, 2004.

87

Rheumatic Manifestations of Systemic Disorders and Sjögren's Syndrome

Andreea Coca, Ghaith Noaiseh

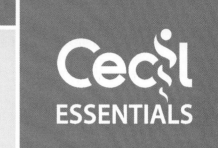

INTRODUCTION

Rheumatologic manifestations may herald a variety of systemic conditions, including malignancy, endocrinopathy, and hematologic disorders (Tables 87.1 and 87.2). Musculoskeletal symptoms can precede or follow the diagnosis of these diseases. Patients may complain of joint or muscle pain, joint swelling, rashes, and many other symptoms.

RHEUMATOLOGIC PARANEOPLASTIC MANIFESTATIONS

Cancer has a myriad of presentations, and paraneoplastic rheumatologic manifestations are not uncommon. They can vary from musculoskeletal conditions to vascular involvement (leukocytoclastic vasculitis), myositis, systemic lupus erythematosus (SLE)–like symptoms, and scleroderma. The pathophysiologic mechanisms of musculoskeletal symptoms in a patient with cancer are often unknown and remain speculative. The association is presumed if there is a close temporal relationship between the diagnosis of a malignancy and the onset of musculoskeletal symptoms or the rheumatic syndrome resolves after successful treatment of the malignancy. In many cases, however, the association may be coincidental.

Cancer may directly invade articular or periarticular structures and mimic rheumatic syndromes, as in chondrosarcoma, giant cell tumor, and osteogenic sarcoma. Musculoskeletal symptoms can occur as paraneoplastic phenomena without direct involvement by the tumor, as in dermatomyositis (DM) in patients with ovarian cancer.

The incidence of malignancy with rheumatic manifestations is unclear, but musculoskeletal symptoms occur more frequently with hematologic malignancies than with solid tumors. No single laboratory test can confirm the diagnosis of a rheumatic illness in a patient with cancer. All patients with rheumatologic syndromes should be evaluated with a thorough history, physical examination, and age-appropriate malignancy screening.

Hypertrophic Osteoarthropathy

Hypertrophic osteoarthropathy (HOA) is characterized by digital clubbing, periostitis of the long bones, and arthritis. Arthritis is most prominent in large joints, and periostitis develops mostly at the distal ends of the femur, tibia, and radius. The primary form of HOA (primary pachydermoperiostosis) is usually a self-limited disease of childhood. The secondary form may be generalized or localized and is mainly associated with lung cancer and suppurative lung disease.

HOA is also associated with cardiovascular disease (e.g., cyanotic congenital heart disease, infective endocarditis), hepatobiliary disorders (e.g., liver cirrhosis, primary biliary cirrhosis), and gastrointestinal disease (e.g., inflammatory bowel disease, celiac disease). Periostitis without digital clubbing can be seen in thyroid acropachy,

hypervitaminosis A, fluorosis, venous stasis, hyperphosphatemia, and sarcoidosis. Isolated chronic digital clubbing, which is mainly associated with pleuropulmonary disease, does not seem to cause HOA.

The pathogenesis of HOA remains elusive, although several possible mechanisms have been proposed, including platelet derived growth factor and vascular derived growth factor.

HOA is usually accompanied by bone and joint pain associated with periarticular periostitis. The pain is usually exacerbated by dependency and relieved with limb elevation. Typical signs of periostitis include periosteal new bone along the distal ends of long bones, which can be seen on plain radiographs. When periostitis is not obvious on plain radiography, a bone scan is useful to demonstrate early evidence of disease. Radiologic evaluation of the thorax is important because of the association between HOA and lung neoplasms.

In many cases, symptomatic management with nonsteroidal anti-inflammatory drugs or other analgesics while treating the underlying disorder provides significant relief of symptoms. In refractory cases, bisphosphonates such as pamidronate and zoledronic acid have been reported to be effective.

Rheumatoid Arthritis–like Polyarthritis

Inflammatory rheumatoid arthritis–like syndrome has been associated with solid neoplasms and hematologic malignancies. Clinical characteristics associated with this paraneoplastic syndrome include acute onset, asymmetrical disease frequently involving the lower extremities, synovitis in large joints that spares the wrists and hands without bony erosion, and negative results for rheumatoid factor and cyclic citrullinated peptide antibody. However, these features are not specific and may be confused with elder-onset rheumatoid arthritis, seronegative rheumatoid arthritis, spondyloarthropathy, and remitting seronegative symmetrical synovitis with pitting edema (RS3PE).

Remitting Seronegative Symmetrical Synovitis With Pitting Edema

RS3PE manifests with sudden onset of polyarthritis, pitting edema, and prominent constitutional symptoms. More than one half of the RS3PE cases are associated with malignancy, including hematologic and solid tumors. The evaluation of the patient presenting with RS3PE should prompt an age-appropriate malignancy work-up.

Eosinophilic Fasciitis

Eosinophilic fasciitis can be easily mistaken for scleroderma, presenting with puffy skin, sometimes indurated, progressing towards significant subcutaneous thickening, with characteristic peripheral eosinophilia. It can be seen in the setting of a variety of hematologic malignant disorders.

TABLE 87.1 Systemic Conditions Associated With Rheumatic Manifestations

Malignancies
Myelodysplasia
Lymphoma
Leukemia

Paraneoplastic Rheumatologic Disorders
RS3PE
Eosinophilic fasciitis
Hypertrophic osteoarthropathy

Hematologic Disorders
Hemophilia
Sickle cell disease
Thalassemia

Endocrinopathies
Diabetes
Hypothyroidism
Hyperthyroidism
Hyperparathyroidism
Acromegaly

Gastrointestinal Disorders
Whipple disease
Hemochromatosis
Primary biliary cirrhosis

Miscellaneous
Multiple myeloma
Amyloidosis
HIV-related rheumatologic disorders
Sarcoidosis

TABLE 87.2 Musculoskeletal Manifestations of Endocrine Disease

Endocrine Disease	Musculoskeletal Manifestations
Diabetes mellitus	Carpal tunnel syndrome
	Charcot arthropathy
	Adhesive capsulitis
	Cheiroarthropathy
	Diabetic amyotrophy
	Diabetic muscle infarction
Hypothyroidism	Proximal myopathy
	Joint effusions
	Carpal tunnel syndrome
	Chondrocalcinosis
Hyperthyroidism	Myopathy
	Osteoporosis
	Thyroid acropachy
Hyperparathyroidism	Myopathy
	Erosive arthritis
	Chondrocalcinosis
Hypoparathyroidism	Muscle cramps
	Soft tissue calcifications
	Spondyloarthropathy
Acromegaly	Carpal tunnel syndrome
	Myopathy
	Raynaud's phenomenon
	Premature osteoarthritis
Cushing syndrome	Myopathy
	Osteoporosis
	Avascular necrosis

Rheumatologic Complications of Checkpoint Inhibitor Immunotherapy

Immune checkpoint inhibitors (ICIs) are the most commonly used type of cancer immunotherapy. They work by blocking inhibitory molecules on the T cells, resulting in heightened T-cell mediated immune response against malignancy. Unfortunately, they have a variety of side effects, the musculoskeletal ones being among the predominant ones.

Inflammatory arthritis can present in a pattern similar to rheumatoid arthritis or a seronegative spondyloarthropathy. Joint damage can be severe and erosions are common. For the most part, the work-up is normal, although inflammatory markers can be elevated. Mild inflammatory arthritis responds to NSAIDs. In cases of severe arthritis, oral corticosteroids are warranted as well as anti-tumor necrosis factor (TNF) agents.

Sjögren's syndrome (SS)–like presentation manifests primarily with significant ocular and mucosal dryness. Most patients do not exhibit autoantibodies. The distinction from SS is based on minor salivary gland biopsy, which demonstrates a diffuse T cell lymphocytic infiltrate and acinar injury, a pattern distinct from SS.

Polymyalgia rheumatica and giant cell arthritis have been described following treatment with ICIs. PMR symptoms are typical, and temporal artery biopsy pathology is under distinguishable between users or nonusers of ICIs.

DM and polymyositis (PM) have also been described, with proximal muscle weakness, elevated muscle enzymes and pathognomonic abnormalities of the electromyography (EMG) and MRI images.

Monotherapy with oral steroids has generally been very effective.

Immune checkpoint inhibitors can also modulate the underlying systemic autoimmune diseases. In patients with rheumatoid arthritis or psoriasis, up to 30% of them can flare during treatment. However, discontinuation of systemic immunosuppression is not recommended, and patients should continue the treatment.

Systemic Autoimmune Diseases and Malignancy
Lupus-like Syndrome
Antinuclear antibodies (ANAs) can be seen in patients with solid neoplasms (e.g., gastric, cervical, and breast carcinomas, testicular seminoma), lymphomas, or myelodysplastic disorders, but the significance of these autoantibodies is poorly understood. It is not clinically indicated to search for an underlying malignancy in a patient with typical SLE. However, lupus-like autoantibodies and unexplained Coombs-positive hemolytic anemia or thrombocytopenia without clinical signs of rheumatic disease warrant further investigation for an occult neoplasm.

Raynaud's Phenomenon and Scleroderma-like Syndrome
The sudden onset of Raynaud's phenomenon and scleroderma-like syndrome can herald an underlying tumor such as hematologic malignancies and carcinomas of the liver, ovary, testis, bladder, breast, or stomach. Scleroderma-like skin changes may also occur in patients with osteosclerotic myeloma with *p*olyneuropathy, *o*rganomegaly, *e*ndocrinopathy, *m*onoclonal gammopathy, and *s*kin abnormalities (i.e., POEMS syndrome) and in those with carcinoid tumors.

Characteristics that suggest secondary Raynaud's phenomenon include age at onset older than 50 years, symptom asymmetry, symptoms that persist year-round, and rapid digital ulceration and necrosis. Secondary Raynaud's is also suggested by scleroderma-like syndromes in patients older than 50 years, rapid progression of skin sclerosis, or a poor response to therapy. The lack of Raynaud's phenomenon can be another distinguishing characteristic of paraneoplastic scleroderma-like syndrome because Raynaud's phenomenon occurs in approximately 95% of cases of systemic sclerosis.

Vasculitides

Vasculitis is rarely associated with malignancy and is most commonly seen in patients with lymphoproliferative disorders and myelodysplastic syndrome. Cutaneous leukocytoclastic vasculitis is the most common manifestation of paraneoplastic vasculitis. Although clinical presentations of paraneoplastic vasculitides are indistinguishable from those of the idiopathic condition, a chronic, relapsing disease with cytopenias and poor response to conventional treatment suggests a hidden malignancy.

Inflammatory Myopathies

The association between inflammatory myopathies and malignancies has been well established. DM and PM have an increased risk for malignancy, primarily solid tumors. Most malignancies are ovarian, lung, and stomach, primarily seen in the Western population. Differentiating between malignancy or not-malignancy-associated DM or PM can be very challenging, because CPK levels and muscle biopsy findings are similar. Immediately after diagnosis, all patients should undergo age-appropriate malignancy screening. This screening should be repeated every 3 to 5 years, regardless of disease activity. The suspicion for malignancy should be significantly increased in treatment-resistant myositis. The association of anti-P1 55/P1 40 antibodies has been described as highly predictive of cancer-associated DM.

Malignancies Associated With TNF Inhibitors

Adalimumab and etanercept have been on the market since the late 1990s and widely used in a variety of systemic and organ-specific autoimmune diseases. The most common malignancy reported was Hodgkin's and non-Hodgkin's lymphomas. There is an increased risk for nonmelanoma skin cancer but no evidence of other malignancies.

HEMATOLOGIC DISORDERS WITH RHEUMATIC MANIFESTATIONS

Hemophilia

Acute, painful hemophilic arthropathy of the knees, elbows, and ankles is the most common manifestation of hemophilia. Repeated episodes of hemarthrosis result in synovial proliferation and chronic inflammation, causing chronic hemophilic arthropathy. This is characterized by joint deformity, fibrous ankylosis, and osteophyte overgrowth. Radiography typically shows degenerative arthritis. Besides prompt administration of factor concentrate replacement, acute hemarthrosis must be treated conservatively with cold applications and joint immobilization followed by a structured physical therapy program. Aspiration (after factor replacement) is needed only if concomitant septic arthritis is suspected or the joint is very tense.

Sickle Cell Disease

Musculoskeletal complications of sickle cell disease include painful crises, arthropathy, dactylitis, osteonecrosis, and osteomyelitis. Sickle cell crisis is the most common musculoskeletal feature, and it can produce painful arthritis of the large joints and noninflammatory joint effusions adjacent to areas of bony crisis. Osteonecrosis of the femoral head, shoulder, and tibial plateau may result from repeated local bone ischemia or infarct.

Dactylitis manifesting as bilateral, painful, swollen hands or feet (i.e., hand-foot syndrome) may be the first manifestation of the disease in infants and young children. It can be associated with fever and leukocytosis, believed to be secondary to local bone marrow ischemia. Treatment is supportive. Increased risk of septic arthritis and osteomyelitis, most often due to *Salmonella* species, has been associated with hemoglobinopathies.

Endocrine Disorders

Endocrine diseases usually manifest with diffuse, poorly defined musculoskeletal symptoms and joint pain that is more often periarticular. Clinical suspicion of endocrinopathy is by far the most important diagnostic step. Routine clinical laboratory tests such as erythrocyte sedimentation rate (ESR), C-reactive protein (CRP), ANA, rheumatoid factor, and uric acid level are usually not helpful. Radiographs often raise the suspicion of an endocrinopathy and are pathognomonic in advanced disease.

Diabetes

One of the most common musculoskeletal complications of diabetes is diabetic cheiroarthropathy (i.e., diabetic hand syndrome). It is characterized by insidious development of waxy thickening of the skin of the fingers and hands and by flexion contractures of the metacarpophalangeal joints and interphalangeal joints. Patients cannot press the palms together completely without a gap with the wrists fully flexed (i.e., prayer sign). Although this syndrome is associated with long duration of diabetes and poor glycemic control, it may develop before the onset of overt diabetes and mimic sclerodactyly.

Dupuytren contracture and stenosing flexor tenosynovitis (i.e., trigger finger) may be identified. People with diabetes are more prone to develop carpal tunnel syndrome. Diabetic periarthritis of the shoulders (i.e., adhesive capsulitis or frozen shoulder) is more common in patients with diabetes, especially in women with a long history of diabetes. Capsulitis is characterized by staged progression of pain and restriction of shoulder motion.

Patients with long-standing, poorly controlled diabetes may develop a painless, swollen, deformed joint known as a Charcot joint or neuropathic arthropathy. Tarsal, metatarsophalangeal, and tarsometatarsal joints are most commonly involved, and it can be confused with osteomyelitis on radiographs.

Diffuse idiopathic skeletal hyperostosis (DISH) is seen in up to 20% of diabetic patients, who are typically obese and older than 50 years. It is associated with neck and back stiffness rather than pain. Lateral radiographic views of the spine show four or more contiguously fused vertebrae, the result of flowing ossification of the anterior longitudinal ligament without involvement of apophyseal (facet) joints.

Diabetic amyotrophy (i.e., diabetic lumbosacral radiculoplexus neuropathy) is remarkable for acute or subacute onset of severe hip, buttock, or thigh pain followed by progressive weakness of the affected extremity. It occurs typically in older male patients who have relatively well-controlled diabetes.

Diabetic muscle infarction occurs in long-standing insulin-dependent diabetes. It presents with sudden onset of pain and swelling in the calf, mimicking deep venous thrombosis. CK levels might be elevated. A biopsy is often necessary to rule out other possible etiologies.

Thyroid Disease

Hypothyroidism is primarily associated with myxedematous arthropathy, primarily affecting the large joints with swelling and stiffness. Synovial fluid analysis reveals a noninflammatory fluid and radiographs are generally normal. Other common rheumatologic manifestations are carpal tunnel, nonspecific arthralgia, and a myositis-like picture with proximal muscle weakness and elevated CK.

Hyperthyroidism is associated with pain and proximal muscle weakness in up to 70% of hyperthyroid patients. Osteoporosis is likely the most common musculoskeletal manifestation of thyroid disease.

Thyroid acropachy is a rare manifestation of Graves' disease presenting with swelling of the hands, digital cramping, and periostitis. It is more likely to occur in patients already having other complications of Graves' disease, primarily ophthalmopathy.

Parathyroid Disease

The most common rheumatologic manifestations of primary hyperparathyroidism include pain, proximal muscle weakness, chondrocalcinosis, tendon ruptures, and osteoporosis. Long-standing uncontrolled hyperparathyroidism leads to osteitis fibrosis cystica, primarily seen in end-stage renal disease. Radiographs are characteristic, with subperiosteal resorption and resorption of the tuft of the distal phalanx. Occasionally, erosions can be seen, making it easy to confuse it with rheumatoid arthritis. Secondary hyperparathyroidism is the leading cause of renal osteodystrophy in chronic kidney disease.

Acromegaly

Acromegaly is often associated with joint pain, mostly secondary to degenerative disease affecting the weight-bearing joints, including the spine. Radiographs are characteristic and include periosteal apposition of tubular bones, deformation of the epiphysis, and chondrocalcinosis. In addition, acromegaly can also be associated with carpal tunnel and proximal muscle weakness. Overgrowth of cartilage initially produces joint space widening, but it may eventually lead to severe osteoarthritis with pain, limited range of motion, and deformity.

GASTROINTESTINAL DISEASES WITH RHEUMATIC MANIFESTATIONS

Whipple Disease

Whipple disease is a rare, multisystem disease that most often affects the gastrointestinal tract, caused by an infection with *Tropheryma whippelii*. Musculoskeletal symptoms can precede the diagnosis by years. Intermittent migratory oligoarthritis of large joints is typical, but some patients may have a florid polyarthritis. Synovial fluid is usually inflammatory with predominant mononuclear cells. Radiographs are often normal.

Hemochromatosis

Hemochromatosis is one of the most common genetic diseases among people of northern European ancestry, and it is frequently associated with osteoarthritis-like arthropathy, chondrocalcinosis, and osteoporosis. The second and third metacarpophalangeal joints of both hands are typically involved, and hook-like osteophytes on the radial side of the metacarpal are characteristic in radiographs, the "iron-fist" sign. Chondrocalcinosis of the wrist and knee is very common in patients with hemochromatosis. Acute attacks of pseudogout can be a predominant clinical manifestation. There is no effective treatment, and regular phlebotomies are not effective.

MISCELLANEOUS DISORDERS

Multiple Myeloma

Rheumatologic manifestations of multiple myeloma include bone pain resulting from lytic bone lesions, pathologic fractures, and osteoporosis. Thoracolumbar pain in the setting of hypercalcemia, renal insufficiency, and anemia suggest the possibility of multiple myeloma.

Multiple myeloma can manifest atypically and mimic specific autoimmune disorders such as SS and SLE.

Amyloidosis

Amyloidosis is a disorder of protein folding in which insoluble fibrillar proteins are deposited in the extracellular space in one or more organs, disrupting tissue structure and function. The clinical manifestations and prevalence depend on the type of amyloidosis. The amyloid protein can be identified as apple green birefringence on Congo red staining of an abdominal fat pad aspiration or rectal mucosal biopsy specimen.

Systemic light-chain (AL) amyloidosis is one of the most common forms of systemic amyloidosis. Amyloid proteins derived from monoclonal light chains can invade the synovium, producing rheumatoid arthritis–like symptoms. Joint stiffness is more pronounced in amyloid arthropathy, and deposition of amyloid protein at the glenohumeral joint produces enlargement of the anterior shoulder, called the *shoulder pad sign*. Amyloid deposition in the blood vessels can manifest as claudication and symptoms similar to those of temporal arteritis. Deposition in the muscles may also lead to weakness or pain, presenting with a myositis-like picture or muscle pseudohypertrophy.

Systemic AA amyloidosis (formerly known as secondary amyloidosis) can complicate any chronic inflammatory disorder. The most common rheumatologic diseases complicated by a systemic AA amyloidosis are rheumatoid arthritis, juvenile idiopathic arthritis and ankylosing spondylitis.

Human Immunodeficiency Virus Infection

There are a plethora of muscular skeletal manifestations associated with human immunodeficiency (HIV), either disease specific or secondary to highly active antiretroviral therapy (ART). They range from arthralgias and arthritis to inflammatory myositis, sarcoidosis, rheumatoid arthritis, SLE, SS, zidovudine-associated myopathy, osteopenia, osteomalacia, and osteomyelitis.

HIV-associated arthritis is seronegative polyarticular noninflammatory arthritis, primarily affecting the weight-bearing joints. It is a self-limiting condition, responding to conservative management. Rarely, it requires NSAIDs or low-dose corticosteroids for symptoms relief.

The incidence of reactive arthritis has been drastically reduced since introduction of ART. The presentation is classical, with enthesopathy, plantar fasciitis, dactylitis, and inflammatory synovial fluid. However, it can be associated with severe erosive arthritis, which is generally not seen in non-HIV-related reactive arthritis.

Muscle involvement in HIV is common. It can present with inflammatory or noninflammatory myopathy. Prior to ART, the patient was more likely to develop PM, nemaline rod (rod like structures in muscle cells) myopathy and HIV wasting syndrome. Posttreatment, mitochondrial myopathy and rhabdomyolysis are more commonly seen. The most common bone diseases seen in HIV patients are osteoporosis and avascular necrosis, especially in patients that have a very low CD4 count.

Sarcoidosis

Clinical features of sarcoidosis can mimic those of many acute and chronic rheumatic diseases. Acute sarcoidosis (also called Löfgren syndrome) manifests with fever, erythema nodosum, hilar lymphadenopathy, and acute polyarthritis, almost invariably involving the ankles and knees. The arthritis is usually self-limited and tends to be nondeforming and nonerosive.

Chronic sarcoid arthropathy is less common and usually associated with active multisystemic disease. Osseous involvement can be focal or generalized and occurs in about 5% of patients with sarcoidosis. Bone cysts are usually asymptomatic, but they can manifest in the phalanges with sausage-like fingers or pseudoclubbing. Focal osteolytic changes can lead to pathologic fractures. Sarcoid muscle involvement is often asymptomatic, but it may manifest with proximal pain, progressive weakness, or atrophy

SJÖGREN'S SYNDROME

Definition and Epidemiology

SS is a chronic systemic autoimmune disease characterized by lymphocytic infiltration of salivary and lacrimal glands that leads to mucosal dryness and salivary gland enlargement, and by autoantibody production. Extra-glandular manifestations occur in 25% to 30% of patients and may occur as the presenting feature or during the evolution of the disease.

Prevalence is approximately 0.1% to 0.6% of the general population. SS is mostly a disease of middle-aged women, but it can affect people of all ages. The female-to-male ratio is at least 9:1. SS can occur as a primary disorder or can be associated with other autoimmune diseases such as rheumatoid arthritis and SLE.

Pathogenesis

The pathogenesis of SS is not fully understood. Autoimmune epithelitis is the most widely accepted model of autoimmunity in SS, in which the glandular epithelial cells (EC) act as a main orchestrator of the inflammatory response and not just an innocent bystander that is damaged by surrounding inflammation. In a genetically predisposed subject (e.g., HLA-DR3-DQ1-positive), outside triggers, such as sialotropic viruses or hormonal factors, activate EC, which then act as nonprofessional antigen presenting cells by expressing MHC I and II molecules and toll-like receptors, secreting cytokines and chemokines necessary to attract other inflammatory cells and activating both innate and adaptive immunity. Altogether, these steps promote a vicious cycle perpetuating immune system activation. Activated macrophages and dendritic cells produce type I interferon, leading to local tissue damage. Inflammatory milieu attracts and activates T and B lymphocytes to form lymphocytic foci. In fact, the presence of lymphocytic infiltration around the epithelial structures of salivary glands and other affected tissues is the histopathologic hallmark of SS.

Additionally, EC are among inflammatory cells that produce B-cell activating factor (BAFF or BLyS), a pivotal molecule that promotes B-cell maturation, proliferation, and survival. B-cell hyperactivity in SS is a key feature of the disease highlighted by presence of specific autoantibodies such as anti-Ro/SSA and anti-La/SSB antibodies, nonspecific hypergammaglobulinemia, presence of monoclonal gammopathy, and development of non-Hodgkin's lymphoma. Moreover, antibody production is essential for the formation of immune complexes (IC), which can lead to complement activation and tissue damage, or vasculitis, when deposited in the capillaries of certain organs such as the skin, kidneys, and peripheral nerves.

To summarize, immunopathogenesis of SS is thought to result from either lymphocytic infiltration of target tissue epithelia leading to progressive functional impairment or IC-mediated complement activation and tissue damage.

Clinical Presentation

Patients typically present with insidious onset of sicca syndrome (persistent dry eyes and dry mouth). Decreased tear flow leads to epithelial damage of cornea and conjunctiva, a condition known as keratoconjunctivitis sicca. Grittiness, foreign body sensation, photophobia, and formation of thick secretions in the inner canthus can occur. Untreated

cases can lead to corneal ulcerations, scarring, bacterial infections, and visual impairment.

Occasionally, patients may deny dry mouth but report difficulty swallowing dry food. Exam may reveal absence of a normal salivary pool under the tongue, dry and sticky mucosa, gingival recession. and dental caries. Atrophic oral candidiasis is a less recognized complication and usually presents with burning mouth syndrome and atrophied papillae on the tongue surface with or without angular cheilitis in the absence of classic whitish exudate. Upper respiratory tract involvement may lead to nasal dryness, recurrent nonallergic rhinitis and sinusitis, and dry cough. Vaginal dryness associated with dyspareunia and dry skin may also occur. Salivary gland enlargement is seen in about 30% to 40% of patients, classically presenting as painless unilateral or bilateral parotid gland enlargement, which spontaneously resolves 2 to 3 weeks later. Other common presentations include arthralgia, myalgia, fatigue, and malaise.

SS can overlap with several nonrheumatic autoimmune diseases, such as Hashimoto thyroiditis and celiac disease. In addition to SS-specific symptoms, patients may have a plethora of extraglandular manifestations, summarized in Table 87.3.

Placental transmission of maternal anti-SSA/Ro and anti-SSB/La may lead to neonatal disease. Female patients with SS or SLE planning a family who have anti-Ro/La antibodies should be counselled about this risk to the neonate, which occurs in approximately 2% to 5% of cases.

Sjögren's Syndrome and Non-Hodgkin Lymphomas

Compared to the general population, SS patients have a 15- to 20-fold increased risk of developing lymphomas, usually mucosa-associated lymphoid tissue (MALT) B-cell lymphoma. Interestingly, lymphoma typically develops in organs where the disease is active, such as salivary glands. Persistent unilateral parotid gland enlargement in SS is alarming and requires additional work-up. Other risk factors associated with lymphoma development include palpable purpura, splenomegaly, lymphadenopathy, positive rheumatoid factor, positive serum cryoglobulins, C4 hypocomplementemia, lymphopenia, and monoclonal gammopathy. Patients who exhibit one or several risk factors need to be closely monitored.

Laboratory Findings

Antinuclear antibodies and rheumatoid factor are seen in up to 80% and 50% of cases, respectively. When present, patients may be erroneously diagnosed with SLE or RA. Anti-SSA/Ro, and anti-SSB/La antibodies are present in 60% to 80% and 30% to 40% of SS patients, respectively. Hypergammaglobulinemia, anemia of chronic disease, and elevated ESR (related to hypergammaglobulinemia) are commonly encountered. CRP is usually normal. Lymphopenia, neutropenia, and thrombocytopenia may also occur. Serum cryoglobulins and monoclonal gammopathy are present in 10% and 15%, respectively. Complement levels C3 and C4 may be decreased as markers of disease activity but low C4 may occasionally be congenital.

Diagnosis

In the clinically appropriate context, such as presence of sicca symptoms or an extraglandular manifestation, the diagnosis is made based on objective demonstration of glandular dysfunction *and* presence of autoimmunity as assessed by elevated serum anti SSA/Ro or a positive minor salivary gland biopsy. Importantly, absence of sicca symptoms does *not* rule out SS.

Various tests are used to assess for glandular dysfunction. To confirm keratoconjunctivitis sicca, the Schirmer test measures tear flow over a 5-minute period using standardized paper strips; 5 mm or less

TABLE 87.3 Systemic Manifestations of Sjögren's Syndrome

System	Clinical Manifestations
Constitutional	Fever
	Fatigue
Cutaneous	Purpura: hypergammaglobulinemic or cryoglobulin- emia-associated leukocytoclastic vasculitis
	Annular erythema (photosensitive, indistinguishable from subacute cutaneous lupus erythematosus)
	Urticaria
	Xeroderma
Musculoskeletal	Arthralgia and myalgia
	Nonerosive arthritis (mimicking rheumatoid arthritis)
	Inflammatory myopathy
Pulmonary	Obstructive pattern on pulmonary function testing
	Interstitial lung disease (nonspecific, usual and lympho- cytic interstitial pneumonia)
	Cryptogenic organizing pneumonia
	Bronchiectasis
Renal	Interstitial nephritis
	Renal tubular acidosis (typically type I, less commonly type II)
	Cryoglobulin-mediated membranoproliferative glomeru- lonephritis
Central nervous system	Multiple sclerosis-like syndrome
	Transverse myelitis
	Cognitive dysfunction
Peripheral ner- vous system	Axonal sensory polyneuropathy
	Sensorimotor polyneuropathy
	Small fiber neuropathy
	Autonomic neuropathy
	Ganglionopathy
	Chronic inflammatory demyelinating polyneuropathy
	Cranial neuropathies (usually trigeminal neuralgia)
	Mononeuritis multiplex (vasculitis-associated)
Hepatobiliary	Autoimmune cholangitis
Vascular	Raynaud's phenomenon (without digital tip ulcerations)
	Vasculitis (affecting small vessels, usually in skin, kidney, and nerves)
Reticuloendo- thelial	Lymphadenopathy
	Splenomegaly
Lymphoprolifer- ative	Non-Hodgkin's lymphoma, usually marginal-zone histo- logic type, particularly mucosa-associated lymphoid tissue (MALT)-related lymphoma

of wetting confirms objective dryness. It is a simple test that can be performed routinely in the clinic. A normal Schirmer test does not rule out dry eyes. Slit-lamp examination of the ocular surface, using vital dye drops such as Lissamine green and fluorescein, assesses severity of ocular damage by staining devitalized spots. Unstimulated salivary flow can be measured by asking the patient to spit into a container for 5 to 15 minutes; a saliva flow rate of 0.1 mL/min or less confirms objective dryness. Diagnostic labial salivary gland biopsy is usually performed by harvesting four to six minor glands from the inner mucosa of the lower lip. The classical histological feature is

focal lymphocytic sialadenitis, which is foci of 50 or more lympho- cytes clustered around normal appearing salivary tissue (periepithe- lial infiltrates) (Fig. 87.1).

Classification Criteria

2016 ACR/EULAR classification criteria are listed in Table 87.4. Although designed for research purposes and not considered diagnos- tic criteria, they can be helpful as a diagnostic framework in patients suspected to have SS. These classification criteria are applicable to any patient with at least one item of the following:

1. A symptom of ocular or oral dryness (persistent dry eyes >3 months, recurrent sensation of sand or gravel in the eyes, using tear substitutes >3 times daily, persistent dry mouth >3 months, or need to drink liquids to aid in swallowing dry food)
2. Suspicion of SS based on presence of a suggestive body organ involvement or abnormal laboratory testing as listed in the ESSDAI (European League Against Rheumatism SS Disease Activity Index) tool. Examples include prominent parotid swelling, recent diag- nosis of axonal sensory polyneuropathy, significant neutropenia, hypergammaglobulinemia, and hypocomplementemia.

Objective dryness testing should be performed after holding anti- cholinergic medications for adequate period of time.

Exclusion criteria include history of head and neck radiation ther- apy, polymerase chain reaction (PCR)–confirmed active hepatitis C infection, AIDS, sarcoidosis, amyloidosis, graft-versus-host disease, and IgG4-related disease.

Differential Diagnosis

The differential diagnosis of SS includes etiologies that can cause sicca symptoms and or lacrimal/salivary gland enlargement. Numerous medications with anticholinergic properties, including over-the- counter products, may lead to dry eyes and mouth. Anxiety, depres- sion or aging may also lead to sicca symptoms. Diffuse infiltrative lymphadenopathy syndrome associated with HIV and infiltrative dis- eases such as sarcoidosis can cause dry mouth and parotid swelling. IgG4-related disease is associated with sicca complaints and persistent lacrimal and salivary gland swelling. Sialadenosis (or sialosis) is a per- sistent, usually painless, bilateral swelling of parotid glands, associated with alcoholism, obesity, diabetes mellitus, chronic liver disease, and eating disorders. Histologic findings include fatty infiltrates and min- imal inflammatory cells. Fibromyalgia syndrome may lead to sicca symptoms, along with fatigue and musculoskeletal pain.

Management

The goal of therapy in SS is to prevent complications and alleviate symptoms. Topical and systemic pharmacologic therapies can improve sicca symptoms, but therapeutic agents able to induce remission or alter the course of the disease are not yet available. Immunosuppressive medications are usually used in patients with severe systemic involve- ment. Treatment of sicca syndrome is summarized in Table 87.5.

Oral disease-modifying antirheumatic drugs (such as azathioprine and methotrexate) do not appear to be effective, although hydroxy- chloroquine is frequently used to treat arthralgia, rashes, and fatigue. Cyclophosphamide may be used with severe body organ involvement such as vasculitic neuropathies or glomerulonephritis. Currently, use of biologic therapies in SS is experimental; however, rituximab has been used in severe thrombocytopenia, interstitial lung disease, vascu- litic neuropathies, and non-Hodgkin's lymphoma.

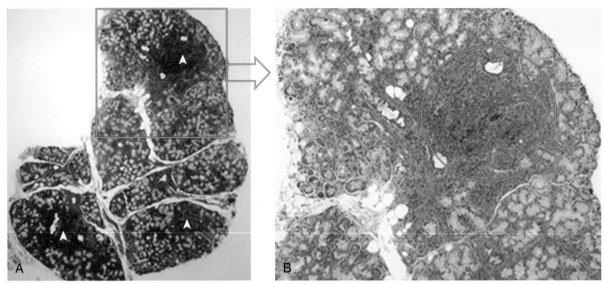

Fig. 87.1 (A) Low magnification. Cross-section of a labial minor salivary gland in SS patient revealing focal lymphocytic sialadenitis. Three lymphocytic foci, each *(triangles)* with >50 lymphocytes adjacent to normal-appearing glandular tissue. (B) High magnification. Several hundred lymphocytes forming a lymphocytic focus.

TABLE 87.4   2016 ACR/EULAR Classification Criteria of Primary Sjögren's Syndrome

Item	Score
Labial salivary gland with focal lymphocytic sialadenitis and focus score of ≥1 foci/4 mm^2	3
Positive anti-SSA/Ro	3
Ocular staining score ≥5 in any eye	1
Schirmer test ≤5 mm/5 min in any eye	1
Unstimulated salivary flow rate ≤0.1 mL/min	1

A score ≥4 points classifies a patient as having SS.

TABLE 87.5   Management of Sicca Syndrome in Patients With Sjögren's Syndrome

Treatment of dry eyes	Avoid dry environment
	Moisture chamber goggles/glasses
	Artificial tears (preservative free if used more than four times daily)
	Lubricating gels (at bedtime)
	Tear drainage duct plugging (reversible) or cautery (irreversible)
	Topical anti-inflammatory therapy (cyclosporine, lifitegrast, corticosteroids)
Treatment of dry mouth	Avoid or discontinue medications with anticholinergic properties, when possible
	Optimize oral hygiene (regular brushing, flossing)
	Sugar-free lozenges (to stimulate saliva)
	Artificial saliva
	Fluoride-based topical products
	Oral secretagogues (pilocarpine, cevimeline)

SUGGESTED READINGS

Brito-Zerón P, Baldini C, Bootsma H, et al: Sjögren syndrome, Nat Rev Dis Primers 2:16047, 2016.

Chakravarty SD, Markenson JA: Rheumatic manifestations of endocrine disease, Curr Opin Rheumatol 25(1):37–43, 2013.

Cordner S, De Ceulaer K: Musculoskeletal manifestations of hemoglobinopathies, Curr Opin Rheumatol 15:44–47, 2003.

Goules AV, Tzioufas AG: Lymphomagenesis in Sjögren's syndrome: predictive biomarkers towards precision medicine, Autoimmun Rev 18(2):137–143, 2019.

Ravindran V, Anoop P: Rheumatologic manifestations of benign and malignant haematological disorders, Clin Rheumatol 30:1143–1149, 2011.

Vivino FB, Bunya VY, Massaro-Giordano G, et al: Sjogren's syndrome: an update on disease pathogenesis, clinical manifestations and treatment, Clin Immunol 203:81–121, 2019.

Infectious Disease

88

Host Defenses Against Infection

Richard Bungiro, Edward J. Wing

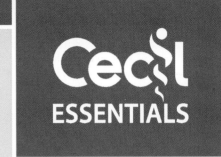

HOST VERSUS PATHOGEN: VICTORY, DEATH, OR COEXISTENCE

Many factors determine whether we coexist peacefully with our normal microbial flora and also whether we live or die in an environment filled with a wide spectrum of potentially pathogenic microbes. Factors such as age, nutritional status, underlying medical conditions (e.g., diabetes mellitus, chronic pulmonary disease), and the nature of the exposure (e.g., microbial virulence, inoculum size) may affect our response to infectious disease, with the outcome ultimately determined by our host defenses, which include anatomic (e.g., skin) and physiologic barriers (e.g., stomach acid), innate immune responses (e.g., phagocytes, microbial pattern receptors), and adaptive responses that include specific antibodies and cell–mediated immunity.

Humans are equipped with a multilayered host defense system to counter infectious organisms, and the interaction between a potential pathogen and a human can lead to one of three basic outcomes: death of the human host, elimination of the pathogen (with or without clinical symptoms), or an ongoing symbiotic relationship whose nature may change with time and under additional biologic pressures. For example, while some healthy humans are colonized by *Streptococcus pneumoniae*, pneumonia or meningitis may be caused by virulent strains, leading to death if the host's defenses cannot eliminate the pathogen in time. Most individuals exposed to *Mycobacterium tuberculosis* are asymptomatic because the adaptive immune response contains the organism in a live but nonreplicating (latent) state. Almost one third of the world's population is so infected, but only about 10% progress to active disease. Immunologic impairment (e.g., as a result of human immunodeficiency virus [HIV] infection) and factors such as age-associated immune senescence increase the risk of progressing from latent to active disease.

The asymptomatic nature of an infection should not automatically be equated with latency or dormancy of the pathogen. For example, chronic HIV infection was initially incorrectly characterized as having a prolonged latent or silent stage before the host developed immunodeficiency and opportunistic infections. However, most untreated HIV-infected individuals harbor actively replicating virus that kill CD4+ T lymphocytes on a daily basis, although the aggregate effects are not appreciated until CD4+ T lymphocyte levels are reduced to below 200 cells/mL, typically after 8 to 10 years of infection without antiretroviral treatment. Infected individuals are contagious to others despite their relatively asymptomatic state, thus treatment (when available) is recommended regardless of CD4+ T lymphocyte levels. Treatment halts viral immune destruction and reduces viral burden in blood and genital secretions, thus decreasing an infected individual's risk of transmitting HIV.

CATEGORIES OF HOST DEFENSES AND RISKS OF INFECTION

The relative importance of the innate and adaptive immune defenses is best illustrated by individuals who are deficient in a particular immunological component. For example, cancer chemotherapy may lead to the depletion of innate cells such as neutrophils, rendering the host more susceptible to bacterial and fungal infections. Congenital deficiency of immunoglobulins increases the risk of infections that are usually thwarted by antibody responses such as those associated with *Streptococcus pneumoniae* and *Haemophilus influenzae*. Pharmacologic inhibition of tumor necrosis factor-α (TNF-α) for the treatment of chronic inflammatory disease such as Crohn's or psoriasis increases the risk of developing active tuberculosis among those with latent infection. In 1981 astute clinicians, recognizing the increased incidence of an atypical pneumonia caused by *Pneumocystis jirovecii* (formerly *P. carinii*) among young men, sounded the alarm that a novel acquired immunodeficiency syndrome (eventually shown to primarily affect CD4+ T lymphocytes) had appeared that was later ascribed to HIV.

Host defenses to infection can be classified as nonimmunologic barriers, innate immunity, and specific or adaptive immunity. Immune defenses against microbial pathogens are composed of cells and molecules located in the blood, peripheral sites such as the skin and submucosal regions, and in secondary lymphoid tissues such as the lymph nodes, tonsils, spleen, and Peyer patches.

For a deeper discussion of these topics, please see Chapters 39 ❖ through 44 in Section VII, "Principles of Immunology and Inflammation," in *Goldman-Cecil Medicine*, 26th Edition.

Nonimmunologic Host Defenses

Nonimmunologic host defenses include anatomic and physiologic barriers that prevent the entry of pathogens into the body. Injuries or devices that damage or bypass anatomic barriers frequently lead to infection. Examples include burns, intravenous catheters, intubation, urinary tract catheters, surgery, and trauma.

The respiratory tract defenses depend on mucus that entraps pathogens and on ciliary action and cough that continuously clear the mucus and organisms from the lungs and upper airways. Respiratory viruses, including influenza, may inhibit ciliary action or denude the mucous membrane completely, allowing bacteria to colonize and cause secondary infection. Stroke, medications, or other causes of reduced cough reflex may lead to poor clearance of secretions, mucus, and pathogens, leading to lung infection. Smoking and exposure to industrial toxins such as silica may similarly reduce lung host defenses, such as by reducing ciliary action and inhibiting alveolar macrophage function respectively. Alveolar macrophages located in the lung parenchyma play an essential role in the initial clearance and killing of pathogens.

Nonimmune gastrointestinal defenses include gastric acidity, which kills many microorganisms, and vomiting and diarrhea, which help to clear pathogens from the gut. Bacteria vary greatly in their susceptibility to gastrointestinal host defenses. For example, as few as 10 *Shigella* sp bacteria can cause infection, whereas 10^5 to 10^8 *Vibrio cholera* bacteria are required for infection.

The urinary tract is protected physically by regular urine flow, the acidity of the urine, and antimicrobial peptides. Conditions that interfere with these factors (e.g., prostatic hypertrophy, renal stones) may lead to stasis and infection. Mechanical injection of bacteria through the urethra into the bladder, as may occur in women during sexual intercourse, can lead to colonization of the bladder and infection. Urinary tract catheters bypass normal mechanical barriers allowing bacteria to enter the bladder retrograde resulting in urinary tract infections.

The normal microbiologic flora on the skin and in the respiratory and gastrointestinal tracts is an important component of host defenses. Normal florae compete with pathogens for nutrients and have antimicrobial activity of their own. To illustrate, certain commensal bacteria of the skin secrete acid that prevents colonization by species more likely to cause disease. Disruption of the normal flora, such as by antibiotic treatment, allows opportunistic organisms such as *Clostridioides difficile* in the gut and *Candida* sp in the mouth or vagina to colonize and cause disease.

Organs that clear organisms from the bloodstream and lymph, including the liver, spleen, and lymph nodes, play an essential role after a pathogen has breached the primary anatomic barriers. Lack of a spleen increases a person's susceptibility to overwhelming sepsis caused by encapsulated bacteria including *S. pneumoniae*, *Neisseria meningitidis*, and *H. influenzae*. Cirrhosis of the liver allows portal vein blood to bypass the liver, increasing susceptibility to infection by gut flora.

Innate Immunity

Innate immunity refers to inborn resistance mechanisms that rapidly recognize pathogens and promote inflammation at the site of infection, thus comprising a critical first line of defense against pathogens. Fig. 88.1 compares the major features of innate and adaptive immunity.

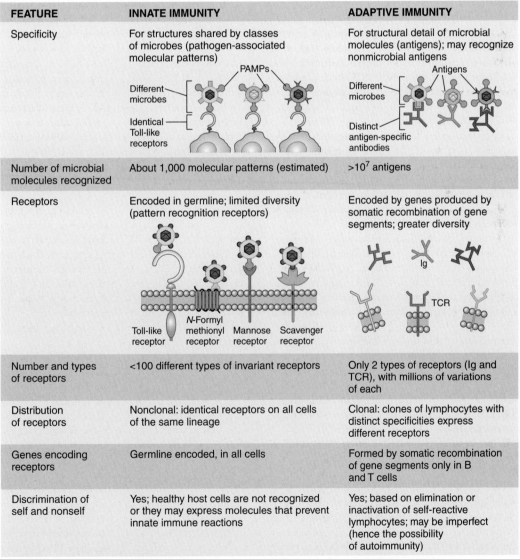

Fig. 88.1 Specificity and receptors of innate immunity and adaptive immunity. This summarizes the important features of the specificity and receptors of innate and adaptive immunity, with select examples illustrated. *Ig,* Immunoglobulin (antibody); *TCR,* T cell receptor. (From Abbas A K, Lichtman A H, Pillai S: Basic immunology: functions and disorders of the immune system, 6th ed. Philadelphia, Elsevier, 2018.)

The response of innate immunity is relatively nonspecific, invariant, rapid, and largely without memory. By contrast, adaptive immunity is highly specific and diverse but relatively slow during a primary infection, typically requiring days or even weeks to reach maximal activation. However, adaptive responses typically lead to the formation of durable memory that can be recalled upon secondary infection with a more rapid, robust response.

The molecules involved in innate immune responses include cytokines, chemokines, integrins, and pattern receptors. Cytokines are soluble proteins that have numerous functions, including promoting cellular growth and activation as well as regulating adaptive immune responses (Table 88.1). Their functions range from stimulating the production of and activating inflammatory cells, including neutrophils, macrophages, and eosinophils, to the direct antiviral action of interferons. Some activate endothelial cells and cause fever, whereas others regulate the inflammatory response.

Concentration gradients of chemokines in tissue attract leukocytes to areas of inflammation. Integrins on the surface of leukocytes allow adhesion to receptors on other types of cells such as vascular endothelium. This is the first step in recruiting and localizing leukocytes to areas of inflammation.

Pathogen pattern recognition receptors on phagocytes include toll-like receptors (TLRs), named for their homology to the toll molecule which was originally identified in the fruit fly, *Drosophila*; nucleotide oligomerization domain–like receptors (often abbreviated as Nod-like receptors, or NLRs); C-type lectin-like receptors (CLRs); and retinoic acid-inducible gene-I-like receptors (RLRs), which are intracellular receptors that detect viral RNA. TLRs, which recognize broad features of microbes such as the lipopolysaccharide (LPS) found in the cell wall of gram-negative bacteria, the peptidoglycan found in the cell walls of gram-positive bacteria, and the nucleic acids of viruses, have been studied extensively. TLRs are located on several immune cell types, including macrophages and dendritic cells. When a pathogen is detected by TLRs on the surface of a cell or associated with endosomes, signaling cascades are initiated that lead to the activation of nuclear transcription factors such as nuclear factor-κB (NF-κB). This stimulates the production of numerous cytokines important in the inflammatory response, including interleukin-1 (IL-1), IL-6, IL-10, IL-15, TNF-α, and growth factors (see Table 88.1). These cytokines amplify the inflammatory response by activating effector cells and by stimulating the production of many other inflammatory factors, including IL-2, interferons, C-reactive protein, complement components, and growth factors.

Complement factors are soluble proteins and enzymes that are produced as inactive precursors in the liver. Complement activation may occur as a result of antigen-antibody immune complex binding by factor C1 (the classical pathway), the binding of mannose-binding lectin (MBL) to microbial glycoproteins containing mannose (the lectin pathway), or the alternative pathway, which can be activated by bacterial cell wall components.

Regardless of how the complement system is activated, the cascade results in the production of C3 convertase, a protein that cleaves C3 into C3a and C3b fragments. This is followed by the production of a C5 convertase, which cleaves C5 into C5a and C5b. C3a and C5a, also known as anaphylatoxins, stimulate histamine release from mast cells leading to vasodilatation, increase vascular permeability and attract activated macrophages. C3b binds to the microbial surface and in conjunction with pathogen-specific immunoglobulin G (IgG) may stimulate phagocytosis. C5b serves as a nucleation point for the assembly of the membrane attack complex (MAC) that consists of C5b, C6, C7, C8 and multiple molecules of C9. MAC assembly results in pore formation that leads to bacterial lysis. Patients deficient in any of the MAC components C5 to C9 appear to be particularly susceptible to organisms such as *Neisseria meningitides* and *N. gonorrhoeae*. The complement system is regulated by numerous factors including soluble C1 inhibitor, which causes breakdown of the C1 complex, as well as the membrane-bound proteins decay-acceleration factor (DAF), which breaks down C3 convertases, and protectin, which inhibits MAC formation. These regulatory factors help to ensure that the complement system is not activated inappropriately against host cells.

The inflammatory response results in the classic clinical signs of inflammation, including erythema, pain, warmth, swelling, and loss of function. It can be initiated by microorganisms in tissue, tissue injury, or dysfunctional adaptive immunity (e.g., autoantibodies). The response includes inflammatory molecules as previously described and tissue and migrating leukocytes. Neutrophils are central to the clinical manifestations of inflammation in tissue, and patients with neutropenia or functional deficits in neutrophil function often lack the signs of inflammation at the site of serious infection.

Neutrophils are bone marrow–derived phagocytes whose production is greatly stimulated by infection through the action of macrophage-produced growth factors, including granulocyte colony-stimulating factor (G-CSF) and granulocyte-macrophage colony-stimulating factor (GM-CSF). Neutrophils circulate in blood (where they are the most abundant white blood cell), are attracted to sites of inflammation, and are activated by chemotactic factors, including formyl peptides derived from bacteria, complement factors C3a and C5a, IL-8, interferon, and leukotrienes, particularly leukotriene B$_4$. Neutrophils migrate from the endovascular space into inflammatory tissue through an integrin-regulated process that includes receptors on neutrophils and vascular endothelial cells. Activated neutrophils then migrate using a chemoattractive (i.e., chemokine) gradient toward the site of inflammation.

Neutrophils are killing machines containing granules that have up to 100 different antimicrobial molecules. The contents of granules are released intracellularly into phagosomes after phagocytosis of a pathogen or released extracellularly in the vicinity of pathogens. Phagocytosis is greatly enhanced by opsonization (i.e., antibody and complement binding) of pathogens. The major microbicidal mechanism of neutrophils is the superoxide burst (i.e., production of superoxide anion catalyzed by NADPH oxidase) and then the dismutation to hydrogen peroxide (H$_2$O$_2$), which may in turn be converted to hypochlorous acid (HClO). Many other granule molecules, such as cathepsins, elastases, defensins, and collagenase contribute to the killing process. Similar mechanisms exist in other phagocytes such as macrophages. More recently it has been found that in addition to phagocytosis and degranulation, activated neutrophils produce neutrophil extracellular traps (NETs), which are webs of chromatin and proteases that can immobilize and kill pathogenic microbes.

Eosinophils, which are found more in tissue than the circulation, are primarily important in host defenses against multicellular parasites such as parasitic worms. Growth and differentiation of eosinophils is promoted by IL-5. Eosinophils are activated and recruited by a variety of mediators, including complement factors and leukotrienes. Eosinophil granules contain specific cationic proteins that are toxic to parasites. Eosinophils also play key roles in the pathogenesis of allergic reactions and diseases such as asthma.

Basophils in blood and mast cells in tissue contain granules with high concentrations of histamine and other inflammatory mediators. Basophils and mast cells express receptors for complement factors and others that bind immunoglobulin E (IgE) produced by B cells. They can be activated by complement factors C3a and C5a and by cross-linking of IgE by antigen on the surface of mast cells. Histamine is a short-acting, low-molecular-weight amine that acts through four

TABLE 88.1 Cytokines

Cytokine and Subunits	Principal Cell Source	Cytokine Receptor and Subunits[a]	Principal Cellular Targets and Biologic Effects
Type I Cytokine Family Members			
Interleukin-2 (IL-2)	T cells	CD25 (IL-2Rα) CD122 (IL-2Rβ) CD132 (γc)	T cells: proliferation and differentiation into effector and memory cells; promotes regulatory T cell development, survival, and function NK cells: proliferation, activation B cells: proliferation, antibody synthesis (in vitro)
Interleukin-3 (IL-3)	T cells	CD123 (IL-3Rα) CD131 (βc)	Immature hematopoietic progenitors: induced maturation of all hematopoietic lineages
Interleukin-4 (IL-4)	CD4+ T cells (Th2, Tfh), mast cells	CD124 (IL-4Rα) CD132 (γc)	B cells: isotype switching to IgE T cells: Th2 differentiation, proliferation Macrophages: alternative activation and inhibition of IFN-γ–mediated classical activation
Interleukin-5 (IL-5)	CD4+ T cells (Th2), group 2 ILCs	CD125 (IL-5Rα) CD131 (βc)	Eosinophils: activation, increased generation
Interleukin-6 (IL-6)	Macrophages, endothelial cells, T cells	CD126 (IL-6Rα) CD130 (gp130)	Liver: synthesis of acute-phase protein B cells: proliferation of antibody-producing cells T cells: Th17 differentiation
Interleukin-7 (IL-7)	Fibroblasts, bone marrow stromal cells	CD127 (IL-7R) CD132 (γc)	Immature lymphoid progenitors: proliferation of early T and B cell progenitors T lymphocytes: survival of naïve and memory cells
Interleukin-9 (IL-9)	CD4+ T cells	CD129 (IL-9R) CD132 (γc)	Mast cells, B cells, T cells, and tissue cells: survival and activation
Interleukin-11 (IL-11)	Bone marrow stromal cells	IL-11Rα CD130 (gp130)	Production of platelets
Interleukin-12 (IL-12): IL-12A (p35) IL-12B (p40)	Macrophages, dendritic cells	CD212 (IL-12Rβ1) IL-12Rβ2	T cells: Th1 differentiation NK cells and T cells: IFN-γ synthesis, increased cytotoxic activity
Interleukin-13 (IL-13)	CD4+ T cells (Th2), NKT cells, group 2 ILCs, mast cells	CD213a1 (IL-13Rα1) CD213a2 (IL-13Rα2) CD132 (γc)	B cells: isotype switching to IgE Epithelial cells: increased mucus production Macrophages: alternative activation
Interleukin-15 (IL-15)	Macrophages, other cell types	IL-15Rα CD122 (IL-2Rβ) CD132 (γc)	NK cells: proliferation T cells: survival and proliferation of memory CD8+ cells
Interleukin-17A (IL-17A) Interleukin-17F (IL-17F)	CD4+ T cells (Th17), group 3 ILCs	CD217 (IL-17RA) IL-17RC	Epithelial cells, macrophages and other cell types: increased chemokine and cytokine production; GM-CSF and G-CSF production
Interleukin-21 (IL-21)	Th2 cells, Th17 cells, Tfh cells	CD360 (IL-21R) CD132 (γc)	B cells: activation, proliferation, differentiation Tfh cells: development Th17 cells: increased generation
Interleukin-23 (IL-23): IL-23A (p19) IL-12B (p40)	Macrophages, dendritic cells	IL-23R CD212 (IL-12Rβ1)	T cells: differentiation and expansion of Th17 cells
Interleukin-25 (IL-25; IL-17E)	T cells, mast cells, eosinophils, macrophages, mucosal epithelial cells	IL-17RB	T cells and various other cell types: expression of IL-4, IL-5, IL-13
Interleukin-27 (IL-27): IL-27 (p28) EBI3 (IL-27B)	Macrophages, dendritic cells	IL-27Rα CD130 (gp130)	T cells: enhancement of Th1 differentiation; inhibition of Th17 differentiation NK cells: IFN-γ synthesis?

Continued

TABLE 88.1   Cytokines—cont'd

Cytokine and Subunits	Principal Cell Source	Cytokine Receptor and Subunits[a]	Principal Cellular Targets and Biologic Effects
Stem cell factor (c-Kit ligand)	Bone marrow stromal cells	CD117 (KIT)	Pluripotent hematopoietic stem cells: induced maturation of all hematopoietic lineages
Granulocyte-monocyte CSF (GM-CSF)	T cells, macrophages, endothelial cells, fibroblasts	CD116 (GM-CSFRα) CD131 (βc)	Immature and committed progenitors, mature macrophages: induced maturation of granulocytes and monocytes, macrophage activation
Monocyte CSF (M-CSF, CSF1)	Macrophages, endothelial cells, bone marrow cells, fibroblasts	CD115 (CSF1R)	Committed hematopoietic progenitors: induced maturation of monocytes
Granulocyte CSF (G-CSF, CSF3)	Macrophages, fibroblasts, endothelial cells	CD114 (CSF3R)	Committed hematopoietic progenitors: induced maturation of granulocytes
Thymic stromal lymphopoietin (TSLP)	Keratinocytes, bronchial epithelial cells, fibroblasts, smooth muscle cells, endothelial cells, mast cells, macrophages, granulocytes and dendritic cells	TSLP-receptor CD127 (IL-7R)	Dendritic cells: activation Eosinophils: activation Mast cells: cytokine production T cells: Th2 differentiation

Type II Cytokine Family Members

Cytokine and Subunits	Principal Cell Source	Cytokine Receptor and Subunits[a]	Principal Cellular Targets and Biologic Effects
IFN-α (multiple proteins)	Plasmacytoid dendritic cells, macrophages	IFNAR1 CD118 (IFNAR2)	All cells: antiviral state, increased class I MHC expression NK cells: activation
IFN-β	Fibroblasts, plasmacytoid dendritic cells	IFNAR1 CD118 (IFNAR2)	All cells: antiviral state, increased class I MHC expression NK cells: activation
Interferon-γ (IFN-γ)	T cells (Th1, CD8+ T cells), NK cells	CD119 (IFNGR1) IFNGR2	Macrophages: classical activation (increased microbicidal functions) B cells: isotype switching to opsonizing and complement-fixing IgG subclasses (established in mice) T cells: Th1 differentiation Various cells: increased expression of class I and class II MHC molecules, increased antigen processing and presentation to T cells
Interleukin-10 (IL-10)	Macrophages, T cells (mainly regulatory T cells)	CD210 (IL-10Rα) IL-10Rβ	Macrophages, dendritic cells: inhibition of expression of IL-12, co-stimulators, and class II MHC
Interleukin-22 (IL-22)	Th17 cells	IL-22Rα1 or IL-22Rα2 IL-10Rβ2	Epithelial cells: production of defensins, increased barrier function Hepatocytes: survival
Interleukin-26 (IL-26)	T cells, monocytes	IL-20R1IL-10R2	Not established
Interferon-λs (type III interferons)	Dendritic cells	IFNLR1 (IL-28Rα) CD210B (IL-10Rβ2)	Epithelial cells: antiviral state
Leukemia inhibitory factor (LIF)	Embryonic trophectoderm, bone marrow stromal cells	CD118 (LIFR) CD130 (gp130)	Stem cells: block in differentiation
Oncostatin M	Bone marrow stromal cells	OSMR CD130 (gp130)	Endothelial cells: regulation of hematopoietic cytokine production Cancer cells: inhibition of proliferation

TNF Superfamily Cytokines[b]

Cytokine and Subunits	Principal Cell Source	Cytokine Receptor and Subunits[a]	Principal Cellular Targets and Biologic Effects
Tumor necrosis factor (TNF, TNFSF1)	Macrophages, NK cells, T cells	CD120a (TNFRSF1) or CD120b (TNFRSF2)	Endothelial cells: activation (inflammation, coagulation) Neutrophils: activation Hypothalamus: fever Muscle, fat: catabolism (cachexia)
Lymphotoxin-α (LTα, TNFSF1)	T cells, B cells	CD120a (TNFRSF1) or CD120b (TNFRSF2)	Same as TNF

TABLE 88.1   Cytokines—cont'd

Cytokine and Subunits	Principal Cell Source	Cytokine Receptor and Subunits[a]	Principal Cellular Targets and Biologic Effects
Lymphotoxin-αβ (LTαβ)	T cells, NK cells, follicular B cells, lymphoid inducer cells	LTβR	Lymphoid tissue stromal cells and follicular dendritic cells: chemokine expression and lymphoid organogenesis
BAFF (CD257, TNFSF13B)	Dendritic cells, monocytes, follicular dendritic cells, B cells	BAFF-R (TNFRSF13C) or TACI (TNFRSF13B) or BCMA (TNFRSF17)	B cells: survival, proliferation
APRIL (CD256, TNFSF13)	T cells, dendritic cells, monocytes, follicular dendritic cells	TACI (TNFRSF13B) or BCMA (TNFRSF17)	B cells: survival, proliferation
Osteoprotegerin (OPG, TNFRSF11B)	Osteoblasts	RANKL	Osteoclast precursor cells: inhibits osteoclast differentiation
IL-1 Family Cytokines			
Interleukin-1α (IL-1α)	Macrophages, dendritic cells, fibroblasts, endothelial cells, keratinocytes, hepatocytes	CD121a (IL-1R1) IL-1RAP or CD121b (IL-1R2)	Endothelial cells: activation (inflammation, coagulation) Hypothalamus: fever
Interleukin-1β (IL-1β)	Macrophages, dendritic cells, fibroblasts, endothelial cells, keratinocyte	CD121a (IL-1R1) IL-1RAP or CD121b (IL-1R2)	Endothelial cells: activation (inflammation, coagulation) Hypothalamus: fever Liver: synthesis of acute-phase proteins T cells: Th17 differentiation
Interleukin-1 receptor antagonist (IL-1RA)	Macrophages	CD121a (IL-1R1) IL-1RAP	Various cells: competitive antagonist of IL-1
Interleukin-18 (IL-18)	Monocytes, macrophages, dendritic cells, Kupffer cells, keratinocytes, chondrocytes, synovial fibroblasts, osteoblasts	CD218a (IL-18Rα) CD218b (IL-18Rβ)	NK cells and T cells: IFN-γ synthesis Monocytes: expression of GM-CSF, TNF, IL-1β Neutrophils: activation, cytokine release
Interleukin-33 (IL-33)	Endothelial cells, smooth muscle cells, keratinocytes, fibroblasts	ST2 (IL1RL1) IL-1 Receptor Accessory Protein (IL1RAP)	T cells: Th2 development ILCs: activation of group 2 ILCs
Other Cytokines			
Transforming growth factor-β (TGF-β)	T cells (mainly Tregs), macrophages, other cell types	TGF-β R1 TGF-β R2 TGF-β R3	T cells: inhibition of proliferation and effector functions; differentiation of Th17 and Treg B cells: inhibition of proliferation; IgA production Macrophages: inhibition of activation; stimulation of angiogenic factors Fibroblasts: increased collagen synthesis

APRIL, A proliferation-inducing ligand; *BAFF*, B cell–activating factor belonging to the TNF family; *BCMA*, B cell maturation protein; *CSF*, colony-stimulating factor; *IFN*, interferon; *IgE*, immunoglobulin E; *ILCs*, innate lymphoid cells; *MHC*, major histocompatibility complex; *NK cell*, natural killer cell; *NKT cell*, natural killer T cell; *OSMR*, oncostatin M receptor; *RANK*, receptor activator for nuclear factor κB ligand; *RANKL*, RANK ligand; *TACI*, transmembrane activator and calcium modulator and cyclophilin ligand interactor; *Th*, T helper; *Tfh*, T follicular helper; *TNF*, tumor necrosis factor; *TNFSF*, TNF superfamily; *TNFRSF*, TNF receptor superfamily; *Treg*, regulatory T cell.

[a]Most cytokine receptors are dimers or trimers composed of different polypeptide chains, some of which are shared between receptors for different cytokines. The set of polypeptides that compose a functional receptor (cytokine binding plus signaling) for each cytokine is listed. The functions of each subunit polypeptide are not listed.

[b]All TNF superfamily (TNFSF) members are expressed as cell surface transmembrane proteins, but only the subsets that are predominantly active as proteolytically released soluble cytokines are listed in the table. Other TNFSF members that function predominantly in the membrane-bound form and are not, strictly speaking, cytokines are not listed in the table. These membrane-bound proteins and the TNFRSF receptors they bind to include OX40L (CD252, TNFSF4):OX40 (CD134, TNFRSF4); CD40L (CD154, TNFSF5):CD40 (TNFRSF5); FasL (CD178, TNFSF6):Fas (CD95, TNFRSF6); CD70 (TNFSF7):CD27 (TNFRSF27); CD153 (TNFSF8):CD30 (TNFRSF8); TRAIL (CD253, TNFSF10):TRAIL-R (TNFRSF10A-D); RANKL (TNFSF11):RANK (TNFRSF11); TWEAK (CD257, TNFSF12):TWEAKR (CD266, TNFRSF12); LIGHT (CD258, TNFSF14):HVEM (TNFRSF14); GITRL (TNFSF18):GITR (CD357 TNFRSF18); and 4-IBBL:4-IBB (CD137).

From Abbas A K, Lichtman A H, Pillai S: Basic immunology: functions and disorders of the immune system, 6th ed. Philadelphia, Elsevier, 2018.

different histamine receptors. Its actions include bronchoconstriction and bronchial smooth muscle contraction, itching, pain, vasodilation, and increased vascular permeability. Histamine also plays a role in gastric acid secretion, motion sickness, and sleep suppression. Commonly used antihistamines counter these effects.

Blood monocytes are produced in the bone marrow and circulate for several days in the blood. Some may migrate into tissues, where they may develop into macrophages that phagocytize pathogens and debris and kill microorganisms when activated by bacterial products such as lipopolysaccharide (LPS), interferon-γ, and other cytokines.

The properties and function of macrophages depend on the tissue. Alveolar macrophages in the lung are continuously exposed to airborne particles and pathogens, whereas microglia in the brain have a very different environment and function. Macrophages clear cellular debris after acute inflammation and thus are the custodians of peripheral tissue. Macrophages produce a variety of cytokines important in the inflammatory process, including IL-1, TNF-α, IL-6, IL-15, and leukocyte growth factors.

Fever during inflammation and infection results from cytokines such as IL-1 and TNF-α that are released by macrophages into the circulation. These molecules increase the level of prostaglandins in the hypothalamus, which elevates the normal temperature set point. This stimulates thermoregulatory mechanisms to elevate the core body temperature, which has antimicrobial effects.

Macrophages play a central role in granuloma formation. For example, macrophages are critical in controlling difficult-to-kill acid-fast mycobacteria such as *M. tuberculosis* or fungi by walling off viable organisms in granulomas. Macrophages also present antigen derived from microbial pathogens to T cells, helping to initiate the adaptive immune response.

Dendritic cells (DCs) are derived from myeloid or lymphocytic precursors. Dendritic cells of the myeloid lineage (also known as conventional DCs or cDCs) are found primarily in tissues where pathogens are likely to enter the body, such as the skin, gastrointestinal tract, spleen, and respiratory tract. These cells have branchlike cytoplasmic extensions (for which they are named), and they phagocytize pathogens in a manner similar to macrophages, then migrate to lymphoid organs where they interact with T cells. They are the major antigen-presenting cells (APCs) in the body and are critical for the initial activation of adaptive immune responses. Dendritic cells of the lymphoid lineage are known as plasmacytoid dendritic cells (pDCs). Like cDCs, pDCs may also present antigen to T cells; however, their major role is to produce copious amounts of interferon-α upon viral infection, providing a critical first line of defense.

Natural killer (NK) cells are large granular lymphocytes that kill abnormal cells, including virus-infected cells and certain tumor cells. NKs do not express immunoglobulins or T-cell receptors but rather employ a system of activating and inhibitory receptors to detect features of stressed cells such as reduction in the expression of major histocompatibility complex (MHC) molecules. Upon activation, NKs kill their targets by releasing granule contents that include the pore-forming protein perforin and various proteases known as granzymes, which may induce target cell death via lysis or apoptosis. NKs are part of the first line of defense against viral infections while adaptive immunity is developing. Patients with NK deficiencies have been shown to be highly susceptible to herpesvirus infection such as varicella-zoster virus.

Adaptive Immunity

The adaptive immune response is capable of producing exquisitely specific protective mechanisms against microbial pathogens (see Fig. 88.1). Adaptive responses to most protein-containing antigens produced by pathogens during a primary exposure leads to the

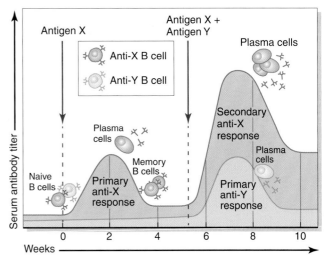

Fig. 88.2 Primary and secondary immune responses. The properties of memory and specificity can be demonstrated by repeated immunizations with defined antigens in animal experiments. Antigens X and Y induce the production of different antibodies (a reflection of specificity). The secondary response to antigen X is more rapid and larger than the primary response (illustrating memory) and is different from the primary response to antigen Y (again reflecting specificity). Antibody levels decline with time after each immunization. The level of antibody produced is shown as arbitrary values and varies with the type of antigen exposure. Only B cells are shown, but the same features are seen with T cell responses to antigens. The time after immunization may be 1 to 3 weeks for a primary response and 2 to 7 days for a secondary response, but the kinetics vary, depending on the antigen and the nature of immunization. (From Abbas A K, Lichtman A H, Pillai S: Basic immunology: functions and disorders of the immune system, 6th ed. Philadelphia, Elsevier, 2018.)

formation of memory B and T cells; secondary exposure to that antigen may recall the memory, leading to adaptive responses that are more rapid, of much greater magnitude, and of higher affinity than before (Fig. 88.2). The capacity of the adaptive immune system to protect against different pathogens is truly astounding. Through a process known as gene rearrangement it has been estimated that B cells can produce 10^{12} different immunoglobulin molecules and that T cells can have up to 10^{18} different T-cell receptors (TCRs) for specific antigens.

Antibodies and B Lymphocytes

Antibodies, also known as immunoglobulins (Igs), are variable glycoproteins produced by B cells that recognize specific structural motifs (epitopes) on the molecules (antigens) produced by microbial pathogens. In antimicrobial defense, binding of an antibody to a pathogen may inhibit (neutralize) the ability of the pathogen to infect a cell (e.g., influenza virus) or the ability of a toxin (e.g., tetanus toxin) to be effective; prompt phagocytosis by phagocytic cells such as neutrophils and macrophages (i.e., opsonization); activate the complement cascade; or kill an infected cell through the process known as antibody-dependent cellular cytotoxicity (ADCC), in which otherwise nonspecific immune cells such as neutrophils or macrophages are able to recognize antibodies bound to target cell surfaces and release cytolytic factors.

Antibody-mediated host defense occurs mainly in the extracellular space, as opposed to T cell–mediated host defenses that act primarily on intracellular pathogens (i.e., those that enter cells and survive intracellularly). The five major isotypes (also known as classes) of antibodies are summarized in Fig. 88.3 (note that IgG and IgA are further divided into subtypes). Effector functions mediated by antibodies include complement activation (IgM and IgG1/2/3),

ISOTYPE OF ANTIBODY	SUBTYPES (H CHAIN)	PLASMA CONCENTRATION (mg/ml)	PLASMA HALF-LIFE (DAYS)	SECRETED FORM	FUNCTIONS
IgA	IgA 1,2 (α1 or α2)	3.5	6	Mainly dimer, also monomer, trimer 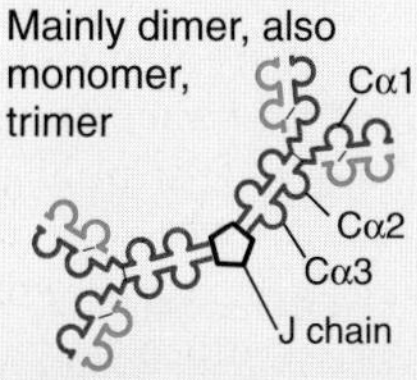	Mucosal immunity
IgD	None (δ)	Trace	3	Monomer	Naive B cell antigen receptor
IgE	None (ε)	0.05	2	Monomer 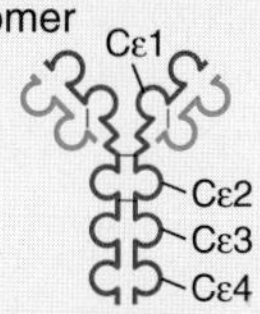	Defense against helminthic parasites, immediate hypersensitivity
IgG	IgG 1-4 (γ1, γ2, γ3 or γ4)	13.5	23	Monomer 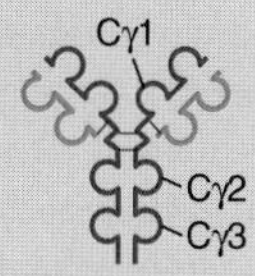	Opsonization, complement activation, antibody-dependent cell-mediated cytotoxicity, neonatal immunity, feedback inhibition of B cells
IgM	None (μ)	1.5	5	Pentamer 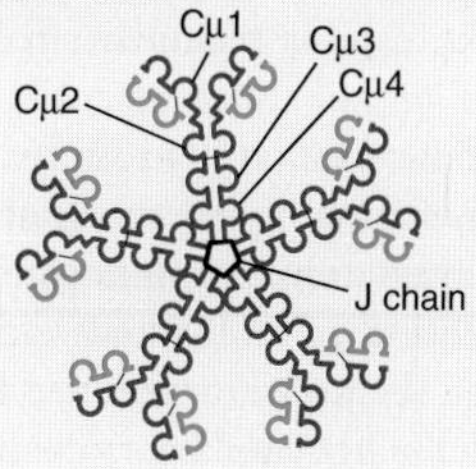	Naive B cell antigen receptor (monomeric form), complement activation

Fig. 88.3 Features of the major isotypes (classes) of antibodies. This figure summarizes some important features of the major antibody isotypes of humans. Isotypes are classified on the basis of their heavy (H) chains; each isotype may contain either κ or λ light chain. The schematic diagrams illustrate the distinct shapes of the secreted forms of these antibodies. Note that IgA consists of two subclasses, called IgA1 and IgA2, and IgG consists of four subclasses, called IgG1, IgG2, IgG3, and IgG4. Most of the opsonizing and complement fixation functions of IgG are attributable to IgG1 and IgG3. The domains of the heavy chains in each isotype are labeled. The plasma concentrations and half-lives are average values in normal individuals. *Ig,* Immunoglobulin. (From Abbas A K, Lichtman A H, Pillai S: Basic immunology: functions and disorders of the immune system, 6th ed. Philadelphia, Elsevier, 2018.)

opsonization (IgG), neutralization (IgM, IgG, and IgA) and mast cell degranulation (IgE) which mediates type I hypersensitivity. IgG antibodies cross the placenta, providing protective immunity to newborns for months after birth. IgA molecules are secretory antibodies that act at mucosal surfaces and are the predominant antibody in external secretions such as mucus, saliva, and breast milk. IgE is responsible for allergic responses and host defenses against parasites. IgM (in monomeric form) and IgD are found on the surface of naïve B cells and function in the initial antigen-mediated activation of these cells.

The basic structural unit of an antibody is composed of two identical "heavy" (H) chains and two identical "light" (L) chains (Fig. 88.4). Each heavy and light chain has constant and variable regions, the latter mediating antigen specificity. The five major types of heavy chains are designated mu, delta, gamma, epsilon and alpha (μ, δ, γ, ε, and α) and define the antibody isotype (IgM, IgD, IgG, IgE and IgA). There are

two types of light chains, kappa and lambda (κ and λ), that may associate with any of the heavy chains. The antigen-binding site of each molecule is composed partly of the variable region of a heavy chain and partly of the variable region of a light chain. There are two such binding sites for each antibody monomer, although secreted antibodies may contain 2, 4, or 10 identical antigen binding sites depending on if they are secreted as a monomer (IgG, IgD, IgE), a dimer (IgA) or a pentamer (IgM) (see Fig. 88.3).

The B-cell receptor (BCR) is composed of the specific immunoglobulin produced by that B cell associated with signaling molecules on the cell surface. Naïve B cells simultaneously express BCRs that contain monomeric IgM or IgD, each with identical antigen specificity. When initially stimulated, B cells typically secrete pentameric IgM antibodies. Later in the immune response, a B cell may undergo a process that allows the isotype of immunoglobulin produced to switch (e.g., from IgM to IgG; see later).

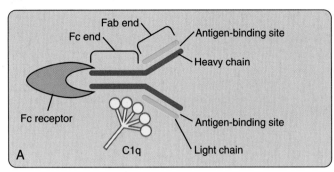
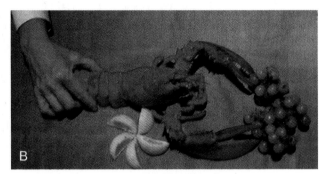

Fig. 88.4 Structure of antibodies. Antibody molecules are composed of two heavy chains *(red lines)* and two light chains *(blue lines)* held together by disulfide bonds. The two heavy chains join to form a tail (Fc end), which can interact with receptors (FcR) on a variety of cells. The heavy and light chains contribute to the Fab end. At the 5′ or amino-terminal end, these chains form two identical antigen-binding sites, much like two lobster claws. Near the hinge region of the antibody, there is a binding site for C1q, the first component of the complement cascade. (From Birdsall H: Adaptive immunity: antibodies and immunodeficiencies. In Bennett JE, Dolin R, Blaser M, editors: Mandell, Douglas, and Bennett's principles and practice of infectious diseases, ed 8, Philadelphia, 2015, Saunders.)

The constant region of the two antibody heavy chains comprises the Fc portion, which can be bound by various Fc receptors (FcRs) on the surface of immune cells (Fig. 88.4), mediating effector functions such as opsonization, ADCC, and degranulation, depending on the isotype and cell type. Soluble complement factors may also bind the Fc portion of antibodies that have bound soluble or surface-associated antigens, activating the classic complement pathway.

Much as a child might produce a large number of unique structures from a small set of building blocks, using a relatively small amount of DNA humans can generate billions of different antibodies. The two major genetic strategies that allow humans to produce antibodies specific to virtually any antigen are known as immunoglobulin gene rearrangement and somatic hypermutation. Immunoglobulin gene rearrangement involves recombination of individual variable (V), diversity (D), and joining (J) gene segments to produce functional genes that encode the immunoglobulin light and heavy chains.

Humans have about 130 functional V segments distributed among the three immunoglobulin gene clusters (heavy chain, kappa light chain, and lambda light chain); each cluster contains four to six functional J segments, with the heavy chain cluster also containing about 25 functional D segments. During B-cell development proteins known as recombination activating genes 1 and 2 (RAG-1/2) mediate random recombination of V, D, and J segments on heavy chain alleles and V and J segments on light chain alleles in a stepwise process. The combinational diversity of V(D)J rearrangement is greatly augmented by flexible joining events that can lead to insertion or deletion of nucleotides at each junction. In this manner, an enormously diverse set of variable chains—perhaps as many as 10^{12}—may be assembled. Further genetic variation arises through a process known as somatic hypermutation, which occurs in proliferating B cells following activation by foreign antigen in lymphoid tissues.

The adaptive humoral response begins with recognition of foreign antigen by specific B cells in secondary lymphoid organs. Before activation, B cells express IgM and IgD with a particular specificity on their membranes; following binding of a protein antigen the B cells internalize and process the antigen, then present peptides derived from it to $CD4^+$ helper T (Th) cells. Interaction with a Th that expresses a TCR specific for peptide derived from the foreign antigen allows a B cell to become activated, proliferate, and differentiate into antibody-secreting plasma cells or memory B cells. Proliferating B cells may begin to express antibody isotypes other than IgM and IgD (e.g., IgG, IgA, IgE) through a process known as isotype switching that is driven by cytokines such as IL-4, IL-10, IL-5 and others produced by T cells. Isotype switching, which does not affect the specificity of the antibody, allows the host to take advantage of the various effector functions mediated by the different isotypes (e.g., complement fixation for IgM, opsonic activity for IgG). As mentioned previously, proliferating B cells may also undergo somatic hypermutation, a process by which point mutations are randomly inserted into the immunoglobulin DNA. While most such mutations are deleterious, those B cells bearing mutations that enhance antigen binding activity (affinity) are selected and expanded, leading to an overall increase in the quality of the antibody response over time—this is known as affinity maturation. Furthermore, T-cell interaction typically drives the generation of a pool of memory B cells that persist for the life of the individual. Such memory cells have the capacity to be reactivated upon subsequent exposure to foreign antigen, leading to secondary antibody responses that are faster, of greater magnitude, and of higher affinity than the primary response (see Fig. 88.2).

Although most protein antigens are said to be T-dependent (i.e., require Th cells for optimal B-cell activation), some antigens can stimulate B cells to proliferate and produce antibody directly without the presence of Th cells (T-independent). T-independent antigens include microbial-derived molecules such as LPS, which bind pattern receptors (e.g., TLRs) on B cells and may stimulate them without regard to antigen specificity. Others, such as microbial-derived polysaccharides that contain repeating epitopes, specifically engage B cells with sufficient strength to bypass the requirement for Th cell interaction. More commonly, however, B cells are stimulated through synergistic action with Th cells. Specific antigen is bound to the surface immunoglobulin of the B cell, triggering endocytosis, degradation of the antigen, and presentation of peptide fragments in association with MHC class II molecules on the cell surface. Th cells with TCRs specific for the MHC-peptide complex interact with the B cell; this interaction is stabilized and strengthened through cell adhesion molecules and costimulatory activation molecules such as CD28 on the T cell and B7-1/2 (also known as CD80/86) on the B cell. Th cells then produce costimulatory molecules such as CD40L (which engages CD40 on the B cell) and cytokines such as IL-4 that drive activation and antibody production by the B cells.

T Lymphocytes

T cell precursors are produced in the bone marrow and migrate to the thymus where they undergo development and selection. At the conclusion of their development most T lymphocytes express either

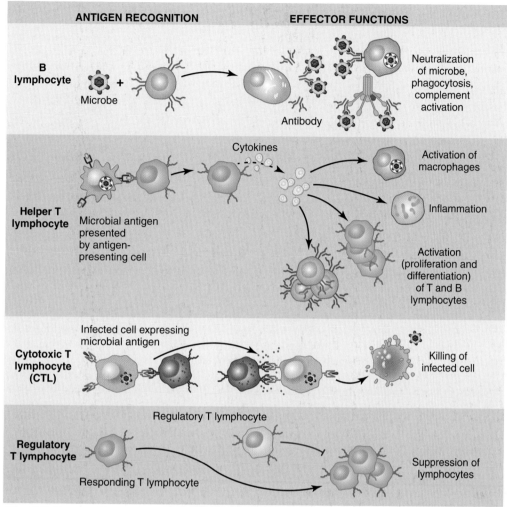

Fig. 88.5 Classes of lymphocytes. B lymphocytes recognize many different types of antigens and develop into antibody-secreting cells. Helper T lymphocytes recognize antigens on the surfaces of antigen-presenting cells and secrete cytokines, which stimulate different mechanisms of immunity and inflammation. Cytotoxic T lymphocytes recognize antigens on infected cells and kill these cells. Regulatory T cells suppress immune responses (e.g., to self antigens). (From Abbas A K, Lichtman A H, Pillai S: Basic immunology: functions and disorders of the immune system, 6th ed. Philadelphia, Elsevier, 2018.)

CD4 or CD8 molecules on their surface along with TCRs specific for a particular combination of antigenic peptide and self MHC. During development, the TCR is produced in a process involving V(D)J gene rearrangement mediated by RAG-1/2 in a manner broadly analogous to that of B cells. Most conventional T cells express TCRs that are a combination of alpha and beta TCR chains, each with constant and variable regions; others express TCRs consisting of gamma and delta TCR chains.

As maturation takes place in the thymus, T cells undergo selection processes that eliminate those whose TCRs have low affinity for self MHC (positive selection) or too high an affinity for self molecules (negative selection). The combination of positive and negative selection thus ensures that T-cell activation requires a combination of self MHC and foreign antigen. Naïve T cells, usually in regional lymph nodes or similar tissues such as Peyer patches in the gut, are sensitized by interaction with an APC such as a dendritic cell or memory B cell. The APC internalizes and processes microbial antigen and then presents peptides derived from that antigen to the associated T cell. Presentation of antigen occurs in association with MHC (also known as human leukocyte antigens, or HLA) class II molecules for CD4+ cells

or MHC class I molecules for CD8+ cells. CD4+ cells are called helper T cells (Th) and develop into Th1, Th2, and Th17 subsets. CD8+ cells are cytotoxic T cells (CTLs; see Fig. 88.5).

CD4+ T cells play a central role in the activation of B lymphocytes, other CD4+ T cells, CD8+ T cells, and phagocytic cells such as macrophages. CD4+ T cells orchestrate host defenses against pathogens that are initially acquired by phagocytic cells during phagocytosis or pinocytosis. Dendritic cells, for example, take up pathogens or antigens by phagocytosis or pinocytosis and then degrade them within phagosomes.

Antigenic peptides, which are produced by proteolytic degradation of protein antigens in phagolysosomes, bind noncovalently to a grove in MHC class II molecules. The complex is then transported to the cell surface for presentation to T cells expressing CD4 molecules on their surface. CD4+ T cells with specificity for the antigen then bind via their TCRs to the MHC class II/antigen complex on the surface of the APC. CD4 also associates with MHC II, stabilizing the interaction between T cell and APC. Accessory molecules, such as the adhesion molecule lymphocyte function–associated antigen 1 (LFA-1) on T cells, which interacts with intercellular adhesion molecule 1 (ICAM-1) on the APC, are necessary to stabilize the interaction. Activating adhesion complexes such as CD28 on T cells and B7-1/2 (also known as CD80/86) on APCs are necessary for activation, proliferation, and activation of T cells. Following activation, T cell proliferation is driven by IL-2, which is produced by the activated T cell and stimulates it in an autocrine loop.

Activated CD4$^+$ Th cells (initially called Th0 cells) can be driven by IL-12 and other cytokines to become Th1 cells or by IL-4 and IL-10 to become Th2 cells. Th17 cell differentiation is driven by transforming growth factor-β (TGF-β), IL-6, and IL-23. Th1 cells mediate host defenses against intracellular pathogens such as viruses, bacteria (e.g., *M. tuberculosis*) or parasites (e.g., *Toxoplasma gondii*). They do so by producing γ-interferon, which activates phagocytic cells such as macrophages that then destroy the invading intracellular pathogen, and IL-2, which activates CTLs to lyse infected cells.

Alternatively, activated CD4$^+$ T cells can be driven by IL-4 to become Th2 cells that mediate processes such as antiparasitic immunity. Th2 cells stimulate B cells to produce antibodies against extracellular pathogens through the production of IL-4, and they stimulate proliferation of eosinophils for activity against parasites (e.g., worms) through the production of IL-5.

Th17 cells are stimulated by IL-23 and produce IL-17, which plays an important role in amplifying the inflammatory response by attracting neutrophils to sites of infection caused by extracellular bacteria and possibly fungi. The complexity of these CD4$^+$ T-cell subsets is still being explored.

CD8$^+$ T cells respond to pathogens that initially enter host cells directly, such as viruses. During intracellular replication, viral proteins are degraded in the cytosol by the immunoproteasome, a variant of the proteasome enzyme complex that is typically involved in cellular protein turnover. Resulting peptide chains of 8 to 10 amino acids are transported into the endoplasmic reticulum where they associate with newly synthesized MHC class I molecules and are routed via the Golgi complex to the cell surface. CD8$^+$ CTLs may then bind to the presented MHC class I/antigen complex and lyse the infected cell through release of the pore-forming molecule perforin and apoptosis-inducing enzymes known as granzymes, or through ligation of Fas ligand on the CTL with Fas on the target cell, which also may induce apoptosis. CTLs are generated from naïve CTL precursors through specific association with a dendritic cell (DC) that has been "licensed" through interaction with a CD4$^+$ Th1 cell. Interaction with the DC stimulates the production of IL-2 by the CD4$^+$ Th1 cell and increases B7-1/2 (CD80/86) expression by the DC. The combination of antigen-specific signaling through the TCR, engagement of CD28 on the CD8$^+$ cell by B7-1/2 on the DC, and Th1-derived IL-2 stimulates the CD8$^+$ T cell to proliferate and differentiate into CTLs, which may then lyse infected target cells as described above.

In addition to effector T cells, populations of regulatory T cells modulate the immune response. Most regulatory T cells (Tregs) express CD4, CD25, and the FOXP3 transcription factor and help to temper immune responses, particularly those related to autoimmune diseases but also some infectious diseases.

HOST DEFENSE RESPONSE TO PATHOGENS

Humans are constantly exposed to microbial pathogens. Organisms such as *Streptococcus pneumoniae*, group A streptococci, and respiratory viruses may colonize the respiratory tract. *Staphylococcus aureus*, fungi, and many other organisms live on the skin. Thousands of microbial species have been identified in the gastrointestinal tract; most are benign, many are beneficial, and some are dangerous.

Host defenses need to react continuously and appropriately to breaches in nonimmunologic host defenses. For example, if a person suffers a puncture wound the skin barrier is breached, and pathogens may be inoculated into the subcutaneous tissues. This stimulates inflammatory responses in which cytokines stimulate the expression of adhesion molecules and chemokines on vascular endothelium. Neutrophils in the bloodstream then bind to the endothelium, traverse the vessel walls, and migrate into tissues, where they are attracted by a chemokine gradient to the site of tissue damage and infection.

A second process that breaches nonimmune host defenses results from infection by respiratory viruses. For example, influenza virus may compromise upper and lower respiratory host defenses by damaging the respiratory epithelium, inhibiting ciliary action and mucus production. Bacterial pathogens, most commonly *S. pneumoniae*, that colonize the respiratory tract in normal hosts may then colonize and invade the lower respiratory tract, leading to pneumonia. Organisms such as *M. tuberculosis* may evade upper respiratory and lower respiratory defenses and lodge in alveolar macrophages in the lung, where they can survive and multiply. Interference with alveolar macrophage function (e.g., silica exposure) may increase susceptibility to tuberculosis.

The innate immune system is critical during the early phases of infection. The response is rapid, albeit relatively nonspecific, and eliminates the pathogen or holds it in check until the adaptive immune system has time to respond. Phagocytes such as tissue macrophages patrol the periphery and detect pathogens through pattern receptors such as TLRs. This activates the phagocyte, induces phagocytosis and killing, and stimulates the production of cytokines and chemokines that initiate the inflammatory response and influence the development of the adaptive response.

Complement may be activated innately by pathogens through the alternative and lectin pathways and produce products to attract neutrophils, opsonize pathogens, lyse pathogens, and degranulate mast cells. Vasodilation results from histamine release, and circulating neutrophils are localized to the vascular endothelium nearest the site of invasion by integrins, pass through the vascular wall, and move down a chemokine gradient to the site of infection. Opsonization helps neutrophils, macrophages, and other immune cells ingest and kill the pathogen. These immediate inflammatory and innate immune responses are initiated immediately and increase over hours to days. These responses are highly effective, buying survival time for the host while more specific responses of the adaptive immune system develop.

Immature dendritic cells in peripheral tissues are sentinels for foreign molecules. Through pinocytosis and phagocytosis initiated by TLRs and other receptors, DCs detect pathogens; once they have acquired foreign antigen, DCs migrate to regional lymph nodes. There the DCs mature, process, and present antigen to T cells, initiating the specific adaptive immune response. The type of response depends on the type of pathogen. Intracellular pathogens such as *M. tuberculosis* stimulate a T cell–mediated response, whereas *S. pneumoniae* stimulates primarily a B-cell, antibody-mediated (humoral) response. Most infections produce components of cellular and humoral responses in various degrees that often act in concert. For example, influenza virus induces B-cell and T-cell responses; antibodies neutralize free virus and prevent further infection of respiratory epithelium and CTLs lyse infected epithelial cells.

Humoral Response

Early in infection, preexisting antibodies and complement factors react to pathogens directly and can initiate lysis, opsonization, and neutralization of pathogens. B cells may be activated by T cell–independent antigens or through interaction with CD4$^+$ T cells for T cell–dependent antigens. B-cell populations proliferate and produce IgM antibodies initially and then with isotype switching produce other types of antibodies, including IgG, IgE, and IgA. Antibodies acting in the extracellular space bind to pathogens or their products, potentially leading to neutralization, agglutination, opsonization, complement fixation, ADCC, and mast cell degranulation.

Cell-Mediated Response

Naïve T cells with specificity for the invading pathogen are activated, proliferate, and produce cytokines. CD4[+] T cells produce cytokines that stimulate other T cells such as CTLs, enhance the overall inflammatory response, activate phagocytes for killing, and stimulate

antibody production. Previously sensitized memory CD4[+] and CD8[+] T cells may react rapidly with activation and proliferation on exposure to previously recognized pathogens.

SUGGESTED READINGS

Bennett JE, Dolin R, Blaser M, editors: Mandell, Douglas, and Bennett's principles and practice of infectious diseases, ed 8, Philadelphia, 2015, Saunders.

Medzhitov R, Shevach EM, Trinchieri G, et al: Highlights of 10 years of immunology in nature reviews immunology, Nat Rev Immunol 11:693–702, 2011.

89

Laboratory Diagnosis of Infectious Diseases

Kimberle Chapin

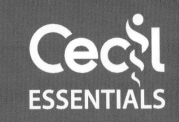

INTRODUCTION

The ability to rapidly and accurately diagnose pathogen-specific infectious diseases and resistance determinants has become the norm in medicine as a result of the continuous introduction of new technologies. In addition, companion diagnostics such as those that assess host-specific biomarker signatures in conjunction with software algorithms to clarify risk (e.g., likelihood of sepsis) or probable pathogen-specific group (e.g., viral vs. bacterial) add a personalized medicine component to infectious disease interpretation.

This chapter highlights significant components of testing for infectious diseases and trends in laboratory medicine and diagnostic technology that affect patient care. The 2018 American Society for Microbiology (ASM) and Infectious Disease Society of America (IDSA) guideline on use of the microbiology laboratory for the diagnosis of infectious diseases is a comprehensive resource summarizing laboratory diagnosis of infectious diseases by basic disease categories (e.g., respiratory, genital) focusing on best-use practice guidelines and containing numerous tables for rapid access of information. The document is well referenced and is updated on a regular basis. Other valued resources exist online for use with uncommonly encountered pathogens, such as the Centers for Disease Control and Prevention (CDC) DPDx (https://www.cdc.gov/dpdx/index.html) for parasitic infections that includes case studies and 360Dx (https://www.360dx.com/) that highlights new infectious diseases technologic advances that are important to track.

DIAGNOSTIC STEWARDSHIP

As infectious disease diagnostic tests and results have become available closer to the time of patient care, the basic concepts of optimal specimen acquisition, test selection, test performance parameters for a given patient population, and result interpretation by providers are admittedly more complex and somewhat overwhelming. Up to 70% of individual patient medical diagnoses are being made with the aid of a laboratory test result. Diagnostic stewardship, a process that promotes a team approach to optimizing microbiology test implementation, provider test choice and interpretation, along with assessment of outcomes to identify value of specific diagnostic tests for patient care have become requisite. For infectious diseases, this includes microbiology diagnostics that have been shown to affect directed patient care, morbidity, mortality, and health care costs. These are now published for a growing list of significant quality measures as shown in Box 89.1.

SPECIMEN COLLECTION AND CANCELLATION OF INAPPROPRIATE SPECIMENS

Collection of the appropriate specimen and its preservation during transportation to a testing site are components of infectious disease

diagnosis that are often overlooked. As part of their accreditation and inspection process, laboratories have collection procedures and criteria for rejection of specimens that are deemed inappropriate to process. These evidence-based protocols ensure that results can be used reliably to treat patients and provide reasons for specimen requests not being performed. Examples include cancellation of a nonliquid stool for *Clostridioides difficile* toxin testing because it is inconsistent for a person with *C. difficile* infection (CDI) that produces watery diarrhea; urine specimens for culture received greater than 2 hours after collection and not refrigerated or in preservative, which allows overgrowth of bacteria and uninterpretable mixed organism results; and blood or genital specimens for molecular-based tests submitted in a device that does not preserve the nucleic acid target.

Liquid Media and Self-Collected Specimens

Specimen collection, including surgical tissue specimens, has recently become decentralized. However, the limitations for samples that require culture have been minimized by the use of flocked swabs placed directly into a liquid matrix that preserve both aerobic and anaerobic organisms and nucleic acid targets (e.g., E-swabs [Copan Diagnostics, Inc.]), and dry swabs for molecular analysis. In addition, patient-collected versus provider-collected specimens have been shown to yield equivalent or better test results, increase patient satisfaction, and encourage appropriate use of health care.

Provider Responsibility for Optimizing Results

All personnel (e.g., physicians, physician assistants, nurses, phlebotomists, patients) collecting specimens should be familiar with the appropriate collection devices, recommended collection techniques, testing requirements, including timeliness of transportation to the laboratory or need of fresh tissue (not in formalin) for culture, to ensure optimal identification of the pathogen.

If the practitioner requests a microbiology test not typically performed, such as anaerobic organisms from a cerebral spinal fluid (CSF) specimen, or a test without standardized interpretive criteria (e.g., antimicrobials not FDA-cleared), a call should be made to the laboratory.

RAPID AND/OR DIRECT FROM SPECIMEN DIAGNOSTIC METHODS

Rapid or *STAT* is no longer a term foreign to direct testing for infectious diseases and the microbiology laboratory. All major areas of diagnostic testing, including direct visualization of organisms in specimens, detection of organism-specific antigens, antibodies, proteins, and nucleic acids, as well as cell counts and biomarkers can be performed in 1 to 4 hours. Results are uploaded automatically upon completion into the electronic medical record (EMR) and are often

- *Clostridioides difficile* toxin molecular testing and infection control practices
- Rapid identification and susceptibility for identification and treatment of sepsis to reduce morbidity and mortality
- Presurgical testing for colonization with methicillin-resistant *Staphylococcus aureus* (MRSA) and *S. aureus* (MSSA), allowing presurgical decontamination and targeted antibiotic therapy in high-risk surgical procedures to reduce surgical site infections
- Rapid organism identification and resistance determinants to aid in successful anti-infective intervention and stewardship programs
- PCR technologies for common infections seen in urgent care settings (e.g., GAS and influenza), allowing appropriate therapy, decreasing wait times, and increasing patient satisfaction
- Multiplex syndromic panels and next-generation sequencing (NGS) allowing rapid identification of public health threats and implementation of risk reduction strategies in outbreak exposures (e.g., GI transmissible pathogens and emerging infections)

available during the time a practitioner is involved with the patient, allowing immediate treatment.

Table 89.1 lists common US Food and Drug Administration (FDA)–cleared or published direct testing methods used in laboratories for primary specimens. Examples include simple stains, such as the Gram stain, to complex nested–polymerase chain reaction (PCR) for syndromic conditions (e.g., infectious disease gastrointestinal panels) and reference tests such as next-generation sequencing (NGS) of cell free DNA.

Direct and *rapid* do not necessarily equate to high predictive values for a true positive or negative test result. Tests commonly used in the past because of ease of use and cost (e.g., viral antigens from throat swabs for influenza and India ink stain in CSF) are not recommended because false-negative and false-positive results, respectively, are common. As well, direct tests that add little value in clarifying the specific diagnosis, such as positive herpes simplex virus 1 and 2 (HSV1/2) antibody in a patient without a vesicle or positive PCR for *C. difficile* toxin in a patient without diarrhea, may in fact be harmful because of misinterpretation about significance.

DIRECT SMEAR INTERPRETATION

A direct smear interpretation can be exceedingly helpful in confirming a suspected infection (e.g., Gram stain of CSF for organisms consistent with pneumococcal meningitis, or fungal elements in tissue) and is performed typically within hours of receipt. Positive sterile specimen smears are reported as critical results. High sensitivity and specificity, however, often depend on specimens being collected appropriately (e.g., obtained before antibiotic administration), providing critical clinical information (e.g., immune status or travel) and experience of the person interpreting the smear.

Special Stains

Specialty staining for a variety of organisms, allowing valuable clinical information, is increasingly being sent off site from clinical care to reference laboratories for either staining or PCR. Most academic medical laboratories still maintain special stain capacity. Fluorescent staining with calcofluor (Fig. 89.1) and auramine have increased sensitivity for direct detection of fungal elements and acid-fast bacilli (AFB), respectively. Direct fluorescent antibody (DFA) staining for *Pneumocystis jirovecii,* more specific and rapid compared with staining of histologic tissue preparations, has some limitations in sensitivity such that

molecular detection is becoming more standard, but when positive, is exceedingly helpful for treatment. Likewise, direct smear interpretation for blood pathogens (e.g., *Babesia* and malaria) is very sensitive for acute disease, but outside of academic medical centers, is typically performed by molecular testing.

CULTURE WITH A BOOST

Despite advances in rapid direct and molecular diagnostics, culture is still a mainstay for infectious disease diagnosis of many specimen types (wounds, urine, blood, tissues), in part because technology to enhance rapid detection and identification of colony growth exist and are cost-effective. Specialized media, such as chromogenic media that are both differential (colony of interest appears a specific color because of added reagents) and selective (incorporated antibiotic allows only desired pathogen to grow), speed detection.

Blood and AFB specimens are incubated in continuously monitoring incubator cabinets that signal when a specimen is positive based on algorithmic growth curves. A positive specimen can be identified at any time of day, pulled and stained immediately after signaling positive, and tested for definitive identification and susceptibility. Many laboratories utilize automated instruments for streaking specimens onto culture plates, allowing consistency better than manual inoculation such that colonies are isolated better and susceptibility can be performed 1 to 2 days earlier. Likewise, incubators that are automated and perform time-lapsed photography on each plate, incorporating comparative differential analysis and artificial intelligence algorithms, can discard "no growth" plates within 24 hours compared to 2 to 5 days. Similarly, rapid identification and antimicrobial susceptibility performed by a combination of fluorescent tagged organisms with specific RNA probes and subsequent time-lapsed photography of organism growth in various antibiotic concentrations allows results 2 days sooner than traditional techniques (Accelerate PhenoTest).

Matrix-Assisted Laser Desorption Ionization–Time of Flight Mass Spectrometry

Many laboratories still rely on automated systems that perform identification from organism growth by biochemical and enzymatic phenotypic methods as well as growth methods for determination of antimicrobial susceptibility. However, because these systems require additional growth for reactions to take place, organism identification is delayed another day and susceptibility an additional day. The increased use of matrix-assisted laser desorption ionization–time of flight mass spectrometry (MALDI-TOF MS) is a significant methodologic change that has become standard in many laboratories. This technique relies on the protein spectral analysis of the organism for identification, takes only minutes rather than days, and is very cost-effective. The technique is described in Fig. 89.2. Direct detection from positive blood broth, after a processing step, is also commonly used and allows a more inclusive organism range than molecular panels.

Table 89.2 lists the most common rapid identification methods used from positive broth cultures (e.g., blood) and from colony growth on a culture plate. Use of specific technologies is dependent on expertise in the laboratory, cost, test performance parameters and patient population.

Antibody and Antigen Tests From Blood and Body Fluids

Serology is valuable for confirmation of vaccination and/or response (e.g., rubella), often when a 4-fold rise in antibody titer is an optimal way to clarify if a disease is present, especially if IgM is nonspecific (e.g., *Bartonella*), or the primary technology for diagnosis (e.g., syphilis). Single antibody measurements are rarely helpful in clarifying the disease state (active or past infection) or the mode of transmission and often can be misinterpreted. (e.g., HSV 1/2 antibody).

TABLE 89.1   Common Methods of Direct Testing From Specimens

Test Methods[a]	Diagnostic Method	Analyte Detected
Smear stain preparations	Gram stain	Bacteria, fungal elements, including yeast and hyphae
	Fluorescence	DFA: *Pneumocystis jirovecii*, viruses[b]
		Auramine: mycobacteria
		Calcofluor: fungi
	Special: acid-fast (Kinyoun), partial acid-fast (PAF), India ink[c]	Smear use determined by laboratory and based on primary stained specimen[d]
	Wright stain	Leukocyte differentiation and count (e.g., *Plasmodium*, *Babesia*)
	Wright-Giemsa	
Antigen-antibody	Latex agglutination	*Legionella* or *Streptococcus pneumoniae* urinary antigen
		Cryptococcal antigen in serum and CSF
	Lateral flow antibody/antigen	GAS, RSV, influenza A or B, *Plasmodium*
	Serology for IgG, IgM, Western blot	Multiple analytes; detection and/or confirmation of immune status and acute disease
	Biomarkers	Single: Procalcitonin,[e] C-reactive protein
		Combination: multiple biomarkers with algorithmic interpretation (e.g., viral vs. bacterial)
Molecular[f]	Hybridization and signal amplification	Yeast, HPV, bacterial vaginosis or vaginitis
	Amplification of RNA or DNA, single analyte, small or large syndromic panels, direct from specimen or from blood, microbiome based and algorithmic interpreted	Single analytes: Enterovirus, GAS, influenza, RSV; small bundle with ≤5 targets: sexually transmitted pathogens (GC, CT, TV, *Mycoplasma genitalium*)
		Multiplex amplification with ≥5 targets: blood sepsis, respiratory, gastrointestinal, meningitis pathogens, microbiome based: vaginosis/vaginitis
		Chip array: Multiple targets, HPV, HCV genotyping
	Amplification with quantification of nucleic acids	HIV, HCV, HBV
Sequencing	Genotyping	Genetic variants of e.g., HIV, HCV, HPV
Next-generation sequencing (NGS)	16S, 18S, ITS or metagenomic cell free DNA	16S rDNA (prokaryotic); 18S rDNA (eukaryotic), ITS (nontranscribed region of fungal reran) targeted or metagenomics, can differentiate multiple species within one pathogen type/selected organism types or unbiased testing that allows discovery of new pathogens, respectively

CSF, Cerebrospinal fluid; *CT*, *Chlamydia trachomatis*; *DFA*, direct fluorescent antibody; *DNA*, deoxyribonucleic acid; *FDA*, US Food and Drug Administration; *GAS*, group A streptococci; *GC*, *Neisseria gonorrhoeae*; *HBV*, hepatitis B virus; *HCV*, hepatitis C virus; *HIV*, human immunodeficiency virus; *HPV*, human papillomavirus; *Ig*, immunoglobulin; *ITS*, internal transcribed spacer; *RNA*, ribonucleic acid; *RSV*, respiratory syncytial virus; *TV*, *Trichomonas vaginalis*.

[a]One-hour, same-day testing.

[b]Direct fluorescent antibody (DFA) is organism specific (e.g., *P. jirovecii*, varicella zoster, herpes simplex 1 or 2, cytomegalovirus), and better than histologic stains (e.g., silver stain) and Tzanck preparations (e.g., nucleated giant cells), which are not specific and can cause confusion by similar appearances for many infectious causes. Most DFA testing for viruses has been replaced with molecular technologies due to same-day turn-around time and increased sensitivity

[c]Cryptococcal antigen from cerebrospinal fluid (CSF) or serum is the recommended test. India ink often yields false-positive results and is used by the laboratory for confirmation of suspected yeast in a Gram stain of CSF or patients positive by cryptococcal antigen.

[d]For example, partial acid-fast testing is performed if the Gram stain shows branching of gram-positive rods and *Nocardia* is suspected; acid-fast testing may be performed if the auramine-stained sample is positive.

[e]Procalcitonin is a single biomarker used in clarifying bacterial sepsis. Newer combination biomarker tests along with machine learning algorithms suggest greater specificity and sensitivity for sepsis as well as clarifying viral or bacterial disease compared to PCT or traditional C-reactive protein.

[f]Common examples of pathogens are listed for each group, but many more analytes are available.

Cryptococcal antigen from cerebrospinal fluid and blood is the standard of care testing for detection of cryptococcal disease. Likewise, *Legionella* urinary antigen (*L. pneumophila* type 1) and *Histoplasma* urinary antigen are rapid and excellent tests for these conditions.

MOLECULAR DIAGNOSTICS

Use of molecular technology for infectious disease diagnosis is standard of care in microbiology because of ease of use (automation) and the tremendous clinical benefits to patient care (sensitive, specific, and rapid detection). Molecular assays may be performed in either microbiology or core laboratories with overlapping specialty responsibilities (e.g., hematology, chemistry.) The basic categories are shown in Table 89.1.

FDA-cleared direct molecular tests include hybridization and amplification methods. The main difference between these methods is that with hybridization methods, the nucleic acid is not multiplied beyond what is already in the sample. For assays that target DNA, the sensitivity is limited because DNA exists as a single copy. For assays that target proteins or RNA, detection sensitivity is somewhat increased because these components are naturally amplified in the microbe. Familiar hybridization assays include fluorescent in situ hybridization (FISH) for targets in tissue and the protein nucleic acid (PNA) smear. Hybridization assay systems can increase their sensitivity by pairing with signal amplification, such as for human papillomavirus (i.e., Qiagen/Digene HPV test), or multiple time point interpretations of probe signal uptake for rapid pathogen identification (i.e., Accelerate PhenoTest).

In contrast, amplification assays increase the original nucleic acid copy number through a variety of processes, including PCR, nested-PCR, transcription-mediated amplification (TMA), and

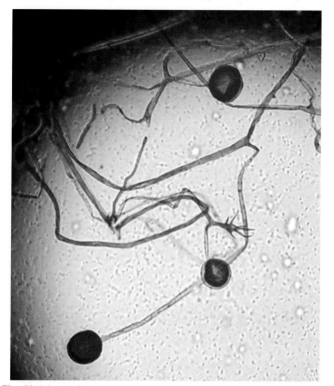

Fig. 89.1 Lactophenol cotton blue depicts fungal hyphae (rhizopus sp.) from a wound specimen.

isothermal loop amplification (LAMP). Real-time PCR refers to amplification and detection occurring simultaneously, enabling the analyte to be detected more quickly. Amplification assays can detect a single analyte (e.g., enterovirus from CSF) or a group of pathogens for a disease entity from a single specimen, such as sexually transmitted infections (e.g., *Chlamydia trachomatis*, *Neisseria gonorrhoeae*, and *Trichomonas vaginalis*). They also allow quantification of the viral load for purposes of long-term treatment and assessment of clearance (i.e., human immunodeficiency virus (HIV), hepatitis B virus, and hepatitis C viral loads).

SYNDROMIC ASSAY PANELS

These assays detect a diverse set of pathogens most commonly associated with a specific syndromic condition as well as multiple resistance determinants, (e.g., acute respiratory disease, methicillin susceptibility genes for *S. aureus*). A single specimen aliquoted into a single cartridge is subsequently tested by amplification for multiple targets (multiplexing). FDA-cleared multiplex assays from 3 to 27 targets exist for respiratory syndromes, acute gastroenteritis, sepsis, STIs, bacterial vaginitis/vaginosis, and meningitis. Providers need to be aware of the syndromic panel in use because multiple manufacturers exist and the pathogens reported can vary widely (Fig. 89.3).

16S, 18S AND METAGENOMIC NEXT-GENERATION SEQUENCING FOR PATHOGEN DETECTION

16S and 16S sequencing for prokaryotic and eukaryotic organism identification are in general limited to specific groups of organisms and used in specialty laboratories. Metagenomic cell free DNA analysis is a hypothesis-free diagnostic approach that has the potential to detect nearly any organism from blood. Sequencing is helpful in patients that are immunocompromised, where uncommon pathogens ranging from

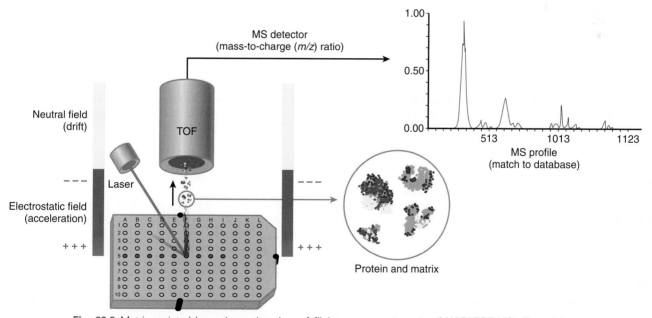

Fig. 89.2 Matrix-assisted laser desorption–time of flight mass spectrometry (MALDI-TOF MS). Bacterial or fungal growth is selected from a culture plate and applied directly onto a MALDI slide. Samples are overlaid with a matrix and dried. Samples are then bombarded by a laser, which results in sublimation and ionization of the sample and the matrix. The ions are separated based on their mass-to-charge ratio in a tube that measures the time it takes the ions to travel. A spectral representation of these ions is generated and analyzed by software that generates a profile that is subsequently compared with a database of reference MS spectra and matched, generating identification. The process takes only minutes. Although the instrumentation is expensive, the technology is US Food and Drug Administration cleared, and it yields rapid, robust, and reliable identification.

bacteria to viruses, fungi, and parasites may be present and potential infection is not being identified by other methods.

POINT-OF-CARE OR NEAR-PATIENT TESTING

Point-of-care (POC) or near-patient testing offers rapid results, typically while the patient is still in the clinical care setting, allowing directed treatment. This arena will continue to grow as patients shift into urgent care and home use venues. In addition, testing options will begin to replace less sensitive antigen tests with molecular-based tests that are more cost-effective (reducing duplicative testing and decreasing repeat visits) and have short turn-around times (minutes). They will also have an increasing menu outside of the usual urgent care pathogens of group A streptococci (GAS), influenza/RSV, and HIV tests to include other common acute care conditions such as sexually transmitted infections (STIs), bacterial vaginosis (BV), urinary tract pathogens, and biomarkers. The difference in testing diagnostics chosen to be performed in these settings (antigen, PCR, syndromic panel) will depend on the clinical severity of the patient. Urgent care assumes less severe disease and fast directed treatment, optimally with test results within an hour before the patient leaves, whereas emergency department providers may be assessing more critical patients, and testing helps decide admission or discharge to home.

Point-of-Care Testing in Resource-Poor Settings

Importantly, point-of-care testing (POCT) has become feasible for resource poor settings with battery-operated molecular systems or low cost microfluidic systems. Systems exist for diagnosis of tuberculosis and resistance determinants, HIV, human papillomavirus, and resistant STIs.

Point-of-Care Testing Quality Issues

Critically, because of cost, any test used in the POC setting should be reliable enough for the provider to have confidence in the directed treatment. Understanding the predictive values of tests being used, no matter the setting, is critical for interpretation of the result.

POCTs are dependent on the specimen type collected (e.g., nasopharyngeal swab is better than a throat swab for influenza A or B testing), the test analyte (e.g., GAS performance is more reliable than HIV oral testing), and the prevalence of disease at the time of testing as related to the technology of the diagnostic (e.g., influenza antigen-based vs. molecular).

For example, data from the novel H1N1 influenza outbreak demonstrated very poor sensitivity for rapid antigen tests (about 50%) compared with molecular tests. When a multiplex viral panel was used, other viral pathogens were identified as the cause of

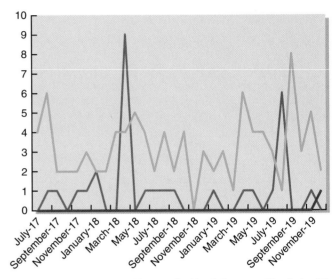

Fig. 89.3 Graph shows results of the parasitic component of a multiplex gastrointestinal PCR panel that identifies pathogens in about 1 hour. Antigen tests are not sensitive and confirmatory parasitic smear or direct fluorescent antibody (DFA) testing takes days to weeks. Two cryptosporidium peaks associated with outbreaks in April 2018 and August 2019 at petting zoos allowed rapid response by the Department of Health, limiting exposures.

TABLE 89.2	Common Rapid Identification Methods From a Positive Culture Broth, Colony, or Tissue[a]				
Method	**Organisms Detected**	**Time**	**Cost**	**Technical Expertise**
PNA fluorescent smear Positive broth	Bacteria, fungi (yeast)	2–4 hr	$$	++
MALDI-TOF MS Colony or positive broth	Bacteria, fungi, mycobacteria	Minutes to 1 hr	$	+
Hybridization probes Colony or positive broth	Bacteria, dimorphic fungi, mycobacteria	4–8 hr	$$$	+++
Amplification[b]	Bacteria, viruses, mycobacteria, parasites	1–4 hr	$$ to $$$$	+ to +++
Next-generation sequencing, whole genome sequencing	Bacteria, fungi, mycobacteria, viruses, environmental	1–3 days	$$$$	+++ to ++++
Combination fluorescent rRNA probe and time-lapsed morphokineteic cellular analysis	Bacterial identification and rapid phenotypic susceptibility	2–8 hr	$$$	++

MALDI-TOF, Matrix-assisted laser desorption ionization–time of flight mass spectrometry; *PLC,* high-pressure liquid chromatography; *PNA,* peptide nucleic acid; *$,* relative cost; *+,* relative level of required expertise.
[a]Rapid methods require 2 to 24 hours. Methods presented are US Food and Drug Administration cleared or have had test performance validated in the clinical laboratory. Due to required technical expertise and cost, some of these assays may not be available in the routine laboratory, and providers should inquire about availability
[b]Includes many different technologies, such as polymerase chain reaction (PCR), transcription-mediated amplification (TMA), and isothermal loop amplification (LAMP).

influenza-like illness in more than 50% of patients admitted to hospitals. As a result, amplified testing assays for influenza, RSV, and GAS have been developed by manufacturers as Clinical Laboratory Improvement Amendment (CLIA)–waived tests for use in POC settings. Syndromic panel use in urgent care settings is unusual, but as more systems achieve CLIA-waived status, syndromic panel use will be more common. But urgent care clinics, especially those that serve patients within a specific health care system with more capacity for testing, will likely be able to incorporate greater POC testing, including receipt of self-collected patient specimens. Costs will be balanced by reducing the number of patients getting their care in costly emergency departments.

TRENDS IN THE DIAGNOSIS OF INFECTIOUS DISEASES

The most significant trend in diagnostics is that rapid change will continue as diagnostics grow to meet the changes in health care systems and the consumer. Relevant components are listed in Box 89.2.

BOX 89.2 Trends in the Diagnosis of Infectious Diseases

- **Guidelines and evidence-based testing:** Continued development of evidence-based guidelines for both patient treatment and test reimbursement. Real-time use of diagnostic stewardship teams and health care system test order algorithms to guide appropriate test implementation, ordering, and interpretation.
- **Testing platforms:** Less reliance on traditional culture-based techniques with culture becoming increasingly automated at the front end (processing), aliquoting for MALDI-TOF identification, as well as the back-end components of reading and interpretation (machine algorithms).
- **Molecular technologies:** Wider availability and adoption of syndromic molecular panel assays as well as genetic resistance determinants due to speed and comprehensive menus. Accepted use of cell-free nucleic acid and next-generation sequencing (NGS) detection for low-yield pathogens (e.g., unusual or unexpected) and/or slow growing culture pathogens (e.g., fungi), especially in immunocompromised patients.
- **Antimicrobial resistance and stewardship:** Standardization of rapid phenotypic antimicrobial susceptibility, providing results 48 hours sooner compared to traditional culture susceptibility, aiding in antimicrobial stewardship initiatives.
- **Emerging infections:** Viruses, mycobacteria, mycology, and specialized pathogen culture and susceptibility will continue to move to specialty reference laboratories and public health until more rapid and user-friendly diagnostics are developed. Worldwide increase in fungal diseases will hasten fungal test development. Emergency use authorization (EUA) test systems will be sought by companies for emerging outbreak infections to aid in global strategizing.
- **Point-of-care testing:** Use of rapid and cost-effective molecular tests (microfluidic or similar), battery-operated (or similar), portable platforms developed for POC, including urgent care clinics and resource poor settings.

SUGGESTED READINGS

Barenfanger J, Graham DR, Kolluri L, et al: Decreased mortality associated with prompt Gram staining of blood cultures, Am J Clin Pathol 130(6):870–876, 2008.

Blauwkamp TA, Thair S, Rosen MJ, et al: Analytical and clinical validation of a microbial cell-free DNA sequencing test for infectious disease, Nat Microbiol 4(4):663–674, 2019.

Buss SN, Leber A, Chapin K, et al: Multicenter evaluation of the BioFire FilmArray™ gastrointestinal panel for the etiologic diagnosis of infectious gastroenteritis, J Clin Microbiol 53(3):915–925, 2015.

Clark AE, Kaleta EJ, Arora A, Wolk DM: Matrix-assisted laser desorption ionization-time of flight mass spectrometry: a fundamental shift in the routine practice of clinical microbiology, Clin Microbiol Rev 26(3):547–603, 2013.

Friedman DZP, Schwartz IS: Emerging fungal infections: new patients, new patterns, and new pathogens, J Fungi (Basel) 5(3), 2019.

Gaydos CA: Let's take a "Selfie": self-collected samples for sexually transmitted infections, Sex Transm Dis 45(4):278–279, 2018.

Gu W, Miller S, Chiu CY: Clinical metagenomic next-generation sequencing for pathogen detection, Annu Rev Pathol 14:319–333, 2019.

Herberg J, Kaforou M, Wright VJ, IRIS Consortium, et al: Diagnostic test accuracy of a 2-transcript host RNA signature for discriminating bacterial vs viral infection in febrile children, J Am Med Assoc 316(8):835–845, 2016.

Kamat IS, Ramachandran V, Eswaran H, et al: Procalcitonin to distinguish viral from bacterial pneumonia: a systematic review and meta-analysis, Clin Infect Dis 70(3):538–542, 2020.

Kozel TR, Burnham-Marusich AR: Point-of-Care testing for infectious diseases: past, present, and future, J Clin Microbiol 55(8):2313–2320, 2017.

Mermel LA, Jefferson J, Blanchard K, et al: Reducing clostridium difficile incidence, colectomies, and mortality in the hospital setting: a successful multidisciplinary approach, Jt Comm J Qual Patient Saf 39(7):298–305, 2013.

Messacar K, Parker SK, Todd JK, Dominguez SR: Implementation of rapid molecular infectious disease diagnostics: the role of diagnostic and antimicrobial stewardship, J Clin Microbiol 55(3):715–723, 2017.

Miller JM, Binnicker MJ, Campbell S, et al: A guide to utilization of the microbiology laboratory for diagnosis of infectious diseases: 2018 update by the Infectious Diseases Society of America and the American Society for Microbiology, Clin Infect Dis 67(6):e1–e94, 2018.

Pritt BS, Patel R, Kirn TJ, Thomson Jr RB: Point-counterpoint: a nucleic acid amplification test for Streptococcus pyogenes should replace antigen detection and culture for detection of bacterial Pharyngitis, J Clin Microbiol 54(10):2413–2419, 2016.

Saenger A. Right test, right patient, right time, wrong interpretation? American association for clinical chemistry (AACC) Clinical Laboratory News, 2014.

Saraswat MK, Magruder JT, Crawford TC, et al: Preoperative Staphylococcus aureus screening and targeted decolonization in cardiac surgery, Ann Thorac Surg 104(4):1349–1356, 2017.

Tansarli GS, Chapin KC: Diagnostic accuracy of the Biofire® FilmArray® meningitis/encephalitis panel: a systematic review and meta-analysis, Clin Microbiol Infect(19):30615–30619, S1198-743X, 2019.

van Houten CB, de Groot JAH, Klein A, et al: A host-protein based assay to differentiate between bacterial and viral infections in preschool children (OPPORTUNITY): a double-blind, multicentre, validation study, Lancet Infect Dis 17(4):431–440, 2017.

Weiss ZF, Cunha CB, Chambers AB, et al: Opportunities revealed for antimicrobial stewardship and clinical practice with implementation of a rapid respiratory multiplex assay, J Clin Microbiol 57(10), 2019.

90

Fever and Febrile Syndromes

Maria D. Mileno

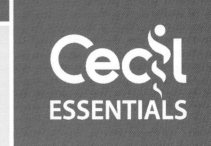

INTRODUCTION

Fever is one of the most common problems requiring medical evaluation. Fever is an elevation in core body temperature greater than normal daily variation, which is 37° C ± 0.4° C (98.6° F ± 0.7° F). Documentation of true fever can be important evidence of infectious processes that warrant investigation. Although fever is characteristic of most infections, it also occurs in noninfectious conditions such as autoimmune and inflammatory diseases, malignancy, and trauma.

This chapter reviews the pathogenesis of the febrile response, the approach to the acutely ill patient with fever, and fever of unknown origin. Fever can be associated with infections, such as those from animal exposures, or with common clinical scenarios in which it may occur as the sole complaint, manifest with rash, or develop with lymphadenopathy. A word of caution about the difference between true and factitious fever is offered at the end of the chapter.

PATHOGENESIS

Thermoregulation of core body temperature is one of the most important mechanisms in mammalian and human physiology. At core temperature the human body's systems work together at their optimum. The hypothalamic heat-regulating set point shifts in response to infection or inflammation mediated primarily by the host's monocytes and macrophages, which are activated as they encounter exogenous bacterial substances, toxins, or the cellular products of trauma.

Monocytes and macrophages produce small proteins called *cytokines,* such as interleukin-1 (IL-1), IL-6, and tumor necrosis factor (TNF). They are collectively known as *endogenous pyrogens* because they actively increase body temperature by increasing the hypothalamic set point, which is the normal temperature for the body that is controlled by the hypothalamus. IL-1 and other endogenous pyrogens are released by macrophages at the site of infection and travel through the bloodstream to the hypothalamus, where they elevate levels of prostaglandin E_2 (PGE_2). Elevated PGE_2 levels increase the set point, and thermoregulatory mechanisms raise the body's core temperature. IL-1 also induces production of PGE_2 in peripheral tissues, which causes the nonspecific myalgias and arthralgias that often accompany fever. Prostaglandin inhibitors such as aspirin or acetaminophen block prostaglandin synthesis and reduce elevated temperatures.

Thermoregulatory control is initiated through sensory neurons in the skin, abdomen, and spinal cord. Central nervous system (CNS) thermoreceptors sense and integrate temperature information. After the hypothalamic set point is raised, the firing rates of neurons in the vasomotor center are altered, causing peripheral vasoconstriction and producing a noticeable cold sensation in the hands and feet. Blood is shunted away from the periphery to the internal organs, and this process is sufficient to raise core body temperature by 1° to 2° C.

Other signaling mechanisms have roles in thermoregulation. The adipocyte-derived hormone leptin actively controls energy homeostasis, and thermogenesis in fat tissue contributes to increasing core temperature. Thermogenesis is important in fighting infection and in responding to cold-induced heat production. Fever has direct antimicrobial effects in some infections such as neurosyphilis and salmonellosis, and elevated temperature augments humoral and cellular immune responses. IL-1 acts independently on two physiologic systems: thermoregulation and iron metabolism. IL-1 can stimulate a wide range of host defenses to conduct a synergistic response to infection.

Fever also can have deleterious effects. It may lead to disorientation and confusion in persons with underlying brain disease and in healthy older individuals. Tachycardia can increase cardiopulmonary work, precipitating congestive heart failure or myocardial infarction in persons with significant cardiopulmonary disease. Fever should be controlled with antipyretics for comfort and to avoid compromising individuals with multiple medical problems. Acetaminophen is preferred for control of fever in children because of the risk of Reye's syndrome with salicylate use.

The terms *fever, hyperthermia,* and *hyperpyrexia* are not synonymous. Although most patients with elevated temperature have fever (>38.3° C or 100.9° F), some conditions can increase the body temperature by overriding or bypassing the normal homeostatic mechanism and may even produce body temperatures in excess of 41° C or 105.8° F (i.e., hyperthermia), which can be rapidly fatal and does not respond to antipyretics. Rapid cooling is critical to the patient's survival in hyperthermic conditions such as heat stroke. Even in otherwise healthy individuals, heat stroke can occur after vigorous exercise and prolonged exposure to high environmental temperatures and humidity. Heat stroke is marked by temperatures greater than 40.6° C (105.1° F), altered sensorium or coma, and cessation of sweating. Treatment includes covering the patient with wet compresses followed by intravenous infusion of fluids appropriate to correct fluid and electrolyte losses.

Severe hyperthermia may be a heritable reaction to anesthetics (i.e., malignant hyperthermia) or a response to phenothiazines (i.e., neuroleptic malignant syndrome). Serotonin syndrome, which often includes fever, is classically associated with the simultaneous administration of two serotonergic agents (e.g., selective serotonin reuptake inhibitors plus tramadol). It can also occur after initiation of a single serotonergic drug that increases the serotonin level of individuals who are particularly sensitive to serotonin. Occasionally, persons with CNS disorders such as paraplegia and persons with severe dermatologic conditions are unable to dissipate heat and can experience hyperthermia.

Hyperpyrexia is the term for extraordinarily high fever (>41.5° C or 106.7° F), which can occur in patients with severe infections but is most commonly observed in persons with CNS hemorrhages.

DIAGNOSTIC APPROACH TO THE ACUTELY ILL PATIENT WITH FEVER

Patterns of fever should be considered when assessing acutely ill, febrile persons. Evaluation includes determining the normal diurnal variation in body temperature, which often persists when patients have fever. Normally, body temperature peaks in the late afternoon or early evening.

Rigors (i.e., bed-shaking chills) often mark the onset of bacterial infection, typically bacteremia, although they may occur in other clinical situations, such as drug-induced fever or transfusion reactions. Wide swings in temperature may indicate an abscess. Malaria should be considered for anyone with fever who has visited or lived in malarious regions or who has relapsing fever accompanied by episodes of shaking chills and high fever separated by 1 to 3 days of normal body temperature and relative well-being. The timing of administration of anti-inflammatory drugs should be assessed because they may alter or blunt the febrile response. Most infectious diseases manifest with fever as an early finding and with subclinical and eventual clinical involvement of specific organ systems.

If fever occurs as the sole complaint or is associated with localized symptoms and signs, the diagnostic approach includes taking a thorough history, including an extensive review of systems, medical and surgical histories, and immunizations, including those from childhood. Antipyretics may be withheld to allow assessment of the fever trajectory. Elderly individuals, persons taking corticosteroids, and patients with chronic liver or renal disease may be less likely to mount a fever. All likely sources of disease, including travel, exposure to *Mycobacterium tuberculosis,* and occupational, hobby, animal, insect, and sexual contacts, should be assessed. Previous itineraries and activities, geographic risks of diseases, and the seasonality and incubation periods of possible disease exposures should be considered in returning travelers.

Viral Infection

Acute febrile illnesses in young healthy adults usually are caused by viral infections, which do not require precise diagnosis because they are self-limited and seldom have therapeutic options. Upper respiratory tract symptoms of rhinorrhea, sore throat, cough, and hoarseness most often result from rhinovirus, coronavirus, parainfluenza virus, and adenoviruses. Adenovirus outbreaks occur among persons living in close quarters such as military barracks or college dormitories. Respiratory syncytial virus, human metapneumovirus, and human bocavirus infections occur in similar conditions and sometimes manifest with pneumonia.

A coronavirus causes the potentially fatal upper respiratory viral infection called *Middle East respiratory syndrome* (MERS). It has caused pneumonia with acute respiratory distress syndrome (ARDS) and death in one half of infected individuals, and it is highly contagious. See Appendix for discussion of COVID-19.

Meningitis symptoms occur predominantly from enterovirus infections during summer months, although the symptom complex warrants urgent treatment of bacterial causes while the diagnostic process occurs. Febrile syndromes without meningitis are more common manifestations of enteroviral infections.

Arthropod-borne viruses such as California encephalitis virus; eastern, western, and Venezuelan equine encephalitis viruses; St. Louis encephalitis virus; and West Nile virus can produce self-limited febrile illnesses and encephalitis. Colorado tick fever is a biphasic illness seen after northwestern and southwestern tick exposures. It is characterized by high fevers and leukopenia. A deer tick virus—Powassan virus—has been associated with numerous cases of fever and encephalitis in New England and the Upper Midwest.

Influenza causes sore throat, cough, myalgias, arthralgias, and headache in addition to fever, and it most often manifests in an epidemic pattern during winter months. It is unusual for fever to persist beyond 5 days in uncomplicated influenza. Prolonged fever in persons with diagnosed influenza warrants investigation and treatment of bacterial superinfection. The epidemics of avian influenza and H1N1 pandemic strains in recent years are sobering reminders that influenza viruses have a remarkable ability to mutate, producing new immune-resistant strains on a regular basis. Preventive yearly influenza vaccination is important.

Mononucleosis syndromes of fever with detectable lymph node enlargement typify infections with Epstein-Barr virus (EBV), cytomegalovirus (CMV), primary human immunodeficiency virus (HIV), and *Toxoplasma gondii* (i.e., toxoplasmosis). Other manifestations of these infections include abnormal liver function test results, respiratory tract symptoms, and neurologic symptoms. Diagnosis of acute HIV infection, which can produce a mononucleosis-like syndrome, is an urgent issue.

Bacterial Infections

Pathogenic bacteria can infect all body parts and can cause a spectrum of localized illness warranting antibiotic therapy. For example, *Staphylococcus aureus* may cause skin abscesses or cellulitis. Highly pathogenic organisms may colonize individuals who have had contact with the health care system. Most concerning is the event of bacteria entering the bloodstream. Obtaining timely blood cultures before administering the antibiotics indicated for presumed bacterial infections in persons with common clinical syndromes can help to identify bloodstream pathogens and define the required course of treatment.

Fever may be the predominant clinical manifestation of *S. aureus* illness. This organism and the methicillin-resistant form (i.e., MRSA) frequently cause sepsis without an obvious primary site of infection. It should be considered in patients undergoing intravenous therapy or hemodialysis and in those who use intravenous drugs or who have severe chronic dermatitis. Bacteremia with staphylococci may cause hematogenous seeding of bones leading to osteomyelitis and heart valves leading to endocarditis in individuals; the bacteremia may also reflect these underlying processes. Other common causes of bacteremia and their sources include *Streptococcus pneumoniae* (i.e., pneumonia), *Escherichia coli* (i.e., urinary tract and gastrointestinal sources), streptococci (i.e., skin), and anaerobes (i.e., gastrointestinal tract).

Listeria monocytogenes bacteremia is seen predominantly in persons with depressed cell-mediated immunity and pregnant women. Although bacteremia is the most common manifestation of listeriosis in these hosts, many with listeriosis may have meningitis and warrant lumbar puncture for cerebrospinal fluid culture. Most cases occur in individuals over age 50.

Typhoid and paratyphoid fever (i.e., enteric fever) are common in many low-income countries. Patients may have fever alone as the primary clinical manifestation. Travelers to six countries account for 80% of US cases: India, Mexico, Philippines, Pakistan, El Salvador, and Haiti. Fever with headache and an insidious onset with an unremarkable physical examination is common, although a faint and transient rash (i.e., rose spots) may appear by the second week of illness. Symptoms may include diarrhea, constipation, vague abdominal discomfort, and sometimes dry cough. Diagnosis depends on the culture of blood or stool.

Fever With Localized Symptoms and Signs

Localized bacterial infection can be apparent, as in cases of abscess, cellulitis, or otitis media, or can be clinically occult. It can develop as

TABLE 90.1   Infections Exhibiting Fever as the Sole or Dominant Feature

Infectious Agent or Source	Epidemiologic Exposure and History	Distinctive Clinical and Laboratory Findings
Viruses		
Rhinovirus, adenovirus, parainfluenza	None (adenovirus in epidemics)	Often URI symptoms; throat and rectal cultures; rapid viral antigen testing
Middle East respiratory syndrome (MERS)	Travel to Arabian Peninsula or contact from Middle East	Pneumonia with ARDS; viral antigen testing of sputum; PCR of normally sterile sites (CDC)
Enteroviruses (non-polioviruses: coxsackie-viruses, echovirus)	Summer, epidemic	Occasionally aseptic meningitis, rash, pleurodynia, herpangina; serologic or nucleic acid testing (PCR)
Influenza	Winter, epidemic	Headache, myalgias, arthralgias; nasopharyngeal culture, rapid viral antigen testing
EBV, CMV	Close personal contact; blood or tissue exposure; occupational or perinatal exposure	Monospot test, EBV specific antibodies; EBV PCR in immuno-compromised; CMV IgM shell vial assay; CMV antigenemia assay; CMV DNA of CSF; culture and histopathology of tissues
Colorado tick fever	Southwest and Northwest regions, tick exposure	Biphasic illness, leukopenia; blood, CSF cultures, serologic or PCR
Powassan virus	New England and Upper Midwest exposure	Altered mentation or encephalitis; serum and CSF IgM (CDC)
Bacteria		
Staphylococcus aureus	IV drug users, IV catheters, hemodialysis, dermatitis	Must exclude endocarditis; blood cultures
Listeria monocytogenes	Depressed cell-meditated immunity	Meningitis may also be present; blood, CSF cultures
Salmonella typhi, Salmonella paratyphi	Food or water contaminated by carrier or patient	Headache, myalgias, diarrhea, or constipation, transient rose spots; blood, marrow, or stool cultures
Streptococci	Valvular heart disease	Low-grade fever, fatigue; blood cultures
Animal Exposure		
Coxiella burnetii (Q fever)	Exposure to infected livestock, parturient animals	Headache, occasionally pneumonitis, hepatitis, culture-nega-tive endocarditis; serologic testing
Leptospira interrogans	Water contaminated by urine From dogs, cats, rodents, small mammals	Headache, myalgias, conjunctival suffusion, biphasic illness, aseptic meningitis; serologic testing

ARDS, Acute respiratory disease syndrome; *CDC,* Centers for Disease Control and Prevention case definition; *CMV,* cytomegalovirus; *CSF,* cere-brospinal fluid; *EBV,* Epstein-Barr virus; *IgM,* immunoglobulin M; *IV,* intravenous; *PCR,* polymerase chain reaction; *URI,* upper respiratory infection.

an undifferentiated febrile syndrome. Careful inspection of mucous membranes and conjunctiva may reveal petechiae, which are clues to meningococcemia or infective endocarditis. Finding heart murmurs in the setting of fever may suggest endocarditis and warrant additional blood cultures. Pulmonary signs in pneumonia include rales and evidence of consolidation, but persons with cryptococcosis, coccidioidomycosis, histoplasmosis, psittacosis, legionellosis, or pneumocystis pneumonia may show few signs. Pyelonephritis and renal abscesses can occur with few localizing signs.

These infections should be suspected based on exposure history and the host's immune status. It is important to assess the size of the liver, spleen, and lymph nodes, particularly in cases of viral infection. A swollen joint may indicate septic arthritis. A complete neurologic examination, including cranial nerves and testing for meningeal signs, may indicate CNS infection.

Malaria, bacterial sepsis, and bacterial infections of the lung, urinary tract, CNS, and intestines with resultant bacteremia warrant urgent initiation of empirical treatment while awaiting final identification and sensitivities. For febrile patients with features suggesting a bacterial infection, evaluation should include complete blood counts with differential and platelet counts, blood smears for those at risk for malaria or babesiosis, urinalysis, throat and blood cultures, and a chest radiograph.

Fevers with rash as a prominent feature warrant exclusion of life-threatening infectious diseases, including meningococcemia, toxic shock syndrome (TSS), and Rocky Mountain spotted fever (RMSF).

Characterization of the rash can help. Clues to some of the common infections exhibiting fever as the sole feature and those causing fever with rash are provided in Tables 90.1, 90.2, and 90.3. Tables 90.4 and 90.5 list common syndromes associated with imported fevers when assessing travelers.

FEVER OF UNKNOWN ORIGIN

Most febrile conditions resolve or are readily diagnosed and treated, but some fevers can persist and remain unexplained. Table 90.6 shows the most common causes of unexplained fevers.

The term *fever of unknown origin* (FUO) identifies a pattern of fever with temperatures greater than 38.3° C (101° F) on several occasions over more than 3 weeks after an initial diagnostic work-up for which the diagnosis remains uncertain. Verifying the presence or absence of fever is important; up to 35% of 347 patients admitted to the National Institutes of Health (NIH) for evaluation of prolonged fever were determined not to have significant fever or had fever of factitious origin. Cases of FUO are categorized as classic FUO, health care–associated FUO, neutropenic (immune-deficient) FUO, and HIV-related FUO. Each of these FUO subtypes can have unique causes.

Classic Fever of Unknown Origin

The most common causes of classic FUO are infections, malignancies, and noninfectious inflammatory disorders; miscellaneous causes and undiagnosed cases account for the remaining categories. Historically,

TABLE 90.2 Differential Diagnosis of Infectious Agents Producing Fever and Rash

Maculopapular, Erythematous Lesions
Enterovirus
EBV, CMV, *Toxoplasma gondii*
Acute HIV infection
Colorado tick fever virus
Salmonella typhi
Leptospira interrogans
Measles virus
Rubella virus
Hepatitis B virus
Treponema pallidum
Parvovirus B19
Human herpesvirus 6

Vesicular Lesions
Varicella-zoster virus
Herpes simplex virus
Coxsackievirus A
Vibrio vulnificus

Cutaneous Petechiae
Neisseria gonorrhoeae
Neisseria meningitidis
Rickettsia rickettsii (Rocky Mountain spotted fever)
Rickettsia typhi (murine typhus)
Ehrlichia chaffeensis
Echoviruses
Streptococcus viridans (endocarditis)

Diffuse Erythroderma
Group A streptococci (scarlet fever, toxic shock syndrome)
Staphylococcus aureus (toxic shock syndrome)

Distinctive Rash
Ecthyma gangrenosum: *Pseudomonas aeruginosa*
Erythema migrans: Lyme disease

Mucous Membrane Lesions
Vesicular pharyngitis: coxsackievirus A
Palatal petechiae: rubella, EBV, scarlet fever (group A streptococci)
Erythema: toxic shock syndrome (*Staphylococcus aureus* and group A streptococci)
Oral ulceronodular lesion: *Histoplasma capsulatum*
Koplik spots: measles virus

CMV, Cytomegalovirus; *EBV,* Epstein-Barr virus; *HIV,* human immunodeficiency virus.

infections have made up the largest category, representing 25% to 50% of cases. Abscesses, endocarditis, tuberculosis, complicated urinary tract infections, and biliary tract diseases have consistently been among the most important. Abscesses account for almost one third of infectious causes, and most are intra-abdominal or pelvic in origin. Perforation of a colonic diverticulum or appendicitis can sometimes lead to large, walled-off abdominal abscesses with few localizing signs.

During the past 50 years, the improvement of imaging studies and their greater accessibility have made abdominal or pelvic abscesses and malignancies more easily detected and less likely to be the cause of prolonged, undiagnosed fever. Malignant neoplasms can induce fever directly through the production and release of pyrogenic cytokines and

indirectly by undergoing spontaneous or induced necrosis or creating conditions conducive to secondary infections. Endovascular infections are usually detectable by blood cultures, although slow-growing or fastidious organisms may make detection difficult.

Infections, including tuberculosis, typhoid fever, malaria, and amebic liver abscesses, remain the most frequent causes of FUO in developing countries. The incidence of some FUOs varies according to geographic location. Classic FUO may occur as familial Mediterranean fever among Ashkenazi Jews; as Kikuchi disease, which is an unusual form of necrotizing lymphadenitis seen primarily in Japan; and as TNF receptor–associated periodic fever (TRAPS), formerly called familial Hibernian fever, which is an inherited periodic fever syndrome described originally in Ireland.

The proportion of FUOs due to noninfectious inflammatory diseases and undiagnosed conditions has risen. Of the connective tissue diseases, juvenile rheumatoid arthritis (i.e., Still disease), other variants of rheumatoid arthritis, and systemic lupus erythematosus predominate among younger patients. Temporal arteritis and polymyalgia rheumatica syndromes are more common among elderly patients.

Fever may be blunted or absent in up to one third of elderly individuals with serious conditions. Older people may more often have atypical clinical presentations of common infectious and noninfectious diseases. For example, elderly persons may have tuberculosis without cough or fever, infective endocarditis with fatigue and weight loss but without fever, and abdominal abscesses with little abdominal tenderness found on physical examination. Leukocytosis and increased band forms are more likely to be associated with a serious infection. HIV should be considered as a possible cause of FUO in older patients, although it is not usually suspected early in the course of FUO.

Fever in returned travelers is most often caused by common infections, such as malaria and respiratory or urinary tract infections. However, fever caused by dengue, typhoid fever, or amebic liver abscess is increasingly identified, especially among international travelers returning from the tropics. Katayama fever is a febrile syndrome occurring after exposure to fresh water schistosomes in endemic areas. It may resolve spontaneously or may require treatment with antiparasitic agents to prevent sequelae that carry severe morbidity. A travel history should be obtained, and it may redirect the entire work-up.

Health Care–Associated Fever of Unknown Origin

Some FUOs are associated with health care practices, including surgical procedures, urinary and respiratory tract instrumentation, intravascular devices, drug therapy, and immobilization. Quality control measures are set up to minimize and avoid bloodstream infections and decubitus ulcers. Drug-related fever, septic thrombophlebitis, recurrent pulmonary emboli, and *Clostridioides difficile* colitis must be considered in the work-up of hospitalized patients who develop fever greater than 38° C (100.4° F) for more than 3 days if it was not present on admission.

Immune Deficiency–Associated Fever of Unknown Origin

Immunosuppressed individuals have the highest incidence of FUO of any group of patients. Due to impaired immune responses, signs of inflammation other than fever are notoriously absent or diminished, producing atypical clinical manifestations and an absence of radiologic abnormalities for what otherwise would be readily diagnosed infections. In patients with impaired cell-mediated immunity, FUO often results from conditions other than pyogenic bacterial infections (e.g., fungi, CMV).

Neutropenia is a dangerous condition that can be considered a subclass of immunodeficiency. Persons with profound neutropenia are at high risk for bacterial and fungal infections. Episodes of fever

TABLE 90.3 Fever and Rash in Viral Infection

Virus	Disease Features	Incubation and Early Symptoms
Coxsackie, ECHO virus	Maculopapular rubelliform, 1–3 mm, faint pink, begins on face, spreading to chest and extremities	Summertime
		No itching or lymphadenopathy
	Herpetiform vesicular stomatitis with peripheral exanthema (papules and clear vesicles on an erythematous base), including palms and soles (hand, foot, and mouth disease)	Multiple cases in household or community-wide epidemic
		Mostly diseases of children
Measles	Erythematous, maculopapular rash begins on upper face and spreads down to involve extremities, including palms and soles. Koplik spots are blue-gray specks on a red base found on buccal mucosa near second molars. Atypical measles occurs in individuals who received killed vaccine and then are exposed to measles. The rash begins peripherally and is urticarial, vascular, or hemorrhagic.	Incubation period 10–14 days
		First, severe upper respiratory symptoms, coryza, cough, and conjunctivitis; then Koplik spots, then rash
Rubella	Maculopapular rash beginning on face and moving down; petechiae on soft palate	Incubation 12–23 days
		Adenopathy; posterior auricular, posterior cervical, and suboccipital
Varicella	Generalized vesicular eruption; pruritic lesions in different stages from erythematous macules to vesicles to crusted; spread from trunk centrifugally; zoster lesions are painful and often dermatomal	Incubation 14–15 days; late winter, early spring
		Herpes zoster is a reactivation, occurs any season
Herpes simplex virus	Oral primary: small vesicles on pharynx, oral mucosa that ulcerates; painful and tender	Incubation 2–12 days
	Recurrent: vermilion border, one or few lesions, genital; may be asymptomatic or appear similar to oral lesions on genital mucosa	
Hepatitis B and C virus	Prodrome in one fifth; erythematous, maculopapular rash, urticaria	Arthralgias, arthritis; abnormal liver function test results; hepatitis B antigenemia
	Leukocytoclastic vasculitis occurs in hepatitis C	
Epstein-Barr virus	Erythematous, maculopapular rash on trunk and proximal extremities	Transiently occurs in 5–10% of patients during first week of illness
	Occasionally urticarial or hemorrhagic	
Human immunodeficiency virus	Maculopapular truncal rash may occur as early manifestation of infection	Associated fever, sore throat, and lymph node enlargement may persist for 2 or more weeks

TABLE 90.4 Common Syndromes and Diseases Associated With Fever in Returned Travelers

Sore Throat	Cough	Abdominal Pain	Arthralgia or Myalgia	Diarrhea
Bacterial pharyngitis	Amebiasis (hepatic)	Amebiasis (intestinal)	Arboviruses	Amebiasis (intestinal)
Diphtheria	Anthrax	Anthrax	Dengue	Anthrax
Infectious mononucleosis	Bacterial pneumonia	Campylobacter enteritis	Yellow fever	Campylobacter enteritis
HIV seroconversion	Filarial fever	Legionnaires disease	Babesiosis	HIV seroconversion
Lyme disease	TPE	Malaria	Bartonellosis	Legionnaires disease
Poliomyelitis	Histoplasmosis	Measles	Brucellosis	Malaria melioidosis
Psittacosis	Legionnaires disease	Melioidosis	Erythema nodosum leprosum	Plague
Tularemia	Leishmaniasis (visceral)	Plague	Hepatitis (viral)	Relapsing fever
Viral hemorrhagic fever (Lassa)	Loeffler syndrome	Relapsing fevers	Histoplasmosis	Salmonellosis
Nonspecific viral URTI	Malaria	Salmonellosis	HIV seroconversion	Schistosomiasis (acute)
	Measles	Schistosomiasis (acute)	Legionnaires disease	Shigellosis
	Melioidosis	Shigellosis	Leptospirosis	Typhoid in children
	Plague	Typhoid fever	Lyme disease	Viral hemorrhagic fevers
	Q fever	Viral hemorrhagic fevers	Malaria	Yersiniosis
	Relapsing fever	Yersiniosis	Plague	
	Schistosomiasis (acute)		Poliomyelitis	
	Toxocariasis		Q fever	
	Trichinosis		Relapsing fevers	
	Tuberculosis		Secondary syphilis	
	Tularemia		Toxoplasmosis	
	Typhoid and paratyphoid		Trichinosis	
	Typhus		Trypanosomiasis (African)	
	Viral hemorrhagic fevers		Tularemia	
	Nonspecific viral URTIs		Typhoid and paratyphoid	
			Typhus	
			Viral hemorrhagic fevers	

HIV, Human immunodeficiency virus; *TPE,* tropical pulmonary eosinophilia; *URTI,* upper respiratory tract infection.
From Beeching N, Fletcher T, Wijaya L: Returned travelers. In Zuckerman JN, editor: Principles and practice of travel medicine, ed 2, Boston, 2013, Wiley-Blackwell, p 271.

TABLE 90.5 Common Clinical Findings and Associated Infections After Tropical Travel

Clinical Findings	Infections
Fever and rash	Dengue, chikungunya, rickettsial infections, enteric fever (skin lesions may be sparse or absent), acute HIV infection, measles, acute schistosomiasis
Fever and abdominal pain	Enteric fever, amebic liver abscess
Undifferentiated fever and normal or low white blood cell count	Dengue, malaria, rickettsial infection, enteric fever, chikungunya
Fever and hemorrhage	Viral hemorrhagic fevers (dengue and others), meningococcemia, leptospirosis, rickettsial infections
Fever and eosinophilia	Acute schistosomiasis; drug hypersensitivity reaction; fascioliasis and other parasitic infections (rare)
Fever and pulmonary infiltrates	Common bacterial and viral pathogens; legionellosis, acute schistosomiasis, Q fever, melioidosis
Fever and altered mental status	Cerebral malaria, viral or bacterial meningoencephalitis, African trypanosomiasis
Mononucleosis syndrome	Epstein-Barr virus, cytomegalovirus, toxoplasmosis, acute HIV infection
Fever persisting >2 weeks	Malaria, enteric fever, Epstein-Barr virus, cytomegalovirus, toxoplasmosis, acute HIV, acute schistosomiasis, brucellosis, tuberculosis, Q fever, visceral leishmaniasis (rare)
Fever with onset >6 weeks after travel	Vivax malaria, acute hepatitis (B, C, or E), tuberculosis, amebic liver abscess

HIV, Human immunodeficiency virus.
Modified from Centers for Disease Control and Prevention: CDC health information for international travel 2012, New York, 2012, Oxford University Press.

are common in patients with neutropenia. Many episodes are short lived because they respond quickly to treatment or are manifestations of rapidly fatal infections.

Bacteremia and sepsis can cause rapid deterioration in neutropenic patients, and empirical, broad-spectrum antibiotics should be administered promptly without waiting for the results of cultures. However, only about 35% of prolonged episodes of febrile neutropenia respond to broad-spectrum antibiotic therapy. If fevers persist after 3 days of treatment with broad-spectrum antibiotics, diagnostic tests to explore fungal causes should be considered along with empirical antifungal treatment.

Human Immunodeficiency Virus–Related Fever of Unknown Origin

The advent of highly active antiretroviral therapy (ART) with the achievable suppression of the HIV viral load has greatly reduced the frequency of FUO in HIV-infected patients. High vigilance is warranted to test for new HIV in a matter-of-fact manner in the primary care setting. The primary phase of HIV infection can be asymptomatic or sometimes be characterized by a mononucleosis-like illness in which fever is a prominent feature (see Chapter 103). After symptoms of the primary phase of HIV infection resolve, patients enter a long period of subclinical infection during which they are usually afebrile. In the later phases of untreated HIV infection, episodes of fever become common, often signifying a superimposed illness. Many of these are potentially devastating opportunistic infections, which tend to manifest in atypical fashion because of the severe immunodeficiency. Patients with untreated acquired immunodeficiency syndrome (AIDS) can have multiple infections simultaneously, which highlights the importance of treating and documenting adherence with ART. After initiating effective ART the HIV viral load is effectively suppressed and the frequency of FUO in HIV-infected patients falls markedly.

Approach to the Patient With Fever of Unknown Origin

Evaluation of a patient with FUO typically includes verification that the patient has fever, consideration of the fever pattern, a comprehensive history, repeated physical examinations, appropriate laboratory investigations, key imaging studies, and invasive diagnostic procedures. The physical examination should scrutinize the patient more closely than usual because key physical abnormalities in patients with FUO are subtle and require repeated examinations to be appreciated.

Work-up of a patient with an FUO should focus on the history, physical examination, and initial laboratory data. In place of rational diagnostic thinking, there is a temptation to order multiple comprehensive laboratory and imaging studies. Rather than leading to a diagnosis, this shotgun approach may result in enormous expense, false-positive results, and unnecessary additional investigations that may obfuscate the true diagnosis.

A fundamental principle in the management of classic FUO is that therapy should be withheld, whenever possible, until the cause of the fever has been determined, so that treatment can be tailored to a specific diagnosis. The exception is in the setting of the immunocompromised host because rapid empirical treatment is most often needed.

If fevers persist after an exhaustive work-up there may be a role for fluorodeoxyglucose positron emission tomography (18 FDG-PET/CT) imaging, if available. This allows enhancement of acute and chronic inflammatory processes by uptake of FDG in all activated leukocytes and provides the necessary spatial resolution that may substantially contribute to finding the cause of FUO. The radiation exposure and cost and the degree of incremental improvement in detection over other methods must be carefully considered.

Cardiac ECHO can be helpful if culture-negative endocarditis or atrial myxoma is suspected in patients with cardiac murmurs. The most invasive tests such as lymph node biopsies, bone marrow biopsies, and temporal artery biopsies should be undertaken only with strong clinical suspicion and based on physical findings or those found on imaging. Persons who reside in the southeastern part of the United States and immigrants from world regions endemic for *Strongyloides stercoralis* should have a *S. stercoralis* titre—whether or not they have a fever—to identify and eradicate risk for overwhelming strongyloidiasis.

SPECIFIC CONDITIONS AND EXPOSURES CAUSING FEVER

Fever After Animal Exposures
Q Fever

Q fever is a widespread zoonotic infection caused by the pathogen *Coxiella burnetii* that has acute and chronic manifestations. The primary source of infection is infected cattle, sheep, and goats. The organism can exist for months in soil and can become airborne. The onset of disease is typically abrupt, and high-grade fever (40° C or 104° F),

TABLE 90.6 Common Causes of Fever of Unknown Origin

Infections
Abscesses
Brucellosis
Catheter infections
Cytomegalovirus
Coccidioidomycosis
Histoplasmosis
Human immunodeficiency virus (HIV) infection
Infective endocarditis
Intra-abdominal, subdiaphragmatic, and pelvic disease
Liver and biliary tract disease
Lyme disease
Mycobacterium tuberculosis
Osteomyelitis
Sinusitis
Toxoplasmosis
Urinary tract infection

Autoimmune Conditions
Adult Still disease
Familial Mediterranean sarcoidosis
Rheumatoid arthritis
Systemic lupus erythematosus
Temporal arteritis

Malignancy
Hepatocellular carcinoma
Leukemia
Metastatic cancers
Pancreatic cancer
Renal cell carcinoma

Miscellaneous Causes
Deep vein thrombosis, pulmonary embolism
Hyperthyroidism
Kikuchi disease
Periodic fever (tumor necrosis factor receptor associated)

fatigue, headache, and myalgias are the most common symptoms. Acute Q fever is usually a mild disease that resolves spontaneously within 2 weeks. Q fever endocarditis usually occurs in patients with previous valvular damage or immunocompromise, and it is often the predominant manifestation of chronic infection.

An immunofluorescence assay is the reference method for the serodiagnosis of Q fever. Consideration of doxycycline therapy is warranted only for patients who are symptomatic.

Leptospirosis

Leptospirosis is a zoonotic infection with protean manifestations caused by the spirochete *Leptospira interrogans*. It is distributed worldwide, but most clinical cases occur in the tropics. The organism infects rodents, cattle, swine, dogs, horses, sheep, and goats, and it is shed in the urine. Humans most often become infected after exposure to environmental sources, such as contaminated water.

Leptospirosis may manifest as a subclinical illness followed by seroconversion, a self-limited systemic infection, or a severe, potentially fatal illness accompanied by multiorgan failure. Acute illness manifests with the abrupt onset of fever, rigors, myalgias, and headache in 75%

to 100% of patients. Conjunctival suffusion in a patient with a nonspecific febrile illness accompanied by lymphadenopathy, hepatomegaly, and splenomegaly points to a diagnosis of leptospirosis.

During the second phase of illness, fever is less pronounced, but headache and myalgias can be severe, and aseptic meningitis is an important manifestation. In some patients with leptospirosis, the clinical course may be complicated by jaundice (although liver failure is rare), renal failure, uveitis, hemorrhage, ARDS, myocarditis, and rhabdomyolysis (i.e., Weil syndrome).

Because the clinical features and routine laboratory findings of leptospirosis are not specific, a high index of suspicion must be maintained. The diagnosis is usually made by serologic testing for *L. interrogans*. Symptomatic individuals warrant treatment with doxycycline.

Brucellosis

Brucellosis is a zoonotic infection caused by *Brucella melitensis*. It is transmitted to humans by contact with fluids from infected animals (e.g., sheep, cattle, goats, pigs) or derived food products such as unpasteurized milk and cheese.

Clinical manifestations of brucellosis include fever, night sweats, malaise, anorexia, arthralgias, fatigue, weight loss, and depression. Patients may have fever and a multitude of complaints but no other objective findings. The onset of symptoms may be abrupt or insidious, developing over several days to weeks. The musculoskeletal and genitourinary systems are the most common sites of involvement. Neurobrucellosis, endocarditis, and hepatic abscesses occur in 1% to 2% of cases.

The diagnosis of brucellosis should be considered for an individual with otherwise unexplained fever and nonspecific complaints who has had a possible exposure. Ideally, the diagnosis is made by culture of the organism from blood or other sites, such as bone marrow. Serologic tests include tube agglutination and enzyme-linked immunosorbent assay (ELISA). For adults with nonfocal disease, treatment with doxycycline and rifampin is suggested.

Fever and Rash

The most concerning diseases associated with fever and rash are meningococcemia, staphylococcal TSS, and RMSF.

Bacterial Meningitis

Neisseria meningitidis is the leading cause of bacterial meningitis in children and young adults in the United States. Recent experience in New York City identified HIV patients as being at increased risk for meningococcal disease.

Manifestations of meningococcal disease can range from transient fever and bacteremia to fulminant disease, with death ensuing within hours of the onset of clinical symptoms. Acute systemic meningococcal disease may manifest as one of three syndromes: meningitis alone, meningitis with accompanying meningococcemia, and meningococcemia without clinical evidence of meningitis.

The typical initial symptoms of meningitis due to *N. meningitidis* consists of the sudden onset of fever, nausea, vomiting, headache, decreased ability to concentrate, and myalgias in an otherwise healthy patient. A petechial rash appears as discrete lesions 1 to 2 mm in diameter, most frequently occurring on the trunk and lower portions of the body. More than 50% of patients have petechiae at clinical presentation. Petechiae can coalesce into larger purpuric and ecchymotic lesions.

Staphylococcal Toxic Shock Syndrome

S. aureus strains produce exotoxins that cause three syndromes: food poisoning, caused by ingestion of *S. aureus* enterotoxin; scalded skin syndrome, caused by exfoliative toxin; and TSS, caused by toxic shock syndrome toxin 1 (TSST-1) and other enterotoxins. About one half of reported TSS cases are menstrual, associated with bacterial growth on highly absorbent tampons. Non-menstrual TSS has been associated with surgical and postpartum wound infections, mastitis, septorhinoplasty, sinusitis, osteomyelitis, arthritis, burns, cutaneous and subcutaneous lesions (especially of the extremities, perianal area, and axillae), and respiratory infections after influenza. Some MRSA strains can produce TSST-1, and patients infected with these strains may develop TSS.

The Centers for Disease Control and Prevention (CDC) case definition for a confirmed case includes several criteria. Patients must have fever greater than 38.9° C, hypotension, diffuse erythroderma, desquamation (unless the patient dies before desquamation can occur), and involvement of at least three organ systems. Although 80% to 90% of TSS patients have *S. aureus* isolated from mucosal or wound sites, the isolation of *S. aureus* is not required for the diagnosis of staphylococcal TSS.

Rickettsial Infections

RMSF is a potentially lethal but usually curable tick-borne disease. Most cases of RMSF occur in the spring and early summer in endemic areas, particularly in the south central and southeastern states, when outdoor activity is most common. The etiologic agent, *Rickettsia rickettsii*, is a gram-negative, obligate intracellular bacterium that is usually transmitted through a tick bite. Up to one third of patients with proven RMSF do not recall a recent tick bite or recent tick contact.

In the early phases of illness, most patients have nonspecific signs and symptoms such as fever, headache, malaise, myalgias, arthralgias, and nausea with or without vomiting. Most patients with RMSF develop a rash between the third and fifth days of illness. The rash typically begins with pink, blanching macules that evolve to a deep red color and then become hemorrhagic. The lesions begin at the wrists, forearms, and ankles and then spread to the arms, thighs, trunk, and face.

The diagnosis of RMSF is based on a constellation of symptoms and signs in an appropriate epidemiologic setting (e.g., endemic area in the spring or early summer). In later illness, the diagnosis can be made by skin biopsy and confirmed serologically.

Murine typhus is a worldwide illness caused by *Rickettsia typhi* organisms that are transmitted by fleas. It produces a moderately severe illness characterized by fever, rash, and headache. Disease in the United States has been reported in Texas and Southern California.

Rickettsia africae, the cause of African tick-bite fever, occurs in travelers returning from East Africa. It produces a large eschar with a febrile syndrome similar to RMSF. Rickettsial infections respond to treatment with doxycycline and warrant rapid initiation of treatment.

Lyme Disease

Lyme disease is a tick-borne illness caused by pathogenic species of the spirochete *Borrelia burgdorferi* in the United States. Other species in Europe and Asia can cause more aggressive presentations. Localized disease includes erythema migrans in 80% of patients and nonspecific findings that resemble a viral syndrome. Erythema migrans is an expanding macule that forms an annular lesion with a clearing middle.

Early disseminated Lyme disease with acute neurologic or cardiac involvement usually occurs weeks to several months after the tick bite and may be the first manifestation of the disease. Nonspecific symptoms (e.g., headache, fatigue, arthralgias) may persist for months after treatment of Lyme disease. There is no evidence that these persistent subjective complaints represent ongoing active infection. Co-infection with *Babesia* and *Ehrlichia* is common, and these infections should be considered in persons diagnosed with Lyme disease.

Human Ehrlichiosis

The principal vector of *Ehrlichia chaffeensis*, the agent that causes human monocytic ehrlichiosis (HME), is the Lone Star tick (*Amblyomma americanum*). Patients typically have an acute illness that has an incubation period of 1 to 2 weeks. Most patients are febrile and have nonspecific symptoms such as malaise, myalgia, headache, and chills.

One feature that may distinguish HME from human granulocytic anaplasmosis (HGA), another tick-borne illness caused by *Anaplasma phagocytophilum*, is a rash (macular, maculopapular, or petechial). This rash occurs in about 30% of patients with HME but is rare in patients with HGA.

The preferred and most widely available diagnostic method for ehrlichiosis is the indirect fluorescent antibody test. The diagnosis should be considered in all patients with Lyme disease or babesiosis. Treatment with doxycycline should be initiated for all patients suspected of having ehrlichiosis or anaplasmosis.

Viral Infections Associated With Rash

The typical manifestations of viral infections associated with rash may unequivocally establish the cause of a febrile syndrome. For example, varicella-zoster virus infection manifests with distinctive lesions of chickenpox or herpes zoster (i.e., shingles). The resurgence of measles mandates the ability to recognize its rash.

Acute onset of high fever characterizes viral hemorrhagic fevers, along with bleeding complications and high mortality rates in some cases. Arthropods often transmit viral infections, including dengue, which is one of the most common causes of fever in returned travelers.

Fever With Lymphadenopathy

Generalized and localized lymphadenopathy can be major manifestations of some infectious diseases, such as in mononucleosis syndromes, tuberculosis, HIV infection, and pyogenic infections.

Infectious mononucleosis is characterized by a triad of fever, tonsillar pharyngitis, and lymphadenopathy. EBV is a widely disseminated herpesvirus that is spread by intimate contact between susceptible persons and EBV shedders. Lymph node involvement in infectious mononucleosis is typically symmetrical and more commonly involves the posterior cervical than the anterior chains. The posterior cervical nodes are deep beneath the sternocleidomastoid muscles and must be carefully palpated. The nodes may be large and moderately tender. Lymphadenopathy may also become more generalized including enlargement of the spleen, which distinguishes infectious mononucleosis from other causes of pharyngitis.

Lymphadenopathy peaks in the first week and then gradually subsides over 2 to 3 weeks. Splenomegaly is seen in 50% of patients with infectious mononucleosis and usually begins to recede by the third week of the illness.

Patients with a clinical picture of infectious mononucleosis should have a white blood cell count with differential and a heterophile (Monospot) test. If the heterophile test result is positive, no further testing is necessary when the clinical scenario is compatible with typical infectious mononucleosis. If the heterophile test result is negative but there is still a strong clinical suspicion of EBV infection, the Monospot test can be repeated because results can be negative early in clinical illness.

If the clinical syndrome is prolonged or the patient does not have a classic EBV syndrome, immunoglobulin M (IgM) and immunoglobulin G (IgG) viral capsule antigen (VCA) and Epstein-Barr nuclear antigen (EBNA) antibodies should be measured. IgG EBNA detected within 4 weeks of symptom onset excludes acute primary EBV infection as an explanation and should prompt consideration of EBV-negative causes of mononucleosis.

Cytomegalovirus

The spectrum of human illness caused by CMV is diverse and mostly depends on the host. CMV infection in the immunocompetent host usually is asymptomatic or may manifest as a mononucleosis-like syndrome. Transmission occurs through multiple routes.

The mononucleosis syndrome associated with CMV infection has been described as typhoidal because systemic symptoms and fever predominate, and signs of enlarged cervical nodes and splenomegaly are not as commonly seen as they are in EBV infection. Diarrhea, fever, fatigue, abdominal pain, and mildly abnormal liver enzymes are common findings. Immunocompromised patients, such as those who have received transplants, may have serious, life-threatening infections such as pneumonitis, hepatitis, colitis, and retinitis. Serology provides indirect evidence of recent CMV infection based on changes in antibody titers at different time points during the clinical illness. Serologies are also helpful in determining past exposure to CMV. This information is particularly relevant for monitoring immunosuppressed hosts at risk for CMV reactivation syndromes.

Primary Human Immunodeficiency Virus Infection

Most cases of new HIV infection are passed asymptomatically, and routine testing of sexually active persons should be performed as part of good primary care. All patients with mononucleosis syndromes should undergo HIV testing. Published series consistently report that the most common findings of acute HIV are fever, generalized lymphadenopathy, sore throat, rash, myalgia or arthralgia, and headache when symptomatic.

Toxoplasmosis

Toxoplasmosis, an infection with a worldwide distribution, is caused by the intracellular protozoan parasite *T. gondii*. Humans can acquire *Toxoplasma* organisms through ingestion of contaminated meat, vertical transmission, blood transfusion, exposure to oocysts from cat feces, or organ transplantation.

Immunocompetent persons with primary infection are usually asymptomatic, but latent infection can persist for the life of the host. When symptomatic infection does occur, the most common manifestation is bilateral, symmetrical, nontender cervical adenopathy. Patients may have headache, fever, and fatigue. Symptoms usually resolve within several weeks. In AIDS patients or other immunocompromised hosts who have been previously infected, *T. gondii* infection may reactivate in the brain, causing abscesses and encephalitis.

Infections Causing Regional Lymphadenopathy

Scrofula (i.e., tuberculous cervical adenitis) develops in a subacute to chronic pattern. Low-grade fever is usually associated with a large mass of matted cervical lymph nodes. In children, *M. tuberculosis* is the etiologic agent, but in adults, *Mycobacterium avium* complex and *Mycobacterium scrofulaceum* are more commonly found. Surgical excision is the treatment of choice.

Cat-Scratch Disease

Cat-scratch disease, a condition caused by *Bartonella henselae*, is characterized by self-limited regional lymphadenopathy after a cat scratch or transmission from another vector. Other manifestations can include visceral organ, neurologic, and ocular involvement. In 85% to 90% of children, cat-scratch disease manifests as a localized cutaneous and lymph node disorder near the site of organism inoculation. In some individuals, the organisms disseminate and infect the liver, spleen, eye, bone, or CNS. Patients with localized disease usually have a self-limited illness, whereas those with disseminated disease can have life-threatening complications. *B. henselae infection* should be considered in the initial evaluation of FUO in children.

The diagnosis of cat-scratch disease is based on typical clinical findings (i.e., lymphadenopathy) associated with probable exposure to cats or fleas. Laboratory testing that supports the diagnosis includes a positive *B. henselae* antibody titer or biopsy of a lymph node with a positive Warthin-Starry stain or polymerase chain reaction (PCR) analysis of tissue.

Pyogenic Infection

S. aureus and group A streptococcal (GAS) infections can produce acute, suppurative lymphadenitis. Enlarged and tender lymph nodes usually are found in the submandibular, cervical, axillary, or inguinal areas. Patients have fever and leukocytosis. Pyoderma, pharyngitis, and periodontal infections are usually the primary sites of infection. Management includes drainage and antibiotics.

Plague

Bubonic plague is a bacterial syndrome caused by *Yersinia pestis* that usually consists of fever, headache, and a large mat of inguinal, axillary, or cervical lymph nodes. Lymph nodes suppurate and drain spontaneously. The diagnosis should be considered for acutely ill patients in the southwestern United States with possible exposure to fleas and rodents. Gram-negative coccobacilli can be seen in lymph node aspirates. The characteristic safety-pin appearance of *Y. pestis* with dark blue staining of polar bodies is seen with Wayson stain.

Sexually Transmitted Diseases

Inguinal lymphadenopathy associated with sexually transmitted diseases can be unilateral or bilateral. In primary syphilis, enlarged nodes are discrete, firm, and nontender. Tender lymphadenopathies with matting are seen in lymphogranuloma venereum. The lymphadenopathy of chancroid is most often unilateral and manifests with pain and fused lymph nodes. Primary genital herpes infection also causes tender inguinal lymphadenopathy.

FACTITIOUS FEVER AND SELF-INDUCED ILLNESS

In most case series, factitious fever or self-induced illness is a relatively uncommon cause of FUO, but it may occur more often than generally appreciated. Patients with these conditions are often young women, and 50% have had training in some aspect of health care. They are often well educated, cooperative, articulate, and manipulative of family and caregivers. Patients can no longer manipulate thermometers because electronic or infrared thermometry is used, and causing factitious fever is difficult. Clues to the factitious fever diagnosis include absence of a toxic appearance despite high temperature readings, lack of tachycardia, and absent diurnal variation. Patients may appear well between episodes of fever.

Genuine fever can be induced if an individual injects or ingests pyrogenic substances such as bacterial suspensions, urine, or feces. Although intermittent polymicrobial bacteremia may suggest a diagnosis of intra-abdominal abscess, it represents self-induced infection. The discovery of needles and substances for injection in the patient's belongings may help in the diagnosis.

In most cases, a psychogenic basis for the behavior is assumed. However, one study with detailed psychological patient analyses found no evidence of major psychiatric diagnoses among individuals with self-induced or simulated illnesses. Munchausen syndrome and Munchausen by proxy are the most extreme forms of factitious fever. Patients often agree stoically to numerous highly invasive procedures to diagnose and treat themselves or their children (i.e., proxy). All of these individuals require objective but complete, tactful, and compassionate assessments and considerable psychiatric care.

SUGGESTED READINGS

Aduan RP, Fauci AS, Dale DC, et al: Factitious fever and self-induced infection: a report of 32 cases and review of the literature, Ann Intern Med 90:230–242, 1979.

Aduan RP, Fauci AS, Dale DC, et al: Prolonged fever of unknown origin (FUO): a prospective study of 347 patients, Clin Res 26:558A, 1978.

Brown I, Finnigan NA: Fever of unknown origin (FUO). In StatPearls [Internet], Treasure Island (FL), 2019, StatPearls Publishing. [Updated 2018 Nov 18]. Available from: https://www.ncbi.nlm.nih.gov/books/NBK532265.

Cannon J: Perspective on fever: the basic science and conventional medicine, Complement Ther Med 21(Suppl 1):S54–S60, 2013.

Osilla EV, Sharma S: Physiology, temperature regulation. In StatPearls [Internet], Treasure Island (FL), 2019, StatPearls Publishing. [Updated 2019 Mar 16]. Available from: https://www.ncbi.nlm.nih.gov/books/NBK507838.

Weber D, Cohen M, Rutala W: The acutely ill patient with fever and rash. In Bennett JE, Dolin R, Blaser M, editors: MandellDouglas and Bennett's principles and practice of infectious diseases, ed 8, Elsevier, 2015, pp 732–747.

91

Bacteremia and Sepsis

Russell J. McCulloh, Steven M. Opal

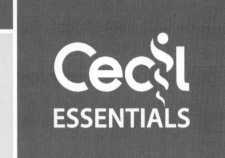

DEFINITION

Sepsis is a leading cause of morbidity and death among hospitalized patients. The disease process results from a complex interplay of host immune responses and infectious microorganisms. In 2016 an international panel of experts released an updated definition of sepsis, specifying it as life-threatening organ dysfunction caused by a dysregulated host response to infection. Manifestations can include fever, altered mental status, and abnormalities in inflammation and coagulation. Severe cases can progress to multiple organ system dysfunction followed by organ failure and death.

Diagnostic criteria for sepsis are provided in Table 91.1. The term "severe sepsis," once recognized as a separate entity defined by more severe organ dysfunction, is now synonymous with the current definition of sepsis and should no longer be used. Septic shock is a combination of sepsis and persistent hypotension and tissue hypoperfusion despite adequate fluid resuscitation or the need to use vasopressors to maintain a mean arterial pressure (MAP) at 65 mm Hg or greater and in addition an elevated serum lactate greater than 2 mmol/L. The continuum of disease manifestations from localized infection to multiorgan failure and refractory septic shock is depicted in Fig. 91.1.

Sepsis is a situation in which the infection-induced systemic inflammatory and coagulopathic responses have become injurious to the host. Sepsis is an infectious process characterized by tissue injury from hypoperfusion and immune dysregulation. *Severe infection* should be used to describe an infection that is accompanied by systemic inflammation but without evidence of organ dysfunction remote from the site of infection (i.e., the former definition of sepsis). Whether these revised definitions can resolve the current confusion in terminology remains to be seen.

Understanding the pathophysiology of sepsis syndrome has proved helpful in differentiating and treating severe inflammatory processes that manifest with symptoms similar to sepsis, including pancreatitis, severe trauma, thermal burns, and certain toxin or environmental exposures. These processes can produce a systemic inflammatory response syndrome (SIRS), but they lack the component of infection needed to establish a diagnosis of sepsis. The remarkable clinical similarity between these severe "sterile" inflammations and septic shock reflects their molecular profiles. Identical signaling pathways for the immune response are activated by highly conserved pathogen-associated molecular patterns (PAMPs), which are molecular motifs recognized by cells of the host's innate immune system. Damage-associated molecular patterns (DAMPs) are molecules released by injured host cells that act as endogenous danger signals to promote the inflammatory response (see "Pathophysiology of Septic Shock" later in this chapter).

EPIDEMIOLOGY

The worldwide incidence of sepsis is difficult to assess due to limited data from developing countries. In industrialized countries, reported rates of sepsis range from 22 to 300 cases per 100,000 people. Sepsis may account for up to 6% of adult deaths. In the United States, more than 750,000 cases of sepsis and 200,000 sepsis-related deaths occur annually. The risk of mortality depends on the severity of illness and multiple host factors (discussed later). Overall, estimates of death from sepsis range from 20% of mild to moderate cases to more than 60% of patients with septic shock.

The financial impact of sepsis cases is immense. Each episode of sepsis costs approximately $50,000 in health care expenditures, for a total of more than $24 billion dollars in 2016 in the United States alone.

Bacterial infections are the most common cause of sepsis. Bloodstream infections due to bacteria account for the largest proportion of hospitalizations. The rates are highest for premature infants, the advanced elderly (especially those older than 85 years of age), and patients with intravenous catheters, implanted devices, or severe medical morbidities such as severe burns or hematologic malignancies.

Pathogens most commonly identified in bloodstream infections include staphylococci (e.g., *Staphylococcus aureus*), group A streptococci, *Escherichia coli*, *Klebsiella* species, *Enterobacter* species, and *Pseudomonas aeruginosa*. Immunocompromised patients and patients with long-term intravascular catheters are at increased risk for fungal bloodstream infections from *Candida* species, and some species may be resistant to commonly used antifungal medications. Given the broad variety of potential pathogens, clinicians face the dual challenges of an accurate and timely diagnosis and choice of appropriate empirical therapy.

Several epidemiologic factors can guide the clinician in cases of sepsis when a source has not been identified. Table 91.2 lists microorganisms that are associated with certain host factors that predispose a patient to infection and sepsis. Host factors associated with worse outcomes include extremes of age, use of immunomodulating medications, and concomitant chronic medical conditions.

Several diagnostic and treatment factors are associated with severity of illness and clinical outcome. Delay in effective antimicrobial therapy correlates with worse outcomes. Infection with multidrug-resistant organisms may cause a delay in effective therapy, and for some organisms, particularly gram-negative enteric rods, the delay may be independently related to worse outcomes. Certain organisms (e.g., *P. aeruginosa*, *Staphylococcus aureus*) are more virulent. The primary infection site also is important; respiratory sites are the most common, and the central nervous system often is the most lethal site of infection. The number of organ systems involved plays a role, with mortality increasing as the number of dysfunctional organ systems increases.

TABLE 91.1 Diagnostic Criteria for Sepsis[a]

General Criteria

Life-threatening organ dysfunction caused by a dysregulated response to infection

Organ Dysfunction Criteria

Change in Sequential (Sepsis-related) Organ Failure Assessment (SOFA)[b] score of ≥2 points. It can be used to measure the severity of organ dysfunction.

SOFA Scoring (Range 0–4 Per Category, 0–24 Total Score Range)

Criterion	0	1	2	3	4
Respiration; Pao_2/Fio_2 (torr)	>400	≤400	≤300	≤200 with respiratory support	≤100 with respiratory support
Platelets (×10³/mm³)	>150	≤150	≤100	≤50	≤20
Bilirubin (mg/dL)	<1.2	1.2–1.9	2.0-5.9	6.0–11.9	>12.0
Glasgow Coma Scale	15	13–14	10–12	6–9	<6
Hypotension[c]	None	MAP <70 mm Hg	Dopamine ≤5 or dobutamine (or any dose of vasopressin)	Dopamine >5 or epi ≤0.1 or norepi ≤0.1 (or phenylephrine 100–300 mcg bolus	Dopamine >15 or epi >0.1 or norepi >0.1 (or phenylephrine>300 mcg bolus
Creatinine (mg/dL) or urine output (mL/day)	<1.2	1.2–1.9	2.0–3.4	3.5–4.9 <500 mL/day	>5.0 <200 mL/day

Septic Shock Criteria

Vasopressor requirement to maintain a mean arterial pressure of 65 mm Hg or greater, AND

Hyperlactatemia (serum lactate >2 mmol/L [>18 mg/dL])

From Singer M, Deutschman CS, Seymour CW, et al: The Third International Consensus Definitions for Sepsis and Septic Shock (Sepsis-3), JAMA 315(8):801-10, 2016.
Fio₂, Fraction of inspired oxygen; *INR*, international normalized ratio; *MAP*, mean arterial pressure; *Pao₂*, partial pressure of oxygen.
[a]The criteria include documented or suspected infection and some of the variables listed.
[b]Assuming baseline SOFA of 0 in most cases.
[c]Adrenergic agents must be administered for at least 1 hour to count; doses are in mcg/kg/min.

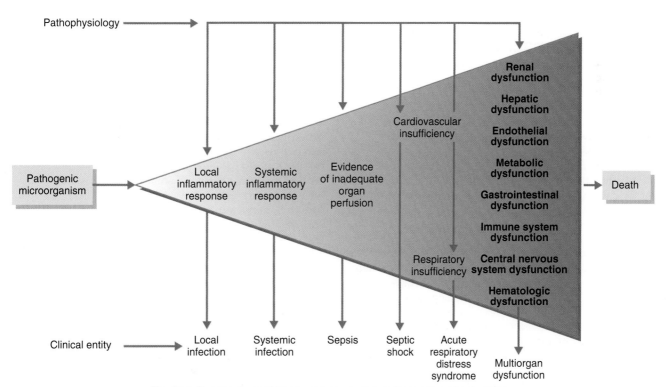

Fig. 91.1 The spectrum of illness and nomenclature for sepsis pathophysiology.

PATHOLOGY AND IMMUNOPATHOGENESIS

The pathologic findings of fatal septic shock are often rather bland on gross examination and even histologic examination of tissue samples.

The most common finding is increased tissue edema in the interstitial spaces and excess lung fluid and pleural fluid. Signs of hyaline membrane formation and fibrin deposition in the alveoli are common and

TABLE 91.2   Microorganisms Commonly Identified in Septic Patients Based on Host Factors

Host Factor	Organisms to Consider
Asplenia	Encapsulated organisms, particularly *Streptococcus pneumoniae, Haemophilus influenzae, Neisseria meningitidis, Capnocytophaga canimorsus*
Cirrhosis	*Vibrio, Salmonella*, and *Yersinia* species; encapsulated organisms, other gram-negative rods
Alcohol abuse	*Klebsiella* species, *S. pneumoniae*
Diabetes	*Mucormycosis, Pseudomonas* species, *Escherichia coli*, group B streptococci
Neutropenia	Enteric gram-negative rods, *Pseudomonas, Aspergillus, Candida, Mucor* species, *Staphylococcus aureus*, streptococcal species
T-cell dysfunction	*Listeria, Salmonella*, and *Mycobacterium* species, herpesviruses (including herpes simplex, cytomegalovirus, varicella-zoster virus)
Acquired immunodeficiency syndrome	*Salmonella* species, *S. aureus, Mycobacterium avium complex, S. pneumoniae*, group B streptococci

indicate the fibroproliferative stage of acute respiratory distress syndrome (ARDS). Occasionally, punctate or macroscopic evidence can be detected in the adrenal tissues. Diffuse petechiae in tissues and mucosal surfaces may indicate disseminated intravascular coagulation (DIC).

The kidneys usually appear normal, and necrosis of kidney tissues is distinctly uncommon. The term *acute tubular necrosis* is a misnomer, and the term *acute kidney injury* (AKI) is more appropriate for describing the functional and usually reversible loss of kidney function found in septic shock without accompanying evidence of glomerular or tubular necrosis.

An important finding at autopsy is identification of the infectious focus that caused septic shock. The focal infection that precipitated sepsis is readily identifiable in most deceased patients despite days to weeks of seemingly appropriate antimicrobial therapy directed against the pathogens. If careful histochemical studies are performed shortly after a patient succumbs to sepsis, excessive apoptosis (but not necrosis) of immune effector cells is identifiable in lung, spleen, lymph nodes, and hepatic tissues. Electron microscopy of tissues after death from sepsis often reveals loss of tight junctions along epithelial and endothelial surfaces. Electron microscopy also demonstrates diffuse mitochondrial swelling and degradation and clearance of intracellular organelles (i.e., autophagy).

PATHOPHYSIOLOGY OF SEPTIC SHOCK

The molecular mechanisms that underlie the basic pathophysiology of septic shock have been determined. Sepsis is triggered when a pathogen or cluster of pathogens breaches the epithelial barriers at a tissue site, evades clearance by humoral and cellular innate immune defenses, and causes an invasive infection. On entry into the host tissues, microbial pathogens are first sensed by myeloid cells of the innate immune system by pattern recognition receptors (e.g., toll-like receptors [TLRs]) on the cell surface and in endosomal compartments. TLRs detect highly conserved molecular motifs of microbes. Examples include lipopolysaccharide (LPS), the endotoxin produced by gram-negative bacteria; bacterial lipopeptides from gram-positive bacteria; β-glucans of the cell wall of fungi; viral RNA genomes and proteins; bacterial flagella; and DAMPs released from injured host cells, including intracellular structures such as histone proteins, mitochondrial DNA, and high-mobility group box 1 (Fig. 91.2).

TLRs and related intracellular pattern recognition receptors, including the inflammasome elements, retinoic acid–inducible gene 1 (*RIG1*)–like helicases, and cytoplasmic microbial TLR4, alert the host to infection. TLR4 is the long-sought-after LPS receptor of the human innate immune system. LPS is released from the cell membrane of gram-negative bacteria on their destruction. LPS is first bound to a

carrier protein, LPS-binding protein, and the LPS monomer is then delivered to a membrane-associated, multiligand, pattern recognition receptor, CD14. LPS monomers are then passed to a soluble protein (i.e., myeloid differentiation factor 2 [MD2]) and bind to the ecto-domain of TLR4. After this LPS/MD2/TLR4 complex is completed and dimerized, intracellular signaling alerts the host to the invasive infectious challenge. The pathway induces a series of phosphorylation events of adaptor proteins and signaling molecules that terminate in the activation and translocation of transcriptional activating factors such as nuclear factor-κB (NF-κB) into the nucleus. The transcription factors bind to promoter sites of the acute phase protein network, resulting in an acute outpouring of inflammatory, host defense, and coagulation components.

Other TLRs, such as TLR5 (i.e., bacterial flagella) and the TLR2/TLR1 and TLR2/TLR6 heterodimers (i.e., bacterial lipopeptides, lipoteichoic acid, and other elements of bacteria and fungi), are expressed on the cell surface of immune effector cells that recognize different molecular patterns. Nucleic acid recognition–specific TLRs reside in endosomal vacuoles, where they detect microbial DNA (TLR9), single-stranded RNA (TLR7 and TLR8), and double-stranded RNA (TLR3).

An array of complement elements, cytokines, chemokines, prostaglandins, vasoactive peptides, platelet-activating factor, and proteases are generated, resulting in activation of neutrophils, neutrophil extracellular traps (NETs), monocytes, macrophages, dendritic cells, lymphocytes, and endothelial cells in a combined effort to wall off the infectious process, clear the pathogens, and begin the process of tissue repair. This defense system efficiently clears pathogens from the host after local injury and the inevitable minor breaches of the epithelial barriers by microorganisms that occur over a lifetime.

If the inflammatory process is unchecked and accompanied by large numbers of pathogens or even a few highly virulent organisms (e.g., plague, tularemia, anthrax, and hemorrhagic fever viruses) to which the host has no preexisting immunity, a generalized, inflammatory, and injurious process known as *sepsis* evolves over a short time, and it can be deleterious or lethal to the host. The same inflammatory response that can be life-saving in localized infection can become life-threatening if it becomes sustained and generalized.

Endothelial membranes throughout the body are activated and become pro-adherent and pro-coagulant surfaces that promote neutrophil and platelet adherence. Neutrophils release proteases, cytokines, NETs, reactive oxygen radicals, and vasoactive prostanoids that damage endothelial cells and their function. Cytokine-inducible nitric oxide synthase is upregulated, resulting in massive generation of nitric oxide (NO). NO is a potent vasodilator, and in combination with other vasoactive peptides and phospholipid mediators, it promotes diffuse opening of capillary beds and increased permeability, with loss of

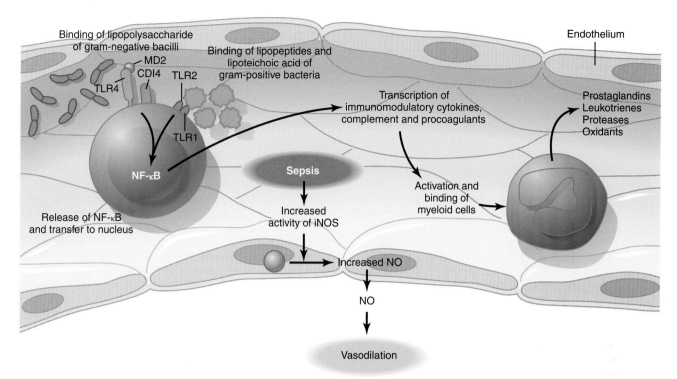

Fig. 91.2 Immunopathogenesis of sepsis. Early recognition of bloodstream infection begins with sensing by pattern recognition receptors: toll-like receptor 4 (TLR4); cluster determinant 14 (CD14); myeloid differentiation factor 2 (MD2) for gram-negative bacterial lipopolysaccharide and TLR2 for lipoteichoic acid and other elements from gram-positive bacteria. Engagement of the TLRs by their ligands signals transcription of the acute phase response genes by nuclear factor-κB (NF-κB). Septic shock is initiated by systemic release of an array of vasoactive mediators, including nitric oxide (NO) produced by cytokine-inducible NO synthase (iNOS).

intravascular fluids into the interstitial spaces. Reactive oxygen species combine with NO to generate highly injurious reactive nitrogen intermediates (e.g., peroxynitrite) that damage mitochondrial function and induce apoptosis. Systemic hypotension rapidly develops, and septic shock ensues. Immediate action by the clinician is mandatory to correct the hemodynamic status and resolve the underlying infection.

CLINICAL PRESENTATION

Despite the vast improvements in understanding the pathophysiologic basis of sepsis, clinical diagnosis remains limited to the medical history, symptomatic assessment, and nonspecific laboratory and hemodynamic criteria. Compounding the problem is the need for prompt institution of appropriate antimicrobial therapy, making early recognition of sepsis critically important. Patients with clinical findings as outlined in Table 91.1 should undergo thorough and prompt evaluation for a possible infectious cause, including bacterial cultures of blood and (when indicated) other body fluids. Localizing signs and symptoms should prompt a thorough physical examination and directed imaging to identify a nidus of infection. Defects of natural defensive barriers, such as transcutaneous devices or intravascular catheters, should be assessed for infection and removed if suspected to be the origin of the septic process. To minimize the potential delay in prompt recognition and management of sepsis resulting from obtaining laboratory data, the Sepsis-3 recommendations included a bedside quick SOFA (qSOFA) scoring system. The qSOFA allows for repeated bedside evaluations of patients at risk for developing sepsis and relies on three clinical criteria, each worth 1 point: (a) Respiratory rate 22/min or greater; (b) altered mentation; and (c) systolic blood pressure

less than 100 mm Hg. A qSOFA score of 2 or greater should prompt further investigation into infectious causes and organ dysfunction as well as initiation or escalation of therapy, as appropriate. Despite its clinical logic and its simplicity, the experience thus far with its predictive value has been mixed. General clinical presentation of sepsis varies widely. Many patients have fever or chills, but older patients and those on immunomodulating medications may not mount a fever. Hypothermia portends a worse prognosis or more severe illness. Tachypnea may be an indicator of respiratory compensation for underlying metabolic acidosis or the early signs and symptoms of ARDS.

Mental status changes can result from metabolic derangements caused by sepsis, hypoglycemia, the underlying infectious process, or concomitant hypotension. This symptom can be difficult to identify in the elderly patient with dementia, and caution should be exercised in the evaluation and treatment of the otherwise stable elderly patient with possible mental status changes.

Skin findings (e.g., cellulitis, abscess) can provide clues to the cause of sepsis and may indicate the state of peripheral systemic perfusion. Several microorganisms can cause specific skin manifestations in systemic infection. *S. aureus* and streptococci can cause diffuse erythroderma, bullous lesions, or generalized desquamation. Bacteremia caused by several gram-negative organisms, including *P. aeruginosa* and enteric organisms, can result in ecthyma gangrenosum, particularly in immunocompromised patients. These lesions are round and 1 to 15 cm in diameter, and they have a central area of necrosis and peripheral erythema. Infection with *Neisseria meningitidis* can result initially in lower extremity petechiae progressing to diffuse purpura, which likely portends septic shock and a high risk of death. A similar clinical presentation can be observed in other unusual infectious diseases, such as overwhelming pneumococcal sepsis in the asplenic host or disseminated neisserial infections in patients with late complement deficiencies.

Hemodynamic instability, particularly hypotension with or without accompanying oliguria, is commonly associated with sepsis. Instability can result from poor cardiac output, intravascular fluid depletion, or low systemic vascular resistance. Hypotension can initially respond to intravenous fluid resuscitation, but in cases of severe sepsis and septic shock, it may require additional support with vasopressors. Intensive cardiac monitoring may be necessary to gauge the relative need for intravenous fluids or vasopressors after initial fluid resuscitation measures are attempted.

Patients in septic shock can be tachycardic and hypotensive. They may have relatively warm extremities (i.e., warm shock or distributive shock), or they may be peripherally vasoconstricted, with mottled and cool extremities (i.e., cold shock). Warm shock is the predominant finding in most adult patients at the onset of septic shock, with evidence of diffuse vasodilation, bounding pulses, and a compensatory high cardiac output despite evidence of diminished myocardial performance. Increased cardiac output is accomplished primarily by increased heart rate in an attempt to maintain blood pressure and perfuse vital organs. If shock is not promptly corrected, myocardial dysfunction ensues and cold shock evolves over the next several hours. Older patients with limited cardiac reserves tolerate shock poorly and are more likely to develop cold shock. Evidence of septic shock at presentation that is refractory to early resuscitation portends a poor prognosis, with mortality rates exceeding 70%.

Besides hypotension, oliguria can represent developing AKI. It can arise from a combination of the disease process, infecting organism, and medications. Inflammatory cytokines, microbial toxins, systemic hypotension, and iatrogenic renal injury from medications can result in AKI. Other causes of renal injury include interstitial injury from infection or medications and immune complex–mediated injury, as seen in cases of endocarditis.

Besides tachypnea, pulmonary symptoms seen in septic patients include marked hypoxia due to interstitial edema, inflammation, or hemodynamic instability. ARDS is defined as an arterial partial pressure of oxygen less than 50 mm Hg despite fractional inspired oxygen of greater than 50%, together with diffuse alveolar infiltrates and a pulmonary capillary wedge pressure of less than 18 mm Hg. ARDS occurs in up to 40% of septic patients. The diffuse pulmonary inflammation in ARDS results in increased pulmonary vascular permeability, which complicates fluid resuscitation efforts because excessive fluid can exacerbate pulmonary edema and hypoxia. Altered mental status and sepsis-related myopathy also result in airway compromise and weak respiratory effort, necessitating invasive ventilatory support.

Patients with sepsis can have marked hematologic changes. They may have neutrophilic leukocytosis, which is often accompanied by increased immature cell counts, or they can be markedly leukopenic (particularly lymphopenic), often in cases of severe septic shock. Transient neutropenia is often seen in the early phase of septic shock and results from activation and adherence of neutrophils along endothelial surfaces in the microcirculation. This is rapidly followed by prolonged neutrophilia as sepsis-induced inflammatory cytokines stimulate bone marrow synthesis of new white blood cells.

Thrombocytopenia and coagulopathy can occur, and patients have petechiae or purpura at presentation. Severe derangements in coagulation can produce DIC, which can lead to thrombin deposition throughout the microcirculation. Excessive activation and degradation of clotting factors can deplete coagulation factors, resulting in diffuse hemorrhage. Excessive mucosal bleeding around airway tubes and prolonged bleeding from venipuncture sites presage internal bleeding events. Massive gastrointestinal hemorrhage can occur, which can cause or exacerbate hypotension and shock.

Derangements in glucose homeostasis can be seen at presentation. This can take the form of hyperglycemia in diabetics receiving glucose-containing fluids or acute metabolic derangement due to infection. Hypoglycemia is more common in patients with underlying liver disease. Increased anaerobic metabolism due to poor tissue oxygenation and coupled with mitochondrial dysfunction and impaired hepatic clearance of lactic acid may result in increased serum lactate levels and metabolic acidosis.

DIAGNOSIS

Accurate diagnosis of sepsis relies on the history, physical examination, and general laboratory investigation. Diagnostic criteria for sepsis in adults based on the Sepsis-3 criteria are listed in Table 91.1.

Accurate and timely identification of the underlying infectious cause is essential. For patients able to provide a history, an assessment of medical comorbidities, potential exposures, prior infections, and immune system abnormalities may help to guide empirical antimicrobial therapy and the laboratory investigation, particularly microbial cultures. Two sets of blood cultures drawn from a fresh venipuncture and from existing indwelling intravascular lines (before initiation of empirical antimicrobial therapy when possible) help to identify the causative organism in many cases. A recent study in over 3000 patients reinforces the value of obtaining diagnostic, pre-antibiotic treatment, blood cultures. The diagnostic yield was nearly 50% higher for blood cultures obtained in the pre-antibiotic treatment group compared to the post-antibiotic treatment blood cultures (sampled up to 120 minutes after the start of antibiotic therapy). Symptomatic assessment and physical examination should suggest a location of focal infection that can help to guide radiologic studies and interventions to drain pus.

Beyond microbial cultures, several other laboratory studies can help to define the severity of illness and provide baseline data for monitoring the response to therapy. Basic laboratory testing, including a complete blood count with differential, chemistries, and creatinine and aminotransferase levels, can help to identify significant organ dysfunction. Oxygen saturation by pulse oximetry should be measured promptly to identify gas exchange capacity and the need for ventilatory support. Coagulation studies should be obtained, particularly for patients with evidence of DIC and those who are thrombocytopenic. For patients with altered mental status or marked respiratory difficulty, arterial blood gas sampling can help define the underlying derangement and physiologic compensation and can indirectly gauge the severity of illness.

Levels of inflammatory markers, including C-reactive protein and procalcitonin, usually are elevated. An elevated procalcitonin level can help to differentiate septic shock from other causes of shock and provide some prognostic data and a measure of response to therapy. In cases of sepsis due to pneumonia, serial measurement of procalcitonin can help to guide the duration of antibiotic therapy.

Other testing should be directed toward identifying the potential cause. Patients with severe diarrhea should undergo testing for antibiotic-associated *Clostridioides difficile* infection. Imaging studies should focus on identifying infectious sources and facilitate drainage of fluid collections or abscesses. Computed tomography may be of use in such circumstances, although for the critically ill patient who is not stable for transport, bedside radiographic studies, especially ultrasound, should be considered.

Multiple tests of physiologic function and advanced microbiologic diagnostic tests are increasingly used in clinical practice. They include polymerase chain reaction (PCR)–based assays for identifying bacteria and viruses and various assays of inflammatory cytokines and other biomarkers alone and in combination as potential diagnostic and prognostic aids.

TABLE 91.3 Recommended Initial Management of Sepsis in Adults

- Start resuscitation immediately in patients with hypotension or serum lactate level >2 mmol/L.
- Obtain appropriate cultures before starting antibiotics if doing so does not significantly delay therapy.
- Evaluate for a focus of infection amenable to source control (e.g., abscess drainage).
- Remove intravascular catheters if potentially infected.
- Begin broad-spectrum antibiotics within the first hour of severe sepsis and septic shock. Initial antibiotic regimen is based on likely source of sepsis, likely pathogens, and local antibiotic susceptibility patterns of common pathogens.
- Begin fluid resuscitation using crystalloids as the first choice. If colloids are used, avoid starches and consider albumin in selected patients who have hypoalbuminemia or require large-volume fluid resuscitation.
- Give fluid challenge of up to 30 mL/kg of crystalloids over 15–30 min in septic patients with suspected volume depletion; larger volumes of fluids may be needed in some patients. The goals for resuscitation should be a central venous pressure of 8–12 mm Hg, a mean arterial pressure (MAP) ≥65 mm Hg, and a superior vena cava oxygen saturation ≥70% or mixed venous oxygen saturation ≥65%.
- Maintain targeted MAP of ≥65 mm Hg; if fluids are not effective in reestablishing adequate blood pressure, begin vasopressors. After hemodynamic parameters are stabilized, limit fluid therapy to prevent pulmonary fluid accumulation and exacerbation of hypoxemia.
- Use norepinephrine, centrally administered, as the vasopressor of choice. Epinephrine is the second choice, followed by vasopressin as salvage therapy. Dobutamine may be useful if an inotrope is needed. Avoid dopamine except for special situations (i.e., low risk of tachyarrhythmia and persistent bradycardia).
- Give red blood cells when the hemoglobin concentration decreases to <7 g/dL; target hemoglobin level is 7–9 g/dL.
- Target a tidal volume of 6 mL/kg in patients with acute respiratory distress syndrome.
- Give low-molecular-weight heparin or unfractionated heparin for deep vein thrombosis prophylaxis; use graduated pressure stockings or intermittent compression devices if heparin therapy is contraindicated.
- Provide stress ulcer prophylaxis using histamine H_2-blockers or a proton pump inhibitor.
- Provide expert supportive care; provide low-dose nutrition for the first week; consider stress-dose steroids if refractory septic shock occurs; maintain blood glucose in the 110-180 mg/dL range.

Data from Dellinger RP, Levy MM, et al: Surviving Sepsis Campaign: international guidelines for the management of severe sepsis and septic shock, 2012, Crit Care Med 41:580-637, 2013.

TABLE 91.4 Initial Antibiotic Recommendations for Adult Patients With Sepsis

Indication	Recommended Dosages[a]
Empirical coverage (source unknown)	Vancomycin 15 mg/kg q12h plus piperacillin-tazobactam[b] 3.375 g IV q6h or imipenem 0.5 g IV q6h or meropenem 1.0 g IV q8h with or without an aminoglycoside (e.g., tobramycin 5 mg/kg IV q24)[c]
Community-acquired pneumonia (CAP)	Ceftriaxone 1 g IV q24h plus azithromycin 500 mg IV q24h or a fluoroquinolone (e.g., moxifloxacin 400 mg IV q24h or levofloxacin 750 mg IV q24h)[d]
Community-acquired urosepsis	Piperacillin-tazobactam 3.375 g IV q6h or ciprofloxacin 400 mg IV q12h
Meningitis	Vancomycin 15 mg/kg IV q6h plus ceftriaxone 2 g IV q12h plus dexamethasone 0.15 mg/kg IV q6h × 2–4 days, preferably before antibiotics; add ampicillin 2 g IV q4h if listeria is suspected.
Nosocomial pneumonia	Vancomycin 15 mg/kg q12h plus piperacillin-tazobactam 4.5 g IV q6h or imipenem 0.5 g IV q6h or meropenem 1 g IV q8h or cefepime 2 g IV q8h plus an aminoglycoside (e.g., amikacin 15 mg/kg IV q24h or tobramycin 5–7 mg/kg IV q24h) or levofloxacin 750 mg IV q24h. Some authorities substitute linezolid 600 mg IV q12h for vancomycin if MRSA is a significant concern or known to be the cause.
Neutropenia	Cefepime 2 g IV q8h; add vancomycin 15 mg/kg IV q12h if a central line is present and infection is a concern. Add antifungal coverage with caspofungin 70 mg IV × 1, then 50 mg IV q24h if fever persists ≥5 days. For suspected or proven invasive aspergillosis, voriconazole 6 mg/kg IV q12h × 2, then 4 mg/kg IV q12h should be used.
Cellulitis and skin infections	Vancomycin 15 mg/kg IV q12h. Add piperacillin-tazobactam 3.375 g IV q6h in diabetics and immunocompromised patients. If necrotizing fasciitis is suspected, add clindamycin 900 mg. IV; surgical debridement is crucial.

IV, Intravenous; *MRSA,* methicillin-resistant *Staphylococcus aureus.*
[a]Assumes normal renal function; dose adjustments are required with impaired creatinine clearance.
[b]Substitute aztreonam 2 g IV q8h if patient is allergic to penicillin.
[c]Monitor drug levels of aminoglycosides (i.e., peak and trough).
[d]Substitute cefepime or a carbapenem and azithromycin ± an aminoglycoside if the patient has severe CAP or health care–associated pneumonia.

TREATMENT

Septic shock is a medical emergency. Immediate attempts to reestablish physiologic hemodynamics, vital organ support, and oxygen delivery to tissues should accompany early diagnosis and treatment of infection. Patients should be transferred to the intensive care unit as soon as possible to receive optimal monitoring, hemodynamic support, and expert supportive care.

Early recognition, prompt resuscitation, and early institution of appropriate antimicrobial agents are the most important determinants of a successful outcome. If appropriate, draining infectious foci (i.e., source control) should be done as soon as possible. Key elements of the 2016 Surviving Sepsis Campaign guidelines are summarized in Table 91.3.

An essential element in the treatment of sepsis is early administration of antibiotics active against the causative pathogen. Treatment is best given within 1 hour of the onset of septic shock, and an empirical, broad-spectrum antimicrobial regimen is usually employed until the results of cultures of blood and the site of infection become available. A suggested initial treatment regimen is provided in Table 91.4. Failing to treat the causative pathogen until its identity and susceptibility profile become available days later is associated with adverse outcomes. After the pathogen is identified, de-escalation to the simplest monotherapy to which it is susceptible is important.

PROGNOSIS

Despite advances in clinical practice and treatment, sepsis mortality rates remain high, ranging from 20% to 30% among relatively healthy adults to more than 80% among the elderly, immunocompromised, and those with significant chronic medical comorbidities. Patients may experience significant weakness, wasting, and debilitation due to severe catabolism, poor nutrition, and prolonged hospitalization. Prolonged rehabilitation in a skilled facility after the initial hospitalization and additional home-based therapy may be required. Patients may have permanent disabilities, including impaired renal function or persistent debilitation from procedures required to treat the underlying infection.

SUGGESTED READINGS

Anand V, Zhang Z, Kadri SS, et al: Epidemiology of quick sequential organ failure assessment criteria in undifferentiated patients and association with suspected infection and sepsis, Chest 156(2):289–297, 2019.

Angus D, van der Poll T: Severe sepsis and septic shock, N Engl J Med 369:840–851, 2013.

Cheng MP, Stenstrom R, Paqette K, et al: Blood culture results before and after antimicrobial administration in patients with severe manifestations of sepsis: a diagnostic study, Ann Intern Med, 2019. https://doi.org/10.7326/M19-1696.

Hotchkiss RS, Coopersmith CM, McDunn JE, et al: The sepsis seesaw: tilting toward immunosuppression, Nat Med 15:496–497, 2009.

Howell MD, Davis AM: Management of sepsis and septic shock, J Am Med Assoc 317(8):317, 2017.

Melamed A, Sorvillo FJ: The burden of sepsis-associated mortality in the United States from 1999 to 2005: an analysis of multiple-cause-of-death data, Crit Care 13:R28, 2009.

Rhee C, Dantes R, Epstein L, et al: Incidence and trends of sepsis in US hospitals using clinical vs claims data, 2009-2014, J Am Med Assoc 318(13):1241–1249, 2017.

Singer M, Deutschman CS, Seymour CW, et al: The third international consensus definitions for sepsis and septic shock (sepsis-3), J Am Med Assoc 315(8):801–810, 2016.

Vincent JL, Opal SM, Marshall JC, et al: Sepsis definitions: time for a change, Lancet 381:774–775, 2013.

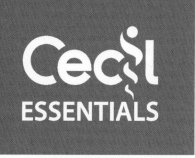

92

Infections of the Central Nervous System

Su N. Aung, Allan R. Tunkel

INTRODUCTION

Infections of the central nervous system (CNS) can be caused by a number of pathogens, including viruses, bacteria, fungi, and parasites (i.e., protozoa and helminths). These infectious agents can penetrate the CNS by direct seeding or hematogenous spread and cause a constellation of symptoms. The clinical presentation of a CNS infection varies depending on the virulence of the offending pathogen, the location of the infection, and underlying host factors. CNS infections can impact structures contained in the cranium or spinal cord and may be associated with significant morbidity and mortality. This chapter focuses on meningitis, encephalitis, and focal intracranial and paraspinal infections, as well as prion diseases.

MENINGITIS

Definition

Meningitis, defined as inflammation of the leptomeninges that cover the brain and spinal cord, is identified by an abnormal increase in the number of white blood cells in cerebrospinal fluid (CSF). Inflammation can be caused by many infectious agents (i.e., bacteria, viruses, fungi, and parasites) and also can occur as a result of non-infectious conditions, including tumors or cysts, medications (e.g., nonsteroidal anti-inflammatory drugs, antimicrobial agents), systemic illnesses (e.g., systemic lupus erythematosus, Behçet disease, sarcoidosis), or neurologic procedures (e.g., neurosurgery, spinal anesthesia, intrathecal injections, retained devices).

The clinical presentation may be acute, subacute, or chronic based on the virulence of the infecting agent and patient characteristics. Acute meningitis is a syndrome characterized by the onset of symptoms within hours to several days, whereas chronic meningitis is usually characterized by abnormal clinical and CSF findings that persist for at least 4 weeks. Acute meningitis is most often caused by bacteria and viruses, whereas chronic meningitis is most often caused by spirochetes, mycobacteria, and fungi. The clinical presentation may also vary depending on the age of the patient, underlying health conditions, predisposing factors (e.g., head trauma, recent neurosurgery, presence of a CSF shunt or other retained devices), and immunosuppression.

Epidemiology and Etiology
Bacterial Meningitis

Bacterial meningitis is associated with high morbidity and mortality and requires prompt clinical recognition and treatment. Over 1.2 million cases of bacterial meningitis are diagnosed each year worldwide with incidence and mortality rates varying by region, pathogen, and age. CSF findings commonly include pleocytosis (CSF white blood cell count in the hundreds to thousands range) usually associated with neutrophilic predominance, low glucose, and elevated protein.

Based on a prior surveillance study in the United States from 2003 to 2007, the most common pathogens causing bacterial meningitis were *Streptococcus pneumoniae* (58% of cases), *Streptococcus agalactiae* (18% of cases), *Neisseria meningitidis* (14% of cases), *H. influenzae* (7% of cases), and *Listeria monocytogenes* (3% of cases). Specific etiologic agents may be identified based on the patient's age and various risk factors (Table 92.1).

In the United States, *S. pneumoniae* is the most common etiologic agent of bacterial meningitis. The incidence has declined since the introduction of pneumococcal conjugate vaccines PCV7 and later PCV13, but mortality remains high, ranging from 18% to 26%. Among survivors, high rates of neurologic sequelae and systemic complications occur, especially in those over 60 years of age. Conditions associated with severe pneumococcal meningitis include asplenia or splenic dysfunction, multiple myeloma, hypogammaglobulinemia, alcoholism, malnutrition, chronic liver or kidney disease, and diabetes mellitus. Patients often have contiguous or distant foci of infection such as pneumonia, otitis media, mastoiditis, sinusitis, and endocarditis. Head trauma, with a CSF leak, is an important risk factor for recurrent pneumococcal meningitis.

The group B streptococcus (i.e., *S. agalactiae*) is a common etiologic agent of meningitis in neonates, with 52% of cases occurring during the first year of life. Mortality in the United States ranges from 7% to 27% with substantial long-term morbidity seen among survivors. Group B streptococcal meningitis can also occur in adults. Risk factors in adults include age older than 60 years, pregnancy or the postpartum state, diabetes mellitus, and other chronic diseases and immunosuppressed states but may also occur in adults without underlying conditions.

Neisseria meningitidis usually causes meningitis in children and young adults. Most cases in the United States are caused by serogroups B, C, and Y; serogroups A and W seldom occur in the United States. Patients with deficiencies in the terminal complement components (C5 to C8, and perhaps C9) and properdin are at increased risk for meningococcal infections, including meningitis with significantly higher rates of neurologic sequelae. Outbreaks of meningitis due to *N. meningitidis* may occur in persons living in close quarters, such as among household members, in daycare centers, college dormitories, and among the incarcerated. One outbreak of serogroup C disease was reported in New York City among men who have sex with men, and outbreaks caused by serogroup B have been reported at college campuses,

TABLE 92.1   Common Bacterial Pathogens and Factors Predisposing to Meningitis

Predisposing Factor	Bacterial Pathogens
Age	
<1 mo	*Streptococcus agalactiae, Escherichia coli, Listeria monocytogenes*
1–23 mo	*S. agalactiae, E. coli, Haemophilus influenzae, Streptococcus pneumoniae, Neisseria meningitidis*
2–50 yr	*S. pneumoniae, N. meningitidis*
>50 yr	*S. pneumoniae, N. meningitidis, L. monocytogenes*, aerobic gram-negative bacilli
Immunocompromised state	*S. pneumoniae, N. meningitidis, L. monocytogenes*, aerobic gram-negative bacilli (including *Pseudomonas aeruginosa*)
Basilar skull fracture	*S. pneumoniae, H. influenzae*, group A β-hemolytic streptococci
Head trauma; post neurosurgery	*Staphylococcus aureus*, coagulase-negative staphylococci (especially *Staphylococcus epidermidis*), aerobic gram-negative bacilli (including *P. aeruginosa*)

From Hasbun R, van de Beek D, Brouwer MC, Tunkel AR: Acute meningitis. In Bennett JE, Dolin R, Blaser M, editors: Mandell, Douglas, and Bennett's principles and practice of infectious diseases, ed 9, Philadelphia, 2020, Saunders.

most recently at the Rutgers University, Columbia University, and University of California San Diego (Centers for Disease Control and Infection [CDC], May 2019). Risk is also increased in patients who are taking eculizumab (inhibits complement).

Prophylaxis is indicated for people in the same household, roommates, young adults exposed in dormitories, travelers who had direct contact with respiratory secretions from an index patient or was seated next to an index patient during a prolonged flight, and individuals who were exposed to oral secretions (e.g., intimate kissing, or health care workers who performed mouth-to-mouth resuscitation or endotracheal intubation on the index patient). Chemoprophylaxis should be administered as soon as possible if indications are met, ideally within 24 hours after identification of the index case, and is usually not beneficial beyond 14 days. Recommended antimicrobials for prophylaxis include rifampin, ciprofloxacin, and ceftriaxone. Currently, there are vaccines that cover serogroups A, C, W, Y (MenACWY) and serogroup B (MenB). Vaccination with the quadrivalent meningococcal vaccine against serogroups A, C, W, and Y is recommended for children ages 11 to 18 years of age and individuals 2 months or older with risk factors including anatomic or functional asplenia, persistent complement deficiency, HIV infection, individuals taking eculizumab, travelling to certain countries where vaccine is recommended (e.g., Saudi Arabia, Mecca, or Hajj), at-risk exposure during outbreaks, and microbiologists who work with the meningococcus bacteria. Two meningococcal B vaccines were approved in 2015 for persons aged 10 to 25 years; the recommendation from the Advisory Committee on Immunization Practices is that adolescents and young adults, ages 16 to 23 years, may be vaccinated for short-term protection against most strains of *N. meningitidis* serogroup B, but that the risk of infection in the United States is currently low.

Among typable strains, *Haemophilus influenzae* serotype b (Hib) was a common cause of meningitis and epiglottis among children prior to the widespread use of the conjugate vaccine against *H. influenzae* type b. The incidence of meningitis due to *H. influenzae* has declined more than 90% since the introduction of vaccination. Isolation of this microorganism in older children and adults suggests certain underlying conditions, such as sinusitis, otitis media, epiglottitis, pneumonia, structural lung disease, diabetes mellitus, alcoholism, splenectomy or asplenic states, head trauma with CSF leak, immune deficiency, hematopoietic stem cell transplantation, and chemotherapy or radiation therapy. In the post-Hib vaccination era, nontypable *H. influenzae* has emerged as a cause of invasive infections, including meningitis, particularly among the elderly and young children.

Meningitis caused by *Listeria monocytogenes* is most common in neonates, adults older than 50 years, alcoholics, immunosuppressed adults, pregnancy, conditions associated with iron overload, and in patients with chronic conditions such as diabetes mellitus, collagen vascular disease, liver disease, and renal disease. Given the likely gastrointestinal portal of entry for this microorganism, outbreaks of *Listeria* infection have been associated with ingestion of contaminated coleslaw, raw vegetables, milk, and cheese. Sporadic cases have been linked to contaminated turkey franks, alfalfa tablets, cantaloupe, diced celery, hog's head cheese, and processed meats. *Listeria* CNS infection has been associated with rhombencephalitis, which refers to inflammation of the hindbrain (brainstem and cerebellum) with concomitant findings on brain imaging and is more commonly seen in immunocompetent persons.

Meningitis caused by aerobic gram-negative pathogens (e.g., *Klebsiella* sp, *Escherichia coli*, *Serratia marcescens*, *Pseudomonas aeruginosa*, *Acinetobacter* sp) are becoming more important as etiologies, particularly in patients with a history of head trauma or neurosurgical procedures. At-risk individuals include neonates, older adults, immunosuppressed patients, those with gram-negative sepsis, and rarely in disseminated strongyloidiasis associated with the hyperinfection syndrome.

Staphylococcus aureus meningitis is usually found in the early period after neurosurgery or recent head trauma, in those with CSF shunts, or in patients with underlying conditions such as diabetes mellitus, alcoholism, chronic kidney disease requiring hemodialysis, injection-drug use, and malignancies. *S. aureus*, particularly methicillin-resistant strains, is most commonly seen in health care–associated ventriculitis and meningitis. Community-acquired *S. aureus* meningitis is found in patients with sinusitis, osteomyelitis, and pneumonia.

Viral Meningitis

Viral meningitis is the most common type of meningitis. The CSF profile of viral meningitis usually includes pleocytosis with elevated WBCs in the tens to hundreds range, lymphocytic predominance, normal glucose, and elevated protein. Overall, meningitis due to a viral etiology is often less severe than bacterial meningitis, and symptoms usually self-resolve. Risk factors for severe infection include young age (less than 5 years) and immunosuppression.

Enteroviruses are the leading identifiable cause of the *aseptic meningitis syndrome*, a term used to define any meningitis (particularly with lymphocytic pleocytosis) for which a cause is not apparent after initial evaluation, routine CSF stains, and cultures. The CDC estimate that 10 to 15 million symptomatic enteroviral infections occur annually in the United States; of these, 30,000 to 75,000 are meningitis cases, although this is likely an underestimation.

Many other viruses can cause the aseptic meningitis syndrome, including mumps virus (in unimmunized populations), human immunodeficiency virus (HIV), several arboviruses (e.g., St. Louis encephalitis virus, the California encephalitis group of viruses, Colorado tick fever virus, West Nile virus), and herpesviruses (including Epstein-Barr virus, the herpes simplex viruses, and varicella-zoster virus). The syndrome of herpes simplex virus (HSV) meningitis is most commonly associated with primary genital infection. The DNA of HSV has been detected in the CSF of patients with the syndrome of recurrent benign lymphocytic meningitis (previously known as Mollaret meningitis), with almost all cases caused by herpes simplex virus type 2 (HSV-2).

Spirochetal Meningitis

The most common spirochetes associated with meningitis are *Treponema pallidum* (the etiologic agent of syphilis) and *Borrelia burgdorferi* (the etiologic agent of Lyme disease). The incidence of syphilitic meningitis is greatest in the first 2 years after initial infection, occurring in 0.3% to 2.4% of untreated cases. The overall incidence of neurosyphilis has increased, with the majority of cases reported in patients with HIV infection. Based on the CDC surveillance data from 2008 to 2015, approximately 12.5% of cases of Lyme disease had neurologic manifestations, including facial palsy (8.4%), radiculoneuropathy (3.8%), lymphocytic meningitis (1.3%), and encephalitis (<1%).

Tuberculous Meningitis

Mycobacterium tuberculosis can lead to pulmonary and extrapulmonary disease, including involvement of the CNS. Tuberculous meningitis accounts for approximately 15% of cases of extrapulmonary tuberculosis in the United States. CNS disease is much more common in less developed areas of the world. Factors associated with reactivation of latent foci and progression to the syndrome of late generalized tuberculosis include advanced age, immunosuppressive drug therapy, HIV/AIDS, transplantation, malignancy, gastrectomy, pregnancy, chronic medical conditions, and close contacts to individuals with active infection. The epidemiology of tuberculosis has been influenced by the advent of HIV infection, in which extrapulmonary disease (including CNS infection) occurs in more than 70% of cases with co-infection.

Fungal Meningitis

The incidence of fungal meningitis has risen dramatically in recent years due to the increasing numbers of immunosuppressed patients and broad usage of immunosuppressive drugs. *Cryptococcus neoformans* is the most common etiologic agent of clinically recognized fungal meningitis, most commonly diagnosed in persons who are immunosuppressed or have chronic medical conditions; HIV-infected patients are in the highest-risk group. Cases have also been documented in immunocompetent healthy individuals.

Coccidioides immitis is a thermal dimorphic fungus that is endemic in the semiarid regions of the Americas and desert areas of the southwestern United States (e.g., California, Arizona, New Mexico, Texas), where about one third of the population is infected. Less than 1% of patients develop disseminated infection, and one third to one half of those with disease have meningeal involvement.

Other fungi less commonly cause CNS infection. *Histoplasma capsulatum* is endemic to fertile river valleys, principally the Mississippi and Ohio River basins. *Blastomyces dermatitidis* is also distributed in the Mississippi and Ohio River basins, as well as regions around the Great Lakes and along the Saint Lawrence River. *Candida* meningitis is uncommon and occurs as a manifestation of disseminated candidiasis, usually in premature neonates, individuals with ventricular drainage devices, and as isolated chronic meningitis.

Clinical Presentation
Acute Meningitis

Adult patients with acute meningitis typically seek medical attention within hours to days of illness. Patients with acute bacterial meningitis classically exhibit fever, headache, meningismus, and signs of cerebral dysfunction (i.e., confusion, delirium, or a declining level of consciousness

ranging from lethargy to coma). The presentation may vary based on age, underlying disease status, and specific pathogen involved. The etiology can be very challenging to distinguish early in the onset of illness. In bacterial meningitis, the meningismus may be subtle, marked, or accompanied by Kernig sign or Brudzinski sign, although the sensitivity of these signs is only 5% in adults. Cranial nerve palsies (especially involving cranial nerves III, IV, VI, and VII) and focal cerebral signs are seen in 10% to 20% of cases. Seizures occur in about 30% of patients. Older adult patients with bacterial meningitis, especially those with underlying conditions (e.g., diabetes mellitus, cardiopulmonary disease), may have disease that manifests insidiously with lethargy or obtundation, no fever, and various signs of meningeal inflammation. Older adult patients may have an antecedent or concurrent bronchitis, pneumonia, or paranasal sinusitis.

Viral meningitis is typically a self-limited illness, but symptoms can be difficult to distinguish from bacterial meningitis, particularly early in the disease course. The clinical manifestations of enteroviral meningitis, the most common etiology of viral meningitis, depend on host age and immune status. In adolescents and adults, more than one half of the patients have nuchal rigidity. Adults usually present with headache, which is often severe and frontal. Photophobia is also common in older patients. Nonspecific symptoms and signs include vomiting, anorexia, rash, diarrhea, cough, upper respiratory findings (especially pharyngitis), and myalgias. Other clues to the diagnosis of enteroviral disease are the time of year (more prevalent in summer and autumn months) and known epidemic disease in the community. The duration of illness of enteroviral meningitis is usually less than 1 week, and many patients report improvement after lumbar puncture, presumably from the reduction in intracranial pressure.

Meningitis associated with HSV-2 infections is usually characterized by stiff neck, headache, and fever. Patients with recurrent benign lymphocytic meningitis characteristically develop a few to 10 episodes of meningitis lasting 2 to 5 days, followed by spontaneous recovery. These patients have acute onset of headache, fever, photophobia, and meningism; about 50% of patients have transient neurologic manifestations, including seizures, hallucinations, diplopia, cranial nerve palsies, or altered consciousness. Unlike HSV encephalitis, HSV meningitis is usually benign and resolves without treatment. The second most common herpesvirus causing aseptic meningitis is varicella-zoster virus (VZV) and can occur in the absence of the typical vesicular rash. Epstein-Barr virus (EBV) meningitis can be seen in the presence of concomitant mononucleosis-like picture with rash, pharyngitis, lymphadenopathy, and splenomegaly.

West Nile virus (WNV) causes neuroinvasive disease in approximately 1% of patients with WNV infections, which is most often seen during summer months in the United States. WNV meningitis symptoms typically include fever, headache, nausea, vomiting, stiff neck, photophobia, and occasionally a maculopapular rash. Patients may experience persistent symptoms and exhibit abnormal neurologic findings for years following the acute infection.

In patients infected with mumps virus, CNS infection causes fever, vomiting, and headache. Fevers are usually high and last for 72 to 96 hours. These symptoms usually occur about 5 days after the onset of parotitis, which can be present in about 50% of cases. In uncomplicated cases, defervescence typically leads to clinical recovery; the total duration of illness is usually 7 to 10 days.

Subacute or Chronic Meningitis

Meningitis caused by spirochetes, mycobacteria, or fungi in the adult patient can linger for weeks to years after clinical presentation. The patient may initially have no overt symptoms, suffer from low-grade headaches and fever, or experience gradual mental status and other neurologic changes.

Syphilitic meningitis (neurosyphilis) caused by *Treponema pallidum* usually manifests in a manner similar to that of other forms of aseptic meningitis. Patients complain of headache, nausea, and vomiting. Other findings include stiff neck, fever, seizures, cranial nerve palsies, and less commonly, other focal neurologic abnormalities (e.g., hemiplegia, aphasia, and mental status changes). Meningovascular syphilis occurs as a result of focal syphilitic arteritis. Most patients experience symptoms including headache, vertigo, personality changes, behavioral changes, insomnia, seizures, or focal neurologic deficits that can last for weeks to months. In rare cases, if untreated, the focal deficits can progress to stroke with irreversible neurologic deficits.

Meningitis is the most important neurologic abnormality of acute disseminated Lyme disease and usually occurs 2 to 10 weeks following erythema migrans. Headache is the most common symptom of Lyme meningitis. Other symptoms include photophobia, nausea, vomiting, and stiff neck. About 50% of patients with Lyme meningitis have mild cerebral symptoms consisting most commonly of somnolence, emotional lability, depression, impaired memory and concentration, and behavioral symptoms. Approximately 50% of patients may exhibit cranial neuropathies, with facial nerve palsy occurring in 80% to 90% of cases.

Patients with tuberculous meningitis experience an insidious prodrome characterized by malaise, lassitude, low-grade fever, intermittent headache, and personality changes. Within 2 to 3 weeks, the meningitic phase manifests as protracted headache, photophobia, stiff neck, vomiting, and confusion. In some adults, the initial prodromal stage may take the form of a slowly progressive dementia, whereas others may have a rapidly progressive meningitis syndrome indistinguishable from pyogenic bacterial meningitis. Fever is an inconstant finding on physical examination (50% to 98% of cases). Meningismus and signs of meningeal irritation are not uniform findings and can be absent in 25% to 80% of patients. Focal neurologic signs frequently consist of unilateral or, less commonly, bilateral cranial nerve palsies; cranial nerve VI is most commonly affected.

The time course of fungal meningitis depends on the clinical setting. Cases may manifest acutely, subacutely, or chronically; some of the fungal meningitides may cause symptoms that persist for years in the absence of antifungal treatment. In contrast, the same organisms can produce severe symptoms and signs within a few days and without clinical signs of meningeal irritation, particularly in the immunocompromised patient. In patients without acquired immunodeficiency syndrome (AIDS), cryptococcal meningitis typically manifests as a subacute process after days to weeks of symptoms. Headache is the most frequent complaint. Fever, stiff neck, photophobia, and personality changes may also occur; confusion, irritability, and other personality changes reflecting meningoencephalitis occur in about 50% of patients. Ocular abnormalities occur in about 40% of patients and include papilledema and cranial nerve palsies.

In AIDS patients, manifestation of cryptococcal meningitis can be subtle, with minimal or no symptoms. AIDS patients may report only headache and lethargy. Although fever is common, meningeal signs occur in a minority of these patients.

Patients with meningeal coccidioidomycosis usually complain of headache, low-grade fever, weight loss, and mental status changes. About one half of patients develop disorientation, lethargy, confusion, or memory loss. Meningeal signs are uncommon. The presenting symptoms of *Histoplasma* meningitis are nonspecific. Symptoms usually include headache and fever. Only about one half of patients have focal neurologic mental status symptoms. Candidal meningitis also manifests with nonspecific findings and is seen as an extension of disseminated disease in at-risk individuals.

Diagnosis

Clinically suspected meningitis is diagnosed by analysis of CSF obtained by lumbar puncture (Table 92.2). Table 92.3 illustrates general CSF

TABLE 92.2 Cerebrospinal Fluid Tests for Patients With Suspected Central Nervous System Infection

Routine Tests
WBC count with differential
RBC count[a]
Glucose concentration[b]
Protein concentration
Gram stain
Bacterial culture

Selected Tests Based on Clinical Suspicion
Viral culture[c]
Smears and culture for acid-fast bacilli
Venereal Disease Research Laboratory (VDRL) test
India ink preparation
Cryptococcal polysaccharide antigen
Fungal culture
Antibody tests (IgM or IgG, or both)[e]
Nucleic acid amplification tests (e.g., PCR)[f]
Cytology[g]
Flow cytometry

From Hasbun R, Tunkel AR: Approach to the patient with central nervous system infection. In Bennett JE, Dolin R, Blaser M, editors: Mandell, Douglas, and Bennett's principles and practice of infectious diseases, ed 9, Philadelphia, 2020, Saunders.
CSF, Cerebrospinal fluid; *IgG,* immunoglobulin G; *IgM,* immunoglobulin M; *PCR,* polymerase chain reaction; *RBCs,* red blood cells; *WBCs,* white blood cells.
[a]Check in the first and last tubes; in patients with a traumatic tap, there should be a decrease in the number of RBCs with continued flow of CSF. The following formula can be used for determining whether the numbers of CSF red blood cells and white blood cells are consistent with a traumatic tap (all units are number of cells/cubic mm):

$$\text{Adjusted WBCs in CSF} = \text{Actual WBCs in CSF} - \frac{\text{WBCs in blood} \times \text{RBCs in CSF}}{\text{RBCs in blood}}$$

[b]Compare with serum glucose concentration measured just before lumbar puncture.
[c]Yield of viral culture may be low.
[e]May be useful for specific causes of meningitis and encephalitis.
[f]Most useful for specific viral causes of encephalitis and causes of chronic meningitis.
[g]In patients with suspected malignancy.

---

findings for patients with meningitis based on cause, and the following sections detail specific methods for establishing an etiologic diagnosis.

Bacterial Meningitis

Gram stain examination of CSF permits rapid, accurate identification of the causative microorganism in 60% to 90% of patients with bacterial meningitis, and it has a specificity of nearly 100%. CSF culture is the gold standard in diagnosis and is positive in 80% to 90% of patients with community-acquired bacterial meningitis if CSF is obtained before the start of antimicrobial therapy. The probability of identifying the organism decreases for patients who received prior antimicrobial therapy. CSF sterilization may occur more rapidly after initiation of parenteral antimicrobial therapy than previously suggested, with complete sterilization of CSF containing meningococcus within 2 hours and the beginning of sterilization of pneumococcus by 4 hours following initiation of antimicrobial therapy.

TABLE 92.3 Cerebrospinal Fluid Findings for Patients With Infectious Causes of Meningitis

Cause of Meningitis	White Blood Cell Count (cells/mm³)	Primary Cell Type	Glucose (mg/dL)	Protein (mg/dL)
Viral	50–1000	Mononuclear[a]	>45	<200
Bacterial	1000–5000[b]	Neutrophilic[c]	<40[d]	100–500
Tuberculous	50–300	Mononuclear[e]	<45	50–300
Cryptococcal	20–500[f]	Mononuclear	<40	>45

From Hasbun R, Tunkel AR: Approach to the patient with central nervous system infection. In Bennett JE, Dolin R, Blaser M, editors: Mandell, Douglas, and Bennett's principles and practice of infectious diseases, ed 9, Philadelphia, 2020, Saunders.
[a]May be neutrophilic early in presentation.
[b]May range from <100 to >10,000 neutrophils/mm³.
[c]About 10% of patients have a cerebrospinal fluid (CSF) lymphocyte predominance.
[d]Should always be compared with a simultaneous serum glucose level; ratio of CSF to serum glucose is ≤0.4 in most cases.
[e]A therapeutic paradox may exist in which a mononuclear predominance becomes neutrophilic during antituberculosis therapy.
[f]More than 75% of patients with acquired immunodeficiency syndrome have <20 cells/mm³.

Several rapid diagnostic tests have been developed to aid in the etiologic diagnosis of bacterial meningitis. Latex agglutination techniques detect the antigens of *H. influenzae* type b, *S. pneumoniae*, *N. meningitidis*, *E. coli* K1, and the group B streptococci. However, because bacterial antigen testing does not appear to modify the decision to administer antimicrobial therapy and false-positive results have been reported, routine use of this modality for rapid determination of the bacterial cause of meningitis is not recommended. It can, however, be considered for patients who have been pretreated with antimicrobial therapy and when CSF Gram stain and culture results are negative.

Nucleic acid amplification tests, such as polymerase chain reaction (PCR), have been used to amplify DNA from patients with meningitis caused by up to 14 meningeal pathogens including bacterial, viral, and fungal agents in one test known as the Meningitis/Encephalitis Panel or BioFire, which has very high sensitivity and specificity. Despite the more comprehensive and rapid identification potential, use of this testing should be reserved for patients with high likelihood of meningitis or encephalitis without an identified pathogen on initial testing. Prior to considering this test, patients should still have CSF sent for routine Gram stain, culture, and testing for other common pathogens (i.e., PCR for herpes simplex viruses and enteroviruses) based on epidemiology, patient risk factors, and season. Therefore, this comprehensive test is commonly reserved for patients with negative initial tests despite clinical correlation or due to prior antimicrobial therapy.

Differentiation of Bacterial From Viral Meningitis

In patients without a positive CSF Gram stain or culture, the diagnosis of acute bacterial meningitis is often difficult to establish or reject. A combination of clinical features, with or without test results, has been assessed to develop models in an attempt to accurately predict the likelihood of bacterial meningitis compared with other potential causes (most often viruses). In a published meta-analysis of bacterial meningitis score validation studies in which 5312 patients were identified from eight studies, 4896 (92%) had sufficient clinical data to calculate the bacterial meningitis score, which identified children with CSF pleocytosis who were at very low risk for bacterial meningitis. Low-risk features were a negative CSF Gram stain, a CSF absolute neutrophil count less than 1000 cells/mm³, a CSF protein level less than 80 mg/dL, and a peripheral absolute neutrophil count less than 10,000 cells/mm³. Despite the potential utility of this meta-analysis and other similar studies, decisions related to empiric therapy should be based on clinical judgment.

Several proteins have been examined for their usefulness in the diagnosis of acute bacterial meningitis. C-reactive protein (CRP) detected in serum or CSF and serum procalcitonin concentrations have been elevated in patients with acute bacterial meningitis and may be useful in discriminating between bacterial and viral meningitis. In patients with meningitis in whom the CSF Gram stain result is negative and analysis of other parameters is inconclusive, serum concentrations of CRP or procalcitonin that are normal or below the limit of detection have a high negative predictive value in the diagnosis of bacterial meningitis.

PCR is the most promising alternative to viral culture for the diagnosis of enteroviral meningitis. Enteroviral reverse transcription PCR (RT-PCR) has been tested in clinical settings and found to be more sensitive than culture for the detection of enterovirus; the sensitivity has ranged from 86% to 100% and specificity from 92% to 100% for the diagnosis of enteroviral meningitis. For patients with HSV-2 meningitis, PCR is the recommended test for diagnosis. In patients with recurrent benign lymphocytic meningitis, detection of HSV-2 has been strongly associated with typical cases in patients without symptoms or signs of genital infection.

Spirochetal Meningitis

For the diagnosis of neurosyphilis, no single routine laboratory test is definitive. The specificity of the CSF Venereal Disease Research Laboratory (VDRL) test for the diagnosis of neurosyphilis is high, but the sensitivity is low (30% to 70%). A reactive CSF VDRL test result in the absence of blood contamination is sufficient to diagnose neurosyphilis; a nonreactive result does not exclude the diagnosis. The diagnosis of neurosyphilis is based on elevated CSF concentrations of white blood cells or protein, or both, in the appropriate clinical and serologic setting.

The best currently available laboratory test for the diagnosis of Lyme disease is demonstration of specific serum antibody to *B. burgdorferi*, and this positive test result for a patient with a compatible neurologic abnormality is strong evidence for the diagnosis. However, these tests are not standardized, and marked variations are seen between laboratories.

Tuberculous Meningitis

The identification of tuberculous organisms in CSF by specific stains is difficult due to the small population of organisms. In many series, less than 25% of specimens were smear positive and less than 50% were culture positive. The technique of PCR for detecting fragments of mycobacterial DNA in CSF specimens appears to be a promising tool. The Gen-Probe technique is based on amplification of ribosomal RNA derived from *Mycobacterium tuberculosis* using a labeled DNA probe. A 5-year retrospective study of the performance of this test found a sensitivity and specificity of 94% and 99%, respectively, for patients with positive CSF cultures.

Fungal Meningitis

Conclusive proof of a fungal etiology for meningitis requires identification of the fungus in CSF, although CSF cultures are not always positive in cases of fungal meningitis. The yield of CSF culture in cryptococcal meningitis is excellent for non-AIDS and AIDS patients. CSF India ink examination remains a rapid, effective test that is positive in 50% to 75% of cases; the yield increases up to 88% among patients with AIDS. In contrast, only 25% to 50% of patients with other causes of fungal meningitis have positive CSF cultures.

Because cultures may be negative or require long periods before yielding positive results for patients with fungal meningitis, adjunctive studies (particularly serologic tests) may be helpful for the diagnosis. The latex agglutination test for cryptococcal polysaccharide antigen is sensitive and specific for the diagnosis of cryptococcal meningitis. Cryptococcal polysaccharide antigen also can be found in the serum and CSF, usually in severely immunosuppressed patients such as those with AIDS. Serologic antibody tests (i.e., coccidioidal and histoplasmal antigens) and antigen urine tests (i.e., histoplasmal antigen) may be useful in other cases of fungal meningitis. Because fungal meningitis is often an indication of disseminated disease, other serologic assays that help in identification of fungal infection, such as galactomannan (component of the cell wall of the mold *Aspergillus* that is released during growth) and 1,3-β-D-glucan (cell wall component of various medically important fungi), may also aid in diagnosis.

Treatment

Initial Treatment of the Patient With Acute Meningitis

Acute bacterial meningitis is a life-threatening illness, and early detection, work-up, and antimicrobial therapy are imperative to reduce morbidity and mortality. The initial management of a patient with presumed bacterial meningitis includes performance of a lumbar puncture to determine whether CSF findings are consistent with the diagnosis (Fig. 92.1). If meningitis is suspected, institution of antimicrobial therapy should be based on the results of Gram staining that suggest an etiologic pathogen (Table 92.4). However, if no etiologic agent can be identified by this means or performance of the lumbar puncture is delayed, institution of empirical antimicrobial therapy after obtaining blood cultures should be based on the patient's age and underlying disease status (Table 92.5).

It is reasonable to proceed with the lumbar puncture without computed tomography (CT) of the head if the patient does not meet any of the following criteria: new-onset seizures, an immunocompromised state, signs that are suspicious for space-occupying lesions (i.e., papilledema or focal neurologic signs, not including cranial nerve palsy), or moderate to severe impairment of consciousness. Patients at risk should undergo CT of the head before lumbar puncture to evaluate for increased intracranial pressure (i.e., result of an intracranial mass lesion or generalized brain edema) due to the potential risk of herniation if a lumbar puncture is performed. In this setting, emergent empirical antimicrobial therapy and adjunctive dexamethasone therapy (if indicated), after obtaining blood cultures, should be initiated before obtaining neuroimaging.

Specific Antimicrobial Therapy for Meningitis

After the infecting meningeal pathogen is isolated and susceptibility testing results are known, antimicrobial therapy can be modified for optimal treatment of patients with bacterial meningitis (Table 92.6). Recommended dosages of antimicrobial agents for adults with infections of the CNS are shown in Table 92.7.

One pathogen requires special discussion. Specific therapy for pneumococcal meningitis depends on the in vitro susceptibility of the organism to penicillin and the third-generation cephalosporins. Based on the reduced susceptibility of meningitis strains of pneumococcus to penicillin (approximately one third of isolates in the United States), penicillin is not recommended as empirical therapy in patients with

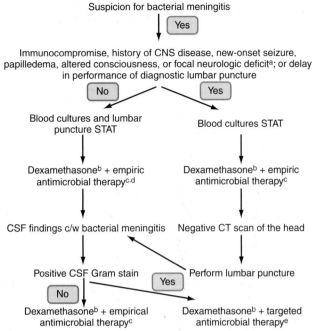

Fig. 92.1 Management algorithm for adults with suspected bacterial meningitis. [a]Palsy of cranial nerve VI or VII is not an indication to delay lumbar puncture. [b]See text for recommendations for use of adjunctive dexamethasone in patients with bacterial meningitis. [c]See Table 92.5. [d]Dexamethasone and antimicrobial therapy should be administered immediately after CSF is obtained. [e]See Table 92.4. *CNS*, Central nervous system; *CT*, computed tomography; *c/w*, consistent with; *STAT*, intervention should be done emergently. (From Tunkel AR, Hartman BJ, Kaplan, SL, et al: Practice guidelines for the management of bacterial meningitis, Clin Infect Dis 39:1267-1284, 2004.)

suspected pneumococcal meningitis. The combination of vancomycin plus a third-generation cephalosporin (i.e., cefotaxime or ceftriaxone) is recommended as an empirical regimen. After susceptibility studies of the isolated pneumococcus are performed, antimicrobial therapy can be modified for optimal treatment (see Table 92.7).

Viral meningitis is usually a benign self-limited illness. Recovery of patients with HSV-2 meningitis is usually complete without neurologic sequelae, and it is not clear whether antiviral treatment alters the course of mild meningitis.

The preferred antimicrobial regimen for the treatment of CNS syphilis is intravenous aqueous crystalline penicillin G at a dosage of 18 to 24 million units daily in divided doses every 4 hours or by continuous infusion for 10 to 14 days. Alternatively, procaine penicillin (2.4 million units intramuscularly daily) plus probenecid (500 mg orally four times daily), both for 10 to 14 days, can be used.

Parenteral antimicrobial therapy is usually needed to treat the neurologic manifestations of Lyme disease, including meningitis. The current recommendation is to treat most patients with Lyme meningitis with intravenous ceftriaxone at a dosage of 2 g daily for 14 days (range, 10 to 28 days); no evidence supports treatment durations longer than 4 weeks.

In patients with tuberculous meningitis, the most important principle of therapy is early initiation on the basis of strong clinical suspicion; it should not be delayed until proof of infection has been obtained. Identification can take weeks due to indolent culture growth. The American Thoracic Society, in conjunction with the CDC and the Infectious Diseases Society of America, recommend 2 months of isoniazid, rifampin, ethambutol, and pyrazinamide, followed by 7 to 10 months of isoniazid and rifampin for patients with drug-sensitive

TABLE 92.4 Recommended Antimicrobial Therapy for Acute Bacterial Meningitis

Microorganism[a]	Antimicrobial Therapy
Haemophilus influenzae type b	Third-generation cephalosporin[b]
Neisseria meningitidis	Third-generation cephalosporin[b]
Streptococcus pneumoniae	Vancomycin plus a third-generation cephalosporin[b,c]
Listeria monocytogenes	Ampicillin or penicillin G[d]

Modified from Tunkel AR, Hartman BJ, Kaplan, SL, et al: Practice guidelines for the management of bacterial meningitis, Clin Infect Dis 39:1267-1284, 2004.
[a]Pathogen presumptively identified by positive Gram stain.
[b]Cefotaxime or ceftriaxone.
[c]Some experts would add rifampin if dexamethasone is also given.
[d]Addition of an aminoglycoside should be considered.

TABLE 92.5 Empirical Therapy for Purulent Meningitis

Predisposing Factor	Antimicrobial Therapy
Age	
<1 mo	Ampicillin plus cefotaxime or cefepime; or ampicillin plus an aminoglycoside
1–23 mo	Vancomycin plus a third-generation cephalosporin[a,b]
2–50 yr	Vancomycin plus a third-generation cephalosporin[a,b,c]
>50 yr	Vancomycin plus ampicillin plus a third-generation cephalosporin[a]
Immunocompromised state	Vancomycin plus ampicillin plus cefepime or meropenem
Basilar skull fracture	Vancomycin plus a third-generation cephalosporin[a]
Head trauma; after neurosurgery	Vancomycin plus ceftazidime, cefepime, or meropenem

Modified from Tunkel AR, Hartman BJ, Kaplan, SL, et al: Practice guidelines for the management of bacterial meningitis, Clin Infect Dis 39:1267-1284, 2004.
[a]Cefotaxime or ceftriaxone.
[b]Some experts add rifampin if dexamethasone is also given.
[c]Add ampicillin if meningitis caused by Listeria monocytogenes is suspected.

tuberculous meningitis. Therapy for tuberculous meningitis may need to be individualized, with longer durations of therapy used for patients with more severe illness or HIV.

Therapy for cryptococcal meningitis in patients with AIDS is usually an amphotericin B preparation (i.e., amphotericin B deoxycholate, liposomal amphotericin B, or amphotericin B lipid complex) plus flucytosine for 2 weeks, followed by consolidation therapy with fluconazole for 8 weeks. For non-AIDS patients with cryptococcal meningitis, the optimal use of fluconazole is less clear.

In a retrospective review of HIV-negative patients with CNS cryptococcosis, the patients were more likely to receive an induction regimen containing amphotericin B and subsequent therapy with fluconazole. Most experts recommend high-dose fluconazole (800 to 1200 mg daily) as first-line therapy for coccidioidal meningitis.

The current recommended treatment for Histoplasma meningitis is liposomal amphotericin B for 4 to 6 weeks, followed by itraconazole for at least 1 year. Amphotericin B, alone or in combination with flucytosine, also is the treatment of choice for Candida meningitis.

Adjunctive Therapy

For adult patients with bacterial meningitis, adjunctive dexamethasone should be administered to those with suspected or proven pneumococcal meningitis. This recommendation is based on a prospective, randomized, double-blind trial enrolling 301 adults with bacterial meningitis. Adjunctive dexamethasone was associated with a reduction in the proportion of patients who had unfavorable outcomes (15% vs. 25%, $P = .03$) and in the proportion of patients who died (7% vs. 15%, $P = .04$). The benefits were most striking for the subgroup of patients with pneumococcal meningitis and those with moderate to severe disease as assessed by the admission Glasgow Coma Scale.

Dexamethasone is administered at a dosage of 10 mg intravenously every 6 hours for 4 days in adults. The first dose should be given concomitantly with or just before the first dose of an antimicrobial agent for maximal attenuation of the subarachnoid space inflammatory response. Adjunctive dexamethasone should not be used in patients who have already received antimicrobial therapy or the meningitis is found not to be caused by S. pneumoniae. Despite the positive benefits of adjunctive dexamethasone for adults with bacterial meningitis described previously, the routine use of adjunctive dexamethasone for patients with bacterial meningitis in the developing world has been controversial.

Tuberculous meningitis is associated with significant morbidity and mortality despite the availability of effective antituberculous chemotherapy. Use of adjunctive corticosteroids has abrogated the signs and symptoms of disease, and early treatment with adjunctive dexamethasone should be used in all patients with tuberculous meningitis.

Patients with cryptococcal meningitis may have increased intracranial pressure or hydrocephalus, or both. For patients with neurologic deficits and evidence of increased intracranial pressure (usually an opening pressure >25 cm H$_2$O), daily lumbar puncture is recommended. Rarely, in cases of persistent opening pressure despite frequent lumbar punctures with removal of CSF, surgical CSF shunting may be required.

ENCEPHALITIS

Definition

Encephalitis is inflammation of the brain parenchyma that is associated with neurologic dysfunction. In the absence of pathologic evidence of brain inflammation, an inflammatory response in the CSF

TABLE 92.6　Antimicrobial Therapy for Patients With Meningitis

Microorganism	Therapy of Choice
Bacteria	
Haemophilus influenzae	
β-Lactamase negative	Ampicillin
β-Lactamase positive	Ceftriaxone or cefotaxime
Neisseria meningitidis	
Penicillin MIC <0.1 µg/mL	Penicillin G or ampicillin
Penicillin MIC 0.1–1.0 µg/mL	Ceftriaxone or cefotaxime
Streptococcus pneumoniae	
Penicillin MIC ≤0.06 µg/mL	Penicillin G or ampicillin
Penicillin MIC ≥0.12 µg/mL	
Ceftriaxone or cefotaxime MIC <1.0 µg/mL	Ceftriaxone or cefotaxime
Ceftriaxone or cefotaxime MIC ≥1.0 µg/mL	Vancomycin[a] plus ceftriaxone or cefotaxime
Enterobacteriaceae[b]	Ceftriaxone or cefotaxime
Pseudomonas aeruginosa	Ceftazidime or cefepime
Acinetobacter baumannii[b]	Meropenem
Listeria monocytogenes	Ampicillin or penicillin G[c]
Streptococcus agalactiae	Ampicillin or penicillin G[c]
Staphylococcus aureus	
Methicillin-sensitive	Nafcillin or oxacillin
Methicillin-resistant	Vancomycin[a]
Staphylococcus epidermidis	Vancomycin[a]
Spirochetes	
Treponema pallidum	Penicillin G
Borrelia burgdorferi	Ceftriaxone or cefotaxime
Mycobacteria	
Mycobacterium tuberculosis	Isoniazid + rifampin + pyrazinamide + ethambutol
Fungi	
Cryptococcus neoformans	Amphotericin B preparation[d] + flucytosine
Coccidioides immitis	Fluconazole
Mucormycosis	Liposomal amphotericin B
Histoplasma capsulatum	Liposomal amphotericin B
Candida species	Amphotericin B preparation[d] ± flucytosine

MIC, Minimum inhibitory concentration.

[a]Addition of rifampin may be considered; see text for indications.

[b]The choice of a specific antimicrobial agent must be guided by in vitro susceptibility testing.

[c]Addition of an aminoglycoside should be considered.

[d]Amphotericin B deoxycholate, liposomal amphotericin B, or amphotericin B lipid complex.

or parenchymal abnormalities on neuroimaging are often used as surrogate markers of brain inflammation; however, encephalitis can occur without significant CSF pleocytosis or demonstrable neuroimaging abnormalities. Encephalitis and meningitis share many features. Both syndromes can manifest with fever, headache, and altered mental status, although the encephalitis patient may suffer from more severe alterations in mental status.

There is also clinical overlap between encephalitis and encephalopathy. Patients with encephalopathy, however, exhibit confusion early in the course of their illness that can quickly progress to obtundation. Causes of encephalopathy include metabolic disturbances, hypoxia, ischemia, intoxications, organ dysfunction, paraneoplastic syndromes, and systemic infections.

Epidemiology and Etiology

Encephalitis is characterized by inflammation of the brain in conjunction with symptoms and signs of neurologic dysfunction. Encephalitis results in substantial morbidity and mortality, and it confers considerable burden on the health care system. The hospital admission rate in one study was 7.3 per 100,000 people. The case-fatality rate among patients with encephalitis varies from 3.8% to 7.4% and is significantly higher among patients also infected with HIV. There is high morbidity among survivors of encephalitis, with resultant loss of productivity, function, and the need for prolonged rehabilitation or skilled nursing care.

Infectious causes of encephalitis are diverse and include viruses (most common), bacteria, fungi, and parasites. Clues in the patient's history that aid identification include seasonal variation, geographic location, prevalence of disease in the local community, travel history, recreational activities, occupational exposures, insect contact, animal contact, vaccination history, and immune status of the patient.

The most commonly identified viral causes of encephalitis in the United States are herpes simplex virus type 1 (HSV-1), West Nile virus, and the enteroviruses, followed by other herpesviruses (e.g., varicella-zoster virus). Other agents may be highly endemic regionally (e.g., La Crosse virus in the Midwest) or internationally (e.g., rabies virus, Japanese encephalitis virus). Bacterial agents, including *Ehrlichia*

TABLE 92.7 Recommended Dosages of Antimicrobial Agents for Meningitis in Adults With Normal Renal and Hepatic Function

Antimicrobial Agent	Total Daily Dose[a]	Dosing Interval (hr)
Amikacin[b]	15 mg/kg	8
Amphotericin B deoxycholate	0.6–1.0 mg/kg	24
Amphotericin B lipid complex	5 mg/kg	24
Ampicillin	12 g	4
Cefepime	6 g	8
Cefotaxime	8–12 g	4–6
Ceftazidime	6 g	8
Ceftriaxone	4 g	12–24
Ethambutol[d]	15 mg/kg	24
Fluconazole	400–800 mg[c]	24
Flucytosine[d,e]	100 mg/kg	6
Gentamicin[b]	5 mg/kg	8
Isoniazid[d,f]	300 mg	24
Liposomal amphotericin B	5–7.5 mg/kg	24
Meropenem	6 g	8
Nafcillin	12 g	4
Oxacillin	12 g	4
Penicillin G	24 million units	4
Pyrazinamide[d]	15–30 mg/kg	24
Rifampin[d]	600 mg	24
Tobramycin[b]	5 mg/kg	8
Sulfamethoxazole-trimethoprim	10–20 mg/kg[g]	6–12
Vancomycin[h]	30–45 mg/kg	8–12
Voriconazole[i]	8 mg/kg	12

[a]Unless indicated, therapy is administered intravenously.
[b]Need to monitor peak and trough serum concentrations.
[c]Dose of 800–1200 mg is recommended for patients with coccidioidal meningitis.
[d]Oral administration.
[e]Maintain serum concentrations of 50–100 µg/mL.
[f]Initiate therapy at a dose of 10 mg/kg.
[g]Dosage based on trimethoprim component; many experts would use a dose of 5 mg/kg every 8 hours.
[h]Maintain serum trough concentrations of 15–20 µg/mL.
[i]IV loading dose of 6 mg/kg every 12 hours for two doses; maintain serum trough concentrations of 2–5 µg/mL.

species and *Rickettsia rickettsii*, are potentially treatable causes of encephalitis, and prompt administration of appropriate antimicrobial therapy may be life-saving.

Perhaps the most challenging aspect of encephalitis is that no pathogen is identified in 50% to 70% of cases. Another difficulty is the relevance of an identification of an infectious agent outside of the CNS in a patient with encephalitis; these agents may cause a systemic illness that also involves neurologic symptoms but does not necessarily invade the CNS directly. Additionally, it may be challenging to distinguish infectious encephalitis from postinfectious or postimmunization encephalitis or encephalomyelitis; the latter process is usually mediated by an immunologic response to a preceding infection or immunization. Up to 10% of patients have a noninfectious cause; examples include paraneoplastic syndromes, vasculitis, or collagen vascular disorders.

Antibody-mediated encephalitis refers to a group of inflammatory brain diseases associated with antibodies against neuronal cell-surface proteins, ion channels, or receptors resulting in neuropsychiatric symptoms. This group of diseases is distinct from traditional autoimmune disorders such as systemic lupus erythematosus. Autoimmune encephalitis may be the third most common cause of encephalitis, and the most common form of autoimmune encephalitis is the type with antibodies against the N-methyl-D-aspartate receptor (NMDAR). In contrast to paraneoplastic syndromes, which are associated with antibodies against intracellular neural antigens, the antibodies bind to extracellular epitopes of cell-surface proteins in autoimmune encephalitis. Common receptors include NMDAR, α-amino-3-hydroxy-5-methyl-4-isoxazolepropionic acid receptor (AMPAR), γ-aminobutyric acid (GABA) receptor, and glioma-inactivated 1 (LG1) receptor. Two potential triggers of autoimmune encephalitis are tumors and viral encephalitis. However, most cases occur with no apparent immunologic triggers, which may suggest a genetic predisposition to these disorders.

Clinical Presentation

Because encephalitis is infrequently confirmed by pathologic means, the signs and symptoms of neurologic dysfunction are used as surrogate markers, and they are often nonspecific. The clinical signs and symptoms of encephalitis are determined by the specific area of the brain involved and by the severity of the infection. Some organisms show neurotropism for particular anatomic sites. HSV-1 infection almost universally involves the temporal lobe, and the clinical presentation typically includes temporal lobe seizures. Associated signs include personality changes, decreasing consciousness, focal neurologic findings (including dysphagia), paresthesias and weakness, and focal seizures. Sudden onset of fever and headache can also accompany these mental status changes.

Diffuse brain involvement is frequently seen with arboviral infections, and it is associated with global impairment in neurologic function and coma. Fever and headache frequently precede the onset of altered mental status, which can range from mild confusion to obtundation. Other neurologic manifestations may include behavioral changes (e.g., psychosis), focal paresis or paralysis, cranial nerve palsies, and movement disorders (e.g., chorea). About 80% of patients infected with West Nile virus are asymptomatic, and about 20% have only fever. Symptomatic patients may have fever, headache, myalgia, and flaccid paralysis. A maculopapular rash is seen in 50% of patients.

VZV is an important cause of acute encephalitis in adults, often associated with viral reactivation and leading to a CNS vasculopathy. Importantly, CNS reactivation may occur in the absence of skin lesions. Children, on the contrary, exhibit CNS symptoms concurrently with varicella or in a postinfectious form.

Evidence of inflammation or infection at sites distant from the CNS may be useful in making a microbiologic diagnosis for patients with encephalitis. For instance, rickettsial diseases, varicella-zoster virus, and West Nile virus often have associated skin manifestations. Stomatitis and ulcerative lesions in the mouth or an exanthem in a peripheral distribution can suggest enterovirus infection. Patients with tuberculous and fungal meningoencephalitis may have suggestive pulmonary findings.

A syndrome frequently misclassified as encephalomyelitis, based on the similar clinical presentation, is post-inflammatory encephalomyelitis. The most widely cited example is acute disseminated encephalomyelitis (ADEM), which is seen primarily in children and adolescents. ADEM is characterized by poorly defined white matter lesions on magnetic resonance imaging (MRI) that enhance after gadolinium administration. Post-inflammatory encephalomyelitis is likely mediated by an immunologic response to an antecedent antigenic stimulus such as infection or immunization. Viral infections associated with ADEM include measles, mumps, rubella, varicella-zoster, Epstein-Barr, cytomegalovirus, herpes simplex, hepatitis A, and coxsackieviruses. Immunizations temporally associated with ADEM include vaccines for Japanese encephalitis, yellow fever, measles, influenza, smallpox, anthrax, and rabies, but a direct causal association with these vaccines is difficult to establish. ADEM usually begins between 2 days and 4 weeks after the antigenic stimulus, and patients develop rapid onset of encephalopathy, with or without meningeal signs. The neurologic features depend on the location of the lesions.

In patients with anti-NMDAR encephalitis, prodromal symptoms, including low-grade fever, headache, and malaise, may occur in approximately 60% of patients. Common clinical features include behavioral changes, psychosis, seizures, memory and cognitive deficits, dysautonomia, abnormal movements, and altered consciousness. Females diagnosed with anti-NMDAR encephalitis will have an ovarian teratoma 50% of the time. Symptoms are more often neurologic in children and psychiatric in adults, but in most cases, symptoms progress to a similar syndrome. In contrast, patients with limbic encephalitis are generally older than 45 years and have symptoms including confusion, seizures, behavioral changes, and distinct memory deficits in which they have trouble forming new memories but old ones are preserved.

Diagnosis

The initial laboratory testing of an individual should include a complete blood count, tests of renal and hepatic function, coagulation studies, and serum and urine toxicology studies. A low white blood cell count, low platelet count, and elevated liver transaminase levels may suggest *Ehrlichia* or *Anaplasma* infection. A baseline chest radiograph should be obtained because a focal infiltrate can suggest particular pathogens (e.g., fungal or mycobacterial infections).

Neuroimaging studies are important to perform for all patients with encephalitis; MRI is more sensitive at detecting abnormalities than CT, and it is the preferred study. Diffusion-weighted MRI is superior to conventional MRI for the detection of early signal abnormalities in viral encephalitis caused by HSV, enterovirus 71, and West Nile virus. In patients with HSV encephalitis, there may be significant edema and hemorrhage in the temporal lobes. Patients with flavivirus (e.g., West Nile virus, Japanese encephalitis virus) encephalitis may display characteristic patterns of mixed-intensity or hypodense lesions on T1-weighted images of the thalamus, basal ganglia, and midbrain. MRI findings with linear T2-weighted regions of high signal involving the internal and external capsules (also termed the "parentheses" sign) has been associated with Eastern equine encephalitis (an arbovirus infection) compared to other viral encephalitides, although the frequency of this finding is unclear given the rarity of this infection. In patients with ADEM, MRI usually reveals multiple focal or confluent areas of signal abnormality in the subcortical white matter and, sometimes, in subcortical gray matter on T2-weighted and fluid attenuation inversion recovery (FLAIR) sequences; the lesions are usually enhancing and display similar stages of evolution. MRI of the head is abnormal in 30% of patients with antibody-mediated encephalitis. Positive findings include increased FLAIR signal involving the cortical, subcortical, or cerebellar regions.

Electroencephalography is rarely specific for a given pathogen in patients with encephalitis, but results can be helpful in identifying the degree of cerebral dysfunction by detecting subclinical seizure activity, and it may provide information about the specific area of the brain involved. In more than 80% of patients with HSV encephalitis, there is a temporal lobe focus with periodic lateralizing epileptiform discharges (PLEDs).

Lumbar puncture with CSF analysis (i.e., cell count and differential, glucose and protein levels) and a measurement of the opening pressure should be performed in all patients with encephalitis unless there is a specific contraindication. Most patients with viral encephalitis have a mononuclear cell pleocytosis with cell counts ranging from 10 to 1000/mm^3. Early in the disease process, CSF pleocytosis may be absent, or there may be an elevation in neutrophils. While lymphocytic predominance is seen with progression of the viral infection, persistent neutrophilic pleocytosis has been observed in patients with West Nile virus encephalitis. The CSF protein concentration is typically elevated, but usually less than 100 to 200 mg/dL, whereas the CSF glucose concentration is typically normal. Patients may have high RBCs in the CSF due to hemorrhagic encephalitis. CSF viral cultures are usually not recommended. Up to 10% of patients with viral encephalitis will have completely normal CSF findings. The presence of eosinophils in the CSF may suggest certain etiologies, specifically encephalitis caused by helminths. A decreased CSF glucose concentration is indicative of bacterial, fungi, or protozoal etiology. CSF profiles of patients with ADEM are similar to patients with viral encephalitis with lymphocytic pleocytosis (though less marked compared to infectious encephalitis), high protein concentration, and normal glucose concentration. Additionally, oligoclonal bands and elevated IgG index and synthesis may be present.

Brain biopsy has largely been replaced by CSF molecular tests. For certain types of infections, however, brain biopsy may be diagnostic. In rabies infections, for example, Negri bodies are a distinctive histopathologic feature. Intranuclear eosinophilic amorphous bodies surrounded by a halo may be seen in diseases such as HSV encephalitis. Biopsy of skin lesions should be performed in encephalitis patients with concomitant rash including maculopapular or petechial lesions, which can be high yield in identifying the responsible agent (e.g., *R. rickettsii*).

Testing for specific agents includes laboratory methods such as antigen detection, culture, serology, and molecular diagnostics. HSV encephalitis is a treatable and relatively common cause of encephalitis, and an HSV PCR should be performed on the CSF of all patients with a clinical diagnosis of encephalitis. False-negative PCR test results can occur within the first 72 hours after onset, and if HSV encephalitis is strongly suspected (e.g., in a patient with temporal lobe involvement), a repeat HSV PCR on a second sample of CSF within 3 to 7 days is recommended. For enterovirus and varicella encephalitis, CSF PCR testing is recommended; however, detection of antibodies to varicella-zoster virus in the CSF appears to have greater sensitivity than detection of viral DNA. Concomitant serum viral studies are sometimes helpful in diagnosing viral encephalitis. In one report of an enterovirus 71 outbreak, only 31% of cases had a positive CSF result with higher yields from throat and stool PCR specimens; viral shedding from the gastrointestinal tract may occur for weeks following infection. Similarly, for Epstein-Barr virus encephalitis, serum serology including antiviral capsid antigens (VCA), immunoglobulin M/immunoglobulin G (IgM/IgG), and anti-Epstein-Barr nuclear antigen (EBNA) are recommended in addition to CSF PCR due to false positive and false negative results associated with the PCR test.

Testing for other agents should be individualized with consideration of the patient's exposures, travel, season of the year, and clinical and laboratory characteristics. Many infections require acute and convalescent (i.e., paired) serum samples to determine a diagnosis. A serum specimen collected during the acute phase of the illness should be stored and tested in parallel when the convalescent serum sample is drawn. Immunoglobulin M (IgM) and immunoglobulin G (IgG) capture enzyme-linked immunosorbent assays (ELISAs) have become useful and widely available for the diagnosis of arboviral encephalitis. Detection of intrathecal IgM antibody is a specific and sensitive method for the diagnosis of West Nile virus infection. There is substantial cross-reactivity among the flaviviruses (e.g., West Nile virus, St. Louis encephalitis virus, Japanese encephalitis virus); plaque-reduction neutralization assays may be helpful in distinguishing which flavivirus is involved in the event of elevated titers.

Serologic testing for *Rickettsia*, *Ehrlichia*, and *Anaplasma* species should be performed for all encephalitis patients during the appropriate season and with travel to or residence in endemic areas, especially because these are treatable causes. In addition to serologies, concurrent serum PCR testing for *Anaplasma* is recommended, because a positive result may be more indicative of an acute infection. Empiric therapy should not be withheld from patients with a compatible clinical presentation because antibodies are not always detectable early in the course of illness.

Identification of NMDAR antibodies confirms the diagnosis of anti-NMDAR encephalitis. Obtaining both serum and CSF antibodies is also recommended. Diagnosis should lead to the search for a tumor in female patients; the tumor is almost always an ovarian teratoma.

Treatment

One of the most important first steps in managing encephalitis is to consider treatable causes. Specific antiviral therapy is usually limited to infections caused by herpesviruses (especially HSV-1 and varicella-zoster virus) and HIV. Therefore, acyclovir (10 mg/kg intravenously every 8 hours in adults with normal renal function) should be administered to patients with encephalitis. Empirical therapy for acute bacterial meningitis should be initiated when clinical and laboratory testing is compatible with bacterial infection. If rickettsial or ehrlichial infections are suspected, empirical doxycycline should be administered. The management of West Nile virus infection is supportive care.

In patients with suspected postinfectious encephalomyelitis (i.e., ADEM), high-dose intravenous corticosteroids (1 g of methylprednisolone intravenously daily for at least 3 to 5 days) are usually recommended, followed by an oral taper for 3 to 6 weeks. In patients with autoimmune encephalitis, the current approach includes immunotherapy and removal of the immunologic trigger. Most patients are treated with glucocorticoids, intravenous immune globulin, or plasma exchange. If there is no clinical response to these treatments, then rituximab or cyclophosphamide may be used. Rituximab may be helpful in reducing the risk of clinical relapse. Additionally, early identification and removal of this trigger is important for achieving a good outcome (i.e., removal of an ovarian teratoma in patients with anti-NMDAR encephalitis). Time to recovery, degree of residual deficit, and risk of relapse vary depending on the type of autoimmune encephalitis. Spontaneous clinical improvement is rare. Prompt institution of immunotherapy is associated with favorable outcomes.

BRAIN ABSCESS

Definition

A *brain abscess* is a focal intracerebral infection that begins as a localized area of cerebritis followed by the formation of a pus collection.

Pathology and Pathophysiology

Brain abscesses produce symptoms and findings similar to those of other space-occupying lesions (e.g., brain tumors), but they often progress more rapidly and affect meningeal structures more frequently than tumors. Brain abscesses may arise from several mechanisms, the most common of which is spread from a contiguous focus of infection; examples include infections of the middle ear, mastoid cells, paranasal sinuses, as well as dental infections. A second mechanism is hematogenous dissemination from a distant focus of infection. Brain abscesses resulting from hematogenous spread are usually multiple and mutiloculated, and they are associated with higher mortality. Original foci of infection include chronic pyogenic lung disease (e.g., lung abscesses, bronchiectasis, empyema, and cystic fibrosis), skin and soft tissue infections, osteomyelitis, intraabdominal infections, infectious endocarditis, cyanotic heart disease, and pulmonary arteriovenous malformations often linked with hereditary hemorrhagic telangiectasia. Traumas, particularly those involving dural breach, and invasive neurosurgical procedures, are also a pathogenic mechanism of brain abscess development. In 10% to 35% of patients, brain abscess is cryptogenic.

The infection is often polymicrobial, and the pathogen(s) involved depend on the mechanism of spread as well as the host characteristics. Commonly isolated pathogens are aerobic and microaerobic streptococci and gram-negative anaerobes such as *Bacteroides* and *Prevotella*. Less common are gram-negative aerobes and *Staphylococcus*. *Actinomyces*, *Nocardia*, and *Candida* are even less prevalent. In immunosuppressed individuals, *Aspergillus* and *Toxoplasma* are important causes of abscesses. Surgical specimens are culture positive in 70% of antibiotic-treated patients and 95% of patients undergoing surgery before antibiotic administration.

Clinical Presentation

The clinical course of brain abscess ranges from indolent to fulminant. The classic clinical picture is composed of signs of systemic infection (e.g., fever), those related to focal brain involvement, and those due to an increased intracranial pressure and mass effect. Elements of one or two categories are often absent in a given case, particularly early in the disease course. For example, almost one half of patients may not have a fever or leukocytosis. The classic triad of fever, headache, and focal neurologic deficit is found only in about 20% of patients on admission. Recent

TABLE 92.8   Location and Clinical Presentation of Brain Abscesses

Location	Clinical Presentation
Frontal lobe	Headache, drowsiness, inattention, deterioration of mental status, hemiparesis with unilateral motor signs, and motor speech disorder
Temporal lobe	Ipsilateral headache and aphasia (dominant side); visual defect
Cerebellum	Ataxia, nystagmus, vomiting, and dysmetria
Brainstem	Fever, headache, facial weakness, hemiparesis, dysphagia, and vomiting

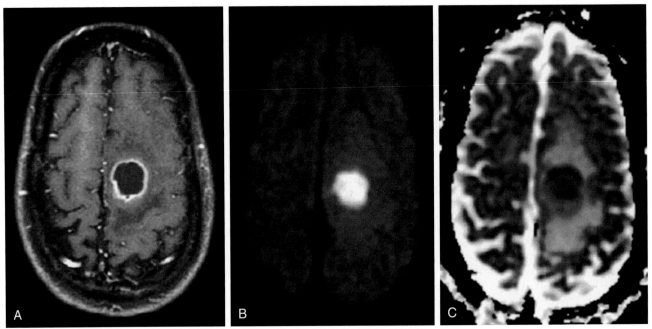

Fig. 92.2 Magnetic resonance imaging features of a brain abscess. (A) Contrast-enhanced scan shows a ring-enhancing lesion in the left frontal lobe. (B) The diffusion-weighted image shows restricted diffusion in the cavity due to viscous pus and cellular material. (C) Corresponding apparent diffusion coefficient map shows dark, viscous material in the cavity and surrounding edema.

onset of a headache is the most common symptom, which may increase in severity associated with focal signs related to the location of the abscess (e.g., hemiparesis, aphasia), followed by obtundation and coma. However, headache may be moderate to severe and hemicranial or generalized but often lacks distinguishing features. Seizures precede the diagnosis in 30% of cases. *Toxoplasma* abscesses are often associated with movement disorders due to their propensity for the basal ganglia. The period of evolution may be as brief as hours or as long as days to weeks with more indolent organisms. The location of the brain abscess can correlate with clinical presentation (Table 92.8). A worrisome complication of brain abscess is rupture. Sudden worsening of a headache with new onset of meningismus may signify rupture of the abscess into the ventricular space. This is associated with a high mortality, up to 85% in some series.

Diagnosis

CSF examination should be avoided; it is seldom diagnostic, and results can be normal. Lumbar puncture in the setting of a mass lesion carries the risk of transtentorial herniation. Because the brain abscess is seeded from a peripheral site of infection, a search for other sites of infection can help to identify the causative organisms and determine appropriate treatment.

MRI with intravenous gadolinium provides better soft tissue visualization than CT and is the imaging of choice in diagnosing brain abscesses. MRI is particularly useful for detecting multiple abscesses and posterior fossa abscesses. It can demonstrate cerebritis, the extent of a mass effect,

and associated venous thrombosis. Repeat or serial imaging can be used to determine response to therapy. In the early cerebritis stage, CT results may be normal, but the MRI FLAIR sequence is very sensitive for visualization of brain edema. On T1-weighted images, the area of cerebritis is seen initially as a low-signal-intensity, ill-defined area. T1-weighted images in the later stages of infection may show the formation of a rim of slightly higher signal intensity and central necrosis. Contrast administration typically shows ring enhancement with central necrosis. This area of central necrosis appears bright on diffusion-weighted images and dark on apparent diffusion coefficient (ADC) images (Fig. 92.2). MRI of tumors shows the opposite features. Differentiating a brain abscess from tumor is important for the stereotactic approach to ring-enhancing lesions before biopsy or surgical excision. An abscess should be drained centrally, whereas a tumor should be biopsied along its rim.

Patient risk factors, location of the brain abscess, and characteristic findings on CT or MRI imaging can help implicate the responsible pathogen. *Nocardia* brain abscesses are often mutilobulated. *Listeria* brain abscesses are often located in the brain stem. Findings of cerebral infarcts that develop into single or multiple brain abscesses usually in the frontal or temporal lobes in a patient with risk factors for invasive aspergillosis should suggest that diagnosis. CT or MRI findings of sinus opacification, erosion of bone, and obliteration of deep fascial planes may indicate rhinocerebral mucormycosis. Rounded isodense or hypodense lesions with ring enhancement seen on contrast imaging are consistent with CNS toxoplasmosis in the appropriate patient.

TABLE 92.9 Predisposing Conditions, Microbiology, and Empiric Treatment[a] of Brain Abscesses

Predisposing Condition	Usual Organism	Antimicrobial Regimen
Otitis media or mastoiditis	Streptococci (anaerobic and aerobic), *Bacteroides* and *Prevotella* sp, Enterobacteraceae	Metronidazole + a third-generation cephalosporin[b]
Sinusitis	Streptococci, *Bacteriodes* sp, Enterobacteriaceae, *Staphylococcus aureus*, *Haemophilus* sp	Vancomycin + a third-generation cephalosporin[b] + metronidazole
Dental infection	Mixed *Fusobacterium*, *Prevotella*, *Actinomyces*, and *Bacteriodes* sp, streptococci	Metronidazole + a third-generation cephalosporin[b]
Lung abscess, empyema, bronchiectasis	*Fusobacterium*, *Actinomyces*, *Bacteriodes*, and *Prevotella* sp, streptococci, *Nocardia* sp	Third-generation cephalosporin[b] + metronidazole + trimethoprim-sulfamethoxazole
Bacterial endocarditis	*S. aureus*, streptococci	Vancomycin[c]
Congenital heart disease	Streptococci, *Haemophilus* sp	Third-generation cephalosporin[b]
Penetrating trauma or invasive neurosurgical procedure	*S. aureus*, streptococci, Enterobacteriaceae, *Clostridioides* sp	Vancomycin + a third- or fourth-generation cephalosporin
Neutropenia	Aerobic gram-negative bacilli, *Aspergillus* sp, Mucorales, *Candida* sp, *Scedosporium* sp	Vancomycin + cefepime; consider antifungals
HIV infection	*Toxoplasma gondii*, *Nocardia* sp, *Mycobacterium* sp, *Listeria monocytogenes*, *Cryptococcus neoformans*	Add pyrimethamine + sulfadiazine; consider isoniazid, rifampin, pyrazinamide, and ethambutol for possible tuberculosis
Transplantation	*Aspergillus* sp, *Candida* sp, Mucorales, *Scedosporium* sp, Enterobacteriaceae, *Listeria monocytogenes*, *Nocardia* sp, *Toxoplasma gondii*, *Mycobacterium tuberculosis*	Add voriconazole + trimethoprim-sulfamethoxazole

[a]Treatment, namely use of targeted antimicrobials, may be modified based on isolation of specific microbes, sensitivities, and patient characteristics (i.e., allergies, risk factors).
[b]Cefotaxime or ceftriaxone.
[c]Additional agents should be added based on other likely microbiologic etiology.

Treatment

A suspected brain abscess requires urgent intervention. MRI or contrast CT should be performed to verify the presence of a brain abscess. Unless the surgical procedure poses a substantial risk, aspiration of the lesion is needed for microbial diagnosis. Corticosteroids should be administered to patients with significant edema, with mass effect causing increased intracranial pressure, or with a predisposition to transtentorial herniation. High-dose intravenous dexamethasone (16 to 24 mg/day in four divided doses) may be used for short periods until surgical intervention is possible. Corticosteroids may retard formation of a capsule around the brain abscess in its early stages and the immune response to infection. Seizures should be controlled because the tonic phase of a generalized seizure may increase intracranial pressure. In a patient with a large abscess, seizures may trigger a brain herniation. Seizure prophylaxis should be initiated in all patients with cortical or temporal lobe abscesses. Anticonvulsants that can be administered intravenously are preferred.

Successful treatment of brain abscesses relies on rapid verification of the abscess, identification of the responsible pathogen, timely surgical intervention, and appropriate antimicrobial therapy. Antibiotic management of brain abscess is based on knowledge of proven or suspected pathogens and antibiotic properties, such as CNS drug penetration capabilities and the spectrum of activity. Empirical antibiotic therapy without surgical intervention may be used if the primary source of infection outside of the CNS is identified, in patients with cerebritis without capsule formation, or in those with multiple, small abscesses or abscesses in basal ganglia or brain stem. If the organism is unknown, empirical therapy may include vancomycin, metronidazole, and a third- or fourth-generation cephalosporin. In brain stem abscesses, the possibility of *Listeria* infection should be considered, and treatment should include intravenous ampicillin. In HIV-infected patients with multiple ring-enhancing lesions, empirical therapy for toxoplasmosis should be initiated even if the patient is seronegative for *Toxoplasma*.

Voriconazole is the recommended antifungal therapy for patients with risk factors and imaging findings concerning for invasive aspergillosis. Recommendations for other causes of fungal brain abscess are shown in Table 92.6. Table 92.9 summarizes the predisposing conditions, microbiology, and recommended empiric treatment of brain abscesses.

Patients undergoing empirical therapy should be followed with repeat CT or MRI. Those who fail to respond should undergo surgical intervention. An important aspect of the management strategy is eradication of the predisposing condition or cause of the brain abscess, such as an oral, ear, cardiac, or pulmonary infection.

PARAMENINGEAL INFECTIONS

Parameningeal infections include infections that produce suppuration in potential spaces covering the brain and spinal cord (i.e., epidural abscess and subdural empyema) and those that produce occlusion of the contiguous venous sinuses and cerebral veins (i.e., cerebral venous sinus thrombosis).

Subdural Empyema
Definition

Subdural empyema refers to infection in the space separating the dura and arachnoid.

Pathology and Pathophysiology

Cranial subdural empyemas account for 15% to 20% of all localized intracranial infections. Two thirds of subdural empyemas result from frontal or ethmoid sinus infections, 20% from inner ear infections, and the remainder from trauma or neurosurgical procedures. The empyema is caused by direct or indirect extension from infected paranasal sinuses through a retrograde thrombophlebitis. Unilateral empyema is most common because the falx prevents passage across the midline, but bilateral or multiple empyemas can occur. Cortical venous thrombosis or brain abscess develops in about 25% of patients. The infection is metastatic in about 5% of patients, primarily from a pulmonary source. In some patients, the subdural empyema may be associated with an epidural abscess or meningitis. These associations occur more often in children than in adults.

Clinical Presentation

The clinical presentation of cranial subdural empyema can be rapidly progressive with signs and symptoms resulting from increased intracranial pressure, meningeal irritation, or focal cortical inflammation. These include fever, intractable headache, vomiting, nuchal rigidity, focal neurologic deficits (e.g., hemiparesis, ocular palsies, dysphasia, dilated pupils, cerebellar signs, or seizures), and varying levels of altered consciousness. If untreated, mental status may decline to obtundation, and the septic mass and swollen underlying brain can lead to venous thrombosis or death from herniation. The clinical presentation of spinal subdural empyema may consist of radicular pain and symptoms of spinal cord compression including saddle anesthesia, lower extremity weakness, and bowel or bladder incontinence. The infection may occur at multiple levels. The presentation can be difficult to differentiate from spinal epidural abscess.

The major differential diagnosis is meningitis. Nuchal rigidity and obtundation occur in meningitis and cranial subdural empyema, but papilledema and lateralizing deficits are more common in cranial subdural empyema.

Diagnosis

Lumbar puncture should be avoided in patients with cranial subdural empyema to prevent cerebral herniation. Contrast-enhanced CT or MRI can be diagnostic of empyema, showing an extra-axial, crescent-shaped mass with an enhancing rim lying just below the inner table of the skull over the cerebral convexities or in the interhemispheric fissures. On MRI, subdural empyema has decreased signal intensity on T1-weighted imaging and increased signal intensity on T2-weighted scans. Similar to brain abscess, subdural empyema has high signal intensity on diffusion-weighted images and low signal intensity on ADC maps.

Treatment

Treatment requires prompt surgical drainage of the empyema cavity and prompt administration of intravenous antibiotics directed at organisms found at the time of craniotomy. Concomitant use of corticosteroids to reduce edema and increased intracranial pressure, as well as anticonvulsants to control seizures, are also important to reduce morbidity and mortality.

SPINAL EPIDURAL ABSCESS

Definition and Epidemiology

A *spinal epidural abscess* is an infection in the epidural space between the dura and the bones of the spine around the spinal cord. It can cause paralysis and death. The incidence is 0.5 to 1.0 cases per 10,000 hospital admissions in the United States, and the frequency is increased among injection drug users.

Pathology and Pathophysiology

Infections of the spinal epidural space originate from contiguous spread or through hematogenous routes from a distant source. Cutaneous infection, particularly in the back, is the most common remote source, especially among injection drug users. Abdominal, respiratory tract,

and urinary sources are also common. As the use of epidural catheters has increased for pain management, epidural abscess and hematoma have been increasingly reported.

The anatomy of the epidural space dictates the location of the abscess. Because the size of the intravertebral canal remains relatively constant but the circumference of the spinal cord changes, abscess formation is maximal in the thoracic and lumbar regions and minimal at the cervical spine. Due to the loose connections between the dura and the bones of the spine, the abscess can extend to multiple levels, causing severe and extensive neurologic manifestations.

Causative organisms can be identified by culture or Gram stain from pus obtained at exploration (90% of patients), blood cultures (60% to 90%), or CSF (20%). *S. aureus* is the most common pathogen, followed by streptococci and gram-negative organisms. Tuberculous abscesses may occur in as many as 25% of patients in high-risk populations. In a previous epidemic, iatrogenic infection occurred with rare fungi after epidural injections of corticosteroids that were contaminated with a plant pathogen, *Exserohilum rostratum*, which rarely infects humans.

Clinical Presentation

The classic triad of fever, back pain, and neurologic deficits may not be identified in all patients, leading to a delay in diagnosis. Patients are usually febrile and have acute or subacute neck or back pain. An important physical finding is focal tenderness over the affected spinous processes. Stiff neck and headache are common. The pain can be mistaken for sciatica, a visceral abdominal process, chest wall pain, or cervical disk disease. If it goes unrecognized at this stage, the symptoms can evolve over a few hours to a few days to weakness, loss of lower extremity reflexes, and paralysis distal to the spinal level of the infection. In this clinical setting, urgent neuroradiologic imaging should be pursued followed by empiric antibiotics with concurrent corticosteroids, and surgical evaluation.

Diagnosis

The diagnosis is made by CT or MRI (Fig. 92.3). The differential diagnosis includes transverse myelitis, intervertebral disk herniation, epidural hemorrhage, and metastatic tumor. These conditions can usually be differentiated by MRI. Epidural abscess is often accompanied by diskitis or osteomyelitis of the vertebral bodies.

Treatment

Unless culture and sensitivities dictate otherwise, a penicillinase-resistant penicillin should be started empirically as antistaphylococcal treatment for presumed bacterial infection. If methicillin resistance is suspected, vancomycin should be used. Considering the severity of the disease, additional gram-negative coverage with a third- or fourth-generation cephalosporin or a fluoroquinolone may be needed. Other empiric agents, including antifungals, can be considered based on clinical suspicion and patient risk factors.

Surgical decompression was previously considered mandatory, but early diagnosis by MRI may allow for effective medical therapy if started before the occurrence of neurologic complications. These patients should be monitored closely, and if signs of neurologic deterioration emerge, surgical intervention may be necessary.

SINUS THROMBOSIS

Septic Cavernous Sinus Thrombosis

Septic cavernous sinus thrombosis usually results from spread of infection from paranasal sinusitis (especially of the sphenoid or ethmoid sinuses) or less commonly from spread of infection from the face and mouth. Symptoms include headache or lateralized facial pain, followed

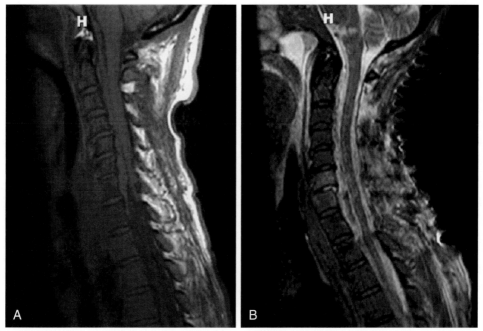

Fig. 92.3 Magnetic resonance imaging shows an epidural abscess due to *Staphylococcus* in the cervical spine of a patient with human immunodeficiency virus infection. (A) Noncontrast T1-weighted image shows an extensive lesion in the epidural space that extends from C2 to C7. Notice straightening of the cervical spine. (B) After a laminectomy from C2 to T1 and fusion, the short tau inversion recovery (STIR) image shows fluid collection in the epidural space as a high-signal-intensity lesion. Normal curvature of the spine is seen.

in a few days to weeks by fever and involvement of the orbit (i.e., proptosis and chemosis due to obstruction of the ophthalmic vein). Paralysis of oculomotor nerves follows rapidly. In some instances, sensory dysfunction occurs in the first and second divisions of the trigeminal nerve along with a decrease in the corneal reflex. Further involvement of the contiguous orbital contents follows, with mild papilledema and decreased visual acuity that sometimes progresses to blindness.

Extension to the opposite cavernous sinus or to other intracranial sinuses with cerebral infarction or increased intracranial pressure due to impaired venous drainage can result in stupor, coma, and death. The CSF is abnormal if there is accompanying meningitis or parameningeal infection. The most common causative organism is *S. aureus*, followed by streptococci and pneumococci; anaerobes and gram-negative bacilli may also be etiologic agents.

Diagnosis of cavernous sinus thrombosis is usually made by MRI with MR venogram. Radiologic evaluation includes imaging of the sphenoidal and ethmoidal sinuses, which may require drainage if infected. Empirical antimicrobial therapy should include an antistaphylococcal agent. An empirical combination therapy with parenteral metronidazole, vancomycin, and a third- or fourth-generation cephalosporin can achieve reasonable CSF and brain penetration and is likely to be active against *S. aureus* and the usual sinus pathogens.

Lateral Sinus Thrombosis

Septic thrombosis of the lateral sinus results from acute or chronic infections of the middle ear, including otitis media and mastoiditis. The infection spreads through emissary veins that connect the mastoid with the lateral venous sinus. It may spread to involve the sigmoid sinus. The symptoms include ear pain followed over several weeks by fever, headache, nausea, vomiting, and vertigo. Mastoid swelling may be seen. Sixth cranial nerve palsies and papilledema can occur, but other focal neurologic signs are rare.

The diagnosis can be established by MRI. Common pathogens of lateral sinus thrombosis include *S. aureus*, streptococci, and *E. coli*; rarely, *Fusobacterium necrophorum* and *Bacteriodes fragilis* have also been reported. Treatment includes an empirical regimen of broad-spectrum intravenous antibiotics to cover staphylococci, gram-negative bacilli, and anaerobes (i.e., vancomycin with metronidazole and a third- or fourth generation cephalosporin). Surgical drainage (i.e., mastoidectomy) may be required.

Septic Sagittal Sinus Thrombosis

Septic sagittal sinus thrombosis is uncommon and occurs as a consequence of purulent meningitis, infections of the ethmoidal or maxillary sinuses spreading through venous channels, face, scalp, subdural space, compound skull fractures, or neurosurgical wound infections (rare). Symptoms include manifestations of elevated intracranial pressure (e.g., headache, nausea, and vomiting) that evolve rapidly to stupor and coma. Motor deficits, nuchal rigidity, and papilledema may be seen. Seizures occur in more than half of these patients. Similar to other sinus thromboses, the likely microorganisms depend on the associated primary condition. Diagnosis and treatment are similar to the lateral venous sinus thrombosis described earlier.

NEUROLOGIC COMPLICATIONS OF INFECTIVE ENDOCARDITIS

Epidemiology

Neurologic complications are among the most common extra-cardiac complications of infective endocarditis and occur in one third of patients with bacterial endocarditis. They are associated with significant morbidity and triple the mortality rate of the disease. Cerebral (but not systemic) emboli from mitral valve endocarditis are increasingly common. Most emboli, regardless of the bacterial cause of the infection, occur before or early in the course of treatment. By 2 weeks of therapy, the risk of embolization decreases dramatically. Mycotic aneurysms in the brain complicate endocarditis in 2% to 10% of patients and are more common in acute than subacute disease.

Pathophysiology

The risk of developing neurologic complications from infective endocarditis depends on a number of characteristics, principally the size and location of the vegetation as well as the duration of antibiotic treatment. Larger, left-sided vegetations involving the mitral valve are more likely to embolize.

Cerebral emboli are distributed in the brain in proportion to cerebral blood flow. Most emboli lodge in the branches of the middle cerebral artery peripherally. Multiple microabscesses can result and cause diffuse encephalopathy. Mycotic aneurysms occur most commonly in the middle cerebral artery, with the aneurysms located distally in the vessel. This differentiates them from congenital berry aneurysms.

Clinical Manifestations

Neurologic complications may be the presenting symptoms of infective endocarditis. Patients may present with severe headache, focal neurologic deficits, altered consciousness, mononeuropathy, or seizures. Embolic stroke is the most common complication. Other complications include ischemic or hemorrhagic stroke, meningitis, brain abscess, spinal epidural abscess, and infected intracranial aneurysm.

Diagnosis

The diagnosis of neurologic involvement from endocarditis is best made with CT or MRI. MRI findings in endocarditis include ischemic lesions, hemorrhagic lesions, subarachnoid hemorrhage, brain abscess, mycotic aneurysm, and cerebral microbleeds. The CSF is abnormal in 70% of patients and simulates purulent meningitis (i.e., polymorphonuclear predominance, elevated protein level, and low glucose level) or a parameningeal infection (i.e., lymphocytic predominance, modest protein elevation, and normal glucose level). If concomitant bacteremia is present, positive blood cultures help identify the causative pathogen.

Multidetector CT angiography may be necessary to diagnose aneurysms. Small brain abscesses may complicate the course of endocarditis, but macroscopic abscesses are rare, with most occurring in the setting of acute rather than subacute endocarditis. Multiple microabscesses may escape detection on CT and are not amenable to surgical drainage.

Treatment

Antibiotic treatment of the primary disease is indicated. Stroke is usually treated conservatively. There are no controlled trials for the management of unruptured mycotic aneurysms, although they may be managed with antibiotics alone. Ruptured aneurysms should be managed with a combination of antibiotics with surgery or endovascular therapy because treatment-related mortality is higher in patients with ruptured aneurysms than unruptured aneurysms. Patients with infective endocarditis who do not respond to conservative medical therapy can have prompt valve replacement despite intracerebral hemorrhage. The balance of risks and benefits should be tailored to each individual patient when considering surgical intervention in the setting of neurologic complications, which can significantly increase the risk of surgical complications. In general, anticoagulation use is not recommended due to the potential risk for hemorrhagic complications and because it does not appear to reduce the risk of embolism in patients with infective endocarditis.

PRION DISEASES

Etiology

Several human diseases have been attributed to a unique infectious protein, the prion. The infectious form of the prion protein is rich in β-sheets, detergent insoluble, multimeric, and resistant to proteinase K treatment.

Prion illnesses (i.e., transmissible spongiform encephalopathies) can be classified as sporadic, hereditary, or acquired. The most common form is sporadic Creutzfeldt-Jakob disease (sCJD). Familial forms include Gerstmann-Sträussler-Scheinker syndrome and familial fatal insomnia.

Acquired forms are caused by the transmission of an abnormal prion protein (PrP) from human to human or from cattle to humans. Accidental transmission of CJD between humans appears to have occurred with cadaveric dura mater grafting, corneal transplantation, receipt of human growth hormone or pituitary gonadotropin, contaminated electroencephalogram electrodes, and contaminated surgical instruments. This form of CJD has been called iatrogenic CJD (iCJD).

The appearance of variant CJD (vCJD) in Great Britain, which was associated with the outbreak of bovine spongiform encephalopathy and the contamination of beef, greatly increased interest in this group of illnesses. Kuru is another transmissible spongiform encephalopathy that was spread in New Guinea by cannibalism, a practice that ceased in the 1950s. The disease is now almost extinct.

Sporadic Creutzfeldt-Jakob Disease
Epidemiology
Illness from sCJD is seen worldwide, with an incidence of 0.5 to 1.0 cases per 1 million people in the general population per year.

Pathology
The pathologic hallmarks of CJD are spongiform or vacuolar changes in the brain without cellular inflammatory infiltrates. The pathogenic isoform of the prion protein can be demonstrated in brain tissue by immunocytochemical staining and by Western blot analysis. The fundamental process involved in human prion propagation is intercellular induction of protein misfolding and seeded aggregation of misfolded prion protein.

Clinical Manifestations

CJD is frequently diagnosed incorrectly initially. Prodromal symptoms include altered sleep patterns and appetite, weight loss, changes in sexual drive, and impaired memory and concentration. Disorientation, hallucinations, depression, and emotional lability are early signs, followed by a rapidly progressive dementia associated with myoclonus (about 90% of patients). Myoclonus is usually provoked by tactile, auditory, or visual startle stimuli. CJD has an abrupt onset in 10% to 15% of patients.

Other distinctive features include seizures, autonomic dysfunction, and lower motor neuron disease, suggesting amyotrophic lateral sclerosis–like characteristics. Cerebellar ataxia occurs in one third of patients.

Diagnosis

The clinical tetrad supporting the diagnosis of CJD consists of a subacute progressive dementia, myoclonus, typical periodic sharp waves on electroencephalography, and normal CSF. FLAIR MRI sequences show extensive curvilinear hyperintensity along the neocortex, called *cortical ribboning*, which affects frontal, parietal, and temporal lobes (in decreasing order of frequency). Routine CSF study is usually normal. A CSF test for the protein 14-3-3, which is released into spinal fluid when brain cells die, in the appropriate clinical context, is supportive for CJD.

Treatment

No effective therapy exits. The disease is inexorably progressive. The median time to death from onset is 5 months, and 90% of patients with sporadic CJD die within 1 year.

Although the illness is not communicable in the conventional sense, a risk exists in handling material contaminated with the prion protein. Gloves should be worn when handling blood, CSF, and other body fluids. Instruments must be disinfected and sterilized appropriately.

❖ For a deeper discussion of these topics, please see Chapter 384, "Meningitis: Bacterial, Viral, and Other"; Chapter 385, "Brain Abscess and Parameningeal Infections"; Chapter 386, "Acute Viral Encephalitis"; and Chapter 387, "Prion Diseases," in *Goldman-Cecil Medicine*, 26th Edition.

SUGGESTED READINGS

Brouwer MC, Thwaites GE, Tunkel AR, et al: Dilemmas in the diagnosis of acute community-acquired bacterial meningitis, Lancet 380:1684–1692, 2012.

Brouwer MC, Tunkel AR, McKhann II GM, van de Beek D: Brain abscess, N Engl J Med 371:447–456, 2014.

Colby DW, Prusiner SB: Prions, Cold Spring Harb Perspect Biol 3: a006833,2011

Dalmau J, Graus F: Antibody-mediated encephalitis, N Engl J Med 378:840–851, 2018.

Darouiche RO: Spinal epidural abscess, N Engl J Med 355:2012–2020, 2006.

Glaser CS, Honarmand S, Anderson LJ, et al: Beyond viruses: clinical profiles and etiologies associated with encephalitis, Clin Infect Dis 43:1565–1577, 2006.

Greenlee JE: Suppurative intracranial thrombophlebitis. In Roos KL, Tunkel AR, editors: Bacterial infections of the central nervous system, Edinburgh, 2010, Elsevier, pp 101–123.

McGill F, Heyderman RS, Panagiotou S, et al: Acute bacterial meningitis in adults, Lancet 388:306–3047, 2016.

Solomon T, Michael BD, Smith PE, et al: Management of suspected viral encephalitis in adults—association of British neurologists and British infection association national guidelines, J Infect 64:347–373, 2012.

Thigpen MC, Whitney CG, Messonnier NE, et al: Bacterial meningitis in the United States, 1998-2007, N Engl J Med 364:2016–2025, 2011.

Tunkel AR, Glaser CA, Block KC, et al: The management of encephalitis: clinical practice guidelines by the Infectious Diseases Society of America, Clin Infect Dis 47:303–327, 2008.

Tunkel AR, Hartman BJ, Kaplan SL, et al: Practice guidelines for the management of bacterial meningitis, Clin Infect Dis 39:1267–1284, 2004.

Tunkel AR, Hasbun R, Bhimraj A, et al: 2017 Infectious Diseases Society of America's clinical practice guidelines for healthcare-associated ventriculitis and meningitis, Clin Infect Dis 64:e34-e65, 2017.

Tyler KL: Acute viral encephalitis, N Engl J Med 379:557–566, 2018.

van de Beek D, Brouwer MC, Thwaites GE, et al: Advances in treatment of bacterial meningitis, Lancet 380:1693–1702, 2012.

Venkatesan A, Michael BD, Probasco JC, et al: Acute encephalitis in immunocompetent adults, Lancet 393:702–716, 2019.

Venkatesan A, Tunkel AR, Bloch KC, et al: Case definitions, diagnostic algorithms, and priorities in encephalitis; consensus statement of the International Encephalitis Consortium, Clin Infect Dis 57:1114–1128, 2013.

93

Infections of the Head and Neck

David Kim, Roberto Cortez, Tareq Kheirbek

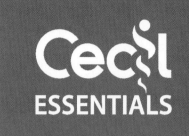

COMMON COLD

Definition and Epidemiology

The common cold is an acute viral syndrome involving the upper respiratory tract with symptoms of sore throat, rhinorrhea, and nasal congestion. It has a considerable economic burden, accounting for over 100 million physician visits annually with approximately 20 million lost workdays and costing $7 billion per year in sick days and lost productivity. The incidence of the common cold decreases with age with children having six to eight colds on average annually, whereas adults have two to three colds per year.

Pathogenesis and Microbiology

Rhinoviruses are the most common pathogen implicated in the common cold and are associated with more than 50% of all colds. However, the syndrome may be caused by over 200 viruses including influenza virus, coronavirus, adenovirus, respiratory syncytial virus, parainfluenza virus, metapneumovirus, and enterovirus. These viruses are transmitted either by direct contact or by aerosols through which they infect the nasal epithelium, thereby stimulating a nonspecific inflammatory response accounting for the associated symptoms.

Clinical Presentation

Onset of symptoms occurs 1 to 3 days following viral infection. The common cold typically manifests with an initial sore throat followed by rhinorrhea, nasal congestion, and sneezing by the third day. Patients may develop a cough later lasting for several days. Symptoms peak between day 3 and 6 and persist for approximately 7 to 10 days. Clinical findings are limited to the upper respiratory tract with increased nasal secretions. Additionally, patients may demonstrate mild oropharyngeal erythema, injected conjunctiva, edematous nasal mucosa, and anterior cervical lymphadenopathy.

Treatment

Treatment is largely symptomatic with rest, oral hydration, and over-the-counter medications including nasal decongestants, nonsteroidal anti-inflammatory drugs, lozenges, and cough suppressants. Antibiotics are not indicated.

ACUTE BACTERIAL RHINOSINUSITIS

Definition and Epidemiology

Acute rhinosinusitis is a common illness with one out of eight adults reporting receiving a diagnosis each year, resulting in more than 30 million patient visits annually. Acute bacterial rhinosinusitis is inflammation secondary to bacterial infection of the nasal cavity and paranasal sinuses lasting less than 4 weeks. Approximately 0.5% to 2% of acute viral rhinosinusitis cases are complicated by bacterial rhinosinusitis.

Pathogenesis and Microbiology

Following an upper respiratory infection, viral inoculation of the nasal cavity and the paranasal sinuses produces an acute viral rhinosinusitis leading to mucosal thickening, edema, and inflammation. Contaminated nasal secretions then enter the typically sterile paranasal sinuses that are normally cleared. However, mucosal inflammation and edema can obstruct sinus drainage and impair mucociliary clearance of bacteria, perpetuating bacterial infection. The most common bacteria associated with acute bacterial rhinosinusitis are *Streptococcus pneumoniae* and *Haemophilus influenzae*.

Clinical Presentation

Symptoms of acute rhinosinusitis may include purulent anterior or posterior nasal discharge, nasal congestion or obstruction, facial congestion or fullness, facial pain or pressure, hyposmia or anosmia, and fever. Patients may complain of headache, ear pain, maxillary tooth pain, cough, and fatigue. Clinical findings may include erythema and swelling of the nasal mucosa, purulent nasal discharge, and sinus tenderness. Clinical history, patterns, and duration of symptoms are helpful in the diagnosis of acute bacterial rhinosinusitis. These include symptoms of nasal congestion, rhinorrhea, and cough persisting greater than 10 days; severe symptoms including fever with purulent nasal discharge for greater than 3 days; or recurrence and worsening of common cold symptoms following a period of initial improvement or "double-sickening." Imaging is not routinely recommended in patients with uncomplicated acute rhinosinusitis.

Treatment

Acute bacterial rhinosinusitis typically resolves with symptomatic management within 2 weeks. Intranasal sterile saline irrigation has been shown to provide symptomatic relief. If symptoms persist in an otherwise immunocompetent patient or if reliable follow-up is unavailable, antibiotics are indicated and should be initiated for a duration of 5 to 7 days. First-line antibiotics are amoxicillin or amoxicillin-clavulanate. Azithromycin and trimethoprim-sulfamethoxazole are not recommended due to high prevalence of antibiotic resistance. Patients should respond to antibiotic therapy within 72 hours with improvement of symptoms. Failure to respond to initial therapy may require high-dose amoxicillin-clavulanate for a duration of 7 to 10 days.

Complications

Patients with acute bacterial rhinosinusitis who fail to respond to high-dose antibiotics warrant a referral to an otolaryngologist for further evaluation. Intracranial and orbital complications may arise from progressing infection (Fig. 93.1). Orbital complications include periorbital cellulitis, orbital cellulitis, and abscess, secondary to acute bacterial ethmoiditis. Intracranial complications include epidural abscess,

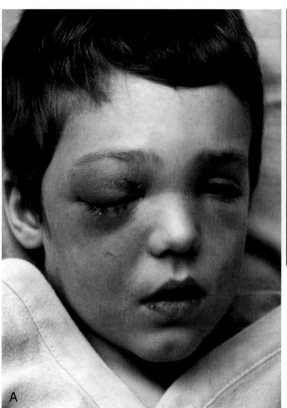
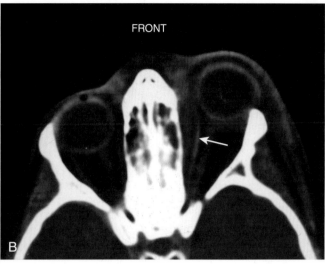

Fig. 93.1 (A) A child has an orbital abscess as a complication of ethmoid sinusitis. Note the marked edema and proptosis. (B) Computed tomography scan of the orbit demonstrates a subperiosteal abscess *(arrow)*. (A, Courtesy Gary Williams, MD; B, From DeMuri GP, Wald ER: Sinusitis. In Bennett JE, Dolin R, Blaser M, editors: Mandell, Douglas, and Bennett's principles and practice of infectious diseases, ed 8, Philadelphia, 2015, Saunders.)

meningitis, cavernous sinus thrombosis, subdural empyema, and brain abscess. In cases of complicated acute rhinosinusitis, evaluation should include computed tomography (CT) or magnetic resonance imaging with appropriate consultations with otolaryngology and/or ophthalmology. Oftentimes, management involves initiating broad-spectrum intravenous antibiotics and urgent surgical intervention in the setting of abscesses.

PHARYNGITIS AND TONSILLITIS

Definition and Epidemiology

Pharyngitis or sore throat is characterized by inflammation of the pharynx from environmental and chemical exposures or from infectious disease. In the United States, more than 10 million patients are diagnosed annually with acute pharyngitis, with incidence peaking in children and in the winter.

Tonsillitis is an inflammatory condition affecting the palatine tonsils, which, in addition to the pharyngeal, tubal, and lingual tonsils, comprise the Waldeyer ring. Tonsillitis refers to infections primarily involving the palatine tonsils, while pharyngitis affects the oropharynx, although they are frequently used interchangeably. Tonsillitis accounts for 1.3% of all outpatient primary care clinic visits with patients aged 5 to 15 years affected most commonly. Early spring and winter months demonstrate a notable up-tick in reported cases. Those afflicted can range from asymptomatic streptococcal carriers to a quinsy or peritonsillar abscess requiring emergent drainage.

Using a combination of history, clinical presentation, and several immediately available laboratory tests, the health care provider may readily distinguish patients with self-limited, viral illnesses from those requiring antibiotic treatment or procedural interventions.

Pathogenesis and Microbiology

Viral causes of pharyngitis account for greater than 70% of cases with common pathogens being rhinovirus, adenovirus, Epstein-Barr virus (EBV), and influenza viruses. The most commonly encountered bacterial pathogen is Group A Streptococcus (GAS), accounting for up to 30% of pharyngitis cases in children and 10% in adults.

The palatine tonsils are pharyngeal lymphoid organs surrounded by overlying respiratory epithelium that invaginate into crypts. These crypts may harbor bacteria and lead to acute or recurrent infections. Most cases of acute tonsillitis represent benign, self-limited episodes of viral origin. Pathogens responsible for the common cold frequently result in self-limited, benign cases of tonsillitis and include rhinovirus, coronavirus, respiratory syncytial virus, and adenovirus. More severe viral cases are less frequent but should raise suspicion for EBV, cytomegalovirus, rubella, and human immunodeficiency virus (HIV).

Difficulty in distinguishing viral from bacterial etiologies frequently results in unnecessary antibiotic therapy. While GAS infections are by far the most common bacterial source requiring antimicrobial therapy, infections yielding *S. aureus*, *S. pneumoniae*, and *H. influenzae* are also possible. Unvaccinated individuals may harbor infections with diphtheria-causing *Corynebacterium species*. A social and sexual history may yield prior or active infections with chlamydia, gonorrhea, HIV, and syphilis, which can also be observed in cases of acute or recurrent episodes of tonsillitis. Tuberculosis should be considered in patients residing in common living quarters, incarcerated facilities, and home-less shelters.

Clinical Presentation

Common presentations include malaise, fever, sore throat, and tender anterior cervical lymphadenopathy. Odynophagia and/or dysphagia warrant further investigation for significant tonsillar swelling and the potential for airway compromise. A thorough history and physical should include onset of symptoms, sick contacts, medical comorbidities, living conditions, prior episodes of tonsillitis, as well as sexual and vaccination history. One must consider the spectrum of illness when navigating diagnostic and management strategies, as this differs greatly when handling benign, minimally symptomatic patients from those demonstrating a toxic appearance with difficulty handling secretions.

The provider should assess the patient's vital signs, paying attention to the presence of a fever, tachycardia, tachypnea, and marginal oxygen saturation levels. Next, a thorough head and neck examination may reveal tonsillar enlargement and exudates, tender cervical lymphadenopathy, and uvular deviation. Both the Infectious Diseases Society of America and the American Society of Internal Medicine recommend the use of scoring systems (i.e., Centor Score), which considers presence of fever, tonsillar exudates and/or enlargement, absence of cough, and tender cervical lymphadenopathy, each of which warrants one point. It has since been modified for age, where patients within age 3 to 15 are given an additional point, and patients 45 years or older have one point subtracted from the overall score. With scores of 0 or 1, no further testing is necessary. With 2 to 3 points, a rapid strep test and throat culture are feasible options. In patients scoring 4 or more points, clinicians should consider testing and beginning empiric antibiotics.

Treatment

Treatment of viral pharyngitis is encouraging symptom control with nonsteroidal anti-inflammatory drugs (NSAIDs) and hydration. First-line treatment of GAS pharyngitis is amoxicillin and penicillin V. For penicillin-allergic patients, first-generation cephalosporins, clindamycin or macrolides are reasonable alternatives. Of note, GAS antibiotic resistance to azithromycin and clindamycin are increasingly common. The recommended duration of treatment using β-lactam antibiotics is 10 days.

Complications include peritonsillar abscess, in which patients may appear ill with muffled speech, foul-smelling breath, uvula displacement, and drooling. Less common complications include contiguous neck space infections or rarely rheumatic fever.

DEEP NECK SPACE INFECTIONS

Definition and Epidemiology

Deep neck space infections most commonly arise from oral cavity or odontogenic origin, and knowledge of cervical anatomy (Fig. 93.2) and the fascial planes is paramount in understanding the infectious etiology and their potential for spread. In addition, the deep cervical fascia creates clinically relevant fascial spaces into which infections can spread rapidly with devastating consequences. Risk factors for developing deep neck space infections include uncontrolled or untreated dental infection, spread of infection from other local structures such as the tonsils, intravenous drug use, diabetes, HIV infection, and local trauma.

Submandibular Space Infection

The submandibular space is defined by the mandible anteriorly and laterally; the hyoid bone posteriorly; the mucosa of the floor of the mouth superiorly; and the superficial layer of the deep cervical fascia inferiorly. Ludwig angina is a severe infection of the submandibular space, typically caused by an infected lower molar tooth. Patients will oftentimes present acutely ill with mouth pain, a swollen, elevated tongue, dysphagia, drooling, stiff neck, and febrile (Fig. 93.3). If left untreated, the infection may spread to the lateral pharyngeal space, resulting in trismus. On exam, the submandibular tissues will appear swollen with woody induration and are generally not fluctuant. Once the disease has been identified, immediate medical and surgical treatment is necessary, which involves initiating broad-spectrum antibiotic therapy as well as surgical decompression through a neck incision and extraction of the infected tooth. Complications of Ludwig angina include death from airway obstruction, aspiration pneumonia, carotid artery erosion, and tongue necrosis.

Retropharyngeal Infection

Defined by the alar fascia anteriorly and the buccopharyngeal layer of the middle layer of cervical fascia covering the pharynx and esophagus posteriorly, the retropharyngeal space extends from the base of the skull to level of T2 approximately, where the two fascial layers fuse. Additionally, there is a distinct prevertebral space that is in between the prevertebral fascia and the vertebral column.

Of note, there is a "danger space" that lies in between the prevertebral space posteriorly and the retropharyngeal space anteriorly, extending from the base of the skull to the diaphragm. This area is of clinical importance because it is continuous with the mediastinum, allowing for infection to spread directly into the thorax and causing mediastinitis.

Many infections can spread into the retropharyngeal space and may develop into abscesses without appropriate treatment. For example, infections in the Waldeyer ring can spread to the retropharyngeal lymph nodes and into this space. Additionally, odontogenic infections that spread to the lateral pharyngeal space can also travel into the retropharyngeal space. Patients will present acutely ill with fever, sore throat, dysphagia, neck stiffness, and dyspnea. Airway obstruction can occur from bulging of the posterior pharyngeal wall anteriorly with supraglottic compression. Definitive treatment requires administration of broad-spectrum antibiotics and oftentimes, surgical drainage of abscess.

Lateral Pharyngeal Space Infection

The lateral pharyngeal space or the parapharyngeal space is located on the lateral aspect of the pharynx, continuous with the retropharyngeal space posteriorly and the submandibular space anteriorly. This space communicates with the submandibular, retropharyngeal, and peritonsillar spaces and is therefore susceptible to both oral cavity and odontogenic infections. Interestingly, *Fusobacterium necrophorum* can cause a rare syndrome called postangina septicemia or Lemierre syndrome, which manifests with severe sore throat and fever. In this syndrome, the lateral pharyngeal space becomes infected with resulting septic thrombophlebitis of the internal jugular vein. The mortality rate can be as high as 50%. Treatment requires prompt initiation of intravenous penicillin and emergent drainage of any abscess.

Bacterial Epiglottitis
Definition and Epidemiology

Epiglottitis is an inflammatory affliction of the epiglottis and nearby structures, which include the arytenoids, aryepiglottic folds, and vallecula. Widespread usage of the *H. influenzae* type b vaccine in children has worked to decrease the incidence of pediatric bacterial epiglottitis by nearly 99%. Prior to widespread vaccination, *H. influenzae* was the leading cause of bacterial meningitis in children and a frequent cause of pneumonia, epiglottitis, and septic arthritis. Health care providers should counsel parents regarding the dangers of *H. influenzae* and

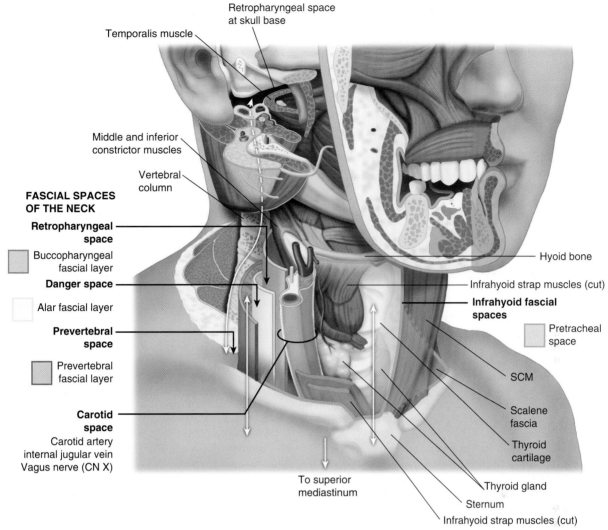

FASCIAL SPACES OF THE NECK

Temporalis muscle

Retropharyngeal space at skull base

Middle and inferior constrictor muscles

Vertebral column

FASCIAL SPACES OF THE NECK

Retropharyngeal space

Buccopharyngeal fascial layer

Danger space

Alar fascial layer

Prevertebral space

Prevertebral fascial layer

Carotid space
Carotid artery
internal jugular vein
Vagus nerve (CN X)

Hyoid bone

Infrahyoid strap muscles (cut)

Infrahyoid fascial spaces

Pretracheal space

SCM

Scalene fascia

Thyroid cartilage

To superior mediastinum

Thyroid gland

Sternum

Infrahyoid strap muscles (cut)

Fig. 93.2 Fascial spaces of the neck. (From Cillo JE: Atlas of oral and maxillofacial surgery, St. Louis, 2016, Elsevier Saunders, Fig. 8-1.)

recommend vaccination starting at 2 months of age. The incidence in adults has remained stable.

Pathogenesis and Microbiology

When compared to adults, the pediatric epiglottis demonstrates a more superoanterior position, more oblique angle, and less rigid structure, which account for increased risk of airway compromise in children compared to adults. Despite vaccination, *H. influenzae* remains the most common infectious cause of pediatric epiglottitis. *S. pyogenes*, *S. pneumoniae*, and *S. aureus* have also been implicated.

Clinical Presentation

Patients may present with fever, toxic appearance, drooling, dysphagia, tripod positioning, and neck hyperextension. Of importance is the sudden onset of symptoms, typically within the preceding 24 hours along with a frequently toxic, alarming appearance. The three D's refer classically to observable drooling, dysphagia, and distress. Inspiratory stridor due to turbulent flow through swollen upper airways represents severe upper airway obstruction and impending respiratory collapse, which should prompt immediate intervention.

Treatment

Airway management is paramount and frequently requires intubation by experienced providers. Edema may present significant challenges with a low threshold to utilize fiberoptic or camera-assisted intubation techniques. After securing the airway, the patient should be admitted to the intensive care unit. Broad-spectrum, empiric antibiotics are initiated and should be narrowed following culture sensitivity and susceptibility results. Although corticosteroids may shorten ICU length of stay, evidence supporting their widespread use is lacking.

Acute Bacterial Otitis Externa

Acute localized otitis externa is usually related to *S. aureus* and represents a localized, superficial infection of the outer ear canal. Oral agents against *Staphylococcus species* are adequate. Acute diffuse otitis externa, also known as swimmer's ear, is typically due to *Pseudomonas aeruginosa*. The infection is brought on by residual water left in the ear canal, which creates a moist environment that promotes bacterial growth. These patients may progress from seemingly benign itching to an erythematous and swollen outer ear canal with pain upon manipulation of the pinna or tragus. Treatment consists of topical antibiotics such as ciprofloxacin or neomycin plus polymyxin. Patients should be

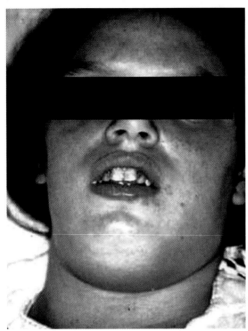

Fig. 93.3 Early appearance of a patient with Ludwig angina, who has a brawny, boardlike swelling in the submandibular spaces. (From Megran DW, Scehifele DW, Chow AW: Odontogenic Infections, Pediatric Infectious Diseases 3:262, 1984.)

counseled to keep ears dry after swimming or bathing and to consider preventative strategies such as acetic acid/isopropyl alcohol mixtures to assist in drying the canal.

Malignant otitis externa is a rare infection more commonly found in elderly diabetic patients. It tends to progress over weeks to months and is characterized by fever, deep ear pain, hearing loss, otorrhea, and granulation tissue on the posterior aspect of the external canal. Inciting agents are typical for the populations involved, which include the elderly, advanced diabetics, chemotherapy patients, and immunosuppressed or immunocompromised individuals. CT scan is the initial imaging modality of choice. The infection can progress to skull-based osteomyelitis and meningitis and has a significant mortality. Treatment consists of prompt surgical débridement and antipseudomonal systemic therapy.

Acute Bacterial Otitis Media
Definition and Epidemiology

Acute otitis media is a bacterial infection of the middle ear that commonly afflicts children with nearly all having at least one episode in the first 10 years of life. In fact, it is the most common pediatric bacterial infection, accounting for one fourth of all office visits, and is the second most common reason for surgery in children, only following circumcision.

Pathogenesis and Microbiology

Compared to adults, young children are more susceptible to otitis media because their eustachian tubes are shorter, wider, and more horizontal. This disease typically progresses from eustachian tube obstruction during or following a viral respiratory tract infection, causing middle ear effusion. Bacteria then colonize the middle ear and cannot be eliminated. The most common bacterial pathogens are *S. pneumoniae*, *H. influenzae*, and *Moraxella catarrhalis*.

Clinical Presentation

Acute bacterial otitis media presents with otalgia in the majority of patients as well as otorrhea and fever. The diagnosis can be difficult in young children because the history may be absent or inaccurate. Physical exam may reveal a middle ear effusion with a bulging tympanic membrane. Additionally, mobility of the tympanic membrane is imperceptible or absent by insufflation. Over time, perforation, drainage, fever, and decreased hearing may develop. Patients may also experience vertigo, tinnitus, and nystagmus. The course of otitis media is usually self-limited with most cases resolving within 1 week.

Treatment

Treatment has been controversial because for most patients otitis media is self-limiting. Inappropriate antibiotic use has resulted in the development of resistant organisms in the United States. Although antibiotics may shorten the course of the disease and may prevent complications such as mastoiditis, facial palsy, abscess, or meningitis, convincing data are lacking because the incidence of these complications is low.

Guidelines recommend the use of antibiotics in otitis media for high-risk patients such as those who are immunocompromised and for patients in whom there is complicated disease. If symptoms persist or worsen over 48 to 72 hours, then antibiotics should be initiated.

Despite higher rates of resistance to penicillin in recent years, amoxicillin or amoxicillin-clavulanate remains first-line therapy. Alternative choices include cephalosporins or macrolide antibiotics. There is no role of prophylactic antibiotics in reducing the frequency of recurrent acute otitis media.

SUGGESTED READINGS

Gallant J, Basem JI, Turner JH, Shannon CN, Virgin FW: Nasal saline irrigation in pediatric rhinosinusitis: a systematic review, Int J Pediatr Otorhinolaryngol 108:155–162, 2018.

Hindy J, Novoa R, Slovik Y, Puterman M, Joshua B: Epiglottic abscess as a complication of acute epiglottitis, Am J Otolaryngol Head Neck Med Surg 34(4):362–365, 2013.

Shulman ST, Bisno AL, Clegg HW, Gerber MA, Kaplan EL, et al: Clinical practice guideline for the diagnosis and management of group a streptococcal pharyngitis: 2012 update by the infectious diseases society of america, Clin Infect Dis 55(10):1279–1282, 2012.

Taub D, Yampolsky A, Diecidue R, Gold L: Controversies in the management of oral and maxillofacial infections, Oral Maxillofac Surg Clin 29(4):465–473, 2017.

Vandelaar LJ, Alava I: Cervical and craniofacial necrotizing fasciitis, Operat Tech Otolaryngol Head Neck Surg 28(4):238–243, 2017.

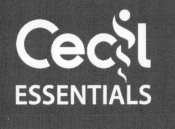

94

Infections of the Lower Respiratory Tract

John R. Lonks, Edward J. Wing

DEFINITION AND EPIDEMIOLOGY

Pneumonia, inflammation of the lung parenchyma, is usually caused by an acute infection. When the disease onset occurs outside of the hospital, it is referred to as community-acquired pneumonia (CAP). CAP ranges in severity from a mild self-limited disease to one that is fatal. CAP is common. Most patients with pneumonia are treated in the outpatient setting. Additionally, pneumonia is one of the most common reasons for hospitalization among all age groups and accounts for approximately 1 million hospitalizations per year. Each year approximately 50,000 people in the United States die from lower respiratory tract infections. Influenza and pneumonia are the leading cause of death due to infection and the eighth most common cause of death overall.

Numerous microorganisms cause pneumonia including bacteria, viruses, mycobacterium, and fungi. These infecting agents range from microorganisms that are part of the normal flora to exogenous microorganisms that are inhaled. Additionally, there are noninfectious diseases that can mimic pneumonia. The incidence of pneumonia is lowest during early adulthood and increases with each decade of life (Fig. 94.1).

PATHOLOGY

Bacterial pneumonia usually causes lobar pneumonia, consolidation of an entire lobe or a large portion of a lobe, or bronchopneumonia, patchy consolidation of the lung. Pneumococcal lobar pneumonia has 4 stages of the inflammatory response: consolidation, red hepatization, gray hepatization and resolution. The initial congestion is characterized by fluid, with some neutrophils and bacteria, filling the alveoli. Red hepatization is characterized by red blood cells along with numerous neutrophils and fibrin filling the alveoli. With gray hepatization there is breakdown of red blood cells and persistence of fibrin and neutrophils. Then the consolidated exudate within the alveolar spaces undergoes resolution.

Pathophysiology

The lower respiratory tract is virtually sterile. Normal host defenses that protect against pneumonia include mucous production and cilia; in combination these form the mucociliary escalator, which removes microorganisms from the lungs. Impairment of host defenses predisposes to the development of pneumonia. Loss or suppression of the cough reflex due to stroke and other neurologic diseases, drugs and alcohol, aging and associated medical illnesses, and environmental factors such as smoking and respiratory irritants impairs ciliary function and increases the likelihood of developing pneumonia. Mechanical obstruction of an airway such as by a tumor or foreign body leads to decreased clearance of microorganisms and may produce

a postobstructive pneumonia. Those infected with HIV virus are at increased risk of developing pneumococcal pneumonia.

The two main mechanisms of entry of microorganisms into the lung are microaspiration of organisms that colonize the upper respiratory tract and inhalation of airborne particles that contain a pathogenic microorganism. When a sufficient inoculum enters the lung and normal host defenses are not able to clear the inoculum, subsequent bacterial replication leads to a lower respiratory tract infection.

Transmission of Respiratory Pathogens

Some pathogens are transmitted from person to person via droplet transmission. Droplets are created when a person coughs, sneezes or talks. Additionally, transmission can occur during medical procedures such as suctioning, endotracheal intubation, cardiopulmonary resuscitation or cough-producing procedures. The greatest distance of transmission is unresolved. Historically, a distance of less than or equal to 3 feet was used for person-to-person droplet transmission. Some data suggest that transmission may occur from as far as 6 feet. Respiratory droplets have also been defined by their size, usually greater than 5 μm in diameter. Pathogens that are transmitted via the droplet route include *S. pneumoniae*, *M. pneumoniae*, and influenza virus. Crowding such as occurs in prisons, barracks, and shelters is associated with increased spread. Infectious agents such as *Mycobacterium tuberculosis*, fungi, and anthrax spores are transmitted via airborne transmission. Microorganisms transmitted in this fashion can be spread over long distances (>6 feet) by air currents and normal airflow. The size of the droplet nucleoli particles that are transmitted via the airborne route are generally less than or equal to 5 μm in diameter.

Specific Etiologic Agents

Many bacteria and viruses cause pneumonia. *Streptococcus pneumoniae* (pneumococcus) is the most common cause of bacterial pneumonia. The classical description of pneumonia is based upon disease caused by *S. pneumoniae*. Hence, *S. pneumoniae* causes "classical" or "typical" pneumonia. Most cases of pneumococcal pneumonia occur between December and April. Pneumococci transiently colonize the upper respiratory tract. Microaspiration leads to entry into the lower respiratory tract. If aspirated in sufficient quantity so that normal host defenses do not clear the bacteria, the patient then develops pneumonia. Pneumococci have a polysaccharide capsule that prevents phagocytosis. Antibodies, acquired from prior exposure or vaccination, against the polysaccharide capsule opsonize pneumococci thus allowing phagocytosis. Other bacteria that can colonize the oropharynx and cause pneumonia when aspirated include *Haemophilus influenzae*, less commonly *Staphylococcus aureus*, and rarely *Streptococcus pyogenes* (group A streptococcus). Similarly, *Moraxella catarrhalis* in patients with chronic obstructive

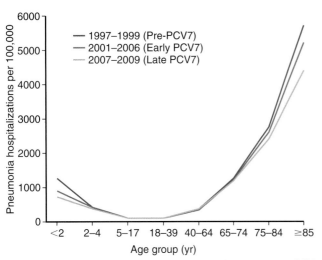

Fig. 94.1 Rate of hospitalization for pneumonia by age group. *PCV7*, Pneumococcus conjugate vaccine. (Data from New England Journal of Medicine 369: 155-63, 2013.)

pulmonary disease (COPD) and the elderly and *Klebsiella pneumoniae* in alcoholics colonize the oropharynx and can cause pneumonia. Most cases of community-acquired pneumonia are monomicrobial.

Patients with pneumococcal pneumonia can develop infections at other sites including empyema, pericarditis, meningitis, endocarditis, and septic arthritis. Approximately one out of five patients with pneumococcal pneumonia have bacteremia.

Mycoplasma pneumoniae usually causes milder disease. Its peak incidence is during the first two decades of life. Patients usually do not required hospitalization; however, some patients can develop severe disease.

Chlamydophila pneumoniae is a common cause of community-acquired pneumonia. It usually causes a milder disease and hence is seen more commonly among patients treated in the outpatient setting.

Legionella, an environmental organism, can cause pneumonia. *Legionella pneumophila* is the most common species to cause pneumonia. Other *Legionella* species such as *L. micdadei, L. bozemanii*, and others can also cause pneumonia. Most cases are sporadic. Outbreaks have occurred from contaminated point sources such as cooling towers and air conditioning units. Transmission is usually due to inhalation of aerosol particles; microaspiration of water containing *Legionella* has also occurred.

Staphylococcus aureus infrequently causes bacterial pneumonia, sometimes as a complication of influenza infection. More recently, community acquired methicillin-resistant strains (MRSA) have caused secondary bacterial pneumonias.

The etiology of CAP requiring hospitalization in adults is changing. More recently, the most commonly identified organisms, in order of decreasing frequency, are human rhinovirus followed by influenza, *Streptococcus pneumoniae*, human metapneumovirus, and respiratory syncytial virus. This change may be due in part to decreased invasive pneumococcal disease after the introduction of the conjugate vaccine, changes in the age distribution of patients and underlying illnesses of the adult population, as well as the ability to detect viral pathogens.

Rapid molecular techniques are now available for the detection of respiratory viral pathogens. The rapid identification of a virus can avoid the unnecessary use of antibiotics. A small subset (approximately 10%) of hospitalized patients with viral pneumonia are coinfected with a bacterium. This may occur because of damage to the respiratory epithelium caused by viral infection. Additionally, dysfunctional innate immune responses caused by a viral infection have been implicated to enhance susceptibility to secondary bacterial infection.

Fungi that cause pneumonia are not part of the normal flora. Certain dimorphic fungi (*Histoplasma capsulatum, Coccidioides immitis*, and

Blastomyces dermatitidis) that reside in the soil cause pneumonia when inhaled. Dimorphic fungi form hyphae at ambient temperatures and yeasts at body temperature. The hyphal form and not the yeast form is the transmissible form of the fungus. The yeast form is not transmissible person to person. These fungi are limited to certain geographic areas: *Histoplasma capsulatum* in the Mississippi, Missouri, and Ohio river valleys; *Coccidioides immitis* in the southwestern United States; and *Blastomyces dermatitidis* in parts of the midwestern, south-central and southeastern regions of the United States. *H. capsulatum, C. immitis*, and *Blastomyces dermatitidis* cause disease in the normal host. *Aspergillus*, a mold ubiquitous in the environment, rarely if ever causes disease in the immunocompetent host. Patients that are immunocompromised or have abnormal airways are at risk of infection with *Aspergillus* and rarely other molds such as Zygomycetes (*Mucorales*). *Pneumocystis jirovecii*, an opportunistic fungus, causes pneumonia in immunocompromised patients such as those with lymphoma or HIV (see Chapter 103 for additional information).

Mycobacterium tuberculosis is not part of the normal flora. It is transmitted via small aerosol particles (<5 μm) that are inhaled directly into the alveolus. *M. tuberculosis* is a slow growing organism and usually causes chronic symptoms; however, it rarely can present acutely.

The normal flora of an acutely ill hospitalized patient is different from a healthy outpatient. Hospitalized patients are more frequently colonized with *S. aureus*, including methicillin-resistant strains, and gram-negative bacilli, including *Pseudomonas aeruginosa*. Hence, when a hospitalized patient aspirates their own oropharyngeal flora leading to hospital-acquired pneumonia (HaP) it may contain one of these organisms.

Some microorganisms almost never cause pneumonia; these include *Candida* species and enterococci.

CLINICAL PRESENTATION

Patients usually present with the acute onset of fever, chills, cough, sputum production, dyspnea, and sometimes pleuritic chest pain. Classically, patients may produce blood-tinged sputum that appears rust-colored specifically when infected with *S. pneumoniae*. Extrapulmonary signs and symptoms may include nausea, vomiting, diarrhea, abdominal pain, headache, confusion, arthralgia, myalgias, and change in mental status. Signs and symptoms can be blunted or absent in the elderly. Rales or rhonchi may be present on auscultation of the chest. Patients usually have a leukocytosis with left shift. Pulmonary signs and symptoms in combination with a new infiltrate on chest radiograph are used to diagnose pneumonia.

DIAGNOSIS

When pneumonia is suspected, the next step is to determine the etiologic diagnosis. Unfortunately, there is no single diagnostic test with a high sensitivity and high specificity. The sputum gram stain provides useful diagnostic information. Although epithelial cells from the upper respiratory tract and oropharyngeal flora may "contaminate" an expectorated sputum sample, careful examination of the sputum gram stain can reveal an area of the specimen that originated from the lower respiratory tract and examination for bacteria in that area can be helpful. Unfortunately, some patients do not produce sputum. Additionally, prior antibiotics can alter sputum results.

S. pneumoniae is a gram-positive coccus that forms pairs and chains; the cocci are sometimes pointed at one end ("lancet-shaped"). *H. influenzae* is a pleomorphic gram-negative rod. *S. aureus* is a gram-positive coccus that forms clusters. *M. catarrhalis* is a gram-negative diplococci. These distinct morphologic features allow for a presumptive diagnosis of a specific etiologic agent when seen on a gram stain of sputum (Fig. 94.2).

Mycoplasma, Legionella, Mycobacterium, and *Chlamydophila* are not seen on sputum gram stain. *Mycobacteria* are seen with special staining (acid fast).

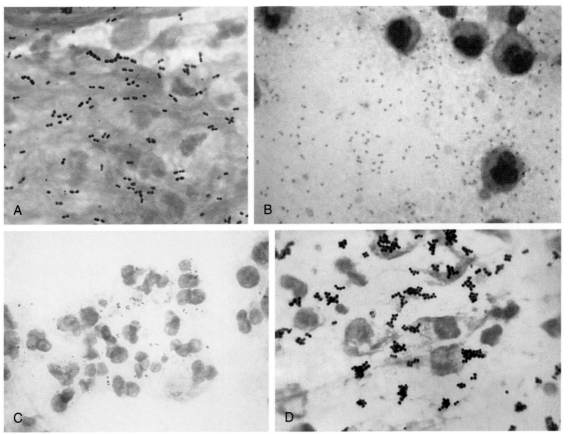

Fig. 94.2 Sputum Gram stain. (A) *Streptococcus pneumoniae.* (B) *Haemophilus influenzae.* (C) *Moraxella catarrhalis.* (D) *Staphylococcus aureus.*

Culture of sputum can reveal the etiologic diagnosis and should be correlated with findings on the sputum gram stain. However, pneumococci are fastidious. A study of patients with bacteremic pneumococcal pneumonia found that only 55% grew pneumococci from their sputum culture. *Mycoplasma*, *Legionella*, *Mycobacterium*, and *Chlamydophila* do not grow on routine agar. Special culture media are required for certain bacteria, such as Lowenstein-Jensen for *Mycobacteria* and buffered charcoal yeast extract (BCYE) for *Legionella*.

Blood cultures can be helpful. However, the ratio of bacteremic to nonbacteremic pneumococcal pneumonia is approximately 1:4. A positive blood culture is very helpful because the etiologic agent is definitely identified and susceptibility data are available to determine appropriate therapy.

Other diagnostic studies used to identify the causative organism include *Legionella* urinary antigen, histoplasmosis urinary antigen, and polymerase chain reaction (PCR) for respiratory viruses, *Mycoplasma*, and *Chlamydophila*.

Chest radiography of patients with pneumococcal pneumonia can show a consolidative lobar infiltrate, a bronchopneumonic (patchy) pattern or, less commonly, an interstitial pattern. A definitive etiologic diagnosis cannot be made based on chest radiograph appearance.

DIFFERENTIAL DIAGNOSIS

Not all patients with fever and a new pulmonary infiltrate have pneumonia. Noninfectious causes of pulmonary infiltrates and fever include pulmonary infarction, vasculitis (granulomatosis with polyangiitis), drug reaction, tumor, congestive heart failure, cryptogenic organizing pneumonia (COP), hypersensitivity pneumonitis, collagen vascular disease, aspiration (macroaspiration) of oropharyngeal or upper gastrointestinal contents, and acute respiratory distress syndrome (ARDS).

TREATMENT

The definitive treatment for pneumonia is to eradicate the infecting microorganism. Antibiotics are used to kill bacteria and hence decrease or stop the spread of infection in the lungs. Normal host responses are needed to repair the inflammatory process in the lungs. Penicillin therapy reduced the mortality rate of bacteremic pneumococcal pneumonia from 84% to 17%. However, antibiotics have little to no effect on mortality during the first 5 days of illness; those destined to die during the first 5 days of illness die whether or not they receive antibiotics.

When an etiologic agent is identified, then the appropriate antibiotic can be given (Table 94.1). When a specific etiologic diagnosis is not made, then empiric treatment with one of many different antimicrobial agents has been recommend. Guidelines are available (IDSA available at https://www.atsjournals.org/doi/full/10.1164/rccm.201908-1581ST).

The decision to admit a patient with pneumonia is based upon clinical prediction rules. These rules use mortality and sometimes other factors to stratify patients. The pneumonia severity index (PSI) stratifies patients into one of five risk groups. Those in a low risk group are treated as outpatients while those in a higher risk group are admitted to the hospital for treatment (see *The New England Journal of Medicine* 336: 243-250, 1997). The CURB-65 score (see *Thorax* 58: 377-382, 2003) is easier to calculate but has not been as rigorously validated as the PSI. Furthermore, psychosocial and other factors that impact the decision to admit a patient are not included by PSI or CURB-65.

Duration of therapy ranges from 3 to 28 days depending on the microorganism and clinical response. The shortest duration (3 days) has been given to patients with pneumococcal pneumonia while 28

TABLE 94.1	Treatment of Pneumonia by Specific Etiologic Agent	
Etiologic Agent	**Preferred Antimicrobial**	**Alternative Antimicrobial**
Streptococcus pneumoniae	Penicillin	Cephalosporin, moxifloxacin, levofloxacin
Haemophilus influenzae	Cefuroxime, ceftriaxone	
Mycoplasma pneumoniae	Macrolide	Moxifloxacin, levofloxacin
Legionella	Macrolide or quinolone	
Staphylococcus aureus		
Methicillin-susceptible	Nafcillin	Cephalosporin
Methicillin-resistant	Vancomycin (IV)	Doxycycline or TMP/SMX (oral)
Moraxella catarrhalis	Amoxicillin/clavulanate, cefuroxime, ceftriaxone, TMP/SMX	

TMP/SMX, Trimethoprim/sulfamethoxazole

days of therapy has been given to patients with *Staphylococcus aureus.* Recent ATS/IDSA guidelines (https://www.atsjournals.org/doi/full/10.1164/rccm.201908-1581ST) recommend no less than 5 days of treatment.

PROGNOSIS

Patients with bacteremic pneumococcal pneumonia have a higher mortality rate (21%) compared to those with nonbacteremic pneumococcal pneumonia (13%). Among patients with bacteremic pneumococcal pneumonia, increased mortality is associated with increasing age (Fig. 94.3), number of lobes involved (one lobe 12% mortality, two lobes 24% and three lobes 63%), leukopenia (mortality 35%), normal peripheral white blood cell count (24%) as compared to patients with leukocytosis (14%). Additionally, mortality rates differ for each capsular type of pneumococcus. For example, the mortality rate among patients infected with type I capsular type is 3% compared to patients infected with capsular type III 22%. Patients who survive usually recover without sequelae.

PREVENTION

Influenza vaccine not only protects against influenza but also bacterial pneumonia since patients who do not have influenza are not at risk of developing secondary bacterial pneumonia. The 23-valent pneumococcal polysaccharide vaccine is recommended for adults 65 years and older (see *Morbidity and Mortality Weekly Report* Supplement/Vol. 62, pages 9-18, February 1, 2013 and *Morbidity and Mortality Weekly Report* Vol. 68, No. 46, pages 1069-1075, 2019). The conjugate pneumococcal vaccine has reduced invasive pneumococcal disease in both the recipients (children) as well as adults (Fig. 94.4). By decreasing carriage in children, there is a reduction in transmission to adults and subsequent adult disease. The pediatric conjugate vaccine has reduced the number of adult admissions for pneumonia (see Fig. 94.1). Additionally, the conjugate vaccine has decreased antibiotic resistance since the capsular types of pneumococci that are more likely to be antibiotic resistant are included in the vaccine.

TUBERCULOSIS

Definition

Tuberculosis (TB) is caused primarily by *Mycobacterium tuberculosis* (MTB), an acid-fast rod that has a slow generation time. Related species include *Mycobacterium bovis* that causes disease in cattle but can infect humans and *Mycobacterium africanum* that causes up to 50% of cases of tuberculosis in Africa. TB primarily causes pulmonary disease but can cause infection in almost any part of the body including

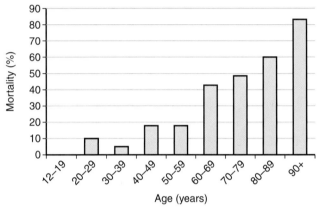

Fig. 94.3 Mortality from bacteremic pneumococcal pneumonia by age group. (Data from *Annals of Internal Medicine* 60: 760-776, 1964.)

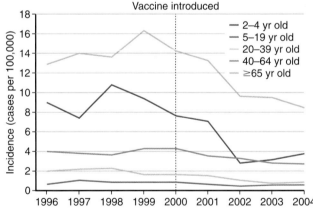

Fig. 94.4 Incidence of penicillin-resistant pneumococci by year for different age groups. (Data from *New England Journal of Medicine* 354: 1455-63, 2006.)

bone, the central nervous system, the gastrointestinal system, and the cardiovascular system. TB is characterized by asymptomatic, lifetime latency for up to 90% of infected individuals. Primary progressive infection typically occurs in 4% to 5% of patients up to 2 years after infection whereas reactivation disease occurs often decades after infection.

Epidemiology

MTB has caused infection in humans throughout history but became widespread during urbanization and industrialization in Europe in the 18th century, causing up to one quarter of all deaths. Rates of tuberculosis began falling in the late 19th and early 20th century and the fall was accelerated by the discovery of effective antibiotics, first streptomycin in 1946, and then isoniazid in 1952. Rates in the United States fell until the 1980s when they increased due to HIV and increased intravenous substance use. With effective antiretroviral therapy, the downward trend returned. For example, the incidence in the United States fell from 25,000 cases in 1993 to 9025 cases in 2018. Seventy percent of cases occurred in non-US-born people and approximately half were diagnosed 10 or more years after arriving in the United States, consistent with reactivation of previously acquired tuberculosis. There is a preponderance of cases in ethnic and racial minorities including Hispanic, American Indian/Alaska native, Asian, and Black individuals. Risk factors include diabetes mellitus, alcohol and substance abuse, HIV, homelessness, and incarceration.

Infection occurs when MTB is aerosolized by coughing, sneezing, shouting or singing from a patient with pulmonary disease and inhaled by a susceptible individual. Small infectious particles 1 to 5 μm in size can persist in the air, particularly in enclosed spaces, and very few infectious particles are required for infection. Household contacts are particularly at risk, with up to 50% becoming infected. Group home settings such as homeless shelters and prisons have been the sites of outbreaks.

Worldwide, TB is among the top ten causes of death and the number one cause of death due to an infection. In 2018, 10 million people contracted tuberculosis and 1.5 million died, including 251 thousand with HIV. Encouragingly, the TB mortality rate fell by 42% from 2000 to 2018. Four hundred eighty four thousand fell ill with drug-resistant tuberculosis (multidrug resistant or MDR defined as resistant to the two most effective drugs, INH and rifampin), and 6.2% of those had XDR-TB (defined as resistant to INH, rifampin, a fluoroquinolone, and second-line injectable drugs). Sixty-six percent of new cases occurred in India, China, Indonesia, the Philippines, Pakistan, Nigeria, Bangladesh, and South Africa. Rapid diagnostic tests (e.g., Xpert MTB/RIF) assays are in widespread use, and the global treatment success in 2017 of newly diagnosed cases was 85%. Newer drugs such as bedaquiline are coming into use for resistant TB. Furthermore, there are currently 14 vaccines in clinical trial.

Microbiology

MTB is an aerobic, nonmotile mycobacteria in the family Mycobacteriaceae with a cell wall content high in high-molecular-weight lipids. It has a slow multiplication time, between 15 to 20 hours, compared to most bacteria, which multiply in less than 1 hour. Humans are the only host. The organism can be identified in sputum by acid-fast staining (Ziehl-Neelsen or Kinyoun) or nucleic acid amplification, which is more common. Xpert MTB/RIF is an automated test that identifies MTB and whether the organism is resistant to rifampin, one of the most commonly used and effective anti-TB drugs. Growth on solid media occurs in 3 to 8 weeks whereas growth in liquid media takes up to 20 days. Culture of the organism is necessary to identify the full susceptibility of an isolate.

Pathobiology

Infection occurs when infectious particles reach the alveoli and are ingested by macrophages. MTB can resist destruction by macrophages and neutrophils and persist within phagosomes and multiply intracellularly, in part due to protective mechanisms such as the production of superoxide dismutase, which can neutralize the production of the bactericidal molecule superoxide anion. In addition, the mycobacteria appear to delay antigen presentation and the onset of immune cell responses mediated by CD4+ T lymphocytes for 4 to 8 weeks. Infected macrophages produce cytokines that attract monocytes, other alveolar

macrophages, and neutrophils. Eventually, delayed hypersensitivity as a measure of specific T cell immunity can be detected. Macrophages activated by T cell–produced cytokines such as gamma interferon result in a tuberculous granuloma containing Langhans giant cells—fused macrophages forming around tuberculous antigen. A form of incomplete necrosis can occur termed "caseous necrosis." If the bacterial replication is not controlled initially at the site of infection, the bacilli enter local draining lymph nodes. This leads to lymphadenopathy, a characteristic manifestation of primary TB. The lesion produced at the initial site of lung infection and lymph node involvement is called the Ghon complex (Fig. 94.5). Further dissemination may occur through the bloodstream.

In 90% of individuals the infection will be contained for their lifetime, although viable organisms persist, and the infection will be labelled latent TB or LTBI (Fig. 94.6). In 4% to 5% of individuals, mycobacteria will continue to multiply and spread within the lung and through the bloodstream to other sites, resulting in symptomatic infection usually within 1 year of infection. This is termed primary infection. In another 5% of people who have LTBI, reactivation will occur years later, sometimes triggered by the development of an immunocompromised state such as HIV or older age. A typical site is the posterior apical region of the lungs. Patients with LTBI have a very low number of organisms and do not transmit to other people.

Diagnosis

The diagnosis of LTBI depends on a positive QuantiFERON-TB Gold test (IGRA), which is an in vitro ELISA interferon release assay to MTB antigens, or a positive tuberculin skin test. The Mantoux skin test is an intradermal injection of 0.1 mL of purified protein derivative (PPD) tuberculin into the forearm. The diameter of induration at the injection site is measured 48 to 72 hours later. Both tests have a high sensitivity to previous infection (approximately 90%), but both may be negative in active disease. The IGRA test has the advantages of not requiring a second visit, not being reactive in individuals who had previously received bacillus Calmette-Guérin (BCG) vaccine, and not being dependent on the subjectivity of measurement.

The diagnosis of active TB depends on the identification of the organism in sputum, other body fluids such as cerebrospinal fluid (CSF) or urine, or in tissue as well as growth of MTB in culture. The mycobacteria can be identified as small, beaded rods that are acid fast by Ziehl-Neelsen or Kinyoun stain. Nucleic acid amplification testing (NAAT) is superseding older staining techniques because of its ease of testing and accuracy. One example is Xpert MTB/Rif testing, which can also give information on resistance. Other helpful clinical information for making the diagnosis includes history (e.g., chronic cough, fever and night sweats, weight loss), potential exposures (e.g., household contact or country of origin), imaging (e.g., chest radiograph showing posterior upper lobe infiltrates with or without cavitation), and laboratory data (e.g., anemia of chronic disease).

Neither tuberculin skin testing nor IGRA distinguish between active disease and latent infection. Additionally, patients with primary infection or reactivation may be anergic and have a negative test. Patients who are latently infected have a positive test but do not have active disease (no signs or symptoms).

Clinical Manifestations
Primary Infection

Primary infection with MTB is usually asymptomatic, although mild symptoms with fever, cough, and mid-lung field infiltrates may occur. With the onset of specific immunity as indicated by conversion of TB skin test or IGRA test, symptoms resolve and the patient may be left with a small parenchymal scar.

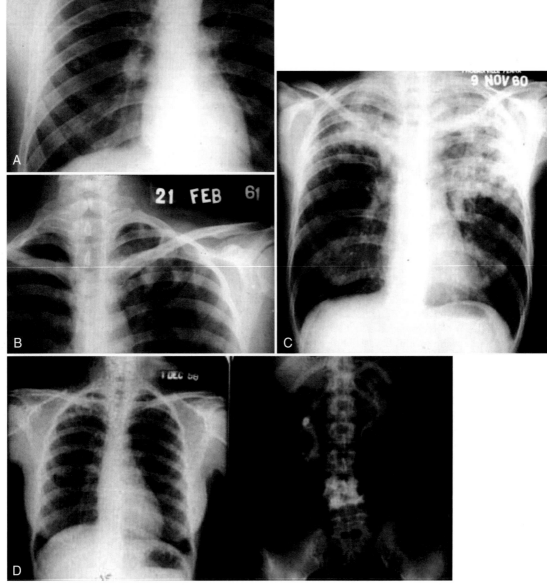

Fig. 94.5 (A) Ghon complex. (B) Moderately advanced pulmonary tuberculosis (TB). (C) Far advanced pulmonary TB. (D) Pulmonary *(left)* and extrapulmonary *(right)* TB.

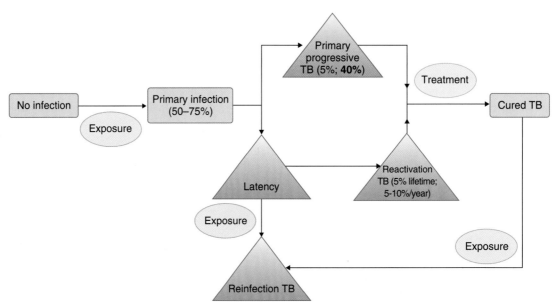

Fig. 94.6 Natural history of TB. The proportion of individuals affected is shown in parentheses. Bolded figures are for HIV infection with severe immunosuppression. A number of medical risk factors besides HIV promote progression from *Mycobacterium tuberculosis* infection to disease.

In approximately 4% to 5% of cases, the infection progresses within 1 to 2 years, manifesting as pulmonary infection either at the original site of infection or in the upper lobe as infiltrates with eventual cavitation. It is termed progressive primary tuberculosis. In high-incidence countries, most cases of pulmonary TB stem from progressive primary infection. In children particularly, hilar or mediastinal lymphadenopathy may be prominent and disseminated disease may occur manifesting as miliary TB or tuberculous meningitis. Young children, the elderly, and those who are immunocompromised (e.g., HIV) are most at risk for progressive primary disease.

Reactivation Infection

After 2 years, but often after decades, despite specific immunity, reactivation of previously latent foci of infection may occur, usually occurring as pulmonary disease. Patients may be asymptomatic with only radiograph findings of upper lobe infiltrates with or without cavitation (see Fig. 94.5) Patients give a history of chronic symptoms, usually greater than 3 weeks, of cough, fever, fatigue, night sweats, and weight loss. Hemoptysis and pleuritic chest pain occur in more advanced disease. Physical examination is often unrevealing. Fine, post-tussive rales may be heard at the apices. Chest radiograph findings are often more extensive than indicated by physical examination. Normocytic, normochromic anemia and hypoalbuminemia are typical for chronic disease. Classically, infiltrates and cavitation are seen in the posterior segment of an upper lobe or the apex of a lower lobe. Initially, cavities are thin walled without fluid but progress to thick-walled cavities. Patients who are immunocompromised, such as those with HIV, may have atypical findings with prominent lymphadenopathy or pulmonary infiltrates throughout the lungs. Patients with TB and cavities are highly infectious and should be placed in isolation immediately.

Extrapulmonary TB

Extrapulmonary TB usually results from a focus of organisms that have spread to extrapulmonary sites by either the bloodstream or lymphatics during initial phases of infection.

Pleural TB usually occurs 3 to 6 months after primary infection when a pleural-based nodule ruptures into the pleural space, producing pleuritic chest pain and a pleural effusion. There are few organisms in the pleural fluid. Pleural TB usually resolves spontaneously within months but is associated with a higher rate of subsequent active TB.

Miliary TB occurs when MTB disseminates widely in the bloodstream, often with nonspecific symptoms of fever, malaise, weight loss, and night sweats without localizing signs. Chest radiograph or CT scan, which has greater sensitivity, may show many small opacities up to 1 mm in size, resembling millet seeds—hence the name miliary—throughout all lung fields. Risk for dissemination is greatest in the very young, very old, and those who are immunocompromised. Physical examination may reveal lymphadenopathy and hepatosplenomegaly. Laboratory abnormalities may include anemia, a leukemoid reaction, and abnormal liver function tests. Mortality is high if the diagnosis and treatment are delayed.

Tuberculous meningitis typically presents over the space of several weeks with fever, stiff neck and headache. Cranial nerve abnormalities such as a VI nerve palsy may be seen. The CSF is characterized by a lymphocytic cell response, low sugar, and high albumin. Mortality is high, particularly if patients present with a prolonged course and have altered consciousness and neurologic findings.

Vertebral TB (also known as Pott disease) involves two adjacent vertebrae with destruction of the intervening disc in the lower thoracic or lumbar spine (see Fig. 94.5). Paraspinal abscess develops frequently. The differential diagnosis includes staphylococcal vertebral osteomyelitis. Bone biopsy may be necessary to establish the diagnosis.

Tuberculous peritonitis is characterized by fever, weight loss, and abdominal pain, either chronic or acute. Peritoneal fluid is exudative but there are few organisms. Mesenteric lymphadenopathy may be prominent. Diagnosis may be made by PCR or biopsy of the peritoneum.

Renal TB is frequently asymptomatic, the only clue being persistent sterile pyuria or hematuria. CT imaging shows cortical scarring and ureteral strictures. Cultures of the urine are positive.

Patients with untreated HIV and low CD4 T cell counts, particularly in endemic regions of the world, are at high risk for acquiring HIV and having disseminated, rapidly advancing TB with high mortality. Clinicians should have a high degree of suspicion for TB and other mycobacterial disease in AIDS patients.

Treatment and Prevention

TB requires prolonged therapy because of the slow multiplication rate of the mycobacteria. Also, multiple drugs are used to treat active TB because of the high rate of resistance each MTB population has to any one drug and because of the increasing rate of resistance of MTB worldwide. Since adherence is critical to successful therapy and prevention of resistance, direct observed therapy (DOT) is recommended for most patients.

Guidelines for treatment can be found at the American Thoracic Society/Centers for Disease Control and Prevention and the Infectious Diseases Society of America: Treatment of Drug-Susceptible Tuberculosis (2016). Initial treatment for most forms of TB in the United States includes isoniazid, rifampin, pyrazinamide, and ethambutol for 2 months and then isoniazid and rifampin for 4 to 6 months longer.

Regimens need to be adjusted for resistance and if there is resistance, it is important to never add one drug to a failing regimen. Treatment of MDR TB is much more difficult and usually includes five drugs to which the isolate is susceptible. This usually includes first-line drugs to which the organism is susceptible, a fluoroquinolone, an injectable such as amikacin, and second-line drugs such as ethionamide or PAS. Newer drugs such as bedaquiline, an ATP inhibitor, have been approved for treatment of MDR-TB. Guidelines for treatment of drug-resistant tuberculosis were published in 2019. Treatment of extensively drug resistant TB (XDR-TB) is based on resistant-based testing and often uses drugs such as linezolid and clofazimine.

Treatment of LTBI requires exclusion of active disease. Prevention is targeted towards those who have recent MTB infection and those with a significant risk factor or comorbidities such as HIV or diabetes. LTBI is treated with a single drug because there are so few organisms within the body that it is unlikely that there is a preexisting spontaneous drug-resistant mutant. Standard regimens include isoniazid alone for 6 or 9 months or rifampin alone for 4 months.

Prognosis

The prognosis for early primary and reactive pulmonary TB with appropriate treatment is excellent. Advanced disease, central nervous system and miliary disease, disease in immunocompromised patients, and disease in those with MDR and XDR-TB have a more guarded prognosis.

SUGGESTED READINGS

American Thoracic Society/Centers for Disease Control and Prevention and the Infectious Diseases Society of America: Treatment of Drug-Resistant Tuberculosis, 2019.

American Thoracic Society/Centers for Disease Control and Prevention and the Infectious Diseases Society of America: Treatment of Drug-Susceptible Tuberculosis, 2016.

Austrian R, Gold J: Pneumococcal bacteremia with especial reference to bacteremic pneumococcal pneumonia, Ann Intern Med 60:760–776, 1964.

Fine M, Auble T, Yealy D: A prediction rule to identify low-risk patients with community acquired pneumonia, N Engl J Med 336:243–250, 1997.

Griffin M, Zhu Y, Moore M: U.S. Hospitalizations for pneumonia after a decade of pneumococcal vaccination, N Engl J Med 369:155–163, 2013.

Kyaw M, Lynfield R, Schaffner W: Effect of introduction of the pneumococcal conjugate vaccine on drug-resistant streptococcus pneumonia, N Engl J Med 354:1455–1463, 2006.

Lim WS, Van der Eerden MM, Laing R: Defining community acquired pneumonia severity on presentation to hospital: an international derivation and validation study, Thorax 58:377–382, 2003.

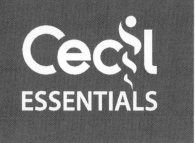

Infections of the Heart and Blood Vessels

Raul Macias Gil, Cheston B. Cunha

95

INFECTIVE ENDOCARDITIS

Definition

Infective endocarditis (IE) is an infection of the endocardium involving one or more cardiac valves or, less commonly, the mural endocardium. The pathologic lesion of IE is the vegetation (infected platelet and fibrin thrombus). The pathologic findings of IE were first described in 1646 by Lazare Rivière, a French physician at the University of Montpellier. At autopsy, Rivière described "small round outgrowths resembling the lungs in texture, the largest of which was about the size of a hazelnut, which blocked the aortic valve." The term *endocarditis* was first used in 1835 by the French physician Jean-Baptiste Bouillaud, but it was not until the 1880s that Sir William Osler was able to synthesize many of the prior clinical, pathologic, and microbiologic findings into a unified description of the disease.

Over the past 6 decades, the epidemiology, risk factors, and treatment of endocarditis have changed significantly. In the pre-antibiotic era, IE was uniformly fatal. Since the advent of antibiotics and valve replacement surgery, IE can be effectively treated and mortality can be significantly reduced, provided the diagnosis is made early. Despite progress, new challenges continue to arise in diagnosis and treatment. As more patients undergo intravascular manipulation, have intracardiac or intravascular devices placed, and harbor more resistant organisms, effective therapy for IE remains a challenge.

Traditionally, IE has been classified, based on the acuteness of onset, as subacute bacterial endocarditis (SBE) or acute bacterial endocarditis (ABE). This classification reflects the virulence of the causative agent: *Staphylococcus aureus* is a common cause of ABE, whereas low-virulence organisms such as viridans streptococci are more likely to be the cause of SBE. IE may also be subdivided according to the nature of the involved valve, as native valve endocarditis (NVE) or prosthetic valve endocarditis (PVE), or by the number of valves involved (multivalvular IE). IE from invasive procedures is classified as health care–associated IE or nosocomial IE. Endocarditis may be further divided according to the causative organism. These categories are often combined (e.g., *S. aureus* tricuspid valve nosocomial ABE).

Epidemiology

SBE is most common in older adults, and over the last 50 years, the average age of patients diagnosed with IE has gradually increased. More than one half of all cases of IE occur in patients older than 50 years of age. Rheumatic heart disease has decreased in the modern era and is now a less common predisposing factor.

While the incidence of IE can have geographic variations in the United States, the overall annual incidence is approximately 12.7 cases per 100,000 persons. A significant increase from prior years has been seen in the elderly, but also in younger patients. Multiple studies have shown that this increase in the incidence of IE could be explained by the alarming numbers of intravenous drug users from the current opioid epidemic in the United States. The age-adjusted hospital admission rate has increased by 2.4% annually, mirroring this increase in incidence. SBE usually involves the mitral valve or, less commonly, the aortic valve. IE of the pulmonic valve is relatively rare, and right-sided ABE occurs primarily in intravenous drug abusers. Individuals with congenital heart disease may be predisposed to IE, depending on the lesion.

Pathogenesis

Normal cardiac endothelium is relatively resistant to bacterial invasion. If the cardiac endothelium is damaged, an uninfected platelet and fibrin thrombus may form. This nonbacterial thrombotic endocarditis may become infected due to bacteremia, forming a vegetation. Endothelial damage may result from degenerative valvular disease, rheumatic heart disease, congenital heart disease, or intracardiac instrumentation or devices.

Predisposing Cardiac Factors

Approximately 15% of patients diagnosed with NVE have underlying congenital heart disease. Of these diseases, tetralogy of Fallot has the highest IE potential. Other lesions that predispose to IE include ventricular septal defect, bicuspid valves, and coarctation of the aorta. Significant mitral valve regurgitation is the most important predisposing factor for IE, with mitral valve prolapse accounting for 20% of NVE cases. Degenerative valvular disease predisposes to SBE in the elderly, and the mitral valve is most frequently involved. Aortic valve IE is rare in hypertrophic cardiomyopathy or asymmetric septal hypertrophy.

Noncardiac Predisposing Factors

Some hosts, particularly intravenous drug abusers, are predisposed to IE. Illicit intravenous drug use can lead to valvular or endothelial damage. Bacteremia with skin, oral flora, or with other organisms contaminating the substance(s) to be injected can develop from the act of injecting the drug(s). Central venous catheters and intracardiac devices can cause endocardial injury, predisposing to IE. The most frequent nosocomial IE pathogens are *S. aureus*, coagulase-negative staphylococci, group D enterococci, and aerobic gram-negative bacilli. Infections with these organisms usually occur less than 1 month after the procedure. Nosocomial IE may affect normal or abnormal valves. Because ABE pathogens are more virulent, nosocomial IE is associated with a high mortality rate.

Low-virulence and noninvasive organisms (e.g., viridans streptococci) are the most common SBE pathogens. The SBE potential of viridans streptococci is directly related to the thickness of the capsule, which permits adherence to damaged cardiac valves. Viridans streptococci are normal inhabitants of the mouth and gastrointestinal tract. Invasive dental procedures frequently cause transient bacteremias that may result in SBE on damaged but not normal cardiac valves. Transient bacteremias of viridans streptococci may form a vegetation in the sterile platelet and fibrin thrombus covering an area of damaged endothelium or intracardiac devices. The gastrointestinal or genitourinary tract is the usual source of bacteremia in cases of native valve SBE due to group D enterococci.

Diagnosis

The clinical diagnosis of IE relies on a combination of clinical, laboratory, and echocardiographic findings. Epidemiologic clues to the potential IE pathogens are outlined in Table 95.1. The most important finding in IE is the demonstration of continuous bacteremia, usually by multiple positive blood cultures. Table 95.2 contains the modified Duke criteria that are frequently used to predict the likelihood that a patient has IE.

Clinical Features

The cardinal clinical features of IE are fever (90% of cases) and heart murmur (85%). In the antibiotic era, fever may not be present if the patient has been taking antibiotics for another reason. Acute versus subacute presentation is determined by the virulence of the IE pathogen. SBE often manifests with sweats, malaise, and anorexia. The course of SBE tends to be more indolent and may be accompanied by back pain, joint pains (>50% of patients), or embolic stroke. As SBE progresses, circulating immune complexes may deposit in the kidney, causing interstitial nephritis, glomerulonephritis, and even renal failure. Osler nodes (painful, subcutaneous nodules on the distal pads of the fingers or toes), Janeway lesions (hemorrhagic, nonpainful macules on the palms and soles), and Roth spots (retinal hemorrhages with small central clearing) are classic findings related to microemboli and SBE immune-mediated vasculitis.

Patients with ABE tend to have a more fulminant course because of the greater virulence of the pathogen. The fever of ABE is usually high (>102° F) and is often accompanied by rigors. If there is mechanical dysfunction of the valve, symptoms of congestive heart failure will predominate. Often, a presenting feature of right-sided ABE is septic pulmonary emboli with pleuritic chest pain. The clinical findings of SBE and ABE are presented in Table 95.3.

Clinically, PVE may be considered as early (<2 months) or late (>2 months) following implantation of the prosthetic valve. Early PVE is caused by virulent pathogens (e.g., *S. aureus*) that infect the prosthetic valve before endothelialization is complete. Endothelialization of a mechanical valve is partially protective against transient bacteremias in late PVE. Over time, bioprosthetic valves have the same IE potential as mechanical ones.

Early PVE pathogens such as *S. aureus* and *Pseudomonas aeruginosa* are typically highly virulent and invasive. Late PVE more closely resembles SBE, is caused by less virulent pathogens, and has a more indolent course. The most common etiologic agents are coagulase-negative staphylococci, but viridans streptococci also cause late PVE.

Nosocomial IE results from invasive intravascular or intracardiac procedures that damage the endothelium or the valves; it can also be caused by direct extension of infection, such as from ABE associated with a pacemaker wire. The organisms causing nosocomial IE originate from the skin (e.g., *S. aureus*, coagulase-negative staphylococci), from gastrointestinal or genitourinary procedures (e.g., group D enterococci), or from central venous catheters, ports, or hemodialysis catheters (e.g., *Candida* spp, aerobic gram-negative bacilli). IE related

to total parenteral nutrition (TPN) is most often caused by *Candida* spp; other TPN-associated fungemias cause IE less frequently. In intravenous drug abusers, tricuspid valve ABE is usually caused by *S. aureus* or *P. aeruginosa* (depending on the geography and drug-related materials).

An otherwise unexplained high-grade or continuous bacteremia and murmur should suggest IE. If blood cultures are negative but a murmur, vegetation, and peripheral manifestations of IE are present, a diagnosis of infectious culture-negative endocarditis (CNE) should be considered. Infectious CNE is caused by organisms that are difficult to culture, such as *Legionella* spp, *Brucella* spp, *Tropheryma whipplei*, and *Coxiella burnetii* (which produces Q fever). Legionnaires disease may cause NVE or PVE. CNE due to *Brucella* spp can be a difficult diagnosis, but an antecedent history of contact with livestock or consumption of unpasteurized dairy products should suggest the diagnosis, and echocardiography often reveals large vegetations. A difficult infectious CNE diagnosis is Q fever. Q fever SBE may be suggested by a history of animal contact. Clinical findings of Q fever are often present, but the diagnosis can be missed because Q fever vegetations are not easily visualized.

Laboratory Findings

The isolation of a microorganism(s) in blood cultures is crucial for the diagnosis and management of IE. At least two sets of blood cultures from two different peripheral veins should be obtained in patients with high suspicion for IE, especially those at high risk (e.g., PVE, intracardiac devices, prior history of IE, etc.). The likelihood of isolating a causative pathogen is higher in patients who are not actively taking or have not received antibiotics 2 weeks prior to collection of blood cultures. Most bacterial and even some fungal organisms can be isolated in standard blood cultures, except for pathogens known to cause CNE.

Diagnosis of *Legionella*-related IE is based on an antecedent pneumonia and elevated titers of urinary antigen. *Brucella*-related IE is confirmed by titers or by polymerase chain reaction or both. A clue to Q fever CNE is enhanced valve uptake on positron-emission tomography (PET) or computed tomography (CT), and such a result should prompt testing for Q fever.

With the advent of sophisticated microbiologic testing, HACEK organisms (*Haemophilus* spp, *Aggregatibacter actinomycetemcomitans* [formerly called *Actinobacillus actinomycetemcomitans*], *Cardiobacterium hominis*, *Eikenella corrodens*, and *Kingella kingae*) grow relatively rapidly and no longer manifest as CNE. Newer molecular-based tests using microbial cell-free DNA sequencing may allow improved diagnosis, and implementation of prompt targeted therapy.

With IE, many nonspecific laboratory abnormalities may occur (Table 95.4); when placed in the appropriate context, these can be a significant aid to diagnosis.

Imaging Studies

Echocardiography is an important element in diagnosis and management; it should be performed for all patients with suspected IE. In those with a low likelihood of having IE or small body habitus, a transthoracic echocardiogram (TTE) may be sufficient. Although TTE is often sufficient to screen for NVE, the "gold standard" remains transesophageal echocardiogram (TEE), which is more sensitive at detecting smaller vegetations, paravalvular abscess, and PVE. If the TTE or TEE demonstrates a vegetation but blood cultures remain negative, the diagnosis of infectious CNE should be considered. A tiered diagnostic approach to such cases is presented in Table 95.5.

Radiologic testing in IE is primarily focused on identifying complications of IE. Although echocardiography is still the preferred method for detecting vegetations, improvements in multislice CT scans have

TABLE 95.1   Clues to the Likely Pathogen in Infective Endocarditis

Epidemiologic Features	Pathogens	Epidemiologic Features	Pathogens
Intravenous drug abuse	*Staphylococcus aureus*	Diabetes mellitus	*S. aureus*
	Pseudomonas aeruginosa		β-Hemolytic streptococci
	β-Hemolytic streptococci		*S. pneumoniae*
	Aerobic GNB	Early PVE	*S. aureus*
	Polymicrobial		Aerobic GNB
	Fungi		Fungi
Indwelling cardiovascular device	*S. aureus*		*Corynebacterium* spp
	CoNS	Late PVE	CoNS
	Aerobic GNB		*S. aureus*
	Corynebacterium spp		Viridans streptococci
Genitourinary disorders,	*Enterococcus* spp		*Enterococcus* spp
infection, manipulation	Group B streptococci (*Streptococcus*		*Corynebacterium* spp
	agalactia)		*Legionella* spp
	Aerobic GNB	Dog or cat exposure	*Bartonella* spp
Chronic skin disorders	*S. aureus*		*Pasteurella* spp
	β-Hemolytic streptococci		*Capnocytophaga* spp
Poor dentition, dental	Viridans streptococci	Contact with contaminated milk or	*Brucella* spp
procedures	Nutritionally variant streptococci	infected farm animals	*Coxiella burnetii* (Q fever)
	(*Abiotrophia* spp, *Granulicatella*		*Erysipelothrix rhusiopathiae*
	spp)	Homelessness	*Bartonella* spp
	Gemella spp	Human immunodeficiency virus	*S. pneumoniae*
	HACEK organisms[a]	infection	*Salmonella* spp
Alcoholic cirrhosis	*Streptococcus pneumoniae*		*S. aureus*
	Bartonella spp	Pneumonia and meningitis[b]	*S. pneumoniae*
	L. monocytogenes	Solid organ transplants	*S. aureus*
	β-Hemolytic streptococci		*Aspergillus fumigatus*
Burns	*S. aureus*		*Enterococcus* spp
	Aerobic GNB		*Candida* spp
	P. aeruginosa	Gastrointestinal lesions	*Streptococcus bovis*
	Fungi		*Enterococcus* spp

Modified from Baddour LM, Wilson WR, Bayer AS, et al: Infective endocarditis: diagnosis, antimicrobial therapy, and management of complications: a statement for healthcare professionals from the Committee on Rheumatic Fever, Endocarditis, and Kawasaki Disease, Council on Cardiovascular Disease in the Young, and the Councils on Clinical Cardiology, Stroke, and Cardiovascular Surgery and Anesthesia, American Heart Association; endorsed by the Infectious Diseases Society of America, Circulation 111:e394-e433, 2005.
CoNS, Coagulase-negative staphylococci; *GNB*, gram-negative bacilli; *PVE*, prosthetic valve endocarditis.
[a]HACEK organisms: *Haemophilus* spp, *Aggregatibacter actinomycetemcomitans*, *Cardiobacterium hominis*, *Eikenella corrodens*, and *Kingella kingae*.
[b]With alcoholic cirrhosis.

allowed chest CT to detect vegetations and valvular abnormalities in addition to the septic emboli seen in right-sided IE. Magnetic resonance imaging (MRI) of the spine is useful in patients with IE who report back pain; it is the preferred method to detect the presence of vertebral osteomyelitis caused by IE. Mental status changes or new focal neurologic signs should prompt CT or MRI imaging of the head to assess for septic emboli to the brain. Although it is less invasive than TEE, cardiac MRI often lacks the special resolution to detect smaller vegetations; however, it may be helpful in identifying aortic root pseudoaneurysms, sinus of Valsalva aneurysms, and embolic vascular lesions.

Differential Diagnosis and Mimics

The diagnosis of SBE is based an otherwise unexplained high-grade or continuous bacteremia caused by a known endocarditis pathogen plus a cardiac vegetation. Depending on the duration before presentation (usually 1 to 3 months), IE may be accompanied by peripheral manifestations such as Osler nodes, Janeway lesions, splinter hemorrhages, or conjunctival hemorrhages. Splenomegaly or embolic phenomena

may also accompany SBE. However, peripheral manifestations that are seen in SBE may also be present in other disorders. Before ascribing peripheral manifestations to SBE, physicians need to rule out other systemic disorders and confirm the diagnosis of SBE.

Clinically, the disorders most likely to mimic SBE are Libman-Sacks endocarditis (associated with systemic lupus erythematosus [SLE]), marantic endocarditis (caused by a malignancy, usually lymphoma, lung cancer, or pancreatic cancer), and atrial myxoma. Myocarditis of any etiology may mimic SBE with fever, murmur, and peripheral embolic phenomena. Cardiomegaly, which is usually present with myocarditis, is typically absent with SBE. Leukopenia and thrombocytopenia may be clues to viral myocarditis, and either finding argues against a diagnosis of SBE. Cardiac echocardiography shows myocarditis but no vegetations, and bacteremia is not present.

SLE, particularly between flares, may mimic SBE with low-grade fevers, murmur, peripheral manifestations, and splenomegaly. Laboratory findings in SLE include the anemia of chronic disease and a mildly to moderately elevated erythrocyte sedimentation rate (ESR). Even if Libman-Sacks vegetations are present, SBE is rare in

TABLE 95.2   Modified Duke Criteria for Diagnosis of Infective Endocarditis

Diagnostic Criteria

Definite IE (any of the following):

Positive findings for IE in the pathology or microbiology of the vegetation

Two major criteria

One major and three minor criteria

Five minor criteria

Possible IE (any of the following):

One major and one minor criteria

Three minor criteria

Not IE (any of the following):

Definite alternative diagnosis or resolution with <4 days of antibiotic therapy

Does not meet the criteria of possible IE

Major Criteria

Positive blood cultures for IE (any of the following):

Typical microorganism for IE from two separate blood cultures:

- Viridans streptococci, *Streptococcus gallolyticus* (formerly *Streptococcus bovis* biotype I), or the nutritional variant strains (*Granulicatella* spp and *Abiotrophia defectiva*)
- HACEK group: *Haemophilus* spp, *Aggregatibacter actinomycetemcomitans*), *Cardiobacterium hominis*, *Eikenella corrodens*, and *Kingella kingae*
- *Staphylococcus aureus*

Community-acquired enterococci, in the absence of a primary focus

Persistently positive blood culture, defined as recovery of a microorganism consistent with IE from any of the following:

Blood cultures drawn more than 12 hr apart

All three or a majority of four or more separate blood cultures, with first and last drawn at least 1 hr apart

[a]Single positive blood culture for *Coxiella burnetii* or antiphase I IgG antibody titer >1:800

Evidence of endocardial involvement

Positive echocardiogram for IE:

[a]TEE is recommended in patients with prosthetic valves rated at least "possible IE" by clinical criteria, or with complicated IE (paravalvular abscess); TTE as first test in other patients

Definition of positive echocardiogram (any of the following):

- Oscillating intracardiac mass, on valve or supporting structures, or in the path of regurgitant jets, or on implanted material, in the absence of an alternative anatomic explanation
- Abscess
- New partial dehiscence of prosthetic valve

New valvular regurgitation (increase in or change in preexisting murmur is not sufficient)

Minor Criteria ([a]Echocardiographic minor criteria have been eliminated)

Predisposition: predisposing heart condition or intravenous drug use

Fever: 38.0° C (100.4° F)

Vascular phenomena: major arterial emboli, septic pulmonary infarcts, mycotic aneurysm, intracranial hemorrhage, conjunctival hemorrhages, Janeway lesions

Immunologic phenomena: glomerulonephritis, Osler nodes, Roth spots, rheumatoid factor

Microbiologic evidence: positive blood culture but not meeting major criterion (excluding single positive cultures for coagulase-negative staphylococci and organisms that do not cause endocarditis) or serologic evidence of active infection with organism consistent with IE

Modified from Li JS, Sexton DJ, Mick N, et al: Proposed modifications to the Duke criteria for the diagnosis of infective endocarditis, Clin Infect Dis 30:633-638, 2000.

IE, Infective endocarditis; *IgG,* immunoglobulin G; *TEE,* transesophageal echocardiography; *TTE,* transthoracic echocardiography.

[a]Represents a change from the previously published Duke criteria.

SLE. A lupus flare may resemble ABE with high fevers (>102° F), tender fingertips (mimicking Osler nodes), and funduscopic findings of cotton-wool spots or Roth spots. Conjunctival and splinter hemorrhages are rare in SLE but common in SBE. Microscopic hematuria is the usual renal manifestation of SBE (i.e., focal glomerulonephritis), but full-blown nephritis with proteinuria and hematuria are typical of SLE renal involvement. Although clinical findings of SLE and SBE may overlap, SBE is ruled out by the absence of high-grade or continuous bacteremia.

Atrial myxomas may mimic SBE with fever, murmurs, and embolic phenomena (e.g., splinter hemorrhages). Highly elevated ESR levels are common with atrial myxomas, but biologically false-positive results on Venereal Disease Research Laboratory (VDRL) testing, elevated rheumatoid factors, and renal involvement are not seen. On TTE or TEE, atrial myxomas appear as masses or vegetations on the atrial surface rather than on a valve as in IE. SBE is ruled out by the absence of bacteremia.

Besides clinical mimics of SBE, there are also echocardiographic mimics, including papillary fibromas, thrombi, calcified valves, myxomatous degeneration, and marantic endocarditis. These disorders are usually unaccompanied by fever or bacteremia. The term *marantic endocarditis* refers to uninfected vegetations with a murmur and negative blood cultures that occur secondary to malignancy. Patients with marantic endocarditis are afebrile unless fever is caused by the underlying malignancy (e.g., lymphoma). The patient with marantic endocarditis due to lymphoma may have fever, splenomegaly, and other manifestations of SBE. Negative blood cultures effectively rule out IE. Infectious CNE (e.g., Q fever) may show little or no visible vegetations. Infectious CNE should be considered if fever, murmur, and vegetation are present along with peripheral manifestations of IE.

Treatment

Effective treatment of IE depends on the antibiotic susceptibility of the pathogen, the penetration of the antibiotic into the vegetation, and the appropriate duration of antibiotic therapy. Antibiotics selected for IE preferably should be bactericidal. In IE, the organisms are deeply embedded in the vegetation, and prolonged therapy is necessary for penetration and sterilization of the vegetation. Early in IE therapy, blood cultures rapidly become negative, but treatment is continued because infection in the vegetation has not been eradicated. Multiplication of bacteria, which is required for bactericidal activity of antibiotics, is reduced within vegetations and is one reason for the requirement for prolonged antibiotics. It is important to note that in cases of *Staphylococcus aureus* endocarditis, blood cultures may not clear rapidly and may remain positive for days despite appropriate antibiotic therapy. Penetration into the vegetation is critical; for example, viridans streptococci are highly susceptible to β-lactam antibiotics but require a prolonged course of antimicrobial therapy to eradicate the pathogens in the vegetation.

Whereas some cases of uncomplicated IE may be treated with 2 weeks of antimicrobial therapy, the usual duration of monotherapy or combination therapy is 4 to 6 weeks, depending on the pathogen.

Current guidelines for the treatment for IE recommend intravenous (IV) antibiotics. However, the POET trial has confirmed what prior evidence had shown, that transition from IV to oral antibiotics showed no inferiority compared to IV antibiotics alone in patients with left-sided IE in patients with *Streptococcus* spp, *Enterococcus faecalis*, *Staphylococcus aureus*, and coagulase-negative *Staphylococcus*. This adds to the significant studies already available, demonstrating the effectiveness of PO therapy for serious systemic infections. As safety and efficacy of oral antibiotic therapy for the treatment of IE is

TABLE 95.3 Clinical Findings for Subacute Bacterial Endocarditis (SBE) and Acute Bacterial Endocarditis (ABE)

Symptoms and Findings[a]	ABE	SBE
Anorexia	–	+
Weight loss	–	±
Myalgias or arthralgias	+	±
Fatigue	–	+
Dyspnea	+	–
Pleuritic chest pain[b]	+	–
Low back pain	+	+
Headache	+	±
Mental status changes	+	±
Acute confusion	+	–
Cerebrovascular accident	–	+
Sudden unilateral blindness	–	+
Left upper quadrant pain	Splenic abscess	Splenic infarct
Fever	>102° F[c]	<102° F
New or changing heart murmur	±	±
Splenomegaly	–	+
Petechiae	+	+
Osler nodes	–	+
Janeway lesions	+	–
Splinter hemorrhages	±	+
Roth spots	–	+
Congestive heart failure (LVF)	+	–

Modified from Cunha BA, Gill MV, Lazar JM: Acute infective endocarditis: diagnostic and therapeutic approach, Infect Dis Clin North Am 10:811-834, 1996.
LVF, Left ventricular fibrillation; *+,* present; *–,* absent; *±,* present or absent.
[a]Otherwise unexplained.
[b]With septic pulmonary emboli from tricuspid valve ABE.
[c]Fever may be <102° F in intravenous drug abusers with ABE.

TABLE 95.4 Nonspecific Laboratory Tests for Infective Endocarditis

Laboratory Findings	Percentage
Anemia	70–90[a]
Leukocytosis	20–30
Elevated ESR	90–100
C-reactive protein (CRP)	100
Histiocytes in blood smear	25
Positive rheumatoid factor (RF)	50[a]
Circulating immune complexes	65–100[a]
Microscopic hematuria	30–50

Data from Brusch JL: Clinical manifestations of endocarditis. In Brusch JL, editor: Infective endocarditis, New York, 2007, Informa Healthcare, pp 143-166.
ESR, Erythrocyte sedimentation rate.
[a]Most consistent with SBE

continued to be proven in future trials, not only would this reduce the morbidity associated with long-term IV catheters, but it would also be ideal for patients who are otherwise not eligible for long-term IV antibiotics. Long-acting lipoglycopeptides (dalbavancin, oritavancin) have been used in a very small number of retrospective studies showing potential promises for treating IE. However, we should be cautious as

TABLE 95.5 Diagnostic Approach to Culture-Negative Endocarditis

Valvular Biopsy Unavailable
1. Q fever and *Bartonella* serology: If negative, then use lysis-centrifugation system for blood cultures and inform microbiology laboratory of concern for fastidious organisms to allow use of special media and culture techniques: thioglycolate-, pyridoxal hydrochloride–, or L-cystine–enriched media for *Abiotrophia*; buffered charcoal yeast extract (BCYE) agar for *Legionella*; prolonged incubation for HACEK organisms[a]
2. Rheumatoid factor (RF), antinuclear antibodies (ANA)
3. PCR for *Bartonella* spp and *Tropheryma whipplei*
4. Nested PCR for fungi, tissue for *Cryptococcus neoformans* capsular antigen, and urine for *Histoplasma capsulatum* antigen: If negative, then obtain serum serology studies for *Mycoplasma pneumoniae, Legionella pneumophila, Brucella melitensis,* and *Bartonella* spp by Western blot

Valvular Biopsy Available
1. Broad-range PCR for bacteria (16S rRNA) and fungi (18S rRNA)
2. Histologic examination with direct staining for *Chlamydia* spp, *Coxiella burnetii, Legionella* spp, fungi, and *T. whipplei*
3. Primer extension enrichment reaction (PEER) or autoimmunohistochemistry (AIHC)

Modified from Fournier PE, Thuny F, Richet H, et al: Comprehensive diagnostic strategy for blood culture-negative endocarditis: a prospective study of 819 new cases, Clin Infect Dis 51:131-140, 2010; and Mylonakis E, Calderwood SB: Infective endocarditis in adults, N Engl J Med 345:1320, 2001.
PCR, Polymerase chain reaction; *rRNA,* ribosomal RNA.
[a]HACEK organisms: *Haemophilus* spp, *Aggregatibacter actinomycetemcomitans, Cardiobacterium hominis, Eikenella corrodens,* and *Kingella kingae.*

failures have been documented, and potential for increasing resistance to standard therapy remains.

Effective antimicrobial therapy does not eliminate suppurative or embolic complications of endocarditis. Therapeutic failure is usually related to valvular destruction, a complication that may require valve replacement. Suppurative intracardiac or extracardiac complications usually require drainage for cure of IE. The overarching principles of IE therapy are presented in Table 95.6, and Table 95.7 provides an outline of specific antibiotic regimens that may be used to treat IE.

Complications of endocarditis may be intracardiac or extracardiac, and they may also be classified by damage mechanism (i.e., immunologic vs. infectious). The infectious intracardiac complications of IE include purulent pericarditis and paravalvular abscess; they manifest clinically with persistent fever or persistent bacteremia despite appropriate antibiotic therapy. Complications may be septic or immunologic; for example, splenic involvement may be immunologic (splenic infarct) or septic (splenic abscess). Embolic events are related to vegetation size. Bland central nervous system emboli (e.g., aseptic meningitis) may complicate SBE, whereas septic emboli (e.g., acute bacterial meningitis) may complicate ABE. Particularly with ABE, there may be valvular perforation or destruction resulting in acute congestive heart failure. It is often these complications that dictate whether and when surgery will occur. The indications for surgical intervention are shown in Table 95.8. As a general principle, paravalvular abscess or intractable congestive heart failure requires urgent surgical intervention. Persistent vegetations or embolic disease that occurs after 1 week of appropriate antibiotic therapy should also prompt surgical consideration.

Prognosis

The prognosis of all forms of IE depends directly on any complications related to the infection. Consequently, early diagnosis and initiation of appropriate antibiotic therapy is the key to limiting mortality. Recent studies have supported the role of early surgical intervention, when appropriate, as a significant aid to decreasing morbidity and mortality, specifically in relation to having fewer embolic events. If treated in a timely fashion and with appropriate antibiotics, the cure rate for viridans streptococci and *S. bovis* is estimated to be 98% in NVE and up to 88% in PVE. Right-sided endocarditis in intravenous drug abusers is usually caused by *S. aureus* and typically has a cure rate of 90% in NVE and 75% to 80% in PVE. However, among non–intravenous drug abusers, cure rates in IE involving *S. aureus* are far lower: 60% to 70% in NVE and 50% in PVE. When gram-negative bacilli or fungal organisms are the causative agent, cure rates are significantly lower (40% to 60%). Increased age, diabetes, aortic valve involvement, and developing complications of IE including congestive heart failure and emboli to the central nervous system are all highly predictive of increased mortality and morbidity.

Infective Endocarditis Prophylaxis

The most recent American Heart Association guidelines state that not all patients require antibiotic prophylaxis and that prophylaxis should be considered only for a specific subset of patients. Antibiotic prophylaxis is indicated for patients with prosthetic heart valves, cardiac transplant recipients with valvular disease, patients with a history of IE, and patients with certain forms of congenital heart disease. Among patients with congenital heart disease, only those with unrepaired or partially repaired lesions and those with prosthetic material should receive prophylactic antibiotics (grade IIa recommendation).

Typically, antibiotic regimens used for prophylaxis against IE prior to invasive procedures above the waist are directed against viridans streptococci. For invasive dental procedures, the recommended prophylactic agent is amoxicillin, 2 g PO as a single dose 30 to 60 minutes before the procedure. In patients with penicillin allergy, clindamycin or a macrolide may be substituted.

ENDARTERITIS AND SUPPURATIVE PHLEBITIS

The term *infectious endarteritis* refers to an intravascular infection of the arteries that affects coarctation of the aorta, aortic valve shunts, or a patent ductus arteriosus, analogous to IE at other sites. As with IE, continuous or high-grade bacteremia in the absence of an intracardiac vegetation should suggest the diagnosis. Imaging studies (e.g., PET scans) delineate the extent of arterial involvement. Treatment is the same as for IE.

The term *suppurative thrombophlebitis* refers to an intravenous infection that is characterized by an intravenular abscess; it is a complication of the use of central venous catheters. Patients have phlebitis with high fevers (>102° F, compared with <102° F in uncomplicated phlebitis with fevers), bacteremia due to a skin organism (e.g., *S. aureus*) and often expressible pus from the catheter site. Treatment consists of a combination of antibiotic therapy and resection of the involved venous segment.

CENTRAL VENOUS CATHETER–RELATED BLOODSTREAM INFECTIONS

Central venous catheter–related bloodstream infections are relatively common, with an annual incidence of approximately

TABLE 95.6   **Principles of Therapy for Infective Endocarditis**
1. Antibiotic selection initially is made empirically on the basis of physical examination and clinical history.
2. Bactericidal antibiotics are prescribed.
3. The MIC and MBC are measured to ensure adequate dosing of the agent.
4. Intermittent dosing provides superior penetration into the thrombus compared with continuous infusion; penetration is directly related to peak serum level.
5. The patient should be treated in a health care facility for the first 1–2 wk.
6. The usual duration of therapy is 4–6 wk.
7. A 4-wk course is appropriate for an uncomplicated case of NVE (a shorter course of 2 wk may be appropriate in some cases); a 6-wk course is required for the treatment of PVE and those infections with large vegetations (i.e., infection by HACEK organisms[a]).

Modified from Brusch JL: Diagnosis of infective endocarditis. In Brusch JL, editor: Infective endocarditis, New York, 2007, Informa Healthcare, pp 241-254.
MBC, Minimal bactericidal concentration; *MIC,* minimal inhibitory concentration.
[a]HACEK organisms: *Haemophilus* spp, *Aggregatibacter actinomycetemcomitans, Cardiobacterium hominis, Eikenella corrodens,* and *Kingella kingae.*

200,000 in the United States. Central venous catheter infection should be suspected if the patient develops fevers, chills, or hypotension without another obvious source of infection. The likelihood of infection increases with the length of time the catheter is in place. In addition to the clinical signs, blood cultures, drawn from the periphery as well as the line, should demonstrate growth of the causative organism. If the culture drawn from the catheter shows growth of bacteria at least 2 hours earlier than the peripheral blood cultures do, infection associated with the central line, rather than bacteremia in the setting of a catheter, should be strongly suspected.

Treatment of catheter-related infections varies depending on what action will be taken with the catheter (i.e., removal, exchange, or salvage). In any case, empirical antibiotic therapy should be initiated against the most likely pathogens. Empirical therapy should cover *S. aureus* and nosocomial gram-negative bacilli. Therapy may then be modified based on the results of blood cultures or catheter tip culture. If a catheter-related bloodstream infection is suspected, immediate removal of the catheter should occur if the infection has led to septic shock or IE. The line also should be removed if blood cultures remain positive for the causative organism for 72 hours longer or if evidence of septic thrombophlebitis develops.

Salvage therapy may be considered in hemodynamically stable patients except when the infection is caused by *S. aureus, P. aeruginosa, Bacillus* spp, *Micrococcus* spp, *Propionibacterium acnes* or other propionibacteria, fungi, or mycobacteria. Salvage therapy relies on concurrent use of systemic antimicrobial agents and antibiotic or ethanol locks.

Guidewire exchange should be reserved for cases in which there is a high risk for complications if the original catheter were to be removed. Guidewire exchange has a lower chance of eliminating the infection than does removal of the catheter.

For a deeper discussion of these topics, please see Chapter 67, ❖ "Infective Endocarditis," in *Goldman-Cecil Medicine,* 26th Edition.

TABLE 95.7 Antimicrobial Treatment of Infective Endocarditis

Causative Organism	NATIVE VALVE		PROSTHETIC VALVE	
	Antibiotic Therapy	Comments	Antibiotic Therapy	Comments
Penicillin-susceptible viridans streptococci, *Streptococcus bovis*, and other streptococci with MIC of penicillin ≤0.1 µg/mL	Penicillin G or ceftriaxone for 4 wk[a]	A 2-wk regimen of penicillin G or ceftriaxone combined with gentamicin may be considered in patients with right-sided NVE without evidence of embolic disease (excluding pulmonary emboli) or other complications.	Penicillin G for 6 wk and gentamicin for 2 wk[a]	Shorter duration of treatment with an aminoglycoside (2 wk) is usually appropriate for PVE due to penicillin-susceptible viridans streptococci, *S. bovis*, or other streptococci with MIC of penicillin ≤0.1 µg/mL.
Relatively penicillin-resistant streptococci (MIC of penicillin >0.1 to 0.5 µg/mL)	Penicillin G for 4 wk and gentamicin for 2 wk[a]		Penicillin G for 6 wk and gentamicin for 4 wk[a]	
Streptococcus species with MIC of penicillin >0.5 µg/mL, *Enterococcus* species, or *Abiotrophia* species	Penicillin G or ampicillin and gentamicin for 4–6 wk[a]	6 wk of therapy is recommended for patients with symptoms lasting >3 mo, myocardial abscess, or selected other complications.	Penicillin G or ampicillin and gentamicin for 6 wk[a]	A study by Fernando-Hidalgo et al. showed that the combination of ampicillin and ceftriaxone is as effective as the combination of ampicillin and gentamicin for treating *Enterococcus faecalis* IE.
Methicillin-susceptible staphylococci	Nafcillin or oxacillin for 4–6 wk, with or without addition of gentamicin for the first 3–5 days of therapy[b]	In the few patients infected with a penicillin-susceptible staphylococcus, penicillin G may be substituted for nafcillin or oxacillin.	Nafcillin or oxacillin with rifampin for 6 wk and gentamicin for 2 wk[b]	It may be prudent to delay initiation of rifampin for 1 or 2 days, until therapy with two other effective antistaphylococcal drugs has been initiated.
Methicillin-resistant staphylococci	Vancomycin, with or without addition of gentamicin, for the first 3–5 days of therapy		Vancomycin with rifampin for 6 wk and gentamicin for 2 wk	If the staphylococcus is resistant to gentamicin, an alternative third agent should be chosen on the basis of in vitro susceptibility testing.
Right-sided staphylococcal NVE in selected patients	Nafcillin or oxacillin with gentamicin for 2 wk	This 2-wk regimen has been studied for infections caused by an oxacillin- and aminoglycoside-susceptible isolate. Exclusions to short-course therapy include any cardiac or extracardiac complications associated with IE, persistence of fever for ≥7 days, and infection with HIV. Patients with vegetations >1–2 cm should probably be excluded from short-course therapy.		
HACEK organisms[c]	Ceftriaxone for 4 wk	Ampicillin and gentamicin for 4 wk is an alternative regimen, but some isolates may produce β-lactamase, thereby reducing the efficacy of this regimen.	Ceftriaxone for 6 wk	Ampicillin and gentamicin for 6 wk is an alternative regimen, but some isolates may produce β-lactamase, thereby reducing the efficacy of this regimen.

Modified from Mylonakis E, Calderwood SB: Infective endocarditis in adults, N Engl J Med 345:1318-1330, 2001.

HIV, Human immunodeficiency virus; *IE,* infective endocarditis; *NVE,* native valve endocarditis; *PVE,* prosthetic valve endocarditis.

[a]Vancomycin therapy is indicated for patients with confirmed immediate hypersensitivity reactions to β-lactam antibiotics.

[b]For patients who have IE due to methicillin-susceptible staphylococci and are allergic to penicillin, a first-generation cephalosporin or vancomycin may be substituted for nafcillin or oxacillin. Cephalosporins should be avoided in patients with confirmed immediate-type hypersensitivity reactions to β-lactam antibiotics.

[c]HACEK organisms: *Haemophilus* spp, *Aggregatibacter actinomycetemcomitans*, *Cardiobacterium hominis*, *Eikenella corrodens*, and *Kingella kingae*.

TABLE 95.8 Echocardiographic Indications for Surgical Intervention in Infective Endocarditis

Vegetation

Persistent vegetation after systemic embolization

Anterior mitral valve leaflet vegetation (particularly if ≥1 embolic events occur during the first 2 wk of antimicrobial therapy)[a]

Increase in vegetation size despite appropriate antimicrobial therapy[a,b]

Valvular Dysfunction

Acute aortic or mitral insufficiency with signs of ventricular failure[b]

Heart failure unresponsive to medical therapy[b]

Valve perforation or rupture[b]

Large abscess or extension of abscess despite appropriate antimicrobial therapy[b]

Paravalvular Extension

Valvular dehiscence, rupture, or fistula[b]

New heart block[b]

Large abscess or extension of abscess despite appropriate antimicrobial therapy[b]

Modified from Baddour LM, Wilson WR, Bayer AS, et al: Infective endocarditis: diagnosis, antimicrobial therapy, and management of complications: a statement for healthcare professionals from the Committee on Rheumatic Fever, Endocarditis, and Kawasaki Disease, Council on Cardiovascular Disease in the Young, and the Councils on Clinical Cardiology, Stroke, and Cardiovascular Surgery and Anesthesia, American Heart Association; endorsed by the Infectious Diseases Society of America, Circulation 111:e394-e433, 2005.

[a]Surgery may be required because of risk of embolization.

[b]Surgery may be required because of failure of medical therapy or heart failure.

SUGGESTED READINGS

Baddour LM, Cha YM, Wilson WR: Clinical practice: infections of cardiovascular implantable electronic devices, N Engl J Med 367:842–849, 2012.

Blauwkamp TA, Thair S, Rosen MJ, et al: Analytical and clinical validation of a microbial cell-free DNA sequencing test for infectious disease, Nat Microbiol 4:663–674, 2019.

Bor DH, Woolhandler S, Nardin R, et al: Infective endocarditis in the U.S., 1998–2009: a nationwide study, PloS One 8(e60033):2013.

Brouqt P, Raoult D: Endocarditis due to rare and fastidious bacteria, Clin Microbiol Rev 14:177–207, 2001.

Fernández-Hidalgo N, Almirante B, Gavaldà J, et al: Ampicillin plus ceftriaxone is as effective as ampicillin plus gentamicin for treating *Enterococcus faecalis* infective endocarditis, Clin Infect Dis 56:1261–1268, 2013.

Fournier PE, Thuny F, Richet H, et al: Comprehensive diagnostic strategy for blood culture-negative endocarditis: a prospective study of 819 new cases, Clin Infect Dis 51:131–140, 2010.

Garcia-Cabera E, Fernandez-Hidalgo N, Almirante B, et al: Neurological complications of infective endocarditis: risk factors, outcome, and impact of cardiac surgery: a multicenter observational study, Circulation 127:2272–2284, 2013.

Iversen K1, Ihlemann N1, Gill SU1, et al: Partial oral versus intravenous antibiotic treatment of endocarditis, N Engl J Med 380(5):415–424, 2019.

Kadri AN, Wilner B, Hernandez AV, et al: Geographic trends, patient characteristics, and outcomes of infective endocarditis associated with drug abuse in the United States from 2002 to 2016, JAHA 8:e12969, 2019.

Kang DH, Kim YJ, Kim SH, et al: Early surgery versus conventional treatment for infective endocarditis, N Engl J Med 366:2466–2473, 2012.

Kiefer T, Park L, Tribouilloy C, et al: Association between valvular surgery and mortality among patients with infective endocarditis complicated by heart failure, J Am Med Assoc 306:2239–2247, 2011.

Li JS, Sexton DJ, Mick N, et al: Proposed modifications to the Duke criteria for the diagnosis of infective endocarditis, Clin Infect Dis 30:633–638, 2000.

Mermel LA, Allon M, Bouza E, et al: Clinical practice guidelines for the diagnosis and management of intravascular catheter-related infection: 2009 Update by the Infectious Disease Society of America, Clin Infect Dis 49:1–45, 2009.

Morrisette T, Miller MA, Montague BT, et al: Long-acting lipoglycopeptides: "Lineless Antibiotics" for serious infections in persons who use drugs, Open Forum Infect Dis 6(7):ofz274, 2019, Published 2019 Jun 5.

Mylonakis E, Calderwood SB: Infective endocarditis in adults, N Engl J Med 345:1318–1330, 2001.

Steele JM, Seabury RW, Hale CM, et al: Unsuccessful treatment of methicillin-resistant Staphylococcus aureus endocarditis with dalbavancin, J Clin Pharm Ther 43:101–103, 2018.

Wilson W, Taubert KA, Gewitz M, et al: Prevention of infective endocarditis: guidelines from the American Heart Association: a guideline from the American Heart Association Rheumatic Fever, Endocarditis, and Kawasaki Disease Committee, Council on Cardiovascular Disease in the Young, and the Council on Clinical Cardiology, Council on Cardiovascular Surgery and Anesthesia, and the Quality of Care and Outcomes Research Interdisciplinary Working Group, Circulation 116:1736–1754, 2007.

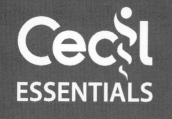

Acute Bacterial Skin and Skin Structure Infections

Sajeev Handa

DEFINITION

Acute bacterial skin and skin structure infections (ABSSSIs) comprise infections of the skin, subcutaneous tissue, fascia, and muscle by a multitude of organisms. The focus of this chapter is on bacterial causes; however, references will be made to select viruses and fungi.

EPIDEMIOLOGY

ABSSSIs are among the most common infections found in all age groups. Although the exact incidence is unknown, several factors predispose to development of ABSSSIs:

- Epidermal breaks caused by trauma, surgical wounds, human or animal bites, or dry and irritated skin with concomitant tinea infection
- Immunosuppressed states caused by malnutrition, diabetes mellitus, or acquired immunodeficiency syndrome (AIDS)
- Chronic venous or lymphatic insufficiency

PATHOLOGY

Infectious Mechanisms

Microbes penetrate the integument after entering through a cut, bite, or hair follicle. Components of the host's defense system, including oxygen radicals, complement, immunoglobulins, macrophages, lymphocytes, and granulocytes, are recruited to the site of invasion through a vast plexus of dermal capillaries.

Bacteria contain proteins whose *N*-terminal amino acid sequence begins with an *N*-formyl-methionine group that is chemoattractive to phagocytes, including macrophages and granulocytes. Other microbial cell wall components, such as the zymosan of yeast, endotoxins of gram-negative bacteria, and the peptidoglycans of gram-positive bacteria, activate the alternative complement pathways, producing serum-derived chemotactic factors. Efflux of phagocytes occurs from the capillary through endothelial cell interstices and follows the gradient of chemotactic factors derived from bacteria and serum to the site of active infection.

Activated endothelial cells also produce chemotactic cytokines such as interleukin-8 (IL-8). Activated granulocytes synthesize leukotriene B_4 from arachidonic acid, a potent chemoattractant for leukocytes. Production of proinflammatory cytokines such as IL-1, IL-6, and tumor necrosis factor augments immune function, inducing fever, priming neutrophils, and increasing antibody production and synthesis of acute phase reactants such as C-reactive protein.

Cytokine-driven stimulation of endothelial cells generates nitric oxide and prostaglandins, both of which cause vasodilatation. The net physiologic effect is greater blood flow to the tissue, causing acute inflammation. As described by Celsus (30 BC to 38 AD), acute inflammation is characterized by rubor (i.e., redness), calor (i.e., increased heat), tumor (i.e., swelling), dolor (i.e., pain), and, as added by Virchow in the 19th century, function laesa (i.e., loss of function). Chapter 88 discusses host defenses against infection in more depth.

Pathologic Manifestations

Impetigo is characterized by thick, crusted lesions with rounded or irregular margins that typically occur on the face. Most cases are caused by *Staphylococcus aureus*, including methicillin-resistant *S. aureus* (MRSA), or by group A streptococci (e.g., *Streptococcus pyogenes*). Certain strains of streptococci causing impetigo have been implicated in the development of poststreptococcal glomerulonephritis.

Folliculitis is a superficial bacterial infection of the hair follicles. Purulent material is found in the epidermis. It manifests as clusters of multiple, small, raised, pruritic, erythematous lesions that are typically less than 5 mm in diameter.

Furuncles (i.e., boils) are infections of the hair follicle. Purulent material extends through the dermis into the subcutaneous tissue, where small abscesses may form. A carbuncle is coalescence of several inflamed follicles into a single inflammatory mass. Purulent drainage exudes from multiple follicles.

Cellulitis is superficial inflammation of the skin and underlying tissues. It is characterized by erythema, warmth, and tenderness of the involved area (Fig. 96.1). Erysipelas ("red skin") is a variant of cellulitis that is predominantly caused by toxin-producing *S. pyogenes*. It manifests as a superficial, spreading, warm, erythematous (fiery red) lesion distinguished by its indurated and elevated margin. Lymphatic involvement and vesicle formation are common. Groups B, C, and D streptococci may also be implicated (Fig. 96.2).

Necrotizing fasciitis is a progressive and rapidly spreading inflammatory reaction deep in the fascia associated with secondary necrosis of the subcutaneous tissues. Thrombosis of the dermal vessels is responsible for tissue necrosis. Necrotizing fasciitis may be polymicrobial (type I), involving aerobic microbes (e.g., streptococci, staphylococci, gram-negative bacilli) and anaerobes (e.g., *Peptostreptococcus*, *Bacteroides*, *Clostridioides* spp), or it may be monomicrobial (type II) and caused by *S. pyogenes* (Fig. 96.3). When involving the scrotum and perineal area, it is known as *Fournier gangrene*.

Pyomyositis is a less serious infection involving the musculature that results from direct inoculation of bacteria. For example, infection can result from injection drug use or from secondary seeding by *S. aureus* or group A β-hemolytic streptococci from an incidental bacteremia or a hematoma caused by non-penetrating trauma.

Ecthyma is an ulcerative pyoderma of the skin that extends into the dermis (unlike impetigo). It is caused by group A streptococci and *Pseudomonas* species.

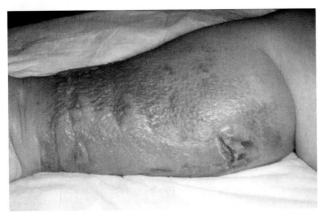

Fig. 96.1 Ill-defined erythema and edema with bullae formation is characteristic of lower extremity cellulitis. (From Pride HB: Cellulitis and erysipelas. In Zaoutis LB, Chiang VW, editors: Comprehensive pediatric hospital medicine, Philadelphia, 2007, Mosby, Fig. 156-1.)

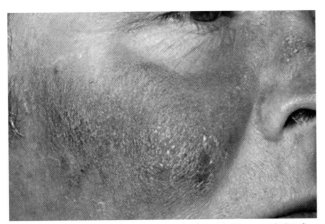

Fig. 96.2 Sharply defined erythema and edema is characteristic of erysipelas. (From Pride HB: Cellulitis and erysipelas. In Zaoutis LB, Chiang VW, editors: Comprehensive pediatric hospital medicine, Philadelphia, 2007, Mosby, Fig. 156-2.)

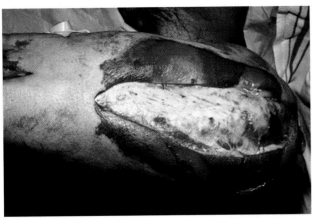

Fig. 96.3 Spontaneous necrotizing fasciitis due to *Clostridioides septicum*. The patient developed sudden onset of severe pain in the forearm. Swelling rapidly ensued, and he sought medical treatment. Crepitus was found on physical examination, and gas in the soft tissue was verified with routine radiographs. Immediate surgical débridement revealed necrotizing fasciitis but sparing of the muscle. Notice the purple-violaceous appearance of the skin. (From Stevens DL, Aldape MJ, Bryant AE. Necrotizing fasciitis, gas gangrene, myositis and myonecrosis. In Cohen J, Powderly WG, Opal SM, editors: Infectious diseases, ed 3, London, 2010, Mosby, Fig. 10-11.)

ETIOLOGY AND CLINICAL PRESENTATION

Causative Organisms

A multitude of organisms can cause ABSSSIs. However, three are most common: *S. pyogenes*, *S. aureus*, and *Streptococcus agalactiae*.

S. pyogenes (i.e., group A β-hemolytic streptococci) is a gram-positive coccus that may cause erysipelas, streptococcal cellulitis, necrotizing fasciitis, myositis, myonecrosis, and streptococcal toxic shock syndrome. Streptococcal cellulitis arises from infection of wounds, burns, or surgical incisions and may progress to involve large areas. Injection drug users and individuals with impaired lymphatic drainage are at high risk. Systemic manifestations include fever, chills, malaise with or without associated lymphangitis, and bacteremia. In contrast to erysipelas, the affected area is not raised, and the demarcation between involved skin and uninvolved skin is indistinct. The lesions tend to be more pink than fiery red.

Streptococcal toxic shock syndrome manifests with hypotension and is associated with acute kidney injury, elevated aminotransferases, rash or soft tissue necrosis, and coagulopathy. It may be complicated by the acute respiratory distress syndrome. Isolation of the organism from a sterile site provides a definite diagnosis.

S. aureus is a gram-positive coccus that is found in the anterior nares of up to 30% of healthy people. It is responsible for a variety of invasive and suppurative infections. Localized ABSSSIs include furuncles, carbuncles, bullous and nonbullous impetigo, mastitis, ecthyma, cellulitis, and wound and foreign body infections. Bacteremia may be complicated by septicemia, endocarditis, pericarditis, pneumonia, empyema, osteomyelitis, and abscesses of the soft tissue, muscle, and viscera.

Staphylococcal toxic shock syndrome is typically associated with tampon use but may occur after childbirth or surgery and can be associated with cutaneous lesions. It manifests with the acute onset of fever, erythroderma, hypotension, and multisystem involvement (e.g., acute kidney injury, elevated levels of aminotransferases, coagulopathy, nausea, vomiting, diarrhea).

Community-associated MRSA is the most common identifiable cause of ABSSSIs in the emergency department. Isolates contain genes encoding for multiple toxins, including cytotoxins that result in leukocyte destruction and tissue necrosis.

S. agalactiae (a group B streptococcus) is a gram-positive diplococcus. It may account for up to one third of ABSSSIs among adults. Cellulitis, foot ulcers, and infection of decubitus ulcers are common manifestations. Cellulitis has been associated with foreign bodies such as breast or penile implants. Less commonly, polymyositis, blistering dactylitis, and necrotizing fasciitis may occur.

Other Organisms

Aeromonas hydrophila, *Aeromonas veronii*, and *Aeromonas schubertii* are gram-negative rods found in salt and fresh water. They may cause mild to severe wound infections after injury, producing cellulitis, myonecrosis, and rhabdomyolysis. Necrotizing fasciitis has been reported with *A. veronii* and *A. schubertii* infections. *Aeromonas* wound infections have also been reported as a result of the medicinal use of leeches.

Arcanobacterium haemolyticum is a gram-positive, weakly acid-fast bacillus. It has been isolated from soft tissue infections, including chronic ulcers, cellulitis, and paronychia.

Bacillus anthracis is a gram-positive bacillus that forms spores. Transdermal inoculation of the spores from even incidental trauma can result in cutaneous anthrax. It manifests initially as a small, pruritic papule that becomes surrounded by painless, nonpurulent vesicles that easily rupture, leaving a black eschar at the base of the ulceration.

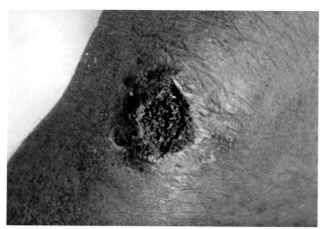

Fig. 96.4 Cutaneous anthrax lesion on the skin of the forearm caused by the bacterium *Bacillus anthracis*. (From Centers for Disease Control and Prevention: Public health image library. Available at http://phil.cdc.gov/Phil/home.asp. Accessed October 31, 2014.)

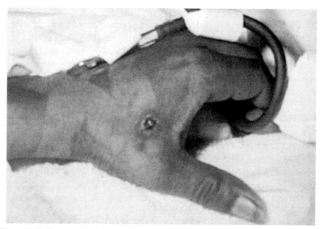

Fig. 96.5 Tularemic ulcer with eschar formation after percutaneous inoculation of *Francisella tularensis*. (From Beard CB, Dennis DT: Tularemia. In Cohen J, Powderly WG, Opal SM, editors: Infectious diseases, ed 3, London, 2010, Mosby.)

Uncomplicated disease heals without scar formation in 1 to 3 weeks. Serious cutaneous disease is marked by extensive edema, worsening inflammation, and toxemia (Fig. 96.4).

Bartonella henselae is a gram-negative bacillus that causes cat-scratch disease. Between 3 and 10 days after a bite or scratch from a cat or other vector, a tender, erythematous papule appears. Lymphadenopathy ipsilateral to the site of inoculation occurs 1 to 3 weeks later, and the patient typically experiences constitutional symptoms. The lymphadenopathy may take months to resolve.

Capnocytophaga canimorsus is a thin, gram-negative bacillus with tapered ends. It is strongly associated with dog (primarily) and cat bites and scratches. Asplenic patients are at particular risk for sepsis due to this organism.

Clostridioides perfringens is an anaerobic, large, gram-positive rod. It can cause cellulitis or life-threatening necrotizing infections of skin, muscle, and other soft tissues. The latter is characterized by rapidly progressive tissue destruction, gas in tissues, shock, and death. Conditions such as trauma or illicit drug injection produce anaerobic tissue conditions that favor the organism. The condition can also develop in patients with bowel carcinoma or neutropenia. Gram stain of tissue or exudate reveals large, gram-positive rods and no inflammatory cells.

Edwardsiella tarda is a gram-negative rod found in fresh water environments. It is associated with wound infections, abscesses, and bacteremia. The mortality rate is high among patients with liver disease and iron overload.

Eikenella corrodens is a gram-negative bacillus that is part of the normal human oral flora. It is an important pathogen in human bite wounds, closed-fist injuries, and infections seen in chronic finger or nail biters. Severe soft tissue infection may occur, leading to septic arthritis and osteomyelitis.

Erysipelothrix rhusiopathiae is a gram-positive rod, but it may appear as gram-negative because of rapid decolorization. Its major reservoir is in domestic swine, and infection occurs by direct cutaneous contact through a cut or abrasion. Disease is characterized as erysipeloid (i.e., subacute cellulitis with vesiculation), as a diffuse cutaneous eruption with systemic symptoms, or as bacteremia that is often associated with endocarditis.

Francisella tularensis is a gram-negative coccobacillus found in rabbits, hares, hamsters, and rodents. Ulceroglandular tularemia occurs 3 to 5 days after humans are inoculated cutaneously during contact with any of these species. A papule is formed initially, followed by ulceration

with enlargement of the regional lymph nodes. Vesicles may be seen. If left untreated, the ulcer remains for weeks before healing, leaving a residual scar. Suppuration of the affected lymph nodes is the most common complication, occurring despite appropriate treatment (Fig. 96.5). *B. anthracis* and *F. tularensis* have been used as agents in bioterrorism.

Mycobacterium marinum is an atypical, acid-fast bacillus; it is the most common atypical mycobacterium that causes infection in humans. After inoculation of a skin abrasion or puncture wound in salt or fresh water (nonchlorinated), lesions appear as papules on an extremity. Lesions progress to shallow ulcers and form scars. Typically, lesions are solitary, but they may take on the appearance of ascending, sporotrichoid-like, nodular lymphangitis that may involve the local joint or tendons.

Mycobacterium leprae is a slow-growing, acid-fast bacillus that cannot be grown in vitro. It is the cause of leprosy (Hansen disease). It is primarily transmitted by the airborne route and causes chronic disfiguring skin lesions and nerve damage.

For a deeper discussion of this topic, please see Chapter 310, ❖ "Leprosy (Hansen Disease)" in *Goldman-Cecil Medicine*, 26th Edition.

Pasteurella multocida is a gram-negative coccobacillus that may occur at the site of a scratch or bite from a dog or cat. Cellulitis results within 24 hours of the injury, producing swelling, erythema, tenderness, serous or purulent discharge with or without regional lymphadenopathy, chills, and fever.

Pseudomonas aeruginosa is a gram-negative rod and primarily a nosocomial pathogen. In the community, serogroup 0:11 may cause folliculitis related to the use of hot tubs, whirlpools, and swimming pools. Typically, the eruption occurs 48 hours after exposure and consists of tender, pruritic papules, papulopustules, or nodules. It is an important pathogen in burn wound infections, which may progress to sepsis.

Vibrio vulnificus is a gram-negative bacillus that is spread by contamination of a superficial wound with warm seawater. It can cause rapidly developing and intense cellulitis, necrotizing fasciitis, and ulcer formation. Aggressive soft tissue infection may occur with necrosis, fever, sepsis, and bullae formation. Ingestion of raw oysters, particularly by immunocompromised patients (e.g., liver cirrhosis, iron overload) may be followed 1 to 3 days later by septicemia associated with necrotizing cutaneous lesions.

Select Fungi and Viruses

Cryptococcus neoformans, *Candida albicans*, *Histoplasma capsulatum*, *Blastomyces dermatitidis*, *Coccidioides immitis*, and opportunistic fungi can have skin manifestations. Opportunistic fungi, including *Aspergillus* species, fungi in the order Mucorales, and *Fusarium* species, can infect the skin of immunocompromised patients. Skin manifestations of fungal infections include papules, nodules, circumscribed erythematous lesions, ulcers, verrucous lesions, and eschars.

Sporothrix schenckii is a dimorphic fungus ubiquitous primarily in the tropical parts of North and South America. Cutaneous inoculation from thorny plants (e.g., rose bushes) is followed by development of a painless papule that enlarges slowly to become a nodular lesion with a violaceous hue or ulceration. Secondary lesions may form along the lymphatic drainage distribution. Exposure to herpes simplex virus types 1 and 2 (HSV-1 and HSV-2) at abraded skin sites allows entry into the epidermis and dermis. Infection typically occurs from sexual contact, but it occasionally occurs at extraoral or extragenital sites, such as the hands of health care workers, producing a painful erythema primarily at the junction of the nail bed and skin (i.e., whitlow). This progresses to a vesicopustular lesion that can mimic a bacterial infection (i.e., paronychia). Sexually transmitted diseases are discussed in Chapter 100.

Primary varicella-zoster virus (VZV) infection occurs by the respiratory route but may occur through contact with infected lesions. Viremia results in crops of papules that primarily occur on the trunk and progress to vesicles and then to pustules, followed by crusting. Zoster or shingles represents reactivation of the latent virus in the sensory neurons of the dorsal root ganglion, resulting in pain that proceeds to a rash in the distribution of the affected dermatome in a few days. The appearance of papules and vesicles in a unilateral dermatomal distribution confirms the diagnosis. Ramsay Hunt syndrome occurs when the VZV infection involves the geniculate ganglia and causes a painful eruption in the ear canal and tympanic membrane that is associated with ipsilateral seventh cranial nerve palsy. Vesicles that appear on the tip of the nose (i.e., Hutchinson sign) may be preceded by development of ophthalmic zoster and involvement of the cornea. Immunosuppressed individuals are at higher risk for disseminated disease.

Table 96.1 provides a classification for the spectrum of skin involvement by bacteria and fungi.

TABLE 96.1   Classification of Bacterial and Mycotic Infections of the Skin

Disease or Disorder	Microorganisms
Primary Pyodermas	
Impetigo	*Staphylococcus aureus*, group A streptococci
Folliculitis	*S. aureus*, *Candida* spp, *Pseudomonas aeruginosa* (diffuse folliculitis), *Malassezia furfur*, *Pityrosporum ovale*
Furuncles and carbuncles	*S. aureus*
Paronychia	*S. aureus*, group A streptococci, *Candida*, *P. aeruginosa*
Ecthyma	Group A streptococci, *Pseudomonas* spp
Erysipelas	Group A streptococci
Chancriform lesions	*Treponema pallidum*, *Haemophilus ducreyi*, *Sporothrix*, *Bacillus anthracis*, *Francisella tularensis*, *Mycobacterium ulcerans*, *Mycobacterium marinum*
Membranous ulcers	*Corynebacterium diphtheriae*
Cellulitis	Group A or other streptococci, *S. aureus*; rarely, various other organisms
Infectious Gangrene and Gangrenous Cellulitis	
Streptococcal gangrene and necrotizing fasciitis	Group A streptococci, mixed infections with Enterobacteriaceae and anaerobes
Progressive bacterial synergistic gangrene	Anaerobic streptococci plus a second organism (*S. aureus*, *Proteus* spp)
Gangrenous balanitis and perineal phlegmon	Group A streptococci, mixed infections with enteric bacteria (*Escherichia coli*, *Klebsiella* spp), anaerobes
Gas gangrene, crepitant cellulitis	*Clostridioides perfringens* and other clostridial species; *Bacteroides* spp, peptostreptococci, *Klebsiella* spp, *E. coli*
Gangrenous cellulitis in immunosuppressed patients	*Pseudomonas*, *Aspergillus* spp, agents of mucormycosis
Preexisting Skin Lesions With Secondary Bacterial Infections	
Burns	*P. aeruginosa*, *Enterobacter* spp, various other gram-negative bacilli, various streptococci, *S. aureus*, *Candida* spp, *Aspergillus* spp
Eczematous dermatitis and exfoliative erythrodermas	*S. aureus*, group A streptococci
Chronic ulcers (varicose, decubitus)	*S. aureus*, streptococci, coliform bacteria, *P. aeruginosa*, peptostreptococci, enterococci, *Bacteroides* spp., *C. perfringens*
Dermatophytosis	*S. aureus*, group A streptococci
Traumatic lesions (abrasions, animal bites, insect bites)	*Pasteurella multocida*, *C. diphtheriae*, *S. aureus*, group A streptococci
Vesicular or bullous eruptions (varicella, pemphigus)	*S. aureus*, group A streptococci
Acne conglobata	*Cutibacterium* (formerly *Propionibacterium*) *acnes*
Hidradenitis suppurativa	*S. aureus*, *Proteus* spp. and other coliforms, streptococci, peptostreptococci, *P. aeruginosa*, *Bacteroides* spp.
Intertrigo	*S. aureus*, coliforms, *Candida* spp
Pilonidal and sebaceous cysts	Peptostreptococci, *Bacteroides* sp, coliforms, *S. aureus*
Pyoderma gangrenosa	*S. aureus*, peptostreptococci, *Proteus* spp and other coliforms, *P. aeruginosa*

TABLE 96.1   Classification of Bacterial and Mycotic Infections of the Skin—cont'd

Disease or Disorder	Microorganisms
Cutaneous Involvement in Systemic Infections	
Bacteremias	*S. aureus*, group A streptococci (and other groups such as D), *Neisseria meningitidis, Neisseria gonorrhoeae, P. aeruginosa, Salmonella typhi, Haemophilus influenzae*
Infective endocarditis	Viridans streptococci, *S. aureus*, group D streptococci, and others
Fungemias	*Candida* spp, *Cryptococcus* spp, *Blastomyces dermatitidis, Fusarium*
Listeriosis	*Listeria monocytogenes*
Leptospirosis (Weil disease and pretibial fever)	*Leptospira interrogans* serotypes
Rat-bite fever	*Streptobacillus moniliformis, Spirillum minus*
Melioidosis	*Burkholderia pseudomallei*
Glanders	*Burkholderia mallei*
Carrión's disease (verruga peruana)	*Bartonella bacilliformis*
Scarlet Fever Syndromes	
Scarlet fever	Group A streptococci, rarely *S. aureus*
Scalded skin syndrome	*S. aureus* (phage group II)
Toxic shock syndrome	Group A streptococci, *S. aureus* (pyrogenic toxin–producing strains)
Parainfectious and Postinfectious Nonsuppurative Complications	
Purpura fulminans (manifestation of disseminated intravascular coagulation)	Group A streptococci, *N. meningitidis, S. aureus*, pneumococcus
Erythema nodosum	Group A streptococci, *Mycobacterium tuberculosis, Mycobacterium leprae, Coccidioides immitis, Leptospira autumnalis, Yersinia enterocolitica, Legionella pneumophila*
Erythema multiforme–like lesions (rarely), guttate psoriasis	Group A streptococci
Other Lesions	
Erythrasma	*Corynebacterium minutissimum*
Nodular lesions	*Candida, Sporothrix, S. aureus* (botryomycosis), *M. marinum, Leishmania brasiliensis*; leprosy due to *M. leprae* can cause popular lesions, nodular, and ulcerative lesions
Hyperplastic (pseudoepitheliomatous) and proliferative lesions (e.g., mycetomas)	*Nocardia* spp, *Scedosporium apiospermum* (formerly *Pseudallescheria boydii*), *Blastomyces dermatitidis, Paracoccidioides brasiliensis, Phialophora, Cladosporium*
Vascular papules/nodules (bacillary angiomatosis, epithelioid angiomatosis)	*Bartonella henselae, Bartonella quintana*
Annular erythema (erythema chronicum migrans)	*Borrelia burgdorferi*

Modified from Mandell GL, Bennett JE, Dolin R, editors: Mandell, Douglas, and Bennett's principles and practice of infectious diseases, ed 9, Philadelphia, 2020, Elsevier.

DIAGNOSIS

A thorough medical history is critical; it should assess the specific risk factors, such as travel history, animal contacts, marine exposures, occupational and avocational hazards (e.g., farming, gardening), and immune status. If an animal bite has occurred, the timing of the bite, circumstances of injury, and health status of the animal should be determined. Human bites are classified as self-inflicted, occlusal (i.e., intentional), or closed-fist injuries.

In addition to wound assessment, evaluation for other transmissible pathogens, including human immunodeficiency virus (HIV), HSV, *Treponema pallidum* (the etiologic agent of syphilis), and hepatitis B and C viruses, should be pursued. A thorough clinical examination should follow. Initial antimicrobial management, if indicated, is directed by the history and physical examination findings.

Evaluation of hospitalized patients should include a complete blood count and a basic metabolic panel. The C-reactive protein level may be useful as a marker for inflammation and guidance for treatment. The creatine phosphokinase concentration may be helpful, but it is not specific for cases of compartment syndrome and necrotizing fasciitis involving the musculature. Cultures are not indicated for uncomplicated common forms of ABSSSIs managed in the outpatient setting. The benefit of blood cultures for cellulitis in hospitalized patients is uncertain because the yield is low. Cultures are indicated for patients who require incision and drainage because of the risk of deep structure and underlying tissue involvement.

The most sensitive and specific test for the diagnosis of HSV and VZV cutaneous lesions is nucleic acid amplification. A sample is scraped from the base of an active dermal lesion with a swab. Direct fluorescent antibody testing is less sensitive. Incision and drainage of these lesions is contraindicated.

Special Diagnostic Considerations
Animal Bites

Blood cultures, tissue biopsy, and aspirates for culture of aerobic or anaerobic organisms are preferred methods in cases of animal bites.

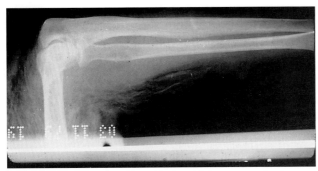

Fig. 96.6 Radiograph of patient with clostridial myonecrosis shows gas in the tissues. (Courtesy J.W. Tomford, MD.)

Human Bites

Wounds swabs may produce misleading information in cases of human bites. A Gram stain should be performed to assess organisms, neutrophils (i.e., inflammation), and squamous epithelial cells (i.e., superficial contamination). If feasible, tissue biopsy or aspiration of the infected site can provide specimens for aerobic and anaerobic culture.

Traumatic Wounds

The optimal time to acquire specimens for cultures is immediately after débridement of the wound site and not within the first 48 hours post-trauma. Analysis of initial cultures should focus on common pathogens, and additional testing should be reserved for uncommon or rare infections associated with unusual circumstances, such as *Vibrio* species after salt water exposure. Tissue biopsy and special stains may be required in certain situations, such as suspected infection with *M. marinum*.

Burn Wounds

Before sampling, the burn area must be clean and devoid of topical antimicrobial agents. Sampling of the burn wound by either surface swab or tissue biopsy for culture is recommended for monitoring the presence and extent of infection. Quantitative evaluation of swab or culture specimens is recommended twice weekly to monitor colonization. Evidence of systemic infection related to the wound should prompt blood cultures.

Diabetic Foot Infections

Superficial swab cultures of ulcerations can be misleading and should be avoided. If surgical débridement is performed, deep tissue specimens should be sent to the microbiology laboratory for evaluation.

Radiographs should be obtained if bone involvement is suspected, and they may also be useful in demonstrating soft tissue gas before crepitus is detected (Fig. 96.6). Magnetic resonance imaging is the most sensitive modality. Chapter 89 discusses the laboratory diagnosis of infectious diseases in more detail.

Differential Diagnosis

Many noninfectious conditions can mimic SSTIs:
- Brown recluse spider bite
- Contact dermatitis
- Gout
- Psoriatic arthritis with distal dactylitis
- Reactive arthritis
- Relapsing polychondritis
- Ruptured Baker cyst
- Mixed cryoglobulinemia due to immune complex disease from chronic hepatitis C or B infection (may have an erythematous rash)
- Pyoderma gangrenosum
- Sweet syndrome (acute febrile neutrophilic dermatosis)
- Venous stasis

TREATMENT

Pharmacologic and Supportive Care

Mild cases of cellulitis may be managed on an outpatient basis with penicillin VK, amoxicillin, or if the patient has a history of a penicillin skin rash and nothing to suggest an IgE-mediated reaction, cephalexin. If clinically unclear whether the infection is due to *S. pyogenes* or *S. aureus*, get cultures and start empiric therapy with amoxicillin or penicillin VK or cephalexin and trimethoprim-sulfamethoxazole (TMP-SMX).

Azithromycin, linezolid, tedizolid or delafloxacin may be used in patients with a past history of IgE-mediated allergic reaction to β-lactam antibiotics. Severe cellulitis should be managed with parenteral penicillin, cefazolin or ceftriaxone. Vancomycin may be used in patients with allergies to penicillin.

Concomitant tinea infection should be treated with a topical antifungal agent such as clotrimazole or terbinafine.

For suspected methicillin-susceptible *S. aureus* (MSSA) (fluctuance or positive Gram stain) dicloxacillin may be used as an outpatient, nafcillin or oxacillin as an inpatient. For MRSA, doxycycline or TMP-SMX may be used as an outpatient, vancomycin as an inpatient. Other inpatient options include daptomycin, telavancin, ceftaroline, clindamycin (watch for inducible resistance), or linezolid. Dalbavancin and oritavancin may be used as alternatives in ABSSSIs for those who are moderately ill and who refuse hospitalization.

Note that neither doxycycline nor TMP-SMX provides adequate streptococcal coverage. A β-lactam antibiotic may be considered for hospitalized patients with nonpurulent cellulitis, with modification to MRSA-active treatment if there is no clinical response. Cellulitis associated with an abscess requires surgical drainage.

In addition to supportive care, urgent surgical consultation should be obtained in the event that crepitus, bullae, rapidly evolving cellulitis, or pain disproportionate to physical examination findings suggests necrotizing fasciitis. Initial parenteral therapy with vancomycin, daptomycin, or linezolid combined with piperacillin-tazobactam or a carbapenem (either meropenem or ertapenem) is appropriate. Type II necrotizing fasciitis due to *S. pyogenes* or clostridial myonecrosis should prompt combined therapy with parenteral penicillin and clindamycin. Clindamycin by virtue of its mechanism of action suppresses streptococcal toxin and cytokine production. The use of intravenous immune globulin in cases of necrotizing fasciitis remains controversial.

Compartment syndrome requires emergent surgical decompression to prevent muscle necrosis and irreversible neuronal damage.

Special Treatment Considerations
Animal Bites

Mild cases of animal bites (dog or cat) may be treated with amoxicillin-clavulanate. Inpatient parenteral agents including ampicillin-sulbactam or piperacillin-tazobactam may be used for those who require hospitalization.

For patients with a penicillin allergy, a fluoroquinolone plus clindamycin may be used in dog bites, doxycycline in cat bites. As with all animal bites, rabies postexposure prophylaxis and vaccination should be considered.

Human Bites

Patients who have human bite wounds without evidence of infection should receive prophylactic treatment with amoxicillin-clavulanate for 3 to 5 days. Closed-fist injuries require radiographic evaluation and consultation with a hand surgeon for possible wound exploration. Parenteral treatment with ampicillin-sulbactam or moxifloxacin is recommended.

Burn Wounds

Systemic therapy with antibiotics and antifungals is reserved for burn patients demonstrating signs of sepsis or septic shock. Infection due to mucormycoses requires liposomal amphotericin B.

Diabetic Foot Infections

Simple infections such as cellulitis are most often caused by group A streptococci or *S. aureus* and should be managed accordingly. If ulcers do not have purulence or inflammation, antimicrobials are not indicated. Severe limb-threatening infections require surgical evaluation and broad-spectrum antibiotic coverage because infection tends to include aerobic and anaerobic organisms. Empirical therapy directed at *P. aeruginosa* is not usually necessary unless the patient has other risk factors. MRSA-active treatment is recommended for patients with a history of MRSA, when the local prevalence of MRSA is high in the community, or if the infection is severe. All wounds require adequate wound irrigation and débridement.

Marine Lacerations and Punctures

The treatment regimen for marine lacerations and punctures should include doxycycline and ceftazidime or a fluoroquinolone to provide adequate coverage for *V. vulnificus*. Treatment of fresh water injuries should also include a third- or fourth-generation cephalosporin (i.e., ceftazidime or cefepime) or a fluoroquinolone. If *M. marinum* is suspected, treatment with clarithromycin, minocycline, doxycycline, sulfamethoxazole-trimethoprim, or rifampin plus ethambutol is appropriate. Aeromonas wound infections may be treated with either ciprofloxacin or levofloxacin.

Others

Cellulitis or wound infections attributed to *A. hemolyticum* may be treated with clindamycin, erythromycin, vancomycin, or tetracycline.

Animal handlers with cutaneous anthrax infection (naturally acquired) require treatment with amoxicillin or penicillin. Cases of suspected bioterrorism, however, must be treated with ciprofloxacin or levofloxacin and must be reported immediately.

Tularemia is treated with streptomycin or gentamicin/tobramycin. Mild cases may be treated with ciprofloxacin or doxycycline. Azithromycin is the drug of choice for cat-scratch disease. For individuals at risk for *E. rhusiopathiae* infection, the treatment of choice is penicillin or amoxicillin for localized skin infection and parenteral penicillin or ceftriaxone for widespread skin infection.

Lymphocutaneous/cutaneous sporotrichosis (*S. schenkii*) may be treated with itraconazole.

HSV and VZV infections are susceptible to acyclovir, famciclovir, or valacyclovir if treatment is indicated.

PROGNOSIS

Full recovery is expected for patients with simple ABSSSIs provided they receive appropriate treatment. For those who develop complications such as necrotizing fasciitis, the estimated mortality rate is between 30% and 70%. The prognosis is guarded for patients with multiple comorbidities and those who are immunosuppressed.

SUGGESTED READINGS

Cohen J, Powderly WG, Opal SM, editors: Infectious diseases, ed 3, London, 2010, Mosby.

Golstein EJ: Bite wounds and infectious, Clin Infect Dis 14:633–640, 1992.

Herchline T: Cellulitis treatment and management. Available at http://emedicine.medscape.com/article/214222-overview. Accessed October 31, 2014.

Lipsky BA, Berendt AR, Cornia PB, et al: Infectious Diseases Society of America clinical practice guideline for the diagnosis and treatment of diabetic foot infections, Clin Infect Dis 54:132–173, 2012, 2012.

Liu C, Bayer A, Cosgrove SE, et al: Clinical practice guidelines by the Infectious Diseases Society of America for the treatment if methicillin-resistant *Staphylococcus aureus* infectious in adults and children, Clin Infect Dis 52:e18–e55, 2011.

Miller JM, Binnicker MJ, et al: A guide to utilization of the microbiology laboratory for diagnosis of infectious diseases: 2018 update by the Infectious Diseases Society of America (IDSA) and the American Society of Microbiology (ASM). Available at http://www.idsociety.org/practice-guideline/laboratory-diagnosis-of-infectious-diseases/.

Spelman D: Cellulitis and skin abscess: clinical manifestations and diagnosis. UpToDate. Available at http://www.uptodate.com/contents/cellulitis-and-skin-abscess-clinical-manifestations-and-diagnosis. Accessed September 16, 2019.

Stevens DL, Bisno AL, Chambers HF, et al: Practice guidelines for the diagnosis and management of skin and soft-tissue infections, Clin Infect Dis 59(2):e10–e52, 2014.

97

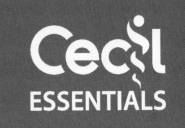

Intraabdominal Infections

Eric Benoit

INTRODUCTION

Intraabdominal infections are common in hospitalized patients, both as a primary indication for admission and as a complication. Although antibiotics play a central role in treatment, many of these patients require source control and warrant surgical consultation to manage complications such as perforation and peritonitis. Intraabdominal infections are usually polymicrobial and are caused by components of bowel flora most commonly including aerobic *Escherichia coli* and other Enterobacteriaceae and anaerobic *Bacteroides fragilis* and streptococci.

SOURCE CONTROL AND TIMING OF ANTIBIOTICS

Early administration of broad-spectrum antibiotics has become standard of care in patients with suspected infection. Mortality increases with every hour delay to antibiotic therapy in septic patients. However, antibiotics alone are not sufficient for most intraabdominal infections, which require an intervention to control the source of infection. Purulence must be drained. This may be surgical removal of the infected tissue as in appendectomy, percutaneous drainage of an abscess by interventional radiology, or endoscopic retrograde cholangiopancreatography (ERCP) to remove obstructing stones in cases of cholangitis. Appropriate source control has been shown to be as important to outcomes as early antibiotics.

The Study to Optimize Peritoneal Infection Therapy (STOP-IT) trial demonstrated that most intraabdominal infections may be treated for 4 days after achieving source control, and this is true even for complicated intraabdominal infections. Furthermore, prolonged antibiotic administration in the setting of intraabdominal infection has been shown to increase the risk of further infections including bacteremia and *Clostridioides difficile* infections as well as increase the rate of in-hospital mortality. Source control and limited duration of antibiotic therapy, therefore, are critical considerations in management of intraabdominal infections.

PERITONITIS

Peritonitis is a disseminated infection of the peritoneal cavity and typically presents with diffuse, rather than localized, tenderness. Primary peritonitis is most often seen in patients with ascites from cirrhosis. It may be managed with antibiotics alone and after therapy may require suppressive antibiotics. Diagnosis is made by sampling peritoneal fluid; the diagnosis is likely if the number of neutrophils is greater than 250/microliter. Cultures may be negative.

Secondary peritonitis is due to an inciting event, such as hollow viscus perforation, ischemia, or a localized abscess that has spread, and is more common than primary peritonitis. Any intraabdominal infection

may progress from localized to diffuse peritonitis. Patients with peritonitis are tachycardic, tachypneic, and acutely uncomfortable. They avoid movement, and merely jostling the bed exacerbates the pain. The patient's abdomen may be rigid due to involuntary tightening of the muscles of the abdominal wall (guarding). The onset of peritonitis is ominous as it may herald the progression to sepsis and septic shock. These cases mandate emergent surgical consultation prior to imaging and almost always require operative exploration. Elderly patients or those with diabetes or on steroids may have a blunted response to peritonitis, and they should therefore be approached with a high degree of suspicion regarding complications of intraabdominal infections.

APPENDICITIS

When the lumen of the appendix is occluded either by a lymphatic tissue or a fecalith, mucosal fluid secretion and bacterial overgrowth cause an increase in pressure within the appendix. This eventually leads to venous outflow obstruction and further increases in pressure until arterial inflow is compromised, and the resulting ischemia leads to perforation. The classic presentation is periumbilical pain that migrates to the right lower quadrant, frequently associated with anorexia and nausea. Patients in whom the appendix has perforated often describe a sudden relief of localized pain followed several hours later by the onset of diffuse peritonitis. Leukocytosis, if present, is often not severe.

CT scan of the abdomen has become the diagnostic tool of choice with both sensitivity and specificity over 90% for detection of acute appendicitis. Findings of dilated appendix, fecalith, and stranding of the fat around the appendix are suggestive of acute appendicitis. CT scan may also detect a phlegmon (inflamed infected tissue) or abscess associated with perforated appendicitis (Fig. 97.1). Ultrasound may be useful in children, and MRI is an alternative imaging modality in pregnant women. Clinical diagnosis of appendicitis can be challenging, but the prevalence of CT scanning has markedly decreased the negative appendectomy rate.

Management of appendicitis is appendectomy, most often performed laparoscopically. Although there is active research into antibiotic therapy alone for appendicitis, this is not standard of care. Those patients who do not undergo appendectomy at initial presentation are often brought back for an interval appendectomy 6 to 8 weeks later. More advanced appendicitis may present with a phlegmon. These patients may be treated with antibiotics until an abscess develops, at which time drainage by interventional radiology is appropriate. Patients who develop signs of physiologic compromise (tachycardia, tachypnea, peritonitis) should instead proceed urgently to the operating room. Patients with perforated appendicitis may require more extensive surgery (e.g., ileo-cecectomy) and have a higher risk of intraabdominal abscess. Appendicitis is a polymicrobial infection with colonic bacteria *E. coli* and *Bacteroides* species being common. Antibiotics should be

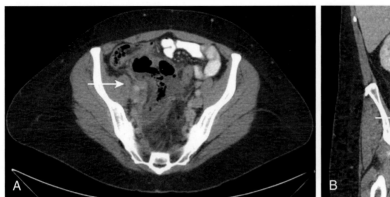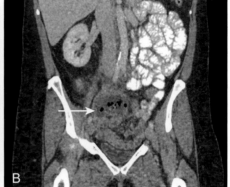

Fig. 97.1 CT scan may detect (A) a phlegmon (inflamed infected tissue) or (B) an abscess associated with perforated appendicitis.

administered until time of operation and may be stopped thereafter in uncomplicated cases. Perforated appendicitis should be treated with antibiotics for 4 days after surgery. Uncomplicated appendicitis has a mortality rate less than 1%, but perforation, particularly in pediatric or elderly patients, increases the risk significantly. Other complications after appendicitis include intraabdominal abscess and wound infection.

DIVERTICULITIS

Diverticula are herniations of the colonic mucosa through naturally occurring openings in the taenia coli through which vessels run (Fig. 97.2). They are most commonly found in the sigmoid colon but may also be present in the right colon. The presence of diverticula (diverticulosis) increases with age, and diet influences their development. Low dietary fiber present in the Western diet contributes to rates of diverticulosis as high as 50% in Americans over the age of 80. Dietary fiber is thought to protect against the development of diverticulosis as demonstrated by lower rates of disease in countries in Asia and Africa. While right-sided diverticular disease is prone to bleeding, sigmoid diverticulosis risks development of diverticulitis, the infection of diverticula. Approximately 10% to 25% of patients with diverticula will develop diverticulosis in their lifetime. The pathophysiology of diverticulitis is similar to appendicitis: occlusion of a diverticulum results in bacterial overgrowth, vascular compromise, ischemia, and perforation.

Diverticulitis can present with varying degrees of severity that are enumerated by the Hinchey classification (Table 97.1). Local infection and inflammation may be self-limited or managed by outpatient antibiotics. More severe cases result in microperforation of diverticula with contained air or abscess within the bowel wall. Complicated diverticulitis results in a distant abscess in the abdomen, pelvis, or retroperitoneum. The most severe cases present with free intraabdominal air and purulent or feculent peritonitis.

Patients with diverticulitis most often present with left lower quadrant pain and tenderness. More severe cases may develop fever and leukocytosis whereas the most critical cases have frank peritonitis and physiologic compromise such as acidosis, acute kidney injury, and hypotension.

Imaging with IV contrast CT scan is standard of care, both to diagnose the presence and severity of diverticulitis and to identify complications such as abscess. However, patients with peritonitis due to suspected diverticulitis should not undergo CT imaging but instead belong in the operating room. An upright chest radiograph may demonstrate free air under the diaphragm in cases of perforation.

Simple diverticulitis may be managed with outpatient antibiotics. More severe cases require admission for intravenous antibiotics, bowel rest, and IV hydration. As the pain and tenderness resolve, the diet may be advanced. Complicated diverticulitis with uncontained abscess requires source control, and these patients should be evaluated for drainage by interventional radiology or laparoscopic drainage by surgery. Patients with free perforation require urgent surgery for control of contamination and resection of perforated bowel. The most common procedure is sigmoid resection with colostomy, although there is increasing evidence to support primary anastomosis with or without a diverting loop ileostomy.

Delayed complications of diverticulitis include abscess, colonic stricture, and fistulae (colovesical, colovaginal or coloenteric). Patients should undergo colonoscopy 6 to 8 weeks after diverticulitis to assess for colorectal cancer. Diverticulitis may recur in up to 20% of patients over 10 years. Although recurrence does make patients more prone to future episodes, the risk of complications such as free perforation does not increase with recurrence. Recurrent diverticulitis does not mandate surgery, but for those patients who wish to avoid future episodes elective sigmoid resection removes the burden of left-sided diverticulosis, effectively eliminating the source of disease. Regardless of treatment plan, patients should be encouraged to pursue a high-fiber diet. Former teaching suggested eliminating such foods as seeds and nuts, but this has not been shown to influence the recurrence of diverticulitis.

Like appendicitis, diverticulitis is a polymicrobial infection with colonic flora such as *E. coli* and bacteroides predominating. Accordingly, broad-spectrum antibiotics such as piperacillin/tazobactam are appropriate, and the duration of therapy is 7 to 10 days. Patients who have resolution of pain while on IV antibiotics may be transitioned to oral agents (such as amoxicillin/clavunate) and complete their course as outpatients.

INFECTIOUS BOWEL DISEASE

Infectious Colitis

Infectious colitis is an infection of the bowel that may be caused by bacteria (*E. coli, Campylobacter, Shigella*), viruses (*norovirus, rotavirus, cytomegalovirus*) or parasites (*Entamoeba histolytica*) (see Chapter 98). These patients present with abdominal pain that is frequently crampy in nature and diarrhea. In older patients particularly, infectious colitis may be difficult to distinguish from ischemic colitis. CT scan with IV contrast demonstrates inflammation of the bowel wall, in contrast to the lack of enhancement seen in ischemic disease. The presence of free fluid is ominous. For many patients with infectious colitis either symptomatic relief or a course of antibiotics directed at potential bacterial

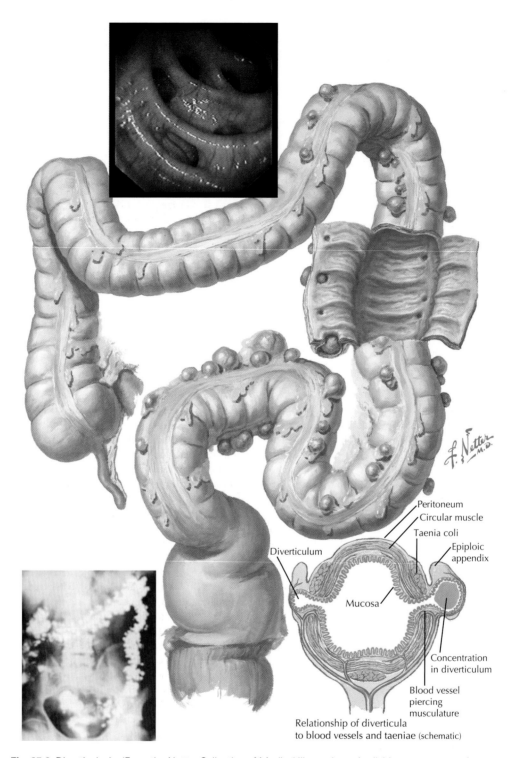

Peritoneum
Circular muscle
Taenia coli
Epiploic appendix
Diverticulum
Mucosa
Concentration in diverticulum
Blood vessel piercing musculature

Relationship of diverticula
to blood vessels and taeniae (schematic)

Fig. 97.2 Diverticulosis. (From the Netter Collection of Medical Illustrations. Available at www.netterimages.com. Accessed October 31, 2014.)

pathogens may be sufficient. Stool samples may aid in diagnosis and treatment of different pathogens. Regardless of etiology these patients require frequent abdominal exams, and in rare cases, should they progress to worsening pain, fever, tachycardia, hypotension or peritonitis, they belong in the operating room for colectomy.

Cytomegalovirus Colitis

Cytomegalovirus is a common, self-limited viral infection, but it may cause colitis in immunocompromised patients, such as transplant patients, those who undergo frequent steroid therapy for ulcerative

colitis or as a complication of acquired immunodeficiency syndrome (AIDS). Diagnosis of CMV colitis requires a high degree of suspicion in the correct clinical context. Colonoscopy may demonstrate ulcerated lesions and CMV immunohistochemistry on biopsy specimens. Antimicrobial therapy is with an antiretroviral agent such as ganciclovir. Surgery is reserved for complications such as perforation.

Clostridioides difficile Colitis

Clostridioides difficile colitis is most often a complication of antibiotic therapy. It occurs when healthy intraluminal bacteria are depleted,

TABLE 97.1   Hinchey Classification of Diverticulitis

Class	Description	Treatment
0	Mild clinical diverticulitis	Oral antibiotics
Ia	Contained pericolic inflammation or phlegmon	IV antibiotics, bowel rest
Ib	Contained pericolic abscess	IV antibiotics, bowel rest
II	Pelvic, distant intraabdominal or retroperitoneal abscess	Percutaneous drainage, IV antibiotics
III	Purulent peritonitis	Operative drainage/resection
IV	Feculent peritonitis	Operative drainage/resection

allowing pathogenic species to predominate. Agents such as cephalosporins, fluoroquinolones, and clindamycin are commonly implicated, but any antibiotic in the preceding several months—even a single dose—increases the risk of *C. difficile* colitis. Hospitalized patients are at greater risk due to exposure, although community strains of *C. difficile* have been identified. Patients most often present with frequent diarrhea as well as abdominal pain. The disease is associated with leukocytosis sometimes as high as 30,000 to 40,000. Diagnosis is ideally sought in those with greater than or equal to three unformed stools in 24 hours. The diagnosis is confirmed by stool studies with PCR for toxin.

Infectious Disease Society Guidelines recommend oral vancomycin or fidaxomicin for 10 days for an initial episode of *C. difficile* colitis. Metronidazole is an alternative if vancomycin or fidaxomicin are not available. Fulminant cases may be treated with oral vancomycin and, if ileus is present, vancomycin enema. Intravenous metronidazole should also be given. First recurrent infection should be treated with oral vancomycin as a tapered and pulsed regimen or a course of fidaxomicin. Fecal microbiota transplant, which aims to repopulate the gut with healthy bacteria, should be considered investigational; while studies have demonstrated utility in patients with recurrent or refractory disease, it carries the risk of disease transmission.

Patients with *C. difficile* colitis remain at high risk of bowel perforation as well as progression to toxic megacolon. Those patients with signs of unremitting inflammation, such as fevers, tachycardia, and tenderness despite antibiotic therapy should be considered for surgery. Patients who progress to perforation often present in shock with hypotension and altered mental state. These patients have a high mortality, and surgery mandates subtotal colectomy, often with vancomycin enemas to the rectal stump.

BILIARY INFECTIONS

Cholecystitis

The gallbladder, like the appendix, is an anatomic cul-de-sac, and the narrow neck of the cystic duct is prone to occlusion by gallstones or edema, preventing drainage of bile and leading to bacterial overgrowth. The undrained, infected fluid present in cholecystitis leads to an increase in pressure that may progress to ischemia of the gallbladder wall, gangrene, and perforation.

Cholecystitis may be distinguished from biliary colic by its duration; biliary colic typically resolves spontaneously and patients are able to eat. Cholecystitis, on the other hand, is marked by prolonged pain and tenderness and is frequently associated with leukocytosis. Patients report right-sided or epigastric pain, often associated with a recent meal. On examination, tenderness is usually localized to the right upper quadrant. However, in cases of gallbladder perforation, infected

bile may flow down the right paracolic gutter, leading to right-sided abdominal or even pelvic tenderness. The classic finding of Murphy's sign is the abrupt cessation of inspiration when palpating the right upper quadrant; the excursion of the diaphragm during inspiration displaces the gallbladder inferiorly to the examiner's hand, resulting in sudden, exquisite pain that interrupts the patient's breathing.

Right upper quadrant ultrasound is the imaging modality of choice in which gallbladder wall thickening, a distended, fluid-filled gallbladder, and pericholecystic fluid are findings consistent with acute cholecystitis. Occasionally the ultrasound will demonstrate air within the gallbladder wall; emphysematous cholecystitis carries a high mortality and these patients warrant urgent surgery. Although CT scan is sensitive and specific for diagnosis of cholecystitis, it exposes patients to radiation and may miss non-cholesterol stones. Laboratory values include leukocytosis and elevated total bilirubin from the blockage of bile drainage.

Treatment of acute cholecystitis is cholecystectomy, most often performed laparoscopically. In patients who are too sick to tolerate operation, percutaneous drainage with a cholecystostomy tube is appropriate to decompress the infected gallbladder. Some of these patients will recover sufficiently to undergo surgery 6 weeks later. Other patients, particularly those who are elderly and frail, may require prolonged cholecystotomy tube drainage.

Acalculous Cholecystitis

Acalculous cholecystitis occurs in critically ill patients, particularly those who have not been receiving enteral nutrition. Diagnosis requires a high index of suspicion, especially in intubated patients. Patients with unexplained fever or leukocytosis without an obvious source should undergo a right upper quadrant ultrasound, which demonstrates a distended gallbladder with a thickened wall. These patients are frequently too sick to tolerate surgical cholecystectomy and instead are referred to interventional radiology for a cholecystostomy tube to decompress the infected bile. Tube drainage is often continued until the patient recovers sufficiently to tolerate cholecystectomy, although for some chronically debilitated patients tube drainage may suffice.

Cholangitis

Cholangitis is an infection due to the blockage of the bile ducts, most commonly from gallstones. These patients present with right upper quadrant or epigastric pain. The classic findings are right upper quadrant pain, fever and jaundice (Charcot's triad) that may progress to include altered mental status and shock (Reynold pentad). These patients have infected bile or pus within the biliary tree, and this is best drained by ERCP with sphincterotomy and stenting. Ascending cholangitis can be an aggressive infection, with patients rapidly progressing to septic shock. Antibiotics alone are not sufficient and source control is mandated. Suspicion of cholangitis should prompt urgent consultation with a gastroenterologist and a surgeon, and these patients often require fluid resuscitation and admission to a critical care unit.

Right upper quadrant ultrasound in cases of cholangitis may demonstrate cholelithiasis without findings of cholecystitis, but a dilated common bile duct as evidence of a stone that has passed out of the gallbladder. Important laboratory values include hyperbilirubinemia, leukocytosis, and an elevated alkaline phosphatase as evidence of bile duct irritation. Patients who undergo ERCP with sphincterotomy may have pneumobilia on subsequent imaging; this is due to retrograde passage of air from the duodenum into the biliary tree and may not indicate infection.

Bacteria associated with biliary infections include *E. coli*, *Klebsiella*, and *Pseudomonas* but may also include *Enterobacter* and *Bacteroides*. Biliary cultures are rarely used to guide therapy and therefore antimicrobial therapy uses broad-spectrum agents such as piperacillin/tazobactam. For patients with uncomplicated acute cholecystitis, antibiotics may be stopped after surgery. For those too sick to undergo surgery, antibiotics are continued for 7 to 10 days, depending on clinical improvement. Patients with cholangitis require broad-spectrum antibiotics and source control in addition to fluid resuscitation.

PANCREATITIS AND PANCREATIC INFECTION

Pancreatitis is usually a self-limited inflammation of the pancreas. A small percentage progress to pancreatic necrosis, which is a risk factor for infected pancreatitis. Percutaneous aspiration of pancreatic fluid collections is not advised due to the risk of seeding sterile collections. The question of prophylactic antibiotics in cases of pancreatic necrosis has been actively debated for decades. In the interest of limiting antibiotic exposure and selecting resistant organisms, we defer antibiotics until there is evidence of infected pancreatic necrosis such as air within the fluid collections. Antibiotic therapy consists of a carbapenem and the duration is dictated by clinical improvement. Patients with infected pancreatic necrosis may undergo percutaneous drainage, but the infected material is often too thick to allow drainage. However, drain placement may be preliminary to creating a tract for videoscopic-assisted retroperitoneal dissection (VARDS) of the necrotic pancreas. Patients with unremitting signs of infection and inflammation may require surgery for drain placement and lavage.

INTRAABDOMINAL ABSCESS

Solid Organ Abscesses

Solid organ abscesses may form in the liver, spleen, and less commonly, the kidneys. The most common causes of hepatic abscess in the United States are biliary tract infection and portal vein bacteremia from diverticulitis, appendicitis or inflammatory bowel disease. Colonic bacteria predominate, including *Klebsiella pneumoniae* as well as anaerobes such as *Bacteroides* spp, *Fusobacterium*, and streptococcal species. Hepatic abscesses present with fevers as well as right upper quadrant pain. Laboratory data may show leukocytosis and an elevated alkaline phosphatase. CT scan is the imaging modality of choice for solid organ abscesses. Hepatic abscesses may be multifocal. Multiple, small abscesses are best treated with antibiotics whereas large, persistent abscesses may require percutaneous drainage. An important but less common cause of liver abscess is due to *Entamoeba histolytica* found frequently in patients from developing countries (see Chapter 105).

Splenic abscesses are seen in patients with infected endocarditis resulting from septic emboli or those who have undergone splenic artery embolization. The resulting ischemia and necrosis of splenic parenchyma serves as a nidus of infection. The presence of a splenic abscess should prompt a search for the source, including an echocardiogram. Patients may be treated with antibiotics and percutaneous drainage. Splenic abscesses may prove difficult to eradicate, in which case splenectomy is an option.

Renal abscesses may occur with recurrent pyelonephritis, particularly in the setting of urinary tract obstruction such as staghorn renal calculi. Source control may require percutaneous nephrostomy tubes to drain infected urine that cannot drain distally, and nephrectomy is indicated in cases of recurrent, fistulizing disease.

Intraabdominal and Intrapelvic

Intraabdominal and intrapelvic abscesses may form as a result of other infections, such as perforated appendicitis or diverticulitis, or after surgery for perforation of the alimentary tract. The omentum may form adhesions around the site of infection, walling it off from the remainder of the peritoneal cavity and allowing an abscess to form. This appears as a rim-enhancing fluid collection on CT scan (with IV contrast). Small abscesses (≈2 cm) in an otherwise healthy patient with a functional immune system may be treated with antibiotics alone. Larger abscesses, however, may require drainage because antibiotics may not penetrate the infected area. Source control may be accomplished with percutaneous drainage, although this warrants a conversation with the interventional radiologist as the location may preclude safe drainage due to surrounding structures. Operative source control may be accomplished by laparoscopic washout and drain placement, although this carries the risk of bowel injury due to the friable nature of the inflamed bowel. Small bowel often forms the wall of deep abscesses and surgical source control often requires bowel resection in these cases.

CONCLUSIONS

Although early administration of broad-spectrum antibiotics remains a mainstay of treatment of intraabdominal infections, source control and early identification of complications such as peritonitis from free perforation or disseminated infection are critical concepts for the clinician to understand. CT scan with intravenous contrast is the imaging modality of choice for most intraabdominal infections. Elderly patients, those with diabetes, those taking steroids, or immunocompromised patients may not mount the same exuberant response of peritonitis, and therefore they must be approached with a high degree of suspicion regarding complications.

SUGGESTED READINGS

Ahmed M: Acute cholangitis—an update, World J Gastrointest Pathophysiol 9(1):1–7, 2018.

Broad JB, Wu Z, Ng J, et al: Diverticular disease management in primary care: how do estimates from community-dispensed antibiotics inform provision of care? PloS One 14(7):e0219818, 2019.

Eid AI, Mueller P, Thabet A, Castillo CF, Fagenholz P: A step-up approach to infected abdominal fluid collections: not just for pancreatitis, Surg Infect (Larchmt) 21(1):54–61, 2020.

Kumar A, Roberts D, Wood KE, et al: Duration of hypotension before initiation of effective antimicrobial therapy is the critical determinant of survival in human septic shock, Crit Care Med 34(6):1589–1596, 2006.

Kumar V, Fischer M: Expert opinion on fecal microbiota transplantation for the treatment of clostridioides difficile infection and beyond, Expert Opin Biol Ther 20(1):73–81, 2020.

Maconi G, Barbara G, Bosetti C, Cuomo R, Annibale B: Treatment of diverticular disease of the colon and prevention of acute diverticulitis: a systematic review, Dis Colon Rectum 54(10):1326–1338, 2011.

Martinez ML, Ferrer R, Torrents E, et al: Impact of source control in patients with severe sepsis and septic shock, Crit Care Med 45(1):11–19, 2017.

Mazuski JE, Tessier JM, May AK, et al: The surgical infection society revised Guidelines on the management of intra-abdominal infection, Surg Infect (Larchmt) 18(1):1–76, 2017.

McDonald LC, Gerding DN, Johnson S, et al: Clinical practice guidelines for clostridium difficile infection in adults and children: 2017 update by the Infectious Diseases Society of America (IDSA) and society for Healthcare Epidemiology of America (SHEA), Clin Infect Dis 66(7):987–994, 2018.

Mourad MM, Evans R, Kalidindi V, Navaratnam R, Dvorkin L, Bramhall SR: Prophylactic antibiotics in acute pancreatitis: endless debate, Ann R Coll Surg Engl 99(2):107–112, 2017.

Podda M, Cillara N, Di Saverio S, et al: Antibiotics-first strategy for uncomplicated acute appendicitis in adults is associated with increased rates of peritonitis at surgery. A systematic review with meta-analysis of randomized controlled trials comparing appendectomy and non-operative management with antibiotics, Surgeon 15(5):303–314, 2017.

Riccio LM, Popovsky KA, Hranjec T, et al: Association of excessive duration of antibiotic therapy for intra-abdominal infection with subsequent extra-abdominal infection and death: a study of 2,552 consecutive infections, Surg Infect (Larchmt) 15(4):417–424, 2014.

Sawyer RG, Claridge JA, Nathens AB, et al: Trial of short-course antimicrobial therapy for intraabdominal infection, N Engl J Med 372(21):1996–2005, 2015.

Schlottmann F, Gaber C, Strassle PD, Patti MG, Charles AG: Cholecystectomy vs. Cholecystostomy for the management of acute cholecystitis in elderly patients, J Gastrointest Surg 23(3):503–509, 2019.

98

Infectious Diarrhea

Awewura Kwara

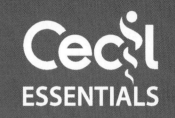

DEFINITION AND EPIDEMIOLOGY

Diarrhea is defined as the passage of three or more unformed stools or more than 250 g of unformed stools per day. Based on duration, diarrhea can be classified as *acute* (less than 14 days), *persistent* (14 to 29 days), or *chronic* (30 or more days). *Infectious diarrhea* is diarrhea that has an infectious etiology and is often associated with symptoms and signs of enteric involvement, such as nausea, vomiting, abdominal cramps, passage of bloody stool (dysentery), or systemic symptoms. Organisms responsible for infectious diarrhea include bacteria, viruses, and parasites.

In the United States (US), acute diarrhea is common, with an estimated annual burden of 179 million outpatient visits, nearly 500,000 hospitalizations, and more than 5000 deaths. The Foodborne Diseases Active Surveillance Network (FoodNet) maintained by the Centers for Disease Control and Prevention (CDC) provides data on pathogen-specific burden of diarrheal diseases in the United States by monitoring cases of laboratory-diagnosed infections caused by eight enteric pathogens transmitted through food in 10 US sites. During 2018, FoodNet identified 25,606 infections, 5893 hospitalizations, and 120 deaths. *Campylobacter*, *Salmonella*, and Shiga toxin–producing *Escherichia coli* (STEC) were the most common identified infections.

PATHOLOGY

Diarrhea is an alteration of movement of ions and water that leads to an increase in water content, volume, or frequency of stools. Under normal conditions, up to 9 L of fluid is passed through the adult gastrointestinal tract daily. Almost 98% of this fluid is absorbed, and only 100 to 200 mL is excreted in stools. Enteric pathogens or microbial toxins that are ingested can overcome host defenses and alter this balance toward a net secretion, leading to diarrhea. A large number of microorganisms are normally ingested with every meal. Host defense mechanisms against enteric pathogens include low gastric pH, rapid transit of bacteria through the proximal small intestine, cellular immune responses, and antibody production. In addition, large numbers of normal bacterial flora inhabit the intestines and prevent colonization by enteric pathogens.

Alteration of the normal defense mechanisms can put individuals at risk for infectious diarrhea. Individuals with gastric resection or achlorhydric states have increased frequency of infection due to *Salmonella*, *Giardia lamblia*, and helminths, whereas some organisms, such as *Shigella* or rotavirus, survive the extreme acidity of the gastric environment. Some viral, bacterial, and parasitic infections are more common in patients with impaired cellular or humoral immunity. More than 99% of the normal colonic flora is made up of anaerobic bacteria; they produce fatty acids and cause acidic pH,

which is important for resistance to colonization. Alteration of the bacterial flora due to broad-spectrum antibiotic therapy predisposes some individuals to the development of *Clostridioides difficile* infection (CDI).

The virulence factors employed by enteric pathogens include inoculum size, adherence factors, toxin production, and invasion. Organisms such as *Shigella*, enterohemorrhagic *Escherichia coli* (EHEC), *G. lamblia*, and *Entamoeba histolytica* need as few as 10 to 100 organisms to produce infection, whereas *Vibrio cholerae* needs 10^5 to 10^8 organisms to cause disease. Infectious diarrhea can be classified as noninflammatory or inflammatory based on pathogenesis. Noninflammatory diarrhea is caused by pathogens that adhere to the mucosa of small intestine, disrupting the absorptive and/or secretory processes without causing inflammation or destruction. Pathogens that cause noninflammatory diarrhea include viruses, enterotoxin-producing organisms, *G. lamblia*, and *Cryptosporidium parvum*. Inflammatory diarrhea is cause by pathogens that target the distal ileum or the colon and cause acute inflammatory reaction by secreting cytotoxins or invading the intestinal epithelium. Cytotoxin-producing bacteria include enteroaggregative *E. coli* (EAEC), EHEC, and *C. difficile* and invasive organisms include *Salmonella*, *Shigella*, and *Campylobacter*.

Enterotoxin-Induced Secretory Diarrhea

Ingested enterotoxin-producing bacteria colonize the small bowel, and then produce enterotoxin, which binds to the mucosa and causes watery diarrhea through hypersecretion of isotonic fluid that overwhelms the absorptive capacity of the colon. *V. cholerae* produces the cholera toxin, a heterodimeric protein composed of a single toxic active A subunit (CTA) and a B subunit pentamer (CTB), which is responsible for binding of the toxin to the intestinal mucosa. The bound toxin through a series of processes activates adenylate cyclase to produce cyclic adenosine monophosphate (cAMP), which causes increased chloride secretion and decreased sodium absorption, leading to hypersecretion of fluid. Enterotoxigenic *E. coli* (ETEC) produces both a heat-labile enterotoxin that acts by the same mechanism as the cholera toxin and a heat-stable enterotoxin that causes secretory diarrhea through activation of guanylate cyclase to produce cyclic guanosine monophosphate (cGMP).

Cytotoxin-Induced Diarrhea

In contrast to enterotoxins, cytotoxins elaborated by enteric pathogens destroy mucosal epithelial cells, causing acute inflammatory reaction and bloody diarrhea (dysentery). *Shigella dysenteriae* produces the Shiga toxin, which causes dysenteric diarrhea in patients with shigellosis. Other toxin-producing bacteria include *Vibrio parahaemolyticus*, *C. difficile*, and STEC.

TABLE 98.1	Epidemiologic and Clinical Characteristics of Common Enteric Pathogens	
Organism	**Epidemiologic Features**	**Common Clinical Features**
Campylobacter jejuni	Consumption of undercooked poultry, travel to tropical and semitropical regions	Acute watery diarrhea, fever, abdominal pain, fecal evidence of inflammation (positive fecal leukocytes or lactoferrin)
Vibrio cholerae	Inadequately cooked seafood, travel to endemic regions	Acute dehydrating watery diarrhea; fever is usually absent
Clostridioides difficile	Antibiotic use, recent hospitalization, elderly patients with coexisting conditions	Diarrhea with fever, fecal evidence of inflammation, marked leukocytosis
Enterotoxigenic *Escherichia coli*	Travel to tropical and semitropical regions	Watery diarrhea, abdominal cramps, nausea and vomiting; leukocytes absent in stools
Nontyphoidal *Salmonella*	Food-borne outbreaks, exposure to animals	Acute watery diarrhea, fever, abdominal pain, evidence of inflammation
Shigella	Person-to-person transmission, daycare center contact	Severe diarrhea with fever, abdominal pain, bloody diarrhea, fecal evidence of inflammation
Shiga toxin–producing *E. coli*	Food-borne outbreaks, undercooked hamburgers, raw seed sprouts, water and wading pool exposure	Abdominal pain, bloody stools, absence of fever, fecal evidence of inflammation
Noncholeraic *Vibrio*	Ingestion of shellfish and undercooked seafood	Watery diarrhea, abdominal cramps, nausea; fever and vomiting are less frequent
Yersinia enterocolitica	Contaminated food or water, inadequately cooked meats, unpasteurized milk	Acute watery diarrhea, fever, abdominal pain, bloody diarrhea
Norovirus	Winter outbreaks in congregate settings, outbreaks on cruise ships	Watery diarrhea, nausea, vomiting, abdominal pain
Cyclospora	Food-borne outbreaks, travel to tropical and subtropical regions (especially Nepal)	Persistent noninflammatory diarrhea
Cryptosporidium	Waterborne outbreaks, travel to tropical and subtropical regions	Persistent noninflammatory diarrhea
Entamoeba histolytica	Travel to tropical regions, recent immigration from endemic regions	Bloody diarrhea, extraintestinal involvement (liver abscess)
Giardia lamblia	Waterborne outbreaks, travel to mountainous areas of North America, Russia	Abdominal pain, persistent watery diarrhea, flatulence, steatorrhea, nausea and vomiting

Invasive Diarrhea

Some bacteria cause dysentery through direct invasion and destruction of intestinal mucosa. *Shigella* and enteroinvasive *E. coli* (EIEC) invade and multiply in epithelial cells and spread to adjacent cells. Diarrhea is often accompanied by fever, abdominal cramps, and small amounts of bloody mucoid stools. Other bacteria, such as *Salmonella typhi* and *Yersinia enterocolitica*, penetrate the mucosa before disseminating into the bloodstream to cause a systemic illness.

Bacterial Food Poisoning

Bacterial food poisoning is caused by ingestion of preformed toxins in food that results in a toxic illness. The toxins may include cytotoxins, enterotoxins, and neurotoxins. Pathogens that cause bacterial food poisoning include *Staphylococcus aureus*, *Clostridioides perfringens*, and *Bacillus cereus*. These organisms grow in food and produce toxins that are ingested directly in the food. Symptoms occur soon after food ingestion, with incubation periods of 1 to 16 hours. The illness is rarely associated with fever, and symptoms usually resolve within 12 to 24 hours after onset.

The staphylococcal and *B. cereus* toxins act on the nervous system to cause vomiting. *S. aureus* causes vomiting and diarrhea within 2 to 7 hours after ingestion of improperly cooked or stored food containing its heat-stable enterotoxin. *C. perfringens* produces secretory and cytotoxin-induced watery diarrhea within 8 to 14 hours after ingestion of contaminated vegetables, meat, or poultry. *B. cereus* often contaminates fried rice, vegetables, or sprouts; it produces one of two toxins that cause disease resembling that of *S. aureus* or *C. perfringens* infection within 1 to 6 hours after ingestion.

SPECIFIC PATHOGENS

The epidemiologic and clinical features of common enteric pathogens and the recommended methods for diagnosis and treatment are summarized in Tables 98.1 and 98.2.

Shigella

Diarrhea due to *Shigella* spp (shigellosis) occurs after ingestion of fecally contaminated food or water. The main strains include *S. dysenteriae*, *S. flexneri*, *S. boydii*, and *S. sonnei*. Ingestion of as few as 10 to 100 microorganisms can lead to infection because the bacteria are relatively resistant to gastric acid. Person-to-person transmission is common, and the attack rate is highest among infants and young children in child-care centers. The incubation period is 6 to 72 hours. Illness may initially manifest as noninflammatory watery diarrhea caused by enterotoxin production or multiplication of bacteria in the small intestines. Invasion of the colonic epithelium and mucosa often manifests as dysentery. Complications of *S. dysenteriae* type 1 shigellosis include hemolytic-uremic syndrome (HUS). Reactive arthritis is associated with *S. flexneri* infection.

Salmonella

Salmonella enterica serovars typhi and paratyphi cause enteric fever whereas nontyphoidal *Salmonella* spp cause diarrhea. Nontyphoidal salmonellosis results from ingestion of contaminated meat, dairy, or poultry products or from direct contact with animals such as birds, pet turtles, snakes, and other reptiles. An oral inoculum of 10^5 to 10^8 organisms is needed but smaller inocula can cause disease in patients

TABLE 98.2   Diagnosis and Recommended Antimicrobial Treatment for Diarrhea With Specific Pathogens in Adults

Organism	Diagnosis	Recommendations
Campylobacter jejuni	Routine stool culture	Azithromycin 500 mg PO daily for 3 days. Alternative ciprofloxacin 500 mg PO bid for 3 days
Vibrio cholerae O1	Stool culture in special salt-containing media (TCBS), test isolate for O1 serotype	Doxycycline 300 mg or azithromycin 1000 mg PO single dose, or tetracycline 500 mg PO qid or TMP-SMZ 160/800 mg PO bid or ceftriaxone 1–2 g IV/IM q24h for 3 days
Clostridioides difficile	Stool test for C. difficile toxin A or B by EIA, or PCR for the B toxin gene	Stop implicated antibiotic. Vancomycin 125 mg PO qid or fidaxomicin 200 mg PO bid for 10 days. For fulminant CDI, vancomycin 500 mg four times daily orally or by NGT is recommended.
Enterotoxigenic Escherichia coli	Stool culture for E. coli, with assay for enterotoxin	Azithromycin 1000 mg PO single dose or 500 mg PO daily for 3 days or ciprofloxacin 500 mg PO bid for 3 days
Nontyphoidal Salmonella	Routine stool culture	Antimicrobials not recommended except for groups at risk of invasive disease. Ciprofloxacin 500 mg bid for 5 to 7 days or ceftriaxone 100 mg/kg/day in one or two divided doses for 5 to 7 days, or longer if endovascular infection or relapsing
Shigella	Routine stool culture	Ciprofloxacin 500 mg bid for 3 days or ceftriaxone 1–2 g IV/IM for 3 days or azithromycin 500 mg PO daily for 3 days
Shiga toxin–producing E. coli	Stool culture with sorbitol-MacConkey agar, followed by serotyping for O157, then H7, with EIA for Shiga toxins	Antibiotics and antimotility drugs should be avoided
Noncholeraic Vibrio	Stool culture in special salt-containing media (TCBS)	Ceftriaxone 1–2 g IV/IM q24h plus doxycycline 100 mg PO bid for 3 days
Yersinia enterocolitica	Stool culture on MacConkey media incubated at 25° to 28° C	Antibiotics usually not required. For severe infection or bacteremia, treat with TMP-SMZ or fluoroquinolone or doxycycline plus aminoglycoside
Cyclospora	Stool trichrome or acid-fast stain for parasites	TMP-SMZ 160/800 mg bid for 7–10 days
Cryptosporidium	Stool trichrome or acid-fast stain for parasites, EIA for Cryptosporidium species	Self-limited in immunocompetent persons. If severe or if patient is immunocompromised, nitazoxanide 500 mg PO bid for 3 to 14 days
Isospora	Stool trichrome or acid-fast stain for parasites	TMP-SMZ 160/800 mg PO bid for 7–10 days
Entamoeba histolytica	Stool examination for ova and parasites, EIA for E. histolytica	Metronidazole 750 mg tid for 5–10 days, plus iodoquinol 650 mg tid for 20 days or paromomycin 500 mg tid for 7 days
Giardia	Stool examination for ova and parasites, EIA for Giardia species	Single dose tinidazole 2 g or nitazoxanide 500 mg bid for 3 days. Metronidazole 250 to 750 mg tid for 5 to 10 days

EIA, Enzyme immunoassay; *PCR,* polymerase chain reaction; *PO,* per oral; *bid,* twice a day; *qid,* four times a day; *TCBS,* thiosulfate-citrate-bile salts-sucrose agar; *tid,* three times a day; *TMP-SMZ,* trimethoprim-sulfamethoxazole.

with impaired gastric acidity or compromised immunity. The organisms invade the distal ileum and cause diarrhea with fever, nausea, or vomiting. Diarrhea usually resolves in 2 to 3 days. Complications include bacteremia and metastatic seeding of atherosclerotic plaques and prostheses. Antibiotic treatment does not shorten the duration of diarrhea and may prolong intestinal carriage in stools. Antibiotics are indicated only for cases of severe disease or extraintestinal involvement.

Campylobacter

Disease caused by *Campylobacter jejuni* usually results from ingestion of undercooked poultry or direct contact with animals. The infective dose is 10^4 to 10^6 organisms, with an incubation period of 1 to 5 days. Acute watery, noninflammatory diarrhea is the most common presentation. Less frequently, acute inflammatory enterocolitis with systemic symptoms may occur. Prodromal symptoms such as fever, myalgia, headache, and malaise may precede diarrhea. Complications include postinfectious irritable bowel syndrome, reactive arthritis, especially associated with the human leukocyte antigen B27 (HLA-B27), and Guillain-Barré syndrome, which can occur 2 to 3 weeks after diarrhea has resolved. Antibiotic therapy shortens the carriage state.

Vibrio

V. cholerae can be divided by the O-antigen of lipopolysaccharide into more than 150 strains. The toxigenic strains *V. cholerae* O1 and O139 produce cholera toxin and are associated with clinical illness. The infectious oral inoculum is about 10^5 to 10^8 organisms, with an incubation period of 6 hours to 5 days. Classic cholera starts with vomiting, abdominal pain, and diarrhea. Diarrhea progresses to voluminous watery stools that have been described as "rice water" because they are clear with flecks of mucus. Massive diarrhea can lead to dehydration and shock within a few hours. The illness may be fulminant, with death occurring 3 to 4 hours after onset. Fever and bacteremia are rare. In endemic areas, the diagnosis is usually made on clinical grounds. Toxigenic *V. cholerae* non-O1, non-O139 produces cholera toxin and has caused sporadic cases of diarrhea or small outbreaks in some parts of the United States through consumption of contaminated seafood or water. *V. parahaemolyticus* has also been reported to cause acute gastroenteritis from consumption of contaminated seafood. The characteristics of noncholeraic *Vibrio* species are covered in Tables 98.1 and 98.2.

Listeria

Listeria monocytogenes is an uncommon cause of diarrhea in the United States. The two major clinical syndromes of *Listeria* infection are gastroenteritis and listeriosis. Outbreaks may be due to ingestion of contaminated ready-to-eat foods such as unpasteurized milk, cheeses, meats, vegetables, and unwashed raw produce. Gastroenteritis is usually mild, noninvasive, and generally self-limiting. Symptoms including diarrhea, fever, chills, headache, joint pains, and myalgia that may occur 9 to 32 (median, 20) hours after ingestion of contaminated food. The diagnosis of gastroenteritis is often missed, as stool is not routinely cultured. In febrile gastroenteritis where traditional pathogens are not isolated using standard media, culture of stools with selective media for *L. monocytogenes* may demonstrate the organism. If diagnosed in a susceptible host, Listeria gastroenteritis may be treated with amoxicillin 500 mg orally three times a day or TMP/SMX 160/800 mg for 7 days.

Listeriosis is a more severe invasive illness, which may manifest as bacteremia, central nervous system disease, or sepsis in pregnant women with fetal loss. Risk factors for listeriosis include extremes of age, pregnancy, and immunocompromised state. In 2019, the FoodNet reported 134 laboratory-diagnosed cases of listeriosis in the United States, of which 131 (98%) were hospitalized and 21 (16%) died. The overall incidence was 0.3 per 100,000 population.

Diarrhea-Causing *Escherichia coli*

There are several types of diarrheagenic *E. coli*, each with a different pathogenesis leading to diarrhea. These include ETEC, STEC, enteropathogenic (EPEC), EIEC, EAEC, and diffusely adherent *E. coli*. ETEC is the most common cause of traveler's diarrhea. EPEC has been associated with epidemic diarrhea in neonates.

EHEC is acquired by eating contaminated food or water. The oral inoculum is 10 to 100 organisms, with an incubation period of 3 to 4 days. Most disease in the United States is caused by *E. coli* O157:H7. Infection with EHEC, including *E. coli* O157:H7 and other STEC serotypes can cause hemorrhagic colitis. It is classically associated with bloody diarrhea, abdominal pain, and fecal leukocytes. Systemic complications include HUS in children and thrombotic thrombocytopenia purpura in adults. Antibiotic therapy may increase the risk of HUS.

Clostridioides difficile

C. difficile infection is the main cause of nosocomial diarrhea among adults in the United States. The main risk factor for CDI is antibiotic use. Advanced age and severe underlying disease contribute to susceptibility. Virtually all antibiotics have been implicated in the development of CDI, but the most common agents are clindamycin, cephalosporins, fluoroquinolones, ampicillin, and amoxicillin. Infection is transmitted by spores, which occur in the environment and are resistant to alcohol-based handwashing solutions. The spores of toxigenic *C. difficile* are ingested, survive gastric acidity, geminate, and colonize the lower intestinal tract, where they elaborate two exotoxins, toxin A (an enterotoxin) and toxin B (a cytotoxin). The toxins disrupt cell and tight junctions, leading to fluid leakage. The cellular toxicity results in neutrophilic colitis and formation of a pseudomembrane in some cases.

The hypervirulent strain referred to as the North American pulsed-field gel electrophoresis type 1 (NAP1/027) strain is associated with a severe course, higher mortality, and increased risk of relapse. Bacterial factors implicated in outbreaks of CDI caused by the NAP1/027 strain include increased production of toxins A and B, fluoroquinolone resistance, and production of a binary toxin. Patients often have abdominal pain and watery diarrhea but may also have bloody stools. Markers of severe or fulminant CDI include pseudomembranous colitis, acute renal failure, marked leukocytosis, hypotension, and toxic megacolon. The indigenous intestinal microbiota is important for colonization resistance and for recovery from antibiotic-associated CDI.

Yersinia enterocolitica

Y. enterocolitica is a zoonosis caused by ingestion of contaminated food or water or undercooked meats. Oral inoculation requires 10^9 organisms for infection, with an incubation period of 3 to 7 days. The illness may mimic acute appendicitis and may be complicated by ileal perforation, mesenteric adenitis, or terminal ileitis. Postinfectious reactive arthritis may occur.

Viral Causes of Diarrhea

Viruses cause diarrhea by adhering to the intestinal mucosa and disrupting the absorptive and secretory processes without causing inflammation. They may invade intestinal villous epithelial cells and cause sloughing of villi. Rotavirus is a common cause of severe diarrhea in children younger than 5 years of age. The incidence of rotavirus disease has fallen in many countries following the introduction of the rotavirus vaccine. Rotavirus still results in greater than 200,000 deaths annually, mostly in low-income countries. Norovirus is highly contagious and is a very common cause of food-borne gastroenteritis in adults and children in the United States. It has been the cause of epidemic diarrhea on cruise ships. Other viruses that cause diarrhea are adenoviruses, sapoviruses, and astroviruses. The incubation period is usually longer than 14 hours, and vomiting may be a prominent feature of diarrheal disease caused by viral agents.

Protozoan Causes of Diarrhea

Important parasitic causes of diarrhea include *G. lamblia*, *C. parvum*, and *E. histolytica*. Contaminated water sources tend to be the cause of outbreaks. *G. lamblia* trophozoites adhere to the epithelium of the upper small intestine and damage the mucosal brush border without invasion. Ingestion of a few organisms can lead to disease. *C. parvum*, *Isospora belli*, and *Cyclospora cayetanensis* occasionally cause self-limited diarrhea in immunocompetent individuals but may cause severe disease in patients with advanced acquired immunodeficiency syndrome (AIDS). *E. histolytica* causes a syndrome ranging from mild diarrhea to fulminant amebic colitis and extraintestinal amebic abscesses.

Traveler's Diarrhea

Traveler's diarrhea affects 10% to 40% of travelers from industrialized countries who visit tropical and semitropical developing countries. The causative agent is identified in about 85% of cases, and 90% of those identified are bacterial pathogens, most often ETEC or EAEC. Less common bacterial causes include EIEC, diffusely adherent *E. coli*, *Shigella* spp, *Salmonella* spp, *Campylobacter* spp, *Aeromonas*, *V. cholerae*, noncholeraic *Vibrio*, and *Plesiomonas*. The viral etiologies include rotavirus and norovirus. Protozoal causes are rare. Travelers to high-risk areas should be counseled to wash hands, avoid uncooked food, and drink bottled water. Patients with traveler's diarrhea should be treated empirically with antibiotics without stool examination.

CLINICAL PRESENTATION

The epidemiologic and clinical characteristics are important to identify the potential etiologic agent and to guide management (see Table 98.1). The initial evaluation should consider the severity of illness, signs of dehydration, and intestinal inflammation indicated by the fever, abdominal pain, blood in stools (dysentery), or tenesmus. Important epidemiologic clues in the history include age, travel history, ingestion of undercooked or raw food and meat, antibiotic use, sexual activity, daycare attendance, and outbreaks involving others with similar exposure (see Table 98.1). Fever (temperature 38.5° C or 101.3° F or higher) is associated with invasive pathogens that cause intestinal inflammation. The examination should determine the severity of dehydration and need for rehydration as well as the likely cause. Signs of dehydration or hypovolemia include lax skin turgor and tenting, dry mucus membranes, decreased urination, tachycardia, and hypotension.

DIAGNOSIS AND DIFFERENTIAL DIAGNOSIS

The approach to diagnosis and management of infectious diarrhea is shown in Fig. 98.1. Most cases of diarrheal illnesses are self-limiting with almost half resolving within 1 day. Therefore, microbiologic investigation is usually not necessary for patients who are seen within 24 hours of the onset of illness unless certain conditions are present.

The indications for stool culture include severe diarrhea (six or more stools per day), diarrhea lasting longer than 1 week, fever, dysentery, hospitalization, inflammatory diarrhea, and multiple cases in a suspected outbreak. Routine stool culture will identify *Shigella*, *Salmonella*, *Campylobacter*, and *Aeromonas*. Polymerase chain reaction (PCR)–based diagnostic tests are now available and include a multiplex approach that allows several bacterial, viral, and parasitic enteropathogens to be detected in a single test simultaneously. The Luminex xTAG Gastrointestinal Pathogens Panel tests for 14 viruses, bacteria, and parasites and the FilmArray Gastrointestinal

panel (Biofire Diagnostics) tests for 22 viruses, bacteria, and parasites. These methods are faster and have higher sensitivity than culture-based methods but they do not distinguish pathogenic and nonpathogenic organisms. If the patient has bloody diarrhea or HUS, stool culture for *E. coli* O157:H7 and tests for Shiga-like toxin (or the genes that encode them) should be performed. If there is a history of recent antibiotic use, hospitalization, or age greater than 65 years with coexisting conditions, immunosuppression, or neutropenia, stool samples should be tested for *C. difficile* toxin. Available tests for *C. difficile* toxin include enzyme immunoassay (EIA), nucleic acid amplification test (NAAT) and glutamate dehydrogenase (GDH plus toxin) test. No single test is suitable as a stand-alone test and often a multistep algorithm testing is used. Consider protozoa, and check stools for ova and parasites (e.g., trophozoites) and/or for *Giardia* antigen test if diarrhea duration is greater than 7 days. If a patient has AIDS, stools should be checked for *Cryptosporidium*, *Microsporidium*, and *Mycobacterium avium* complex.

TREATMENT

Initial therapy should include fluid and electrolyte repletion with or without antimicrobial therapy. Oral rehydration is often adequate unless the patient is comatose or severely dehydrated. Nutritional support with continued feeding improves outcomes in children.

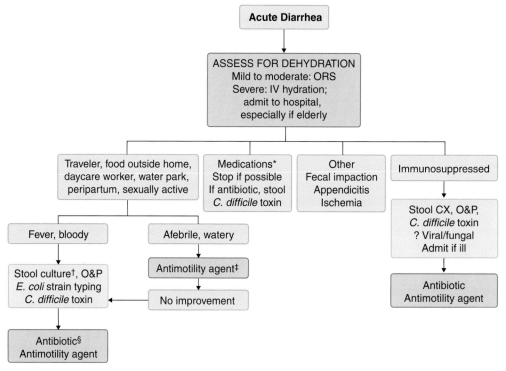

Report to Public Health and save blood/stool.

Fig. 98.1 Approach to the diagnosis and management of acute infectious diarrhea. *More than 700 medications cause diarrhea, including furosemide, caffeine, protease inhibitors, thyroid preparations, metformin, mycophenolate mofetil, sirolimus, cholinergic drugs, colchicine, theophylline, selective serotonin reuptake inhibitors, proton pump inhibitors, histamine-2 blockers, 5-ASA derivatives, angiotensin-converting enzyme inhibitors, bisacodyl, senna, aloe, anthraquinones, and magnesium- or phosphorus-containing medications. †Specifically request culture for *Yersinia*, *Plesiomonas*, enterohemorrhagic *Escherichia coli* serotype O157:H7, and *Aeromonas* if suspected. ‡If high suspicion for *Clostridioides difficile* or invasive bacterial infection, wait for stool culture and toxin studies before starting. Racecadotril has antisecretory effects without paralyzing intestinal motility and can be used if available. §Not recommended for patients with bloody diarrhea due to *E. coli* O157:H7. *CX*, Culture; *IV therapy*, intravenous rehydration; *O&P*, ova and parasites; *ORS*, oral rehydration solution. (From Goldman L, Schaefer AI: *Goldman-Cecil Medicine*, 25th ed. Philadelphia, Elsevier, 2016, Fig. 140-1.)

Oral Fluid Therapy

In most patients with diarrhea, fluid repletion can be achieved with oral rehydration therapy using isotonic fluids containing glucose and electrolytes. An effective solution can be prepared by the addition of 2 tablespoons of sugar, one fourth of a teaspoon of salt (NaCl), and one-fourth of a teaspoon of baking soda ($NaHCO_3$) to 1 L of boiled drinking water. In the United States, fluids such as Pedialyte or Rehydrolyte solutions are recommended. Fluid should be administered in large quantities until there is clinical evidence that fluid balance is restored and then as maintenance therapy. Oral rehydration therapy can be life-saving for patients in developing countries with severe diarrhea.

Intravenous Fluid Therapy

Massive fluid loss due to diarrhea should be rapidly replaced by the administration of intravenous fluids. Lactated Ringer's solution is the fluid of choice because the composition is similar to electrolyte loss during diarrhea. The rate of fluid administration and maintenance should be guided by clinical signs including vital signs, appearance of the mucosa, neck veins, and skin turgor.

Antimicrobial Therapy

Most cases of infectious diarrhea do not require antimicrobial therapy. However, antibiotics may decrease the volume of diarrhea (e.g., in cholera) or the duration and severity of the illness. Antibiotics are effective in the treatment of shigellosis, traveler's diarrhea, and *Campylobacter* infection. In uncomplicated salmonellosis, antibiotics may prolong the shedding of *Salmonella*. The choice and dose of antimicrobials for specific pathogens are described in Table 98.2. For traveler's diarrhea in adults, empiric therapy with azithromycin 500 mg daily, or ciprofloxacin 500 mg twice a day, or trimethoprim-sulfamethoxazole (TMP-SMZ) 160/800 mg twice a day, for 3 days is adequate. For antibiotic-associated *C. difficile* colitis, broad-spectrum antibiotics should be discontinued, if possible. Preferred therapy for an initial episode of CDI is oral vancomycin 125 mg four times a day or fidaxomicin 200 mg twice daily for 10 days. If those antibiotics are not available, metronidazole 500 mg three times daily for 10 days is an alternative therapy. Fecal microbiota transplantation may be indicated for patients with multiple recurrences of CDI who have failed appropriate antibiotic treatments. Antibiotics must be avoided in patients with STEC O157 or other STEC that produce Shiga toxin.

Symptomatic Therapy

Antidiarrheal agents such as loperamide and bismuth subsalicylate can be used in some instances for symptomatic relief. Loperamide inhibits intestinal peristalsis and has some antisecretory properties. When used with or without antibiotics in cases of traveler's diarrhea, it may reduce the duration of diarrhea by about 1 day. Antimotility agents should be avoided in patients with bloody or suspected inflammatory diarrhea. The use of these agents has been implicated in prolonging the duration of fever in shigellosis, development of toxic megacolon in CDI, and development of HUS in children with STEC infection.

PROGNOSIS

The prognosis is generally good but is variable depending on the etiology and the severity of illness. Most patients recover completely within 3 to 5 days. However, serious complications, including death, can be seen in individuals who become severely dehydrated, infants, elderly patients, and those with underlying medical conditions or immunosuppression. Untreated severe dehydration may lead to shock, renal failure, and death. Postinfectious reactive polyarthritis can complicate cases due to *Yersinia*, *Campylobacter*, and *Shigella*, and Guillain-Barré syndrome may occur after diarrhea caused by *Campylobacter*.

SUGGESTED READINGS

DuPont HL: Acute infectious diarrhea in immunocompetent adults, N Engl J Med 370:1532–1540, 2014.

DuPont HL: Persistent diarrhea: a clinical review, J Am Med Assoc 315:2712–2723, 2016.

McDonald LC, Gerding DN, Johnson S, et al: Clinical practice guidelines for clostridium difficile infection in adults and children: 2017 update by Infectious Diseases Society of America (IDSA) and Society for Healthcare Epidemiology of America (SHEA). Clin Infect Dis 66:987-994.

Shane AL, Mody RK, Crump JA, et al: 2017 infectious Diseases Society of America clinical practice guidelines for diagnosis and management of infectious diarrhea, Clin Infect Dis 65:e45–e79, 2017.

99

Infections Involving Bone and Joints

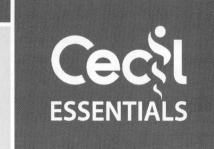

Jerome Larkin

DEFINITION

Osteomyelitis refers to infection of any component of the bony skeleton, whereas *septic arthritis* refers to that of native or prosthetic joints. Tendons, ligaments, and bursae can also become infected, especially if they involve prosthetic or bio-grafted material. Osteomyelitis and septic arthritis can occur by seeding during bacteremia, due to extension from a contiguous focus of infection in an adjacent tissue or structure, as a consequence of vascular insufficiency or as a complication of trauma. In the case of hematogenous infection, the bacteremia itself may be relatively transient and of little clinical consequence. Hematogenous osteomyelitis is common in children but accounts for only 20% of osteomyelitis in adults. The vertebrae and pelvis are the most commonly involved sites of hematogenous osteomyelitis in adults. Peripheral vascular disease leading to tissue hypoxia and related to diabetes, hypertension, hyperlipidemia, and smoking is the biggest risk factor for the development of osteomyelitis in adults older than 50. There is often preceding soft tissue infection or destruction as a result of vascular insufficiency and neuropathy. It is most common in the lower extremities, particularly in the feet, and often occurs in diabetics. Trauma, especially when it involves open fracture with its attendant disruption of the bony architecture and vascular supply, is a second major risk factor for the development of osteomyelitis and septic arthritis. This is particularly true when an open fracture, as may be experienced in a fall or motor vehicle accident, is heavily contaminated with soil or other environmental materials. Such fractures often require internal fixation (i.e., the placement of rods, screws, and other metal devices to stabilize the bone). The presence of such internal fixation provides a nidus for bacteria and other microorganisms including fungi to elude the immune system and incubate. Chronic osteomyelitis is a possible complication of such injuries and is often a result of multiple or unusual organisms. It may occur despite aggressive débridement and prophylactic antibiotic treatment at the time of injury and can arise months or even years afterwards. Individuals who experience prolonged periods of immobility such as those suffering from paraplegia are also at risk for osteomyelitis. Infection typically involves the pelvis, sacrum, and lower spine corresponding to areas of unrelieved pressure as a result of the immobility.

Osteomyelitis may be conceptualized as acute or chronic. The former is typically hematogenous, associated with signs of inflammation in the overlying soft tissue and with an onset over the course of days to a week. Radiographs are usually normal at presentation. Chronic osteomyelitis is more indolent with onset over the course of months, is more likely to exhibit bony destruction on plain radiograph at the time of presentation, and is often associated with a draining sinus tract. Sequestra (areas of dead bone) and involucra (new bone formed around sequestra) may also be seen. Whereas acute osteomyelitis may require a 6-week course of antibiotics alone to effect cure, chronic osteomyelitis more typically requires surgical intervention and a prolonged (3 or more months) course of antibiotic therapy.

PATHOPHYSIOLOGY

Aspects of the vascular supply of the bone as well as properties of the most common pathogen, *Staphylococcus aureus*, may combine to lead to infection. Although bone is generally resistant to infection, the vasculature of the metaphysis contains capillary loops composed of a single layer of discontinuous endothelial cells, which may allow bacteria to enter the extracellular matrix. These capillary beds lack functionally active phagocytes. *S. aureus* can elaborate proteins expressed on its surface that promote adherence to tissues of the extracellular matrix. When engulfed by osteoblasts, *S. aureus* can survive for prolonged periods of time in an almost spore-like state leading to potential recurrences of infection. Finally, many bacteria can elaborate biofilms that allow them to elude clearance by the immune system. Prosthetic material such as in joint replacements and other grafts can serve as a platform for the formation of such biofilms.

In the case of septic arthritis there is usually some underlying abnormality in the joint, but this abnormality may be as mundane as osteoarthritis. It is hypothesized that relatively trivial injury, which may in fact go unnoticed or unremembered by the patient, leads to minor bleeding into the joint, which in turn provides a hospitable environment for bacteria to incubate.

CLINICAL PRESENTATION AND DIAGNOSIS

Patients with osteomyelitis will often present with pain at the site of infection. The overlying soft tissue may have signs of inflammation or tissue destruction, the latter often seen in diabetics with soft tissue ulceration. Historically, the diagnosis of osteomyelitis relied on the presence of lucency on plain radiograph of the affected area. Diagnosis could be confirmed histologically by bone biopsy with culture to identify the pathogenic organism. Currently, diagnosis is typically made by MRI with gadolinium, which demonstrates marrow edema with or without bony destruction. Alternatively, diagnosis may be made by three-phase bone scan or CT. These may be especially helpful in patients with renal insufficiency who cannot undergo gadolinium-enhanced studies due to the risk of nephrogenic systemic fibrosis. An elevated C-reactive protein (CRP) or erythrocyte sedimentation rate (ESR) supports the diagnosis. Microbiologic diagnosis is made either by positive blood cultures or bone biopsy and culture. Culture of cutaneous ulcers is typically not helpful because results of such studies usually demonstrate multiple colonizing organisms and do not correlate with organisms isolated on bone culture. An exception is the isolation of *S. aureus* or *Salmonella* from a draining fistula or on occasion *Pseudomonas* from an ulcer. In the former case, the bacterium can then be presumed to be the pathogen; in the latter, a decision would then need to be made to include coverage for this organism in an empiric antibiotic regimen. If cultures of bone obtained by noninvasive techniques under radiographic guidance are negative, either the procedure should be repeated or an open biopsy with culture performed.

Septic arthritis of native joints typically will present with the cardinal features of inflammation (i.e., erythema, swelling, warmth, and pain) when involving joints of the extremities. Fever may often be present and septic arthritis is more likely to present with an associated bacteremia. Septic arthritis of the spine, pelvis, and hip may require imaging, usually MRI, because these may be difficult to assess by examination alone. Persistent back, pelvic or hip pain that is otherwise unexplained should prompt radiographic evaluation even in the absence of fever. Diagnosis ultimately relies on joint aspiration with débridement. Such procedures should occur prior to the administration of antibiotics. Fluid should be sent for cell count with differential, crystal analysis, Gram stain, anaerobic culture, and fungal and acid-fast stains and cultures. Positive stains and/or cultures are taken as evidence of infection in most cases in which an appropriate clinical syndrome is also present. White blood cell (WBC) counts higher than 50,000 cells/mL are suggestive of infection. In cases that are difficult to diagnose or instances where antibiotics have been given prior to aspiration, it may be appropriate to have cultures held for up to 14 days. Specialized culture techniques for fastidious organisms such as anaerobes and nutritionally deficient streptococci may be required. Ultimately, tagged WBC scans may help to clarify the presence or absence of septic arthritis in difficult cases. Evolving molecular technologies such as PCR, especially microarray assays that detect multiple pathogens, and 16-S ribosomal sequencing may offer alternative and more rapid and precise diagnosis in the future.

Prosthetic joint infections (PJI) are defined by their timing following implantation: acute (less than 3 months), delayed (3 to 12 months) or late (12 months). Early PJI presents similarly to native joint infections. Delayed and late infections are more indolent, presenting with pain, decreased function, and evidence of loosening of the prosthesis on plain films. More overt signs of inflammation or systemic infection may be subtle or absent altogether. Diagnosis relies on the presence of either a draining sinus tract that communicates with the prosthesis or two or more periprosthetic cultures harboring the same organism. Minor criteria have been proposed with three or more of the following used to diagnose PJI: elevated CRP or ESR, synovial fluid WBC greater than 3000, elevated synovial polymorphonuclear cells (PMNs), a single positive culture or greater than five PMNs per high-power field on examination of periprosthetic tissue. A point scoring system as advanced by Parvizi and colleagues may increase the sensitivity of the use of minor criteria or be used as a tool in more diagnostically obscure cases.

Most cases of osteomyelitis and septic arthritis are due to *Staphylococcus, Streptococcus*, and aerobic gram-negative bacilli, although virtually any pathogenic microorganism can cause such infections in the appropriate circumstance. Infecting staphylococci include both *S. aureus* and coagulase-negative staphylococci. Coagulase-negative staphylococci are often implicated in prosthetic joint infections or infections associated with orthopedic hardware. *Streptococcus* spp causing bone and joint infections include groups A, B, C, G and F as well as *Abiotrophia* and *Gemella* (formerly termed nutritionally deficient streptococci). Gram-negative organisms account for as much as 30% of hematogenous infections. Gram-negative infections are seen more commonly in the elderly as a result of urinary tract infections with associated bacteremia. Isolated species include *Escherichia coli, Haemophilus influenza*, and *H. parainfluenza*. Infections with *Serratia marcescens* and *Pseudomonas* are associated with exposure to water and are usually nosocomial or related to intravenous drug use. Fungi such

as *Candida, Aspergillus*, and *Zygomycetes* may cause bone and joint infections, particularly in immune-compromised patients, diabetics or those who have suffered trauma. *Nocardia* and other acid-fast organisms may be seen following trauma or in association with prosthetic joints and may require several attempts at débridement before being isolated. *Cutibacterium acnes* is often isolated from shoulder infections, especially those involving prosthetic joints. The variety of potential pathogens underscores the need to obtain appropriate specimens for culture prior to the administration of antibiotics.

Infection with *Borrelia burgdorferi*, the causative agent of Lyme disease, can lead to a multifocal or monoarticular septic arthritis. Fluid analysis is consistent with bacterial septic arthritis but is negative for typical organisms on culture. Associated findings of erythema migrans, diffuse myalgias and arthralgias, cranial nerve palsies, fever, and aseptic meningitis may also be present. Polymerase chain reaction of joint fluid has a reported sensitivity of between 30% and 75%. Diagnosis relies on serology and associated findings in patients who reside in endemic areas. Later-stage disease may present with a less inflammatory-appearing effusion, often without any other symptoms. Treatment is with either doxycycline or ceftriaxone depending on the stage of disease.

Neisseria gonorrhea may cause a solitary or multifocal septic arthritis. It is usually seen in sexually active younger adults. Culture of the joint fluid may be negative but testing of specimens from the pharynx, urethra or rectum are usually positive by nucleic acid amplification. The treatment of choice is ceftriaxone.

DIFFERENTIAL DIAGNOSIS

The differential diagnosis of both osteomyelitis and septic arthritis includes other noninfectious inflammatory disorders such as gout, pseudogout, rheumatoid arthritis, inflammatory bowel disease, and other inflammatory and autoimmune disorders. Occasionally, neoplasms such as sarcomas or metastatic lesions may present similarly to osteomyelitis. Several viruses such as rubella, parvovirus B19, Chikungunya and hepatitis B can cause arthritis. Chronic recurrent multifocal osteomyelitis is a noninfectious inflammatory lesion of bone thought to be autoimmune in nature and characterized by findings on MRI similar to osteomyelitis. It is culture-negative and unresponsive to antibiotics. It is a diagnosis of exclusion often made only after several attempts at diagnosing and treating presumed bacterial osteomyelitis. Although typically seen in children, with peak incidence between 7 and 12 years of age, it can also occur in adults.

TREATMENT

Treatment of osteomyelitis involves débridement of appropriate infected and/or necrotic tissue as well as the administration of antibiotics. It is critically important to remove all necrotic or devitalized tissue, which may serve as a nidus of chronic or recurrent infection if not removed. In this regard, it is often necessary to remove any fixating hardware, plastic devices, bone grafts or other donor tissue if infection has been present for greater than one month or is recurrent. Cadaveric donor tissue infections often are caused by atypical organisms such as *Clostridioides* spp. Historically, sequestra developed in the site of chronically infected bone. These are produced by the action of the immune system and histologically are characterized by granulomatous tissue that serves to isolate the infection. While effective in containing infection, they also represented a risk for recurrence as well as an area of bone weakening. When present, they should be surgically excised. Infection that occurs in the immediate postoperative period (i.e., within 1 month after placement of hardware and grafts) and that appears to only involve the soft tissue may be treated with débridement and antibiotics alone with a reasonable chance of success. Occasionally, infected hardware must be left in place in order to stabilize the bone while a fracture is healing. In this instance, it may be necessary to continue antibiotic treatment until hardware removal can be accomplished. Infected spine hardware that must remain in place may require prolonged antibiotic treatment, at times indefinitely. The addition of rifampin for staphylococcal infections with retained hardware to which the infecting organism is susceptible improves overall cure rates.

Septic arthritis requires serial débridement of the joint until active purulence has resolved. This is indicated by decreasing cell count and sterilization of joint fluid cultures. Prosthetic joint infection typically requires removal of the infected prosthesis with placement of an antibiotic spacer for 4 to 6 weeks while antibiotics are administered. This is followed by placement of a new prosthesis once all signs and symptoms of infection have resolved. Selected infections with coagulase-negative staphylococci and *Streptococcus* infections may be treated with débridement, joint retention, and a 6-week or longer course of antibiotics. Consideration should then be given to chronic suppressive antibiotic therapy, assuming an appropriate agent is available.

Antibiotic treatment should be with agents active against the infecting organism if culture and susceptibility data are available. β-Lactams are the preferred agent in most cases. Therapy with quinolones for Enterobacteriaceae and in combination with rifampin for staphylococci may be considered. These drugs have the advantage of high oral bioavailability that approaches or equals tissue levels when given intravenously. Care should be taken regarding drug interactions with rifampin and the risk of *Clostridioides difficile* colitis and Achilles tendon rupture with quinolones. Recent literature also indicates a small increased risk of aortic aneurysm or dissection with this class of antibiotics. In the face of negative cultures, empiric therapy with an agent active against typical pathogens, including methicillin-resistant *S. aureus*, is reasonable. Vancomycin remains the standard agent for empiric therapy. Prior administration of antibiotics may lead to negative cultures even in cases of unequivocal infection. In this situation, empiric therapy should be based on the activity of the agents previously administered, as well as on potential pathogens based on exposure history. In all cases, the clinical response to infection should be monitored and should inform subsequent decision making regarding the need for additional débridement or changes in antibiotic therapy. Monitoring inflammatory markers such as CRP or ESR is helpful in determining the adequacy of response to treatment. If elevated at the start of treatment they should fall to normal or near normal by the time treatment is finished. Signs and symptoms of inflammation at the site of infection should have also resolved at the cessation of treatment.

There are few randomized, controlled trials comparing different durations of antimicrobial therapy. Acute osteomyelitis should be treated for 4 to 6 weeks. Continuing treatment in a patient who is improved but who has failed to resolve elevated inflammatory markers or local signs of inflammation is reasonable. Such patients should be closely monitored and evaluated for the need for additional débridement or other measures aimed at diagnosis and source control. Chronic osteomyelitis may require 12 or more weeks of therapy, and treatment is usually individualized based on the clinical situation. Patients on therapy should also be monitored weekly for toxicity to antibiotics. Assessment of renal and hepatic function, complete blood count, and drug levels are typically followed depending on the specific agent used. In the case of aminoglycosides, renal function and peak and trough levels should be followed twice weekly. Long-acting glycopeptides such as dalbavancin and oritavancin are promising alternatives to daily antibiotic dosing.

A recent open-label study of the treatment of osteomyelitis that included over 1000 randomized patients demonstrated a lack of inferiority of oral therapy when compared with intravenous therapy. Costs were reduced and patient satisfaction was higher in the orally treated group. The incidence of serious side effects and adverse reactions was similar between the two groups. Oral therapy was largely with quinolones. The study encompassed a heterogenous population so, although promising, application of the findings to particular patients should be done thoughtfully. Adjunctive therapies such as bone grafting, revascularization procedures, and the placement of muscle flaps to cover and protect exposed bone may be utilized in the appropriate clinical situation.

Native joint septic arthritis may be treated with a 4-week course of antibiotics; prosthetic joint infections are typically treated for 6 or more weeks. Monitoring for toxicity and response to treatment is similar to that for osteomyelitis.

PROGNOSIS

The prognosis for osteomyelitis and septic arthritis is excellent, assuming adequate diagnosis, débridement, and antimicrobial therapy. The most common complication is residual pain and/or decreased function of the affected bone or joint. These are relatively rare and relatively minor. An exception involves prosthetic joint infections, in which 25% to 50% of patients experience some loss of function as a result of the infection. Recurrence rates for chronic osteomyelitis, especially in diabetics, may be as high as 30%. In more complex cases such as open contaminated fractures or infected hardware that requires retention, complications include nonunion, prosthesis failure, and chronic osteomyelitis. Infections that cannot be controlled may lead to the need for amputation and its attendant loss of function and mobility. Occasionally, bone or joint infections can lead to dissemination to other joints or the bloodstream. Such cases usually involve infection with *S. aureus* and fortunately remain the exception.

SUGGESTED READINGS

American Academy of Orthopedic Surgeons: Diagnosis and prevention of periprosthetic joint infections clinical practice guidelines. March, 2019.

Lew DP, Waldvogel FA: Osteomyelitis, Lancet 364:369–379, 2004.

Li HK, Rombach I, Zambellas R, et al: Oral versus intravenous antibiotics for bone and joint infection, N Engl J Med 380:425, 2019.

Parvizi J, Tan TL, Goswami K, et al: The 2018 definition of periprosthetic hip and knee infection: an evidence-based and validated criteria, J Arthroplasty 33:1309, 2018.

Rappo U, Puttagunta S, Shevchenko V, et al: Dalbavancin for the treatment of osteomyelitis in adult patients: a randomized clinical trial of efficacy and safety, Open Forum Infect Dis 6:331, 2018.

Shuford JA, Steckelberg JM: Role of oral antimicrobial therapy in the management of osteomyelitis, Curr Opin Infect Dis 16:515–519, 2003.

Spielberg B, Lipsky BA: Systemic antibiotic therapy for chronic osteomyelitis in adults, Clin Infect Dis 54:393, 2012.

Stengel D, Bauwens K, Sehouli J, et al: Systematic review and meta-analysis of antibiotic therapy for bone and joint infections. Lancet Infect Dis 201 1: 175-188.

Tande AJ, Steckelberg JM, Osmon DR, Berbari EF: Osteomyelitis. In Bennett JE, Dolin R, Blaser MJ, editors: Principles and practice of infectious diseases, 9th ed, Philadelphia, 2020, Elsevier.

Tice AD, Hoaglund PA, Shoultz DA: Outcomes of osteomyelitis among patients treated with outpatient parenteral antimicrobial therapy, Am J Med 114:723–728, 2003.

Waldvogel FA, Medoff G, Swartz MN: Osteomyelitis: a review of clinical features, therapeutic consideration and unusual aspects, N Eng J Med 282:316–322, 1970.

Wunsch S, Krause R, Valentin T, et al: Multicenter clinical experience of real life dalbavancin use in gram-positive infection, Int J Infect Dis 81:210, 2019.

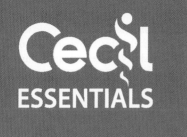

100

Urinary Tract Infections

Abdullah Chahin, Steven M. Opal

DEFINITION AND DIAGNOSIS

The term *urinary tract infection* (UTI) refers to significant bacteriuria in a patient with symptoms or signs attributable to the urinary tract and no alternative diagnosis. UTI includes asymptomatic bacteriuria, urethritis, cystitis, pyelonephritis, catheter-associated UTI, prostatitis, and urosepsis. This chapter focuses primarily on the two major forms of UTI, cystitis and pyelonephritis.

A practical classification divides these infections into uncomplicated and complicated UTI. Uncomplicated UTIs are episodes of cystitis and mild pyelonephritis occurring in healthy, premenopausal, sexually active, nonpregnant women with no history suggestive of abnormalities in the urinary tract. All other episodes of UTI are deemed to be potentially complicated and deserving of further evaluation.

The term *asymptomatic bacteriuria* refers to isolation of bacteria in an appropriately collected urine specimen from an individual who describes no symptoms for urinary tract infection. In women, asymptomatic bacteriuria is defined as two consecutive voided midstream urine specimens with isolation of the same bacterial strain at levels of at least 10^5 colony-forming units (CFU) per milliliter from patients without genitourinary symptoms. In men, a single clean-catch, midstream voided urine specimen with one bacterial species at a concentration greater than 10^5 CFU/mL defines asymptomatic bacteriuria. The diagnosis of asymptomatic bacteriuria is also established in both women and men from a single catheterized urine specimen (not an indwelling catheter) with one bacterial species isolated at concentrations greater than 10^2 CFU/mL. Although infants and toddlers infrequently have asymptomatic bacteriuria, the incidence increases with age, owing to the incomplete bladder emptying from various obstructive urologic conditions that develop with advanced age, reaching up to 15% or greater in women and men age 65 to 80 years and as high as 50% after age 80. Asymptomatic bacteriuria is therefore commonly encountered in clinical practice, and it frequently poses a challenge in determining the exact source of infection in elderly patients presenting with sepsis. Asymptomatic bacteriuria is a common cause for unnecessary use of antibiotics and the array of complications that can result from antibiotic misuse, ranging from mild adverse reactions to devastating complications such as antibiotic-associated *Clostridioides difficile* infections.

The presence of asymptomatic bacteriuria therefore should not be considered as equivalent to UTI except in neutropenic patients and individuals with anatomic or functional defects in the urinary tract. Asymptomatic bacteriuria in pregnancy has been an indication for treatment. However, the most recent Systematic Review for the US Preventive Services Task Force in September of 2019 showed that screening and treatment for asymptomatic bacteriuria during pregnancy was associated with reduced rates of pyelonephritis and low birth weights, but the available evidence was not current, with only one study conducted in the past 30 years. It is difficult to define asymptomatic bacteriuria in the patient who has undergone renal transplantation, and bacteriuria in such patients often indicates the need to treat for UTI.

To increase the sensitivity of urinalysis and culture, *significant bacteriuria* is defined as greater than 10^2 CFU/mL of urine in a woman with symptoms of uncomplicated cystitis and pyuria (≥5 white blood cells per milliliter of urine per high-power field). Among women with symptoms of uncomplicated pyelonephritis and men with UTI, significant bacteriuria is defined as greater than 10^4 CFU/mL plus pyuria. In patients with complicated UTI, a concentration of 10^5 CFU/mL or higher is required for the definition of significant bacteriuria independently of pyuria.

In order for these definitions to be valid, the urine must remain in the bladder for at least 2 hours, and after urine collection the sample should be incubated immediately. If urine is not incubated immediately, it can be refrigerated for up to 8 hours before proper incubation.

Although the presence of bacteriuria is vital for the establishment of the diagnosis of UTI, clinical symptomatology is the hallmark of UTI. The presence of dysuria, increased frequency of urination, suprapubic tenderness, and hematuria associated with bacteriuria or pyuria on urinalysis is unequivocally consistent with the diagnosis of cystitis. Back or flank pain, nausea, vomiting, and the presence of fever or rigors suggest infection of the upper urinary tract, although it is not easy to distinguish cystitis from pyelonephritis on clinical grounds alone. The diagnosis of UTI gets more difficult when patients cannot ascribe symptoms to the urinary tract (e.g., patients with paraplegia or neurogenic bladder, confused elderly or sedated patients) or when they have atypical symptoms, such as changes in mental status, agitation, or hypotension. Sometimes patients have urinary symptoms without bacteriuria (the pyuria-dysuria or "urethral syndrome" commonly caused by *Chlamydia trachomatis* or other difficult-to-culture genitourinary pathogens).

With the widespread utilization of indwelling catheters, *catheter-associated urinary tract infection* (CAUTI) remains a challenge in health care and one of the most common nosocomial infections. Essentially, CAUTI has similar symptoms to a typical UTI but requires the presence of an indwelling urinary catheter for the term to apply. The standard Centers for Disease Control and Prevention (CDC) National Healthcare Safety Network (NHSN) CAUTI definition is complex and subjective. Moreover, it can be difficult to diagnose in patients who are already hospitalized due to the resemblance of the potential signs and symptoms of CAUTI with many other acute disorders that were part of the original reason for hospitalization.

LABORATORY FINDINGS

Young, sexually active women with typical symptoms of UTI have a high pretest probability for UTI. Therefore, no laboratory test is indicated. In this population, pretreatment urine analysis and culture are indicated only if the diagnosis is not straightforward or if an antibiotic-resistant organism is suspected. Urinalysis and culture are indicated in all cases of suspected complicated UTI. The presence of white blood cell casts in urinalysis indicates pyelonephritis, and this finding suggests a complicated UTI with possible obstructive lesions within the kidney or collecting system (e.g., papillary necrosis). Blood cultures are mandatory for patients with suspected pyelonephritis. *Staphylococcus aureus* bacteriuria should prompt work-up for *S. aureus* bacteremia and for renal abscesses in non-catheter-related UTIs, particularly in those who are hospitalized and have laboratory evidence of infection. *S. aureus* UTI may also occur without hematogenous seeding in cases of indwelling catheters, with frequent instrumentation, or in the presence of hardware in the genitourinary tract. Candida is a commonly isolated organism on urine cultures (candiduria). Yeasts can be detected in contaminated samples during collection, in patients who have bladder or indwelling catheter colonization, and rarely in patients who have upper urinary tract infection that developed either from retrograde spread from the bladder or hematogenous spread from a distant source. The presence of pyuria and quantitative cultures of urine in cases of candiduria have proved to be of little use in separating infection from colonization. Therefore, clinical symptoms are of great importance, because diagnosing UTI with *Candida* might necessitate an extensive work-up to assess for invasive fungal infections (Candidemia or perinephric abscesses). Imaging studies are indicated if kidney stones, malignancy, obstructive uropathy, and urologic malformations are suspected.

EPIDEMIOLOGY

At the extremes of age, men are more prone to UTI than women. In young boys, urethral malformation is commonly the cause, and in older men, UTI is usually caused by bladder neck obstruction secondary to prostatic hypertrophy. Homosexual men are at increased risk for acquiring UTIs. Teenage girls and sexually active women have more UTIs than their male counterparts. A higher than expected incidence of UTI among young girls might suggest sexual abuse. Sexually active women have the highest rate of UTI. Postmenopausal women have increased prevalence of UTI due to estrogen deficiency and age-related pelvic relaxation with poor bladder emptying.

The most common etiologic agent in patients with uncomplicated UTI is *Escherichia coli* (90% of cases), followed by *Staphylococcus saprophyticus*. Other agents include *Klebsiella* spp, *Enterococcus faecalis*, *Enterococcus faecium*, *Proteus* spp, *Providencia stuartii*, and *Morganella morganii*. In patients with complicated UTI, *E. coli* is still the most frequent uropathogen, but at a lower rate than in uncomplicated UTI. Other causative organisms are *Pseudomonas aeruginosa*, *Acinetobacter baumannii*, *Enterobacter* spp, *Serratia marcescens*, *Stenotrophomonas maltophilia*, *Enterococcus* spp, and *Candida* spp.

Anaerobic agents are infrequent causes of UTI; when present, they represent fistulae between the digestive tract and the urinary tract. *Staphylococcus aureus* UTI most often represents bacteremia with bacteriuria resulting from clearance of bloodstream bacteria by the kidney. Whereas 1% of individuals with a UTI get pyelonephritis, 20% to 40% of pregnant women with a UTI develop pyelonephritis, and 30% of patients with pyelonephritis have bacteremia. In diabetic and transplanted patients with UTI, the incidence of bacteremia is higher.

PATHOGENESIS

There are at least three routes by which bacteria can enter the bladder or kidney: ascending, hematogenous, and lymphatic. Lymphatic spread is the least common route. The hematogenous route is important for gram-positive organisms such as *S. aureus* or *Candida* spp but unimportant for gram-negative bacilli. The ascending route is the most important for enteric bacteria, and this mechanism is supported by higher frequency of UTI in women, given the shorter length of the female urethra, and in individuals with an indwelling Foley catheter.

Before reaching the urinary bladder or kidney, the microorganism must colonize the external part of the urinary tract. Probably the most important aspect in the establishment of UTI is the interaction between host factors (e.g., secretor phenotype, P1 blood group, uroplakin I and II) and bacterial virulence factors (the adhesins, P fimbriae, and type I fimbriae [pili]). The urinary bladder is normally covered by a glycosaminoglycan surface that prevents binding of bacteria that transiently enter the bladder. P-fimbriated uropathogenic *E. coli* bind to alpha 1-4 linked, galactose-galactose disaccharide moieties found on uroepithelial cells, and these gal-gal glycolipids are also expressed on the P1 blood group. People with P1 blood group are overrepresented among individuals with either recurrent UTI or pyelonephritis. Also, people who lack P1 blood group are less prone to complicated UTI.

Studies have shown that P-fimbriated *E. coli* is present in 60% to 100% of isolates from patients with UTI. Ascending UTI infection can be inhibited experimentally by epithelial cell surface receptor analogues. Type I fimbriae bind to glycoprotein uroplakin I and II. *E. coli* expressing type I fimbriae are responsible for most cases of cystitis.

Once *E. coli* is attached to uroepithelial cells, both mechanical and biochemical factors facilitate the development of full-blown UTI. The local trauma and mechanical massage of the urethra during sexual intercourse help deliver bacteria into the bladder and, if vesicoureteral reflux or another ureteral anatomic defect is present, into the kidney. Urinary catheter placement also helps to propel bacteria into the bladder, and all patients with a long-term indwelling catheter in place will eventually develop asymptomatic UTI. All uropathogenic organisms have the ability to multiply in the urine.

From the standpoint of the host, other factors associated with the development of UTI are a new sex partner (within 1 year), use of diaphragms and spermicides, family history of UTI in a first-degree relative, and lower expression of CXCR1, an interleukin 8 receptor. Pathogenic factors associated with the development of UTI are flagellae, diverse adhesins, siderophores, toxins, polysaccharide coating, and the ability to cause a deleterious inflammatory response.

Patient behaviors that are not associated with UTI include precoital or postcoital voiding patterns, daily beverage consumption, frequency of urination, delayed voiding habits, wiping patterns, tampon use, douching, use of hot tubs, and type of underwear.

TREATMENT

The goal of treatment in uncomplicated UTI is to decrease symptoms and prevent complications. Treatment should be guided by two important principles: the prevalence of resistant genitourinary pathogens in the community and collateral damage to ecologic microbiota (i.e., the risk of propagation of resistant organisms). First-line agents for uncomplicated UTI are nitrofurantoin, trimethoprim-sulfamethoxazole (TMP-SMX), and fosfomycin trometamol; alternative agents are the fluoroquinolones (except moxifloxacin) and the β-lactams (Table 100.1).

Treatment of complicated UTI should be based on culture results and the other comorbidities that are present. Recurrent UTI in sexually active women can be prevented with postcoital TMP-SMX 40/200 mg single dose (if the patient has more than two UTIs per year related to coitus) or with daily, every other day, or weekly antibiotic. If the patient has a UTI unrelated to coitus or there are fewer than two UTIs per year related to coitus, the prevention of the UTI recurrence can be achieved with patient-initiated therapy. Daily topical application of intravaginal estriol can be helpful in postmenopausal women. After completion of the treatment, urine culture is indicated for pregnant women and on an individualized basis for other patients with complicated UTI.

❖ For a deeper discussion on this topic, please see Chapter 268, "Approach to the Patient with Urinary Tract Infection," in *Goldman-Cecil Medicine*, 26th Edition.

COMPLICATIONS

Unrecognized and untreated UTIs can quickly develop grave complications. Recurrent infections, structural damage of the urinary tract and scar tissue formation, loss of renal function, increased risk of delivering low-birthweight or premature infants in pregnant women, and septic shock could all develop in untreated UTI cases. Serious complications include renal abscesses which usually present with fever, back and abdominal pain and may include urinary tract symptoms. Abscesses are usually due to ascending urinary tract infection often with an obstructive process. *E. coli* or other enteric aerobic rods are typical organisms. Renal abscess can also be due to hematogenous spread of *S. aureus*. Prolonged antibiotic therapy directed at the offending organism is usually curative. Perinephric abscess results from rupture of an intrarenal abscess into the perinephric space between the renal capsule and Gerota's fascia. Treatment is drainage and antibiotics. Some other serious complications of urinary tract infections are listed in Table 100.2.

TABLE 100.1 Therapy for Uncomplicated Urinary Tract Infections

Antimicrobial Agent	CYSTITIS			PYELONEPHRITIS		
	Useful Therapeutically	Dose and Duration	Comments	Useful Therapeutically	Dose and Duration	Comments
Nitrofurantoin monohydrate macrocrystals	[a]Yes, first line	100 mg bid for 5 days	Cheap, well tolerated SE: N, H Low impact on microbiome	No	NA	Reduced renal tissue penetration
Trimethoprim-sulfamethoxazole	[a]Yes, first line	160/800 mg bid for 3 days	If resistance is known to be <20% SE: rash, urticaria, N, V	Yes	160/800 mg bid for 14 days	[a]If organism susceptibility is known [c]If not, give an initial LA IV agent
Fosfomycin trometamol	[a]Yes, first line	3 g single-dose sachet	May be less efficient SE: N, D, H	No	NA	Active against MRSA ESBL, VRE
Fluoroquinolones (ciprofloxacin levofloxacin)	[b]Yes, second line	3-day regimen 250 mg bid 250 mg qd	High collateral damage SE: N, V, D, H, tendinitis	[a]Yes, first line	Dose varies; 7–14 days	If resistance is known to be <10%
β-Lactams	[c]Yes, second line	Dose varies by agent; 5–7 days	Less effective, increased side effects SE: N, V, D, rash, urticaria	[c]Yes Use cautiously Less efficient	Dose varies; 10–14 day regimen	[c]Give an initial LA IV agent

Data from Gupta K, Hooton TM, Naber KG, et al: International clinical practice guidelines for the treatment of acute uncomplicated cystitis and pyelonephritis in women: a 2010 update by the Infectious Diseases Society of America and the European Society for Microbiology and Infectious Diseases—executive summary, Clin Infect Dis 52:561-564, 2011.
D, Diarrhea; *ESBL*, extended-spectrum β-lactamase; *H*, headache; *IV*, intravenous; *LA*, long acting; *MSRA*, methicillin-resistant *Staphylococcus aureus*; *N*, nausea; *NA*, not applicable; *SE*, side effects; *V*, vomiting; *VRE*, vancomycin-resistant enterococci.
[a]AI level of evidence from current guidelines.
[b]AIII level of evidence from current guidelines.
[c]BI level of evidence from current guidelines.

TABLE 100.2 Complications of Urinary Tract Infections

Complications	Pathophysiology	Diagnostic Methods/Likely Pathogens	Treatment
Cortico-medullary abscess	Focal abscesses can occur with ascending, generalized pyelonephritis, often occur with anatomic abnormalities of the GU tract	CT scanning is the study of choice. Ultrasound findings are less specific. Likely pathogens are gram-negative bacilli.	Antibiotics alone for lesions <3 cm. Drainage and antibiotics for larger lesions.
Cortical abscess (Renal carbuncle)	Focal abscess within the kidney parenchyma from hematogenous blood stream infection	Ultrasound or CT scanning. *Staphylococcus aureus*, enteric gram-negative bacteria.	Treat source of bacteremia, large lesions need drainage
Septic shock	Urinary tract infections are a common source of gram-negative bacteremia sepsis and septic shock	Blood cultures, imaging studies for possible urinary obstruction/enteric gram-negative bacteria	Urgent antibiotic therapy, urinary drainage if needed, IV fluids and vasopressors
Perinephric abscess	Insidious purulent collection between the kidney capsule and Gerota fascia; secondary to urinary tract obstruction and/or hematogenous spread	CT scan or renal ultrasonography. Fifty percent have accompanying pleural effusion or lung pathology. Gram-negative bacterial pathogens.	Percutaneous drainage and antibiotics. Septation of the perinephric space makes drainage more difficult.

Continued

TABLE 100.2   Complications of Urinary Tract Infections—cont'd

Complications	Pathophysiology	Diagnostic Methods/Likely Pathogens	Treatment
Emphysematous pyelonephritis	Rapid onset, severe infection of the kidney with accumulation of gas in the tissues. Seen in uncontrolled diabetes and impaired host immunity.	Detection of air surrounding the kidney by chest radiography or CT scan. *E. coli* accounts for most cases.	Intravenous antibiotics and drainage; urgent nephrectomy often needed
Papillary necrosis	Necrosis of the renal medullary pyramids and papillae secondary to vascular impairment. Can occur with infectious and noninfectious processes.	CT scanning or intravenous urography (IVU). Associated with a variety of enteric gram-negative and gram-positive bacteria.	Treat the underlying cause and ameliorate the ischemia with hydration and alkalization
Xanthogranulomatis pyelonephritis	Chronic, insidious, and destructive disease of the kidney marked by a granulomatous inflammatory response with lipid-laden macrophages	Rare chronic, infectious, inflammatory disease of the kidney seen in diabetes, lipid storage diseases, obstructive uropathy. *Proteus* sp is the most common bacterial pathogen.	Treat underlying cause, mass effects from kidney can form fistula tracts and be confused for neoplastic disease

SUGGESTED READINGS

Gupta K, Hooton TM, Naber KG, et al: International clinical practice guidelines for the treatment of acute uncomplicated cystitis and pyelonephritis in women: a 2010 update by the Infectious Diseases Society of America and the European Society for Microbiology and Infectious Diseases—executive summary, Clin Infect Dis 52:561–564, 2011.

Gupta K, Trautner B: In the clinic: urinary tract infection [review], Ann Intern Med 156:ITC3-1–ITC3-15, quiz ITC-13–ITC-16, 2012.

Henderson JT, Webber EM, Bean SI: Screening for asymptomatic bacteriuria in adults: updated evidence report and systematic review for the US preventive Services Task Force, J Am Med Assoc 322(12):1195–1205, 2019. https://doi.org/10.1001/jama.2019.10060.

Hooton TM: Clinical practice: uncomplicated urinary tract infection [review], N Engl J Med 366:1028–1037, 2012.

Hooton TM, Bradley SF, Cardenas DD, et al: Diagnosis, prevention, and treatment of catheter-associated urinary tract infection in adults: 2009 International clinical practice guidelines from the infectious Diseases society of America, Clin Infect Dis 50:625–663, 2010.

Nicolle LE, Bradley S, Colgan R, et al: Infectious Diseases Society of America guidelines for the diagnosis and treatment of asymptomatic bacteriuria in adults, Clin Infect Dis 40:643–654, 2005.

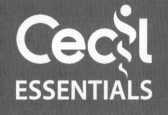

101

Health Care–Associated Infections

Paul G. Jacob, Thomas R. Talbot

INTRODUCTION

A health care–associated infection (HAI) is an infection that did not exist or was not incubating at the time of admission to the health care facility. These infections can occur in all types of health care settings, including acute care units, long-term care facilities, rehabilitation facilities, outpatient dialysis clinics, and outpatient surgical centers. Surgical site infections (SSI), central line–associated bloodstream infections (CLABSI), and catheter-associated urinary tract infections (CAUTI) are common examples.

HAIs cause a substantial degree of morbidity and mortality. A 2018 study of 199 hospitals found a prevalence rate of 3.2% among a population of 12,299 patients in 2015. Extrapolating from this data, researchers concluded there were approximately 687,200 HAIs in US acute care hospitals in 2015. The Centers for Disease Control and Prevention (CDC) estimates that on any given day, approximately 1 in 31 hospitalized patients has an HAI. Beyond the extensive morbidity and mortality they cause, HAIs are costly, with costs ranging from $896 per catheter-associated urinary tract infection to $45,814 per central line–associated bloodstream infection. These costs are likely to be underestimated because of incomplete estimation of the outpatient costs of parenteral antibiotics, skilled nursing care, physical rehabilitation, and lost work days.

As of January 2011, the Centers for Medicare and Medicaid Services (CMS) required public reporting of certain facility-specific HAI outcomes as part of value-based purchasing. As of August 2019, the following acute care–related HAIs are required for reporting by CDC's National Healthcare Safety Network (NHSN): catheter-associated urinary tract infections and central line–associated bloodstream infections in all adult, pediatric, and neonatal intensive care units (ICU) and from all patient care locations meeting the NHSN definition for adult and pediatric medical, surgical or combined medical/surgical wards, colon and abdominal hysterectomy SSIs, hospital-onset *Clostridioides difficile* infections (CDIs), and hospital-onset methicillin-resistant *Staphylococcus aureus* (MRSA) bacteremias. The importance of preventing HAIs has never been more apparent.

The major types of HAIs include the infections reported to CMS, hospital-acquired pneumonia (HAP) or ventilator-associated pneumonia (VAP), health care–associated respiratory viral infections (e.g., influenza and respiratory syncytial virus acquired within a health care facility) and other multidrug-resistant organisms (MDROs). MDROs are pathogens with resistance to various important antibiotics (e.g., MRSA, vancomycin-resistant *Enterococcus* (VRE), antibiotic-resistant gram-negative bacilli). This chapter reviews the major classes of HAIs, with a focus on prevention, diagnosis, and treatment.

HEALTH CARE EPIDEMIOLOGY AND INFECTION PREVENTION

In the age of increasing MDROs, shortage of new antibiotics, and public reporting of HAIs, the importance of efforts to prevent HAIs is growing. The fields of health care epidemiology and infection prevention focus on the practices of tracking HAIs in a systematic fashion (i.e., surveillance) to implement evidence-based HAI prevention practices.

Although HAIs were once thought to be the cost of being critically ill and receiving care in a hospital, several key events have occurred during the past 20 years that have shifted that perception. In 2006, Pronovost and colleagues implemented a "simple and inexpensive intervention" in 103 ICUs in the state of Michigan while participating in the Michigan Health and Hospital Association Keystone ICU project. This landmark study showed a reduction in the median rate of CLABSIs from 2.7 per 1000 catheter days to zero. These results shifted the discussion from merely controlling HAIs to preventing them. Other major events have included the recognition and effectiveness of using bundles of evidence-based practices to reduce HAIs; the recognition of the HAI burden in nonacute, non-ICU settings (including ambulatory clinics, long-term care facilities, and other venues where healthcare is delivered); and the importance of quality improvement science in reducing HAIs.

The prevention of HAIs has become increasingly possible, and various types of prevention interventions can reduce the HAI burden dramatically. In 2010, Wenzel and Edmund described these interventions as horizontal and vertical strategies (Table 101.1). Horizontal infection prevention strategies are broad practices (e.g., hand hygiene, isolation precautions) aimed at preventing many or all types of HAIs, regardless of the specific pathogen, procedure, or device. Vertical HAI prevention strategies are directed at specific types of HAIs or target a specific organism. Vertical strategies include using procedural checklists or standardized bundles and MRSA decolonization.

CATHETER-ASSOCIATED URINARY TRACT INFECTIONS

CAUTIs were the third most common device-related infection according to a survey performed in 2018. In comparison to data in 2011, the percentage of patients with an HAI due to CAUTI in 2015 declined from 23.6% to 18.7%. The additional cost of a CAUTI, according to a 2013 meta-analysis, has been estimated at approximately $896 (range: $603 to $1189) per episode.

CAUTI complications include cystitis, pyelonephritis, and in up to 4%, bacteremia. Although urinary catheter–associated bacteremias are rare, they are an underappreciated cause of health care–associated bacteremias and have been estimated to cost an additional $3744 per episode. Though surveillance of CAUTI has long been emphasized in the ICU, efforts have increasingly focused on understanding its impact in non-ICU settings. A 2013 study of 506 CAUTIs among 15 hospitals revealed 72% occurred in non-ICU settings.

Most health care–associated urinary tract infections are catheter associated. A catheterized patient's daily risk of developing bacteriuria is about 3% to 10%. Indwelling urinary catheters disrupt several mechanisms of the natural defense against infection, including urine flow, length of the urethra, and micturition to prevent attachment of potential pathogens to the uroepithelium. Tamm-Horsfall proteins, the most abundant soluble proteins in the urine, play a significant role by binding uropathogenic bacteria, facilitating wash out, and lowering the threshold for activating local innate immunity. These soluble proteins are prevented from entering the lower urinary tract by the catheters.

An indwelling catheter allows colonization, attachment, and biofilm formation by certain microorganisms. Most of the organisms causing CAUTIs arrive by ascending the urethra from the meatus and perineum. The most common uropathogens identified in CAUTIs are *Escherichia coli, Candida* spp, *Klebsiella* spp, *Pseudomonas aeruginosa,* and *Enterococcus* spp (Fig. 101.1).

Common symptoms of a urinary tract infection (e.g., dysuria, urinary frequency) may not be useful in diagnosing a patient with an indwelling catheter. However, the most common clinical manifestations of a CAUTI are fever (≥38° C) and bacteriuria. Other signs and symptoms of a CAUTI can include rigors, altered mental status, pelvic or suprapubic pain, costovertebral angle tenderness, and acute onset of hematuria without another underlying cause. One of these signs or symptoms plus a positive urine culture with a known uropathogen (>10^5 colony-forming units) strongly suggests a CAUTI. Pyuria (>5 leukocytes/mL of urine) is not always a reliable indicator for infection in patients with indwelling catheters; pyuria and asymptomatic bacteriuria are not necessarily indications for treatment. Risk factors for CAUTI acquisition include duration of catheterization, underlying fatal illness, age older than 50 years, having a nonsurgical underlying illness, and nonadherence to proper catheter care (E-Table 101.1).

The most effective method of preventing CAUTIs is to avoid placing urinary catheters unless absolutely necessary and to restrict catheter use to institutionally accepted indications. Proper insertion and care of urinary catheters are paramount (see Table 101.1). Maintenance of unobstructed flow with the collection bag below the bladder, use of a closed catheter system (even when sampling urine), and discontinuation of the catheter as soon as appropriate are key elements for preventing a CAUTI. Nurse-directed discontinuation protocols in which frontline personnel have defined parameters for removing catheters without requiring a provider's order are increasingly used to eliminate unnecessary catheters. The routine use of antimicrobial-coated catheters is not recommended except when infection rates remain elevated despite proper adherence to all other prevention strategies.

Treatment of asymptomatic bacteriuria usually is not recommended, with exception of pregnant women and patients who will undergo urologic procedures. Treatment of CAUTI is based on current Infectious Disease Society of America (IDSA) guidelines, and the choice of antimicrobial regimen should be based on the local antibiogram and identified syndrome (e.g., pyelonephritis). Before treatment, urine culture and sensitivity results are used to evaluate a resistant organism and tailor an empirical antimicrobial regimen. To ensure accurate diagnosis of urinary tract infections, many hospitals have adopted algorithms that will only allow for cultures if there is pyuria demonstrated on urinalysis (also known as reflexive culture).

Most clinicians prefer to replace or discontinue the catheter after a urinary tract infection is diagnosed. Guidelines recommend replacement if it has been in place for more than 2 weeks. There is good evidence based on review by expert committees that duration of treatment can be 7 days if symptoms quickly resolve or 10 to 14 days if resolution is delayed. In nonpregnant women younger than 65 years of age, a 3-day course of antibiotic therapy can be considered after the urinary catheter has been removed.

HOSPITAL-ACQUIRED AND VENTILATOR-ASSOCIATED PNEUMONIA

Pneumonia remains one of the most common HAIs, following *C. difficile* infection. Both HAP and VAP are included in the surveillance of HAIs. As of the most recent American Thoracic Society and IDSA guidelines in 2016, the term "health care–associated pneumonia (HCAP)" has been retired due to overlap with HAP and VAP. Other definitions are given in Table 101.2.

The incidence of HAP or VAP is difficult to determine due to the various definitions that have been used for surveillance and the subjective nature of these diagnoses. Some studies have estimated that the incidence of VAP ranges from 2 to 16 cases per 1000 ventilator days. VAP is associated with an increased length of hospital stay (10 days in one study), costs (approximately $40,000), and mortality (attributable mortality rate of 13%, highest among surgical patients).

Risk factors for VAP include conditions that lead to increased aspiration or impairment of host defenses and bacterial colonization of the respiratory and upper gastrointestinal tracts (see E-Table 101.1). In a ventilated patient, the body's natural mechanical defense mechanisms (e.g., ciliated epithelium, mucus, cough) are interrupted, leading to colonization of the lower airways by potentially pathogenic organisms. The most significant source of these organisms tends to be the patient's own oropharynx and upper gastric contents.

The most commonly implicated respiratory pathogens are *S. aureus* and *P. aeruginosa,* followed by several Enterobacteriaceae species and *Acinetobacter baumannii* (see Fig. 101.1). Colonization with MDROs correlates with an increasing duration of hospitalization. Guidelines argue that late (>4 days after admission) compared with early HAP may be the most useful factor when determining empirical antimicrobial therapy. Although bacteria play the largest role in HAP, fungi and viruses also must be considered in immunosuppressed patients.

One definition of HAP or VAP includes clinical, radiographic, and microbiologic criteria. Signs and symptoms indicating an infection include fever (≥38° C), peripheral leukocytosis, purulent sputum, and worsening respiratory status. A tracheal aspirate for Gram stain and culture provides the last piece of diagnostic information. When several of these signs and symptoms exist in the absence of a pulmonary infiltrate, alternative diagnoses should be considered, including ventilator-associated tracheobronchitis.

The greatest risk factor for the prediction of MDRO-related pneumonia is prior intravenous antibiotic therapy, whether for HAP or VAP (see Table 101.2). Longer duration of hospitalization increases the risk for acquisition of multidrug resistant pathogens, though the concept of early- and late-onset pneumonia has been challenged by more recent studies. Prior intravenous antibiotic therapy within the last 90 days is an independent risk factor for both MRSA and MDR *Pseudomonas aeruginosa.* Additional risk factors in VAP include septic shock, acute respiratory distress syndrome (ARDS), 5 or more days prior to occurrence, and prior receipt of acute renal replacement therapy.

INFECTIONS ASSOCIATED WITH VASCULAR CATHETERS

The NHSN collects data on CLABSIs, and public reporting is required for CLABSIs in ICUs and certain non-ICU inpatient units. In 2011, the incidence of CLABSIs ranged from 0 to 3.7 cases per 1000 catheter days. In 2015, CLABSIs made up a smaller percentage of HAIs (16.9%) than in 2011 (18.8%). Although CLABSIs have the lowest prevalence

TABLE 101.1 Strategies for Preventing Health Care–Associated Infections

Horizontal Strategies (to Prevent All or Many Types of HAIs)
1. Standard precautions
   - Hand hygiene
   - Use of appropriate PPE
   - Respiratory hygiene and cough etiquette
   - Appropriate environmental cleaning and waste disposal
2. Chlorhexidine bathing in all ICU patients and in non-ICU acute inpatients with central lines[a]
3. Isolation precautions appropriate for pathogen
4. Steps to prevent needlestick injuries
5. Education of health care workers on IC/IP protocols

Vertical Strategies (Specific to HAI Type)
CAUTI
Urinary catheter placed only for appropriate indications:
   Urinary retention or obstruction
   Need for accurate UOP measurement in critical illness
   Incontinence and perineal or sacral wounds
   Comfort care use for terminal illness
Consider alternatives:
   Condom catheters
   Intermittent catheterization
Proper insertion and maintenance:
   Maintain aseptic technique
   Properly secure catheter to patient
   Maintain closed drainage system
   Maintain unobstructed flow
Urinary catheter premeditated stop order or RN-initiated discontinuation policy
Anti-infective catheters if infection rates remain high
Reflexive culture testing algorithms to reduce false diagnosis of urinary tract infection

VAP
Use noninvasive ventilation when able
On intubation:
   Semirecumbent position (30–45 degrees) unless contraindicated
   Hypopharyngeal suctioning
   Avoid gastric overdistention
   Use cuffed ET tube
   Oral care, tooth brushing
   Keep ventilatory circuit closed unless changing for soiling or malfunctioning
   Daily targeted sedation management
   Spontaneous breathing trial if screening finds applicable
Use weaning protocols to minimize duration of ventilation

CLABSI
Use checklist for device insertion:
   Bundle supplies
   All present use at least face mask, then proceduralist uses sterile gown and gloves, mask, and head cap
   Avoid femoral line placement if possible
   Skin antisepsis with alcohol and >0.5% chlorhexidine
   Use of chlorhexidine-impregnated dressing or sponge at insertion site
   Empower personnel to stop nonemergent insertion if improper technique is followed
Maintenance:
   Access as infrequently as feasible
   Scrub the access hub or port with antiseptic
   Daily bathing with chlorhexidine and intranasal antiseptic with mupirocin or povidone-iodine
Daily audits for assessment of device need and potential discontinuation
Interventions to reduce blood culture contamination that may be falsely assessed as true bacteremia

SSI
Preoperative strategies:
   Nonirritative hair removal with clippers on the day of surgery (not razors)
   Eradicate remote infection
   Decolonization of *Staphylococcus aureus*
   CHG bathing
   Smoking cessation
   Glucose control, hemoglobin A_{1c} <7% if possible
   Avoid immunosuppressive medication in perioperative period
   Identify and address malnutrition
Intraoperative strategies:
   In OR: proper ventilation, minimize traffic, proper attire, and surgical scrub
   Proper skin preparation (chlorhexidine plus alcohol or povidone plus alcohol) and draping
   Antimicrobial prophylaxis; proper timing, dosing, and intraoperative redosing
   Maintain normothermia
   Glucose control
   Tissue oxygenation, preoperative and postoperative supplementation

CDI
Prevention of acquisition:
   Antimicrobial stewardship
Prevention of transmission:
   Contact precautions (e.g., empiric placement for those suspected of CDI before confirmation of diagnosis)
   Hand hygiene with soap and water before leaving the patient's room
   Continue contact precautions
Appropriate environmental cleaning with bleach-containing agents

CAUTI, Catheter-associated urinary tract infection; *CDI, Clostridioides difficile* infection; *CHG*, chlorhexidine gluconate; *CLABSI*, central line–associated bloodstream infection; *ET*, endotracheal; *HAI*, health care–associated infection; *IC/IP*, infection control or prevention; *ICU*, intensive care unit; *MDRO*, multidrug-resistant organism; *OR*, operating room; *PPE*, personal protective equipment; *RN*, registered nurse; *SSI*, surgical site infection; *UOP*, urine output; *VAP*, ventilator-associated pneumonia.
[a]Current data are not strong for prevention of CAUTI, VAP, and CDI by this method.

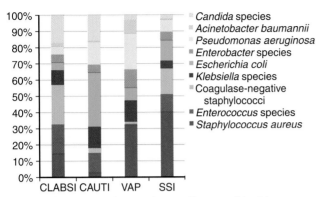

Fig. 101.1 Causative pathogens by specific type of health care–associated infection as reported to the Centers for Disease Control and Prevention National Healthcare Safety Network. *CAUTI,* Catheter-associated urinary tract infections; *CLABSI,* central line–associated bloodstream infections; *SSI,* surgical site infections; *VAP,* ventilator-associated pneumonia. (Modified from Sievert DM, Ricks P, Edwards JR, et al: Antimicrobial-resistant pathogens associated with healthcare-associated infection: summary of data reported to the National Healthcare Safety Network at the Centers for Disease Control and Prevention, 2009-2010, Infect Control Hosp Epidemiol 34:1-14, 2013.)

TABLE 101.2	Definitions of Types of Health Care–Associated Pneumonia	
Pneumonia Type	**Definition**	
Hospital-acquired pneumonia (HAP)	Pneumonia that occurs at least 48 hours after admission and that was not incubating at the time of admission	
Ventilator-associated pneumonia (VAP)	Pneumonia that arises 48–72 hours after endotracheal intubation	

Data from American Thoracic Society, Infectious Diseases Society of America: Guidelines for the management of adults with hospital-acquired, ventilator-associated, and healthcare-associated pneumonia, Am J Respir Crit Care Med 171:388-416, 2005.
IV, Intravenous; *LTCF,* long-term care facility; *NH,* nursing home.

among HAIs, the cost per episode and morbidity rate remain high. The estimated additional cost of an infection related to an intravenous catheter has been estimated at $45,814 (95% confidence interval [CI]): $30,919 to $65,245) per episode. The attributable increase in length of stay has been between 6.5 and 22 days, and the attributable mortality rate is about 10% among hospitalized patients.

The most common pathogens that cause primary CLABSIs are flora arising at the percutaneous insertion site or from contamination of the catheter hub. Hematogenous seeding from a gastrointestinal or other endovascular source occurs but is less likely. The most common pathogens that cause CLABSIs are coagulase-negative staphylococci, *Candida* species, *S. aureus,* and *Enterococcus* spp (see Fig. 101.1). The risk factors for CLABSI are provided in E-Table 101.1. The rising proportion of infections caused by *Enterococcus* and *Candida* spp since the 2006 to 2007 period suggests that skin colonization is being adequately addressed by the adoption of evidence-based prevention strategies and that an increasing fraction of CLABSIs are caused by secondary hematogenous seeding. Patients who are more severely ill, are neutropenic, have burns, or are on total parenteral nutrition are also at increased risk for candidemia. Other types of catheter-related infections include phlebitis, exit site infection, and pocket infection, tunnel infection, and septic thrombophlebitis.

Many CLABSIs are preventable through the use of evidence-based prevention practices for line insertion and maintenance. Strategies include appropriate decolonization of the skin before insertion with chlorhexidine plus alcohol, use of maximal sterile barriers (i.e., proceduralist wears sterile gloves and gown, cap, and mask, and a large barrier drape is placed over the patient), hand hygiene, and sterile technique (see Table 101.1). Appropriate maintenance of the central line mandates scrubbing the hub with an antiseptic and discontinuing the catheter as soon as it is not needed. Additional strategies with evidence for prevention of CLABSIs in the ICU include daily chlorhexidine bathing and nasal decolonization with mupirocin or povidone-iodine.

For a patient with a fever or systemic symptoms who has a central venous catheter, a bloodstream infection should be suspected. The diagnostic evaluation should begin with paired peripheral and catheter blood samples for culture before initiation of antimicrobial therapy. In a suspected case of bloodstream infection, the exudate at the exit site should be cultured.

The type of device (e.g., peripheral vs. central, short term vs. long term), associated infectious complications, and the implicated organism all play a role in treatment. For CLABSIs associated with short-term, nontunneled catheters and no complicating factors (e.g., suppurative thrombophlebitis, endocarditis, intravascular hardware), it may be appropriate to treat for 7 to 14 days after removal of the catheter. However, for long-term catheters, salvage may be attempted with systemic plus antibiotic lock therapy (as indicated by only a moderate amount of evidence from well-designed clinical trials or cohort or case series). Salvage of catheters associated with *S. aureus* bacteremia and fungemia have largely been unsuccessful, and it is not recommended. In the setting of an endovascular complication, removal of the catheter is strongly recommended, and systemic antibiotic therapy should be prolonged (i.e., 4 to 6 weeks). In many cases, septic thrombophlebitis may require surgical attention. Tunnel and pocket infections may also require débridement, but after the catheter is removed, 7 to 14 days of antimicrobial therapy should be sufficient.

SURGICAL SITE INFECTIONS

Standard definitions of SSIs classify them as superficial incisional, deep incisional (involving fascia or muscle), and organ space depending on the depth of tissue involvement. Most SSIs occur within 30 days of the operation, but some may develop later, especially in the setting of implanted foreign bodies (e.g., arthroplasty). The 2015 HAI Prevalence study from the CDC estimated an annual national burden of over 110,800 SSIs among hospitalized adult patients, a figure that does not include those patients with an SSI that did not require hospitalization. A patient who develops an SSI while hospitalized has a greater than 60% risk of being admitted to the intensive care unit, is 15 times more likely to be readmitted to the hospital within 30 days after discharge, and incurs an attributable extra hospital course of 6.5 days, leading to a direct cost of an additional $3000 per infection.

Endogenous seeding from the patient's skin flora is the most common avenue of infection. *S. aureus* and coagulase-negative *Staphylococcus* cause more than 40% of SSIs. In clean-contaminated operations, including open abdominal surgeries, gram-negative bacilli are predominant. An SSI should be suspected when postoperative patients have wound-associated purulent drainage, pain, tenderness, swelling, or redness. Positive culture growth from an aseptically obtained specimen is most convincing.

Many practices are used to prevent SSIs (see Table 101.1). One of the earliest and most effective strategies has been active surveillance and subsequent reporting of infection rates to the surgeons and staff. Much of the reduction in rates was attributed to the Hawthorne effect (i.e., active monitoring changes the behaviors of those being monitored). Other important interventions designed to reduce SSIs include

TABLE 101.3	Pathogenic Isolates Resistant to Selected Antimicrobial Agents According to the NHSN, 2014				
Organism	Antimicrobial	CLABSI	CAUTI	VAP[a]	SSI
Staphylococcus aureus	Oxacillin, methicillin, cefoxitin	50.7%	52.0%	42.4%	42.6%
Enterococcus faecium	Vancomycin	82.2%	85.1%	n/a	58.4%
Klebsiella pneumoniae	Ceftriaxone, ceftazidime, cefotaxime, or cefepime	24.1%	22.5%	21.0%	11.3%
	Carbapenems	10.9%	9.5%	10.1%	3.3%
Escherichia coli	Ceftriaxone, ceftazidime, cefotaxime, or cefepime	22.2%	16.1%	16.7%	15.3%
	Fluoroquinolones	49.3%	34.8%	30.8%	30.9%
Enterobacter spp	Ceftriaxone, ceftazidime, cefotaxime, or cefepime	36.1%	40.5%	26.9%	27.5%
	Carbapenems	6.6%	6.5%	3.2%	3.4%
Pseudomonas aeruginosa	Fluoroquinolones	30.2%	32.6%	31.9%	11.5%
	Piperacillin-tazobactam	18.4%	15.5%	19.4%	7.4%
	Cefepime, or ceftazidime	24.2%	22.5%	25.7%	9.9%
	Carbapenems	25.8%	23.9%	28.4%	7.7%
Acinetobacter baumannii	Carbapenems	46.6%	64.0%	55.5%	33.3%

Modified from Weiner LM, Webb AK, Limbago B, et al. Antimicrobial-resistant pathogens associated with healthcare-associated infections: summary of data reported to the National Healthcare Safety Network at the Centers for Disease Control and Prevention, 2011-2014. Infect Control Hosp Epidemiol. 2016;37(11):1288-1301.

CAUTI, Catheter-associated urinary tract infection; *CLABSI,* central line–associated bloodstream infection; *NHSN,* National Healthcare Safety Network; *SSI,* surgical site infection; *VAP,* ventilator-associated pneumonia.

[a]2012.

antimicrobial prophylaxis (i.e., the right drug at the right dose and right time), appropriate skin antisepsis, and maintenance of glucose control (see Table 101.1).

Management of SSIs often involves opening of the incision, evacuation of infected tissue, and allowing the wound to heal by second intention. The decision for initiating antibiotics is made on an individual basis and depends on the appearance of the wound, systemic signs of infection, depth of the infection, host's immune system, and type of surgery. Culture and Gram stain results help to dictate antibiotic coverage. For SSIs from a clean operation, empirical therapy covering *S. aureus* and *Streptococcus* species is recommended. For procedures involving the perineum, intestinal tract, or urogenital tract, broader coverage is needed to address gram-negative and anaerobic pathogens. When the SSI occurs within 48 hours of the index operation, *Streptococcus pyogenes* and *Clostridioides* spp are often implicated.

CLOSTRIDIOIDES DIFFICILE INFECTION

CDI is defined as diarrhea or toxic megacolon with detection of the *C. difficile* organism or toxin A or B, or both, in the stool or evidence of pseudomembranous colitis detected endoscopically, surgically, or histopathologically. This colonic infection is often accompanied by fever and leukocytosis.

C. difficile is the most common pathogen responsible for HAIs, approximating 12.1% of all HAIs. The incidence and severity of CDIs had been steadily increasing until more recently. Most reports have implicated the emerging BI/NAP1/027 strain, antibiotic overuse, and the aging population of hospitalized patients, who are disproportionately affected by CDI. Virtually every antibiotic has been associated with increasing the risk of CDI. Intensive efforts to combat CDI have also focused on several avenues: accurate diagnosis, reducing vectors for transmission, and judicious use of antimicrobials. Diagnosis of CDI must correctly identify infection versus colonization. The strategy of diagnostic stewardship aims to employ proper testing algorithms to ensure only patients exhibiting clear signs and symptoms receive diagnostic evaluation. Transmission prevention has focused on efforts to reduce the environmental burden of pathogens through environmental cleaning and hand hygiene as well as through the use of transmission-based precautions (e.g., contact precautions).

The continued rise of CDI, increasing resistance to antimicrobials by many different pathogens, and lack of antimicrobials with novel mechanisms of action underscore the importance of antimicrobial stewardship. Antimicrobial stewardship is a strategy that emphasizes optimal selection, dose, and duration of antimicrobial therapy, producing the best clinical outcome while decreasing the risk of subsequent complications.

The consequences of poor stewardship include the emergence of resistance, CDI, and excessive drug expenditures. Antimicrobials have different probabilities of invoking resistance or CDI. Strategies implemented by antimicrobial stewardship programs include provider education and guidelines, de-escalation or tailoring of empirical therapy when possible, use of more appropriate empirical treatments, and front-end restriction of certain antibiotics.

For a deeper discussion of these topics, please see Chapter 267, ❖ "Approach to the Patient with Suspected Enteric Infection," and Chapter 280, "Clostridial Infections," in *Goldman-Cecil Medicine*, 26th Edition.

MULTIDRUG-RESISTANT PATHOGENS

MDROs are organisms that are resistant to more than one class of antimicrobial agents, although the names of some (e.g., MRSA, VRE) imply resistance to only one drug. According to NHSN data reported from the 2011 to 2014 period, high rates of resistance persist for a multitude of common bacterial pathogens (Table 101.3).

Infections caused by MDROs lead to increased length of hospitalization, health care costs, and mortality rates for patients compared with those who are infected by antimicrobial-susceptible organisms. Kollef and colleagues found that patients who received inadequate antimicrobial therapy for their HAIs had an infection-related mortality rate 2.37 times that of those in the ICU who received adequate coverage. The principal reason for inadequate coverage was multidrug resistance.

The predominant gram-positive MDRO pathogens are MRSA and VRE. Methicillin resistance in *S. aureus* is caused by the production of an alternative penicillin-binding protein (PBP2A) that has a low affinity for β-lactam antibiotics and forms stable peptidoglycan products in the presence of adequate levels of the β-lactam. MRSA infections tend to have worse outcomes compared with methicillin-susceptible *S. aureus* (MSSA), but the typical health care–acquired strains are not necessarily more virulent. However, community-acquired MRSA, the most prevalent of which is the USA-300 strain, tends to be more virulent, and many of these isolates produce the Panton-Valentine leukocidin toxin, which is associated with greater leucocyte destruction and tissue necrosis. The largest reservoirs of MRSA are patients with the greatest contact with the health care system, and most carriers are asymptomatic.

Vancomycin resistance in *S. aureus* is another concern. Vancomycin intermediate-resistant strains, vancomycin heteroresistant strains, and vancomycin-resistant strains have been detected. The intermediate resistance or decreased susceptibility to vancomycin is thought to result from cell wall and biomatrix thickening, making the drug target more difficult to reach. Complete vancomycin resistance occurs by acquisition of the *vanA* gene from VRE. VRE, unlike many MRSA strains, is almost entirely a health care–associated phenomenon. Clusters of *vanA* or *vanB* genes are carried on mobile genetic elements that are readily transmitted between strains. These genes encode peptidoglycan precursors that have a low affinity for vancomycin.

Gram-negative MDROs have a greater tendency to form resistance to multiple antimicrobials, and new antimicrobials to target these pathogens are not available. The Enterobacteriaceae are gram-negative bacteria that usually reside in the gastrointestinal tract, are glucose fermenters, and account for about 29% of HAIs. These organisms tend to be the most common pathogens in SSIs associated with abdominal operations. The non–glucose fermenting organisms, including *P. aeruginosa*, *Acinetobacter baumannii*, and *Stenotrophomonas maltophilia*, account for about 9% of HAIs.

Multidrug-resistant gram-negative bacteria are making their way into the limelight largely due to the emergence of isolates that are resistant to most or all available antimicrobials (e.g., MDROs that exhibit β-lactamases, extended-spectrum β-lactamases (ESBL), carbapenem and fluoroquinolone resistance). The emergence of carbapenem-resistant Enterobacteriaceae (CRE) has become particularly concerning. The predominant carbapenem-resistance mechanisms are the loss of OprD, an outer membrane protein, *Klebsiella pneumoniae* carbapenemases (KPCs), and the metalo-β-lactamases (MBLs), which hydrolyze carbapenems. The New Delhi metalo-β-lactamase 1 (NDM1) is one of the first MBLs to cause outbreaks in the United States. The carbapenemases and MBLs are easily transmissible and tend to be associated with other genes encoding mechanisms of resistance to other antimicrobial classes. Fluoroquinolone resistance can occur by efflux pumps or mutations in genes encoding the drug targets DNA gyrase and topoisomerase IV. Emerging resistance among fungi (e.g., *Candida* spp) is an additional concern. In particular, *Candida auris* has led to outbreaks in ICUs and often harbors high rates of resistance to first- and second-line antifungal agents as well as some routine disinfectants.

Limiting the spread of MDROs in the health care setting should be a comprehensive and system-wide program at any institution. Infection prevention programs should include optimized surveillance practices to identify emerging MDROs and appropriate intervention strategies. The mainstay of these programs includes use of evidence-based prevention practices and antimicrobial stewardship programs. Prevention also necessitates increased communication between hospitals and public health institutions to limit the spread of MDROs, conduct proper surveillance, and implement infection control actions.

SUGGESTED READINGS

Ban KA, Minei JP, Laronga C, et al: American College of Surgeons and Surgical Infection Society: Surgical Site Infection Guidelines, 2016 update, J Am Coll Surg 224(1):59–74, 2017.

Hooton TM, Bradley SF, Cardenas DD, et al: Diagnosis, prevention, and treatment of catheter-associated urinary tract infection in adults: 2009 International Clinical Practice Guidelines from the Infectious Diseases Society of America, Clin Infect Dis 50:625–663, 2010.

Kalil AC, Metersky ML, Klompas M, et al: Management of adults with hospital-acquired and ventilator-associated pneumonia: 2016 Clinical Practice Guidelines by the Infectious Diseases Society of America and the American Thoracic Society, Clin Infect Dis 63(5):e61–e111, 2016.

Kollef MH, Hamilton CW, Ernst FR: Economic impact of ventilator-associated pneumonia in a large matched cohort, Infect Control Hosp Epidemiol 33:250–256, 2012.

Magill SS, O'Leary E, Janelle SJ, et al: Changes in prevalence of health care-associated infections in U.S. Hospitals, N Engl J Med 379(18):1732–1744, 2018.

O'Grady NP, Alexander M, Burns LA, et al: Guidelines for the prevention of intravascular catheter-related infections, Clin Infect Dis 52(9):e162–e193, 2011.

Pronovost P, Needham D, Berenholtz S, et al: An intervention to decrease catheter-related bloodstream infections in the ICU, N Engl J Med 355:2725–2732, 2006.

Scott RD II: The direct medical costs of healthcare-associated infections in U.S. hospitals and the benefits of prevention. Available at: http://www.cdc.gov/hai/pdfs/hai/scott_costpaper.pdf. Accessed November 1, 2014.

Stevens DL, Bisno AL, Chambers HF, et al: Practice guidelines for the diagnosis and management of skin and soft tissue infections: 2014 update by the Infectious Diseases Society of America, Clin Infect Dis 59(2):e10–52, 2014.

Wenzel RP, Edmond MB: Infection control: the case for horizontal rather than vertical interventional programs, Int J Infect Dis 14(Suppl 4):S3–S5, 2010.

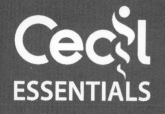

102

Sexually Transmitted Infections

Philip A. Chan, Susan Cu-Uvin

INTRODUCTION

Sexually transmitted infections (STIs) encompass a wide variety of organisms that have been causing human disease for thousands of years. Recognition of STIs can be challenging due to the heterogeneous nature and multiple symptoms of a single disease. Diagnosis and management of STIs is further complicated by underlying social bias and hesitancy by medical providers and patients to discuss issues related to sexuality and disease transmission.

The diagnosis of STIs should be based on a detailed history with special attention to sexual orientation and behaviors, a physical examination, and laboratory confirmation when appropriate. Professional and respectful attitudes by medical providers are essential to obtaining an accurate clinical history pertinent to STIs. Patients often deny risky behavior because of embarrassment or social stigma. Patients may also underestimate risky behaviors, and the diagnosis of STIs should therefore be based on a combination of history, epidemiology, clinical examination, and diagnostic testing.

A detailed sexual history should be obtained from all individuals with a suspected STI. They should be informed that the information is necessary to appropriately diagnose and manage STIs. The history should include sexual preferences for male or female partners; gender identity; the number of main, casual, and one-time partners; the use of condoms, drugs, and alcohol; and use of preexposure prophylaxis (PrEP) for human immunodeficiency virus (HIV) prevention as well as last HIV/STI testing. The history of partners should be elicited, including current symptoms and diagnosed STIs. If possible, counseling and education should be incorporated during the encounter. Prevention topics include abstinence, routine testing, disclosure of STIs to partners, behavior modification (i.e., avoiding risky sexual activities), condom use, prophylactic treatment for STI exposures, and PrEP.

Because of the diverse nature of STIs, it is useful to categorize the infections into a few major groups. There is overlap between different categories, and clinical judgment must be used to accurately diagnose STIs. For example, STIs that typically manifest with an ulcer may occasionally manifest with urethritis. Importantly, many STIs are asymptomatic or have symptoms that go unnoticed. When an individual has one STI, other STIs should be considered. The main categories of STIs are urethritis and cervicitis, genital ulcer disease, and genital warts. Symptomatic individuals with an STI usually fit into one of these categories.

URETHRITIS AND CERVICITIS

Urethritis and cervicitis are characterized by dysuria, burning, and urethral discharge. The discharge may range from barely noticeable to watery or frank pus. Urethritis has been categorized as gonococcal (i.e., caused by *Neisseria gonorrhoeae* and visible on Gram stain) or nongonococcal (i.e., commonly caused by *Chlamydia trachomatis*). Nongonococcal urethritis can be caused by other organisms, many of which are rarely tested for. Urethritis has historically been classified as gonococcal or nongonococcal because *N. gonorrhoeae* can easily be visualized on Gram stain. Most patients with symptomatic urethritis should be treated empirically with antibiotics directed against gonorrheal and chlamydial organisms without waiting for test results.

Chlamydia
Definition and Epidemiology
Chlamydia is the most prevalent bacterial STI in the United States and the world. The infection is caused by the bacterium *C. trachomatis*, which causes 30% to 40% of nongonococcal urethritis and cervicitis cases. In the United States, approximately 1.8 million cases were reported to the Centers for Disease Control and Prevention (CDC) in 2018, with an estimated number of infections that is more than twice the number of reported cases.

Age is a factor. Chlamydia has a 5% to 10% prevalence among adolescents and young adults. Other risk factors include having multiple sex partners, having condomless sex, or living in a lower socioeconomic area. In men, chlamydia is uncommonly associated with complications. In women, untreated chlamydia is associated with potentially severe complications, including pelvic inflammatory disease (PID), ectopic pregnancy, and infertility.

The CDC and USPTF recommends all sexually active women age 24 years or younger and other at-risk women be screened for chlamydia. Screening should also be considered for individuals who have a history of chlamydia or other STIs, have new or multiple sex partners, or exchange sex for drugs or money. All pregnant women should be screened. Men who have sex with men (MSM) should be screened at least annually and more frequently if there are ongoing risk factors such as multiple partners. The rationale for screening men is to prevent symptomatic epididymitis, proctitis, and urethritis. Importantly, MSM should also be screened at sites of exposure, which may include oropharyngeal and rectal screening for men that perform oral sex or have receptive anal sex, respectively. Screening MSM only for urogenital infection will miss up to 80% of chlamydia and gonorrhea infections. The presence of a rectal STI is a notable risk factor for HIV infection.

Pathology
C. trachomatis is an obligate intracellular, gram-negative bacterium that is evolutionary distinct from other bacteria. Several serovars of *C. trachomatis* are associated with human disease. They include serovars A-C (i.e., trachoma or ocular disease), D-K (i.e., anogenital disease), and L1-L3 (i.e., lymphogranuloma venereum [LGV]). *C. trachomatis* exists as an extracellular elementary body before attachment to susceptible epithelial cells and subsequent endocytosis. On entering the cell, the elementary form of *C. trachomatis* reorganizes into a reticulate

body within vacuoles that is functionally active, leading to growth and replication of the organism.

Clinical Presentation

Chlamydia may manifest with signs and symptoms ranging from none (most common) to life-threatening PID in women. When individuals have symptoms, the most common is urethritis in men and cervicitis in women. The incubation period varies but is usually 7 to 14 days after exposure.

Among men, 40% to more than 90% of chlamydia cases may be asymptomatic. Urethritis usually manifests as dysuria or discharge. *C. trachomatis* and *N. gonorrhoeae* infections are common causes of epididymitis in younger men. The infection typically manifests with unilateral testicular pain, swelling, and tenderness. *C. trachomatis* infection may also cause prostatitis and proctitis; the latter is typically found in MSM. The symptoms of proctitis in MSM should raise the possibility of LGV. The rates of transmission from infected men to women are as high as 65%.

In women and men, more than 85% of infections are asymptomatic. When symptomatic, *C. trachomatis* infection in women can be difficult to diagnose due to the nonspecific nature of symptoms. The classic manifestation is cervicitis, which can cause discharge, bleeding, pelvic pain, cervical friability, and ulcers. Complications of chlamydia include chronic pelvic pain, infertility, ectopic pregnancy, and PID. The lifetime prevalence of PID due to *C. trachomatis* infection depends on the population studied but is approximately 4%. PID usually manifests as abdominal or pelvic pain, cervical motion tenderness, and uterine or adnexal tenderness. Infection may also cause perihepatitis (i.e., Fitz-Hugh–Curtis syndrome), which is inflammation of the liver capsule. It occurs in 5% to 15% of PID cases. Chlamydia is the leading cause of preventable infertility worldwide.

Chlamydia may cause conjunctivitis and ocular trachomatis, the most common cause of preventable blindness worldwide. The disease also may manifest with pharyngitis and LGV. Classically a disease endemic in Africa, Southeast Asia, and the Caribbean, LGV has been identified in the United States and Europe, particularly among MSM with symptoms of proctitis. Typically, LGV manifests with genital ulceration and inguinal lymphadenopathy. Recognition of LGV is important given the longer duration of treatment.

Diagnosis and Differential Diagnosis

C. trachomatis cannot be routinely cultured on growth media, which has made diagnosis difficult. The introduction of nucleic acid amplification testing (NAAT) was a major advance and is now the standard diagnostic test. NAAT encompasses several laboratory methods including polymerase chain reaction (PCR), transcription-mediated amplification, and strand displacement amplification. The reported sensitivity of NAAT is 80% to 90%, with a specificity of 99%. The test may be performed on urine and vaginal or urethral (men) endocervical swab specimens. NAAT may also be performed on rectal and pharyngeal swab specimens.

Individuals who test positive and are treated for chlamydia should not be retested for at least 3 weeks after treatment. NAAT may remain positive during this time due to remnant material that does not signify persistent infection. Repeat testing to demonstrate cure should be performed for pregnant women or those with a concern about persistent infection. Individuals are usually retested at 3 months and then periodically depending on risk behaviors. Having had an STI places individuals at risk for becoming infected again. For individuals with multiple partners, including MSM, general STI testing that includes chlamydia is recommended every 3 to 6 months.

Treatment

Standard treatment regimens for urethritis or cervicitis due to chlamydia are azithromycin (1 g taken once orally) or doxycycline (100 mg twice daily for 7 days). These two medications are effective and cure more than 95% of infections. Azithromycin should be used in situations where adherence is a concern given the simplicity of dosing, which facilitates adherence. However, doxycycline may be more effective in achieving cure. Azithromycin can also be used in pregnancy. Other drugs that are effective in treating chlamydia include quinolones and penicillin. Sulfonamides (e.g., Bactrim) and cephalosporins should not be used. Doxycycline, ofloxacin, and levofloxacin are contraindicated in pregnant women.

Epididymitis due to chlamydia should be treated with doxycycline (100 mg taken orally twice per day for 10 days). Treatment for LGV proctitis depends on the severity of symptoms and should include doxycycline (100 mg orally twice each day for up to 3 weeks). In women, PID should be treated with ceftriaxone (250 mg given once intramuscularly) to cover gonorrhea and doxycycline (100 mg taken orally twice each day for 14 days) for chlamydia. Women who have concerning symptoms should be hospitalized and started on intravenous antibiotics, including cefoxitin (2 g given intravenously every 6 hours) or cefotetan (2 g given intravenously every 12 hours) and doxycycline (100 mg taken orally every 12 hours) (if not pregnant). Alternative treatment regimens include clindamycin (900 mg given intravenously every 8 hours) and gentamicin (2-mg/kg loading dose followed by 1.5 mg/kg every 8 hours). The duration depends on clinical improvement but is usually 2 weeks.

Prognosis

The natural history of untreated *C. trachomatis* infection varies. Individuals may remain asymptomatic for long periods, and the infection may resolve spontaneously or progress to symptoms and complications. Approximately 20% of individuals diagnosed with chlamydia but without symptoms may clear the infection before returning for treatment. Infection does not translate to protective immunity, and reinfection is common (10% to 20%). Therefore treatment of sex partners is important. In many areas, expedited partner therapy is allowed, and medical providers may prescribe treatment for sex partners without seeing them.

Gonorrhea
Definition and Epidemiology

Gonorrhea is caused by the bacterium *N. gonorrhoeae* and is the second most common reportable STI in the United States behind chlamydia. Similar to chlamydia, gonorrhea is a significant cause of urethritis in men and cervicitis in women and has the same complications. In the United States, the rate of gonorrhea declined in 2009 to a nadir of 98.1 cases per 100,000 people. Much of this was attributed to screening and treatment programs. Since 2009, however, cases of gonorrhea have increased each year to 104.2 cases per 100,000, with almost 600,000 cases reported in 2018.

Most individuals diagnosed with gonorrhea are adolescents or young adults. Cases among males are now more common than among females. MSM have also emerged as an important at-risk group. Risk factors for infection include younger age, multiple sexual partners, race or ethnicity, low socioeconomic status, and previous STIs. African Americans and Hispanic/Latinos have significantly higher rates of gonorrhea than white individuals in the United States.

Pathology

N. gonorrhoeae is a gram-negative bacterium with an outer membrane, peptidoglycan cell wall, and cytoplasmic membrane. Several components contribute to the virulence of the organism. Attachment to columnar epithelial cells is facilitated by pili, which extend from the cell surface and allow entry into the host cell by endocytosis. Organisms without pili are thought to be noninfectious. Gonococci are able to replicate within host epithelial cells and phagocytes. After mucosal infection, immune activation of neutrophils produces significant inflammation and exudate as pus.

Clinical Presentation

Gonorrhea is transmitted during sex with an infected partner. The risk of infection ranges from 20% to 50% per single act of sexual intercourse and increases with multiple acts. The incubation period is 2 to 7 days. When symptomatic, individuals with gonorrhea tend to have more purulent discharge than individuals with nongonococcal urethritis. In men, urethritis is the most common symptom at clinical presentation. Ten percent of men may be asymptomatic. Other manifestations of gonorrhea include epididymitis, proctitis, and pharyngitis. Rare but severe complications include abscesses and urethral strictures.

Between 50% and 80% of women with gonorrhea are asymptomatic. Typical symptoms include those of cervicitis, such as pelvic or adnexal pain, discharge, dysuria, and abnormal bleeding. As in men, gonorrhea can cause proctitis and pharyngitis in women. Most of these infections are asymptomatic. The most common complication of gonorrhea is PID. It may result in severe infection, chronic pelvic pain, and infertility. Infection during pregnancy may lead to complications such as premature labor, rupture of membranes, and spontaneous abortions.

Gonorrhea infection may also be associated with perihepatitis (Fitz-Hugh–Curtis syndrome). In less than 3% of individuals, disseminated gonococcal infection can lead to a classic triad of tenosynovitis (i.e., affecting multiple tendons), dermatitis (i.e., painless, few transient pustular lesions), and polyarthralgias (i.e., nonpurulent forms). Alternatively, individuals with disseminated infection may have purulent arthritis alone. Clinical presentation usually includes fever and other nonspecific systemic symptoms.

Diagnosis and Differential Diagnosis

N. gonorrhoeae is a gram-negative diplococci that can be visualized easily on Gram stain of purulent material. However, the most common method of diagnosis is NAAT, which has more than 98% sensitivity. NAAT testing can be performed on urethral, cervical, oropharyngeal, and rectal specimens. The major disadvantage of NAAT is the inability to evaluate antibiotic susceptibilities. *N. gonorrhoeae* can also be cultured from swab specimens from the rectum, urethra, pharynx, or cervix. Samples often contain many different microorganisms. Selective media such as modified Thayer-Martin media (with vancomycin, colistin, nystatin, and trimethoprim) is used to inhibit growth of indigenous flora. The sensitivity of cultures varies from 65% to 95%. When drug resistance is a concern, cultures should be sent for sensitivity testing.

Treatment

Antibiotic resistance of *N. gonorrhoeae* continues to be a worldwide problem. In the last decade, treatment of gonorrhea has been complicated by an increase in higher minimum inhibitory concentrations (MICs) for commonly used antibiotics, including first-line cephalosporins. The resistance patterns of gonorrhea vary by region.

To address the concern of antibiotic resistance, uncomplicated urogenital gonorrhea should be treated with dual therapy; one agent should be ceftriaxone (250 mg given once intramuscularly)

and the other azithromycin (1 g taken once orally). This regimen is 99% effective in curing gonorrhea. Azithromycin can also treat concurrent chlamydia. Alternatively, doxycycline (100 mg taken orally twice each day for 7 days) may be given instead of azithromycin. High resistance rates (10% to 20%) limit the use of tetracyclines. Cefixime (400 mg taken once orally) should be reserved only if ceftriaxone is unavailable and given with azithromycin (1 g taken once orally). Cefixime may be less effective in the treatment of pharyngeal gonorrhea. In patients allergic to ceftriaxone, dual treatment with single doses of gentamicin (240 mg intramuscular once) and azithromycin (2 g taken orally once) may be used cautiously. Gastrointestinal side effects are common with the higher dose of azithromycin.

Other antibiotics with activity against gonorrhea include spectinomycin. Antibiotics that should not be used to treat gonorrhea due to resistance include penicillins and fluoroquinolones. Disseminated or complicated gonococcal infections should be treated with intravenous ceftriaxone and doxycycline or azithromycin. The duration of these regimens depends on the clinical course and response to therapy.

Prognosis

Gonorrhea is curable with proper antibiotic therapy. Untreated disease often resolves over several weeks, but prompt treatment halts transmission and prevents complications.

Vaginitis
Definition and Epidemiology

The term *vaginitis* refers to disorders of the vagina characterized by inflammation or irritation of the vulva and an abnormal vaginal discharge. Although a separate entity from urethritis, there is significant overlap of symptoms and the organisms that cause vaginitis and urethritis. The three main types of infectious vaginitis are *Candida* vulvovaginitis, bacterial vaginosis, and trichomoniasis. The latter two are strongly associated with sexual transmission.

Trichomoniasis is the most common nonviral STI worldwide. In the United States, 3.1% of women between the ages of 14 and 49 years are infected with *Trichomonas vaginalis*. Screening is recommended for trichomoniasis in women who are at high risk for other STIs as determined by commonly accepted measures (i.e., having new or multiple partners). Screening for bacterial vaginosis in pregnant women is a controversial topic.

Pathology

Candida albicans and *Candida glabrata* are the most common organisms responsible for *Candida* vulvovaginitis. These species may colonize asymptomatic women but their presence does not necessarily mean infection. Symptomatic cases are caused by an overgrowth of the species and penetration of the superficial vaginal epithelial cells. Overgrowth can result from increased estrogen levels or suppression of other vaginal flora by antibiotics.

Trichomoniasis is caused by the protozoan *T. vaginalis*, which infects the squamous epithelium in the urogenital tract. *T. vaginalis* is not normally present in the vagina and has an incubation period of a few days.

Bacterial vaginosis is caused by a variety of organisms flourishing in the vaginal ecosystem in conjunction with a reduction of normally occurring lactobacilli. The bacterium *Gardnerella vaginalis* is especially prominent in cases of bacterial vaginosis and is thought to infect the vaginal epithelium, creating a biofilm to which other bacteria may adhere. *G. vaginalis* is also the organism thought to play the most likely role in sexual transmission of bacterial vaginosis.

Clinical Presentation

Symptoms of vaginitis may include pruritus (i.e., primary feature of *Candida* vulvovaginitis); a change in the volume, color, or odor of discharge; burning; irritation; erythema; dyspareunia; spotting; and dysuria. In the case of trichomoniasis and bacterial vaginosis, infection is often asymptomatic but can be associated with sex. Symptomatic trichomoniasis in women most commonly includes a purulent vaginal discharge, erythema, and irritation of the vulva. An abnormal odor is also often associated with infection.

Bacterial vaginosis manifests with milder symptoms of irritation and erythema and is rarely associated with dysuria or dyspareunia. Patients with bacterial vaginosis most commonly have a notably fishy odor in the vaginal discharge, which may also be abnormally colored or textured.

Diagnosis and Differential Diagnosis

Laboratory testing and microscopy are needed for a diagnosis of vaginitis. Examination of vaginal pH can be a helpful differentiating tool. *Candida* vulvovaginitis typically does not cause a change in vaginal pH, whereas bacterial vaginosis and trichomoniasis do increase the pH up to 6. The identification of *Candida* organisms on a wet mount or culture of discharge from women with characteristic clinical symptoms indicates *Candida* vulvovaginitis.

The diagnosis of trichomoniasis may be based on laboratory testing (NAAT), motile trichomonads on a wet mount, or positive culture results. NAAT testing for vaginitis is also available that evaluates for *Candida*, trichomoniasis, and bacterial vaginosis. Amsel criteria or Nugent criteria may be used to diagnose bacterial vaginosis when Gram stain or microscopy is not available.

Treatment

Vaginitis is curable with proper antibiotic therapy. Trichomoniasis is treated with metronidazole (500 mg orally twice each day for 7 days or 2 g taken orally once) or tinidazole. Pregnant women can be treated with 2 g of metronidazole in a single dose at any stage of pregnancy. The safety of tinidazole has not been fully established.

Treatment of all recent sexual partners is recommended because trichomoniasis is almost exclusively transmitted by sexual contact. The same twice-daily regimen of 500 mg of oral metronidazole is the primary treatment for bacterial vaginosis; however, the single 2-g oral dose is *not* recommended for treatment of bacterial vaginosis. Treatment of *Candida* vulvovaginitis with a single 150-mg dose of fluconazole is highly effective. Use of a topical agent depends on whether the case is considered complicated or uncomplicated. Only topical azole therapies, applied for 7 days, are recommended for use by pregnant women.

Prognosis

Bacterial vaginosis is treatable with various antibiotics, but the primary concern is failure of normal *Lactobacillus* flora to reestablish colonization in the vagina. This leads to repeated infections and necessitates prolonged treatment. Oral and vaginal administration of *Lactobacillus* bacteria is sometimes recommended. Bacterial vaginosis increases risk of infection with HIV, herpes simplex virus type 2 (HSV-2), and *N. gonorrhoeae*, making treatment critical for the management of other STIs.

Other Causes of Nongonococcal Urethritis

There are several other known causes of urethritis and cervicitis and likely more that are unknown. Significant causes may include *Mycoplasma genitalium*, HSV-1/2, *Treponema pallidum*, adenovirus, and *Ureaplasma urealyticum*. *U. urealyticum* can be part of the normal flora, and its role in urethritis has not been validated.

The most common of these organisms is *M. genitalium*. It is a bacterium that lacks a cell wall, cannot be Gram stained, and is very difficult to grow in culture. The organism accounts for 15% to 25% of men with nongonococcal urethritis in the United States and is thought to be a cause of cervicitis and PID in women. NAAT testing of urine, urethral, vaginal, and cervical specimens for *M. genitalium* is available and is the recommended diagnostic test. Testing for *M. genitalium* should be considered for individuals with persistent urethritis or cervicitis. Treatment of *M. genitalium* is complicated by concerns of emerging resistance across the world. Empirical treatment of symptomatic individuals includes azithromycin (1 g taken orally once or a 500-mg dose followed by 250 mg daily for 4 days; a longer duration of azithromycin may be more effective). Moxifloxacin (400 mg daily for 7 to 14 days) is also effective and should be used if individuals have persistent symptoms.

GENITAL ULCER DISEASE

Genital ulcers are a major manifestation of several STIs. Genital ulcers are best classified as painful (e.g., HSV, chancroid) or nonpainful (e.g., syphilis). LGV due to *Chlamydia* also manifests with ulcerations. Ulcers may be classified as single (e.g., syphilis, chancroid) or multiple or grouped (e.g., HSV-1/2). All of these STIs manifest with diverse signs and symptoms, and clinical examination alone may be inadequate for accurate diagnosis (Table 102.1).

Syphilis
Definition and Epidemiology

Syphilis is caused by the spirochete *T. pallidum*, which can result in a wide spectrum of clinical disease. At the beginning of the 20th century, it was thought that an astounding 10% of the general population in the United States had syphilis. The CDC began reporting rates of syphilis in 1941. The rates peaked in the early 1940s at almost 600,000 cases and subsequently reached a nadir in 2000 with a rate of 2.1 cases per 100,000 people in the general population. However, since that time, the number of reported syphilis cases has been increasing. The major at-risk group is MSM, but the disease is observed in people across all ages, genders, sexual orientations, socioeconomic status, and racial and ethnic classes.

The resurgence of a generalized syphilis epidemic among MSM with HIV infection has had important consequences. Clinicians at STI clinics and those treating individuals with HIV need to be aware of guidelines for the diagnosis and treatment of syphilis in this population. Furthermore, clinicians need to be aware of less common presentations of syphilis and have a high degree of suspicion. Given the increasing number of MSM living with HIV, it is not uncommon to see coinfection in this population. All MSM, regardless of HIV status, should be considered for syphilis screening on an annual basis and more frequently if they have other risk factors.

Pathology

T. pallidum organisms are thinly coiled bacteria that move in a corkscrew motion. *T. pallidum* cannot be easily cultured, hindering diagnosis and study of the organism. *T. pallidum* infects and penetrates mucosal membranes, resulting in the classic chancre lesion. The organism then infects local lymph nodes and disseminates systemically. The median incubation period is approximately 3 weeks. In more than 60% of infected individuals, syphilis does not progress to tertiary stages. Immune host factors are thought to contribute to the development of tertiary syphilis.

Clinical Presentation

Primary syphilis classically involves the genitals, although lesions may also be observed in the rectum or oropharynx. The estimated risk of

TABLE 102.1 Differential Diagnosis of Genital Ulcer Disease

Disease	Primary Lesion	Adenopathy	Systemic Features	Diagnosis and Treatment
Genital herpes (HSV-1/2)				
Primary	Incubation 2-7 days; multiple, painful vesicles on erythematous base; lasts 7-14 days	Tender, soft, and usually bilateral	Fever, malaise	Viral cultures, DFA, antibody testing, Tzanck smear
Recurrent	Grouped, painful vesicles on erythematous base; lasts 3-10 days	None	None	Tx: acyclovir, famciclovir, or valacyclovir for 7-10 days (shorter for recurrent cases)
Primary syphilis *(Treponema pallidum)*	Incubation 10-90 days (average, 21) Chancre: painless papule that ulcerates with firm, raised border and smooth base; usually single; may be genital or almost anywhere; heals in 3-6 weeks without treatment	1 week after chancre appears; bilateral or unilateral; firm, discrete, no overlying skin changes, painless, nonsuppurative	During later stages	Nontreponemal tests (RPR, VDRL), treponemal tests (FTA-ABS), darkfield microscopy; cannot be cultured Tx: see Table 102.3
Chancroid *(Haemophilus ducreyi)*	Incubation 3-5 days; vesicle or papule to pustule to ulcer; soft, not indurated; very painful	1 week after primary in 50%; painful, unilateral in two thirds; suppurative	None	Gram stain and culture. Tx: azithromycin, ceftriaxone, ciprofloxacin
Lymphogranuloma venereum *(Chlamydia trachomatis* serovars L1, L2, L3)	Incubation 5-21 days; self-limited, painless papule, vesicle, or ulcer; lasts 2-3 days; found in only 10-40%	5-21 days after primary; one third bilateral, tender, matted iliac or femoral groove sign; multiple abscesses; coalescent, caseating, suppurative; thick yellow pus; sinus tracts; fistulas; strictures; genital ulcerations	Fever, arthritis, pericarditis, proctitis, meningoencephalitis, keratoconjunctivitis, preauricular adenopathy, erythema nodosum	NAAT for *Chlamydia*. Samples can be sent to the CDC to evaluate for LGV specific serotypes. Tx: incision and drainage, doxycycline
Granuloma inguinale (donovanosis)	Incubation 9-50 days; at least one painless papule that gradually ulcerates; ulcers are large (1-4 cm), irregular, nontender, with thickened; rolled margins and beefy red tissue at base; older portions of ulcer show depigmented scarring, white areas; advancing edge contains new papules	No true adenopathy; in one fifth of patients, subcutaneous spread through lymphatics leads to indurated swelling or abscesses of groin (pseudobuboes)	Metastatic infection of bones, joints, liver	Wright or Giemsa staining with short, plump, bipolar staining pattern, Donovan bodies in macrophage vacuoles Tx: doxycycline
Condyloma acuminatum (genital warts)	Characteristic large, soft, fleshy, cauliflower-like excrescences around vulva, glans, urethral orifice, anus, perineum	None	None	Clinical diagnosis, biopsy if necessary Tx: topical podophyllin, surgery, others

DFA, Direct fluorescent antibody test; *FTA-ABS,* fluorescent treponemal antibody absorption test; *HSV,* herpes simplex virus; *NAAT,* nucleic acid amplification test; *RPR,* rapid plasma reagin; *Tx,* treatment; *VDRL,* venereal disease research laboratory.

transmission from an individual with primary syphilis to an uninfected individual is 30% per sexual act. Syphilis may also be transmitted to others sites (i.e., rectum, oropharynx) through exposure with any contact of a primary lesion. Inoculation of the organism by surgeons through needlesticks has been well documented and typically does not result in a chancre at the site of infection (i.e., syphilis d'emblee).

The four classic stages of syphilis are primary, secondary, latent, and tertiary. Staging is best thought of as a continuum rather than as discrete stages of infection. The states can manifest individually, but individuals often have symptoms consistent with primary and secondary symptoms. The primary and secondary stages of syphilis are extremely

infectious, and cases of transmission during the tertiary stage have been reported.

It can be very difficult to diagnose primary syphilis based solely on the physical examination. The primary chancre is generally described as a painless, clean-based, indurated ulcer. The borders are firm and raised. However, the presentation of a primary chancre may vary and any dermatologic manifestation in the right clinical setting (i.e., sexually active MSM) should be tested for syphilis. The chancre is teeming with spirochetes and should be considered extremely infectious. It is rare for a primary chancre to be absent, but it may go unnoticed. The chancre spontaneously heals without treatment over several weeks.

Secondary syphilis usually manifests as a diffuse, maculopapular rash that classically involves the palms and soles. However, a wide range of early skin manifestations exists, including macular, papular, pustular, vesicular, or any combination of these. Vesicular lesions may easily be confused with other STIs, including HSV-1/2. Syphilis may also have late skin manifestations, including nodular, squamous, or gummous appearances.

The rash typically develops a few weeks after the chancre and results from dissemination of the organism. Up to 80% of patients have some cutaneous manifestations of disease. The rash is usually symmetrical and pink, with no pain or burning, and it usually spares the face. It resolves on its own over weeks to months and may be confused with pityriasis rosea, erythema multiforme, drug rashes, tinea, measles, and seborrheic dermatitis. The maculopapular rash of secondary syphilis is considered noninfectious, although lesions in axillary or inguinal folds or other regions exposed to chaffing may erode and become infectious.

Syphilis then enters a latent stage, during which an infected individual has no symptoms but does have positive serologic test results (Table 102.2). Tertiary syphilis may then develop at any point from years to decades after the initial infection.

Approximately 30% to 40% of individuals with untreated syphilis infection develop tertiary disease, which can include neurosyphilis, cardiovascular syphilis, and gummatous disease. Neurosyphilis has classically been thought of as a complication of tertiary syphilis. However, *T. pallidum* may invade and cause symptoms of the central nervous system at the time of initial infection. Early neurosyphilis may be characterized by signs and symptoms of meningitis and milder symptoms, including headache. Other manifestations of neurosyphilis include otosyphilis (i.e., hearing loss) and ocular syphilis, which is classically characterized as posterior uveitis. Late neurosyphilis may manifest with general paresis (i.e., progressive dementia, forgetfulness, psychiatric disease, and personality change), Argyll-Robertson pupils (i.e., no response to light but normal accommodation), and tabes dorsalis (i.e., ataxia and lancinating pains). The most common finding in late neurosyphilis is irregular pupils.

Gummas, a result of immune system activation, may develop in any tissue or organ in the body. Classic cardiovascular symptoms of syphilis include aortitis, which often affects the ascending thoracic aorta causing a tree-bark appearance with dilation and aortic valve regurgitation.

Diagnosis and Differential Diagnosis

The diagnosis of syphilis is limited by the inability of *T. pallidum* to grow on standard laboratory media. Diagnostic testing for syphilis relies on the direct and indirect measurement of antibodies against treponema. Nontreponemal tests such as the rapid plasma reagin (RPR) and venereal disease research laboratory (VDRL) test rely on anticardiolipin antibodies, which usually resemble antibodies against treponema. These tests are usually sensitive but nonspecific, and false-positive results are relatively common, especially in individuals with other autoimmune diseases or who are pregnant. Nontreponemal tests report antibodies in terms of dilutions; a titer of 1:2 is extremely low compared with a titer of 1:1024. This measurement can be used as a general representation of spirochete load in the patient. With treatment, nontreponemal test results may revert to nonreactive. However, some individuals may not have a serologic response (12%) or may have persistent nontreponemal titers ("serofast"; 35% to 44%) despite appropriate treatment.

Treponemal tests such as the fluorescent treponemal antibody absorption (FTA-ABS) test rely on antibodies that directly target the organism and are therefore more specific. Test results may be positive or negative, and a positive result usually remains so for life. The normal testing algorithm employs the sensitive, nontreponemal tests, followed by a more specific treponemal test to confirm the diagnosis. However, the "reverse" algorithm, which employs a treponemal test first followed by a nontreponemal test, is also commonly used. In the case of a discordant result (i.e., a positive treponemal test and a negative nontreponemal test), a third different treponemal test is used (*Treponema pallidum* particle agglutination assay, TP-PA). The inherent limitation of antibody testing results in many cases of unclear diagnoses.

Several mistakes may be made by clinicians in the diagnosis of syphilis. In primary syphilis, the initial nontreponemal test result may be negative up to 30% of the time. A patient with a lesion suspicious for syphilis should undergo repeat testing or empirical treatment regardless of the serologic results. In the event of a recent exposure, a patient should be counseled that a syphilis and HIV antibody test may be negative. A patient who is treated early in the course of disease may never develop an antibody response and may therefore never have a positive test result.

After successful treatment, patients with an initial episode of syphilis should see a 4-fold decrease in nontreponemal titers at approximately 6 to 12 months. Titers may never return to normal and should be followed periodically. For MSM, CDC guidelines suggest yearly STI testing and more frequent testing (3 to 6 months) for patients with multiple partners, anonymous partners, or other risk factors for infection.

TABLE 102.2 Serologic Testing for Syphilis

Features	Nontreponemal	Treponemal
Technique	Antibody to cardiolipin-lecithin (RPR, VDRL)	Antibody to *Treponema pallidum* (FTA-ABS, EIA)
Indications	Screening and assessing response to therapy; should be quantified by diluting serum and reporting in titers	Confirmatory test; usually remains positive for life; may be used as a screening test
Positive for syphilis		
Primary	77%	86%
Secondary	98%	100%
Early latent	95%	99%
Late latent	73%	96%
False positives	1-2% of the population may have a false-positive RPR/VDRL; common in pregnancy, recent immunization, autoimmune diseases, acute infectious illness, HIV, chronic liver disease, prozone reaction (negative result due to high antibody titers)	Borderline positive is common in pregnancy, and test should be repeated

EIA, Enzyme immunoassay; *FTA-ABS,* fluorescent treponemal antibody absorption test; *HIV,* human immunodeficiency virus infection; *RPR,* rapid plasma reagin; *VDRL,* venereal disease research laboratory test.

Treatment

Despite the classic staging of syphilis as primary, secondary, latent, or tertiary, the disease is best thought of in terms of early infection (<1 year) or late infection (≥1 year) when considering treatment. Early infection consists of primary, secondary, and early latent stages. Late infection consists of late latent and tertiary disease. *T. pallidum* remains sensitive to penicillin. Individuals with early syphilis can be treated with a single intramuscular injection of benzathine penicillin G (Bicillin), which achieves high and prolonged serum concentrations. Individuals with late syphilis or disease of unknown duration should be treated with three weekly injections of intramuscular benzathine penicillin G (Table 102.3). This cures most patients. Importantly, other formulations of penicillin are less effective and should not be used.

Although penicillin remains the drug of choice, doxycycline may also be used in individuals who have severe allergies to penicillin. However, every effort should be made to use penicillin because of the sensitivity of the organism. For pregnant women who are allergic to penicillin, penicillin desensitization should occur in collaboration with a pharmacist and an allergist specialist. As a result of treatment, individuals may experience a febrile reaction (i.e., Jarisch-Herxheimer reaction). Symptoms are caused by killing of the spirochetes and should not be confused with an allergic reaction.

The co-epidemic of syphilis and HIV has led to an increase in individuals with manifestations of neurosyphilis. In cases of syphilis with neurologic symptoms, a lumbar puncture and CSF examination is warranted to rule out neurologic involvement. Any pleocytosis or increase in protein concentration warrants treatment for neurosyphilis. A cerebrospinal fluid (CSF) sample should be sent for VDRL testing, but the test lacks sensitivity (50%), and a negative test result does not rule out neurosyphilis. Usually, HIV-negative individuals with syphilis without neurologic symptoms should not undergo a lumbar puncture. Many HIV-infected individuals with syphilis, however, have asymptomatic neurosyphilis. The clinical implications of this are unclear, but these individuals may fail intramuscular therapy at a high rate. Some experts recommend CSF examination in all HIV-infected individuals with a CD4+ count lower than 350 cells/µL or a nontreponemal titer greater than 1:32. These criteria capture almost everyone with asymptomatic neurosyphilis.

Individuals with neurosyphilis should be treated with intravenous penicillin G for 10 to 14 days. In tertiary disease with manifestations of neurologic disease, treatment with intravenous penicillin halts disease progression but does not reverse existing structural damage. Ocular disease or other similar neurologic manifestations should be treated as neurosyphilis. Nontreponemal titers should be followed to ensure an appropriate response. Repeat treatment may be necessary in a small number of cases.

Prognosis

Although penicillin is the treatment of choice for syphilis, it has not been validated in clinical trials but is based on a long history of clinical use. However, a significant number of individuals with syphilis do not respond with the recommended decline in nontreponemal titer. Individuals who do not respond should be retreated.

For a deeper discussion of these topics, please see Chapter 303, "Syphilis," in *Goldman-Cecil Medicine*, 26th Edition.

Herpes Simplex Virus
Definition and Epidemiology

HSV-1/2 cause a wide variety of clinical disease. HSV-1 is historically the cause of herpes labialis (i.e., cold sores), and HSV-2 is the cause of genital herpes, although there is overlap. After infection occurs, HSV-1/2 enters a latent state and may later reactivate to cause disease in a subset of individuals.

The overall prevalence of HSV-1 and HSV-2 in the population is approximately 60% and 20%, respectively. However, the incidence of HSV-1 infection approaches 90% to 100% among middle-aged adults. Seroprevalence of HSV-2 is associated with a patient's sexual activity, including number of partners and history of other STIs, and with age, gender (women are at higher risk than men), and race or ethnicity. More than 50 million people in the United States are infected with genital HSV-1/2, and most are asymptomatic. CDC guidelines do not recommend routine screening for HSV-1/2 in people without symptoms. There is no evidence that screening for HSV-1/2 reduces its spread or has an impact on the disease. HSV-1/2 is not a reportable disease in the United States.

Pathology

HSV-1 and HSV-2 are two of eight double-stranded DNA human herpesviruses. Others include varicella-zoster virus (VZV), cytomegalovirus (CMV), Epstein-Barr virus (EBV), and human herpesviruses 6, 7, and 8. Infection with one type of HSV does not prevent or increase the chances of infection with other types. After initial infection, HSV-1/2 enters a latent state within neuronal cells of sensory or autonomic peripheral ganglia. Reactivation can occur at any time and is mediated in part by immune factors. HSV-1 most commonly infects the trigeminal ganglia and HSV-2 the sacral nerve root ganglia (S2-S5).

Clinical Presentation

Transmission of HSV-1/2 is through skin-to-skin contact, including sexual contact at mucosal surfaces such as the oropharynx, vagina, rectum, cervix, and conjunctivae. Importantly, transmission may occur in the absence of symptoms.

TABLE 102.3	**Syphilis Treatment**	
Clinical Category	**Regimen of Choice**	**Alternative[a]**
Early syphilis (<1 year)	Benzathine penicillin, 2.4 million units IM, given once	Penicillin desensitization Doxycycline, 100 mg PO bid for 14 days Tetracycline, 500 mg PO qid for 14 days Azithromycin 2 g PO qd
Late syphilis (≥1 year) or unknown duration	Benzathine penicillin, 2.4 million units IM, given once each week for 3 wk	Penicillin desensitization Doxycycline, 100 mg PO bid for 28 days Tetracycline, 500 mg PO qid for 28 days
Neurosyphilis	Penicillin G, 4 million units IV q4h or 24 million units by continuous infusion qd for 10-14 days	Penicillin desensitization Ceftriaxone 2 g qd IM or IV for 10-14 days

[a]If patient has a penicillin allergy.

The stages of HSV-1/2 infection include primary, latent, and recurrent. Primary infection of genital HSV-1/2 may include fever, headache, other systemic symptoms, and the classic local symptoms of painful genital vesicles or ulcers (multiple) and lymphadenopathy. Oral infections of HSV-1 may include gingivostomatitis and pharyngitis. Symptoms may vary from none to serious and require hospitalization. HSV-1/2 then enters a latent state. Reactivation occurs in a subset of individuals with symptoms less severe than those of primary infection. Some individuals have no reactivation, and others have multiple reactivations per year.

Complications of HSV-1/2 infection include meningitis and proctitis. Recurrent episodes of meningitis (i.e., Mollaret meningitis) may be caused by HSV-1/2. Other manifestations of HSV-1/2 include herpetic whitlow (e.g., infection of a finger of a health care worker), herpes gladiatorum (e.g., HSV-1/2 skin infections in athletes such as wrestlers), and ocular disease (e.g., keratitis, acute retinal necrosis). HSV-1/2 infection may rarely be associated with erythema multiforme, hepatitis, and encephalitis.

Diagnosis and Differential Diagnosis

The diagnosis of HSV-1/2 is typically made clinically. If possible, lesions should be tested for HSV-1/2 using viral culture (50% sensitivity), PCR, or direct fluorescent antibody (DFA) testing. Alternatively, serology testing for immunoglobulin M (IgM) and immunoglobulin G (IgG) antibodies is available. This test should be reserved for individuals with suspected primary infection or to document chronic infection, and it should usually not be used for screening purposes.

Treatment

Recommended regimens for primary HSV-1/2 infection include acyclovir (400 mg orally three times per day for 7 to 10 days or 200 mg orally five times per day for 7 to 10 days), famciclovir (250 mg orally three times each day for 7 to 10 days), or valacyclovir (1 g orally twice each day for 7 to 10 days). Treatment can also be used for reactivation disease: acyclovir (400 mg orally three times each day for 5 days, 800 mg orally twice each day for 5 days, or 800 mg orally three times each day for 2 days), famciclovir (125 mg orally twice each day for 5 days or 1000 mg orally twice each day for 1 day or 500 mg once followed by 250 mg twice each day for 2 days), or valacyclovir (500 mg twice each day for 3 days or 1 g orally once each day for 5 days).

Individuals with frequent recurrences may be candidates for suppressive therapy. Severe disease should be treated with intravenous acyclovir (5 to 10 mg/kg intravenously every 8 hours). Duration and transition to oral medication should be based on clinical improvement. Total treatment duration is usually at least 10 days. The safety of systemic acyclovir, valacyclovir, and famciclovir therapy in pregnant women is not established.

Prognosis

Although HSV-1/2 infection cannot be cured, most people are asymptomatic, and suppressive therapy is available. Individuals with HSV-1/2 infection should be educated regarding the disease, including transmission and available treatments. They should be encouraged to discuss their status with sexual partners, including the possibility that transmission may occur in the absence of symptoms. Individuals should abstain from sex during an outbreak.

Chancroid

Chancroid is a rare cause of genital ulceration in the United States. The infection is caused by the gram-negative rod *Haemophilus ducreyi* and is endemic in parts of Africa and the Caribbean. Classic symptoms include a single or multiple painful, nonindurated genital ulcers and inguinal lymphadenopathy. Growth of the organism in cultures requires hemin-containing media, and it may appear as a school of fish on Gram stain. PCR may be available in certain areas.

Testing for HSV-1/2 and syphilis should always be performed. Recommended treatment regimens include azithromycin (1 g orally once), ceftriaxone (250 mg intramuscularly once), or ciprofloxacin (500 mg orally twice each day for 3 days). Ciprofloxacin is contraindicated in pregnant and lactating women.

Granuloma Inguinale

Granuloma inguinale is also known as donovanosis. It is caused by the gram-negative bacterium *Klebsiella granulomatis*. The disease is rare in the United States but endemic in regions of Africa, India, Oceania, and the Caribbean. Clinical manifestations include painless, ulcerative genital lesions with erythema. Classic Donovan bodies may be observed on histopathology.

The recommended treatment regimen is doxycycline (100 mg orally twice each day for at least 3 weeks). Alternative regimens include azithromycin, ciprofloxacin, and sulfamethoxazole-trimethoprim. Azithromycin may be useful for treating granuloma inguinale during pregnancy. Doxycycline and ciprofloxacin are contraindicated in pregnant women.

Other Causes of Genital Ulcers

Other causes of genital ulcers should be considered when the results of routine testing are negative. Noninfectious causes include trauma, Behçet's disease, malignancy, and drug-mediated disease.

OTHER SEXUALLY TRANSMITTED INFECTIONS

Genital Warts

Human papillomavirus (HPV) is responsible for a spectrum of cutaneous and mucosal disease, ranging from genital warts to invasive cancer. HPV has been linked to cervical, anal, and oropharyngeal cancer. There are more than 100 types of HPV. Sexually transmitted HPV infection is responsible for genital warts and anogenital carcinoma. More than 80% of sexually active adults acquire HPV infection in their lifetime. Genital warts tend to be benign and asymptomatic, and 90% are caused by HPV types 6 and 11. The HPV types most often linked to anogenital carcinoma are 16 and 18; HPV-16 is the most common.

Warts are usually described as flat and papular in the genital regions. Diagnosis of genital warts is usually made by clinical examination. If unclear, a biopsy may be performed. Treatment of genital warts may include podofilox (0.5% solution or gel), imiquimod (5% cream), sinecatechins (15% ointment), cryotherapy, podophyllin resin (10% to 25% concentration), trichloroacetic acid (TCA), and surgical excision.

HPV vaccination is available with Gardasil (quadrivalent vaccine) and Cervarix (bivalent vaccine). The main objective of vaccination is to prevent cervical and other cancers. The vaccines are also effective in preventing genital warts. The vaccines are most effective before sexual debut. Guidelines suggest vaccination of males and females between the ages of 11 to 26 years. Vaccines may be administered to individuals as young as 9 years old. HPV vaccination is approved for men and women up to 45 years of age. In several countries including the United States, there has been a decline in anogenital warts in adolescents, young women, older women, heterosexual men, as well as men who have sex with men.

Pubic Lice

Pubic lice (i.e., *Pediculosis pubis*) may spread from the genitalia to other areas of the body. The most common symptom is pruritus. Small macules and localized lymphadenopathy may occur. Diagnosis of this STI is made by light microscopy of the organism.

Treatment includes permethrin (1% cream applied to affected areas, rinsed off in 10 minutes) or pyrethrins (similar application). Alternative medications include malathion (0.5% lotion) or ivermectin. Clothing, bed sheets, and other linens should be thoroughly washed.

Scabies

Scabies is caused by the skin mite *Sarcoptes scabiei*. Transmission occurs by skin contact, and among adults, it is usually sexual. Clinical presentation usually includes pruritus and small erythematous papules that are classically present on the wrists, forearms, fingers, and genital areas.

Diagnosis is usually based on clinical presentation and examination of skin scrapings. Recommended treatment regimens include permethrin (5% cream applied from the neck down and washed off after 8 to 14 hours) or ivermectin.

SUGGESTED READINGS

Centers for Disease Control and Prevention: Sexually transmitted diseases surveillance 2012, Atlanta, 2013, U.S. Department of Health and Human Services.

Cook RL, Hutchison SL, Østergaard L, et al: Systematic review: noninvasive testing for *Chlamydia trachomatis* and *Neisseria gonorrhoeae*, Ann Intern Med 142:914–925, 2005.

Geisler WM, Lensing SY, Press CG, et al: Spontaneous resolution of genital *Chlamydia trachomatis* infection in women and protection from reinfection, J Infect Dis 207:1850–1856, 2013.

Jensen JS: *Mycoplasma genitalium*: the aetiological agent of urethritis and other sexually transmitted diseases, J Eur Acad Dermatol Venereol 18:1–11, 2004.

Platt R, Rice PA, McCormack WM: Risk of acquiring gonorrhea and prevalence of abnormal adnexal findings among women recently exposed to gonorrhea, J Am Med Assoc 250:3205–3209, 1983.

Rockwell DH, Yobs AR, Moore Jr MB: The Tuskegee study of untreated syphilis: the 30th year of observation, Arch Intern Med 114:792–798, 1964.

Schroeter AL, Lucas JB, Price EV, et al: Treatment for early syphilis and reactivity of serologic tests, J Am Med Assoc 221:471–476, 1972.

Vall-Mayans M, Caballero E, Sanz B: The emergence of lymphogranuloma venereum in Europe, Lancet 374:356, 2009.

103

Human Immunodeficiency Virus Infection

Joseph Metmowlee Garland, Timothy Flanigan, Edward J. Wing

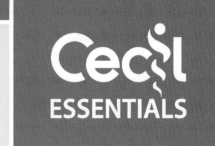

HISTORY

Human immunodeficiency virus (HIV) infection was first diagnosed in 1981 in the United States, when it was recognized as an immunodeficiency syndrome in young gay men and people who inject drugs. Soon after, the disease was recognized in patients with hemophilia, others who had received blood transfusions, previously healthy women, and rarely, health care workers. Patients with the syndrome were susceptible to unusual opportunistic infections such as *Pneumocystis jirovecii* pneumonia and unusual tumors such as Kaposi's sarcoma. Tragically, once patients had clinically identified disease, mortality over several years was very high. Patients developed recurrent infections, progressive tumors such as Kaposi's sarcoma and B cell lymphoma, wasting, and progressive neurologic syndromes including dementia. The immunodeficiency was characterized by weakened cell-mediated immunity marked by low CD4 T cells in the peripheral blood. Subsequently this disease was labeled the acquired immunodeficiency syndrome, or AIDS. In 1983, the causative agent, the human immunodeficiency virus, was identified by Luc Montagnier in France (winner of the Nobel Prize in Medicine) and Robert Gallo in the United States. By 1985, there was a serum test to identify the virus. Transmission in the United States was primarily through sex, particularly anal sex in men who had sex with men (MSM), through sharing needles during injection drug use, and through infusion of blood products.

The effect on a generation of young people was devastating. Initially, the cause was unknown, the modes of transmission uncertain, and the infectivity unclear. There was no treatment available, other than specific therapy for the opportunistic infections and tumors. All classes, races, and ethnic groups were affected. The incidence of the disease rose to greater than 50,000/year, and the number infected in the United States increased to over 1 million. Discrimination against people living with HIV (PLWH) was widespread. The government's response was slow. The early epidemic is poignantly described in Randy Shilts' book *And The Band Played On*. In 1987 the first drug, zidovudine or AZT, was approved for use against HIV and heralded a new era of virus-directed treatment. Unfortunately because of the virus' ability to mutate, resistance developed in most patients after several months of use. Other drugs with other mechanisms were developed over the next decade so that by 1995, with the discovery and approval of protease inhibitors, widespread use of effective combinations of antiretroviral therapy (ART) became available (initially called highly active antiretroviral therapy [HAART] or combination ART [cART]). This transformed HIV from a progressive disease to a manageable chronic condition in those diagnosed and engaged in treatment. Even patients

with severe end-stage AIDS could resolve their opportunistic infections and recover CD4 T cell counts.

Once the virus was identified, there was a vigorous search for the geographic and animal origins of the virus. By the late 1980s, AIDS was recognized as a worldwide pandemic. Because early cases had been identified in Africa, particularly West Africa, and because HIV was closely related to endemic simian viruses, early samples from West Africa were sought and tested. The earliest human case was identified retrospectively from serum taken from a sailor in 1959 in Kinshasa, now in the Democratic Republic of Congo. Because the virus mutates at a very fast rate, a retrospective "molecular clock" technique with mathematical modeling was used to project that the origin of HIV occurred in the early 20th century during several cross-species transmission events from chimpanzees, which harbor simian immunodeficiency virus (SIV), to humans, likely in southeast Cameroon. Such transmission occurred presumably in hunters during the killing and butchering of primates for food. Sexual transmission between humans followed, and the disease progressed along rivers and highways in West Africa during a time of social change and development in the early 20th century. Spread throughout the world eventually occurred due to increased international travel and interaction.

Subsequent virologic studies of HIV have demonstrated that HIV-1 can be divided into four groups that include group M (90% to 95% of all infections) and groups N, O, and P that account for much small numbers. Group M is further divided into subgroups or clades labeled A through D, F through N, and J and K. Clade B is the most frequent in the United States and Europe, whereas C and A are found in Africa, where they account for 50% and 12% of all HIV cases, respectively. A separate distinct retrovirus, HIV-2, was identified in 1986. Confined primarily to West Africa, it causes a less severe form of AIDS.

EPIDEMIOLOGY

The course of the HIV epidemic in the United States is shown in Fig. 103.1. Stage 3 (AIDS) classification refers to those with CD4 count less than 200 or with specific opportunistic infections/tumors. As can be seen, the incidence of HIV/AIDS rose until 1993, and the death rate until 1995. Subsequently, both fell dramatically with the widespread use of multidrug effective ART. From 1998 onward, there was a leveling off, with little change in the death rate but a slow decline in number of AIDS diagnoses. Overall there has been a linear increase in the prevalence, that is, in PLWH.

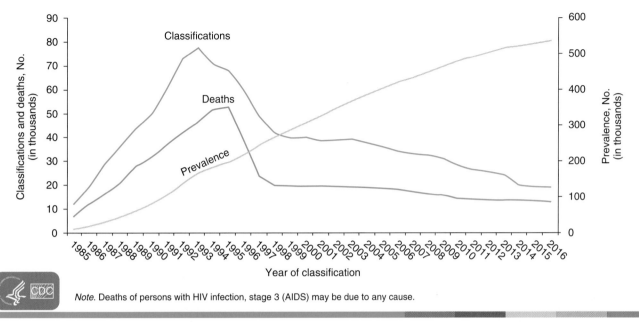

Classifications

Deaths

Prevalence

Note. Deaths of persons with HIV infection, stage 3 (AIDS) may be due to any cause.

Fig. 103.1 Stage 3 (AIDS) classifications, deaths, and persons living with diagnosed HIV infection ever classified as stage 3 (AIDS) 1985–2016: United States and six dependent areas. (From the Centers for Disease Control and Prevention; National Center for HIV/AIDS, Viral Hepatitis, STD, and TB Prevention Division of HIV/AIDS Prevention. *Trends in HIV Infection Stage 3 [AIDS]*. https://npin.cdc.gov/publication/trends-hiv-infection-stage-3-aids. Accessed January 23, 2019.)

In 2017, there were 38,739 new cases of HIV infection in the United States, a rate that has been unchanged since 2012. In 2017 it was estimated that 1.2 million people were living with HIV in the United States and 86% had been diagnosed. Sixty-three percent of those who had been diagnosed had a suppressed viral load. Geographically, the rates of new HIV diagnoses are highest in the South followed by the Northeast, the West, and finally the Midwest. Those at greatest risk remain MSM, accounting for 66% of all HIV diagnoses in 2017. The risk of acquiring HIV is 22 times higher than in the general population in men who have sex with men. Women are at risk primarily through heterosexual contact (17% of new diagnoses), with African American women being at greatest risk. Minority populations, particularly African American and Hispanic individuals are at greater risk for HIV compared to other races/ethnicities. In 2017 African Americans accounted for 43% of new HIV diagnoses, though they accounted for only 13% of the entire population. Hispanic individuals accounted for 26% of new diagnoses but were only approximately 17% of the total population.

Though still considered a traditional risk factor, injection drug use has fallen markedly as a cause of HIV transmission, largely through the use of syringe exchange programs and other harm reduction practices among people who inject drugs. In 2017, injection drug use accounted for only 9% of new HIV diagnoses in the United States. The risk of acquiring HIV is 22 times higher in those who inject drugs and 21 times higher in sex workers. Unfortunately, in 2018, only 18% of persons at high risk with indications had been prescribed medications for preexposure prophylaxis (PrEP, see later section) for prophylaxis.

Since the 1980s, HIV infection has become a worldwide pandemic and HIV continues to spread throughout all continents. Since the late 1990s, rapid transmission has occurred throughout Africa, India, Southeast Asia, the former Soviet Union, and some parts of Eastern Europe. Today, approximately 70% of PLWH live in Africa; the Americas and South-East Asia account for slightly more than 9% each, and Europe accounts for 6%. Because of latency between HIV infection and the development of AIDS-associated illnesses, the clinically recognized epidemic of AIDS has lagged 6 to 8 years behind the spread of the virus into new populations.

Since the start of the epidemic, according to UNAIDS, 74.9 million people have become infected with HIV and 32 million people have died from HIV. In 2018 it was estimated that 37.9 million people globally were living with HIV and of those, 1.7 million people were younger than 15 years of age. In that year 1.7 million people were newly infected and 770,000 people died from HIV. In 2018, 23.3 million people living with HIV were taking ART. As a result of increasing availability of ART, the number of new infections has been reduced by 40% since 1997 and AIDS-related deaths have been reduced by more than 56% since 2004. With more access to ART worldwide and increasing efforts at availability and adherence, incidence and mortality rates should continue to fall. Tuberculosis remains the leading cause of death among PLWH, accounting for approximately one in three deaths due to HIV. It is estimated that almost half of people infected with HIV and TB are unaware of their coinfection and therefore are not receiving appropriate care.

VIROLOGY

HIV contains two single-stranded copies of the viral RNA genome, together with the virus-encoded enzymes reverse transcriptase, protease, and integrase (Fig. 103.2). Surrounding the structural (p24 and p18) proteins is a lipid bilayer derived from the host cell, through which protrude the transmembrane (gp41) and surface (gp120) envelope glycoproteins. The HIV envelope glycoproteins have a high affinity for the

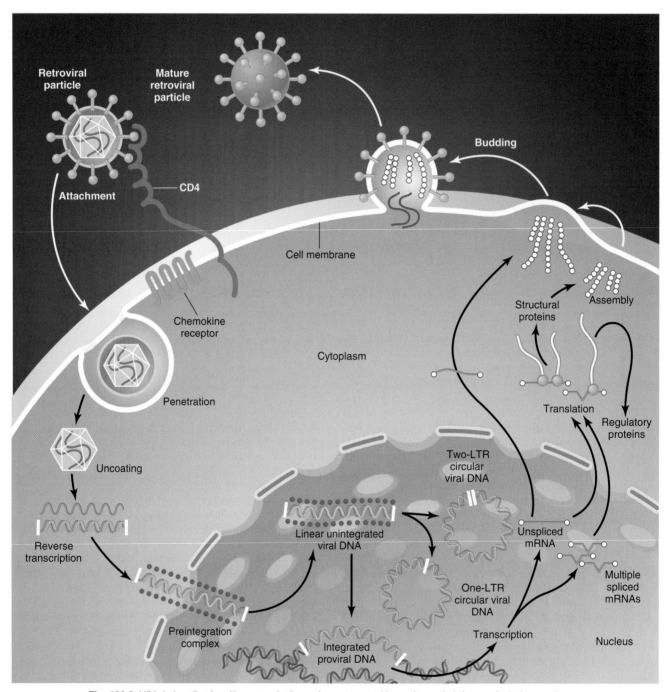

Fig. 103.2 HIV viral replication. Key steps in the pathway targeted by antiretroviral therapy include membrane binding and fusion, reverse transcription, integration of proviral DNA, and protein synthesis. *LTR,* Long terminal repeat; *mRNA,* messenger RNA. (Modified from Furtado MR, Callaway DS, Phair JP, et al: Persistence of HIV-1 transcription in patients receiving potent antiretroviral therapy, N Engl J Med 340:1614–1622, 1999.)

CD4 molecule on the surface of T-helper lymphocytes and other cells of monocyte-macrophage lineage. After HIV binds to the CD4 molecule, the envelope undergoes a conformational change that facilitates binding to another cellular coreceptor; the most important of these are the chemokine receptors CCR5 and CXCR4. This second binding event promotes a major conformational change that causes approximation of the viral and cellular membranes; fusion of these membranes is mediated by insertion of the newly exposed fusion domain of the envelope gp41 into the host cell membrane.

As a result of these processes, the HIV nucleoprotein complex enters the cytoplasm, where the RNA viral genome undergoes reverse transcription by the virally encoded reverse transcriptase. The resulting double-stranded viral DNA enters the nucleus, where proper localization of the viral pre-integration complex is mediated by host proteins, and integration of the DNA provirus into the host chromosome is catalyzed by the retroviral integrase. Latently infected resting memory CD4 lymphocytes serve as reservoirs of persistent infection for the life of the patient even with effective ART (see later discussion). However, the bulk of viral replication takes place in activated T cells, which are both more susceptible to HIV infection and more capable of supporting productive HIV replication.

When a CD4+ lymphocyte is activated, expression of HIV messenger RNA (mRNA) is enhanced. Core proteins, viral enzymes, and envelope proteins are encoded by the *gag, pol,* and *env* genes of HIV, respectively. More than 100 host proteins, in addition to the viral proteins,

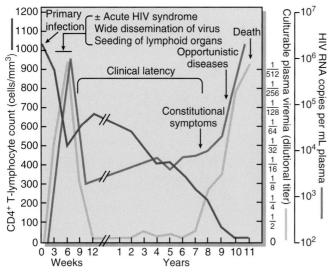

Fig. 103.3 The natural progression of HIV disease. (From Bennett JE, Dolin R, Blaser MJ. Mandell Douglas and Bennett's Principles and Practice of Infectious Diseases, 9th ed. Figure 122.1, page 1659.)

may be important for viral replication. Viral particles are assembled at the cell membrane, each containing two copies of unspliced mRNA within the core as the viral genome, and virions are released from the cell by budding. Productive viral replication is lytic to infected lymphocytes. A number of other host cells, including macrophages and certain dendritic cells, are also infected by HIV, but viral replication does not appear to be lytic to these cells.

Following acute infection, high-level viral multiplication occurs in mucosal lymphoid tissues of the gut and in other lymphatic sites. Plasma HIV RNA levels (i.e., the plasma viral load [PVL]) often exceed 1 million copies per milliliter during the second to fourth weeks after infection. Almost all instances of acute HIV infection are caused by R5 tropic viruses, viruses that use the chemokine receptor CCR5 for cellular entry. During subsequent weeks, the PVL decreases, often rapidly. This decrease in viremia results largely from a partially effective immune response. After 6 to 12 months, the PVL typically stabilizes at a level denoted the viral *set point*, and it may remain at approximately that level for several years, entering a period of clinical latency (Fig. 103.3). The set point, assessed as the PVL at 6 to 12 months after infection, is a significant predictor of the subsequent rate of progression of HIV disease but accounts for only half of the population variability in disease progression rates.

After recovery from the acute retroviral syndrome, the patient may feel entirely well for several years, but even in the asymptomatic individual, more than 100 billion new virions may be produced daily. Rapid production and turnover of circulating CD4+ cells also occurs throughout the course of HIV infection, and a progressive decline in circulating CD4+ cells occurs in most individuals. Cell lysis associated with HIV replication accounts only partially for this progressive loss of CD4 cells. During the years of clinical latency, virions are present in large numbers in the follicular dendritic processes of the germinal centers of the lymph nodes, which undergo both hyperplasia and progressive fibrosis. As HIV disease progresses over several years, the lymphatic tissue atrophies and plasma viremia intensifies. In later-stage HIV disease, a more dramatic CD4 cell decline is observed, following a sharp rise in the PVL (see Fig. 103.3).

The decline in the number of CD4 cells is accompanied by profound functional impairment of the remaining lymphocyte populations. Anergy may develop early in HIV infection and eventually occurs in almost all persons with AIDS. T-helper lymphocyte proliferation in

response to antigenic stimuli is dramatically impaired, T cell cytotoxic responses are diminished, and natural killer cell activity against virus-infected cells is greatly impaired. Decrease in function as well as number of CD4 cells is central to the immune dysfunction, and this impairment partly underlies the failure of B-lymphocyte function, as measured by impaired capacity to synthesize antibody in response to new antigens.

IMMUNOLOGY AND INFLAMMATION

Acute HIV infection results in massive destruction of T cells in lymphoid tissue throughout the body, particularly in the intestinal wall, and the decrease can be easily quantified in the peripheral blood. Partial recovery of T cell numbers and partial control of HIV viral load occurs due to the initial immune response in which both CD4 and CD8 cell clones react to HIV antigens (see Fig. 103.3). Robust inflammatory responses to initial infection occur. Within weeks to months, this response decreases but persists above baseline compared to the inflammation in the age-matched general population. One of the hallmarks of HIV infection is the continuous slow destruction of the CD4 T cell population with eventual loss of antigenic reactivity. Continuous stimulation of the CD8 cell population results in a reversal of the usual CD4:CD8 ratio. Eventually there is an increase in the CD8 phenotype termed (CD28−, CD57+) that is reactive towards viruses, particularly cytomegalovirus. This phenotype is termed senescent and secretes proinflammatory cytokines. In late stages, destruction of lymph tissue architecture inhibits normal immune cell interaction, furthering immunodeficiency. In addition, there is hemopoietic progenitor cell loss and thymic dysfunction, both reducing T lymphocyte homeostasis.

Cells of the monocyte/macrophage and dendritic lineage are also infected by HIV but are not destroyed. This includes macrophages in tissues such as adipose tissue and brain microglia. Because of gut immunodeficiency and microbial translocation, as well as stimulation by HIV and other viruses, chronic activation of macrophages occurs, as indicated by elevated levels of soluble CD14 and soluble CD163 in serum, with resultant secretion of proinflammatory cytokines. HIV itself can stimulate immune responses through stimulation of toll-like receptors 7, 8, and 9 on antigen presenting cells with subsequent production of interferons. As a result, cytokine levels, particularly IL-6 and type I interferons among others have been shown to be elevated in PLWH.

ART markedly decreases HIV viral replication (and hence serum viral load) and allows recovery and stabilization of CD4 T cell numbers. However, even with effective ART, decreased immune reactivity and low-level chronic inflammation persist in PLWH. This decreased reactivity depends roughly on the level of CD4 T cells on stable ART. For example, decreased immunity to *Streptococcus pneumoniae* persists in PLWH on ART even in those with recovered CD4 T cell numbers and suppressed viral loads.

Persistent chronic inflammation in people living with HIV, even in those on effective ART, is presumed to be multifactorial in etiology including: (1) low levels of HIV replication; (2) gut immunodeficiency allowing continuous exposure to microbial antigens resulting in macrophage activation; (3) reactivation of herpes viruses, particularly CMV and EBV; and (4) cytokine production by cells including macrophages and senescent CD8 T cells. This low-level inflammation is linked in part to increased risk for chronic diseases including cardiovascular, bone, kidney, and other morbidities associated with aging.

CLINICAL DIAGNOSIS OF HIV

Since 2013, the US Preventive Services Task Force has recommended routine HIV testing in all persons ages 15 to 65, to be offered in primary care settings. Despite this recommendation, almost a quarter of new

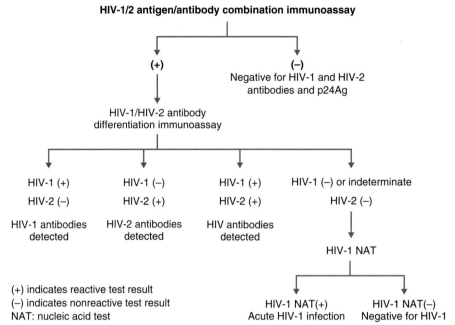

HIV-1/2 antigen/antibody combination immunoassay

(+)

(−)
Negative for HIV-1 and HIV-2
antibodies and p24Ag

HIV-1/HIV-2 antibody
differentiation immunoassay

HIV-1 (+)
HIV-2 (−)

HIV-1 antibodies
detected

HIV-1 (−)
HIV-2 (+)

HIV-2 antibodies
detected

HIV-1 (+)
HIV-2 (+)

HIV antibodies
detected

HIV-1 (−) or indeterminate
HIV-2 (−)

HIV-1 NAT

(+) indicates reactive test result
(−) indicates nonreactive test result
NAT: nucleic acid test

HIV-1 NAT(+)
Acute HIV-1 infection

HIV-1 NAT(−)
Negative for HIV-1

Fig. 103.4 Recommended HIV testing algorithm (CLSI).

HIV diagnoses are made when the patient already has an AIDS diagnosis (CD4 count <200 or AIDS-defining condition), indicating late diagnosis and missed opportunities for earlier testing remain an issue. All pregnant women should be offered HIV testing as well. Standard testing for HIV in the United States is through use of a fourth-generation immunoassay for HIV-1 and HIV-2 antibodies and an HIV early antigen (p24). Confirmation is by an HIV-1 and HIV-2 antibody differentiation immunoassay and nucleic acid testing if these are both negative or indeterminate (Fig. 103.4). The "window period" from disease acquisition to test positivity has greatly reduced as compared with earlier generations of the test; fourth-generation testing is usually positive within 18 to 45 days. Rapid point-of-care testing methods also exist and may play an important role in HIV testing in many clinical and community settings. These rapid tests are lateral-flow (immunochromatographic) or vertical-flow (immunofiltration) assays that detect the presence of HIV-1/2 antibodies and/or HIV p24 antigen and can be performed on oral fluid or a drop of serum ("finger stick") to provide results within 30 minutes. They do require confirmation by serum antibody-based tests. If HIV is diagnosed, it is important to pursue further testing to characterize the stage of disease, including a CD4 count and PVL.

Identification of persons with HIV and linkage to effective care are critical public health priorities. Early identification of infection affects prognosis; patients who have AIDS at diagnosis have a lower predicted life expectancy than those with higher CD4 counts. Further, studies have demonstrated that patients who are diagnosed and treated with effective ART do not transmit virus to others once their serum viral load is undetectable, therefore HIV treatment is also a cornerstone of HIV prevention efforts.

Any discussion of HIV diagnosis raises the important question of disclosure. Respect for patients' right to confidentiality is important to remember at all points of contact with the health care system, particularly given the often-stigmatized nature of HIV infection in society. Communication of a new diagnosis, and any subsequent discussion of treatment, prognosis, transmission, or other aspects of care, must be performed in a confidential setting. Whether and how to disclose to partners or family members is a patient decision, and disclosure should be done by the patient or by the patient with the provider's assistance. State-by-state laws differ on the legality of disclosing patients' HIV status without their consent, but best practices generally discourage this practice because it will damage the patient-provider relationship and increases the risk of losing the patient to care entirely. After establishing a relationship with a patient, providers should also discuss designating a health care proxy (HCP) and gain an understanding of what the HCP knows about the patient's health, so that the patient's wishes around confidentiality can be respected even in the setting of incapacitation.

THE NATURAL PROGRESSION OF HIV DISEASE

Acute Retroviral Syndrome

Up to 50% of PLWH report a mononucleosis-like syndrome (acute retroviral syndrome) occurring 2 to 6 weeks after initial infection. The symptoms may include fever, sore throat, gastrointestinal symptoms, diffuse lymph node enlargement, rash, arthralgias, and headache that usually persist for several days to 3 weeks (Table 103.1). The rash is typically maculopapular and short-lived and usually affects the trunk or face. Ten percent of infected individuals experience an acute, self-limited, aseptic meningitis, which on lumbar puncture can be characterized by cerebrospinal fluid (CSF) pleocytosis with detectable HIV in the CSF; however, this syndrome is often not recognized. Rarely, patients may present with opportunistic infections during this period, most commonly thrush (*Candida* pharyngitis). The acute retroviral syndrome is often sufficiently severe that the patient seeks medical attention, though it is uncommon to require hospitalization. During acute infection, the plasma viral load can be extremely high, often greater than 1 million copies per mL, and the CD4 count will dip lower than where it will eventually settle (see Fig. 103.3). It is critical to maintain a high index of suspicion for acute HIV retroviral syndrome because the very high plasma HIV RNA level during this period confers a high likelihood of HIV transmission to sexual or needle-sharing partners, or from mother to infant (e.g., during breast-feeding).

Natural Clinical Progression of Untreated Disease

Untreated HIV infection usually results in a slow, nonlinear progression to severe immunodeficiency over the course of years. However, the progression of disease varies greatly among individuals. Within

TABLE 103.1 Symptoms and Signs of Acute Retroviral Syndrome in 209 Patients

Symptom or Sign	No. With Finding	Frequency (%)
Fever	200	96
Adenopathy	154	74
Pharyngitis	146	70
Rash	146	70
Myalgia or arthralgia	112	54
Thrombocytopenia	94	45
Leukopenia	80	38
Diarrhea	67	32
Headache	66	32
Nausea, vomiting	56	27
Elevated aminotransferase levels	38	21
Hepatosplenomegaly	30	14
Thrush	24	12
Neuropathy	13	6
Encephalopathy	12	6

Modified from Niu MT, Stein DS, Schnittman SM. Primary human immunodeficiency virus type 1 infection: review of pathogenesis and early treatment intervention in human and animal retrovirus infections. J Infect Dis 1993;168:1490-1501.

TABLE 103.2 Progressive Complications of HIV Infection by CD4 Count

CD4 Count (cells/mm³)	Opportunistic Infection or Neoplasm
>500	Herpes zoster
	Tuberculosis
200-500	Oral hairy leukoplakia
	Candida pharyngitis (thrush)
	Kaposi's sarcoma, mucocutaneous
	Bacterial pneumonia, recurrent
	Cervical or anal neoplasia
100-200	*Pneumocystis jirovecii* pneumonia
	Histoplasmosis capsulatum infection, disseminated
	Kaposi's sarcoma, visceral
	Progressive multifocal leukoencephalopathy
	Lymphoma, non-Hodgkin's
<100	*Candida* esophagitis
	Cytomegalovirus retinitis
	Mycobacterium avium-intercellulare
	Toxoplasma gondii encephalitis
	Cryptosporidium parvum enteritis
	Cryptococcus neoformans meningitis
	Herpes simplex virus, chronic, ulcerative
	Cytomegalovirus esophagitis or colitis
	Primary central nervous system lymphoma

10 years after infection, approximately 50% of untreated individuals will develop AIDS, 30% will have milder symptoms, and fewer than 20% will be entirely asymptomatic (see Fig. 103.3). Children and adolescents progress to AIDS at a slower rate than older persons. The rate of progression of immunodeficiency is not influenced by the route of HIV transmission and appears mostly to be inherent to characteristics of the individual rather than the transmitted virus. In the long term, disease does not appear to differ by gender, although typically women with HIV infection tend to experience more rapid disease progression with lower levels of HIV in plasma.

Clinically recognized lymph node enlargement occurs in 35% to 40% of asymptomatic HIV-infected persons but is not significantly associated with either rate of progression of immunodeficiency or with subsequent development of lymphoma. During early HIV infection, thrombocytopenia, probably caused by autoimmune platelet destruction, is common. Most PLWH remain asymptomatic until their CD4 count falls to less than 200 cells/mm³, a fact that contributes to the late diagnosis of disease.

Patients with moderate immunodeficiency (CD4 counts between 200 and 500 cells/mm³) exhibit diminished antibody response to protein and polysaccharide antigens, as well as decreased cell-mediated immune function. These functional impairments are manifested clinically by a 3-fold to 4-fold increase in the incidence of bacteremic pneumonias caused by common pulmonary pathogens (especially *Streptococcus pneumoniae* and *Haemophilus influenzae*) and by a marked increase in incidence of active pulmonary tuberculosis in endemic areas (Table 103.2). Mucocutaneous lesions may be the first manifestations of immune dysfunction; these include reactivation of varicella zoster (shingles), recurrent genital herpes simplex virus (HSV) infections, oral or vaginal candidiasis, and oral hairy leukoplakia (see later discussion). Women living with HIV show an increased prevalence of high-grade squamous intraepithelial lesions on Papanicolaou (Pap) smear. Both men and women may show similarly increased rates of dysplasia or neoplasia on anal Pap smear.

With advanced immunodeficiency, indicated by CD4 counts lower than 200 cells/mm³, patients are at high risk for development of opportunistic diseases, including infections and malignancies (see Table 103.2). Prior to the advent of antiretroviral therapy, time from diagnosis of AIDS to death was on average 1.3 years; death was generally due to opportunistic disease, including *Pneumocystis jirovecii* pneumonia and *Toxoplasma* meningitis, among many others. CD4 counts lower than 50 cells/mm³ indicate profound immunosuppression and, in the absence of effective ART, are associated with a high mortality rate within the subsequent 12 to 24 months. Cytomegalovirus (CMV) retinitis, which can lead rapidly to blindness, and disseminated *Mycobacterium avium* complex (MAC) infection occur frequently in the absence of therapy at these low CD4 counts. They respond adequately to specific therapy only if it is accompanied by effective control of viral replication.

Opportunistic Infections
Candida Infections
Perhaps one of the earliest indications of HIV disease in many patients is the development of *Candida* disease. Both oropharyngeal and esophageal candidiasis are common in PLWH. Angular cheilosis may also be a manifestation of *Candida* infection. Typically, but not exclusively, caused by *Candida albicans*, oropharyngeal candidiasis may manifest as painless, creamy white, plaque-like lesions on the buccal surface, classically on an erythematous base. Esophageal disease is often symptomatic, usually presenting with odynophagia and/or retrosternal burning pain. In women living with HIV, *Candida* vulvovaginitis usually presents with white adherent vaginal discharge and a burning or itching sensation. *Candida*-associated disease may occur at any CD4 count, but esophageal disease is generally associated with lower CD4 counts. Treatment with oral fluconazole is as effective as or superior to localized topical therapy and is generally better tolerated and therefore preferred. Primary and secondary prophylaxis against *Candida* infection is generally not recommended unless patients have severe or frequent recurrences because therapy for acute disease is rapidly effective, mortality is extremely low, therapy is costly, and potential for development of resistance is of concern.

TABLE 103.3   Primary Antimicrobial Prophylaxis for Adults Living With HIV and a Low CD4 Count

Opportunistic Infection	Treatment	When to Start	When to Stop
Pneumocystis jirovecii	TMP/SMX 1 DS *or* SS daily *Alt:* TMP/SMX 1 DS TIW *Alt:* Dapsone 100 mg daily or 50 mg BID *Alt:* Nebulized pentamidine 300 mg monthly *Alt:* Atovaquone 1500 mg daily	CD4 <200 *or* CD4% <14%	CD4 >200 for >3 mo (AI) *or* CD4 between 100-200 if HIV VL is undetectable >3 mo (BII)
Toxoplasma gondii	TMP/SMX 1 DS daily *Alt:* TMP/SMX 1 DS TIW *Alt:* TMP/SMX 1 DS daily *Alt:* Dapsone-pyrimethamine + leucovorin *Alt:* Atovaquone 1500 mg daily	CD4 <100	CD4 >200 for >3 mo (AI) *or* CD4 between 100-200 if HIV VL is undetectable >3 mo (BII)
Mycobacterium avium complex	Azithromycin 1200 mg weekly Clarithromycin 500 mg BID *Alt:* Rifabutin	Not recommended if effective ART initiated immediately. Recommended for those who are not on fully suppressive ART, after ruling out active disseminated MAC disease	CD4 >100 for >3 mo
Mycobacterium tuberculosis	Isoniazid (INH) 300 mg daily × 9 months *Alt:* Rifapentine + INH 900 mg once weekly for 12 weeks *Alt:* Rifampin 10 mg/kg/day (600 mg max) × 4 months	Positive screening test for LTBI with no evidence of active TB, and no prior treatment for active TB or LTBI	Stop after completion of recommended LTBI treatment duration
Histoplasmosis	Itraconazole 200 mg daily	CD4 <150 if high-risk environmental or occupational exposure exists	CD4 >150 for >6 mo
Cryptococcosis	Fluconazole	Not recommended in United States	

Pneumocystis Pneumonia

Pneumocystis jirovecii is a ubiquitous yeast in the environment. It is not associated with disease except in the setting of immunocompromise. Before the widespread use of ART and prophylactic medications, *Pneumocystis jirovecii* pneumonia (PJP or PCP; both abbreviations are still used) occurred in 70% of patients with AIDS, and the course of treated PCP was still associated with 20% to 40% mortality. The typical presentation is subacute, with progressive fever, shortness of breath, and weight loss over weeks. Profound desaturation with exertion is a common clinical sign, as is a substernal catch on inspiration. Hypoxemia is the most common laboratory abnormality. A serum LDH greater than 500 is common, and a serum 1,3-β-D-glucan is commonly elevated as well. Both of these can be helpful diagnostically. Definitive diagnosis can be made on sputum sample; induced sputum may be positive, though often bronchoscopic sampling for DFA and/or PCR testing is needed. Radiographic findings are classically described as diffuse, bilateral, symmetrical "ground-glass" interstitial infiltrates emanating from the hila in a "butterfly" pattern. However, it is important to remember that 10% of patients will have a normal radiograph, and 30% will have nonspecific findings. Atypical findings such as nodules, blebs, or cysts, can occur, as can spontaneous pneumothorax. Early initiation of treatment is crucial, and treatment should not be delayed while waiting for diagnostic results in patients with a high index of suspicion. First-line therapy is trimethoprim-sulfamethoxazole 15 to 20 mg/kg/day in divided doses over a 21-day course. Steroids should be added in patients with moderate or severe disease, generally defined as a PO_2 of less than 70 or an Aa gradient of 35 mm Hg or greater. Alternative treatments for mild-to-moderate disease include primaquine with clindamycin, dapsone with trimethoprim, or atovaquone. Alternative treatments for moderate-to-severe disease include primaquine with clindamycin or intravenous pentamidine. Due to the high prevalence of *Pneumocystis*, prophylaxis with trimethoprim-sulfamethoxazole is recommended for all patients with a CD4 count less than 200. Alternatives include dapsone, atovaquone, or inhaled pentamidine. In patients with a CD4 count between 100 and 200, prophylaxis can be discontinued once the serum HIV viral load is undetectable for 3 to 6 months. See Table 103.3 for prophylaxis guidelines.

Cryptococcal Disease

Cryptococcus neoformans is a yeast that generally affects immunocompromised individuals. It enters the body through the lungs, though pulmonary disease is often asymptomatic. Meningitis is the most common clinical presentation of cryptococcal disease, but cutaneous manifestations, classically presenting as umbilicated papules, may be present in 10% of patients. Cryptococcal meningitis occurs in about 1 million cases per year worldwide, with an estimated 600,000 deaths annually. Classic meningeal symptoms occur in only 25% of patients; more commonly, patients present with progressive headache, lethargy progressive to encephalopathy, personality changes, memory loss, coma, and death. A serum cryptococcal antigen test is generally positive, but a lumbar puncture must be performed both for diagnosis and for therapeutic purposes to evaluate CSF pressure (and relieve it, if elevated). CSF studies will generally show an elevated total protein and low glucose, and CSF cryptococcal antigen testing will be positive. India ink staining of the CSF, though uncommon now in the United States, will show encapsulated yeast forms. CSF lymphocyte counts may be elevated or may be normal. A minimal inflammatory response is common; in fact, 55% of patients with AIDS-related cryptococcal meningitis have a CSF lymphocyte count of less than 10 cells/mL. This lack of immunologic response is associated with a poorer prognosis. Treatment is focused on (1) management of CSF pressures through serial lumbar puncture with removal of CSF until pressures return to normal range and (2) antifungal therapy. Therapy is generally divided into three phases: induction, consolidation, and maintenance. Induction therapy is with amphotericin B and flucytosine. Once CSF cultures have cleared and patients have completed at least 2 weeks of therapy, consolidation with high-dose oral fluconazole is continued for 8 additional weeks. Maintenance therapy is with oral fluconazole 200 mg daily for a minimum of 1 year.

Toxoplasma Encephalitis

Toxoplasma gondii is an obligate intracellular protozoan that most commonly causes encephalitis in patients with AIDS, though it may also present with retinitis or in skeletal muscle or myocardium. Primary infection occurs from eating undercooked meat containing tissue cysts or ingesting oocysts that have been shed in cat feces and sporulated into the environment. Clinical disease in PLWH is usually due to reactivation. Patients present with a focal encephalitis with headache, confusion, motor weakness, and fever. In the absence of treatment, disease will progress to seizures, stupor, coma, and death. Imaging is usually the means of diagnosis, with contrast-enhanced MRI showing multiple contrast-enhancing lesions in the gray matter of the cortex or basal ganglia, often associated with edema. Because disease is usually due to reactivation of latent disease, patients may have a positive serum anti-toxoplasma IgG. CSF testing for toxoplasma PCR may be positive as well. Treatment is initiated based on high clinical suspicion rather than definitive diagnosis. If repeat imaging in 1 to 3 weeks does not show response to treatment in all visualized lesions, brain biopsy may be necessary. In this scenario, biopsy is important to rule out alternative diagnoses such as CNS lymphoma, progressive multifocal leukoencephalopathy (PML), or tuberculosis, among others. Treatment consists of pyrimethamine and sulfadiazine with leucovorin to reduce hematologic toxicity. Treatment is for a minimum of 6 weeks; then patients should be put on chronic maintenance therapy until the CD4 has been greater than 200 for over 6 months. Primary prophylaxis for *Toxoplasma* with trimethoprim-sulfamethoxazole should be initiated in any patient with a CD4 count less than 100, with atovaquone as an alternative. See Table 103.3 for prophylaxis guidelines.

Mycobacterium Tuberculosis

Tuberculosis is the most common opportunistic infection seen worldwide in people living with HIV disease and in fact is the leading cause of death due to infectious disease worldwide. PLWH may either acquire acute disease through inhaling droplet nuclei or suffer reactivation disease due to impaired cellular immunity. The annual risk of reactivation tuberculosis disease in people living with HIV is estimated to be 3% to 16% per year. Reactivation can occur at any CD4 count but is higher risk the more significant the immunodeficiency. The greatest risk in people living in the United States is birth or residence outside the United States because global rates of tuberculosis are much higher than in the United States itself. Clinical presentations of people living with HIV are generally not different than in people who do not have HIV, but presentations of severe systemic disease and disseminated disease are more common. Clinical manifestations can be protean, but classic symptoms of fever, cachexia, and night sweats remain common. Pulmonary disease is still the most common presentation. Chest radiographs in patients may show features of primary tuberculosis, including hilar adenopathy, lower or middle lobe infiltrates, miliary pattern, or pleural effusions, as well as classic patterns of reactivation with upper lobe disease. Less common presentations include pericarditis, pericardial effusions, meningitis, CNS lesions, and bony disease. Diagnosis is determined in the same manner as in HIV-negative patients, and treatment does not differ, though careful review of medications is important to avoid significant drug/drug interactions that can occur between antiretrovirals and antituberculous medications. See Chapter 94 for more details.

Nontuberculous Mycobacterial Disease

A number of different nontuberculous mycobacteria are associated with advanced HIV disease, though far and away the most common is *Mycobacterium avium* complex (MAC). The incidence of MAC in patients with severe AIDS-associated immunosuppression is 20% to 40% in the absence of effective ART or chemoprophylaxis. Disease tends to occur with a CD4 count less than 50 and a high HIV viral load (usually greater than 100,000). MAC often presents as a disseminated disease with fever, night sweats, weight loss, diarrhea, and abdominal pain. On physical examination, hepatosplenomegaly and lymphadenopathy are common. Laboratory testing is often initially nonspecific, though anemia and an increased alkaline phosphatase are common. Diagnosis is usually made on a compatible clinical syndrome and isolation of MAC on culture or AFB stain on tissue with confirmation on culture. Cultures can be sent from blood, lymph node biopsy, bone marrow, or other tissues or fluids felt to be infected. Treatment is with two or more drugs, usually clarithromycin or azithromycin with ethambutol. Rifabutin may be added as a third agent in some cases. Treatment is for a minimum of 12 months and may then be discontinued when patients are asymptomatic and have a CD4 count greater than 100 for over 6 months. Prophylaxis against MAC is no longer recommended routinely for those who are immediately initiating ART, based on literature demonstrating no added benefit when ART is initiated promptly. Prophylaxis is therefore only recommended in those with a CD4 count less than 50 who are not receiving ART or who are not on fully suppressive ART, and only once active MAC disease has been ruled out based on clinical assessment, including a baseline AFB blood culture. Prophylaxis is generally with azithromycin 1200 mg once weekly.

Progressive Multifocal Leukoencephalopathy

PML is an opportunistic infection of the CNS caused by JC virus, a polyoma virus that causes focal demyelination. JC virus is common throughout the world and demonstrates a seroprevalence of 39% in healthy adults. PML is a disease that occurs with profound immunosuppression in people with HIV (CD4 <50) or in people receiving certain immunomodulatory humanized antibodies (e.g., natalizumab, rituximab). Prior to the advent of ART, PML developed in 3% to 7% of patients with advanced AIDS. PML manifests with focal neurologic deficits, usually of slow and insidious onset, that become progressive. Seizures occur in 20% of patients. Patients do not have headache or fever. Diagnosis is suspected based on MRI findings of distinct nonenhancing white matter lesions in areas of the brain corresponding to clinical deficits. Confirmation of diagnosis is usually through testing of the CSF for JC virus DNA by PCR, which is positive in 70% to 90% of patients. In some patients, however, brain biopsy is required to establish the diagnosis. There are no specific therapies for treating JC virus or PML. Initiation of antiretroviral therapy is the cornerstone of treatment; over 50% of patients will experience remission, though some neurologic deficits often persist.

Cytomegalovirus Disease

Cytomegalovirus (CMV) is a ubiquitous DNA virus. In patients with advanced AIDS and a CD4 count less than 50, it may present with end-organ disease. Before the advent of ART, 30% of patients with advanced AIDS developed CMV retinitis. Retinitis often begins unilaterally but then progresses to bilateral disease. This may be asymptomatic or present with floaters, scotomata, or visual field deficits. Ophthalmologic exam is generally diagnostic, with fluffy, yellow-white retinal lesions with or without intraretinal hemorrhage, and absent or minimal vitreous inflammation. Other manifestations of CMV can occur, including colitis, esophagitis, and CNS disease. CMV pneumonitis is extremely uncommon in patients with HIV. For these other manifestations, diagnosis based on biopsy is still necessary. An elevated CMV viral load in serum may be present but does not confirm disease. Treatment is oral valganciclovir or intravenous ganciclovir.

Varicella-Zoster Disease

Varicella-zoster is a ubiquitous virus known to have infected over 95% of adults in the United States. Reactivation varicella (termed herpes zoster, or "shingles") occurred at a 15-fold higher rate in PLWH prior to the advent of ART, and rates remain elevated in PLWH. Varicella reactivation can occur at any CD4 count, but reactivation is strongly associated with CD4 counts less than 200 and with active HIV viremia. Herpes zoster, or reactivation varicella virus, manifests as a painful vesicular eruption on the skin in a dermatomal distribution; 50% are in thoracic dermatomes, but cranial nerves and cervical nerves are also common, and any nerve distribution can be involved. The probability of a recurrence within 1 year is 10% in PLWH. If the eye is involved, acute retinal necrosis (ARN) or progressive outer retinal necrosis (PORN) can occur; both are associated with high rates of vision loss. In patients with CD4 counts less than 200, disseminated herpes zoster can also occur, including with CNS involvement that may manifest with CNS vasculitis, multifocal leukoencephalitis, ventriculitis, myelitis, optic neuritis, cranial nerve palsies, focal brainstem lesions, or aseptic meningitis. Diagnosis of varicella reactivation can be made based on clinical exam demonstrating classic dermatologic manifestations; VZV PCR of an unroofed vesicle can assist with diagnosis of unclear cases. PCR can also be performed on CSF or vitreous humor to help diagnose disease in those locations. Treatment of uncomplicated herpes zoster is similar to HIV-negative patients with use of oral valacyclovir, famciclovir, or acyclovir for 7 to 10 days. Intravenous acyclovir is recommended for treatment of severe or complicated varicella disease. Ophthalmologic disease should be managed by an experienced ophthalmologist. Current recommendations regarding primary vaccination (in patients with no reported history of childhood illness or vaccination) and to prevent reactivation disease are addressed in Table 103.6.

Other Opportunistic Infections

A number of other infections are considered opportunistic in patients living with HIV disease. These infections include bacterial and parasitic intestinal infections (including *Cryptosporidium*, *Cystoisospora*, and *Microsporidia* spp). Other bacterial infections, such as *Bartonella* spp, syphilis, and bacterial pneumonias, also occur at increased rates in patients living with HIV. Systemic fungal infections, including endemic fungi such as *Coccidioides*, *Histoplasma*, and *Talaromyces* infections, occur regionally. Viral diseases, including hepatitis B, hepatitis C, HSV, and HPV, are associated with worsened disease in PLWH, as is reactivation of varicella virus (herpes zoster).

HIV and Malignancy

Early in the HIV epidemic, rates of certain cancers were noted to be high in PLWH. Kaposi's sarcoma (KS) and non-Hodgkin's B-cell lymphoma were recognized as markers of the disease. Other AIDS-defining tumors, including invasive cervical cancer and primary central nervous system lymphoma, were also detected early. These AIDS-defining tumors were associated with viral coinfections, and the interplay of the immune dysregulation of advanced HIV disease and other viruses with potential for oncogenesis raise the risk of an opportunistic malignancy.

Kaposi's Sarcoma

In the early days of the HIV epidemic, rates of KS, a rare angiogenic cutaneous tumor found previously in elderly men, were present at rates 1000 times that of the general population. In the United States, KS occurred predominantly in young MSM infected with HIV and human herpes virus 8 (HHV-8). In Africa, rates of KS were particularly high in people living with HIV, accounting in some series for as much as 40% of all cancers in men. Ninety-five percent of patients with KS will have

skin lesions characterized as violaceous, red macules or nodules with a wide distribution. Thirty percent will also have oral lesions and 40% will have gastrointestinal disease. Pulmonary disease and rarely visceral disease can also occur. Rates of KS have fallen dramatically with the widespread use of ART, although they remain significantly higher than in the non-HIV population. The mainstay of treatment is initiation of ART. Of note, paradoxical worsening of disease after initiation of ART is well described (see section on Immune Reconstitution Inflammatory Syndrome). Radiotherapy and intralesional chemotherapy may be used for skin disease, and chemotherapy, usually with liposomal doxorubicin, is used for widespread disease.

Non-Hodgkin's Lymphoma

The incidence of non-Hodgkin's B-cell lymphoma (NHL) early in the epidemic was 100 times the incidence seen in the general population. This has fallen significantly with the use of ART. Similar to other AIDS-defining malignancies, lymphoma in PLWH is usually associated with a viral coinfection, in this instance, Epstein-Barr virus (EBV). The most common types of lymphoma in patients living with HIV in decreasing order of prevalence include diffuse large B-cell lymphoma, Burkitt's lymphoma, and primary CNS lymphoma. Primary CNS lymphoma complicates advanced HIV infection in 3% to 6% of cases and is almost invariably associated with detectable EBV DNA in the CSF. Lesions may be single or multiple and are often weakly ring enhancing. Irradiation often provides remission, which may be sustained as immune function is restored by effective ART. Treatment for other types of lymphoma in HIV is with standard chemotherapy and radiation regimens.

HPV-Associated Cancers

Cervical and anal cancers appear at increased rates in people living with HIV. This is related to both HPV persistence and the degree of immunodeficiency. It appears that ART decreases the persistence of cervical HPV and the rate of invasive cervical cancer. Screening for cervical cancer with Pap smear and/or high-risk HPV according to guidelines for cervical cancer remains very important for HIV-positive women throughout their lives (see recommendations later). Anal cancer is also increased in both men and women with HIV. At this time, no national recommendations exist for screening for anal cancer, though the Infectious Disease Society of America (IDSA) HIV Primary Care Guidelines do recommend anal Pap smear testing. Treatment for both cervical and anal cancer, if found, is per guidelines, and treatment is not different for people living with HIV disease. Rates for oropharyngeal cancer, related to both smoking and HPV, are also increased in PLWH.

Non-AIDS–Defining Cancers

Non-AIDS–defining cancers (NADC) in PWLH include lung, liver, renal, colorectal, and oropharyngeal cancer, as well as Hodgkin's disease. The incidence of many of these malignancies has historically been increased for PLWH and although they have fallen recently with the use of ART, many persist with higher incidence than in the general population.

- *Lung cancer* is increased 2 to 3 times in PLWH compared with the general population, primarily because of high rates of smoking (42% to 59% of PLWH smoke), though the risk for lung cancer in PLWH is increased even when smoking is controlled for. Non–small cell carcinoma is the most common form of lung cancer in PLWH, as with the general population. Treatment follows guidelines for the general population, but it should be noted that protocols for lung cancer therapy have historically excluded PLWH, and thus data do not exist specifically for this population. The effect of ART on lung cancer risk or prognosis is not clear. Unfortunately, survival for PLWH and lung cancer is poorer than the general population.

- *Colorectal cancer* is the third leading cause of cancer death in the United States in the general population. HIV has historically not been associated with increased rates of colorectal cancer, but of concern, the rates of colorectal cancer in PLWH appear to be increasing and occurring at a younger age. Both screening rates for colorectal cancer, and as a result survival rates, are lower for PLWH. Future efforts will need to focus on appropriate screening and treatment for this increasingly common and lethal malignancy, particularly as the population ages.
- Rates of *liver cancer*, particularly hepatocellular carcinoma, are increased in PLWH in part due to the increased rates of hepatitis B and C virus coinfection and increased alcohol use leading to cirrhosis. In addition, with increasing rates of obesity in people living with HIV, the risk for cirrhosis due to nonalcoholic steatohepatitis (NASH) and subsequent malignancy will rise as well. Treatments for viral hepatitides are now available and treatment is recommended for all PLWH. Similarly, identifying and then treating NASH remains a priority.
- Rates of *skin cancer*, including squamous cell carcinoma and malignant melanoma, are increased in PLWH and skin screening is an important part of primary care.
- Rates of *prostate and breast cancer* are not increased in PLWH. Screening recommendations and treatment guidelines do not differ for this population.

As the population of PLWH ages, rates of all malignancies will increase. Unfortunately, cancer-related mortality is predicted to increase along with increased rates. Screening and appropriate treatment for both AIDS-defining malignancies and NADC are essential in this at-risk population.

Immune Reconstitution Inflammatory Syndrome

The immune reconstitution inflammatory syndrome (IRIS) is a syndrome strongly associated with HIV, though the phenomenon is not specific to HIV and has been seen in association with other conditions, most notably tuberculosis. HIV-associated IRIS occurs after initiation of ART, usually in patients with low CD4 counts, and manifests as either a paradoxical worsening of treated opportunistic infections, called paradoxical IRIS, or an unmasking of a previously subclinical (untreated) infections, called unmasking IRIS. In both of these syndromes, patients are initiated on ART but subsequently develop a clinical decline, generally 2 weeks to several months later. Fever is extremely common with IRIS. Paradoxical IRIS will often present with fever and a clinical worsening of a known OI that is being treated. Unmasking IRIS usually presents as new-onset fevers and tachycardia, sometimes with localizing symptoms suggestive of a previously undiagnosed OI (e.g., headache and obtundation in the setting of cryptococcal disease, or abdominal pain in the setting of MAC). The frequency of IRIS in patients with HIV disease demonstrates a broad range; a meta-analysis found a rate in the published literature of around 13%, with differences by disease process: highest with CMV retinitis, cryptococcal meningitis, PML, and tuberculosis. IRIS is a clinical diagnosis, and there is no specific diagnostic test. Clinicians should have a suspicion for IRIS in the setting of recent ART initiation, particularly in patients with baseline low CD4 counts in which either a known OI appears to worsen, or a patient appears to worsen clinically despite evidence of immune reconstitution. There is significant morbidity to IRIS; up to 50% of IRIS cases require hospitalization, and patients often require extensive testing and both diagnostic and therapeutic procedures. Diagnostic work-up is driven by clinical presentation but generally would involve blood cultures, mycobacterial isolators on serum, sputum for bacterial and AFB

staining and culture if respiratory symptoms or radiographic findings are suggestive, imaging such as CT abdomen and pelvis or brain imaging if symptoms are suggestive, a retinal exam if any eye symptoms are present, a lymph node biopsy if any lymphadenopathy is notable, and further additional work-up as dictated by symptoms. Management of IRIS focuses on management of the identified opportunistic infection and use of corticosteroids and/or NSAIDs to calm the immunologic response. In all but life-threatening cases, ART should be continued. Steroid treatment is often prolonged, generally for 4 weeks or more, with gradual tapering as symptom management tolerates.

CO-OCCURRING DISEASE AND MULTIMORBIDITY WITH HIV

Neurologic Disease in HIV

Nervous system complications ultimately occur in most persons with untreated HIV infection. They range from mild cognitive disturbances or peripheral neuropathy to severe dementia and life-threatening central nervous system (CNS) infections. As with other lentiviruses, HIV enters microglial cells of the CNS early in the course of infection. Both direct neuronal destruction and effects of viral proteins on neuronal cell function may contribute to nervous system disease in AIDS. Infection in the CNS can be documented by CSF viral load and elevated immune markers. ART generally suppresses viral load in the CNS as well as the peripheral blood, although rarely elevated viral loads can occur in the CSF while the PVL remains suppressed; this is termed "CSF viral escape." CNS penetration by ART is variable depending on the drug, and treatment of CNS HIV infection is an area of active research.

Before effective ART therapy, a variety of severe neurologic complications were noted in patients with AIDS, including progressive dementia (termed the AIDS dementia complex), focal CNS disease, and peripheral neuropathy. ART has dramatically decreased the incidence of neurocognitive complications of HIV but has led to recognition of more subtle neurologic manifestations on the spectrum of what is now described as HIV-associated neurocognitive disorder (HAND), which includes asymptomatic neurologic impairment (ANI), mild cognitive dysfunction (MCD), and HIV-associated dementia (HAD). Approximately 40% of people living with HIV will have some abnormalities based on careful neuropsychological testing. Most of these patients will be asymptomatic (ANI), but 12% will have minor manifestations (MCD), and 2% severe disorders (HAD). Patients may have memory deficits, decreased executive function, and flattened affect, all of which may markedly affect quality of life. Screening tools such as the Montreal Cognitive Assessment (MoCA) test and the Frontal Assessment Battery test can be used to diagnose HAND. MRI findings may show diffuse cerebral atrophy, which correlates with symptoms. Risk factors for developing HAND include age at seroconversion, low CD4 count, comorbidities such as hepatitis C virus, other CNS infections, and trauma. Neurologic manifestations in PLWH on ART generally seem to be nonprogressive or very slowly progressive, and thus adherence to ART is critical. Interestingly, therapy early after initial infection may lower the CNS reservoir for the virus and result in less immune activation compared to those initiated on treatment later in chronic infection.

Focal Lesions of the Central Nervous System

A large variety of neurologic problems can occur in patients with low CD4 T-cell counts. A neuroanatomic classification of these manifestations is presented in Table 103.4. Some of the more frequent or treatable problems are discussed here and in the next section.

Several opportunistic complications of HIV infection produce focal CNS lesions, as mentioned previously. Patients with focal neurologic signs, seizures of new onset, or recent onset of rapidly progressive cognitive impairment should undergo magnetic resonance imaging (MRI) or CT of the brain. Toxoplasmosis, CNS lymphoma, and PML are the most common causes of CNS focal lesions in this setting (Table 103.5). A more detailed review of these opportunistic diseases was discussed previously.

Central Nervous System Diseases Without Prominent Focal Signs

Evaluation of PLWH with fever and headache is difficult because of the often subtle manifestations of serious CNS lesions in immunocompromised patients. Bacterial meningitis management is the same as for non-immunocompromised patients. Meningeal diseases in PLWH fall into the broad categories of aseptic meningitis, chronic meningitis, and meningoencephalitis.

A brief review of these conditions is as follows:

- *Aseptic Meningitis:* Patients with aseptic meningitis, which can be a manifestation of the acute retroviral syndrome, complain most often of headache. Their sensorium is generally intact, and findings on neurologic examination are normal. In the individual with established HIV infection, aseptic meningitis may result from several potentially treatable causes.
- *Chronic Meningitis:* As discussed previously, *Cryptococcus* followed by tuberculosis are the most common causes of chronic meningitis in PLWH. Patients with an AIDS diagnosis with chronic meningitis characteristically have headache, fever, difficulty in concentrating, or changes in sensorium. Neurosyphilis in PLWH is more common than in uninfected patients and may manifest earlier after infection.
- *Meningoencephalitis:* Patients with meningoencephalitis manifest alterations in sensorium varying from mild lethargy to coma. Patients may be febrile, and neurologic examination often shows evidence of diffuse CNS involvement. MRI may show only nonspecific abnormalities, whereas electroencephalography often is consistent with diffuse disease of the brain. CMV, HSV, and HIV itself are possible causes.

Distal symmetrical peripheral neuropathy (PN) is a common neurological complication of HIV. In addition to the direct effect of the virus itself, older ART drugs, particularly stavudine and didanosine, were associated with PN. Distressing pain, hyperesthesia, or hypesthesia, occurring most commonly in the lower extremities and worse at night, were previously common and were difficult to treat. With newer drugs and earlier treatment of all patients with HIV, new diagnoses of PN are becoming less common. Treatment consists of removing potentially neurotoxic drugs and, depending on symptoms, typically initiating gabapentin therapy.

Gastrointestinal Diseases

Patients with advanced HIV disease have a variety of potential gastrointestinal complications, whereas those with elevated CD4 counts and suppressed viral loads on ART have far less risk. Thus, in the pre-ART era, gastrointestinal complications ranging from severe oral stomatitis and esophagitis caused by *Candida* infections, to acalculous cholecystitis, severe chronic hepatitis, and chronic diarrhea caused by protozoal parasites, were common. In the ART era, these complications in diagnosed and treated patients are far rarer.

Mouth and Esophagus

Thrush, or *Candida* pharyngitis, and *Candida* esophagitis have been some of the historic markers of HIV, although many other causes of immunodeficiency can also put people at risk for these infections (see prior section on *Candida* disease). Other causes of ulcerations in the mouth and esophagus include aphthous ulcers and herpes virus reactivation, including HSV-1 and CMV. In patients with AIDS, KS frequently occurs in the mouth and may also occur in the stomach and liver.

Large and Small Intestines

The lower GI tract was previously the site of chronic infection due to a variety of microorganisms, including *Cryptosporidium, Cystoisospora*

TABLE 103.4   Neuroanatomic Classification of Neurologic Complications of HIV Infection

Category	Condition
Meningitis and headache	Aseptic meningitis
	Cryptococcal meningitis
	Tuberculous meningitis
	Neurosyphilis
Diffuse brain diseases	
With preservation of consciousness	AIDS dementia complex
	Neurosyphilis
With decreased arousal	*Toxoplasma* encephalitis
	Cytomegalovirus encephalitis
Focal brain diseases	Tuberculous brain abscess
	Primary central nervous system lymphoma
	Progressive multifocal leukoencephalopathy
	Cerebral toxoplasmosis
	Neurosyphilis
Myelopathies	Subacute or chronic progressive vacuolar myelopathy
	Cytomegalovirus myelopathy
Peripheral neuropathies	Predominantly sensory polyneuropathy
	Toxic neuropathies
	Autonomic neuropathy
	Cytomegalovirus polyradiculopathy
Myopathies	Noninflammatory myopathy
	Zidovudine myopathy

TABLE 103.5   Neurologic Complications of HIV Infection

Condition	CLINICAL ONSET			NEURORADIOLOGIC FEATURES		
	Time	Alertness	Fever	Number of Lesions	Characteristics of Lesions	Location of Lesions
Cerebral toxoplasmosis	Days	Reduced	Common	Usually multiple	Spherical, ring enhancing	Basal ganglia, cortex
Primary CNS lymphoma	Days to weeks	Variable	Absent	One or few	Irregular, weakly ring enhancing	Periventricular
PML	Weeks to months	Variable	Absent	Often multiple	Multiple lesions visible on MRI	White matter

MRI, Magnetic resonance imaging; *PML,* progressive multifocal lymphoma.

belli, Microsporidia spp, CMV, and mycobacteria. These infections caused chronic diarrhea leading to inanition and wasting. In the era of ART, these infections are much less common and have been superseded in frequency by *Clostridioides difficile* infection due to frequent antibiotic exposure in PLWH. Additionally, increased risk of anal cancer has been recognized in PLWH. With the aging population of PLWH, colon cancer risk is also on the rise (see prior section on HIV and malignancy).

Hepatobiliary Disease

Abnormalities on liver function testing are common in HIV disease and often are nonspecific. Elevations of serum alanine aminotransferase and aspartate aminotransferase may represent chronic active viral hepatitis B or C but may also reflect hepatic inflammation caused by alcohol or medications, including trimethoprim-sulfamethoxazole or antiretroviral agents. Alcohol use is highly prevalent among PLWH and may contribute, as can use of other drugs such as MDMA ("ecstasy"). Marked elevations in serum alkaline phosphatase levels may reflect infiltrative disease of the liver (e.g., MAC, CMV, tuberculosis, tumor) but also may occur in patients with acalculous cholecystitis, cryptosporidiosis, AIDS-associated sclerosing cholangitis, or syphilitic hepatitis.

Viral hepatitides, particularly hepatitis C, are an important cause of morbidity and mortality among PLWH. More than 80% of persons with HIV who have a history of injection drug use are coinfected with hepatitis C, and the risk of progression to end-stage liver disease is greater for those with HIV and hepatitis C coinfection. Recently, therapy of hepatitis C has been revolutionized by combination directly acting agents (DAAs), which achieve hepatitis C cure rates of over 95%. Response rates among PLWH appear to be similar to those among HIV-negative persons. In contrast, treatment of hepatitis B is rarely curative; however, very effective suppression can be achieved utilizing combination therapy. Common agents used for HIV ART, such as tenofovir, emtricitabine, and lamivudine, have potent hepatitis B antiviral activity, and an ART regimen that treats both HIV and hepatitis B coinfection is easily possible. Occult hepatitis infections (antibody negative but with detectable virus on RNA/DNA testing) have been described for both hepatitis C and hepatitis B, particularly in the context of advanced immunodeficiency. Hepatocellular carcinoma is a complication of both hepatitis B and C infection. Regular screening with liver imaging is indicated for all patients with hepatitis C and known cirrhosis, all patients with hepatitis B who are at increased risk, namely those with active hepatitis (elevated serum ALT) and/or high viral load (>20,000 IU/mL), those with a family history of hepatocellular carcinoma, Asian males over 40, Asian females over 50, and all Africans and African Americans.

Cardiovascular Disease

Before ART, patients with HIV with low CD4 counts were at risk for myocarditis, pericardial effusion, and dilated cardiomyopathy, but at present these conditions are markedly less common. What has become apparent, however, is an increased risk for cardiovascular disease, including both myocardial infarction and stroke. In a landmark study from the US Veteran Affairs system in 2013, PLWH were found to have a 50% increase in acute myocardial infarction compared to HIV-uninfected patients, even after controlling for traditional risk factors such as smoking and diabetes. In a more recent review in 2018, a relative risk of 2.16 for cardiovascular (CV) disease in PLWH was noted. Unlike HIV-negative patients, there is an increased rate (up to 50%) of type II myocardial infarction (vasospasm, endothelial dysfunction) compared to type I (thromboembolic) infarction, suggesting different etiologic processes. Longitudinal studies have shown that the risk for stroke and, more recently, congestive heart failure are similarly elevated.

Several additional features of CV disease are worth noting. Long-term studies from the Kaiser Permanente system in California and from Europe initially demonstrated increased rates of CV disease in PLWH but found that more recent data in selected populations saw a convergence of rates with HIV-negative patients, perhaps due to improvements in CV prevention, such as the widespread use of HMG co-A reductase inhibitors ("statins"). It is also worth noting that PLWH do have a higher prevalence of some risk factors for CV disease, particularly smoking, diabetes mellitus, renal disease, metabolic syndrome, and hypertension. The risk conveyed by these factors in total is of a much larger magnitude than that contributed by HIV itself. Thus, addressing these risk factors is particularly important in this population that has a baseline elevated CV risk due to HIV. Proven interventions include smoking cessation and the use of antihypertensives and statins, which should be prescribed following American College of Cardiology/American Heart Association guidelines. Improving diet and exercise also are important, especially for patients as they age.

The effect of certain antiretrovirals on CV risk remains an area of controversy. Protease inhibitors (PIs) are known to have an adverse effect on the metabolic profile, including inducing hyperlipidemia, when compared to newer classes of ART drugs such as integrase inhibitors. Risk is not necessarily uniform across the class; a recent cohort analysis specifically identified darunavir to be associated with increased risk when compared to atazanavir. In addition, several studies have shown that abacavir increases CV risk, but these findings have not been confirmed in others. Integrase inhibitors and newer reverse transcriptase inhibitors have a lesser effect on patients' lipid profiles, although integrase inhibitors have been associated with more weight gain than other classes, which itself may raise the risk of other diseases that raise CV risk (e.g., diabetes, hypertension).

Renal Disease

In the early years of the HIV epidemic, a new form of progressive renal disease was identified, termed HIV-associated nephropathy (HIVAN). It was characterized by rapidly progressive renal failure and nephrotic-range proteinuria. This disease was found to be more common in African Americans. The incidence of HIVAN rose until the mid-1990s and then fell with the advent of effective ART. Although HIVAN has become uncommon, the incidence of chronic renal disease in PWHV remains significantly higher than in the general population. The prevalence of stage III chronic kidney disease (glomerular filtration rate of 30 to 59 mL/min) has ranged from 3.5% to 9.7%. PLWH are more than 16 times more likely to need renal replacement therapy.

The etiology of renal disease in PLWH is multifactorial; risk factors include low CD4 counts, high viral loads, hypertension, diabetes mellitus, cardiovascular disease, African American race, hepatitis C coinfection, and prior exposure to certain ART drugs such as tenofovir. Patients are also at risk of acute kidney injury, particularly in the setting of dehydration, infection, and polypharmacy. In addition, patients may develop immune complex kidney disease and thrombotic microangiopathy. Most important in prevention and treatment of renal disease is the use of effective ART and consistent monitoring of renal function. Controlling both hypertension and diabetes are also essential in preventing the progression of renal disease.

Osteoporosis and Bone Disease

PLWH have increased rates of osteopenia and osteoporosis and consequently longitudinal controlled studies have shown an almost 3-fold rate of fractures compared to that of the general population. Risk factors for decreased bone density are usually multiple and include effects of ART, particularly protease inhibitor– and tenofovir disoproxil fumarate–containing regimens; low body weight; vitamin D deficiency;

alcohol use; hypogonadism; opiate exposure; smoking; and effects of HIV itself. Patients should be assessed for vitamin D deficiency and other risk factors and treated and counseled appropriately. Bone density assessment by dual-energy x-ray absorptiometry (DXA) is recommended for all men with HIV who are over 50, all postmenopausal women, those with a history of fragility fractures, patients on chronic corticosteroids, and patients at high risk for fall. Risk of fragility fracture should be assessed primarily using the Fracture Risk Assessment Tool (FRAX). ART regimens should be reviewed for osteopenia and osteoporosis risk. Patients diagnosed with osteopenia or osteoporosis should be treated following established guidelines.

Endocrine Disorders
Metabolic Syndrome

PLWH are at increased risk for metabolic syndrome, which includes central obesity, insulin resistance, hypertension, and hypertriglyceridemia. Some classes of ART such as protease inhibitors seem to increase the risk for metabolic syndrome, and this risk translates into increased risk for CV disease. Treatment with weight loss and exercise, anti-hypertensives, and diabetic medications if diabetes is diagnosed, are recommended.

Diabetes Mellitus

The risk for diabetes mellitus (DM) in PLWH patients was not initially appreciated but has become apparent in more recent years. One estimate is that the relative risk for DM in PLWH is 2.4 when compared to the general population. This risk is compounded by the rates of metabolic syndrome, obesity, and adverse lifestyle (such as poor diet and low rates of exercise). In addition, a diagnosis of DM markedly increases the risk for CV disease, including stroke and peripheral vascular disease, as well as renal disease. Screening PLWH with a hemoglobin A_{1c} or fasting blood sugar on an annual basis is important, particularly as the population ages. Treatment for patients at risk for DM and those with DM should follow established guidelines for management of diabetes.

Other Endocrine Disorders

Other endocrine disorders that disproportionately affect PLWH, particularly those with low CD4 counts, include adrenal insufficiency (AI), hypogonadism, and male gynecomastia. In the pre-ART era, adrenal gland pathology caused by CMV and mycobacteria was frequent, but clinical AI characterized by malaise, orthostatic hypotension, weight loss, hyponatremia, and hypoglycemia, was uncommon. Clinical AI remains rare. Hypogonadism is common in men with HIV and may manifest as erectile dysfunction and loss of libido but may also occur more subtly with low energy, depression, or inability to gain muscle mass. Screening with serum testosterone may indicate hypogonadism that can be treated with androgen replacement therapy. Gynecomastia in men with HIV may also occur and be due to hypoandrogenism, liver disease, medication side effects, or as a part of normal aging.

Nonalcoholic Fatty Liver Disease

Nonalcoholic fatty liver disease (NFLD) ranges from simple hepatic steatosis (or fatty liver) to NASH and hepatic fibrosis that can lead to cirrhosis. The rates of steatosis and NASH in PLWH are increasing and appear to be greater than in the general population, perhaps because of the increased rates of obesity, metabolic syndrome, and diabetes mellitus. NASH and subsequent cirrhosis pose a significant risk for PLWH and emphasize the importance of preventative measures including weight control.

Obesity

In the early years of the HIV epidemic, advanced AIDS was associated with low weight, and in fact one of the characteristics of the disease was wasting and inanition. Effective ART prevented and even reversed this manifestation of infection, even in end-stage AIDS. Now with PLWH on ART, a new problem has arisen—obesity. In countries like the United States, the rates of obesity in PLWH (20% to 31%) match the rates in the general population. Rates of complications related to obesity in PLWH, such as diabetes mellitus and cardiovascular disease, are nearly twice the rates in uninfected patients. Rates of obesity in PLWH may be related to a combination of factors including poor diet quality, greater food insecurity, lack of exercise, and genetics. Perhaps most important, however, has been the lack of awareness of the consequences of obesity and also the best approaches to losing weight. Although there has been a dearth of research in the treatment of obesity in PLWH, behavioral weight loss programs focusing on behavior change, diet, and exercise have been shown to be effective for this population. In addition, bariatric surgery for morbidly obese patients has been an effective strategy in individual cases.

Aging and HIV

The average age of the first 1000 cases of HIV reported in 1983 was 34 years. With the advent of effective ART, the age of PLWH has steadily increased so that by the year 2015, it was estimated that 50% of PLWH were over the age of 50, and by the year 2030 it is estimated that 70% will be over the age of 50. Similar trends, although delayed, are being observed worldwide in low- to medium-income countries. Despite this increase in the age of PLWH, mortality remains elevated compared to the general population, although there is great heterogeneity. Individuals with risk factors such as low CD4 count, elevated viral loads, drug use, hepatitis coinfections, and other comorbidities have increased mortality rates, whereas subgroup analysis of population studies have shown that individuals with CD4 counts greater than 350 cells/microliter at diagnosis, consistent viral suppression, and an absence of other risk factors have a life expectancy similar to uninfected individuals. Nonetheless, most population studies comparing PLWH to the general population, controlling for risk factors, have shown a decrease in life expectancy of anywhere from 2 to 13 years depending on the subpopulation.

Whether HIV infection accelerates the aging process has been a controversial subject and continues to be investigated. It is known, however, that HIV is associated with chronic inflammation at levels that are similar to older individuals. Inflammation is presumed to be driven by ongoing low-level viral replication, even in virally suppressed individuals, and by the effect of the initial damage to the immune system during acute HIV infection (e.g., injury to gut immune tissue). Elevated markers of inflammation include elevated levels of IL-6, elevated markers of microbial translocation, and elevated levels of macrophage activation. In addition, immune dysregulation and immune senescence as evidenced by decreased pools of CD4 T cells, increased senescent CD8 T cells that secrete cytokines, and an inability to respond robustly to new antigens, all occur in PLWH as well as elderly noninfected people. Increased inflammation and immune dysregulation are part of the normal aging process but appear to occur earlier in PLWH. In addition, as discussed previously, PLWH are at increased risk for a variety of comorbidities, some of which are associated with increased inflammation, such as cardiovascular disease.

Compared to age-matched controls, PLWH have higher rates of geriatric syndromes including falls, urinary incontinence, difficulty with activities of daily living, slow gait, decreased vision and hearing, and frailty. As a result, they are at increased risk for associated morbidity. In addition, PLWH are more likely to develop frailty early. Frailty is defined several ways, but Fried's criteria are commonly used and include decreased strength, endurance, activity, and walking speed, as well as weight loss. Patients with frailty are at significant risk for poor outcomes including hospitalization and death. Risks for frailty in PLWH include low current and nadir CD4 counts as well as other comorbidities and geriatric syndromes. As the population of PLWH ages, recognizing and addressing both geriatric syndromes and frailty will be increasingly important in their care.

Finally, aging patients in general face a number of challenges to their health and well-being including comorbidities, increasing physical impairments, loss of partners, and family and social isolation. PLWH are particularly at risk for some of these challenges and in addition many face challenges such as poverty, housing and/or food insecurity, and concern for safety. The loss of friends and community is particularly stressful and has been described by one aging PLWH as "a shrinking kind of life." It is important for physicians caring for PLWH to be aware of these issues.

Mental Health

As HIV has changed to a chronic and manageable illness, the emphasis of mental health treatment has shifted from managing acute syndromes to helping patients live well. Depression and anxiety, as well as other mental illnesses, are very common among PLWH. Often patients will not feel comfortable acknowledging the need for mental health care. For many PLWH, their HIV physician may be their only health care provider, and therefore it is crucial for providers to offer routine screenings for mental health concerns such as depression and anxiety. Screenings will also offer opportunities for physicians to facilitate referrals for additional mental health evaluation and appropriate behavioral and psychiatric care. Trauma is not uncommon and treatment of PTSD can be very helpful.

Substance Use Disorder

Substance/alcohol use and substance/alcohol use disorders are common among PLWH. Alcohol use (e.g., problematic and binge drinking) may also co-occur with the use of substances (e.g., cocaine, methamphetamine). Both alcohol use and substance use have been associated with higher rates of risk-taking behaviors (e.g., condomless sex with multiple partners) and have also been associated with decreased adherence to ART. It is also important to note that many individuals who use substances maintain high levels of adherence to ART; thus, the existence of substance or alcohol use should not prevent physicians from prescribing ART. There are many factors that contribute to or exacerbate substance and alcohol use. For instance, among methamphetamine users, there exists a high correlation between methamphetamine use and chemsex behaviors. Other common factors that may perpetuate continued use include co-occurring mental health diagnoses (e.g., PTSD, anxiety, ADHD), minority stress, and environmental instability. Many studies have shown that treatment of opiate use disorders with medication assisted therapy, such as buprenorphine, can be done in conjunction with HIV treatment. Likewise, treatment of alcohol use disorders can be done in conjunction with HIV treatment. Whereas pharmacotherapy for stimulant use disorders is lacking, the patient-physician relationship can still play an important role in facilitating referral for evidence-based behavioral care for stimulant use. Importantly, patient-centered HIV care cannot focus solely on HIV viral suppression but must proactively address mental health and substance use concerns to promote the goal of patients living meaningful lives with the chronic disease of HIV. Routine screening for substance abuse treatment (i.e., at regular follow-up visits) is recommended. Co-locating substance abuse treatment with HIV care (i.e., one stop shopping) is preferred.

Sexually Transmitted Infections

Rates of sexually transmitted infections (STIs) continue to rise in the United States, reaching an all-time high in 2018 (the last available reported data at the time of this publishing), with no sign of leveling

off in the coming years. The presence of STIs increases the risk of HIV transmission from partner to partner, particularly syphilis and herpes simplex disease. In people living with HIV, rates of STIs have also increased. As "undetectable = untransmittable" becomes a more commonly understood concept among patients, education about protecting themselves from acquiring STIs is important as patients make informed decisions about condom use. Annual STI screening, or more frequent depending on risk behavior, is important in sexually active patients. Treatment of these STIs is the same in HIV-negative as in HIV-positive persons and the response to treatment is good.

HIV MANAGEMENT AND TREATMENT

Initial Counseling and Ambulatory Evaluation

Once HIV is diagnosed, the health care provider should talk to the patient about the clinical course and treatment of HIV infection and the use of immunologic and virologic studies (e.g., CD4 counts, PVL assays) to guide therapy. Stigma related to HIV remains an important concern and a key barrier to engagement in care. Addressing this as part of post-test counseling and intake to care is key to retention in care for persons newly diagnosed. The patient should be educated about modes of HIV transmission through unprotected sex or sharing of needles. The benefit of "U=U" (undetectable = untransmittable) should be discussed with patients so they understand that initiating treatment and achieving an undetectable viral load is both important for their own health as well as their partners.

The initial evaluation should include both an HIV-oriented review of systems and a complete physical examination. In particular, the skin must be examined for HIV-associated rashes and Kaposi's sarcoma. Examination of the oral cavity may reveal thrush, gingivitis, hairy leukoplakia, superficial ulcers caused by HSV, aphthous ulcers, or lesions characteristic of Kaposi's sarcoma. In persons with very advanced disease, the optic fundi may have hemorrhagic lesions characteristic of CMV retinitis. Lymph node enlargement, hepatomegaly, splenomegaly, and any genital lesions should be carefully noted. Neurologic examination for both peripheral neuropathy and decreased global cognition deserves close attention.

Laboratory Monitoring

The CD4 count and the PVL should be measured at the first visit, and the patient should be shown the results. Graphic illustrations of the interaction between PVL and CD4 can be useful to increase patient understanding. HIV genotyping to assess for drug resistance should also be performed. The PVL is a key measure of treatment adherence and is repeated at regular intervals, generally 2 to 8 weeks after initiation of therapy and every 3 to 6 months once patients are stably on treatment. Once a patient is stable on treatment with suppressed virus (<200 copies) and CD4 counts higher than 200 cells/mL, the value of CD4 monitoring is less clear, and guidelines allow for extending the monitoring interval to yearly. If a patient's count is greater than 500 for greater than 1 year, CD4 monitoring becomes optional, as long as the PVL remains undetectable.

An initial assessment of basic chemistries (including a creatinine), hepatic function testing, a complete blood count with differential, a random or fasting glucose, and a urinalysis should be performed to establish a baseline. Women should have a pregnancy test. Once patients are initiated on ART, they should have a basic chemistry panel and hepatic function testing (along with a PVL as noted previously) repeated between 2 to 8 weeks after starting therapy. Patients stably on ART should have these same labs repeated every 6 months, to monitor for toxicity and changes that might affect dosing. A yearly complete

TABLE 103.6   Recommended Vaccinations in Adults With HIV

Vaccine	Recommendation
Influenza vaccination (inactivated or recombinant)	Recommended annually
Influenza vaccination (live attenuated)	Not recommended
Tdap (tetanus, diphtheria, pertussis) or Td	Recommended primary series then every 10 years
MMR (measles, mumps, rubella)	Not recommended if CD4 <200; recommended if nonimmune and CD4 >200
Varicella primary vaccination (Varivax)	Not recommended if CD4 <200; recommended if nonimmune and CD4 >200
Recombinant zoster vaccination (RZV; Shingrix)	No recommendation at this time[a]
Live attenuated varicella vaccination (ZVL; Zostavax)	Not recommended if CD4 <200; no recommendation at this time[a] if CD4 >200
Human papillomavirus (HPV) vaccination	Three-dose series recommended through age 26
PCV-13 (pneumococcal conjugate)	One lifetime dose recommended, at least 8 weeks prior to, or 1 year following PPS-23
PPS-23 (pneumococcal polysaccharide)	Recommended once, with a repeat dose at least 5 years later, and 1 dose after age 65
Hepatitis A	Recommended two-dose series, or three-dose HAV/HBV combined vaccine for all patients
Hepatitis B	Recommended two- or three-dose series for all patients
Meningitis ACYW135	Recommended two-dose series at least 8 weeks apart; repeat every 5 years
Meningitis B	Recommended only if additional risk factors exist (e.g., asplenia, complement deficiency)
Hib	Recommended only if additional risk factors exist (e.g., asplenia, hematopoietic stem cell transplant)

[a]Current ACIP guidelines do not recommend for or against RZV due to limited data. DHHS guidelines state that "given that risk of herpes zoster is high among persons with HIV, and the vaccine appears safe, experts recommend administration of RZV to persons with HIV aged ≥50 years following the FDA-approved schedule for persons without HIV (IM dose at 0 and 2 months)."

blood count is recommended in all patients. A urinalysis every 6 months is also recommended in patients on tenofovir-based regimens.

Screening for Associated Infections
Tuberculosis
Tuberculin skin test (TST) or blood interferon-γ release assays (IGRA) testing should be performed early in the course of HIV management. Induration of 5 mm or more on the TST should be considered positive. IGRA testing will provide an interpretation based on patient results. Any patient with a positive tuberculous test result should be evaluated for the presence of active tuberculosis with a thorough physical exam, chest radiograph, and symptom screen. If no active disease is present, the patient should receive 9 months of prophylaxis with isoniazid or combination drug therapy for a shorter period (see Chapter 94). If active tuberculosis is identified, multidrug therapy should be initiated after careful consideration of possible interactions with ART. It is important to remember that false-negative TB testing, both TSTs and IGRAs, can occur in patients with HIV, especially those with CD4 count less than 200.

STIs
Serologic testing for syphilis should be followed by prompt treatment if the patient is confirmed to be positive. Syphilis infections are common within many populations highly impacted by HIV, and coinfection with syphilis increases the risk of transmission of HIV to others. Gonorrhea and chlamydia testing of any potentially exposed orifice is recommended, and "triple-point testing" (oral, rectal, and urine PCR testing) should be offered whenever appropriate. All women should be tested for vaginal trichomonas as well. Following initial screening, annual STI screening is recommended. (See Chapter 102.)

Viral Hepatitis
Liver disease is an important cause of morbidity and mortality for PLWH. Screening for hepatitis B and C at baseline is recommended and vaccination offered if appropriate. Hepatitis C is highly prevalent among persons who acquired HIV from injection drug use, and MSM populations are also at higher risk due to sexual transmission. Given the lack of an effective vaccine for hepatitis C, regular screening is recommended for persons with ongoing risk of exposure.

Other Infections
Screening for antibodies to *Toxoplasma gondii* should be considered for persons with low CD4 counts who are potentially in need of prophylaxis. Persons from endemic areas may be screened for histoplasmosis and coccidiomycosis and considered for prophylaxis if positive.

Immunization
Antibody responses to polysaccharides are better among patients with higher CD4 counts, though the optimal timing of immunization is uncertain. For persons with low CD4 counts, many physicians provide initial immunization and reimmunization for certain vaccines after immune reconstitution occurs. Live vaccines should be avoided in persons with CD4 counts lower than 200 cells/mm³. The US Centers for Disease Control and Prevention (CDC) recommends ensuring routine childhood vaccination (e.g., tetanus series, measles, mumps, rubella, varicella vaccination or reported history of disease). The following vaccines are additionally recommended in PLWH (Table 103.6).

Streptococcus pneumoniae Vaccination
All persons with HIV should receive a single lifetime dose of PCV13 (Prevnar13), followed by a dose of PPV23 (Pneumovax) at least 8 weeks later. If previously vaccinated with PPV23, the patients should receive PCV13 at least 1 year after PPV23. Patients should have a CD4 cell count greater than or equal to 200/microliter. A second PPV23 dose is recommended 5 years after the first PPV23, and again after the age of 65.

Influenza Virus Vaccination
PLWH have excess morbidity and mortality associated with influenza and its complications. They should receive seasonal influenza vaccination yearly.

Human Papillomavirus Vaccination
The CDC recommends use of the human papillomavirus (HPV) vaccine in boys or girls at age 11 or 12 regardless of HIV status, in MSM, and in persons with immune compromise, including those with HIV, up to the age of 26 if not previously vaccinated. Vaccination is now FDA-approved through age 45.

Hepatitis A and B Viruses Vaccination

PLWH should be assessed by serology for prior exposure to hepatitis B. All PLWH who are not immune to hepatitis B should receive immunization. All PLWH should receive immunization against hepatitis A. Antibody testing prior to vaccination is reasonable in patients likely to have had childhood exposure (e.g., immigrants from endemic countries).

Neisseria meningitidis Vaccination

Due to a higher incidence of meningococcal meningitis in PLWH, the CDC recommends all PLWH receive the quadrivalent conjugate meningitis A, C, Y, W-135 vaccine (MCV4). This vaccine can be administered as two doses spaced 8 weeks apart, with boosters given every 5 years.

Other Health Screening
Cervical Cancer

Women living with HIV should be screened for cervical cancer with a Pap smear. Due to the increased risk for cervical cancer in PLWH, screening guidelines are more aggressive for women living with HIV. Women with normal cytology with no high-risk HPV on Pap smear are recommended to have repeat screening in 3 years (whereas HIV-negative women undergo repeat screening at 5 years).

Anal Cancer

As discussed previously, HPV is associated with an increased risk of anal cancer in both men and women living with HIV. At this time, no national recommendations exist for routine screening for anal cancer, though the IDSA HIV Primary Care Guidelines do recommend anal Pap smear testing in MSM, women with a history of receptive anal intercourse or abnormal cervical Pap smears, and all patients with genital warts. The quality of supporting evidence is low and no specific timing interval for repeat testing is suggested. Despite clear national guidelines, anal Pap smear testing is commonly performed in clinical practice due to an acknowledgement of the increased risk of anal cancer in PLWH.

ANTIRETROVIRAL TREATMENT

The goal of ART is to ensure that all PLWH can lead symptom-free, productive lives. Currently available therapy makes achieving this goal possible in almost all individuals. Treatment guidelines in the United States and worldwide recommend that all patients be offered ART regardless of CD4 count, as early treatment has been demonstrated to have significant health benefit to the individual regardless of CD4 count; further, treatment is prevention because patients who are undetectable are do not transmit to others ("U=U"). This confers a significant public health benefit in addition to the benefit to the health of the individual.

Current Antiretrovirals

Currently available antiretrovirals fall into five classes:

1. **The nucleotide/nucleoside reverse transcriptase inhibitors (NRTIs):** These are nucleotide or nucleoside analogs that lack a 3′-hydroxyl group on the deoxyribose moiety, causing chain termination of viral DNA and inhibition of viral reverse transcriptase. Examples include tenofovir alafenamide, tenofovir disoproxil fumarate, lamivudine, emtricitabine, abacavir, and zidovudine.
2. **Non-nucleotide reverse transcription inhibitors (NNRTIs):** NNRTIs are also inhibitors of the reverse transcriptase enzyme, but they are not nucleotide analogs and do not bind at the nucleotide binding site of the enzyme. These agents have "-vir-" in their names. Agents available in this class include efavirenz, nevirapine, etravirine, rilpivirine, and doravirine.
3. **PIs:** PIs are inhibitors of the virally encoded protease, an enzyme necessary for proteolytic cleavage of protein precursors necessary for the production of an infectious viral particle. These agents end with the suffix "-navir." Examples include darunavir, atazanavir, and lopinavir.
4. **Entry Inhibitors:** "Entry inhibitors" is an "umbrella" grouping of agents that block viral entry into CD4+ cells through a variety of mechanisms. This grouping includes attachment inhibitors (fostemsavir), fusion inhibitors (enfuvirtide), entry inhibitors (ibalizumab, a monoclonal antibody that binds to CD4), and CCR5 antagonists (maraviroc); none of these agents is first-line, and all are only used in salvage regimens.
5. **Integrase Inhibitors** *or* **Integrase Strand Transfer Inhibitors (InSTIs):** InSTIs are drugs that inhibit the viral integrase, which is responsible for integrating reverse-transcribed viral DNA into the host genome of infected cells. These agents end with the suffix "-tegravir." Agents in this class are raltegravir, elvitegravir, dolutegravir, and bictegravir.

Some agents, including all protease inhibitors and the integrase inhibitor elvitegravir, are paired with "boosters," agents that serve as cytochrome P450 3A4 enzymatic inhibitors. This inhibition slows the metabolism of the antiviral drug to decrease the needed dose and lower toxicity and slow metabolism to allow once-daily dosing. The two boosters utilized today are ritonavir and cobicistat. Both can be given independently or co-formulated into combination tablets. Boosting agents must be used with caution as they also affect the metabolism of a number of other drugs as well.

Treatment Guidelines

Since 1996, treatment of HIV has utilized the concept of "combination antiretroviral therapy," which involves treating patients with multiple agents targeting multiple steps in the viral replication cycle. This multitargeted approach overcomes the virus' ability to mutate and evolve resistance to single agents. A complete regimen is generally composed of three active agents (three drugs to which the virus is not believed to harbor resistance), though there are clinical situations in which fewer (two) or more agents are used. Co-formulations are common, as they are simpler for patients and improve adherence. The US Department of Health and Human Services (DHHS) and the International AIDS Society-USA (IAS-USA) both issue HIV treatment guidelines that are considered standard-of-care for HIV providers in the United States. They are available online at https://aidsinfo.nih.gov/guidelines and https://www.iasusa.org/resources/guidelines/, respectively. Both are updated frequently. The World Health Organization (WHO) also publishes treatment recommendations for resource-limited settings, which delineate first- and second-line regimen recommendations. The last decade has seen a major shift in recommended treatment guidelines such that a combination of NRTIs plus an InSTI are now recommended as the components of all first-line therapies for patients initiating HIV treatment.

Tables 103.7A and 103.7B review the current first-line recommended regimens of the DHHS and IAS-USA. Decisions on which regimen to recommend to patients should be made in cooperation with the patient and should take into consideration any known resistance, drug/drug interactions, coexisting conditions (e.g., hepatitis B, cardiovascular disease, renal disease), patient preference about time of day and taking the medication with or without food, and insurance coverage.

Resistance Testing

Approximately 16% of treatment-naïve patients have detectable baseline mutations that confer resistance in the genome of their HIV.

TABLE 103.7A   Recommended Initial Regimens for Most People With HIV (DHHS)

Drug Combination	Restrictions	Strength
Bictegravir/tenofovir alafenamide/emtricitabine (Biktarvy)		AI
Dolutegravir/abacavir/lamivudine (Triumeq)	Only for patients who are HLA-B*5701 negative and without chronic hepatitis B coinfection	AI
Dolutegravir (Tivicay) *plus* emtricitabine *or* lamivudine *plus* tenofovir alafenamide *or* tenofovir disoproxil fumarate		AI
Dolutegravir/lamivudine (Dovato)	Except for individuals with HIV RNA >500,000 copies/mL, HBV coinfection, or in whom ART is to be started before the results of HIV genotypic resistance testing for reverse transcriptase or HBV testing are available	AI
Raltegravir (Isentress) *plus* emtricitabine *or* lamivudine *plus* tenofovir alafenamide *or* tenofovir disoproxil fumarate		BI for TDF BII for TAF

TABLE 103.7B   Generally Recommended Initial Regimens (IAS-USA)

Drug Combination	Details	Strength
Bictegravir/tenofovir alafenamide/emtricitabine (Biktarvy)		AIa
Dolutegravir/abacavir/lamivudine (Triumeq)	Testing for HLA-B*5701 allele should be performed before abacavir use (evidence rating AIa); patients who test positive should not be given abacavir (evidence rating AIa). Because it typically takes several days or longer to obtain results for HLA-B*5701 testing, tenofovir-containing regimens should be used when starting ART on the same day as HIV diagnosis or until HLA-B*5701 testing results are available. In patients with or at high risk for cardiovascular disease, a tenofovir-containing regimen, rather than an abacavir-containing regimen, should be used if possible.	AIa
Dolutegravir (Tivicay) *plus* emtricitabine/tenofovir alafenamide (Descovy)	In settings in which TAF/emtricitabine is not available or if there is a substantial cost difference, TDF (with emtricitabine or lamivudine) is effective and generally well tolerated, particularly if the patient does not have, or is not at high risk for, kidney or bone disease	AIa

Because of this, baseline resistance testing is recommended prior to initiation of ART. Treatment does not necessarily need to be delayed until results are available, as resistance testing can take several weeks to result. If treatment is initiated empirically, adjustments should be made promptly if resistance is discovered. Repeat resistance testing should be considered in the setting of treatment failure to help determine whether the patient's virus has developed resistance to the current regimen, or whether medication adherence, drug/drug interactions, absorption, or another issue is the reason for virologic failure.

Resistance testing can be performed in three major ways. The most common method is HIV-1 RNA genotyping. This involves direct sequencing of viral genes that encode the drug target proteins (i.e., reverse transcriptase, protease, and integrase). Genes are sequenced and compared to the wild-type genotype and previously determined resistance mutations. A second method for identifying resistance is by performing HIV-1 phenotype testing. This involves replication of the virus in culture when exposed to various antivirals. This provides a direct measure of viral resistance in vitro; growth would be expected to occur in the presence of a drug if the virus harbors resistance mutations to that agent. Finally, cellular-associated DNA genotyping allows for resistance testing even in the setting of patients with undetectable PVLs. This testing involves sequencing of archived HIV-1 proviral DNA that has been integrated into infected host cells during virus replication. The choice of a resistance test depends on the patient's viral load and the desired information.

In patients determined to have resistance, several resources are available to help choose a new regimen. The IAS-USA has developed a useful catalog of resistance mutations that is available online at https:// www.iasusa.org/resources/hiv-drug-resistance-mutations/. Stanford University also maintains an interactive web-based database of known HIV resistance mutations, which is also freely available online at https://hivdb.stanford.edu. Its interactive format allows the user to input specific mutations and it will generate a predicted susceptibility profile of all available drugs. Use of these resources and expert consultation with an HIV specialist experienced in treatment of resistant virus is recommended.

Future Directions of Antiretroviral Treatment

Current antiretroviral therapy has made leaps and bounds from the early regimens, which involved multiple drugs with high toxicity given multiple times per day. Today, most patients can be treated with a small number of pills—usually one—dosed once or twice a day. Still, treatment is advancing. Several new regimens are challenging the "triple-therapy" paradigm, including two-drug combinations that demonstrate noninferiority when compared to traditional three-drug first-line regimens. More are sure to come. A few other treatment options that are likely close on the horizon include the following:

1. **Injectable regimens:** Clinical trials of injectable therapy have been completed, showing high efficacy and patient acceptance of once-monthly injectable treatments. Some issues of concern with these regimens include the need for more frequent appointments, how to provide oral "bridge" therapy to patients missing an appointment, how to deal with adverse reactions of medications with long half-lives, and concern over the subtherapeutic tail that follows discontinuation of an injectable depot-type regimen. Even so, these regimens present an exciting new direction for therapy.

2. **Implantable slow-release medications:** Similar to implantable contraceptive devices, implantable antiretroviral-delivery devices offer an attractive approach to infrequent (once-monthly or even longer) dosing. The minor surgery needed for placement of the device is a concern, as is any complication of removal.

3. **Oral agents with longer half-lives:** Several oral agents are in development that might be able to be dosed once weekly or longer. As with injectable regimens, concerns remain about how to deal with adverse reactions of medications with long half-lives and the subtherapeutic tail that follows discontinuation.

4. **New drug classes:** Several new drug classes with novel mechanisms of action are in development and provide hope for patients with complex resistance patterns, patients who struggle with side effects of current regimens, and those seeking new delivery methods or dosing intervals. Classes currently in development include attachment inhibitors, nucleoside reverse transcriptase translocation inhibitors (NRTTIs), maturation inhibitors, monoclonal antibodies to CCR5, capsid inhibitors, and broadly neutralizing antibodies.

HIV CURE RESEARCH

Thus far, there have only been two documented cases of HIV cure. The first case, described as the "Berlin patient," was reported in 2009. He was a man with refractory AML who had HIV infection with a CCR5-tropic virus. He received two hematopoietic stem cell transplants, the second from a CCR5-negative donor. He also received total body irradiation and anti-thymocyte globulin. The second case, the "London patient," was reported in 2019. This patient had refractory Hodgkin's lymphoma and HIV with CCR5-tropic virus and received a stem cell transplant from a CCR5-negative donor. The patient did not receive irradiation, and T-cell depletion was achieved with an anti-CD52 agent. Both patients had mild graft-versus-host disease (GVHD). Both patients have had no recurrence of HIV viremia and no isolation of active virus from any tissue samples despite remaining off of antiretroviral therapy. These cases both illustrate extreme examples of potential routes to a cure—stem cell transplants carry a very high mortality, and GVHD is a lifelong disease that can have significant morbidity. However, the cases do demonstrate that the possibility of a cure is more than just theoretical, and ongoing studies for a cure to HIV is an area of intense research.

As a retrovirus, HIV integrates into the host genome, and latently infected cells are the primary reason that ART is not curative. All current ART targets viral proteins involved in viral replication; therefore, they are ineffective at removing the viral reservoir of latent disease, as the target viral proteins are not active in latently infected cells. Stopping ART always results in a recurrence of viremia over time in PLWH, as latent cells awaken and replication resumes. Thus the problem of finding a cure for HIV is largely a problem of determining how to cure latently infected cells. Further, currently ART is highly effective and very well tolerated, resulting in an essentially normal life expectancy. Ethically, the "cure" cannot be worse than treatment; this poses a high bar for researchers. A safe, effective, scalable, well-tolerated, and cost-effective intervention that is fully curative, or that allows for long-term viral control without the use of ART, is still many years away, but the groundwork has now been laid.

HIV PREVENTION, PEP AND PREP

Three broad approaches have had a major impact on reducing HIV transmission: harm reduction and behavioral modification, ART for "treatment as prevention," and the use of medications for pre- and postexposure prophylaxis. All of these activities are supported by expanded testing and improved linkage to care.

Harm reduction and behavior modification are broad categories of public health interventions to prevent HIV transmission. An example is the adoption of safer sexual practices, especially the use of condoms during sexual activity to prevent HIV transmission. Other interventions, such as those targeted toward people who inject drugs, including syringe exchange programs, safe injection facilities, and community methadone and buprenorphine programs, have also had a marked effect on reducing risk of HIV transmission. Many other approaches in the appropriate clinical and societal context can also have significant impact, such as male circumcision in highly impacted communities.

Treatment as prevention is the cornerstone of efforts to control the worldwide HIV epidemic, and widespread access to ART is a key goal of HIV prevention efforts today. Antiretroviral treatment of HIV-infected pregnant women and their infants in the peripartum period has decreased maternal-child transmission from 25% to less than 5% in North America. If a pregnant woman maintains viral suppression during pregnancy and during breast-feeding, the risk of transmission to her infant is less than 1%. Among sexually active individuals, a number of studies across thousands of individuals have demonstrated that patients who are on treatment and undetectable cannot transmit HIV to their sexual partners, regardless of condom use. The strength of these data are robust and results are consistent across multiple large studies in different populations across multiple countries, including in both heterosexual and MSM populations. In fact, none of the studies demonstrated a single case of transmission from an undetectable patient to their partner. The power of treatment as prevention has led to the popular educational campaign of "U=U" or "undetectable = untransmittable."

The use of ART has also been shown to be an effective tool for HIV prevention as postexposure prophylaxis after both occupational exposures to HIV (termed "PEP") and after unprotected sexual exposures (termed "nPEP"). Guidelines for PEP and nPEP recommend treatment as early as possible, within 72 hours at the most after an exposure. The treatment regimen should be based on the source patient's resistance pattern, if known, or if unknown, is generally with two NRTIs (tenofovir disoproxil fumarate and emtricitabine) and an integrase inhibitor (either raltegravir or dolutegravir) for 28 days. Occupational PEP is highly effective, and post exposure seroconversion of health care workers is virtually nonexistent since implementation of PEP. Guidelines for both PEP and nPEP are available through the CDC at: https://www.cdc.gov/hiv/risk/pep/index.html.

The use of ART for PrEP in HIV-negative individuals at high risk for HIV exposure has demonstrated excellent efficacy across multiple studies and populations. In individuals at high risk for sexual exposure, including MSM, individuals in serodiscordant relationships, sex workers, and individuals with multiple sexual partners, the daily use of either tenofovir disoproxil fumarate with emtricitabine (the combination tablet Truvada) or tenofovir alafenamide with emtricitabine (Descovy) has been shown to reduce risk of HIV transmission by 99% if taken with consistent adherence. PrEP has also been shown to be effective in people who inject drugs, with a 74% reduction with consistent daily use. Studies have been performed and others are ongoing to evaluate more risk-based, intermittent dosing. Additionally, studies are underway to look at other potential medications and delivery methods (e.g., injectable drugs, implantable devices).

Universal linkage, retention, and access to high-quality, culturally appropriate, and affordable HIV treatment should be the central goals of both HIV treatment and prevention, because effective treatment *is* effective prevention. Individuals should also be supported to protect themselves, and harm reduction techniques and behavior modification interventions play an ongoing important role in HIV prevention for at-risk populations, with both PEP and PrEP offering additional pharmacologic aids to the universal goal of bringing an end to new HIV infections.

SUGGESTED READINGS

Aberg JA, Gallant JE, Ghanem KG, et al: Primary care guidelines for the management of persons infected with HIV: 2013 update by the HIV Medicine Association of the Infectious Diseases Society of America, Clin Infect Dis 58:e1–34, 2014.

International Antiviral Society–USA: Antiretroviral Drugs for Treatment and Prevention of HIV Infection in Adults: 2018 Recommendations of the International Antiviral Society–USA Panel. Available at: https://www.iasusa.org/resources/guidelines/. Accessed January 2020.

International Antiviral Society–USA: HIV Drug Resistance Mutations. Available at: https://www.iasusa.org/resources/hiv-drug-resistance-mutations/. Accessed January 2020.

Stanford University: HIV Drug Resistance Database. Available at: https://hivdb.stanford.edu. Accessed January 2020.

U.S. Center for Disease Control and Prevention: Post-Exposure Prophylaxis. Available at: https://www.cdc.gov/hiv/risk/pep/index.html. Accessed January 2020.

U.S. Department of Health and Human Services: Guidelines for the Prevention and Treatment of Opportunistic Infections in Adults and Adolescents with HIV. Available at: https://aidsinfo.nih.gov/guidelines/html/4/adult-and-adolescent-opportunistic-infection/0. Accessed January 2020.

U.S. Department of Health and Human Services: Guidelines for the Use of Antiretroviral Agents in Adults and Adolescents with HIV. Available at: https://aidsinfo.nih.gov/guidelines. Accessed January 2020.

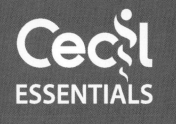

104

Infections in the Immunocompromised Host

Dimitrios Farmakiotis, Ralph Rogers

INTRODUCTION

Individuals with an impaired immune system are at risk for infections due to typical pathogens and less virulent organisms that usually do not cause illness. Diagnosis can be challenging due to atypical disease manifestations. The pace and severity of illness in tenuous patients demands that complicated treatment decisions are made early, despite lack of diagnostic certainty. This chapter aims to provide a clinically oriented framework for diagnosis and management of infections in immunocompromised hosts, excluding patients with HIV/AIDS (Figs. 104.1 and 104.2).

EPIDEMIOLOGY

The population of immunocompromised individuals is rapidly growing and becoming more diverse, including patients with primary (congenital) immunodeficiencies, some of which are newly recognized; individuals with hematologic malignancies (HM), who are now surviving longer; solid organ (SOT) and hematopoietic cell transplant (HCT) recipients; and finally, patients being treated with newly developed immunomodulatory medications (TNF-α inhibitors, monoclonal antibodies, ibrutinib) that expose more and more individuals to potential infectious complications.

PATHOGENESIS

Not all immunocompromised individuals are at equal risk for every possible infection. Instead, "immunocompromised hosts" are a heterogenous group, in which specific immune deficits come with distinct risks (see Fig. 104.1 and Tables 104.1 and 104.2).

Neutropenia

Neutrophils are the primary defense against bacterial and fungal infections. Neutropenia associated with increased risk for infection is defined as absolute neutrophil count less than 500/μL. Primary immunodeficiency syndromes such as congenital neutropenia (inadequate production), chronic granulomatous disease (ineffective microbial killing), and leukocyte adhesion deficiency (ineffective recruitment to sites of infection) are associated with increased number and severity of infections, usually caused by typical bacterial (e.g., *Staphylococcus*, *Streptococcus*, Enterobacteriaceae) and fungal (e.g., *Candida*) colonizers of skin, gastrointestinal, genitourinary, and respiratory tracts.

Neutropenia is common with HM, due to decreased neutrophil production from both bone marrow infiltration and cytotoxic chemotherapy. Cytotoxic chemotherapy acts primarily on rapidly dividing

cells, thus in addition to its desired effect it also has negative impact on the rapidly dividing cells of the gastrointestinal tract lining (mucositis). This decrease in an anatomic barrier in combination with decreased neutrophil defense can lead to rapidly progressive infections from microbial translocation. Therefore, "neutropenic fever" is a medical emergency, and such patients need prompt and broad antimicrobial therapy against typical enteric pathogens and *Pseudomonas* (which is associated with high mortality).

Cell-Mediated and Humoral Immune Deficits

The adaptive immune response provided by the cell-mediated and humoral components of the immune system allows for effective intracellular and extracellular microbial killing and is critical against viral infections, while also contributing to antibacterial and antifungal defenses. Many primary immunodeficiency syndromes affect cellular and humoral immunity, each causing increased susceptibility to various bacterial, fungal, and viral infections. Severe combined immunodeficiency (underdevelopment of both T cells and B cells) predisposes infants to serious infections from common viruses (e.g., Herpesviridae), bacteria, and fungi (e.g., *Pneumocystis*). DiGeorge syndrome (thymic hypoplasia leading to underdevelopment of T cells) and hyperimmunoglobulin-E syndrome (impaired T cell differentiation and function) predispose individuals to recurrent bacterial skin or sinopulmonary infections. X-linked agammaglobulinemia (underdevelopment of B cells) predisposes patients to bacterial infections with encapsulated organisms (pneumococcus, *Haemophilus influenza*, *Neisseria meningitidis*) and common viral pathogens (e.g., Enteroviridae). Secondary causes of hypogammaglobulinemia (e.g., chronic lymphocytic leukemia [CLL], protein-losing enteropathy, nephrotic syndrome) may also lead to increased risk for viral and bacterial infections.

Asplenia and Complement Deficits

Functional or anatomic asplenia leads to increased risk for severe infections due to encapsulated bacteria and blood-borne parasites (e.g., *Plasmodium*, *Babesia*) since the spleen is the primary site that filters out parasitized red blood cells. The complement system acts by opsonization of pathogens allowing for subsequent phagocytosis and can also act on its own to eliminate pathogens via the membrane attack complex. Complement deficiencies lead to an increased risk for infections due to encapsulated bacteria, especially *N. meningitidis*. They can be congenital or from eculizumab, a monoclonal antibody that is effective treatment for atypical hemolytic uremic syndrome by inhibiting terminal complement.

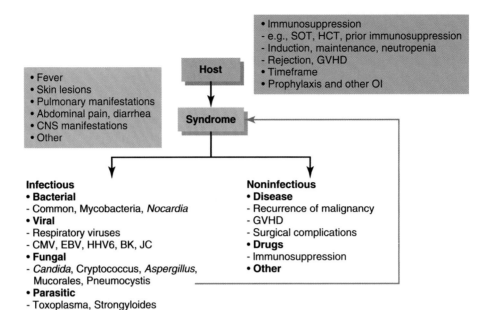

Fig. 104.1 Algorithmic approach to the diagnosis of syndromes suspicious for infection in the immuno-compromised host. Continuous reassessment is paramount. For a discussion of abbreviations and specific pathogens see "Specific Pathogens" section below.

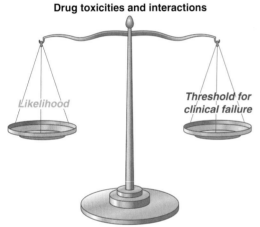

Fig. 104.2 Management decisions should be based on the balance between the likelihood of a diagnosis and the clinical consequences of not treating immediately, given the toxicities and drug-drug interactions of antimicrobials.

Hematologic Malignancies

Neutropenia is the main risk factor for infection in patients with acute leukemia. At the time of diagnosis, an individual may have already been neutropenic for an extended time and thus at risk for infection by environmental molds, such as *Aspergillus* or the Mucorales. After induction chemotherapy, patients stay profoundly neutropenic for several weeks, leading to increased risk for infection as outlined previously. Lymphoma patients usually do not experience extended periods of neutropenia from chemotherapy, which is, nonetheless, profoundly lymphocyte-depleting. Risk for infection sometimes depends on dosing (e.g., there is increased risk for *Pneumocystis* with R-CHOP-14, i.e., bi-weekly, due to more frequent administration of steroids). CLL is a chronic leukemia that is often monitored but not treated given its indolent course. However, these patients frequently have hypogammaglobulinemia and may be at increased risk for bacterial or viral sinopulmonary infections.

TABLE 104.1	**Primary Immunodeficiency Syndromes**
Syndrome	**Description**
Defects in Phagocytes	
Congenital neutropenia	Inadequate neutrophil production
Chronic granulomatous disease	Ineffective microbial killing by phagocytes due to decreased NADPH oxidase activity
Leukocyte adhesion deficiency	Ineffective recruitment of phagocytes to sites of infection
Defects in Cellular and Humoral Immunity	
Severe combined immunodeficiency	T- and/or B-cell deficiency or absence
ZAP-70 deficiency	Defects in T-cell proliferation and activation
DiGeorge syndrome	Thymic hypoplasia leading to defects in T-cell maturation
Idiopathic CD4 lymphopenia	Inadequate CD4+ T-cell production
Hyper-IgE syndrome	Defect in JAK/STAT signaling pathway leading to multiple immune deficits
Hyper-IgM syndrome	Defect in class-switch recombination leading to inadequate IgG/IgA/IgE production
X-linked agammaglobulinemia	Defect in B-cell maturation leading to decreased or absent immunoglobulin production
Common variable immunodeficiency	Defective immunoglobulin production
Defects in Innate Immunity	
NK cell deficiency	Absent or defective NK cells
Complement deficiencies	Absent or defective complement components

Solid Organ Transplantation

SOT is a life-saving procedure, but unless the transplanted organ (allograft) is coming from the recipient's identical twin, the transplant recipient must take immunosuppressive medications in order to prevent their immune system from rejecting the allograft as "nonself."

TABLE 104.2 Immunosuppressive Medications

Class	Examples
Cytotoxic agents	Bleomycin
	Cisplatin
	Cyclophosphamide
	Cytarabine
	Doxorubicin
	Etoposide
	Fluorouracil
	Methotrexate
	Paclitaxel
	Vincristine
Lymphocyte depleting agents	Alemtuzumab
	Anti-thymocyte globulin
	Basiliximab
	Belatacept
	Rituximab
TNF-α inhibitors	Adalimumab
	Etanercept
	Infliximab
Corticosteroids	Prednisone
Common antirejection medications	Azathioprine
	Cyclosporine
	Mycophenolate
	Sirolimus
	Tacrolimus
Other monoclonal antibodies and signal transduction inhibitors associated with increased risk for infection	Eculizumab
	Ibrutinib
	Idelalisib
	Natalizumab
	Ruxolitinib
	Tocilizumab

TABLE 104.3 Infections After Solid Organ Transplantation

Risk Category	Examples
Early Infections	
Anatomic disruption	Anastomotic leak
	Surgical site infection
Donor derived	Bacterial: *Mycobacterium tuberculosis*
	Fungal: *Aspergillus*
	Viral: CMV, EBV, HBV, HCV, HIV, HSV, LCMV, VZV
	Parasite: *Toxoplasma*
Hospital acquired	Catheter-related infection
	Clostridioides difficile colitis
	Ventilator-associated pneumonia
Middle Infections	
Reactivation of latent pathogens	Bacterial: *M. tuberculosis*
	Fungal: *Candida*
	Viral: BKPyV, CMV, HBV, HCV, HSV, VZV
	Parasite: *Strongyloides, Toxoplasma*
Opportunistic infections	Bacterial: *Nocardia*
	Fungal: *Aspergillus, Pneumocystis*
	Parasite: *Microsporidia*
Late Infections	
Community acquired	Pneumonia
	Urinary tract infection
Post-prophylaxis reactivation	CMV
	HSV
	VZV

SOT recipients are given potent immunosuppressive medications to prevent acute rejection at the time of their transplant (induction) and thereafter stay on two to three immunosuppressants (maintenance). The risks for specific types of infection differ, depending on the time since transplantation (Table 104.3). Infections early on are related to the transplant surgery itself (anastomotic leak, surgical site infection) or are hospital acquired (catheter infection, *C. difficile colitis*); early infections can also be donor derived (i.e., present in the donor at the time of transplant, then transferred to the recipient with the allograft). Infections in the "middle period" are often due to reactivation of pre-existing latent infections (CMV, hepatitis B or C, *Toxoplasma*) or to opportunistic pathogens (*Pneumocystis, Aspergillus*). Late infections are usually community acquired (e.g., pneumonia) and organ specific (recurrent urinary tract infections in kidney transplant recipients, cholangitis in liver transplant recipients, late aspergillosis in lung transplant recipients). Augmented immunosuppression for rejection increases the risk for infection. So does "immunosenescence," and elderly SOT recipients sometimes present with opportunistic infections many years after transplantation.

Hematopoietic Cell Transplantation

Hematopoietic (stem) cell transplantation (HCT) involves replacing the bone marrow and immune system with a new, healthier one. This life-saving procedure is associated with many infectious and noninfectious post-transplantation complications. HCT recipients are given high doses of cytotoxic medications and/or radiation therapy to destroy their old immune system (conditioning) and thus are at risk for many infections while waiting for their new hematopoietic cells to populate the bone marrow and begin functioning (engraftment). A common complication after HCT is graft-versus-host disease (GVHD), where the donor immune system recognizes recipient organs (mostly the skin and gastrointestinal tract) as "nonself" and mounts a potentially devastating immune response. Additional immunosuppressive medications are given to prevent or treat GVHD, adding to the risk for infection. Further, GVHD is itself an immunosuppressive condition given that it acts to slow immune expansion after HCT.

As in individuals receiving SOT, risks for specific types of infection differ depending on the time since transplantation and presence of GVHD (Table 104.4). Early on, infections are related to profound neutropenia and mucositis from the conditioning regimen. Functional neutrophils are newly present after engraftment, but other arms of adaptive and innate immunity are slowly reconstituted thereafter, first NK-cells, then CD8+ T cells, and finally B cells and CD4+ T cells, sometimes years later. This process can be delayed by both GVHD and immunosuppressive medications for it (see Table 104.4).

Novel Immunomodulatory Medications

The number and variety of immunomodulatory medications has dramatically increased in recent years, leading to newly recognized syndromes. Examples are invasive fungal infections with ibrutinib (a tyrosine kinase inhibitor used to treat lymphoid malignancies),

TABLE 104.4   Infections After Hematopoietic Cell Transplant

Risk Category	Examples
Pre-engraftment	
Neutropenia	Bacterial: skin/GI/GU flora
Mucositis	Fungal: *Candida, Aspergillus*
	Viral: HSV, VZV
Hospital acquired	Catheter-related infection
	Clostridioides difficile colitis
	Ventilator-associated pneumonia
Early Post-engraftment	
Reactivation of latent pathogens	Bacterial: *Mycobacterium tuberculosis*
	Fungal: *Candida*
	Viral: adenovirus, BKPyV, CMV, HBV, HCV, HHV-6, HHV-8, HSV, JCPyV, VZV
	Parasite: *Strongyloides, Toxoplasma*
Opportunistic infections	Bacterial: *Nocardia*
	Fungal: *Aspergillus, Mucorales, Pneumocystis*
	Parasite: *Microsporidia*
Late Post-engraftment	
Community acquired	Pneumonia
	Sinusitis
	Urinary tract infection
Post-prophylaxis reactivation	CMV
	HSV
	VZV

progressive multifocal encephalopathy (PML) with natalizumab (selective adhesion molecule inhibitor used to treat multiple sclerosis), hepatitis B reactivation or rituximab (anti-CD20+ monoclonal antibody used for treatment of B-cell lymphomas), and mycobacterial infections and histoplasmosis with TNF-α inhibitors (see Table 104.2).

CLINICAL PRESENTATION

Central Nervous System Infection

Headache, neck stiffness, photophobia, encephalopathy, or new focal neurologic deficits, with or without fever, may be indicative of central nervous system (CNS) infection. Clinical symptoms of meningitis and cerebrospinal fluid (CSF) pleocytosis may be dampened in the setting of immunosuppression. In addition to typical pathogens (pneumococcus, enterovirus, herpes simplex virus [HSV]), one should consider other bacterial (*Listeria, Nocardia*), viral (e.g., arbovirus, astrovirus, CMV, Epstein-Barr virus [EBV], lymphocytic choriomeningitis [LCMV], varicella zoster virus [VZV]), fungal (e.g., *Cryptococcus*), and parasitic (*Toxoplasma*) etiologies. CNS infection can be part of a systemic syndrome, and dysfunction of other organs may give a clue to the etiology (e.g., severe pneumonia with adenovirus meningitis, *Nocardia* lung nodules). CNS imaging is paramount and can aid in diagnosis (e.g., multiple ring-enhancing lesions with *Toxoplasma* encephalitis, multifocal white matter changes with PML [Fig. 104.3]).

Pneumonia

Although fever and productive cough are the hallmark sign and symptom of pneumonia, both may be muted in immunocompromised hosts. Alternatively, pneumonia may be rapidly progressive and fulminant.

Beyond typical bacterial and viral etiologies, pneumonia in immunocompromised patients can be caused by atypical bacterial (*Legionella, Nocardia, Mycobacterium tuberculosis* or nontuberculous mycobacteria), viral (adenovirus, CMV, HSV, VZV), fungal (*Aspergillus, Cryptococcus*, dimorphic fungi, non-*Aspergillus* molds, *Pneumocystis*), and parasitic (*Toxoplasma, Strongyloides* hyperinfection) etiologies. Associated nonpulmonary manifestations (e.g., cryptococcal meningitis) can help make the diagnosis. Computed tomography (CT) and bronchoscopy are often necessary to better define the infectious process.

Diarrhea

Clinicians should consider bacterial (*Clostridioides difficile, Salmonella*), viral (adenovirus, CMV, enterovirus, norovirus), and parasitic (*Cryptosporidium, Giardia*) etiologies. Stool PCR panels can be useful but sometimes cannot differentiate between colonization and infection for some organisms, such as enteropathogenic *E. coli*. A careful exposure history can help narrow the possible diagnoses, especially for infections with regional endemicity. Colonoscopy with tissue biopsy may be necessary to make a definite diagnosis. At our institution, multiplex PCR, *C. difficile* toxin in the stool, and CMV viral load in the blood are standard protocol for SOT recipients with diarrhea. Leading noninfectious causes are medications, especially mycophenolate (an antimetabolite used for maintenance immunosuppression), and GVHD.

Skin Manifestations

Skin lesions in the immunocompromised patient can be a sign of localized ("outside-in") or disseminated ("inside-out") infection. Necrotic lesions raise concern for angioinvasive mold, although they can also be seen with severe bacterial infections and neutropenia, due to toxin effect with minimal inflammation. The most classic lesion is ecthyma gangrenosum, a painful eschar in neutropenic sepsis caused by *Pseudomonas*, but also other gram-negative or gram-positive (*S. aureus*) bacteria. Disseminated candidiasis can present with diffuse maculopapular rash and *Fusarium* sepsis with painful nodules. Vesicular lesions always raise concern for herpetic infection, although HSV (especially resistant or HSV2) can also cause large ulcerated lesions. "Sporotrichoid lesions" (cordlike clusters of inflammatory nodules) can be due to *Sporothrix, S. aureus, Nocardia* or atypical mycobacteria. Noninfectious causes are very common, such as drug rash, primary skin cancer (the most common malignancy after SOT), skin metastases and leukemia cutis, GVHD, neutrophilic eccrine hidradenitis, and Sweet syndrome (febrile neutrophilic dermatosis, an inflammatory reaction to tumors and chemotherapy that is best treated with corticosteroids). For accurate diagnosis, a skin biopsy with cultures is often necessary.

Fever of Unknown Origin

Persistent fever in an immunocompromised host without a clear etiology or any focal signs or symptoms is a relatively common clinical scenario. History and physical examination will often reveal subtle signs or symptoms integral to steering further diagnostic efforts. Careful attention to the mouth (Fig. 104.4), skin, and perineal area is imperative, because each may provide easily overlooked clues. Perineal infection can manifest with rectal pain alone. Beyond typical screening studies such as blood and urine cultures and a chest radiograph, an algorithmic approach to further investigation may involve stepwise additional testing including fungal markers, PCR-based testing for viruses (CMV, EBV, HHV-6), and cross-sectional imaging of the chest, abdomen, and pelvis. Advanced laboratory tests (e.g., cell-free DNA sequencing, an emerging technology that detects and identifies nonhuman DNA fragments in a clinical sample) and

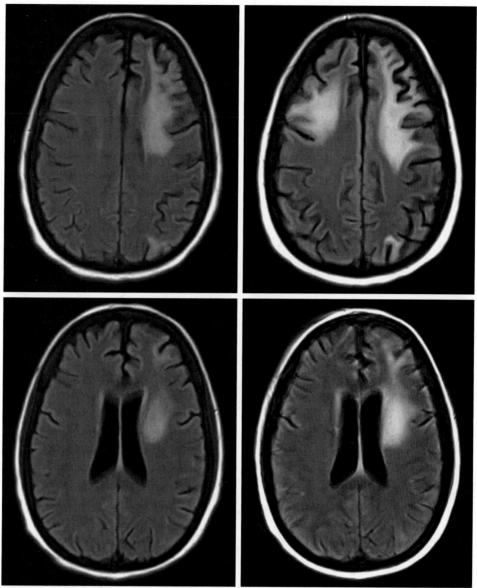

Fig. 104.3 Progressive multifocal encephalopathy (PML) in an immunocompromised patient with severe combined immunodeficiency (SCID) and autoimmune hemolytic anemia requiring many cycles of rituximab and high-dose corticosteroids. MRI shows significant progression of white matter abnormalities after 3 months.

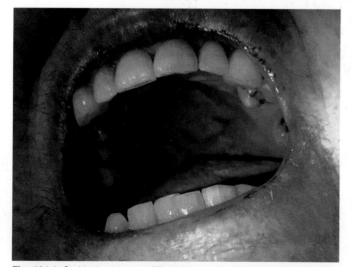

Fig. 104.4 Oral lesions in an HCT recipient with GVHD on high-dose steroids who developed disseminated HSV1 infection with fulminant hepatitis.

imaging studies (positron emission tomography-PET) may be useful adjuncts depending on the clinical scenario.

DIAGNOSIS

The pace and breadth of diagnostic testing is best driven by the pace and severity of a patient's underlying illness. Although there is a vast number of potential pathogens that may be the cause of an individual's presenting illness, the history the patient gives along with their physical examination is usually enough to dramatically narrow the differential diagnosis. Although most patients present with a single unifying diagnosis, it is not uncommon for immunocompromised patients to present with multiple ongoing processes. Therefore, we favor a structured approach, frequently revisiting the initial or new clinical manifestations (see Fig. 104.1).

Host Considerations

First, one should understand the host, mainly the immune deficits specific to the individual patient: How long has the patient been neutropenic and what potential pathogens has the patient been exposed to while neutropenic? How long has it been since SOT and what is the immunosuppression? For HCT recipients, are they pre- or post-engraftment, do they have GVHD, and what immunosuppressive medications are they on? What prophylactic antimicrobials are they taking, and for how long? What previous chemotherapy have they received? Previous and concomitant opportunistic infections often speak for the host.

Syndrome Considerations

Next, one identifies the syndrome using presenting complaints. Often there is a single clinical syndrome such as pneumonia or diarrhea. At other times, the signs and symptoms are less focal, and instead the presenting syndrome may simply be fever and fatigue; more than one clinical syndrome can be present. One structured way to construct a broad differential diagnosis for the host and the syndrome is to first consider infectious versus noninfectious causes and then build a differential diagnosis by pathogen kingdom (bacterial, fungal, viral, parasitic) and noninfectious causes (underlying disease, GVHD, medication toxicities, unusual causes) (see Fig. 104.1).

Laboratory Testing

In immunocompromised hosts, direct tests for pathogens (antigen or PCR-based testing) are much more useful than antibody assays, which mainly indicate past exposure, and because the measured immune response may be absent. Fungal markers are components of the fungal cell wall that can be detected in blood or other body fluids and help make the diagnosis of fungal infections. The most commonly used are serum and CSF cryptococcal antigen, serum, bronchoalveolar lavage (BAL) or CSF *Aspergillus* galactomannan, and serum or CSF 1,3-β-D-glucan, which is a broad fungal marker that can aid in the diagnosis of invasive aspergillosis, candidiasis, and pneumocystis pneumonia. However, fungal markers can be falsely elevated (e.g., false-positive 1,3-β-D-glucan in patients receiving hemodialysis or intravenous immunoglobulin [IVIG]) and should be interpreted in context. Peripheral blood cultures (including standard bacterial cultures and those facilitating growth of acid-fast bacilli and fungi) and cultures from more invasive procedures (BAL) may provide a diagnosis and also give a measure of antimicrobial susceptibility. Invasive tissue biopsy may at times be necessary for a definitive diagnosis and to help differentiate between colonization and infection.

Diagnostic Imaging

Imaging studies are also important in the diagnostic process. As with laboratory testing, the lack of inflammation can lead to misleading imaging findings (e.g., relatively normal abdominal imaging despite ongoing acalculous cholecystitis). Some findings can be suggestive of specific diagnoses when interpreted in the context of a specific syndrome in an at-risk immunocompromised host (e.g., the halo sign [ground-glass opacities surrounding a pulmonary nodule] suggestive of invasive pulmonary aspergillosis [Fig. 104.5] versus the reversed halo sign [ground-glass opacity surrounded by a ring of consolidation] suggestive of mucormycosis).

TREATMENT

General Principles

Choosing an appropriate empiric treatment regimen for an immunocompromised patient can be challenging. Waiting for test results may not be wise given the potentially rapid progression of infection in this population. Medication toxicities and drug-drug interactions

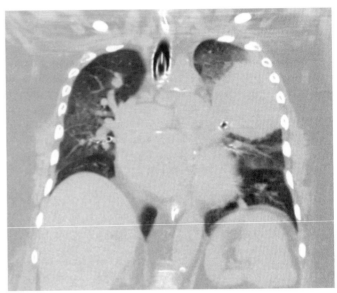

Fig. 104.5 Invasive aspergillosis in a patient receiving high-dose corticosteroids. Chest CT shows dense consolidation and surrounding "halo sign" (i.e., hazy, ground-glass-like opacities surrounding a nodule or mass), which represents hemorrhage and is typically seen in invasive aspergillosis. Blood and BAL cultures grew *A. fumigatus*; the value of *Aspergillus* antigen (galactomannan) in the blood was great than the assay cut off.

(DDI) are often a determining factor in the clinical outcome. Early and aggressive treatment is often necessary, though given the breadth of potential infectious etiologies, treating every possible pathogen is not feasible. Instead, when considering empiric treatment, the unlikeliness of a specific diagnosis should be balanced against the potential consequences of not treating. As a rule, broad coverage is in order while the patient's clinical presentation is unfolding, with de-escalation of therapy to prevent toxicities after further diagnoses are ruled out and as the patient improves (see Fig. 104.2).

Source Control

Control of the source of infection is imperative. In immunosuppressed patients, antimicrobials alone are often insufficient to combat infection. Given the diminished clinical reserve and lack of expected immune response, an undrained abscess or an infection due to a biofilm-forming agent on a blood stream or unremoved intravascular catheter or urinary catheter can be devastating.

Adjusting Immunosuppression

Reducing immunosuppression can be life-saving. With neutropenia in particular, granulocyte colony-stimulating factor (G-CSF) administration can help early ANC recovery. In SOT, acute rejection can develop after reducing immunosuppression, but it is very unusual to have simultaneous acute rejection and overwhelming infection given the polarization of an already impaired immune system towards fighting infection. There is also the possibility of developing immune reconstitution inflammatory syndrome (IRIS) (i.e., increased inflammation from reduction of immunosuppression), which often needs to be treated with corticosteroids. Further, some immunosuppressive medications have desirable adjuvant properties (e.g., antifungal effect of calcineurin inhibitors [CNI]). Specifically, in cryptococcal infections, CNI discontinuation leads to increased risk for IRIS and unfavorable outcomes. Immunosuppression adjustments are thus individualized. Reinstitution of immunosuppressive therapy may be indicated as infection resolves.

Drug-Drug Interactions

It is imperative to check for DDI with immunosuppressive or other medications every time any antimicrobial is started and stopped (see Fig. 104.2). For instance, triazole antifungal medications predictably increase the serum concentration of CNI (via triazole-mediated inhibition of their metabolism by cytochrome P-450), and thus empiric dose adjustments of CNI are usually indicated when stopping or starting a triazole.

PREVENTION

Lifestyle Precautions

While in the hospital, neutropenic patients often have specific measures in place to reduce the risk of acquisition of new infections by ingestion (bottled water, avoidance of foods with potential for bacterial or fungal colonization), inhalation (air filtration and positive pressure ventilation, no flowers or plants, avoidance of nearby heavy construction or remodeling activities), or mucosal translocation (avoidance of hard food that can cause oral trauma). Many of these commonsense precautions can also be implemented at home. For immunocompromised patients, close contact with other individuals with viral infection should be avoided, and thorough evaluations before travel are advised.

Immunizations

The best time to give immunizations is prior to the onset of immunosuppression, which allows for the most robust immune response. Otherwise, most vaccines are administered 1 year post-transplant. Live vaccines are generally contraindicated in immunocompromised individuals, out of concern for clinical illness caused by the vaccine strain. Immunization of household contacts and health care workers is mandated.

Antimicrobial Prophylaxis

At many centers, individuals with acute leukemia undergoing induction chemotherapy and patients receiving HCT are given a fluoroquinolone (levofloxacin) and a yeast-only (fluconazole) or mold-active (voriconazole, posaconazole) triazole. Antiviral prophylaxis with acyclovir protects against reactivation of latent herpesviruses (e.g., HSV, VZV).

Fluconazole is used sometimes in liver transplant recipients and anti-*Aspergillus* prophylaxis in lung transplant recipients. Antiviral prophylaxis active against CMV ([val]ganciclovir) is given to many SOT patients. Given the potential myelotoxicity of (val)ganciclovir, alternative strategies are used to prevent CMV infection in HCT (close monitoring of viral load or alternative antivirals such as letermovir). Prophylaxis against *Pneumocystis* is indicated in SOT and HCT recipients for 6 to 12 months after transplant and in patients receiving prolonged high-dose corticosteroids. Some HCT recipients with severe GVHD receive antibacterial prophylaxis active against encapsulated bacteria and antifungal prophylaxis.

SPECIFIC PATHOGENS

HSV and VZV

HSV1/2 cause mainly mucocutaneous disease (oral or genital lesions), but in immunocompromised patients they can more frequently disseminate, cause CNS infection, multiorgan failure, predominantly fulminant hepatitis, and protean manifestations (e.g., pneumonia) (see Fig. 104.4). VZV can also cause disseminated disease and various CNS syndromes, including vasculitis. The treatment of choice for severe infections is intravenous acyclovir. (Val)acyclovir and (val)ganciclovir are effective prophylaxis; (val)acyclovir administration in very immunosuppressed patients can lead to resistance, mostly in HSV1. Resistant herpetic infections are treated with foscarnet.

CMV

Similar to other herpesviruses, CMV remains dormant after primary infection and can reactivate, causing disease. The highest-risk patients are SOT recipients who are not immune to CMV and receive it from the donor (D+/R−), as well as lymphocyte-depleted and D−/R+ HCT recipients (because they adopt the immune system of their donor). CMV causes fever and infectious mononucleosis-like symptoms and signs, gastrointestinal disease (esophagitis, gastritis, colitis) and pneumonia (mostly in lung and HC transplant recipients). Retinitis is rare in HIV-negative patients. Treatment of choice is (val)ganciclovir and foscarnet for resistant CMV. Multidrug-resistant CMV is rare but an emerging threat. Prophylaxis with (val)ganciclovir is used in most SOT recipients for the first few months after transplant. The main toxicity of (val)ganciclovir is bone marrow suppression, whereas foscarnet can cause nephrotoxicity and electrolyte abnormalities.

Other Herpesviruses

EBV can manifest as lytic infection (directly caused by proliferating virus, such as infectious mononucleosis or CNS infection). However, it is mainly associated with post-transplant lymphoproliferative disorder (PTLD) (progressive transformation of EBV-infected B-lymphocytes to lymphoma). Treatment is reduction of immunosuppression to allow for cytotoxic T-cell surveillance of the abnormal EBV-infected B cells. For the same reason, rituximab is often used early on, even preemptively with rising EBV viremia in HCT recipients.

Other pathogenic human herpesviruses include HHV-6, which typically causes CNS infection in HCT recipients (PALE: Post-transplant acute limbic encephalopathy) treated with ganciclovir or foscarnet, and HHV-8, which causes Kaposi's sarcoma.

Polyomaviruses

In addition to patients with AIDS, JC virus causes PML in a variety of hosts (SOT, HCT recipients, and patients with HM) (see Fig. 104.3). PML manifests with progressive cognitive decline, focal neurologic deficits, and characteristic MRI findings; it overall has poor prognosis. BK virus causes renal allograft dysfunction in kidney transplant recipients, hemorrhagic cystitis in HCT or (less commonly) other severely T-cell depleted individuals; BK can rarely cause PML and disseminated infection. The cornerstone of management for polyomavirus infections is decrease in immunosuppression. A promising recent approach to the management of PML and other refractory viral infections is infusion of virus-specific active T cells (adoptive immunity).

As a rule, laboratory diagnosis of viral infections in immunocompromised patients is based on detection of the virus by quantitative PCR and, sometimes, histopathology.

Candida

Candida albicans is the most common fungal pathogen in the Western world and an important commensal of the normal skin, oral, gastrointestinal, and vaginal flora. Non-albicans *Candida* species can be resistant to antifungal drugs, therefore an important threat with rising frequency in patients receiving antifungal prophylaxis. *Candida auris* has recently emerged as the first virulent fungus that exhibits multidrug resistance and the potential for nosocomial transmission, which is considered a public health emergency.

Candida species cause mucocutaneous (dermatitis, thrush, esophagitis or vaginitis) and invasive candidiasis. Neutropenia, corticosteroids, and abdominal pathology are the main risk factors. Indwelling catheters are an important source of candidemia, given the strong propensity of this organism to form biofilms (Fig. 104.6). Therefore, central line removal is strongly advised for the successful management of candidemia. Echinocandins (caspo/mica/anidulafungin) are the treatment of choice for severe invasive candidiasis, except for urinary, eye or CNS infections given their poor penetration in these compartments. Amphotericin-B and azoles have activity against most *Candida* species; the latter can be used for mild infections and as step-down oral therapy.

Cryptococcus

Cryptococcus can cause meningitis, encephalitis, pneumonia, sepsis-like syndrome, and atypical infections (such as cellulitis) in patients with significant T-cell immunosuppression (SOT or HCT recipients, lymphoma patients). Diagnosis is made by culture, detection of cryptococcal antigen in blood or CSF, and histopathology. Severe infections, including meningitis, are treated with amphotericin-B and flucytosine, followed by many months of fluconazole. Decrease in immunosuppression without discontinuation of CNI should be individualized. Fluconazole and other azoles, often used as antifungal prophylaxis in immunosuppressed patients, decrease the risk for cryptococcosis.

Aspergillus

Unlike *Candida*, molds such as *Aspergillus* and the Mucorales are not part of normal flora but inhaled from the environment. In the setting of impaired immune (especially neutrophil) defenses, they grow and invade tissues, causing invasive sinopulmonary or even disseminated mold infections. Individuals with prolonged neutropenia, those receiving high-dose corticosteroids, and lung

transplant recipients are the highest risk groups, especially with exposure to high inocula (e.g., construction). *Aspergillus* can often be a colonizer (saprophytic aspergillosis), without causing invasive disease, such as in the absence of radiographic abnormalities, or as an isolated aspergilloma (Fig. 104.7). Fungal markers (*Aspergillus* galactomannan, 1,3-β-D-glucan), with careful review of imaging findings (see Fig. 104.5), host factors, and clinical presentation, can help differentiate between colonization and infection.

An interesting entity at the intersection of saprophytic and invasive disease is chronic necrotizing (also known as cavitary or semi-invasive) aspergillosis. It affects "immunomodulated" patients, such as elderly patients with chronic obstructive pulmonary disease (COPD), often with negative fungal markers but positive anti-*Aspergillus* antibodies, and warrants antifungal treatment (Fig. 104.8).

The treatment for the majority of aspergilloses is voriconazole, with close follow-up of drug levels and dose adjustments of other medications that have significant DDI. Alternative agents include isavuconazole, amphotericin, or the echinocandins; the latter are static and not preferred as monotherapy.

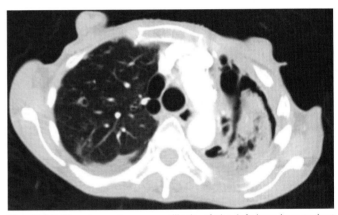

Fig. 104.8 Chronic cavitary aspergillosis of the left lung in a patient with severe COPD. *A. fumigatus* antibodies were positive, galactomannan negative, BAL cultures grew *A. fumigatus*. The lesions on CT progressed over months.

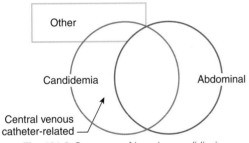

Fig. 104.6 Spectrum of invasive candidiasis.

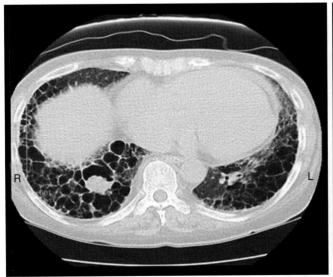
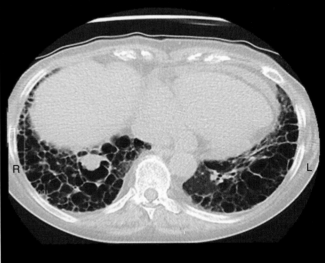

Fig. 104.7 Aspergilloma (saprophytic aspergillosis) in a patient with emphysema. Chest CT shows a mobile mass (*Left:* supine, *right:* prone) within a small cavity.

Mucorales and Other Fungi

Clinical syndromes caused by molds of the order Mucorales (e.g., *Rhizopus, Mucor, Rhizomucor, Cunninghamella, Lichtheimia,* and *Apophysomyces* spp) are rare, aggressive infections with the potential for rapid progression and high mortality. The most common manifestations are sinus and pulmonary infections in neutropenic patients, those receiving high-dose corticosteroids, diabetics, and even immunocompetent individuals when there is high inoculum exposure (e.g., in natural disasters and trauma with significant soil inhalation or contamination of deep wounds). These organisms are highly angioinvasive, and necrotic tissue is an important clue on physical exam. The "reversed halo" sign on CT is considered suggestive of pulmonary mucormycosis. The Mucorales do not have significant amounts of 1,3-β-D-glucan or galactomannan, therefore fungal markers will typically be negative. In vitro culture can be challenging. Therefore, the diagnosis of mucormycoses is elusive and often made by tissue histopathology with visualization of aseptate, broad-angled hyphae. In contrast, *Aspergillus* hyphae are narrow branching at 45° angles and septate (Fig. 104.9). Surgical débridement, when possible, and timely initiation of appropriate treatment with amphotericin-B are paramount. Posaconazole and isavuconazole have activity against the Mucorales, but voriconazole and the echinocandins do not.

Immunocompromised patients are at risk for endemic infections from dimorphic fungi (histoplasmosis, blastomycosis, and coccidiomycosis); preemptive testing and/or prophylaxis might be indicated in certain geographic areas. Histoplasmosis in particular has been associated with TNF-α inhibition.

Pneumocystis infection can manifest as typical interstitial or focal ("granulomatous") pneumonia, almost exclusively in patients not receiving prophylaxis. Treatment is similar to patients with AIDS (first line: trimethoprim/sulfamethoxazole [TMP/SMX]).

Microsporidia, now classified as fungi, can cause diarrhea, CNS, and multiorgan infections (including donor-derived outbreaks), for which albendazole is the treatment of choice.

Nocardia

Nocardia species are abundant in soil and cause subacute pulmonary, CNS or skin infections in patients with impaired cellular immunity, mainly SOT/HCT recipients and those on high-dose corticosteroids. Most species are sensitive to TMP/SMX. Initial combination of at least two antibiotics (TMP/SMX with a carbapenem, linezolid or minocycline)

is usually indicated given distinct susceptibilities of different *Nocardia* species. Targeted treatment should be continued for many months.

Mycobacteria

Individuals with latent tuberculosis (LTB) are at high risk for reactivation after TNF-α inhibition or T-cell immunosuppression, such as SOT/HCT. In immunosuppressed patients, active TB is often disseminated and its treatment challenging due to medication toxicities and DDI. Therefore, candidates for SOT, HCT, or TNF-α inhibitors are tested for LTB by protocol and if positive treated with isoniazid or an alternative regimen, prior to or shortly after onset of immunosuppression.

Atypical (nontuberculous) mycobacteria (NTM) cause diverse clinical syndromes, mainly pulmonary, skin, and catheter-related infections. The immune deficits predisposing to such infections are similar to TB. NTM are frequent colonizers of the respiratory tract. Treatment regimens are often complicated, with multiple toxicities and DDI; therefore, it is important to differentiate infection from colonization and treat, when indicated, in a timely manner, especially lung transplant candidates and recipients.

Parasites

Immunocompromised patients (especially heart transplant recipients) are at risk for donor-derived or reactivation of toxoplasmosis. TMP/SMX is effective prophylaxis. Toxoplasmosis can manifest as CNS lesions, pneumonia, or fever of unknown origin (FUO) and severe sepsis, the latter mainly in HCT recipients who are not on prophylaxis prior to engraftment, given concern for bone marrow suppression from TMP/SMX. Sulfamethoxazole with pyrimethamine or high-dose TMP/SMX are effective treatments.

Strongyloides hyperinfection is rare but devastating and can be recipient- or donor-derived. It develops usually weeks after onset of T-cell immunosuppression (e.g., transplant, high-dose steroids) with diarrhea, and, as the larvae translocate from the bowel and disseminate to different organs, ileus, pulmonary infiltrates, skin lesions, and gram-negative sepsis from intestinal bacterial co-translocation. Diagnosis is made by visualization of *Strongyloides* larvae in the stool, BAL or tissue. The treatment for hyperinfection is oral or parenteral veterinary ivermectin for days. Mortality is very high. Transplant candidates and donors from endemic areas are typically screened by serology (antibody) and, if positive, receive 1 to 2 days of ivermectin.

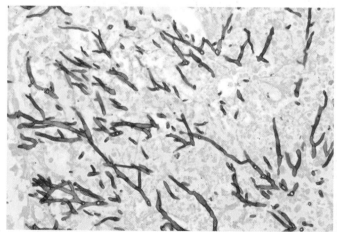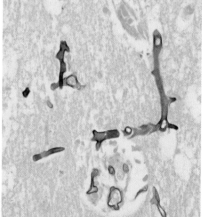

Fig. 104.9 *Aspergillus* (*left*: narrow-angled, septate) and *Lichtheimia* (*right*: wide-angled, aseptate) hyphae on Gomori-methenamine silver (GMS) stains of lung and heart tissue, respectively, from the autopsy of a patient with CLL on high-dose steroids. In immunocompromised patients, Ockham's razor doesn't always apply and multiple infections can coexist. (Tsikala-Vafea M, Weibiao C, Olszewski AJ, et al. Fatal mucormycosis and aspergillosis in an atypical host: What do we know about mixed invasive mold infections? Case Rep Infect Dis 2020:8812528, 2020.)

Intestinal parasites *(Giardia lamblia, Entamoeba histolytica, Cryptosporidium parvum)* can cause acute or chronic diarrhea in immunocompromised patients. *Giardia* in particular affects patients with IgA deficiency. Free-living amoebas can cause severe meningoencephalitis with almost 100% mortality.

SUGGESTED READINGS

Bousfiha A, Jeddane L, Picard C, et al: The 2017 IUIS phenotypic classification for primary immunodeficiencies, J Clin Immunol (38):129–143, 2018.

Denning DW, Cadranel J, Beigelman-Aubry C, et al: Chronic pulmonary aspergillosis: rationale and clinical guidelines for diagnosis and management, Eur Respir J 47(1):45–68, 2016.

ESCMID Study Group for Infections in Compromised Hosts (ESGICH) Consensus Document on the safety of targeted and biologic therapies: an infectious diseases perspective, Clin Microbiol Infect (24), 2018, Supplement 2.

Farmakiotis D, Kontoyiannis DP: Emerging issues with diagnosis and management of fungal infections in solid organ transplant recipients, Am J Transplant 15(5):1141–1147, 2015.

Farmakiotis D, Ross J, Koo S: Chapter 201: Candida and Aspergillus. In McKean SC, Ross JJ, Dressler DD, Scheurer DB, editors: Principles and practice of hospital medicine, ed 2, McGraw-Hill, 2017, pp 1618–1624.

GarciaCadenas I, Rivera I, Martino R, et al: Patterns of infection and infection-related mortality in patients with steroid-refractory acute graft versus host disease, Bone Marrow Transplant 52(1):107–113, 2017.

Guidelines from the American Society of Transplantation Infectious Diseases Community of Practice, Clin Transplant, 2019.

Li X, Jevnikar A: Transplant immunology, West Sussex, 2016, John Wiley & Sons.

Mehta H, Malandra M, Corey S: G-CSF and GM-CSF in neutropenia, J Immunol 195(4):1341–1349, 2015.

Pizzo P: Management of patients with fever and neutropenia through the arc of time: a narrative review, Ann Intern Med 170(6):389–397, 2019.

Qian C, Wang Y, Reppel L, et al: Viral-specific T-cell transfer from HSCT donor for the treatment of viral infections or diseases after HSCT, Bone Marrow Transplant 53(2):114–122, 2018.

Simner P, Miller S, Carroll K: Understanding the promises and hurdles of metagenomic next-generation sequencing as a diagnostic tool for infectious diseases, Clin Infect Dis 66(5):778–788, 2018.

Taplitz R, Kennedy E, Bow E, et al: Antimicrobial prophylaxis for adult patients with cancer related immunosuppression: ASCO and IDSA clinical practice guideline update, J Clin Oncol 36(30):3043–3054, 2018.

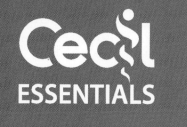

105

Infectious Diseases of Travelers: Protozoal and Helminthic Infections

Jessica E. Johnson, Rebecca Reece

INTRODUCTION

Medical advice for overseas travelers, recommended protective measures, and the diagnosis and treatment of common parasitic diseases endemic in the United States and abroad are reviewed in this chapter.

PREPARATION OF TRAVELERS

Americans made more than 70 million international trips in 2015, and this number continues to increase every year. If we look at a breakdown of where these travels occur, 75% were to a malaria-endemic country. Increases in international travel are associated with exposures to infectious diseases worldwide and bring the issues of prevention and management of health problems in travelers into the office of every physician. The risk of becoming ill while traveling internationally depends on the destination and duration of the trip, the underlying health and age of the traveler, and activities/exposures that occur while abroad. Major issues to be addressed before traveling include required and recommended immunizations, malaria prophylaxis, and traveler's diarrhea, as well as measures to prevent tick and mosquito bites. Information about health risks in specific geographic areas, updated weekly, can be obtained from the US Centers for Disease Control and Prevention (CDC) through its publications or website (www.cdc.gov/travel/destinations/list).

Immunizations

All international travelers should ensure they are up-to-date on routine vaccinations. Only yellow fever vaccination may be required by law for international travel, but other immunizations are often strongly recommended, depending on the destination, type, and duration of travel. Before immunization, a thorough history should be obtained to determine the safety of immunizations and any allergies to eggs or chick embryo cells. Pregnant women and individuals who are immunocompromised by human immunodeficiency virus (HIV), malignancy, or chemotherapy pose specific and important concerns requiring review before receiving vaccinations.

Hepatitis A

In the United States, one of the most frequently identified risks for hepatitis A infection is travel. The risk varies with living conditions, length of stay, and incidence of hepatitis A in the area visited. In some areas, the disease affects an estimated 1 of every 500 to 1000 travelers on a 2- to 3-week trip. Therefore, hepatitis A vaccination is recommended for all susceptible persons traveling to or working in countries with intermediate or high endemicity of infection. Hepatitis A vaccine should be given at least 2 weeks before departure but remains effective if given up until the time of travel. A single dose provides protection for 1 to 2 years; a booster 6 to 18 months later is required for long-lasting immunity (at least 20 years and possibly lifelong).

Influenza

Although influenza is not necessarily considered a travel-related illness, it is the most common vaccine-preventable disease in travelers. The influenza vaccine should be considered in the panel of vaccines offered to the traveler. Influenza seasons can occur at different times of the year in different parts of the world. If a patient cannot be immunized, a course of the antiviral medication oseltamivir can be provided to take at the first sign of a flu-like illness.

Japanese Encephalitis

Japanese encephalitis (JE) virus is closely related to the West Nile and Saint Louis encephalitis viruses and is transmitted to humans through the bite of an infected mosquito. JE virus is the most common vaccine-preventable cause of encephalitis in Asia. It occurs throughout most of Asia and parts of the western Pacific. The overall incidence of JE among people from non-endemic countries traveling to Asia is estimated to be less than 1 case per 1 million travelers. However, expatriates and travelers who stay for prolonged periods in rural areas with active JE virus transmission are likely to be at similar risk as the susceptible resident population (i.e., 5 to 50 cases per 100,000 children per year). Even during brief trips, travelers might be at increased risk if they have extensive outdoor or nighttime exposure in rural areas during periods of active transmission. Short-term (<1 month) travelers whose visits are restricted to major urban areas are at minimal risk for JE. The inactivated JE vaccine, a two-dose series given 28 days apart, is approved for individuals 2 months old and up.

Measles

In the United States, most measles cases result from international travel, and measles remains a common disease in many parts of the world. A large outbreak in 2015 originating from Disney parks in California demonstrated how imported diseases can spread widely to unvaccinated individuals. Currently, measles vaccination is recommended at 15 months of age, with a second vaccination after age 5. Individuals born after 1956 who have no physician-documented record of immunization or who have not received a booster after early childhood should have a one-time booster before travel.

Meningococcal Meningitis

Vaccination for meningococcal disease is recommended to persons who travel to or reside in countries in which the bacterium *Neisseria meningitidis* is hyper-endemic or epidemic, particularly if they will be in close contact with the local population. Vaccination is recommended for travelers to Saudi Arabia during the Hajj, along the "meningitis belt" of sub-Saharan Africa, and in other locations for which travel advisories have been issued (information available on the CDC website). The meningococcal conjugate vaccine (MCV4) is preferred for people age 9 months through 55 years, and the meningococcal polysaccharide vaccine (MPSV4) is the recommended vaccine for persons older than 55. Serogroup B vaccine was approved in the United States in 2015; however, there are no specific recommendations for travelers because serogroup B is rare internationally. It should be considered in the setting of a reported outbreak or in those with certain risk factors.

Polio

Polio remains endemic in only three countries since 2016: Nigeria, Pakistan, and Afghanistan. Before traveling to areas where poliomyelitis cases are still occurring, travelers should ensure that they have completed the recommended age-appropriate polio vaccine series and have received a booster dose with the inactivated polio vaccine as an adult.

Typhoid

International travelers are at greatest risk for contracting typhoid in the Indian subcontinent, Central America, western South America, and sub-Saharan Africa. Vaccination is recommended for travel to endemic areas where exposure to contaminated food and water is likely. Both a live oral vaccine (four enteric-coated capsules given over 7 days) and an injectable vaccine (single-dose) are available; they are essentially equivalent in effectiveness, which ranges from 50% to 70%.

Yellow Fever

The yellow fever vaccine is a live, attenuated virus vaccine that is recommended for persons traveling to areas in South America and Africa where yellow fever is endemic. Proof of vaccination is required for entry into several countries in these regions unless the traveler meets medically exempt criteria. Since 2016, the World Health Organization (WHO) has lifted the recommendation of a booster every 10 years, stating that a single vaccination is protective for life except in three situations: pregnancy, bone marrow transplant, and HIV infection. Severe adverse events are rare and include yellow fever vaccine–associated viscerotropic and neurologic disease, both of which are more common in elderly persons and in those with thymus disease. Because the adverse events occur more commonly in people older than 60 years of age, a careful assessment of risks and benefits for these travelers should be made before vaccination.

Other Vaccines

Some individuals live for prolonged periods in developing countries or are at special risk for contracting certain highly contagious diseases. Consideration should be given to immunization against hepatitis B, cholera, plague (not commercially available in United States), and rabies. Tetanus vaccinations should be up to date: for travel, a tetanus booster within the previous 5 years is recommended. The cholera vaccine became approved in the United States as of 2016 as a single-dose oral vaccine. Immunity is not long-lasting, with protection less than 80% at 3 months. Given this and limited travel to areas of active cholera transmission, it is not routinely recommended for travelers in the United States, but standard cholera prevention and control measures are emphasized.

Malaria Prophylaxis

Malaria infection is associated with significant morbidity and mortality, particularly if the causative agent is *Plasmodium falciparum*. Worldwide, over 200 million cases occur per year, with increasing numbers of cases among travelers. The need for, as well as the type

of, malaria prophylaxis depends on known resistance patterns and the exact itinerary within a given country because the risk of transmission is regional. In general, travelers to areas where chloroquine-sensitive *P. falciparum* strains are exclusively found (i.e., parts of Central America, the Caribbean, and some countries in the Middle East) should take chloroquine phosphate (300 mg base or 500 mg salt) weekly, starting 1 week before travel to malarious areas and continuing during the trip and for 4 weeks after leaving the area.

Travelers to Southeast Asia, sub-Saharan Africa, South America, and South Asia, where chloroquine-resistant *P. falciparum* is common, may take mefloquine (Lariam), atovaquone-proguanil (Malarone), or doxycycline. Mefloquine may be associated with neurologic side effects (dizziness, tinnitus, and vivid dreams) and, rarely, with significant neuropsychiatric side effects. A US Food and Drug Administration (FDA) black box warning issued in 2013 indicated that the neurologic side effects can occur at any time and persist indefinitely; this has lent some caution to the prescription of mefloquine. Mefloquine is also not completely effective in Myanmar, rural Thailand, or some parts of East Africa, where resistance is a growing problem. Mefloquine is taken once weekly for prophylaxis, so is an attractive option for long-term travelers, but must be taken for 4 additional weeks on return. Atovaquone-proguanil and doxycycline are effective in Southeast Asia and may be used in other areas of chloroquine resistance. Atovaquone-proguanil is well tolerated but must be taken every day and extended for 1 week on return. Daily doxycycline can be associated with photosensitivity, esophagitis, and, occasionally, vaginal candidiasis. Doxycycline must also be taken for 4 additional weeks on return from travel.

Where it is approved, primaquine can be used for primary prophylaxis in areas with higher rates of *Plasmodium vivax* or *Plasmodium ovale* infection. It has the advantage of both preventing acute infection from all malaria parasites and preventing the later recurrent infections of *P. vivax* and *P. ovale*. This is taken as a daily dose and continued for 4 weeks on return. It cannot be used in individuals with glucose-6-phosphate dehydrogenase (G6PD) deficiency. Tafenoquine is a newer agent that also prevents acute infection and the later recurrent disease of *P. vivax* and *P. ovale*, as in primaquine, but must be avoided in those with G6PD deficiency. Emphasis must also be given to the use of mosquito bite prevention measures, including netting, screens, permethrin for clothing, and insect repellents, because this can help prevent malaria as well as other vector-borne diseases.

Traveler's Diarrhea

Each year between 30% and 75% of international travelers develop diarrhea. Bacterial infections such as enterotoxigenic *Escherichia coli* are most common, causing more than 80% of traveler's diarrhea; other causes include parasites (i.e., *Giardia*) and viruses (i.e., Norovirus). The average duration of an episode of traveler's diarrhea is 3 to 6 days, but about 10% of episodes last longer than 1 week. The diarrhea may be accompanied by abdominal cramping, nausea, headache, low-grade fever, vomiting, or bloating. Travelers with fever greater than 101° F (38° C), bloody stools, or both should see a physician at once (see Chapter 98).

Diarrheal illness can be avoided by taking precautions with regard to food and beverages. All water and ice should be presumed to be unsafe. Salads are often contaminated by protozoal cysts; along with street vendor foods, they are the most dangerous foods encountered by most travelers. Food should be well cooked, and unpasteurized dairy products should be avoided.

Prophylactic antibiotics are not generally recommended. Diphenoxylate (Lomotil) and loperamide (Imodium) may provide symptomatic relief of mild diarrhea. Oral rehydration is recommended in all cases regardless of severity and serves as an adjunct to antibiotics in moderate and severe disease. First-line treatment includes fluoroquinolones, although increasing resistance is being seen in South and Southeast Asia, as well as other destinations. Alternative to quinolones is azithromycin. Updated guidelines by the International Society of Travel Medicine recommends a single-dose antibiotic regimen (of either choice above) as treatment for traveler's diarrhea.

Special Problems
Pregnant Women

Although travel is rarely contraindicated during a normal pregnancy, complicated pregnancies require special consideration and may warrant a recommendation that travel be delayed. The risk of obstetric complications is highest during the first and third trimesters.

Most live-virus vaccines are contraindicated during pregnancy. Yellow fever vaccine, for which pregnancy is considered a precaution by the Advisory Committee on Immunization Practices (ACIP), should be avoided if possible. If travel is unavoidable and the risks for yellow fever virus exposure are believed to outweigh the risks of vaccination, a pregnant woman should be vaccinated. Pregnant women should avoid or delay travel to malaria-endemic areas because no prophylactic measures provide complete protection. If travel is unavoidable, pregnant women should take utmost precautions to avoid mosquito bites; for chemoprophylaxis, chloroquine and mefloquine are the drugs of choice for destinations with chloroquine-sensitive and chloroquine-resistant malaria, respectively.

Zika virus has been shown to cause congenital brain abnormalities including microcephaly as seen in the 2015-2016 outbreak throughout the Americas and Pacific Islands. Though WHO declared an end of the epidemic in November 2016, pregnant women should be counseled to avoid travel to areas with active local transmission. If travel is unavoidable, pregnant women should be counseled on mosquito prevention methods to reduce their risk. Zika virus can also be sexually transmitted, and barrier precaution with condoms, or abstinence, should be advised throughout pregnancy.

Acquired Immunodeficiency Syndrome

Several countries continue to have policies that bar entry to persons with human immunodeficiency virus (HIV)/acquired immunodeficiency syndrome (AIDS). Several countries require serologic testing for HIV from all travelers applying for visas lasting longer than 3 months; official documentation is required well in advance of travel. Patients with HIV infection need special preparation before travel to developing countries because of their increased susceptibility to certain illnesses (e.g., pneumococcal infection, tuberculosis). Risk of HIV infection and other sexually transmitted diseases should be discussed, especially with young, sexually active adults.

The Returning Traveler

The most common medical problems encountered by travelers after their return home are diarrhea, fever, respiratory illnesses, and skin lesions. A detailed history should focus on the traveler's exact itinerary, including dates of travel, exposure history (e.g., food indiscretions, drinking-water sources, freshwater contact, sexual activity, animal contact, insect bites), style of travel (urban vs. rural), immunization history, and use of antimalarial chemoprophylaxis.

Diarrhea

Traveler's diarrhea is an acute condition that usually resolves within 2 weeks. If the traveler's diarrhea is not responsive to empiric antibiotic treatment, a work-up should be performed to evaluate for *Giardia lamblia* (see later discussion). Three stool specimens for ova and parasites and a stool culture are indicated (E-Fig. 105.1). If *Giardia* tests are

negative, an empirical trial of metronidazole for treatment of a possible infection with *Giardia* or other protozoan (e.g., amebiasis) should be considered. Noninfectious causes such as temporary lactose intolerance, irritable bowel syndrome, and, less commonly, inflammatory bowel disease should also be in the differential diagnosis.

Fever

Malaria should be the first diagnosis considered in a febrile traveler who has returned from a malarious area. *P. falciparum* malaria can be fatal if it is not diagnosed and treated promptly. Detection of the *Plasmodium* species on Giemsa-stained blood smears by light microscopy is the standard tool for diagnosis of malaria. Rapid diagnostic tests for detection of malaria parasite antigens are becoming increasingly important tools in resource-limited endemic settings because of their accuracy and ease of use.

Travelers with chloroquine-sensitive *P. falciparum* malaria should be treated with chloroquine. Reasonable agents for uncomplicated malaria caused by chloroquine-resistant *P. falciparum* include atovaquone-proguanil, artemisinin derivative combinations (if available) and mefloquine- or quinine-based regimens. Quinine- and mefloquine-based regimens are more frequently associated with adverse effects, and mefloquine should not be used to treat *P. falciparum* malaria acquired in the Thai-Myanmar-Cambodia area because of high resistance rates.

Severe malaria is defined as acute malaria with major signs of organ dysfunction or a high level of parasitemia (>5%) or both. It should be treated with intravenous quinidine for 7 days with close monitoring of the QTc interval. In many parts of the world, intravenous artesunate is used, but it may be associated with high rates of relapse.

Other important causes of fever after travel include viral hepatitis (hepatitis A and E), typhoid fever, bacterial enteritis, arboviral infections (e.g., dengue, chikungunya, Zika), rickettsial infections, and, in rare instances, leptospirosis, acute HIV infection, and amebic liver abscess (see also Chapter 90).

Skin Diseases

Sunburn, insect bites, skin ulcers, and cutaneous larva migrans are the most common skin conditions affecting travelers after their return home. Persistent skin ulcers should prompt a work-up for cutaneous leishmaniasis, mycobacterial infection, or fungal infection. Careful, complete inspection of the skin is important in detecting the rickettsial eschar in a febrile patient or the central breathing hole in a "boil" caused by myiasis.

PROTOZOAL INFECTIONS

Protozoal infections, though endemic to certain regions, can be encountered all around the world, partly because of the increase in travel and migration (Table 105.1). They cause a tremendous burden of disease in the tropics and subtropics as well as more temperate climates. Immunosuppression associated with various conditions, particularly HIV infection, leads to more severe manifestations. Of all protozoal diseases, malaria causes the most deaths globally, approximately 1 million people each year.

Protozoal Infections in the United States
Giardiasis

Giardiasis is a common cause of nonbloody diarrhea in returning travelers. *G. lamblia* and *G. intestinalis* are found worldwide, including in the United States. However, giardiasis is most commonly diagnosed in travelers returning from Latin America, Southeast Asia, or the Middle East. Transmission is by the fecal-oral route in the setting of contaminated

TABLE 105.1   Protozoal Infections

Protozoan	Setting	Vectors	Diagnosis	Special Considerations	Treatment
Endemic in the United States					
Babesia microti	New England	Ixodid ticks, transfusions	Thick or thin blood smear	Severe disease in asplenic persons	Quinine and clindamycin
Giardia lamblia	Mountain states	Humans, small mammals	Microscopic examination of stool or duodenal fluid	Common in homosexual men, travelers, children in daycare centers	Quinacrine, nitazoxanide, or metronidazole
Toxoplasma gondii	Ubiquitous	Domestic cats, raw meat	Clinical; serologic confirmation	Pregnant women, immunosuppressed host (AIDS)	Pyrimethamine and sulfadiazine
Entamoeba histolytica	Southeast	Human	Microscopic examination of stool or touch preparation from ulcer	Common in homosexual men, travelers, institutionalized persons	Metronidazole
Cryptosporidium species	Ubiquitous	Human	Acid-fast stain of stool	Severe in immunosuppressed hosts (AIDS)	Nitazoxanide
Trichomonas vaginalis	Ubiquitous	Human	Wet preparation of genital secretions	Common cause of vaginitis	Metronidazole
Primarily Seen in Travelers and Immigrants					
Plasmodium species	Africa, Asia, South America	*Anopheles* mosquito	Thick and thin blood smears	Consider in returning travelers with fever	Dependent on regional resistance pattern (see text)
Leishmania donovani	Middle East	Sandfly	Tissue biopsy	Consider in immigrants with fever and splenomegaly	Sodium stibogluconate
Trypanosoma species	Africa, South America	Reduviid bugs, transfusion	Direct examination of blood or CSF	Very rare in travelers, transfusion associated	Dependent on species and stage of disease

AIDS, Acquired immunodeficiency syndrome; *CSF,* cerebrospinal fluid.

food or water or public swimming areas, or by person-to-person contact in certain risk populations such as men who have sex with men. It is usually a self-limited diarrheal illness that lasts 2 to 4 weeks but may persist longer. Rarely, individuals have associated fevers, nausea, or vomiting. The diagnosis is made by microscopic examination of stool for cysts or trophozoites or by an antigen detection test. Treatment options include metronidazole, tinidazole, or nitazoxanide.

Amebiasis

Amebiasis is another diarrheal illness that occurs in travelers. Like *Giardia, Entamoeba histolytica* is found worldwide, and transmission is by the fecal-oral route. However, most infected individuals (80%) are asymptomatic. The presentation in those acutely infected includes bloody or watery diarrhea with abdominal cramping lasting up to 4 weeks. In immunocompromised individuals, a severe invasive infection can occur with risk of necrotizing colitis or bowel perforation. Extraintestinal amebiasis can occur as well, particularly liver abscesses. The diagnosis can be made by microscopic examination of stool for ova and parasites or by antigen detection tests of stool or serum. Treatment is with metronidazole or tinidazole in symptomatic individuals, followed by paromomycin or iodoquinol. Asymptomatic patients should also be treated with iodoquinol or paromomycin to prevent spread or later disease development.

Protozoal Infections Common in Travelers and Immigrants
Leishmaniasis

Leishmaniasis is transmitted by the sandfly and can manifest with cutaneous, mucocutaneous, or visceral involvement. The skin finding is a persistent ulcer with raised edges in a traveler returning from the Middle East (Old World: *Leishmania major, Leishmania tropica*) or Latin America (New World: *Leishmania braziliensis, Leishmania*

peruviana, others). Diagnosis is by tissue biopsy. Visceral leishmaniasis can have hepatic, splenic, or bone marrow involvement and is more commonly identified in immigrants from Asia (*Leishmania donovani*) or South America (*Leishmania chagasi*). Diagnosis is by tissue biopsy or culture of the involved organ.

Treatment varies based on severity of presentation and resistance characteristics. Most cutaneous lesions are self-limited, but treatment options include sodium stibogluconate (Pentostam) or paromomycin. For visceral involvement, treatment includes sodium stibogluconate, amphotericin B, or a combination of these two agents.

African Trypanosomiasis

African trypanosomiasis, or African sleeping sickness, is a protozoal infection caused by *Trypanosoma rhodesiense* (East Africa) or *Trypanosoma gambiense* (Central and West Africa), which is transmitted by the tsetse fly. Presenting symptoms include fever, headache, and central nervous system involvement. The disease is rarely reported in travelers returning from sub-Saharan Africa but should be considered in immigrants from these areas. Frequently, the patient remembers a chancre at the site of the insect bite (E-Fig. 105.2). The diagnosis is made by microscopic examination of blood, lymph, or cerebrospinal fluid for the parasite (E-Figs. 105.3 and 105.4). Treatment varies by species and is highly toxic. Consultation with an expert in infectious disease or tropical medicine is recommended.

American Trypanosomiasis

American trypanosomiasis, or Chagas' disease, is caused by *Trypanosoma cruzi* and is endemic in Central and South America. Transmitted by contact with feces of reduviid bugs (kissing bugs) (E-Fig. 105.5), it can also be acquired through blood transfusion or organ transplantation from an infected individual. The risk to travelers is extremely low but increases with prolonged stays in poor-quality housing. The presentation has an acute phase of 3 months followed by a chronic infection for life. The classic acute presentation involves swelling and erythema of the eyelid and ocular tissue at the entry site of infection, known as the Romaña sign. However, most individuals are asymptomatic throughout the infection and are identified only at the time of blood donation. Between 20% and 30% of individuals develop manifestations of chronic infection decades later that can include cardiomegaly and heart failure, megaesophagus, or megacolon.

Diagnosis in the acute phase is by microscopic examination of peripheral blood (E-Fig. 105.6). In the chronic phase, various serologic analyses are available to aid in diagnosis. Treatment is recommended early because it may prevent chronic manifestations. In the United States, antitrypanosomal drugs are available through the CDC in consultation with an expert in the field. For most chronic manifestations, however, treatment is supportive.

HELMINTHIC INFECTIONS

Infestation by nematodes, or roundworms, is the most common parasitic infection in the world. The intestinal nematodes *Ascaris* and *Trichuris* are the two most prevalent types. Other important helminths include *Strongyloides*, *Enterobius*, schistosomes, and tapeworms (see later discussion). Although most helminths are found worldwide, they disproportionately affect the developing world and pose potential risk to travelers to those areas (Table 105.2).

Helminthic Infections Common in the United States
Pinworm

Enterobiasis is common in the United States and worldwide. Children are predominantly infected, and transmission is by the fecal-oral route. The clinical presentation is perianal pruritus. Diagnosis is made by the tape test, in which transparent tape is applied to the perianal skin overnight and then examined microscopically for ova on the tape. Treatment is with mebendazole or albendazole.

Roundworm

Ascaris lumbricoides is found worldwide, including in the United States, but mostly affects people in the developing world. Although affected individuals are usually asymptomatic, some develop pulmonary infiltrates during the migration phase of the worm or obstruction of the biliary, pancreatic, or intestinal tract. These manifestations usually occur in the setting of high worm burden. Diagnosis is by stool examination for ova and parasites (E-Fig. 105.7). Treatment is with mebendazole or albendazole.

Whipworm

Trichuris trichiura are called whipworms because of their characteristic shape in the adult form. Like *Ascaris*, this is an intestinal nematode that infects mostly children. It is usually asymptomatic except in the setting of heavy worm burden, which can lead to rectal prolapse and bloody diarrhea among children in the developing world. Diagnosis is made by stool examination for ova and parasites or by endoscopy revealing colitis and the presence of adult worms. The treatment of choice is mebendazole or albendazole.

Hookworm

Ancylostoma duodenale and *Necator americanus* (hookworms) are similar to roundworms in their worldwide distribution and are common among immigrants from Asia and sub-Saharan Africa. Infection occurs through direct penetration of the skin by the larvae, which travel through the lymphatics and the bloodstream to the lungs and are then swallowed. Infected individuals may be asymptomatic, or they

may develop pruritic dermatitis at the site of entry. As with the roundworm, pulmonary infiltrates can occur during the migration phase; this is known as Löffler syndrome. Chronic iron deficiency anemia associated with heavy hookworm infection can be severe and debilitating. Eosinophilia is common. The diagnosis is made by stool examination for ova and parasites (E-Fig. 105.8). The treatment is mebendazole or albendazole.

Helminth Infections Common in Travelers and Immigrants
Strongyloidosis

Strongyloides stercoralis is a helminthic parasite that is found worldwide, although more commonly in the tropics. Infection occurs from contact with contaminated soil; the larva penetrates the skin, migrates to the lungs, and is then swallowed by the individual. The infection is usually asymptomatic, but infection can persist into the chronic phase decades later. Those with symptoms usually have gastrointestinal complaints of bloating, diarrhea, and abdominal pain. Eosinophilia is a common finding in these individuals. In immunocompromised individuals, a hyperinfection syndrome with dissemination of the organism can occur. Hyperinfection syndrome has a higher mortality rate and occurs usually in immigrants who become immunosuppressed as a result of chemotherapy, use of steroids, or illness. Diagnosis is made by stool examination (approximately 30% to 50% sensitivity) (E-Fig. 105.9) or by serology but this does not distinguish between chronic and acute disease. Treatment is with ivermectin for 2 days; in the setting of hyperinfection, a longer course is required.

Schistosomiasis

Schistosomiasis is found throughout the tropics and the developing world. Also known as blood flukes, schistosomes use freshwater mollusks as their intermediate host and penetrate the skin of individuals, leading to infection. The three major species are: *Schistosoma mansoni* (Africa, Middle East, South America), *Schistosoma haematobium* (Africa, Middle East), and *Schistosoma japonicum* (China, Philippines, and Southeast Asia). Acute infection can manifest with dermatitis, although most cases are asymptomatic. Chronic infection develops from the immune response to egg deposition. *S. haematobium* can lead to urinary obstruction or hematuria and is associated with an increased risk of bladder cancer. *S. mansoni* and *S. japonicum* can lead to hepatosplenomegaly, hepatic fibrosis, obstruction of portal blood flow, and varices. *S. japonicum* can infect the central nervous system causing ring enhancing lesions and seizures. Diagnosis is by examination of stool or urine for schistosome eggs in individuals from endemic areas, who have a high egg burden; among travelers, in whom the egg burden is usually low, serology is used for diagnosis. The treatment of choice is praziquantel.

Lymphatic Filariasis (Elephantiasis)

Wuchereria bancrofti and *Brugia malayi* are found throughout the tropics; they are lymph-dwelling filariae that cause elephantiasis. The presentation can vary from acute lymphadenitis, to asymptomatic microfilaremia, filarial fevers, or tropical pulmonary eosinophilia. Lymphadenitis can involve both upper and lower extremities with both of these filarial species, but scrotal involvement only occurs with *W. bancrofti*. The diagnosis is made by examination of a peripheral blood smear for microfilariae obtained between 10 PM and 4 AM because these organisms are nocturnally periodic.

Diethylcarbamazine is used for lymphatic filariasis to eradicate the microfilariae and the adult worms. However, the management of chronic lymphatic obstruction remains a challenge because it is not fully reversible and requires supportive therapy.

TABLE 105.2   **Helminthic Infections**

Helminth	Setting	Vectors	Diagnosis	Treatment
Endemic in the United States				
Pinworm (enterobiasis)	Ubiquitous	Human	Direct examination for ova	Mebendazole, albendazole
Ascaris lumbricoides	Southeast	Human	Stool examination for ova	Mebendazole, albendazole
Trichuris trichiura	Southeast	Human	Stool examination for ova	Mebendazole, albendazole
Hookworm	Southeast	Human	Stool examination for ova	Mebendazole, albendazole
Common in Travelers and Immigrants				
Strongyloides stercoralis	Developing world	Human	Stool examination for larvae	Thiabendazole, ivermectin
Schistosoma species	Developing world	Snails	Stool or urine examination for ova	Praziquantel
Wuchereria and *Brugia* species	Asia, some parts of Africa	Mosquitoes	Nocturnal blood examination	Ivermectin
Onchocerca volvulus	Africa, South and Central America	Black flies	Biopsy	Ivermectin
Loa loa	Africa	Tabanid flies	Blood examination, clinical setting	Diethylcarbamazine or ivermectin
Clonorchis sinensis	Asia	Undercooked fish and snails	Stool examination for ova, radiology	Praziquantel
Echinococcus species	Worldwide	Canines and livestock	Radiology, serology, biopsy	Surgery, supportive therapy
Taenia solium (cysticercosis)	Developing world	Humans, pigs	Radiology, serology	Surgery, albendazole
T. solium, Taenia saginata, Diphyllobothrium latum (tapeworms)	Worldwide	Pigs, bovine, fish	Stool examination for ova or proglottids	Praziquantel

Loa loa (Eyeworm)

Loiasis is caused by the eyeworm *(Loa loa)* and is found in West and Central Africa. Presentation can vary and may include pruritus, subcutaneous swellings, joint manifestations, or neurologic symptoms. In the rarest presentation, the adult worm can be seen in the anterior chamber of the individual's eye. Diagnosis is confirmed by the presence of microfilariae in blood samples or isolation of the adult worm. Treatment is as for lymphatic filariasis, with diethylcarbamazine.

River Blindness

Onchocerca volvulus infection mostly occurs in regions of West and Central Africa but also in South and Central America. Pruritic dermatitis is the most common presentation; but involvement of the eye is the most serious presentation. Ocular involvement occurs in endemic areas in individuals with heavy worm burden. The complications can begin with conjunctivitis and photophobia. Corneal involvement with the microfilariae causes an inflammatory reaction leading to sclerosing keratitis and blindness. River blindness is the most common cause of blindness in Africa. The diagnosis is made by examination of skin snips for microfilariae. Ivermectin is the drug of choice; an initial single dose is followed by a repeat dose at 3 or 6 months to suppress any further microfilariae because this does not eliminate the adult worm.

Clonorchiasis

Clonorchis sinensis is the Chinese liver fluke. This is an important infection to consider in Asian immigrants who have symptoms consistent with biliary tract disease, including right upper quadrant pain, anorexia, and weight loss. Though the disease is uncommon, untreated infections can lead to cholangiocarcinoma. Treatment is curative with praziquantel in 85% of cases.

Cysticercosis

Cysticercosis is caused by the pork tapeworm, *Taenia solium.* Individuals report new-onset seizures or headaches. Head computed

tomographic (CT) scans show ring enhancing lesions. The diagnosis is usually based on the history and imaging findings, and confirmation can be made by immunoblot assay. Treatment depends on the site of infection and symptoms. It may include antiparasitic treatment, antiseizure medications, and surgical removal. The antiparasitic drug of choice is praziquantel or albendazole. Expert consultation before treatment is recommended because of the risk of increasing focal cerebral edema and seizure activity.

Intestinal Tapeworms

Tapeworms that commonly infect humans include *Taenia solium* (from raw pork), *Taenia saginata* (raw beef), and *Diphyllobothrium latum* (raw fish). Most infections are asymptomatic except in the case of invasive disease with *T. solium*, as discussed earlier (see Cysticercosis). Praziquantel is the treatment of choice for all three tapeworms.

Echinococcus

The tapeworm *Echinococcus granulosus* causes hydatid disease with production of a cystic liver mass. This occurs in immigrants from sheep-raising parts of the world such as South America, Central Asia, and the Middle East. The characteristic appearance of the cyst includes a calcified wall with a dependent hydatid on CT scans. This appearance and the supporting history help to make the diagnosis; the serologic testing available can be falsely negative. Treatment often includes percutaneous drainage or surgical removal. Care must be taken to avoid rupture or spillage of the contents, which can result in life threatening anaphylaxis. Albendazole is usually given before surgical removal.

Less common is *Echinococcus multilocularis*, which causes alveolar cyst disease. This more aggressive infection leads to liver lesions as well as brain and lung involvement. Treatment includes resection of liver lesions in combination with antiparasitic therapy with mebendazole or albendazole. However, these agents are not parasiticidal, so the mortality rate remains high. Other potential therapies, such as amphotericin B and nitazoxanide, are being explored.

FUTURE DIRECTIONS

The field of travel medicine is constantly changing as infectious diseases do not always follow a historical pattern. With the increasing globalization of travel, we can see outbreaks and epidemics develop in new areas such as the West Africa Ebola outbreak in 2014-2015, the Zika epidemic 2015-2016, and the ongoing MERS-CoV outbreak in the Middle East that alter our guidance to patients and our management of returning travelers from these areas. As a physician caring for travelers, we must stay informed of the changing landscape of infectious diseases across the world.

SUGGESTED READINGS

Arguin P: Approach to the patient before and after travel. In Goldman L, Schafer A, editors: Cecil textbook of medicine, ed 24, Philadelphia, 2012, Saunders, pp 1800–1803.

Centers for Disease Control and Prevention: CDC health information for international travel 2018, New York, 2017, Oxford University Press2017.

Freedman DO, Chen LH, Kzoarsky PE: Medical considerations before international travel, N Eng J Med 375:247–260, 2016.

Jeronimo S, de Queiroz Sousa A, Pearson R: Leishmaniasis. In Guerrant RL, Walker DH, Weller PF, editors: Tropical infectious diseases: principles, pathogens, and practices, ed 3, Philadelphia, 2011, Saunders, pp 696–706.

Kirchoff L: Trypanosoma species (American trypanosomiasis, Chagas' disease): biology of trypanosomes. In Mandell GL, Bennett JE, Dolin R, editors: Principles and practice of infectious diseases, ed 7, Philadelphia, 2010, Churchill Livingstone, pp 3481–3488.

Leder K, Torresi J, Libman M, et al: GeoSentinel surveillance of illness in returned travelers, 2007-2011, Ann Intern Med 158:456–468, 2013.

Neurologic Disease

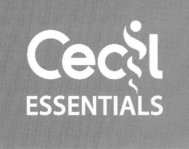

106

Neurologic Evaluation of the Patient

Frederick J. Marshall

INTRODUCTION

To arrive at an accurate neurologic diagnosis, the clinician generates and tests hypotheses about the location and the mechanism of injury to the nervous system. Hypotheses are refined as the clinician progresses from the interview to the physical examination to the laboratory assessment of the patient. The focus is first placed on entities that are common, serious, and treatable. Common presentations of common diseases account for roughly 80% of cases, rare presentations of common diseases account for roughly 15%, typical presentations of rare diseases roughly 5%, and rare presentations of rare diseases less than 1% of cases. Focus your energy on common diseases but learn the rare disorders too.

TAKING A NEUROLOGIC HISTORY

The clinician should strive to determine the location, quality, and timing of symptoms. Encourage the patient to report the progression of symptoms rather than a list of diagnostic procedures and specialty evaluations. Establish when the patient last felt normal, whether the progression has been relentless or remitting, and whether it has been chronic, subacute or acute. This information substantially constrains the differential diagnosis. Ambiguous descriptors such as *dizzy* should be rejected in favor of evocative descriptors such as *light-headed* (which may implicate cardiovascular insufficiency) or *off balance* (which may implicate cerebellar or posterior column dysfunction).

Family members and other witnesses should corroborate historical information when appropriate. Historical information should include the medical and surgical histories; current medications; prior responses to efforts at treatment; allergies; family history; review of systems; and social history, including the patient's level of education, work history, possible toxin exposures, substance use, sexual history, current life circumstance, and overall function.

Clues to localization are sought during the interview. For example, pain is usually caused by a lesion of the peripheral nervous system, whereas aphasia (i.e., disordered language processing) indicates an abnormality of the central nervous system. Because sensory and motor functions are anatomically relatively distant in the cerebral cortex but progressively closer together as fibers converge in the brain stem, spinal cord, roots, and peripheral nerves, the coexistence of sensory loss and motor dysfunction in a limb implies a large lesion at the level of the cortex or a smaller lesion lower down in the neuraxis. Small lesions in areas of high traffic such as the spinal cord or brain stem can result in widespread neurologic dysfunction, whereas small lesions elsewhere may be asymptomatic.

Table 106.1 lists the potential localizing values of common neurologic symptoms to help address the issue of lesion localization. Tables 106.2 and 106.3 list symptoms that are commonly associated with lesions at specific locations in the nervous system. Some symptoms can result from a lesion at any of several levels of the nervous system. For example, double vision can result from a focal lesion in the brain stem, peripheral nerves (cranial nerve III, IV, or VI), neuromuscular junction, or extraocular muscles; or it can be nonfocal and result from an increase in intracranial pressure. Associated symptoms (or their lack) may lead the interviewer to reject certain hypotheses that at first seemed most likely. Table 106.4 lists the most important types of neuropathologic conditions and provides examples of diseases in each category.

Some neuroanatomic locations point to a specific diagnosis or a limited number of diagnoses. For example, disease of the neuromuscular junction is usually caused by an autoimmune process such as myasthenia gravis (common) or Eaton-Lambert myasthenic syndrome (uncommon). The exceptions—botulism and congenital myasthenic disorders—are rare. Alternatively, some areas of the nervous system (e.g., the cerebral hemispheres) are vulnerable to practically any of the categories of disease outlined in Table 106.4.

The pace and temporal order of symptoms are important. Degenerative diseases usually progress gradually, whereas vascular diseases (e.g., stroke, aneurysmal subarachnoid hemorrhage) progress rapidly. Certain symptoms such as double vision almost invariably develop abruptly, even if the underlying disorder has been developing gradually over days to weeks.

NEUROLOGIC EXAMINATION

Performance of the main elements of a general screening neurologic examination is imperative (Table 106.5), but the examination should be tailored to confirm or disprove the clinical hypotheses generated from the patient's history. Unexpected signs must be explained, often with a return to the history for further clarification. The goal of the exam is to determine whether the cause is diffuse, focal or multifocal.

The examination is approached as if only one of two possible injuries has occurred—the final common pathway to a structure is disrupted, or the input to that pathway is disrupted (Fig. 106.1). In the case of the motor system, the *final common pathway* is the motor unit and includes the anterior horn cells giving rise to axons in a nerve, the nerve itself, the neuromuscular junction, and the muscle. Injury to any of these structures results in dysfunction of the muscle. Conversely, if these structures are intact, observing the muscle function may be possible under the right circumstances. If all modes of engaging the final common pathway fail to elicit a response, the clinician can conclude that the lesion is located somewhere within the final common pathway.

For example, a man with paralysis of facial movement on one side that is caused by a lesion of cranial nerve VII cannot smile voluntarily, close his eye, or wrinkle his forehead on the affected side. Spontaneous laughter or smiling as an automatic response to a joke also fails to move the paretic side. If the problem is central, however, facial movement with involuntary (spontaneous) smiling may be preserved or increased. This observation is common in patients with facial weakness caused by a stroke.

Central input to a final common pathway in the nervous system is usually tonically inhibitory. Damage to this input typically results in overactivity of the involved muscle group. Signs of damage to central inhibitory systems include spasticity and hyperreflexia (i.e., motor cortex, subcortical white matter, or corticospinal pathways in the brain stem and spinal cord); dystonia, rigidity, tremor, and tic (i.e., basal ganglia or extrapyramidal systems); and ataxia and dysmetria (i.e., cerebellum). An exception is hypotonia, which may be seen in cerebellar disease.

TECHNOLOGIC ASSESSMENT

Laboratory investigations and special testing should be used to confirm a clinical suggestion and to finalize the diagnosis. Testing should be selectively performed because of expense, risk, and discomfort to the patient. Frequently helpful tests are discussed in subsequent sections. Diagnostic tests should never be ordered without a specific differential diagnosis firmly in mind. Many neurodiagnostic tests disclose incidental abnormalities unrelated to a patient's symptomatic disease process.

Lumbar Puncture

Investigation of the cerebrospinal fluid (CSF) is indicated in a small number of specific circumstances, usually infections, malignancy, or inflammatory/immune mediated conditions (Table 106.6). When taken, a CSF specimen should be routinely sent for laboratory testing to determine cell and differential counts, protein and glucose levels, and bacterial cultures. The CSF should also be examined for its color and clarity. Cloudy or discolored CSF should be centrifuged and examined for xanthochromia in comparison with water. Additional, special studies may be obtained as appropriate, including Gram stain; fungal, viral, and tuberculous cultures; cryptococcal and other antigens; tests for syphilis; Lyme titers; malignant cytologic patterns; paraneoplastic and other specific protein antibodies; and oligoclonal bands. Polymerase chain reaction for specific viruses may also be appropriate. Assessment of specific CSF proteins such as tau, phosphorylated tau, and amyloid-β in selected patients at risk for dementia may be considered. The 14-3-3 protein, found in Creutzfeldt-Jakob disease, may be found in patients with rapid-onset dementia.

Recording the opening and closing pressures is important. Tissue infection in the region of the puncture site is an absolute contraindication to lumbar puncture. Relative contraindications include known or probable intracranial or spinal mass lesion, increased intracranial pressure as a result of mass lesions, coagulopathy caused by thrombocytopenia (usually correctable), anticoagulant therapy, and bleeding disorders.

Rare but severe complications of lumbar puncture include transtentorial or foramen magnum herniation, spinal epidural hematoma, spinal abscess, herniated or infected disk, meningitis, and adverse reaction to a local anesthetic agent. More common and relatively benign complications include headache and backache.

Tissue Biopsies

In selected specialty centers, a diagnostic biopsy is performed on various tissues, including brain, peripheral nerve (see Chapter 123),

TABLE 106.2 Symptom Localization in the Central Nervous System

Sign or Symptom	Location
Cerebral Hemispheres	
Unilateral weakness or sensory complaints	Contralateral cerebral hemisphere
Language dysfunction	Left hemisphere (frontal and temporal)
Spatial disorientation	Right hemisphere (parietal and occipital)
Anosognosia (lack of insight into deficit)	Right hemisphere (parietal)
Hemivisual loss	Contralateral hemisphere (occipital, temporal, and parietal)
Flattening of affect or social disinhibition	Bihemispheric (frontal and limbic)
Alteration of consciousness	Bihemispheric (diffuse)
Alteration of memory	Bihemispheric (hippocampus, fornix, amygdala, and mammillary bodies)
Cerebellum	
Limb clumsiness	Ipsilateral cerebellar hemisphere
Unsteadiness of gait or posture	Midline cerebellar structures
Basal Ganglia	
Slowness of voluntary movement	Substantia nigra and striatum
Involuntary movement	Striatum, thalamus, and subthalamus
Brain Stem	
Contralateral weakness or sensory complaints in the body with ipsilateral weakness or sensory complaints in the face	Midbrain, pons, and medulla
Double vision	Midbrain and pons
Vertigo	Pons and medulla
Alteration of consciousness	Midbrain, pons, medulla (reticular formation)
Spinal Cord	
Weakness and spasticity (ipsilateral) and anesthesia (contralateral) below a specified level	Corticospinal and spinothalamic tracts
Unsteadiness of gait	Posterior columns
Bilateral (can be asymmetrical) weakness and sensory complaints in multiple contiguous radicular distributions	Central cord

TABLE 106.1 Potential Localizing Value of Common Neurologic Symptoms

Potential Localizing Value	Sign or Symptom
High	Focal weakness, sensory loss, or pain
	Focal visual loss
	Language disturbance
	Neglect or anosognosia
Medium	Vertigo
	Dysarthria
	Clumsiness
Low	Fatigue
	Headache
	Insomnia
	Dizziness
	Anxiety, confusion, or psychosis

TABLE 106.3 Symptom Localization in the Motor Unit[a]

Sign or Symptom	Location
Anterior Horn Cell	
Weakness and wasting with muscle twitching (fasciculation) but no sensory complaints	Anterior horn of spinal cord (diffuse or segmental)
Spinal Root	
Weakness and sensory loss confined to a known radicular distribution (pain, a common feature, may spread)	Cervical, thoracic, lumbar, and sacral
Plexus	
Pain, weakness, and sensory loss in a limb; not limited to a single radicular or peripheral nerve distribution	Brachial and lumbosacral (may also be caused by polyradiculopathy)
Nerve	
Pain, distal weakness, and/or sensory changes confined to a single peripheral nerve distribution	Peripheral nerves (mononeuropathy)
Pain, distal weakness, and/or sensory changes affecting both sides symmetrically (usually starting in feet)	Peripheral nerves (polyneuropathy)
Pain, distal weakness, and/or sensory changes affecting scattered single peripheral nerve distributions	Peripheral nerves (mononeuropathy multiplex)
Unilateral special sensory loss	Cranial nerves I, II, V, VII, VIII, and IX
Unilateral facial weakness involving entire one half of face	Cranial nerve VII (ipsilateral)
Neuromuscular Junction	
Progressive weakness with repeated use of a muscle; no sensory complaints	Ocular, pharyngeal, and skeletal
Muscle	
Proximal weakness; no sensory complaints	Diffuse and various patterns

[a]Anterior horn cell and the peripheral nervous system.

TABLE 106.4 Categories of Neurologic Disease

Disease Category	Example
Genetic	
Autosomal dominant	Huntington's disease
Autosomal recessive	Friedreich's ataxia
X-linked recessive	Duchenne muscular dystrophy
Mitochondrial	Progressive external ophthalmoplegia
Sporadic	Down syndrome
Neoplastic	
Intrinsic	Glioblastoma
Extrinsic	Metastatic melanoma
Paraneoplastic	Cerebellar degeneration
Vascular	
Stroke	Thrombotic, embolic, lacunar, hemorrhagic
Structural	Arteriovenous malformation
Inflammatory	Cranial arteritis
Infectious	
Bacterial	Meningococcal meningitis
Viral	Herpes encephalitis
Protozoal	Toxoplasmosis
Fungal	Cryptococcal meningitis
Helminthic	Cysticercosis
Prion	Creutzfeldt-Jakob disease
Degenerative	
Central	Parkinson's disease
Central and peripheral	Amyotrophic lateral sclerosis
Autoimmune	
Central demyelinating	Multiple sclerosis
Peripheral demyelinating	Guillain-Barré syndrome
Neuromuscular junction	Myasthenia gravis
Toxic and Metabolic	
Endogenous	Uremic encephalopathy
Exogenous	Alcoholic neuropathy
Other Structural	
Trauma	Spinal cord injury
Hydrodynamic	Normal pressure hydrocephalus
Psychogenic	Hysterical paraparesis

muscle (see Chapter 124), and skin. Occasionally, biopsy provides the only means of arriving at a definitive diagnosis.

Electrophysiologic Studies

Electrophysiologic studies include electroencephalography, electromyography, nerve conduction studies, and evoked potentials. These studies are helpful in situations in which the patient cannot be examined or interviewed adequately.

Electroencephalography is most often used to investigate seizures (see Chapter 120). It can document encephalopathy, in which case the background electrical activity of the brain is slowed, and it is also used in the evaluation of brain death.

Electromyography is useful in the differential diagnosis of muscle disease, neuromuscular junction disease, peripheral nerve disease, and anterior horn cell disease. Nerve conduction studies (see Chapters 123 and 124) may show decreased amplitude (characteristic of axonal neuropathy) or decreased velocity (characteristic of demyelinating neuropathy).

Visual-evoked potential studies are commonly used in the evaluation of possible multiple sclerosis (see Chapter 122). Asymmetrical slowing of the cortical response to visual pattern stimulation suggests demyelination in the optic nerve or central optic pathways. Brain stem auditory-evoked potential studies are useful in the diagnosis of diseases affecting cranial nerve VIII or its central projections. Lesions at the cerebellopontine angle and the brain stem cause abnormal delay in conduction. Brain stem auditory-evoked potentials are helpful in the diagnosis of deafness in infants. Somatosensory-evoked potentials are used to identify a slowing of central sensory conduction that results from demyelinating disease, compression, or metabolic derangements. They are also used to evaluate spinal cord–mediated sensory abnormalities.

Imaging Studies

Magnetic resonance imaging (MRI) and computed tomography (CT) are high-resolution imaging techniques that provide extraordinary

TABLE 106.5   Elements of a General Screening Neurologic Examination

Systemic Physical Examination

Head (trauma, dysmorphism, and bruits)

Neck (tone, bruits, and thyromegaly)

Cardiovascular (heart rate, rhythm, and murmurs; peripheral pulses and jugular venous distention)

Pulmonary (breathing pattern, cough and cyanosis)

Abdomen (hepatosplenomegaly)

Back and extremities (skeletal abnormalities, peripheral edema, and straight-leg raising)

Skin (neurocutaneous stigmata and hepatic stigmata)

Mental Status

Level of consciousness (awake, drowsy, and comatose)

Attention (coherent stream of thought, serial 7s)

Orientation (temporal and spatial)

Memory (short and long term)

Language (naming, repetition, comprehension, fluency, reading, and writing)

Visuospatial skills (clock drawing and figure copying)

Judgment, insight, thought content (psychotic)

Mood (depressed, manic, and anxious)

Cranial Nerves

Olfactory (smell in each nostril)

Optic (afferent pupillary function, funduscopic examination, visual acuity, visual fields, and structural eye findings)

Oculomotor, trochlear, and abducens (smooth pursuit and saccadic eye movements, nystagmus, efferent pupillary function, and eyelid opening)

Trigeminal (jaw jerk, facial sensation, afferent corneal reflex, and muscles of mastication)

Facial (efferent corneal reflex, facial expression, eyelid closure, nasolabial folds, and power and bulk)

Vestibulocochlear (nystagmus, speech discrimination, Weber test, and Rinne test)

Glossopharyngeal and vagus (afferent and efferent gag reflex and uvula position)

Spinal accessory (power and bulk of sternocleidomastoid and trapezii muscles)

Hypoglossal (position, bulk, and fasciculations of tongue)

Motor Examination

Pronator drift (subtle corticospinal lesion)

Tone and bulk of muscles (basal ganglia lesion yields rigidity, cerebellar lesion yields hypotonia, corticospinal lesion yields spasticity, nonspecific bihemispheric disease yields paratonia [inability to relax muscles], hypertrophy indicates dystonia, pseudohypertrophy indicates muscle disease, and atrophy indicates lower motor neuron disease)

Adventitious movements (tremor, tic, dystonia, and chorea indicate disease of the basal ganglia; asterixis and myoclonus may indicate toxic metabolic process)

Power of major muscle groups (scale 0-5)

Upper extremities: deltoids, biceps, triceps, wrist extension and flexion, finger extension and flexion, and interossei

Lower extremities: hip flexion, extension, abduction, and adduction; knee extension and flexion; ankle dorsiflexion, plantar flexion, inversion, and eversion; toe extension and flexion

Sensory Examination

Light touch (posterior columns)

Pinprick (spinothalamic tract)

Temperature (spinothalamic tract)

Joint position sense (posterior columns)

Vibration (posterior columns)

Graphesthesia (cortical sensory)

Double simultaneous stimulation (cortical sensory)

Two-point discrimination (posterior columns and cortical sensory)

Reflex Examination

Standard reflexes (grades 0-4)

Biceps

Triceps

Brachioradialis

Knee jerk

Ankle jerk

Pathologic reflexes

Babinski sign (if present)

Myerson sign (glabellar sign) (if present)

Snout (if present)

Jaw jerk (if brisk)

Palmomental (twitch of chin muscles when palm is stroked) (if present)

Hoffmann sign (thumb or index finger flexion when nail of middle finger is flicked) (if brisk)

Coordination and Gait

Finger-nose-finger (action tremor suggesting cerebellar disease)

Rapid alternating movements (dysdiadochokinesia suggesting cerebellar disease)

Fine motor movements (slowness and small amplitude suggesting basal ganglia or corticospinal tract abnormalities)

Heel-to-shin (ataxia suggesting cerebellar disease)

Arising from chair with arms folded across chest (inability in advanced basal ganglia, cerebellar, corticospinal, or muscle disease)

Walking naturally (look for decreased arm swing, spasticity, broad base, festination (quickening and shortening of normal gait), waddle, footdrop, start hesitation, and dystonia)

Tandem gait (look for ataxia)

Walking with feet everted or inverted (look for latent dystonia)

Hopping on each foot separately (look for latent dystonia)

Stand with feet together and eyes open, eyes closed (sensory ataxia and cerebellar disease)

Response to retropulsive stress (loss of postural righting mechanisms)

---

diagnostic precision for central nervous system lesions. Most neurologic diseases, however, can have normal CT and MRI findings. Moreover, many abnormal findings on CT and MRI bear no relation to the diagnosis responsible for the patient's symptoms.

Table 106.7 compares CT with MRI. MRI is used for most purposes, although CT has the advantage of wider accessibility, greater speed of acquisition, and better tolerability by the patient. CT detects acute hemorrhage and is preferred for emergencies. MRI provides more detail and simultaneously obtains images in the horizontal,

vertical, and coronal planes. Contrast media for CT or MRI are useful in the diagnosis of tumors, abscesses, and other processes that derange the blood-brain barrier. MRI can be used for functional imaging and spectroscopy; both techniques have great promise for the evaluation of cognitive and metabolic disorders, epilepsy, multiple sclerosis, and many other conditions.

MR- and CT-angiography allow noninvasive visualization of the major vessels of the head and neck. Conventional angiography with an intra-arterial injection of contrast agent is used for evaluation of

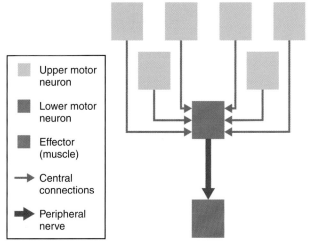

Fig. 106.1 The nervous system can be conceptually reduced to a series of higher-order inputs that converge on final common pathways. For example, upper motor neurons converge on lower motor neurons, whose axons form the final common pathway to an effector muscle.

Legend for figure:
- Upper motor neuron
- Lower motor neuron
- Effector (muscle)
- → Central connections
- ➤ Peripheral nerve

TABLE 106.6 Indications for Lumbar Puncture

Urgent (Do Not Wait for Brain Imaging)

Acute central nervous system infection in the absence of focal neurologic signs

Less Urgent (Wait for Brain Imaging)

Vasculitis, subarachnoid hemorrhage, or cryptic process

Increased intracranial pressure in the absence of mass lesion on magnetic resonance imaging or computed tomography

Intrathecal therapy for fungal or carcinomatous meningitis

Symptomatic treatment for headache from idiopathic intracranial hypertension or subarachnoid hemorrhage

TABLE 106.7 Magnetic Resonance Imaging Versus Computed Tomography

Magnetic Resonance Imaging (MRI)

Resolution 1-2 mm (higher with newer 3-Tesla magnets)

Gadolinium contrast relatively safe, except in severe renal insufficiency

Unaffected by bone; multiple planes of imaging available; functional (physiologic) imaging capacity

Computed Tomography

Resolution >5 mm

Iodine contrast associated with anaphylaxis and rash

Faster acquisition than MRI

Metallic objects such as pacemaker or aneurysm clip preclude MRI

Acute hemorrhage well visualized

Better tolerated by patients who are severely ill or claustrophobic

many intracranial vascular abnormalities, including small aneurysms and arteriovenous malformations, and inflammation of small blood vessels.

Noninvasive ultrasonography of the carotid and vertebral arteries can define stenotic vessels. It has been supplemented by transcranial Doppler technology, which allows characterization of blood flow in intracranial arteries.

TABLE 106.8 Some Neurologic Conditions for Which Genetic Tests Are Commercially Available

- Neuromuscular diseases: nerve (Charcot-Marie-Tooth disease); muscle (myotonic dystrophy, Duchenne-Becker muscular dystrophy); spinal muscular atrophy, familial amyotrophic lateral sclerosis
- Movement disorders: ataxia (spinal cerebellar ataxias, Friedreich ataxia); dystonia, parkinsonism, chorea
- Dementias: Alzheimer's disease, frontotemporal dementia, hereditary prion disease
- Mental retardation (fragile X syndrome)
- Mitochondrial diseases: *mitochondrial encephalomyelopathy, lactic acidosis, and stroke-like symptoms* (MELAS syndrome); *myoclonus epilepsy with ragged red fibers* (MERRF syndrome)

Single-photon emission CT (SPECT) is useful for the evaluation of intracranial blood flow. The development of iodine-123 ioflupane injection (DaTscan) makes it possible to visualize the dopamine transporter to follow cell loss in patients with Parkinson's disease.

Positron-emission tomography (PET) is a functional imaging technology that can demonstrate specific metabolic derangements. It is useful for evaluating local abnormalities of glucose and oxygen metabolism. PET is of particular value in defining the site of origin of focal seizures. Customized ligands can be used to identify specific pathologic processes. Examples include three FDA-approved agents for estimating β-amyloid neuritic plaque density in Alzheimer's disease and fluorodopa F18 in Parkinson's disease.

Genetic and Molecular Testing

There are more neurologic diseases than diseases of all other systems combined. Discoveries have revolutionized the diagnostic approach to many of these diseases, and new genetic tests are discovered every year. Table 106.8 outlines the tests that are commercially available.

Genetic testing for a disorder requires the clinician to perform a thoughtful and caring evaluation of the patient, usually with input from and evaluation of the patient's family. Important ethical issues surround the use of genetic tests, including the ability to ensure privacy, to ensure adequate psychological and social support for patients who may be given devastating news, and to address adequately the appropriateness of prenatal screening or presymptomatic testing when no treatment is available.

PROSPECTS FOR THE FUTURE

Novel imaging techniques and molecular diagnostic studies are beginning to shed light on the pathogenesis of neurologic conditions that have been identifiable only by clinical phenomenology. Studies of previously untreatable neurodegenerative disorders are now targeting presymptomatic individuals in the hope that earlier intervention can modify disease outcomes. Despite these and foreseeable future advances, the clinical aspects of neurologic disease remain fundamentally important in understanding the impact of disease on patients and their families.

SUGGESTED READINGS

Biller J, editor: Practical neurology, ed 4, Philadelphia, 2012, Lippincott Williams & Wilkins.

DeLuca GC, Griggs RC: Approach to the patient with neurologic disease. In Goldman L, Schafer AI, editors: Goldman-Cecil medicine, ed 26, 2020, pp 2298–2304, (Philadelphia..

Ropper, AH, Samuels MA, Leine JP, Prasad S, editors: Adams and victor's principles of neurology, ed 11, New York, McGraw Hill.

107

Disorders of Consciousness

Leah Dickstein, Paul M. Vespa

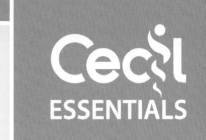

INTRODUCTION

Coma is a state in which the patient is unresponsive and the eyes remain closed even with vigorous stimulation. A poorly responsive state in which the eyes are spontaneously open, or an agitated and confused state, or delirium is not coma but may represent early stages of the same disease processes and should be investigated in the same manner.

Consciousness requires that the brain stem reticular activating system and its cortical projections be intact and functioning. The reticular formation begins in the mid pons and ascends through the dorsal midbrain to synapse in the thalamus; it then innervates higher centers through thalamocortical connections. Knowledge of this anatomic substrate provides the short list of regions to be investigated in the search for a structural cause of coma: Brain stem or bihemispheric dysfunction, be it medication or lesion-related, is typically needed to impede consciousness, whereas structural lesions elsewhere are not the cause of the patient's unconsciousness. In addition to structural lesions, meningeal inflammation, metabolic encephalopathy, sedation, and seizures diffusely affect the brain and complete the differential diagnosis for the patient in coma.

PATHOPHYSIOLOGIC FACTORS

Meningeal irritation caused by infection or blood in the subarachnoid space is an essential early consideration in coma evaluation because its cause requires immediate attention (especially with purulent meningitis) and may not be diagnosed by computed tomography (CT).

Hemispheric mass lesions result in coma either by expanding across the midline laterally to compromise both cerebral hemispheres or by impinging on the brain stem to compress the rostral reticular formation. These processes—*lateral herniation* (lateral movement of the brain) and *transtentorial herniation* (vertical movement of the brain)—most commonly occur together. At the bedside, clinical signs of an expanding hemispheric mass evolve in a level-by-level, rostral-caudal manner (Fig. 107.1). Hemispheric lesions of adequate size to produce coma are readily seen on CT.

Brain stem mass lesions produce coma by directly affecting the reticular formation. Because the pathways for lateral eye movements—the pontine gaze center, medial longitudinal fasciculus, and oculomotor (third nerve) nucleus—traverse the reticular activating system, impairment of reflex eye movements is often the critical element of diagnosis of a brain stem lesion. A comatose patient without impaired reflex lateral eye movements does not have a mass lesion compromising brain stem structures in the posterior fossa. CT is not able to show some lesions in this region. Posterior fossa lesions may block the flow of cerebrospinal fluid from the lateral ventricles, resulting in the dangerous situation of *noncommunicating hydrocephalus.*

Metabolic abnormalities are caused by deficiency states (e.g., thiamine, glucose), by derangements of metabolism (e.g., hyponatremia), or by the presence of *exogenous toxins* (e.g., drugs) or *endogenous toxins* (e.g., organ system failure). Metabolic abnormalities result in diffuse dysfunction of the nervous system; therefore, with rare exceptions, they produce no localized signs such as hemiparesis or unilateral papillary dilation. The diagnosis of *metabolic encephalopathy* means that the examiner has found no focal anatomic features on examination or neuroimaging studies to explain coma but that a specific metabolic cause has not been established. Drugs have a predilection for affecting the reticular formation in the brain stem and for producing paralysis of reflex eye movement on examination. *Multifocal structural disorders* may simulate metabolic coma (Table 107.1).

In the late stages of status epilepticus, motor movements may be subtle even though *seizure activity* is continuing throughout the brain (nonconvulsive status epilepticus). Once seizures stop, the so-called *postictal state* can also cause unexplained coma.

DIAGNOSTIC APPROACH

The history and examination are essential in the diagnosis and are not replaced by brain imaging (Table 107.2). A history of a premonitory headache supports a diagnosis of meningitis, encephalitis, or intracerebral or subarachnoid hemorrhage. A preceding period of intoxication, confusion, or delirium points to a diffuse process such as meningitis or endogenous or exogenous toxins. The sudden apoplectic onset of coma is particularly suggestive of ischemic or hemorrhagic stroke affecting the brain stem or of subarachnoid hemorrhage or intracerebral hemorrhage with intraventricular rupture. Lateralized symptoms of hemiparesis or aphasia before coma occur in patients with hemispheric masses or infarctions.

The physical examination is critical, quickly accomplished, and diagnostic. The issues are three: (1) Does the patient have meningitis? (2) Are signs of a mass lesion present? and (3) Is this condition a diffuse syndrome of exogenous or endogenous metabolic etiology? Emergency management should then be instituted accordingly (Table 107.3).

Identification of Meningitis

Signs of meningeal irritation are not invariably present and have differing sensitivities depending on the cause: They are extremely common with acute pyogenic meningitis and subarachnoid hemorrhage and less common with indolent, fungal meningitis. Nevertheless, the presence of these signs on examination is the central clue to the diagnosis. Missing these signs results in time-consuming additional tests such as brain imaging and the potential loss of a narrow window of opportunity for directed therapy.

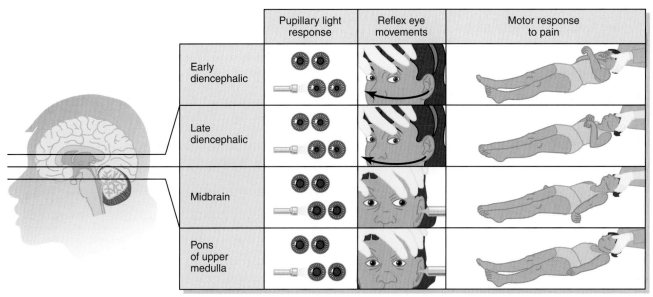

Fig. 107.1 The evolution of neurologic signs in coma from a hemispheric mass lesion as the brain becomes functionally impaired in a rostral-caudal manner. The terms *early diencephalic* and *late diencephalic* refer to levels of dysfunction just above and just below the thalamus, respectively. (From Aminoff MJ, Greenberg DA, Simon RP: Clinical neurology, Stamford, Conn., 1996, Appleton and Lange.)

TABLE 107.1	Multifocal Disorders Indicating Metabolic Coma
Disseminated intravascular coagulopathy	
Sepsis	
Pancreatitis	
Vasculitis	
Thrombotic thrombocytopenic purpura	
Fat emboli	
Hypertensive encephalopathy	
Diffuse micrometastases	

Passive neck flexion should be tested (Fig. 107.2) in all comatose patients unless a history of head trauma exists. When the neck is passively flexed by attempting to bring the chin within a few fingerbreadths of the chest, patients with irritated meninges reflexively flex one or both knees. This sign, called the *Brudzinski reflex*, is usually asymmetrical and not dramatic, but any evidence of knee flexion during passive neck flexion mandates that the cerebrospinal fluid be examined.

Is CT required before lumbar puncture in this setting? In the absence of lateralized signs (e.g., hemiparesis) supporting a superimposed mass lesion, a spinal puncture should be performed immediately. Although rare cases of herniation after lumbar puncture have been reported in children with bacterial meningitis, the urgency of diagnosis and treatment at the point of coma is paramount. The time required for CT may result in a fatal therapeutic delay. An alternative approach involves obtaining blood cultures and immediately initiating antibiotic therapy with subsequent lumbar puncture. With this approach, the cerebrospinal fluid cell count, glucose determination, and protein content are unchanged, and Gram stain and culture often remain positive despite a short period of antibiotic treatment. Bacterial antigens in the cerebrospinal fluid or blood can also be detected.

Separation of Structural From Metabolic Causes of Coma

The goal of this differential diagnosis is achieved by neurologic examination. Because the evaluation and potential treatments for structural and metabolic coma are widely divergent and the disease processes in both categories are often rapidly progressive, initiating prompt medical and surgical evaluation may be life-saving. Identification of a structural versus a metabolic cause is accomplished by focusing on three features of the neurologic examination: the *motor response* to a painful stimulus, *pupillary function*, and *reflex eye movements*.

Motor Response

Asymmetrical or reflex function of the motor system provides the clearest indication of a mass lesion. Elicitation of a *motor response* requires that a painful stimulus be applied, to which the patient will react. The patient's arms should be placed in a semiflexed posture, and a painful stimulus should be applied to the head or trunk. Strong pressure on the supraorbital ridge or pinching of the skin on the anterior chest or inner arm is the most useful method; finger nail bed pressure is also used, but it makes the interpretation of upper limb movement difficult.

The neurologic examination of a patient with an expanding hemispheric mass lesion is shown in Fig. 107.1. Hemispheric masses in their *early diencephalic* stage (i.e., compromising the brain above the thalamus) produce appropriate movement of one upper extremity—that is, movement toward the painful stimulus. The attenuated contralateral arm movement reflects a hemiparesis. This lateralized motor response in a comatose patient establishes the working diagnosis of a hemispheric mass. As the mass expands to involve the thalamus (*late diencephalic* stage), the response to pain becomes reflex arm flexion associated with extension and internal rotation of the legs (*decorticate posturing*); asymmetry of the response in the upper extremities is seen. With further brain compromise at the midbrain level, the reflex posturing in the arms changes such that both arms and legs respond by extension (*decerebrate posturing*); at that level, the asymmetry tends to

TABLE 107.2   Causes of Coma With Normal Computed Tomography Scan

Meningeal disorders
  Subarachnoid hemorrhage (uncommon)
  Bacterial meningitis
  Encephalitis
  Subdural empyema
Exogenous toxins
  Sedative drugs and barbiturates
  Anesthetics and γ-hydroxybutyrate[a]
  Alcohol
  Stimulants
  Phencyclidine[b]
  Cocaine and amphetamine[c]
Psychotropic drugs
  Cyclic antidepressants
  Phenothiazines
  Lithium
  Anticonvulsants
  Opioids
  Clonidine[d]
  Penicillins
  Salicylates
  Anticholinergics
  Carbon monoxide, cyanide, and methemoglobinemia
Endogenous toxins, deficiencies, derangements
  Hypoxia and ischemia
  Hypoglycemia
  Hypercalcemia
Osmolar causes
  Hyperglycemia
  Hyponatremia
  Hypernatremia
Organ system failure
  Hepatic encephalopathy
  Uremic encephalopathy
  Pulmonary insufficiency (carbon dioxide narcosis)
Seizures
  Prolonged postictal state
  Spike-wave stupor
Hypothermia or hyperthermia
Brain stem ischemia
Basilar artery stroke
Pituitary apoplexy
Conversion or malingering

[a]General anesthetic, similar to γ-aminobutyric acid; used as a recreational drug and body building aid. It has a rapid onset and rapid recovery, often with myoclonic jerking and confusion. It causes deep coma lasting 2 to 3 hours (Glasgow Coma Scale score = 3) with maintenance of vital signs.
[b]Coma associated with cholinergic signs: lacrimation, salivation, bronchorrhea, and hyperthermia.
[c]Coma after seizures or status epilepticus (i.e., a prolonged postictal state).
[d]An antihypertensive agent that is active through the opiate receptor system; overdose is frequent when used to treat narcotic withdrawal.

be lost. At this point, the pupils become mid-position in size, and the light reflex is lost, first unilaterally and then bilaterally. With further progression to the level of the pons, the most frequent finding is no response to painful stimulation, although spinal-mediated movements of leg flexion may occur.

TABLE 107.3   Emergency Management

1. Ensure airway adequacy.
2. Support ventilation and circulation.
3. Obtain blood for glucose, electrolytes, hepatic and renal function, prothrombin and partial thromboplastin times, complete blood count, and drug screen.
4. Administer 100 mg of thiamine intravenously (IV).
5. Administer 25 g of dextrose IV (typically 50 mL of 50% dextrose) to treat possible hypoglycemic coma.[a]
6. Treat opiate overdose with naloxone (0.4-2 mg IV repeated every 2-3 minutes as needed).
7. The specific benzodiazepine antagonist flumazenil (0.2 mg IV every 1 min, ×1-5 doses; max is 1 mg) should be given for reversal of benzodiazepine-induced coma or conscious sedation.[b]

[a]The glucose level is poorly correlated with the level of consciousness in hypoglycemia; stupor, coma, and confusion are reported with blood glucose concentrations ranging from 2 to 60 mg/dL.
[b]Not recommended in coma of unknown origin because seizures may be precipitated in patients with polydrug overdoses that include benzodiazepines with tricyclic antidepressants or cocaine.

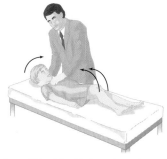

Fig. 107.2 Elicitation of Brudzinski sign of meningeal irritation, as seen in infectious meningitis or subarachnoid hemorrhage. (From Aminoff MJ, Greenberg DA, Simon RP: Clinical neurology, Stamford, Conn., 1996, Appleton and Lange.)

The classic postures illustrated in Fig. 107.1, and particularly their asymmetry, strongly support the presence of a mass lesion. However, these motor movements, especially early in coma, are most frequently seen as fragments of the fully developed, asymmetrical flexion or extension of the arms (illustrated as decorticate and decerebrate postures in Fig. 107.1). A small amount of asymmetrical flexion or extension of the arms in response to a painful stimulus carries the same implications as the full-blown postures of decortication or decerebration.

Metabolic lesions do not compromise the brain in a progressive, level-by-level manner as do hemispheric masses, and they rarely produce the asymmetrical motor signs typical of masses. Reflex posturing may be seen, but it lacks the asymmetry of decortication seen with a hemispheric mass, and it is not associated with the loss of pupillary reactivity at the stage of decerebration.

Pupillary Reactivity

In metabolic coma, one feature is central to the examination: Pupillary reactivity is present. This reactivity is seen both early in metabolic coma, when an appropriate motor response to pain may be retained, and late in coma, when no motor responses can be elicited. The pupillary reaction in metabolic coma is lost only when coma is so deep that the patient requires ventilatory and blood pressure support.

Reflex Eye Movements

The presence of inducible lateral eye movements reflects the integrity of the pons and midbrain. These reflex eye movements (see Fig. 107.1) are brought about with the use of passive head rotation to stimulate the semicircular canal input to the vestibular system (so-called *doll's eyes maneuver*) or by inhibiting the function of one semicircular canal by infusing ice water against the tympanic membrane (caloric testing).

In metabolic coma, reflex eye movements may be lost or retained. Lack of inducible eye movements with the doll's eyes maneuver, in the setting of preserved pupillary reactivity, is virtually diagnostic of drug toxicity. With metabolic coma of non–drug-induced origin, such as organ system failure, electrolyte disorders, or osmolar disorders, reflex eye movements are preserved.

Brain stem mass lesions are most commonly caused by hemorrhage or infarction. Reflex lateral eye movements, the pathways for which traverse the pons and midbrain, are particularly affected, and the reflex postures of decortication and decerebration typical of brain stem injury are common. Lesions restricted to the midbrain (e.g., embolization from the heart to the top of the basilar artery) cause sluggish pupillary reflexes or their absence, with or without impaired medial eye movements; both are controlled by the third cranial nerve. With lesions restricted to the pons (e.g., intrapontine hypertensive hemorrhage), pupils are reactive but very small (pinpoint or pontine pupils), reflecting focal impairment of sympathetic innervations; pinpoint pupils are rare. Ocular bobbing (spontaneous symmetrical or asymmetrical rhythmic vertical ocular oscillations) is most often a manifestation of a pontine lesion.

Seizures occurring in a patient with acute brain injury (such as that resulting from encephalitis, hypertensive encephalopathy, hyponatremia, hypernatremia, hypoglycemia, or hyperglycemia) or chronic brain injury (such as dementia or mental retardation) often result in prolonged postictal coma. The examination shows reactive pupils and inducible eye movements (in the absence of overtreatment with anticonvulsants), and often up-going toes or focal signs are observed (Todd paresis).

Nonconvulsive status epilepticus should be considered as a diagnosis even if there are no obvious seizure movements. Nonconvulsive seizures can cause coma and also can complicate other etiologies of coma, including infectious and metabolic disorders. Nonconvulsive seizures should be suspected in patients with (1) a seemingly prolonged "postictal state" after generalized convulsive seizures or prolonged alteration of alertness after an operative procedure or neurologic insult; (2) acute onset of impaired consciousness or fluctuating mentation interspersed with episodes of normal awareness; (3) altered mental status or consciousness associated with facial myoclonus or nystagmoid eye movements; or (4) episodic blank staring, aphasia, automatisms (e.g., lip-smacking, fumbling with fingers), or acute-onset aphasia without an acute structural lesion. The diagnosis is made by electroencephalography (EEG) (see Chapter 120). EEG provides information about brain electrical activity even when brain function is depressed and cannot be evaluated otherwise, as in comatose patients. EEG is essential to detect electrical seizures and document their duration as well as the response to therapy and to improve coma prognostication.

Current evidence suggests that the presence of nonconvulsive seizures or periodic discharges, delay to diagnosis, and duration of nonconvulsive status in patients with or without acute brain injury are independent predictors of worse outcome.

PROGNOSIS IN COMA AFTER CARDIAC ARREST

Historically, prognostication after cardiac arrest was solely based on neurologic examination. Pupillary, corneal, and motor responses are

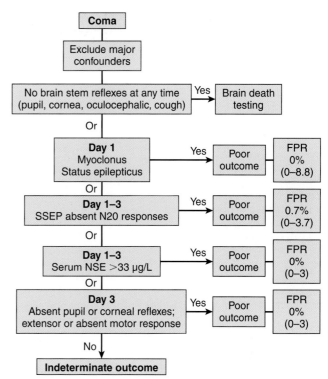

Fig. 107.3 Decision algorithm for use in prognostication of comatose survivors after cardiopulmonary resuscitation (CPR). The numbers in parentheses show the exact 95% confidence intervals. *FPR*, False-positive rate; *N20*, a negative peak at 20 ms on SSEP; *NSE*, neuron-specific enolase; *SSEP*, somatosensory evoked potential. (Data from Wijdicks EFM, Hijdra A, Young GB, et al: Practice parameter: prediction of outcome in comatose survivors after CPR [an evidence-based review]: report of the Quality Standards Subcommittee of the American Academy of Neurology, Neurology 67:203-210, 2006.)

the best clinical indicators of prognosis that can be assessed at bedside. Such responses reflect the functionality of the brain stem, which is the most resilient portion of central nervous system (Fig. 107.3).

Although the neurologic exam is still the cornerstone of prognostication, there has been extensive work using other modalities to better predict prognosis. Current guidelines endorse using EEG to guide prognostication in comatose survivors of cardiac arrest. The absence of normal background activity or reactivity predicts a poor prognosis. Conversely, continuous background activity and the presence of reactivity are among the few reliable predictors of good neurologic recovery. Somatosensory evoked potentials (SSEPs), another electrophysiologic marker of cortical responsiveness, are most helpful for predicting which patients will remain in a persistent coma. By 24 hours after cardiac arrest, bilateral absence of the N20 cortical response (a negative peak at 20 ms) to median nerve stimulation predicts a grave outcome. The early onset of generalized myoclonic status is an ominous sign. Neuron-specific enolase (NSE) is the most promising of several serum biomarkers that have been evaluated. NSE level greater than 30 ng/mL predicts persistent coma. Despite tremendous potential, the role of neuroimaging as a prognostic tool after hypoxic-ischemic injury from cardiac arrest has yet to be clearly defined. Severe reductions in the apparent diffusion coefficient (ADC), as well as bilateral hippocampal hyperintensities on magnetic resonance imaging (MRI), suggest severe global damage and extensive ischemic injury and are predictive of poor neurologic recovery.

Therapeutic hypothermia has been demonstrated to improve neurologic outcomes in patients who have return of spontaneous circulation

TABLE 107.4   Locked-In Syndrome

Clinical features
  Eye opening
  Reactive pupils
  Volitional vertical eye movements in response to command
  Muteness
  Quadriparesis
  Sleep-wake cycles
Causes
  Pontine vascular lesions (common)
  Head injury, brain stem tumor, pontine myelinolysis (rare)
Recovery possible
  Onset over 1-12 wk (vascular)[a] *or*
  Onset over 4-6 mo (nonvascular)[a]
Prognosis favorable
  Normal CT scan[a]
  Early recovery of lateral eye movements[a]

CT, Computed tomography.
[a]Implications for care.

but remain comatose after cardiac arrest. The use of therapeutic hypothermia quite likely influences the clinical examination and ancillary test findings. There are a scarcity of data about the utility of physical examination, EEG, and evoked potentials in predicting outcomes among cardiac arrest patients with induced hypothermia. It is well accepted that one should consider observation for longer than 72 hours before prognosticating outcome in patients treated with hypothermia.

COMA-LIKE STATES

Patients with *locked-in syndrome* have a lesion (usually a hemorrhage or an infarct) that transects the brain stem at a point below the reticular formation (thereby sparing consciousness) but above the ventilatory nuclei of the medulla (thereby maintaining cardiopulmonary function) (Table 107.4). Such patients are awake, with eye opening and sleep-wake cycles, but the descending pathways through the brain stem that are necessary for volitional vocalization or limb movement have been transected. Voluntary eye movement, especially vertically, is preserved, and patients can open and close their eyes or produce appropriate numbers of blinking movements in answer to questions. The EEG is usually normal, reflecting normal cortical function.

Psychogenic unresponsiveness is a diagnosis of exclusion. The neurologic examination shows reactive pupils and no reflex posturing in response to pain. Eye movements during the doll's eyes maneuver show volitional override rather than the smooth, uninhibited reflex lateral eye movements of coma. Ice water caloric testing either arouses the patient because of the discomfort produced or induces cortically mediated nystagmus rather than the tonic deviation typical of coma. The slow, conjugate roving eye movements of metabolic coma cannot be imitated and therefore rule out psychogenic unresponsiveness. Likewise, the slow, often asymmetrical, and incomplete eye closure seen after passive eye opening in a comatose patient cannot be feigned. In contrast, conscious patients usually exhibit some voluntary muscle tone in the eyelids during passive eye opening. The EEG in psychogenic unresponsiveness is that of normal wakefulness, with reactive posterior rhythms on eye opening and eye closing. In patients with catatonic stupor, lorazepam administration may produce awakening.

Unresponsive wakefulness syndrome, previously called vegetative state (VS), is exhibited by patients with eye opening and sleep-wake cycles. The reticular activating system of the brain stem is intact to produce wakefulness, but the connections to the cortical mantle are interrupted, precluding awareness.

A VS is termed *persistent* after 3 months if the brain injury was ischemic in nature or after 12 months if the brain injury was traumatic in nature. The determination as to when *persistent* equals *permanent* cannot be stated absolutely. Prediction early in VS of which patients will remain persistently vegetative is particularly difficult in cases of trauma. Lesions of the corpus callosum and dorsolateral brain stem seen on MRI 6 to 8 weeks after trauma correlated with persistence of VS at 1 year. A combined analysis of morphologic MRI studies and post-traumatic brain stem spectroscopy can be a predictor of persistent vegetative states (PVS) and minimally conscious states (MVS). In rare cases, patients show late improvement, but they do not return to normal. Bilateral absence of SSEPs in the first week predicts death or VS.

Patients in a PVS open their eyes diurnally and in response to loud sounds; blinking occurs with bright lights. Pupils react and eye movements occur both spontaneously and with the doll's eyes maneuver. Yawning, chewing, swallowing, and, uncommonly, guttural vocalizations and lacrimation may be preserved. Spontaneous roving eye movements (very slow, with constant velocity) are particularly characteristic and distressing to the patient's visitors because the patient appears to be looking about the room. The brain stem origin of the eye movements is documented by their being readily redirected by the oculocephalic (doll's eyes) reflex. The limbs may move, but motor responses are only primitive; pain usually produces decorticate or decerebrate postures or fragments of these movements.

Minimally conscious state (MCS) is a newly described entity in which patients do not meet criteria for PVS. Both patients in PVS and those in MCS demonstrate severe alteration in consciousness. In contrast to PVS, subjects with MCS exhibit evidence of limited interaction with the environment by visually tracking, following simple commands, answering yes or no (not necessarily reliably), or having intelligible verbalization or restricted purposeful behavior. It is estimated that the rate of misdiagnosis between the VS and MCS is about 40%.

Novel applications of functional neuroimaging in patients with disorders of consciousness may aid in differential diagnosis, prognostic assessment, and identification of pathophysiologic mechanisms. In one study, authors prospectively evaluated cortical activation in response to a familiar voice in seven patients in VS and four subjects in MCS. All four of the MCS patients and only two of the VS patients showed activation that extended beyond the primary auditory cortex to hierarchically higher-order associative temporal areas. Over the course of 3 months, these two VS patients improved clinically to MCS.

Brain death characterizes the *irreversible cessation* of brain function. Therefore, death of the organism can be determined based on death of the brain. Although local laws may dictate some details, the standard definition permits a diagnosis of brain death based on documentation of irreversible cessation of all brain function, including function of the brain stem (Table 107.5). Documentation of *irreversibility* requires that the cause of the coma is known, that the cause is adequate to explain the clinical findings of brain death, and that exclusionary criteria are absent (Table 107.6). Confirmatory tests are sometimes used but are not required for diagnosis (Table 107.7). Brain death results in asystole, usually within days (mean, 4 days), even if ventilatory support is continued. Recovery after appropriate documentation of brain death has never been reported. Removal of the ventilator results in terminal rhythms (most often complete heart block without ventricular response), junctional rhythms, or ventricular tachycardia. Purely spinal motor movements may occur in the moments of terminal apnea (or during apnea testing in the absence of passive administration of oxygen); these may include arching of the back, neck turning, stiffening of the legs, and upper extremity flexion.

TABLE 107.5 Criteria for Cessation of Brain Function[a]

Anatomic Region Tested	Confirmatory Sign
Hemispheres	Unresponsive and unreceptive to sensory stimuli including pain[b]
Midbrain	Unreactive pupils[c]
Pons	Absent reflex eye movements[d]
Medulla	Apnea[e]

CO_2, Carbon dioxide; Pco_2, partial pressure of carbon dioxide.

[a]Sequential testing is necessary for a clinical diagnosis of brain death; it should be done at least every 6 hours in all cases and at least every 24 hours in the setting of anoxic-ischemic brain injury.

[b]The patient does not rouse, groan, grimace, or withdraw limbs. Purely spinal reflexes (deep tendon reflexes, plantar flexion reflex, plantar withdrawal, and tonic neck reflexes) may be maintained.

[c]Most easily assessed by the bright light of an ophthalmoscope viewed through its magnifying lens when focused on the iris. Unreactive pupils may be either midposition, as they will be in death, or dilated, as they often are in the setting of a dopamine infusion.

[d]No eye movement toward the side of irrigation of the tympanic membrane with 50 mL of ice water. The oculocephalic response (doll's eyes maneuver) is always absent in the setting of absent oculovestibular testing.

[e]No ventilatory movements in the setting of maximum CO_2 stimulation (≥60 mm Hg); with apnea, Pco_2 passively rises 2 to 3 mm Hg/min). Disconnect the ventilator from the endotracheal tube and insert a cannula with 6 L of oxygen per minute.

TABLE 107.6 Exclusionary Criteria for Brain Death

Seizures
Decorticate or decerebrate posturing
Sedative drugs
Hypothermia (<32.2° C)
Neuromuscular blockade
Shock

TABLE 107.7 Confirmatory Tests for Brain Death

EEG isoelectricity	Deep coma from sedative drugs or hypothermia (temperature <20° C) can produce EEG flattening.
Nuclear medicine	The most common radionuclide modality for brain imaging uses the tracer HMPAO. Absence of isotope uptake ("hollow skull phenomenon") indicates no brain perfusion and supports the diagnosis of brain death.
Transcranial Doppler	Findings of small systolic peaks without diastolic flow or a reverberating flow pattern suggest high vascular resistance and support the diagnosis of brain death. No cerebral blood flow is the most definitive confirmatory test.
CT angiography	Nonopacification of the cortical segments of MCAs and ICVs appears to be highly sensitive for confirming brain death, with a specificity of 100%. Lack of opacification of the ICVs is the most sensitive sign.

CT, Computed tomographic; EEG, electroencephalogram; HMPAO, 99mTc-labeled hexamethylpropyleneamine oxime; ICV, internal cerebral vein; MCA, middle cerebral artery.

SUGGESTED READINGS

Bernard SA, Gray TW, Buist MD, et al: Treatment of comatose survivors of out-of-hospital cardiac arrest with induced hypothermia, N Engl J Med 346:557–563, 2002.

Bernat JL: Chronic disorders of consciousness, Lancet 367:1181–1192, 2006.

Fins JJ, Master MG, Gerber LM, et al: The minimally conscious state: a diagnosis in search of an epidemiology, Arch Neurol 64:1400–1405, 2007.

Greer DM, Scripko PD, Wu O, et al: Hippocampal magnetic resonance imaging abnormalities in cardiac arrest are associated with poor outcome, J Stroke Cerebrovasc Dis 22:899–905, 2013.

Laureys S, Celesia GG, Cohadon F, et al: Unresponsive wakefulness syndrome: a new name for the vegetative state or apallic syndrome, BMC Med 8:68, 2010.

Laureys S, Schiff ND: Coma and consciousness: paradigms (re)framed by neuroimaging, Neuroimage 61(2):478–491, 2012.

Meaney PA, Bobrow BJ, Mancini ME: Cardiopulmonary resuscitation quality: improving cardiac resuscitation outcomes both inside and outside the hospital–a consensus statement from the American Heart Association, Circulation 124:417–435, 2013.

Peberdy MA, Callaway CW, Neumar RW, et al: Cardiac arrest care: 2010 American Heart Association guidelines for cardiopulmonary resuscitation and emergency cardiovascular care, Circulation 122(18 Suppl 3):S768–S786, 2010. [Errata in Circulation 123:e237, 2011, and Circulation 124:e403, 2011.].

Plum F, Posner JB: The diagnosis of stupor and coma. Contemporary Neurology Series, vol. 71, ed 3, New York, 2007, Oxford University Press.

Rodriguez RA, Nair S, Bussiere M, et al: Long-lasting functional disabilities in patients who recover from coma after cardiac operations, Ann Thorac Surg 95:884–891, 2013.

Rossetti AO, Rabinstein AA, Oddo ML: Neurological prognostication of outcome in patients in coma after cardiac arrest, Lancet Neurol 15(6):597–609, 2016.

Wijdicks EFM: The diagnosis of brain death, N Engl J Med 344:1215–1221, 2001.

Wijdicks EFM, Hijdra A, Young GB, et al: Practice parameter: prediction of outcome in comatose survivors after cardiopulmonary resuscitation (an evidence-based review), Neurology 67:203–210, 2006.

Wu O, Soresnen AG, Benner T, et al: Comatose patients with cardiac arrest: predicting clinical outcome with diffusion-weighted MR imaging, Radiology 252:173–181, 2009.

Young GB: Neurologic prognosis after cardiac arrest, N Engl J Med 361:605–611, 2009.

Zandbergen EGJ, Hijdra A, Koelman JH, et al: Prediction of poor outcome within the first 3 days of postanoxic coma, Neurology 66:62–68, 2006.

108

Disorders of Sleep

Sagarika Nallu, Selim R. Benbadis

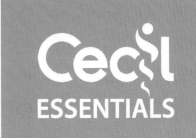

INTRODUCTION

The *International Classification of Sleep Disorders* (ICSD-3) groups disorders with sleep into six major categories: insomnia, sleep-related breathing disorders, central disorders of hypersomnolence, circadian rhythm sleep-wake disorders, parasomnias, and sleep-related movement disorders. From a practical point of view, sleep disorders are better classified by their clinical presentation, which is the approach taken here. This chapter focuses on primary sleep disorders rather than sleep disturbances that result from self-evident medical or psychiatric diseases.

DISORDERS OF EXCESSIVE DAYTIME SLEEPINESS

History and Examination

Evaluating patients with sleep disorders should include a thorough sleep history and physical examination that includes the respiratory, cardiovascular, and neurologic symptoms. The majority of the patients with sleep disorders present with excessive daytime somnolence (EDS) as their chief symptom. A careful history is the starting point and often uncovers the likely causes (e.g., insufficient sleep time with sleep deprivation, lifestyles, circadian rhythm disorders, medications, systemic illnesses). Most of these causes do not require any diagnostic interventions. To subjectively quantify EDS, various scales have been developed. The most validated and useful in the clinical practice is the Epworth Sleepiness Scale (ESS). The ESS consists of a brief questionnaire on the likelihood of dozing off in eight situations. This yields a score between 0 and 24 (Table 108.1). Scores of 10 or above warrant investigation.

Sleep Studies

Polysomnography (PSG) is an all-night sleep study that measures multiple parameters such as sleep staging, respiration, leg movements, and electrocardiographic patterns. The limited channel sleep monitoring version is also called portable home sleep testing (HST) and is used in patients with high probability of obstructive sleep apnea (OSA). The multiple sleep latency test (MSLT) and the maintenance of wakefulness test (MWT) are used to measure and quantify EDS. They consist of a series of daytime naps during which sleep latency is measured and sleep stages are determined. MSLT must be performed with a prior night PSG.

SLEEP-DISORDERED BREATHING

Definition and Epidemiology

Sleep-disordered breathing encompasses a spectrum of chronic conditions in which partial or complete cessation of breathing occurs multiple times throughout sleep. This group includes the most common disorders: OSA, central sleep apnea, and sleep-related hypoventilation.

Respiratory events are classified as apneas and hypopneas; apneas are further subdivided into obstructive, central or mixed. Obstructive apneas are episodes of complete upper airway collapse, defined as a greater than 90% drop in the airflow/thermal sensor in the presence of continued respiratory effort lasting at least 10 seconds. Hypopnea is defined as a 30% or more drop in the nasal pressure signal lasting for at least 10 seconds, associated with a 3% or more oxygen desaturation or an arousal. In contrast, central apnea is defined as a greater than 90% drop in the airflow/thermal sensor accompanied by absent respiratory effort that lasts for at least 10 seconds. The severity of sleep apnea is based on the polysomnographic scoring and is defined by the apnea-hypopnea index (AHI), a ratio of the sum of all respiratory events to the total hours of sleep on the PSG or HST.

The estimated prevalence rates of obstructive sleep apnea have increased substantially over the last two decades, most likely due to the obesity epidemic. It is now estimated that 26% of adults between the ages of 30 and 70 years have sleep apnea.

Pathophysiology

The pathophysiology of OSA is recurrent upper airway closure/collapse with resulting oxygen desaturation leading to arousals. The sleep fragmentation caused by arousal is responsible for sleep deprivation and EDS.

Clinical Manifestation

OSA patients typically present with at least one of these symptoms: snoring, waking up with gasping/choking or witnessed apneas in sleep by their bed partners. EDS, nonrestorative sleep, fatigue, and insomnia also have comorbid conditions such as hypertension, coronary artery disease (CAD), mood disorders, cognitive dysfunction or type 2 diabetes. Risk factors for OSA are both modifiable and nonmodifiable. Modifiable risk factors include sedative medication, alcohol, tobacco use, obesity, endocrine disorders (e.g., hypothyroidism, polycystic ovary syndrome, acromegaly) and nasal obstruction/congestion. Nonmodifiable factors include genetic predisposition, craniofacial anomalies and congenital syndromes (e.g., Down, Pierre Robin, and Treacher Collins syndromes).

Treatment and Prognosis

Depending on the severity, treatment modalities of OSA include positive airway pressure therapy (PAP), oral appliance therapy, surgical modifications of upper airway, weight loss, and positional measures to prevent sleeping supine (positional therapy). Initial treatment of OSA requires close monitoring and early identification of difficulties with PAP use (including troubleshooting and monitoring of objective efficacy and usage data to ensure adequate treatment and adherence). Success over the first few days to weeks has been shown to predict long-term adherence.

TABLE 108.1 Epworth Sleepiness Scale

How likely are you to doze off or fall asleep in the following situations in contrast to just feeling tired? The situations refer to your usual way of life. Even if you have not done some of these things recently, try to work out how they would have affected you. Use the following scale to choose the most appropriate number for each situation.

0 = would never doze
1 = slight chance of dozing
2 = moderate chance of dozing
3 = high chance of dozing

What is your chance of dozing in the following situations?

Sitting and reading	_____
Watching TV	_____
Sitting and inactive in a public place (theater or meeting)	_____
As a passenger in a car for an hour without a break	_____
Lying down to rest in the afternoon when possible	_____
Sitting and talking to someone	_____
Sitting quietly after lunch (without alcohol)	_____
In a car while stopped for a few minutes in traffic	_____
Total	_____

Modified from Johns MW: A new method for measuring daytime sleepiness: the Epworth Sleepiness Scale, Sleep 14:540-545, 1991.

TABLE 108.2 Agents Promoting Wakefulness

Drug	Dose Range (mg)
Amphetamine (Dexedrine, Desoxyn, Adderall, Adderall XR)	5-60
Methylphenidate (Ritalin, Metadate, Methylin, Concerta)	10-60
Modafinil (Provigil)	200-400
Armodafinil	150-250

Central sleep apnea (CSA) is seen in a variety of settings, including periodic breathing in infancy, healthy adults at altitude, and Cheyne-Stokes respirations in heart failure. In most cases of CSA, the cyclic absence of effort is a paradoxical consequence of hypersensitive ventilatory chemo reflex responses that oppose changes in airflow, producing elevated loop gain and leading to overshoot/undershoot ventilatory oscillations. Therapies for CSA affect loop gain by improving lung volumes (PAP therapy), reducing the alveolar-inspired Pco_2 difference (stimulants) and lowering chemosensitivity (supplemental oxygen). CSA is further differentiated by a hypercapnic (e.g., brain stem lesions, opioids, obesity hypoventilation syndrome, congenital central alveolar hypoventilation syndrome, neuromuscular disorders, chest wall deformities) or hypocapnic response (e.g., Cheyne-Stokes respiration).

NARCOLEPSY

Narcolepsy is a complex sleep disorder that can manifest in childhood or adolescence. It is the most common cause of excessive daytime sleepiness and can occur in isolation or in combination with other symptoms such as cataplexy, hypnogogic/hypnopompic hallucinations, disturbed nocturnal sleep, and sleep paralysis. Cataplexy distinguishes type 1 (narcolepsy with cataplexy) from type 2 narcolepsy (narcolepsy without cataplexy). Cataplexy is reported by 60% to 75% of patients with narcolepsy and is defined as a transient, sudden-onset loss of skeletal muscle tone with retained consciousness. It is often in seen in response to a strong emotion (e.g., laughter, startle, anger). Hypnagogic or hypnopompic hallucinations are vivid, dreamlike sensations that an individual feels, hears or sees and that occur near the onset of sleep (hypnogogic) or upon waking up from sleep (hypnopompic). Sleep paralysis is defined as temporary inability to move or speak while being conscious and that occurs when a person is falling asleep or waking up from sleep.

Pathophysiology

Genetic and environmental factors reportedly play a role in the etiology of narcolepsy. Evidence suggests that the loss of hypocretin is highly associated with its development. Hypocretin, a neuropeptide found in the lateral and posterior hypothalamus, targets monoaminergic and cholinergic areas. The loss of hypocretin neurons results in characteristic symptoms of narcolepsy including the inability to sustain long periods of wakefulness and frequent lapses into sleep. Evidence suggests a link between HLA DQB1*06:02 and narcolepsy, indicating an autoimmune basis for narcolepsy that is mediated by hypocretin neurons.

Diagnosis and Differential Diagnosis

Diagnosis of narcolepsy requires a detailed clinical history and diagnostic studies such as an overnight PSG followed by an MSLT. An MSLT with sleep latency of 8 minutes or less and two or more sleep-onset REM periods and the exclusion of other sleep disorders on PSG provide a definitive diagnosis of narcolepsy. The PSG performed the night prior to MSLT is important for excluding other primary sleep disorders such as sleep apnea and periodic limb movement disorder. Abnormal MSLT findings are not specific for narcolepsy and may be produced by other sleep disorders such as sleep apnea, circadian misalignment, other mental or medical conditions, medications or substance use or sleep deprivation. An alternative criterion for diagnosis is a CSF hypocretin level 110 pg/mL or less.

Treatment

Narcolepsy treatment includes a multimodal approach with both nonpharmacologic and pharmacologic components. Pharmacologic therapy includes stimulant therapy, which aims to improve alertness and functioning (Table 108.2). Wake-promoting medications such as modafinil and armodafinil are considered first-line therapy for excessive daytime sleepiness. Sodium oxybate (Xyrem), a precursor for GABA, is the only treatment for cataplexy that has been approved by the FDA. Tricyclic antidepressants (e.g., clomipramine), selective serotonin reuptake inhibitors (e.g., fluoxetine), and serotonin and norepinephrine reuptake inhibitors (e.g., venlafaxine) have all been used to treat cataplexy. Nonpharmacologic treatments include scheduled brief naps, practicing good sleep hygiene, and regular exercise during the day to improve alertness.

IDIOPATHIC HYPERSOMNIA

Definition and Epidemiology

Idiopathic hypersomnia (IH) is a chronic neurologic disorder that manifests as pathologic daytime sleepiness with or without prolonged sleep durations. Etiology of IH is presently unknown, although a genetic predisposition is suggested by the strong family history of similar symptoms. Patients report unrefreshed (i.e., sleep inertia) nocturnal sleep and long daytime naps, and they can have prolonged states of fogginess despite long sleep hours (i.e., sleep drunkenness).

Diagnosis and Differential Diagnosis

Diagnosis of IH involves a careful history, with particular attention to the possibility of other disorders with similar symptomatology, and objective testing with sleep studies. Other causes of EDS must be excluded, and the PSG should be normal with no sleep-disordered breathing. MSLT confirms sleep latency of less than 8 minutes but without sleep-onset REM.

Treatment and Prognosis

There are no FDA-approved treatments for IH symptoms, which are typically treated with off-label use of medications approved for narcolepsy.

KLEINE-LEVIN SYNDROME

Kleine-Levin syndrome is a rare, recurrent or cyclic hypersomnia with a prevalence of 1 case per 1 million people. Its cause is unknown. Its onset is usually in the second decade of life.

These episodes of hypersomnia are also associated with other symptoms including hyperphagia, hypersexuality, confusion and hallucinations. Episodes can last days to weeks and reoccur every few months, and at least once a year. Lithium is the choice of medication along with other stimulants and wake-promoting agents (see Table 108.2).

Other symptomatic causes of EDS must be excluded. With time, episodes tend to become less severe, less prolonged, and less frequent.

RESTLESS LEGS SYNDROME, PERIODIC LIMB MOVEMENTS IN SLEEP, AND PERIODIC LIMB MOVEMENT DISORDER

Restless legs syndrome (RLS), also known as Willis-Ekbom disease, is a common neurologic sensorimotor disorder that manifests as an irresistible urge to move the body to relieve the uncomfortable sensations. These sensations always occur during resting, sitting or sleeping. Symptoms commonly worsen at night, causing difficulties with initiating sleep. It is more prevalent in females, and a family history of RLS was detected in 90.9% of the patients with RLS, indicating high heritability.

Periodic limb movements in sleep (PLMS) are polysomnographic findings and are characterized by stereotypical jerks lasting between 0.5 to 10 seconds and occurring at 15- to 40-second intervals. PLMS are present in approximately 80% of patients with RLS. A periodic limb movement index of 15 or greater, when associated with a sleep complaint not accountable by any other sleep disorder, may suggest a periodic limb movement disorder (PLMD).

Clinical Manifestations

Leg movements may be reported by the bed partner, and the patient may report EDS, insomnia, or symptoms of RLS (i.e., urge to move legs or walk due to unpleasant "creepy-crawly" sensations at rest). Most patients with RLS have PLMD, but the reverse is not true.

Treatment and Prognosis

The management of RLS and PLMD involves both nonpharmacologic and pharmacologic approaches. Secondary causes that can aggravate both RLS and PLMD symptoms should be investigated, which includes polyneuropathy, spinal cord disease, pregnancy, iron and B_{12} deficiencies, uremia, sleep deprivation, irregular sleep schedules, caffeine, nicotine, alcohol, and certain medications (e.g., antihistamines, serotonergic antidepressants, neuroleptics).

Dopamine agonists and alpha2delta calcium-channel ligands are considered first-line treatments, but these treatments have very

TABLE 108.3	Treatments for Restless Legs Syndrome	
Drug	**Dose Range (mg)**
Levodopa or carbidopa (Sinemet)	50-200
Ropinirole (Requip)	0.25-4.0
Pramipexole (Mirapex)	0.125-0.5
Rotigotine (Neupro) transdermal patch	1-3

different side effect profiles that should be taken into consideration. Doses of dopamine agonists used for RLS treatment are much lower than typical doses in patients with Parkinson's disease and are timed to be taken approximately 2 hours before typical symptom onset. The starting dose of ropinirole is 0.25 mg/d, then is titrated as follows: 0.25 mg for 2 days, then 0.5 mg for 5 days, then may increase by 0.5-mg increments every week until an effective or maximum dose is achieved, whichever comes first. Doses above 4 mg/d should be avoided in patients with RLS whenever possible. The pramipexole starting dose is 0.125 mg/d, and it may be increased by 0.125-mg increments every 4 to 7 days until symptom control or maximum dose is reached. The maximum recommended RLS dose of pramipexole is 0.75 mg/d (although this is an expert consensus recommendation that differs from the FDA labeling of 0.5 mg/d). Rotigotine is the only dopamine agonist that is dosed via daily transdermal patch, which is initiated at 1 mg/d, and may be escalated to 2 mg/d or 3 mg/d in increments of 1 mg/d every week (Table 108.3).

For a deeper discussion of these topics, please see Chapter 382, "Other Movement Disorders," in *Goldman-Cecil Medicine*, 26th Edition.

INSOMNIA

Definition and Epidemiology

Insomnia is the most common sleep complaint in the United States, affecting as many as 30 million people in the general population. A diagnosis of insomnia can be present either with or without a comorbid mental or physical disorder. Insomnia is defined as persistent difficulty with sleep initiation, duration, and consolidation, or sleep quality that occurs despite adequate opportunity and circumstances for sleep, and results in some form of daytime impairment. Individuals who report these sleep-related symptoms in the absence of daytime impairment are not regarded as having insomnia disorder that warrants clinical attention other than education and reassurance. The three diagnostic categories for insomnia include chronic insomnia, short-term insomnia, and other insomnia disorder.

Pathophysiology

Acute or short-term insomnia is caused by identifiable factors and can become a chronic, persistent problem. Chronic insomnia results from predisposing (genetic), precipitating (environmental), and perpetuating (behaviors) factors. With the exception of rare conditions such as the prion disease of fatal familial insomnia, insomnia alone is almost never the symptom of a neurologic disease.

Clinical Manifestations

Insomnia may manifest as the inability to fall asleep (i.e., onset insomnia) or to stay asleep (i.e., maintenance insomnia). In addition to nighttime symptoms, the diagnosis demands daytime symptoms considered to be the consequence of insomnia (e.g., fatigue, EDS, poor concentration, altered mood, headache).

TABLE 108.4 Sleep Hygiene

1. Maintain a regular schedule each day.
2. Wake at the same time each morning.
3. Exposure to natural light entrains the circadian rhythm.
4. Exercise in the morning or early afternoon; avoid vigorous exercise in the evening.
5. Avoid napping during the day, especially after 3 PM.
6. Avoid stimulants such as caffeine and nicotine and avoid alcohol close to bedtime.
7. Avoid large meals close to bedtime.
8. Maintain regular and relaxing routines at bedtime.
9. Maintain a comfortable sleep environment.
10. Reserve the bed for sleep; avoid other activities (e.g., TV, radio, reading).
11. Sleep only when sleepy.
12. Try to resolve worries (or list for future thought) before sleeping.
13. Get out of bed if not sleeping in 20 minutes.

Adjustment insomnia is an acute reaction to some type of stress. When the trigger combines with a propensity for poor or fragile sleep, the condition can become chronic (>1 month) and lead to maladaptive behaviors and a conditioned arousal associated with sleep. This is known as *psychophysiologic insomnia,* and it is by far the most common insomnia syndrome. A vicious cycle is created by poor sleep habits that worsen the insomnia. Because of its chronicity, it is typically associated with poor sleep habits, multiple treatment trials, and anxiety about sleep. If there was no trigger at onset, there may be a lifelong history of poor sleep (i.e., idiopathic insomnia) with the same end result of psychophysiologic insomnia.

Paradoxical insomnia and *sleep-state misperception* are terms applied to patients who claim to not sleep. However, when studied objectively, they have normal sleep amounts and architecture.

Diagnosis and Differential Diagnosis

The diagnosis is based on the history, which should include a sleep diary. Identifiable medical, psychiatric, or drug-related disease and other sleep disorders (e.g., OSA) require exclusion. Sleep studies (PSG and MSLT) are occasionally helpful.

Treatment and Prognosis

Nondrug treatments include commonsense sleep hygiene recommendations (e.g., avoiding caffeine, exercising late in the day) (Table 108.4) and behavior modifications to avoid the conditioned arousal responses associated with sleep (e.g., using the bedroom only for sleep and sex). Other strategies include cognitive behavior therapy specifically for insomnia (CBT-I), relaxation techniques, biofeedback, and behavioral changes such as sleep restriction therapy and stimulus control therapy.

The principles of the pharmacologic treatment of insomnia include using the lowest effective dose, intermittent (not daily) use, using the appropriate (i.e., short or intermediate half-life) drug based on the type of insomnia (i.e., onset or maintenance), and limiting the duration of treatment. Treatment should be tapered to avoid rebound. Medications should be used only in combination with nondrug (i.e., behavioral) treatments. Behavioral treatment has been effective.

Over-the-counter sleep aids (usually antihistamines) are typically safe, but use is limited by anticholinergic and hangover effects. Melatonin may promote sleep and be used for circadian rhythm disorders, including jet lag. The selective melatonin agonist ramelteon is helpful for sleep-onset insomnia.

Prognosis is usually good with the combination of drug and nondrug treatments. Behavior modification may be limited by the willingness of patients to participate.

PARASOMNIAS

Parasomnias are undesirable phenomena that occur in sleep or during transition to or from sleep. They may occur in REM or NREM sleep. They usually consist of complex and seemingly purposeful behaviors, sometimes dramatic, of which the patient is not aware. They are often classified by the sleep stage in which they arise.

NREM Parasomnias

NREM-related parasomnias include confusional arousals, sleep walking (somnambulism), and sleep terrors (pavor nocturnus), and arise as a result of incomplete arousals from deep sleep. They tend to begin in childhood and a family history of similar symptoms is common. The events usually occur during the first third of sleep when delta sleep predominates. Episodes are often triggered by precipitants such as intercurrent illness, sleep deprivation, alcohol use, and stress. Sleep walking episodes typically begin as confusional arousals. These patients often start with sitting up in bed and looking about in a confused manner. Sleep terrors differ from sleep walking in that episodes are more dramatic, with abrupt arousal, a scream or cry and autonomic hyperactivity (e.g., mydriasis, diaphoresis, flushing, piloerection, tachycardia). The child appears terrified and is inconsolable.

Diagnosis and Differential Diagnosis

The main differential diagnosis is nocturnal seizures, which requires video-monitored electroencephalogram (EEG) for diagnosis. Nocturnal seizures tend to be more stereotyped than parasomnias, and they often include tonic or clonic motor activity. Treatment consists of reassurances and measures to avoid injuries during these episodes. Other sleep disorders such as OSA can precipitate these episodes and should be ruled out as part of the treatment. For severe episodes with injurious behaviors, low-dose benzodiazepines such as clonazepam are often recommended.

Treatment and Prognosis

Reassurance and measures to avoid injuries usually are sufficient. For episodes with injurious behaviors, low-dose benzodiazepines (clonazepam, 0.5 to 1 mg) are often effective. Prognosis is good, and most patients do not require treatment.

Rapid Eye Movement Behavior Disorder
Definition and Epidemiology

REM behavior disorder (RBD) is a disorder of REM sleep regulation in which there is a dissociation of REM features with loss of the muscle atonia, leading to patients acting out their dreams. RBD typically affects patients after the age of 50 (usually older) and the male-to-female ratio is 10:1.

Pathophysiology

REM inhibition is lost due to bilateral degeneration of REM atonic neurons in the pons. RBD occurs with α-synucleinopathies (i.e., Parkinson's disease, multiple system atrophy, and dementia with Lewy bodies), and RBD typically heralds these neurodegenerative diseases, sometimes by 10 to 15 years.

Clinical Manifestations

Typically, the episodes are reported by the bed partner and consist of high-amplitude, flailing, injurious behaviors during sleep. When awakened, the patient typically recalls the dream. As is typical of REM arousals, the patient is alert and coherent immediately (unlike slow-wave sleep arousal). Medications, especially psychotropics, can exacerbate RBD.

Diagnosis and Differential Diagnosis

The diagnosis can usually be made by the history alone, and PSG is not needed. When performed, PSG shows a lack of REM atonia or increased phasic and tonic REM. Like slow-wave parasomnias, the main differential diagnosis is nocturnal seizure, and this occasionally requires epilepsy monitoring. Home video (cell phone) recordings can be useful.

Treatment and Prognosis

Low-dose clonazepam (0.5 to 2 mg) is usually effective. Symptoms initially respond to treatment, but a neurodegenerative disease is likely to become evident.

❖   For a deeper discussion of these topics, please see Chapter 377, "Sleep Disorders," in *Goldman-Cecil Medicine*, 26th Edition.

SUGGESTED READINGS

Berry RB, Wagner MH: Sleep medicine pearls, ed 3, 2014, Elsevier/Saunders.

Ebisawa T: Analysis of the molecular pathophysiology of sleep disorders relevant to a disturbed biological clock, Mol Genet Genomics 288:185–193, 2013.

Handbook of sleep disorders. In Thorpy MJ, editor: Neurological disease and therapy, New York, 1990, Taylor & Francis.

International Classification of Sleep Disorders: ed 3, Darien, IL USA, 2014, American Academy of Sleep Medicine.

Kryger MH, Rosenberg R, Kirsch D: Kryger's sleep medicine review E-Book: a problem-oriented approach, ed 3, 2019, Elsevier.

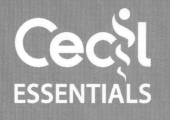

109

Cortical Syndromes

Sinéad M. Murphy, Timothy J. Counihan

FUNCTIONAL ANATOMY

The cerebral cortex consists of two hemispheres connected by a large band of white matter fibers, the *corpus callosum.* Each hemisphere consists of four anatomically and functionally distinct regions: the frontal, temporal, parietal, and occipital lobes (Fig. 109.1). It is worth considering in some detail the regional functionality of specific brain regions, as they can provide valuable localizing information in assessing patients with cerebral dysfunction syndromes.

- Frontal Lobe: Motor control of the opposite side of the body, attention, executive function, social cognition, language production
- Temporal Lobe: Memory, emotion, speech comprehension
- Parietal Lobe: Sensation for the opposite side of the body, spatial perception
- Occipital Lobe: Vision

Although the two cerebral hemispheres share a number of behavioral and sensorimotor tasks, certain functions, particularly language, manual dexterity, and visuospatial perception are strongly lateralized to one hemisphere. Language function is lateralized to the left hemisphere in 95% of the population; although 15% of people are left-handed, the right hemisphere is dominant for language in only about 10%. Visuospatial perception is largely a function of the right (nondominant) hemisphere. On either side of the central sulcus lie the pre- and post-central gyri; in these regions, cortical representations of the different parts of the body are arranged as the motor (frontal lobe) and sensory (parietal lobe) homunculi (Fig. 109.2). It is worth noting that the juxtaposition of facial and hand representation in the homunculus accounts for the facio-brachial predominant pattern of weakness in syndromes affecting the cerebral lateral convexity such as is seen in many patients with ischemic stroke. Similarly, motor or sensory signs confined to the lower extremities may suggest a parasagittal lesion.

CLINICAL ASSESSMENT

Although lesions in specific regions of the cerebral cortex can result in well-defined syndromes, it is important to be aware of potential pitfalls in interpreting symptoms and signs of cortical origin.

- Patients with lesions of the nondominant hemisphere are often unaware of the extent of their deficit.
- Symptoms and signs caused by cortical lesions may be less consistent than deficits caused by lesions of the spinal cord or more peripheral nerves.

REGIONAL SYNDROMES

Table 109.1 summarizes some of the more common syndromes associated with damage to individual cerebral lobes.

Aphasia

Aphasia or *dysphasia* refers to a loss or impairment of language function as a result of damage to the specific language centers of the dominant hemisphere. It is distinct from dysarthria, which is a disturbance in the articulation of speech. The principal types of aphasia are summarized in Table 109.2.

Clinical assessment for aphasia requires testing of fluency, comprehension, repetition, naming, reading, calculation, and writing. *Anomia* refers to difficulty in the naming of objects. Patients may

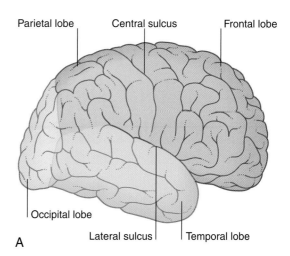

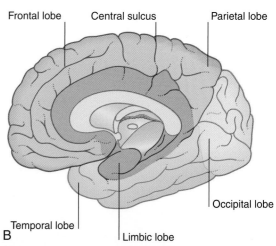

Fig. 109.1 Lateral (A) and medial (B) views of the cerebral hemispheres. (From FitzGerald MJT, editor: Clinical neuroanatomy and neuroscience, ed 6, Philadelphia, 2011, Saunders, Fig. 2-1.)

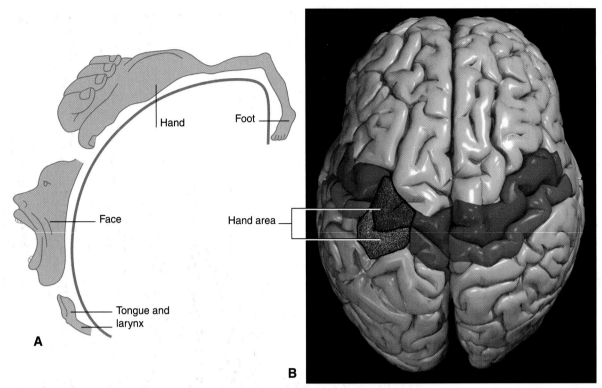

Fig. 109.2 (A) Homuncular arrangement shows the correlations with the primary motor cortex lying anterior to the central sulcus and the somatosensory cortex posteriorly (B). (Modified from Kretschmann HJ, Weinrich W: Neurofunctional systems: 3D reconstructions with correlated neuroimaging: text and CD-ROM, New York, 1998, Thieme.)

TABLE 109.1 Cortical Syndromes and Their Localization

Function	Location	Clinical Signs
Frontal Lobe		
Executive function	Dorsolateral prefrontal cortex	Motor sequencing
Motor function	Primary motor cortex (prefrontal gyrus)	Contralateral weakness
Language	Broca area (inferior frontal cortex)	Expressive aphasia
Behavior	Cingulate (medial frontal lobe)	Obsessive-compulsive traits
	Orbitofrontal	Disinhibition apathy
Oculomotor (frontal eye fields)	Middle frontal gyrus	Forced contralateral eye deviation
Temporal Lobe		
Hearing	Superior temporal gyrus	Auditory hallucinations
Smell	Uncus of temporal lobe	Olfactory hallucinations
Emotion	Amygdala of temporal lobe	Irrational fear
Memory	Hippocampus (medial temporal lobe)	Amnesia; déjà vu
Language	Posterior superior temporal lobe	Wernicke aphasia
Parietal Lobe		
Sensation	Post-central gyrus	Contralateral sensory loss
Visuo-spatial	Posterior parietal lobe	Constructional apraxia
Language	Inferior parietal lobe	Gerstmann syndrome (acalculia, finger agnosia, agraphia, left-right disorientation)
Occipital Lobe		
Vision	Calcarine cortex of occipital lobe	Cortical blindness; visual hallucinations; contralateral homonymous hemianopia

TABLE 109.2   Principal Types of Aphasia

Type	Lesion Site	Fluency	Comprehension	Repetition	Naming	Other Signs
Broca (expressive)	Inferior frontal lobe	↓	Good	↓	↓	Contralateral weakness
Wernicke (receptive)	Posterior superior temporal lobe	Good	↓	↓	↓	Homonymous hemianopia
Transcortical motor	Inferior frontal gyrus	↓	Good	Good	May be normal	May be contralateral weakness
Transcortical sensory	Middle temporal gyrus, thalamus	Good	↓	Good	Usually normal	May be normal
Conduction	Supramarginal gyrus	Good	Good	↓	↓	None
Global	Frontal lobe (large)	↓	↓	↓	↓	Hemiplegia

↓, Reduced.

have difficulty with the correct identification of common items such as a watch, often using a word that either sounds like the intended word ("a spotch"—a literal paraphasic error) or a word with a broadly similar meaning ("a clock"—a semantic paraphasic error). There are two broad types of aphasia depending on the anatomic site of the lesion: anterior (Broca) aphasia and posterior (Wernicke) aphasia.

Broca aphasia is characterized by a severe disruption in the fluency of speech, with profound impairments of expression in both speech and writing. Comprehension may be mildly affected. The language disturbance is almost invariably accompanied by contralateral face and arm weakness as a result of the proximity of the motor homunculus to the Broca speech area in the inferior frontal lobe.

Wernicke aphasia is characterized by an inability to comprehend spoken or written language. Affected patients speak fluently, but the content is meaningless. The lesion is located in the posterior superior temporal area and may be associated with a homonymous hemianopic visual field deficit.

Conduction aphasia is characterized by normal comprehension and fluent speech but a striking inability to repeat a phrase. The responsible lesion lies in the arcuate fasciculus connecting the Broca and Wernicke areas. *Global aphasia* results from large lesions of the frontal lobe; all aspects of language are affected. Lesions of the language areas of the nondominant hemisphere result in *dysprosody*. For instance, patients with lesions in the inferior frontal lobe of the nondominant hemisphere, analogous to the Broca area, speak with a monotonous voice, losing the ability to add emotional cadence to their speech. Similarly, lesions affecting the nondominant Wernicke area result in patients failing to pick up on the emotional inflexions (such as anger) of what is said to them.

Writing is almost invariably affected in patients with disturbances of language (Fig. 109.3). An exception to this occurs in the syndrome of *alexia without agraphia*, which results from a lesion in the dominant occipital lobe and splenium of the corpus callosum (usually caused by infarction in the territory of the posterior cerebral artery). The patient's language center is "disconnected" from the contralateral (unaffected) visual cortex. Such patients can write a sentence but are unable to read what they have written.

Agnosia and Apraxia

Agnosia is the inability to recognize a specific sensory stimulus despite preserved sensory function. For instance, visual agnosia is the inability to recognize a visual stimulus despite normal visual acuity. Other agnosia syndromes include the inability to recognize sounds (auditory agnosia), color (color agnosia), or familiar faces (prosopagnosia). Usually, the responsible lesions are located in the occipitotemporal region.

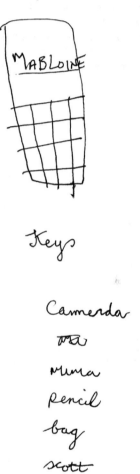

Fig. 109.3 Neologisms written by a patient with aphasia who was attempting to name cell phone, keys, camera, watch, pen, bag, and boots.

Apraxia refers to an inability to perform learned motor tasks despite sufficient sensorimotor function to physically execute the movement; it is a disorder of motor planning (Fig. 109.4). The responsible lesions are usually in the dominant inferior parietal lobe. A simple test of apraxia is to ask the patient to perform a pantomime (e.g., combing the hair, blowing out a candle). Lesions of the nondominant parietal lobe often result in *hemispatial neglect*: the patient does not attend to stimuli in the contralateral (usually the left) visual field or on the contralateral side of the body. In a milder form of neglect, called *extinction*, patients can attend to stimuli contralateral to the side of the brain with the lesion (typically the right hemisphere), but

Copy this cube:

Draw a clock, fill in the numbers and put the time at ten after 2:

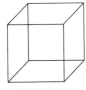

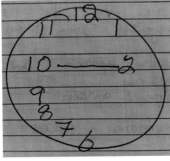

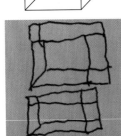

Fig. 109.4 Attempts to copy a cube and draw a clock by patients with neurodegenerative disorders demonstrate constructional apraxia and right-sided neglect.

when presented with bilateral stimuli simultaneously, they respond to stimuli only on the right hemibody side. *Anosognosia*, or the lack of awareness of one's deficit, frequently accompanies hemispatial neglect. In severe cases, patients may even deny that the affected limb belongs to them. Patients with anosognosia may present a challenge to rehabilitation therapists.

PROSPECTUS FOR THE FUTURE

Recent advances in neuroimaging technology have added to our understanding not only of the structural and functional anatomy of the brain but also its metabolic activity. Functional magnetic resonance imaging (fMRI) permits mapping of the metabolic anatomy of subcortical gray and white matter structures, such as the basal ganglia, and their roles in conditions such as dystonia. Furthermore, a modality known as diffusion tensor imaging allows for the mapping of white matter tracts (tractography) in great detail.

Several new strategies are emerging in an attempt to reverse the deficit in self-awareness in patients with neglect or anosognosia resulting from degenerative or ischemic lesions of the nondominant hemisphere. The development of virtual reality computer interface programs has opened the possibility to generate a variety of computer-based simulation environments to provide patients with detailed feedback options to improve self-awareness as part of a rehabilitation program.

SUGGESTED READINGS

Brazis PW, Masdeu JC, Biller J: Localization in clinical neurology, ed 7, Philadelphia, 2016, Wolters Kluwer.

Fitzgerald MJT, Gruener G, Estomih M: Clinical neuroanatomy and neuroscience, ed 6, Saunders, 2011.

Muratore M, Tuena C, Pedroli E, Cipresso P, Riva G: Virtual reality as a possible tool for the assessment of self-awareness, Front Behav Neurosci 13:62, 2019. https://doi.org/10.3389/fnbeh.2019.00062.

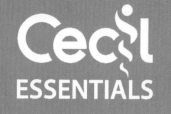

Dementia and Memory Disturbances

Frederick J. Marshall

MAJOR DEMENTIA SYNDROMES

Dementia places an enormous burden on the patient, family, and society. A third of older adults in the United States die of Alzheimer disease (AD) or other form of dementia, but only one in six older adults receives routine cognitive screening. The annual direct and indirect expenditure for AD and other dementias in the United States was $290 billion in 2019.

The term *dementia* refers to a syndrome of progressive cognitive decline leading to the loss of fully independent function in daily life. Memory loss is the most common central feature, and specific dementia syndromes characteristically cause particular forms of memory impairment. Different dementias produce specific abnormalities of cognition in language, spatial processing, praxis (the ability to execute learned motor behaviors), and executive function (the ability to plan and sequence thoughts and activities), and many have associated non-cognitive features. *Cortical dementia* and *subcortical dementia,* although older terms, remain helpful for subdividing the dementias (Table 110.1).

Neurodegeneration is the most common underlying cause of dementia. Table 110.2 provides the differential diagnosis of neurodegenerative causes of dementia. Table 110.3 outlines other causes of dementia.

Most causes of dementia are currently untreatable. Potentially correctable causes account for less than 5% of dementia cases. Structural processes or infections must be considered, along with metabolic and nutritional diseases. Every patient with dementia should have tests of serum electrolytes and vitamin B_{12} and assessments of liver, renal, and thyroid function. Serologic studies for syphilis, human immunodeficiency virus (HIV), and Lyme exposure should be done if risk factors are identified. Chronic infections (see Chapter 92), normal-pressure hydrocephalus (NPH), and autoimmune encephalopathies should be considered. Brain imaging should be performed.

Neuropsychological testing characterizes the pattern of cognitive and memory impairments and is helpful in the differential diagnosis. The Montreal Cognitive Assessment (MoCA) (Table 110.4) is a standard test that can be used as a bedside or office screening tool for identifying patients with dementia. It typically takes about 10 minutes to administer. This examination is superior to the Mini-Mental Status Examination (MMSE) in that it is more sensitive to abnormalities in a wider array of cognitive domains, including visual-spatial or executive function, naming, attention, fluency; abstract reasoning, short-term memory encoding and retrieval, and orientation.

In addition to the MoCA, patients with dementia should have tests of praxis (e.g., show how you would comb your hair; show how you would blow out a match) and neglect (e.g., testing of double-simultaneous extinction to visual, tactile, and auditory stimuli). Depending on the results of these screening procedures, more detailed neuropsychological studies can be pursued.

Alzheimer Disease

AD accounts for approximately 70% of dementia cases among older adults. There is widespread confusion among the lay population about the relationship between the terms *Alzheimer disease, senility,* and *dementia.* Patients and their family members often need clarification. Alzheimer *disease* (a specific diagnosis) is only one possible cause (albeit by far the most common cause) of *dementia* (a syndrome). Nearly six million persons in the United States are affected, and this number is estimated to approach 14 million by 2050 as the population ages. The disease occurs in 32% to 47% of persons older than 80 years of age. Incidence at age 65 is one in 200 people per year. Incidence at age 80 is one case per 10 people per year. More than 50% of caregivers develop depression or a major medical illness. Deaths from heart disease decreased 9% between 2000 and 2017, while deaths from AD increased 145%.

AD has many causes, but none is fully defined. All causes produce similar clinical and pathologic findings. The disease is characterized by the progressive loss of cortical neurons and the formation of amyloid plaques and intraneuronal neurofibrillary tangles. β-Amyloid (Aβ) is the major component of the plaques, while hyperphosphorylated tau protein is the major constituent of the neurofibrillary tangles. The process starts in the hippocampus and entorhinal cortex and spreads to involve diffuse areas of association cortex in the temporal, parietal, and frontal lobes. The relative deficiency of cortical acetylcholine (resulting from the loss of neurons in the nucleus basalis) provides the rationale for symptomatic treatment of the disease with centrally acting acetylcholinesterase inhibitors.

Pathogenesis

AD is often categorized as a young-onset hereditary or familial form, which is rare (≈5% overall) and for which three specific genetic abnormalities have been determined, or as a common (≈95% overall), sporadic form that typically occurs in persons older than 65 years of age (Table 110.5).

The autosomal dominant early-onset forms of AD have in common abnormalities of Aβ production and processing that have provided clues to the molecular pathogenesis of sporadic AD. Abnormal processing of amyloid precursor protein into the amyloidogenic peptide Aβ (1-42) is thought to be important in the pathogenesis of AD. It is thought to provoke downstream abnormalities of tau protein processing, with hyperphosphorylation of tau yielding intraneuronal tangles.

The apolipoprotein E (Apo E) gene *(APOE)* is a susceptibility locus for sporadic AD in late-onset familial AD pedigrees. The gene is

TABLE 110.1 Distinguishing Characteristics of Cortical and Subcortical Dementias

Cortical Dementia

Symptoms: major changes in memory, language deficits, perceptual deficits, praxis disturbances

Affected brain regions: temporal cortex (medial), parietal cortex, and frontal lobe cortex

Examples: Alzheimer disease, diffuse Lewy body disease, vascular dementia, frontotemporal dementias

Subcortical Dementia

Symptoms: behavioral changes, impaired affect and mood, motor slowing, executive dysfunction, less severe changes in memory early on in the course

Affected brain regions: thalamus, striatum, midbrain, striatofrontal projections, subcortical white matter

Examples: Parkinson's disease, progressive supranuclear palsy, normal-pressure hydrocephalus, Huntington's disease

TABLE 110.2 Etiologic Diagnosis of Neurodegenerative Dementia in Adults

Alzheimer disease[a] (AD)

Parkinson's disease[a] (PD)

Diffuse Lewy body disease[a] (DLBD)

Progressive supranuclear palsy (PSP)

Corticobasal ganglionic degeneration (CBGD)

Striatonigral degeneration

Huntington's disease[a]

Frontotemporal dementias (FTD)

Frontotemporal dementia without characteristic neuropathology

Frontotemporal dementia with motor neuron disease

Neurodegeneration with brain iron accumulation

Dentatorubral-pallidoluysian atrophy (DRPLA)

Spinal-cerebellar ataxias (SCAs)

[a]Denotes conditions for which symptomatic pharmacologic treatment is available.

TABLE 110.3 Other Causes of Progressive Dementia in Adults

Structural Disease or Trauma

Normal-pressure hydrocephalus (NPH)[a]

Neoplasms[a]

Dementia pugilistica (multiple concussions in boxers)

Chronic traumatic encephalopathy (CTE)

Vascular Disease

Vascular dementia[b] (also called multi-infarct dementia)

Vasculitis[a]

Heredometabolic Disease

Wilson's disease[a]

Neuronal ceroid lipofuscinosis (Kufs disease)

Other late-onset lysosomal storage diseases

Demyelinating or Dysmyelinating Disease

Multiple sclerosis[b]

Metachromatic leukodystrophy

Infectious Disease

Human immunodeficiency virus type 1[a]

Tertiary syphilis[a]

Creutzfeldt-Jakob disease

Progressive multifocal leukoencephalopathy

Whipple disease[a]

Chronic meningitis[a]

Cryptococcal meningitis[a]

Others

Metabolic or Nutritional Disease

Vitamin B_{12} deficiency[a]

Thyroid hormone deficiency or excess[a]

Thiamine deficiency[a] (Korsakoff syndrome)

Alcoholism[b]

Psychiatric Disease

Pseudodementia from depression[a]

[a]Denotes conditions for which preventive or corrective treatment is available.

[b]Denotes conditions for which symptomatic treatment is available.

polymorphic (ε2, ε3, ε4), and first-degree relatives of AD patients who inherit both ε4 alleles have a greater than 60% lifetime risk of developing AD. Apo E-ε4 interacts selectively with Aβ and with tau protein, but how Apo E-ε4 increases the risk of AD remains unknown.

Clinical Features

AD begins gradually and affects memory, orientation, language, visuospatial processing, praxis, judgment, and insight. Depression is common early in AD, and psychosis with agitation and behavioral disinhibition often occur in advanced stages. Patients become dependent on others for all activities of daily living. The rate of progression of AD varies but usually takes 5 to 15 years to progress from presentation to advanced illness.

Diagnostic criteria are outlined in Table 110.6. Although a definitive diagnosis of AD requires biopsy (rarely done) or autopsy confirmation, these diagnostic criteria establish the diagnosis with more than 85% specificity in moderately demented patients.

There are now three different positron emission tomography (PET) ligands that bind to Aβ plaques approved by the US Food and Drug Administration (FDA) for use in the clinical diagnosis of AD.

These compounds are costly, however, and not universally approved by insurances, limiting their utility in clinical practice. Cerebral amyloid accumulation is largely completed at a relatively early stage of AD when patients may be asymptomatic or have only isolated impairment of memory but no overt loss of independent function in daily life (a stage known as *mild neurocognitive disorder*). Research efforts are underway to find disease modifying approaches that ameliorate plaque and possibly prolong the time to patients' loss of independence.

Another protein, known as *tau*, plays an important role in the stabilization of microtubules involved in the transport of nutrients and other substances within the neuron. In AD, tau becomes hyperphosphorylated and forms intraneuronal neurofibrillary tangles that cannot be effectively disposed of by the cell. Smaller forms of tau (oligomers) are known to circulate among neurons and interfere with their function and can be found in AD brains more than a decade prior to symptom onset. Because tau continues to accumulate throughout the course of AD, it is a potentially useful marker of disease progression. The FDA has recently approved a PET ligand that binds to tau.

TABLE 110.4 Elements of the Montreal Cognitive Assessment

Cognitive Domain	Items	Score
Visual-spatial or executive	Complete a trail-making task, copy a cube, draw a clock	5
Naming	Name three depicted animals	3
Attention	Recall five digits forward, three digits backward, maintain letter vigilance, subtract 7s serially	6
Language	Repeat two phrases, generate a list of words starting with a specific letter	3
Abstraction	Identify the similarity between nouns (train/bicycle; watch/ruler)	2
Delayed recall	Recall five words rehearsed twice previously (face, velvet, church, daisy, red)	5
Orientation	Identify the date, month, year, day, place, and city	6
Total possible score		30

A score of 26 or greater is considered normal.
From Nasreddine ZS, Phillips NA, Bedirian V, et al: The Montreal Cognitive Assessment, MoCA: a brief screening tool for mild cognitive impairment, J Am Geriatr Soc 53:695-699, 2005.

TABLE 110.5 Familial Versus Sporadic Alzheimer Disease

Chromosome and Gene	Age at Onset (Yr)	% of All FAD Cases	% of All SAD Cases
Familial Alzheimer Disease[a]			
Chromosome 1, *PSEN2* (presenilin 2)	40-80	5-10	<0.5
Chromosome 14, *PSEN1* (presenilin 1)	30-60	70	<1
Chromosome 21, *APP* (amyloid-β precursor protein)	35-65	5	<0.5
Sporadic Alzheimer Disease[b]			
No single determinant gene[c]	Usually >60	—	98

[a]Familial Alzheimer disease (FAD) has early onset and is autosomal dominant.
[b]Sporadic Alzheimer disease (SAD) has late onset and may be polygenetic and/or environmental.
[c]Apolipoprotein E-ε4 allele on chromosome 19 increases the risk compared with the ε2 or ε3 allele.

TABLE 110.6 Diagnostic Criteria for Probable Alzheimer Disease

Progressive functional decline and dementia established by clinical examination and mental status testing and confirmed by neuropsychological assessment
Insidious onset
Clear-cut history of worsening cognition by report or observation
Initial and most prominent cognitive deficits evident on history and examination in one of the following categories:
  Amnestic presentation (plus at least one other domain)
  Nonamnestic presentations (plus deficits in other domains): language, visuospatial, executive dysfunction
No evidence of vascular dementia, dementia with Lewy bodies, frontotemporal dementias, or other concurrent active neurologic or non-neurologic medical comorbidity or use of medication that could have a substantial effect on cognition

Tau has been implicated in several other neurodegenerative diseases, but the abnormal tau in these diseases is not identical. Along with AD, these diseases are sometimes referred to as *tauopathies*. These include: chronic traumatic encephalopathy (CTE), corticobasal-ganglionic degeneration (CBGD), frontotemporal dementia with parkinsonism-17 (FTDP-17), Pick disease, and progressive supranuclear palsy (PSP) (see later for further discussion).

Analysis of cerebrospinal fluid (CSF) for Aβ, total-tau, and phosphorylated-tau protein levels has been commercialized as an aid to diagnosis. Because amyloid plaques accumulate extraneuronally and sequester soluble Aβ, the level of Aβ found in CSF samples from patients with AD is lower than normal. Alternatively, tau is intraneuronal and is released into the CSF when neurons die, thereby increasing the level of tau in CSF from patients with AD and a variety of other diseases that involve neuronal cell death. In AD, the ratio of CSF tau to

CSF Aβ goes up. Because of the invasive nature of the testing (involving a spinal tap) and the relatively high pretest probability of AD in older individuals with dementia who meet diagnostic criteria, CSF analysis is more commonly performed in young-onset patients.

Treatment

Although their benefits are modest, the cholinesterase-inhibiting drugs donepezil (Aricept), rivastigmine (Exelon), and galantamine (Razadyne) represent important advances. These drugs may be given in once-daily formulations. Rivastigmine is also available as a transdermal patch.

In clinical trials, cholinesterase inhibitors benefited less than 50% of patients. They have not been shown to prevent AD in patients with mild cognitive impairment (MCI), a condition in which the memory or another domain of cognition is impaired in the absence of meaningful dysfunction in daily life. Approximately 12% of patients with MCI go on to develop AD per year, with roughly two thirds of patients with MCI developing clinical AD within 5 years of symptom onset.

The glutamate antagonist memantine (Namenda) has been shown to prolong daily function in patients with moderate to advanced AD.

Treatment strategies in clinical trials over the past decade have included decreasing Aβ peptide production by blocking α-secretase or β-secretase or upregulating cleavage of the amyloid precursor protein at the α-secretase site. Studies of active and passive immunization have been designed to lower brain Aβ levels. However, these approaches have failed to deliver on the promise of disease modification, necessitating a wide-reaching reassessment of current theories of disease pathogenesis.

Nursing services provide oversight of hygiene, nutrition, and medication compliance. Antipsychotics, antidepressants, and anxiolytics are useful for patients with behavioral disturbances, which are the most common cause of nursing home placement. Patients and families can be referred to a local Alzheimer's Association chapter for further information on available community support.

Prevention

There is relatively strong epidemiologic evidence, but no well controlled prospective randomized clinical trial evidence, that the following five things lower the lifetime incidence of dementia in populations: (1) alcohol in moderation (no more than one drink per day), (2) cardiovascular risk-factor mitigation, (3) regular socialization, (4) Mediterranean diet, and (5) regular exercise (three times weekly to the point of sweating). There is some epidemiologic evidence that statin medications and fish oil lower the risk of AD in populations (though there are individuals for whom statins may provoke encephalopathy). There is randomized clinical trial evidence that *gingko biloba* does not have benefit in AD. There is a moderate level of scientific evidence that conjugated equine estrogen with methyl-progesterone increases the risk of AD. There is a low level of scientific evidence that some nonsteroidal anti-inflammatory drugs, depressive disorder, diabetes mellitus, hyperlipidemia in midlife, current tobacco use, traumatic brain injury, pesticide exposure, and relative social isolation increase the risk of AD.

Diffuse Lewy Body Disease

Lewy bodies are pathologic intraneuronal alpha-synulcein inclusions that are the hallmark of Parkinson's disease when they are restricted to the brain stem (see Chapter 116). Patients with diffuse Lewy body disease have clinical parkinsonism (i.e., slow movement, rigidity, and balance problems) combined with early and prominent dementia. Pathologically, Lewy bodies are found in the brain stem, limbic system, and cortex. Visual hallucinations and cognitive fluctuations are common, and patients are unusually sensitive to the adverse effects of neuroleptic medication.

Diffuse Lewy body disease may represent the second most common cause of dementia after AD. However, the common concurrence of the pathologic features of diffuse Lewy body disease with the classic neuritic plaques and neurofibrillary tangles of AD complicates the identification of the cause of dementia in a given patient.

Vascular Dementia

Approximately 10% to 20% of older patients with dementia have radiographic evidence of focal stroke on magnetic resonance imaging (MRI) or computed tomography (CT), combined with focal signs on the neurologic examination. When the dementia syndrome begins with a stroke and progression of the illness is stepwise (suggesting recurrent vascular events), the diagnosis of vascular dementia is likely.

Patients typically develop early incontinence, gait disturbances, and flattening of affect. A subcortical dementing process attributed to small vessel disease in the periventricular white matter has been referred to as *Binswanger disease,* but it may be a radiographic finding rather than a true disease. Appropriate treatment of risk factors for vascular disease—blood pressure control, smoking cessation, diet modification, and anticoagulation (in select settings such as atrial fibrillation)—is mandatory and may be of benefit.

Frontotemporal Dementias

Patients with the behavioral variant of frontotemporal dementia (FTD) are frequently socially disinhibited, but they may also be lethargic and lack motivation and spontaneity. Patients with the progressive nonfluent aphasia variant of FTD have loss of speech fluency with poor articulation and syntactic errors but relative preservation of comprehension. Those with the semantic dementia variant of FTD remain fluent with normal phonation but have progressive difficulty with naming and word comprehension. Memory and spatial skills and praxis are relatively preserved early on in all of these forms, whereas executive function, emotional regulation, and conduct are relatively impaired.

There are several frontotemporal lobar degenerations (FTLDs), including Pick disease (now referred to as FTLD-tau). In some families, a mutation in the microtubule-associated protein tau gene *(MAPT)* on chromosome 17 causes tau-positive frontotemporal dementia with parkinsonism (FTDP-17). Transactive response DNA-binding protein (TDP-43) pathology accounts for 40% of FTD with or without motor neuron disease. Although mutations in the fused sarcoma gene *(FUS)* had previously been identified as a cause of familial amyotrophic lateral sclerosis (ALS), some also give rise to 5% to 10% of clinically diagnosed FTD (typically the behavioral variant). Hexanucleotide repeat expansions in *C9orf72* cause neurodegeneration in FTD and ALS. RNA processing is abnormal in both conditions.

As in AD, all forms of FTD progress over years. No intervention slows the inevitable decline of these patients. Approximately 50% of patients have a family history of the disease.

Parkinson's Disease

The majority of patients with Parkinson's disease (see Chapter 116) become demented in the later stages of illness. The dementia of Parkinson's disease affects executive function out of proportion to its impact on language. Thought processes appear to slow down *(bradyphrenia)*, analogous to the slowing of movement *(bradykinesia)*.

Because dementia occurs relatively late in the progression of Parkinson's disease, most patients are taking drugs to improve their movement disorder by enhancing dopaminergic neurotransmission. These drugs can induce psychosis. Dose reductions should be attempted before the diagnosis of underlying dementia is made for these patients. Acetylcholinesterase inhibition has been helpful for patients with dementia caused by Parkinson's disease, and the FDA has specifically approved rivastigmine for this indication.

Normal-Pressure Hydrocephalus

The triad of dementia (typically subcortical), gait instability, and urinary incontinence suggests the possibility of normal-pressure hydrocephalus. These patients appear to walk with their feet stuck to the floor, without lifting up the knees and with a broad base. Symptoms evolve over the course of weeks to months, and brain imaging reveals ventricular enlargement out of proportion to the degree of cortical atrophy.

Numerous diagnostic tests have been described, including radionuclide cisternography and MRI flow studies. The most important test remains the clinical response to removal of large volumes of CSF through serial lumbar punctures or the temporary placement of a lumbar drain, followed by examination of the patient's gait and cognitive function. Neurosurgical placement of a permanent ventriculoperitoneal shunt may correct the problem. Patients likely to benefit from shunt placement have a clear response to the removal of 30 to 40 mL of spinal fluid, with improved gait and alertness within minutes to hours of the procedure. The cause of normal-pressure hydrocephalus is a derangement of the CSF hydrodynamics. Shunt placement is most likely to be effective if normal-pressure hydrocephalus occurs after severe head trauma or subarachnoid hemorrhage.

Prion Infection, Chronic Meningitis, and Dementia Related to Acquired Immunodeficiency Syndrome

Creutzfeldt-Jakob disease (CJD) is a subacute, dementing, transmissible illness with typical onset between 40 and 75 years of age and an incidence of one case per 1 million people (see Chapter 92). The disease causes spongiform degeneration and gliosis in widespread areas of the cortex. Clinical variants of the disorder are differentiated by the relative predominance of cerebellar symptoms, extrapyramidal hyperkinesias, or visual agnosia and cortical blindness (*Heidenhain variant*).

Ninety percent of patients with CJD have myoclonus, compared with 10% of patients with AD. Patients with all forms of the disease share a relentlessly progressive dementia and disruption of personality over weeks to months. The electroencephalogram shows characteristic abnormalities, including diffuse slowing and periodic sharp waves or spikes.

The transmissible agent, a prion protein, is invulnerable to routine modes of antisepsis. CSF can be tested for the 14-3-3 protein, although this test is not as sensitive or specific for CJD as once hoped. Real-time quaking-induced conversion (RT-QuIC) assays are currently considered more sensitive and specific but can be adversely effected if the protein, red or white cell count in the CSF sample studied is elevated.

Certain infectious agents can cause the subacute or chronic development of subcortical dementia. These chronic meningitides are discussed in Chapter 92.

Human immunodeficiency virus accesses the central nervous system through monocytes and the microglial system and causes associated neuronal cell loss, vacuolization, and lymphocytic infiltration. The dementia associated with this infection is characterized by bradyphrenia and bradykinesia. Patients have executive dysfunction, impaired memory, poor concentration, and apathy. Treatment of the underlying viral infection with effective antiretroviral therapy may slow the progression of the dementia (see Chapter 103).

There is increasing recognition of the potential for abnormal production of antibodies misdirected against brain epitopes to cause encephalopathy that can sometimes mimic classical dementia. Waxing and waning mental status rather than insidious progression of cognitive decline should prompt consideration of this category of illness as should cancer comorbidity, a history of autoimmune disease, or seizures in a patient presenting with cognitive changes. CSF should be sent for analysis to centers specializing in this emerging area of neuroimmunology.

OTHER MEMORY DISTURBANCES

Structure of Memory

Memory function is divided into introspective processes (i.e., declarative, explicit, aware memories) and processes that are not accessible to introspection (i.e., nondeclarative, implicit, procedural memories). Short-term memory (e.g., words on a list) is a form of declarative memory. Other forms include the conscious recall of episodes from personal experience (i.e., episodic memory) and factual knowledge

(i.e., semantic memory) that can be consciously recalled and stated (i.e., declared). Declarative memory involves consciously *knowing that…* Patients with amnesia resulting from lesions of the medial temporal lobes or midline diencephalic structures have deficits of declarative memory.

Nondeclarative memory encompasses several distinct and neuroanatomically less clearly localized functions related to the performance of specific learned motor, cognitive, or perceptual tasks. Nondeclarative (procedural) memories involve unconsciously *knowing how…* Deficits in nondeclarative memory may involve various areas of association neocortex, depending on the nature of the task (e.g., parietal-temporal-occipital junction cortex for visual perceptual tasks, frontal association cortex for motor tasks). Patients with amnesia resulting from lesions of the medial temporal lobes tend to perform normally on tests of nondeclarative memory.

Anterograde amnesia is the inability to learn new information. It commonly occurs after brain injury or in association with dementia. The inability to recollect prior information is retrograde amnesia. Both types of amnesia usually occur together in brain injury syndromes, although the extent of one type or the other may vary. The degree of anterograde amnesia after head injury correlates with the severity of the injury.

Isolated Disorders of Memory Function

Memory can be impaired in relative isolation as a consequence of head injury, thiamine deficiency (i.e., Korsakoff syndrome), benign forgetfulness of aging, transient global amnesia, or psychogenic disease.

Head injury typically results in retrograde amnesia in excess of anterograde amnesia, with both forms stretching out over time from the discrete event. As time passes, these disrupted memories gradually return, although rarely to the point at which the events immediately surrounding the trauma are recalled.

Korsakoff syndrome is characterized by the near-total inability to establish new memory. Patients often confabulate responses when they are asked to convey the details of their current circumstance or to relay the content of a recently presented story. Deficiency of thiamine and other nutritional deficiencies in the context of chronic alcoholism are the most common underlying causes. Thiamine is a necessary cofactor in the metabolism of glucose, and thiamine must be replenished at the same time glucose is administered whenever a comatose patient is seen in the emergency department.

Aging is associated with mild loss of memory, exhibited by difficulty in recalling names and by forgetfulness for dates. Population-based assessments of neuropsychological function have demonstrated that poor performance on delayed-recall tasks is the most sensitive indicator of cognitive change with advancing age. Verbal fluency, in contrast, remains intact with advancing age, and vocabulary may increase with time, even into old age.

Transient global amnesia is a dramatic memory disturbance that affects older patients (>50 years). Patients usually have only one episode; occasionally, episodes recur over the course of several years. Patients have complete temporal and spatial disorientation; orientation for person is preserved. Near-total retrograde and anterograde amnesia persists for various periods, typically 6 to 12 hours. Patients are often anxious and may repeat the same question over and over again. Transient global amnesia may be confused with psychogenic amnesia, fugue state, or partial complex status epilepticus. Transient global amnesia is thought to reflect underlying vascular insufficiency to the hippocampus or midline thalamic projections.

Unlike patients with organic memory disturbances, patients with psychogenic amnesia typically have inconsistent loss of recent and remote memory, relatively more loss of emotionally charged memory (rather than relatively less loss of such memory in organic disease), and an apparent indifference to their own plight; they ask few questions. Most characteristically, patients with psychogenic amnesia tend to express disorientation to person (asking, *Who am I?*), a phenomenon seldom seen in organic memory disturbance.

Patients with severe depression may exhibit pseudodementia. Vegetative signs, including changes in appetite, weight, and sleep pattern, are common, whereas signs of cortical impairment, such as aphasia, agnosia, and apraxia, are rare. Memory and bradyphrenia improve with antidepressant therapy. Depression often coexists with other causes of dementia, such as AD, Parkinson's disease, and vascular dementia.

❖ For a deeper discussion on this topic, please see Chapter 374, "Cognitive Impairment and Dementia," in *Goldman-Cecil Medicine*, 26th Edition.

SUGGESTED READINGS

Femminella GD, Thayanandan T, Calsolaro V, Komici K, Rengo G, Corbi G, Ferrara N: Imaging and molecular mechanisms of Alzheimer's disease: a review, Int J Mol Sci 19(12):3702, 2018.

Gomperts SN: Lewy body dementias: dementia with lewy bodies and Parkinson disease dementia, Continuum 22:435–463, 2016.

Hane FT, Robinson M, Lee BY, Bai O, Leonenko Z, Albert MS: Recent progress in Alzheimer's disease research, Part 3: diagnosis and treatment, J Alzheimers Dis 57:645–665, 2017.

Jack Jr CR, Bennett DA, Blennow K, Carrillo MC, Dunn B, Elliott C, et al: NIA-AA research framework: towards a biological definition of Alzheimer's disease, Alzheimer Dement 14:535–562, 2018.

O'Brien JT, Thomas A: Vascular dementia, Lancet 386:1698–1706, 2015.

Sivasathiaseelan H, Marshall CR, Agustus JL, Benhamou E, Bond RL, van Leeuwen JEP, Hardy CJD, Rohrer JD, Warren JD. Frontotemporal dementia: a clinical review. Semin Neurol 2019;266:2075-2086.

Villain N, Dubois B: Alzheimer's disease including focal presentations, Semin Neurol 39:213–226, 2019.

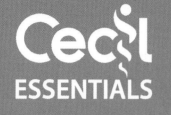

111

Major Disorders of Mood, Thoughts, and Behavior

Jeffrey M. Lyness, Jennifer H. Richman

CLASSIFICATION OF MENTAL DISORDERS

Mental (psychiatric) disorders are alterations in thoughts, feelings, or behaviors that produce substantive subjective distress or affect the patient's functional status. Many mental disorders are caused by the direct effects of drugs, systemic disease, or neurologic disease on brain physiology. They may be broadly considered as secondary psychiatric disorders, as opposed to the primary or idiopathic psychiatric disorders. The distinguishing feature of neurocognitive disorders is impairment in intellectual functions such as level of consciousness, orientation, attention, or memory; however, these disorders also often include disruption of mood, thoughts, and behaviors similar to that seen in other psychiatric syndromes. Neurocognitive disorders are the focus of Chapter 126.

The noncognitive secondary syndromes by definition cause psychiatric phenomena similar to their idiopathic counterparts. During the evaluation of any patient with new or worsened psychiatric symptoms, it is essential to conduct a thorough evaluation for other medical causes, including a careful history and physical examination (with a screening neurologic examination) that often are supplemented by laboratory evaluations. Table 111.1 outlines important causes of psychiatric syndromes. Although some conditions are likely to produce certain psychiatric syndromes, many manifest as any of several psychiatric syndromes. Conversely, a psychiatric syndrome may be caused by a wide range of conditions.

Because the cause of primary psychiatric disorders is unknown, approaches to classification depend on reliable empirical observations of phenomena clustered into recognizable syndromes. Table 111.2 shows the most important psychiatric syndromes and the disorders in which they may manifest. Table 111.3 shows the major idiopathic disorders, excluding addictive disorders (see Chapter 128). Many psychiatric disorders manifest with multiple syndromes. For example, major depression with psychotic features manifests with a depressive syndrome and a psychotic syndrome. In evaluating a patient with new or worsened psychiatric symptoms, the clinician must construct a differential diagnosis based on syndromes alongside the differential diagnosis based on potential secondary causes.

DEPRESSIVE AND BIPOLAR DISORDERS

Depressive and bipolar disorders are characterized by idiopathic episodes of depression alone (i.e., unipolar) or mania and depression (i.e., bipolar). The core symptoms of depressive episodes include emotional symptoms (e.g., dysphoria, irritability, anhedonia, loss of interests), ideational symptoms (e.g., thoughts with hopeless, worthless, guilty, or suicidal themes), and neurovegetative symptoms and signs (e.g., anergia; psychomotor slowing or agitation; decreased concentration; altered sleep, appetite, and weight).

Major depressive disorder is defined by episodes of a least five symptoms, including depressed mood, anhedonia, or loss of interests, that occur almost every day for at least 2 consecutive weeks, sufficient to cause significant distress and affect functional status. Other prominent symptoms may include associated anxiety, somatic worry, or new somatic symptoms, and in the most severe cases, psychotic symptoms, including nihilistic or self-deprecatory (i.e., mood-congruent) delusions.

Major depression is common, with a 12-month prevalence of approximately 7% and a lifetime prevalence of up to 10% among men and 20% to 25% in women. New depressive episodes have an annual incidence of approximately 3%. First onset may occur at any age but is most common in the third through fifth decades of life. Whereas most episodes of major depression fully remit spontaneously or with treatment, the lifetime risk of recurrence is at least 50% to 70%, and up to 20% of patients may experience chronic symptoms over many years. Major depression is a leading correlate of disability worldwide, is an important determinant of death by suicide, and is associated with increased risk of death from comorbid physical illnesses. Major depression also causes significant economic burden, costing approximately 210.5 billion inflation-adjusted dollars in the United States alone in 2010. Persistent depressive disorder (i.e., dysthymia) is a condition defined by chronic depressive symptoms, often of insufficient severity to meet criteria for major depression.

Depressive disorders are heterogeneous, with many potential pathogenic mechanisms. Genetic factors, such as polymorphisms of the serotonin transporter protein, affect vulnerability to depressive episodes in the face of psychosocial stressors. Depression is polygenic and multifactorial, with genetic factors accounting for about 40% of the risk. Alterations in the functioning of brain serotonergic and noradrenergic systems and of the hypothalamic-pituitary-adrenal axis are found in depression. Neuroimaging studies show smaller hippocampal volumes and altered metabolic activity in several regions, including the anterior cingulate cortex. However, the information in these studies is not sufficient for making the clinical diagnosis, which depends on identification of the clinical syndrome. Dysfunctional, negativistic patterns of thinking, impaired social relationships, and stressful life events also contribute to depression.

Mild to moderate forms of major depression respond to focused psychotherapies or antidepressant medications (Table 111.4). More severe forms of depression do not respond to psychosocial interventions alone. Severe or refractory depression may be treated safely and effectively with electroconvulsive therapy. Other evidence-based somatic therapies include light therapy (for depression with a seasonal component) and vagal nerve stimulation. Data suggest that the dissociative anesthetic ketamine, an *N*-methyl-D-aspartate (NMDA)

TABLE 111.1   Important Causes of Psychiatric Syndromes

Central Nervous System Conditions
Tumor
Toxins
Vascular disorders
Seizure
Infection
Genetic disorders
Congenital malformation
Demyelinating conditions
Degenerative conditions
Hydrocephalus

Systemic Diseases
Cardiovascular diseases
Pulmonary diseases
Cancer
Infection
Nutritional disorders
Endocrine disorders
Metabolic disorders
Autoimmune disorders

Drugs
Drug intoxication
Drug withdrawal

receptor antagonist, may rapidly improve patients with treatment-resistant depression, although the general clinical applicability of ketamine remains to be determined.

Bipolar disorder (i.e., bipolar I) is characterized by recurrent episodes of mania, usually with episodes of major depression. Manic episodes include elevated (euphoric) or irritable mood, goal-directed hyperactivity (often for pleasurable activities with poor judgment leading to substantial adverse consequences such as sexual, spending, or gambling sprees), pressured speech, increased energy level with a decreased need for sleep, and distractibility.

Compared with unipolar depression, bipolar disorder has a lower 12-month prevalence (approximately 0.6%) and a younger average age of onset (typically late teens to 20s). Unlike unipolar depression, bipolar disorder is slightly more common among males. Most patients return to baseline functioning between acute mood episodes, but some have a deteriorating course, and others have frequent debilitating episodes (i.e., rapid cycling of four episodes per year).

Genetic factors play a greater role in the pathogenesis of bipolar disorder than in major depressive disorder, accounting for approximately 50% of the risk and representing a greater than 50-fold increase over the population base rate. Bipolar disorder is polygenic and has been linked in individual families to different loci. The pathogenesis is unclear but likely involves dysregulation of frontostriatal systems. Structural neuroimaging studies show increased ventricular-to-brain ratios, suggesting parenchymal atrophy. Psychosocial stressors often play a role in precipitating episodes of mania and depression.

The mainstay of treatment for bipolar disorder is mood stabilizer medications (e.g., lithium, anticonvulsants such as valproic acid and

TABLE 111.2   Important Psychiatric Syndromes

Syndrome	Main Symptoms and Signs	Disorders
Neurocognitive	Impairment in intellectual functions (e.g., level of consciousness, orientation, attention, memory, language, praxis, visuospatial, executive functions)	Neurocognitive disorders Intellectual disability (if onset in childhood)
Mood	Depressive: lowered mood, anhedonia, negativistic thoughts, neurovegetative symptoms Manic: elevated or irritable mood; grandiosity; goal-directed hyperactivity with increased energy; pressured speech; decreased sleep need	Neurocognitive disorders Mood disorders (bipolar or depressive) (primary or secondary) Trauma- and stressor-related disorders Psychotic disorders (schizoaffective disorder)
Anxiety	All include anxious mood and associated physiologic signs and symptoms (e.g., palpitations, tremors, diaphoresis) May include various types of dysfunctional thoughts (e.g., catastrophic fears, obsessions, flashbacks) and behaviors (e.g., compulsions, avoidance behaviors)	Neurocognitive disorders Mood disorders (bipolar or depressive) (primary or secondary) Psychotic disorders (primary or secondary) Anxiety disorders (primary or secondary) Obsessive-compulsive and related disorders Trauma- and stressor-related disorders
Psychotic	Impairments in reality testing: hallucinations, thought process derailments	Neurocognitive disorders Mood disorders (bipolar or depressive) (primary or secondary) Psychotic disorders
Somatic symptom syndromes	Somatic symptoms with associated distressing thoughts, feelings, or behaviors	Mood disorders (bipolar or depressive) (primary or secondary) Anxiety disorders (primary or secondary) Obsessive-compulsive and related disorders Trauma- and stressor-related disorders Somatic symptom disorders
Personality pathology	Dysfunctional enduring patterns of emotional regulation, thought patterns, interpersonal behaviors, impulse regulation	Neurocognitive disorders Personality change due to another medical condition Personality disorders

Data from American Psychiatric Association: Diagnostic and statistical manual of mental disorders, ed 5, Washington, D.C., 2013, American Psychiatric Association.

TABLE 111.3 Major Idiopathic (Primary) Disorders of Mood, Thoughts, and Behavior

Mood Disorders
Depressive (Unipolar)
Major depressive disorder
Persistent depressive disorder (dysthymia)

Bipolar
Bipolar disorder
Cyclothymic disorder
Bipolar II disorder (bipolar disorder not otherwise specified)

Anxiety Disorders
Panic disorder (without or with agoraphobia)
Generalized anxiety disorder
Social phobia
Specific phobia

Other Conditions With Anxiety as a Prominent Feature
Obsessive-compulsive disorder
Acute stress disorder, post-traumatic stress disorder

Psychotic (Schizophrenia and Related) Disorders
Schizophrenia
Schizophreniform disorder
Brief psychotic disorder
Schizoaffective disorder
Delusional disorder

Somatic Symptom Disorders
Somatic symptom disorder
Illness anxiety disorder
Conversion (functional neurologic symptom) disorder
Psychological factors affecting physical condition
Factitious disorder (i.e., Munchausen syndrome)

Personality Disorders
Cluster A: Odd Eccentric
Schizoid personality disorder (detachment from social relationships, restricted emotional expression)
Schizotypal personality disorder (social and emotional deficits, cognitive or perceptual distortions, eccentric behavior)
Paranoid personality disorder (pervasive distrust and suspiciousness)

Cluster B: Dramatic or Emotional
Borderline personality disorder (instability of interpersonal relationships, self-image, and affects, and impulsivity)
Narcissistic personality disorder (grandiosity, need for admiration, lack of empathy)
Antisocial personality disorder (disregard for and violation of the rights of others)
Histrionic personality disorder

Cluster C: Anxious or Fearful
Avoidant personality disorder (social inhibition, feelings of inadequacy, hypersensitivity to criticism)
Dependent personality disorder (pervasive and excessive need to be taken care of, leading to submissive and clinging behavior and fears of separation)
Obsessive-compulsive personality disorder (preoccupation with orderliness, perfectionism, and mental and interpersonal control, at the expense of flexibility, openness, and efficiency)

Data from American Psychiatric Association: Diagnostic and statistical manual of mental disorders, ed 5, Washington, D.C., 2013, American Psychiatric Association.

carbamazepine) for acute episodes and maintenance therapy. The anticonvulsant lamotrigine may be particularly useful for bipolar depression. Antipsychotic medications are useful for acute manic episodes and may have a role in maintenance therapy. Benzodiazepines may be used to treat acute agitation and aggression while waiting for more definitive antimanic therapies to take effect. Antidepressants have long been used for depressive episodes, although they may precipitate manic episodes.

Electroconvulsive therapy is effective for refractory mania and depression. Psychosocial treatments alone do not effectively treat mania and may be less effective for bipolar depression, but psychoeducation and support to manage psychosocial stressors and encourage medication compliance improve longer-term outcomes.

A spectrum of less severe bipolar disorders includes conditions marked by episodes of hypomania (i.e., low-level manic symptoms without psychosis or significant impairment in functioning). They include bipolar II disorder, characterized by episodes of hypomania and major depression, and cyclothymic disorder, characterized by hypomania and low-level depression not meeting criteria for major depression. Because patients with bipolar II disorder are most likely to seek care during depressive episodes, it is important to inquire about a history of manic symptoms to avoid precipitating mania with the use of antidepressant medications. The pathogeneses of these less severe mood disorders is unclear.

DISORDERS WITH ANXIETY AS A PROMINENT FEATURE

The idiopathic anxiety disorders manifest with troublesome thoughts and somatic symptoms (Table 111.5) along with the emotional sensation of anxiety. A panic attack is a transient episode of crescendo anxiety, catastrophic thoughts (e.g., fears of dying, going insane, losing self-control), and somatic symptoms. If panic attacks or other clinically significant anxiety symptoms occur only in predictable response to environmental stimuli, the anxiety disorder is known as a *phobia*, which may further be classified as agoraphobia (i.e., anxiety about being in places from which escape may be difficult or embarrassing such as being alone, in crowds, in tunnels, or on bridges), social phobia (i.e., anxiety in interpersonal situations), and specific phobia (i.e., anxiety provoked by other situations or objects such as blood, animals, or heights). *Panic disorder* manifests with recurrent panic attacks, some of which are unexpected and unpredictable, along with anticipatory anxiety (i.e., fear of having another attack) and avoidance behaviors (i.e., avoiding situations that may provoke a panic attack or in which having an attack is perceived to be embarrassing or dangerous). Other disorders may not cause discrete panic attacks. Enduring anxiety in various domains that the individual finds difficult to control is classified as *generalized anxiety disorder*. Those with generalized anxiety disorder may also experience physical symptoms such as feeling keyed up, muscle tension or fatigue; however, they are not in discrete episodes.

Obsessive-compulsive disorder is characterized by recurrent obsessions (i.e., thoughts, impulses, or mental images that are anxiety-producing, perceived as intrusive and inappropriate, and resistant to attempts to suppress or neutralize them) and compulsions (i.e., repetitive behaviors or mental acts performed in response to obsessions or other rigid rules). Recognizing its distinct pathogenesis involving striatofrontal function and central serotonergic systems, it has been classified separately from the anxiety disorders.

Individuals exposed to severely stressful events (typically involving the actual or threatened loss of life or limb) may experience any of a wide variety of psychiatric sequelae. If the sequelae include symptoms of intrusion (e.g., intrusive memories, dreams, flashbacks,

TABLE 111.4	**Psychotherapies for Depression and Antidepressant Medications**
Name	**Approach or Mechanism of Action**
Psychotherapy	
Cognitive psychotherapy	Identify and correct negativistic patterns of thinking
Interpersonal psychotherapy	Identify and work through role transitions or interpersonal losses, conflicts, or deficits
Problem-solving therapy	Identify and prioritize situational problems; plan and implement strategies to deal with top-priority problems
Commonly Used Antidepressants	
Selective serotonin reuptake inhibitors (SSRIs)	Inhibit presynaptic reuptake of serotonin
Citalopram and escitalopram	
Fluoxetine	
Fluvoxamine	
Paroxetine	
Sertraline	
Serotonin and norepinephrine reuptake inhibitors (SNRIs)	Inhibit presynaptic reuptake of serotonin and norepinephrine
Duloxetine	
Venlafaxine and desvenlafaxine	
Milnacipran and levomilnacipran	
Tricyclic antidepressants (TCAs)	Inhibit presynaptic reuptake of serotonin and norepinephrine (in various proportions depending on the specific TCA)
Amitriptyline	
Desipramine	
Doxepin	
Imipramine	
Nortriptyline	
Monoamine oxidase inhibitors (MAOIs)	Inhibit monoamine oxidase, the enzyme that catalyzes oxidative metabolism of monoamine neurotransmitters
Isocarboxazid	
Phenelzine	
Selegiline	Selective MAO-B inhibitor
Tranylcypromine	
Other drugs	
Bupropion	Unknown, although it is weak inhibitor of presynaptic reuptake of norepinephrine and dopamine
Mirtazapine	Serotonin (5-hydroxytryptamine [5-HT]) antagonist at α_2 and 5-HT2 receptors
Trazodone	Inhibits presynaptic reuptake of serotonin; antagonist at 5-HT2 and 5-HT3 receptors
Vilazodone	Inhibits presynaptic reuptake of serotonin; agonist at 5-HT1A receptors
Vortioxetine	Inhibits the reuptake of serotonin (5-HT); antagonist at 5-HT3, 5-HT1D, and 5-HT7 receptors; agonist at 5-HT1A receptors; 5-HT1B receptor partial agonist

intense distressing responses to reminders of the trauma), avoidance of distressing memories or external reminders, negative cognitions and mood (e.g., amnesia for aspects of the event, negativistic thoughts about oneself in general or self-blame for the event, diminished interests or activities, feelings of detachment), and alterations in arousal and reactivity, the disorder is called *acute stress disorder* (duration up to 1 month) or *post-traumatic stress disorder* (duration is more than 1 month). These disorders also have been classified separately, as in addition to anxiety symptoms, they can present with prominent dysphoric symptoms, externalizing aggressive symptoms, or dissociative symptoms.

These disorders are common, with point prevalence of 1% to 2% each for panic disorder and obsessive-compulsive disorder and up to 10% for phobias. Although there are fewer data on long-term outcome than for mood disorders, many of these disorders tend to have a chronic waxing and waning course. Most of these disorders have a first onset in the teens, 20s, and 30s. Although new-onset anxiety is common in later life, the cause is rarely a late-onset primary anxiety disorder (see Table 111.2).

The pathogeneses of most anxiety disorders may be understood as inappropriate activation of the stress response system involving a variety of neuroendocrine and autonomic outputs and coordinated

by the central nucleus of the amygdala and other brain structures. The amygdala receives excitatory glutamatergic inputs from cortical sensory areas and the thalamus and has outputs to the major monoaminergic centers (e.g., noradrenergic neurons of the locus coeruleus, dopaminergic neurons of the ventral tegmental area, and serotonergic neurons of the raphe nuclei), which project to the many brain regions subserving the symptoms of anxiety.

The identification and correction of dysfunctional patterns of thinking (i.e., cognitive therapy) and the extinction of pathologic behaviors and positive reinforcement of more functional behaviors (i.e., behavior therapy) are evidence-based psychotherapies useful in most anxiety disorders. They are the sole therapies for specific phobias and may be the sole or primary therapy for most other anxiety disorders or combined with pharmacotherapy.

Antidepressant, anxiolytic, and other drug therapies are used in treatment. Increasingly, antidepressant medications have replaced anxiolytics as the mainstay of pharmacotherapy for panic disorder, post-traumatic stress disorder, generalized social phobia, and generalized anxiety disorder. For obsessive-compulsive disorder, only antidepressant agents with pronounced activity on the serotonergic system (i.e., clomipramine and selective serotonin reuptake inhibitors [SSRIs]; see Table 111.4) are efficacious.

PSYCHOTIC DISORDERS

Psychosis is a loss of reality testing, manifested as hallucinations (i.e., false sensory perceptions), delusions (i.e., fixed false beliefs), and thought process derailments. Schizophrenia is the prototypic psychotic disorder; it includes acute episodes of psychosis (i.e., positive symptoms) and often declining overall functioning over time related to the negative symptoms such as affective flattening, abulia, apathy, and social withdrawal.

The lifetime prevalence of schizophrenia is slightly less than 1%, and its chronic, debilitating course takes a considerable toll on patients, families, and society. Peak onset is in late adolescence to young adulthood, with slightly younger ages for males than females. The annual incidence is approximately 15 cases per 100,000 people, but with marked variability across study samples and populations. The condition is slightly more common in males than females.

The pathogenesis of schizophrenia remains unknown, but it is clearly multifactorial. Genetic factors account for up to 50% of the risk, with multiple loci implicated. Studies of postmortem brains indicate a nongliotic neuropathologic process with subtle disruptions of cortical cytoarchitecture. It is likely that psychosocial factors and neurodevelopment interact with a nonlocalizable brain lesion present at birth or acquired early in life. Dopaminergic mesocortical and mesolimbic pathways are important in the production of psychotic symptoms.

Antipsychotic medications, often with adjunctive benzodiazepines, are used to treat acute psychotic episodes (Table 111.6). Although maintenance antipsychotic medications help reduce the severity and frequency of acute psychotic episodes, comprehensive psychosocial rehabilitation programs are required to help patients manage interpersonal and other stressors and to improve overall clinical outcomes. Adjunctive cognitive-behavioral therapy also may improve outcomes for some patients. Second-generation (atypical) antipsychotic medications have replaced first-generation antipsychotics in common US practice because of their lower rates of extrapyramidal side effects, including tardive dyskinesia. However, second-generation drugs contribute to an increase in obesity and metabolic syndrome.

Schizoaffective disorder is a chronic, recurrent disorder with a prevalence slightly lower than that of schizophrenia. It is characterized by episodes of non-mood psychosis and mood episodes (i.e., manic or depressed) with psychotic features. Its diagnosis therefore cannot be based on the patient's clinical findings at any one point in time but requires knowledge of the overall course. The outcomes of schizoaffective disorder are heterogeneous but on average are intermediate between schizophrenia and mood disorders. Treatment is symptomatic, using antipsychotic, mood stabilizing, and antidepressant medications to target specific psychotic and mood symptoms.

Delusional disorder is characterized by delusions in the absence of thought process disorder, prominent hallucinations, or the negative symptoms of schizophrenia. The delusions may be potentially

---

TABLE 111.5 Common Somatic Symptoms of Anxiety

Cardiorespiratory
Palpitations
Chest pain
Dyspnea or sensation of being smothered

Gastrointestinal
Sensation of choking
Dyspepsia
Nausea
Diarrhea
Abdominal bloating or pain

Genitourinary
Urinary frequency or urgency

Neurologic or Autonomic
Diaphoresis
Warm flushes
Dizziness or presyncope
Paresthesia
Tremor
Headache

TABLE 111.6 Commonly Used Antipsychotic Medications

Name	Mechanism of Action/Side Effect Profile
First Generation ("Typical")	Blocks D2 receptors in addition to some level of muscarinic, histaminic and alpha-adrenergic blockade; tend to have higher rates of neurologic side effects
Chlorpromazine	High blockade of histaminic, alpha adrenergic receptors, higher likelihood of sedation and anticholinergic effects, "low potency"
Fluphenazine	
Haloperidol	Higher blockade of D2 receptors with little blockade of others, higher likelihood of extrapyramidal side effects, "high potency"
Perphenazine	
Thioridazine	
Thiothixene	
Trifluorophenazine	
Second Generation ("Atypical")	Blocks D2 receptors and 5HT2A receptors; higher rates of metabolic side effects
Aripiprazole	Partial D2 agonist
Asenapine	
Brexpiprazole	
Cariprazine	
Clozapine	
Iloperidone	
Lurasidone	

plausible (i.e., not bizarre). Delusional disorder has a lifetime prevalence of approximately 0.2%. It often is only partially responsive to antipsychotic medications, but patients' functioning may be largely unimpaired if they are able with the aid of antipsychotics and psychotherapy to avoid acting on their delusions. The pathogeneses of the non-schizophrenic primary psychotic disorders remain largely unknown.

SOMATIC SYMPTOM DISORDER AND RELATED DISORDERS

Formerly called *somatoform disorders*, these conditions include somatic symptoms and associated thoughts, feelings, or behaviors that are distressing and disabling. Prominent types include somatic symptom disorder (i.e., excessive thoughts, feelings, or behaviors associated with one or more somatic symptoms), illness anxiety disorder (i.e., illness preoccupation and health-related behaviors disproportionate to somatic symptoms), conversion (i.e., functional neurologic symptom) disorder (i.e., neurologic somatoform symptoms incompatible with recognized neurologic or general medical conditions), and psychological factors affecting physical conditions. Factitious disorder (i.e., Munchausen syndrome) is a mental disorder in which patients consciously produce stigmata of disease (e.g., simulated or artificially induced fever or hypoglycemia) for the unconscious gain of assuming the sick role.

Although identifiable physical disease is insufficient to fully explain the patient's presentation, in all these conditions other than factitious disorder, the patient's distress and dysfunction are *not* consciously produced and are just as distressing to patients as would be similar symptoms produced by other medical conditions. Malingering is the conscious feigning of illness for conscious gain and therefore is not a mental disorder.

PERSONALITY DISORDERS

Personality is defined as the repertoire of enduring patterns of inner mental experience and behavior, including affect and impulse regulation, defense and coping mechanisms, and interpersonal relatedness. Personality traits must be distinguished from time-limited states. For example, a patient who exhibits dependent features solely while acutely depressed does not have a dependent personality.

A personality disorder is diagnosed when personality traits lead to pervasive (if variable) subjective distress or dysfunction in a broad range of situations. The major personality disorders are listed in Table 111.3. Personality and personality disorders are the result of complex interactions among genetic, environmental, and developmental factors. Approaches to patients with personality disorders depend on the specific type, but in most clinical circumstances other than long-term psychotherapy, the realistic goal is not to alter fundamental personality structure but to help the patient maximize use of personality strengths (e.g., optimal defense mechanisms) while minimizing the harmful effects of emotional dysregulation, unhelpful defenses, and destructive behaviors.

Although not the mainstay of most treatments for personality disorders, pharmacotherapy can be useful in selected patients (e.g., antipsychotics to target escalating paranoia in paranoid personality disorder, mood stabilizers or antidepressants to target emotional dysregulation in borderline personality disorder). Patients with personality disorders are also prone to mood, anxiety, eating, addictive, and other treatable psychiatric disorders.

PROSPECTUS FOR THE FUTURE

Advances in neuroscience will lead to not only better pharmacologic and other somatic therapies, but may hold the key to more accurate diagnosis of psychiatric illness. In the future, precision medicine in psychiatry will allow us to use information such as genomics and brain imaging to more accurately define, diagnose, and treat illness. Although not ready to be used clinically, the National Institute of Mental Health (NIMH) has initiated the Research Domains Criteria in order to test a framework of mental illness that goes beyond the traditional syndrome-based diagnosis by aligning more closely with underlying neural systems. The recent approval of two drugs with different mechanisms of action from previous antidepressants, intranasal esketamine and brexanolone, exemplifies the potential to discover new ways to treat mood and other psychiatric disorders. What is particularly exciting regarding these new medications is that they appear to work more quickly than other antidepressants. It remains to be seen how they will be optimally deployed among other therapeutic choices. Prevention remains an important area of growth in psychiatry, albeit an area that historically had lagged behind many other medical specialties. Promising data showing that early intervention teams for patients suffering from first onset psychosis improve long-term outcomes is a step in the right direction. Evidence is also growing that late-life depression can be prevented by cost-effective preventive interventions in at-risk patients in primary care and several specialty settings. Advances in prevention, diagnosis, and treatment will contribute to a new understanding of mental illness and lead to a future in which the global burden of mental illness can be decreased.

SUGGESTED READINGS

American Psychiatric Association: Diagnostic and statistical manual of mental disorders, ed 5, Arlington, VA, 2013, American Psychiatric Association.

Batelaan NM, Bosman RC, Muntingh A, et al: Risk of relapse after antidepressant discontinuation in anxiety disorders, obsessive compulsive disorder and post-traumatic stress disorder: systematic review and meta-analysis of relapse prevention trials, BMJ 358:j3927, 2017.

Bateman AW, Gunderson J, Mulder R: Treatment of personality disorder, Lancet 385:735–743, 2015.

Cipriani A, Furukawa TA, Salanti G, et al: Comparative efficacy and acceptability of 21 antidepressant drugs for the acute treatment of adults with major depressive disorder: a systematic review and network meta-analysis, Lancet 391:1357–1366, 2018.

Grande I, Berk M, Birmaher B, Vieta E: Bipolar disorder, Lancet 387:1561–1572, 2016.

Leucht S, Cipriani A, Spineli L, et al: Comparative efficacy and tolerability of 15 antipsychotic drugs in schizophrenia: a multiple-treatments meta-analysis, Lancet 382:951–962, 2013.

Lieberman JA, First MB: Psychosis, N Engl J Med 379:270–280, 2018.

Malhi GS, Mann JJ: Depression, Lancet 392:2299–2312, 2018.

O'Neal MA, Baslet G: Treatment for patients with a functional neurologic disorder (conversion disorder): an integrated approach, Am J Psychiatry 175:307–314, 2018.

Sanacors G, Frye MA, McDonald W, et al: A consensus statement on the use of ketamine in the treatment of mood disorders, JAMA Psychiatry 74:399–405, 2017.

Slee A, Nazareth I, Bondarek P, et al: Pharmacological treatments for generalized anxiety disorder: a systematic review and network meta-analysis, Lancet 393:768–777, 2019.

Stroup TS, Gerhard T, Crystal S, et al: Comparative effectiveness of clozapine and standard antipsychotic treatment in adults with schizophrenia, Am J Psychiatry 173:166–172, 2016.

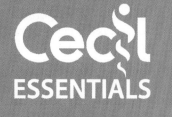

112

Autonomic Nervous System Disorders

William P. Cheshire, Jr.

DEFINITION AND EPIDEMIOLOGY

The autonomic nervous system reaches throughout the body and governs all visceral activity. Its central network and peripheral sympathetic and parasympathetic divisions integrate complex organ functions, maintain internal homeostasis in response to environmental change, modulate the flight-or-fight physiologic response to stress, and enable circulation, digestion, and procreation.

Benign dysautonomias are common. Neurally mediated syncope and situational reflex syncope in response to emotional distress, carotid sinus stimulation, micturition, defecation, coughing, straining, or other factors occur in about 20% of people during a lifetime and account for 1% to 3% of all emergency room visits. Hyperhidrosis of the palms and soles affects about 1% of the population. Anhidrosis can contribute to increased mortality rates during severe heat stress.

One of the most disabling manifestations of autonomic failure is orthostatic hypotension, the prevalence of which increases with age, physical inactivity, and in diseases that impair sympathetic adrenergic nerves. Orthostatic hypotension affects about 5% to 20% of the elderly.

Diabetes mellitus is the most common cause of autonomic neuropathy in industrialized nations. About 30% of diabetics develop autonomic neuropathy, and symptomatic orthostatic hypotension occurs in 5% of patients. Other features of autonomic neuropathy include constipation in 40% to 60% of diabetics, gastroparesis in 20% to 40%, bladder dysfunction in 30% to 80%, and erectile impotence in more than 30% of men.

❖ For a deeper discussion of these topics, please see Chapter 22, "Common Clinical Sequelae of Aging," and Chapter 216, "Diabetes Mellitus," in *Goldman-Cecil Medicine*, 26th Edition.

PATHOLOGY

Many brain, spinal cord, peripheral nerve, and systemic disorders that impair autonomic nerves can cause autonomic dysfunction or failure. They include a wide range of degenerative, traumatic, cerebrovascular, autoimmune, genetic, metabolic, toxic, and pharmacologic conditions.

Small-caliber peripheral autonomic nerves are unmyelinated or thinly myelinated, and small-fiber peripheral neuropathies that cause distal sensory loss may also involve sympathetic or parasympathetic nerves. Diabetic autonomic neuropathy results from microvascular damage to autonomic nerves. Several hereditary, infectious, metabolic, toxic, and drug-induced sensory and autonomic neuropathies are recognized causes.

Accumulation of abnormal proteins distinguishes some of the degenerative dysautonomias. Oligodendroglial cytoplasmic inclusions composed of aggregates of misfolded α-synuclein are pathognomonic of multiple system atrophy. Abnormally folded sympathetic neuronal accumulation of α-synuclein occurs in Lewy body disorders such as Parkinson's disease. Peripheral autonomic nerve deposition of β-pleated sheet amyloid protein causes a severe autonomic

neuropathy, which is frequently seen in primary amyloidosis, immunoglobulin light chain–associated disease, and hereditary amyloidosis, although rarely in reactive amyloidosis.

Other dysautonomias have an autoimmune basis. Autonomic instability has long been recognized in Guillain-Barré syndrome, which is an acute inflammatory, demyelinating polyradiculoneuropathy associated with antiganglioside antibodies (e.g., anti-GM_1, anti-GM_3). The list of autoimmune autonomic neuropathies includes acute autonomic ganglionopathy; patients with acute pandysautonomia have antibodies against the nicotinic acetylcholine receptor in autonomic ganglia, which is sometimes associated with lung cancer or thymoma. Additional paraneoplastic autonomic neuropathies include those associated with antineuronal nuclear antibody type 1 (i.e., ANNA-1 or anti-Hu) and antibodies against collapsing response mediator proteins (i.e., CRMP-5 or anti-CV2). Lambert-Eaton myasthenic syndrome is associated with antibodies to voltage-gated calcium channels. Antibodies to voltage-gated potassium channels cause autoimmune neuromyotonia and dysautonomia with hyperhidrosis and orthostatic intolerance.

Pharmacologic agents frequently alter autonomic function. Diuretics, sympatholytic drugs, α-adrenoreceptor blockers, and vasodilators can cause or contribute to orthostatic hypotension. Anticholinergics and carbonic anhydrase inhibitors decrease sweating, whereas opioids and selective serotonin reuptake inhibitors increase sweating. Opioids slow intestinal transit. Anticholinergics, tricyclic antidepressants, and antihistamines may cause urinary retention.

Functional dysautonomias are medical conditions in which autonomic function is impaired in the absence of a known structural neurologic deficit. Some psychological disorders may manifest with autonomic symptoms because emotional and autonomic centers are closely linked in the limbic system.

❖ For a deeper discussion of these topics, please see Chapter 392, "Peripheral Neuropathies," Chapter 179, "Amyloidosis," and Chapter 41, "Mechanisms of Immune-Mediated Tissue Injury," in *Goldman-Cecil Medicine*, 26th Edition.

CLINICAL PRESENTATION

Clinical manifestations of autonomic disorders vary according to which nerves are involved and how severely. Autonomic signs and symptoms may be benign or serious, paroxysmal or continuous, or localized or generalized, and they may represent hypofunction or hyperfunction.

Afferent autonomic lesions that separate central autonomic nuclei from incoming information needed to gauge an appropriate response may cause excessive or erratic autonomic outflow. An example of afferent dysautonomia is the volatile hypertension in carotid arterial baroreceptor failure after irradiation to treat laryngeal carcinoma. Spinal cord injuries above the level of sympathetic outflow at T5 can cause autonomic dysreflexia, a condition of paroxysmal sympathetic surges with hypertension, diaphoresis, flushing, and headache. Catastrophic brain disorders such as subarachnoid hemorrhage, trauma, or hydrocephalus may also cause autonomic storms if hypothalamic circuits are released from cortical inhibition.

More common are efferent autonomic lesions, which cause failure of outflow to neuroeffector junctions, resulting in inadequate excitatory or inhibitory autonomic responses. An example of efferent dysautonomias is autonomic peripheral neuropathy, which may accompany distal sensory loss and decreased Achilles tendon jerks.

Cardiovascular adrenergic failure impairs the cardiac and peripheral vascular response needed to maintain blood pressure during orthostatic stress. Patients present with orthostatic hypotension and may report lightheadedness or fatigue on standing that is relieved by sitting.

Vagal failure impairs cardiac parasympathetic tone that may protect against arrhythmogenic sympathetic activity. Patients have a fixed heart rate that does not vary with respiration.

Sudomotor failure (failure to stimulate the sweat glands) with extensive anhidrosis may coexist with tonic pupils (sluggish response to light) and areflexia (i.e., Ross syndrome), and it can increase the risk of heat exhaustion or heat stroke. A dramatic example of regional sudomotor failure is harlequin syndrome, in which hemifacial cutaneous sympathetic denervation divides the pale and dry denervated half of the face from the intact half that flushes red in response to heat stress. Horner syndrome (i.e., unilateral ptosis, miosis, and anhidrosis) may be identified.

The clinical hallmark of generalized autonomic failure is severe orthostatic hypotension without pulse acceleration. In at least one half of patients, it is accompanied by supine and nocturnal hypertension, a reversal of the normal diurnal decrease in blood pressure during sleep. In addition to vagal and sudomotor failure, patients with generalized autonomic failure may have constipation, gastroparesis, bladder dysfunction, male erectile dysfunction, dry mouth, or dry eyes. Some have postprandial hypotension, in which a large meal high in carbohydrate content causes a reduction in blood pressure.

One of the most severe autonomic disorders is multiple system atrophy, which is a sporadic, progressive, ultimately fatal neurodegenerative disorder in which autonomic failure occurs in combination with parkinsonism or cerebellar ataxia. Bladder hypotonia with overflow incontinence and nocturnal respiratory stridor may occur. The parkinsonian phenotype (i.e., Shy-Drager syndrome) tends to respond poorly to levodopa. Orthostatic hypotension is also common in Lewy body disorders such as Parkinson's disease. Pure autonomic failure consists of widespread autonomic failure without other neurologic features.

In contrast to autonomic failure, neurally mediated syncope occurs in patients with a functioning autonomic nervous system in which there is a reversal of normal autonomic outflow. Prodromal features typically include pallor, sweating, nausea, abdominal discomfort, mydriasis, increased respiratory rate, and cognitive slowing, which may progress to transient loss of consciousness if the patient continues in an upright posture. Withdrawal of peripheral sympathetic vasomotor tone (i.e., vasodepressor syncope) or an increase in parasympathetic tone (i.e., vasovagal syncope) causes a fall in blood pressure, heart rate, and cerebral perfusion.

Orthostatic intolerance refers to a heterogeneous group of conditions in which patients have difficulty sustaining the autonomic outflow needed to maintain blood pressure during the gravitational stress of prolonged standing. Some patients experience a gradual decline in blood pressure, but others experience an abnormal increase in heart rate without a drop in blood pressure.

❖ For a deeper discussion of these topics, please see Chapter 56, "Approach to the Patient with Suspected Arrhythmia," Chapter 70, "Arterial Hypertension," Chapter 127, "Disorders of Gastrointestinal Motility," and Chapter 381, "Parkinsonism," in *Goldman-Cecil Medicine*, 26th Edition.

DIAGNOSIS AND DIFFERENTIAL DIAGNOSIS

A careful history and discerning physical examination are essential for reaching a diagnosis. The astute clinician inquires about the time course of symptoms and the circumstances that provoke or modify them. How long have they been present? Are they stable, improving, or worsening? Do they occur consistently or episodically? Orthostatic disorders are typically worse in the early morning, in heat, and after physical exercise or a large meal. How well the patient tolerates standing in line or taking a warm shower are helpful clues to identifying orthostatic intolerance.

Physical signs of autonomic dysfunction may include pupillary asymmetry or sluggishness, ptosis, or mucosal dryness. An acutely distended bladder may be suspected by percussion. Asymmetrical sweating may be visible or palpable.

The most important part of the examination, but one that is frequently omitted, is measurement of orthostatic blood pressure (Fig. 112.1). Blood pressure and heart rate should be assessed when the patient is resting supine and again after standing for 1 to 3 minutes. Correlation with symptoms is key. Patients with orthostatic

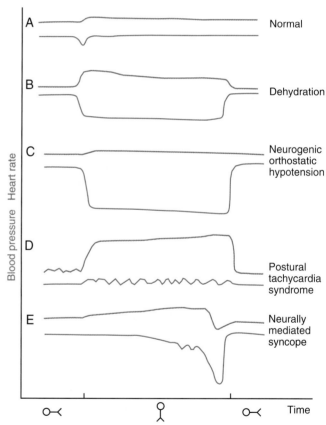

Fig. 112.1 Orthostatic blood pressure profiles. (A) The normal response to standing or head-up tilt is no change or a small decrease in blood pressure that recovers within half a minute and a small increase in heart rate. (B) Dehydration causing intravascular hypovolemia may cause a fall in blood pressure accompanied by reflex tachycardia. (C) Neurogenic orthostatic hypotension may cause a more profound drop in blood pressure. Hypotension occurs immediately and is sustained without recovery during standing and often without adequate compensatory tachycardia. (D) Postural tachycardia syndrome is characterized by an abnormal increase in heart rate without orthostatic hypotension. (E) Neurally mediated syncope develops after standing for some time, may be preceded by oscillations in blood pressure, and may be accompanied by bradycardia with loss of consciousness in about 7 seconds if cerebral perfusion is not restored.

hypotension may appear less alert, or they may shift weight from one leg to the other to improve venous return, lower the head to bring the cerebral circulation closer to the level of the heart, or exhibit lower extremity rubor if cutaneous vasomotor function is impaired.

Orthostatic hypotension is a reduction in systolic blood pressure of at least 20 mm Hg or a reduction in diastolic blood pressure of at least 10 mm Hg, with or without symptoms, within 1 to 3 minutes of assuming an erect posture. Neurogenic orthostatic hypotension, a cardinal manifestation of sympathetic adrenergic failure, is typically sustained with continued standing and may lack the reflex tachycardia seen when hypotension is caused by blood loss, dehydration, or excessive venous pooling.

Orthostatic intolerance is difficulty tolerating the upright posture because of symptoms that resolve when supine. These patients do not have orthostatic hypotension but may have a sustained increase in postural heart rate (postural tachycardia syndrome) of more than 30 beats per minute in adults (40 in adolescents).

Laboratory testing of autonomic responses under controlled conditions is useful to determine the presence, severity, and distribution of autonomic failure and to distinguish neurogenic from other causes of orthostatic hypotension. Clinical autonomic testing typically evaluates beat-to-beat blood pressure and heart rate responses to the Valsalva maneuver, upright tilt, and periodic deep breathing, along with quantitative assessment of axons that produce sweating responses. Ambulatory blood pressure testing is useful for the assessment of episodic or postprandial hypotension, nocturnal hypertension, and the volatile hypertension of autonomic storms.

TREATMENT

Treatment options for orthostatic hypotension are outlined in Table 112.1. The goal is to enable the patient to stand long enough to engage in daily activities without symptoms. Medication is not always needed and can potentially exacerbate recumbent hypertension. Orthostatic intolerance was shown in a randomized controlled trial to improve after endurance exercise training.

Generalized hyperhidrosis may be reduced by oral anticholinergic agents such as 1 to 2 mg of glycopyrrolate taken one to three times daily. Topical glycopyrrolate reduces regional gustatory sweating. Subdermal botulinum toxin injections are helpful for some forms of focal hyperhidrosis, and palmar hyperhidrosis may respond to tap water iontophoresis or, in severe cases, to endoscopic thoracic sympathotomy.

For a deeper discussion of these topics, please see Chapter 390, ❖ "Autonomic Disorders and Their Management," in *Goldman-Cecil Medicine*, 26th Edition.

PROGNOSIS

Orthostatic intolerance and neurally mediated syncope are frequently benign, manageable, and improve or recover with time. Autonomic failure, in contrast, can signify a more serious prognosis, depending on the nature and extent of its pathophysiology. Persistent or severe orthostatic hypotension carries a worse prognosis.

Diabetic cardiovascular autonomic neuropathy doubles the risk for silent myocardial ischemia and overall mortality. Amyloid autonomic neuropathy is especially grave, with a median survival of less than 1 year if the patient has orthostatic hypotension. Pure autonomic failure may remain stable for many years, although some patients with this phenotype eventually develop signs of multiple system atrophy, which denotes a life expectancy of 7 to 9 years after diagnosis.

Regular physical exercise can reverse the autonomic deconditioning that comes from inactivity. In the elderly, it may compensate for some age-associated decline in autonomic function.

For a deeper discussion of these topics, please see Chapter 390, ❖ "Autonomic Disorders and Their Management," in *Goldman-Cecil Medicine*, 26th Edition.

TABLE 112.1 Treatment of Orthostatic Hypotension

Intervention	Rationale	Dosage
Avoid prolonged bed rest and increase time spent upright	Reverses physiologic deconditioning	
Liberalize fluid intake	Expands plasma volume	2-2.5 L/day
Increase sodium intake	Expands plasma volume	Salt 10-20 g/day
Compressive leg garments and abdominal binder	Reduces venous pooling	20-40 mm Hg (10 mm Hg for abdominal binder)
Physical counter-maneuvers	Tensing limb muscles augments venous return	Isometric contractions for 30 sec
Water bolus treatment	Sympathetic reflex increases blood pressure for 1-2 hr	16 oz. plain water
Elevate head of bed 4 inches	Decreases nocturnal natriuresis and nocturnal hypertension	
Avoid large meals high in carbohydrate content	If patient is subject to postprandial hypotension	
Discontinue or decrease dose of blood pressure–lowering drugs		
Midodrine	α-Adrenergic agonist, constricts capacitance vessels	5-10 mg tid
Droxidopa	Norepinephrine prodrug, stimulates sympathetic nerves	100-600 mg tid
Fludrocortisone	Retains sodium and sensitizes peripheral vascular α-adrenergic receptors	0.1-0.4 mg/day
Pyridostigmine	Stimulates sympathetic ganglionic transmission	30-60 mg bid or tid

SUGGESTED READINGS

Cheshire WP: Syncope, Continuum 23:335–358, 2017.

Cheshire WP, Goldstein DS: Autonomic uprising: the tilt table test in autonomic medicine, Clin Auton Res 29:215–230, 2019.

Cheshire WP, Goldstein DS: The physical examination as a window into autonomic disorders, Clin Auton Res 28:23–33, 2018.

Eschlböck S, Wenning G, Fanciulli A: Evidence-based treatment of neurogenic orthostatic hypotension and related symptoms, J Neural Transm 124:1567–1605, 2017.

Feldstein C, Weder AB: Orthostatic hypotension: a common, serious and under-recognized problem in hospitalized patients, J Am Soc Hypertens 6:27–39, 2013.

Figueroa JJ, Basford JR, Low PA: Preventing and treating orthostatic hypotension: as easy as A, B, C, Cleve, Clin J Med 77:298–306, 2010.

Goldstein DS, Cheshire WP: The autonomic medical history, Clin Auton Res 27:223–233, 2017.

Guzman JC, Armaganijan LV, Morillo CA: Treatment of neurally mediated reflex syncope, Cardiol Clin 31:123–129, 2013.

Karayannis G, Giamouzis G, Cokkinos DV, et al: Diabetic cardiovascular autonomic neuropathy: clinical implications, Expert Rev Cardiovasc Ther 10:747–765, 2012.

Koike H, Watanabe H, Sobue G: The spectrum of immune-mediated autonomic neuropathies: insights from the clinicopathological features, J Neurol Neurosurg Psychiatry 84:98–106, 2013.

Spallone V, Ziegler D, Freeman R, et al: Cardiovascular autonomic neuropathy in diabetes: clinical impact, assessment, diagnosis, and management, Diabetes Metab Res Rev 27:639–653, 2011.

Stewart JM: Common syndromes of orthostatic intolerance, Pediatrics 131:968–980, 2013.

Wenning GK, Geser F, Krismer F, et al: The natural history of multiple system atrophy: a prospective European cohort study, Lancet Neurol 12:264–274, 2013.

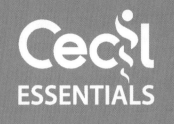

113

Headache, Neck and Back Pain, and Cranial Neuralgias

Shane Lyons, Timothy J. Counihan

HEADACHE

Definition and Epidemiology

Headache is caused by irritation of pain-sensitive intracranial structures, including the dural sinuses; the intracranial portions of the trigeminal, glossopharyngeal, vagus, and upper cervical nerves; the large arteries; and the venous sinuses. Many structures are insensitive to pain, including the brain parenchyma, the ependymal lining of the ventricles, and the choroid plexuses. The insensitivity of the brain parenchyma to pain accounts for the common clinical observation of patients who, despite having large intracerebral lesions (such as a hematoma or a brain tumor), complain of little or no headache. The term "cervicogenic" headache is sometimes used to indicate that the source of headache (usually occipital in location) arises from an abnormality in the cervical spine.

Classification of Headache

Headache is generally classified into primary, secondary, and cranial neuralgia syndromes (Table 113.1, Table 113.2, Table 113.3). It is essential that the clinician make every effort to make an accurate clinical diagnosis of the presenting headache syndrome; Table 113.4 provides some key questions in the assessment of the patient with headache.

Migraine

Definition. Migraine is a common episodic neurologic disorder characterized by disabling headache and reversible neurologic and systemic symptoms. Migraine may be heralded by a premonitory phase of fatigue and neck stiffness, which precedes attacks by hours or days. One third of patients with migraine experience various combinations of neurologic, gastrointestinal, and autonomic phenomena (termed the "aura"). The diagnosis is based on the headache's characteristics and associated symptoms. Results of the physical examination as well as the laboratory studies are usually normal.

Every year, up to 18% of women and 6% of men experience a migraine attack. It is estimated that 28 million Americans have disabling migraine headaches. All varieties of migraine may begin at any age from early childhood on, although peak ages at onset are adolescence and early adulthood.

Several subtypes of migraine are described (Table 113.5). The two most common are migraine without aura and migraine with aura; migraine without aura accounts for 70% of patients. Migraine auras are focal neurologic symptoms that precede, accompany, or, rarely, follow an attack. The aura usually develops over 5 to 20 minutes, lasts less than 60 minutes, and can involve visual, sensorimotor, language, or brain stem disturbances. The most common aura is typified by positive visual phenomena (such as scintillating scotomata [zig zag, shimmering or colored lines] or fortification spectra [more complex images sometimes resembling a fortress]) that often precede the headache. Auras may also occur in the absence of headache (acephalgic migraine), particularly later in life. Migraine auras are stereotyped and a sudden change in a previously predictable aura pattern should prompt evaluation for an aura mimic.

The differential diagnosis of an aura includes a focal epileptic seizure arising from the visual cortex of the occipital lobe, a transient ischemic attack (TIA), or "amyloid spells" occurring in the context of cerebral amyloid angiopathy. In the latter, there is no evolution of symptoms, and the symptoms themselves are typically "negative" (such as a hemianopia) rather than the "positive" visual phenomenon of phosphenes that is characteristic of the migrainous aura. Amyloid spells are associated with evolving and "positive" symptoms and may be difficult to accurately distinguish clinically from migraine aura. The pain of migraine is often pulsating, unilateral, frontotemporal in distribution, exacerbated by movement, and usually accompanied by anorexia, nausea, and, occasionally, vomiting. In characteristic attacks, patients are markedly intolerant of light (photophobia) and seek rest in a dark room. There may also be intolerance to sound (phonophobia) and occasionally to odors (osmophobia). The diagnosis of migraine requires the presence of at least one of these features, particularly in the absence of gastrointestinal symptoms. The presence of these symptoms results in a syndrome that is invariably disabling for the patient, to the extent that for the duration of the attack he or she is unable to function normally. Following resolution of headache, a postdromal phase characterized by asthenia, fatigue, poor concentration, and nausea may persist for hours. In children, migraine is often associated with episodic abdominal pain, motion sickness, vertigo, and sleep disturbances. Onset of typical migraine late in life (older than age 50) is rare, although recurrence of migraine that had been in remission is not uncommon. Recurrent migraine headache associated with transient hemiparesis or hemiplegia occurs rarely as a clearly genetically determined (mendelian) disease, most commonly due to mutations of the *CACNA1A* gene (*familial hemiplegic migraine*).

Migraine with basilar aura is unusual and occurs primarily in childhood. Severe episodic headache is preceded, or accompanied by, signs of bilateral occipital lobe, brain stem, or cerebellar dysfunction (e.g., diplopia, bilateral visual field abnormalities, ataxia, dysarthria, bilateral sensory disturbances, other cranial nerve signs, and occasionally coma). *Vestibular migraine* is characterized by symptoms of vertigo with or without the other typical migraine symptoms. A number of episodic syndromes have been identified that bear similarities to migraine; these include cyclical vomiting, abdominal migraine, benign paroxysmal vertigo, and benign paroxysmal torticollis.

Complications of migraine. *Status migrainosus* refers to a severe migraine lasting greater than 72 hours. *Migrainous infarction* is a rare complication of migraine with aura. The term *migralepsy* has been suggested for patients in whom an aura triggers a seizure.

TABLE 113.1 Primary Headache Syndromes

Migraine
Tension-type headache
Trigeminal autonomic cephalgias
- Cluster
- Paroxysmal hemicrania
- SUNCT

Other primary headache syndromes
- Primary stabbing headache
- Exertional/sex headache
- Primary thunderclap headache
- Hemicrania continua

SUNCT, Sudden-onset unilateral neuralgiform (headache with) conjunctival tearing.

TABLE 113.2 Secondary Headache Syndromes

Post-traumatic
Vascular
- Subarachnoid hemorrhage
- Vasculitis
- Arterial Dissection (carotid or vertebral)

Nonvascular
- Idiopathic intracranial hypertension (pseudotumor cerebri)
- Low CSF pressure (e.g., post lumbar puncture or CSF leak)
- Tumor
- Chiari malformation

Infection
- Meningitis
- Abscess
- Sinusitis

Disordered Homeostasis
- Hypoxia or hypercapnia (e.g., obstructive sleep apnea)
- Dialysis-associated headache
- Hypoglycemia

Medication
- Side effects (e.g., dipyridamole, nitrates, cyclosporine)
- Withdrawal

Syndrome of Transient Headache and Neurological Deficits With CSF Lymphocytosis (HANDL)
Cervicogenic

CSF, Cerebrospinal fluid.

TABLE 113.3 Common Cranial Neuralgias and Related Disorders

Trigeminal neuralgia
Glossopharyngeal neuralgia
Occipital neuralgia
Other cranial branch neuralgias (e.g., superior orbital neuralgia)
Central facial pain syndromes (e.g., cold-stimulus headache)

TABLE 113.4 Key Questions in the Assessment of Headache

1. For how long have you been having headaches?
2. What were they like when they first began? Were they intermittent, daily persistent, or progressive from the beginning?
3. What is the length of time from the start of the headache until its peak intensity?
4. Are there any warning symptoms (e.g., aura)?
5. Does the headache interfere significantly with normal activity (e.g., work, school)?
6. What aggravates the headache (e.g., light, noise, odors)?
7. What do you do for relief from the headache (e.g., rest, move around, take medication)?
8. What time of day are the headaches most likely to occur? Do they regularly awaken you from sleep?
9. Are you aware of any specific triggers (e.g., foods, stress, lack of sleep, menstrual cycle)?
10. Does anyone else in the family have headaches?

TABLE 113.5 Classification of Migraine

Migraine without aura
Migraine with aura
Migraine variants
- Hemiplegic migraine
- Migraine with basilar aura
- Vestibular migraine
- Retinal migraine

family history is reported in 65% to 91% of cases. Three distinct ion channel gene mutations have been identified in patients with familial hemiplegic migraine (FHM), including a mutation in the *P/Q* type calcium channel on chromosome 19 (FHM 1) and a gene encoding a Na/K– ion pump on chromosome 1 (FHM 2). These findings lend support to the theory that migraine may be a true channelopathy in which mutations of diverse channels result in a common phenotype. The etiology of migraine in the majority of patients remains unknown.

The migrainous aura is likely caused by a "cortical spreading depression," corresponding to a wave of neuronal depolarization spreading over the cortex from posterior to anterior. One of the key structures in the mechanism of pain in migraine is the trigeminal vascular system. Stimulation of the trigeminal nucleus caudalis can activate serotonin receptors and nerve endings on small dural arteries and result in a state of neurogenic inflammation. Activation of the trigeminal ganglion nociceptive (pain) neurons results in the release of calcitonin gene-related peptide (CGRP), a vasoactive peptide that is strongly implicated in the generation of migraine. The critical role of CGRP in migraine has been demonstrated through the induction of migraine by infusing CGRP, while treatment with potent CGRP inhibitors can abort an acute migraine attack. It is postulated that these processes, in turn, stimulate perivascular nerve endings, with resultant orthodromic (normal direction) stimulation of trigeminal nerve and pain referred to its territory. Furthermore, positron emission tomographic (PET) studies have demonstrated activation of brain stem neuromodulatory structures, including the periaqueductal gray matter, locus coeruleus, and raphe nuclei during a migraine attack.

Treatment of migraine. The goals of treatment are (1) making an accurate and confident diagnosis of migraine to reassure the patient that there is no more sinister cause for the headache; (2) relieving acute attacks; and (3) preventing pain and associated symptoms

Pathophysiology of migraine. A migraine attack is the end result of the interaction of a number of factors of varying importance in different individuals. These factors include a genetic predisposition, a susceptibility of the central nervous system to certain stimuli, hormonal factors, and a sequence of neurovascular events. A positive

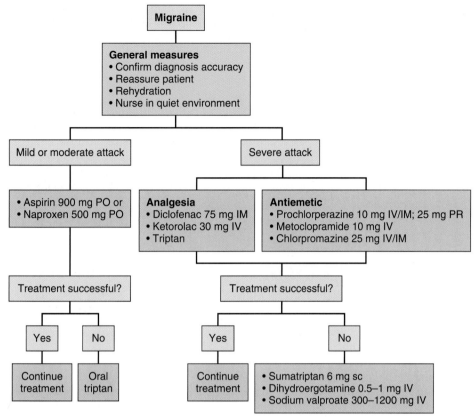

Fig. 113.1 Algorithm for the treatment of migraine. *DHE,* Dihydroergotamine; *IM,* intramuscular; *IV,* intravenous; *NS,* normal saline; *NSAIDs,* nonsteroidal anti-inflammatory drugs; *SC,* subcutaneous.

of recurrent headaches. The first step is to inform the patient that he or she has a migraine. The benign nature of the disorder and the patient's central role in the treatment plan should be emphasized. It is important that the patient keep a headache diary, which serves to help identify covert headache triggers, assists in monitoring headache frequency and response to treatment, and actively involves the patient in the management of the condition. A sustained pain-free therapeutic response should aim to have the patient pain-free at 2 hours with no recurrence and no need for subsequent rescue medication.

Acute migraine attack. Acute attacks are best alleviated using a stratified, rather than stepped care approach, using single agents or varying combinations of drugs as well as with behavioral modification therapy. Many attacks of migraine respond to simple analgesics, such as acetaminophen, aspirin, or nonsteroidal anti-inflammatory agents (NSAIDs). Opioid drugs and butalbital should not be used in the routine management of patients with migraine. Overuse of analgesics is particularly frequent in headache patients; therefore, one of the most important aspects of therapy is the monitoring of amounts of analgesic used to avoid both side effects and the emergence of medication-associated headache. In patients who are nauseated, it is often helpful to prescribe an antiemetic agent early in an attack. Phenothiazine drugs have antiemetic, prokinetic, and sedative properties, but they can produce involuntary movements as an acute adverse effect (acute dystonic reaction) or with prolonged use (tardive dyskinesias).

A number of *migraine-specific* serotonin agonist drugs have become available. These agents, commonly referred to as "triptans," are useful in the acute treatment of migraine, having a rapid onset of action. The increasing availability of non-oral (parenteral, inhaled, and transdermal) preparations has largely circumvented the problem of emesis and gastroparesis in migraine patients resulting in greater efficacy. For instance, sumatriptan, available as a subcutaneous preparation, results

in a headache response rate of close to 70% (Fig. 113.1). Although triptans are highly effective in alleviating migraine, patients must be carefully instructed in their appropriate use. Moreover, a response to these medications does not confirm a diagnosis of migraine.

Treating acute migraine in the emergency room. Migraine is one of the most common reasons for emergency room visits and presents some treatment challenges; typically migraine is more difficult to treat once it is fully established. It is essential to confirm that the diagnosis is accurate, even in patients with an established history of migraine. Patients will usually be aware that the headache will have started as their typical migraine, although it may be more severe than usual. In patients who state that the new headache is different than their usual headache, consideration should be given to exclude a more sinister cause. Thereafter the core principles of treatment include reassurance that the headache can be treated effectively, hydration, pain control, and relief of accompanying symptoms such as nausea and photophobia. The majority of patients presenting with acute migraine as an emergency will have already tried some form of abortive therapy, and they are likely to be dehydrated. In this setting parenteral therapy with an NSAID, a triptan, and an antiemetic is often effective. 5-HT1F receptor agonists (ditans), such as lamiditan, may offer similar benefits to triptans without the vasoconstrictive effect of triptans.

Migraine prevention. Several agents have a strong evidence base for efficacy in the prevention of migraine (Table 113.6). The use of these agents should be restricted to patients who have frequent attacks (usually more than four per month) and who are willing to take daily medication. With any of the medications, an adequate trial period should be given, using adequate doses, before it is declared ineffective. Combination therapy is occasionally required but is not routinely prescribed. For a preventative drug to be considered successful, it should reduce the headache frequency rate by at least

TABLE 113.6   Preventive Therapies for Migraine

Drug Class	Agent	Dose Range	Adverse Effects
β-Adrenoceptor blockers	Propranolol	80-240 mg	Contraindicated in asthma, syncope
	Metoprolol	50-150 mg	
	Timolol	10-20 mg	
Antiepileptic drugs	Divalproex sodium	200-1500 mg	Weight gain, thrombocytopenia, tremor
	Topiramate	25-150 mg	Renal calculi, weight loss, amnesia, glaucoma, dysequilibrium
	Gabapentin	300-1800 mg	
Antidepressants	Amitriptyline	10-150 mg	Somnolence
	Nortriptyline	25-100 mg	Insomnia, hypertension
	Venlafaxine	37.5-150 mg	
Calcium-channel blockers	Verapamil	180-480 mg	Constipation, hypotension, edema
	Flunarizine[a]	5-10 mg	Weight gain, depression
Other	Onabotulinum toxin A	Variable	Discomfort, ecchymosis
CGRP monoclonal antibodies	Erenumab	70-140 mg every 4 week, subcut	Injection site reactions, muscle spasm, hypersensitivity reaction.
	Fremanezumab	225 mg monthly or 675 mg 3-monthly, subcut	Hypersensitivity and injection site reactions
	Galcanezumab	120 mg monthly subcut	Injection site reactions, vertigo, pruritus, constipation

[a]Not available in the United States.

50%. Other medications commonly used for migraine prevention include gabapentin, cyproheptadine, methysergide, and clonidine, but these have limited evidence to support their use as first-line therapy. Magnesium supplementation, the plant extract feverfew, butterbur, and high-dose riboflavin (vitamin B$_2$) have been effective in some patients.

Recent years have seen the emergence of the first medications specifically designed to treat migraine based on pathophysiologic understanding of migraine; monoclonal antibodies directed against CGRP. A number of medications targeting the CGRP cascade in migraine have been developed, including small molecule CGRP antagonists (gepants) and monoclonal antibodies directed against both the CGRP receptor and the CGRP molecule itself. Three CGRP monoclonal antibodies have been approved for the prevention of migraine (erenumab, fremanezumab, and galcanezumab). They are administered by infusion or subcutaneous injection and in trials improved headache by 75% in one third of patients.

A variety of interventional procedures including greater occipital nerve blockade, botulinum toxin injection to the scalp and cervical musculature, and sphenopalatine ganglion (SPG) blockade are deployed in the management of severe and chronic migraine. Neuromodulation, by means of noninvasive vagal nerve stimulation, external trigeminal nerve stimulation, and transcranial magnetic stimulation represents a novel, nonpharmacologic method of migraine management.

Cluster Headache

Clinical features. Cluster headache is the prototypic trigeminal autonomic cephalgia, entirely distinct from migraine, although there may be some clinical overlap. It is uncommon, occurring in less than 10% of all patients with headache. Unlike migraine, it is much more common in men than in women, and the mean age at onset is later in life. Also, unlike migraine, cluster headache rarely begins in childhood, and there is less often a family history. The pain in cluster headache is extremely intense, is strictly unilateral, and is associated with congestion of the nasal mucosa and injection of the conjunctiva on the side of the pain. Increased sweating of the ipsilateral side of the forehead and face may occur. There may be associated ocular signs of

Horner syndrome: miosis, ptosis, and the additional feature of eyelid edema. Attacks often awaken patients, usually 2 to 3 hours after the onset of sleep ("alarm-clock headache"). In contrast to migraineurs, the pain is not relieved by resting in a dark, quiet area; on the contrary, patients sometimes seek activity that can distract them. The duration of headache is usually around 1 hour, although it may recur several times in a day, paroxysmally (in *clusters*) for several weeks.

These periods of frequent headaches are separated by headache-free periods of varying duration, often several months or years. Attacks have a striking tendency to be precipitated by even small amounts of alcohol. There are rare variants of cluster headache: a "chronic variety" in which remissions are brief (less than 14 days); *chronic paroxysmal hemicrania,* in which attacks are shorter and strikingly more prevalent in women; and *hemicrania continua,* in which there is continuous, moderately severe, unilateral headache. The cause of all these syndromes is unknown, although the distribution of the pain suggests dysfunction of the trigeminal nerve.

Treatment. Therapy for cluster headache may be abortive for acute headache or prophylactic to prevent headache. Acute headache may respond to oxygen by mask (7 to 10 L/min for 15 minutes), which is effective within several minutes in 70% of patients. Sumatriptan and dihydroergotamine are also effective. Preventive medications include lithium, divalproex sodium, verapamil, methysergide, melatonin, and corticosteroids. Noninvasive vagal nerve stimulation is now licensed for the acute treatment of episode cluster headache and has evidence to support its use in prevention. Emerging treatments include galcanezumab and SPG stimulation. Paroxysmal hemicrania and related syndromes are often strikingly responsive to indomethacin.

Tension-Type Headache

In contrast to migraine, tension-type headache is featureless. The pain is usually not throbbing, but rather steady and often described as a "pressure feeling" or a "viselike" sensation. It is usually not unilateral and may be frontal, occipital, or generalized. There is frequently pain in the neck area, unlike in migraine. Pain commonly lasts for long periods of time (days) and does not rapidly appear and disappear in attacks. There is no "aura." Photophobia and phonophobia are not prominent. Although tension-type headache may be related by the patient to occur or be exacerbated at times of particular emotional stress, the pathophysiology may relate to sustained craniocervical muscle contraction; hence, a more useful term for this syndrome is *muscle-contraction headache.*

A careful evaluation should be made of the patient's psychosocial milieu and the presence of anxiety or depression. The tricyclic antidepressant drugs in low doses have proven the most useful for prevention of tension-type headache. Although the best documented is amitriptyline, newer agents with fewer side effects may be equally effective. Nonpharmacologic therapies such as relaxation therapy, massage, physiotherapy, or acupuncture may be useful in refractory cases. Intramuscular botulinum toxin injections have been used both in migraine and tension-type headache but are of established benefit only in patients with chronic migraine.

Other Defined Primary Headache Syndromes

Other acute short-lasting headache syndromes need to be differentiated from migraine, cluster, or tension headache. These include primary "thunderclap" headache, *primary stabbing headache, primary exertional headache,* and coital headache. The latter may be indistinguishable from the headache of intracranial aneurysm rupture and requires computed tomography (CT) and lumbar puncture to exclude subarachnoid hemorrhage (SAH). All of these headache syndromes are more common in migraineurs. Two additional rare, short-lasting headache syndromes deserve mention: short-lasting unilateral neuralgiform headache with conjunctival tearing (SUNCT) and *hypnic* headache. The latter refers to multiple episodes of very brief headache that awaken the patient (typically an older woman) from sleep. The syndrome of SUNCT causes multiple very brief (seconds to minutes) episodes of cluster-like headache and autonomic disturbance.

Chronic daily headache is defined arbitrarily as headache lasting for more than 4 hours on more than 15 days in the month for more than 3 months. In clinical practice this means that the patient has a headache more often than not. In these cases it is important to establish whether the headache syndrome began as an episodic disorder (as in migraine or tension-type headache) or whether it consists of new daily persistent headaches.

New daily persistent headache. New daily persistent headache needs to be distinguished from tension-type or migraine headaches that have transformed into chronic daily headache and necessitates investigation to exclude a secondary cause.

Headache may be a manifestation of underlying structural brain disease (see Table 113.2). Headache can be seen in all forms of cerebrovascular disease, including infarction, intracerebral hemorrhage, and SAH, although headache is rarely prominent in cerebral infarction. In contrast, the headache in SAH is usually extremely severe and often described by the patient as "the worst headache of my life." Nuchal rigidity, third nerve palsy (usually involving the pupil), and retinal, preretinal, or subconjunctival hemorrhages may be found. CT of the head usually shows subarachnoid, intraventricular, or other intracranial blood.

Certain symptoms raise suspicion for a structural brain lesion (Tables 113.7 and 113.8).

The patient with headache and fever presents a common diagnostic problem in the emergency department. Neck stiffness is a common symptom. Meningismus is confirmed by eliciting Brudzinski and Kernig signs. Vomiting occurs in about 50% of patients. Suspicion for meningitis should prompt immediate investigation, including a lumbar puncture. If the patient shows focal signs, papilledema, or profound alteration in level of consciousness, CT of the head before

TABLE 113.7 **Differential Diagnosis of Acute Headache: Major Causes**
Migraine
Cluster headache
Stroke
• Subarachnoid hemorrhage
• Intracerebral hemorrhage
• Cerebral infarction
• Arterial dissection (carotid or vertebral)
Acute hydrocephalus
Meningitis or encephalitis
Giant cell arteritis (often chronic)
Tumor (usually chronic)
Trauma

TABLE 113.8 **Clinical Features of Headaches Suggesting a Structural Brain Lesion**
Symptoms
Worst of the patient's life
Progressive
Onset >50 years
Worse in early morning—awakens patient
Marked exacerbation with straining
Focal neurologic dysfunction
Signs
Nuchal rigidity
Fever
Papilledema
Pathologic reflexes or reflex asymmetry
Altered state of consciousness

lumbar puncture is required to rule out focal disease such as an abscess or subdural empyema. These lesions, however, are rare.

Acute sinusitis. Head and face pain is the most prominent feature of sinusitis. Malaise and low-grade fever are usually present. The pain is dull, aching, and nonpulsatile; is exacerbated by movement, coughing, or straining; and is improved with nasal decongestants. The pain is most pronounced on awakening or after any prolonged recumbency and is diminished with maintenance of an upright posture.

The location of the pain depends on the sinus involved. Maxillary sinusitis provokes ipsilateral malar, ear, and dental pain with significant overlying facial tenderness. Frontal sinusitis produces frontal headache that may radiate behind the eyes and to the vertex of the skull. Tenderness to frontal palpation may be present with point tenderness on the undersurface of the medial aspect of the superior orbital rim. In ethmoidal sinusitis, the pain is between or behind the eyes with radiation to the temporal area. The eyes and orbit are often tender to palpation, and, in fact, eye movements themselves may accentuate the pain. Sphenoidal sinusitis causes pain in the orbit and at the vertex of the skull and occasionally in the frontal or occipital regions. Given that the trigeminal nerve mediates pain perception from the sinuses, many patients who complain of "sinus headaches" are probably suffering from the trigeminovascular disturbance of migraine, rather than sinusitis. Chronic sinusitis is seldom a cause of headache.

Brain tumors. Posterior fossa tumors (particularly of the cerebellum) frequently produce headache, especially if hydrocephalus occurs because cerebrospinal fluid (CSF) flow is partially obstructed. Supratentorial tumors, however, are less likely to cause headache and are more frequently heralded by altered mental status, focal deficits, or seizures. Although increased intracranial pressure is often associated with headache, it is usually not the primary mechanism because uniform pressure elevations do not usually produce distortions of pain-sensitive structures.

Idiopathic intracranial hypertension. Idiopathic intracranial hypertension (IIH), also called *benign intracranial hypertension,* is defined as a syndrome of elevated intracranial pressure without evidence of focal lesions, hydrocephalus, or frank brain edema. It usually occurs between the ages of 15 and 45 years and is more frequent in obese women. The disorder is characterized by headache with features of raised intracranial pressure. The headache is usually insidious in onset, is typically generalized, is relatively mild in severity, and is often worse in the morning or after exertion (e.g., straining or coughing).

At times, patients have visual disturbances, such as restricted peripheral visual fields, enlarged blind spots, visual blurring *(obscurations),* or diplopia secondary to abducens nerve palsies. Funduscopic examination shows papilledema, which is often more impressive than the clinical picture. IIH is usually a benign and self-limited disorder, but it may lead to visual loss, including blindness. IIH often coexists with other disorders, including polycystic ovary syndrome, sleep apnea, anxiety, and cognitive dysfunction.

The condition has been associated with drugs—vitamin A intoxication, nalidixic acid, danazol (Danocrine), and isotretinoin (Accutane)—as well as corticosteroid withdrawal and systemic disorders such as hypoparathyroidism and lupus.

CT scans are usually normal but can show small ventricles and an "empty sella"; in some cases flattening of the posterior aspect of the ocular globe, tortuosity of the optic nerve, and distension of the perioptic subarachnoid space may be seen. CSF opening pressure is elevated, usually in the range of 250 to 450 mm of water, with the pressure fluctuating markedly when monitoring occurs over a prolonged period. Some cases of IIH are caused by cerebral venous sinus occlusion. These cases can occur in hypercoagulable states, including peripartum, in association with the combined oral contraceptive pill, and in association with antiphospholipid antibody syndrome. After secondary causes of IIH have been eliminated, the patient should have dietary counseling for weight loss; up to 15% weight loss is required to put IIH into remission. Carbonic anhydrase inhibitors (acetazolamide) and corticosteroids have proved useful in headache control. As a second-line agent, furosemide also acts to lower CSF production. In cases where the headache has migrainous features (68%), acute and preventative treatments for migraine may be useful. Topiramate can prevent headache and may facilitate weight loss. Serial lumbar punctures are understandably unpopular with patients even though transient headache relief is obtained. CSF shunting procedures (ventriculoperitoneal shunt) are occasionally necessary. For patients with progressive visual loss, optic nerve sheath fenestration preserves or restores vision in 80% to 90% of cases and provides headache relief in a majority. Patients should be followed for visual acuity, pupil examination, formal visual field assessment, dilated fundal examination to grade papilledema, and BMI monitoring.

Idiopathic intracranial hypotension. Also known as *low pressure headache,* idiopathic intracranial hypotension is commonly encountered as a sequela of lumbar puncture, resulting from leakage of CSF through the dural sac. Low pressure headaches may also occur spontaneously as a result of rupture of subarachnoid cysts. The headache is initially characteristically positional, being severe on standing but relieved rapidly on lying down. Occasionally the headache

is associated with focal or "false localizing" signs, especially abducens nerve palsies.

Post-traumatic headache. Headache following trauma has no specific quality and is associated with irritability, concentration impairment, insomnia, memory disturbance, and lightheadedness. Anxiety and depression are present to variable degrees. Multiple treatment options are available, and amitriptyline and nonsteroidal anti-inflammatory agents are useful. Occasionally, muscle relaxants and anxiolytics are beneficial. Training is occasionally associated with the onset of typical migraine.

Medication-associated headache. Medication overuse of "rebound" headache accounts for a significant portion of the headache burden in the population and in headache clinics. The term describes a chronic (≥15 days/month) headache that occurs in patients with a preexisting headache syndrome (most commonly migraine or tension-type headache) who use analgesic medication. Opioids, such as codeine, are particularly apt to give rise to this syndrome, but triptans, NSAIDs, and even paracetamol may have the same effect. Treatment involves the reduction or cessation of analgesic medication with a "washout" period of several weeks, during which time the headaches may worsen. Nonpharmacologic methods of pain management play a crucial role in this period. A range of other medications and substances, such as nitrous oxide, carbon monoxide, cocaine, alcohol, and phosphodiesterase inhibitors have also been reported to induce headache.

Giant cell arteritis. Headache occurs in 60% of patients with giant cell arteritis, a granulomatous vasculitis of medium and large arteries. Over 95% of patients are 50 years of age or older. Malaise, fever, weight loss, and jaw claudication occur early, in addition to headache. Polymyalgia rheumatica, a syndrome of painful stiffness of the neck, shoulders, and pelvis, is found in half the patients. Visual impairment secondary to ischemic optic neuritis may occur. The headache is usually described as aching and is exacerbated at night and after exposure to cold. The superficial temporal artery is frequently swollen, tender, and may be pulseless. The erythrocyte sedimentation rate is usually elevated; the mean is 100 mm/hr. Anemia is frequently present. Doppler ultrasound of the temporal arteries demonstrates a hypoechoic "halo sign" around the lumen of affected arteries. Temporal artery biopsy usually confirms the diagnosis, but, because the arteritis is segmental, large or multiple sections may be required. Prednisone therapy is often dramatically effective and must be given promptly to preserve vision on the affected side. Tocilizumab, a monoclonal antibody directed against the interleukin-6 receptor, is now available for the treatment of GCA, particularly in refractory or relapsing disease.

Evaluation of the Patient With Acute Headache

It is important to distinguish benign from ominous causes of headache. A detailed history (the quality, location, duration, and time course of the headache) helps in determination of which patients have a symptomatic structural intracranial lesion (see Table 113.7, Table 113.8, Table 113.4). Pain intensity is not of much diagnostic value, except for the patient who complains of the acute onset of the worst headache of his or her life. The quality of pain ("throbbing," "pressure," "jabbing") and the location may also be helpful, especially if the pain is of extracranial origin, such as temporal in temporal arteritis. Posterior fossa lesions cause occipitocervical pain, occasionally associated with unilateral retro-orbital pain. In general, multifocal pain usually implies a benign cause. It is most important to clarify the acuity of onset of the headache; patients who describe the onset of pain as "like being hit on the head with a bat" should be suspected of having the sentinel headache of subarachnoid headache. Equally important is to establish the time course of the headache. Is this paroxysmal, nonprogressive headache (typical of migraine or tension-type headache)? Or is the headache daily persistent (such as in temporal arteritis) or progressive (suggesting the presence of a structural brain lesion)? Patients should be asked about any known triggers for the headache, such as menses, particular foods, caffeine, alcohol, or stress. Positional headache (headache that is maximal in the upright position and disappears rapidly on lying down) is characteristic of intracranial hypotension (low pressure headache). Diurnal variation in headache severity may give a clue to cause; morning headache or headache that awakens a patient from sleep may indicate raised intracranial pressure or sleep apnea as a cause. The presence of associated symptoms such as visual disturbances, nausea, or vomiting should be noted. The history should include inquiries about medications, especially use of analgesics and over-the-counter remedies. Information regarding the patient's past medical history as well as family history should also be taken into consideration. In the majority of patients with headache, the physical and neurologic examination findings are normal, although special attention may be directed toward examination of the eyes for papilledema, as well as the temporal arteries for a palpable nonpulsatile artery. Assessment of the patient with acute nontraumatic headache in the emergency room can be challenging; it is essential to establish how the headache evolved. Acute-onset severe headache should prompt investigation to exclude SAH, intracranial hemorrhage, acute obstructive hydrocephalus, and meningitis (see Table 113.7). Appropriate initial investigations should include brain imaging with CT or magnetic resonance imaging (MRI). Patients with suspected meningitis without focal neurologic signs or impaired consciousness should not have their lumbar puncture delayed unnecessarily before imaging. All patients should have standard blood tests, including blood cultures if bacterial meningitis is suspected.

A wide variety of systemic diseases have headache as a prominent symptom; some of the more prevalent disorders are summarized in Table 113.2.

CRANIAL NEURALGIAS

Neuralgias are differentiated from other head pains by the brevity of the attacks (usually 1 to 2 seconds or less) and by the distribution of the pain (see Table 113.3).

Trigeminal Neuralgia

In trigeminal neuralgia (tic douloureux), stabbing, spasmodic pain occurs unilaterally in one of the divisions of the trigeminal nerve. It lasts seconds, but it may occur many times a day for weeks at a time. It is characteristically induced by even the lightest touch to particular areas of the face, such as the lips or gums. Trigeminal neuralgia is the most frequent neuralgia of the elderly and is thought to be caused by compression of the trigeminal nerve root in the pons by an aberrant arterial loop. A small minority of cases are caused by multiple sclerosis, cerebellopontine angle tumors, aneurysms, or arteriovenous malformations, although in these cases (unlike "true" trigeminal neuralgia) there are usually objective signs of neurologic deficit, such as areas of diminished sensation. In these cases of "symptomatic" neuralgia, the pain is often atypical. MRI is indicated in patients who have sensory loss, those who are under 40, and those with bilateral or atypical symptoms. Trigeminal neuralgia may be life threatening when it interferes with eating. Neuralgic pain is often responsive to treatment with standard doses of an anticonvulsant such as phenytoin, carbamazepine, gabapentin, pregabalin, and, occasionally, baclofen. Antidepressant drugs such as amitriptyline and, more recently, duloxetine may also be useful in this setting. Combination therapy, including an antidepressant, anticonvulsant, and opiate analgesic, has been shown to have synergistic effects.

If medical treatments are unsuccessful, surgical treatment may be indicated: microvascular decompression or radiofrequency lesioning of the sensory portion of the trigeminal nerve. The latter occasionally gives rise to the complication of anaesthesia dolorosa, in which the loss of sensation resulting from the procedure is experienced as being extremely unpleasant.

Glossopharyngeal Neuralgia

Glossopharyngeal neuralgia is less common than trigeminal neuralgia. Brief paroxysms of severe, stabbing, unilateral pain radiate from the throat to the ear or vice versa and are frequently initiated by stimulation of specific "trigger zones" (e.g., tonsillar fossa or pharyngeal wall). Swallowing often provokes an attack; yawning, talking, and coughing are other potential triggers. Microvascular decompression is necessary if medical treatment is ineffective.

Postherpetic Neuralgia

Herpes zoster produces head pain by cranial nerve involvement in one third of cases. In some cases a persistent intense burning pain follows the initial acute illness. The discomfort may subside after several weeks or persist (particularly in the elderly) for months or years. The pain is localized over the distribution of the affected nerve and associated with exquisite tenderness to even the lightest touch. The first division of the trigeminal nerve is the most frequent cranial nerve involved (ophthalmic herpes) and is occasionally associated with keratoconjunctivitis. When the seventh nerve is affected ("geniculate herpes"), the pain involves the external auditory meatus and pinna. Occasionally, concomitant facial paralysis may occur (Ramsay Hunt syndrome).

Occipital Neuralgia

Occipital neuralgia is a syndrome that includes occipital pain starting at the base of the skull and often provoked by neck extension. Physical examination shows tenderness in the region of the occipital nerves and altered sensation in the C2 dermatome. Treatment includes the use of a soft collar, muscle relaxants, physical therapy, and local injections of analgesics and anti-inflammatory agents. The term *cervicogenic headache* is often used to describe headache associated with myofascial trigger points in the neck. Importantly, cervical spondylosis (discussed next) is not usually typically associated with headache.

CERVICAL SPONDYLOSIS

Cervical spondylosis is a degenerative disorder of the cervical intervertebral disks leading to osteophyte formation and hypertrophy of adjacent facet joints and ligaments. In contrast to the lumbar spine, herniation of cervical intervertebral disks (nucleus pulposus) accounts for only 20% to 25% of cervical root irritation. Cervical spondylosis is one of the most common pathologies seen in office practice and is present radiographically in over 90% of the population older than 60 years. For unknown reasons, the degree of anatomic abnormality is not directly correlated with the clinical signs and symptoms. Clinical disease may represent a combination of normal, age-related, degenerative changes in the cervical spine and a congenital or developmental stenosis of the cervical canal; the process may be aggravated by trauma. Cervical spinal myelopathy results from a combination of degenerative disc disease, spondylosis aggravated by biomechanical instability, as well as stiffening and buckling of the ligamentum flavum. It may manifest as a painful stiff neck, with or without symptoms or signs of cervical root irritation or spinal cord compression. Patients with root irritation (cervical radiculopathy) complain of pain and paresthesias radiating down the arm roughly in the dermatomal distribution of the affected nerve root. More typically, the pain radiates in a myotomal

TABLE 113.9 Common Cervical Root Syndromes

Disk Space	Root Affected	Muscles Affected	Distribution of Pain	Distribution of Sensory Symptoms	Reflex Affected
C4-5	C5	Deltoid; biceps	Medial scapula; shoulder	Shoulder	Biceps
C5-6	C6	Wrist extensors	Lateral forearm	Thumb; index finger	Triceps
C6-7	C7	Triceps	Medial scapula	Middle finger	Brachioradialis
C7-T1	C8	Hand intrinsics	Medial forearm	Fourth and fifth fingers	Finger flexion

pattern, whereas numbness and paresthesias follow a dermatomal distribution. Discrete sensory loss is uncommon and less prominent than symptoms (Table 113.9). For relief, patients often adopt a position with the arm elevated and flexed behind the head. Pain is exacerbated by turning the head, ear down, to the side of the pain (Spurling maneuver). Objective neurologic findings may be limited to reflex asymmetry because weakness may be obscured by pain. Patients who have some degree of spinal cord compression demonstrate gait and bladder disturbances and evidence of spasticity on examination of the lower extremities. These patients require investigation with MRI. Plain radiographs of the cervical spine add little information except in patients with rheumatoid arthritis in whom basilar invagination or atlantoaxial subluxation is suspected.

Cervical spondylosis is so common in the general population that it may be present coincidentally in a patient with another disease of the spinal cord. Among other diseases that may mimic cervical spondylosis are multiple sclerosis, amyotrophic lateral sclerosis, and, less commonly, subacute combined system disease (vitamin B_{12} deficiency). Conservative treatment includes the use of anti-inflammatory medication, cervical immobilization, and physical therapy for isometric strengthening of neck muscles once pain has subsided. Surgery should be considered if there is progression of the neurologic deficit, especially the emergence of signs of cervical cord compression. There is some evidence to suggest that cervical spondylosis is an active degenerative disease rather than simply the process. Furthermore, early studies with the glutamate antagonist riluzole suggest a potential role in reducing disease progression.

ACUTE LOW BACK PAIN

Low back pain without sciatica (radiating radicular pain) is common, with a reported point prevalence of up to 33%. Acute low back pain lasting several weeks is usually self-limiting, with a low risk for serious permanent disability. Risk factors for prolonged disability include psychological distress, compensation conflict over work-related injury, and other coexistent pain syndromes. The evaluation of patients with acute low back pain should focus on distinguishing pain of mechanical origin from neurogenic pain caused by nerve root irritation. The same pathologic changes that affect the cervical spine may also affect the lumbar spine. Because the spinal cord ends at the level of the first lumbar vertebra, lumbar canal stenosis from intervertebral disk disease and degenerative spondylosis will affect the roots of the cauda equina. The most common levels for lumbar degenerative disk disease are at L4 to L5 and L5 to S1, resulting in the common complaint of sciatica caused by irritation of the lower lumbar roots. Pain tends to improve with sitting or lying down, in contrast to the pain from spinal or vertebral tumors, which is aggravated by prolonged recumbency. Examination shows loss of the normal lumbar lordosis, paraspinal muscle spasm, and exacerbation of pain with straight leg rising, owing to stretching of the lower lumbar roots. About 10% of disk herniations occur lateral to the spinal canal, in which case the more rostral root is compressed. Percussion of the spine may elicit focal tenderness of one of the vertebrae, suggesting bony infiltration by infection or tumor.

Spinal stenosis of the lumbar region may manifest as "neurogenic claudication," which is usually described as unilateral or bilateral buttock pain that is worse on standing or walking and relieved by rest or flexion at the waist. Patients may have pain that is worse when walking downhill, in contrast to patients with vascular claudication, whose pain is maximal when walking up an incline.

MRI in many patients with isolated low back pain shows nonspecific findings; MRI assessment early in the course of an episode of low back pain does not improve clinical outcome. MRI should be limited to patients with back pain who have associated neurologic symptoms or signs, especially new-onset disturbances of bladder or bowel continence or perineal sensory symptoms suggestive of a *cauda equina syndrome*. Patients with risk factors for malignancy, infection, or osteoporosis, as well as those with pain maximal at rest (or nocturnal pain) require imaging. Patients with primary and metastatic tumor can present with acute back pain. Moreover, developmental anomalies are often associated with pain (see Chapter 117).

Treatment strategies for lumbar pain are similar to those for cervical pain, with surgery reserved for patients with neurologic signs and clear pathologic processes seen on imaging studies. Most cases of acute low back pain, even with rupture of an intervertebral disk, can be treated conservatively with a short period of rest, muscle relaxants, and analgesics. Prolonged bed rest is recommended only for patients in severe pain. Patient education regarding proper posture and appropriate back exercises is helpful, as is a formal physical therapy program. Chiropractic manipulation should not be performed for patients who have evidence of neurologic injury or spine instability.

For a deeper discussion on this topic, please see Chapter 370, ❖ "Headaches and Other Head Pain," in *Goldman-Cecil Medicine*, 26th Edition.

SUGGESTED READINGS

Bronfort G, Evans R, Anderson AV, et al: Spinal manipulation, medication, or home exercise with advice for acute and subacute neck pain: a randomized trial, Ann Intern Med 156:1–10, 2012.

Cherkin DC, Sherman KJ, Kahn J, et al: A comparison of the effects of 2 types of massage and usual care on chronic low back pain: a randomized, controlled trial, Ann Intern Med 155:1–9, 2011.

El Barzouhi A, Vleggeert-Lankamp CL, Lycklama à Nijeholt GJ, et al: Magnetic resonance imaging in follow up assessment of sciatica, N Engl J Med 368:999–1007, 2013.

Fehlings MG, Tetreault LA, Wilson JR, et al: Cervical spondylitic myelopathy. Current state of the art and future directions, Spine 38:S1–S8, 2013.

Gelfand AA, Goadsby PJ: A neurologist's guide to acute migraine treatment in the emergency room, Neurohospitalist 2:51–59, 2012.

Headache Classification Subcommittee of the International Headache Society: The international classification of headache disorders: 3rd edition, Cephalalgia 33:629-808, 2013. Available at: http://ihs.classification.org/en/.

Rana MV: Managing and treating headache of cervicogenic origin, Med Clin North Am 97:267–280, 2013.

Rizzoli PB: Acute and preventive treatment of migraine, Continuum 18:764–782, 2012.

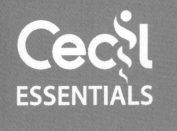

114

Disorders of Vision and Hearing

Eavan Mc Govern, Timothy J. Counihan

DISORDERS OF VISION AND EYE MOVEMENTS

Examination of the Visual System

Visual Acuity

The clinical examination of visual function begins with testing visual acuity.

Examination technique.
- Use a Snellen chart at a distance of 20 feet (Fig. 114.1).
- If applicable, test visual acuity with a patient's corrective lenses.
- Examine each eye separately.
- Record the smallest line the patient can read. This is the visual acuity for the eye tested; for instance, acuity of 20/40 refers to letters that the patient sees maximally at 20 feet, which a normal individual can see at 40 feet.
- If a patient is unable to read the largest letter, visual acuity is recorded using finger counting or light perception.

Clinical clues. When errors of refraction are responsible for decreased visual acuity, vision may be improved by having the patient look through a pinhole. Corrected vision in one eye of less than 20/40 suggests damage to the lens (cataract) or retina or a disorder of the anterior visual (prechiasmal) pathway. Color vision should be tested using Ishihara color plates to detect an acquired unilateral or bilateral cause of color loss. Patients with optic nerve lesions with normal visual acuity can report that colors appear "washed out" in the affected eye (color desaturation).

Visual Fields

Confrontational examination of visual fields is helpful when localizing lesions interrupting the afferent visual system (Fig. 114.2).

Examination technique.
- The examiner's head should be level with the patient's head.
- Test each eye separately, by initially asking the patient to cover the other eye.
- Visual fields should be tested in all four quadrants using finger counting by comparing the patient's field with that of the examiner.
- Use a white pin to map peripheral visual fields and a red pin to assess for the presence of a central area of visual field loss (referred to as a scotoma).

Examination tips. Finger counting is more sensitive than presenting moving objects in detecting visual field deficits. The field should be tested first unilaterally and then bilaterally. A defect (particularly in the left hemifield) with bilateral testing only (extinction) suggests visual neglect and a lesion in the contralateral parietal lobe.

Clinical clues. The following questions are helpful to help localize the lesion within the visual afferent system.
- Is the defect monocular or binocular? Monocular lesions localize the defect to the retina or to the optic nerve. A binocular lesion localizes posterior to and including the optic chiasm.

- Is the defect central or peripheral? *Scotomas* are areas of partial or complete visual loss and may be central or peripheral. Central scotomas result from damage to the macula. A scotoma affecting one half of a visual field is known as a *hemianopia*. Field defects are said to be *homonymous* if the same part of the visual field is affected in both eyes; a homonymous hemianopia implies a postchiasmal lesion.
- Is the defect congruous or incongruous? A homonymous defect may be *congruous* (the visual defect is identical in each hemifield) or *incongruous* (the visual defect is not identical in each hemifield). The closer the visual field defect to the occipital lobe the more congruous the defect.
- Does the defect involve the superior, inferior or bitemporal visual fields? Quadrantanopsias are smaller defects in the visual field and may be superior (which suggests a temporal lobe lesion) or inferior (which suggests a parietal lobe lesion). Bitemporal hemianopia implies a lesion at the chiasm, such as a pituitary tumor. An altitudinal hemianopia occurs with vascular damage to the retina.
- Is the visual defect associated with positive symptoms? Scintillating scotomas are hallucinations of flashing lights. If they are monocular, they may be caused by retinal detachment; binocular scintillations suggest occipital oligemia (as in migraine) or seizure.

Any suspicious findings on bedside confrontation testing warrant formal visual field testing using perimetry (Fig. 114.3).

Pupils

Pupil constriction is mediated by the parasympathetic system of the oculomotor (third cranial) nerve, whereas dilation is mediated by the sympathetic system. If the balance of these systems is disrupted, *anisocoria* (unequal pupil size) results.

Examination technique.
- Observe the pupillary size and shape at rest.
- Examine the pupils in both dim and bright light.
- Note the direct and consensual light responses for each eye. This is best tested using the "swinging light test," in which the light is moved quickly from one eye to the other.
- Test for accommodation by asking the patient to first look at a distant object and then at the examiner's fingers, held 12 inches away.

Clinical clues. If the degree of anisocoria increases going from dim to bright light, this suggests that the larger lesion is failing to constrict due to a lesion of the parasympathetic system. Similarly, if the degree of pupillary asymmetry is maximal in a dimly lit environment, this suggests that the smaller pupil fails to dilate appropriately due to a lesion of the sympathetic nervous system. *Physiologic anisocoria* is characterized by pupillary asymmetry that is unchanged irrespective of the ambient light intensity; this occurs in approximately 20% of the population. When light is shone into one eye, both eyes should

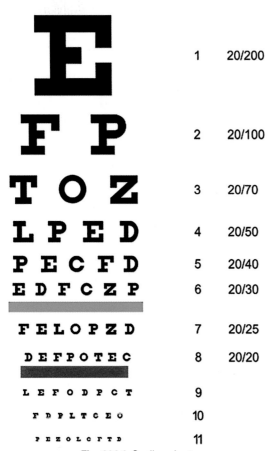

Fig. 114.1 Snellen chart.

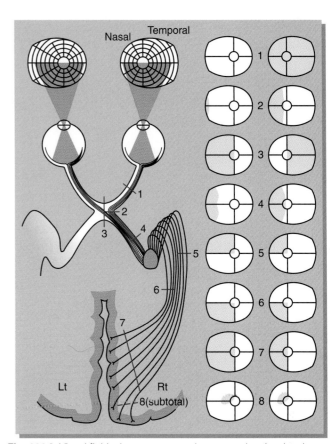

Fig. 114.2 Visual fields that accompany damage to the visual pathways. *1,* Optic nerve: unilateral amaurosis. *2,* Lateral optic chiasm: grossly incongruous, incomplete (contralateral) homonymous hemianopia. *3,* Central optic chiasm: bitemporal hemianopia. *4,* Optic tract: incongruous, incomplete homonymous hemianopia. *5,* Temporal (Meyer) loop of optic radiation: congruous partial or complete (contralateral) homonymous superior quadrantanopia. *6,* Parietal (superior) projection of the optic radiation: congruous partial or complete homonymous inferior quadrantanopia. *7,* Complete parieto-occipital interruption of optic radiation: complete congruous homonymous hemianopia with psychophysical shift of foveal point often sparing central vision, giving "macular sparing." *8,* Incomplete damage to visual cortex: congruous homonymous scotomas, usually encroaching at least acutely on central vision. (From Baloh RW: Neuro-ophthalmology. In Goldman L, Bennett JC, editors: Cecil textbook of medicine, ed 21, Philadelphia, 1998, WB Saunders, p 2236.)

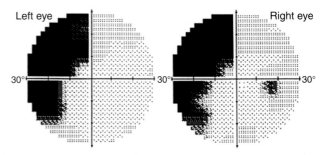

Fig. 114.3 Humphrey visual fields demonstrating an incongruent homonymous hemianopia.

constrict simultaneously. When the light source is shone from a normal eye to an affected, relative dilatation of both pupils is observed. This abnormality is referred to as an *afferent pupillary defect* and indicates severe retinal disease or an optic neuropathy. *Argyll-Robertson pupils* are small, irregular pupils that constrict to near vision (accommodation reflex) but not in response to light. They are associated with neurosyphilis, diabetes, and other disorders. This so-called *light-near dissociation* may also occur in rostral dorsal midbrain lesions, in which there may be associated abnormalities of vertical gaze, eyelid retraction, and convergence retraction nystagmus (Parinaud syndrome). This constellation of clinical findings is occasionally found in patients with lesions of the pineal gland.

The presence of drooping of the eyelid (ptosis) should be noted. A large, unreactive pupil with complete ptosis indicates a lesion of the oculomotor nerve *(third cranial nerve palsy)* interrupting the parasympathetic nerve supply to the pupil. The associated paralysis of the medial and inferior rectus and inferior oblique muscles (see later discussion) results in distortion of the eye (inferolaterally, "*down and out*") and a subjective complaint of diplopia by the patient. Common causes of a third nerve palsy include compression by an aneurysm of the posterior communicating artery, by transtentorial herniation, or from ischemia, usually in the setting of diabetes or vasculitis. A third cranial nerve palsy caused by ischemia often spares the pupil but results in complete paralysis of the oculomotor and eyelid levator muscles. Acute painful third nerve palsy should be treated as an emergency, with the need to investigate for an intracranial aneurysm.

A small, poorly reactive pupil with associated partial ptosis is known as *Horner syndrome* and results from damage to the sympathetic fibers to the pupil, which may occur anywhere along their course from the hypothalamus, brain stem, and ascending sympathetic chain from the superior cervical ganglion to the orbit. There may be associated unilateral anhidrosis resulting from damage to sympathetic fibers. Horner syndrome may be the first sign of an apical lung tumor (Pancoast) or may occur in diseases affecting the carotid artery such as dissection.

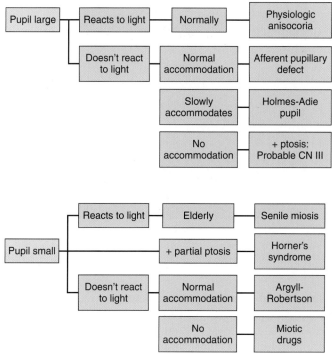

Fig. 114.4 Algorithm for the approach to unequal pupils (anisocoria).

Tonic (Adie) pupils constrict slowly and incompletely in response to light. This is usually an incidental finding on examination but may be associated with areflexia (Holmes-Adie syndrome). Reaction to accommodation is preserved, and it has been suggested that the disorder is a result of parasympathetic denervation. *Hippus* refers to pupillary unrest with synchronous oscillation of the pupil size; it is considered a normal phenomenon. Fig. 114.4 summarizes common pupillary abnormalities and their associated features.

Eye Movements

Abnormalities in ocular motility may arise from lesions of the cerebral hemisphere, brain stem, cranial nerves and ocular muscles. The ability to localize lesions disrupting binocular vision can provide valuable diagnostic information for the clinician.

Examination technique. First note the position of the head and eyes with the eyes in primary gaze. Next, the four components of oculomotor function should be tested:

1. Pursuit eye movements: Smooth pursuit eye movements allow fixation on a moving object. Ask the patient to follow a moving target such as a pin in all directions of gaze.
2. Saccadic eye movements: These movements allow rapid switching of gaze from one target to another. Both horizontal and vertical saccadic movements should be checked.
3. Vestibulo-ocular reflex: This reflex enables fixation on an object even if the head is moving. It is assessed by using the *doll's eye maneuver.*
4. Convergence response: This tests the ability of the eyes to track an object as it is brought close to the limit of accommodation. Ask the patient to look into the distance and then at your finger held close to their eyes.

Both smooth pursuit and (voluntary) saccadic eye movements in horizontal and vertical directions are checked to determine whether the movements are conjugate or dysconjugate.

Clinical clues from history. The following questions from the clinical history can be helpful in evaluating the patient with diplopia.

- Is the diplopia primarily horizontal or vertical, or is it greater looking to the right or to the left?
- Is there diurnal variation? Double vision that varies during the day suggests myasthenia gravis.
- Is the diplopia maximal with near or distant vision? Greater difficulty with near vision suggests impairment of the medial rectus, oculomotor nerve, or convergence system, whereas abducens nerve weakness results in horizontal diplopia when objects are viewed at a distance. Diplopia that worsens on going down stairs may suggest a fourth nerve lesion.
- Is the diplopia monocular or binocular? Monocular diplopia is usually caused by an optical problem (i.e., diseases of the retina or lens). It is corrected by having the patient look through a pinhole, unless the cause is psychogenic. Binocular diplopia suggests ocular misalignment that is a disorder of the brain stem (at the level of the ocular motor nuclei or their connections), the peripheral nerves (cranial nerves III, IV, or VI), the neuromuscular junction (myasthenia gravis or botulism) or individual eye muscles (ocular myopathy). A large deficit in the range of eye movements may provide sufficient diagnostic information. However, in many cases, although the patient complains of diplopia, no clear misalignment is visible on testing eye movements. The corneal reflection test may help identify misalignment in these cases. The patient is instructed to look at a light shining directly at the eyes. If the eyes are normally aligned, the light reflection will be about 1 mm nasal to the center of the cornea. If one eye is deviated medially, the reflection will be displaced outward; the reflection will be displaced inward if the eye is deviated outward.

When assessing eye movements, it is important to know the cranial nerves and muscles involved in eye movement. The abducens (sixth cranial) nerve supplies the lateral rectus muscle. The trochlear (fourth cranial) nerve subserves the superior oblique muscle, which intorts the eye as well as depresses the eye in adduction (such as when a patient tries to look downstairs). All other muscles are supplied by the oculomotor nerve (Fig. 114.5). Abnormalities of the cranial nerves in the brain stem are usually accompanied by other signs, such as weakness, ataxia, or dysarthria. The abducens nerve has a long ascending course through the posterior fossa, where it is prone to compression at multiple sites and as a result of raised intracranial pressure; hence, a sixth nerve palsy may be a false localizing sign. Conjugate eye movement is regulated by supranuclear pathways from the cerebral hemisphere to the medial longitudinal fasciculus in the brain stem. A lesion in the cerebral hemisphere resulting from hemorrhage, infarction, or tumor disrupts conjugate gaze to the contralateral side, so that the eyes "look away" from the hemiplegia. Lesions of the brain stem cause conjugate paralysis to the ipsilateral side (eyes looking toward the side of the hemiplegia). Lesions of the medial longitudinal fasciculus, which connects the nuclei of the oculomotor and abducens nerves, lead to *internuclear ophthalmoplegia.* In this case, horizontal gaze results in failure of adduction in one eye and nystagmus in the abducting eye. The lesion is on the side of failed adduction; bilateral lesions are frequently seen in multiple sclerosis. Table 114.1 lists the major causes of acute ophthalmoplegia.

Funduscopy

The retina should be carefully examined in each patient by direct ophthalmoscopy, which provides a magnified view of the fundus without the necessity for dilation of the pupil (Fig. 114.6).

Examination technique.
- The examiner's head should be level with the patient's head.
- The examiner's right eye should be used to examine the patient's right eye.

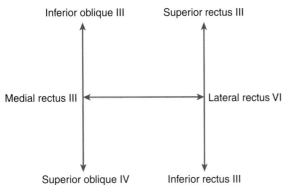

Inferior oblique III   Superior rectus III

Medial rectus III ⟷ Lateral rectus VI

Superior oblique IV   Inferior rectus III

Fig. 114.5 Movements of eye muscles and their innervation.

TABLE 114.1 Major Causes of Acute Ophthalmoplegia

Condition	Diagnostic Features
Bilateral	
Botulism	Contaminated food; high-altitude cooking; pupils involved
Myasthenia gravis	Fluctuating degree of paralysis; responds to edrophonium chloride (Tensilon) IV
Wernicke encephalopathy	Nutritional deficiency; responds to thiamine IV
Acute cranial polyneuropathy	Antecedent respiratory infection; elevated CSF protein level
Brain stem stroke	Other brain stem signs
Unilateral	
P Comm aneurysm	Third cranial nerve, pupil involved
Diabetic-idiopathic	Third or sixth cranial nerve, pupil spared
Myasthenia gravis	As above
Brain stem stroke	As above

CSF, Cerebrospinal fluid; *IV,* intravenous; *P Comm,* posterior communicating artery.

- Locate the red reflex in both eyes. While focusing on one eye, move closer until the retina comes into view.
- While focusing on the retina, follow the vessels toward the patient's nose to locate the optic disc.
- To view the macula, ask the patient to look directly at the light.
  Clinical clues from patient history. In eliciting the history the most important thing to establish is whether the visual loss is monocular or binocular.

Monocular Visual Loss

Loss of vision in one eye localizes to the prechiasmatic visual pathway (i.e., the eye itself or the optic nerve). Causes include lesions of the cornea, lens, vitreous, retina, or optic nerve. Loss of the red reflex suggests a lesion of the anterior chamber. Careful funduscopic examination will usually reveal ocular and retinal lesions, but acute lesions of the optic nerve (optic neuritis) may not be associated with abnormalities of the optic nerve head.

Optic neuritis is characterized by inflammation of the optic nerve accompanied by non-homonymous visual defects. Optic neuropathies acutely associated with a normal appearing optic disk on funduscopic examination are posterior or *retrobulbar optic neuritis* ("the doctor sees nothing and the patient sees nothing"). Those with a swollen disk on funduscopic examination are anterior optic neuropathies. In

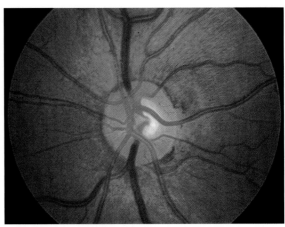

Fig. 114.6 A normal optic disk on funduscopic examination.

most cases of optic neuropathy, the optic disc becomes pale after 4 to 6 weeks.

Clinical Clues From Patient Examination

In assessing a patient presenting with an optic neuropathy the following features are important to identify on clinical examination and can be helpful in guiding the differential diagnosis:

- Visual acuity
- Color vision
- Visual field
- The presence or absence of a relative afferent pupillary defect (RAPD)
- Optic nerve head appearance on funduscopic examination

The patient with optic neuritis complains of difficulty with vision in the affected eye. Loss of vision may be insidious and recognized only when the unaffected eye is accidentally occluded. Patients often complain of periorbital pain on eye movement on presentation. The evolution of visual loss is highly variable, progressing over a period ranging from less than a day to several weeks, although most patients will have reached their maximal visual deficit in 3 to 7 days.

At the time the patient is first examined, visual acuity may range from almost 20/20 to the extreme of total blindness. Patients may describe their vision as blurred or dim, and colors may appear less bright than usual or "gray." Red desaturation may occur with optic neuritis and may be detected using Ishihara color plates. Examination of the visual field shows defects within the central 25 degrees, with central and paracentral scotomas being the most common types. An afferent pupillary defect is frequently present. The funduscopic examination is abnormal in only about one half of the cases. The disc may appear hyperemic with blurred margins, and hemorrhages, when present, are few and found only on the disc or in the area immediately surrounding the disc.

There are many causes of optic neuropathy. Broadly speaking, the causes may be divided into inflammatory, vascular, or compressive/infiltrative. Treatment is directed at the underlying cause. Inflammatory causes usually result in subacute painful loss of central vision. In this instance, high-dose intravenous corticosteroids should be used to shorten time to recovery. The most common cause of inflammatory optic neuritis is multiple sclerosis. Bilateral optic neuritis is much less common and may coincide with longitudinally extensive transverse myelitis, known as *neuromyelitis optica* (NMO) or *Devic disease.* The recent discovery of antibodies directed toward aquaporin 4 (a water channel present on astrocytes and vascular endothelial cells), associated with NMO, has identified this as a separate disease entity, with a different treatment regimen emerging for it. The NMO antibody is the first sensitive and specific biomarker associated with a central demyelinating disorder.

The optic nerve may be compressed by tumors that originate in the nerve itself or in the region of the optic chiasm. Compressive/infiltrative causes typically cause progressive visual loss, color desaturation, and no pain on eye movement. Headache may result in the presence of raised intracranial pressure. Proptosis and diplopia occurs with orbital lesions. Cranial nerve palsies result with lesions involving the cavernous sinus. Causes may be broadly divided into neoplastic and non-neoplastic causes such as thyroid eye disease.

Ischemic optic neuropathy (ION) is the most common cause of acute optic neuropathy in patients over 50 years. The posterior ciliary artery, a branch of the ophthalmic artery, supplies the optic nerve. Due to its anatomic arrangement, optic nerve ischemia results in superior or inferior segmental optic nerve atrophy and clinically manifests as altitudinal defects. ION occurs in two forms. The *atherosclerotic* variety occurs mostly between the ages of 50 and 70 years, and typically no evidence of systemic disease is present. The *arteritic* form is usually a manifestation of giant cell arteritis. There may be systemic manifestations of the disease, including headache, scalp tenderness, and generalized myalgias. Laboratory evaluation shows anemia and elevated erythrocyte sedimentation rate in almost every case. Patients with arteritis should be treated with high doses of corticosteroids to prevent permanent loss of vision.

Acute transient monocular blindness is usually the result of embolization to the central retinal artery from an atheromatous plaque in the carotid artery *(amaurosis fugax)*. Any complaint of transient visual loss constitutes an emergency, and steps must be taken to prevent permanent loss of vision by making a prompt diagnosis and initiating appropriate therapy. Examples of sight-saving procedures include corticosteroid therapy for cranial arteritis, reduction of intraocular pressure for acute glaucoma, and carotid surgery, anticoagulation, or antiplatelet therapy for embolic cerebrovascular disease.

Binocular Visual Loss

Binocular visual loss usually suggests retro-chiasmatic pathology. Gradual bilateral visual loss caused by optic nerve lesions is rare. Causes include Leber hereditary optic neuropathy and a toxic nutritional–deficiency state. Acute transient bilateral visual loss (visual obscuration) may be a symptom of raised intracranial pressure caused by a brain tumor or idiopathic intracranial hypertension (IIH); papilledema is often severe. IIH, formerly known as *pseudotumor cerebri*, requires prompt investigation and treatment to prevent potential bilateral visual failure. It is often associated with a high body mass index (BMI) and is more common in young females. Vitamin A and tetracycline ingestion have been associated with the condition. Unilateral or bilateral lateral rectus palsy may be present. It is one of the few situations in which, after imaging, performance of a lumbar puncture is safe in the setting of marked bilateral papilledema. Cerebral venous sinus thrombosis may mimic IIH and should be screened for with neuroimaging.

Bilateral damage to the optic radiations or visual cortex results in cortical blindness. The pupillary light reflex is normal, as are the funduscopic examination findings, and the patient may occasionally be unaware that he or she is blind *(Anton syndrome)*. Patients are often misdiagnosed as having a conversion reaction. Transient cortical blindness occurs most often in basilar artery insufficiency but is also seen in hypertensive encephalopathy. Positive visual phenomena (e.g., phosphenes, scintillating scotomas) are characteristic of migrainous aura and probably reflect oligemia to the occipital lobes from vasoconstriction. Arteriovenous malformations, tumors, and seizures may produce similar symptoms and should be distinguished from migraine

with aura by a careful history and examination as well as by imaging in appropriate cases.

Visual hallucinations are visual sensations independent of external light stimulation; they may be either simple or complex, may be localized or generalized, and may occur in patients with a clear or clouded sensorium. Visual illusions are alterations of a perceived external stimulus in which some features are distorted. The simplest visual phenomena consist of flashes of light (photopsias), blue lights (phosphenes), or scintillating zigzag lines, which last a fraction of a second and recur frequently or which appear to be in constant motion. These can arise from dysfunction within the optic pathways at any point from the eye to the cortex. Glaucoma, incipient retinal detachment, retinal ischemia, or macular degeneration can cause simple visual hallucinations. Lesions of the occipital lobe are often associated with simple hallucinations; classic migraine is by far the most common condition of this type. Complex visual hallucinations such as seeing objects as people, animals, landscapes, or various indescribable scenes occur most frequently with temporal lobe lesions or parieto-occipital association areas. Visual hallucinations of epileptogenic origin are typically stereotyped.

HEARING AND ITS IMPAIRMENTS

Symptoms of Auditory Dysfunction

The two main symptoms of lesions affecting the auditory system are hearing loss and tinnitus. Hearing loss can be classified as conductive, sensorineural, mixed, or central, based on the anatomic site of pathology (Figs. 114.7 and 114.8). Tinnitus can be either subjective or objective. Conductive hearing loss results when there is difficulty transferring sound waves from the external to the middle ear. Any lesion along this pathway can cause conductive hearing loss. Patients with conductive loss have particular difficulty hearing low-frequency sounds and hear better in noisy backgrounds than in quiet environments. Patients often report frequently ear fullness as if their ear is blocked.

Sensorineural hearing loss usually results from lesions of the cochlea or the auditory division of the vestibulocochlear (eighth cranial) nerve. The cochlea analyzes the frequency of sounds and activates appropriate sensory cells depending on the frequency. Patients with sensorineural hearing loss often have difficulty hearing speech that is mixed with background noise and may be annoyed by loud speech. Low tones are better heard than high-frequency ones. Distortion of sounds is common with sensorineural hearing loss. Central (retrocochlear) hearing disorders are rare and result from bilateral lesions of the central auditory pathways, including the cochlear and dorsal olivary nuclear complexes, inferior colliculi, medial geniculate bodies, and auditory cortex in the temporal lobes. Damage to both auditory cortices may result in pure word deafness, in which patients are selectively unable to discriminate language but may be able to hear nonverbal sounds.

Tinnitus is the perception of a noise or ringing in the ear that is usually audible only to the patient (subjective), although, rarely, an examiner can hear the sound as well. The latter, so-called *objective tinnitus,* can be heard when the examining physician places a stethoscope against the patient's external auditory canal. Tinnitus that is pulsatory and synchronous with the heartbeat suggests a vascular abnormality within the head or neck. Aneurysms, arteriovenous malformations, and vascular tumors can produce this type of tinnitus.

Subjective tinnitus, heard only by the patient, can result from lesions involving the external ear canal, tympanic membrane, ossicles, cochlea, auditory nerve, brain stem, and cortex. The character of the tinnitus does not usually aid in determining the site of the disturbance. For this, one must rely on associated symptoms and signs. When tinnitus results from a lesion of the external or middle ear, it is usually accompanied by a conductive hearing loss. The patient may complain that his or her voice sounds hollow and that other sounds are muffled. Because the masking effect of ambient noise is lost, the patient may be disturbed by normal muscular sounds such as chewing, tight closure of the eyes, or clenching of the jaws. The characteristic tinnitus associated with Meniere's syndrome is low pitched and continuous, although fluctuating in intensity. Often the tinnitus becomes very loud immediately preceding an acute attack of vertigo and then may disappear after the attack. Tinnitus resulting from lesions within the central nervous system is usually not associated with hearing loss but is nearly always associated with other neurologic symptoms and signs. High-dose salicylates frequently result in tinnitus.

Examination of the Auditory System
Examination Technique
Hearing is first tested in the speech range to observe the response to spoken commands at different intensities (whisper, conversation, and shouting). The examiner must be careful to prevent the patient from reading his or her lip movement. A high-frequency stimulus such as a watch tick should also be used because sensorineural disorders often

involve only the higher frequencies. Tuning fork tests permit a rough assessment of the hearing level for pure tones of known frequency. The Rinne test compares a patient's hearing by air and by bone conduction. A 512-cps tuning fork is first held against the mastoid process until the sound fades. It is then placed 1 inch from the ear. Normal subjects can hear the fork about twice as long by air conduction as compared with bone conduction. If hearing by bone conduction is longer than by air conduction, a conductive hearing loss is suggested. The Weber test compares the patient's hearing by bone conduction in the two ears. The fork is placed at the center of the forehead, and the patient is asked where he or she hears the tone. Normal subjects hear it in the center of the head, patients with unilateral conductive loss hear it on the affected side, and patients with unilateral sensorineural loss hear it on the side opposite the loss. Otoscopic examination may reveal impacted cerumen as a cause of conductive hearing loss.

Causes of Hearing Loss
Presbycusis is bilateral hearing loss associated with advancing age. It is not a distinct disease entity. It represents multiple effects of aging on

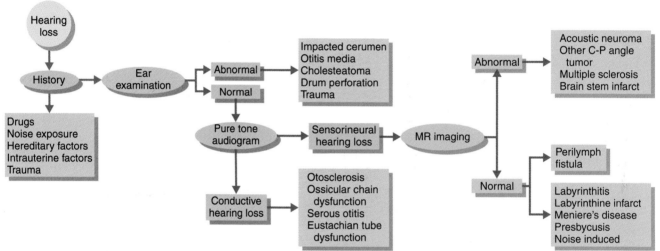

Fig. 114.7 Evaluation of deafness (unilateral and bilateral). *C-P,* Cerebellopontine; *MR,* magnetic resonance. (Modified from Baloh RW: Hearing and equilibrium. In Goldman L, Bennett JC, editors: Cecil textbook of medicine, ed 21, Philadelphia, 1998, WB Saunders, p 2250.)

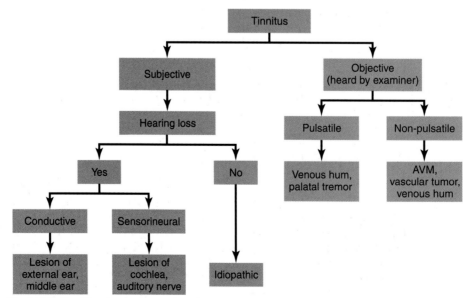

Fig. 114.8 Algorithm for the approach to the patient with tinnitus. *AVM,* Arteriovenous malformation.

the auditory system. Presbycusis may include conductive and central dysfunction, although the most consistent effect of aging is on the sensory cells and neurons of the cochlea; as a result, higher tones are lost early.

Otosclerosis is a disease of the bony labyrinth that usually manifests itself by immobilizing the stapes, thereby producing a conductive hearing loss. Seventy percent of patients with clinical otosclerosis notice hearing loss between the ages of 11 and 30. A family history of otosclerosis is observed in approximately 50% of cases. *Stapedectomy*, a procedure in which the stapes is replaced with a prosthesis, is effective in correcting the conductive component of hearing loss.

A lesion of the cerebellopontine angle, such as a vestibular schwannoma, causes slowly progressive unilateral hearing loss (Table 114.2). Symptoms are caused by compression of the nerve in the narrow confines of the canal (Fig. 114.9). The most common symptoms associated with vestibular schwannomas are slowly progressive hearing loss and tinnitus from compression of the cochlear nerve. Vertigo occurs in fewer than 20% of patients, but approximately 50% complain of imbalance or disequilibrium. Next to the auditory nerve, the cranial nerves most commonly involved by compression are the seventh (facial weakness) and fifth (sensory loss). Loss of the corneal reflex on the affected side is often the first clinical sign. Diagnosis is confirmed with gadolinium-enhanced MRI brain imaging. Treatment in most cases is surgical removal.

TABLE 114.2   Cause of Acute Unilateral Sensorineural Deafness

Cochlear
Idiopathic (85%)
Trauma
Meniere's disease
Lyme disease
Syphilis
Autoimmune disease
Retrocochlear
Demyelination
Vestibular schwannoma (usually gradual onset)
Stroke

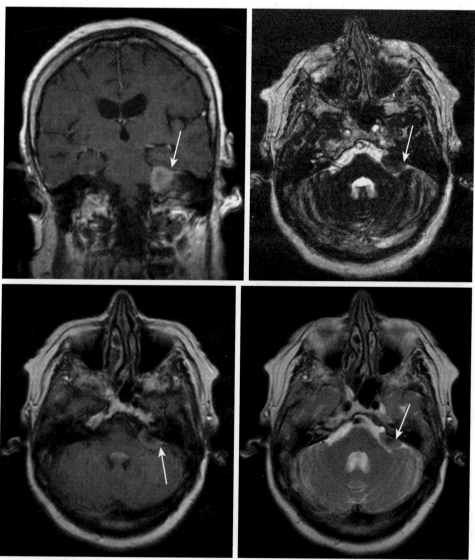

Fig. 114.9 Magnetic resonance imaging scan of the brain showing coronal and axial views of a tumor of the left cerebellopontine angle, consistent with a schwannoma.

Meniere's syndrome presents with a clinical triad of fluctuating hearing loss, tinnitus, and episodic vertigo. It is thought to be caused by endolymphatic hydrops in the lymphatic system of the inner ear. Typically the patient develops a sensation of fullness and pressure, along with decreased hearing and tinnitus in one ear. Vertigo rapidly follows, reaching a maximum intensity within minutes and then slowly subsiding over the next several hours. The patient is usually left with a sense of unsteadiness and dizziness for days after the acute vertiginous episode. In the early stages the hearing loss is completely reversible, but in later stages a residual hearing loss remains. Up to 50% of patients with idiopathic Meniere's syndrome have a positive family history, suggesting genetic predisposing factors. The key to the diagnosis of Meniere's syndrome is to document fluctuating hearing levels in a patient with the characteristic clinical history. Medical therapy for endolymphatic hydrops includes dietary sodium restriction and oral diuretics.

Acute unilateral deafness usually results from damage to the cochlea and may be caused by viral or bacterial labyrinthitis or vascular occlusion in the territory of the anterior inferior cerebellar artery. Perilymphatic fistulas may also cause abrupt unilateral deafness, usually in association with tinnitus and vertigo.

Drugs that cause acute irreversible bilateral hearing loss include aminoglycosides, cisplatin, and furosemide. Salicylates may cause reversible hearing loss and tinnitus.

Treatment of Hearing Loss

The best treatment is prevention, particularly by the appropriate use of earplugs for those working in a noisy environment. Hearing aids help patients with conductive hearing loss, and developments with cochlear implants may help patients with sensorineural hearing loss.

Prospectus for the Future

Ophthalmology has experienced significant advances in imaging modalities that evaluate the retina. Optical coherence tomography (OCT) is one such technique that provides high-resolution images of retina and optic nerve. Cross section images of the retina, optic nerve, and peripapillary areas are produced. It is helpful at detecting macular disease that is not readily detected on funduscopic examination. In addition, OCT is helpful for monitoring disease activity in various optic neuropathies. OCT angiography is a noninvasive imaging technique that uses OCT technology to visualize retinal and choroidal vasculature. This assists with diagnosis and provides insight into the vascular contribution of various retinal diseases.

For a deeper discussion on this topic, please see Chapter 395, "Diseases of the Visual System," and Chapter 396, "Neuro-Ophthalmology," in *Goldman-Cecil Medicine*, 26th Edition.

SUGGESTED READINGS

Margolin E: The swollen optic nerve; an approach to diagnosis and management, Practical Neurol 19(4):302–309, 2019.
Toosy AT, Mason DF, Miller DH: Optic neuritis, Lancet Neurol 13:83–99, 2014.

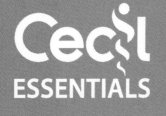

115

Dizziness and Vertigo

Jonathan Cahill

DEFINITIONS AND EPIDEMIOLOGY

Vertigo is defined as the sensation of self-motion in the absence of motion or the sensation of distorted self-motion during normal movement. Traditionally, vertigo is described as a spinning sensation, though other descriptions such as a rising, sinking, or floating sensation may also be vertiginous. Dizziness has a less specific definition and has often been further categorized into sensations of vertigo, disequilibrium, lightheadedness, or presyncope. Patients with dizziness frequently describe multiple different and simultaneous symptoms, and their descriptions of symptoms are frequently inconsistent, which makes accurate diagnosis challenging. Throughout this chapter, the terms *vertigo* and *dizziness* will be used almost interchangeably.

Dizziness is a very commonly reported symptom. As a chief complaint, dizziness accounts for 3% of adult primary care clinic visits and 4% of adult emergency department visits. Approximately 30% of the general population reports having had some type of bothersome dizziness.

THE VESTIBULAR SYSTEM AND BRAIN STEM CIRCUITRY

The sense of balance is maintained by a complicated network of afferent (vestibular, visual, and proprioceptive) and efferent (motor, cerebellar, and oculomotor) systems. The vestibular system consists of the vestibular labyrinth in the temporal bone of the inner ear and its projections to the vestibular portion of the eighth cranial nerve. The eighth cranial nerve projects to the vestibular nuclear complex in the brain stem, which in turn projects widely to the cerebellum, other brain stem nuclei, thalamus, and cerebral cortex.

The paired vestibular systems (left and right) maintain balanced tonic input to the brain. Perturbation of any portion of the circuit by focal lesions or aberrant stimulation can lead to dizziness. The connection of the vestibular system to the oculomotor system, demonstrated by the vestibulo-ocular reflex (VOR), is vital in maintaining clear vision during movement. In many cases, vestibular system abnormalities can be detected by examination of eye movements and the VOR. Nystagmus, alternating fast and slow rhythmic eye movements, is a characteristic sign of vestibular system dysfunction. The type and pattern of nystagmus can assist in more accurately localizing the vestibular disorder. Table 115.1 summarizes common patterns of nystagmus observed in patients with vestibular disorders.

DIFFERENTIATING CENTRAL FROM PERIPHERAL

Most causes of dizziness and vertigo are benign. But it is important to consider the rare more serious causes, such as brain stem infarct or a posterior fossa mass, and to understand the strengths and limitations of available diagnostic testing. The goal of most diagnostic tests is to differentiate causes of vertigo localized to the peripheral (e.g., vestibule, labyrinth, or vestibular nerve) or central (e.g., vestibular nuclear complex, other brain stem connections, cerebellum) vestibular systems.

Computed tomography (CT) scan of the brain is sensitive to rule out acute intracerebral hemorrhage but has limited sensitivity for other etiologies of vertigo. The contents of the posterior fossa (brain stem, cerebellum, and supporting structures) are not well imaged with CT. Furthermore, acute intracerebral hemorrhage commonly presents with additional symptoms and signs and is rarely confused for the other etiologies considered here. Magnetic resonance imaging (MRI) of the brain has better sensitivity for acute ischemic stroke, but in the posterior fossa MRI can miss 15% to 20% of acute ischemic strokes, especially in cases of small (<1 cm) infarctions and when MRI imaging is performed within 24 to 48 hours of symptom onset.

In cases of acute onset dizziness and vertigo, the acute vestibular syndrome, a three-step bedside oculomotor examination is more sensitive than MRI for acute ischemic stroke. The Head-Impulse—Nystagmus—Test-of-Skew (HINTS) examination can be performed in less than 1 minute and can lead to accurate diagnosis in many cases. Table 115.2 summarizes the possible findings of the HINTS examination. It is important to recognize that the HINTS examination findings can only be interpreted when the examination is performed in symptomatic patients.

CLINICAL PRESENTATION PATTERNS

For patients presenting with dizziness, the traditional approach had been to specify the nature or quality of the dizziness as vertigo, imbalance, lightheadedness, or presyncope. The differential diagnosis would then be informed by the specific symptom type. This approach, however, does not lead to accurate diagnosis in many cases and has been replaced by a focus on the timing and triggers of symptoms, rather than the quality of dizziness.

There are four patterns of dizziness presentation: (1) acute persistent, (2) episodic-spontaneous, (3) episodic-triggered, and less commonly, (4) chronic/progressive. It is important to note that no pattern is definitively associated with a particular diagnosis but that the examination and additional testing can be used to home in on a specific disorder and rule out others.

The three most common peripheral vestibular disorders can be thought of as prototypes for most pathology involving the peripheral vestibular system. Each of these three disorders (vestibular neuronitis, Meniere's disease, and benign-paroxysmal positional vertigo [BPPV]) can be diagnosed using the tests described previously and after consideration of possible red flag symptoms. The timing of symptom onset and the triggers of symptoms are the most important features to consider. Table 115.3 summarizes the symptom onset, triggers, and

TABLE 115.1 Nystagmus Patterns

	Pattern	Localization	Principal Causes
Spontaneous	Unidirectional, horizontal > torsional	Vestibular nerve, less commonly brain stem	Vestibular neuronitis, less commonly stroke
	Downbeat, upbeat, or pure torsional	Brain	Stroke, brain stem mass, brain stem demyelination
Gaze-evoked (Video 115.1)	Unidirectional (Video 115.2)	Vestibular nerve	Vestibular neuronitis
	Bidirectional	Brain	Stroke, cerebellar syndrome, medication side effect
Positional	Burst of upbeat torsional with Dix-Halpike maneuver	Semicircular canal of labyrinth	Benign-paroxysmal-positional vertigo (BPPV) (Video 115.3)
	Horizontal with supine positional testing	Semicircular canal of labyrinth, less commonly brain stem	BPPV, brain stem lesion
	Persistent downbeat	Brain	Chiari malformation, cerebellar degeneration

TABLE 115.2 HINTS Examination

	Technique	Findings Suggestive of Central Etiology	Findings Suggestive of Peripheral Etiology
Head-Impulse	Patient attempts to maintain visual fixation while the examiner quickly turns the patient's head 5-10 degrees horizontally	Normal fixation, no corrective saccade (rapid eye movements that change the point of fixation)	Abnormal corrective horizontal saccade when the head is turned toward the affected ear
Nystagmus	Extraocular movements examined for nystagmus	Direction changing nystagmus, pure vertical nystagmus	Unidirectional horizontal nystagmus, with some rotary component, worst with gaze in the direction of the fast phase nystagmus
Test-of-Skew	Alternate eye cover testing while patient maintains fixation	Vertical skew with corrective saccade upon uncovering of the eye	Normal, no skew or corrective saccade

TABLE 115.3 Acute Persistent, Episodic-Spontaneous, and Episodic-Triggered Acute Vestibular Syndromes

	Acute Persistent	Episodic-Spontaneous	Episodic-Triggered
Primary consideration	Vestibular neuronitis	Meniere's disease	BPPV
Key features	Constant vertigo, unidirectional horizontal nystagmus, HINTS suggestive of peripheral etiology	Vertigo lasting hours, no specific triggers, unilateral auditory symptoms	Positionally triggered, brief (<1 min) attacks, upbeat torsional nystagmus
Other considerations	Stroke, metabolic disorder, brain stem lesion (mass, demyelination)	TIA, vestibular migraine, panic/anxiety	Orthostatic hypotension
Red flags	Abnormal neurologic examination, HINTS suggestive of central etiology	HINTS (during symptoms) suggestive of central etiology	Prolonged duration of symptoms. Neurologic symptoms other than vertigo.

examination findings for these three common presentations of the acute vestibular syndrome.

DIFFERENTIAL DIAGNOSIS

For vestibular syndromes, the determination of a peripheral or central etiology and the pattern of presenting symptoms serve as the framework for generating the differential diagnosis. In addition to the peripheral and central causes of vertigo and dizziness considered here, there are several other general medical conditions that can present with symptoms mimicking a vestibular syndrome. And despite careful history, examination, and diagnostic testing selection, many cases of dizziness and vertigo remain idiopathic.

The three common causes of a peripheral vestibular disorder (see Table 115.3) are vestibular neuronitis, Meniere's disease, and BPPV. Vestibular neuronitis, caused by a viral infection of the vestibular

nerve, typically presents with abrupt onset vertigo (acute-persistent pattern) and nausea, most commonly lasting for several days. The vertigo attacks of Meniere's disease are shorter in duration, typically hours, and accompanied by nausea and prominent auditory symptoms of hearing loss, ear fullness, and tinnitus. The auditory symptoms of Meniere's disease become more prominent as the disease progresses and can occur outside of specific vertigo attacks. Meniere's disease attacks occur without provocation (episodic-spontaneous), unlike the attacks of BPPV (episodic-triggered). BPPV is caused by otoliths entering the semicircular canals of the inner ear and causing aberrant stimulation of the vestibule and vestibular nerve. In BPPV, sudden movement of the head, such as rolling over in bed or turning one's head to the side, can provoke severe vertigo and nausea, which lasts typically for less than 1 minute if the head is held still. Despite the short duration of vertigo in BPPV, the symptoms can be severe and disabling.

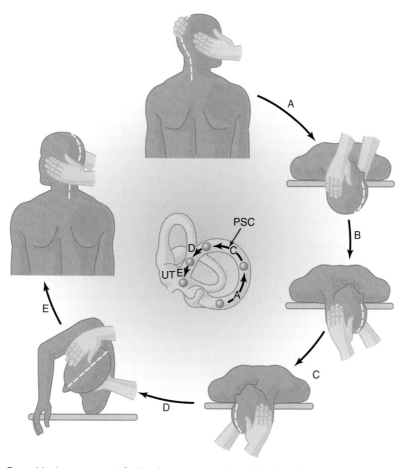

Fig. 115.1 Repositioning treatment for benign paroxysmal positional vertigo designed to move endolymphatic debris out of the posterior semicircular canal (PSC) of the right ear and into the utricle (UT). The patient is seated, and the patient's head is turned 45 degrees to the right (A). The head is then lowered rapidly to below the horizontal (B). The examiner shifts hand positions (C), and the patient's head is rotated rapidly 90 degrees in the opposite direction, so it now points 45 degrees to the left, where it remains for 30 seconds (D). The patient then rolls onto the left side without turning the head in relation to the body and maintains this position for another 30 seconds (E) before sitting up. The treatment is repeated until nystagmus is abolished. The procedure is reversed for treating the left ear. (Modified from Foster CA, Baloh RW: Episodic vertigo. In Rakel RE, editor: Conn's Current Therapy, Philadelphia, 1995, WB Saunders.)

Central causes of vertigo include numerous pathologies that cause structural or functional disturbance of the brain stem and cerebellum. For acute vestibular syndromes, ischemic stroke and/or transient ischemic attack (TIA) should be considered, especially in cases where the HINTS examination is concerning or there are other neurologic symptoms or signs in addition to vertigo and dizziness. Migraine may be one of the most common central causes of vertigo, with up to 40% of migraine patients reporting some accompanying vertigo with their migraine attacks. Both vestibular migraine and migraine with brain stem aura can have vertigo as a prominent symptom, though it is usually not the lone symptom. Space occupying lesions in the brain stem or cerebellum (neoplasm, abscess) should be considered in patients with risk factors. And unlike acute ischemic stroke, which can be missed by MRI up to 20% of the time, mass lesions of the brain stem or cerebellum will typically be seen on MRI. Hydrocephalus, which can be readily diagnosed on CT or MRI imaging, may cause symptoms of dizziness, but more typically it would present with a gait ataxia in the absence of dizziness. Degenerative disorders of the cerebellum can cause vertigo, but the pattern of symptoms would not be confused with that of stroke or other AVS.

A wide array of other general medical conditions can cause dizziness or vertigo as well. Dizziness as a side effect of medications is probably the most common. Dizziness can also be a prominent symptom of panic and anxiety. Symptomatic anemia can cause lightheadedness and dizziness. And following significant head trauma, a post-traumatic dizziness can last for several weeks.

TARGETED TREATMENT

Because most causes of vertigo are benign and the symptoms typically resolve spontaneously in hours to days, conservative treatments are most often appropriate. Symptomatic relief of vertigo can be achieved with antihistamines, benzodiazepines, or antiemetics, but their side effects in the long term and in older patients limit their use. More specific, targeted treatment to the underlying cause of vertigo is preferable.

Vestibular rehabilitation as directed by a physical therapist is the most helpful treatment for prolonged vertigo, such as with vestibular neuronitis. Meniere's disease is commonly treated with a low salt diet or diuretics to reduce the frequency of attacks. The Epley maneuver (Fig. 115.1) for repositioning semicircular canal otoliths is highly effective for BPPV, especially in the most common circumstance where the posterior semicircular canal is affected. For central causes of vertigo, both stroke and migraine have specific treatments proven to be effective as both abortive and preventative therapies.

SUGGESTED READING

Kattah JC, Talkad AV, Wang DZ, Hsieh YH, Newman-Toker DE: HINTS to diagnose stroke in the acute vestibular syndrome, Stroke 40:3504–3510, 2009.

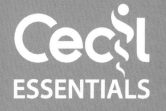

116

Disorders of the Motor System

Ruth B. Schneider, Adolfo Ramirez-Zamora, Christopher G. Tarolli

INTRODUCTION

The motor system is broadly divided into the pyramidal and extrapyramidal systems. The pyramidal system functions to execute motor activity, while the extrapyramidal system provides feedback to the pyramidal system, allowing selection of wanted patterns of movement and suppression of unwanted patterns. The pyramidal system is a two-neuron system, which originates in the primary motor cortex of the frontal lobes and, with white matter projections, coalesces to form the internal capsule; it then traverses the brain stem (as the cerebral peduncles in the midbrain, the basis pontis in the pons, and the pyramids in the medulla where the majority of neurons decussate to form the corticospinal tracts) and ultimately synapses on the lower motor neurons in the anterior horn of the spinal cord. The extrapyramidal system consists primarily of the basal ganglia and the cerebellum and provides coordinating and integrating information to the pyramidal tract system under the influence of various afferent feedback loops. The components and pathways of the basal ganglia (Fig. 116.1) and cerebellum (Fig. 116.2) influence and modulate voluntary motor activity of the motor cortex.

Disorders of the motor system affect the components of the pyramidal and extrapyramidal systems. The approach to the patient with motor dysfunction depends on the ability to accurately localize the neuroanatomic region affected through a careful history and focused examination. Disorders of the pyramidal system (central and peripheral) will be described in other chapters of this text (Chapters 109, 119, 123, and 125). Here, we will focus on disorders of the extrapyramidal system, which present with a variety of disorders of movement.

INTRODUCTION TO MOVEMENT DISORDERS

Movement disorders are a heterogeneous group of disorders associated with basal ganglia dysfunction. Movement disorders refer to a broad group of conditions leading to involuntary or abnormal movement as a prominent feature. In contrast to most seizures, the involuntary movements occur when the patient is conscious but are absent during sleep (with very few exceptions).

Movement disorders can be classified as either hyperkinetic or hypokinetic. Hyperkinetic phenomena include tremor, chorea, dystonia, tics, myoclonus, and other involuntary movements (Table 116.1). Hypokinetic disorders encompass the parkinsonian disorders characterized by a paucity of spontaneous movement (akinesia), slow movements (bradykinesia), and low amplitude movements (hypokinesia). The term bradykinesia is commonly used to encompass all three of these phenomena. While this classification strategy is a valuable means for approaching the patient with abnormal movements, many movement disorders display a combination of both hyperkinetic and hypokinetic phenomena. Idiopathic Parkinson's disease is the prototypical hypokinetic movement disorder, but it is associated with the hyperkinetic phenomenon of tremor in over 60% of patients. Similarly, Huntington's disease, a traditionally hyperkinetic disorder, is associated with bradykinesia.

Parkinsonism

Parkinsonism is characterized by bradykinesia, rigidity, tremor, and postural instability. It can be caused by a wide variety of degenerative disorders, medications, toxins, and systemic diseases. Table 116.2 summarizes the differential diagnosis of parkinsonism.

Idiopathic Parkinson's Disease

Idiopathic Parkinson's disease (PD), which is the most common cause of parkinsonism, is a progressive, neurodegenerative disorder characterized by a constellation of motor and nonmotor symptoms. The prevalence of PD increases with age and it affects approximately 1% to 2% of individuals over the age of 60. Beyond advancing age, some risk factors for PD include male sex, pesticide exposure, solvent exposure, and family history of PD. The motor symptoms of PD result from the selective loss of dopaminergic neurons in the substantia nigra-pars compacta that project to the striatum. The pathological hallmark of PD is the presence of eosinophilic cytoplasmic neuronal inclusions known as Lewy bodies containing α-synuclein.

Clinically, PD is most commonly recognized by its motor phenomena: rigidity, bradykinesia, rest tremor, and postural instability. Functionally, patients may describe difficulty with fine motor tasks (such as doing buttons), difficulty getting dressed, trouble getting up from a chair, a lack of facial expression, changes in speech (softening or hoarseness), decreased arm swing, poor balance, or tremor at rest or when holding a newspaper. Motor symptoms typically present unilaterally and remain asymmetric over time. Parkinsonian gait is characterized by a flexed and stooped posture, with a slow shuffling quality and decreased stride length and heel strike. Patients can also display festination, a phenomenon in which the stooped posture and hypometric stepping results in the center of gravity being located in front of the feet. Some experience freezing of gait, which refers to a brief and sudden inability to initiate or continue walking. Nonmotor manifestations include autonomic dysfunction (orthostatic hypotension, constipation, urinary symptoms, and impaired temperature regulation), psychiatric features (depression, anxiety, apathy, and psychosis), cognitive changes (mild cognitive impairment and dementia), sleep disorders (insomnia, excessive daytime sleepiness, restless legs syndrome, rapid eye movement [REM] sleep behavior disorder), and a myriad

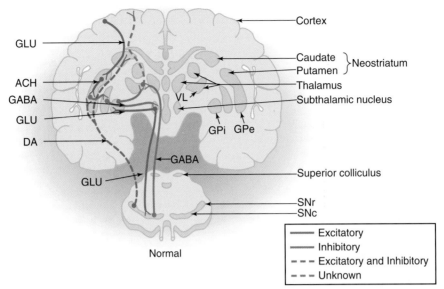

Fig. 116.1 Anatomy of the basal ganglia and their connections. The feedback loop proceeds from cerebral prefrontal areas to the basal ganglia and eventually back from the basal ganglia to the thalamus to the motor cortex. This ultimately regulates the descending corticospinal motor system. *ACH,* Acetylcholine; *DA,* dopamine; *GABA,* γ-aminobutyric acid; *GLU,* glutamate; *GP,* globus pallidum (e, external; i, internal); *SN,* substantia nigra (c, compacta; r, reticulate); *VL,* ventrolateral. (From Jankovic J: The extrapyramidal disorders: Introduction. In Goldman L, Bennett JC, editors: Cecil Textbook of Medicine, ed 21, Philadelphia, 2000, Saunders, p 2078.)

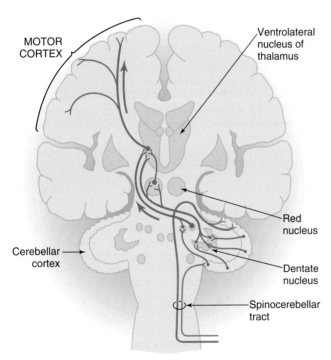

Fig. 116.2 Corticocerebellar loop. The major cerebellar input is from the spinocerebellar tract. Outflow is to the motor cortex via the mesencephalon and thalamus.

of other symptoms (pain, sexual dysfunction, vision changes, fatigue, micrographia, and decreased sense of smell).

PD is a clinical diagnosis based on the presence of gradual progression of characteristic motor symptoms and signs as well as a robust and sustained response to levodopa therapy. While the diagnosis of PD is made on the basis of the presence of a characteristic motor syndrome, it is now recognized that there are earlier stages of PD: preclinical

PD (neurodegeneration in the absence of symptoms or signs) and prodromal PD (symptoms and signs, often nonmotor, insufficient to meet diagnostic criteria). Certain "red flags" on history or examination might suggest an atypical or secondary cause of parkinsonism (Table 116.3). Dopamine transporter (DaT) SPECT imaging can assist in distinguishing neurodegenerative forms of parkinsonism from drug-induced parkinsonism and essential tremor with parkinsonian features. The dopamine transporter is responsible for re-uptake of dopamine into presynaptic terminals and is, therefore, an indirect measure of nigro-striatal neuronal density. In PD, nigro-striatal neurons are lost asymmetrically; on dopamine transporter imaging, this is characterized by asymmetric reduction in dopamine transporter signal in the striatum. With drug-induced parkinsonism and essential tremor, dopamine transporter imaging is normal. Dopamine transporter imaging does not distinguish PD from other degenerative forms of parkinsonism.

PD is a slowly progressive disorder associated with accumulating disability. No medications have been proven to slow progression; however, exercise may slow the progression of disease. Treatments of the motor symptoms can reduce disability and improve function. The mainstay of treatment is levodopa, the precursor to dopamine, given with a dopa-decarboxylase inhibitor (e.g., carbidopa) to maximize CNS penetration of levodopa and minimize systemic side effects. Other symptomatic treatments stimulate dopamine receptors in the brain (dopamine agonists) or inhibit the breakdown of levodopa and dopamine (monoamine oxidase type B inhibitors and catechol-O-methyltransferase inhibitors). This approach to symptom management is effective early in the course of the disease; however, as the disease continues to progress, it may be complicated by the development of motor complications, including motor fluctuations and dyskinesias (which manifest as chorea and/or dystonia). Surgical approaches to treatment of motor complications include deep brain stimulation (DBS) and continuous intestinal infusion of levodopa-carbidopa. Unfortunately, some motor features, such as postural instability, are

TABLE 116.1 Definition of Common Movement Phenomena

Movement	Definition
Parkinsonism	Generic term referring to some combination of features including a paucity of spontaneous movement (akinesia), slow movements (bradykinesia), and low amplitude movements (hypokinesia) as well as tremor (at rest), rigidity, and postural instability.
Tremor	Rhythmic oscillatory movement of a body part. Rest tremor occurs at rest. Action tremor encompasses postural tremor (present during maintenance of a posture), kinetic tremor (which occurs with voluntary movement), and intention tremor (when the tremor worsens upon approaching a target).
Chorea	Irregular, purposeless, abrupt, rapid, brief, arrhythmic, unsustained movements that flow randomly from one part of the body to another.
Dystonia	Sustained or intermittent muscle contractions causing abnormal, often repetitive movements, postures, or both. Dystonic movements are typically patterned, twisting, sustained at the peak of the movement, and may be tremulous.
Tics	Abrupt, usually brief, suppressible, "jerky" and often repetitive and stereotyped movements, which vary in intensity and are repeated at irregular intervals. Key features of tics are the presence of a premonitory urge that is usually temporarily relieved following the movement.
Ataxia	Impairment in coordination of voluntary movement, which may manifest as incoordination of limb movements, gait impairment, eye movement abnormalities, or speech impairment.
Akathisia	Sensorimotor disorder defined by a subjective sense of restlessness affecting all or part of the body with a marked difficulty staying still.
Myoclonus	Simple, rapid, involuntary movement causing movement of a part of the body across a joint. While it can be similar in appearance to a tic, myoclonus is typically a simpler movement fragment and is not associated with a premonitory urge or post-movement sense of relief.

TABLE 116.2 Differential Diagnosis of Parkinsonism

Degenerative/inherited causes	Idiopathic Parkinson's Disease
	Multiple system atrophy
	Progressive supranuclear palsy
	Dementia with Lewy body
	Corticobasal degeneration
	Frontotemporal dementia with Parkinsonism
	Huntington's disease
	Wilson disease
	Dopa-responsive dystonia
	Pantothenate kinase–associated neurodegeneration
Secondary causes	Dopamine receptor blocking medications (e.g., antipsychotics, metoclopramide, prochlorperazine)
	Presynaptic dopamine depleting medications (tetrabenazine)
	Other medications (e.g., valproic acid, calcium-channel blockers, lithium)
	Cerebrovascular disease
	Toxins (MPTP, manganese, carbon monoxide)

MPTP, 1-Methyl-4-phenyl-1,2,3,6-tetrahydropyridine.

unresponsive to medical or surgical therapy. Rehabilitative therapies play an important role throughout the disease course.

A number of monogenic causes of Parkinsonism have been identified. Mutations in α-synuclein *(SNCA)* and leucine-rich repeat kinase 2 *(LRRK2)* are associated with autosomal dominant parkinsonism. Autosomal dominant causes account for less than 2% of all adult-onset Parkinson's disease cases with higher frequencies in certain populations due to founder effects. Autosomal recessive monogenic causes include mutations in genes encoding parkin *(PRKN)*, PTEN-induced kinase 1 *(PINK1)*, and DJ-1 *(PARK7)* and are relatively common in familial cases with onset before the age of 45. Mutations in glucocerebrosidase (GBA) are the most commonly identified mutations in PD. An improved understanding of these genetic causes suggests an important role of impairment in lysosomal pathways and protein degradation in PD pathogenesis.

Atypical Parkinsonism

The atypical parkinsonian or "Parkinson plus" syndromes refer to a heterogeneous group of sporadic neurodegenerative disorders characterized by parkinsonism, reduced or absent response to dopaminergic therapy, and characteristic nonmotor features. The most common are the synucleinopathies: multiple system atrophy and dementia with Lewy bodies; and the tauopathies: progressive supranuclear palsy and corticobasal syndrome.

Multiple system atrophy (MSA), formerly termed olivopontocerebellar degeneration, striatonigral degeneration, or Shy-Drager syndrome, is a neurodegenerative syndrome characterized by prominent autonomic dysfunction in combination with parkinsonism and/or cerebellar ataxia. MSA has an estimated prevalence of 2 to 5/100,000. Current nomenclature subdivides patients with MSA based on their predominant motor feature: MSA with predominant parkinsonism (MSA-P) and MSA with predominant cerebellar ataxia (MSA-C), but a mixed phenotype is common. Bradykinesia and rigidity are prominent features of the parkinsonism in MSA-P, though these tend to be symmetric, compared to the asymmetry of early idiopathic PD. Both forms of MSA have prominent autonomic dysfunction manifesting as orthostatic hypotension, urinary retention, delayed gastrointestinal motility, or erectile dysfunction in men. Patients may have a transient response to dopaminergic therapy for motor symptoms, though it is often incomplete; limited interventions are available for management of the associated ataxia. Symptomatic therapy can be utilized to manage orthostatic hypotension, constipation, and urinary symptoms

TABLE 116.3 "Red Flags" in the Diagnosis of Parkinson's Disease

Clinical or Historical "Red Flag"	Suggested Diagnosis
Early postural instability and falls	PSP, MSA, CBD, DLB, vascular
Early dysphagia	PSP, CBD
Early or spontaneous hallucinations	DLB
Early dementia or dementia predating PD	DLB
Early or severe dysautonomia	MSA
Pyramidal tract and/or cerebellar signs	MSA
Antipsychotic exposure	Tardive or drug-induced
Acute onset and/or non-progressive	Vascular

CBD, Corticobasal degeneration; *DLB*, dementia with Lewy body; *MSA*, multiple system atrophy; *PSP*, progressive supranuclear palsy.

(see Chapter 112). Death typically occurs around 6 to 8 years after the onset of motor symptoms, most often due to respiratory dysfunction or complications of swallowing difficulties.

Dementia with Lewy bodies (DLB) is characterized by the presence of parkinsonism, early dementia (preceding or within 1 year of the onset of motor symptoms), spontaneous visual hallucinations, and fluctuating levels of alertness. Unlike Alzheimer disease, DLB tends to affect visuospatial and executive domains of cognitive function with relative sparing of memory early in the course. The motor symptoms of DLB may be indistinguishable from PD, and patients can have a reasonable response to dopaminergic therapy; however, cautious use is appropriate, given the risk for worsening psychotic symptoms. Patients are also characteristically sensitive to antipsychotics, though atypical antipsychotics with low potency D2 receptor blockade (quetiapine, clozapine, pimavanserin) can generally be used to manage psychotic symptoms. Rivastigmine and other cholinesterase inhibitors are frequently used to treat the cognitive symptoms of PD; these may also offer some benefit for the treatment of hallucinations.

Progressive supranuclear palsy (PSP) is characterized by eye movement abnormalities, early postural instability and falls, axial parkinsonism, dysphagia, dysphonia, and dementia. The supranuclear palsy refers to the characteristic eye movement abnormalities in PSP with a vertical greater than horizontal gaze palsy and preserved oculocephalic reflex; early ocular features can include delayed saccadic initiation (rapid eye movement to focus of interest), slowed vertical eye movements, and the loss of the fast phase of optokinetic nystagmus. There is prominent axial parkinsonism in PSP with truncal rigidity and hyperextension and relatively symmetric appendicular bradykinesia and rigidity; these are typically unresponsive to dopaminergic therapy. Patients may also have prominent dystonia, including frontalis dystonia with associated lid lag giving patients a characteristic surprised appearance. PSP can be rapidly progressive with death often within 5 years of motor symptom onset related to dysphagia, falls, or complications of dementia.

Finally, corticobasal syndrome (CBS) is a rare and heterogeneous disorder characterized by the presence of strikingly asymmetrical parkinsonism, dystonia, and/or myoclonus with associated cortical signs including upper motor neuron features, apraxia, neglect, cortical sensory changes (e.g., agraphesthesia), alien limb phenomena, and dementia. Patients may additionally have oculomotor features that overlap with progressive supranuclear palsy or cognitive features that overlap with frontotemporal dementia. The disease is rapidly progressive, and treatment is symptomatic; motor features do not typically respond to dopaminergic therapy.

Secondary Parkinsonism

There are many causes of secondary parkinsonism, including medications, toxins, and cerebrovascular disease (see Table 116.2).

Medications associated with parkinsonism include any medication that reduces dopaminergic tone in the brain, either through direct blockade of postsynaptic dopamine receptors (e.g., antipsychotics and certain antiemetics) or through depletion of presynaptic dopamine stores (e.g., vesicular monoamine transporter-2 inhibitors). Metoclopramide, a medication commonly used to treat gastroparesis, is a frequent cause because its dopamine blocking effects may be overlooked. Although classically characterized by symmetrical parkinsonism and absence of rest tremor, drug-induced parkinsonism can be clinically indistinguishable from PD. Hyposmia, which is common in PD, may be a helpful clue in distinguishing between drug-induced parkinsonism and PD but it should be recalled that hyposmia is also common among the elderly population. Treatment consists of withholding the offending agent, recognizing that it may take months for the symptoms to resolve. Even then, patients exposed to dopamine blocking agents may develop a tardive parkinsonism (i.e., a drug-induced parkinsonism that persists even after the offending agent is removed). DAT SPECT imaging can be useful in distinguishing drug-induced or tardive parkinsonism from a neurodegenerative parkinsonism.

Cerebrovascular disease is a common cause of secondary parkinsonism. Tremor is uncommon in vascular parkinsonism; lower extremity bradykinesia and gait difficulties dominate the clinical picture. Patients may have a history of clinical strokes with acute deteriorations followed by plateaus; however, many patients have vascular risk factors and a history of gradual decline. Neuroimaging is helpful in these cases.

Tremor

Tremor is characterized by a rhythmic oscillatory movement of a body part. Tremor is classified based on location and state (rest or action). Rest tremor is present when the affected body part is fully supported and not actively contracting; however, it is absent during sleep. Types of action tremor include postural tremor, kinetic tremor, and intention tremor. Postural tremor is present during maintenance of a posture against gravity, such as when extending the arms horizontally. Kinetic tremor is present with voluntary movement of the body part. An intention tremor refers to worsening of tremor on approach of a target (e.g., finger to nose) and is characteristic of cerebellar disease. Tremor has multiple etiologies, including medications, alcohol and drug intoxication and withdrawal, systemic disease (e.g., hyperthyroidism), structural brain lesions, or as a component of a neurodegenerative disease.

Essential Tremor

Essential tremor is among the most common movement disorders and the most common cause of tremor. Essential tremor has a worldwide prevalence of 2% to 4% with increasing incidence with aging. While essential tremor is often familial with an apparent autosomal dominant pattern of inheritance, no causative genetic mutation has

TABLE 116.4	Treatment Options for Essential Tremor
First line	Propranolol
	Primidone
Second line	Topiramate
	Zonisamide
	Benzodiazepines
	Other β-blockers
	Gabapentin/Pregabalin
Medication failure	Botulinum toxin injections
	Deep brain stimulation

TABLE 116.5 Medications Associated With Tremor

Asthma Medications	Neuroactive Medications
β-Agonists (albuterol)	Lithium carbonate
Theophylline	Stimulants (prescribed and illicit)
Antiseizure Medications	Selective serotonin reuptake inhibitors
Valproic acid	Tricyclic antidepressants
Phenytoin	**Other**
Carbamazepine	Levothyroxine
Immunomodulators	Caffeine
Corticosteroids	
Cyclosporine	
Tacrolimus	

been identified, and there are other non-monogenic causes of essential tremor. Cerebellar dysfunction has been implicated in the pathogenesis of essential tremor. Clinically, it is a heterogeneous disorder characterized by relatively symmetric 4- to 12-Hz postural and kinetic tremor of the upper extremities. It may cause functional impairment (e.g., difficulty with handwriting, drinking, or using utensils) and may even be disabling. Involvement of the head and voice are common. Tremor tends to improve with alcohol ingestion. Cognitive dysfunction, psychiatric manifestations (e.g., depression, anxiety), and balance impairment can also be seen. Mild parkinsonian features (e.g., tremor at rest, rigidity with activation) may develop and can make distinguishing incipient PD challenging. Propranolol and primidone are first-line treatments for essential tremor and are of similar benefit (Table 116.4).

Other Tremors

Beyond essential tremor and parkinsonian tremor, there are a number of other less common etiologies of tremor and tremor syndromes. All individuals may have some fine physiologic shaking of the hands or fingers with posture or action. At times when this tremor becomes visibly or functionally notable, it is termed enhanced physiologic tremor. Enhanced physiologic tremor is most commonly due to an underlying physical or psychological stressor. Common causes include anxiety, hyperthyroidism, excessive caffeine intake, stimulant or corticosteroid use, beta agonist use (e.g., albuterol), and valproic acid use among other medications (Table 116.5). Appropriate screening for medications and contributing medical or psychiatric causes should be undertaken in anyone presenting with suspected enhanced physiologic tremor. Enhanced physiologic tremor may be clinically indistinguishable from mild or early essential tremor. If no causative etiologies can be identified or mitigated, the approach to treatment is similar with β-blockers such as propranolol being used most commonly.

Tremor is also commonly seen in association with other movement phenomena including dystonia and cerebellar features. Dystonic tremor is irregular and is associated with abnormal posturing. Cerebellar tremor is an intention tremor that is characteristically low frequency, high amplitude, and worsens as one approaches a target. The distribution of tremor is dependent upon the cause with common locations of both dystonic and cerebellar tremors including the head/neck, trunk, and limbs. The presence of dystonia or cerebellar features is necessary to diagnose a dystonic or cerebellar tremor, and treatment typically focuses on management of the alternative movement. These movements and their associated differential diagnoses are discussed elsewhere in this chapter.

Chorea

Chorea is characterized by purposeless, abrupt, rapid, brief, arrhythmic, unsustained movements that flow randomly from one part of the body to another. The term "choreoathetosis" describes the combination of chorea and athetosis, a slow form of chorea manifested by writhing movements predominantly involving distal extremities. *Ballism* is a severe form of chorea with large amplitude, flinging movements usually affecting the proximal musculature. Chorea is often associated with a variety of secondary clinical features detailed in Table 116.6.

The differential diagnosis for chorea is broad, reflecting a wide variety of processes affecting the basal ganglia network and specifically the striatum. Generally, chorea either represents the primary manifestation of an inherited disorder or is acquired secondary to basal ganglia insults due to various comorbid medical conditions, medications or toxins, or structural abnormalities. Table 116.7 summarizes the differential diagnosis of chorea categorized by genetic and acquired causes.

Huntington's Disease

Huntington's disease (HD) is an autosomal dominant, progressively disabling, and fatal neurodegenerative disease; it is the most common cause of inherited adult-onset chorea. The causative mutation is an expansion of an unstable cytosine-adenine-guanine (CAG) trinucleotide repeat of the IT-15 gene (also known as the HTT or HD gene) on the short arm of chromosome 4, which results in production of abnormal *huntingtin* protein. The neuropathology of HD is characterized by selective neuronal vulnerability, particularly involving the caudate and putamen of the striatum. Microscopically, the pathologic hallmark of the disease is the preferential loss of medium-sized spiny neurons projecting from the striatum to the external pallidum.

The motor symptoms of HD may start at any age, with the peak incidence between 35 and 40 years of age with death occurring 10 to 20 years after development of manifest symptoms. Age of onset and rate of progression of the disease are inversely associated with CAG repeat length with the longest repeats associated with juvenile-onset disease and a more rapid disease progression.

HD is characterized clinically by the triad of a movement disorder, progressive cognitive decline (dementia), and psychiatric features. Chorea is the prototypical motor manifestation of HD occurring in 90% of patients. Other motor manifestations include dystonia, bradykinesia, and rigidity. Cognitive impairment is invariable in HD and typically progresses from selective deficits in psychomotor, executive, and visuospatial abilities to more global impairment with higher cortical functions usually spared. Psychiatric manifestations include depression, irritability, apathy, anxiety, and obsessive-compulsive symptoms.

The juvenile variant of HD, in which motor symptoms start before age 20, typically has an akinetic-rigid phenotype and only rarely chorea; patients may also have seizures. Paternal inheritance of the HD gene is the rule for onset before the age of 10 and paternal inheritance predominates (about 3:1 paternal:maternal) for onset before the age of 20. This can be explained by a phenomenon called anticipation; the

TABLE 116.6   Secondary Features Associated With Chorea

Athetosis	Slow, writhing movements of distal limbs
Ballism	Rapid, flinging movements of proximal limbs
Parakinesis	Incorporation of an involuntary movement into a voluntary movement (e.g., crossing and uncrossing of legs, adjusting glasses)
Motor impersistence	Inability to maintain tongue protrusion, "milk maid's grip"
Partially suppressible	Brief ability to voluntary reduce the severity of movements
Deep tendon reflex changes	"Hung up" or "pendular" reflexes
Gait disorders	Irregular or dancelike gait

TABLE 116.7   Differential Diagnosis of Chorea

Genetic disorders	Autosomal dominant	Huntington's disease
		Spinocerebellar ataxia (SCA 17 >1-3)
		DRPLA
		Neuroferritinopathy
		Benign hereditary chorea
	Autosomal recessive	Neuroacanthocytosis
		Wilson's disease
		Ataxia (Friedreich, ataxia-telangiectasia, ataxia with oculomotor apraxia)
		Disorders associated with brain iron accumulation (PKAN)
	X-linked	McLeod syndrome
		Lesch-Nyhan syndrome
Acquired/sporadic	Medications	Direct side effects (e.g., levodopa)
		Tardive dyskinesia
	Immune mediated	Sydenham chorea
		Systemic lupus erythematosus
		Anti-phospholipid antibody syndrome
		Vasculitis
		Paraneoplastic (*CRMP5* gene, anti-Hu)
	Infectious	HIV/AIDS
		Variant CJD
		Neurosyphilis
	Endocrine	Hyperthyroidism
		Chorea gravidarum
	Metabolic	Hyperglycemia
		Electrolyte disturbances
		Acquired hepatocerebral degeneration
	Vascular	Basal ganglia infarcts/hemorrhage
	Miscellaneous	Polycythemia vera
		Post-cardiac bypass pump
		Multiple sclerosis
		Sporadic neurodegenerative disorders

CJD, Creutzfeldt-Jakob disease; *DRPLA*, dentatorubropallidoluysian atrophy; *PKAN*, pantothenate-kinase-associated neurodegeneration; *SCA*, spinocerebellar ataxia.

CAG trinucleotide repeat is unstable and with paternal transmission the number of repeats tends to expand.

Treatment of HD is currently symptomatic. Vesicular monoamine transporter-2 inhibitors and antipsychotic drugs can be used for the management of chorea. No disease modifying treatments have been identified; *huntingtin* lowering approaches are currently under study.

Other Choreas

Beyond HD, the differential diagnosis of chorea remains quite broad with other inherited etiologies and a number of acquired causes (see Table 116.7). Approximately 10% of individuals with an autosomal dominant HD-like disorder will not carry the causative mutation for HD. Among these "phenocopies," only a small minority will have an identifiable genetic mutation. The most common genetic causes in the Caucasian population include spinocerebellar ataxia (SCA) 17, Friedreich's ataxia, HD-like 2, and familial prion disease (HD-like 1). Alternative diagnoses include dentatorubropallidoluysian atrophy (DRPLA), SCA 1-3, Wilson's disease (described elsewhere in this chapter), neuroacanthocytosis syndromes, and neuroferritinopathy. Young-onset, nonprogressive chorea, particularly in the setting of a family history and the absence of cognitive or behavioral changes, should raise concern for benign hereditary chorea, caused by a mutation in the *NKX2* gene; beyond chorea, the condition is associated with an increased risk of pulmonary and thyroid cancers.

Medication side effects are likely the most common acquired and overall cause of chorea. Levodopa-induced dyskinesias can be seen in patients with degenerative parkinsonian syndromes, and tardive dyskinesia can be encountered in patients on chronic antidopaminergic therapy. These entities are described elsewhere in the chapter.

Sydenham chorea is the most common acquired cause of chorea in children and follows a throat infection with group A streptococcus. Chorea typically develops within a few weeks of the pharyngeal infection, though can be delayed by more than 6 months. Though the chorea may be generalized, the face and tongue are most commonly involved. Psychiatric symptoms are also common and can include irritability, emotional lability, or obsessive-compulsive symptoms. Various biomarkers including elevated antistreptolysin O (ASO) and anti-deoxyribonuclease B titers are associated with Sydenham chorea but are not required to make a diagnosis. The behavioral and motor symptoms associated with Sydenham disease are typically mild and self-limited. Symptomatic treatment of chorea can be considered; corticosteroids may also be considered in moderate to severe cases and likely shorten the duration of symptoms. Chorea is a major criterion for acute rheumatic fever, and all patients with suspected Sydenham chorea should be evaluated for carditis. Definitive antibiotic therapy to treat the GAS pharyngeal infection is recommended even if there are no ongoing signs or symptoms of pharyngitis. Chronic prophylactic antibiotic therapy is recommended for all patients with Sydenham chorea until age 21; treatment for 10 years or until the age of 40 is generally recommended in those with residual cardiac disease following rheumatic fever.

Other acquired forms of chorea include chorea gravidarum in pregnancy, paraneoplastic chorea, and autoimmune etiologies. Paraneoplastic chorea is most commonly associated with CRMP-5 antibodies in the setting of small-cell lung cancer. Autoimmune causes of chorea include the antiphospholipid antibody syndrome and systemic lupus erythematous. In these cases, identification of the underlying etiology and initiation of appropriate therapy represent the definitive management.

Wilson's Disease

Wilson's disease (WD) is a rare, autosomal recessive disorder of impaired copper metabolism resulting in copper accumulation, neurologic dysfunction, and hepatic dysfunction. Typically, neurologic symptoms in WD begin in the second or third decade although late onset can occur. Patients develop a variety of abnormal movements including chorea, dystonia, parkinsonism, and tremor. The most common form of tremor in WD is an irregular, and somewhat jerky, dystonic tremor. A classical "wing-beating tremor" or "flapping tremor" in combination with dysarthria strongly suggests the diagnosis of WD. Dysarthria is frequently combined with slow tongue movements and orofacial dyskinesia including "risus sardonicus," which is characterized by involuntary grimacing with the mouth open and the upper lip contracted. Beyond abnormal movements, patients may also have seizures, cognitive impairment, and psychiatric features including abnormal behavior (typically increased irritability or disinhibition), personality changes, anxiety, and depression.

WD can present with acute liver failure or chronic liver disease that may clinically be indistinguishable from other hepatic conditions. The absence of clinical or biochemical evidence of liver disease does not exclude WD. A history of jaundice, a positive family history of neuropsychiatric disease, and increased sensitivity to neuroleptics can be diagnostic clues for WD in such patients. Untreated it is invariably fatal; early treatment is associated with better clinical outcomes; therefore, a high level of suspicion should be maintained. Diagnosis is confirmed by the presence of Kayser-Fleischer corneal rings in the setting of increased urinary copper excretion or elevated copper on liver biopsy. Bilateral symmetric high signal intensity in the putamen, caudate, thalamus, and midbrain on T2-weighted MR images can be seen

and the classic imaging sign is the "face of the giant panda" (Fig. 116.3). Serum ceruloplasmin is usually low in symptomatic patients, but this is not definitive, and confirmatory testing with ophthalmologic screen, 24-hour urinary copper, liver biopsy, or genetic testing for homozygous mutations in the *ATP7B* gene is necessary. Treatment consists of drugs that facilitate copper excretion, such as zinc, and the copper chelators D-penicillamine, trientine, and tetrathiomolybdate.

Drug-Induced Movement Disorders

The term *tardive dyskinesia (TD)* was initially coined to describe patients with rhythmic, repetitive (stereotypic), persistent movements after long exposure to antipsychotic drugs. Over time, other abnormal, persistent, involuntary movements have been reported after exposure to these drugs and other dopamine receptor blocking agents (DRBAs). Because of differences in treatment and approach, it is helpful to use the term TD to refer to the classic description of rhythmic, repetitive, stereotypic movements of the face, mouth, and tongue manifesting as lip smacking, chewing motions, and tongue protrusion. The term *tardive syndrome* more broadly refers to other phenomena, including rocking movements, tremor, myoclonus, and other forms of dystonia. Akathisia refers to the inability to remain still with an urge to move, giving the appearance of restlessness. It is a sensory phenomenon and a common and disabling form of tardive syndrome. Common movements seen in patients include repetitive self-touching, marching in place, rocking from one leg to the other, pumping the legs up and down, and crossing and uncrossing the legs.

TD and tardive syndromes are characterized by the late appearance of abnormal movements after prolonged exposure to a DRBA. Whenever the diagnosis is suspected, a careful and comprehensive review of treatment history should be done. Risk factors for the development of tardive syndromes include advancing age, female gender, and the use of high-potency antipsychotics. While removal of the offending agent is critical to prevent worsening, symptoms might persist in up to two thirds of patients and treatment can be challenging. Dopamine depleting agents can be considered for treatment and two vesicular monoamine transporter-2 inhibitors have recently been approved for the treatment of TD.

Dystonia

Dystonia is a heterogenous group of disorders that are defined by sustained or intermittent muscle contractions causing abnormal, often repetitive movements, postures, or both. Dystonic movements are typically patterned, twisting, and may be tremulous.

Dystonia may involve nearly any region of the body, emerge at any age, appear static or progressive, and can co-occur with other neurologic or medical problems. The classification of dystonia is challenging. Newer classification systems address the different clinical manifestations with four dimensions: body region affected, age at onset, temporal aspects, and any associated symptoms. Classification according to the presence or absence of associated features addresses whether dystonia occurs by itself (isolated dystonia, previously known as primary dystonia) or is part of a more complex syndrome that combines other features (combined dystonia, previously known as secondary dystonia or dystonia-plus). This new classification system provides a more clinically useful approach for diagnosis than previously used strategies.

Adult-onset focal dystonias are by far the most common. Cervical dystonia is the most common type of focal dystonia, followed by focal dystonias involving the face and jaw muscles (blepharospasm, oromandibular dystonia or the combination); laryngeal and limb dystonias are rare. Adult-onset limb dystonias are usually task-specific with dystonic contraction only occurring during specific voluntary actions (e.g., writer's cramp, musician's dystonia). However, this task

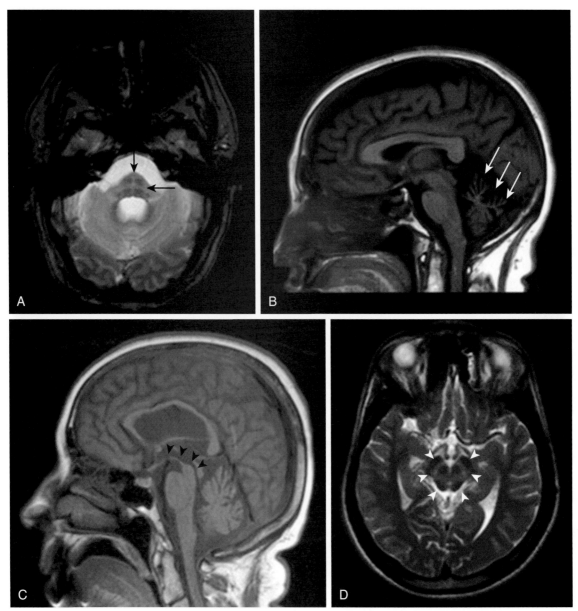

Fig. 116.3 Representative MRI findings of different movement disorders. (A) "Hot cross bun" in multiple system atrophy (MSA) *(black arrows)*. (B) Marked cerebellar and vermis atrophy in spinal cerebellar atrophy (SCA) 6 *(white arrows)*. (C) "Hummingbird" sign in progressive supranuclear palsy (PSP) due to prominent midbrain atrophy *(black arrowheads)*. (D) "Face of giant panda" sign in Wilson's disease *(white arrowheads)*.

specificity may be lost over time and even occur at rest. Focal adult-onset limb dystonia that is not task specific can be the earliest manifestation of parkinsonism and Parkinson's disease.

Recent advances in our understanding of the genetics of dystonia syndromes allow for unique classification and prognosis. Mutations in the *TOR1A* gene *(DYT1)* encoding torsinA are the most common cause of early onset generalized dystonia. Patients present with childhood-onset limb dystonia that often progresses to generalized dystonia within a few years. DYT1 is an autosomal dominant disorder with reduced penetrance (30%).

Dopa-responsive dystonia is a rare but important cause of childhood onset dystonia. It is inherited in autosomal dominant fashion with reduced penetrance (30%) with females more commonly affected than males. It is characterized by lower extremity dystonia, parkinsonism, and diurnal variability with the symptoms worsening as the day progresses and improving with sleep. As the name suggests, it is

exquisitely sensitive to levodopa therapy. The condition is often misdiagnosed and untreated; therefore, patients with childhood-onset dystonia should have a trial of levodopa. Other autosomal dominant disorders characterized by dystonia include myoclonus dystonia syndrome and rapid-onset dystonia parkinsonism. In addition, multiple other genetic causes of dystonia have been identified.

Treatment of dystonia consists of a combination of oral medications including anti-epileptics, anticholinergics, benzodiazepines, GABAergic drugs, and botulinum toxin injections for focal or segmental dystonia. Deep brain stimulation is commonly used for refractory cases.

Tics and Tourette Syndrome

Tics are rapid, repetitive, nonrhythmic, and typically briefly suppressible movements or vocalizations associated with a premonitory urge to perform the action and a post-event sense of relief. Tics are quite common, affecting up to 20% of school-age children, though the vast majority will have transient tics, lasting less than 12 months. Tics are broadly subdivided into motor tics, which involve movement of one or more parts of the body or musculature, and vocal tics, which involve creation of a sound. These can be further subdivided into simple tics (e.g., excessive blinking, head turning, grunting, and throat clearing) and complex tics (e.g., jumping, moving, and complex vocalizations or patterns of movement).

Tourette syndrome (TS) is the most common chronic tic disorder and involves a combination of motor and vocal tics, present daily, and for at least 1 year. Patients may have comorbid psychiatric diagnoses including attention-deficit/hyperactivity disorder, obsessive-compulsive disorder, or anxiety, which are often more disabling than the tics themselves. Tics commonly improve in late adolescence and in the majority of individuals there is partial or complete resolution of symptoms by adulthood. Treatment of tics can be considered when they are bothersome, functionally impairing, or causing harm to the individual. A combination of behavioral approaches (comprehensive behavioral intervention for tics), oral medications (α-adrenergic agonists, antipsychotics, and vesicular monoamine transporter-2 inhibitors), and botulinum toxin injections can be effective at minimizing the impact of symptoms.

Paroxysmal Dyskinesias

The paroxysmal dyskinesias are a group of rare hyperkinetic movement disorders characterized by recurrent, stereotyped episodes of abnormal involuntary movements (most commonly dystonia, chorea, or a combination of both). The three classically recognized types, paroxysmal kinesigenic dyskinesia (PKD), paroxysmal non-kinesigenic dyskinesia (PNKD), and paroxysmal exercised-induced dyskinesia (PED), were defined on the basis of triggers. Several causal genetic mutations have recently been identified. However, cases may also be secondary to structural abnormalities, and seizures should always be considered in the differential. PKD episodes are triggered by sudden movement, are often preceded by a premonitory sensation, last seconds, and occur with high frequency. The most common genetic cause is a mutation in the *PRRT2* gene. PKD is typically responsive to low-dose carbamazepine. PNKD episodes are triggered by caffeine, alcohol, and stress, may be preceded by a premonitory sensation, last minutes to hours, and occur less frequently than PKD episodes. The most common genetic cause is a mutation in the MR-1 gene. Treatment of PNKD includes avoidance of identified triggers and treatment with benzodiazepines. With both PKD and PNKD, onset typically occurs in childhood and boys are more likely to be affected. PED episodes are triggered by sustained exercise, last minutes to hours, and typically involve the lower extremities. The most common genetic cause is a mutation in the *SLC2A1* gene and when such a mutation is identified, symptoms may be responsive to the ketogenic diet.

Restless Leg Syndrome

Restless leg syndrome (RLS) is a common sensorimotor disorder that predominantly, but not exclusively, affects the legs. RLS is characterized by an urge to move the legs, predominantly when at rest, accompanied by leg discomfort that improves with ambulation. There are diurnal fluctuations with symptoms typically present initially only at night. The prevalence of RLS is variable and highest among European populations (5% to 12%). It is strongly heritable, with one half of patients having at least one affected first-degree relative. The three conditions most strongly associated with RLS are pregnancy, iron deficiency, and end-stage renal disease. Most patients with RLS also have periodic limb movements of sleep, which are periodically recurring limb movements that occur during sleep.

Although the mechanism of the disease is incompletely understood, a hypodopaminergic pathology is suspected in RLS based on the clinical observation that dopaminergic medications improve symptoms. Treatment includes the use of nonpharmacologic strategies like exercise and removal of offending drugs (e.g., antidepressants). Iron replacement should be undertaken when indicated. If medical management is needed, dopamine agonists or alpha-2-delta calcium-channel ligands (gabapentin, pregabalin, and gabapentin enacarbil) can be considered as first-line treatment. The use of opioids and/or benzodiazepines can be entertained in certain refractory cases.

Cerebellar Ataxias

The ataxias are a heterogeneous group of conditions reflecting impaired cerebellar function or impairment in cerebellar afferent and efferent pathways. Clinically, patients may present with incoordination, disorganized gait, poor balance, falls, dysarthria, impaired hand coordination, tremor, swallowing difficulties, and eye movement abnormalities. Comprehensive assessment is critical in elucidating potential etiologies and must include an understanding of the rate of onset/progression, ascertainment of family history, thorough examination for specific diagnostic signs, and brain magnetic resonance imaging (MRI). The presence of associated neurologic features can be useful for differentiating ataxic etiologies and guiding additional investigations. Structural lesions affecting the cerebellum or its connections can present with ataxia including abnormalities of brain development, stroke, tumor, infection, trauma, and inflammatory and demyelinating diseases. Table 116.8 summarizes the differential diagnosis of the ataxic disorders divided by genetic and acquired causes.

Inherited/Genetic Ataxias

Progressive ataxia in coordination and gait disturbance are the cardinal features of the inherited ataxias. Autosomal dominant SCAs may present with a pure cerebellar syndrome or be associated with parkinsonism, spasticity, cognitive, or behavioral features. They are usually adult-onset disorders with variable genetic mutations, including trinucleotide repeats, mutations in noncoding regions, and point mutations. Genetic testing is available for many of the common spinocerebellar ataxias and new mutations are being identified in a rapid and ongoing basis. Currently there are no treatments to address disease progression and symptomatic treatment is limited.

The fragile X mental retardation (*FMR1*) gene contains a CCG trinucleotide repeat expansion of greater than 200 in the fully penetrant mutation associated with mental retardation in boys. Recently a premutation associated with repeats of 55-200 in the *FMR1* gene has been found to be the cause of the adult-onset neurodegenerative disorder, fragile X–associated tremor/ataxia syndrome (FXTAS). Clinically, affected males have a progressive cerebellar tremor and ataxia. Fragile X–associated tremor/ataxia syndrome has been under-recognized and may be the most common genetic cause of late-onset ataxia. Treatment is largely symptomatic and the disease results in progressive disability.

Autosomal recessive ataxias are rare conditions with onset in childhood. Friedreich ataxia (FA) is the most common and best characterized of these disorders. It results from an unstable GAA expansion on chromosome 9. Clinically it is characterized by childhood-onset gait ataxia and clumsiness. The ataxia reflects a combination of spinocerebellar degeneration and peripheral sensory loss. Overt weakness secondary to pyramidal tract dysfunction is a late complication. Non-neurologic manifestations include cardiomyopathy, diabetes mellitus, and skeletal deformities, which add to the morbidity and mortality of the disease. Since identification of the mutation, late-onset forms of the disease with less systemic involvement and milder symptoms have

TABLE 116.8 Differential Diagnosis of Cerebellar Ataxia

Genetic disorders	Autosomal dominant	Spinocerebellar ataxias
		Episodic ataxia
		DRPLA
	Autosomal recessive	Friedreich ataxia
		Ataxia-telangiectasia
		Ataxia with oculomotor apraxia
		Ataxia with vitamin E deficiency
	X-linked	Fragile X–associated tremor/ataxia syndrome
	Mitochondrial	Polymerase gamma (POLG)
Acquired/ sporadic	Medications/toxins	Alcohol
		Phenytoin
		Fluorouracil
		Heavy metals
		Carbon monoxide
	Developmental	Chiari malformations
		Dandy-Walker malformations
		Pontocerebellar hypoplasia
	Immune mediated	Paraneoplastic (anti-Hu/Yo/Ri)
		Pediatric postviral
		Behçet's disease
	Infectious	HIV/AIDS
		PML
		CJD
		Lyme disease
	Metabolic	Thiamine deficiency (Wernicke encephalopathy)
		Vitamin E/B_{12} deficiency
		Thyroid disease
	Vascular	Cerebellar stroke/hemorrhage
	Neoplastic	Primary and metastatic tumors
		Paraneoplastic (anti-Hu/Yo/Ri)
	Miscellaneous	MSA-cerebellar
		Multiple sclerosis

CJD, Creutzfeldt-Jakob disease; *DRPLA,* dentatorubropallidoluysian atrophy; *MSA,* multiple system atrophy; *PML,* progressive multifocal leukoencephalopathy.

been identified. Therefore, Friedreich ataxia should be considered in the differential of adult-onset sporadic ataxias.

Ataxia with vitamin E deficiency is a childhood-onset ataxia with a Friedreich ataxia phenotype. Treatment with high-dose vitamin E may slow the progression of neurologic symptoms. Ataxia with vitamin E deficiency should be considered in any child with signs and symptoms of Friedreich ataxia that do not carry the Friedreich ataxia mutation. Abetalipoproteinemia and Refsum disease may resemble Friedreich ataxia and because of the availability of directed testing, they should be considered in the differential. Mitochondrial disorders, ataxia telangiectasia, and ataxia with oculomotor apraxia are other common causes of early-onset ataxia with cerebellar atrophy.

Sporadic/Acquired Ataxias

Insidious onset of cerebellar ataxia without a family history can be a diagnostic challenge. Alcohol abuse, toxins, chronic infections, multiple system atrophy, and mitochondrial disorders are diagnostic considerations. Sporadic autoimmune ataxias amenable to treatment include glutamic acid decarboxylase (GAD) ataxia and steroid-responsive encephalopathy associated with autoimmune thyroiditis.

Acute or subacute onset ataxia is most often associated with cerebrovascular disease, demyelinating illness, or direct or indirect effects of cancer. Paraneoplastic cerebellar degeneration is one of the more common paraneoplastic syndromes usually associated with gynecologic, breast, lung cancer, or lymphoma. A variety of antineuronal antibodies have been implicated; however, anti-Hu/Yo/Ri are most frequently seen. The cerebellar syndrome often predates the identification of the cancer. Treatment of the underlying cancer and plasma exchange are sometimes beneficial.

Vitamin B_{12} and vitamin E deficiency secondary to malabsorption can present with ataxic gait as a result of posterior column sensory deficits. In the appropriate clinical situation, Wernicke encephalopathy due to thiamine deficiency needs to be considered as an acute cause of gait ataxia.

Superficial siderosis is characterized by deposition of free iron and hemosiderin along the pial and subpial structures of the brain and spinal cord, resulting in damage to the cerebellar cortex, cochlear nerves, cerebral cortex, and spinal cord. Patients present with the triad of sensorineural hearing loss, cerebellar ataxia, and spasticity.

Functional Movement Disorders

Functional movement disorders (FMD), which fall into the broader category of functional neurologic disorders, are a heterogeneous group of abnormal involuntary movements that do not adhere to the physiologic characteristics of the other movement phenomena described in this chapter. FMD have traditionally been considered *conversion disorders,* where the body converts an underlying psychological stressor into a physical symptom. However, while there is clearly a link between psychological stressors and prior trauma with the development FMD, this traditional understanding is likely an oversimplification of the pathophysiology, which is not well understood. The prevalence of FMD is not well established, though it has been reported to be as high as 10% of patients seen in movement disorders specialty clinics.

Patients with FMD can present with movements that mimic any of the phenomena described in this chapter (e.g., tremor, dystonia, myoclonus). However, the examination will also typically demonstrate features inconsistent with other causes and suggestive of FMD, including variability (e.g., in the distribution, type of movement, amplitude), entrainment (where the frequency of the abnormal movement entrains to match that of an alternative volitional movement), and distractibility. Abrupt onset of symptoms, the presence of a triggering event, and rapid onset may also be suggestive of a diagnosis of FMD. A clinical diagnosis of FMD can be made based on the presence of these typical features. Electrodiagnostic testing can be helpful in identifying functional tremor and functional myoclonus.

Management of FMD can be challenging but generally starts with patient and family education and requires a multidisciplinary approach. Cognitive-behavioral therapy with counseling is the best evidence-based approach for the management of FMD. Rehabilitative therapies have a role for most patients. Pharmacotherapy has a limited role in the management of FMD though can be useful in the treatment of any comorbid psychiatric conditions.

Acknowledgment

We gratefully acknowledge the contributions of the previous-edition chapter author, Kevin Biglan, to this chapter.

SUGGESTED READINGS

Abdo WF, van de Warrenburg BP, Burn DJ, et al: The clinical approach to movement disorders, Nat Rev Neurol 6:29–37, 2010.
Albanese A, Bhatia K, Bressman SB, et al: Phenomenology and classification of dystonia: a consensus update, Mov Disord 28:863–873, 2013.

Bandmann O, Weiss KH, Kaler SG: Wilson's disease and other neurological copper disorders, Lancet Neurol 14(1):103–113, 2015.

Caron NS, Dorsey ER, Hayden MR: Therapeutic approaches to huntington disease: from the bench to the clinic, Nat Rev Drug Discov 17(10): 729–750, 2018.

Ferreira JJ, Mestre TA, Lyons KE, et al: MDS evidence-based review of treatments for essential tremor, Mov Disord 34(7):950–958, 2019.

Hallett M: Functional (psychogenic) movement disorders—clinical presentations, Parkinsonism Relat Disord 22(Suppl 1):S149–152, 2016.

McColgan P, Tabrizi SJ: Huntington's disease: a clinical review, Eur J Neurol 25(1):24–34, 2018.

McFarland NR: Diagnostic approach to atypical parkinsonian syndromes, Continuum (Minneap Minn) 22(4 Movement Disorders):1117–1142, 2016.

Postuma RB, Berg D, Stern M, et al: MDS clinical diagnostic criteria for Parkinson's disease, Mov Disord 30(12):1591–1601, 2015.

Pringsheim T, Okun MS, Müller-Vahl K, et al: Practice guideline recommendations summary: treatment of tics in in people with Tourette syndrome and chronic tic disorders, Neurology 92(19):896–906, 2019.

Ramirez-Zamora A, Zeigler W, Desai N, et al: Treatable causes of cerebellar ataxia, Mov Disord 30(5):614–623, 2015.

Schuepbach WM, Rau J, Knudsen K, et al: Neurostimulation for Parkinson's disease with early motor complications, N Engl J Med 368(7):610–622, 2013.

Seppi K, Weintraub D, Coelho M, et al: The movement disorder society evidence-based medicine review update: treatments for the non-motor symptoms of Parkinson's disease, Mov Disord 26(Suppl 3):S42–S80, 2011.

Verschuur CVM, Suwijn SR, Boel JA, et al: Randomized delayed-start trial of levodopa in Parkinson's disease, N Engl J Med 380(4):315–324, 2019.

Winkelmann J, Allen RP, Högl B, et al: Treatment of restless legs syndrome: evidence-based review and implications for clinical practice (revised 2017), Mov Disord 33(7):1077–1091, 2018.

117

Congenital, Developmental, and Neurocutaneous Disorders

Kristin A. Seaborg, Jennifer M. Kwon

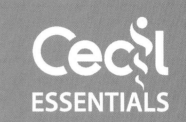

INTRODUCTION

This chapter describes some important congenital nervous system malformations, neurodevelopmental disorders, and neurocutaneous syndromes. Advances in imaging and molecular genetic testing have improved our understanding of these disorders. Neuroimaging facilitates early diagnosis and management of malformations of the brain and spinal cord. Advances in genetic sequencing and microarray analysis are improving our understanding of single-gene disorders, such as fragile X syndrome and neurofibromatosis, as well as genetically complex disorders, such as autism and attention-deficit/hyperactivity disorder (ADHD).

CONGENITAL MALFORMATIONS

Malformations of the central nervous system develop during fetal life. Table 117.1 summarizes the timeline of early neural and cortical development and the defects that may occur during these stages. Malformations developing early in embryogenesis can be more severe than those arising after the basic structures of the nervous system are in place.

Disorders of Dorsal Induction
Definition/Embryology

Dorsal induction is when neural tube closure occurs at 18 to 26 days post-conception. The central portion closes first, then the rostral and caudal portions. Failure to completely close the neural tube can occur anywhere along the neuro axis, leading to neural tube defects (NTDs) in 6.5/10,000 live births, the prevalence varying by geography, and genetic and environmental factors. Use of folic acid at the time of conception and during pregnancy can significantly reduce NTD rates.

If the rostral end of the neural tube fails to close, anencephaly can result, characterized by incomplete development of the brain and skull, and affected infants may not survive. If the caudal end of the neural tube fails to close, the result is spina bifida, described next.

Spina Bifida

Definition/epidemiology. Failure of complete closure of the caudal end of the neural tube during the 24th to 26th days post-conception results in spina bifida, the most common type of NTD, occurring in 3.5 of 10,000 live births. Abnormal caudal closure with overlying bony and skin defects can cause "open" NTDs, such as myelomeningocele (MMC). MMC is the most severe form of spina bifida and is characterized by the protrusion of the spinal cord and meninges through a defect in the vertebral column. "Closed" defects of the caudal spinal cord, or spina bifida occulta, are associated with malformation of one or more vertebrae and typically have limited neurologic symptoms.

Pathology. The deficits associated with meningomyelocele are not only secondary to the abnormal caudal closure of the neural tube but also from the ongoing exposure and chemical damage of the neural tube contents to amniotic fluid, trauma, and leakage of CSF. CSF leak through the open meningomyelocele impairs rostral vesicle expansion, leading to underdevelopment of the posterior fossa with cerebellar tonsil herniation into the upper spinal canal, called the Arnold-Chiari or Chiari 2 malformation.

Clinical presentation. Many of the stigmata of MMC can be detected on first trimester fetal ultrasound. MMC causes severe distal spinal cord dysfunction, including paralysis and sensory loss in the lower extremities as well as bowel and bladder dysfunction. Progressive loss of neurologic function and development of congenital clubfoot is commonly observed during pregnancy. Nearly all children with MMC have a Chiari 2 malformation and obstructive hydrocephalus.

Children with spina bifida occulta, or a "closed" caudal neural tube defect, may have symptoms including lower extremity spasticity and bladder abnormalities and the overlying skin may show nevi, lipomas, abnormal dimples, or whorls of hair. The most common location for spina bifida is within the lumbosacral region.

Diagnosis. Prenatal diagnosis of MMC cannot be reliably determined by ultrasound until the second trimester of pregnancy. Maternal serum testing for α-fetoprotein (AFP), which is secreted from an open spinal dysraphism (incomplete fusion), can be done in conjunction with second trimester ultrasound. Further evaluation of specific characteristics of the fetal anomaly can be done with fetal MRI.

Treatment/prognosis. Previously, infants born with MMC had surgical closure of the defect within the first 2 days of life to minimize neurologic complications. In 2011, the Management of Meningomyelocele Study (MOMS) demonstrated that prenatal surgery for MMC repair decreased the rate of enlarged cerebral ventricles and ventriculoperitoneal shunting by 1 year of age by 42% and improved the rate of independent ambulation by 21%. This study represented a turning point in management of MMC and subsequently led to affected fetuses with normal karyotype, isolated spina bifida with upper border between T1 and S1, and evidence of hindbrain herniation to be referred for prenatal closure of MMC during the second trimester of pregnancy.

Chiari Malformation Type I

Definition/epidemiology. Though not technically a disorder of ventral induction or a neural tube defect, Chiari I malformation (CM1) is the consequence of similar pathologic processes occurring during formation of the posterior fossa. CM1 is characterized by cerebellar tonsils that are downwardly displaced more than 5 mm past the foramen magnum. CM1 is much more common (1/1000 births) than Chiari 2 and associated with fewer neurologic sequelae.

TABLE 117.1	Stages of Prenatal Neural Development (Simplified)			
	Stage	Structures Forming	Post-Conceptual Age	Anomalies Seen[a]
Neural tube, brain vesicle development	Dorsal induction	Neural tube closure	18-26 days (3-5 weeks)	Anencephaly, spina bifida, myelomeningocele, Chiari 2 malformation
	Ventral induction	Brain vesicle and face development	5-10 weeks	Holoprosencephaly agenesis of the corpus callosum, septo-optic dysplasia
Cortical development	Proliferation	Development of neuroblasts and glioblasts	2-4 months (neuroblasts)	Microcephaly, megalencephaly
	Migration	Formation of six cortical layers	Peak occurrence at 2-4 months, though occurs from 8 weeks to 8 months	Lissencephaly, periventricular heterotopias
	Post-migrational organization	Cortex formed		Polymicrogyria, schizencephaly

[a]Some anomalies (such as microcephaly, polymicrogyria) can arise from different stages. So even though it may seem intuitive to think of microcephaly as a disorder of neuronal proliferation, there are some forms of microcephaly that develop well after migration.

Pathology. CM1 results from underdeveloped bones of the skull base and reduced volume of the posterior fossa. This leads to displacement of cerebellar tonsils into the spinal canal. Obstruction of CSF outflow through the tight foramen magnum may lead to development of fluid-filled cavities in the spinal cord called syringomyelia (see later). Symptoms can occur with compression of brain stem structures.

Clinical presentation. The clinical presentation of CM1 is variable. Eighty percent of patients report occipital headaches or posterior neck pain. Younger patients can have symptoms from compression of the brain stem, including disordered sleep, vertigo, dysphagia, tinnitus, and ocular symptoms. Some CM1s are found incidentally during MRI evaluation for other reasons. Incidentally found CM1s are less likely to develop syringomyelia, intractable symptoms, or progressive neurologic findings (10%).

Diagnosis/differential. MRI is the most effective method for diagnosis. CSF flow studies may be helpful to establish clinical significance of the CM1. Since any cause of increased intracranial pressure can lead to tonsillar herniation, it is important to exclude idiopathic intracranial hypertension and CNS mass lesions.

Treatment. Asymptomatic patients without syringomyelia may be managed by observation. If patients have severe headaches, neurologic deficits, or syringomyelia, posterior fossa decompression with or without duraplasty is indicated to reestablish CSF flow across the craniovertebral junction.

Prognosis. CM1 is generally not disabling and outcome after surgical decompression leads to resolution of clinical symptoms in over 80% of patients. For symptomatic patients, posterior fossa bone-only decompression without dural opening is associated with a lower rate of complications.

Syringomyelia

Definition/epidemiology. Syringomyelia or syrinx is a cystic cavitation in the parenchyma of the spinal cord or is a dilation in the central spinal canal (hydromyelia). The estimated prevalence of 8/100,00 is likely an underestimate. Syrinx is a common and important neurologic sequela of CM1 in up to 30 to 70% of pediatric patients.

Pathology. Syringomyelia may occur as either a congenital or acquired condition. Congenital syrinx is associated with a neural tube defect and forms during embryogenesis. Acquired syringomyelia is caused by disruption of the normal CSF circulation and is seen with CM1, tethered cord syndrome, spinal cord tumors, or trauma.

Clinical. The classic presentation is a dissociated sensory loss (loss of pain and temperature sensation with preservation of light touch and proprioception) in the neck, arms, or legs. A cervical lesion produces a capelike dissociated sensory loss of the arms and shoulders, atrophy of the hands and arms, with increased tone in the legs. Scoliosis is a common finding in patients with a terminal syrinx.

Diagnosis/differential. Diagnosis is confirmed by MRI, which will also differentiate syrinx from neoplasms, infections, and other spinal cord lesions. MRI of the lumbo-sacral spine should be included to rule out tethered cord.

Treatment. Surgical correction of the cause—CM1, CM2, neoplasm, tethered cord—is the most effective way to treat syringomyelia. A small syrinx may be an asymptomatic incidental finding on MRI and can be observed without intervention.

Prognosis. Syringomyelia is most often a chronic, slowly progressive condition with periods of symptom exacerbation and remission. Patients typically experience symptomatic improvement after corrective surgery. Conservative treatment without surgical correction may be considered in young children and asymptomatic patients.

Disorders of Ventral Induction
Definition/Epidemiology

Ventral induction is the second phase of central nervous system development; the brain vesicles and the face begin to form between the fifth week after conception and mid-gestation. Insults during this phase affect brain and facial development.

Common malformations that arise during this period include holoprosencephaly (HPE), agenesis of the corpus callosum (ACC), agenesis of septum pellucidum, and septo-optic dysplasia (SOD). ACC is most commonly seen. The prevalence in the general population is 0.7% and higher in those with developmental disabilities. The estimated incidence of HPE and SOD are both 1 in 10,000.

Pathology/Embryology

Ventral induction ensues with the cleavage and formation of three primary brain vesicles: prosencephalon, mesencephalon, and rhombencephalon. By embryonic day 49 or gestational week 8, the prosencephalon cleaves into the telencephalon and diencephalon and then the telencephalon subsequently divides into two hemispheres.

Abnormal prosencephalon cleavage leads to HPE, a spectrum of abnormalities ranging from alobar HPE (cortex with a single ventricle)

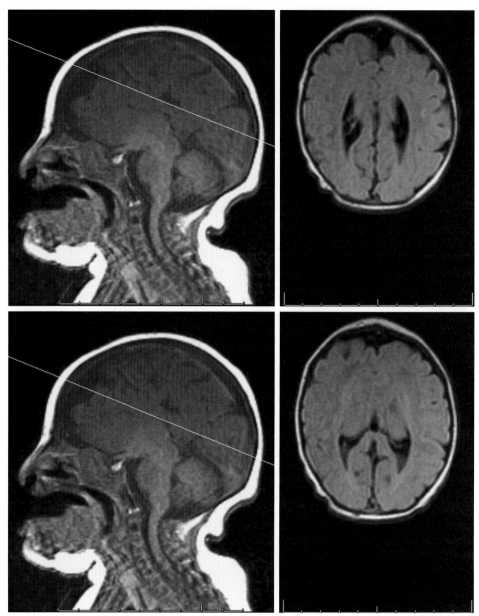

Fig. 117.1 Semilobar HPE. MRI (sagittal T1 image taken at midline paired with an axial FLAIR image whose location is indicated by the scout line) of 13 day old with hypotelorism and microcephaly. There is presence of partial fusion of the frontal lobes with lack of interhemispheric fissure/falx and septum pellucidum. The body and genu of corpus callosum is likewise poorly formed. There is appropriate separation of the thalami.

to semilobar and lobar HPE (cerebral hemispheres are mostly separated except for the frontal lobes) (Fig. 117.1). In all cases, there is some fusion between the two cerebral hemispheres, often accompanied by facial anomalies. ACC and SOD represent more discrete abnormalities localized to specific midline structures and occur later in prosencephalic development.

Clinical Presentation

Children with HPE, ACC, and SOC have varying degrees of developmental disability and other congenital anomalies. Because prosencephalon cleavage occurs at the same time as facial formation, facial anomalies ranging in severity can occur, including hypotelorism, solitary median incisor, cleft palate, proboscis, or cyclopia.

The clinical spectrum of SOD includes optic nerve hypoplasia, pituitary hypofunction, and midline brain abnormalities. Individuals with SOD often present for evaluation of visual abnormalities, poor growth, hypoglycemia, or precocious puberty. Seizures and developmental delay are the most common neurologic manifestations of SOD.

ACC may occur either in isolation or in association with other congenital syndromes. When present in isolation, individuals with ACC may be neurologically intact. If associated with other brain malformations, there may be developmental delay and intellectual disability.

Diagnosis/Differential

Neuroimaging is the primary method for diagnosing HPE, ACC, and SOD. The diagnosis of HPE can be made by prenatal ultrasound between 10 and 14 weeks' gestation. Ophthalmology exam can detect hypoplastic optic nerves in SOD. Because HPE, ACC, and SOD are associated with a number of genetic syndromes, genetic testing is indicated to guide management.

TABLE 117.2 Complications and Management of Severe Neurologic Impairment

Complication	Management
Epilepsy	Antiepileptic medications, vagal nerve stimulation, ketogenic diet
Dysphagia	Thickened feeds or enteral feeds via G tube
Respiratory insufficiency	Positive pressure ventilation while asleep, tracheostomy and mechanical ventilation if necessary
Spasticity	Physical therapy, intramuscular or intrathecal baclofen, oral benzodiazepines
Musculoskeletal	Serial monitoring for neuromuscular scoliosis, hip dislocations, and joint contractures. Often requires orthopedic surgeries.
Cognitive impairment	Individualized education plans, therapies

Treatment

Surgical treatment can improve craniofacial anomalies (e.g., cleft lip, choanal atresia [blockage of the back of the nasal passages]) in HPE and hormone replacement can treat pituitary insufficiency in SOD. Table 117.2 shows additional complications and management of the associated complications of severe neurologic impairment.

Prognosis

Prognosis for affected individuals depends on the degree of medical impairment and associated comorbidities. Most fetuses with alobar HPE die perinatally, but those with semilobar and lobar HPE have improved survival with aggressive management of associated problems such as dysphagia and epilepsy.

Children with SOD have variable outcomes depending on the presence of comorbid brain abnormalities. Prognosis for individuals with ACC depends upon whether ACC is an isolated defect (excellent prognosis) or associated with a neurologic or genetic syndrome.

Malformations of Cortical Development

Definition/Epidemiology

Malformations of cortical development (MCD) are a group of disorders that are characterized by disrupted migration and organization of neuronal progenitor cells, resulting in the abnormal appearance of cortical sulci and gyri.

The primary categories of MCD include lissencephaly (refers to smooth appearance of the brain surface), polymicrogyria, schizencephaly, focal cortical dysplasia (FCD), and periventricular nodular heterotopia. The recognized incidence of MCD is increasing with the use of MRI in children with epilepsy and congenital neurologic deficits. It is estimated that 25% to 40% of medication-resistant childhood epilepsy is secondary to MCD. The more severe forms of lissencephaly occur in approximately 1.2/100,000 births. All other forms of MCD are more common than lissencephaly.

Pathology

Neuronal migration is a complex, highly regulated process integral to formation of normal cortical architecture that occurs throughout gestation but peaks from 2 to 4 months. More than 100 genes play various roles in neuronal migration.

Schizencephaly is characterized by the presence of a cleft in the brain that extends from the surface of the pia mater to the cerebral ventricles that may occur as a consequence of a defect in neuronal migration, a genetic mutation, or a structural CNS insult in utero.

Focal cortical dysplasia (FCD) is typically the least severe type of MCD and often is clinically silent until patients present with focal seizures. FCD most often occurs as a postmigrational defect leading to cortical disorganization and focal lesions.

Clinical Presentation

MCD can have highly variable clinical presentations depending on postconceptual timing of cortical disruption and degree of cortical involvement. Lissencephaly has a severe presentation with marked motor disability and seizures, including infantile spasms. Polymicrogyria and schizencephaly, depending on the extent and location, can have less severe presentations. Most children with severe MCD present early in infancy with microcephaly, seizures, feeding difficulties, and developmental delays. The most common presentation of FCD is onset of focal seizures in early childhood.

Diagnosis/Differential

Neuroimaging is the primary method of diagnosing all types of MCD. Moderate- to high-resolution MRI scans are used for diagnosis in infants and young children. Prenatal ultrasound or fetal MRI may identify early features of some MCD. Most MCD are associated with genetic syndromes and warrant further genetic testing.

Treatment

Seizures are treated with antiepileptic medications and, when indicated, epilepsy surgery. Severe neurologic impairment leads to other complications (see Table 117.2)

Prognosis

Children with severe lissencephaly syndromes have a severe course and high mortality rates. Long-term prognosis for all other types of MCD depends on the degree of neurologic impairment and underlying etiology.

DEVELOPMENTAL DISORDERS

Autism Spectrum Disorder

Definition/Epidemiology

Autism spectrum disorder (ASD) is characterized by impaired social communication and interactions and restricted and repetitive behaviors. Approximately 1 in 69 children are affected by ASD with an incidence four times higher in boys than girls. The early symptoms of ASD can be identified between 1 and 3 years of age.

Pathology

A combination of genetic and epigenetic factors are thought to increase the risk of developing ASD. Many genetic syndromes, such as fragile X syndrome and Rett syndrome (see later), have autistic features as part of their clinical presentation. In addition, environmental factors such as advanced maternal or paternal age, maternal diabetes mellitus, or low birthweight increase the risk of ASD.

Clinical Presentation

The early symptoms of ASD are apparent during early childhood and a reliable diagnosis can be obtained by age 2 years. Patients usually present with delayed language development or language regression and limited social interaction. Children with ASD have impaired joint attention and often display repetitive, stereotypic behaviors.

Diagnosis/Differential

Several rating scale instruments and standardized interview tools have been developed to help diagnose ASD. The most commonly used tools are the Autism Diagnostic Observation Schedule (ADOS) and the Autism Diagnostic Interview-Revised (ADI-R). Both use standardized questions and observation scores based on the DSM-5 criteria for ASD.

Treatment

Prompt diagnosis and early initiation of intensive behavioral interventions such as applied behavioral analysis (ABA) and early childhood therapies are among treatments for ASD. In addition, some individuals with ASD require treatment for comorbid ADHD, anxiety, or epilepsy.

Prognosis

In 2014, a review of all studies examining the effectiveness of ABA intervention demonstrated that ABA delivered over an extended time leads to improvement in cognitive ability, language, and adaptive skills. Approximately 10% of children with ASD may develop skills for independent living and work. Early diagnosis and prompt referral to intensive ABA therapy are associated with improved prognostic outcomes.

Attention-Deficit/Hyperactivity Disorder
Definition/Epidemiology

ADHD is a common neurodevelopmental disorder occurring in 5% of children and 2.5% of adults. It is three times more common in males than females and often associated with additional neurodevelopmental and psychiatric disorders. ADHD is marked by inattention, impulsivity, and hyperactivity causing impaired functioning.

Pathology

There are no consistent pathologic brain findings or neurotransmitter abnormalities found in individuals with ADHD. However, ADHD is a highly heritable disorder. Several genetic disorders are associated with ADHD, including fragile X syndrome and 22q11 microdeletion (DiGeorge syndrome).

Environmental factors are known to play a role. Low birthweight, prematurity, and in utero exposure to maternal cigarette smoking, alcohol, and illicit substances are associated with a higher ADHD risk.

Clinical Presentation

Patients with ADHD typically present before age 12 years with complaints of 6 months or more of developmentally inappropriate behaviors, hyperactivity, inappropriate inattention, and impulsivity resulting in significant impairment in at least two different settings (e.g., home, school, work, or with peers).

On neuropsychiatric testing, patients with ADHD often have deficits in response inhibition, vigilance, working memory, and planning. These patients often struggle in school and have a history of behavioral outbursts due to poor impulse control.

Diagnosis/Differential

The diagnosis of ADHD can be made with the help of standardized rating scales that assess for symptoms of inattention, hyperactivity, and impulsivity in several different settings. The Vanderbilt Assessment Scale and Connors' Parent and Teacher Rating Scales are examples of standardized tools that help distinguish ADHD from inattention due to learning disability, hearing impairment, or mood disorders.

Treatment

Stimulant medications such as methylphenidate and amphetamines are the primary class of medication used in ADHD. They can improve cognition, executive and nonexecutive function, and memory. Other nonstimulant medications such as atomoxetine, guanfacine, and clonidine can be used when stimulant side effects are bothersome or when comorbid treatment of anxiety or sleep disorders is desired.

Prognosis

ADHD generally responds to treatment but there are often residual school difficulties. Core symptoms of childhood ADHD generally persist into adulthood, leading to higher risk of adverse occupational, economic, and social outcomes. Improvement in symptoms depends on age at diagnosis, associated intellectual disability, and effectiveness of clinical follow-up.

Rett Syndrome
Definition/Epidemiology

Rett syndrome is an X-linked dominant disorder caused by a mutation of the methyl-cytosine binding protein (MECP2), a transcriptional repressor. It is the second most common cause of severe intellectual disability in girls after Down syndrome, affecting 1 in 9000 to 10,000 girls. In boys, MECP2 mutations are lethal or result in severe encephalopathy.

Pathology

The loss of MECP2 function prevents regulation of gene expression during critical developmental periods in infancy.

A few patients who meet clinical criteria for Rett syndrome do not have MECP2 mutations. Other genes, such as *CDKL5*, *FOXG1*, and *MEF2C*, have been associated with Rett syndrome, and, like MECP2, encode proteins that are essential for early brain development.

Clinical Presentation

Patients with classic Rett syndrome develop normally during their first 6 to 18 months and then have stagnation in development, followed by loss of communication skills and deceleration in head growth. Other findings are "wringing" hand movements at midline, hyperventilation, air swallowing, abdominal distension, and chronic constipation. Between 60% and 80% develop seizures.

Diagnosis/Differential

Diagnosis can be confirmed by MECP2 mutational testing. As noted previously, other genes can cause Rett or Rett-like syndrome. Angelman syndrome, mitochondrial disorders, and neuronal ceroid lipofuscinosis may also present similarly.

Treatment

Girls with Rett syndrome usually require a multidisciplinary approach to address the complications associated with their severe neurologic impairment (see Table 117.2). Comorbidities often seen in Rett syndrome include seizures, spasticity with joint contractures, and prolonged QTc interval.

Prognosis

Most girls survive into adulthood but will not acquire speech or functional skills and will remain dependent for their care.

Fragile X Syndrome
Definition/Epidemiology

Fragile X syndrome (FXS) is an X-linked disorder caused by expanded CGG triplet repeats in the first exon of the fragile X mental retardation gene *(FMR1)*. An X-linked recessive disorder, girls can be symptomatic though they may have milder intellectual disability compared to boys. FXS is the most common single-gene cause of inherited cognitive disability and affects 1.4/10,000 females and 1.9/10,000 males. The prevalence of the female carrier status is estimated to be as high as 1 in 250 to 300.

Pathology

A normal *FMR1* gene contains between 6 and 44 CGG trinucleotide repeats and produces fragile X mental retardation protein (FMRP), which is important in brain development. Affected individuals have greater than 200 repeats, which causes silencing of *FMR1* gene transcription with loss of FMRP.

Clinical Presentation

Boys with FXS typically have moderate to severe cognitive disability and typical facies with relative macrocephaly, long and narrow face, high-arched palate, and prominent ears. Other physical features include pubertal macro-orchidism, joint hypermobility, hypotonia, and pes planus.

Some with FXS have comorbid epilepsy, with onset between 2 and 10 years of age. Other common findings are sleep disturbances, anxiety, and ADHD. Approximately 30% of males and 25% of females with fragile X have a comorbid diagnosis of autism.

Individuals with the "premutation" range of 55 to 200 CGG repeats often develop ataxia, tremor, and cognitive dysfunction in adulthood at a median age of onset of 60 years (fragile X associated tremor/ataxia syndrome or FXTAS).

Diagnosis/Differential

Diagnosis is confirmed by identifying increased CGG repeats in the *FMR1* gene. Other conditions can be mistaken for FXS, including Sotos syndrome, Prader-Willi syndrome, and Klinefelter syndrome. Adult-onset disorders presenting like FXTAS include parkinsonism, other ataxia syndromes, and tremor.

Treatment

Treatment focuses on management of comorbid conditions such as epilepsy, autism, ADHD, and disordered sleep. Use of stimulants or selective serotonin reuptake inhibitors (SSRIs) may effectively decrease inattention, hyperactivity, and psychiatric symptoms. Behavioral and educational services validated for autism are helpful in FXS. Earlier diagnosis and earlier developmental interventions may improve outcomes.

Prognosis

Patients with FXS respond to training and education over time, but their intellectual disability may make it difficult for them to live independently. FXTAS is associated with gradual and progressive neurologic deterioration over many years.

NEUROCUTANEOUS DISORDERS

Neurocutaneous disorders are congenital, often hereditary disorders characterized by pathognomonic cutaneous and central nervous system lesions that uniquely distinguish each disease. Many neurocutaneous disorders are associated with abnormal, noncancerous growth of tissues, often in a disorganized manner. Here we discuss neurofibromatosis 1 and 2 and tuberous sclerosis complex.

Neurofibromatosis 1
Definition/Epidemiology

Neurofibromatosis type 1 (NF1) is an autosomal dominant disorder caused by mutations in the *NF1* gene on chromosome 17. NF1 is characterized by altered skin pigmentation, tumors, and abnormalities of bones, connective tissue, and brain (Fig. 117.2). It is the most common neurocutaneous disorder, occurring in 1/2500 to 1/3000 individuals worldwide.

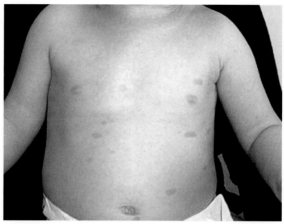

Fig. 117.2 Multiple café-au-lait spots in a child with neurofibromatosis type 1. (From Shah KN: The diagnostic and clinical significant of café-au-lait macules, Pediatr Clin N Am 57:1131-1153, 2010, Fig. 3.)

Pathology

The *NF1* gene codes for neurofibromin, which regulates tissue growth and tumor formation, explaining the occurrence of cutaneous neurofibromas, plexiform neurofibromas, and gliomas in NF1. Malignant tumors can occur secondary to malignant transformation of previously benign tumors. Approximately 50% of NF1 cases are due to spontaneous mutations.

Clinical Presentation

Patients can present with NF1 variably. All NF1 patients can be diagnosed before 20 years of age based on clinical criteria shown in Table 117.3. Patients can have learning disabilities, macrocephaly, and epilepsy. Important complications of NF1 include scoliosis, gastrointestinal neurofibromas, pheochromocytomas, and renal artery stenosis.

Diagnosis/Differential

The diagnostic criteria outlined previously are highly sensitive and specific. *NF1* DNA testing for mutations in NF1 can confirm the diagnosis. Schwannomatosis and neurofibromatosis type 2 may be mistaken for NF1.

Treatment

Regular multidisciplinary surveillance is recommended with frequent skin exams and assessment of neurocognitive development. Ophthalmology exams are strongly recommended until age 8 years because the risk of optic pathway gliomas is highest during this time. Many optic pathway tumors can be followed conservatively without surgery unless there are visual changes, when treatment with chemotherapeutic agents is recommended.

Large cutaneous neurofibromas and smaller fibromas can be removed but often recur. Subcutaneous plexiform neurofibromas grow along nerves and extend into surrounding tissue, causing pain or deformities. They have a high lifetime risk of malignant transformation and should be excised if possible. Drugs that target the biological pathways involved in tumor growth are being actively investigated.

Neurofibromatosis 2
Definition/Epidemiology

Neurofibromatosis type 2 (NF2) is a rare autosomal dominant adult-onset disease affecting 1/33,00 individuals and characterized by bilateral vestibular schwannomas and nonmalignant brain tumors.

TABLE 117.3	**NIH Diagnostic Criteria for NF1 and NF2**
NF1	**NF2**

Clinical diagnosis based on presence of two of the following:
 1. Six or more café-au-lait macules over 5 mm in diameter in prepubertal individuals and over 15 mm in greatest diameter in postpubertal individuals
 2. Two or more neurofibromas of any type or one plexiform neurofibroma
 3. Freckling in the axillary or inguinal regions
 4. Two or more Lisch nodules (iris hamartomas)
 5. Optic glioma
 6. A distinctive osseous lesion such as sphenoid dysplasia or thinning of long bone cortex, with or without pseudarthrosis
 7. First-degree relative (parent, sibling, or offspring) with NF1 by the above criteria
	The criteria are met by an individual who satisfies condition 1 or 2:
	 1. Bilateral masses of the eighth cranial nerve seen with appropriate imaging techniques (e.g., CT or MRI)
	 2. A first-degree with NF2 and either:
	     a. Unilateral mass of the eighth cranial nerve, or
	     b. Two of the following:
	       • Neurofibroma
	       • Meningioma
	       • Glioma
	       • Schwannoma
	       • Juvenile posterior subcapsular lenticular opacity

Pathology

The *NF2* gene on chromosome 22q12 is a tumor suppressor gene so mutations lead to loss of the protein merlin and a predisposition for tumor formation. Approximately 50% with NF2 have sporadic mutations.

Clinical Presentation

NF2 is characterized by multiple nonmalignant nervous system tumors including meningiomas, ependymomas, and gliomas. Bilateral vestibular schwannomas are the characteristic tumors of NF2, affecting 95% of patients. NF2 is typically diagnosed around 20 to 30 years with the onset of hearing loss and identification of unilateral or bilateral vestibular schwannomas.

Individuals with NF2 can have café au lait lesions, but rarely in the size or numbers noted in NF1. Many with NF2 have ophthalmologic findings including cataracts, retinal changes, and amblyopia.

Diagnosis/Differential

Like NF1, patients with NF2 are initially diagnosed based on highly specific clinical criteria (see Table 117.3). Molecular testing can confirm the diagnosis.

NF2 is frequently misdiagnosed as NF1, especially if there are café-au-lait spots. Patients with NF2 may also be misdiagnosed as having an isolated meningioma or unilateral vestibular schwannoma if other findings are not sought.

Treatment

Removal of the schwannomas and other tumors is usually indicated later in life when the tumors are larger and causing significant symptoms. There may be postsurgical complications and tumors may recur.

While traditional treatment has focused on surgical interventions, as described in NF1, attention has turned to development of drugs targeting tumor growth pathways.

Tuberous Sclerosis Complex
Definition/Epidemiology

Tuberous sclerosis complex (TSC) is an autosomal dominant disorder of early cellular differentiation, proliferation, and migration. TSC results in hamartomatous lesions involving multiple organs at different stages. The incidence of TSC is 1/6000. Mutations in two genes, *TSC1* and *TSC2*, are known to cause TSC in the majority of cases, and about 70% of cases are sporadic.

Pathology

TSC1 and *TSC2* are on different chromosomes but both encode proteins (hamartin and tuberin, respectively) that act as tumor suppressors, inhibiting the mammalian target of rapamycin (mTOR) pathway, which is essential in cell growth and proliferation. Mutations of these genes lead to unregulated growth and proliferation.

Clinical Presentation

The skin findings of TSC are common. Ninety percent have hypomelanotic macules, or "ash leaf spots." Facial angiofibromas are benign 1- to 5-mm dome-shaped skin-colored papules that first appear between 2 and 5 years of age. Shagreen patches are large plaques in the lumbosacral region with an "orange-peel" texture to the skin and are specific to TSC.

CNS involvement affects almost all individuals with TSC. Common conditions are epilepsy, autism, developmental delay, and intellectual disability. Brain imaging may reveal subcortical tubers, subependymal nodules, and subependymal giant cell astrocytomas (SEGAs) in some. Forty percent to 50% of infants develop a severe form of seizures called infantile spasms.

Diagnosis/Differential

The diagnosis of TSC is confirmed by identifying a pathogenic mutation of TSC1 or TSC2. Because 10% to 25% of affected patients have no mutation, identified clinical criteria have been established as well.

The spectrum of tumors seen in TSC may also be seen in isolation. Biopsy may be needed to distinguish facial angiofibromatomas from acne and other skin lesions.

Treatment

Treatment is primarily directed toward the sequelae of TSC-associated conditions. Several studies have shown that infants with TSC and infantile spasms have a superior response to treatment with vigabatrin.

SEGAs are typically slow growing, benign lesions that may be monitored with serial neuroimaging if asymptomatic. However, SEGAs located near the foramen of Monro can lead to obstructive hydrocephalus. Surgical intervention with gross total resection may be curative, but treatment with mTOR inhibitors such as everolimus is often helpful.

Prognosis

TSC associated with *TSC1* mutations is more often familial and has a milder clinical phenotype. Patients with *TSC2* mutations are more likely to have a sporadic mutation with more severe clinical complications. The variability in outcome depends on the extent and type of presenting symptoms. Patients with refractory seizures, developmental delays, and CNS lesions have a poorer prognosis. The development of renal angiolipomas, especially multiple tumors, is also associated with poorer outcome.

Sturge-Weber Syndrome
Definition/Epidemiology

Sturge-Weber syndrome (SWS) is a vascular malformation syndrome characterized by vascular lesions of the skin, brain, and eyes. It occurs in 1/20,000 to 1/50,000 live births with no clear evidence of heritability. SWS is the third most common neurocutaneous syndrome after NF1 and TSC.

Pathology

SWS is caused by somatic mutations in the *GNAQ* gene that plays an important role in vascular development. The gain-of-function mutation in *GNAQ* is found in affected tissues associated with vascular lesions. Leptomeningeal vascular malformations are ipsilateral to the port-wine birthmark and are associated with cortical injury secondary to venous stasis and insufficient tissue perfusion.

Clinical Presentation

SWS is characterized by leptomeningeal angiomatosis of the posterior hemisphere, facial cutaneous vascular malformations known as port-wine birthmarks, choroid angioma of the eye, seizures, and glaucoma.

Diagnosis/Differential

The diagnosis is usually made by observing a port-wine birthmark in the distribution of the ophthalmic branch of the trigeminal nerve, with neuroimaging confirmation of the intracranial abnormality. While 10% to 35% of children with a facial port-wine birthmark on the forehead or upper eyelid will have SWS, as many as 80% of children with a port-wine birthmark do not have intracranial lesions. SWS should be distinguished from other disorders involving abnormal intracranial vessels and seizures, including moyamoya disease, other vascular malformations, and tuberous sclerosis.

Treatment

Aggressive treatment of seizures with antiepileptic medications and consideration for surgical excision of epileptogenic areas may be indicated. Facial birthmarks may be treated with laser ablation for cosmetic purposes. Careful screening and treatment for glaucoma is necessary.

The use of daily aspirin to prevent strokes is controversial.

Prognosis

Prognosis for patients with SWS depends on the degree of underlying intellectual and developmental disability, control of seizures, and extent of visual impairment usually due to glaucoma.

SUGGESTED READINGS

Adzik NS, Thom EA, Spong CV, et al: A randomized trial of prenatal versus postnatal repair of myelomeningocele, N Eng J Med 364:993–1004, 2011.

Alexander H, Tsering D, Myseros JS, et al: Management of Chiari I malformations: a paradigm in evolution, Childs Nerv Syst 35(10):1809–1826, 2019.

Ardern-Homes S, Fischer G, North K: Neurofibromatosis type 2: presentation, major complications, and management, with a focus on the pediatric age group, J Child Neurol 32(1):9–22, 2017.

Calloni SF, Caschera L, Triulzi FM: Disorders of ventral induction/spectrum of holoprosencephaly, Neuroimag Clin N Am 29:411–421, 2019.

Ciaccio C, Fontana L, Milani D, Tabano S, Miozzo M, Esposito S: Fragile X syndrome a review of clinical and molecular diagnoses, Ital J Pediatr 43, 2017.

Fakhoury M: Autistic spectrum disorders: a review of clinical features, theories, and diagnosis, Int J Devl Neuroscience 43:70–77, 2015.

Gold W, Krishnaraju R, Ellaway C, Christodoulou J: Rett syndrome: a genetic update and clinical review focusing on comorbidities, ACS Chem Neurosci 9:167–176, 2018.

Guerrini R, Dobyns W: Malformations of cortical development: clinical features and genetic causes, Lancet Neurol 13:710–726, 2014.

Hirbe A, Gutmann D: Neurofibromatosis type 1: a multidisciplinary approach to care, Lancet Neurol 13:834–843, 2014.

Kabagambe S, Jensen G, Chen Y, et al: Fetal surgery for myelomeningocele: a systematic review and meta-analysis of outcomes in fetoscopic versus open repair, Fetal Diagn Ther 43:161–174, 2018.

Perlman S: Von Hippel-Lindau disease and Sturge-Weber syndrome, Handbook of Child Neurology 148, 2018, Neurogenetics, Part II.

Raspa M, Wheeler A, Riley C: Public Health Literature Review of Fragile X syndrome, Pediatrics 139:S153, 2017.

Rosenberg R, Kiely Law J, Yenokyan G, McGready J, Kaufmann W, Law PA: Characteristics and concordance of autism spectrum disorders among 277 twin pairs, Arch Pediatr Adolesc Med 163(10):907–914, 2009.

Rosser R: Neurocutaneous disorders, Continuum 24(1, Child Neurology): 96–129, 2018.

Thapar A, Cooper M: Attention deficit hyperactivity disorder, Lancet 387:1240–1250, 2015.

Vandertop WP: Syringomyelia, Neuropediatrics 45:3–9, 2014.

Weitlauf AS, McPheeters ML, Peters B, et al: Therapies for children with autism spectrum disorder: behavioral interventions update. AHRQ Comparative Effectiveness Reviews. Report no. 14-EHC036-EF, Agency for Healthcare Research and Quality, 2014.

118

Cerebrovascular Disease

Mitchell S. V. Elkind

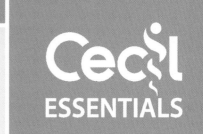

INTRODUCTION

Stroke is a major public health problem throughout the world due to its high prevalence and mortality and its association with significant disability among survivors. Stroke is the fifth leading cause of death in the United States and a leading cause of death in other countries, particularly in Asia. It is the leading cause of serious disability and results in enormous costs measured in both health care dollars and lost productivity. Major strides have been made in understanding the epidemiology, etiology, and pathogenesis of cerebrovascular disease, which have led to dramatic change in the approach to diagnosis and treatment of stroke in the past decade.

DEFINITIONS AND EPIDEMIOLOGY

The term *cerebrovascular disease* encompasses a host of disorders that share pathology localized to the vessels of the brain and spinal cord, including ischemic stroke, transient ischemic attack (TIA), intracerebral hemorrhage (ICH), subarachnoid hemorrhage (SAH), cerebral venous and sinus thrombosis, and disorders of the vessels themselves unassociated with cerebral injury (Table 118.1). Strokes, the major type of cerebrovascular disease, may be classified as either ischemic (i.e., due to lack of blood flow) or hemorrhagic. With widespread use of sensitive brain imaging, such as diffusion-weighted MRI (DWI), cerebral injury from ischemia can be seen among patients whose symptoms last only a few minutes. The definition of a transient ischemic attack has thus evolved from one in which symptoms lasted less than 24 hours, to one in which the duration of symptoms is not as relevant, and the focus is instead on whether there is evident brain injury on imaging (or pathology in those instances in which a patient dies). A definition from an expert panel in 2013 defined an *ischemic stroke* as "an episode of neurological dysfunction caused by focal cerebral, spinal, or retinal infarction." A *stroke due to ICH* was defined as "rapidly developing clinical signs of neurologic dysfunction due to a focal collection of blood within the brain parenchyma or ventricular system which is not due to trauma."

Because advanced imaging techniques permit the detection of abnormalities consistent with infarction or microhemorrhage that are unassociated with any clinical symptoms, the current definitions distinguish between "stroke," which involves clinical symptoms, and "cerebral infarction" and "microhemorrhages" (or "microbleeds"), which need not be associated with symptoms of cerebral injury. So-called "silent strokes," however, are not so silent; they can be associated with cognitive decline, dementia, gait disorders, functional disability, and an increased risk of clinical strokes. Because subclinical infarcts are approximately five times more common than clinically evident strokes, including them (and microbleeds) within the rubric of *cerebrovascular*

disease substantially increases the recognized burden of cerebrovascular pathology.

Ischemic strokes may be further classified into etiologic subgroups, based on the mechanism of the ischemia and the type and localization of the vascular lesion. Cardioembolism as the source occurs in 15% to 30% of cases, large vessel atherosclerotic infarction varies from 14% to 40%, and small-vessel lacunar infarcts account for 15% to 30%. Stroke from other determined causes, such as arteritis or dissection, account for less than 5% of cases. In 30% to 40% of ischemic infarcts the cause cannot be determined. Intracranial hemorrhage may also be subdivided into subtypes, based on the site and vascular origin of the blood: subarachnoid, when the bleeding originates in the subarachnoid spaces surrounding the brain; and intracerebral, when the hemorrhage is into the brain parenchyma. Other forms of intracranial bleeding, such as subdural hemorrhage and epidural hemorrhage, are generally associated with trauma and not usually considered manifestations of stroke.

In the United States, there are 6.4 million stroke survivors (prevalence of 3%), and there are approximately 600,000 new (incident) and 200,000 recurrent strokes per year. Of these strokes, about 87% are ischemic infarctions, 10% primary hemorrhages, and 3% SAHs. Among adults age 65 to 74, stroke incidence is 670 to 970/100,000 per year. Stroke incidence rates are approximately twice as high for African Americans as for white individuals. In northern Manhattan, Caribbean Hispanic individuals had an incidence rate intermediate between that of white individuals and African Americans. Temporal trends in stroke incidence suggest that stroke incidence and mortality rates have declined since 1950; however, disparities in stroke incidence and mortality have persisted. Stroke rates in the young have also increased. From 1995 to 2012, stroke hospitalization rates for men age 18 to 44 years have doubled. Overall, due to the graying of the global population and the increased prevalence of stroke risk factors in younger people, the mean global lifetime risk of stroke has increased almost 9% over the past 25 years (through 2016) to 25%, meaning that 1 in 4 people will experience a stroke at some point during their lifetime.

Stroke incidence increases with age, but strokes do occur in young adults and children and may be missed if the diagnosis is not considered. Although stroke incidence rates are higher for men than women at most ages, among young adults the rates are similar or higher among women, probably related to pregnancy, hormonal contraception, and other hormone-related differences. At older ages, incidence rates among women are again greater, and because women tend to live longer than men, overall about 55,000 more women than men have a stroke each year.

MODIFIABLE RISK FACTORS

Well-established modifiable stroke risk factors include hypertension, cardiac disease (particularly atrial fibrillation), diabetes,

TABLE 118.1 Common Forms of Cerebrovascular Disease

Ischemic cerebrovascular disease
  Symptomatic
  - Ischemic stroke
    - Cerebral infarction
    - Spinal cord infarction
    - Retinal infarction
  - Transient ischemic attack
  - Transient monocular blindness *(amaurosis fugax)*
  Asymptomatic
  - Cerebral infarction/spinal cord infarction/retinal infarction
Hemorrhagic cerebrovascular disease
  - Intracerebral hemorrhage
  - Subarachnoid hemorrhage
  - Intraventricular hemorrhage
  - Subdural hemorrhage
  - Epidural hemorrhage
  - Cerebral microbleeds
Other forms of cerebrovascular disease
  - Cerebral vein thrombosis
  - Dural sinus thrombosis
Disorders of cerebral autoregulation
  - Posterior reversible encephalopathy syndrome
  - Hypertensive encephalopathy
  - Reversible cerebral vasoconstriction syndrome
Vascular abnormalities
  - Aneurysms
  - Arteriovenous malformations
  - Cavernous malformations
  - Fibromuscular dysplasia

TABLE 118.2 Stroke Risk Factors

Nonmodifiable risk factors	Age
	Sex
	Race/ethnicity
	Family history
	Genetic disorders
Well-established modifiable risk factors	Hypertension/blood pressure
	Diabetes mellitus/hyperglycemia
	Cardiac disorders
	Atrial fibrillation
	Valvular heart disease
	Recent myocardial infarction
	Cardiomyopathy/heart failure
	Bacterial endocarditis
	Hyperlipidemia
	Cigarette smoking
	Carotid stenosis
	Transient ischemic attack (TIA)
	Physical inactivity
	Hypercoagulable states (e.g., antiphospholipid antibody syndrome, cancer-associated hypercoagulopathy)
	Alcohol abuse
	Substance abuse (e.g., cocaine, intravenous drug abuse)
Other potential risk factors	Migraine
	Sleep apnea
	Cardiac disorders
	Paroxysmal supraventricular tachycardia
	Patent foramen ovale/atrial septal aneurysm
	Aortic atheroma
	Atrial cardiopathy
	Infections (e.g., varicella zoster virus, influenza)
	Inflammation
	Others

hyperlipidemia, cigarette use, physical inactivity, alcohol abuse, asymptomatic carotid stenosis, and a history of TIAs (Table 118.2).

Hypertension is the most powerful modifiable stroke risk factor and is associated with both ischemic and hemorrhagic strokes. Risk of stroke decreases with lower systolic and diastolic blood pressures, and this graded decrement in risk persists down to levels as low as 115/75 mm Hg. There is no clearly defined threshold level below which stroke risk levels off.

Cardiac disease is associated with an increased risk of ischemic stroke. Atrial fibrillation (AF) is the cardiac disease most often associated with stroke risk and accounts for up to 24% of cerebral infarction in the elderly. Other cardiac diseases, including valvular heart disease, myocardial infarction (MI), coronary artery disease (CAD), and congestive heart failure (CHF) are also associated with stroke risk. Recent evidence also suggests that other atrial arrhythmias, such as paroxysmal supraventricular tachycardia, may also increase risk of stroke, even in the absence of atrial fibrillation. Other possible sources of cardiac emboli include patent foramen ovale, aortic arch atherosclerotic disease, atrial septal aneurysms, and valvular strands.

Hyperlipidemia is a stroke risk factor, though its relationship to stroke is more complicated than for heart disease, primarily because of the many types of stroke. Lipid abnormalities, such as elevations in low-density lipoprotein (LDL) and decreased levels of high-density lipoprotein, are strongly associated with ischemic stroke of atherosclerotic origin. Somewhat paradoxically, however, low levels of LDL are associated with an increased risk of hemorrhagic stroke.

The role of alcohol as a stroke risk factor also depends on stroke subtype, as well as the quantity consumed. Alcohol consumption has been shown to be a risk factor for both ICH and SAH in a linear fashion, whereas a J-shaped relationship exists between alcohol and ischemic stroke, such that modest consumption (up to two drinks daily in men, and one daily in women) may be protective against stroke and heavy consumption (five or more drinks per day) increases risk.

Asymptomatic carotid artery disease, particularly with 70% or greater stenosis, is associated with increased stroke risk (approximately 2% per year). The risk of stroke also depends, however, on the rate of progression of the stenosis, collateral circulation, and the stability of the atherosclerotic plaque.

TIAs are a strong predictor of subsequent stroke. The first several days after a TIA have the greatest stroke risk, with clinical series demonstrating a 5% risk at 2 days and 10% risk at 90 days. Patients with transient monocular blindness *(amaurosis fugax)* have a better outcome than those with hemispheric ischemic attacks. The stroke risk after TIA depends on the underlying cause of the ischemia, including the presence and severity of underlying atherosclerotic disease or AF. Age, hypertension, the presence of diabetes, clinical syndromes including aphasia and hemiparesis, and duration of at least 10 minutes predict TIA patients at higher risk of stroke. Patients with TIA with evidence of infarction on MRI are also at higher risk. Other potential stroke risk factors include migraine, oral contraceptive use, drug abuse, sleep apnea, infection, and inflammation.

PATHOLOGY

Understanding the pathology of cerebrovascular disease requires an appreciation of the vascular anatomy of the brain, the vascular pathologies that can affect brain vessels, and the response of brain tissue to ischemia and hemorrhage.

Clinical Implications of Vascular Anatomy

The brain is perfused by four major vessels, the paired carotid and vertebral arteries. These originate extracranially as branches off the aorta and great vessels and course through the neck and base of the skull to reach the intracranial cavity (Fig. 118.1). The carotid and its branches constitute the anterior circulation and the vertebral arteries and its branches the posterior circulation. Anterior and posterior circulations communicate with one another through the posterior communicating arteries. The left and right sides of the anterior circulation communicate with each other through the anterior communicating artery. The major vessels at the base of the brain and these communicating vessels constitute the circle of Willis, the anastomotic network that allows for collateral blood flow when individual vessels are stenotic or occluded. Because variants in the circle of Willis are common, collateral flow may not be sufficient in many cases of blockage, and the risk of ischemic stroke therefore depends on a patient's individual anatomy.

The right common carotid artery usually begins as a branch from the innominate artery, whereas the left common carotid artery originates directly from the aortic arch. The common carotid arteries bifurcate into the internal and external carotid arteries, usually at the level of the fourth cervical vertebra. The internal carotid arteries have no branches in the neck and face and enter the cranium through the carotid canal. There are four main segments of each internal carotid artery: cervical, petrous, cavernous, and supraclinoid. The siphon is the term used to describe the hairpin turn made by the cavernous and supraclinoid segments, and it is at this level that the ophthalmic artery originates, providing the first major branch of the internal carotid artery and supplying blood flow to the optic nerve and retina. Thus, internal carotid artery disease commonly causes ocular ischemia, leading to a transient ischemic attack (*amaurosis fugax*) or infarction of the optic nerve or retina, a warning sign of impending cerebral stroke. The internal carotid arteries then give off the superior hypophyseal, posterior communicating, and anterior choroidal arteries, before terminating intracranially by dividing into the middle and anterior cerebral arteries. In addition to the eye, the paired carotid systems supply approximately 80% of the hemispheric blood flow, including the frontal, parietal, and anterior temporal lobes. In up to 15% of individuals, the posterior cerebral artery (PCA) also arises directly from the internal carotid artery (the so-called fetal origin PCA), so that the entire hemisphere including the occipital lobe is supplied by the internal carotid artery. The anterior choroidal artery supplies a number of structures in addition to the choroid plexus, including the inferior portion of the posterior limb of the internal capsule, the hippocampus, and portions of the globus pallidus, posterior putamen, lateral geniculate, amygdala, and ventrolateral thalamus.

The middle cerebral artery (MCA) is the largest branch of the internal carotid artery. Its first portion, or stem, is often referred to as the M1 segment, and this usually bifurcates into superior and inferior divisions or, less often, trifurcates into three major divisions (upper, middle, and lower). The MCA stem gives rise to the medial and lateral

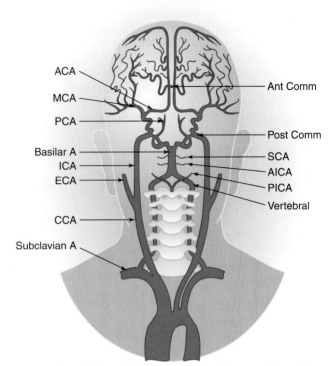

Fig. 118.1 Coronal view of the extracranial and intracranial arterial supply to the brain. Vessels forming the circle of Willis are highlighted. *A,* Artery; *ACA,* anterior cerebral artery; *AICA,* anterior inferior cerebellar artery; *Ant Comm,* anterior communicating artery; *CCA,* common carotid artery; *ECA,* external carotid artery; *ICA,* internal carotid artery; *MCA,* middle cerebral artery; *PCA,* posterior cerebral artery; *PICA,* posterior inferior cerebellar artery; *Post Comm,* posterior communicating artery; *SCA,* superior cerebellar artery. (Modified from Lord R: Surgery of occlusive cerebrovascular disease, St. Louis, 1986, Mosby.)

lenticulostriates, which supply the extreme capsule, claustrum, putamen, most of the globus pallidus, part of the head and the entire body of the caudate, as well as the superior portions of the anterior and posterior limbs of the internal capsule. The divisions of the MCA supply almost the entire lateral cortical surface of the brain, including the insula, operculum, and frontal, parietal, temporal, and occipital cortices.

The anterior cerebral artery (ACA) also has a proximal, or A1, segment, which ends at the junction with the anterior communicating artery. The ipsilateral ACA then continues as the distal, or A2, segment. An important branch is the recurrent artery of Heubner, which supplies the head of the caudate nucleus, and several cortical branches supply the medial and orbital surfaces of the frontal lobe.

The vertebral arteries generally originate from the subclavian arteries, course through the transverse foramina of the cervical vertebrae, pierce the dura, and enter the cranial cavity through the foramen magnum. The two vertebral arteries join to form the basilar artery at the level of the pontomedullary junction. Anterior and posterior spinal arteries and the posterior inferior cerebellar artery (PICA), which supplies the inferior surface of the cerebellum, arise from the distal segments of the vertebrals. The lateral medulla is supplied by the multiple, perforating branches of PICA or the direct penetrating branches of the vertebral artery. Occlusion of the distal vertebral artery may, therefore, cause infarction of the lateral medulla (Wallenberg syndrome), characterized by vertigo, imbalance, Horner syndrome, dysphagia, and sensory loss.

After originating as the union of the right and left vertebral arteries, the basilar artery travels up the ventral pons. Paramedian and circumferential penetrating arteries exit the basilar to dive into the pontine parenchyma. Proximally, the basilar gives off the paired anterior inferior cerebellar arteries (AICAs), and more distally the superior cerebellar arteries (SCAs); these perfuse the ventrolateral aspect of the cerebellar cortex. An internal auditory (labyrinthine) artery arises either directly from the basilar or from the AICA to supply the cochlea, labyrinth, and part of the facial nerve. Ischemia in the basilar territory may, therefore, cause hearing loss and vertigo, sometimes as an isolated symptom.

The basilar artery terminates in the right and left posterior cerebral arteries (PCAs). A series of penetrators arise from the posterior communicating and posterior cerebral arteries to supply the hypothalamus, dorsolateral midbrain, lateral geniculate, and thalamus. The posterior cerebral artery supplies the inferior temporal lobe and the medial and inferior surfaces of the occipital lobe. In some patients a single large penetrating vessel at the midline of the terminal basilar artery may supply medial aspects of both thalami (the artery of Percheron); emboli occluding this vessel may, therefore, cause bilateral thalamic infarcts, with a decrease in alertness and vertical gaze abnormalities, without significant motor deficit.

The brain's anastomotic network includes not only the connections through the circle of Willis, but also intercommunicating systems extracranially and more distal connections intracranially through meningeal anastomoses that cover the cortical and cerebellar surfaces (pial-pial collaterals). These networks all protect the brain from ischemia by providing alternative routes to circumvent obstructions in the main arteries.

Venous anatomy is more variable than arterial. Superficial veins drain into the transverse, superior sagittal, and cavernous sinuses. The deep venous drainage is via the great vein of Galen, which drains into the straight sinus, and in turn drains into the torcula along with the sagittal sinus. Blood drains from the torcula to the transverse sinus, then to the sigmoid sinus, and thereafter the jugular vein. Anterior venous drainage is via the cavernous sinus, which communicates with the contralateral cavernous sinus, the transverse sinus via the superior petrosal sinus, and the inferior petrosal sinus, which drains directly into the jugular bulb.

Vascular Pathogenesis

There are multiple mechanisms leading to brain ischemia. Hemodynamic infarction occurs as a result of reduced perfusion, usually in the setting of arterial stenosis due to atherosclerosis. In some cases, stenosis may be due to arterial dissection, vasculitis, fibromuscular dysplasia, or other arteriopathies. Embolism occurs when a thrombus originating from a more proximal source (e.g., arterial or cardiac) travels through the arteries and occludes a cerebral artery. Paradoxical embolism occurs when a thrombus crosses from the venous circulation to the left side of the heart through a patent foramen ovale or, less commonly, an intrapulmonary arteriovenous shunt. Other particles that may embolize include neoplasms, fat, air, or other foreign substances. Air emboli can follow injuries or procedures involving the lungs, the dural sinuses, or jugular veins. Fat embolism usually results from a bone fracture. Septic emboli arise from bacterial endocarditis.

Intracranial hemorrhage results from the rupture of a vessel anywhere within the cranial cavity. Intracranial hemorrhages may be classified by location (e.g., extradural, subdural, subarachnoid, intracerebral, intraventricular), by the type of ruptured vessel (e.g., arterial, capillary, venous), or by cause (e.g., primary, secondary). Trauma is often involved in the generation of extradural hematoma from laceration of the middle meningeal artery or vein, and subdural hematomas from traumatic rupture of veins that traverse the subdural space.

Intracerebral, or intraparenchymal, hemorrhage is characterized by bleeding into the substance of the brain, usually originating from a small penetrating artery. Hypertension has been implicated as the cause of weakening in the walls of arterioles and the formation of microaneurysms (i.e., Charcot-Bouchard aneurysms). The most common sites for hypertensive arterial hemorrhage are the putamen, pons, cerebellum, and thalamus. Blood under arterial pressures destroys or displaces brain tissue. Amyloid angiopathy, due to the vascular deposition of β-amyloid protein similar to that seen in Alzheimer disease has been implicated as an important cause of lobar hemorrhage in elderly patients. Other causes of intracerebral hemorrhage include arteriovenous malformations, infectious aneurysms, cavernous angiomas, moyamoya disease, bleeding disorders, anticoagulation, illicit drug abuse, trauma, and tumors.

Subarachnoid hemorrhage occurs when blood is localized to the surrounding membranes and cerebrospinal fluid. It is most frequently caused by leakage of blood from a cerebral aneurysm. The combination of congenital and acquired factors leads to a degeneration of the arterial wall and the release of blood, under arterial pressures, into the subarachnoid space and cerebrospinal fluid. Aneurysms may be distributed at different sites throughout the base of the brain, particularly at the origin or bifurcations of arteries of the circle of Willis. Other secondary causes that may lead to SAH include trauma, arteriovenous malformations, bleeding disorders or anticoagulation, amyloid angiopathy, or cerebral sinus thrombosis.

The most common intrinsic disorder of the cerebral blood vessels is atherosclerosis, which shares similarities in pathology with atherosclerosis throughout the body. Arteriosclerotic plaques may develop at any point along the carotid artery and the vertebrobasilar system, but the most common sites are the bifurcation of the common carotid artery, the origins of the MCAs and ACAs, and the origins of the vertebral from the subclavian arteries (Fig. 118.2). In the past it was thought that intracranial atherosclerotic disease required significant stenosis (>50%) to cause symptoms. However, recent pathologic and radiologic studies provide evidence that substenotic lesions can also cause strokes due to plaque rupture and acute thrombosis, as is the case elsewhere in the body.

Small-vessel disease refers to the occlusion of a penetrant branch of a larger artery, usually due to microatheroma or to lipohyalinosis, a degenerative disorder of the vessel characterized by deposition of fatty and proteinaceous material. Hematologic disorders and coagulopathies, including leukemia, Waldenström's macroglobulinemia, polycythemia, primary and secondary antiphospholipid antibody syndrome, and genetic defects of the coagulation cascade, may also lead to occlusive thrombi and emboli.

The cerebral circulation differs from the systemic circulation in some important ways. The brain is protected by the anastomoses described previously. In addition, cerebral autoregulation maintains a constant cerebral perfusion pressure over a range of systemic blood pressures (Fig. 118.3). Cerebral arterioles have a well-developed muscular coat that allows constriction in response to increased blood pressure and dilation with hypotension. The arterioles are also exquisitely sensitive to changes in peripheral arterial concentrations of carbon dioxide ($Paco_2$) and oxygen (Pao_2). When the partial pressure of CO_2 decreases, such as during hyperventilation, the arterioles constrict and blood flow is reduced. In healthy individuals, cerebral autoregulation maintains a constant cerebral blood flow over mean arterial pressures of 60 to 140 mm Hg. In patients with chronic hypertension, the autoregulatory curve is shifted to the right, so that even minor reductions in blood pressure may not be tolerated. At blood pressures above these limits, moreover, as in severe hypertension, autoregulatory capacity may be overwhelmed, leading to breakthrough edema and hemorrhage.

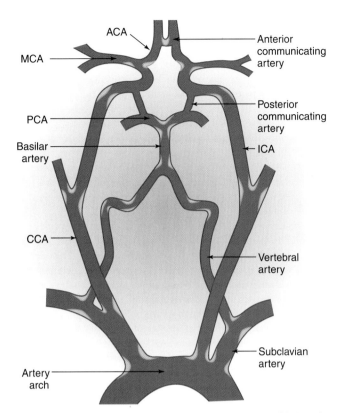

Fig. 118.2 Sites of predilection for atheromatous plaque. *ACA,* Anterior cerebral artery; *CCA,* common carotid artery; *ICA,* internal carotid artery; *MCA,* middle cerebral artery; *PCA,* posterior cerebral artery. (From Caplan LR: Stroke: a clinical approach, ed 2, Boston, 1993, Butterworth-Heinemann.)

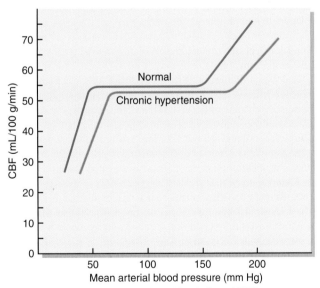

Fig. 118.3 Autoregulatory cerebral blood flow (CBF) response to changes in mean arterial pressure in normotensive and chronically hypertensive persons. Note the shift of the curve toward higher mean pressures with chronic hypertension. (From Pulsinelli WA: Cerebrovascular diseases-principles. In Goldman L, Bennett JC, editors: Cecil textbook of medicine, ed 21, Philadelphia, 2000, Saunders, p 2097.)

In the setting of infarction or hemorrhage, cerebral autoregulation is also impaired, resulting in cerebral dependence on systemic blood pressure to maintain adequate perfusion. Thus, decreasing the blood pressure in the setting of acute ischemia may be hazardous.

Specific disorders may originate from autoregulatory dysfunction: posterior reversible encephalopathy syndrome (PRES) and the reversible cerebral vasoconstriction syndrome (RCVS). In posterior reversible encephalopathy syndrome, there is loss of autoregulatory control with leakage of fluid across the blood-brain barrier, primarily in the posterior regions of the brain. Patients present with elevated blood pressures, headaches, seizures, and loss of visual function. Reversible cerebral vasoconstriction syndrome, a recently recognized syndrome, remains incompletely characterized, and shares features with posterior reversible encephalopathy syndrome. The two disorders overlap in 10% or more of cases. Patients with RCVS are typically young women who present with acute, severe headache, have minimal or no neurologic deficits, and may have evidence of non-aneurysmal, superficial SAH as well as vasospasm of the cerebral arteries. Sympathetic innervation of the vessels is also less in the posterior circulation than anteriorly, leading to a reduced ability of the posterior circulation to adapt to changes in blood pressure, and may contribute to the propensity for edema to form in the occipital lobes during hypertensive crises.

In addition, focal cerebral activity, such as occurs when activating brain regions responsible for moving a limb, is accompanied by increased metabolic activity in the appropriate region, and is accommodated by slight increases in local blood flow and oxygen delivery. Exploitation of this increased local energy demand and delivery is what allows imaging of functional brain activity using MRI, which can detect subtle changes in regional cerebral blood flow. These changes in blood flow are mediated by the neurovascular unit, a complex structure characterized by the local interaction of neural, glial, and vascular elements in the brain. Intracerebral capillaries also lack adventitia, with astrocytes serving as the vascular component of the neurovascular unit. Tight junctions at the capillary level play an important role in the blood-brain barrier, which limits permeability between the vascular compartment and the brain tissue.

Injury to Brain Tissue

The adult brain weighs about 1500 g, or 2% of total body weight, but accounts for 20% of the total body oxygen consumption. Because the brain cannot store much energy, dysfunction results after only a few minutes of deprivation when either oxygen or glucose content is reduced below critical levels. In the resting state, normal total cerebral blood flow is 50 mL/min per 100 g of brain tissue.

Neuronal dysfunction occurs at cerebral blood flow levels below 50 mg/dL, and irreversible neuronal injury begins at levels below 30 mg/dL. Both the degree and duration of reductions in cerebral blood flow are related to the likelihood of permanent neuronal injury. When blood supply is completely interrupted for 30 seconds, brain metabolism is altered; after 1 minute, neuronal function may cease. After 5 minutes, anoxia initiates a chain of events that may result in cerebral infarction; however, if oxygenated blood flow is restored quickly enough, the damage may be reversible, as with a TIA.

Research into the cellular basis of cerebral ischemia has led to the concept of the "ischemic cascade." As perfusion of the brain decreases, a chain of events at the neuronal level begins with failure of the membrane sodium/potassium (Na/K) pump, the depolarization of the neuronal membrane, the release of excitatory neurotransmitters such as glutamate and glycine that hyperstimulate their receptors, and the opening of calcium channels. Calcium enters the neuron through various voltage-sensitive and receptor-mediated channels (e.g., the *N*-methyl-D-aspartate receptor). The influx of calcium is at the root of further neuronal injury, leading to damage to organelles and further destabilization of neuronal metabolism and function. These events may lead to neuronal death, which may be delayed, even after restoration of blood flow, and are a target of experimental neuroprotective strategies.

Recent research has distinguished between the "core" infarct and an "ischemic penumbra," or shadow. The core represents a central region of necrosis, or tissue that dies very quickly after blood flow ceases. The penumbra represents the surrounding region of brain tissue, in which neurons are dysfunctional but potentially salvageable. Recanalization of occluded vessels with blood flow into infarcted tissue, particularly when delayed, results in "reperfusion injury." Increased use of MRI has shown that petechial hemorrhagic infarction is very common, occurring in the majority of strokes, even when not suspected clinically.

CLINICAL PRESENTATION

The signs and symptoms of strokes are varied and depend on the type of stroke, the region of the nervous system affected by the lack of flow or hemorrhage, and the patient's handedness (Table 118.3). In general, embolic ischemic strokes are characterized by the sudden onset of a neurologic deficit, usually painless. Thrombotic strokes may have a stuttering or progressive course due to fluctuating hypoperfusion and gradual occlusion. Arterial dissections, as well as hemorrhages, are more often associated with headaches than ischemic stroke of other causes. Hemorrhagic strokes and large hemispheric infarcts can lead to decrease in consciousness due to increased intracranial pressure.

Most emboli occur in the territory of the MCAs. Lesions of the dominant (almost always left) hemisphere are characterized by variable combinations of right hemiparesis, right hemisensory loss, right visual loss, impaired gaze to the right side of space, and language disturbance. When the superior division of the MCA is affected, the language impairment is predominantly motor: the patient either cannot speak or produces sparse, agrammatic speech, despite an ability to fully comprehend spoken and written material. When the inferior division is affected, the patient may produce fluent, prosodic (normal stress and intonation), but nonsensical speech and be unable to follow instructions. Larger infarcts of the dominant hemisphere produce a total loss of language function, leaving the patient mute and uncomprehending.

Lesions of the nondominant (right) hemisphere produce deficits of the left side of the body. Language is preserved but the patient may demonstrate impaired attention, particularly to the left side of space; fail to appreciate the presence of people or objects to their left; and may even fail to recognize the left side of their own body (asomatognosia). This neglect phenomenon may extend even to a lack of awareness of any deficit of function on their part (anosognosia). These patients may thus be found at home, lying on the floor paralyzed yet unaware that anything is the matter; their unawareness can delay their presentation to the hospital for treatment and similarly limit their participation in rehabilitation. Lesions in the right hemisphere may also cause dysprosody, the nondominant equivalent of aphasia, which is characterized by a lack of the emotional and gestural components of speech, despite preservation of its semantic content; many of these patients have a flat affect or appear to be depressed.

Infarcts in the territory of the anterior cerebral arteries often cause weakness limited to the legs, due to location of the representation of the legs in the medial part of the hemispheres. They may have incontinence, lack initiative (abulia), and have gaze palsies. In some cases their deficits may be more extensive and mimic those of MCA infarctions. Posterior cerebral artery infarcts lead to visual loss, often without any motor deficit. With involvement of the medial temporal lobes supplied by the PCAs, there may also be behavioral disturbances, including delirium and amnesia.

Brain stem infarcts cause specific syndromes due to the affected neural pathways and nuclei. Midbrain infarcts often produce vertical gaze deficits and impaired consciousness if the reticular activating system is involved.

TABLE 118.3 Clinical Manifestations of Ischemic Stroke

Occluded Vessel	Clinical Signs
ICA	Ipsilateral blindness (variable), MCA syndrome
MCA	Contralateral hemiparesis, hemisensory loss (face or arm more than leg)
	Aphasia (dominant) or anosognosia (nondominant)
	Homonymous hemianopsia (variable)
ACA	Contralateral hemiparesis, hemisensory loss (leg more than arm)
	Abulia (especially if bilateral)
VA or PICA	Ipsilateral facial sensory loss, hemiataxia, nystagmus, Horner syndrome
	Contralateral loss of temperature or pain sensation
	Dysphagia
SCA	Gait ataxia, nausea, vertigo, dysarthria
BA	Quadriparesis, dysarthria, dysphagia, diplopia, somnolence, amnesia
PCA	Contralateral homonymous hemianopsia, amnesia, sensory loss

ACA, Anterior cerebral artery; *BA,* basilar artery; *ICA,* internal carotid artery; *MCA,* middle cerebral artery; *PCA,* posterior cerebral artery; *PICA,* posterior inferior cerebellar artery; *SCA,* superior cerebellar artery; *VA,* vertebral artery.

Many cerebral infarctions do not cause weakness and may therefore be missed by the less astute clinician who assumes that a stroke always leads to paralysis. These syndromes include fluent (or Wernicke) aphasia, cortical visual loss, and Wallenberg syndrome (lateral medullary syndrome caused by occlusion of the vertebral or posterior inferior cerebellar artery). Because the inferior division of the MCA supplies the lateral temporal lobe and parietal lobes, including the Wernicke area, occlusion of that vessel may cause a prosodic, fluent speech with multiple paraphasic errors and poor comprehension, while sparing the motor strip in the frontal lobe. Emboli traveling up the basilar artery may lead to significant infarction in the territory of both PCAs, causing complete blindness, sometimes without awareness of the deficit on the part of the patient, due to infarction of both occipital lobes (the "top of the basilar syndrome"). Behavioral abnormalities, memory loss, and eye movement abnormalities may also occur, due to involvement of the medial temporal lobe structures and the midbrain eye movement centers. Small emboli to branches of the superior division of the MCA may cause focal weakness of the hand, particularly fine finger movements, simulating a peripheral compression neuropathy.

In patients presenting with dizziness, it is particularly difficult to distinguish stroke from vestibular neuronitis or Meniere's disease (see Chapter 115). The presence of a normal head-thrust test, skew deviation, or direction-changing nystagmus are all signs of stroke, rather than a peripheral cause. Patients in the emergency ward should not be discharged until they can walk without imbalance; patients with nausea and vomiting due to cerebellar infarction may develop fatal brain stem compression due to swelling (so-called "fatal gastroenteritis").

The signs and symptoms of *subarachnoid hemorrhage* differ from other stroke types due to the absence of focal deficits. Instead, patients present with abrupt onset of severe headache (i.e., "the worst headache of my life"), vomiting, altered consciousness, and sometimes coma, typically without localizing signs.

Thrombosis of cerebral veins or the larger draining dural sinuses present with a combination of headache due to elevated intracranial pressure, seizures, and focal deficits due to hemorrhage. Rarely the

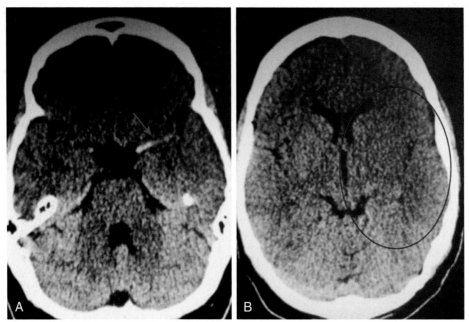

Fig. 118.4 Early signs of infarction on computed tomography of the brain. (A) Hyperdense middle cerebral artery sign *(red arrow)*, and (B) hypoattenuation of the left caudate and lentiform nuclei, loss of the insular ribbon, and sulcal effacement *(outlined in red)*.

syndrome of *thunderclap headache*, or sudden severe headache without any focal signs similar to that occurring in SAH, may be due to venous thrombosis. Occlusion of the cerebral venous sinuses may occur in association with hyperviscosity or a hypercoagulable state, including pregnancy or hormonal contraceptive use. Imaging findings include bilateral hemorrhagic infarctions in a parasagittal distribution and extensive white matter edema. Contrast-enhanced CT may demonstrate the *empty delta* sign, indicating a filling defect in the sagittal sinus. Magnetic resonance venography (MRV) and T1-weighted MRI images confirm the presence of thrombus; cerebral angiography is seldom needed to confirm the diagnosis.

DIAGNOSIS AND DIFFERENTIAL DIAGNOSIS

The potential benefit of thrombolytic therapy within 4.5 hours of onset of acute ischemic stroke requires urgent differentiation of ischemic stroke from hemorrhage and other causes of sudden neurologic symptoms. Headache, vomiting, seizures, and coma are more common in hemorrhagic stroke, though these are never reliable enough to preclude imaging. The distinction is straightforward in most cases once a head CT is performed. The hyperdense signal of blood in the parenchyma on CT almost invariably distinguishes hemorrhage from ischemia. In exceptional cases the typical hyperdensity of ICH is absent owing to severe anemia or to its subacute state, during which blood may be indistinguishable from brain tissue. Certain imaging findings on initial CT further support a presumed diagnosis of infarction, such as a hyperdense vessel sign indicative of thrombus in the vessel, or loss of the gray-white junction and sulci in the cortex, and loss of the demarcation of the insular cortex and deep gray nuclei, both of which are early indicators of ischemia and edema (Fig. 118.4). CT angiography often identifies the site of vascular occlusion.

Imaging in the setting of suspected acute ischemia does not definitively diagnose ischemia but rather excludes hemorrhage; if clinical symptoms are consistent with cerebral ischemia, then thrombolytic treatment is indicated within the appropriate time window. Primary stroke centers must perform and interpret CT scans within 30 minutes of the arrival of a patient with suspected stroke. MRI can also effectively

exclude acute hemorrhage, and diffusion-weighted imaging sequences are more sensitive to the earliest changes of ischemia (Fig. 118.5), but the speed and availability of CT make it the initial imaging modality of choice at most centers. MRI scanning may then be used to provide additional information. Specific MRI sequences have greater sensitivity to blood than CT and may identify hemorrhagic infarction missed by CT.

Clinical features at stroke onset may suggest a subtype of cerebral infarction but require confirmatory laboratory data. Cerebral embolism is suggested by sudden onset and a syndrome of circumscribed focal signs attributable to cerebral surface infarction, such as pure aphasia or pure hemianopia. Unless the source of embolization is obvious on hospital admission, blood cultures, electrocardiographic monitoring, and echocardiography are indicated.

A diagnosis of atherosclerotic infarction is suggested if there were previous TIAs, particularly when the symptoms are stereotypical. Doppler ultrasonography, CT angiography or magnetic resonance angiography can usually identify the stenosis. In equivocal cases, conventional angiography may be needed. Small penetrating vessel infarcts, or *lacunar infarcts*, usually spare cortical functions, such as language and cognition, but cause loss of elementary neurologic function, such as strength, sensation, and coordination. Up to 25% of patients with lacunar infarcts have large-vessel disease or a cardioembolic source, so it is important to carry out a complete etiologic evaluation in all stroke patients.

Up to 50% of patients with transient deficits lasting less than 24 hours have evidence of infarction on imaging, and the risk of stroke and other vascular events is as high after TIA as after completed stroke. In the acute setting, when decisions about thrombolysis must be made, it is virtually impossible to know which patients with ischemia will have symptoms resolve without infarction (thus, having a TIA) and which will have a completed infarction. Patients with either stroke or TIA need immediate attention to secondary prevention strategies. In terms of choosing treatments, the important issue is to identify the cause of the cerebral ischemia, rather than its duration. Entities other than cerebral ischemia can masquerade as strokes and TIAs. Among patients diagnosed with stroke in emergency departments, 20% or

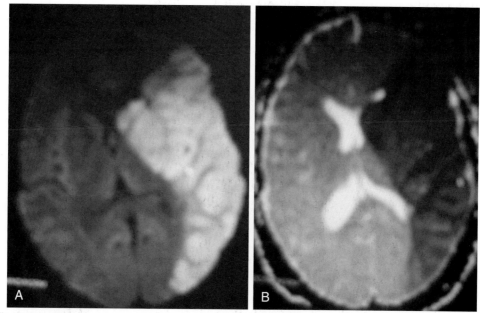

Fig. 118.5 Magnetic resonance imaging scan of the brain of the same patient shown in Fig. 118.4. (A) Diffusion-weighted image shows bright signal in the left middle cerebral artery territory. (B) Apparent diffusion coefficient shows dark signal in the same area, confirming acute infarction.

more have a stroke *mimic*, including seizure, migraine, systemic infection, brain tumor, and toxic-metabolic encephalopathy. Other sources of misdiagnosis are listed in Table 118.4.

In patients with a prior history of cerebral infarct or hemorrhage, new *metabolic derangements*, including infections, may precipitate a recrudescence of the original stroke syndrome. Hypoglycemia, hyponatremia, urinary tract infection, pneumonia, and initiation of a psychotropic medication can each precipitate this phenomenon. The patient returns to normal over hours to days when the new insult is treated or reversed. Such metabolic and infectious causes of neurologic deterioration should be excluded in patients with a history of earlier brain injury before diagnosing a new stroke. Focal signs may also occur with metabolic disturbances in patients without prior history of stroke.

External signs of injury are usually present in brain *trauma*, but they need not be present after acceleration-deceleration injury, such as from a motor vehicle accident. The most frequent sites of brain contusions are the frontal and temporal poles, which are not typical locations for strokes.

Seizures may occasionally complicate acute stroke, but they may also mimic stroke. Unlike stroke, seizures are often characterized by obtundation, an amnestic state, clonic activity, incontinence, or tongue biting. The postictal deficit, often called a *Todd paralysis*, resembles stroke because weakness or language and other cortical deficits may occur. The deficits after seizure usually resolve within hours after the seizure but occasionally persist for up to a week, making the distinction from stroke difficult. Seizures may also develop months or years after an infarct or hemorrhage, and the postictal state in these patients may recapitulate the initial stroke syndrome.

Migraine with persistent aura often mimics stroke or TIA. Aura alone, without headache (i.e., acephalgic migraine), is sometimes experienced by those who previously suffered from migraine with aura. Migraine aura typically produces a visual disturbance that marches across the vision of both eyes as an advancing, enlarging blind spot that takes 20 to 30 minutes to resolve. Subsequent unilateral, pounding headache suggests the diagnosis but may not occur. Less often, migrainous auras take the form of sensory symptoms. The speed of the march is generally slower than the rapid spread of symptoms in stroke.

As many as 10% of *brain tumors* present with acute transient symptoms reflecting intratumoral hemorrhage or focal seizures. Seizures

TABLE 118.4 Stroke Mimics and Differential Diagnosis

Common Mimics
Metabolic encephalopathy (e.g., hypoglycemia, hyponatremia)
Systemic infection
Seizure
Migraine
Brain tumors

Other Mimics
Transient focal neurologic symptoms associated with amyloid angiopathy
Positional vertigo
Cardiac events
Syncope
Trauma (especially acceleration-deceleration without evidence of external injury)
Subdural hematoma
Herpes simplex virus encephalitis
Transient global amnesia
Dementia
Demyelinating disease
Cervical spine disease/radiculopathy/fracture
Myasthenia gravis
Parkinsonism
Hypertensive encephalopathy
Conversion disorder
Intoxication/substance abuse

often precede focal signs. Imaging usually demonstrates an enhancing mass even when symptoms are mild.

TREATMENT

Stroke prevention and treatment are directed toward: (1) preventing the first stroke (primary prevention); (2) limiting damage from the stroke; (3) optimizing functional recovery following stroke; and (4) avoiding recurrence (secondary prevention). Specific measures for treatment and prevention depend on the patient's risk factors and stroke mechanism. The diagnostic evaluation of the stroke patient dictates optimal therapy.

Primary Prevention of Stroke

Randomized trials have demonstrated that specific interventions prevent first stroke among patients with specific risk factors (Table 118.5). Treatment of hypertension, for example, is associated with up to a 45% reduction in the risk of stroke. Among patients with atrial fibrillation, the use of warfarin is associated with a 60% to 70% relative reduction in risk of stroke, though younger patients without any accompanying heart disease, hypertension, or diabetes may be managed with antiplatelet agents alone. Hydroxymethylglutaryl-coenzyme A (HMG-CoA) reductase inhibitors, or statins, have been shown in some primary prevention studies, and in studies of patients with heart disease, to reduce the risk of a first stroke as well as that of heart disease. The effects on stroke risk are more modest than the effects on heart disease, possibly reflecting the greater heterogeneity among causes of stroke compared to heart disease. For patients with asymptomatic carotid stenosis of at least 60%, carotid endarterectomy reduces the risk of stroke, though the effect is much more modest than in symptomatic patients, and the number of patients needed to treat to prevent one stroke is greater. Because many of the large randomized trials of endarterectomy for asymptomatic patients were conducted in the era before the current recommended use of statins and antiplatelet agents, it is no longer clear that surgery is superior to medical therapy. New trials are therefore addressing medical versus surgical and endovascular treatment in patients with asymptomatic stenosis.

Antiplatelet therapy is not of established benefit for prevention of a first stroke. In a large primary prevention study, for example, aspirin use was associated with an increased risk of both ischemic and hemorrhagic stroke, despite reducing the risk of ischemic heart disease. However, other studies have shown that aspirin reduces the risk of ischemic stroke among women over the age of 45.

The Mediterranean diet also protects against cardiovascular disease, including stroke. It is characterized by high intake of fruits, vegetables, and legumes; olive oil as the principal source of fat; moderate consumption of fish and poultry, with minimal intake of red meat and dairy; and an option of mild to moderate consumption of red wine, mostly with meals. Compared to a low-fat diet, this combination of nutrients decreased 5-year stroke risk by approximately 30% in a randomized trial.

Observational studies provide evidence that certain behaviors prevent stroke. Smoking cessation leads to a reduction by 5 years in stroke risk to levels similar to nonsmokers. Consumption of alcohol in moderation, up to two drinks daily for men and one daily for women, is associated with a lower level of stroke risk than in those who do not drink. Physical activity, weight loss when appropriate, and management of diabetes are also recommended.

Acute Treatment of Ischemic Stroke

For patients with ischemic stroke evaluated within 3 hours of symptom onset with no evidence of hemorrhage on a brain CT or MRI, recombinant tissue plasminogen activator (rt-PA), a thrombolytic agent, improves functional outcomes at 3 months compared to placebo. Among the 624 ischemic stroke patients treated within 3 hours in the original landmark study, the proportion of patients achieving normal or near-normal neurologic and functional status by 3 months was significantly higher among those receiving rt-PA, though there was no definite benefit at 24 hours. The proportion of patients who achieved independence in their performance of activities of daily living was

TABLE 118.5 Evidence-Based Primary Prevention of Ischemic Stroke

Risk Factor	Treatment
Hypertension	Anti-hypertensives
Myocardial infarction	HMG-CoA reductase inhibitors
Hyperlipidemia	HMG-CoA reductase inhibitors
Atrial fibrillation	Anticoagulation (warfarin, other agents)
	Left atrial exclusion (selected patients)
Diabetes mellitus/vascular disease	ACE inhibitor
Diabetes mellitus type II, obesity	Metformin
	Bariatric surgery
Asymptomatic carotid stenosis (60-99%)	Carotid endarterectomy
Diet	Mediterranean diet
High vascular risk populations	Antiplatelet therapy
	HMG-CoA reductase inhibitors

HMG-CoA, Hydroxymethylglutaryl-coenzyme A.

increased from 38% to 50%, an absolute benefit of 12%. The absence of an immediate (24-hour) benefit, coupled with the finding of a benefit at 3 months, is consistent with the hypothesis that thrombolytic treatment works to reduce the size of the infarct penumbra by reperfusing tissue before permanent infarction of the entire territory occurs, despite some irreversible injury to a core component.

Patients treated with rt-PA had a 10-fold increase in incidence of hemorrhagic conversion of the infarction (from 0.6% in placebo-treated patients to 6.0% in rt-PA–treated patients). Overall, however, the rates of neurologic deterioration and mortality within the first day after stroke were similar between the groups. Rt-PA was approved for patient use by the US Food and Drug Administration (FDA) in 1996, and it is now considered standard of care for ischemic stroke patients presenting within 3 hours. Specific guidelines for eligibility and exclusion must be met when using rt-PA to reduce the risk of complications (Table 118.6).

Because of the potential to reduce cerebral perfusion below the limits permitted by autoregulation in the setting of acute brain injury, current guidelines recommend that blood pressure not be reduced acutely after ischemic stroke, and systolic blood pressure levels as high as 220 mm Hg are allowed. Before and following thrombolytic treatment, however, systolic blood pressure should be kept below 180 mm Hg to reduce the risk of hemorrhagic conversion. In addition, antiplatelet and anticoagulant medications must be withheld for 24 hours after rt-PA.

Subsequent meta-analyses and individual trials have demonstrated that the benefit of thrombolytic therapy decreases as the time interval between symptom onset (the presumed beginning of ischemia) and treatment increases, but that the therapeutic time window persists as long as 4.5 hours after stroke in selected patients (i.e., those under age 80 years without a combined history of prior ischemic stroke and diabetes mellitus).

In considering the duration of stroke symptoms, neurologists use the time that the patient was last known to be well as the time of onset of the stroke, rather than the time that the patient was discovered to have stroke symptoms. Because stroke is usually painless, patients may not be aware of the onset of symptoms. In patients with aphasia, anosognosia, or diminished consciousness, the patient may not be able to provide details regarding the time of onset of their symptoms, and a witness is required. In patients who wake with stroke,

TABLE 118.6 Eligibility and Exclusion Criteria for Treatment of Acute Ischemic Stroke With Intravenous Rt-PA

Eligibility

Age ≥18 years

Diagnosis of ischemic stroke causing measurable neurologic deficit

Well-documented onset of symptoms <4.5 hours before beginning treatment

Major Exclusion Criteria

Stroke or head trauma within the preceding 3 months

Major surgery within the preceding 2 weeks

History of intracerebral hemorrhage

Systolic blood pressure >185 mm Hg

Diastolic blood pressure >110 mm Hg

Rapidly improving or minor neurologic symptoms and signs

Symptoms suggestive of subarachnoid hemorrhage

Gastrointestinal or urinary tract bleeding within 3 weeks

Arterial puncture at a noncompressible site within 1 week

Platelet count <100,000/mm^3

INR >1.7

Relative Exclusion Criteria (Must Weigh Risks and Benefits)

Seizure at stroke onset

Myocardial infarction within 6 weeks

Infective endocarditis

Hemorrhagic eye disorder

Blood glucose <30 mg/dL (2.7 mmol/L)

Blood glucose >400 mg/dL (21.6 mmol/L)

Patients requiring very aggressive therapy for blood pressure reduction

---

moreover, it is difficult if not impossible to determine the time at which the symptoms started, and so the time that the patient went to bed is usually considered the starting point of the time window to decide eligibility for thrombolytic therapy. Recent clinical trials, however, provide evidence that when advanced imaging techniques are used, patients can be selected for treatment with intravenous rt-PA up to 9 hours after last known well. In one study, when the MR DWI showed changes consistent with ischemia but the fluid attenuated inversion recovery (FLAIR) sequences did not, the duration of ischemia was presumed to be less than 4.5 hours, and patients were considered eligible for randomization to rt-PA or placebo; among those treated with IV rt-PA, outcomes were significantly better. Another trial used the mismatch between areas of permanent injury and those of diminished perfusion, representing "at risk" tissue, from CT or MRI, to establish an ischemic penumbra that could be salvaged up to 9 hours after onset.

Interventional techniques to revascularize occluded vessels have also been demonstrated to benefit selected patients with ischemic stroke. For patients with MCA occlusions presenting up to 6 hours after symptom onset, there is evidence that intra-arterial thrombolytic agents delivered via catheter into the face of the occluding thrombus can improve functional outcomes, despite an increase in risk of hemorrhage similar to that seen with intravenous rt-PA. More recently, the FDA has approved the use of mechanical devices called stent-retrievers specifically engineered to facilitate clot extraction in the setting of ischemic stroke in the middle cerebral artery in selected patients. These devices, used during an angiographic procedure, provide a wire mesh that can surround the thrombus in the vessel and then be used to pull the clot out. They may be used up to 24 hours after stroke onset and

can achieve a recanalization rate of up to 80%. Patients are selected for the procedure by using infarction-perfusion mismatch imaging to identify those with areas of uninfarcted, salvageable brain tissue. Meta-analyses of several randomized trials in these patients have shown marked benefits, with about two to three patients needed to treat to achieve clinically significant functional improvement.

Treatment with heparin and various heparinoids for acute stroke are not of benefit and are not recommended in acute stroke. In some patients with massive hemispheric strokes, surgical decompression (hemicraniectomy) can be life-saving with acceptable functional outcomes, particularly for younger patients.

Since stroke is characterized by a cascade of events that can cause further neuronal injury for hours or days after stroke, experimental animal stroke studies have tested strategies that might limit this injury (i.e., neuroprotection), including drugs targeting N-methyl-D-aspartate (NMDA) receptors, glycine receptors, calcium channels, adhesion molecules, free radicals, albumin, inflammation, and membrane constituents. However, none of these have been of benefit in human clinical trials.

Treatment of Intracerebral Hemorrhage

Treatment of ICH is primarily supportive. Many patients require management in the intensive care setting to manage elevated blood pressure and secondary complications, such as respiratory failure, aspiration, and hemodynamic instability in severely neurologically compromised patients. In many cases, patients also require management of intracranial pressure using osmotic agents, such as mannitol or hypertonic saline, or therapeutic hyperventilation. In some patients, surgical evacuation of hematomas may be life-saving, although trials have thus far failed to show that most ICH patients benefit from surgical decompression. Among more than 1000 participants randomized in a large international study, there was no evidence of benefit of surgical over medical therapy, apart from a potential benefit in the subgroup of patients with small superficial hemorrhages. Most hemorrhages that occur deep within the hemispheres probably cause the majority of their damage immediately after the ictal hemorrhage, so that evacuation does not save tissue and may introduce further damage.

One of the major recent insights into the pathogenesis of cerebral injury associated with ICH has been the recognition that a large proportion of hemorrhages continue to expand during the early hours after onset. As a result, there has been increased interest in the use of prothrombotic agents to reduce this expansion and to limit secondary cerebral injury. Though preliminary studies on the potential benefits of infusing factor VII as a prothrombogenic agent showed promise, subsequent and more definitive studies did not confirm a benefit in the majority of patients, although it remains possible that subgroups of patients, including those with warfarin-associated hemorrhage, may benefit.

For cerebellar hemorrhages, surgical decompression may be life-saving, and it is essential to recognize the signs and symptoms of incipient brain stem compression and herniation (i.e., headache, vertigo, nausea, vomiting, and truncal ataxia without focal weakness, declining sensorium, and gaze-palsy). Neuroimaging studies that support the need for surgical decompression include hematoma greater than 3 cm, fourth ventricular shift, cisternal obliteration, and ventricular enlargement. Lumbar puncture is contraindicated with ICH, particularly with cerebellar hemorrhages, because life-threatening tonsillar herniation and midbrain compression may occur. Great caution must be taken in these patients subjected to ventriculostomy for the purposes of reducing intracranial pressure because upward cerebellar herniation may occur.

The management of aneurysmal SAH is complicated, and recurrent bleeding risks and mortality are high. Antifibrinolytic agents, such as ε-aminocaproic acid, used to preserve the thrombus around an aneurysm and thereby prevent rebleeding, have been unsuccessful. Therefore, definitive therapy is elimination of the ruptured aneurysm. This may be accomplished surgically or with interventional embolization techniques, such as with coils deposited in the aneurysm. Even after securing the aneurysmal site of bleeding, however, several other complications may ensue, of which vasospasm leading to cerebral infarction is one of the most common. Vasospasm appears to represent a reaction of the blood vessels to the blood in the surrounding subarachnoid space. Transcranial Doppler screening may be used daily to detect early changes of vasospasm; continuous EEG monitoring and multimodality monitoring of vital signs are other emerging ways to detect cerebral dysfunction while still reversible. The calcium-channel antagonist nimodipine, which crosses the blood-brain barrier, has become standard of care in SAH patients for up to 3 weeks after hemorrhage. It improves outcomes, although it is not clear that this is through a reduction in vasospasm, as originally hypothesized. Hydration, hyperosmolar therapy, hypertensive therapy, and angioplasty of vascular spasm may also be used to reduce risk of infarction. Other complications of SAH include cerebral edema, seizures, ventricular dilatation, the syndrome of inappropriate ADH secretion (SIADH), and cardiac failure. Hydrocephalus may require ventricular shunting.

Rehabilitation and Recovery

A team approach to stroke rehabilitation, starting with a stroke recovery unit with experienced physiatrists and physical therapists, has proven beneficial for the optimum recovery of patients. A specialized stroke unit is particularly helpful in avoiding complications such as infections, contractures, and decubiti, and in maximizing independence for patients. Speech and occupational therapists help patients improve their swallowing, communication, and daily living skills.

Constraint-induced therapy is a specific type of physical therapy that involves having a hemiparetic patient wear a large mitt to prevent use of the unaffected limb for several hours daily, forcing the patient to use the affected limb for most tasks. In a randomized trial, constraint-induced therapy with intensive task-directed therapy was associated with functional improvement compared to standard physical therapy. It remains unclear, however, whether the use of constraints or the intensive nature of the therapy itself was responsible for the improvements in function. Intensive task-directed therapy is both difficult for the patient and expensive, however, and may not be practical for large numbers of patients. Recent studies have suggested that home therapy, guided by therapists using videoconferencing with patients (i.e., "telerehabilitation") may be more feasible for patients.

Depression is a frequent accompaniment of stroke, reflecting both the physical disability and altered brain chemistry. Depression may respond to selective serotonin reuptake inhibitors (SSRIs) and tricyclic antidepressants. Escitalopram administered prophylactically to stroke patients was effective in preventing the development of depression, though other studies have not confirmed this. There is also evidence from other trials that SSRI treatment facilitates functional recovery after stroke.

Secondary Stroke Prevention

The optimal secondary prevention strategy for an individual patient depends on the stroke mechanism. For stroke or TIA caused by carotid stenosis of 70% or more of the vessel diameter, carotid endarterectomy (CEA) by a skilled surgeon with an acceptable complication rate (<5%) is preferable to medical therapy in good surgical candidates. For patients at high risk of surgical complications, including those over age 80, those with cardiac or pulmonary disease, or those with radiation-induced arteriopathy, stenting reduces the risks of cardiac

complications. Trials that tested whether carotid angioplasty and stenting are more effective or safer than carotid endarterectomy in patients at low surgical risk have not demonstrated any benefit over open surgery. Among patients with symptomatic intracranial stenosis (lesions not amenable to surgery), a recent randomized trial demonstrated that best medical therapy, including aggressive risk factor control, was associated with a lower recurrence risk.

Anticoagulation is indicated in patients with definite cardioembolic sources of stroke, such as mechanical valves or atrial fibrillation. In patients with atrial fibrillation, anticoagulation with warfarin was superior to aspirin, with a relative risk reduction of about 68%. Recommended options for secondary prevention among patients with atrial fibrillation now include warfarin with an INR between 2.0 and 3.0, or use of one of the newer antithrombotic agents, such as dabigatran, rivaroxaban, edoxaban, or apixaban, which are associated with a lower risk of bleeding complications. For patients who cannot tolerate anticoagulants because of a risk of ICH or bleeding elsewhere, newer treatment modalities, including interventions to exclude the left atrial appendage from the circulation using a device delivered endovascularly has been approved after a clinical trial demonstrated that it was as effective at preventing stroke as anticoagulation with warfarin, with a low risk of bleeding or other complications.

Recent evidence suggests that some patients with unexplained stroke may have cardiac emboli from conditions related to atrial dysfunction but without frank atrial fibrillation; this entity has been labelled *atrial cardiopathy* and may be detected using cardiac biomarkers such as an enlarged heart on echocardiography, frequent ectopy on monitoring, P wave abnormalities on the electrocardiogram, or serum biomarkers. An ongoing clinical trial is testing whether patients with unexplained stroke and atrial cardiopathy would benefit from anticoagulation just as patients with atrial fibrillation do.

Other causes of cardiogenic emboli require different treatments. Closure of patent foramen ovale using umbrella-like devices has now been shown in several randomized trials to reduce the risk of recurrent stroke in selected patients (younger patients without other stroke risk factors). Among patients with patent foramen ovale, there is limited evidence that anticoagulation is any more effective than antiplatelet agents such as aspirin, and anticoagulation is not routinely recommended in the absence of a known hypercoagulable disorder or evidence of thrombi elsewhere. Infected prosthetic valves need replacement if emboli persist on antibiotics, there are large valvular vegetations, or if patients develop heart failure. Emboli from myxomatous tumors of the atria frequently require surgical removal of tumor. The need for anticoagulation among patients with other less well-established sources of emboli, such as calcific valvular disease or aortic arch plaque, is unproven, and current guidelines do not support its use in this setting.

All patients with ischemic stroke without a definite indication for anticoagulation, and in whom no contraindication is present, should receive long-term antiplatelet therapy, which reduces the risk of recurrence by 20% to 25%. Agents currently approved for this purpose include aspirin, dipyridamole, and clopidogrel, a thienopyridine derivative ADP receptor inhibitor. Head-to-head trials have failed to demonstrate a benefit of one of these agents over another; the combination of aspirin and dipyridamole was more effective than either agent alone, but long-term treatment with the combination of aspirin and clopidogrel was no more effective than aspirin alone and increased the risk of significant bleeding. More recent trials suggest that there may be benefit to the combination of aspirin and clopidogrel when used for up to approximately 30 days after stroke or TIA. The benefits to dual antiplatelet agents after about 30 days, however, are outweighed by the increased risk of significant bleeding. Aspirin doses as low as 30 mg daily appear effective and have fewer side effects, such as gastrointestinal bleeding, than higher doses, although there is some evidence that the efficacious dose of aspirin may depend on body weight. The FDA recommends doses between 50 and 325 mg daily for stroke prevention.

Clinical trials provide evidence for increased use of anti-hypertensive agents in patients with stroke and TIA. There are theoretical concerns about lowering blood pressure in patients with existing cerebrovascular disease due to the possibility that in patients with arterial disease of cerebral vessels and reduced autoregulation, a reduction in blood pressure could worsen perfusion and precipitate clinical events or affect cognition. Randomized trials provide evidence, however, that blood pressure reduction among patients with cerebrovascular disease reduces risks of recurrent stroke by 28% independently of a history of hypertension. Guidelines currently focus on the use of blood pressure agents to achieve recommended target blood pressure levels, rather than on specific agents, which should be individualized depending on a patient's comorbidities.

Trials using hydroxymethylglutaryl-coenzyme A (HMG-CoA) reductase inhibitors, or statins, among cardiac and other vascular disease high-risk patients have demonstrated benefits in stroke risk reduction. The Stroke Prevention by Aggressive Reduction in Cholesterol Levels (SPARCL) trial provided more direct evidence of the benefit of statin therapy in secondary prevention of stroke among patients presenting with stroke or TIA. SPARCL randomized patients with recent stroke or TIA to atorvastatin 80 mg daily or placebo. Over 5 years, atorvastatin reduced the risk of the primary outcome, recurrent stroke, from 13.1% to 11.2%, an absolute risk reduction of about 2%. More recently, the Treat Stroke to Target trial demonstrated that among patients with ischemic stroke and atherosclerotic disease, those treated to an LDL level of less than 70 mg/dL had a lower risk of recurrent cardiovascular events.

Among those with diabetes, diet and exercise, oral hypoglycemic drugs, and insulin are recommended to obtain glycemic control. Although glycemic control reduces risks of microvascular complications, the benefit in reducing macrovascular complications is less certain. In one trial, tight glycemic control of a prospective cohort of newly diagnosed diabetics was not found to significantly reduce stroke risk. The peroxisome proliferator-activated receptor-γ (PPAR-γ) agonist pioglitazone, a potent insulin-sensitizing agent, was shown in another trial to reduce risk of recurrent stroke among patients with stroke or TIA and insulin resistance, although an increase in weight gain and fractures has limited its use. Recent evidence also suggests that bariatric surgery, a way to reduce obesity and treat the metabolic syndrome, reduces risks of cardiovascular events, including stroke.

Behavioral risk factors are difficult to control but are also important. Smoking is addictive, and cessation may necessitate psychologic counseling and medical aids, such as nicotine patches or varenicline. Physical activity should be encouraged, because a sedentary lifestyle is associated with elevations in blood pressure and stroke risk. Alcohol consumption in excess of two drinks daily should be discouraged, though there is evidence that moderate alcohol consumption may have protective effects against stroke risk. It should be noted, however, that there is only limited evidence that control of these risk factors reduces recurrent stroke risk.

PROGNOSIS

The immediate period after an ischemic stroke carries the greatest risk of death, with fatality rates ranging from 8% to 20% in the first 30 days. Age and stroke severity are the most important predictors of prognosis. Case fatality rates are worse for hemorrhagic strokes, ranging from 30% to 80% for intracerebral hemorrhage and 20% to 50% for subarachnoid hemorrhage.

Stroke survivors continue to have a 3- to 5-fold increased risk of death, compared with the age-matched general population. Annual aggregate estimates of death have been 5% for minor stroke and 8% for major stroke. Survival is influenced by age, hypertension, cardiac disease, and diabetes. Patients with lacunar infarcts appear to have a better long-term survival than do those with the other infarct subtypes.

Recurrent stroke is frequent. The immediate period after a stroke carries the greatest risk for early recurrence; rates range from 3% to 10% during the first 30 days. Thirty-day recurrence risks vary by infarct subtypes; the greatest rates are in patients with atherosclerotic infarction and the lowest rates in patients with lacunes. After the early phase, the risk of stroke recurrence continues to threaten the quality of life of a stroke survivor. Long-term stroke recurrence rates range in different studies from 4% to 14% per year, with aggregate annual estimates of 6% for minor stroke and 9% for major stroke. These rates have been decreasing with the advent of the improved protection strategies outlined previously. Recurrent stroke contributes to the burden of dementia and functional decline after stroke. Importantly, cardiac events are also increased in stroke survivors, and pose a major threat of death.

For a deeper discussion on this topic, please see Chapter 58, ❖ "Supraventricular Cardiac Arrhythmias," in *Goldman-Cecil Medicine*, 26th Edition.

SUGGESTED READINGS

Albers GW, Marks MP, Kemp S, et al: Thrombectomy for stroke at 6 to 16 hours with selection by perfusion imaging, N Engl J Med 378:708–718, 2018.

Amarenco P, Bogousslavsky J, Callahan 3rd A, et al: The Stroke Prevention by Aggressive Reduction in Cholesterol Levels (SPARCL) investigators. High-dose atorvastatin after stroke or transient ischemic attack, N Engl J Med 355:549–559, 2006.

Amarenco P, Kim JS, Labreuche J, et al: A comparison of two LDL Cholesterol targets after ischemic stroke, N Engl J Med 382:9–19, 2020.

GBD Lifetime Risk of Stroke Collaborators, Feigin VL, Nguyen G, et al: Global, regional, and country-specific lifetime risks of stroke, 1990 and 2016, N Engl J Med 379:2429–2437, 2018.

George MG, Tong X, Bowman BA: Prevalence of cardiovascular risk factors and strokes in younger adults, J Am Med Assoc Neurol 74:695–703, 2017.

Goyal M, Menon BK, van Zwam WH, et al: Endovascular thrombectomy after large-vessel ischaemic stroke: a meta-analysis of individual patient data from five randomised trials, Lancet 387:1723–1731, 2016.

Hemphill 3rd JC, Greenberg SM, Anderson CS, et al: Guidelines for the management of spontaneous intracerebral hemorrhage: a guideline for healthcare professionals from the American Heart Association/American Stroke Association, Stroke 46:2032–2060, 2015.

Holmes Jr DR, Kar S, Price MJ, et al: Prospective randomized evaluation of the watchman Left atrial appendage closure device in patients with atrial fibrillation versus long-term warfarin therapy: the PREVAIL trial, J Am Coll Cardiol 64(1):1–12, 2014.

Howard G, Lackland DT, Kleindorfer DO, et al: Racial differences in the impact of elevated systolic blood pressure on stroke risk, J Am Med Assoc Intern Med 173:46–51, 2013.

Kamel H, Elkind MSV, Bhave PD, et al: Paroxysmal supraventricular tachycardia and the risk of ischemic stroke, Stroke 44:1550–1554, 2013.

Kamel H, Okin P, Elkind MSV, Iadecola C: Atrial fibrillation and mechanisms of stroke: time for a new model, Stroke 47(3):895–900, 2016.

Johnston SC, Easton JD, Farrant M, et al: Clopidogrel and aspirin in acute ischemic stroke and high-risk TIA, N Engl J Med 379:215–225, 2018.

Kernan WN, Ovbiagele B, Black HR, et al: Guidelines for the prevention of stroke in patients with stroke and transient ischemic attack: a guideline for healthcare professionals from the American Heart Association/American Stroke Association, Stroke 45:2160–2236, 2014.

Lackland DT, Elkind MSV, D'Agostino R, et al: Inclusion of stroke in cardiovascular risk prediction instruments: a statement for healthcare professionals from the American Heart Association/American Stroke Association, Stroke 43:1998–2027, 2012.

López-López JA, Sterne JAC, Thom HHZ, et al: Oral anticoagulants for prevention of stroke in atrial fibrillation: systematic review, network meta-analysis, and cost effectiveness analysis, BMJ 359:j5058, 2017.

Ma H, Campbell BCV, Parsons MW, et al: Thrombolysis guided by perfusion imaging up to 9 hours after onset of stroke, N Engl J Med 380:1795–1803, 2019.

Mayer SA, Brun NC, Begtrup K, et al: Efficacy and safety of recombinant activated factor VII for acute intracerebral hemorrhage, N Engl J Med 358:2127–2137, 2008.

Mendelow AD, Gregson BA, Fernandes HM, et al: Early surgery versus initial conservative treatment in patients with spontaneous supratentorial intracerebral haematomas in the International Surgical Trial in Intracerebral Haemorrhage (STICH): a randomised trial, Lancet 365:387–397, 2005.

Nogueira RG, Jadhav AP, Haussen DC, et al: Thrombectomy 6 to 24 hours after stroke with a mismatch between deficit and infarct, N Engl J Med 378:11–21, 2018.

Powers WJ, Rabinstein AA, Ackerson T, et al: 2018 Guidelines for the early management of patients with acute ischemic stroke: a guideline for healthcare professionals from the American Heart Association/American Stroke Association, Stroke 50:e344–e418, 2019.

Robinson RG, Jorge RE, Moser DJ, et al: Escitalopram and problem-solving therapy for prevention of poststroke depression: a randomized controlled trial, J Am Med Assoc 299:2391–2400, 2008.

Ropper AH: Tipping point for patent foramen ovale closure, N Engl J Med 377:1093–1095, 2017.

Rothwell PM, Eliasziw M, Gutnikov SA, et al: Analysis of pooled data from the randomised controlled trials of endarterectomy for symptomatic carotid stenosis, Lancet 361:107–116, 2003.

Saver JL, Fonarow GC, Smith EE, et al: Time to treatment with intravenous tissue plasminogen activator and outcome from acute ischemic stroke, J Am Med Assoc 309:2480–2488, 2013.

Singhal AB, Biller J, Elkind MS, et al: Recognition and management of stroke in young adults and adolescents, Neurology 81:1089–1097, 2013.

SPS3 Study Group, Benavente OR, Coffey CS, et al: Blood-pressure targets in patients with recent lacunar stroke: the SPS3 randomised trial, Lancet 382(9891):507–515, 2013.

Thomalla G, Simonsen CZ, Boutitie F, et al: MRI-guided thrombolysis for stroke with unknown time of onset, N Engl J Med 379:611–622, 2018.

Winstein CJ, Stein J, Arena R, et al: Guidelines for adult stroke rehabilitation and recovery: a guideline for healthcare professionals from the American Heart Association/American Stroke Association, Stroke 47:e98–e169, 2016.

Yan G, Wang J, Zhang J, et al: Long-term outcomes of macrovascular diseases and metabolic indicators of bariatric surgery for severe obesity type 2 diabetes patients with a meta-analysis, PloS One 14(12):e0224828, 2019.

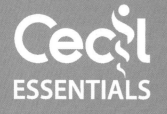

119

Traumatic Brain Injury and Spinal Cord Injury

Geoffrey S.F. Ling, Jeffrey J. Bazarian

INTRODUCTION

Traumatic brain injury (TBI) and traumatic spinal cord injury (TSCI) are leading causes of traumatic death and disability. It is estimated that almost 60 million people worldwide sustain a TBI each year. According to the World Health Organization, TBI is projected to become the third largest cause of disease burden worldwide by the year 2020. In the United States, TBI results in over 2.5 million emergency department (ED) visits; the vast majority (over 80%) are mild TBI or concussion. However, approximately 52,000 patients in the United States die from severe TBI as a direct consequence, making it the leading cause of traumatic death and disability. Furthermore, yearly, about 11,000 patients are severely disabled by TSCI. The vast majority are due to falls, motor vehicle accidents, sports-related occurrences, and assaults. Among the almost 5.5 million TBI and TSCI survivors, most require prolonged rehabilitation.

TYPES OF INJURY

Certain lesions require neurosurgical intervention while others do not. TBI conditions for which emergency neurosurgery is needed are penetrating wounds, intracerebral hemorrhage with mass effect including subdural and epidural blood, and bony injury such as displaced fracture and vertebral subluxation. However, focal, hypoxic-anoxic, diffuse axonal and diffuse microvascular injuries typically do not require surgery.

MANAGEMENT

Traumatic Brain Injury

Patients with mild TBI typically recover quickly and fully. To optimize outcome, it is critical to first remove the TBI victim from play or work to prevent further injury. Diagnosis of mild TBI or concussion begins simply with identifying affected patients. This is often difficult because these patients suffer transient alteration of consciousness with only a minority completely losing consciousness. Most have memory impairment. As a result, patients are typically unaware that they are injured. Thus, it is important that colleagues, coaches, athletic trainers, parents, and other observers have a heightened suspicion when a potential head injury event occurs. If so, then a sideline point-of-injury screening tool should be administered, such as the standardized assessment of concussion (SAC) or sports concussion assessment tool version 5 (SCAT 5). SAC is a neuropsychological battery that tests orientation, immediate memory, concentration, and memory recall. An abnormal score is less than 25. If the SAC score is abnormal, the patient is at high risk for having suffered a concussion and thus should be brought to medical attention for further evaluation, diagnosis, and treatment. The SCAT-5 includes the SAC and also other neurologic tests such as balance.

In the early stage of management, it is important that patients at risk of having incurred a mild TBI or concussion have a provider skilled in managing TBI perform a detailed history, physical examination, and neurologic examination, especially assessment of cognitive function. The history should determine the duration of altered sensorium, amnesia or loss of consciousness a patient may have suffered.

The decision to obtain neuroimaging is based on the index of suspicion of intracranial hemorrhage or skull fracture. Both CT and MRI are inadequate in ruling out mild TBI, which is a clinical diagnosis. If a patient lost consciousness or has persistent altered mentation, abnormal Glasgow Coma Score (GCS), focal neurologic deficit or is clinically deteriorating, then neuroimaging should be obtained.

In general, patients with mild TBI do not require hospitalization; almost all do well after adequate convalescence. It is essential that patients have adequate time for recovery; they should not return to play or work until fully recovered. A second head injury before full recovery may be catastrophic due to the "second impact syndrome" (SIS), which leads to worse clinical outcome, including death.

The patient must be allowed to rest with minimal cognitive burden. There are no specific medications to foster recovery. Treatment is focused on ameliorating symptoms according to published evidence-based guidelines, such as VA/DoD Clinical Practice Guidelines for the Management of Concussion/mild TBI. In general, headache, the most common complaint, can be treated with acetaminophen or a nonsteroidal anti-inflammatory agent. Triptans can be considered if there are features of migraine. Dizziness can be treated with physical therapy. Meclizine should be reserved only for symptoms that are severe enough to impair activities of daily function. Insomnia can be treated with proper sleep hygiene. A sedative can be used acutely and should be limited to non-benzodiazepine agents such as zolpidem. Visual and auditory symptoms should be evaluated by appropriate medical specialists.

The patient is able to return to play or work after at least 24 hours of recovery and when cleared to do so by an advanced practice health care provider experienced in the management of concussion. In many states, statutes specify these requirements. In general, patients are able to return to play when their symptoms no longer require treatment. At this point, many practitioners will subject the patient to provocative testing such as having the patient perform exertion (e.g., run) followed by cognitive testing. If this does not cause symptoms to recur and the patient performs well cognitively, then he/she is allowed to return to full activity.

For moderate to severe TBI the initial care goals are the "ABCs" of airway, breathing, and circulation. Next is "D" for disability

TABLE 119.1 Glasgow Coma Score

Best Eye Response	Best Verbal Response	Best Motor Response
1 = No eye opening	1 = No verbal response	1 = No motor response
2 = Eye opening to pain	2 = Incomprehensible sounds	2 = Extension to pain
3 = Eye opening to verbal command	3 = Inappropriate words	3 = Flexion to pain
4 = Eyes open spontaneously	4 = Confused	4 = Withdrawal from pain
	5 = Orientated	5 = Localizing pain
		6 = Obeys commands

GCS = Eye Response + Verbal Response + Motor Response.

(neurologic). Every patient should undergo a detailed neurologic examination to ascertain the level of neurologic disability. An initial GCS should be assigned to each patient. The GCS (Table 119.1) categorizes patients with TBI and provides a quantifiable measure of impairment.

Patients with severe TBI are those who present with GCS scores of eight or less. To optimize outcome, medical management should adhere to currently accepted clinical guidelines such as the Brain Trauma Foundation "Clinical Guidelines for Severe TBI." An important early intervention is airway protection, usually by endotracheal intubation. If elevated intracranial pressure (ICP) is suspected, elevate the patient's head to 30° and keep it midline, ideally with a rigid neck collar (at least until the cervical spine can be evaluated for stability). Mannitol should be given intravenously at a dose of 0.5 to 1.0 g/kg. Hyperventilation may also be used with a goal of Pco_2 34 to 36 mm Hg. ICP should be kept less than 20 mm Hg with the cerebral perfusion pressure (CPP) greater than 60 mm Hg. A head CT without contrast should be done as soon as possible to identify lesions that will require surgery and to determine the extent of injury.

If ICP remains poorly controlled, one can consider administering an intravenous bolus of 23% hypertonic saline (50 cc) followed by continuous infusion of 2% or 3% hypertonic saline (75 to 125 cc/hr) through a central venous catheter. If these interventions are unsuccessful, pharmacologic coma or surgical decompression should be considered. Pharmacologic coma can be induced with pentobarbital. This is given as a loading dose of 5 mg/kg intravenously, followed by an infusion of 1 to 3 mg/kg/hr. Alternatively, propofol can be used, which is administered as a loading dose of 2 mg/kg intravenously, followed by an infusion up to 200 μg/min. Continuous EEG monitoring is helpful as the limit of drug induced coma is achieving ICP control or cerebral electrical burst-suppression. Persistently elevated ICP after all these efforts is ominous. Consideration should be given to frontal or temporal lobe decompression and hemicraniectomy.

To meet CPP goals, patients must first be adequately hydrated. The goal of TBI fluid management is to increase the osmolar gradient between systemic vasculature and brain, not dehydration. For this purpose, hyperosmolar intravenous solutions are used, such as normal saline. Other options are hypertonic saline (e.g., 3% sodium solutions). If meeting CPP goals is difficult with intravenous fluids alone, vasoactive pharmacologic agents such as norepinephrine and phenylephrine can be administered. These two agents are preferred because they are considered to have the least effect on cerebral vasomotor tone. Since barbiturates and propofol are myocardial depressants, aggressive cardiovascular management will probably be necessary when pharmacologic coma is induced.

Agitation can be treated with dexmedetomidine, lorazepam or haloperidol. If inadequate, then infusions of midazolam or propofol may be used. Pain should be controlled. Acetaminophen and nonsteroidal anti-inflammatory agents are adequate for mild discomfort. However, for moderate to severe pain, narcotic analgesics such as fentanyl or morphine should be used. A benefit of opioids is that they can be reversed by naloxone to allow reassessment of neurologic status.

Hypoxia, seizures, and fever must be avoided. Maintaining Po_2 at approximately 100 mm Hg is sufficient. An antiepileptic drug (AED), such as phenytoin or levetiracetam, is administered for the first 7 days after injury as it will reduce early onset seizures. After 7 days it should be stopped. It can be restarted if seizures recur. Fever should be reduced with antipyretics such as acetaminophen, using a cooling blanket if needed. Other important management considerations include prevention of gastric stress ulcer, deep vein thrombosis (DVT), and decubitus ulcers. Feeding should be instituted as soon as practical to maintain nutrition.

After the initial few hours, efforts should be made to reduce hyperventilation, which is indicated only for initial emergency management. After 12 hours, metabolic compensation negates the ameliorative effects of respiratory alkalosis caused by the hypocapnic state induced by hyperventilation.

Repeated neurologic examination and continuous ICP and CPP measurement are indicated. Generally, the peak period of cerebral edema is from 48 to 96 hours after TBI. Thereafter, the edema resolves spontaneously and clinical improvement should follow.

A complication of TBI is post-concussive syndrome (PCS). Diagnosis can be made using the Post-Concussion Symptom Scale (PCSS) and Graded Symptom Checklist (GSC). The most common symptoms of PCS are headache, difficulty concentrating, appetite changes, sleep abnormalities, and irritability. PCS has a variable presentation and duration depending on the patient and the severity of TBI. In general, PCS lasts for a few weeks post-injury. However, uncommonly, it can persist beyond a year or more. Treatment is symptomatic. For headache, nonsteroidal anti-inflammatory agents, migraine drugs, and biofeedback can be effective. For cognitive dysfunction, neuropsychological testing may be helpful in determining appropriate intervention, which may include cognitive-behavioral therapy.

Traumatic Spinal Cord Injury

The emergency management of traumatic injury to the spinal cord has greatly improved with adherence to the American Association of Neurological Surgeons "Guidelines for the Management of Cervical Spine and Spinal Cord Injuries." Therapy begins with the "ABCs" of airway, breathing, and circulation. A secure airway is absolutely vital. In patients suffering from high cervical lesions, spontaneous ventilation will be lost. Lesions below C5 may also impair ventilatory capability. If the airway or ventilatory efforts are compromised, emergency intubation is required. In a patient in whom cervical spine trauma has not been assessed, the preferred method is nasotracheal intubation using fiberoptic guidance. Other approaches are nasotracheal (blind) or orotracheal intubation, so long as cervical spine alignment is maintained by traction.

Maintaining intravascular volume is essential in TSCI. Hypotension may be due to either neurogenic shock or hypovolemia. For neurogenic shock, vasopressive pharmacologic agents such as phenylephrine may be needed. If tachycardia is present, then hypovolemia is the more likely etiology and fluid resuscitation with normal saline is the appropriate initial management.

After addressing the "ABCs," a neurologic history and examination should be obtained. An accompanying TBI must be considered. Up to 50% of TSCI patients have an associated TBI. Neuroimaging is often indicated, but not all patients need radiographic study. A normal neurologic assessment obviates the need for imaging studies. However, a complaint of burning hands or of pain over the spine, numbness, tingling or weakness indicates spinal cord injury. A detailed neurologic examination is needed to identify the level of the injury and the completeness of any deficits and to document the degree of neurologic dysfunction at the earliest time possible. The level of the injury is the lowest spinal cord segment with intact motor and sensory function. The prognosis for neurologic improvement is better if the lesion is incomplete rather than complete. Following the acute injury, serial examinations must be made frequently.

If spinal cord injury is suspected, the patient should be immediately and appropriately immobilized with a rigid collar or backboard or both. Radiologic evaluation should begin with plain radiographs of the bony spine. Abnormalities on radiographs should lead to further neuroimaging. Bony vertebrae should be examined with CT and the spinal cord with MRI. Intervertebral and paravertebral soft tissue are best studied with MRI. A chest radiograph should also be obtained in order to visualize the lower cervical and thoracic vertebrae. Presence of a pleural effusion in the setting of a possible thoracic spine injury suggests a hemothorax.

If the C-spine radiographs are normal but the patient complains of neck pain, then ligamentous injury may be present. Ligamentous injury is evaluated by flexion-extension C-spine radiographs. However, in the acute period, pain may prevent an adequate study. These patients should be kept in a rigid cervical collar for a few days until the pain and neck muscle spasm resolves. At that time, imaging may be performed. If abnormal, the patient will need surgical evaluation.

Spinal Cord Syndromes

There are three main spinal cord syndromes: anterior cord, Brown-Sequard, and central cord. Anterior cord syndrome is associated with deficits referable to bilateral anterior and lateral spinal cord columns. There is loss of touch sensation, pain, temperature, and motor function below the level of the lesion. The posterior column functions of proprioception and vibratory sensation remain intact. In Brown-Sequard syndrome, the deficits are due to injury to a lateral half of the cord. There is functional loss of ipsilateral motor, touch, proprioception and vibration, and contralateral pain and temperature. Central cord results in a "man in a barrel" syndrome: motor paralysis of both upper extremities with sparing of the lower extremities. Weakness is greater proximally than distally. Pain and temperature sensations are generally reduced but proprioception and vibration are spared.

Spinal Shock

Spinal shock may occur after acute injury causing a temporary loss of spinal reflexes below the level of injury. Neurologic examination will reveal loss of muscle stretch reflexes, bulbocavernosus reflex (testing anal sphincter tone in response to stimulating the glans penis or clitoris), and the anal wink. In high cervical injuries, the lower reflexes (bulbocavernosus and anal wink) may be preserved. There may also be the "Schiff-Sherrington" phenomenon, in which reflexes are affected above the level of injury. Additionally, there may be loss of autonomic reflexes leading to neurogenic shock, ileus, and urinary retention.

Acute and Subacute Management

In the intensive care unit, the patient will need continued treatment. TSCI patients require close cardiovascular and respiratory monitoring. Other issues are genitourinary, bowel, infectious disease, nutrition, skin, and prophylaxis against ulcers and deep vein thrombosis formation.

Patients suffering from spinal cord injury are at risk for neurogenic shock and dysautonomia with resulting peripheral vasodilation and hypotension. Lesions at T3 or above compromise sympathetic tone with hypotension accompanied by bradycardia: the classic neurogenic shock triad of bradycardia, hypotension, and peripheral vasodilation.

Dysautonomia is treated by ensuring adequate circulating volume. The goal is to fluid resuscitate to a euvolemic state. Blood can be used if the patient is anemic (i.e., hematocrit less than 30). If blood is not required, then either colloid (e.g., albumin solutions) or crystalloid (e.g., normal saline) may be used. Central venous pressure (CVP) should be maintained at 4 to 6 mm Hg. Hypervolemia should be avoided, as this will exacerbate peripheral edema. Once an adequate circulating volume has been achieved, vasopressive agents can be used (e.g., phenylephrine, norepinephrine or dopamine). The mean arterial pressure (MAP) should be 85 mm Hg or greater. Symptomatic bradycardia can be treated with atropine.

Patients with TSCI are at risk for ventilatory compromise. Patients whose injuries are at C5 or higher typically require mechanical ventilation with an appropriate tidal volume (6 to 10 mL/kg), F_{IO_2} and mandatory machine driven rate. The F_{IO_2} inspired oxygen concentration should give a P_{O_2} between 80 and 100 mm Hg. The rate should be set to give a P_{CO_2} of 40 mm Hg. Positive end-expiratory pressure (PEEP) should also be used to minimize atelectasis. If the patient does not show signs of ventilatory recovery within 2 weeks of intubation, a tracheostomy should be considered. Lesions below C5 may also be associated with inadequate spontaneous ventilation. Mid-cervical lesions may be associated with intact but compromised diaphragm function. If suspected, a "sniff" test under fluoroscopy can be performed to determine if both hemidiaphragms are functioning properly. If not, intubation/tracheostomy with volume-controlled ventilation may be needed. If intact, then pressure support (PS) ventilation sufficient to maintain an appropriate tidal volume with oxygenation and PEEP should be set as described previously.

Patients with cervical lesions at C6 and below, including the thoracic cord, do not require mechanical ventilation. However, their ventilatory effort may be inadequate because the thoracic cord innervates intercostal muscles, which are accessory muscles of respiration. Such patients have decreased cough and inability to increase ventilation when needed, leading to atelectasis and inability to clear secretions, which can cause pneumonia. Such patients need assistance with clearing their airway: chest percussion, suctioning, and encouragement in coughing.

Thromboembolic disease is a leading cause of morbidity and mortality in patients with TSCI: up to 80% will develop DVT without prophylaxis. All patients with TSCI should receive anticoagulation and have mechanical compression devices applied to their legs. As soon as possible, sequential compression devices (SCD) or compression stockings should be placed on patients. As soon as hemostasis is assured, low-molecular-weight heparin (LMWH) should be initiated. Unfractionated heparin may also be used in conjunction with SCD but LMWH is preferred. An inferior vena cava filter may be placed in those patients in whom anticoagulation therapy is contraindicated but should not be the primary means of preventing DVT.

Mid-low thoracic spinal cord injury can lead to ileus. A nasogastric tube should be placed to decompress the stomach. Parental nutrition should be started as soon as possible. Enteral feeding should be delayed until gastrointestinal motility returns, usually 2 to 3 weeks. Pharmacologic agents that promote motility are metoclopramide, erythromycin, and cisapride. Gastric ulcer should be prevented with medication: H2 receptor antagonists, proton pump inhibitors, antacids or sucralfate. Pancreatitis and trauma-related bowel perforation occur: loss of abdominal muscle tone and visceral sensation may mask usual clinical findings of pain, guarding, or rigidity.

Bladder tone may be lost due to spinal shock. A Foley catheter should be placed and maintained for a minimum of 5 to 7 days to

TABLE 119.2 American Spinal Injury Association Impairment Scale

Grade	Injury Type	Definition
A	Complete	No motor or sensory function below the lesion
B	Incomplete	Sensory but no motor function
C	Incomplete	Some motor strength (<3)
D	Incomplete	Motor strength >3
E	None	Sensory & motor normal

drain the bladder and to evaluate circulatory volume and renal status. Once spinal shock resolves, autonomic dysreflexia may occur from bladder distention: skin flushing and hypertension. Clinical examination by palpation and percussion will reveal a distended bladder, which can be treated with intermittent catheterization or bladder training. Phenoxybenzamine may be helpful in this condition. Urinary tract infection is a significant risk of Foley catheters and should be monitored for, particularly if spinal cord injury affects normal sensation.

Nutrition should be given. Until enteral feeding can begin, parenteral nutrition should be used. A caloric level of 80% of the Harris-Benedict prediction should be used for quadriplegic patients. The full Harris-Benedict predicted amount should be used for patients with thoracic spine injuries and below. Skin care is essential to prevent decubitus ulcers. Mechanical kinetic beds, regular log rolling (every 2 hours), and padded orthotics are all useful in minimize this complication.

Orthotics, physical therapy, and occupational therapy (for cervical cord injury) are useful. Therapy should begin as soon as the spine is stabilized, with the goal of minimizing contractures and beginning the rehabilitation. Once therapy begins, energy expenditure will increase requiring additional nutrition. If intermittent compression devices need to be removed during therapy, heparin dose may need to be increased.

PROGNOSIS

Traumatic Brain Injury

The most useful prognostic indicator following TBI is the neurologic exam at presentation. Clearly, the better the neurologic exam, the higher the likelihood of improved recovery. The initial GCS score is a very reliable prognostic indicator. The lower the initial GCS score, the less likely it is that a patient will have meaningful neurologic or functional recovery. However, some patients with very low presenting GCS scores can have a meaningful recovery.

Traumatic Spinal Cord Injury

For TSCI, the completeness of the injury is the most useful prognosticator. The American Spine Injury Association Impairment Scale grades spinal cord injury on the basis of completeness (Table 119.2). A grade "A" or complete motor and sensory deficit below the lesion is the most ominous prognosis. If such a lesion persists greater than 24 hours, there is little reasonable likelihood of meaningful recovery. On the other hand, partial injuries, even severe, have substantial probability of recovery.

FUTURE

TBI and TSCI are serious neurologic conditions with significant implications on society. Prevention remains the most effective way of reducing the incidences of these diseases. Introduction of practice guidelines have contributed to improved outcome from TBI and TSCI. Sadly, morbidity remains a serious problem. Medical management is largely confined to supportive efforts primarily directed towards minimizing secondary injury, optimizing perfusion and oxygenation, and preventing nonneurologic morbidity. Surgical intervention helps restore structural stability, minimize further injury, and reduce the lesion. However, neither reverses neuronal death nor fully prevents secondary injury processes. There are significant medical research efforts to improve our understanding of the pathogenesis of these diseases and find ways to mitigate them. As new pharmacologic, medical, and surgical approaches are introduced, there will be increasing opportunities to restore these patients.

SUGGESTED READINGS

Carney N, Totten AM, O'Reilly C, et al: Guidelines for the management of severe traumatic brain injury, fourth edition, Neurosurgery 80:6–15, 2017.

Department of Veteran Affairs. Management of concussion-mild traumatic brain injury (mTBI). 2016. VA/DoD clin practice guidelines[Internet]. 2016 Sep 22 [cited 2016 Sep 24]. Available from http://www.healthquality.va.gov/guidelines/Rehab/mtbi/.

Marshall S, Bayley M, McCullagh S, et al: Updated clinical practice guidelines for concussion/mild traumatic brain injury and persistent symptoms, Brain Inj 29:688–700, 2015.

McCrory P, Meeuwisse W, Dvorak J, et al: Consensus statement on concussion in sport—the 5th international conference on concussion in sport held in Berlin, October 2016, Br J Sports Med, bjsports-2017, 2017.

Waters BC, Hadley MN, Hurlbert RJ, et al: Guidelines for the management of acute cervical spine and spinal cord injuries: 2013 update, Neurosurgery 60(Suppl 1):82–91, 2013.

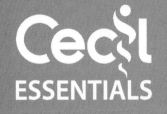
Epilepsy

Andrew S. Blum

DEFINITIONS AND EPIDEMIOLOGY

Epileptic seizures are defined as transient signs and/or symptoms, often including changes in behavior, due to abnormal neuronal activity (often excessively synchronous) in the brain. A wide range of symptoms accompanies seizures depending upon the CNS networks involved, including involuntary movements, abnormal sensations and behaviors, and impaired consciousness.

Seizures often occur amidst many acute medical or neurologic illnesses that compromise brain function (Table 120.1). Common secondary causes of seizures include metabolic derangements (e.g., hypoglycemia or hyponatremia), intoxications (e.g., alcohol, cocaine), withdrawal states (e.g., alcohol, benzodiazepine), acute traumatic brain injury, and hypoxic-ischemic conditions (e.g., cardiac arrest, embolic stroke). Such *provoked* seizures are usually self-limited and generally do not recur after the underlying disorder abates. Thus, provoked seizures do not constitute epilepsy.

Epilepsy, by contrast, is a chronic CNS disease characterized by a predisposition to *spontaneous* epileptic seizures. The diagnosis of epilepsy is applied when there are at least two unprovoked seizures occurring longer than 24 hours apart or one unprovoked seizure and a presumed high probability of further seizures based upon additional data, such as an epileptiform electroencephalography (EEG) or brain imaging revealing a likely structural substrate for recurrent seizures. Individuals with epilepsy have increased seizure susceptibility (lowered seizure threshold). Epilepsy represents a highly heterogeneous set of distinct epilepsy syndromes, with differing etiologies. Genetic factors and prior CNS injury (of diverse mechanisms) account for many of the causes of epilepsy. There have been successive efforts to classify both seizures and epilepsies over the past 5 decades. Classification of epilepsy syndromes depends upon many factors, including seizure type, etiology, genetics, EEG findings, neuroimaging, and response to therapy. The diagnosis of epilepsy encompasses its neurobiological, cognitive, psychological, and social consequences.

Epilepsy presents a host of challenges for patients and their families. Most seizures in people with epilepsy occur unpredictably. This aspect worsens quality of life for patients with epilepsy. When functionally impairing seizures occur during waking hours (diurnal seizures), then activity restrictions may ensue, including restriction from driving, operating heavy machinery, climbing heights, and unobserved swimming or bathing. These activity restrictions erode independence. The psychological impact of intermittent involuntary loss of bodily control and its aftermath, and the dependence imposed by activity restrictions contribute to the increased incidence of comorbid depression and anxiety in people with epilepsy (up to 50%).

In many people with epilepsy, seizures predominate in sleep due to increased synchronization of neuronal activity. Seizures that occur exclusively in sleep constitute nocturnal epilepsy. In women with epilepsy (WWE), seizures sometimes occur more often during the week around menses or at ovulation (catamenial epilepsy). Sleep deprivation, alcohol consumption, intercurrent infections, certain medications, and marked emotional stress can further lower the seizure threshold and increase the risk of seizures in people with epilepsy (see Table 120.1).

As indicated earlier, provoked seizures are highly prevalent, accompanying many acute medical or neurologic conditions. Ten percent of the population in developed countries will have a seizure at some time during their lifetime. In contrast, approximately 1% of the population has current epilepsy (prevalence) and 3% to 4% have epilepsy at some time during their life (lifetime prevalence). In the United States, there are approximately 125,000 new cases of epilepsy diagnosed each year (incidence). Epilepsy occurs across the age spectrum. However, its incidence and prevalence are biphasic, more common in childhood (primarily because of perinatal injury, infections, and genetic factors) and with advancing age (because of stroke, tumors, and dementia) (Fig. 120.1). In developing countries, the frequency of epilepsy is higher, largely due to the increased burden of CNS infections such as neurocysticercosis.

PATHOLOGY

Prior to the 1990s, the underlying cause of a patient's epilepsy was frequently unsolved. The advent of MRI and, more recently, genetic and immunologic investigations has substantially improved our ability to identify the causes of many epilepsies. About 70% of adults and 40% of children with new-onset epilepsy have focal onset seizures, usually implying a focal cerebral injury or lesion. In parallel with the diversity of seizure types and epilepsies, there is a similarly wide variety of epilepsy-associated pathologies. The most common lesions are hippocampal sclerosis, neuronal and glial tumors, vascular malformations, neuronal migration disorders (e.g., cortical dysplasia), hamartomas, encephalitis, paraneoplastic and related autoimmune mechanisms, cerebral trauma, embolic stroke, and hemorrhage.

Hippocampal sclerosis (sometimes referred to as mesial temporal sclerosis) remains one of the more common and distinctive pathologies and can occur in isolation or secondary to another coincident epileptogenic lesion (dual pathology). It consists of loss of pyramidal cells and gliosis in several hippocampal subfields. Hippocampal sclerosis is associated with temporal lobe epilepsy and often with short-term memory dysfunction. The group of neuronal migration disorders has also been brought to light with wider use of brain imaging, especially MRI. Focal cortical dysplasia (FCD) represents one of the more common examples of such pathologies. These involve zones of dystrophic gray matter located out of place such as in the subcortical white matter, often with distorted neuronal architecture. Microscopy sometimes reveals atypical cells that exhibit both glial and neuronal markers (e.g.,

TABLE 120.1   Causes of Symptomatic Seizures[a]

Acute Electrolyte Disorders
Acute hyponatremia (<120 mEq/L)
Acute hypernatremia (>155 mEq/L)
Hyperosmolality (>310 mOsm/L)
Hypocalcemia (<7 mg/dL)
Hypomagnesemia (<0.8 mEq/L)
Hypoglycemia (<30 mg/dL)
Hyperglycemia (>450 mg/dL)

Drugs
Quinolone antibiotics, isoniazid, carbapenems, penicillins (in renal insufficiency)
Theophylline, aminophylline, ephedrine, phenylpropanolamine, terbutaline
Tramadol, lidocaine, meperidine (in renal insufficiency), fentanyl
Tricyclic antidepressants (especially clomipramine), bupropion, clozapine, neuroleptics
Cyclosporine, chlorambucil
Cocaine (crack), phencyclidine, amphetamines; alcohol withdrawal, benzodiazepine and barbiturate withdrawal

Central Nervous System Disease
Hypertensive encephalopathy, eclampsia
Hepatic and uremic encephalopathy
Sickle cell disease, thrombotic thrombocytopenic purpura
Systemic lupus erythematosus
Meningitis, encephalitis, brain abscess
Acute head trauma, stroke, brain tumor

[a]The metabolic derangements and drugs listed in here also lower the seizure threshold in people with epilepsy.

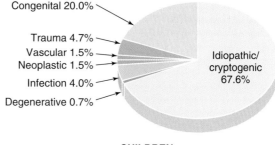

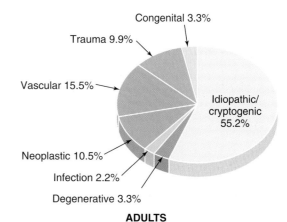

Fig. 120.1 Etiology of epilepsy, according to age, in all newly diagnosed cases in Rochester, Minnesota, 1935-1984. (Modified from Hauser WA, Annegers JF, Kurland LT: Incidence of epilepsy and unprovoked seizures in Rochester, Minnesota: 1935-1984, Epilepsia 34:453-468, 1993.)

balloon cells of type IIb FCDs). Not all patients with cerebral lesions develop epilepsy nor do all lesions in a single patient equally contribute to the epileptic phenotype; how or why a particular lesion becomes epileptogenic remains poorly understood.

Hereditary influences have long been associated with epilepsy. During the past several decades, many gene mutations have been linked with specific epilepsy syndromes, including those with either focal or generalized seizure types. Many such gene mutations affect ion channel proteins, which, not surprisingly, lead to neuronal dysfunction and epilepsy. These have been collectively termed channelopathies. Two important examples of channelopathies are genetic (generalized) epilepsy with febrile seizures plus (GEFS+) and Dravet syndrome. These genetically related syndromes have markedly different phenotypes. GEFS+ is typically associated with a partial loss of function mutation in the voltage-gated sodium channel gene, *SCN1A*, whereas a complete loss of function mutation in the same gene results in Dravet syndrome. Less commonly, mutations in other ion channel genes can also lead to the same phenotypes. GEFS+ can begin at any age, although it is usually evident in childhood, with various seizure types in different affected family members; some have febrile seizures after age 6 years (febrile seizures plus), whereas others may have myoclonic, absence, or partial seizures. In contrast, Dravet syndrome typically presents at 6 to 8 months of age with prolonged hemi-clonic seizures associated with an intercurrent fever. Children with Dravet syndrome often develop cognitive deficits, spasticity or ataxia, and occasionally nocturnal clonic seizures plus other seizure types.

The newly recognized group of paraneoplastic and autoimmune epilepsies constitute a very different etiologic process and pathology. These conditions arise either in the context of a systemic malignancy that triggers an aberrant immune attack on specific CNS targets or arise spontaneously (autoimmune). In many cases, MRIs may show multifocal signal changes in various cortical and limbic CNS regions. These syndromes can increasingly be diagnosed by serum or CSF assays for specific antibodies reactive to specific CNS antigens. Some antigens are intracellular (e.g., Hu), while others are membrane bound (e.g., the NMDA receptor).

CLASSIFICATION AND CLINICAL MANIFESTATIONS
Seizures

Various classification strategies have been used over decades to help sort out the diversity of seizure types and epilepsies. In 2017, the International League Against Epilepsy (ILAE) published their most recently revised seizure and epilepsy classification, which makes salient changes to its predecessors, including changes to core terminology. The new system offers important advantages, but since several terms from earlier systems persist in common clinical use, this section will occasionally reference both sets of terms, new and old, where felt helpful.

Seizure classification will be addressed first. Seizures are classified by their clinical symptoms and signs. The manifestations of a seizure depend upon whether its onset includes broad bilateral cortical regions or only a part of the cerebral cortex and reflect the functions of the involved cortical areas and the subsequent pattern of spread within the brain. Seizures are now initially subdivided into three broad types: those with onset limited to a specific region of cerebral cortex (*focal seizures*), those with onset involving the cerebral cortex diffusely and bilaterally (*generalized seizures*), and a new third group in the 2017 classification for *seizures of unknown onset*. (Note that in the 1981 classification, focal seizures were also called partial seizures. The term

TABLE 120.2 Localization of Seizures by Symptoms and Ictal Manifestations

Locus	Manifestation
Temporal Lobe	
Uncus/amygdala	Foul odor
Middle/inferior temporal gyrus	Visual changes: micropsia, macropsia
Parahippocampal-hippocampal area	Déjà vu; jamais vu
Amygdala-septal area	Fear, pleasure, anger, dreamy sensation
Auditory association cortex	Voices, music
Insular, anterior temporal cortex	Lip smacking, drooling, abdominal symptoms, cardiac arrhythmia
Frontal Lobe	
Motor cortex	Contralateral clonic movements of face, fingers, hand, foot
Premotor cortex	Contralateral arm extension, hypermotor behaviors
Language areas	Speech arrest, aphasia
Lateral cortex	Contralateral eye deviation
Bifrontal	Absence-like seizure
Parietal lobe cortex	Sensory symptoms
Occipital lobe cortex	Visual hallucinations (often in color), teichopsias, metamorphopsias

"partial seizure" has been set aside in the updated version, though this descriptor is still frequently encountered in practice.) Among focal seizure types, the next criterion relates to the retention or impairment of awareness. (In the 1981 version, "simple partial seizure" was used to indicate a *focal seizure with retained awareness*, the currently used term. Similarly, a "complex partial seizure" in 1981 parlance now corresponds to a *focal seizure with impaired awareness*.)

The next criterion relates to specific focal seizure related symptoms, motor or nonmotor, that predominate early on (Table 120.2), reflecting the distinct functions of the various CNS regions that are engaged. Focal seizures are dynamic, with evolving patterns of spread within the brain. Thus, focal seizures with preserved awareness (previously "simple partial seizures" or "auras") often progress into more widespread focal seizures with impaired awareness (previously "complex partial seizures") and can spread further still to become *focal to bilateral tonic-clonic seizures* in the 2017 nomenclature (previously "secondarily generalized tonic-clonic seizures").

Generalized seizures at onset are subdivided into those with motor or nonmotor symptoms. Seizures of unknown onset are also subdivided in similar fashion. If the information is insufficient or if the seizure can't be classified, then it can be designated as "unclassified."

In an individual, seizures are typically stereotyped, although some patients have more than one seizure type and a specific seizure type often has varying intensities. The behaviors that occur during the seizure are termed the *seizure semiology*. The seizure itself is referred to as the *ictus* and the period of the actual seizure is termed the *ictal phase*. The period after the seizure has ended until the patient is fully recovered is the *postictal phase* (usually minutes to hours, but occasionally days to rarely 1 to 2 weeks) and the time between seizures (which can be seconds to years) is the *interictal phase*. Most routine outpatient EEGs are performed during the interictal phase. Long-term video-EEG monitoring, however, may also record examples of the ictal and early postictal phases. Specific seizure types are further illustrated later, followed by a description of several attendant epilepsy syndromes.

Focal Seizures

In some focal seizures, the abnormal neuronal firing may be so confined to a small non-eloquent patch of cortex that there is no clinical manifestation of the seizure, which can only be detected with EEG. This is termed a *subclinical* or *electrographic seizure*.

Focal Seizures With Preserved Awareness (Previously Simple Partial Seizures)

This seizure type occurs when the electrical discharge involves a small but clinically functional area. This manifests as a symptom without impairment of consciousness. The symptom may be a sensation, an autonomic symptom (e.g., nausea or other epigastric sensation), abnormal thought (e.g., fear, déjà vu), or involuntary movement. This type of seizure is also commonly called an *aura* and can serve as a warning symptom to the patient that a more intense seizure may follow. Auras occur in about 60% of patients with focal epilepsy. During a focal seizure with preserved awareness, the patient can interact normally with the environment except for any limitations imposed by the seizure itself on specific functions. Thus, some subdivide this category into subgroups with impairment (e.g., a jerking limb) or without impairment (e.g., only an internal sensation). Those focal seizures with preserved awareness but with impairment may be more apt to impede safe driving.

Focal Seizures With Impaired Awareness (Previously Complex Partial Seizures)

The degree of impaired awareness within this category varies considerably. The patient's eyes are almost always open during the ictus. The eyes may close after the seizure ends and the patient typically experiences some degree of postictal confusion, fatigue, and sometimes headache (often ipsilateral to the seizure focus). Focal seizures with impaired awareness typically last 1 to 2 minutes with a postictal state lasting a few minutes up to several hours. The specific signs and symptoms that occur during such a focal seizure characteristically reflect the location of seizure onset (see Table 120.2). The location of the focus is important because it can predict the nature of the pathology and directs diagnostic testing. As well, surgical treatment options are largely governed by the location of the seizure focus.

Focal to Bilateral Tonic-Clonic Seizures (Previously Secondarily Generalized Tonic-Clonic Seizures)

A focal-onset seizure that spreads throughout the brain leading to a convulsion is termed a *focal to bilateral tonic-clonic seizure*. Typically, the tonic phase consists of extensor posturing lasting 20 to 60 seconds followed by progressively longer periods of CNS inhibition manifesting as the clonic phase that lasts up to another minute before resolving. In some patients, a few clonic jerks precede the tonic-clonic sequence; in others, only a tonic or clonic phase occurs.

As a focal seizure transitions into a bilateral tonic-clonic seizure, the arm contralateral to the seizure focus may extend first, while the ipsilateral arm flexes at the elbow. This is termed the *figure-4 sign* and can aid in lateralization of the seizure focus. A loud *tonic-cry* may occur at the onset of a convulsion as air is forcibly expelled through tightly contracted vocal cords. The eyes are open and commonly described to roll upward. During a convulsion, breathing stops and cyanosis may develop. Foaming at the mouth may occur. Oral trauma, especially tongue laceration, is typical; this most commonly affects the lateral aspect of the mid-tongue. Urinary incontinence is common. Fecal incontinence is less so. First aid involves turning the patient onto their side as the seizure ends to allow saliva to drool from the mouth, decreasing the likelihood of aspiration. The tonic-clonic phase rarely lasts longer than 2 minutes, though witnesses commonly describe such convulsions as lasting 5 to 10 minutes or even longer. The CNS mechanisms that terminate such seizures are a matter of great research interest. Failure of seizure termination leads to convulsive status epilepticus. The postictal phase is marked by a transient deep stupor, followed in 15 to 30 minutes by a lethargic, confused state. Occasionally, this period of immediate post convulsive stupor is accompanied by profound suppression of EEG activity (postictal generalized EEG suppression, PGES). As recovery progresses, many patients complain of headache, muscle soreness, mental dulling, lack of energy, or mood changes lasting hours to days. Rarely, patients may report feeling not fully back to normal for 1 to 2 weeks. Convulsions result in many striking, transient physiologic changes, including hypoxemia, lactic acidosis, elevated catecholamine levels, and increased serum concentrations of creatine phosphokinase, prolactin, corticotropin, and cortisol. Complications include oral trauma, vertebral compression fractures, shoulder dislocation, aspiration pneumonia, and, very rarely, sudden death, which may relate to acute pulmonary edema, cardiac arrhythmia, or respiratory failure. Recent research has explored whether transient PGES may predict a greater risk of sudden unexplained death in epilepsy (SUDEP). The contributors and mechanisms of SUDEP are still incompletely understood.

Focal seizures of all intensities may be followed by transient neurologic dysfunction reflecting postictal depression of the epileptogenic cortical area. Thus, focal weakness may follow a focal motor seizure or numbness may follow a sensory seizure. These reversible neurologic deficits are collectively referred to as *Todd paralysis* and last minutes to hours, rarely more than 48 hours. Examination of a patient immediately after a seizure may show transient focal abnormalities that help implicate the site or side of seizure origin.

Generalized Seizures

Generalized seizures begin diffusely and involve both cerebral hemispheres simultaneously from the outset. Generalized seizures should be distinguished from focal to bilateral tonic-clonic seizures because, while in many instances they have similar clinical features, they may respond better to different treatments. These are subdivided into motor and nonmotor categories.

Nonmotor generalized seizures include *typical absence seizures* (historically termed "petit mal"). These occur mainly in children and are characterized by sudden, momentary lapses in awareness with staring. Sometimes eye fluttering occurs with a slight loss of neck tone. Many absence seizures last less than 15 seconds. If the absence lasts longer than 20 seconds, automatisms are usually present, making differentiation from focal seizures with impaired awareness and motor automatisms difficult. The EEG has a characteristic pattern of generalized 3-per-second spikes and slow waves (Fig. 120.2) during a typical absence seizure. Behavior and awareness typically return to normal immediately after the seizure ends. There is no postictal period and usually no recollection that a seizure occurred.

Atypical absence seizures somewhat clinically resemble typical absence seizures (discussed previously). These also involve staring or mental slowing but instead are associated with a slower generalized spike and slow wave discharge (2.5 Hz or less) on EEG. Also, atypical absence seizures may last longer than typical absence seizures, up to many minutes. Fluctuating levels of awareness, gradual onset and offset, and occasional hypotonia are notable features of atypical absence seizures that differentiate them from typical (3 Hz) absence seizures.

Among the motor group of generalized onset seizures, several patterns will be highlighted, including myoclonic, tonic-clonic, tonic, and atonic seizures. *Myoclonic seizures* manifest as rapid, recurrent, brief muscle jerks that can occur unilaterally or bilaterally, synchronously or asynchronously, without loss of consciousness. Myoclonic seizures may affect the limbs, face, eyes or eyelids and may be of variable amplitude. Myoclonic seizures have a corresponding discharge on EEG. Other types of noncortical myoclonus that lack an EEG correlate, such as benign nocturnal (hypnic) jerks, or subcortical and spinal myoclonus, are not considered epileptic seizures. Repeated myoclonic seizures may crescendo and evolve into a generalized tonic-clonic seizure (called myoclonic-tonic-clonic seizures). Although myoclonic seizures can occur at any time, clusters of such shortly after awakening are typical.

Generalized onset tonic-clonic seizures may begin with a few myoclonic jerks or abruptly with a tonic phase lasting 20 to 60 seconds, followed then by a clonic phase of similar duration, then by a postictal state. Although there are usually no focal features, head turning occasionally occurs; this movement does not suggest a specific localization. If the onset of this seizure type is missed, it is often impossible to clinically distinguish a generalized onset tonic-clonic seizure from a focal to bilateral tonic-clonic seizure.

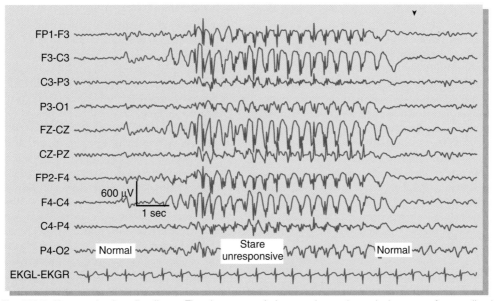

Fig. 120.2 Absence (petit mal) epilepsy. The electroencephalogram shows the typical pattern of generalized 3-Hz spike-wave complexes associated with a clinical absence seizure.

Tonic Seizures, Atonic Seizures, and Epileptic Spasms

Generalized onset *tonic seizures* are characterized by a sudden marked increase in tone, usually involving bilateral limbs and torso. They are more apt to occur during sleep and are typically brief, under 20 seconds. If standing, these seizures may lead to falls with associated injuries, including head injuries. Generalized onset *atonic seizures* are denoted by a sudden loss of tone affecting the head, limbs or torso. If standing, the patient may fall due to loss of tone, with associated risk of injuries. Head protective gear may be helpful. Such seizures are brief, usually less than 15 seconds. They are often referred to as drop attacks or drop seizures. *Epileptic spasms* are very brief attacks that may cluster and are classically denoted by sudden flexion of the trunk and simultaneous flexion or extension of the limbs. Epileptic spasms manifest as flexor or extensor tonus, myoclonus, or a mixed pattern. The spasms last 1 to 20 seconds each and often occur in clusters for up to 20 minutes. Epileptic spasms often occur in infancy with several forms of early life epilepsies (see later).

EPILEPSIES

Epilepsy classification is governed by the seizure type(s) expressed by that form of epilepsy. This is primarily driven on clinical grounds but is supported by EEG findings, imaging or other metrics. The epilepsies are now divided into four major categories: focal epilepsy, generalized epilepsy (also known as idiopathic or genetic generalized epilepsy), combined generalized and focal epilepsy, and unknown epilepsy. Within each category are epilepsy syndromes. Reflex epilepsy syndromes may reside in either the generalized or the focal epilepsies. Epilepsy syndromes involve a cluster of features such as seizure types, EEG findings, imaging findings, age of onset, prognosis, comorbidities, family history, and genetics. Epilepsy etiology is a major feature in epilepsy classification. There are six main etiologies: structural, genetic, infectious, metabolic, immune, and unknown. Examples of structural epilepsies include post-stroke epilepsy, post-traumatic, tumor-related, postinfectious, and cortical maldevelopment. Genetic causes of epilepsy are being rapidly discovered. While some do run in pedigrees, many are found de novo in the affected patient. Absence of a clear family history does not exclude a genetic etiology. One family of genetic causes relates to channelopathies, or mutations in ion channels or receptors that regulate neuronal excitability. Another subset refers to gene mutations that disrupt neural development. Another subset relates to genes that disrupt metabolism (e.g., glucose transporter, or mitochondrial genes). The immune etiologies are some of the most recently recognized. Assays for various autoantibodies targeting distinct CNS antigens, both intracellular and cell surface, are becoming more commonplace in the work-up of certain acquired epilepsies. While some of these conditions are paraneoplastic in nature, others are more purely autoimmune in origin. These often have seizures as one principle facet of a symptom complex, which may also include neuropsychiatric, dystonic, or cognitive symptoms. These may be quite fulminant in presentation (e.g., the anti-NMDA receptor antibody syndrome). Some examples of common, distinctive, or illustrative epilepsy syndromes follow.

Focal Epilepsy

Focal epilepsies are characterized by recurrent focal seizures. As discussed previously, six etiologic categories aid our understanding of the epilepsies and are germane to classification. One group of self-limited focal epilepsies is thought to be due to genetic developmental anomalies that manifest in childhood and remit during puberty. Among the several syndromes of this type, the most common is *childhood epilepsy with centrotemporal spikes* (previously called benign epilepsy with centrotemporal spikes [BECTS] or benign rolandic epilepsy [BRE]).

Seizures usually begin between the ages of 3 and 12 years in an otherwise normal child. The seizures are focal and consist of brief hemifacial motor or sensory events with preserved awareness. Typically, there is twitching of one side of the face, speech arrest, drooling, and paresthesias of the face, gums, tongue, or inner cheeks. The affected child often points to their face and goes to a parent and holds on until it is over; the child then quickly resumes normal activity. Seizures may progress to include hemiclonic movements or hemitonic posturing. Focal to bilateral tonic-clonic seizures occasionally occur, usually during sleep. The parents may report only the convulsions, as the focal onset can be missed unless the child is carefully questioned. The EEG reveals distinctive, stereotyped epileptiform discharges over the central and midtemporal regions that are dramatically activated by sleep with a normal underlying background. Prognosis for this syndrome is good, as it is for most of the other self-limited focal epilepsy syndromes; the seizures disappear and the EEG normalizes by mid to late adolescence. Outcome is unaffected by treatment, but antiepileptic drugs (AEDs) can prevent recurrent attacks.

Another example within this group is the Panayiotopoulos syndrome (also known as early onset occipital epilepsy). This self-limited syndrome is associated with focal autonomic seizures, classically involving pallor, hypersalivation, and vomiting, occasionally with eye deviation and tonic-clonic activity. Most seizures arise from sleep, often within the first hour of sleep. Seizures are lengthy, 20 to 60 minutes. The EEG in the Panayiotopoulos syndrome shows high amplitude and sleep activated, unilateral or bilateral occipital spikes. Seizures may continue for 2 to 3 years after presentation but then abate. Prognosis is good.

Many focal epilepsies can be understood by their specific locale of focal seizure onset. Temporal lobe epilepsy is an example, as is frontal lobe epilepsy. Within each of these designations, one may be able to define the epilepsy further, as in mesial temporal lobe epilepsy, or supplementary motor frontal lobe epilepsy. Distinct etiologies may account for individual forms but the seizure semiology may be similar if the seizure onset zone is shared. For instance, a structural mesial temporal lobe epilepsy secondary to a ganglioglioma may involve identical seizures as would hippocampal sclerosis associated with long-standing mesial temporal lobe epilepsy. These acquired focal epilepsies are often classified based upon the cerebral lobe involved during the initial phase of the seizure. Temporal lobe epilepsy is the most frequent, followed by frontal, then by rarer cases of parietal and occipital lobe epilepsies. Most cases of focal epilepsy entail a single seizure focus. However, the focus can sometimes involve a large, multilobar circuit. Some patients have multiple foci, each associated with a different seizure semiology.

Temporal lobe epilepsy (TLE) is the most common epilepsy syndrome of adults, accounting for at least 40% of epilepsy cases. There is a history of childhood febrile seizures in a subset. Most patients have focal onset seizures with impaired awareness, some of which evolve to focal to bilateral tonic-clonic seizures. Medial temporal lobe seizures involve the hippocampus and/or amygdala. A rising epigastric sensation or vague cephalic sensation is the most commonly reported aura. Less frequently, the classical symptoms of a foul smell, déjà vu, or other stereotyped altered thinking may occur. Olfactory auras have been called uncinate seizures because of their origin in or near the uncus of the medial temporal lobe. In lateral (neocortical) temporal lobe seizures, language impairment (dominant hemisphere), recurring vocalizations (nondominant hemisphere), eye blinking, or formed visual or auditory hallucinations can occur. As a temporal lobe seizure spreads to involve the dominant temporal lobe or bilateral temporal lobe structures, including the limbic system, the seizure evolves to impair awareness. A blank stare is often described by witnesses. Automatic motor behaviors, termed *automatisms*, are common in seizures that involve the limbic system (usually in the temporal lobe). Automatisms include oroalimentary signs (e.g., lip-smacking, repetitive swallowing) and repetitive hand movements (manual automatisms).

Frontal lobe epilepsy (FLE) can be more difficult to diagnose because the scalp EEG may be normal or not reveal a classic epileptic discharge, even with ictal recordings. There are at least four different premotor frontal lobe seizure semiologic patterns, with differing localization. *Supplementary motor* seizures (superior frontal gyri, posterior aspect) consist of contralateral versive posturing of the head and arms in a so-called "fencer posture"; the contralateral arm is extended, the head is turned strongly to that side, and the ipsilateral arm is flexed and held either up above the head or across the chest. *Lateral frontal* seizures manifest as contralateral head and eye deviation. *Hypermotor* seizures (frontal, poorly localized) consist of wild asynchronous movements and are often confused with psychogenic nonepileptic attacks. Almost all hypermotor seizures last less than 40 seconds and typically occur one to five times per night during sleep and less often during waking. *Frontal absence* seizures are rare and due to diffuse, bisynchronous frontal epileptic activity. These consist of staring and mimic typical or atypical absence seizures. Seizures arising in the posterior frontal lobe motor cortex (precentral gyrus) are classically clonic with a Jacksonian march.

Reflex epilepsies are distinguished by seizures that are precipitated by a specific stimulus such as touch, a musical tune, a specific movement, reading, flashing lights, or certain complex visual images. Apart from the photosensitive response in juvenile myoclonic epilepsy (see later), which is relatively common, reflex seizures are rare and are classified as a type of parietal or occipital lobe epilepsy because these regions mediate sensory functions.

Focal post-traumatic epilepsy is a common etiologic type of structural epilepsy. The likelihood of developing post-traumatic epilepsy relates directly to the severity of the head injury. The relative risk for developing epilepsy after a penetrating wound to the brain (e.g., bullet or shrapnel) is up to 600 times that of the general population. Severe closed head injuries result in epilepsy in 20% of patients. Severe closed head injuries are defined by the presence of intracranial hemorrhage of various types, unconsciousness or amnesia lasting more than 24 hours, or persistent abnormalities on neurologic examination, such as hemiparesis or aphasia. Although most patients with epilepsy following severe traumatic brain injury develop seizures within 1 to 2 years of their head injury, new-onset epilepsy may appear after 20 years or longer from the insult. Mild closed head injuries (uncomplicated brief loss of consciousness, no skull fracture, absence of focal neurologic signs, and no contusion or hematoma) may minimally increase the risk of seizures. Post-traumatic epilepsy is always focal or multifocal.

Idiopathic or Genetic Generalized Epilepsy

Both terms, "idiopathic" and "genetic," for this subset of the generalized epilepsies have advocates and critics among experts. *Idiopathic* in this context is meant to imply "self or genetic" in origin. Genetic often suggests that these forms of epilepsy are inherited and track within a family tree. However, often there is no helpful family history and so some of these instances probably arise de novo in affected individuals. The idiopathic (or genetic) generalized epilepsies (IGEs) are likely polygenic, resulting from a combination of mutations and polymorphisms in genes involved in thalamocortical circuitry. Different members within a family carrying these traits often exhibit dissimilar phenotypes. However, only rare IGE genes have been identified. A person with IGE has a 10% chance of passing the condition to a child. Most people with IGE have normal intelligence. Four entities comprise this group and are described later.

Childhood absence epilepsy (CAE; pyknolepsy, petit mal epilepsy) begins between 4 and 10 years of age with a peak at 7 years. Children with CAE have frequent absences (often dozens per day) and are sometimes initially thought to have attentional problems or to be day-dreamers. The absences occur throughout the day. Some children with CAE have occasional generalized tonic-clonic seizures (GTCs). CAE is usually self-limited and seizures and EEG abnormalities resolve by young adulthood in most. The absence seizures of CAE are typically provoked by hyperventilation, a useful procedure in the office setting and during an EEG. The ictal EEG findings of CAE include abrupt and bilaterally synchronous 3-Hz spike and wave discharges, lasting 4 to 20 seconds with loss of responsiveness. Interictal EEGs show brief generalized spike and wave discharges in isolation or in brief bursts lasting a few seconds. Occipital intermittent rhythmic delta activity (OIRDA) is a less frequent finding.

Juvenile myoclonic epilepsy (JME) begins between ages 5 to 34 years old, with peak onset in the mid-teens, and is highly prevalent. JME exhibits a distinctive age-related expression of diverse seizure types, some of which have a clear nonrandom relationship to the sleep-wake cycle. As the name suggests, myoclonic seizures are a core feature; essentially all with JME have myoclonic seizures, though they may be occasionally subtle. Clusters of myoclonic seizures occur most commonly in the morning, usually soon after awakening. The clustered myoclonic seizures typically persist for up to 30 minutes. Myoclonic jerks predominantly affect the arms and last less than 1 second each. Consciousness is preserved with these events. Affected patients may often fail to mention their morning jerks unless specifically asked. Generalized tonic-clonic seizures often occur as well, often arising a bit later in adolescence or into the early 20s. This seizure type often brings the patient to neurologic attention. In JME, GTC seizures are more common after sleep deprivation or alcohol consumption the prior night. People with JME are usually photosensitive. That is, the seizures and EEG discharges are activated by flickering lights between 5 to 20 Hz (*photoparoxysmal* or *photoconvulsive* responses). This is a type of reflex seizure. Between 20% and 40% of patients with JME also have absence seizures. Absences in JME arise several years prior to the appearance of myoclonic seizures. The EEG in JME is like that of CAE, but the generalized discharges are slightly faster (classically 4 to 6 Hz) and often have polyspike components over a normal waking background rhythm. Unlike CAE, seizures in JME persist into adulthood and can be lifelong.

Less common IGE phenotypes include *juvenile absence epilepsy (JAE)* and epilepsy with *generalized tonic-clonic seizures alone (EGTCS)*. In JAE the predominant seizure type is absence with peak onset in the early teenage years and, unlike CAE, persists into adulthood. Absences are numerous. GTC seizures occur frequently as well, but myoclonic seizures are less common in JAE. In EGTCS, the predominant seizure type is a GTC seizure. These GTCs often occur within 1 to 2 hours of awakening but can occur anytime. EGTCS arises between 5 and 40 years of age, most often in the teens, and is not a self-limited epilepsy.

Combined Generalized and Focal Epilepsy

This category includes those epilepsies in which patients may have both focal and generalized seizures. Similarly, EEGs of these patients may exhibit both focal and generalized epileptiform patterns. This new epilepsy category includes a subgroup presently called developmental and epileptic encephalopathies, that were previously termed the symptomatic generalized epilepsies (ILAE, 1989 classification). Individuals with these epilepsies have multifocal or diffuse brain dysfunction since early in life. There is an associated encephalopathy with variable developmental delay. Important examples of the developmental and epileptic encephalopathies are Lennox-Gastaut syndrome (LGS), infantile spasms, and Dravet syndrome.

LGS is a more common form of combined generalized and focal epilepsy. LGS presents from 2 to 10 years of age. It is characterized by the presence of multiple seizure types, usually a combination of tonic or atonic seizures, myoclonic seizures, and atypical absences, and with a characteristic EEG pattern of 2.5 Hz or slower generalized spike and slow wave discharges, in the setting of intellectual disability. Sixty percent have preexisting encephalopathy and developmental delay and up to 25% had infantile spasms earlier in their course. Tonic-clonic and focal seizures also occur. Sleep EEG recordings reveal bursts of diffuse 10- to 20-Hz rhythms with or without coincident tonic seizures. LGS is a chronic condition requiring supervision; many patients ultimately live in group homes. If drop seizures are present, and the patient is ambulatory, a protective helmet should be considered.

Infantile spasms are often a precursor to LGS. Infantile spasms usually begin during the first year of life, rarely beyond 18 months. *West syndrome* is the combination of epileptic spasms in infancy, hypsarrhythmia (a chaotic, disorganized epileptiform EEG pattern), and arrest of psychomotor development. The term infantile spasms is often used synonymously with West syndrome. Numerous etiologies can give rise to infantile spasms. Diagnostic evaluation may uncover an etiology in up to two thirds of cases. Common etiologies include CNS malformations such as cortical dysplasia, neurocutaneous disorders such as tuberous sclerosis complex, various metabolic disorders of infancy (e.g., phenylketonuria), congenital infections, genetic causes (e.g., chromosomal disorders, specific genetic abnormalities), plus other peri- and postnatal CNS insults. Infantile spasms have a poor prognosis with over 90% developing intellectual disability and most progressing to LGS; a small percent of usually cryptogenic cases have a more favorable outcome.

Dravet syndrome (previously severe myoclonic epilepsy of infancy) is both a genetic epilepsy and a developmental and epileptic encephalopathy. Children with Dravet syndrome have refractory epilepsy including multiple seizure types. Seizures commonly present within the first year of life, rarely during the second year. Affected children have normal development up to their presentation with seizures but then experience neurodevelopmental delay. Their initial seizure is typically a prolonged febrile tonic-clonic seizure, either unilateral or bilateral. More often, this is in the context of a febrile illness or recent vaccination, or less frequently with bathing. No precipitants are found in one third. Within weeks to months of this first seizure, more seizures follow, febrile or afebrile, often including bouts of status epilepticus. These may include hemiclonic seizures amongst others; these can even alternate sides. Seizures can be readily triggered by a variety of stimuli. Treatment-resistant seizures are accompanied by psychomotor impairment beginning months after the sentinel seizure. Cognitive, behavioral, language, gait, and other motor impairments accrue. EEGs show both focal and generalized epileptiform patterns and may vary with age. Mutations in the voltage-gated sodium channel, alpha-1 gene (SCN1A) are responsible for this syndrome in 70% to 80% of cases. Recognition of Dravet syndrome is important because voltage-gated sodium channel blocking AEDs (e.g., lamotrigine, phenytoin) can cause clinical deterioration, whereas others are particularly beneficial (e.g., topiramate, levetiracetam, valproate, benzodiazepines).

Other Seizure Conditions

Febrile seizures affect 3% to 5% of children younger than the age of 6 years. About 30% of children have more than one episode; recurrence is more likely if the first seizure occurs before 1 year of age or there is a family history of febrile seizures. Several distinct gene mutations predispose to febrile seizures. Although most affected children have no long-term consequences and appear to outgrow this age-restricted trait, febrile seizures increase the risk of later epilepsy. This risk is low for most children (2% to 3%) but increases to 10% to 15% in those with prolonged or focal febrile seizures (*complicated febrile seizures*), a family history of nonfebrile seizures, or neurologic abnormalities that predate their first febrile seizure.

DIAGNOSIS

Accurate diagnosis is the cornerstone of epilepsy care. The diagnostic evaluation has three objectives: (1) to determine whether the patient's spell(s) are epileptic seizures, (2) to identify a specific underlying cause, and (3) to establish if the seizures are provoked and isolated, or if epilepsy is present and, if so, to determine the type of epilepsy, ideally the specific epilepsy syndrome.

History and Examination

The patient's and witnesses' descriptions of the events are central to diagnosis. The patient's recall of their seizure may be spotty due to associated amnesia surrounding the episode, and so the witnesses' descriptions are often more helpful. Attention should be paid to details of the patient's behavior before, during, and after the seizure. The setting of the seizure can suggest acute causes such as drug withdrawal, CNS infection, trauma, stroke, or other contributing or provoking factors. Recent-onset seizures in an adult may suggest a new intracranial process. A prior history of seizures suggests epilepsy. Any focal feature before, during, or after the seizure may suggest a possible structural brain lesion requiring appropriate investigation. The pattern of the seizures and the patient's age are often important clues to the seizure and epilepsy type.

The physical examination is normal in most patients with epilepsy. Examination should seek overt or subtle focal neurologic signs: slight unilateral lower facial paresis, clumsy fine finger movements, or mild hyperreflexia. These can be present in patients with epilepsy with a contralateral seizure focus. Careful skin examination is indicated to detect features of neurocutaneous syndromes such as a facial port-wine stain involving the upper eyelid in Sturge-Weber syndrome, hypopigmented macules (ash-leaf spots), shagreen patch (pink, elevated skin nodules with "orange peel" appearance found in the lumbar area), facial angiofibromas in tuberous sclerosis, and café-au-lait spots and axillary freckling in neurofibromatosis. Asymmetry in the size of the hands, feet, or face may signify a long-standing abnormality of the cerebral hemisphere contralateral to the smaller side. Absence seizures can be triggered during an office examination in untreated children with CAE with hyperventilation for 2 to 3 minutes.

Laboratory Tests—EEG

EEG is the most helpful diagnostic test for seizures and epilepsy. EEG findings help confirm the diagnosis, classify the seizures, identify the epilepsy syndrome, and impact therapeutic decisions. Epilepsy remains a largely clinical diagnosis, informed by EEG and other test findings. In combination with suitable clinical findings, *epileptiform* EEG discharges, termed *spikes* or *sharp waves*, strongly support a diagnosis of epilepsy. In patients with recurrent seizures, focal epileptiform discharges are consistent with epilepsies with focal onset seizures, whereas generalized epileptiform activity usually indicates a generalized form of epilepsy (associated with seizures of generalized onset). Most EEGs are obtained between seizures, and such interictal abnormalities alone cannot prove or disprove a diagnosis of epilepsy. Up to 50% of patients with epilepsy show epileptiform abnormalities on their initial EEG. The chance of capturing epileptiform activity is enhanced by sleep deprivation the night before the test, which increases the likelihood of recording drowsiness and light sleep during the EEG. Serial EEGs also increase the yield of a positive test. Some neurologists rely on prolonged EEG monitoring studies to record much more data including more sleep samples. Supplemental T1 and T2 electrodes can occasionally benefit the yield of the EEG. A small proportion of patients with epilepsy have normal interictal EEGs despite all efforts to record an abnormality.

The interpretation of the interictal EEG is confounded by two factors. Epileptiform discharges occur in about 2% of normal people; many of these may be asymptomatic markers of a genetic trait, especially in children. Also, the interpretation of the EEG is subjective. Normal benign variant waveforms and artifacts can be occasionally misinterpreted as epileptiform activity and erroneously considered to indicate seizure susceptibility.

Epilepsy can be definitively established by recording a characteristic ictal discharge during a representative clinical attack. This is uncommon during routine EEGs but can often be accomplished with *video-EEG long-term monitoring (LTM)*. This can be performed in the outpatient setting (ambulatory video-EEG LTM) or in the inpatient setting at many epilepsy centers throughout the world. The inpatient setting permits AED tapering as needed in a safe setting to increase the odds of eliciting one or more seizures for characterization, whereas this is not the case for ambulatory LTM. Inpatient video-EEG monitoring is indicated in people who have ongoing seizures despite treatment with appropriate AEDs. About one third of patients admitted for LTM are found not to have epilepsy. The majority of these patients have psychogenic nonepileptic attacks. A much smaller subset of patients with nonepileptic seizures have other physiologic mimics of epileptic seizures (e.g., certain movement disorders). In the approximately 30% of people with treatment-resistant epilepsy (those with seizures despite trials of multiple AEDs, alone or in combination), inpatient video-EEG monitoring to more precisely define the seizure focus is a critical step toward determining candidacy for various epilepsy surgery options. Phase I LTM involves scalp EEG recordings. A subset of patients require phase II LTM studies in which electrodes are neurosurgically implanted in or on the brain to more precisely localize the seizure onset zone and map critical functional cortical regions nearby. Recently, stereotactically placed depth leads have been gaining popularity for such investigations in many tertiary epilepsy centers in the United States.

Laboratory Tests—Neuroimaging

Brain MRI complements EEG findings by identifying structural pathology that is causally related to the development of epilepsy. MRI is the best test to detect epileptogenic cerebral lesions including hippocampal sclerosis, neuronal migration disorders, tumors, focal atrophy, arteriovenous malformations, and cavernous malformations. It is important to obtain a complete imaging study that includes T1-weighted, T2-weighted, and inversion-recovery sequences in coronal and axial planes. Contrast can also be helpful for some epilepsy pathologies. Imaging in the coronal plane perpendicular to the long axis of the hippocampus has improved detection of hippocampal atrophy and increased T2 signal, findings that correlate with the pathologic finding of hippocampal sclerosis and an epileptogenic temporal lobe. Additional sequences that should be routine include T2-weighted gradient echo (GRE), to detect hemosiderin indicating prior hemorrhage associated with vascular malformations or trauma, and diffusion-weighted images (DWI) for cytotoxic edema, sometimes present with acute cerebral injury from prolonged seizures or status epilepticus. In 2019, many tertiary centers in the United States offered 3T MRI. This provides improved resolution over lower strength MRIs and can aid in detecting smaller lesions such as very small cortical dysplasias.

An MRI should be obtained in all patients with suspected epilepsy with the exception that many pediatric epileptologists view MRI as optional for patients with definite childhood epilepsy with centrotemporal spikes or definite generalized genetic epilepsies (e.g., CAE and JME). CT scan with contrast is an alternative study for those who cannot have MRI but has lower resolution than MRI for detecting small lesions. Any patient with seizures and abnormal neurologic findings or focal slow-wave abnormalities on EEG should have neuroimaging. Repeat neuroimaging should be considered if there is an unexplained change in seizure pattern, to evaluate for a new lesion, or in those with possible low-grade neoplastic lesions.

Positron emission tomography (PET) and single-photon emission computed tomography (SPECT) use physiologically active, radiolabeled tracers to image the brain's metabolic activity and are useful adjunctive imaging methods for certain patients seeking a surgical treatment option for their epilepsy. SPECT is most useful when an ictal and interictal study are combined to identify an extratemporal seizure focus. Abnormalities on PET or SPECT can be present when brain MRI is normal and thus add value in that scenario. PET has been most useful in treatment-resistant, MRI-negative, temporal lobe epilepsy.

Other Tests

Routine blood tests rarely offer diagnostic assistance in otherwise healthy patients with epilepsy. Serum electrolytes, liver function tests, and complete blood count are useful with acute new-onset seizures and as baseline studies before AED therapy is started. A mildly increased serum WBC count without a marked "left shift" is a common, but nonspecific, transient finding after convulsive seizures or status epilepticus. Serum CPK can also transiently increase postictally but is also nonspecific and no longer commonly obtained outside of the setting of suspected myonecrosis or rhabdomyolysis. Adolescents and adults with unexplained seizures should be screened for substance abuse (especially cocaine) with blood or urine studies. Genetic testing should be considered in specific cases with suspected phenotypes, especially if a positive genetic test would alter therapy, such as in SCN1A-associated epilepsies (e.g., Dravet syndrome). Lumbar puncture is indicated if there is a suspicion of meningitis, encephalitis, autoimmune or paraneoplastic process, or a CNS glucose transporter abnormality. Repeated generalized seizures and status epilepticus can increase cerebrospinal fluid protein measures slightly and produce a mild pleocytosis for 24 to 48 hours; cerebrospinal fluid pleocytosis should be attributed to seizures only in retrospect after excluding an intracranial inflammatory process. An electrocardiogram (ECG) should be obtained in any young person with a first generalized seizure if there is a family history of arrhythmia, sudden unexplained death, or episodic unconsciousness. An ECG should also be obtained in any patient with a personal history of cardiac arrhythmia or valvular disease.

DIFFERENTIAL DIAGNOSIS

Not every paroxysmal event is a seizure, and misidentification of other conditions leads to ineffective, unnecessary, and potentially harmful treatments plus delay to reach the correct diagnosis. Misdiagnosis accounts for a subset of patients who have not responded to AED treatment. The conditions confused with epilepsy depend on the age of the patient and the nature and circumstances of the attacks (Table 120.3). Nonepileptic paroxysmal disorders that are confused with epileptic seizures have sudden, discrete abnormal behaviors, variable responsiveness, changes in muscle tone, and various postures or movements.

Psychogenic nonepileptic seizures (PNES) frequently are misdiagnosed as intractable epilepsy in adults. PNES are felt to be due to unconscious emotional conflicts impacting the patient's physical state, mimicking a seizure (i.e., a somatoform manifestation of psychologic distress). Roughly 10% of patients with PNES also have epilepsy.

TABLE 120.3 Nonepileptic Episodic Disorders That May Resemble Seizures

Movement disorders: tic disorders, subcortical myoclonus, paroxysmal choreoathetosis, episodic ataxias, hyperekplexia (startle disease)

Migraine: confusional, vertebrobasilar, visual auras

Syncope (particularly convulsive syncope)

Behavioral and psychiatric: psychogenic nonepileptic seizures, hyperventilation syndrome, panic/anxiety disorder, dissociative states

Cataplexy (usually associated with narcolepsy), parasomnias

Transient ischemic attack (especially aphasic or limb-shaking)

Alcoholic blackouts

Hypoglycemia

Definitive diagnosis requires video-EEG documentation, although a history of atypical and nonstereotyped attacks, emotional or psychological precipitants, psychiatric illness, lack of response to AEDs, and repeatedly normal interictal EEGs suggests PNES as an alternate consideration. A substantial fraction of patients with PNES have experienced prior physical or sexual abuse. PNES are more common in females than in males and occur across a broad range of ages.

Panic attacks (anxiety attacks) with hyperventilation can superficially resemble focal seizures with affective, autonomic, or special sensory symptoms. Hyperventilation typically causes perioral and fingertip tingling. Prolonged hyperventilation results in muscle twitching or spasms (tetany); affected patients may faint.

Syncope refers to the symptom complex associated with a transient reduction in global cerebral perfusion associated with cardiovascular dysfunction. Loss of consciousness typically lasts only a few seconds, uncommonly a minute or more, and recovery is usually rapid. If the cerebral ischemia is sufficiently severe, the syncopal episode may include tonic posturing of the trunk or clonic jerks of the arms and legs and even incontinence (*convulsive syncope*). Convulsive syncope is a form of syncope, not seizure; it is a frequent mimic of epileptic seizures.

Some forms of *migraine* can be mistaken for seizures, especially if the headache is atypical or mild and/or when confusion occurs. The visual aura, present in some migraineurs, is typically black, gray, and white; a colored aura more often indicates an epileptic seizure. Basilar artery migraine, usually in children and young adults, can include lethargy, mood changes, confusion, disorientation, vertigo, bilateral visual disturbances, and loss of consciousness. This uncommon form of migraine may also mimic a seizure.

TIAs can occasionally mimic seizure and vice versa. The postictal phase of a seizure can be quite stroke-like in nature and typically resolves as do TIA-related symptoms. Seizures involving the language cortex often produce speech arrest—aphasia—as is more commonly encountered in association with TIA/stroke.

TREATMENT

If the cause of a provoked seizure is corrected, AEDs are usually not necessary. Adults with a single, unprovoked seizure and normal clinical, EEG, and imaging findings frequently do not have subsequent seizures. AEDs are usually not indicated if only one seizure has occurred in those instances. However, patients with abnormal focal findings on neurologic exam or abnormal radiologic or EEG findings are at higher risk for repeated seizures and may therefore be more often recommended AED treatment. In individual patients, social considerations may dictate treatment after a single seizure. Patients who have had repeated unprovoked seizures (>24 hours apart) are recommended for AED prophylaxis.

Medication Therapy

The goal in epilepsy care is complete seizure freedom. In the United States, as of 2019, there were 22 AEDs in standard use for epilepsy with several other medications sometimes used adjunctively. There is no ideal AED; all have potential toxic side effects and idiosyncratic reactions. For over one half of people with epilepsy, the appropriate AED for their type(s) of seizures can be highly effective and well tolerated. However, for 25% to 30% of people with epilepsy, no AED alone or in combination is completely effective (termed treatment-resistant or medically refractory epilepsy). Once the seizure type and epilepsy syndrome are determined, an initial and, if needed, subsequent AED, should be chosen based on both anticipated efficacy and toxicity profiles. All AEDs can cause sedation, cognitive dysfunction, and/or incoordination in some patients, especially at high blood levels. Various rare, sometimes life-threatening, reactions can occur with all the AEDs. Some common scenarios follow.

Genetic Generalized Epilepsy (CAE, JME, and Others)

- In all genetic generalized epilepsies, valproate or lamotrigine are first-line agents and result in complete seizure control in 85% to 90% of patients.
  - Valproate may promote weight gain in many patients and has been associated with hair loss in approximately 5%. It causes tremor in many in a dose-related manner. It poses an increased risk of teratogenicity relative to other AEDs. It can be associated with hyperammonemia and rare thrombocytopenia and liver function test abnormalities.
  - Lamotrigine has a small but significant risk of a severe rash (e.g., toxic epidermal necrolysis, Stevens Johnson syndrome [SJS]) for about the first several months after initiation. A slow dose escalation substantially lowers this risk. Much less severe allergic reactions (e.g., rash) can occur in 3% to 5%. Lamotrigine's metabolism is substantially inhibited by valproate, so in combination, lower doses of lamotrigine are required. Occasionally lamotrigine worsens myoclonus, but it is effective in most cases of JME.
- Second-line options include clobazam, topiramate, levetiracetam, and zonisamide. Levetiracetam is often used as an early option for JME, given its efficacy in myoclonic seizures.
- In childhood absence epilepsy with exclusively absence seizures, ethosuximide should be the first treatment choice. If any convulsions have occurred, valproate or lamotrigine should be used.
- If there is a history of more than 5 minutes of crescendo absences or myoclonus (often described as a "foggy" state) culminating in a convulsion, then oral benzodiazepines (lorazepam or diazepam) can occasionally help abort the cluster and prevent an impending convulsion.
- Absences and myoclonus can be exacerbated by carbamazepine, oxcarbazepine, and GABAergic compounds including gabapentin, pregabalin, and tiagabine. These AEDs should be avoided in the genetic generalized epilepsies.

Focal Epilepsy

- Almost all of the AEDs (except ethosuximide) can be effective in focal epilepsy. The choice of the first AED should be mainly guided by individualized side effect considerations, teratogenicity where appropriate, and pharmacokinetics.
- Phenytoin remains one of the most commonly used AEDs in focal epilepsy in developed countries. Patients presenting with initial seizures or status epilepticus to the emergency room are commonly "loaded" intravenously with phenytoin and subsequently continued. However, phenytoin has substantial short- and long-term

toxicity and its levels are difficult to regulate due to saturation kinetics and multiple drug interactions. Its toxicities include hirsutism, coarsening of features, and gingival hyperplasia, especially in children and adolescents. Long-term risks include osteomalacia, peripheral neuropathy, and cerebellar degeneration with risk of permanent incoordination. Peak level toxicities include nystagmus, ataxia, lethargy, and, if the level rises above 50, acute cerebellar degeneration and cardiac arrhythmias. Phenytoin poses an allergic risk to a subset, including the rare risk of SJS.

- Carbamazepine, oxcarbazepine, topiramate, levetiracetam, lamotrigine, and zonisamide are currently used as first-line therapy for partial seizures. Carbamazepine and oxcarbazepine can cause hyponatremia and allergic reactions, rarely severe in type (SJS). Topiramate can lead to weight loss but also has undesirable dose-dependent cognitive side effects and predisposes to renal stones (1%). Levetiracetam can cause undesirable mood changes, sometimes only transiently, sedation, and rare allergic risk, but is usually well tolerated. Lamotrigine needs to be titrated slowly due to its allergic risk (discussed previously). Zonisamide, which also can cause weight loss and predisposes to renal stones, has a long half-life (48 to 72 hours) so is a good option for less consistently compliant patients or those less successful with more than once-daily dosing. It can cause allergic reactions (including rarely severe ones).
- Patients of Asian ancestry should be tested for the HLA-B*1502 allele and patients of Northern European ancestry tested for the HLA-A*3101 allele prior to initiating treatment with carbamazepine, oxcarbazepine, and eslicarbazepine. Patients with these alleles are at increased risk of SJS and toxic epidermal necrolysis when exposed to these drugs.
- Adjunctive treatments for focal seizures include clobazam, valproate, pregabalin, lacosamide, gabapentin, perampanel, and primidone. The proportion of gabapentin that is absorbed decreases with increasing dose, limiting its effectiveness. For most, pregabalin may be a better choice.
- Phenobarbital is the most widely used AED in the world due to its low cost. However, it causes sedation, cognitive impairment, and poses a risk of bone loss and therefore should probably be avoided except in difficult to control epilepsy. The exception is in neonatal seizures where it remains one of the most commonly accepted AEDs.

Developmental and Epileptic Encephalopathies

- All AEDs have a role in the treatment of this category of epilepsies, but seizure freedom is rarely achieved. At a minimum, control of the more severe seizures, including drop seizures and convulsions, should be a central goal of therapy. AED polytherapy is usually required.
- Valproate is commonly the initial medication instituted.
- Added efficacy can occur with clobazam, lamotrigine, topiramate, levetiracetam, rufinamide, and zonisamide.
- Felbamate may be effective, but its use should be limited to epileptologists due to its significant risk of fatal aplastic anemia and liver failure.
- The vagus nerve stimulator (see later) has a specific role in reducing the severity of seizures in these conditions.
- Dravet syndrome and possibly the related syndrome of GEFS+ respond best to topiramate, levetiracetam, and benzodiazepines. Some voltage-gated sodium channel blocking AEDs, including lamotrigine and phenytoin, worsen Dravet syndrome.

Dosing of AEDs must be done with great care. Only a few AEDs are safe to load or start at a full therapeutic dose. Most should be started with a gradual dose escalation. Management guidelines are: (1) the type of seizures and epilepsy should be defined and the preferred medication for such should be given in usual starting doses and then increased until seizure control is complete or side effects occur (Table 120.4); (2) If seizures persist despite toxic levels, or if major side effects occur, another AED should be tried; (3) Do not stop one agent until another has been added (overlap during transitions). Otherwise, status epilepticus may occur; (4) If seizures persist after one to two AEDs have been given to toxic levels, consider referral to a specialized epilepsy center for further evaluation and treatment; (5) Toxic levels of some AEDs (e.g., phenytoin and carbamazepine) can cause seizures; (6) Extended release and longer acting AEDs are preferred for most patients; (7) Patients should be counseled to adhere to the medication regimen. Pill boxes should be encouraged. Medication noncompliance is a leading cause of poor seizure control.

Epilepsy Surgery

In most patients, epilepsy is controlled with AEDs. When seizures cannot be controlled by adequate trials of two appropriate single agents and/or by the combination of two agents, the epilepsy is termed

---

TABLE 120.4 Frequently Prescribed Antiepileptic Drugs

Nonproprietary AED Name	Adult Total Dose Per Day	Dose Frequency (in Hours)	"Therapeutic" Concentrations
Carbamazepine	600-1400 mg	6-8 (12 for sustained release)	4-12 µg/mL
Clobazam	10-40 mg	12	Unknown
Ethosuximide	500-1500 mg	8-12	40-100 µg/mL
Gabapentin	900-3600 mg	6-8	2-20 µg/mL
Lacosamide	200-600 mg	12	Unknown
Lamotrigine[a]	100-800 mg	12	2-18 µg/mL
Levetiracetam	500-3000 mg	12	10-45 µg/mL
Oxcarbazepine	900-2400 mg	8-12	10-35 µg/mL
Phenobarbital	60-240 mg	24	15-40 µg/mL
Phenytoin	200-600 mg	24	10-20 µg/mL
Pregabalin	100-600 mg	12	Unknown
Topiramate	50-400 mg	12	2-20 µg/mL
Valproate	500-5000 mg	8 (12-24 for sustained release)	50-125 µg/mL
Zonisamide	100-600 mg	24	10-40 µg/mL

[a]Slow initial dose titration mandatory for lamotrigine and often indicated for other agents. Daily dose targets are adjusted depending on co-administered AEDs.

treatment resistant (or *medically refractory*), a situation encountered in 25% to 30% of patients with epilepsy. Such patients are at risk for many consequences: inability to drive; stigmatization by schools, employers, and society; and threats to personal educational and occupational goals, possible cognitive or memory loss over time, plus seizure-related morbidity and mortality including risk of SUDEP. In appropriately selected cases, epilepsy surgery can abolish seizures with restoration of normal neurologic function. The accurate localization of a safely resectable seizure focus requires intensive investigation at a specialized epilepsy center.

A variety of surgical approaches are presently available. These range from lesionectomies, to lobectomies, to (rarely) hemispherectomies. Palliative approaches such as transection of the corpus callosum can help those with drop attacks. The surgical options are tailored to the needs of each individual patient, depending on the nature of their epileptogenic lesion and proximity to cortical regions that cannot be resected without causing unacceptable neurologic deficits (so-called "eloquent cortex"). Recently, laser-mediated ablative techniques have permitted surgical approaches for certain pathologies, with much less risk to the surrounding normal brain near the surgical target. Laser interstitial thermal therapy (LITT) can permit smaller surgical approaches, shorter inpatient stays, and faster postoperative recoveries. Outcomes seem to approach those of conventional resective approaches, though longer-term outcome data are still needed.

Dietary Therapy

The *ketogenic diet* is a very high fat diet with markedly restricted carbohydrates and adequate protein carefully designed to cause a ketotic state, while still supplying adequate nutrition. It is mainly used in children with developmental and epileptic encephalopathies who have an unsatisfactory response to AED treatment. The ketogenic diet can be effective in these most refractory forms of epilepsy, resulting in seizure freedom in 15% to 20%. However, the diet is hard to maintain and requires a dedicated, cooperative caregiver and a specially trained dietician.

The *modified Atkins diet* (MAD) and *low glycemic-index diet* are scaled-down versions of the ketogenic diet with mainly carbohydrate restriction. These diets are more palatable than the ketogenic diet and can be tolerated by adults. The slight ketosis achieved sometimes results in dramatic seizure reduction in many forms of epilepsy.

Neurostimulators

The *vagal nerve stimulator (VNS)* is a surgically implanted device. The stimulating electrode is placed on the left vagus nerve in the neck. The current version of this device has three treatment modes. Routine round-the-clock stimulation occurs intermittently according to programmed settings. Standard settings deliver stimuli lasting 30 seconds every 5 minutes. However, one can program the VNS to deliver stimuli in a more rapid cycling pattern (greater duty cycle) and/or alter the intensity of the stimulation by modifying other parameters. Swiping a magnet over the device gives an extra "on-demand" stimulation that can sometimes abort a seizure. A third mode called autostimulation delivers stimulation based upon detected tachycardias of sufficient magnitude, since a significant percentage of seizures foster an associated tachycardia. Preapproval studies found that approximately 45% of recipients had a greater than 50% reduction in their seizure frequency (the responder rate) and seizure intensity was also often decreased in many. Postapproval long-term follow-up studies suggest an even more robust response to VNS therapy.

Deep brain stimulation (DBS) of bilateral anterior nuclei of the thalami also has been approved in the United States since 2018 for treatment-resistant epilepsy involving bilateral limbic regions. Like the VNS, this method also relies on preset, round-the-clock, intermittent stimulation to modulate the epileptic circuitry and decrease seizure burden. Studies show that it can lead to a 60% responder rate with several years of follow-up.

Another newer strategy for medically refractory focal epilepsy is *responsive neurostimulation (RNS)*, approved in the United States since 2013. Chronically implanted electrodes at or near the seizure foci are used to rapidly detect seizure onset and treat the seizure and its supporting circuitry within seconds by delivering electrical stimulation directly to the seizure focus. This method can use implanted depth electrodes or strips of electrodes to access either cortical or deeper targets (e.g., hippocampi) and provides a means to treat patients with greater than one seizure focus, thereby offering a non-resective option for patients who would not otherwise be appropriate resective surgical candidates. Detection and stimulation algorithms are tailored to the patient's electrocorticography samples collected over time to improve its performance. Studies have reported a 72% responder rate with 5-year follow-up.

All three neuromodulatory methods appear to variably thwart seizures as they initiate and spread and, perhaps more importantly, gradually reduce the propensity of the epileptic circuitry to generate seizures. These treatments seem to improve clinical outcomes in a slower manner than is commonly seen with AEDs. However, unlike AEDs, the neuromodulatory treatments so far appear to exhibit sustained improved outcomes over years, do not seem to lose efficacy, are nonsedating, and spare neurocognitive function versus most resective surgical methods.

The process by which tertiary epilepsy programs assess the candidacy of medically refractory patients for the above dietary, surgical, or neuromodulatory methods involves careful analysis of several streams of clinical data. Patients' EEG and LTM results are aligned with their brain imaging and neuropsychological test results. Concordant data more strongly implicate the localization of the seizure focus or foci. This is then matched with the most appropriate treatment options in a highly individualized manner.

Status Epilepticus

Status epilepticus can occur with focal or generalized seizure types and is defined as prolonged or rapidly recurring seizures without full intervening recovery. *Acute repetitive seizures* are defined as a cluster of seizures over minutes to hours with intervening recovery.

Convulsive status epilepticus is a medical emergency. Prolonged and continuous generalized convulsive epileptic activity can lead to irreversible brain injury. The most frequent cause is abrupt withdrawal of AEDs (e.g., noncompliance) in a person with epilepsy. Other precipitants include acute withdrawal from alcohol, benzodiazepines or barbiturates, cerebral infections such as encephalitis, trauma, hemorrhage, and brain tumor.

Nonconvulsive status epilepticus includes two main types. *Focal status epilepticus* (also known as complex partial status epilepticus) may resemble a sustained confusional state often associated with motor and autonomic automatisms. Some instances produce bizarre behaviors or stupor. These bouts can even last for hours or days. Occasionally, this is preceded by an overt convulsive seizure that may have incompletely resolved, with or without AED treatment. This can be diagnostically challenging, as the semiology overlaps with a myriad of other forms of encephalopathy or delirium. EEG is crucial for diagnosis and shows nearly continuous epileptiform activity predominating in a brain region or regions, often the temporal lobes.

The other main form of nonconvulsive status epilepticus is *absence status epilepticus* (or petit mal status). This resembles focal status epilepticus and consists of a similar confusional state with some automatisms. EEG reveals continuous runs of generalized 3- to 4-Hz spike and slow wave activity. This usually occurs in children or young adults with known absence epilepsy.

With the current widespread use of ICU EEG monitoring in neurocritically ill patients, there is a burgeoning subset whose EEGs show less sustained and less rapid epileptiform discharges than in typical status epilepticus, though often periodic and abundant, with a waxing and waning quality. Such epileptiform discharges may be lateralized or generalized. These patterns fall short of the status epilepticus patterns described previously but may follow recent bouts of status epilepticus, as they resolve. Recently, these patterns have been categorized as falling within the "ictal-interictal continuum." Their clinical significance is less clear and is a current focus of investigation.

Focal motor status epilepticus (or *epilepsy partialis continua, [EPC]*) ranges from highly focal, clonic movements of the face or hand to jerks involving a limb or half the body. The clonus frequency can vary from 0.3 to 3.0 Hz. It is less common. Causes include stroke, trauma, neoplasm, encephalitis, and marked hyperglycemia (e.g., glucose > 450 mg/dL as in nonketotic hyperglycemic states) and in Rasmussen encephalitis, a very rare, usually pediatric epilepsy syndrome. Status epilepticus related to profound hyperglycemia can produce refractory focal status epilepticus that often resolves once hyperglycemia is corrected.

Postanoxic myoclonic status epilepticus is often accompanied by generalized polyspike and slow wave epileptiform discharges on EEG but may be less responsive to common AED treatments for status epilepticus. It typically reflects significant and extensive cortical injury, often associated with a poor prognosis.

Once status epilepticus is diagnosed, treatment is urgent. The longer status epilepticus lasts, the more difficult it is to terminate and the more likely it is to cause brain damage. Aggressive therapy is mandatory for convulsive status epilepticus (Table 120.5). If initial therapy is not rapidly effective, anesthetic agents requiring intubation and ventilation should be used within an hour of onset. Focal status epilepticus can also result in permanent neuronal injury and should also be treated expeditiously, although therapeutic choices are often made to try to stop focal status epilepticus with agents that do not cause respiratory depression to avoid intubation. Absence status is unlikely to result in permanent sequelae and usually responds promptly to benzodiazepine treatment. Investigation into the cause of status epilepticus should be undertaken during its treatment and continued after seizures stop.

GENETIC COUNSELING AND PREGNANCY

Heredity

Patients with epilepsy should be advised about the hereditary risks to their children, although in most people with epilepsy, it does not influence their decision about having children. The most common genetic generalized epilepsies have complex inheritance patterns with about 10% of children of an affected parent developing seizures. There are over 200 mendelian-inherited syndromes with epilepsy, all rare. Screening for genetic causes of epilepsy has become more useful for certain subgroups of patients, particularly those with unknown etiology under the age of 2 years. Gene microarray assays have become more effective tools and have added to older less precise genetic assays such as karyotype or FISH assays. Genetics counselors provide valuable diagnostic and educational assistance in the care of patients who may have a genetic form of epilepsy or who may have specific concerns about the potential risk for their children.

TABLE 120.5	**Treatment of Convulsive Status Epilepticus**
Time (Min)	**Steps**
0-5 (Stabilize, ABCs)	Give O$_2$; ensure adequate ventilation
	Monitor: vital signs, ECG, oximetry, seizure duration
	Establish intravenous access;
	Obtain finger stick blood glucose level, If <60 mg/dL, then:
	Adults: 100 mg thiamine IV, then 50 mL D50W IV
	Children ≥2 years: 2 mL/kg D25W IV
	Children <2 years: 4 mL/kg D12.5W IV
	Collect complete blood cell count, electrolytes, Ca, Mg, toxins, and AED levels
5-20 Initial therapy (benzodiazepine)	Choose one of the following 3 options:
	1. Intravenously administer lorazepam 0.1 mg/kg/dose, max: 4 mg/dose, may repeat dose once, or
	2. Intravenously administer diazepam 0.15-0.2 mg/kg/dose, max: 10 mg/dose, may repeat dose once, or
	3. Intramuscularly administer midazolam 10 mg for >40 kg, 5 mg for 13-40 kg, single dose.
	If none of the above are available, then choose one of the following:
	1. IV phenobarbital 15 mg/kg/dose, single dose. Note that IV phenobarbital following a benzodiazepine ventilatory assistance is usually required.
	2. Rectal diazepam 0.2-0.5 mg/kg, max: 20 mg/dose, single dose
	3. Intranasal midazolam, buccal midazolam
20-40 (Second therapy)	If status epilepticus persists, administer one of the following:
	1. IV fosphenytoin[a] 20 mg PE/kg, max: 1500 mg PE/dose, 1 dose
	2. IV valproic acid 40 mg/kg, max: 3000 mg/dose, 1 dose
	3. IV levetiracetam 60 mg/kg, max: 4500 mg/dose, 1 dose
	If none of the above are available, and if not already given, administer IV phenobarbital 15 mg/kg, max dose.
	(Alternative to fosphenytoin above, may use phenytoin at 1 mg/kg/min up to 50 mg/min max rate in adults in a proximal IV. Monitor carefully for hypotension, arrhythmia, local extravasation.)
40-60 (Third therapy)	If the seizures do not stop after the above, choices include repeating second-line therapies not previously given, or intravenous anesthetic doses of thiopental, midazolam, or propofol, with intubation and with continuous EEG monitoring. Vasopressors or supplemental IV fluids are often necessary.

ABCs, Airway, breathing, and circulation; *AED,* antiepileptic drug; *ECG,* electrocardiogram; *EEG,* electroencephalograph.
[a]Always dosed in phenytoin-equivalents (PE).

Teratogenicity

Children of mothers taking AEDs have a birth defect rate of 2% up to 9%, which is up to five times that of the general population. However, seizures, especially convulsive seizures, also pose a substantial risk to both the mother and fetus. Thus, AEDs should not be stopped during pregnancy. There is significant variation in the relative teratogenic risk of the available AEDs and in their specific effects on fetal development. Two AEDs, valproate and carbamazepine, have been incriminated in neural tube closure defects. Since the neural tube closes by 28 days of fetal development, this defect develops before the mother may be aware that she is pregnant. Phenytoin, phenobarbital, primidone, and topiramate have been associated with a spectrum of neurodevelopmental abnormalities. Topiramate has been associated with higher risk of low birthweight and increased oral cleft risk. Large registries suggest that the newer AEDs have less teratogenic risk, but the data are incomplete for some of these newer AEDs. Lamotrigine and levetiracetam are presently associated with the lowest rates of major congenital malformations in these registries (approximately 2%). By contrast, valproate has the worst profile with an approximately 9% incidence. Use of two or more AEDs (polytherapy) increases the teratogenic risk. Pregnancies in women with epilepsy should be planned. During the year prior to conception, an attempt should be made to minimize the teratogenic potential of the AED regimen by considering a change to AEDs with significantly superior teratogenic risk where appropriate, to monotherapy from polytherapy, or tapering off AEDs, if there are reasons to believe that seizures will not recur (see later). The lowest effective dose of the AEDs should be used, but this must be balanced with the risk of breakthrough seizures. Folic acid deficiency is an established risk factor for neural tube defects in the general population. There is little evidence that additional folic acid in a well-nourished woman with epilepsy decreases the AED effects on neural tube closure. However, it is shared practice to advise women with epilepsy of childbearing age to take supplemental folic acid (1 mg per day) as prophylaxis against neural tube defects. Once pregnancy is planned or recognized, the dose of folic acid is commonly increased to 4 mg per day.

Management During and After Pregnancy

Women with epilepsy have generally a 1- to 1.7-fold increased rate of complications of pregnancy, including prematurity, preeclampsia, preterm labor, placental abruption, fetal death, bleeding, and poor fetal growth, except for a 10-fold higher rate of maternal mortality than the general population. They should be managed as high-risk pregnancies. High-quality level 2 ultrasound (and possibly 3D ultrasound), maternal serum α-fetoprotein level (elevated in neural tube closure defects), and amniocentesis for chromosomal analysis are used to identify fetal malformations.

During pregnancy, AED serum levels decrease due to increased hepatic and renal clearance and increased plasma volume. The free fraction of highly protein-bound AEDs (e.g., phenytoin and valproate) typically increases due to decreased albumin concentration and increased competition for binding sites by sex steroids. Thus, it is essential to monitor AED levels (free levels for highly protein-bound AEDs) prior to conception and at regular intervals throughout pregnancy (generally every 4 weeks). Hormonal changes associated with pregnancy lead to progressive induction of hepatic glucuronidation pathways that dramatically reduce lamotrigine levels, sometimes requiring doubling or even tripling the lamotrigine dose over the course of pregnancy to maintain prepregnancy levels. In light of these expected AED level changes, it is very helpful to have prepregnancy baseline AED levels, especially those corresponding to periods of good seizure control, in women aiming for pregnancy.

Emesis, a common problem during early pregnancy, can result in missed and partial doses of AEDs. The pregnant woman should be instructed to retake a full or partial dose of her AEDs if vomiting occurs after medications are taken. After the child is born, the dose of AEDs should be tapered to prepregnancy doses over 3 to 6 weeks, beginning approximately 3 days postpartum, but the duration of taper may vary according to the AED's route of clearance (renal or glucuronidation pathways—3 weeks; cytochrome pathways—6 weeks). The AED levels can be checked 1 to 2 weeks after completing the taper to confirm they are at the patient's baseline. In general, breast-feeding is not contraindicated in women taking AEDs.

During the postpartum period the mother with epilepsy may be at increased risk of seizures, especially if her seizures are activated by sleep deprivation. To lessen this risk, a support person should perform at least one of the newborn's nighttime feedings. Patients whose seizure semiology would put the infant at risk (e.g., dropping or excessively clutching the baby) require childcare modification and/or supervision.

PSYCHOSOCIAL CONCERNS

Ongoing epileptic seizures often have major emotional consequences for the patient and family. Comorbid depression is present in up to 30% to 50% of patients with refractory epilepsy and 20% of patients with controlled epilepsy. Anxiety disorders accompany epilepsy in 15% to 20%. Both are often unrecognized and untreated. In people with epilepsy, quality of life impairment better correlates with depression than with seizure frequency. The unpredictable nature of seizures and the necessary activity restrictions cause dependence, decreased self-worth, embarrassment, stigma, underemployment, and helplessness. Reduced libido and hyposexuality are common in patients with epilepsy and often unrecognized.

Family dynamics may also be disrupted by the presence of epilepsy. Patients and their families often fear seizures (seizure phobia). Family members may think their loved one is dying when they convulse, especially for the first time. Patients with epilepsy are helped most by seizure freedom, but reassurance and optimistic support from family and friends aids immeasurably. Once seizure control is achieved, people with epilepsy should be encouraged to live as normal and full a life as possible, using common sense as a guide. Although activity restrictions may eventually be lifted, patients with past epilepsy (with the exception of CAE and childhood epilepsy with centrotemporal spikes, which completely remit) should be advised to avoid head contact sports and activities or occupations that may prove catastrophic were a seizure to recur (e.g., swimming alone, working at great heights, weapon use).

All states grant automobile driver's licenses to patients with epilepsy provided that no seizures impairing consciousness or bodily control have occurred for specified periods of time (typically 3 months to 1 year). Life and health insurance policies can generally be obtained. The American with Disabilities Act (ADA) provides protection from loss of employment on the basis of disability and this pertains to those with epilepsy. Reasonable accommodations to patients should be made in the workplace setting, although there are several important caveats to these rules. Epilepsy foundations and local social service organizations can assist patients with case coordination, including social and vocational concerns.

PROGNOSIS

Two thirds of those with epilepsy achieve a 5-year remission of seizures within 10 years of diagnosis. About half of these patients can eventually become seizure-free without AEDs. Factors favoring remission include specific genetic generalized forms of epilepsy, a normal neurologic examination, and onset in early to middle childhood (excluding neonatal seizures). Approximately 30% of patients continue to have seizures and never achieve a permanent remission despite one or more AEDs. Such treatment-resistant (or medically refractory) patients should be evaluated at an epilepsy center to ensure diagnostic accuracy and to explore the full gamut of available treatments. Seizures are occasionally associated with significant morbidity and mortality. Injuries due to seizures are common. These can include traumatic injuries such as lacerations and fractures, head injuries, aspiration, drowning, and burns, among others. Such injuries can infrequently be life-threatening. Accidental deaths related to seizures (e.g., motor vehicle collisions) further increase the death rate. Aspiration with convulsions is common but can be prevented by turning the head to one side as the convulsion ends. A growing literature suggests that some types of repeated seizures, especially prolonged seizures and status epilepticus, may be associated with certain forms of cognitive decline such as memory impairment, over the lifetime of a patient.

SUDEP occurs in approximately 1 per 1000 patients per year, taking all forms of epilepsy together. In the most refractory epilepsies, the SUDEP rate may approach 10 per 1000 patients per year. SUDEP may result from transient autonomic nervous system dysfunction, which may occur during or immediately after an unwitnessed seizure (often during sleep) with resultant cardiac arrhythmia or respiratory dysfunction (central and/or peripheral forms of apnea). Suffocation can occur after an unwitnessed convulsion if the patient is prone with face down in a pillow or bedding. Whether some patients have a still unknown genetic predisposition toward SUDEP is a current active area of investigation, as are new monitoring technologies to help detect nocturnal seizures or their autonomic sequelae and alert caregivers.

DISCONTINUING ANTIEPILEPTIC DRUGS

Many patients with epilepsy become seizure-free on AED therapy for an extended time. Some patients can successfully discontinue AEDs without relapse. Successful drug withdrawal is most likely with shorter duration of epilepsy before achieving remission, with a longer seizure-free interval before antiseizure drug withdrawal (minimum of 2 years is advised but many advocate for at least 5 years), fewer seizures before achieving remission (≥10 carries higher relapse risk), history of a self-limiting epilepsy syndrome (e.g., absence epilepsy, childhood epilepsy with centrotemporal spikes), and no epileptiform abnormalities on EEG before withdrawal. Other factors of possibly lesser statistical import that may also increase the risk of relapse upon AED taper include an abnormal neurologic exam, brain MRI revealing a pertinent structural correlate, intellectual disability, family history of epilepsy, history of multiple seizure types, or if seizure control was difficult to establish and required polytherapy. Ultimately, this decision is highly individualized as the perceived burden of continuing AED treatment versus the impact of a seizure relapse may vary among individual patients with differing goals and life circumstances.

Acknowledgments

The author would like to acknowledge the work of Michel J. Berg, who contributed this chapter to the previous edition.

SUGGESTED READINGS

Berg AT, Coryell J, Saneto RP, et al: Early-life epilepsies and the emerging role of genetic testing, JAMA Pediatr 171(9):863–871, 2017.

Berg AT, Scheffer IE: New concepts in classification of the epilepsies: entering the 21st century, Epilepsia 52:1058–1062, 2011.

Fazel S, Wolf A, Langstrom N, et al: Premature mortality in epilepsy and the role of psychiatric comorbidity: a total population study, Lancet 382:1646–1654, 2013.

Fisher RS, Cross JH, French JA, et al: Operational classification of seizure types by the International League against epilepsy: position paper of the ILAE commission for classification and terminology, Epilepsia 58(4):522–530, 2017.

French JA, Pedley TA: Clinical practice. Initial management of epilepsy, N Engl J Med 359:166–176, 2008.

Glauser T, Shinnar S, Gloss D, et al: Evidence-based guideline: treatment of convulsive status epilepticus in children and adults: report of the guideline Committee of the American epilepsy society, Epilepsy Curr 16(1):48–61, 2016.

Harden CL, Hopp J, Ting TY, et al: Practice parameter update: management issues for women with epilepsy—focus on pregnancy (an evidence-based review): obstetrical complications and change in seizure frequency, Neurology 73(2):126–132, 2009.

Harden CL, Meador KJ, Pennell PB, et al: Practice parameter update: management issues for women with epilepsy—focus on pregnancy (an evidence-based review): teratogenesis and perinatal outcomes, Neurology 73:133–141, 2009.

Krumholz A, Wiebe S, Gronseth GS, et al: Evidence-based guideline: management of an unprovoked first seizure in adults, Neurology 84(16):1705–1713, 2015.

Kumada T, Miyajima T, Hiejima I, et al: Modified Atkins Diet and Low Glycemic Index Treatment for Medication-Resistant Epilepsy. Current Trends in Ketogenic Diet, J Neurol Neurophysiol S2:007, 2013.

Pack AM: Epilepsy overview and revised classification of seizures and epilepsies, Continuum (Minneap Minn) 25(2):306–321, 2019.

Proposal for revised classification of epilepsies and epileptic syndromes: Commission on classification and terminology of the international League against epilepsy, Epilepsia 30(4):389–399, 1989.

Proposal for revised clinical and electroencephalographic classification of epileptic seizures: From the commission on classification and terminology of the international League against epilepsy, Epilepsia 22(4):489–501, 1981.

Scheffer IE, Berkovic S, Capovilla G, et al: ILAE classification of the epilepsies: position paper of the ILAE Commission for Classification and Terminology, Epilepsia 58(4):512–521, 2017.

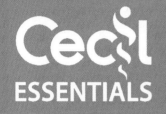

121

Central Nervous System Tumors

Bryan J. Bonder, Lisa R. Rogers

DEFINITION/EPIDEMIOLOGY

Central nervous system (CNS) tumors are of two types, primary or metastatic. Primary tumors arise from a variety of cell types within the parenchyma of the brain, spinal cord or the meninges. Metastatic tumors result from spread of systemic cancer to the brain, spinal cord, or meninges and represent the majority of central nervous system tumors. This chapter reviews both primary and metastatic brain tumors.

The incidence of primary malignant and nonmalignant brain tumors in the United States increases with age and is 5.65/100,000 in persons age 0 to 14, 11.2/100,000 in persons age 15 to 39, and 44.47/100,000 in persons older than 40. High-grade gliomas and meningiomas are the most common types of adult primary brain tumors. Meningiomas are the most common benign intracranial tumor and account for approximately one third of benign brain tumors. The incidence of primary CNS lymphoma (PCNSL) is increasing in all age groups, accounted for only in part by CNS lymphoma associated with HIV and immunocompromised states such as solid organ transplant.

Brain metastases are one of the most common neurologic complications of cancer with an incidence of up to 17%. Because incidence rates are based on tumor registries and many patients with brain metastasis do not undergo surgery, they may be underrepresented in these statistics.

Primary brain tumors are the second most common cancers in children. Medulloblastomas are the most common malignant pediatric brain tumor. In the United States, approximately 300 new cases of pediatric medulloblastomas are diagnosed each year. The cause of most primary CNS tumors is unknown. Aside from exposure to ionizing radiation, no environmental agents are known to be causative. Hereditary syndromes that are associated with an increased risk of CNS tumors include neurofibromatosis 1 and 2, tuberous sclerosis, von Hippel-Lindau disease, Li-Fraumeni syndrome, and Turcot syndrome, but these account for less than 1% of primary CNS tumors. Although the chromosomal abnormalities associated with many of these syndromes are known, the specific mechanisms leading to CNS neoplasia have not been defined.

PATHOLOGY

The most recent World Health Organization classification from 2016 defines brain tumors based on the cell of origin and molecular signature and includes a grading system, which is of use in predicting the biological behavior of the tumor. Most adult primary brain tumors are of neuroepithelial origin and result from neoplastic transformation of astrocytes, oligodendrocytes, or ependymocytes. Astrocytomas are the most common primary parenchymal brain tumor in adults. Meningiomas derive from arachnoidal cap cells in the meningeal covering of the brain. They most frequently occur in older adults. Common locations of meningioma are the cerebral convexity, falx and parasagittal area, olfactory groove, sphenoid wing, and posterior fossa. They are comprised of heterogeneous histopathology patterns, and careful neuropathological assessment is needed for accurate grading.

Primary central nervous system lymphoma is a rare form of non-Hodgkin's lymphoma, typically of B cell origin. It presents within the white matter of the cerebral hemispheres, often in a periventricular location, and is often multiple.

Brain metastasis develops when tumor cells gain access to the systemic circulation and embolize to the brain. Metastases occur most commonly from solid tumors arising in the breast, lung, kidneys, colon, and skin (melanoma). Lung cancer, both non–small and small cell type, is one of the most common tumors to metastasize to the brain and constitutes up to 50% of cases of brain metastasis. In women, breast cancer is the most common source. Malignant melanoma is a less common systemic cancer but carries a high risk of brain metastasis; up to 50% of stage IV melanoma patients develop brain metastasis.

Medulloblastomas are of primitive neuro-ectodermal origin and are highly cellular. Homer Wright rosettes (arrangement of tumor cells around a central area filled with neurofibrillary processes) can be identified in resected specimens in up to 40% of cases. Medulloblastomas are grade IV tumors as they are invasive and rapidly growing, with a tendency to disseminate through the cerebrospinal fluid (CSF).

CLINICAL PRESENTATION

Symptoms and signs caused by brain tumors typically result from compression or invasion of adjacent neural tissue by the tumor or from vasogenic edema resulting from disruption of the blood-brain barrier which can be caused by cerebral vessel compression/invasion from tumor or from "leaky" blood vessels present within the tumor. Neoangiogenesis associated with tumor growth is typically comprised of embryonic vessels that lack a normal blood-brain barrier. Because of the uncompromising rigidity of the cranial vault, both histologically benign and malignant tumors may cause symptoms, even when they are small. Symptoms caused by low-grade primary brain tumors tend to be slowly progressive whereas those in mid- and high-grade histology are acute or subacute (over weeks to months). The exception is the clinical presentation of a low-grade glioma with seizure. Metastatic tumors often present in a subacute fashion but may present acutely when hemorrhage into the tumor occurs. Hemorrhage into metastatic brain tumors is most common with renal cell, lung, papillary thyroid carcinomas, melanoma, and choriocarcinomas.

The clinical symptoms and signs depend on the location of tumor. In most pediatric patients with brain tumors, tumors arise in the posterior fossa and result in diplopia, ataxia, dysphagia, or nausea/vomiting. Most adult brain tumors arise in the cerebral hemispheres and present with symptoms and signs related to the supratentorial structure involved: unilateral limb weakness, aphasia, and speech abnormality or memory loss are common. Tumors in either location may present with generalized symptoms arising from increased intracranial pressure or meningeal irritation. Headache occurs in up to two thirds of patients as a presenting sign. There are no unique characteristics to this headache, but useful clinical clues include a new or different headache pattern, a progressively worsening headache, and one that occurs at night or on awakening. The pain may localize to the side of the tumor in patients with supratentorial tumors, whereas patients with infratentorial tumors frequently describe pain in the retro-orbital, retroauricular, or occipital region. Other generalized symptoms include changes in mood or personality, a decrease in appetite, and nausea. Projectile vomiting, while common in children with posterior fossa tumors, is rare in adults. Meningiomas generally grow slowly; they may also be found incidentally during the evaluation of unrelated neurologic symptoms. Seizures may develop over the course of the illness in up to 15% of patients with any type of primary tumor, often in association with tumor progression.

DIAGNOSIS/DIFFERENTIAL

All patients suspected of having a brain tumor should undergo a contrast-enhanced magnetic resonance imaging (MRI) brain scan. If MRI is not available or is contraindicated because of a non-MRI-compatible pacemaker or other condition, brain computed tomography (CT) with contrast should be obtained. Brain MRI is preferred because it is more useful in imaging the temporal and posterior fossae and it is more sensitive in detecting the extent of parenchymal involvement by tumor of any type. In addition, advanced sequences such as diffusion, perfusion, and spectroscopy can add to the diagnostic accuracy of imaging. Vasogenic edema resulting from leakage of intravascular fluid through a disrupted blood-brain barrier is easily visible on MRI.

High-grade gliomas typically appear as irregularly shaped contrast-enhancing masses surrounded by edema. Central necrosis is characteristic of glioblastoma (Fig. 121.1). Anaplastic gliomas appear similarly, except for less frequent regions of necrosis. Although there are exceptions, most low-grade gliomas do not enhance after intravenous contrast injection (Fig. 121.2). Meningiomas typically demonstrate smooth and homogeneous enhancement originating from the extra-axial space and may also compress adjacent brain. Primary CNS lymphomas typically present as multiple contrast-enhancing lesions within the white matter but in rare instances do not show contrast enhancement. Brain metastases are often located at the gray-white junction of the brain and demonstrate homogeneous enhancement or peripheral enhancement surrounding a necrotic or cystic center. When solitary, a brain metastasis cannot be accurately distinguished from other neoplasm or nonneoplastic entities. Medulloblastomas are usually large by the time they are identified and demonstrate homogeneous enhancement within or superior to the floor of the fourth ventricle (Fig. 121.3). They are often accompanied by hydrocephalus. The desmoplastic variant of medulloblastomas can be located lateral to the fourth ventricle.

The differential diagnosis of contrast-enhancing lesions includes brain abscess, but infection is a consideration only in rare clinical situations. Diffusion-weighted magnetic resonance images can be useful in distinguishing tumor from infection. Low-grade gliomas can be misdiagnosed as cerebral infarction, especially on brain CT. Periventricular enhancement in PCNSL can sometimes be confused with active multiple sclerosis lesions or with brain metastasis. Dural pathologies such as sarcoidosis, meningeal infection, or dural metastasis can mimic a meningioma. Posterior fossa ependymomas in children can mimic medulloblastomas.

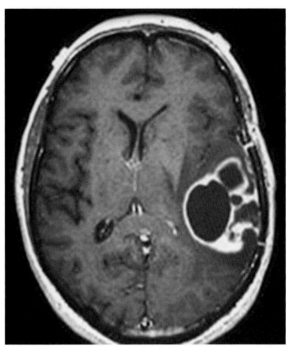

Fig. 121.1 Contrast-enhanced T1-weighted MRI demonstrates irregular contrast enhancement with central necrosis in the left temporal lobe. There is adjacent vasogenic edema and mass effect on midline structures characteristic of a high grade glioma.

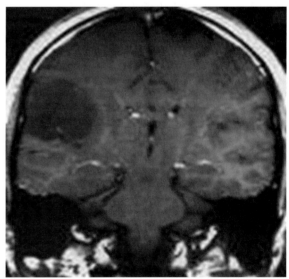

Fig. 121.2 Coronal T-weighted MRI following contrast injection in a low-grade astrocytoma shows low signal intensity and no contrast enhancement, typical of a low-grade glioma.

Leptomeningeal metastasis can be suspected in cancer patients with multiple cranial nerve deficits, asymmetrical limb weakness, unexplained headaches or seizures. Evaluation typically includes imaging of the entire neuraxis with contrast-enhanced MRI. Leptomeningeal tumor will appear as diffuse or nodular enhancement arising from the leptomeninges of the brain or spinal cord. Cranial nerves, when involved, may enhance and appear thickened. The diagnosis can be made by MRI in the appropriate clinical setting, but definitive diagnosis is established by demonstration of tumor cells in cytology examination of CSF. In patients with lymphoma, flow cytometry is preferable to cytology. A large volume (>10 mL) lumbar puncture is frequently

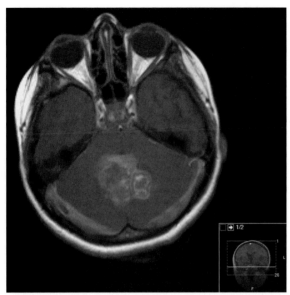

Fig. 121.3 Contrast-enhanced T1-weighted MRI shows a large enhancing tumor in the midline of the cerebellum with compression of the fourth ventricle.

required in order to make the diagnosis. If the initial cytology is negative and suspicion is high, additional lumbar puncture can be considered. Findings of elevated CSF protein and white blood cell count or low glucose should raise suspicion.

In the majority of cases, biopsy or resection is the preferred method to establish the histology and grade of primary brain tumors. Exceptions include patients suspected to have PCNSL; a search for malignant cells in the CSF or by vitreous biopsy can be attempted to avoid surgery. Additionally, surgery is typically avoided in brain stem gliomas because the MRI appearance is characteristic and biopsy is considered dangerous.

TREATMENT

Surgical resection is the initial goal for most patients with benign and malignant primary brain tumors. Surgical resection provides tissue for analysis and often relieves neurologic symptoms; maximal surgical resection, when feasible, improves outcome. One exception is PCNSL, in which clinical deterioration can result from resection. Biopsy alone is adequate unless significant symptoms of mass effect from the tumor are present. In addition, small meningiomas can often be observed.

Standard therapy for newly diagnosed glioblastoma is maximal resection and focal external beam radiation of 60 Gy in combination with temozolomide followed by adjuvant temozolomide for 6 months. In a prospective randomized trial of newly diagnosed glioblastoma patients, the median survival with radiation and temozolomide was 14.6 months versus 12.1 months with radiation alone. In addition, the 2-year survival rate was superior with the combined regimen (26.5%) versus radiation alone (10.4%). O-6-methylguanine DNA methyltransferase (MGMT) is a DNA repair gene that reduces the efficacy of temozolomide and other DNA-damaging treatments for cancer. Methylation of the MGMT promoter in tumor tissue silences this gene and results in improved survival in glioblastoma. There is evidence that tumors harboring isocitrate dehydrogenase (IDH) 1and 2 mutations are correlated with a superior outcome compared with wild-type IDH. The discovery of molecular "drivers" may lead to identification of additional targets for therapy. New approaches using next-generation sequencing and DNA-methylation fingerprinting are being evaluated in trials of glioblastoma.

The introduction of "targeted agents" that are designed to deactivate oncogenic pathways or angiogenesis is a major advance in cancer treatment. Bevacizumab, a monoclonal antibody to vascular endothelial growth factor, is associated with a high response rate and reduction in neurologic symptoms in recurrent glioblastoma, although the effect on overall survival is not significant. Because current treatment results are unsatisfactory, it is suggested that patients with glioblastoma be referred for clinical trial.

Anaplastic gliomas, most commonly anaplastic astrocytoma and anaplastic oligodendroglioma, are treated by maximal surgical resection, followed by focal external beam radiation in association with chemotherapy. However, there is increasing reliance upon the molecular markers of MGMT and IDH1 status to predict survival and to dictate the utility of adding chemotherapy in poor prognosis patients. One type of anaplastic glioma exquisitely sensitive to chemotherapy is the anaplastic oligodendroglioma with co-deletions of 1p and 19q.

The long-term progression-free survival and overall survival of low-grade glioma (grade 2) patients is better than those with glioblastoma or anaplastic glioma, but malignant transformation occurs in up to 50% of such patients and close monitoring with serial MRIs is required. Most patients with low-grade gliomas should be treated initially with maximal safe surgical resection. When grade 2 patients undergo resection, adjuvant therapy with radiation and chemotherapy is reserved for those who are older than 40 years of age or in whom the resection was subtotal. Characterizing low-grade gliomas by molecular markers such as IDH1 and chromosomal analysis for co-deletion of 1p and 19q mutations and (IDH) mutation predicts prognosis. Regardless of the treatment modality selected, serial monitoring for progression with regular MRIs is indicated. If there is disease progression or recurrence, repeat surgery, RT, and chemotherapy are all potential options depending on individual patient characteristics.

The type of therapy selected for a meningioma depends on patient characteristics, tumor features, potential for harm if untreated, and consideration of side effects of the treatment. Maximal surgical resection is important to reduce the risk of relapse. When complete removal is not possible, radiation therapy should be considered postoperatively, especially for grade 2 tumors. Radiation therapy is recommended regardless of the extent of resection for malignant (grade 3) meningiomas. Chemotherapy for this disease has not been proven to be effective.

Symptoms and imaging abnormalities associated with PCNSL often improve with the administration of corticosteroids because of the cytotoxic effects of steroids on lymphoma cells. However, administration of steroids before brain biopsy reduces the yield of tissue biopsy and can confound diagnosis. Therefore, delaying steroids prior to surgery is appropriate in suspected PCNSL because resection is often associated with neurologic deterioration and because there is no clear evidence that resection improves prognosis. A high-dose methotrexate-based regimen incorporating an alkylating agent and rituximab is the preferred induction therapy. Consolidation therapy may include other chemotherapies or low-dose whole brain radiation. High-dose radiation following chemotherapy should be avoided because of the risk of white matter damage. Up to a quarter of patients have ocular or CSF involvement at the presentation of CNS lymphomas, and staging by performing lumbar puncture and consultation with ophthalmology is appropriate prior to beginning therapy.

Contemporary management of brain metastases is individualized and is often best accomplished by a multidisciplinary team including medical oncology, neuro-oncology, radiation oncology, and neurosurgery. Initial systemic evaluation for a suspected new brain metastasis should include contrast-enhanced CT scans of the chest, abdomen, and pelvis and additionally a mammogram if the patient is female. If the lesions are multiple and the underlying diagnosis is not known, tissue from the safest and most readily accessible site should be obtained. Standard therapy for patients with a single brain metastasis is complete resection if the tumor is resectable and the patient has a good performance status and has limited extracranial disease. Some patients with limited systemic cancer show a survival benefit with resection of up to three metastatic tumors. Resection is typically followed by whole brain radiation or stereotactic surgery to the tumor margin. Radiosurgery to all lesions, avoiding resection, is also an option. The addition of whole brain radiation therapy (WBRT) after resection or radiosurgery provides better control of tumor in the brain but does not result in increased survival, and its use should be determined based on the individual clinical circumstances.

Patients presenting with more than three brain metastases should be considered for WBRT. Novel approaches to preserving memory in patients undergoing WBRT include sparing the hippocampus during radiation and/or adding memantine. If the patient does not receive WBRT, close observation with periodic MRI scans is indicated to assess for recurrence at the original site or at other sites in the brain. A variety of systemic treatments show therapeutic efficacy in newly diagnosed and recurrent brain metastasis, depend upon the sensitivity of the brain metastasis to the agent. Examples include small molecule targeted agents for non–small cell lung cancer, immunotherapy for malignant melanoma, and chemotherapy with or without targeted agents for breast cancer.

Leptomeningeal metastasis is treated based on the underlying pathology and the performance status of the patient. Options include radiation to symptomatic sites or bulky disease in the brain or spine on MRI, systemic chemotherapy, or intrathecal chemotherapy.

The extent of resection is prognostic in medulloblastomas. Staging evaluations for the extent of disease include postoperative MRI of the brain and spine and lumbar CSF sampling. Prospective randomized trials and single-arm trials suggest that adjuvant chemotherapy administered during and after craniospinal radiation improves the progression-free survival and overall survival in both average and poor risk groups. The therapy for children younger than 3 years of age excludes craniospinal radiation therapy because of the long-term deleterious effects and includes surgery and chemotherapy alone. Distinct subgroups of medulloblastomas have been identified, and profiling of these subgroups reveals distinct genomic events, some of which represent actionable targets for therapy.

Vasogenic edema associated with parenchymal and meningeal tumor causes neurologic symptoms and signs and can be life-threatening. Treatment with corticosteroids often reduces edema and improves neurologic function. Dexamethasone is the preferred steroid because of its long half-life and low mineralocorticoid activity. Patients with symptoms related to vasogenic edema often improve within 48 hours of dexamethasone administration. Doses used for treatment of tumor-related edema are typically 4 to 24 mg/day of dexamethasone given in divided doses (two to four times daily). Because steroids can be associated with a variety of adverse effects, the lowest dose and duration of administration should be sought. In patients with severe neurologic signs related to brain edema, an intravenous bolus of 10 mg dexamethasone should be considered. If the neurologic signs are life-threatening, including signs of brain herniation, mannitol and dexamethasone should be administered and urgent neurosurgical consultation obtained. Seizures should be aggressively managed with antiepileptic drugs. Liver nonenzyme-inducing antiepileptic drugs (e.g., phenytoin) are favored because of a better safety profile than liver enzyme-inducing drugs and because of the lack of interaction with other medications prescribed to treat the tumor, including steroids and chemotherapy. Prophylactic antiepileptic

drugs are generally not recommended for patients with a primary or metastatic brain tumor. One exception is melanoma brain metastases in which patients with multiple supratentorial brain metastases, especially those with hemorrhage, have a high risk of seizures.

PROGNOSIS

The grade of glioma, performance status, and age are important predictors of prognosis. Glioblastoma has the worst prognosis, with a median survival of just over 1 year even with aggressive therapy. Favorable prognosis patients can live more than 2 years. Data from the nationwide Surveillance, Epidemiology, and End Results registry identified an overall median survival of 15 months and 42 months for patients with anaplastic astrocytomas and anaplastic oligodendrogliomas, respectively. This analysis did not include the status of 1p19q chromosomal loss, and the more favorable survival of patients with co-deletions was thus not demonstrated. Low-grade gliomas have a median survival of approximately 5 years, but there is individual variation depending on age, size of tumor, and extent of resection. The incorporation of molecular markers will allow for more specific prognostication in these tumors.

Recurrence rates in meningioma depend upon grade and vary from greater than 25% in grade 1 to greater than 90% in grade 3. Risk factors for recurrence include incomplete resection, higher tumor grade, young age, specific subtypes, brain infiltration, and high proliferative rate.

Median survival in PCNSL has improved with the introduction of high-dose methotrexate regimens in contrast to whole brain radiation that was used decades ago. Depending upon a variety of clinical factors, most importantly age and performance status, it ranges from 1 to 8 years. Elderly patients (>70 years) fare the worst.

Performance status, age, status of the extracranial tumor, and number of brain metastases are some of the factors that predict prognosis in patients with brain metastasis. The prognosis of patients with brain metastases has become increasingly individualized. As newer targeted therapies become available, the particular genetic mutations driving the cancer are also becoming important for determination of prognosis. The median survival ranges from 3 to 6 months in patients with multiple metastases treated with whole brain radiation therapy. Patients with a single metastasis with limited extracranial disease who undergo surgical resection and whole brain radiation therapy have significantly improved survival (40 weeks) as compared with those who undergo whole brain radiation therapy alone (15 weeks). Importantly, the improved survival is accompanied by a longer period of functional independence.

The 5-year progression-free survival in medulloblastomas is 70% to 85%. However, more than one third of patients experience recurrence, and there is no standard therapy at the time of recurrence. Median survival after recurrence is usually less than 1 year.

The advent of molecular markers in the diagnostic evaluation of primary brain tumors, especially gliomas, has significantly altered the approach to predicting prognosis and treatment response. In addition, multi-institution trials have provided robust information regarding the optimal therapy for subgroups of glioma, subdivided by important clinical factors such as patient age, performance status, degree of surgical resection, and incorporation of molecular markers. It is anticipated that prospectively designed trials, stratified on these factors, will yield additional information to aid the clinician in treatment recommendations. Significant advances in the treatment of systemic cancer are providing additional therapies when those cancers spread to the central nervous system.

SUGGESTED READINGS

American Cancer Society: www.cancer.org. Accessed October 22, 2013.

Backer-Grøndahl T, Moen BH, Torp SH: The histopathological spectrum of human meningiomas, Int J Clin Exp Pathol 5:231–242, 2012.

Barnholtz-Sloan JS, Yu C, Sloan AE, et al: A nomogram for individualized estimation of survival among patients with brain metastasis, Neuro Oncol 14:910–918, 2012.

Buckner, et al: Radiation plus procarbazine, CCNU, and vincristine in low-grade-glioma, NEJM 374:1344–1355, 2016.

CBTRUS: Primary Brain and Central Nervous System Tumors Diagnosed in the United States in 2004–2007, Central Brain Tumor Registry of the United States statistical Report, 2011.

De Braganca KC, Packer RJ: Treatment options for medulloblastoma and CNS primitive neuroectodermal tumor (PNET), Curr Treat Options Neurol 15:593–606, 2013.

Nuño M, Birch K, Mukherjee D, et al: Survival and prognostic factors in anaplastic gliomas, Neurosurgery 73:458–465, 2013.

Olson JJ, Paleologos NA, Gaspar LE, et al: The role of emerging and investigational therapies for metastatic brain tumors: a systematic review and evidence-based clinical practice guideline of selected topics, J Neuro Oncol 96(1):115–142, 2010.

Patil CG, Pricola K, Sarmiento JM, et al: Whole brain radiation therapy (WBRT) alone versus WBRT and radiosurgery for the treatment of brain metastases, Cochrane Database Syst Rev 9:CD006121, 2012.

Rutkowski S, von Hoff K, Emser A, et al: Survival and prognostic factors of early childhood medulloblastoma: an international meta-analysis, J Clin Oncol 28:4961–4968, 2010.

Stupp R, Mason WP, van den Bent MJ, et al: Radiotherapy plus concomitant and adjuvant temozolomide for glioblastoma, N Engl J Med 352(10):987–996, 2005.

Tawbi, et al: Combined nivolumab and ipilimumab in melanoma metastatic to the brain, NEJM 379:722–730, 2018.

van den Bent MJ, Brandes AA, Taphoorn MJ, et al: Adjuvant procarbazine, lomustine, and vincristine chemotherapy in newly diagnosed anaplastic oligodendroglioma: long-term follow-up of EORTC brain tumor group study 26951, J Clin Oncol 31:344–350, 2013.

Wang Z, Bao Z, Yan W, et al: Isocitrate dehydrogenase 1 (IDH1) mutation-specific microRNA signature predicts favorable prognosis in glioblastoma patients with IDH1 wild type, J Exp Clin Cancer Res 32:59, 2013.

122

Demyelinating and Inflammatory Disorders

Anne Haney Cross

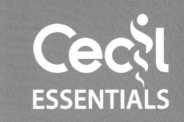

INTRODUCTION

In demyelinating CNS disorders, previously normal myelin is lost due to an acquired, typically inflammatory disease. The prototypic CNS demyelinating disorder is multiple sclerosis (MS). Other disorders of this type include neuromyelitis optica (NMO), acute disseminated encephalomyelitis (ADEM), acute transverse myelitis (TM), and optic neuritis (ON).

MULTIPLE SCLEROSIS

Definition/Epidemiology

Recent data indicate that MS affects between 600,000 and 900,000 people in the United States and over 2.3 million worldwide. Though presumed to be autoimmune, its exact etiology is still not fully understood. MS begins as a relapsing remitting disease in greater than 80% of patients and ultimately becomes progressive in greater than 50% of patients with untreated relapsing-remitting MS (RRMS). Progressive MS patients accumulate neurologic disability unassociated with relapses (although relapses may be superimposed). MS is more common in females, with the current female to male ratio in North America and in Europe estimated at 2:1 to 4:1. An exception is primary progressive MS (see Clinical Presentation), where the female to male ratio is 1:1.

MS is most common in persons of northern European ancestry. Recent genome-wide association studies indicate that many genes affect the risk of MS, although most confer only a small risk of disease (odds ratios less than 1.5). Alleles within the HLA-DR region (DRB1*15:01 > DRB1*13:03 > DRB1*03:01) are the most well established and confer the greatest risk with odds ratios between 1.5 and 4 for most populations of northern European ancestry.

Environmental factors can confer risk for MS, including modifiable factors such as low vitamin D blood level, high body mass index during adolescence/young adulthood, and smoking cigarettes. Seropositivity to the Epstein-Barr virus increases the risk of MS; a symptomatic case of infectious mononucleosis confers greater risk than seropositivity alone. Though relatively high at 1/1000 to 1/500, MS incidence appears to be relatively stable in North America, the United Kingdom, and Europe. Incidence of MS may be increasing in several regions where MS was not previously prevalent, such as Iran, Turkey, Sicily, and South Africa. These reports of increasing incidence may reflect a real increase, improved recognition, or both.

Pathology

Classically, MS causes demyelinating CNS white matter lesions with relative sparing of axons. The most common pathology of active lesions in white matter is perivascular mononuclear cell infiltration (monocyte/macrophages, lymphocytes), with a variable presence of antibody and activated complement. Acutely active white matter lesions display blood-brain barrier breakdown, manifest on MRI by gadolinium enhancement. Despite its categorization as a "white matter disease," gray matter is also damaged in MS. Gray matter MS lesions have been under-recognized because they are difficult to see by MRI and are often not appreciated pathologically without special stains. Such gray matter lesions may occur in the deep gray structures such as the thalamus and in the cerebral cortex. Cortical gray matter lesions can be subpial, extend into cortex from underlying white matter (leukocortical), or wholly within the cortex (intracortical). Cortical lesions are characterized by activated microglia and relatively fewer infiltrating lymphocytes and macrophages than white matter MS lesions. Ectopic lymphoid tissue containing components of secondary lymphoid tissues (B cells, follicular helper T cells, dendritic cells, CXCL13) has been observed in meninges of people with MS, especially those with progressive MS, and is associated with poor prognosis.

Clinical Presentation

MS may manifest with a variety of symptoms and signs. Common presentations include: optic neuritis, diplopia (often caused by internuclear ophthalmoplegia due to a propensity of MS to affect the medial longitudinal fasciculus), other brain stem syndromes, partial transverse myelitis, sensory disturbances, and weakness. Less frequent presentations include seizures, cognitive problems, bladder control problems, and pain. Pain in MS is often of a burning, tingling, or electrical nature. Clinically isolated syndrome (CIS) refers to a single attack that is likely due to CNS demyelination. CIS may be acute or subacute in onset and may involve a single or more than one CNS region. CIS presentations may look identical to MS attacks, but a formal diagnosis of MS cannot be made without dissemination of lesions in space and time. New MS diagnostic criteria allow positive spinal fluid findings (CSF-restricted oligoclonal bands) to substitute for dissemination in time. Ultimately, most CIS patients with typical demyelinating syndromes develop MS. In one study, over 85% of CIS patients with even one silent abnormality on brain or spinal cord magnetic resonance imaging (MRI) eventually developed clinically definite MS.

Three main clinical subtypes of MS are defined based on clinical course: relapsing remitting, secondary progressive, and primary progressive. RRMS is characterized by clinical stability between individual attacks from which the person may or may not fully recover. Secondary progressive MS (SPMS) patients have gradual neurologic deterioration and may also have superimposed attacks ("active" SPMS). Secondary progressive MS develops following an initial relapsing-remitting course in a substantial proportion of individuals with RRMS. This proportion may be declining with the advent of disease-modifying therapies.

TABLE 122.1 The 2017 Revised McDonald Criteria

Clinical[a]	Lesions With Objective Clinical Evidence	Additional Data Needed for MS Diagnosis
≥2 attacks	≥2	None
≥2 attacks	1 lesion, plus clear cut historical evidence of a prior attack in a different anatomic location	None
≥2 attacks	1	DIS demonstrated by an additional clinical attack implicating a different anatomic location, or >1 new T2w lesion in at least one other region typical of MS (periventricular, cortical or juxtacortical, brain stem/cerebellar, spinal cord)
1 attack	≥2 lesions	DIT demonstrated by a 2nd clinical attack, or new T2w and/or gad+ lesion on follow-up MRI, or simultaneous presence of gad+ and nonenhancing lesion on MRI at any time, or positive cerebrospinal fluid findings (oligoclonal bands restricted to CSF)
1 attack	1 lesion (CIS)	DIS demonstrated by a 2nd clinical attack implicating a different CNS region, or ≥1 new T2w lesion in MS-typical region of CNS; DIT demonstrated by a 2nd clinical attack plus either new T2w MRI lesion *or* CSF-restricted oligoclonal bands
Gradual neurologic progression suggestive of MS (PPMS)	1 year or more of disease progression plus two of three of following criteria: evidence for DIS in the brain based on ≥1 T2w lesions characteristic of MS, evidence of DIS in the spinal cord based on ≥2 T2w cord lesions, positive CSF (elevated IgG index or oligoclonal bands not present in serum)	

[a]These criteria were developed in Caucasian adults aged 18 to 50 years with CIS presentations typical of CNS inflammatory demyelinating disease. Care should be taken when applying these criteria to persons not fitting this description. Alternative diagnoses that might better explain the disorder must always be considered and reasonably excluded.
DIS, Dissemination in space; *DIT,* dissemination in time.
Modified from Thompson AJ, Banwell BL, Barkhof F, et al: Diagnosis of multiple sclerosis: 2017 revisions of the McDonald Criteria, Lancet Neurol 17:162–173, 2018.

About 10% of MS patients have primary progressive MS (PPMS), which from onset is characterized by gradual downhill progression without any clinical attacks. The International Advisory Committee on Clinical Trials of MS has proposed additional clinical descriptors that include disease activity (based on relapse rate and new imaging findings) and progression over the prior year.

Diagnosis

The diagnosis of MS requires dissemination of CNS disease in time and in space, and no other disease should provide a better explanation. MRI, spinal fluid analyses, evoked potentials (EPs) and ocular coherence tomography (OCT) are tools that may aid in the diagnosis. The latest McDonald criteria (Table 122.1) allow CSF-restricted oligoclonal bands to substitute for dissemination in time in the diagnosis of MS in the setting of a CIS typical of demyelination. The new diagnostic criteria allow more rapid diagnosis of MS and earlier treatment.

MRI

The finding of classic imaging features on brain and spinal cord MRI greatly aids the certainty of diagnosis. MS lesions are characterized by increased intensity on T2-weighted (T2w) and T2-FLAIR (fluid attenuated inversion recovery) images (Fig. 122.1A). Lesions are usually ovoid and often localize to the periventricular or juxtacortical regions, the corpus callosum, the brain stem, and the cervical spinal cord. On sagittal images, lesions in the corpus callosum are usually flame-shaped (Fig 122.1C). On T1w images, MS lesions may be isointense or hypointense. T1w hypointensity in a chronic inactive lesion denotes underlying tissue damage, including axonal loss (Fig.122.1D). Enhancement of lesions following administration of gadolinium containing contrast agents indicates blood-brain barrier breakdown; such a lesion is considered to be active (Fig. 122.1B). Enhancing lesions are also often T1w hypointense, but this hypointensity resolves more than 50% of the time. A ring pattern (often an incomplete ring) of enhancement is common. Most enhancing MS lesions display no mass effect. Occasional "tumefactive" MS lesions are difficult to distinguish from tumors and may require biopsy.

Spinal Fluid Analysis

Evidence of increased intrathecal immunoglobulin synthesis is present in more than 90% of people with MS. Elevated concentrations of CSF IgG and IgM, CSF-restricted oligoclonal bands of immunoglobulin (Fig. 122.2), and a high intrathecal IgG synthesis rate are seen. The IgG index, which is derived from the ratio of CSF to serum IgG and takes BBB integrity into account, is elevated in MS. A mild lymphocytic pleocytosis is frequently seen in CSF during MS relapses.

Evoked Potentials

EPs detected by surface electrode recording were used in the past to detect subclinical demyelination in the brain stem (auditory EPs), spinal cord (somatosensory EPs), and optic nerves (visual EPs). The advent of high-resolution MRI has led to far less use of EPs to aid MS diagnosis.

Optical Coherence Tomography

OCT is a safe and rapid means to image the retina and detect evidence of prior optic neuritis. OCT uses infrared light to measure thickness of the retinal nerve fiber layer (RNFL), which contains axons that form the optic nerve. A thinned temporal region of the RNFL can be used as evidence of prior subclinical optic neuritis.

Differential Diagnosis

The diagnosis of MS requires the exclusion of diseases that might better explain the clinical scenario. The differential diagnosis of MS is broad (Table 122.2). Some diseases that can mimic MS have relapses and others display progressive courses. "Red flags" that are atypical for MS, such as systemic (arthritis, rash, mouth or genital sores, or pulmonary) symptoms, bilateral hearing loss, peripheral neuropathy, or

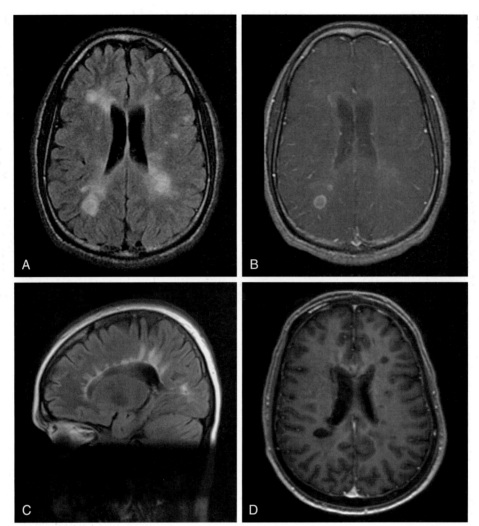

Fig. 122.1 (A) Axial fluid-attenuated inversion recovery (FLAIR) image of the brain from a person with MS revealing classical periventricular and deep white matter high-signal intensity lesions. (B) Axial T1-weighted image following gadolinium contrast administration in the same patient as A. Enhancing lesions after gadolinium contrast administration, indicating loss of integrity of the blood-brain barrier that is seen with active MS lesions. One enhancing lesion in the right parietal region is ring enhancing. (C) Sagittal FLAIR image of the brain of a person with MS demonstrating classical flame-shaped pericallosal lesions radiating outward from the ventricle. (D) Axial T1-weighted image showing areas of T1 low signal intensity ("black holes").

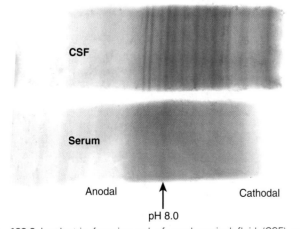

Fig. 122.2 Isoelectric focusing gel of cerebrospinal fluid (CSF) and serum of a patient with multiple sclerosis. The CSF *(upper lane)* shows oligoclonal bands cathodal to the pH 8.0, which are not seen in the serum *(lower lane).*

atypical age of onset (early childhood or after age 50) should lead the clinician to seek further support for the diagnosis of MS.

Prognosis of Multiple Sclerosis

MS is highly variable. It is occasionally "benign," in which case the disease has little impact on quality of life. It can also be severe with considerable disability or early death. Most people with MS fall in between these extremes. It is currently not possible to predict the future course of MS in an individual patient with full accuracy. Poor prognostic indicators at onset of MS include primary progressive course, male gender, frequent attacks, prominent motor or cerebellar findings, and high initial MRI lesion burden. Expected lifespan of people with MS is reduced overall by 7 to 14 years. Suicide rate is 1.7 to 7.5 times that of the general population. The use of disease modifying therapies likely improves not only relapse rate but also long-term disability and even mortality. In one nonrandomized study, early initiation of disease modifying therapies within a year of symptom onset was associated with better long-term outcomes.

TABLE 122.2 Differential Diagnosis of Demyelinating Diseases

Disease Category[a]	Examples of Disorders[b]
Immune-mediated/autoimmune	Multiple sclerosis, neuromyelitis optica (NMO), anti-MOG disorder, acute demyelinating encephalomyelitis (ADEM), idiopathic optic neuritis, CRION, idiopathic transverse myelitis, Behçet's disease
Infectious	Progressive multifocal leukoencephalopathy (PML), HTLV-I, HIV, CNS abscess, Lyme disease, Whipple disease, neurosyphilis
Metabolic	Vitamin B_{12}, vitamin E or copper deficiency, central pontine and extrapontine myelinolysis
Neurodegenerative	Spinocerebellar ataxias, spine disease (e.g., compressive cervical spondylopathy, central canal stenosis)
Rheumatologic	Sarcoidosis, systemic lupus erythematosus, antiphospholipid antibody syndrome, Sjögren's syndrome
Genetic disorders	Adrenoleukodystrophy/adrenomyeloneuropathy, hereditary spastic paraparesis, CADASIL (a hereditary stroke disorder), Leber optic neuropathy, Perlizeus-Merzbacher, Wilson's disease
Neoplastic/paraneoplastic	CNS lymphoma, meningeal carcinomatosis, paraneoplastic CRMP-5 IgG, anti-amphiphysin-1 Abs
Vascular	CNS vasculitis (e.g., giant cell arteritis, primary CNS vasculitis), spinal dural fistula, Susac syndrome
Iatrogenic	TNF inhibitors, CNS irradiation, immune checkpoint inhibitors

[a]Several of the disorders listed could be placed in more than one category.
[b]This list is not comprehensive.

❖ For a deeper discussion of these topics, please see Chapter 383, "Multiple Sclerosis and Demyelinating Conditions of the Central Nervous System," in *Goldman-Cecil Medicine*, 26th Edition.

Treatment

MS treatment can be divided into three categories: treatment of symptoms (e.g., spasticity, fatigue, or depression), treatment of acute relapses, and disease modifying therapies. The following discussion will be limited to the latter categories. However, Table 122.3 lists some frequent MS symptoms and their therapies.

Relapses that alter function or cause severe pain are usually treated with corticosteroids. Severe relapses are often managed with high-dose corticosteroids, such as intravenous methylprednisolone at 500 to 1000 mg daily for 3 to 5 days, followed by a short oral taper. Lower dosed corticosteroid courses may be used for mild relapses. Blood pressure, serum electrolytes and glucose, and patient mood should be monitored during corticosteroid therapy. Based on the multicenter Optic Neuritis Treatment Trial (ONTT), this regimen will lead to more rapid recovery from the attack but is unlikely to alter the degree of eventual recovery.

For severe relapses that do not respond to high-dose IV corticosteroids, a small randomized study showed that plasma exchange can be effective. Rapid functional improvement in over 40% of patients occurred with early initiation of plasma exchange. Subjects in this trial likely included patients with NMO and ADEM, in addition to MS.

MS is one of only a handful of chronic neurologic disorders with effective disease modifying therapies. The beta-interferons (BIFNs) and glatiramer acetate (GA) are US Food and Drug Administration (FDA)-approved for the treatment of patients with relapsing forms of MS to decrease the frequency of clinical exacerbations and delay the accumulation of physical disability. The BIFNs and GA all reduced annualized relapse rate by about 30% in early pivotal studies. Most have been shown in randomized trials to delay progression to definite MS in those with CIS who are at high risk for developing MS.

As of mid-2020, 19 different disease modifying therapies, plus several generics versions of these, with 10 different mechanisms of action are available for MS (Table 122.4). The approved agents have distinct risk profiles. As there are currently no biomarkers that direct the choice of disease modifying therapies for an individual patient, selection of the disease modifying therapy for an individual is based on disease course and severity, comorbidities, and patient preferences.

Five BIFNs are approved for use in relapsing MS and CIS in the United States. They differ in dosage, mode of administration, side

TABLE 122.3 Selected MS Symptoms and Their Management

Symptom/Sign	Treatment(s)
Stiffness/cramps/spasms/spasticity	Baclofen, tizanidine
Fatigue	Amantadine, modafinil, armodafinil
Depression	Selective serotonin reuptake inhibitors, cognitive behavioral therapy
Pain/paresthesias/trigeminal neuralgia	Gabapentin, carbamazepine, oxcarbazepine, pregabalin, amitriptyline
Gait impairment	Fampridine SR
Nystagmus, with visual impairment	Gabapentin
Dizziness/vertigo	Meclizine, dimenhydrinate, benzodiazepines
Urinary urgency/incontinence/neurogenic bladder	Mirabegron, oxybutynin, tolterodine, other anticholinergics, BOTOX injection
Impotence/erectile dysfunction	Sildenafil, tadalafil, testosterone supplementation if low
Tonic spasms	Phenytoin, carbamazepine

effects, and incidence of neutralizing antibody induction. Three are identical to human BIFN-1a. Polyethylene glycol has been covalently attached to one of the three for longer duration of effect. The other two are BIFN-1b, which differs by one amino acid from BIFN-1a. BIFNs are immunomodulators whose exact mechanism of action in MS is not fully established. BIFN therapy is associated with increased circulating soluble VCAM-1, and increased IL-10, an immunoregulatory cytokine. Hepatic transaminases and CBC should be monitored in those taking BIFNs. Common side effects include a "flu-like" feeling for several hours after a dose, which can be lessened by nonsteroidal anti-inflammatory medications or acetaminophen. BIFNs are administered by injection and, as with any injectable drug, skin infection can occur. Although the risk of taking BIFNs during pregnancy and lactation are thought to be minimal, it is recommended that BIFNs be discontinued before conception.

Glatiramer acetate is given as a subcutaneous injection at 20 mg per day or 40 mg three times per week. This drug is a random polymer of four amino acids that are abundant within myelin basic protein, a major protein in CNS myelin. It is considered immunomodulatory not immunosuppressive, although its mechanism of action is not

TABLE 122.4 Disease Modifying Medications for MS

Drug (Brand Name), Dosing	Approved	MS Indication	Mechanism of Action
Interferon-β-1b (Betaseron, Extavia), 250 µg SQ qod	1993, 2009	RRMS, CIS	Inhibits "pro-inflammatory" cytokines, such as interferon (IFN)-γ, tumor necrosis factor-α, and lymphotoxin. Increases IL-10. Adhesion molecule and class II MHC induction reduced.
Interferon-β-1a (Avonex) 30 µg IM weekly	1996	RRMS, CIS	
Interferon-β-1a (Rebif) 22 or 44 µg SQ 3×/wk	2002	RRMS	
Interferon-β-1a (Plegridy) 125 µg SQ every 14 days	2014	Relapsing forms of MS	
Glatiramer acetate (Copaxone) 20 mg SQ daily, or 40 mg SQ 3×/wk	1996, 2014	RRMS, CIS	Alters T cell cytokine profile toward that of Th2 immunomodulatory cells
Mitoxantrone (Novantrone) 12 mg/m² IV q 3 months	2000	Worsening RRMS, relapsing SPMS, PRMS	Anthracenedione chemotherapeutic agent
Natalizumab (Tysabri) 300 mg IV q 4 weeks	2004/2006 (removed briefly from market)	Relapsing forms of MS	Monoclonal antibody targeting the alpha-4-integrins, part of the VLA-4 adhesion molecule
Fingolimod (Gilenya) 0.5 mg po daily	2010	Relapsing MS, including children	Modulates sphingosine1-phosphate receptors 1,3,4, and 5; lymphocytes unable to migrate out of lymphoid tissue. May have direct effects in CNS.
Teriflunomide (Aubagio) 7 mg or 14 mg po daily	2012	Relapsing MS	Inhibits dihydroorotate dehydrogenase, thus inhibiting proliferation of activated lymphocytes
Dimethyl fumarate (Tecfidera) 240 mg po BID;	2013	Relapsing forms of MS, including active SPMS and CIS	Activates nuclear factor erythroid 2-related factor 2 (Nrf2) pathway that enhances response to oxidative stress
Diroximel fumarate (Vumerity) 231 mg po BID;	2020		
Monomethyl fumarate (Bafiertam) 95 mg po BID	2020		
Alemtuzumab (Lemtrada) IV infusion	2014	Relapsing forms of MS	Monoclonal antibody that lyses cells expressing CD52
Ocrelizumab (Ocrevus) IV infusion 600 mg every 24 weeks	2017	Relapsing forms of MS, primary progressive MS	Lytic monoclonal antibody targeting B cells expressing CD20
Oral cladribine (Mavenclad) 1.75 mg/kg po yearly ×2	2019	Relapsing forms of MS, including active SPMS	Cytotoxic to T and B lymphocytes through impairment of DNA synthesis
Siponimod (Mayzent) usually 2 mg po daily;	2019	Relapsing forms of MS, including active SPMS and CIS	Modulates sphingosine 1-phosphate receptors 1 and 5, lymphocytes are unable to migrate out of lymphoid tissue. May have direct effects in CNS.
Ozanimod (Zeposia) 0.92 mg po daily	2020		
Ofatumumab (Kesimpta) 20 mg SQ monthly	2020	Relapsing forms of MS, including CIS and active SPMS	Human lytic monoclonal antibody targeting B cells expressing CD20

fully understood. Glatiramer acetate has no known drug interactions. Laboratory monitoring is not needed. Side effects include injection site reactions and a tachycardia reaction that occurs infrequently and seemingly randomly, but always soon after an injection. Lipoatrophy at injection sites may develop with prolonged use. Glatiramer acetate is considered the safest MS disease modifying therapy to use in women who may become pregnant. No increase in risks for malformations or fetal/neonatal toxicity or pregnancy loss has been noted in those who were exposed to branded glatiramer acetate, although exposure has been mostly limited to the first trimester.

Mitoxantrone is an anthracenedione chemotherapeutic agent that is FDA approved for secondary progressive MS, progressive relapsing MS, or worsening relapsing-remitting MS. It is administered by IV infusion every 3 months. Due to dose-limiting cardiotoxicity and drug-induced leukemia (the latter in approximately 1% of MS patients receiving it), mitoxantrone is rarely used any more.

Natalizumab is a humanized monoclonal antibody targeting the α-4-integrins, part of the VLA-4 adhesion-related heterodimer. The dose is 300 mg infused intravenously every 4 weeks. A 2-year phase 3 trial of natalizumab showed 68% reduction in annualized relapse rate, 42% reduction in sustained disability, and over 90% reduction in gadolinium-enhancing lesions compared with placebo. Natalizumab was temporarily removed from the market in 2005 due to its association with progressive multifocal leukoencephalopathy

(PML), a severe and sometimes fatal viral disorder caused by the JC virus. Because of its association with PML, this drug is recommended mainly in cases of an inadequate response or intolerance of an alternative MS therapy. Patients should be tested for serum antibodies to the JC virus prior to initiating therapy with natalizumab and, if positive, treatment should proceed with caution. Enrollment in a risk-mitigation program is required, and the drug can only be infused at a certified infusion center. Infusion reactions are not uncommon, and neutralizing antibodies to natalizumab develop in some patients. It is not recommended that natalizumab be used during pregnancy or during breast-feeding.

Fingolimod, an oral disease modifying therapy, is indicated for those with relapsing forms of MS, including CIS, RRMS, and active SPMS MS patients 10 years of age and older. This daily 0.5-mg capsule reduces annualized relapse rate in adults with RRMS by about 50% and disability progression by about 25% versus placebo. Fingolimod modulates sphingosine 1-phosphate receptors 1, 3, 4, and 5 and is believed to work in relapsing MS primarily by the sequestration of lymphocytes in secondary lymphoid tissues. Fingolimod affects several organ systems. Adverse effects include macular edema, pulmonary dysfunction, bradycardia, and increased infection rate (including opportunistic infections such as herpetic and cryptococcal infections and PML). Patients who are varicella zoster virus antibody-negative should be vaccinated prior to initiation. Fingolimod is contraindicated in the setting of recent myocardial infarction, stroke, uncontrolled heart failure, unstable angina, stroke, transient ischemic attack, or if baseline QTc interval on ECG is 500 ms or greater. Fingolimod can interact with a number of other drugs; it should not be initiated in those taking class IA and class III antiarrhythmic drugs. Medical monitoring for potential bradycardia for at least 6 hours after the first dose is required. Fingolimod may cause fetal harm. Women of childbearing age should use contraception during fingolimod use and for 2 months after its discontinuation.

Siponimod is a second-generation sphingosine 1-phosphate receptor modulator that was FDA-approved in 2019 for adults with relapsing forms of MS, including active SPMS, RRMS, and CIS. Siponimod is more specific than fingolimod, primarily modulating sphingosine 1-phosphate receptors 1 and 5. The maintenance dose is 2 mg per day by mouth but should be reduced to 1 mg/day for those with CYP2C9*1/*3 or *2/*3 genotype, and it is contraindicated for those who are CYP2C9*3/*3 homozygous. In a study of SPMS patients who were notably older (mean age 48 years) and more disabled (median EDSS 6.0) compared with most other MS clinical trials, siponimod reduced 3-month confirmed disability progression by a statistically significant 21% ($P = 0.013$) versus placebo. First-dose monitoring should be done in people with sinus bradycardia, first- or second-degree atrioventricular block, history of myocardial infarction or heart failure. Women of childbearing age who take siponimod should undergo effective contraception, as siponimod has potential for a serious risk to the fetus. Several other sphingosine 1-phosphate receptor modulators are currently being studied in MS.

Ozanimod is a second-generation sphingosine 1-phosphate receptor 1 and 5 modulator that was FDA-approved in 2020 for adults with relapsing forms of MS. In two trials enrolling over 800 subjects with active relapsing MS each, ozanimod was compared to BIFN 1a 30 g IM weekly, showing 48% and 38% relative reductions (each $P < 0.0001$) in annualized relapse rate versus active comparator. As with fingolimod and siponimod, patients should have baseline bloodwork to include CBC and liver function tests, an electrocardiogram to assess for preexisting conduction abnormalities, and baseline and follow-up ophthalmic assessments to assess for macular edema. If live attenuated vaccine immunizations are needed (such as for varicella zoster), these should be administered at least 1 month prior to starting ozanimod (or fingolimod or siponimod). Several other sphingosine 1-phosphate receptor modulators are currently being studied in MS with at least one of these expected to be approved in 2021.

Teriflunomide is a once-daily oral tablet of 7 mg/day or 14 mg/day. Two phase 3 studies in patients with relapsing forms of MS found that the 14-mg/day dose significantly reduced annualized relapse rate by over 30% and disability progression by around 30%. The 7-mg dose had a lesser beneficial effect. Teriflunomide can cause hepatotoxicity, and liver blood work monitoring should continue monthly for 6 months after initiation. Based on animal data, teriflunomide may cause major birth defects and thus pregnancy must be avoided during treatment. If necessary, teriflunomide can be rapidly eliminated from the body using cholestyramine; otherwise, it persists for long periods. Teriflunomide may reactivate latent tuberculosis, is associated with peripheral neuropathy, and can increase blood pressure. Teriflunomide is closely related to the drug leflunomide, approved for rheumatoid arthritis in 1998.

Dimethyl fumarate is an oral medication taken twice daily and is indicated for all relapsing forms of MS. In phase 3 trials, it reduced MS relapse rates by 44% to 53% and improved MRI outcomes. The white blood cell count may drop and should be monitored. In late 2014, the FDA issued a warning regarding the association of PML with this medication, and since then over 20 people have developed PML in

the setting of dimethyl fumarate use. The risk of PML may be greater in those with persistent low lymphocyte counts and those over age 50. Adverse effects include flushing, gastrointestinal side effects, and rash. Dimethyl fumarate should be discontinued prior to conception. Several related fumarates with improved side effect profiles are under investigation for use in MS.

Diroximel fumarate and *monomethyl fumarate* are two second-generation oral fumarates each approved in 2020 by the FDA for relapsing forms of MS. These oral fumarates have similar efficacy and safety to dimethyl fumarate, but fewer gastrointestinal side effects.

Alemtuzumab is a lytic monoclonal antibody targeting cells expressing CD52, which includes T and B lymphocytes, monocytes, and other mononuclear white blood cells. In the United States, it is indicated for people with relapsing forms of MS and, because of its health risks, is reserved for those with inadequate response to two or more disease-modifying drugs for MS. In the CARE-MS I and II studies in RRMS patients, alemtuzumab infusions were compared to 44 µg BIFN-1a given subcutaneously three times per week. Patients treated with alemtuzumab had a lower annualized relapse rate (by 49% and 53.8%) and disability progression (by 28% and 42%). Alemtuzumab leads to a profound drop in the white blood cell count, which may last for months or even years. In trials, secondary autoimmune diseases developed in a sizeable proportion of alemtuzumab-treated subjects, with autoimmune thyroid disease being most common. Alemtuzumab may increase risk of malignancies, including thyroid cancer, melanoma, and lymphoproliferative disorders. Infusion reactions are common and can be life-threatening. Alemtuzumab is available only through clinicians and infusion centers that have been certified to use it. Women of childbearing potential should use effective contraceptive measures when receiving a course of alemtuzumab and for 4 months following that course of treatment.

Ocrelizumab is a fully humanized lytic monoclonal antibody targeting CD20, a cell surface antigen found on B lymphocytes. Ocrelizumab was FDA-approved in 2017 for patients with relapsing or primary progressive forms of MS. Ocrelizumab is given as an intravenous infusion of 600 mg every 24 weeks. In the phase 3 studies, those in the ocrelizumab group had almost 50% reduction in annualized relapse rate and a 40% reduction in 12-week confirmed disability progression compared to relapsing MS patients given subcutaneous BIFN-1a at 44 micrograms three times per week. In the phase 3 ORATORIO study in primary progressive MS, those receiving ocrelizumab had 24% reduction in 3 month confirmed progression versus placebo. Side effects include infusion reactions, increased infection rate (including herpetic infections) and a possible increased risk of cancers, including breast cancer. Patients should screen negative for hepatitis B before commencing use of ocrelizumab. Risks associated with ocrelizumab in pregnant women are unclear, but transient B cell depletion and lymphocytopenia have been reported in infants born to mothers exposed to other anti-CD20 antibodies during pregnancy. Being of immunoglobulin G1 subtype, ocrelizumab is expected to cross the placental barrier. Women of childbearing potential should use contraception while receiving ocrelizumab and for 6 months after the last infusion.

Ofatumumab is a human monoclonal antibody that targets and lyses cells expressing CD20. It is administered monthly, subcutaneously. In two clinical trials of over 900 relapsing MS patients each, ofatumumab was compared to teriflunomide 14 mg/day po. Annualized relapse rate reductions of 51% and 59% (both $P < 0.001$) were observed in the ofatumumab groups relative to teriflunomide groups. The combined studies showed ofatumumab to confer a 34.4% relative reduction in three-month confirmed disability progression ($P = .002$) versus teriflunomide. Potential risks and side effects are similar to those for ocrelizumab and include infections, injection reactions, and reduced response to vaccinations.

Oral cladribine was approved by the FDA in 2019 for the treatment of relapsing forms of MS in adults, including RRMS and active SPMS. This drug is recommended for patients who have had an inadequate response to, or are unable to tolerate, an alternative disease modifying treatment of MS. Oral cladribine is a purine antimetabolite that destroys certain immune cells. It is given at a cumulative dosage of 3.5 mg/kg divided into two treatment courses at 1.75 mg/kg per treatment course given a year apart. Oral cladribine may increase the risk of malignancy, and it is contraindicated in those with concurrent malignancy. Patients should be screened for HIV, tuberculosis, and hepatitis B and C prior to use. Varicella zoster virus antibody-negative persons should be vaccinated before initiation. Oral cladribine is contraindicated in pregnant or breast-feeding women and in both women and men of reproductive potential who do not plan to use effective contraception because of risk of fetal harm.

NEUROMYELITIS OPTICA SPECTRUM DISORDER (DEVIC DISEASE)

Definition/Epidemiology

Neuromyelitis optica spectrum disorders (NMOSD) comprise a spectrum of inflammatory CNS disorders causing both demyelination and necrosis that are clinically characterized by attacks of optic neuritis and longitudinally extensive TM that are not necessarily concurrent. Only rarely is NMOSD monophasic. In most cases serum autoantibodies to the aquaporin 4 (AQP4) water channels are found. AQP4 channels are strongly expressed by astrocytes. AQP4 is also expressed outside of the CNS in the kidney, stomach, and other tissues, but curiously no pathology has been recognized in the non-CNS organs expressing AQP4.

NMOSD is much less common than MS, with estimates by the Guthy-Jackson Charitable Foundation of 15,000 patients in the United

States. It is even more female-preponderant than MS, with female to male ratio estimated at 7:1. Children and adults both develop NMO. Unlike MS, NMO is *not* associated with HLA-DRB1*15:01, and it affects those of Asian, African, Hispanic, and Polynesian ancestry disproportionately.

Clinical Presentation

NMO presents clinically as an acute attack of optic neuritis and/or TM; it often takes a relapsing course. Gradually progressive NMO is exceedingly rare (helping to distinguish progressive MS from NMO). Other autoimmune diseases often occur together with NMOSD including Sjögren's syndrome, systemic lupus erythematosus, Hashimoto disease, and myasthenia gravis.

Diagnosis/Differential

In 2004, researchers first reported the presence of a serum IgG autoantibody targeting aquaporin 4 in NMO. NMO-IgG/AQP4-IgG is highly specific (>90%) and moderately sensitive (≈75%) for NMOSD. Fulfilling two out of three of the following criteria is reported to be 99% sensitive and 90% specific in the setting of optic neuritis and TM: (1) longitudinally extensive spinal cord lesion, which is greater than or equal to three segments in length (Fig. 122.3); (2) NMO-IgG (anti-AQP4) positivity; and (3) brain MRI not typical or diagnostic for MS.

For a deeper discussion of these topics, please see Chapter 383, ❖ "Multiple Sclerosis and Demyelinating Conditions of the Central Nervous System," in *Goldman-Cecil Medicine*, 26th Edition.

Pathology

Histopathologic changes in NMOSD are mostly in the spinal cord and optic nerves; the brain is less involved. Lesions affect both white and gray matter. In the brain, lesions are most common in the hypothalamus and around the fourth ventricle. NMO lesions center on blood vessels where IgG, IgM, and complement activation products are seen. The vessels are abnormally thickened and hyalinized. Active

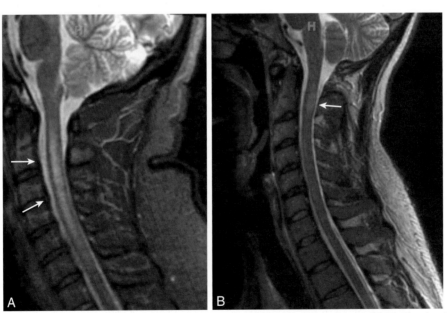

Fig. 122.3 (A) Sagittal T2w image of the upper spinal cord in a 37-year-old female with NMO. She developed quadriparesis over several days and was AQP4-IgG seropositive. Two years later she had right eye optic neuritis, which left her with visual acuity of only 20/200. The spinal cord lesion *(arrows)* had mild mass effect and was contiguous over six vertebral segments. (B) Sagittal T2w image of the upper spinal cord in a 24-year-old male with MS shows a lesion *(arrow)* in the posterior cord at C2. This patient had moderate vibration loss in the legs but was otherwise asymptomatic.

NMO lesions show infiltration by mononuclear cells (lymphocytes, monocytes), neutrophils, and eosinophils. Older lesions display demyelination, axon loss, and death of oligodendroglia and neurons. Accumulating data indicate that AQP4-IgG itself is pathogenic, causing complement- and antibody-mediated damage.

Treatment

Acute relapses are treated with high-dose corticosteroids. If these are not quickly effective, plasma exchange is performed. Although NMO is rare, several multicenter randomized, controlled trials of disease modifying therapies have been completed recently with notably positive results.

Eculizumab, a monoclonal antibody that inhibits the complement cascade, was compared to placebo in a randomized, double-blind, multicenter trial in adult NMOSD patients. The trial was stopped early when it showed that relapses occurred in only 3% in the eculizumab group versus 43% in the placebo group (hazard ratio, 0.06; 95% confidence interval, 0.02 to 0.20; $P < 0.001$). Upper respiratory tract infections and headaches were more common in the eculizumab group and a death from pulmonary empyema occurred in this group.

Inebilizumab, a monoclonal antibody to CD19 that depletes B cells, was compared to placebo in adults with NMOSD in a randomized, double-blind, multicenter study. Primary end point was time to onset of an NMOSD attack. This study too was stopped before complete enrollment because of a clear demonstration of efficacy. Twelve percent of 174 participants receiving inebilizumab had an attack versus 39% those receiving placebo (hazard ratio 0.272 [95% confidence interval 0.150 to 0.496]; $P < 0.0001$). Serious adverse effects were no higher in the active treatment group than in the placebo group.

Satralizumab, a monoclonal antibody targeting the IL-6 receptor and thereby inhibiting IL-6 activity, has been reported to show positive results in NMOSD, particularly in those with positive ant-AQP4 antibodies. Notably, beta-interferons are *not* effective for NMOSD and may actually increase the rate of attacks.

Prognosis

NMOSD typically displays worse outcomes than MS. Seropositive NMO patients tend to have more frequent and severe relapses than AQP4-IgG negative patients. The death rate in a retrospective study covering 1950 to 1997 was over 30%. Less than 10% mortality was reported in a more recent retrospective study of Caucasian NMO patients. Death is often due to respiratory failure.

ANTI-MYELIN OLIGODENDROCYTE GLYCOPROTEIN DISORDER

A CNS demyelinating disease identified by its association with serum antibodies to the CNS myelin component, myelin oligodendrocyte glycoprotein (MOG), was recently described. Diagnosis is based on positive serum IgG1antibodies to MOG using cell-based assays, as well as the absence of anti-AQP4 antibodies, and absence of CSF-restricted oligoclonal bands. Anti-MOG disorder shares features with both MS and classical NMO. Anti-MOG disorder occurs in children and adults and affects males and females in similar proportion. In adults, anti-MOG disorder is often characterized by optic neuritis and transverse myelitis (which may occur separately), but the disease is usually less severe than AQP4 antibody positive NMOSD and is often monophasic. An acute disseminated encephalomyelitis-like presentation is common in children. The spectrum of anti-MOG disorder is still being determined, as is the optimum treatment strategy.

ACUTE DISSEMINATED ENCEPHALOMYELITIS

ADEM is an acute, inflammatory, presumed immune-mediated disorder of the CNS that is encountered primarily in children but may occur in adults. An antecedent viral infection or vaccination is common. ADEM presents with multifocal neurologic symptoms and signs. These can include encephalopathy, which may manifest as reduced level of consciousness (even coma) or as behavioral changes (e.g., confusion or irritability). Fever is common. Seizures, optic neuritis, and spinal cord involvement can all occur. Males and females are about equally affected. ADEM is usually monophasic, although relapsing ADEM has been described. On MRI, both white and gray matter CNS regions are affected. Gray matter involvement can include the basal ganglia, a region not typically affected in MS. The periventricular white matter region is often spared, unlike MS. When present, enhancement with gadolinium occurs in all lesions simultaneously. CSF often shows pleocytosis and an elevated protein but no infection. Findings typical of MS, such as oligoclonal bands, are unusual. No randomized prospective treatment trials for acute disseminated encephalomyelitis are reported. Intravenous methylprednisolone followed by a prednisone taper is typically administered with usually good response. Over 80% of cases recover. Because ADEM is only rarely recurrent, long-term immunomodulatory/immunosuppressive therapy is not indicated. A rare hemorrhagic form of ADEM (Weston Hurst syndrome) is more severe and can lead to death or severe disability.

ACUTE TRANSVERSE MYELITIS

TM is an inflammatory spinal cord syndrome presenting with abrupt or subacute onset of motor and/or sensory loss below a specific spinal level. Control of bladder and bowel is often affected, as is autonomic function below the level. Back pain and paresthesias may be prominent. Many cases of acute TM are idiopathic, but treatable causes must be ruled out. An urgent MRI with and without gadolinium should be obtained to look for compressive etiologies needing immediate treatment. After a compressive etiology has been ruled out, a lumbar puncture to assess CSF for cell count, glucose, and protein and cultures and PCRs for infectious causes should be done. The usual tests for MS should be performed, and CSF should be analyzed for evidence of neoplastic cells. Serum AQP4-IgG, anti-MOG using cell-based assays, paraneoplastic panels, and chest CT should be considered. CSF may also be tested for NMO-IgG, angiotensin converting enzyme, and paraneoplastic antibodies when no etiology is forthcoming.

Acute TM can be the presenting episode for MS (in which case the TM is generally incomplete and asymmetrical) or NMO (where the TM affects ≥3 spinal cord segments). Acute TM can also be caused by spinal cord infarction due to occlusion of the anterior spinal artery. Infections by viruses can cause acute or subacute TM. The most common viruses associated with acute TM are varicella zoster, herpes virus type 2, and cytomegalovirus. The retroviruses HTLV-I and HIV can each cause a myelopathy that is usually subacute. West Nile virus can cause a myelopathy that resembles poliomyelitis, with flaccid paralysis due to infection and death of anterior horn cells. Subacute TM may be caused by vitamin B_{12} or copper deficiency or infiltrating or compressive syndromes such as tumors or abscesses. Nitrous oxide anesthesia can precipitate an acute-onset myelopathy in the case of borderline vitamin B_{12} deficiency. Rheumatologic disorders such as Sjögren's disease, systemic lupus erythematosus, and Behçet's disease can all cause TM. Paraneoplastic syndromes associated with anti-CRMP-5 and anti-amphiphysin can cause a tract-specific myelopathy. The history and physical examination should be performed with these disorders in mind.

Treatment is determined by the most likely etiology. Idiopathic TM is treated much like TM in MS or NMO, with intravenous methylprednisolone at 500 mg to 1000 mg/day, usually followed by a short oral prednisone taper. When response to intravenous methylprednisolone is suboptimal, plasma exchange should be considered.

IDIOPATHIC ACUTE OPTIC NEURITIS

Inflammatory demyelinating optic neuritis can occur as part of MS or NMO, or as an idiopathic entity. Classically, optic neuritis presents over hours with loss of vision together with pain exacerbated by eye movement. Vision loss may range from subclinical to frank blindness. Color vision and contrast sensitivity are disproportionately affected. On examination, a relative afferent pupillary defect is seen in unilateral optic neuritis. Acute demyelinating optic neuritis is often retrobulbar without papillitis. On MRI, the optic nerve can be swollen and enhance after gadolinium contrast. After recovery from the acute episode, the optic disk may appear pale, and the relative afferent pupillary defect may persist. Transient worsening of vision when the body temperature rises due to exercise or fever (Uhthoff phenomenon) may occur following recovery. The differential diagnosis includes other causes of acute monocular or binocular vision loss, such as Leber hereditary optic neuropathy, giant cell arteritis, and acute nonarteritic anterior ischemic optic neuropathy.

The Optic Neuritis Treatment Trial studied patients with acute optic neuritis (either idiopathic or due to MS) who were randomized to one of three treatments, intravenous methylprednisolone versus oral prednisone taper versus oral placebo. Visual acuity initially recovered faster in the intravenous methylprednisolone group, but by 6 months later there was no difference among the three groups. Recovery of vision was good. Patients from this trial were examined 10 years later and acuity in the affected eyes was 20/20 or better in 74% and less than 20/200 in only 3%. However, recurrence of optic neuritis was common and had occurred in either eye in 35% of the patients. Recurrences were more frequent in those who had MS than in those with idiopathic optic neuritis ($P < .001$).

CHRONIC RELAPSING INFLAMMATORY OPTIC NEUROPATHY

First described in 2003, chronic relapsing inflammatory optic neuropathy (CRION) is an inflammatory optic neuropathy characterized by acute relapses, often with more severe visual loss than idiopathic optic neuritis or optic neuritis associated with MS. CRION can commence at any age and has been described worldwide. Prevalence rates and epidemiology are still unclear. As in other types of optic neuritis, eye pain at onset is frequent. Five diagnostic criteria for CRION have been suggested: (1) optic neuritis with at least one relapse, (2) visual loss, (3) AQP4-IgG seronegativity, (4) contrast enhancement on MRI of acutely inflamed optic nerve, and (5) response to immunosuppressive treatment and relapse on withdrawal. Other diseases that might present similarly, such as sarcoidosis and giant cell arteritis, should be ruled out. Acute CRION is treated similarly to other causes of optic neuritis, with high-dose methylprednisolone. Relapses are common upon corticosteroid discontinuation. Successful long-term treatment with "steroid sparing" agents such as methotrexate, azathioprine, or mycophenolate mofetil has been reported. The underlying pathology is not yet known, but the disease appears inflammatory based on clinical presentation, imaging, and specific medication response. Eventual visual outcomes are often poor. One report indicated that visual acuity was less than 20/200 in one third of CRION patients.

SUGGESTED READINGS

Correale J, Gaitán MI, Ysrraelit MC, Fiol MP: Progressive multiple sclerosis: from pathogenic mechanisms to treatment, Brain 140:527–546, 2017.

Kim SH, Huh SY, Lee SJ: A 5-year follow-up of rituximab treatment in patients with neuromyelitis optica spectrum disorder, JAMA Neurol 70:1110–1117, 2013.

Klaver R, De Vries HE, Schenk GJ, et al: Grey matter damage in multiple sclerosis: a pathology perspective, Prion 7:66–75, 2013.

Langer-Gould A, Brara SM, Beaber BE, et al: Incidence of multiple sclerosis in multiple racial and ethnic groups, Neurology 80:1734–1739, 2013.

Lublin FD, Reingold SC, Cohen JA, et al: Defining the clinical course of multiple sclerosis: the 2013 revisions, Neurology 83:277–286, 2014.

Petzold A, Plant GT: Chronic relapsing inflammatory optic neuropathy: a systematic review of 122 cases reported, J Neurol 261:17–26, 2014.

Pittock SJ, Berthele A, Fujihara K, et al: Eculizumab in aquaporin-4-positive neuromyelitis optica spectrum disorder, N Engl J Med 381:614–625, 2019.

Reindl M, Di Pauli F, Rostásy K, Berger T: The spectrum of MOG antibody-associated demyelinating disorders, Nat Rev Neurol 9:455–461, 2013.

Thompson AJ, Banwell BL, Barkhof F, et al: Diagnosis of multiple sclerosis: 2017 revisions of the McDonald criteria, Lancet Neurol 17:162–173, 2018.

West TW, Hess C, Cree BA: Acute transverse myelitis: demyelinating, inflammatory, and infectious myelopathies, Semin Neurol 32:97–113, 2012.

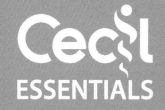

123

Neuromuscular Diseases: Disorders of the Motor Neuron and Plexus and Peripheral Nerve Disease

Carlayne E. Jackson, Ratna Bhavaraju-Sanka

INTRODUCTION

Neuromuscular diseases are classified into four groups, according to which portion of the motor unit is involved (Table 123.1). Motor neuron and peripheral nerve diseases are considered in this chapter; myopathies are considered in Chapter 124, and neuromuscular junction diseases are considered in Chapter 125. The symptoms and signs of the neuromuscular diseases are at times indistinguishable. However, some useful general rules apply to assist with localization based on the distribution of weakness, presence or absence of sensory symptoms, reflex abnormalities, and specific associated clinical features (Table 123.2).

Electromyography and Nerve Conduction Studies

Electromyography (EMG) and nerve conduction studies can also be useful diagnostic tools in localizing the lesion in a patient with a suspected neuromuscular disease. The measurement of electrical activity arising from muscle fibers is performed by inserting a needle electrode percutaneously into a muscle. Normal muscle is electrically silent at rest. Spontaneous activity during complete relaxation occurs in myotonic disorders, in inflammatory myopathies, and in denervated muscles. Spontaneous activity of a single muscle fiber is called a *fibrillation*, and such activity of part of or an entire motor unit is called a *fasciculation*. In myotonia, repeated muscle depolarization and contraction occur despite voluntary relaxation. Abnormalities in motor unit potentials occur during the course of denervation; with the development of reinnervation, the remaining motor units increase in amplitude and become longer in duration and polyphasic (E-Fig. 123.1). Conversely, in muscle diseases such as the muscular dystrophies and other diseases that destroy scattered fibers within a motor unit, the motor unit action potentials are of lower amplitude and shorter duration and are polyphasic. A reduced recruitment (interference) pattern from maximum voluntary effort occurs in denervation. Conversely, in patients with primary muscle disease, submaximal voluntary effort produces a full recruitment pattern despite marked weakness.

Nerve conduction is studied by stimulating a peripheral nerve (e.g., the ulnar) with surface electrodes placed over the nerve or muscle. The resulting action potential is recorded by electrodes placed over the nerve more proximally in the case of large sensory nerve fibers and over the muscle distally in the case of motor nerve fibers in a mixed motor sensory nerve. For sensory nerves, the sensory nerve action potential (SNAP) is quantitated, and for motor nerves, the compound muscle action potential (CMAP) is quantitated. Abnormalities in sensory and motor nerve studies are suggestive of a peripheral neuropathy while abnormalities in motor nerve studies with normal sensory studies can indicate a myopathy, motor neuronopathy, pure motor neuropathy or radiculopathy.

DISEASES OF THE MOTOR NEURON (ANTERIOR HORN CELL)

Amyotrophic Lateral Sclerosis

Definition and Epidemiology

The most common *acquired* motor neuron disease, amyotrophic lateral sclerosis (ALS), is a progressive, typically fatal disorder. The incidence is approximately 2 to 5 per 100,000 population, and there is a slight male predominance. The peak age of onset is in the sixth decade, although the disease can occur at any time throughout adulthood. The cumulative lifetime risk is about 1 in 400. Epidemiologic studies have incriminated risk factors for ALS including exposure to insecticides, smoking, participation in varsity athletics, and military service in the Gulf War. The cause of ALS is largely unknown, with 95% of cases considered "sporadic," and 5% related to an autosomal dominant disease (familial ALS [FALS]). FALS is an adult-onset disease that is clinically and pathologically indistinguishable from sporadic ALS. FALS is caused by mutations in many genes, including the *C9orf72, SOD1, TARDBP, FUS, ANG, ALS2, SETX,* and *VAPB* genes. Mutations in the *C9orf72* gene are responsible for 30% to 45% of FALS in the United States and Europe. Mutations in *C9orf72* also cause sporadic ALS (E-Table 123.1).

Pathology

ALS results from degeneration of the cortical motor neurons originating in layer five of the motor cortex and descending via the pyramidal tract (resulting in upper motor neuron signs and symptoms) and from degeneration of the anterior horn cells in the spinal cord and their brain stem homologues innervating bulbar muscles (resulting in lower motor neuron signs and symptoms) (Table 123.3).

Clinical Presentation

Clinical symptoms relating to the upper motor neuron degeneration include loss of dexterity, slowed movements, muscle weakness, stiffness, and emotional lability. Signs on neurologic examination that confirm an upper motor neuron lesion include pseudobulbar affect, pathologic hyperreflexia, spasticity, and extensor plantar responses (Babinski sign). Lower motor neuron signs and symptoms caused by anterior horn cell degeneration include weakness, muscle atrophy, fasciculations, and cramps. Fasciculations in the absence of associated muscle atrophy or weakness are usually benign and may be aggravated by sleep deprivation, stress, and excessive caffeine ingestion. Muscle weakness in patients with ALS usually begins distally and asymmetrically and may manifest as a monoparesis, hemiparesis, paraparesis, or quadriparesis. It may also be limited initially to the bulbar region, resulting in difficulty with swallowing, speech, and movements of the face and tongue. For unclear reasons, ocular motility is spared until the very late stages of the illness. Bowel and bladder function and sensation remain spared throughout the course of the disease although patients may develop symptoms of bladder urgency. Up to 60% of patients with ALS may also have a component of frontotemporal dementia characterized by executive dysfunction, poor insight, personality changes (disinhibition, impulsivity, apathy), abnormal eating habits, poor hygiene, and language dysfunction.

Diagnosis/Differential

The diagnosis of ALS remains one of "exclusion," in which other potential causes must be ruled out through a variety of neuroimaging, laboratory, and electrodiagnostic investigations (E-Table 123.2). For example, compression of the cervical spinal cord or cervicomedullary junction from tumors or cervical spondylosis can produce weakness,

atrophy, and fasciculations in the upper extremities and spasticity in the lower extremities, closely resembling ALS.

Treatment

Specialized multidisciplinary clinic referral should be considered for patients with ALS to optimize health care delivery and prolong survival. The first US Food and Drug Administration (FDA)–approved therapy for ALS was riluzole 50 mg twice per day, which in clinical trials prolonged survival by 2 to 3 months. The mechanism of this effect is not known with certainty; however, riluzole may reduce excitotoxicity by diminishing presynaptic glutamate release. Edaravone was also recently FDA approved based on studies suggesting a slowing of the rate of functional decline by 33% (measured by the ALS Functional Rating Scale-Revised). Initiation of noninvasive ventilation (NIV) on a spontaneous timed mode has also been shown to prolong survival up to 20 months, to slow the rate of forced vital capacity (FVC) decline (level B) and to improve quality of life. NIV should be initiated when the FVC is less than 50%, the maximal inspiratory pressure is less than −60 cm, or when patients report symptoms that suggest nocturnal hypoventilation (daytime fatigue, frequent arousals, supine dyspnea, morning headaches). A cough-assist device can be used to assist with clearing upper airway secretions and has been shown to minimize the risk of pneumonia in clinical trials. A percutaneous gastrostomy (PEG) tube should be considered for prolonging survival and stabilizing body weight in patients with impaired oral food intake. Symptomatic therapy for spasticity, pseudobulbar affect, muscle cramping, and sialorrhea is also essential in maintaining patient dignity and quality of life (Table 123.4). Augmentative speech devices can assist patients with communication and computer access.

TABLE 123.1 Classification of Neuromuscular Diseases

Site of Involvement	Typical Examples
Anterior Horn Cell	
Without upper motor neuron involvement	Spinal muscular atrophy
	Progressive muscular atrophy
	Bulbospinal muscular atrophy
	Poliomyelitis
	West Nile virus
With upper motor neuron involvement	Amyotrophic lateral sclerosis
	Primary lateral sclerosis
Peripheral Nerve	
Mononeuropathy	Carpal tunnel syndrome
	Ulnar palsy
	Meralgia paresthetica
Multiple mononeuropathies	Mononeuritis multiplex (e.g., polyarteritis nodosa), leprosy, sarcoidosis, amyloidosis
Polyneuropathies	Diabetic neuropathy
	Charcot-Marie-Tooth disease
	Gullain-Barré syndrome
Neuromuscular Junction	
	Myasthenia gravis
	Lambert-Eaton syndrome
Muscle	
	Duchenne muscular dystrophy
	Dermatomyositis

TABLE 123.3 Symptoms and Signs Associated With Amyotrophic Lateral Sclerosis

Symptoms	Signs
Upper Motor Neuron Degeneration	
Loss of dexterity	Pathologic hyperreflexia
Slowed movements	Babinski response
Weakness	Hoffman response
Stiffness	Jaw jerk
Pseudobulbar affect	Spasticity
Lower Motor Neuron Degeneration	
Weakness	Muscle atrophy
Fasciculations	Fibrillation potentials on electromyography
Cramps	Neurogenic atrophy on muscle biopsy

TABLE 123.2 Clinical Features of the Neuromuscular Diseases

Clinical Feature	Anterior Horn Cell	Peripheral Nerve	Neuromuscular Junction	Muscle
Distribution of weakness	Asymmetrical limb or bulbar	Symmetrical, usually distal	Extraocular, bulbar, proximal limb	Symmetrical, proximal limb
Atrophy	Marked and early	Mild, distal	None (or very late)	Slight early; marked later
Sensory involvement	None	Dysesthesias, loss of sensation	None	None
Reflexes	Variable (depending on degree of upper motor neuron involvement)	Decreased out of proportion to weakness	Normal in myasthenia gravis, depressed in Lambert-Eaton syndrome	Decreased in proportion to weakness
Characteristic features	Fasciculations, cramps	Combined sensory and motor abnormalities	Fatigability	Usually painless

TABLE 123.4 Symptom Management for Motor Neuron Diseases

Respiratory Insufficiency
Noninvasive ventilation
Cough-assist devices
Dysarthria
Augmentative speech device
Dysphagia
Percutaneous endoscopic gastrostomy (PEG) placement
Suction machine
Sialorrhea
Amitriptyline 25-75 mg qhs
Glycopyrrolate 1-2 mg q8h
Botulinum toxin
Spasticity
Baclofen 10-20 mg QID
Dantrium 25-100 mg QID
Pseudobulbar Affect
Serotonin reuptake inhibitors
Amitriptyline 25-75 mg QHS
Dextromethorphan/quinidine 20/10 mg BID
Weakness
Ankle-foot orthosis
Wheelchair
Elevated toilet seat

TABLE 123.5 Clinical Spectrum of Motor Neuron Diseases[a]

Upper and Lower Motor Neuron Involvement
Sporadic amyotrophic lateral sclerosis
Familial amyotrophic lateral sclerosis
Upper Motor Neuron Involvement
Primary lateral sclerosis
Hereditary spastic paraparesis
Lower Motor Neuron Involvement
Motor neuronopathy related to malignancy or paraproteinemia
Poliomyelitis
West Nile virus
Postpolio syndrome
Hexosaminidase deficiency
Progressive muscular atrophy
Spinal muscular atrophy
   Type I: Infantile onset (Werdnig-Hoffmann disease)
   Type II: Late infantile onset
   Type III: Juvenile onset (Kugelberg-Welander disease)

[a]Italicized disorders are hereditary.

Prognosis

Mean survival from onset of symptoms is 2 to 5 years, with 10% of patients surviving beyond 10 years. The majority of deaths are related to respiratory muscle failure and aspiration pneumonia.

Other Acquired Motor Neuron Diseases

Other motor neuron diseases involve only particular subsets of motor neurons (Table 123.5). Progressive muscular atrophy (PMA) is a pure lower motor neuron disease that accounts for 8% to 10% of patients with motor neuron disease. Weakness is typically distal and asymmetrical, and bulbar involvement is rare. Patients with PMA generally have a better prognosis than those with ALS, with a survival of 3 to 14 years. Primary lateral sclerosis (PLS) is a pure upper motor neuron syndrome in which patients demonstrate either a slowly progressive spastic paralysis or dysarthria. This is a rare disorder, accounting for 2% of all motor neuron cases. Survival is generally years to decades.

Spinal Muscular Atrophy

Spinal muscular atrophy (SMA) is a hereditary form of motor neuron disease in which only the lower motor neuron is affected. It is an autosomal recessive disorder that may begin in utero, in infancy, in childhood, or in adult life and represents the first class of neurologic disorders in which a developmental defect in neuronal apoptosis most likely produces the disease. The most common forms of SMA are due to a defect in the survival motor neuron 1 *(SMN1)* gene localized to 5q11.2-q13.3. All affected individuals with SMA have mutations in both copies of the *SMN1* gene causing little or no SMN (survival motor neuron) protein production from this gene. The *SMN2* gene can help replace some of the missing SMN protein. Patients who have multiple copies of the *SMN2* gene are usually associated with later onset and less severe disease. Nusinersen was recently approved for intrathecal use and has been shown to significantly slow functional decline and increase life expectancy. It is an antisense oligonucleotide targeted to increase the proportion of SMN2 mRNA transcripts, leading to translation of more full-length SMN protein. In May of 2019 the FDA also approved onasemnogene abeparvovec-xioi (Zolgensma), the first gene therapy to treat children less than 2 years of age with SMA.

Bulbospinal muscular atrophy (BSMA) or Kennedy disease is an X-linked recessive disorder in which the mean age at onset is 30 years; the range is from 15 to 60 years. BSMA is a trinucleotide repeat disorder with a CAG expansion encoding for a polyglutamine tract in the first exon of the androgen receptor gene, on chromosome Xq11-12. The mechanism by which disruption of the androgen receptor gene alters the function of bulbar and spinal motor neurons is not known. An inverse correlation exists between the number of CAG repeats and the age of onset of the disease. Affected individuals exhibit chin fasciculations, midline furrowing and atrophy of the tongue, and proximal weakness. Dysphagia and dysarthria are common, and up to 90% of patients demonstrate gynecomastia and infertility. Two findings distinguishing this disorder from ALS are the absence of upper motor neuron signs and in some patients the presence of a subtle sensory neuropathy.

DISORDERS OF THE BRACHIAL AND LUMBOSACRAL PLEXUS

The roots within the cervical, lumbar, and sacral regions organize into the cervical, lumbar, and sacral plexuses before giving rise to individual peripheral nerves. Diseases of these plexuses (plexopathies) tend to be *focal* in symptoms and signs, whereas many diseases of the peripheral nerves and muscles are *generalized*.

Brachial Plexopathy

The brachial plexus is constituted by mixed nerve roots from C5 to T1 that fuse into upper, middle, and lower trunks above the level of the clavicle and redistribute into lateral, posterior, and medial cords below that landmark (E-Fig. 123.2). Symptoms include weakness, pain, and sensory loss in the shoulders or arms. Upper trunk lesions may be due to birth injury, trauma, and idiopathic brachial plexitis (see later). Lower trunk lesions may result from birth injury, malignant tumor invasion, thoracic outlet syndrome, or as a complication of sternotomy. If the entire plexus is involved, radiation injury, trauma, and late metastatic disease are the most common causes.

Acute Autoimmune Brachial Neuritis

Acute autoimmune brachial neuritis (or neuralgic amyotrophy or Parsonage-Turner syndrome) is characterized by the abrupt onset of severe pain, usually over the lateral shoulder, but at times extending into the neck or entire arm. The acute pain generally subsides after a few days to a week; by this time, weakness of the proximal arm becomes apparent. The serratus anterior, deltoid, and supraspinatus are the most commonly affected muscles, but other muscles of the shoulder girdle may also be affected. In rare cases, most of the patient's arm and even the ipsilateral diaphragm are involved. Sensory loss is usually slight and generally involves the axillary nerve distribution. Weakness lasts weeks to months and will be accompanied by severe atrophy of the shoulder girdle. No therapy has been shown to alter or shorten the clinical course, although steroids and analgesics may reduce pain. Most patients recover within several months to 3 years. The disorder frequently follows an upper respiratory infection or an immunization, but in many instances no antecedent illness occurs. It is bilateral in one third of cases but is always asymmetrical; it may recur in 5% of patients. Recurrent brachial plexopathies that are painless may be related to an autosomal dominant disorder with mutation in the *SEPTIN9* gene on chromosome 17q25 or hereditary neuropathy with liability to pressure palsies (HNPP), caused by a deletion or point mutation of PMP-22 protein (chromosome 17p).

Lumbosacral Plexopathy

The lumbosacral plexus is formed from the ventral rami of spinal nerves T12 to S4. These divide within the plexus into ventral and dorsal branches that form the femoral, sciatic, and obturator nerves. The plexus is located within the substance of the psoas major muscle. Clinical features include proximal pain and weakness in anterior thigh muscles (femoral) or posterior thigh muscles and the buttocks. Bowel and bladder dysfunction may also occur. Diabetes, malignant invasion, radiation therapy, infection (herpes zoster), psoas abscess, trauma, and retroperitoneal hemorrhage are common causes. An autoimmune form is much less frequent than brachial neuritis.

DISORDERS OF THE PERIPHERAL NERVES

Definition and Epidemiology

Peripheral neuropathy refers to a large group of disorders that can produce focal (mononeuropathy or multiple mononeuropathies) or generalized nerve dysfunction (polyneuropathies) (Table 123.6). Peripheral neuropathies are prevalent neurologic conditions, affecting 2% to 8% of adults, with the incidence increasing with age. They range in severity from mild sensory abnormalities, found in up to 70% of patients with long-standing diabetes, to fulminant, life-threatening paralytic disorders such as Guillain-Barré syndrome (GBS) or acute inflammatory demyelinating polyradiculoneuropathy (AIDP).

Mononeuropathies are disorders in which only a single peripheral nerve is affected. The most common cause is nerve entrapment such as median nerve compression resulting in carpal tunnel syndrome or peroneal nerve injury causing foot drop (Table 123.7). When more than one peripheral nerve is involved, the term *mononeuropathy multiplex* or *multiple mononeuropathies* is often used. Multiple mononeuropathies are most commonly seen in diabetes mellitus and vasculitis but also occur in leprosy, vasculitis, sarcoidosis, hereditary neuropathy with predisposition to pressure palsies, and amyloidosis.

Polyneuropathies are a group of disorders affecting the motor, sensory, and autonomic nerves. These disorders may predominantly affect the nerve axon (axonal neuropathies), myelin sheath (demyelinating neuropathies), or the small- to medium-sized blood vessels supplying

TABLE 123.6 Classification and Causes of Peripheral Neuropathy

Type of Neuropathy	Examples
Mononeuropathies	
Compressive	Carpal tunnel syndrome, ulnar palsy
Hereditary	Hereditary neuropathy with predisposition to pressure palsies
Inflammatory	Bell's palsy
Multiple mononeuropathies	Vasculitis (mononeuritis multiplex), diabetes, leprosy, sarcoidosis, amyloidosis
Polyneuropathies	
Hereditary	Charcot-Marie-Tooth disease, familial amyloid polyneuropathy
Endocrine	Diabetes, hypothyroidism
Metabolic	Uremia, liver failure
Infections	Leprosy, diphtheria, human immunodeficiency virus, Lyme disease
Immune mediated	Guillain-Barré syndrome, chronic inflammatory demyelinating polyneuropathy
Toxic	Lead-, arsenic-, alcohol-, drug-induced
Paraneoplastic	Lung cancer

the nerves (vasculitic neuropathies). The clinical features of the polyneuropathies reflect the pathology of the underlying process.

Pathology

In the symmetrical *axonal* polyneuropathies, the underlying pathology is usually a slowly evolving type of axonal degeneration that involves the ends of long nerve fibers first and preferentially. With time, the degenerative process involves more proximal regions of long fibers, and shorter fibers are affected. This pattern of distal axonal degeneration or *dying back* of nerve fibers results from a wide variety of metabolic, toxic, and endocrinologic causes.

In the *demyelinating* polyneuropathies, the underlying pathology involves the myelin sheath. Demyelination of a peripheral nerve at even a single site can block conduction, resulting in a functional deficit identical to that seen after axonal degeneration. In contrast to repair by regeneration, however, repair by remyelination can be rapid. Autoimmune attack on the myelin sheath occurs in the inflammatory demyelinating neuropathies (GBS/AIDP and chronic inflammatory demyelinating polyneuropathy [CIDP]) and some neuropathies associated with paraproteinemias (see later). Inherited disorders of myelin such as Charcot-Marie-Tooth (CMT) disease comprise the other major category of demyelinating neuropathies. Other causes include toxic, mechanical, and physical injuries to nerves. Although these examples have nearly pure demyelination, many neuropathies have both axonal degeneration and demyelination. This mixed pathologic abnormality reflects the mutual interdependency of the axons and the myelin-forming Schwann cells. Vasculitic neuropathies occur as a result of disease of the small or medium-sized blood vessels that leads to ischemia and infarction of isolated peripheral nerves. The term *mononeuritis multiplex* is also used to describe this clinical situation, in which there is multifocal involvement of individual nerves.

Clinical Presentation

The clinical picture of an *axonal* polyneuropathy includes early loss of muscle stretch reflexes at the ankle and weakness that initially involves the intrinsic muscles of the feet, the extensors of the toes, and the dorsiflexors at the ankle. The motor signs are usually mild in

TABLE 123.7 Common Mononeuropathies

	Precipitating Factors	Motor Signs and Symptoms	Sensory Signs and Symptoms	Treatment
Median Nerve Entrapment at the wrist (carpal tunnel syndrome)	Repetitive wrist flexion or sleep	Weakness in thenar muscle	Numbness, tingling, and/or pain in thumb, index finger, middle finger, and medial half of ring finger. Tinel and Phalen signs	Neutral wrist splint, carpal tunnel injections or surgery
Ulnar Nerve Entrapment at the elbow	External compression in condylar groove, fracture of humerus	Weakness or atrophy of the interossei and thumb adductor	Sensory loss in the little finger and contiguous half of the ring finger	Elbow pads; ulnar nerve transposition or decompression of cubital tunnel
Radial Nerve Entrapment at the spiral groove	Prolonged sleeping on arm after drinking excessive amounts of alcohol: "Saturday night palsy"	Wrist drop with sparing of elbow extension; weakness of finger and thumb extensors	Sensory loss on dorsum of hand	Spontaneous recovery; wrist splint
Femoral Nerve	Abdominal hysterectomy, hematoma, prolonged lithotomy position, diabetes	Weakness and atrophy of quadriceps	Sensory loss in anterior thigh and medial calf	Physical therapy
Lateral Femoral Cutaneous Nerve Meralgia paresthetica	Obesity, pregnancy, diabetes, constrictive belts	None	Sensory loss, pain, or tingling over anterolateral thigh	Weight loss; spontaneous recovery
Peroneal Nerve Entrapment at the fibular head	Habitual leg crossing, knee casts, prolonged squatting, profound weight loss	Weakness of ankle dorsiflexors or evertors and toe extensors	Sensory loss in anterolateral leg and dorsum of foot	Ankle-foot orthosis; remove source of compression
Sciatic Nerve	Injection injury, fracture or dislocation of hip	Weakness of hamstrings, ankle plantar flexors or dorsiflexors	Sensory loss in buttock, lateral calf, and foot	Ankle-foot orthosis; physical therapy
Tibial Nerve Entrapment in tarsal tunnel	External compression from tight shoes, trauma, tenosynovitis	None	Sensory loss and tingling in sole of foot	Tarsal tunnel injection, eliminate source of compression, medial arch support

contrast to the sensory abnormalities, which may include numbness, tingling, and burning sensations (dysesthesias). The sensory symptoms usually begin symmetrically in the toes and feet and then ascend proximally to the legs in a "stocking" distribution. When the sensory abnormalities reach the level of the knees, the symptoms begin in the hands, in a "glove" distribution. Truncal and abdominal dysesthesias may develop once the sensory abnormalities ascend to the level of the elbows.

The prominent clinical feature of an acquired *demyelinating* polyneuropathy is weakness that affects not only the distal muscles but also the proximal and facial muscles. Unlike in an axonal neuropathy, sensory loss is rarely the presenting symptom. Patients generally have diffuse hyporeflexia or areflexia.

Vasculitic neuropathies typically present with acute or subacute asymmetrical, predominantly distal weakness and sensory loss associated with severe pain.

Diagnosis/Differential

Neuropathic disorders can be broadly divided into those that are acquired and those that are hereditary (Table 123.8). Acquired disorders are the more common and have many causes: metabolic or endocrine disorders (diabetes mellitus, renal failure, porphyria); immune-mediated disorders (GBS, CIDP, multifocal motor neuropathy, anti-myelin-associated glycoprotein neuropathy); infectious causes (human immunodeficiency virus [HIV], Lyme disease, cytomegalovirus [CMV], syphilis, leprosy, diphtheria); medications (HIV drugs, chemotherapies); environmental toxins (heavy metals); or paraneoplastic processes. Diabetes mellitus and alcoholism are the most common causes of polyneuropathy in developed countries. As many as one third of acquired neuropathies are cryptogenic in which the etiology can never be identified. Causes of mononeuritis multiplex include systemic vasculitis (rheumatoid arthritis, systemic lupus erythematosus, Wegener granulomatosis, Churg-Strauss syndrome, polyarteritis nodosa) and primary peripheral system vasculitis (25% of cases).

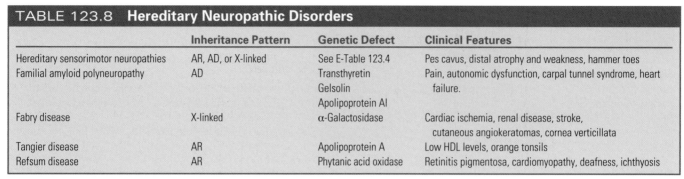

TABLE 123.8   Hereditary Neuropathic Disorders

	Inheritance Pattern	Genetic Defect	Clinical Features
Hereditary sensorimotor neuropathies	AR, AD, or X-linked	See E-Table 123.4	Pes cavus, distal atrophy and weakness, hammer toes
Familial amyloid polyneuropathy	AD	Transthyretin Gelsolin Apolipoprotein AI	Pain, autonomic dysfunction, carpal tunnel syndrome, heart failure.
Fabry disease	X-linked	α-Galactosidase	Cardiac ischemia, renal disease, stroke, cutaneous angiokeratomas, cornea verticillata
Tangier disease	AR	Apolipoprotein A	Low HDL levels, orange tonsils
Refsum disease	AR	Phytanic acid oxidase	Retinitis pigmentosa, cardiomyopathy, deafness, ichthyosis

AD, Autosomal dominant; *AR,* autosomal recessive; *HDL,* high-density lipoprotein.

TABLE 123.9   Differential Diagnosis of Neuropathic Disorders Based on Symptoms

Motor Symptoms Only	Sensory Symptoms Only	Autonomic Symptoms
Porphyria	Cryptogenic sensory polyneuropathy	Amyloid neuropathy
Charcot-Marie-Tooth	Metabolic, drug-related, or toxic neuropathy	Diabetic neuropathy
Chronic inflammatory demyelinating polyneuropathy	Paraneoplastic sensory neuropathy	Fabry disease
Guillain-Barré syndrome		Guillain-Barré syndrome
Lead neuropathy		Hereditary sensory or autonomic neuropathy
Motor neuron disease		Porphyria

Because of the many causes, it is important to approach the patient with neuropathy systematically, beginning with the patient's history and physical examination. It is essential to determine which nerves are involved (motor, sensory, or autonomic) and in what specific combination (Table 123.9). Small-fiber neuropathies often manifest with unpleasant or abnormal sensations such as a burning pain, electric shock–like sensations, cramping, tingling, pins and needles, or prickly feelings such as the limb "feeling asleep." Large-fiber neuropathies can manifest as numbness, tingling, or as gait ataxia. Symptoms suggesting motor nerve involvement include muscle weakness that typically involves the distal foot muscles. Autonomic nerve involvement is suggested by symptoms of orthostatic hypotension, impotence, cardiac arrhythmia, or bladder dysfunction.

The distribution of muscle weakness is important. In axonal neuropathies, the weakness predominantly involves the distal lower extremity muscles, and in demyelinating neuropathies the weakness can involve both proximal and distal muscles as well as facial muscles. Most neuropathies result in *symmetrical* weakness. If asymmetry is present, motor neuron disease, radiculopathy, plexopathy, compressive mononeuropathies, or mononeuritis multiplex should be considered. The intensity and distribution of painful dysesthesias can also be informative. Although many axonal neuropathies are associated with a burning sensation in the feet, pain as the chief complaint suggests specific causes of neuropathy (Table 123.10). A neuropathy that manifests with acute, asymmetrical weakness and severe pain suggests vasculitis.

In patients with severe, asymmetrical proprioceptive deficits, with sparing of motor function, the site of the lesion is usually the sensory neuron/dorsal root ganglion. This specific syndrome has a relatively limited differential diagnosis, including paraneoplastic process with anti-Hu antibodies, Sjögren's syndrome, cisplatinum toxicity, vitamin B$_6$ toxicity, and HIV infection.

Most neuropathies are relatively insidious in onset, particularly those associated with metabolic or endocrine disorders. Acute neuropathies may be caused by a vasculitic process, toxin exposure, porphyria, or GBS. GBS

TABLE 123.10   Neuropathies Associated With Pain

Alcoholic neuropathy
Amyloidosis
Cryptogenic sensorimotor neuropathy
Diabetic neuropathy
Fabry disease
Guillain-Barré syndrome
Heavy metal toxicity (arsenic, thallium)
Hereditary sensory or autonomic neuropathy
HIV sensorimotor neuropathy
Radiculopathy or plexopathy
Vasculitis

HIV, Human immunodeficiency virus.

is commonly preceded by a viral illness, immunization, or a surgical procedure. The neurologic history must thoroughly explore potential toxic exposures such as prior medications and alcohol use (E-Table 123.3).

Because many neuropathies are hereditary, it is essential to obtain a detailed family history, specifically inquiring about a history of gait instability, use of adaptive equipment, or skeletal deformities of the feet. Hereditary neuropathies may be autosomal recessive, autosomal dominant, or X-linked. In some situations, it may be helpful to actually examine family members because the severity of disease may vary considerably from one generation to the next. The most common hereditary neuropathy is Charcot-Marie-Tooth disease (see later).

A complete neurologic examination should always be performed in a patient complaining of numbness. If the patient shows evidence of upper motor neuron involvement in addition to the sensory loss, vitamin B$_{12}$ or copper deficiency should be considered, even in the absence of apparent anemia. An elevated methylmalonic acid or homocystine level can also help confirm the diagnosis of B$_{12}$ deficiency in patients

TABLE 123.11 Peripheral Neuropathy Laboratory Studies

Standard Tests	Tests Indicated in Selected Cases
B$_{12}$	Anti-Hu antibody
Complete blood count (CBC)	ESR, ANA, RF, SS-A, SS-B
Glucose tolerance test	Genetic studies for Charcot-Marie-Tooth
RPR	Human immunodeficiency virus (HIV)
Chem 20	Lyme antibody
Serum protein electrophoresis	Phytanic acid
(SPEP) and immunofixation	Copper level
electrophoresis (IFE)	
Thyroid function tests	24-hr urine for heavy metals
Nerve conduction studies or	Quantitative sensory testing
electromyogram (EMG)	Lumbar puncture
	Nerve biopsy
	Skin biopsy
	Tilt table testing

with borderline levels. The presence of weakness and upper motor neuron signs without associated sensory loss suggests ALS.

If the neuropathy is associated with mental status abnormalities, then pyridoxine intoxication or deficiencies of thiamine, niacin ("dementia, diarrhea, dermatitis"), and vitamin B$_{12}$ should be considered in the differential diagnosis. Lyme disease (see Chapter 90) may result in both peripheral nervous system symptoms (facial nerve palsies, paresthesias, weakness) and central nervous system symptoms (dementia, headache). Acquired immunodeficiency syndrome (AIDS) can also affect both the central and the peripheral nervous systems. GBS and CIDP usually occur at the time of HIV seroconversion, whereas sensory neuropathy, mononeuritis multiplex, and CMV polyradiculopathy generally occur in the context of low CD4 counts in the later stages of the disease. Older antiretroviral drugs (e.g., stavudine) were associated with a significant rate of neuropathy.

Once a preliminary differential diagnosis is developed based on the history and neurologic examination findings, laboratory studies can confirm the diagnosis. Laboratory tests to identify potentially treatable causes of neuropathy are included in Table 123.11. Additional studies can be ordered based on the suspected diagnosis. An impaired glucose tolerance test is found in more than half of patients with cryptogenic sensory peripheral neuropathy and is more sensitive than tests of fasting glucose or hemoglobin A$_{1c}$ (HbA$_{1c}$). In a patient with acute, asymmetrical weakness and sensory loss, screening for an inflammatory process (ESR, ANA, RA, SS-A, SS-B) is appropriate. In addition, genetic testing is now available for most patients with CMT disease. If a monoclonal protein is identified on serum protein electrophoresis, a skeletal survey, urine immunofixation electrophoresis, and bone marrow biopsy should be ordered to rule out an underlying lymphoproliferative disorder. If the patient has a monoclonal protein associated with autonomic dysfunction, congestive heart failure, or renal insufficiency, a biopsy (rectal, abdominal fat, or sural nerve) should be considered for diagnosis of amyloidosis. Amyloidosis can be acquired or familial with mutations in the transthyretin (TTR) gene. CIDP can be associated with a monoclonal gammopathy, and in this situation patients should be treated with immunosuppressive therapy. Monoclonal gammopathies observed in patients with an axonal peripheral neuropathy are frequently benign (monoclonal gammopathy of unknown significance) and do not necessarily warrant therapy.

A lumbar puncture is indicated only if an acquired demyelinating neuropathy such as GBS or CIDP is being considered. In these cases,

one expects to find an "albuminocytologic dissociation" with an elevation in cerebrospinal fluid (CSF) protein and a relatively normal white blood cell (WBC) count. If the CSF WBC count is greater than 50, Lyme disease, HIV-associated disease, or a paraneoplastic process must be considered.

Electrodiagnostic studies consisting of nerve conduction testing and EMG can be a helpful extension of the physical examination. These studies are useful in defining whether the neuropathic process is caused by a primarily axonal or demyelinating process. In general, axonal degeneration decreases the amplitude of the compound muscle action potential out of proportion to the degree of reduction in peripheral nerve conduction velocity, whereas demyelination produces prominent reduction in conduction velocities. Nerve conduction testing can help determine, in the case of a demyelinating neuropathy, whether the process has an acquired or hereditary cause. A uniform slowing of nerve conduction usually suggests a hereditary cause while focal demyelination causing conduction block suggests an acquired demyelinating neuropathy. Electrodiagnostic studies can identify subclinical neuropathy (in patients receiving potentially neurotoxic medications) and can quantitate the extent of axon loss. Finally, these studies can localize the lesion in the case of radiculopathies, dorsal root ganglionopathies, plexopathies, and multiple mononeuropathies.

Sensory nerve biopsies should be obtained for diagnosis of a vasculitic neuropathy because treatment involves potentially toxic medications. Performing a muscle biopsy in addition to the nerve biopsy may improve the diagnostic yield and should be considered because the inflammation is random and focal and easily missed. Nerve biopsies are not indicated in "cryptogenic" neuropathies, diabetic neuropathy, or motor neuron disease. If nerve conduction studies are normal, skin biopsies allow quantification of the number of intraepidermal nerve fibers. A length-dependent decrease in the number of these fibers can help confirm a small-fiber neuropathy.

Treatment

Despite a very thorough history, examination, and laboratory studies, the cause of as many as one third of neuropathies remains unknown. In this situation, the focus of management is pain control. Patients with neuropathy frequently report a burning, searing, and aching sensation in their feet and hands that interferes with sleep. Neuropathic pain is difficult to treat but may respond to various medications having different mechanisms of action (Table 123.12). It is important to "start low and taper slow" and to treat for a minimum of 4 weeks before concluding that an agent is ineffective. In patients with a vasculitic neuropathy, therapy with corticosteroids in addition to a cytotoxic agent can stabilize and, in some cases, improve the neuropathy.

Prognosis

Peripheral neuropathies caused by axonal degeneration are generally progressive unless the underlying cause can be identified and treated. Recovery from axonal degeneration requires nerve regeneration, a process that often requires 2 to 3 years. Prognosis of demyelinating and vasculitic neuropathies is extremely variable, depending on the cause.

COMMON MONONEUROPATHIES

Common mononeuropathies are explored in Table 123.7.

Carpal Tunnel Syndrome

Carpal tunnel syndrome results from compression of the median nerve at the wrist as it passes beneath the flexor retinaculum. Precipitating factors include activities that require repetitive wrist movements:

TABLE 123.12 Symptomatic Treatment for Neuropathic Pain

Tricyclic Antidepressants
Amitriptyline 10-150 mg qhs
Nortriptyline 10-150 mg qhs
Imipramine 10-150 mg qhs
Desipramine 10-150 mg qhs
Venlafaxine 75-225 mg qd

Anticonvulsants
Gabapentin 300-1200 mg tid
Carbamazepine 100-200 mg tid
Topiramate 150-200 mg bid
Duloxetine 60-120 mg qd
Pregabalin 150-600 mg qd
Sodium valproate 250-500 mg bid

Alternative Treatments
Tramadol 50-100 mg qid
Lidoderm patches
Capsaicin cream
Transcutaneous nerve stimulation
Acupuncture

mechanical work, gardening, house painting, and typing. Predisposing causes include pregnancy, diabetes, acromegaly, rheumatoid arthritis, chronic renal failure, thyroid disorders, and primary amyloidosis.

Symptoms usually begin in the dominant hand but commonly involve both hands over time. Patients typically report numbness, tingling, and burning sensations in the palm and in the fingers supplied by the median nerve: the thumb, index finger, middle finger, and medial one half of the ring finger. Some patients report that all fingers become numb. Pain and paresthesias are most prominent at night and often interrupt sleep. The pain is prominent at the wrist but may radiate to the forearm and occasionally to the shoulder. Shaking the hand relieves both pain and paresthesias. Percussion of the median nerve at the wrist provokes paresthesias in a median nerve distribution in 60% of patients (Tinel sign), and flexion of the wrist for 30 to 60 seconds provokes pain or paresthesias in 75% of cases (Phalen sign).

The diagnosis is based on clinical symptoms and signs. Electrodiagnostic studies may demonstrate prolongation of the sensory or motor latencies across the wrist in up to 85% of patients. In more severe cases, EMG may demonstrate evidence of denervation in the abductor pollicis brevis.

Treatment initially includes avoidance of repetitive wrist activities and the use of a neutral wrist splint. If these conservative measures fail, injections of lidocaine and methylprednisolone can be given into the carpal tunnel or surgical treatment by section of the transverse carpal ligament can effectively decompress the nerve. Indicators that have been shown to predict failure with conservative management include age older than 50, disease duration longer than 10 months, constant paresthesias, and a positive Phalen sign in less than 10 seconds.

Ulnar Palsy

The ulnar nerve may become entrapped at the elbow because of external compression in the condylar groove. Injury may also occur years after a malunited supracondylar fracture of the humerus with bony overgrowth. Contrary to the findings in carpal tunnel syndrome, muscle weakness and atrophy characteristically predominate over sensory symptoms and signs. Patients notice atrophy of the first dorsal

interosseous muscle and difficulty performing fine manipulations of the fingers. Numbness of the little finger, the contiguous one half of the ring finger, and the ulnar border of the hand may be present. Ulnar nerve compression can be confirmed with electrodiagnostic studies demonstrating slowed motor conduction velocity across the elbow. Treatment includes the use of elbow pads to avoid compression or surgical procedures including transposition of the ulnar nerve or decompression of the cubital tunnel.

Peroneal Neuropathy

The peroneal nerve can become compressed as it wraps around the fibular head and passes into the fibular tunnel between the peroneus longus muscle and the fibula. Compression may occur as a result of habitual leg crossing, prolonged bed rest, knee casts, prolonged squatting, anesthesia, or profound weight loss. The nerve can also be compressed as a result of Baker cysts, fibular fractures, blunt trauma, tumors, or hematomas at the knee. Symptoms include "foot drop" with selective weakness of the ankle dorsiflexors and evertors as well as the toe extensors. Reflexes remain normal, and sensory loss generally involves the anterolateral leg and dorsum of the foot. Electrodiagnostic studies demonstrate slowing of the peroneal conduction velocity across the fibular head and may demonstrate denervation if axonal injury is present. Compressive injuries usually resolve spontaneously within weeks to months. Magnetic resonance imaging (MRI) and surgical exploration should be considered if symptoms are progressive.

SPECIFIC ACQUIRED POLYNEUROPATHIES

Guillain-Barré Syndrome: Acute Inflammatory Demyelinating Polyneuropathy

Since the advent of polio vaccination, GBS has become the most frequent cause of acute flaccid paralysis throughout the world. GBS is an immune-mediated disorder that follows an identifiable infectious disorder in approximately 60% of patients. The best-documented antecedents include infection with *Campylobacter jejuni*, infectious mononucleosis, CMV, herpesvirus, and mycoplasma. *C. jejuni* is often associated with more severe axonal cases.

The initial symptoms of GBS often consist of tingling and pins-and-needles sensations in the feet and may be associated with dull low-back pain. By the time of presentation, which occurs hours to 1 to 2 days after the first symptoms, weakness has usually developed. The weakness is usually most prominent in the legs, but the arms or cranial musculature may be involved first. Muscle stretch reflexes are lost early, even in regions where strength is retained. Cutaneous sensory deficits (loss of pain and temperature) are relatively mild; however, large-fiber functions (vibration and proprioception) are more severely impaired. Other clinical features include pain (20%), paresthesias (50%), autonomic symptoms (20%), facial weakness (50%), ophthalmoparesis (9%), bulbar weakness, and respiratory failure (25%). Symptoms associated with GBS typically evolve over a 2- to 4-week period, with approximately 90% of patients showing no evidence of progression beyond 4 weeks. For this reason, patients who are seen within several weeks from onset continue to require hospitalization for close observation. Respiratory muscle strength should be monitored with bedside measurements of the FVC and negative inspiratory function (NIF). Intubation should be initiated when the FVC falls below 15 mL/kg or NIF is less than −20 cm of H_2O.

Treatment may include either intravenous gammaglobulin (0.4 g/kg/day × 5 days) or plasmapheresis—the exchange of the patient's plasma for albumin (200 mL/kg over 7 to 10 days). Clinical studies have confirmed equal efficacy between these two therapies, with no additional benefit conferred with combination therapy. Corticosteroids are not effective in GBS. Indications for therapy include inability to ambulate independently, impaired respiratory function, or rapidly progressive weakness.

Clinical features predicting a poor prognosis or prolonged recovery time include rapidly progressive weakness, need for mechanical ventilation, and low-amplitude CMAPs. The mortality rate remains 5% to 10%, usually due to respiratory complications, cardiac arrhythmia, or pulmonary embolism. With appropriate supportive care and rehabilitation, 80% to 90% of patients recover with little or no disability.

Chronic Inflammatory Demyelinating Polyneuropathy

CIDP has been considered the "chronic form" of GBS, because by definition the symptoms must progress for at least 8 weeks. The clinical features include proximal and distal weakness, areflexia, and distal sensory loss. Autonomic dysfunction, respiratory insufficiency, and cranial nerve involvement can occur but are much less common than in GBS. Treatment for CIDP includes the use of oral immunosuppressive agents such as prednisone, cyclosporine, mycophenolate mofetil, and azathioprine. Intravenous immune globulin and plasmapheresis are also indicated for severe or refractory cases.

Diabetic Neuropathy

Diabetes mellitus is the most frequent cause of peripheral neuropathy worldwide. The diabetic neuropathies take many clinical forms, including symmetrical polyneuropathies and a wide variety of individual plexus or nerve disorders.

Diabetes mellitus often causes a slowly progressive, distal, symmetrical sensorimotor polyneuropathy (DSPN). DSPN is uncommon at the time of diagnosis of diabetes, but its prevalence increases with duration of diabetes with a lifetime prevalence of 55% for type 1 and 45% for type 2. The precise pathogenesis is not defined, but, similar to the ocular and renal complications, diabetic neuropathy can be reduced in incidence and in severity by maintaining blood glucose levels close to normal.

Initial symptoms may consist of numbness, tingling, burning, or prickling sensations affecting the feet and toes. Mild distal weakness and gait instability may subsequently develop. The sensory symptoms can then slowly progress to involve a "stocking-glove pattern." The small-fiber dysfunction often produces spontaneous neuropathic pain in which unpleasant sensations can be evoked by normally innocuous stimuli, such as the bed sheets on the toes at night. Continuous burning or throbbing pain may occur, and prolonged walking is often distressing. In severe cases, patients may develop foot ulcers in insensitive areas that necessitate amputation. Autonomic dysfunction is also frequently associated with DSPN including impotence, nocturnal diarrhea, sweating abnormalities, orthostatic hypotension, and gastroparesis.

Other less common neuropathies associated with diabetes include cranial neuropathies (the sixth, third, and rarely fourth nerves), mononeuropathies, mononeuropathy multiplex, radiculopathies, and plexopathies. Diabetic amyotrophy (also known as *diabetic lumbosacral polyradiculoplexopathy*) is a distinctive disorder characterized by severe thigh pain followed by proximal greater than distal lower extremity weakness that progresses over a period of months. The onset is invariably unilateral, but the condition may progress to involve both lower extremities. Physical therapy and effective pain management are essential; treatment with immune modulators is controversial.

Toxic-Induced Neuropathies

Toxic neuropathies constitute a large number of disorders caused by alcohol, drugs, heavy metals, and environmental substances (see E-Table 123.3). The majority of toxic neuropathies manifest as a distal sensorimotor axonal neuropathy that chronically progresses over time unless the offending agent is eliminated. Clinical evaluation should focus on the temporal relationship between exposure and the onset of sensory or motor symptoms as well as symptoms of systemic toxicity.

Critical Illness Polyneuropathy

Critical illness polyneuropathy (CIP) is a common cause of failure to wean from a ventilator in a patient with associated sepsis and multiorgan failure. Clinical features include generalized or distal flaccid paralysis, especially involving the lower extremities, depressed or absent reflexes, and distal sensory loss with relative sparing of cranial nerve function. The diagnosis can be confirmed with nerve conduction studies showing evidence of a severe, generalized axonal neuropathy. CSF protein should be normal and, in addition to conduction studies, distinguishes CIP from GBS.

SPECIFIC HEREDITARY POLYNEUROPATHIES

Charcot-Marie-Tooth Disease

CMT identifies a group of heritable disorders of peripheral nerves that share clinical features but differ in their pathologic mechanisms and the specific genetic abnormalities (E-Table 123.4). CMT is the most common heritable neuromuscular disorder, with an incidence of 17 to 40 cases per 100,000.

CMT disease usually manifests during the first to second decades with symptoms related to insidious foot drop: frequent tripping and inability to jump well or run as fast as other children. Over time, distal upper extremity weakness develops, resulting in difficulty with buttoning, handling keys, and opening jars. Examination reveals distal weakness and wasting of the intrinsic muscles of the feet, the peroneal muscles, the anterior tibial muscles, and the calves ("inverted champagne bottle" legs). A variable degree of impaired large-fiber sensory function is reflected in reduced vibratory sensation at the toes. Muscle stretch reflexes are lost, first at the ankles. Typically, a foot deformity exists, with high arches (pes cavus) and hammer toes, reflecting long-standing muscle imbalance in the feet. Most patients with CMT disease have nearly normal occupational and daily activities, and they have a normal life span. Although no specific treatment has been developed, the foot drop can be treated by appropriate bracing of the ankle with ankle-foot orthoses. Genetic counseling and education of affected patients and their families are important, both for reassurance and to preclude unnecessary diagnostic evaluation of affected members in future generations.

Demyelinating forms of CMT are classified as CMT1 and axonal forms as CMT2. CMT is usually transmitted as an autosomal dominant trait; however, X-linked dominant transmission is responsible for approximately 10% of cases. Rare autosomal recessive forms are designated CMT4, and these patients tend to have an earlier onset and more severe phenotype. CMT1A is the most common form and accounts for 90% of CMT1 and 50% of all CMT cases. CMT1A is associated with the 17p11.2-p12 duplication in the *PMP22* gene expressed by Schwann cells. A deletion or a point mutation of the *PMP22* gene produces a different phenotype, HNPP, which is characterized by recurrent episodes of focal entrapment with attacks of weakness and numbness in the peroneal, ulnar, radial, and median nerves (in descending order of frequency) or in a brachial plexus distribution.

FAMILIAL AMYLOID NEUROPATHIES

Amyloid neuropathy is an autosomal dominant disorder caused by extracellular deposition of the fibrillary protein amyloid in peripheral nerve and sensory and autonomic ganglia, as well as around blood vessels in nerves and other tissues. The age of onset varies from 18 to 83 years. In all forms of amyloidosis, the initial and major abnormalities affect the small sensory and autonomic fibers. Involvement of small fibers responsible for pain and temperature sensibilities leads to loss of the ability to perceive mechanical and thermal injuries and to an increased risk of tissue damage. As a result, painless injuries present a major hazard of this disorder; in advanced stages, they can lead to chronic infections or osteomyelitis of the feet or hands and the necessity for amputation. Amyloid deposition in the heart can lead to cardiomyopathy. Mutations in transthyretin, apolipoprotein A1, or gelsolin are responsible. Early recognition is essential, as liver transplantation has been shown to halt disease progression. Recently, the FDA approved two new medications, inotersen and patisiran, for treatment of transthyretin-associated familial amyloid polyneuropathy.

SUGGESTED READINGS

Alport AR, Sander HW: Clinical approach to peripheral neuropathy: Anatomic localization and diagnostic testing, Continuum Lifelong Learning Neurol 18(1):13–38, 2012.

Al-Zaidy, SA, Mendell JR: From clinical trials to clinical practice: Practical considerations for gene replacement therapy in SMA type 1. Pediatr Neurol 100:P3–11, 2019.

Bril V, England J, Franklin GM, et al: Evidence-based guideline: treatment of painful diabetic neuropathy, Muscle Nerve 43:910–917, 2011.

Bromberg MB: An approach to the evaluation of peripheral neuropathies, Semin Neurol 25(2):153–159, 2005.

Brown RH, Al-Chalabi: Amyotrophic lateral sclerosis, N Engl J Med 377:162–172, 2017.

Camdessanche JP, Jousserand G, et al: The pattern and diagnostic criteria of sensory neuronopathy: a case-control study, Brain 132(7):1723–1733, 2009.

Chiriboga CA: Nusinersen for the treatment of spinal muscular atrophy, Expert Review of Neurotherapeutics 17(10):955–962, 2017.

Ludolph AC, Brettschneider J, Weishaupt JH: Amyotrophic lateral sclerosis, Curr Opin Neurol 25(5):530–535, 2012.

Mauermann ML, Burns TM: The evaluation of chronic axonal polyneuropathies, Semin Neurol 28(2):133–151, 2008.

Miller RG, Jackson CE, Kasarkis EJ, et al: Practice parameter update: the care of the patient with amyotrophic lateral sclerosis: drug, nutritional, and respiratory therapies (an evidence-based review): report of the Quality Standards Subcommittee of the American Academy of Neurology, Neurology 73(15):1218–1226, 2009.

Miller RG, Jackson CE, Kasarksi EJ, et al: Practice parameter update: the care of the patient with amyotrophic lateral sclerosis: multidisciplinary care, symptom management, and cognitive/behavioral impairment (an evidence-based review): report of the Quality Standards Subcommittee of the American Academy of Neurology, Neurology 73(15):1227–1233, 2009.

Oskarsson B, Gendron TF, Staff NP: Amyotrophic lateral sclerosis: an update for 2018, Mayo Clin Proc 93(11):1617–1628, 2018.

Turner MR, Hardiman O, Benatar M: Controversies and priorities in amyotrophic lateral sclerosis, Lancet Neurol 12(3):310–322, 2013.

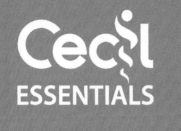

124

Muscle Diseases

Johanna Hamel, Jeffrey M. Statland

INTRODUCTION

Skeletal muscle fibers are the effector cells of the nervous system, turn thoughts into actions, and are the means by which we interact with our environment. Myopathies are primary diseases of the muscle and can be both inherited and acquired (Table 124.1). Myopathies can result in weakness and muscle wasting, myalgias, cramps, muscle breakdown, or contractures. Inherited disorders affect muscle proteins involved in transmission of signals from the neuromuscular junction, proteins involved in energy production or metabolism, or structural proteins that anchor and transmit force from the contractile apparatus to the extracellular matrix. They do this either by mutations directly to the muscle proteins or by mutations altering cell regulation of transcription or splicing. Acquired myopathies are caused by external factors and can be due to metabolic derangements, toxic exposures or drugs, infections, or autoimmune dysfunction often resulting in inflammation in the muscle. Acquired myopathies can improve with treatments geared towards eliminating or ameliorating the precipitating factors.

With recent advances in our understanding of the genetic and molecular mechanisms in hereditary myopathies, coupled with advances in drug development targeting DNA and RNA, efforts to develop targeted therapies for hereditary muscle diseases accelerated and increased exponentially. The first treatment targeting the underlying genetic mechanism of a muscle disease (Duchenne muscular dystrophy) was approved by the US Food and Drug Administration (FDA) in 2016. Many more disease-specific treatments targeting genetic mechanisms of muscle diseases are currently in clinical trials with a subset expected to become available to patients in the future. This change in paradigm, from supportive to disease-modifying therapies, targeting patients' DNA or RNA that will alter the trajectory of progression, will change the landscape of how we care for patients with muscle diseases. One technology worth mentioning here due to imminent clinical trials and the possibility for transformational change in inherited myopathies is systemic gene replacement therapies. The three concepts that make up systemic gene therapy are: (1) the vector, which is a virus, serotypes of which can specifically target muscle or the heart; (2) the construct, which is the gene that will be packaged into the virus vector; the size can be limited by the capsid size, and so for large genes like dystrophin new engineered genes (i.e., microdystrophin) are used; and (3) the promotor, the on and off switch for the gene, which can also be tissue specific. The first such systemic gene replacement therapy was approved for spinal muscular atrophy, and several companies have phase 3 studies starting for muscular dystrophies. With these fundamental advances on the horizon, early recognition and diagnosis of these rare diseases will be important to achieve the greatest benefit from these treatments. Physicians administering the therapies not only need to be familiar with the disease and its complications but with molecular and genetic mechanisms that are being targeted. These advances provide abundant opportunities and challenges.

ORGANIZATION AND STRUCTURE OF NORMAL MUSCLE

Each muscle is enclosed in a connective tissue sheath made up of collagen and extracellular matrix proteins called the epimysium, which merges at either end to form the tendons, which attach muscle to bone. The epimysium divides internally into the perimysium, which separates the muscle into individual bundles of muscle fibers called fascicles. The endomysium surrounds and provides support for the individual fibers. Each muscle fiber is a single multi-nucleated syncytial cell and can be as long as 10 cm. On cross section, muscle fibers appear polygonal in shape and in adults range from 40 to 80 micrometers in diameter. Medium size arterioles and veins run in the perimysium, with capillaries between the individual muscle fibers. On hematoxylin and eosin stains, cytoplasm appears pink and the nuclei blue (Fig. 124.1A). Each individual muscle fiber has multiple nuclei, which are found beneath the sarcolemma membrane on the periphery of the cell.

The plasma membrane around the muscle fiber is called the sarcolemma, and inside there are a large number of myofibrils made of thick (myosin) and thin (actin) filaments, which make up 70% to 80% of the volume of the cell, and when activated, create force. Electrochemical signals carry the signal from the nerve, through the neuromuscular junction, into the muscle fiber along the sarcolemma and t-tubule system. Muscle ion channels line this network and carry electrochemical signals. Mitochondria and enzymes involved in glycolysis and fatty acid metabolism provide energy for muscle. A network of proteins, the dystrophin-glycoprotein complex (DGC), anchors the myofibrils to the subsarcolemma cytoskeleton and connects to the extracellular matrix (Fig. 124.2). Many inherited myopathies are caused by mutations in these ion channels, metabolic enzymes, or structural anchoring proteins.

SYMPTOMS OF MUSCLE DISEASE

The most common symptom of a patient with muscle disease is a loss of function caused by weakness (for an overview of symptoms see Table 124.2). Other common symptoms, like fatigue, exercise intolerance or myalgias (muscle pain), are less specific than muscle weakness. Muscle cramping is more commonly caused by disorders of the nerves, and not the muscle.

EXAMINATION

The physical examination uses a standard modified Medical Research Council scale of motor strength to determine the pattern and degree of involvement of various muscles (Table 124.3). But just as important as isolated strength testing are functional

Hereditary Myopathies
Muscular dystrophies
Congenital myopathies
Metabolic/mitochondrial myopathies
Channelopathies

Acquired Myopathies
Inflammatory myopathies
Myopathy with HMGCR antibodies
Endocrine myopathies
Systemic illness/infectious myopathies
Toxic/drug-induced myopathies

motor tasks, particularly in children. Muscles should be inspected for atrophy or hypertrophy and range of motion around the joints for evidence of tendon contractures. Ten broad patterns of muscle weakness occur in myopathies (Table 124.4). Most myopathies have the proximal, limb-girdle pattern. There are other, highly distinctive, patterns. Weakness that is asymmetric and includes the face, proximal arms and shoulders, and distal lower extremities is characteristic of facioscapulohumeral muscular dystrophy. Weakness that starts in the distal finger flexors (patients cannot curl fingers when making a fist) and proximal lower extremities (the quadriceps) is virtually pathognomonic for sporadic inclusion body myositis. A patient in middle age who presents with ptosis and difficulty swallowing is highly characteristic for oculopharyngeal muscular dystrophy.

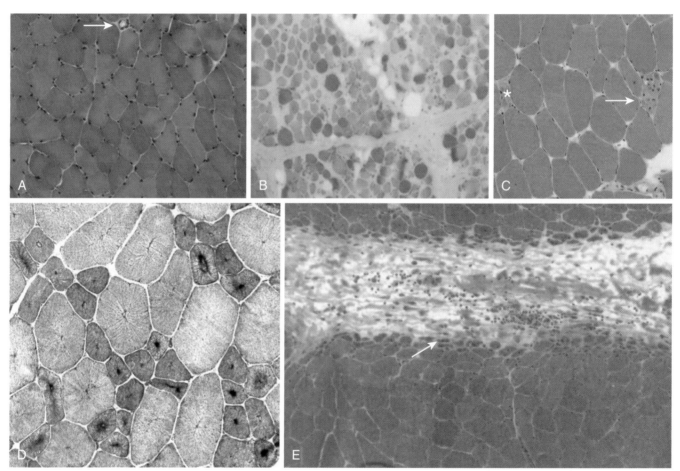

Fig. 124.1 Muscle biopsies hematoxylin and eosin staining. When assessing the health of muscle tissue, the pathologist evaluates the size, shape and internal architecture of muscle fibers, presence of inflammation and mitochondrial dysfunction, and amount of connective tissue. In a chronic myopathic muscle, the muscle fibers are typically more variable in size, rounded, and have central nuclei. Connective tissue can be increased. In an active myopathy, necrotic fibers undergoing phagocytosis and regenerating fibers can be seen. (A) **Normal adult muscle,** medium power. Notice polygonal muscle fibers arranged in fascicles with blue staining nuclei on the periphery. A small arteriole is visible *(white arrow)*. (B) **Chronic myopathy,** Duchenne muscular dystrophy low power. Note the variability in fiber size with rounding of fibers, increase in connective tissue, and fatty deposition. (C) **Acute myopathy,** necrotizing myopathy with HMGCR antibodies. Necrotic fiber *(white arrow)* undergoing phagocytosis and regenerating fiber (*) with plump nuclei. Examples for disease characteristic findings on muscle pathology. (D) **Centronuclear congenital myopathy.** The NADH reaction shows numerous fibers with spoke-like, radial projections with central nuclei. Also notable fiber size variability, identified as moderate type 1 fiber atrophy on other stains. (E) **Dermatomyositis** on low power. Notice the prominent pathognomonic perifascicular atrophy *(white arrow)* of fibers, and perivascular inflammatory infiltrates.

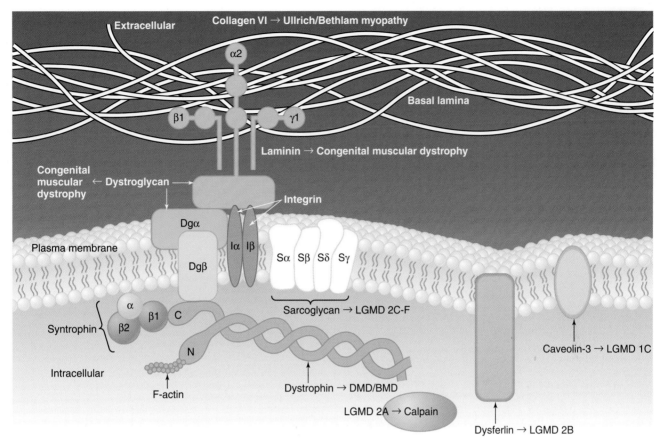

Fig. 124.2 The dystrophin-glycoprotein complex. Muscle structural proteins connect the contractile apparatus to the internal cytoskeleton and the extracellular matrix. Mutations in proteins from the extracellular matrix to the anchoring proteins, which connect the extracellular matrix to the internal cytoskeleton, and mutations to proteins, which attach the internal cytoskeleton to the contractile apparatus, are all involved in the inherited muscular dystrophies and myopathies.

DIAGNOSTIC TESTING

The work-up of a patient with a suspected myopathy is a staged process, outlined in Table 124.2. A useful initial laboratory test is the serum creatine kinase (CK), which is elevated commonly in acquired and often in inherited myopathies. Despite the obvious localizing value of elevated muscle enzymes it is important to remember not all elevations in serum CK are due to myopathy and a normal CK does not exclude a myopathy (Table 124.5). Furthermore, CK levels can vary depending on physical activity, gender, and race.

Electrodiagnostic testing can help distinguish between neurogenic and myopathic causes for weakness (see Table 124.2). Genetic testing is the initial test when a specific hereditary disease is suspected. Muscle biopsies can be important in patients whose family history and physical examination does not suggest a particular myopathic diagnosis and can help resolve variants of uncertain significance on genetic testing. Characteristic morphologic changes (see Fig. 124.1) are hallmarks of the congenital myopathies (e.g., centronuclear myopathy in Fig. 124.1D), inflammatory myopathies (dermatomyositis in Fig. 124.1E), and metabolic myopathies (glycogen storage disorders), but most myopathies result in nonspecific muscle changes, which confirms the localization (muscle), but not the cause.

INHERITED MYOPATHIES

Muscular Dystrophies

The muscular dystrophies are inherited myopathies characterized by progressive weakness. Typically the muscular dystrophies are divided into the dystrophinopathies, the myotonic dystrophies, facioscapulohumeral muscular dystrophy, Emery-Dreifuss muscular dystrophy, and the limb-girdle dystrophies (Tables 124.6, 124.7, and E-Table 124.1). The limb-girdle muscular dystrophies (LGMD) are a diverse group of diseases due to mutations in more than 20 genes. The LGMDs are inherited in either autosomal dominant or recessive fashion and present anywhere from childhood after achieving independent walking to later in life, with elevated CK and proximal muscle weakness (see E-Table 124.1). Another group of patients who have dystrophic changes in the muscle from birth, often with accompanying changes in the brain on MRI, include congenital muscular dystrophies (see Table 124.7). The traditional distinction between dystrophies and other inherited myopathies is becoming blurred as our genetic understanding advances because mutations for different diseases are often allelic.

Dystrophinopathies
Definition and Epidemiology

Dystrophinopathies are X-linked recessive disorders resulting from mutations of the large dystrophin gene located at Xp21. The incidence of Duchenne muscular dystrophy is 1 in 5300 male births; one third of the cases result from a new mutation. Becker muscular dystrophy is a milder form of dystrophinopathy and is less common than the Duchenne form, with an incidence of 5 per 100,000.

Genetics and Pathology

The majority of patients have deletions or duplications in the dystrophin gene. In the remaining patients, mutations can be small insertions

TABLE 124.2   Evaluation for a Patient With Suspected Myopathy

Feature	Description
History	
Age of onset	Congenital, childhood, adult
Acute/subacute or chronic	Hereditary myopathies are usually chronic with gradual onset, acquired myopathies can occur more acutely
Progressive or episodic	Dystrophies are usually progressive; congenital static; metabolic/channelopathies episodic
Triggers	Exercise, foods, temperature
Myotonia	Delayed relaxation of muscle: e.g., difficulty letting go when shaking hands, opening doorknobs, myotonia can also affect tongue movements (speech) and chewing. Myotonia improves with repetition (warm-up phenomenon) and gets worse in cold temperature.
Family History	It can be helpful to draw out a pedigree to determine the pattern of inheritance, which can be dominant, recessive, or no family history. Questions about whether family members require assistive devices to walk or wheelchairs, and asking about extra-muscular manifestation of muscular dystrophies can be useful, specifically as diseases may not have been recognized.
Weakness on Exam	
Proximal	Difficulty lifting objects, climbing stairs, getting up from chair, scapular winging, waddling gait, Gower sign
Distal	Difficulty making a tight fist, fastening buttons, opening jars, wrist drop, foot drop
Facial	Difficulty squeezing the eyes shut, transverse smile, inability to pucker or blow out cheeks, inability to whistle
Oculopharyngeal	Ptosis, restricted extra-ocular movements, coughing after drinking, and difficulty swallowing
Respiratory	Shortness of breath with activity, with lying flat, use of accessory muscles
Other Features	
Myotonia	Action Myotonia: Delayed hand opening after making a tight fist, or eye opening after tight closure
	Percussion Myotonia: With percussion of the extensor digitorum muscle in the forearm, the finger extensors relax with delay. Same can be observed with percussion of the thenar eminence
Cardiac	Cardiac conduction defects, cardiomyopathy
Multiorgan involvement	E.g., joint deformities, skin (rash), GI symptoms, eye (cataract), hearing loss, CNS involvement
Laboratory	
Creatine kinase (CK)	Dystrophies/inflammatory myopathy increased >10× normal; congenital 3–5× normal; metabolic >10× normal during attacks
Thyroid/Parathyroid	High TSH, low T4, low PTH, Ca^{2+}
Antibodies	Patients with myositis:
	Myositis specific antibodies: Anti-Jo-1, antisynthetase antibodies, signal recognition particle (SRP) antibodies, Mi-2 antibodies, anti hPMS-1, anti-MDA-5 antibody, anti-p140, anti-p155/140.
	Inclusion Body myositis: Cytoplasmic 5′-nucleotidase 1A (cN1A)
	Patients with proximal muscle weakness of unknown etiology or necrotizing myopathies: Antibodies to 3-hydroxy-3-methylglutaryl coenzyme A reductase (HMGCR)
Genetic Testing	Patients with family history and/or examination suggestive of a hereditary myopathy. A positive test can be confirmatory and avoid additional diagnostic testing.
Electrodiagnostic Studies	Nerve conduction studies are typically normal in muscle diseases. On electromyography, irritated muscle shows fibrillations and positive sharp waves; myopathic motor units are brief, low amplitude, and polyphasic; electrical myotonia is a repetitive muscle fiber potential discharge with waxing and waning frequency and amplitude with characteristic sound similar to an accelerating, decelerating motorcycle engine.
Muscle Biopsy	Chronic: Changes in muscle fiber shape and composition of fiber types, central nuclei, increased amount of connective tissue
	Acute: Necrotic muscle fibers, regenerating fibers
	Other: Presence of inflammatory cells, number or morphology of mitochondria, or abnormal deposits of fat or glycogen

or deletions, point mutations, or splice site variants. Dystrophin is a large subsarcolemmal cytoskeletal protein that, along with the other components of the dystrophin-glycoprotein complex, provides support to the muscle membrane during contraction. Mutations in dystrophin can result in a spectrum of dystrophin dysfunction, from a severely truncated protein that is rapidly degraded, as in Duchenne muscular dystrophy, to a semi-functional protein still expressed such as in the milder form, Becker's muscular dystrophy, or mild dysfunction such as in female carriers. Muscle biopsies are typically not required for diagnosis (example depicted in Fig. 124.1B).

Clinical Presentation

Duchenne muscular dystrophy manifests as early as age 2 to 3 years with delays in motor milestones and difficulty running. Patients can have marked pseudo-hypertrophy of the calf muscles. And when asked to get up from the floor, boys use a Gower maneuver (use hands to push up). The average age of diagnosis is around 4 years of age. The proximal muscles are the most severely affected, and the course is relentlessly progressive. Patients begin to fall frequently by age 5 to 6, have difficulty climbing stairs by age 8 years, and are usually confined to a wheelchair in their early teens. Patients have a reduced life expectancy due to cardiac (dilated cardiomyopathy) and respiratory muscle weakness. The average IQ of boys with Duchenne muscular dystrophy is low, reflecting central nervous system involvement.

Diagnosis and Differential Diagnosis

Diagnosis is based on clinical history, physical examination, serum CK, and is confirmed by genetic testing. Other differential considerations are congenital myopathies, muscular dystrophies, and limb-girdle muscular dystrophies.

Treatment

Care for children with Duchenne muscular dystrophy involves a multidisciplinary team along with pulmonologists, orthopedists, and cardiologists, with monitoring of cardiac and respiratory function as well as scoliosis. Prednisone and deflazacort (a synthetic derivative of prednisolone) improve strength and motor function, pulmonary function, and prolong the ability to walk and survival in children with Duchenne muscular dystrophy.

About 15% of patients with Duchenne muscular dystrophy carry a mutation on exon 51. Eteplirsen is a drug that binds to exon 51 and induces "exon skipping," resulting in production of a truncated, but potentially functional dystrophin protein. The drug was approved in the United States by the FDA in 2016 and current trials are carried out to demonstrate a clinical benefit. Subsequently, two therapies were approved for patients with pathogenic variants on exon 53 (about 8% of patients with Duchenne muscular dystrophy). These therapies, golodirsen and vitolarsen, target RNA and result in exon 53 skipping. Ataluren is approved in countries outside of the United States for children with nonsense mutation. The drug allows read-through of premature stop mutations with the goal to produce a more functional dystrophin protein but with mixed results on functional outcome measures. Continued efforts and studies focus on strategies to make the cell produce some form of dystrophin, by targeting RNA or utilizing gene therapy targeting DNA. While these therapies will likely change the trajectory of DMD and care practices, new challenges will arise, such as costs, access (due to the genetic variability of DMD, therapies will target a subset of patients), duration of effect, and long-term safety concerns.

There are no guidelines for the treatment of Becker muscular dystrophy and clinical presentation is highly variable, but monitoring for cardiac and respiratory involvement is warranted. Some female carriers of dystrophin mutations may become symptomatic later in life and may have severe cardiomyopathy.

Prognosis

Patients with Duchenne muscular dystrophy die of respiratory complications in their 20s unless they are provided with respiratory support. Emerging targeted therapies will likely change this trajectory. Congestive heart failure and arrhythmias can occur late in the disease.

TABLE 124.3 Modified Medical Research Council Motor Strength Testing Scale

Grade	Degree of Strength
5	Normal strength through entire range of motion and against resistance
5−	Equivocal, barely detectable weakness
4+	Able to move against gravity and resistance, but examiner can break
4	Able to move against gravity and some resistance
4−	Able to resist gravity but only minimal resistance
3+	Able to overcome gravity and transient resistance, but then quickly gives out
3	Able to overcome gravity but no resistance
3−	Able to resist gravity but not through full range of motion
2	Able to move through range of motion with gravity eliminated
1	Trace muscle contraction
0	No contraction

TABLE 124.4 Characteristic Patterns of Muscle Weakness and Associated Myopathies

Pattern	Weakness	Diseases
Proximal limb-girdle	Symmetrical, pelvic and shoulder girdle muscles. Distal muscles to lesser extent. ±Neck flexor/extensor	Nonspecific: Duchenne muscular dystrophy; limb-girdle muscular dystrophy; inflammatory myopathies; Myopathy with HMGCR antibodies; myotonic dystrophy type 2
Distal	Symmetrical, distal upper or lower extremity. Proximal muscles to lesser degree	Nonspecific: Miyoshi myopathy (calves); Welander myopathy (wrist and finger extensors); Nonaka and Markesbery/Udd myopathy (tibialis anterior); rule out neuropathy
Proximal arm/distal leg	Scapuloperoneal distribution: periscapular muscles (proximal arm) and anterior compartment distal leg (tibialis anterior). Scapular winging. Can be asymmetrical.	When face involved highly suggestive of facioscapulohumeral muscular dystrophy; with elbow contractures Emory-Dreifuss dystrophy; scapuloperoneal dystrophies; certain limb-girdle dystrophies; congenital myopathies
Distal arm/proximal leg	Distal forearm muscles (distal finger flexors) and proximal leg (quadriceps). Other muscles variable. Often asymmetrical.	Highly suggestive of sporadic inclusion body myositis; also consider myotonic dystrophy type 1 with distal leg, neck flexion, respiratory and facial weakness
Ptosis ± ophthalmoparesis	Restriction of eye movements often without diplopia. Often with pharyngeal weakness and variable extremity weakness.	Ocular and pharyngeal weakness highly suggestive of oculopharyngeal muscular dystrophy; mitochondrial myopathies
Neck extensor weakness	Neck extensors, "dropped head syndrome." Variable neck flexor. ±Extremity weakness.	Inflammatory myopathies, in isolation consider isolated neck extensor myopathy; rule out amyotrophic lateral sclerosis and myasthenia gravis
Bulbar weakness	Tongue and pharyngeal weakness	Certain myopathies (e.g., oculopharyngeal muscular dystrophy); significant overlap with neuromuscular junction and motor neuron disease
Episodic pain, weakness, and myoglobinuria	May be triggered by exercise or metabolic stress	Metabolic myopathies; may also occur in deconditioning
Episodic weakness delayed or unrelated to exercise	May be triggered by food, stress, rest after exercise	Characteristic of periodic paralyses
Stiffness and decreased ability to relax	May be episodic, triggered by cold	Characteristic of myotonic disorders

Modified from Jackson CE, Barohn RJ: A pattern recognition approach to myopathy, Continuum (Minneap Minn) 19(6 Muscle Diseases): 1674-1697, 2013.

TABLE 124.5	Causes for Elevated Serum CK

Myopathies
Muscular dystrophies/Duchenne carrier state
Congenital myopathies
Metabolic myopathies
Inflammatory myopathies

Channelopathies
Motor Neuron Disease (ALS, SMA)
Neuropathies (GBS, CIDP)
Viral Illness

Medications
Statins
Fibric acid derivatives
Chloroquine
Colchicine

Endocrine Abnormalities (Thyroid/Parathyroid)
Surgery
Trauma
Strenuous Exercise
Increased Muscle Mass
Idiopathic—Ethnic Variability

Myotonic Dystrophy
Definition and Epidemiology

Myotonic dystrophies are the most common muscular dystrophies in adults of European ancestry with autosomal dominant inheritance. There are two types of myotonic dystrophy, type 1 (DM1) and type 2 (DM2). The frequency of DM1 in Europe is estimated at 1 in 8000. While DM1 and DM2 are equally frequent in Europe, DM2 seems less common in the United States.

Genetics and Pathology

DM1 is caused by a CTG repeat expansion on the *DMPK* gene whereas DM2 is caused by a CCTG repeat expansion on the *CNBP* gene. Both diseases share the same mechanism of RNA toxicity. Expanded CUG/CCUG repeats accumulate in nuclear foci and sequester important proteins that typically regulate RNA splicing. Loss of function of these proteins results in missplicing of various RNAs of multiple genes, resulting in wide transcriptome changes and multisystemic disease. In DM1, some but not all of the variability in age of symptom onset is explained by repeat length, with earlier onset typically associated with greater disease severity and longer repeat length. The CTG repeat is unstable and increases in somatic tissue throughout a persons' life (somatic instability) and tends to increase from generation to generation (anticipation). Genetic testing confirms the diagnosis and muscle biopsies are not required but characteristic findings

TABLE 124.6	Prevalent Muscular Dystrophies				
Disease	**Inheritance**	**Mutations**	**Age of Onset**	**Phenotypes**	**Treatment**
Dystrophinopathies	X-linked recessive	Xp21; ≈75% deletion or duplication	Duchenne diagnosis by age 4; Becker variable	Limb-girdle pattern. Duchenne: severe progressive and life limiting. Becker: progressive but not as severe, more variable. Calf pseudo-hypertrophy; isolated cardiomyopathy.	For Duchenne: Prednisone (or deflazacort), Eteplirsen, golodirsen, and vitolarsen; surveillance for respiratory, cardiac, and orthopedic problems
Myotonic dystrophy type 1	Autosomal dominant	19q13; CTG expansion >50 repeats	Any age with marked variability; congenital at birth	Marked clinical variability but typically muscle weakness and wasting affecting face, neck flexion, respiratory and distal muscles (finger flexion, ankle dorsiflexion); myotonia; temporal wasting, frontal balding; multisystemic disease manifestations (e.g., with cognitive deficits, hypersomnolence, cataracts); cardiac conduction deficits	Mexiletine for symptomatic myotonia; yearly surveillance for ocular and respiratory involvement and cardiac conduction deficits
Myotonic dystrophy type 2	Autosomal dominant	3q13; CCTG expansion >75 repeats	30s and older	Limb-girdle pattern; myalgia; myotonia; multisystem involvement (e.g., cataracts, cardiac conduction deficits); diabetes	Mexiletine for symptomatic myotonia; surveillance for ocular, cardiac, and respiratory involvement
Facioscapulohumeral muscular dystrophy	Autosomal dominant	95%: 4q35 (FSHD1), 5% digenic mutation affecting methylation (FSHD2)	Any age	Scapuloperoneal pattern with facial involvement; can have marked asymmetry; significant axial involvement	Screening for extramuscular manifestation
Emery-Dreifuss muscular dystrophy	X-linked recessive; autosomal dominant or recessive	≈70% Xq28 Emerin or FHL1 mutation; 1q21 lamin A/C, both dominant and recessive mutations reported	Joint contractures childhood; progressive weakness 20s–30s	Scapuloperoneal pattern; early joint contractures, particularly at elbows, marked cardiac involvement	Yearly surveillance for cardiac and respiratory involvement; orthopedic evaluation for symptomatic contractures
Oculopharyngeal muscular dystrophy	Autosomal dominant and recessive	14q11 PABPN1 GCG repeats >11 repeats	40s (range 20s–60s)	Ptosis dysphagia; limb-girdle pattern weakness	Swallow study; blepharoplasty for ptosis, cricopharyngeal myotomy for severe swallowing difficulty

TABLE 124.7   Congenital Muscular Dystrophies

Name/AKA	Gene	Inheritance	Phenotype	CNS Involvement
Merosin-deficient	6q22; laminin alpha-2	Autosomal recessive	Hypotonia; contractures; scoliosis or rigid spine; respiratory involvement; external ophthalmoplegia	MRI diffuse white matter changes; 20%–30% seizures
Bethlem myopathy/ Ullrich muscular dystrophy	21q22; 2q37; COL6 (collagen 6 spectrum disorders)	Autosomal dominant or recessive	Hypotonia; contractures; distal joint laxity; keloid; respiratory involvement	
Dystroglycanopathy	9q34 (POMT1); 14q24 (POMT2); 9q31 (fukutin); 19q13 (FKRP); 22q12 (LARGE); 1q32 (POMGnT1); 7p21 (ISPD)	Autosomal recessive	Spectrum of disorders but characteristic intellectual, eye, and brain involvement; motor early death, to acquiring ambulation	Walker-Warburg syndrome: severe eye involvement, cobblestone lissencephaly, hypoplastic cerebellum and brain stem. Muscle eye brain syndrome: common eye involvement, pachygyria/polymicrogyria, hypoplastic cerebellum and brain stem. Fukuyama: mild eye involvement, cortex mild changes, hypoplastic cerebellum but normal brain stem
SEPN1-related myopathy	1q36 (SEPN1)	Autosomal recessive	Cervicoaxial weakness, rigid spine syndrome, early nocturnal hypoventilation, medial thigh wasting	
LMNA related	1q22 (lamin A/C)	Autosomal dominant and recessive	Cervicoaxial weakness, dropped head, rigid spine syndrome, respiratory and cardiac involvement	

include pyknotic clumps (result of severe fiber atrophy), ring fibers, and type 1 fiber predominance.

Clinical Presentation

DM1 is one of the most variable monogenetic diseases and can present at any age. The wide spectrum of disease ranges from infants with hypotonia, respiratory weakness, and clubfeet at birth (congenital myotonic dystrophy) to late onset of disease at old age with minimal symptoms or signs. Typical features include facial weakness with temporalis muscle wasting, frontal balding, ptosis, and neck flexor weakness. Speech can be dysarthric with bulbar weakness resulting in dysphagia. Inspiratory (difficulty lying flat) and expiratory (weak cough) muscle weakness may be present. Extremity weakness usually begins distally and progresses slowly to affect the proximal limb-girdle muscles. In conjunction with myotonia (see Table 124.2), this phenotype is nearly pathognomonic of DM1. DM2 is considered milder because age of onset occurs typically in the late 30s and there is no congenital or childhood form of the disease. The pattern of weakness predominantly affecting proximal muscles and less facial involvement is different than in DM1. Pain is commonly described by patients with DM2. Both disorders affect multiple organ systems, such as early cataracts (<55 years), cardiac conduction abnormalities, and smooth muscle involvement with symptoms mimicking irritable bowel syndrome. *DMPK* is expressed in the brain and patients with DM1 can experience cognitive deficits including visuospatial and executive dysfunction, apathy, as well as hypersomnolence, which can be one of the most bothersome symptom in some individuals. Central nervous system involvement is thought to be less severe in DM2.

Diagnosis and Differential Diagnosis

The diagnosis is based on clinical examination, demonstration of myotonia clinically and electromyographically, and is confirmed by genetic testing. The classic phenotype and multisystemic presentation typically distinguishes myotonic dystrophy from other adult onset muscular dystrophies and non-dystrophic myotonic disorders.

Treatment

Annual surveillance for cardiac (ECG) and respiratory involvement (pulmonary function testing) is recommended. A sleep study can identify the presence of sleep apnea. Noninvasive ventilation is recommended for respiratory weakness and sleep apnea. With advanced heart block, a pacemaker may need to be placed. Mexiletine, a type IB anti-arrhythmic medication, effectively treats myotonia but is contraindicated in patients with severe arrhythmia. There is currently no treatment to halt disease progression but many therapies targeting the toxic RNA or releasing the sequestered proteins are under investigation.

Prognosis

Patients with DM1 have a reduced life expectancy due to respiratory and cardiac involvement, which on average appears to be less severe in DM2.

Facioscapulohumeral Muscular Dystrophy
Definition and Epidemiology

Facioscapulohumeral muscular dystrophy (FSHD) is the second most common adult muscular dystrophy with an estimated prevalence of 1:15,000.

Genetics and Pathology

FSHD is caused by *DUX4* expression, a gene that is typically silenced but is toxic to muscle when expressed. *DUX4* is expressed when the segment on chromosome 4q35 carrying the gene is hypomethylated. In most patients hypomethylation occurs due to a deletion/contraction of the segment on 4q35 (FSHD1), but in about 5% of patients it is caused by a mutation in a different gene regulating methylation (FSHD2). Both forms are clinically indistinguishable. FSHD1 has an autosomal dominant inheritance whereas FSHD2 as a digenic disease requires mutations on two genes, and sporadic occurrences occur in both. Muscle biopsy is typically not required for the diagnosis but shows nonspecific myopathic changes and inflammatory infiltrates in up to 30% of biopsies.

Clinical Presentation

Although FSHD can affect people at all ages, most patients present in their late teens or early twenties with weakness in a characteristic pattern, often with dramatic side-to-side asymmetry: typically first in the face, shoulders, and arms, and later involving the trunk and distal lower extremities. Patients are unable to squeeze their eyes shut, have a transverse smile, scapular winging, loss of proximal muscle mass with often preserved forearm muscles, and a positive Beevor sign (movement of the umbilicus up or down when asked to tense the abdominal muscles). Extramuscular manifestations of FSHD are rare: retinal vascular changes, which can occasionally lead to symptomatic retinal vasculopathy termed Coat syndrome, high-frequency hearing loss, and atrial arrhythmias.

Diagnosis and Differential Diagnosis

Diagnosis is based on clinical examination and family history and is confirmed by genetic testing. The differential diagnosis includes other myopathies such as inclusion body myositis, limb-girdle muscular dystrophies and acid maltase deficiency.

Treatment

There are currently no pharmacologic disease-modifying therapies available. However, several therapy approaches are being studied with the unifying goal to suppress DUX4. One drug is currently being tested in a multisite clinical trial. In the interim, treatment is supportive with ankle bracing and assistive devices. In selected patients surgical fixation of the scapular can improve function. Monitoring for retinal disease, hearing loss, and respiratory function is indicated.

Prognosis

FSHD is not life limiting, but approximately 20% over the age of 50 will require a wheelchair.

CONGENITAL MYOPATHIES

Congenital myopathies are defined by their appearance on biopsy (E-Table 124.2; and see Fig. 142.1C) and have a large number of genetic mutations associated with them. They are usually present at birth with hypotonia and subsequent delayed motor development. If the child survives the perinatal period, most congenital myopathies are relatively nonprogressive and may not be diagnosed until the second or third decade. Clinical findings common in the congenital myopathies are reduced muscle bulk, slender body build, a long and narrow face, skeletal abnormalities (high-arched palate, pectus excavatum, kyphoscoliosis, dislocated hips, and pes cavus), and absent or reduced muscle stretch reflexes.

METABOLIC MYOPATHIES

Metabolic myopathies are muscle diseases due to mutations in enzymes responsible for energy production including glycogen, lipid, and mitochondrial metabolism (E-Table 124.3). Classically, these disorders present in older children or adults with episodes of exercise intolerance, muscle cramping, myalgia, and recurrent rhabdomyolysis associated with myoglobinuria. Newborns and infants can present with severe multisystem disorders that are often fatal.

Glucose and Glycogen Metabolism Disorders
Definition and Epidemiology

Glucose, and its storage from glycogen, is essential for the short-term, predominantly anaerobic energy requirements of muscle (see E-Table 124.3). Disorders of glucose and glycogen metabolism (called glycogenesis) have two distinct syndromes: (1) static symptoms of fixed weakness without exercise intolerance or myoglobinuria and (2) dynamic symptoms of exercise intolerance, pain, cramps, and myoglobinuria. Acid maltase deficiency (Pompe disease) is an example of the first and is treatable with enzyme replacement therapy, which is life extending for the childhood variant. McArdle disease is an example of the second. The incidence varies between region and ethnic group. For example, acid maltase deficiency has an incidence as high as 1:14,000 in African Americans. The prevalence of McArdle disease is approximately 1:100,000.

Genetics and Pathology

All are due to mutations in enzymes responsible for glucose or glycogen metabolism. Muscle biopsies usually show subsarcolemmal accumulation of glycogen.

Clinical Presentation

Acid maltase disease typically has a severe infantile form with respiratory and cardiac involvement and a slowly progressive adult myopathy, which can present with respiratory muscle weakness as the initial symptom. McArdle disease presents with severe episodes of muscle cramping and contractures associated with exercise and a fixed myopathy later in life. Many patients note a "second wind" phenomenon, which means that after a brief period of rest patients can resume physical activity with improved tolerance.

Diagnosis and Differential Diagnosis

Diagnosis is made by characteristic appearance on muscle biopsy with subsequent study of the enzyme activity or by searching for specific genetic mutations. The differential diagnosis includes other glycogen storage disorders, disorders of lipid metabolism, or mitochondrial disorders.

Treatment

The only glycogen storage disorder with a therapy approved by the FDA is enzyme replacement for infantile or adult-onset acid maltase deficiency. Therapies targeting the genetic mechanism of acid maltase deficiency are expected to enter clinical trials in the near future.

Prognosis

The spectrum is wide from severe fatal infantile diseases to milder symptoms in adults.

DISORDERS OF FATTY ACID METABOLISM

Disorders of lipid metabolism differ from glucose and glycogen disorders in that the metabolic derangement is in the enzymatic breakdown of fatty acids (see E-Table 124.3). Many present in childhood with episodes of encephalopathy precipitated by fasting with hypoketotic hypoglycemia. Serum fatty acid profiles often show reduced carnitine and increased longer chain fractions, depending on whether the mutation is in very long chain, long chain, or medium chain fatty acid metabolism. Adults typically show exercise intolerance and myoglobinuria and may develop a mild limb-girdle pattern myopathy. The most prevalent disorder of fatty acid metabolism is carnitine palmitoyltransferase II (CPT II) deficiency. This disease ranges from a lethal neonatal form to an adult form with muscle pain and recurrent myoglobinuria, often precipitated by exercise, febrile illness, or fasting. The diagnosis is usually made by detection of reduced CPT II activity in skeletal muscle with confirmatory genetic testing.

MITOCHONDRIAL MYOPATHIES

Definition and Epidemiology

Mitochondrial myopathies can present at any age, with varying degrees of severity or weakness, affect multiple organ systems, and have any pattern of inheritance (see E-Table 124.3). Mutations affect enzymes necessary for normal mitochondrial function and can be mitochondrial or nuclear. The overall prevalence for mitochondrial disorders is thought to be approximately 1:8500; however, the prevalence of individual mitochondrial syndromes is much lower and ranges from just a handful of cases, to 1 to 6 per 100,000.

Genetics and Pathology

Mutations can occur in both mitochondrial DNA (in which case inheritance is maternal) and nuclear DNA (autosomal dominant, recessive, or X-linked). Mitochondrial disorders produce biochemical defects proximal to the respiratory chain (involving substrate transport and usage) or within the respiratory chain. On muscle biopsy, muscle fibers contain abnormal mitochondria. Pathologically, these fibers have a "ragged red" appearance on biopsy stains (trichrome) and fail to react for cytochrome C oxidase.

Clinical Presentation

Despite the diversity, certain patterns are characteristic for mitochondrial disorders, including slowly progressive myopathy and myalgias, which worsen with exertion or illness, and ptosis and/or ophthalmoplegia. E-Table 124.3 lists common clinical mitochondrial syndromes.

Diagnosis and Differential Diagnosis

The diagnosis is based on clinical history with recognition of multisystemic involvement, serum lactate levels, which can be elevated at rest, and characteristic findings on muscle biopsy. Diagnosis is confirmed by mitochondrial or nuclear genetic testing.

Treatment

Treatment is largely supportive and includes identification of other multisystem involvement, including diabetes, cardiac and ophthalmologic involvement, and hearing loss. Many agents have been tried in mitochondrial diseases, including coenzyme Q10, creatine, and carnitine. Aerobic exercise may reduce fatigue and improve muscle function, although there are no large trials of efficacy for either supplements or exercise.

Prognosis

The severity and prognosis depend partially on the load of abnormal mitochondrial DNA as well as the degree of multisystem involvement. Certain clinical syndromes with more predictable prognosis have been described (see E-Table 124.3).

MUSCLE CHANNELOPATHIES

The muscle channelopathies are a spectrum of disorders due to mutations in muscle ion channels commonly divided into the nondystrophic myotonias and periodic paralyses. Most are inherited in an autosomal dominant fashion, with episodic symptoms, often triggered by temperature or certain foods.

Nondystrophic Myotonias
Definition and Epidemiology
Nondystrophic myotonias are due to dysfunction of sodium or chloride channels resulting in hyperexcitable muscle and myotonia. The overall worldwide prevalence for nondystrophic myotonias is 1:100,000.

Genetics

Nondystrophic myotonias are caused by mutations in the muscle chloride (CLCN1) or sodium (SCN4A) channel genes causing alterations of depolarization and hyperpolarization of the muscle fiber membrane.

Clinical Presentation

As the name implies, patients have myotonia (see Table 124.2). Chloride channel mutations have a characteristic warm-up of myotonia with repetition. Sodium channel myotonias typically have more eye closure myotonia and can demonstrate a paradoxical worsening of myotonia with activity (paramyotonia). Symptoms usually start in the first decade, and patients can have a characteristic muscular build.

Diagnosis and Differential Diagnosis

Diagnosis is based on family history, clinical examination, and electrodiagnostic testing. It is confirmed by genetic testing. The differential diagnosis includes myotonic dystrophy and secondary causes of myotonia (other myopathies and drugs associated with myotonia—e.g., statins, fibric acid derivatives, and colchicine).

Treatment

Treatment for nondystrophic myotonias consists of non-mutation–specific sodium-channel blockade: mexiletine, a class IB antiarrhythmic, is the first-line therapy, but ranolazine, phenytoin, procainamide, and flecainide can be considered. Certain sodium-channel myotonias respond to the carbonic anhydrase inhibitor acetazolamide.

Periodic Paralyses
Definition and Epidemiology
The periodic paralyses are disorders that present with episodic weakness often triggered by exercise or food. Overall prevalence for the primary periodic paralyses varies between conditions from 1:100,000 to 1:1,000,000.

Genetics and Pathology

Periodic paralysis is caused by mutations in the calcium (CACN1AS), sodium (SCN4A), and potassium-channel (KCNJ2) genes that result in depolarized but inexcitable sarcolemma and episodes of paralysis. Hyperkalemic periodic paralysis is due to sodium-channel mutations that lead to persistent inward sodium current causing both myotonia and paralysis. Hypokalemic periodic paralysis can be caused by calcium-, sodium-, and potassium-channel mutations and is due to an anomalous gating pore current that, in low potassium conditions, produces a depolarizing current larger than hyperpolarizing potassium currents. Andersen-Tawil syndrome is due to loss of function in a potassium inward rectifier.

Clinical Presentation

Common to all are attacks of weakness first presenting in childhood or early adulthood, often brought on by rest after exercise, or in the mornings, and associated with changes in extracellular potassium. Hyperkalemic periodic paralysis is associated with either high or normal extracellular potassium, triggered by potassium-rich foods. In hypokalemic periodic paralysis attacks are associated with low extracellular potassium and are triggered by carbohydrates, stress, alcohol, or rest after exercise. Andersen-Tawil syndrome is characterized by the clinical triad of attacks of flaccid paralysis, dysmorphic features (wide-set eyes, narrow mandible, low-set ears, bent fifth finger, and common origin for the second and third toes), and polymorphic ventricular tachyarrhythmias.

Diagnosis and Differential Diagnosis

Diagnosis is based in family history and clinical history, supported by electrodiagnostic testing and confirmed by genetic testing.

Treatment

In all of the periodic paralyses disorders mild exercise at onset of weakness can abort attacks of paralysis. Treatment for acute attacks consists of carbohydrates (hyperkalemic periodic paralysis) or potassium supplementation (hypokalemic periodic paralysis). Prophylactic treatment for all the periodic paralyses consists of carbonic anhydrase inhibitors.

ACQUIRED MYOPATHIES

Unlike the inherited myopathies, the acquired myopathies are typically secondary to another process: toxic, autoimmune, inflammatory, or infectious. Pathologic changes can be distinctive and are not due to mutations in muscle-related proteins. Clinically, symptoms appear acutely or subacutely.

Inflammatory Myopathies

The idiopathic inflammatory myopathies can be divided into dermatomyositis/polymyositis and sporadic inclusion body myositis (Table 124.8).

Dermatomyositis/Polymyositis

Definition and epidemiology. Dermatomyositis/polymyositis (DM/PM) are acquired idiopathic diseases of muscle characterized by inflammation and variable symmetrical proximal muscle weakness, associated with elevated serum creatine kinase and irritable features on electromyography. The overall annual incidence is approximately 1 in 100,000.

Pathology. Dermatomyositis shows a pathognomonic pattern on muscle biopsy of perifascicular atrophy and perivascular inflammatory infiltrates and positive pericapillary membrane attack complex staining (see Fig. 124.1D). In contrast, polymyositis shows endomysial inflammatory infiltrates with invasion of non-necrotic fibers.

Clinical presentation. Dermatomyositis can occur at any age with an acute to insidiously progressive onset of symmetrical proximal muscle weakness with characteristic skin changes, which include heliotrope rash, shawl sign (maculopapular violaceous rash in V-shape around neck), Gottron nodules (erythematous papular rash on the extensor surfaces of the hands or fingers), and mechanic's hands (dry, cracked skin on the dorsal or ventral hands). In contrast, polymyositis is largely a diagnosis of exclusion, occurring in adults without associated skin changes. Myalgias are more common in polymyositis. Both DM/PM can be associated with respiratory weakness, interstitial lung disease, difficulty swallowing, or cardiomyopathy. Both DM/PM can be associated with underlying malignancy (dermatomyositis more frequently than polymyositis), so screening for malignancy is recommended especially in patients over age 40.

Diagnosis and differential diagnosis. Diagnosis is based on clinical history and examination findings in conjunction with irritable changes on electromyography (e.g., fibrillation potentials and positive sharp waves) and characteristic muscle biopsy. In about 30%, both DM/PM can be associated with myositis specific autoantibodies (see Table 124.2). Antibodies can help define a clinical syndrome and guide treatment. For example, patients with anti-Jo-1 antibodies can have interstitial lung disease and methotrexate may need to be avoided due to pulmonary toxicity. Patients may be at higher risk to develop malignancy with antibodies to transcription intermediary factor (TIF)-1gamma (anti-p155, anti-p155/140) and to nuclear matrix protein (NXP)-2 (anti-MJ or anti-p140). Muscle biopsy can help differentiate from other inflammatory myopathies associated with systemic disease (e.g., sarcoidosis).

Treatment. For both DM/PM the first line of treatment is prednisone. Steroid-sparing immunosuppressive therapies (e.g., methotrexate, azathioprine) are often added for those patients requiring long-term therapy in order to reduce the required dose of prednisone or to replace prednisone completely. In patients who do not respond to conventional therapy or have severe symptoms, intravenous immunoglobulin is used. Rituximab may also be effective.

Prognosis. Most patients respond to immunosuppressive therapies.

Sporadic Inclusion Body Myositis

Definition and epidemiology. Sporadic inclusion body myositis (s-IBM) is an idiopathic, slowly progressive muscle condition in older adults (occurring in more men than women), associated with inflammation and characteristic pathologic changes on muscle biopsy. It is the most common inflammatory muscle disease in patients over 50, affecting 3.5 per 100,000.

Pathology. Muscle biopsies resemble polymyositis with endomysial inflammatory infiltrates and invasion of non-necrotic fibers. Distinctive for IBM are vacuoles rimmed by mitochondria, secondary mitochondrial changes, and electron microscopy, which shows 15- to 18-nm tubulofilamentous inclusions.

Clinical presentation. S-IBM causes slowly progressive, often asymmetric weakness. It occurs usually after 50 years of age in an initially distinctive pattern, including distal forearm muscles (distal finger flexors) and quadriceps wasting and weakness. This can progress to involve almost any muscle and can affect swallowing in up to 70% of patients.

Diagnosis and differential diagnosis. Diagnosis is based on clinical history and examination and characteristic muscle pathology. In clinically challenging cases autoantibody levels directed against cytoplasmic 5′-nucleotidase 1A (anti-cN1A) can be helpful, with an estimated specificity around 90%. The main differential diagnosis is other idiopathic inflammatory myopathies or late-onset inherited

TABLE 124.8	**Idiopathic Inflammatory Myopathies**					
Myopathy	Sex	Typical Age at Onset	Pattern of Weakness	Creatine Kinase	Muscle Biopsy	Response to Immunosuppressive Therapy
Dermatomyositis	Women > men	Childhood and adult	Proximal > distal, respiratory weakness, dysphagia	Increased (up to 50× normal)	Perifascicular atrophy, inflammation, complement deposition on capillaries	Yes
Polymyositis	Women > men	Adult	Proximal > distal	Increased (up to 50× normal)	Endomysial inflammation; invasion of non-necrotic fibers	Yes
Sporadic inclusion body myositis	Men > women	Elderly (>50 yr)	Proximal and distal; predilection for finger and wrist flexors, knee extensors	Increased (<10× normal)	Endomysial inflammation, rimmed vacuoles; electron microscopy: 15- to 18-nm tubulofilaments	No

myopathies. The prominent hand weakness can be misinterpreted as neurogenic (e.g., amyotrophic lateral sclerosis) and electrodiagnostic studies can help differentiate the two.

Treatment. Unlike the other inflammatory myopathies, IBM does not respond to immunosuppression. Treatment is supportive.

Prognosis. Most patients with s-IBM progress to needing a wheelchair over 10 to 15 years. Swallowing difficulty can be life-threatening.

Myopathy With HMGCR Antibodies

Patients typically present with proximal greater than distal symmetric weakness and myalgia. Most patients, but not all, report concurrent or prior exposure to statins. The CK is usually high. EMG can show muscle fiber irritability with myotonic discharges. Laboratory testing is positive for autoantibodies against 3-hydroxy-3-methylglutaryl coenzyme A reductase (HMGCR). Muscle biopsy shows a necrotizing myopathy. Treatment includes discontinuation of statin therapy and corticosteroids or IVIG. With early recognition and treatment, patients can recover markedly.

Infectious Myositis

An acute viral myositis can occur in the setting of viral infections. Patients develop muscle pain, proximal weakness, and elevated CK levels. The disorder is self-limited but when severe can be associated with myoglobinuria and occasionally with renal failure.

An inflammatory myopathy can occur in the setting of human immunodeficiency virus infection, either in early or in later acquired immunodeficiency syndrome. The clinical presentation resembles polymyositis. The patient's condition may improve with corticosteroid therapy. The disorder must be distinguished from the toxic myopathy caused by zidovudine, which responds to dose reduction. Although rarely seen, tuberculosis can present with muscle abscess (pyomyositis) either in the setting of pulmonary or disseminated disease or in isolation.

Myopathies Caused by Endocrine and Systemic Disorders/Corticosteroid Myopathy

Thyroid studies should be part of the evaluation in any adult with muscle weakness. Patients with hyperthyroidism often have some degree of proximal weakness but this is rarely the presenting manifestation of thyrotoxicosis. Hypothyroid myopathy is associated with proximal weakness and myalgias, muscle enlargement, slow relaxation of the reflexes, and marked (up to 100-fold) increase of the serum CK level.

Excess corticosteroids can result from endogenous Cushing's syndrome; however, muscle weakness is rarely the presenting manifestation of Cushing's syndrome.

The most common endocrine myopathy is an iatrogenic **corticosteroid myopathy**, due to exogenous glucocorticoid administration. CK is typically low or normal and EMG normal. Muscle biopsy can show type 2 fiber atrophy. Therapy consists of reducing the corticosteroid dose to the lowest possible level, exercise, and adequate nutrition.

Toxic Myopathies

Many drugs, for example hydroxychloroquine, have been associated with muscle damage, proximal weakness, elevated CK levels, myopathic EMG readings, and abnormalities on muscle biopsy. Symptoms generally improve after stopping the medication.

Critical illness myopathy, also termed acute quadriplegic myopathy, develops in a patient in the intensive care setting and is often discovered when a patient is unable to be weaned off a ventilator. The cause of the diffuse weakness is the prolonged daily use of either high-dose intravenous glucocorticoids or nondepolarizing neuromuscular blocking agents, often both. Patients often have had sepsis and multiorgan failure. The diagnosis of critical illness myopathy is often clinical but can be confirmed by muscle biopsy, which shows the loss of myosin-thick filaments on electron microscopic examination. Treatment is discontinuation of the offending agents and early intensive physical therapy.

SUGGESTED READINGS

Amato AA, Griggs RC: Overview of the muscular dystrophies, Handb Clin Neurol 101:1–9, 2011.

Hamel J, Tawil R: Facioscapulohumeral muscular dystrophy: update on pathogenesis and future treatments, Neurotherapeutics 15(4):863–871, 2018.

Hehir MK, Logigian EC: Electrodiagnosis of myotonic disorders, Phys Med Rehabil Clin N Am 24:209–220, 2013.

Jackson CE, Barohn RJ: A pattern recognition approach to myopathy, Continuum (Minneap Minn) 19(6 Muscle Disease):1674–1697, 2013.

Lemmers RJ, Tawil R, Petek LM, et al: Digenic inheritance of an SMCHD1 mutation and an FSHD-permissive D4Z4 allele causes facioscapulohumeral muscular dystrophy type 2, Nat Genet 44(12):1370–1374, 2012.

Mammen AL: Statin-associated autoimmune myopathy, N Engl J Med 374:664–669, 2016.

Matthews E, Fialho D, Tan SV, et al: The non-dystrophic myotonias: molecular pathogenesis, diagnosis and treatment, Brain 133(Pt 1):9–22, 2010.

McGrath ER, Doughty CT, Amato AA: Autoimmune myopathies: updates on evaluation and treatment, Neurotherapeutics. 15(4):976–994, 2018.

Pfeffer G, Majamaa K, Turnbull DM, et al: Treatment for mitochondrial disorders, Cochrane Database Syst Rev (4):CD004426, 2012.

Statland JM, Bundy BN, et al: Mexiletine for symptoms and signs of myotonia in nondystrophic myotonia: a randomized controlled trial, J Am Med Assoc 308(13):1357–1365, 2012.

Statland JM, Tawil R: Facioscapulohumeral muscular dystrophy: molecular pathological advances and future directions, Curr Opin Neurol 24(5):423–428, 2011.

Thornton CA, Wang E, Carrell EM: Myotonic Dystrophy: approach to therapy, Curr Opin Genet Dev 44:135–140, 2017.

Wheeler TM, Leger AJ, Pander SK, et al: Targeting nuclear RNA for in vivo correction of myotonic dystrophy, Nature 488(7409):111–115, 2012.

125

Neuromuscular Junction Disease

Emma Ciafaloni

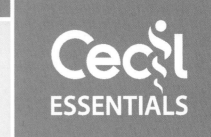

Neuromuscular junction diseases are caused by abnormal neuromuscular transmission of the action potential from the nerve terminal to the muscle, and they can be autoimmune (myasthenia gravis, Lambert-Eaton syndrome), hereditary (congenital myasthenic syndromes), or toxic (botulism, organophosphate intoxication).

MYASTHENIA GRAVIS

Definition/Epidemiology/Pathology

Myasthenia gravis (MG) is a rare autoimmune disease caused by antibodies against the postsynaptic acetylcholine receptors (AChR Ab) in the neuromuscular junction. All ages are affected but incidence is higher in women younger than 40 and in men older than 50. Prevalence is approximately 20 in 100,000. Transient neonatal MG occurs in about 12% of newborns of myasthenic mothers and is caused by transplacental passive transfer of antibodies from the mother to the fetus. Thymoma is found in 10% of patients with MG and thymic hyperplasia is present in 65%.

Clinical Presentation

MG is characterized by fluctuating, fatigable weakness either isolated to the ocular muscles (ocular MG) or involving ocular as well as limb, bulbar, and respiratory muscles (generalized MG). The majority of patients present first with ocular symptoms (blurred vision, double vision, droopy eyelids), but about 15% of cases present with bulbar symptoms first (dysarthria, dysphagia, shortness of breath) or limb weakness. Ptosis is usually asymmetric. Myasthenia crisis is a true neurologic emergency that occurs in 15% to 20% of patients and consists of severe dysphagia or respiratory failure requiring ventilator support and/or tube feeding in an ICU setting.

Diagnosis and Differential Diagnosis

The diagnosis of MG is based on a combination of clinical history, physical examination, and confirmatory tests. The ice pack test is a simple and relatively sensitive test to differentiate ptosis caused by MG from other causes of ptosis. In this test an ice pack is applied to the ptotic eye for 2 minutes and an improvement of 2 mm or more in ptosis supports MG.

Edrophonium chloride (Tensilon) is a short-acting acetylcholinesterase inhibitor administered intravenously to demonstrate symptom improvement in patients with MG. A positive Tensilon test is defined as an unequivocal improvement in strength in an affected muscle after 2 to 5 minutes from administration of 2 mg incremental doses up to 10 mg. Atropine should be available during a Tensilon test because bradycardia and hypotension are possible side effects. Edrophonium testing can be positive in other disorders.

Electrodiagnostic testing with 3 Hz repetitive nerve stimulation (RNS) demonstrates a compound muscle action potential

(CMAP) decrement more than 10% in about 50% to 75% of patients with generalized MG but is abnormal in less than 50% of patients with purely ocular symptoms. Single fiber electromyography (SFEMG) is the most sensitive test in the diagnosis of MG and reveals increased jitter and blocking in 99% of patients with generalized MG and in 97% of those with purely ocular MG when a weak muscle is tested. SFEMG is usually available only in specialized EMG laboratories.

Serum antibody testing for AchR Ab (binding antibody) is positive in about 80% of patients with generalized MG and 50% of patients with purely ocular symptoms. Muscle specific tyrosine kinase (Anti MuSK) antibody is detected in a portion of seronegative patients, more frequently women.

Chest CT should be performed to rule out thymoma, found in approximately 10% of seropositive myasthenic patients. Thyroid function should be evaluated because thyroid disease is commonly associated with MG. Electrodiagnostic and serum antibody testing help with differentiating MG from motor neuron disease, Lambert-Eaton myasthenic syndrome (LEMS), and Guillain-Barré syndrome (GBS).

Treatment

Pyridostigmine 30 to 60 mg every 4 hours improves symptoms in most patients with MG; it is used alone to treat purely ocular and generalized cases with only minimal or mild weakness, or in combination with immunosuppressant drugs in patients with more severe manifestations. Prednisone is effective in improving muscle weakness in a short period of time, but long-term use is associated with side effects. Azathioprine and mycophenolate mofetil are used for long-term treatment and as steroids-sparing agents. Eculizumab is a complement inhibitor recently approved for patients with generalized MG with positive AChR antibody. Plasmapheresis and IVIG are used for cases with severe bulbar or generalized weakness, respiratory crisis, and in refractory patients who do not respond to oral immunomodulating medications. Thymoma resection is indicated in all patients with MG and thymoma. Thymectomy is also recommended in patients with nonthymomatous autoimmune MG to increase the probability of remission or improvement. Thymectomy is usually not recommended in patients over age 60. Some medications may exacerbate the symptoms of MG or precipitate the initial signs and symptoms of the disease (Table 125.1).

Prognosis

Most patients with MG who are optimally treated experience improvement or remission of their symptoms. About 10% of patients with MG experience refractory symptoms despite optimal treatment. Mortality is currently less than 5%.

TABLE 125.1 Drugs to Be Avoided or Used With Caution in Myasthenia Gravis

- D-penicillamine
- Penicillins
- Telithromycin
- Interferon-α
- Aminoglycoside antibiotics
- Fluoroquinolones
- Nitrofurantoin
- Tetracyclines
- Sulfonamides
- Botulinum toxin
- Magnesium, magnesium salts contained in some laxatives and antacids
- Neuromuscular blocking agents such as succinylcholine and vecuronium should only be used by an anesthesiologist familiar with MG
- Quinine, quinidine or procainamide
- β-blockers (propranolol; timolol maleate eyedrops)
- Calcium-channel blockers
- Iodinated contrast agents
- Checkpoint inhibitors: pembrolizumab
- Anesthetics: Methoxyflurane, succinylcholine

LAMBERT-EATON MYASTHENIC SYNDROME

Definition/Epidemiology/Pathology

LEMS is an acquired, presynaptic neuromuscular transmission disorder caused by antibodies against the P/Q type voltage-gated calcium channel (VGCC). P/Q VGCC antibodies cause reduced Ca^+ influx into the presynaptic nerve terminal, resulting in decreased acetylcholine release and neuromuscular transmission failure. LEMS is associated with cancer, usually small cell lung carcinoma, in 60% of cases. LEMS may predate tumor detection by up to 3 years. LEMS is very rare and more common in men (3:1).

Clinical Presentation

LEMS should be suspected whenever the triad of muscle weakness, dry mouth, and decreased or absent reflexes is present. Patients have fluctuating weakness and fatigability of proximal limb and trunk muscles, with the lower limbs more severely affected than the upper ones. Difficulty walking is a common symptom. Dysphagia, dysarthria, and ocular symptoms (ptosis, blurred vision, and diplopia) are less common than in MG. Tendon reflexes are hypoactive or absent and may increase following short exercise of the muscle. Autonomic manifestations (dry mouth, impotence, decreased sweating, orthostatic hypotension, and slow pupillary reflexes) occur in 75% of patients.

Diagnosis and Differential Diagnosis

Serum antibodies against P/Q VGCCs are found in nearly all cases of paraneoplastic LEMS and in about 90% of non-paraneoplastic cases. Electrodiagnostic testing can help confirm the diagnosis by demonstrating reduced CMAP amplitudes in distal hand muscles; CMAP facilitation of at least 100% after 10″ maximal voluntary contraction or high frequency RNS (post-tetanic facilitation); and CMAP decrement greater than 10% with low frequency RNS. Patients diagnosed with LEMS should be screened and monitored with chest CT for lung cancer, especially if they are smokers and over age 50. LEMS and MG can be differentiated with electrodiagnostic and antibody testing.

Treatment

Symptomatic treatment with 3,4 diaminopyridine (3,4-DAP) 5 to 10 mg every 3 to 4 hours and up to a maximum daily dose of 80 to 100 mg is most effective in improving muscle strength in patients with LEMS. Side effects at doses up to 60 mg per day are rare. Acral and perioral paresthesias occur within minutes from a dose and resolve in about 15 minutes. It is contraindicated in patients with seizures. Pyridostigmine 60 mg every 4 hours is also used to improve symptoms. In patients in whom symptoms are not adequately controlled with 3,4-DAP and pyridostigmine, immunomodulation with prednisone, azathioprine, or mycophenolate mofetil is used. Severe weakness is treated with plasmapheresis or IVIG. The underlying cancer should be treated.

Prognosis

In paraneoplastic LEMS the prognosis is determined by the underlying cancer. The presence of LEMS in patients with small cell lung cancer (SCLC) is associated with longer survival from the malignancy. Non-paraneoplastic LEMS, when optimally treated, has an excellent prognosis and normal life expectancy, although patients may continue to experience various degrees of muscle weakness.

BOTULISM

Definition/Epidemiology/Pathology

Botulism is a rare, potentially lethal, paralytic illness caused by the neurotoxin produced by the anaerobic, spore-forming bacterium *Clostridioides botulinum*. Botulinum toxin blocks voluntary and autonomic cholinergic neuromuscular junctions by binding irreversibly to the presynaptic nerve endings where it inhibits the release of acetylcholine. Human forms of the disease include food-borne botulism most commonly caused by home-canned food, wound botulism with most cases occurring among "black tar" heroin users, and infant botulism occurring usually in the second month of life due to intestinal colonization. Outbreaks of food-borne botulism occur in prison inmates due to ingestion of pruno, an alcoholic drink made illicitly in prison. About 145 botulism cases are reported each year in the United States; approximately 15% are food-borne, 65% are infant, and 20% are wound botulism.

Clinical Presentation

The disease is characterized by symmetric descending flaccid paralysis starting with blurred or double vision, ptosis, dysphagia, dry mouth, dysarthria, and muscle weakness. Symptoms usually start 18 to 36 hours after ingesting contaminated food.

Botulism should be suspected in any infant with poor feeding and sucking, constipation, dilated pupils, weak cry, poor tone, and respiratory distress. Sensory examination and mental status are normal.

Diagnosis and Differential Diagnosis

All suspected cases of botulism need to be reported to public health authorities immediately. Local health department and CDC laboratories can confirm the diagnosis by detecting the toxin in serum, stool, or gastric or wound aspirate specimens. Electrodiagnostic testing can also confirm the diagnosis by demonstrating persistent post-tetanic facilitation of CMAP of at least 20%, a decremental response greater than 10% with slow RNS, and increased jitter and blocking on SFEMG. Electrodiagnostic tests are also helpful in differentiating botulism from Guillain-Barré syndrome and myasthenia gravis.

Treatment

Prompt intensive care support with mechanical ventilation and parenteral feeding as needed are crucial in reducing mortality. Timely administration of equine antitoxin within the first 24 hours may arrest the progression of paralysis and decrease the duration of illness. The antitoxin is provided by the CDC through the local health departments. Children younger than 12 months old should not be fed honey because it can contain *Clostridioides botulinum*.

Prognosis

The proportion of patients with botulism who die has fallen from 50% to between 3% and 5% in the past 50 years. Recovery of muscle strength may take several months. Mortality in untreated botulism is 60%.

ORGANOPHOSPHATE POISONING

Organophosphorus compounds (OPs) are used as pesticides and developed for chemical warfare. Exposure to even small amounts of an OP can be fatal and death is usually caused by respiratory failure. OPs cause inhibition of acetylcholinesterase (AChE) resulting in accumulation of acetylcholine at the cholinergic receptor sites, producing continuous stimulation of cholinergic fibers throughout the nervous system. A combination of an antimuscarinic agent (e.g., atropine), AChE reactivator, such as one of the pyridinium oximes (i.e., pralidoxime, trimedoxime, obidoxime, and HI-6), and diazepam are used for the treatment of OP poisoning in humans.

❖   For a deeper discussion on this topic, please see Chapter 394, "Disorders of Neuromuscular Transmission," in *Goldman-Cecil Medicine*, 26th Edition.

SUGGESTED READINGS

Palace J, Newsom-Davis J, Lecky B: A randomized double-blind trial of prednisolone alone or with azathioprine in myasthenia gravis, Neurology 50:1778–1783, 1998.

Pascuzzi RM, Coslett HB, Johns TR: Long-term corticosteroid treatment of myasthenia gravis: report of 116 patients, Ann Neurol 515:291–298, 1984.

Passaro DJ, Werner SB, McGee J: Wound botulism associated with black tar heroin among injecting drug users, J Am Med Assoc 279(11):859–863, 1998.

Sanders DB, Wolfe GI, Benatar M, et al: International consensus guidance for management of myasthenia gravis, Neurology 87(4):419–425, 2016.

Sobel J, Tucker N, Sulka A: Foodborne botulism in the United States, 1990-2000, Emerg Infect Dis 10:1606–1611, 2004.

Tim R, Massey J, Sanders D: Lambert-Eaton myasthenic syndrome: electrodiagnostic findings and response to treatment, Neurology 54:2176–2178, 2000.

Underwood K, Rubin S, Deakers T: Infant botulism: a 30 year experience spanning the introduction of botulism immune globulin intravenous in the intensive care unit at Children's Hospital Los Angeles, Pediatrics 120(6):1380–1385, 2007.

Vugia DJ, Mase SR, Cole B: Botulism from drinking pruno, Emerg Infect Dis 15:69–71, 2009.

Wirtz P, Lang B, Graus F: P/Q-type calcium channel antibodies, Lambert-Eaton myasthenic syndrome and survival in small cell lung cancer, J Neuroimmunol 164:161–165, 2005.

Wolfe GI, Kaminski HJ, Aban IB, et al: Randomized trial of thymectomy in myasthenia gravis, N Engl J Med 375:511–522, 2016.

Geriatrics

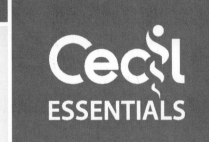

126

The Aging Patient

Laura A. Previll, Mitchell T. Heflin, Harvey Jay Cohen

INTRODUCTION

The aging of the world's population compels all health care team members to gain competency in geriatrics, the clinical science of assessment, prevention, and treatment of illness in older adults. A basic grasp of geriatrics requires understanding at epidemiologic, biologic, and clinical levels. The provider must appreciate the impact of aging on presentation of and predisposition to certain conditions, must identify goals of care, and must select appropriate treatment strategies. Moreover, care of older adults demands a multifaceted approach, accounting for individual, family, and community resources. Finally, the practice of geriatrics requires an appreciation for systems of care that include interprofessional teams working in a variety of settings ranging from home to hospital to long-term care to community settings. This chapter will provide an introduction to geriatrics and the essentials of caring for older adults.

Over the last century, the number of Americans over the age of 65 years increased from 3 million to nearly 51 million in 2016, accounting for 16% of the population. During the same period the population over age 85 grew rapidly, expanding from 100,000 in 1900 to nearly 6.4 million in 2016. By 2030, the number of adults over age 65 will likely reach 74 million, or 21% of the total population. Ten million of those people will be over age 85 (Fig. 126.1). A report from the National Institute on Aging and the US State Department points out that this phenomenon is not isolated to the United States. Around the globe, the percentage of the population over 65 years of age will increase by 25% to 50% over the next 25 years and by 140% in developing nations.

EPIDEMIOLOGY OF AGING

Most experts believe that the rapid growth of the population of older adults reflects the many health care successes of the twentieth century. Fries, in his landmark paper, attributes the extension of the human lifespan to "the elimination of premature death, particularly neonatal mortality." Improvements in other aspects of public health, including adequate nutrition and housing, safe drinking water, immunizations, and antibiotics, have led to lower rates of mortality throughout childhood and early adulthood, affording an opportunity for more people to survive to late life. Examination of survival curves across the twentieth century demonstrates a marked change in the shape of the overall graph from nearly linear in 1900 to rectangular in the 1990s, with much of the mortality compressed into late life (Fig. 126.2). However, despite advances in public health, life expectancy at birth continues to vary by race and gender and social drivers of health affect the ability to achieve old age for many. As of 2016, the greatest average life expectancy at birth by ethnicity was in Hispanic females compared to non-Hispanic

black males who average 10 years fewer (E-Fig. 126.1). Although the overall average population life expectancy at birth rose dramatically in the 20th century from 47 years to nearly 77 years with up to 10% of the birth cohort surviving to age 95, the maximum lifespan defined as the age of the oldest surviving humans has remained remarkably stable at around 114 years.

THE BIOLOGY OF AGING

The relatively static nature of the maximum lifespan reflects the human body's limits at the cellular, tissue, and organ level in dealing with the stresses of aging. Across cell types and organ systems, certain consistent age-related alterations in physiologic function exist. Variability in tissue and organ function decreases, as evidenced by less fluctuation in heart rate or hormone secretion. Organ systems also exhibit predictable declines in function over time Table 126.1. These changes are most evident at times of stress, and ultimately these systems are slower to react and recover. The overall result is an impaired ability to deal with any demands within a narrow range. This progressive restriction in the capacity to maintain homeostasis can be depicted as a steady tapering in the reserve available in multiple organ systems as time progresses (Fig. 126.3). In this situation an individual may function within the normal range in the absence of crisis, but stress such as acute illness may exceed his or her capacity to restore function and recover health. The result at best may be a decline in health and ability, and at worst, death.

THEORIES OF AGING

Scientific research provides a number of plausible theories of aging, which can be grouped into two major categories. *Error* or *damage theories* propose that aging occurs because of persistent threats from damaging agents derived from environmental stressors and an ever-declining ability to respond to or repair this damage. *Program theories* postulate that genetic and developmental factors most significantly determine the biologic life course and the maximal age of the organism. In actuality, biologic aging may reflect a complex combination of many types of events. In a landmark paper outlining specific "Hallmarks of Aging," Lopez-Ortin suggests nine possible molecular or genetic mechanisms through which physiologic systems age. This section provides an introduction to some of these theories (Fig. 126.4). The end of the chapter also describes the emerging field of geroscience related to these criteria.

The free radical theory of aging proposes that oxidative metabolism results in an excess of highly reactive byproducts, called *oxygen free radicals*, which damage proteins, DNA, and lipids. Molecular injury eventually leads to cell dysfunction and ultimately to tissue and organ

Millions

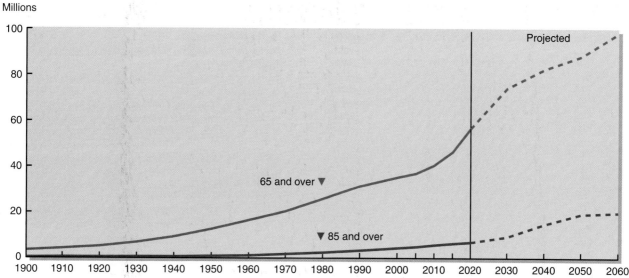

Fig. 126.1 Population age 65 and over and age 85 and over, selected years, 1900-2014, and projected years, 2020-2060. (From Federal Interagency Forum on Aging-Related Statistics: Older Americans 2016: key indicators of well-being. Federal Interagency Forum on Aging-Related Statistics, Washington, D.C., 2016, U.S. Government Printing Office.)

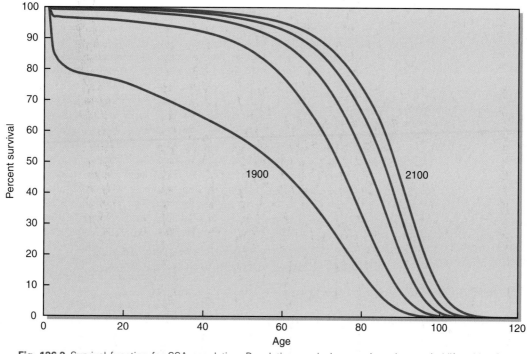

Fig. 126.2 Survival function for SSA population. Population survival curves based on period life tables for: 1900, 1950, 2000 and projected years 2050 and 2100. (From Bell, F.C. and Miller, M. L. Actuarial Study No. 120. Life Tables for the United States Social Security Area 1900-2100. [2005]. https://www.ssa.gov/oact/NOTES/as120/LifeTables_Body.html.)

disrepair. A second theory asserts that the accumulation of glucose-related molecules on proteins contributes to their dysfunction and degradation. These "glycosylated" molecules become more abundant over time and lead to impaired function at the tissue and organ level. Theory proponents point to the many chronic problems that routinely arise in patients with diabetes mellitus as proof of the significance of this phenomenon.

A different line of reasoning asserts that human lifespan and aging result from genetic-based timing mechanisms. Older theories suggest

that evolutionary pressures are biased for traits that promote health and reproduction in early adulthood, possibly at the expense of health and function in late life. Furthermore, little selective pressure exists against negative traits that emerge in late life, leaving humans prone to the ill effects of aging. Geneticists have identified, among species of fruit flies and certain nematodes, specific genes that result in a significant prolongation in the organism's lifespan. Further exploration of specific modification to gene expression, also called epigenetics, has led to improved understanding of the influence of environmental factors

TABLE 126.1 Changes in Physiologic Function With Age

Organ System	Age-Related Decline in Function
Special senses	Presbyopia
	Lens opacification
	Decreased hearing
	Decreased taste, smell
Cardiovascular	Impaired intrinsic contractile function
	Increased ventricular stiffness and impaired filling
	Decreased conductivity
	Increased systolic blood pressure
	Impaired baroreceptor function
Respiratory	Decreased lung elasticity
	Decreased maximal breathing capacity
	Decreased mucus clearance
	Decreased arterial Po_2
Gastrointestinal	Decreased esophageal and colonic motility
Renal	Decreased glomerular filtration rate
Immune	Decreased cell-mediated immunity
	Decreased T-cell number
	Increased T-suppressor cells
	Decreased T-helper cells
	Loss of memory cells
	Decline in antibody titers to known antigens
	Increased autoimmunity
Endocrine	Decreased hormonal responses to stimulation
	Impaired glucose tolerance
	Decreased androgens and estrogens
	Impaired norepinephrine responses
Autonomic nervous	Impaired response to fluid deprivation
	Decline in baroreceptor reflex
	Increased susceptibility to hypothermia
Peripheral nervous	Decreased vibratory sense
	Decreased proprioception
Central nervous	Slowed speed of processing and reaction time
	Decreased verbal fluency
	Increased difficulty learning new information
Musculoskeletal	Decreased muscle mass

Po_2, Partial pressure of oxygen.

such as chronic inflammation that impact gene expression and ultimately lifespan.

Study of the enzyme telomerase has also generated much interest among theorists on aging. In a process called apoptosis, cells undergo programmed death to be replaced by younger cells. These divisions and replacements are limited by the number of generations intrinsic to a specific cell line (the Hayflick phenomenon). As telomeres located on the ends of chromosomes are depleted, cell aging and demise eventually occur. The enzyme telomerase prevents telomere shortening and may increase a cell's number of allotted replications and thereby extend the lifespan of the organism. Of course, this advantage must be weighed against the price of "immortality," namely the increased risk of malignancy. Both apoptosis and cellular senescence are considered protective mechanisms against malignancy. The accumulation of senescent cells contributes to the biology of aging through secretion of various proteins that serve as inhibitory factors for halting cellular growth and division. In this way, regenerative capacities diminish when senescent cells shift the balance of cellular communication.

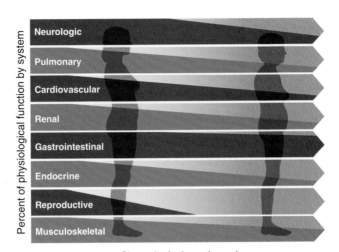

Fig. 126.3 Relative decline by organ system. (From Khan SS, Singer BD, Vaughan DE. [2017]. Molecular and physiological manifestations and measurement of aging in humans. *Aging Cell*, 16[4], 624-633.)

ASSESSMENT OF FRAILTY

Biologic changes of aging portend the increased vulnerability of humans to illness and functional decline in late life—a state commonly referred to as "frailty." The definition of frailty moves beyond traditional components of chronologic age, comorbidity, and disability to identify a unique clinical entity with independent predictive capacity. Two prevailing models of frailty have emerged—one focused more exclusively on a set of physiologic changes occurring in a cyclical pattern (the frailty phenotype) and the other that includes measures of both physiologic markers as well as disease burden (cumulative deficit frailty). System-specific changes over time lend a specific phenotype of frailty, including weight loss, weakness, poor endurance, slowness, and inactivity. Frailty, defined as three or more of these phenotypic conditions, independently predicts falls, declines in mobility, loss of ability to perform activities of daily living (ADLs), hospitalization, and death. This definition seems to provide a defined link between aging-related disease and disability and, perhaps, a target for interventions to prevent the onset of functional decline.

Alternatively, the impact of multiple external factors over time allows "deficits to accumulate" and impact multiple facets of overall health, cognitive, psychological, and physical function (Fig. 126.5). Many believe that the phenotypic model remains difficult to recognize or measure in the clinical setting. The other definition conceives of frailty as a result of accumulation of problems (or deficits) that ultimately exceeds an individual's ability to maintain function and health. This count of deficits generates an index predictive of disability and death. To some degree both models capture different aspects of complex and heterogeneous phenomena of vulnerability to declines in health and function with aging.

CLINICAL CARE OF OLDER ADULTS

Caring for older adults requires a strong foundation in the basics of internal medicine or family medicine integrated with an appreciation for the complexity and heterogeneity of the impact of aging on health and well-being. The clinician must possess strong diagnostic skills, given that older adults may have unique presentations or multiple comorbid conditions and functional decline. In addition, the clinician must monitor for a number of nonspecific conditions, such

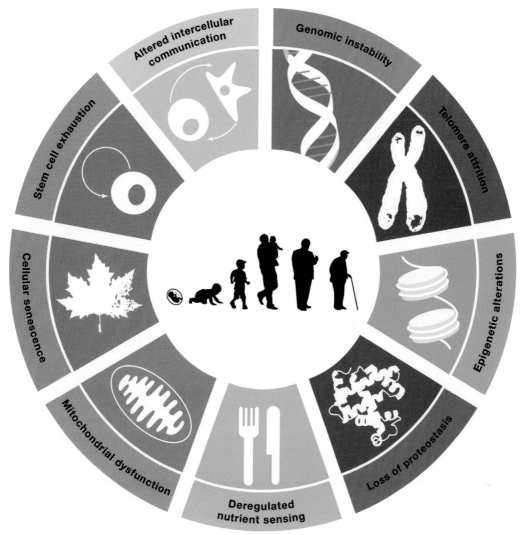

Fig. 126.4 The hallmarks of aging. (From López-Otín C, Blasco MA, Partridge L, et al [2013]. The Hallmarks of Aging. Cell, 153[6], 1194-1217.)

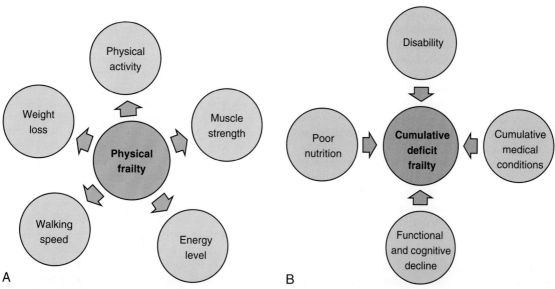

Fig. 126.5 Two major frailty theories. (A) Physical frailty or phenotypic frailty and (B) cumulative deficit frailty. (From Walston, J, Bandeen-Roche, K, Buta, B, et al. Moving frailty toward clinical practice: NIA Intramural Frailty Science Symposium Summary. J Am Geriatr Soc, 67: 1559-1564, 2019.)

TABLE 126.2	The Geriatric 5-M's
Mind	Mentation, dementia, delirium, depression
Mobility	Impaired gait and balance, fall injury prevention
Medications	Polypharmacy, de-prescribing, optimal prescribing, adverse medication effects and medication burden
Multi-Complexity	Multi-morbidity, complex bio-psycho-social situations
Matters Most	Each individual's own meaningful health outcome goals and care preferences

as problems with mobility, mood, or mentation that affect self-care capacity and safety. Treatment strategies present unique challenges as well, often requiring a balance of pharmacologic and nonpharmacologic interventions with careful consideration of the individual's goals for care. Tinetti and colleagues capture these tenants of geriatrics as the five M's: "Mind, Mobility, Medications, Multi-complexity, and Matters Most to Me" (Table 126.2). This section presents the core components of the comprehensive assessment of the older patient.

COMORBID CONDITIONS, FUNCTION, AND LIFE EXPECTANCY

With advancing age and declines in reserve, older adults experience high rates of chronic illness and often related functional decline. Eighty percent of those over age 65 years have at least one chronic illness, and 50% have two or more comorbid conditions. Some of these conditions contribute directly to increased rates of mortality, including the leading causes of death among older adults—heart disease, cancer, stroke, lung disease, and Alzheimer's disease. Many common diseases, however, primarily threaten function and result in disability and institutionalization. Arthritis, hearing loss, and vision impairment are all important problems in this respect. The presence of multiple comorbid conditions compounds the disabling effects of individual diseases and further complicates management. In the era of evidence and guidelines, a clinician caring for a patient with several common chronic conditions, such as diabetes mellitus, coronary artery disease, and osteoporosis, may feel compelled to prescribe six or seven medications to remain in compliance with current recommendations. This practice can result in "polypharmacy" (described later), adding significant cost to the patient with limited accounting for risks, benefits, and individual preferences. In addition to considering the discrete management of individual diseases, care of the older adult requires assessment of the overall impact of treatment on symptoms, function, and life expectancy. To address this common clinical challenge, the American Geriatrics Society maintains publication of guiding principles on care of older persons with multiple comorbid conditions that highlights the importance of accounting for complex interactions between conditions, risks, and benefits of various treatment options, overall prognosis, and patient goals and preferences.

Function, defined formally by Reuben et al., is "a person's ability to perform tasks and fulfill social roles across a broad range of complexity"—more succinctly, self-care capacity. Assessing this ability provides the clinician with a means of understanding the impact of illness, assessing quality of life, identifying care needs, and estimating progress and prognosis. Comprehensive assessment of function should include questions about self-care capacity as well as objective measures of cognition and mobility (see later sections for details about the latter two). Self-care capacity is most often divided into basic, instrumental, and advanced ADLs. Basic ADLs include those actions that maintain personal health and hygiene, including transferring, bathing, toileting, dressing, and eating. Instrumental ADLs (IADLs)

include activities necessary for living independently, specifically driving or using public transportation, cooking, shopping, managing medications and finances, using the telephone (or other communication device), and doing housework. Advanced ADLs include social or occupational functions associated with activities such as hobbies, employment, or caregiving. Approximately 30% of adults over age 65 and 78% of those over age 85 have difficulty with IADLs or one or more basic ADLs. Predictably, as the incidence of disability rises, so does the rate of dependence and placement in skilled facilities. Long-term care in skilled facilities increases from 2% among those aged 65 to 74 to 14% among those older than 85 years. Impairment in ADLs is also associated with an increased risk of falls, depression, and death in the affected elder. Among older adults the assessment of self-care capacity provides key health status information independent of age and comorbid conditions.

For clinicians, navigating the myriad options for management of multiple chronic conditions requires individualized assessment of risks, benefits, and specific goals of various therapies. Estimates of life expectancy, integrating the impact of age, comorbid illness, and function, have been generated to assist in medical decision making. These estimates assist clinicians in predicting median survival and thus can help in estimating the potential life remaining, which can impact treatment decision making (E-Fig. 126.2). For example, the options offered to a frail 85-year-old man with less than 3 years left to live may be quite different from those presented to his healthy counterpart of the same age with a median life expectancy of 5 to 7 years. In addition, any decision should take into account the individual patient's goals and preferences. A variety of prognostic tools exist to assist clinicians with estimating survival in different populations and care circumstances (Table 126.3). These tools can be accessed online in an interactive fashion for clinicians at http://eprognosis.ucsf.edu/.

PRESENTATION OF DISEASE IN THE OLDER ADULT

Competent care of the frail older adult starts with recognition of disease, even in the absence of signs and symptoms typically present in younger people. Presentation of disease among older adults may differ dramatically from that expected in younger patients; manifestations of distress may be subtle or nonspecific, and improvement is less obvious and slower. These phenomena occur for a number of reasons. As noted previously, older adults experience high rates of comorbid illness, which may confound the clinician's ability to diagnose a problem accurately. For example, a patient with heart disease and chronic obstructive pulmonary disease who visits the office because of dyspnea may be experiencing a flare of his or her pulmonary disease or an atypical presentation of ischemic heart disease or both. Reporting of symptoms may also be affected by psychosocial factors, including limited access to the health care system, cognitive problems, or minimization of symptoms as "normal aging." Likewise, health care professionals may minimize complaints by older adults with complex medical illness or frail health.

Variable presentations for certain conditions can be seen in older adults (Table 126.4). Hyperthyroidism can manifest with apathy, malaise, depression, and fatigue, while lacking classic symptoms of tremor, tachycardia, or sweating. It can also manifest with heart failure and is highly prevalent among older adults with new-onset atrial fibrillation. Likewise, older patients with hypothyroidism may atypically demonstrate failure to thrive, weight loss, cognitive decline, or depression. In the presence of infection, older adults may not reliably mount fever or experience localized symptoms. Studies have demonstrated that lowering the threshold definition of fever can improve the diagnostic utility of body temperature as a sign of bacterial infection. Although

TABLE 126.3   Clinical Decisions Influenced by Life Expectancy

Life Expectancy	Clinical Decision Examples
Short-term, <2 years	Minimize major, invasive surgical procedures
	Discuss goals of care and when to consider hospice care
	Discontinue statin therapy
Mid-term, 2–3 years	Aggressive blood pressure and lipid management in the setting of diabetes less likely to prevent microvascular complications
Long-term	Discontinue colon cancer screening if <7 years
	Limited benefit to A_{1C} target <8.0% if <5 years
	Discontinue prostate cancer screening if <10 years
	Limit breast cancer screening if <5 years

Adapted from Yourman LC, Lee SJ, Schonberg MA, et al. Prognostic indices for older adults: a systematic review. JAMA. 2012;307(2):182-192.

TABLE 126.4   Presentations of Disease in Older Adults[a]

Diagnosis	Potential Presenting Symptoms and Signs
Myocardial infarction	Altered mental status
	Fatigue
	Fever
	Functional decline
Infection	Altered mental status
	Functional decline
	Hypothermia
Hyperthyroidism	Altered mental status
	Anorexia
	Atrial fibrillation
	Chest pain
	Constipation
	Fatigue
	Weight gain
Depression	Cognitive impairment
	Failure to thrive
	Functional decline
Electrolyte disturbance	Altered mental status
	Falls
	Fatigue
	Personality changes
Malignancy	Altered mental status
	Fever
	Pathologic fracture
Pulmonary embolus	Altered mental status
	Fatigue
	Fever
	Syncope
Vitamin deficiency	Altered mental status
	Ataxia
	Dementia
	Fatigue
Fecal impaction	Altered mental status
	Chest pain
	Diarrhea
	Urinary incontinence
Aortic stenosis	Altered mental status
	Fatigue

[a]This table represents only a limited list of select disease processes and presentations; it is not meant to serve as an exhaustive reference for use during patient care activities.

chest pain remains the most common and important symptom of ischemic heart disease, dyspnea in the absence of chest pain is a commonly reported symptom, particularly in older adults and those with multiple comorbidities.

In truth, any medical illness may manifest nonspecifically among older adults, particularly those in frail health. Nonspecific symptoms related to an underlying illness include changes in mentation, difficulty with balance and falls, new urinary incontinence (UI), and a general change in functional ability. These presentations are often referred to as the "geriatric syndromes" and are detailed later. A lack of understanding of how disease presentation differs among older adults can lead to delays in diagnosis and treatment and result in worse outcomes. Research indicates that altered presentation predicts not only suboptimal care, but future functional decline and increased mortality.

MEDICATIONS

Medication-related problems are very common in older adults. In the United States, outpatients over age 65 take a median of four prescription medications daily, and nearly 40% are on five or more. Although medications may be indicated for specific medical conditions, use of multiple medications or polypharmacy increases the risk for drug-drug interactions and associated adverse drug events. Altered pharmacokinetics and pharmacodynamics contribute to adverse drug events, which are a common cause of hospitalization and morbidity in older persons. It is for this reason that certain medications can be considered "potentially inappropriate" in older adults. Common changes in pharmacokinetics include changes in body composition, with increased fat stores and decreased body water. Fat-soluble medications, such as benzodiazepines, have a prolonged duration of effect because of this phenomenon. Age-related declines in glomerular filtration rates result in decreased clearance of many medications, including such drugs as gabapentin, nitrofurantoin, and direct oral anticoagulants. Accurate calculations of creatinine clearance will inform drug choice and dosing and improve prescribing safety. Pharmacodynamic changes include decreased sensitivity to certain commonly prescribed drugs, such as β-blockers, and increased sensitivity to other agents, such as narcotics and warfarin.

Given the risks of medication use in older adults, health care professionals and systems must employ strategies to improve both the effectiveness and safety of prescribing as well as when to "de-prescribe" certain medications. Evidence-based recommendations include the following:

- Maintain an up-to-date medication list, including over-the-counter medications and herbal supplements.
- Comprehensively review medications at each visit with special attention at the time of transitions between care settings (e.g., after hospitalization). A clear indication for each medication, and documentation of response to therapy (particularly for chronic conditions) should be included.
- Assess for duplication and drug-drug or drug-disease interactions. Using a drug information database will help with this process.
- Assess adherence and affordability and inquire about the patient's system for administering medications (e.g., a pillbox).
- Assess for specific classes of medications commonly associated with adverse events: antiplatelet agents, anticoagulants, analgesics

(particularly narcotics and nonsteroidal anti-inflammatory drugs [NSAIDs]), antihypertensives (particularly angiotensin-converting enzyme [ACE] inhibitors and diuretics), insulin and hypoglycemic agents, and psychotropics.

- Be suspicious that new symptoms arise from adverse effects of current drugs, not new disease.
- Minimize or avoid use of anticholinergic medications, which present specific risks.

In addition to following these general principles, prescribing clinicians also benefit from consulting lists of potentially inappropriate medications. The Beers List of Potentially Inappropriate Medications (PIMs) provides an evidence-based guide to drugs that should be avoided if possible or used with caution in older adults. A clear and rational approach to prescribing and ongoing management of medications that accounts for indication, interactions, and adherence may reduce the risk of common adverse events.

COGNITION

Dementia

The prevalence of dementia increases with age, with estimates ranging from 20% to 50% after age 85. The most common forms of dementia include Alzheimer's disease, Lewy body dementia, and vascular dementia. The latter is commonly present in combination with Alzheimer's disease in a condition termed *mixed etiology dementia*. Dementia is characterized by impairment in one or more cognitive domains severe enough to disrupt function or occupation. Mild cognitive impairment (MCI) is present when an individual has discernible cognitive limitations without apparent deficits in IADLs. Patients with MCI develop dementia at a rate of approximately 15% per year. Dementia is associated with a higher risk of falls, functional impairment, institutionalization, and death. Caregivers of demented individuals also face increased rates of stress and health problems. Clinicians diagnose dementia through symptom and functional history (often including the input of caregivers), cognitive assessment, and physical examination. A number of instruments, including the MOCA (see Chapter 110), clock-drawing test, and the Mini-Cog, are validated screening tools. The time-tested Mini Mental State Examination (MMSE) offers an assessment of multiple cognitive domains but does not provide adequate measure of executive function. It is also prone to lack of sensitivity in individuals with high premorbid intelligence and lack of specificity in those with low levels of education. Validated assessments of executive function include the clock-drawing test, verbal fluency test, and the Trail Making test part B. Instruments also exist for collecting data regarding patient function from a relative or caregiver. In patients suspected of having dementia, personal safety with respect to firearms, driving, and the home environment should be assessed. A careful medication review and physical examination, including vital signs, complete neurologic assessment, including gait and balance, are, of course, essential in evaluating for dementia to reveal findings that point to a specific cause.

Delirium

The differential diagnosis for cognitive problems other than dementia is broad, and includes delirium, mood disturbance, and drug effects. The differentiation of dementia and delirium may present the most significant challenge, particularly in hospitalized elders (Table 126.5). Delirium is characterized as an abrupt change in global cognitive function, whereas dementia is chronic and affects specific cognitive domains over time. Differentiation often hinges on history, which may be lacking at presentation. Delirium, sometimes called "altered mental status," affects more than 2 million hospitalized persons each year. Its incidence is variably estimated at 25% to 60% among patients

TABLE 126.5 Features of Delirium Versus Dementia

Feature	Delirium	Dementia
Onset	Acute	Insidious
Course	Fluctuating, lucid at times	Generally stable
Duration	Hours to weeks	Months to years
Alertness	Abnormally low or high	Usually normal
Perception	Illusions and hallucinations common	Usually normal
Memory	Immediate and recent impaired	Recent and remote impaired
Thought	Disorganized	Impoverished
Speech	Incoherent, slow, or rapid	Word-finding difficulty
Physical illness or medication causative	Frequently	Usually absent

in acute care settings and results in extra hospital days and related expenditures. Delirium is also associated with prolonged hospital stay, increased costs, increased readmission rates to the hospital (12% to 65% at 6 months), higher in-hospital and 1-year mortality, and incident dementia. The Confusion Assessment Method (CAM) offers a validated framework for identifying delirium (https://consultgeri.org/try-this/general-assessment/issue-13.pdf). Per the CAM, delirium is likely present if the patient has both an acute onset of confusion with fluctuating course and inattention and either disorganized thinking or altered level of consciousness. According to Inouye and colleagues, key vulnerability factors for delirium include older age, cognitive impairment, comorbid illness, and impairments in vision and hearing. Precipitating factors related to acute illness include hypoxia, electrolyte abnormalities, dehydration, and malnutrition as well as medications and alcohol withdrawal. Delirium can also be a presenting sign for a number of serious medical conditions (see Table 126.2). Although treatment of delirium is difficult and revolves around the underlying medical issues, controlled trials have demonstrated that a multimodal intervention is effective in reducing rates of delirium in high-risk patients. There is evidence that the use of physical restraints in combative or confused older adults leads to increased morbidity and mortality. Nonpharmacologic management strategies include reorientation and preservation of sleep patterns, family or caregiver presence at the bedside, and early mobilization. "Chemical restraint" use, such as prescribing low dose antipsychotics, similarly has limited benefit. The use of pharmacologic agents, specifically neuroleptics, should be reserved for patients in whom nonpharmacologic strategies do not help and the patient presents a risk of harm to self or others.

MENTAL HEALTH

Older adults commonly experience depressive symptoms, with prevalence estimates as high as 15% to 19% among those over age 75, although in community-dwelling elders, major depressive disorder is actually less common than in younger adults. The presence of comorbid illness and grief often confound the presentation of depression. As a result, it can remain undetected despite its significant adverse impact on quality of life, morbidity, and mortality. Suicide rates are almost twice as high among older persons when compared with the general population, with the rate highest for white men over 85 years of age. Among older adults, depression can present with cognitive, functional, or sleep problems, as well as complaints of fatigue or low energy. Several instruments have been developed and validated for screening for depression in elders. Asking two simple questions about mood and anhedonia ("Over the past 2 weeks have you felt down, depressed, or hopeless?" and "Over the past 2 weeks have you felt little interest or pleasure in doing things?") may be as effective as using longer instruments. Longer screening questionnaires, such as the Geriatric Depression Screen (GDS) or Patient Health Questionnaire (PHQ-9), are also useful tools in the ambulatory setting. Any positive screening test result should trigger a full diagnostic interview. When screening for depression in elders, it is particularly important to have systems in place to provide feedback of screening results, a readily accessible means of making an accurate diagnosis, and a mechanism for providing treatment and careful follow-up. Randomized trials indicate that the addition of counseling to pharmacologic therapy confers additional benefit for older, frail patients with depression. Anxiety is more common than depression among older adults and may similarly result in physical and cognitive symptoms, insomnia, agitation, psychosis, and isolation. Clinicians should consider a diagnosis of generalized anxiety, panic, or agoraphobia in older adult patients with any of these symptoms.

SLEEP

Sleep disorders are present in more than 50% of older adults and have a negative impact on health and quality of life. Sleep disorders or disturbance are associated with cognitive impairment, poor health status, functional decline, and increased mortality. This may stem in part from changes in sleep structure with aging such as decreased deep (stage N3) sleep, longer sleep latency, and decreased sleep efficiency. Moreover, a variety of comorbid factors present in later life have adverse effects on sleep quality, including medical conditions, medications, psychosocial factors, and disruptive or disabling symptoms such as pain or nocturia. This includes drug and alcohol use as well as use of prescription and over-the-counter sedative hypnotics, which can cause sleep fragmentation and rebound insomnia. Additionally, medications commonly prescribed for insomnia, such as benzodiazepines and non-benzodiazepine hypnotics, are linked with cognitive impairment and falls. The mainstay of treatment for insomnia among older adults is careful attention to addressing the variety of comorbid factors and behaviors that lead to sleep disruption. The following is a sleep hygiene resource: https://www.nhlbi.nih.gov/files/docs/public/sleep/healthy_sleep.pdf). Strong evidence supports cognitive-behavioral therapy for insomnia (CBT-I) and other nonpharmacologic approaches including stimulus control, sleep restriction, and relaxation techniques. Older adults also suffer higher rates of other primary sleep disorders, including sleep apnea, periodic leg movements of sleep, and REM sleep behavior disorder. Eliciting a history of daytime somnolence and/or sleep partner complaints characteristic of these disorders should lead to completion of a diagnostic polysomnogram, which then guides initiation of appropriate therapies.

MOBILITY

Problems with mobility are common among older persons. Among those over age 65, 20% of men and 32% of women report difficulty with one or more of five specific physical activities (stooping or kneeling, reaching overhead, writing, lifting 10 pounds, or walking two to three blocks). Among these, respondents cite problems with walking most commonly. Difficulties with balance and gait present significant risks for older adults. Approximately 30% of community-dwelling elders fall each year. The annual incidence of falls approaches 50% in patients over 80 years of age. Five percent of falls in older adults result in fracture or hospitalization. According to the CDC, the rate

of deaths from falls among persons aged 65 years or older increased 31% from 2007 to 2016. Risk factors for falls include a history of falls, fear of falling, decreased vision, cognitive impairment, medications (particularly anticholinergic, psychotropic, and cardiovascular medications), peripheral neuropathy, diseases causing problems with strength and coordination, and environmental factors. Effective interventions for people with a history of falls or who are at risk for falling involve addressing multiple contributing factors. Clinicians and health care professionals should regularly inquire about recent falls or a fear of falling in older patients. For patients who report falling, the assessment should include review of circumstances of the fall(s), measure of orthostatic vital signs, visual acuity testing, cognitive evaluation, and gait and balance assessment. A brief physical examination maneuver called the "Timed get up and go" (TUG) has the patient arise from a sitting position, walk 10 feet, turn, and return to the chair to sit. A time of more than 12 seconds to complete the process, or observation of postural instability or gait impairment, suggests an increased risk of falling. Gait speed, an additional measure of mobility, predicts changes in ability and health status in older adults. Gait speed is measured over a 10-meter span with the patient walking at a comfortable pace. A speed of less than 1.0 m/sec is associated with increased mortality; 0.8 m/sec predicts difficulty navigating outside the home; and a speed of less than 0.6 m/sec predicts a high risk of falls and functional decline. For those found to be at risk for falls, providers should ask about possible causative agents and provide education about home safety. High-risk patients should be referred for evaluation by a physical therapist and consideration should be given to the utility of assistive devices and a supervised exercise program (Table 126.6).

VISION AND HEARING

Problems with vision and hearing are very common among older adults and frequently complicate the management of comorbid conditions and accelerate functional decline. Significant vision loss occurs in 16% to 18% of adults over age 65. Common causes include glaucoma, cataracts, age-related macular degeneration, and retinopathy from hypertension and diabetes. Decreased visual acuity increases fall risk and has been associated with all-cause mortality in older adults. Such problems may be detectable with regular testing via bedside tools such as the Snellen or Jaeger eye chart. Given the implications of vision loss for function and safety, a general ophthalmologic examination every 1 to 2 years is recommended for all older adults. Fortunately, many ophthalmologic centers recognize the multifaceted challenges faced by older adults with vision impairment. They offer specialized low vision clinics providing care from optometrists, occupational therapists, and social workers with a focus on improving quality of life and maintaining independence.

Hearing loss affects an estimated 40% to 66% of those over age 75. It is associated with depression, social isolation, poor self-esteem, cognitive decline, and functional disability. Pure tone audiometry is the reference standard for screening for hearing loss, but a simple whispered voice test is also highly sensitive and specific. Ideally, all older adults would undergo annual hearing screen by questionnaire and handheld audiometry. Unfortunately, the lack of reimbursement for hearings aids under most insurance plans, including Medicare, presents a major barrier for many older adults.

CONTINENCE

UI affects up to 30% of community-dwelling older adults and at least half of those residing in skilled nursing facilities. It occurs more frequently in women, but this gender disparity narrows as the rate of UI

TABLE 126.6 Recommended Components of Clinical Assessment and Management for Older Persons Living in the Community Who Are at Risk for Falling

Assessment and Risk Factor	Management
Circumstances of previous falls[a]	Change in environment and activity to reduce the likelihood of recurrent falls
Medication use • High-risk medications (e.g., benzodiazepines, other sleep medications, neuroleptics, antidepressants, anticonvulsives, or Class IA antiarrhythmics—including quinidine, procainamide, and disopyramide)[a,b,c] • Four or more medications[c]	Review and reduction of medications
Vision[a] • Acuity <20/60 • Decreased depth perception • Decreased contrast sensitivity • Cataracts	Ample lighting without glare; avoidance of multifocal glasses while walking; referral to an ophthalmologist
Postural blood pressure (after ≥5 min in a supine position, immediately after standing, and 2 min after standing)[c] • ≥20 mm Hg (or ≥20%) drop in systolic pressure, with or without symptoms, either immediately or after 2 min of standing	Diagnosis and treatment of underlying cause, if possible; review and reduction of medications; modification of salt restriction; adequate hydration; compensatory strategies (e.g., elevating head of bed, rising slowly, or performing dorsiflexion exercises); pressure stockings; pharmacologic therapy if the above strategies fail
Balance and gait[b,c] • Patient's report or observation of unsteadiness • Impairment on brief assessment (e.g., the "get up and go" test or performance-oriented assessment of mobility)	Diagnosis and treatment of underlying cause, if possible; reduction of medications that impair balance; environmental interventions; referral to physical therapist for assistive devices and for gait, balance, and strength training
Targeted neurologic examinations • Impaired proprioception[a] • Impaired cognition[a] • Decreased muscle strength[b,c]	Diagnosis and treatment of underlying cause, if possible; increase in proprioceptive input (with an assistive device or appropriate footwear that encases the foot and has a low heel and thin sole); reduction of medications that impair cognition; awareness on the part of caregivers of cognitive deficits; reduction of environmental risk factors; referral to physical therapist for gait, balance, and strength training
Targeted musculoskeletal examinations of legs (joints and range of motion) and examination of feet[a]	Diagnosis and treatment of underlying cause, if possible; referral to physical therapist for strength, range-of-motion, and gait and balance training, and for assistive devices; use of appropriate footwear; referral to podiatrist
Targeted cardiovascular examination[b] • Syncope • Arrhythmia (if there is known cardiac disease, abnormal electrocardiogram, and syncope	Referral to cardiologist; carotid-sinus massage (in case of syncope)
Home-hazard evaluations after hospital discharge[b,c]	Removal of loose rugs and use of nightlights, nonslip bathmats, and stair rails; other interventions as necessary

Adapted from Tinetti ME: Clinical practice. Preventing falls in elderly persons, N Engl J Med 348(1):42-49, 2003.

[a]Recommendation of this assessment is based on observations that the finding is associated with an increased risk of falling.

[b]Recommendation of this assessment is based on one or more randomized controlled trials of a single intervention.

[c]Recommendation of this assessment is based on one or more randomized controlled trials of a multifactorial intervention strategy that included this component.

in men increases after age 85. The impact of UI on health ranges from increased risk of skin irritation, pressure wounds, and falls, to social isolation, functional decline, and depression. For caregivers of older adults, UI complicates physical care and can contribute to decisions for placement in skilled nursing facilities. Common comorbid conditions include diabetes mellitus, heart failure, arthritis, and dementia.

A systematic approach to the investigation of UI can often reveal a cause and potential solution. It is important to first determine if the incontinence is acute or chronic in nature. Acute causes of incontinence are often attributable to specific medical problems, including infection, metabolic disturbance, or medication effects. The pneumonic DIAPERS recalls the various potential acute causes of UI (*D*, delirium; *I*, infection; *A*, atrophic vaginitis; *P*, pharmaceuticals; *E*, excess urine output from congestive heart failure [CHF] or hyperglycemia; *R*, restricted mobility; and *S*, stool impaction). If the UI is chronic, then further history can characterize the nature of the symptoms from among four types. Urge incontinence from detrusor overactivity is the

most common type. Patients with this problem will complain of urinary frequency, nocturia, and a sudden onset of urge to void. Stress incontinence occurs with incompetence of pelvic musculature or urethral sphincter and is characterized by small amounts of leakage with laughing, sneezing, coughing, or even standing. Overflow incontinence results from urinary retention, often related to prostatic hyperplasia in men or bladder atony in patients with diabetes or spinal cord injury. Patients often have constant dribbling or leakage without a true sense of needing to void. Finally, functional incontinence results from comorbid conditions that limit a patient's ability to act on or interpret the need to void, mobility problems such as arthritis, and weakness or cognitive problems. Table 126.7 describes the various types of incontinence and suggested approaches. Of course, older adults with multiple comorbid conditions often have incontinence that results from a combination of chronic and/or acute causes.

Continence problems are frequently treatable but are often not raised by patients as a concern. A targeted history and physical

TABLE 126.7 Causes, Types, and Treatment of Urinary Incontinence

Type	Definition	Cause	Treatment
Stress	Leakage associated with increased intra-abdominal pressure (coughing, sneezing)	Hypermobility of the bladder base, frequently caused by lax perineal muscles	Pelvic muscle exercise, timed voiding, α-adrenergic drugs, estrogens, surgery
Urge	Leakage associated with a precipitous urge to void	Detrusor hyperactivity (outflow obstruction, bladder tumor, detrusor instability), idiopathic (poor bladder), compliance (radiation cystitis), hypersensitive bladder	Bladder training, pelvic muscle exercise, bladder-relaxant drugs (anticholinergics, oxybutynin, tolterodine, imipramine)
Overflow	Leakage from a mechanically distended bladder	Outflow obstruction, enlarged prostate, stricture, prolapsed cystocele, acontractile bladder (idiopathic, neurologic [spinal cord injury, stroke, diabetes])	Surgical correction of obstruction, intermittent catheter drainage
Functional	Inability or unwillingness to void	Cognitive impairment, physical impairment, environmental barriers (physical restraints, inaccessible toilets), psychological problems (depression, anger, hostility)	Prompted voiding, garment and padding, external collection devices

examination can often identify the cause of UI and lead to appropriate intervention. Asking about and documenting the presence or absence of UI should be done biannually, as well as determining whether the UI, if present, is bothersome to the patient or caregiver. In addition to a history of acute and chronic causes, a targeted physical examination should include an assessment for fluid overload, genital and rectal examination, and neurologic evaluation. Urine and blood tests are indicated to evaluate for infection, metabolic causes, and renal dysfunction. In addition, for patients suspected of having urinary retention, catheterization or ultrasound can help define the postvoid residual and determine any need for catheter placement and further urologic evaluation. Many institutions now offer more specialized evaluation and care through incontinence clinics, which offer a multidisciplinary approach to management, addressing both pharmacologic and nonpharmacologic options. Effective nonpharmacologic options include scheduled toileting, bladder training, and biofeedback. Use of these strategies may avoid the use of medications with frequent adverse effects, such as anticholinergic medications for detrusor overactivity.

Like UI, fecal incontinence (FI) is an underreported and undermanaged issue among older adults with multiple factors contributing to etiology. FI is present in 45% or more of nursing home residents and is much more common in those with impaired mobility, dementia, chronic constipation or diarrhea. Ensuring prevention of constipation and associated overflow diarrhea is essential in management. Issues with muscular weakness that commonly contribute to fecal incontinence have excellent potential for treatment with specific types of physical therapy targeting pelvic floor muscles.

NUTRITION

Older adults experience high rates of malnutrition related to multiple causes, including medical illness, dental problems, or access issues related to limited mobility, cost, or cognitive problems. Approximately 15% of older outpatients and half of hospitalized elders are malnourished and have associated increases in morbidity and mortality. The utility of general laboratory testing is limited, but a combination of serial weight measurements and inquiries about changing appetite can reveal nutritional problems in the older adults. Vulnerable elders with an involuntary weight loss of 10% or more in 1 year or less should undergo further evaluation for undernutrition. This includes assessment of medical or medication-related causes, dental status, problems with acquiring or preparing food, appetite and intake, swallowing ability, and previous directions for dietary restrictions. Obese older adults suffer from high rates of malnutrition, but it is often unrecognized. They should also be screened routinely for nutrition concerns.

SOCIAL AND LEGAL ISSUES

Evaluation of the social history for older persons includes assessment of resources for direct caregiving and financial support available. These issues become particularly important for frail older adults, given their physical and economic vulnerability.

Caregiving

The clinician should always inquire about who is providing care for the older patient, including both personal care with ADLs and help with IADLs, such as transportation, medications, food preparation, finances, and housekeeping. This list should include both formal caregivers, such as home health professionals or hired aides, and informal caregivers, such as family members, neighbors, or friends. The majority of elder care provided in the United States is delivered by informal caregivers. Over 34 million people in the United States provide informal care for older adults and, of these, 15.7 million are caring for persons suffering from dementia. Seventy-five percent of informal caregivers are women and 39% are over age 65. The stress of providing daily care can have serious deleterious effects on the caregiver's health. Studies have demonstrated adverse effects on blood pressure and immune function and increased rates of cardiovascular disease and death. In addition, caregivers have alarmingly high rates of psychological illness, with symptoms of depression reported in up to 50%. This problem is particularly prevalent in those providing care for patients with dementia. The presence of mental illness further raises the risk of verbal or physical abuse or neglect of the patient. The clinician must recognize caregiver problems early and consider referral to a social worker, patient resource manager, or, when available, a geriatric assessment team. Key risk factors for caregiver stress include a frail family caregiver; a patient with cognitive impairment, emotional disturbance, substance abuse, sleep disruption, or behavioral problems; low income or financial strain; and acute illness or hospitalization. Heath care professionals should recognize signs and symptoms of physical or mental strain and regularly inquire about caregiver burden with an offer to talk apart from the patient if need be.

A number of resources exist to support caregivers and provide strategies for problem solving and self-care. Community-based programs provide assistance with meals, transportation, and respite care options through volunteer organizations or subsidized programs. Counseling on both the physical and emotional aspects of care has been demonstrated to reduce health risks to the caregiver and delay institutionalization, including in-home or institutional respite stays to provide caregivers with precious time off. Studies consistently demonstrate that such services are underused by caregivers. One resource that provides resources and supportive information about caregiving is https://eldercare.acl.gov/Public/Resources/Topic/Caregiver.aspx#UsefulLinks.

Mistreatment

Older adults are particularly vulnerable to mistreatment due to poor health, functional dependence, and social isolation. Mistreatment is defined as either elder abuse (harm caused by others) or self-neglect. Self-neglect is thought to be the most common form of mistreatment, but true rates are difficult to estimate. Risk factors include cognitive impairment and recent functional decline. Elder abuse has been reported in 3% to 8% of the older adult population in the United States, although this is likely an underestimate due to underreporting by patients and lack of recognition by health care providers. Abuse assumes many forms including psychological, financial, physical, sexual, and neglect. Studies have demonstrated that neglect and abuse are associated with higher rates of nursing home placement and mortality among older adults. Signs of physical abuse include contusions, burns, bite marks, genital or rectal trauma, pressure ulcers, or unexplained weight loss. Other forms of abuse may be more difficult to discern on examination but can be improved with direct questions such as "Has anybody hurt you?"; "Are you afraid of anybody?"; or "Is anyone taking or using your money without your permission?" Any suspicion of abuse or neglect should be reported to Adult Protective Services. Of note, 44 states and the District of Columbia have laws mandating reporting of suspected elder abuse and the U.S. Department of Justice has a growing network of resources (https://www.justice.gov/elderjustice/about-eji).

Finances

The older adult population in the United States varies widely in measures of wealth. Although the overall rate of poverty among adults over age 65 has declined over the last 50 years, 9.3% of older adults still live at or below the poverty line, and the percentage is higher among African Americans (18.7%) and Hispanic individuals of any race (17.4%). Members of the health care team including providers should screen for financial problems because these issues have direct implications for health status and well-being. Older adults with limited means are more likely to have problems affording medications, meals, and basic amenities. Referrals to community resource networks can help identify options for help with basic needs, including housing options and congregate meals. Information on agencies and services in specific locales can be identified at https://eldercare.acl.gov/Public/Index.aspx.

Advance Care Planning

Advance directives come in a number of different forms and serve a variety of purposes. Ideally, these documents articulate a person's preferences for care in the event of serious illness or incapacitation. Often they will describe limits on care and circumstances in which life-sustaining or restoring measures may be withheld or even withdrawn. Traditionally, advance directives have included a living will and health care power of attorney. The living will often addresses situations in which the patient has a terminal illness, persistent vegetative state, or progressive neurologic condition and can include explicit directions for care management including withdrawal or withholding of specific measures, including artificial nutrition and hydration. Living wills are ideally paired with a companion document, the health care power of attorney, which designates the person's preferred decision maker, or proxy, in the event of an incapacitating illness. For patients who have not created a health care power of attorney, typically the spouse or other first-degree relative is the default decision maker. If no proxy is designated and no next of kin is available, guardianship may be obtained.

Guardianship is a legal proceeding whereby the court appoints a surrogate decision maker. The physician's responsibility includes determination of a person's capacity for independent decision making in the event of altered sensorium or progressive cognitive impairment. This involves an assessment of his or her ability to understand the situation, ask questions, weigh options and render an opinion and, in certain situations, may require a full geriatric or neuropsychological assessment. Traditional advance directives, particularly the living will, have been criticized as having limited utility in conveying specific preferences. Recently, more detailed forms have emerged to record very specific preferences and limits for measures such as hydration, nutrition, hospitalization, and resuscitation. Examples include the Medical Orders for Scope of Treatment (MOST) and Physician's Orders for Life Sustaining Treatment (POLST) forms https://polst.org/programs-in-your-state/. Of course, effective completion and application of any of these forms should include a goals of care conversation conducted with the primary care provider, ideally involving family caregivers. In addition, as preferences change over time depending on health status, health care providers should encourage older adults to revisit and renew their advance directives on an annual basis.

CONTEXTS OF CARE: SPECIAL CONSIDERATIONS

The Hospitalized Patient

Millions of older adults are hospitalized in the United States each year for a variety of acute illnesses and elective procedures. Fortunately, in the United States, Medicare Part A covers much of the cost associated with acute care, including hospitalization and short-term rehabilitation. While in the hospital, however, older adults can become vulnerable to myriad complications related to both their compromised health state and problems inherent to the acute care environment itself. As noted previously, delirium afflicts hospitalized elders at a very high rate and increases risk of prolonged hospital stays, nursing home admission, and death. Hospitalized older adults also experience the effects of immobilization, with loss of muscle strength and deconditioning. Acutely, these factors increase the risk of falls and impair function and ability to provide self-care. In addition, poor oral intake may result in malnutrition, and illness-related fluid losses may cause dehydration. As a result, hypotension and protein-calorie malnutrition are common problems. Immobility and malnutrition both predispose the acutely ill patient to the development of pressure wounds, which can develop in under 2 hours. All these problems worsen in the presence of delirium or depressed mood. Environmental factors also contribute to problems, including tethers such as catheters and intravenous lines (which increase risk of falls), noisy wards, and frequent tests and procedures that further disrupt diurnal rhythms and sleep. Up to one third of hospitalized older adults experience a decline in their ability to perform ADLs in the course of their hospitalization. Patients who experience declines in function during hospitalization have higher rates of rehospitalization, prolonged institutionalization, and mortality after discharge, and many (41%) never return to their preadmission level of function. To combat these problems, some hospitals have created specialized inpatient geriatric care units, often termed *acute care for elders (ACE) units*. These units incorporate adaptations in the physical environment and specially trained staff to provide safe, patient-centered care designed to maximize restoration of function and prevent common complications of hospitalization. In randomized trials, ACE units and their consultative counterpart, the mobile ACE (or MACE), have reduced lengths of stay, improved care transitions, and lowered readmissions. Likewise, geriatric evaluation and management (GEM) units (described later) offer specialized, team-based postacute care with an emphasis on rehabilitation and return to prior level of function.

Care Transitions

As noted previously, older adults experience high rates of complications during acute illness and require prolonged periods of time and sometimes admission for rehabilitation in various types of facilities in order to recover. For this reason, management in the postacute period represents a critical and complex time. Specifically, older adults with acute illness often find themselves transferred among different care settings and providers. Nearly one quarter of hospitalized older adults are discharged to skilled nursing facilities, and another 12% are discharged with home health care. Of those discharged to skilled facilities, about one fifth will return to the hospital within 30 days. Transitions in care represent high-risk episodes, and evidence shows that patients and caregivers frequently experience miscommunication, medication errors, and missed essential laboratory tests or appointments during this period. Recent trials have demonstrated a reduction in rehospitalization through a structured discharge and transition of care plan. This includes interdisciplinary team communication, medication reconciliation before and after discharge, careful planning for laboratory and appointment follow-up, communication with patients and caregivers about expectations and preferences, and specific coaching for patients and caregivers in symptom management. More information on care management in transitions is available at www.caretransitions.org.

SYSTEMS OF CARE

Ambulatory and Home Care

The majority of care for older adults occurs in the outpatient setting. Much of the cost of this care, including visit fees, laboratory tests, radiograph studies, and vaccinations, is covered under Medicare Part B, for which patients pay a monthly premium. Outpatient visits may occur with the physician, physician assistant, nurse practitioner, or clinical nurse specialists, depending on the nature of the problem and the structure of the setting. Other key members of the care team include social workers, pharmacists, psychologists, and physical and occupational therapists. Most assessments discussed in this chapter can be performed in outpatient settings, including functional assessments, cognitive and mood screening, gait and balance assessment, medication review, eye and ear examinations, and continence evaluations. Interview of a caregiver can augment the information collected. Care in this setting can be complicated, though, by problems with transportation and ineffective or inefficient communication among multiple providers, particularly for patients with multiple specialists.

Over the last several years, home care has reemerged as an effective means of providing health care for older adults. As with the outpatient setting, Medicare Part B will reimburse providers in part for services rendered in the home. In addition, if a rehabilitative or skilled service is needed (i.e., home nursing care or home physical therapy) Medicare Part A provides coverage. Patients receiving services in the home must be "homebound," implying that they are significantly functionally impaired and travel with assistance out of the home infrequently and usually only for medical purposes. Services rendered in the home include a full range of evaluations by teams of health care professionals depending on needs. Social workers often lead these visits and perform case management, assessing financial and other resource needs. Nurses, clinical nurse specialists, and/or nurse practitioners provide skilled services when necessary, including health education, symptom monitoring, or wound care. Physical and occupational therapy can assess mobility and home safety and greatly enhance function and independence. Furthermore, examination of a person's home environment can reveal much about his or her safety and nutrition and can facilitate education or intervention in these areas. Physicians may serve as medical directors of such programs but may also perform visits themselves to learn more about a given patient's health status. If significant concerns exist about a patient's safety, particularly in the setting of cognitive impairment, a home visit may provide information about the need for more urgent interventions, including referrals to Adult Protective Services. Research has demonstrated that coordinated home care programs can improve management of chronic disease, including dementia, diabetes mellitus, and congestive heart failure, as well as to reduce rehospitalization in patients with congestive heart failure. One home care model that began pushing the traditional boundaries of home care prior to 2001 is the hospital at home (HaH) program, which provides home-based acute care for older adults with specific illnesses identified in the ED. High quality care and patient satisfaction continue to aid in the spread of this model of care throughout the United States.

Long-Term Care

The phrase *long-term care* describes the array of services available to provide care for people with disability from chronic and acute conditions. This definition includes the services offered in the outpatient and home settings described previously. Most associate the term, however, with the system of nursing facilities providing personal and medical care for disabled adults of all ages. Skilled nursing facilities provide long-term care for those with permanent disabilities from chronic illness or short rehabilitative stays after acute illness (e.g., stroke) or procedures (e.g., joint replacement). The scope of services may also include end-of-life care in conjunction with a hospice care team. Facility staff includes licensed nurses who give 24-hour supervision, with much of the personal care provided by certified nursing assistants. Each facility also has a medical director overseeing various aspects of medical care. An attending physician, who may or may not be the medical director, performs scheduled patient visits every 30 to 60 days. Most SNFs also employ advanced practice providers (physician assistants or nurse practitioners), physical, occupational, and speech therapists for rehabilitation care, dietitians, social workers, and recreational therapists. Patients with moderate or severe dementia constitute approximately 60% of patients living in skilled nursing facilities. Although Medicare Part A provides payment for rehabilitative stays of 100 days or less (with a copayment for days 21 to 100), it does not finance long-term stays. Such patients pay out of pocket, through long-term care insurance, or through Medicaid, a joint federal and state assistance program. Medicaid constitutes between 45% and 65% of all payment sources for skilled nursing facility care in the United states.

For patients with less complex care needs, assisted living facilities or domiciliary care homes provide an alternative arrangement for long-term care. Although these facilities vary dramatically in their size and structure, most provide nonskilled care for patients who need some assistance with activities of daily living. Licensed nurses may be present during some specified periods of time, and other professions may visit the facility intermittently to provide services such as physical therapy. Assisted living facilities do not have medical directors, and patients normally continue to see a primary care provider in the outpatient setting. Unlicensed staff, including nursing aides, provide most of the personal care and assistance. Medicare does not cover the cost of assisted living. Medicaid provides some reimbursement for this type of care, but the majority of residents pay out of pocket or through other assistance programs, such as Social Security. For those with adequate means, a living option has emerged that combines independent living, assisted living, and skilled care in one location. Continuing care retirement communities allow residents to live within the same community while moving through or between levels of care. They offer residents convenient central resources, such as recreational and dining facilities, transportation, and onsite health care.

Program of All-Inclusive Care for the Elderly

In the 1970s, a group providing care for older Chinese adults in San Francisco developed a model of long-term care centered in the community. Proponents of this model, entitled the Program of All-inclusive Care for the Elderly (PACE), believed that the community (rather than the institution) provided a better location to meet the chronic care needs of older adults. From its start as a community-based effort in California, the PACE model has grown with the support of private foundations and Medicare demonstration projects; now PACE is a benefit for older adults who qualify for both Medicare and Medicaid. Reimbursement is at 95% of the cost of nursing home care in the area where the patient lives. Participants must be over 55 and certified by the state to be eligible for nursing home care. The PACE program then uses combined Medicare and Medicaid funds otherwise slated to pay for the individual's long-term care to provide care in the community. Much of it is coordinated through senior centers offering an array of resources and services, including the following:

- Adult day care, offering nursing; physical, occupational, and recreational therapies; meals; nutritional counseling; social work; transportation; and personal care
- Medical care provided by a PACE physician familiar with the history, needs, and preferences of each participant
- Home health care and personal care
- All necessary prescription drugs
- Social services
- Medical specialists such as audiology, dentistry, optometry, podiatry, and speech therapy
- Respite care

When necessary, PACE participants are admitted to the hospital or nursing home. These services are provided under the auspices of the PACE program as part of the care package, and the program bears full financial risk. The benefits of care for older adults, particularly those of limited means, appear to be substantial.

See the National PACE Association website at www.npaonline.org for more information.

Geriatric Care

In caring for frail older adults with complex care needs, consultation with a geriatrician or geriatrics-focused interprofessional team can often provide highly useful information. The team can assist in the assessment and management of the specific conditions or situations described earlier. The geriatrician can advise on appropriate level or setting of care for an older adult as difficult decisions related to treatment options in the context of limited life expectancy occur. Geriatricians complete a minimum of 1 year of fellowship after residency training in internal medicine or family practice. After training they are eligible for board certification and qualified to work in a number of different settings, including the hospital, long-term care, home care, and outpatient clinics. Comprehensive assessment by a geriatrician or geriatrics team includes components detailed previously, including evaluation of the patient's medical condition, function, and social support. Normally the consultant will work with an interprofessional team that may include a nurse case manager, physician assistant and/or nurse practitioner, social worker, physical or occupation therapist, pharmacist, psychologist, and others. The outcome of the geriatric assessment is a comprehensive plan for safely restoring the patient to optimal function with mutually agreeable and realistic goals of care.

In the setting of acute illness, geriatricians also provide important services. As described earlier, ACE units can improve patient care and prevent iatrogenic complications. Similarly, once patients are medically stable, transfer to a specialized geriatrics care unit, often termed a geriatric evaluation and management unit, may be possible in some

institutions, to provide a comprehensive medical assessment and plan for transition of care. Early consultation with a geriatrician and an interprofessional, transdisciplinary team in the acute care setting can help in the management of complex medical illness and with communication with patients and caregivers about post-hospitalization options. After hospitalization, locating facilities or services that offer comprehensive care by a geriatrician and interdisciplinary team is ideal, including a coordinated approach that uses specific strategies to manage transitions of care.

For a deeper discussion on this topic, please see Section IV, "Aging ❖ and Geriatric Medicine," in *Goldman-Cecil Medicine*, 26th Edition.

FUTURE DIRECTIONS: GEROSCIENCE, AN EMERGING FIELD

Frameworks of aging theory described previously provide a foundation for the emerging field of geroscience. The nine "hallmarks of aging" (see Fig. 126.4) introduced previously are considered a theoretical framework through which to study interventions that have the potential to influence the biology of aging and delay the emergence of most chronic diseases that appear to be driven by this mechanism. Through study of molecular mechanisms of aging, evidence is increasing to suggest ways humans can influence *healthspan*, which can be thought of as an overall delay of onset of chronic disease. Caloric restriction (CR), or the purposeful reduction of food intake, is the only intervention that has been shown to reproducibly extend maximal lifespan in certain laboratory animal models. In rats, lifespan increases an average of 20 months with a 40% reduction in calories. Rhesus monkeys enrolled in a trial of caloric restriction appear to have improvements in metabolic markers and a lower disease burden than controls after 15 years but have had no definitive extension in lifespan. The mechanism is not well understood but may be metabolically mediated. In observational studies in humans, those with lower average body temperature, lower insulin levels, and higher dehydroepiandrosterone sulfate (DHEAS) levels (all changes found in calorically restricted monkeys) appeared to survive longer. Current research is focused on similarly influencing the cellular biology of healthspan in human subjects and discovering chemical agents that mimic or mediate these metabolic effects.

Emergence of Geroscience Guided Therapies

Potential molecular targets that allow for the delayed onset of human disease are well described in animal models of cardiovascular, pulmonary, and musculoskeletal systems. Animal studies have shown delayed onset of aging with inhibition of mTOR pathway in multiple species. In recent years, translational clinical trials in humans evaluating geroscience guided therapies (GGTs) have begun to occur. The trials demonstrate promise toward impacting the trajectory of certain chronic diseases. The first human trial using senolytic therapy to ablate senescent cells showed potential for improvement in physical function in people with idiopathic pulmonary fibrosis. The emergence of translational geroscience as a multidisciplinary field has the potential to influence medical practice and outcomes in the coming years.

SUGGESTED READINGS

Boyd C, Smith CD, Masoudi FA, et al: Decision making for older adults with multiple chronic conditions: executive summary for the American geriatrics Society guiding principles on the care of older adults with Multimorbidity, J Am Geriatr Soc 67:665–673, 2019.

Campisi J: Aging, cellular senescence, and cancer, Annu Rev Physiol 75:685–705, 2013.

Cesari M, Gambassi G, Abellan van Kan G, Vellas B: The frailty phenotype and the frailty index: different instruments for different purposes, Age Ageing 43:10–12, 2014.

Fries JF: Aging, natural death, and the compression of morbidity, N Engl J Med 303:130–135, 1980.

Goode PS, Burgio KL, Richter HE, et al: Incontinence in older women, J Am Med Assoc 303:2172–2181, 2010.

Gooneratne NS, Vitiello MV: Sleep in older adults: normative changes, sleep disorders, and treatment options, Clin Geriatr Med 30(3):591–627, 2014.

Khan SS, Singer BD, Vaughan DE: Molecular and physiological manifestations and measurement of aging in humans, Aging Cell 16(4):624–633, 2017.

Kim CS, Flanders SA: In the clinic: transitions of care, Ann Intern Med 158: ITC3-1, 2013.

Kirkland JL, Tchkonia T, Zhu Y, Niedernhofer LJ, Robbins PD: The clinical potential of senolytic drugs, J Am Geriatr Soc 65:2297–2301, 2017.

Li RM, Iadarola AC, Maisano CC, editors: Why population aging matters: a GlobaPerspective. A booklet prepared in follow-up to the 2007 Summit on global aging hosted by the U.S. State Department and the national Institute on aging, National Institute on Aging and the National Institutes of Health, March 2007.

López-Otín C, Blasco MA, Partridge L, Serrano M, Kroemer G: The hallmarks of aging, Cell 153(6):1194–1217, 2013.

Marcantonio ER: In the clinic. Delirium, Ann Intern Med 154, 2011:ITC6-1, 2011.

Mosqueda L, Dong X: Elder abuse and self-neglect: "I don't care anything about going to the doctor, to be honest…," J Med Assoc 306:532–540, 2011.

Reuben DB: Medical care for the final years of life: "When you're 83, it's not going to be 20 Years," J Am Med Assoc 302:2686–2694, 2009.

Reuben DB, Wieland DL, Rubenstein LZ: Functional status assessment of older persons: concepts and implications, Facts Res Gerontol 7:232, 1993.

Salzman B, Beldowski K, de la Paz A: Cancer screening in older adults, Am Fam Physician 96:659–667, 2016.

Steinman MA, Hanlon JT: Managing medications in clinically complex elders: "There's got to be a happy medium," J Am Med Assoc 304:1592–1601, 2010.

The 2019 American Geriatrics Society Beers Criteria® Update Expert Panel. American Geriatrics Society 2019 Updated AGS Beers Criteria® for Potentially Inappropriate Medication Use in Older Adults, J Am Geriatr Soc 67(4):674–694, 2019.

Tinetti M, Huang A, Molnar F: The geriatrics 5M's: a new way of communicating what we do, J Am Geriatr Soc 65(9):2115, 2017.

Wald HL, Ramaswamy R, Perskin MH, Roberts L, Bogaisky M, Suen W: The case for mobility assessment in hospitalized older adults: American geriatrics Society white paper executive summary, J Am Geriatr Soc 67:11–16, 2019.

Yourman LC, Lee SJ, Schonberg MA, Widera EW, Smith AK: Prognostic indices for older adults: a systematic review, J Am Med Assoc 307(2):182–192, 2012.

Palliative Care

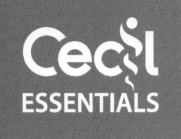

127

Palliative Care

Brandon J. Wilcoxson, Erin M. Denney-Koelsch, Robert G. Holloway

INTRODUCTION

Palliative care is both a philosophy of care and an area of specialization within several medical fields. The primary goal of palliative care is to minimize suffering and to support the best possible quality of life for patients and their families. Patients with serious and debilitating illness need and deserve excellent symptom control, assistance with difficult medical decisions, effective communication and collaboration among their providers, addressing of psychosocial problems, and an empathetic presence that fosters hope and healing relationships. Palliative care affirms life by supporting the patients' goals for the future in light of a full understanding of their medical condition, potentially including their hopes for cure, life-prolongation, relief from suffering, as well as preparation for death when time is short. This process includes exploring which life goals would be left undone if treatment does not go as hoped, who should make medical decisions for the patient if decision-making capacity is lost, and what limits might be set on aggressive therapy.

Palliative care provides an organized, structured system for delivering care by an interdisciplinary team, including physicians, nurses, social workers, chaplains, and counselors, as well as other health care professionals. Palliative care should be integrated within various health care settings including the hospital, emergency department, nursing home, home care, assisted living facilities, and outpatient settings. Palliative care remains very unevenly available, so many patients and families needlessly suffer, having either no, limited, or delayed access to appropriate palliative care. There is no evidence to suggest that early integration of palliative care shortens survival, yet many patients and health care professionals share an unspoken concern that it may hasten death. This common misconception, along with the misconception that palliative care is equivalent to end-of-life care, denies patients and families access to palliative care until late in the illness trajectory. Several prospective randomized controlled trials have compared early integration of specialty palliative care with standard care. These trials, primarily conducted in patients with advanced cancer, have shown improvements in important end points, including patient quality of life, rates of depression or anxiety, patient or caregiver satisfaction, and utilization of health services at the end of life. Two trials have also reported longer survival when palliative care is proactively integrated earlier than routine referral. Fig. 127.1 shows a visual concept of early integration of palliative care into a patient's disease course.

Basic palliative care should be part of the tool kit for all physicians who care for seriously ill patients. Specialty palliative care should be available for the more challenging symptom management, as well as the complex medical decision making that occurs in serious illness.

COMMON ILLNESS TRAJECTORIES AND PALLIATIVE CARE

There are four distinct trajectories of functional decline before dying (E-Fig. 127.1). These trajectories have major implications for palliative care and health care delivery. Patients and families will also have different physical, psychological, social, and spiritual needs depending on the trajectory of their illness before they die. Being aware of these trajectories can help providers deliver appropriate care that integrates both disease-directed and palliative treatments.

Trajectory 1: Short Period of Evident Decline Before Death

Cancer typifies this trajectory. Function is preserved until rather late, followed by a predictable and precipitous decline over weeks to months. The onset of decline usually suggests metastatic tumor. A more predictable decline in function can assist in anticipating care needs, transitioning away from curative treatments toward a more exclusive emphasis on palliation, and eventually into hospice care. Not all malignancies follow this trajectory (e.g., prostate, breast) and some nonmalignant conditions (e.g., rapidly progressive dementias, amyotrophic lateral sclerosis) may follow this course.

Trajectory 2: Chronic Illness With Exacerbations and Sudden Dying

Congestive heart failure (CHF), chronic obstructive pulmonary disease (COPD), end-stage liver disease, and AIDS typify this trajectory. These organ system diseases represent chronic illnesses with occasional, acute exacerbations (e.g., physiologic stress that overwhelms the body's reserves), often requiring hospital admission. Patients can have a return of function after an exacerbation, but often not to the level of their baseline. They also may die suddenly during an exacerbation, but it is difficult to predict in advance. Prognosticating is very challenging in this trajectory. When patients choose to forego or stop aggressive life support, planning for aggressive symptom relief during a future exacerbation is essential.

Trajectory 3: Prolonged Dwindling

Dementia and frailty typify this trajectory. These patients have a prolonged course of physical and/or cognitive decline and become increasingly frail. Additional diagnoses include other neurodegenerative conditions (e.g., Parkinson's disease) and patients with multiple moderate to severe comorbidities (e.g., arthritis, visual impairment, past mild strokes, diabetes with neuropathy). Gradual decline in function, weight loss, fatigue, and low levels of activity are core features. Caregiver burden is usually immense. Prognosticating survival is

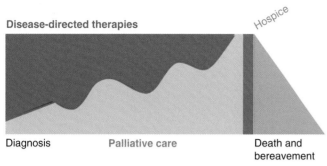

Disease-directed therapies

Hospice

Diagnosis   Palliative care   Death and bereavement

Fig. 127.1 Palliative care and hospice.

difficult and complications, such as pneumonia and fractures, may be terminal events. The benefits and burdens of artificial nutrition and hydration must be balanced in the late stages.

Trajectory 4: Severe Acute Brain Injury

Sudden impairment trajectories are those that stem from sudden neurologic injury that can lead to profound cognitive and functional impairment. These include the causes of severe acute brain injury: stroke, hypoxic ischemic encephalopathy, and traumatic brain injury. The vast majority of deaths occur either early after the event, when treatments are withheld or withdrawn, or in the chronic stage in survivors who have accumulating debility. The diagnoses in this trajectory represent the leading cause of adult disability. At the extremes of impairment are chronic disorders of consciousness (vegetative and minimally conscious states) and locked-in syndrome. But there is a vast spectrum of severe impairments short of these extremes that raise questions about how to manage potentially severe debility with little or uncertain chances of improvement. This trajectory requires a health care system responsive to negotiating goals of treatment with patients and surrogates who may consider these future health states to be "worse than death."

INTRODUCING PALLIATIVE CARE TO PATIENTS AND FAMILIES

Patients with serious, potentially life-threatening illnesses and their families are very vulnerable and initially may be frightened about the prospect of receiving palliative care. This fear develops from the association of palliative care with end-of-life care and some have even used the term "supportive care" to avoid this negative association. Such concerns, however, can be addressed by reinforcing that palliative care is intended to augment the usual treatment plan and that the integration of palliative care is designed to meet several objectives: (1) to ensure that pain and symptom control, psychosocial distress, spiritual issues, and practical needs are addressed throughout the continuum of care; (2) to make certain that patients and families obtain the information they need in an ongoing and comprehensible manner to understand their prognosis and treatment options. This process incorporates their values and preferences, and is sensitive to changes in the patient's condition over time; (3) palliative care seeks to provide seamless care coordination across settings with high-quality communication among providers; and (4) for those patients who are not going to recover, palliative care prepares patients and families, to the extent possible, for the dying process and for death, including options for hospice care, opportunities for personal growth and bereavement support.

SUFFERING AND SYMPTOM MANAGEMENT

Palliative care aims to relieve suffering, which is defined as severe distress related to events that threaten the stability of personhood or

interconnectedness of the physical, psychological, spiritual, and social aspects of self. Beginning with simple, open-ended screening questions, such as *In what ways are you suffering most?* and following with more domain-related screening questions (e.g., physical, psychological, spiritual, social) may allow for more probing and multidimensional inquiries to better understand the various sources of and contributions to an individual's suffering.

One of the first steps in the care of any seriously ill patient is to control pain and other forms of physical suffering. There are striking similarities between the burden of symptoms experienced in patients dying of cancer and noncancer conditions. Although the profile of symptoms may differ, each disease carries with it troubling symptoms that can potentially be addressed and managed.

Physical Symptoms
Pain

Uncontrolled pain dominates all other experiences, and most pain can be relieved using basic pain management strategies. This includes a detailed history and physical examination, categorizing the likely type or types (i.e., somatic, visceral, neuropathic) and severity (rated on a 0-10 scale) of pain, knowledge about proper opioid dosing strategies, and judicious use of consultations and invasive interventions (e.g., nerve blocks, epidural analgesia). The overarching three-tiered approach is to use nonopioids (e.g., acetaminophen, nonsteroidal antiinflammatory drugs) for mild pain, weak opioids (e.g., hydrocodone or codeine) for mild-to-moderate pain, and strong opioids (e.g., morphine, hydromorphone, fentanyl, methadone) for moderate to severe pain.

Developing an opioid regimen. Most seriously ill patients with chronic moderate to severe pain should be initially started on around-the-clock dosing using a short-acting opioid. Table 127.1 shows the equianalgesic dosing, usual starting doses, half-lives, and durations for the commonly available opioid agents. Once the total daily dosing has been determined (sum of all scheduled and as-needed doses), the patient may be switched to a long-acting opioid to cover the baseline requirements. As-needed opioids for breakthrough pain should be approximately 10% of the total daily dose every 1 to 2 hours orally or every 30 to 60 minutes subcutaneously or intravenously. If a patient is requiring more than four to six breakthrough doses per day, he/she should be in contact with the prescribing clinician for reevaluation of dosing. Continuous intravenous or subcutaneous infusions of opioids may be needed for rapid control of severe pain.

There are additional opioid selection recommendations for patients with renal insufficiency (avoid morphine and codeine; use hydromorphone and oxycodone with caution; methadone and fentanyl are optimal) and hepatic insufficiency (cautiously use fentanyl, hydromorphone, oxycodone, or methadone; avoid or decrease dose of morphine). Methadone is useful in palliative care because of its excellent oral bioavailability, lack of active metabolites in renal impairment, low cost, flexible route of administration (PO, IV, SC), and possible effect on both neuropathic and somatic pain. However, it does have a dose-dependent, progressively long half-life and arrhythmogenic potential; therefore, an ECG should be considered prior to starting.

Opioid adverse effects. Adverse effects with opioids exist and can be serious. Constipation occurs with all opioids, and it should be anticipated and treated by starting the patient on an appropriate bowel regimen. In refractory cases, one may consider use of methylnaltrexone, if all other methods have been exhausted.

Respiratory depression with opioid use is rare, as long as the opioid is dosed appropriately and proportionately to the severity of symptoms. Therefore, respiratory diseases, such as congestive heart failure, chronic obstructive pulmonary disease, and lung cancer should not

TABLE 127.1 Equianalgesics for Adults

Pain	Medication	EQUIANALGESIC DOSE (FOR CHRONIC DOSING)		USUAL STARTING DOSES ADULT >50 KG; FOR OPIOID NAÏVE PATIENTS (◆ ½ DOSE FOR ELDERLY, OR SEVERE RENAL OR LIVER DISEASE)				Relative Generic Cost
		IM/IV Onset 15–30 min	PO Onset 30–60 min	Parenteral	PO	Half-Life	Duration	
Moderate to severe	Morphine	10 mg	30 mg	2.5–5 mg IV/SC q3–4h (◆ 1.25–2.5 mg)	5–15 mg q3–4h (IR or oral solution) (◆ 2.5–7.5 mg)	1.5–2 h (includes active metabolites)	3–7 h	$ (IR tablet) $$ (solution) $$ (ER generic) $$$$ (ER brand)
	Oxycodone	Not available	20 mg	Not available	5–10 mg q3–4h (◆ 2.5 mg)	3–4 h	4–6 h	$$ (comb. w/APAP) $$ (IR tablet) $$ (solution) $$$ (ER brand)
	Hydromorphone	1.5 mg	7.5 mg	0.2–0.6 mg IV/SC q2–3h (◆ 0.2 mg)	1–2 mg q3–4h (◆ 0.5–1 mg)	2–3 h	4–5 h	$ (tablet) $$$ (solution) $$$$ (ER tablet)
	Methadone	Oral:IV 2:1	24 h oral morphine dose	1.25–2.5 mg q8h (◆ 1.25 mg)	2.5–5 mg q8h (◆ 1.25–2.5 mg)	15–190 h (N.B. large variation)	6–12 h	$ (tablet) $ (solution)
			Oral morphine:methadone ratio					
			<30 mg ... 2:1					
			31–99 mg ... 4:1					
			100–299 mg ... 8:1					
			300–499 mg ... 12:1					
			500–999 mg ... 15:1					
			1000–1200 mg ... 20:1					
			>1200 mg ... Consider consult					
	Fentanyl (Duragesic Patch)	100 µg (single dose) (T1/2 life and duration of parenteral doses variable)	24 h oral morphine dose ... Initial patch dose	25–50 µg IV q1–3h (◆ 12.5–25 µg)	12.5 µg/hr q72h (transdermal) (◆ Not recommended for opioid naïve)	7 h (lozenge) 12–22 h (buccal) 13–22 h (transdermal)	60+ min (lozenge) 120+ min (buccal; not well studied) 48–72 h (transdermal)	$$$ (transdermal) $$$$ (buccal) $$$$ (buccal)
			30–59 mg ... 12.5 µg/hr					
			60–134 mg ... 25 µg/hr					
			135–224 mg ... 50 µg/hr					
			225–314 mg ... 75 µg/hr					
			315–404 mg ... 100 µg/hr					
Mild to moderate	Codeine	130 mg (IM only)	200 mg	15–30 mg IM/SC q4h (◆ 7.5–15 mg) IV contraindicated	30–60 mg q3–4h (◆ 15–30 mg)	3 h	4–6 h	$$ (combination with APAP)
	Hydrocodone	Not available	30 mg	Not available	5 mg q3–4h (◆ 2.5 mg)	3 h	4–6 h	$$$ (tablet) $$ (comb. with ibuprofen) $ (combination with APAP)

exclude opioid use in these patients. In fact, opioids can provide these patients with the additional benefit of relieving dyspnea. Furthermore, respiratory depression is almost always preceded by sedation. Therefore, if sedation develops, decreasing the dose of the opioid usually prevents respiratory depression.

Other predictable but less common side effects include nausea, myoclonus, urinary retention, pruritus, and delirium. Some of these side effects are time-limited with initiation and can be managed by dose reduction or opioid rotation.

If patients have had severe adverse effects from opioids in the past, the particular opioid associated with the adverse effects should be avoided, and other opioids should be used with caution (start with a very low dose). To avoid precipitating adverse effects in elderly and debilitated patients, recommended starting doses should be reduced by approximately 50%. Naloxone should be rarely used unless a clear overdose is suspected or if life-threatening complications occur.

Opioid crisis and abuse. The United States is currently facing a public health crisis related to opioid abuse/misuse. According to the National Institute on Drug Abuse, in 2017, more than 47,000 Americans died as a result of an opioid overdose, including prescription opioids, heroin, and illicitly manufactured fentanyl, a powerful synthetic opioid. That same year, an estimated 1.7 million people in the United States suffered from substance use disorders related to prescription opioid pain relievers, and 652,000 suffered from a heroin use disorder. Given this escalating problem, risk factors for potential opioid abuse or misuse should be screened for, including any lifetime personal or family history of substance abuse, as well as certain psychosocial characteristics (e.g., history of psychiatric illness or poor socioeconomic status) before initiating an opioid regimen. When patients with such risk factors develop painful, potentially life-limiting medical conditions, they deserve adequate pain treatment, but with extreme caution because of the risk of reactivating or aggravating abuse behavior. If risk factors are present, special precautions should be taken to minimize the risk of abuse, including clearly defined and adhered to prescribing contracts. These contracts outline an agreement with the patient, ensuring face-to-face encounters for all renewals, placing limits on opioid dosing (max daily amount) and requiring that dose adjustments can only be made after direct conversation with the prescriber. One single prescriber should be responsible for all opioid prescriptions and renewals, and one pharmacy should be used. If clinicians are inexperienced with such prescribing or there is difficulty with contract compliance, formal consultation with specialists in palliative care and/or addiction medicine should be considered.

Evidence abounds that pain is under-treated in many medical settings, including those patients who are severely and even terminally ill (especially women, the elderly, the cognitively impaired, and those from underrepresented groups). Some under-treatment stems from fears about addiction as well as concerns about the possibility of hastening death. When patients with prior addiction problems are excluded, the incidence of new addictive behavior when opioids are used to treat pain in those with a well-defined, serious illness is rare. Similarly, there are very little data to suggest that properly prescribed opioids hasten death. In fact, current evidence supports the idea that opioids may prolong life in these patients and enhance quality of life in those with advanced illness and major pain or dyspnea.

Adjuvant analgesia. Adjuvant analgesia includes both pharmacologic and nonpharmacologic therapies that may be effective in treating pain. The World Health Organization recommends that adjuvant medications be considered in all cases of pain management. Adjuvants should be tried before opioids in cases of chronic, nonmalignant pain. For malignant, moderate to severe pain, combination therapy with an opioid and an adjuvant has been shown to

achieve better pain relief with less toxicity than continued escalation of the opioid alone. Adjuvants should be targeted to the particular type of pain (somatic, neuropathic, and visceral). For somatic pain, NSAIDS, acetaminophen, bisphosphonates, and corticosteroids have proven effective. For neuropathic pain, antidepressants (tricyclic and selective serotonin and norepinephrine reuptake inhibitors), anticonvulsants, and even topical analgesics (e.g., lidocaine patch) have provided relief. For visceral pain, anticholinergics have been used effectively. For a list of examples of commonly prescribed adjuvants, along with usual starting doses, please refer to Table 2.3 in Quill et al. *Primer of Palliative Care,* 7th edition. Prescribers who are unfamiliar with the use of these medications for pain management are encouraged to consult further with specialists in palliative care or pain management.

Other Symptoms

There are numerous non-pain physical symptoms that can dominate and overwhelm the clinical picture in any given patient. These include dyspnea, nausea and vomiting, constipation, anorexia-cachexia, fatigue, bleeding, agitation, apathy, myoclonus, pruritus, and specific functional deficits. Each symptom requires a structured approach to the history and physical examination with a full exploration of the potential etiologies and treatment options informed by the prognosis and preferences of the patient and family. A few of these are discussed in more detail here, but for practical information geared toward basic management of symptoms in palliative care refer to Quill et al., *Primer of Palliative Care,* 7th ed.

Dyspnea. Dyspnea is defined by the American Thoracic society as "a subjective experience of breathing discomfort." It is a common symptom at the end of life, experienced by patients suffering from diseases such as cancer, COPD, CHF, and pulmonary fibrosis. Dyspnea is very distressing, and when severe, requires urgent intervention.

The first step in management is identification of the underlying cause/disease, followed by treatment directed towards the particular etiology. After the underlying etiology is addressed, if dyspnea remains a prominent symptom, there are several general measures which can be done. These include reducing the need for exertion, repositioning the patient to a more upright position, keeping the compromised lung down in unilateral disease and improving air circulation by opening windows/doors or using a bedside fan.

Opioids are the preferred agents for symptomatically treating dyspnea because they effectively suppress awareness of the sensation of shortness of breath. Most routes of administration are effective except the use of nebulized opioids. There is emerging evidence that low-dose, sustained-release morphine may provide lasting relief of dyspnea, mainly in COPD patients. Some providers avoid the use of opioids for dyspnea out of fear of causing respiratory depression. However, in the absence of preexisting carbon dioxide (CO_2) retention, respiratory depression is uncommon in patients who are on carefully titrated dosages of opioids.

Anxiety and dyspnea frequently exacerbate one another. It is important to treat an anxious dyspneic patient with opioids first to reduce breathlessness and then follow with a benzodiazepine if anxiety persists.

Nausea and vomiting. Nausea and vomiting are some of the most distressing symptoms for patients. Studies have shown that these symptoms are experienced by up to 78% of patients with advanced cancer at some point during their disease course. They also occur in other advanced illnesses, including end-stage cardiac, renal, and liver disease. Persistent nausea and vomiting can affect appetite, pain management, and the quality of interactions with family members or friends.

When evaluating patients with nausea and vomiting, it is important to first consider whether the symptoms are a result of intra-abdominal factors (e.g., gastroparesis, ileus, gastric outlet obstruction, bowel obstruction) or extra-abdominal factors (drugs, electrolyte abnormalities, central nervous system metastases). The goal is to identify and treat underlying reversible causes first.

In most cases, empiric pharmacologic treatment is necessary to immediately control symptoms. There are a number of pharmacologic agents that have been shown to be useful for nausea/vomiting, depending on the etiology. One of the most useful is haloperidol. When nausea and vomiting are due to increased intracranial pressure, a steroid such as dexamethasone is useful. Metoclopramide may be useful in situations of delayed gastric emptying or early satiety. When nausea and vomiting are due to inner-ear pathology or motion sickness, antihistamines can help manage vertigo.

In addition, high dosages of a combination of agents may be required for adequate control of symptoms. Treating patients with a scheduled dose of antiemetics can often prevent recurrent nausea. If the patient is too nauseated to tolerate oral medications, consider SC, IV, or PR routes.

Constipation. Palliative care patients are at particularly high risk for developing constipation due to a combination of factors, including decreased PO intake, impaired mobility and use of opioid analgesics.

Pharmacologic options for management of constipation include stool softeners (docusate sodium), stimulants (Senokot and bisacodyl), and osmotic agents (polyethylene glycol, lactulose, magnesium hydroxide, magnesium citrate). The key to adequate management of constipation in the palliative care setting is prevention, which involves initiation of a maintenance bowel regimen. If the patient has a history of constipation, the preferred maintenance regimen should be the patient's regular home regimen. If constipation has never been a problem in the past, starting with senna can be a good option. Docusate may also be used initially; however, the efficacy of docusate alone is limited, and most patients will require addition of a bowel stimulant, like senna or bisacodyl. Osmotic agents, such as polyethylene glycol or lactulose, are effective additions to most bowel regimens but may also bring about adverse effects such as bloating and flatulence. Rectal suppositories and enemas may be necessary when constipation is severe. Avoid bulk-forming agents (psyllium, methylcellulose) in palliative care patients, as these agents can lead to impactions with inadequate fluid intake.

All of the above medications may be used in combination when managing constipation. However, maximizing the dose/frequency of current bowel medications will typically provide desired effects and should be done prior to addition of other medications.

Medical Marijuana

Cannabis has several beneficial health effects although clinical data are limited because of restrictions on research.

The body contains an endogenous network known as the endocannabinoid system, which involves two receptors, CB1 and CB2. As endocannabinoids interact with these receptors, they impact many physiologic processes, including gastrointestinal (GI) function, appetite, metabolism, pain, memory, movement, immunity, and inflammation. Cannabis contains phytocannabinoids, Δ-tetrahydrocannabinol (THC) and cannabidiol (CBD), which interact with these receptors much the same way that endocannabinoids do, thereby providing the various medicinal effects that are observed with cannabis use.

THC is the primary psychoactive constituent of cannabis. Observed effects include impairments of learning, memory, spatial orientation, and attention. However, patients also report benefits including antiemetic, analgesic, and anti-inflammatory properties. CBD lacks the THC-induced intoxicating properties, and the presence of CBD in a cannabis product is actually believed to counteract the psychosis-inducing effects of THC. CBD has reported benefits of anticonvulsant, anxiolytic, anti-inflammatory, and neuroprotective properties; however, none of these have been verified. Synthetic cannabinoids currently marketed are dronabinol, a biochemically identical form of THC, and nabilone, a THC analogue. Both can be prescribed clinically for nausea and/or vomiting, appetite stimulation, pain, and spasticity.

The National Academies of Sciences, Engineering, and Medicine (NASEM) published a comprehensive literature review on the health effects of cannabis and concluded that there is substantial evidence that cannabis is effective (1) for the treatment of chronic pain, (2) as an antiemetic in chemotherapy-induced nausea and vomiting, and (3) for muscle spasticity syndromes in MS. As far as adverse effects, the NASEM concluded that there is substantial evidence for an association between cannabis smoking and respiratory disease, motor vehicle collisions (MVCs), lower birthweight offspring, and schizophrenia or other psychoses.

Medicolegal realities surrounding medical cannabis are rapidly evolving in the United States. As of publication of this book, 33 US states and the District of Columbia have programs authorizing cannabis use for specific medical conditions. Because cannabis is illegal under federal law, clinicians cannot prescribe it and pharmacies cannot dispense it as they would with other pharmaceuticals. States require health care professionals to be registered in order to certify patients for cannabis use. Cannabis is then supplied to patients through state-licensed medical cannabis dispensaries, in various forms, including vaporized oils or plant material, sublingual tinctures, and oral capsules.

Psychological Distress

Depression, anxiety, and delirium are all common in the palliative care setting. They are frequently under-recognized and under-treated, although appropriate diagnosis and treatment can have significant improvement in a patient's quality of life.

Depression and Anxiety

Almost all patients in palliative care and their families experience normal sadness/grief as illness advances. Depression, however, is more enduring, persistent, intense, and may be associated with hopelessness, helplessness, worthlessness, and guilt. Two questions, found to have high sensitivity for depression screening, include: "*Are you depressed?*" and "*Do you have much interest and pleasure in doing things?*" A more formal exploration is indicated if the patient gives a positive answer to either of these questions. One should be cautious about overusing somatic symptoms to diagnose depression (e.g., fatigue, anorexia, sleep disturbance) because they frequently overlap with physiological changes associated with advanced disease. Terminally ill patients with depression are at higher risk of suicide and suicidal ideation, and they may have increased desires and requests for hastened death.

Anxiety symptoms may be triggered by a range of medical transitions, such as the initial diagnosis of serious illness, a recurrence of illness, treatment side effects/failure, or discussion of hospice. The patient may also have underlying fears related to their disease and end-of-life, including uncontrolled pain, isolation, abandonment, loss of control, worry about family members or even the idea of death/dying.

Regarding treatment of depression and anxiety, first recognize and address contributions from physical symptoms (e.g., uncontrolled pain), medical causes (e.g., hypothyroidism, hyperthyroidism), and medications. Effective pharmacologic and nonpharmacologic treatments exist for both depression and anxiety, though treatment selection depends on symptom intensity, patient prognosis, and treatment benefits and burdens. Other members of the interdisciplinary team (social worker, chaplain, and psychologist) often play a critical role in assessment and ongoing management.

Delirium

Delirium, an acquired and fluctuating disorder of consciousness and cognition, occurs commonly in the palliative care setting. The level of psychomotor activity can vary from hyperactive ("agitated" delirium) to hypoactive ("quiet" delirium). Nearly 80% of the delirium in the palliative care setting is the hypoactive variant. As a result, it is often under-diagnosed or misdiagnosed as depression and fatigue. The most common causes of delirium in palliative care include medications (e.g., opioids), metabolic disorders due to progressive organ failure, and infection. Meticulous attention to the history from collateral sources (e.g., nurses, caregiver) and a detailed medication history are essential for an accurate diagnosis. While delirium may reverse if an obvious cause is identified and removed, frequently it represents an important marker of progressive illness; therefore, cognitive improvements may be transient and incomplete. In addition to etiology-specific treatment (e.g., change or stop medications, treat infection, oxygen, hydration, bisphosphonates), environmental interventions are recommended for all patients (e.g., quiet reassurance, gentle reorientation, optimize sensory input, minimize night disruptions). Pharmacologic management should be used sparingly and cautiously and may include antipsychotic medications, benzodiazepines, and psychostimulants (for the hypoactive variant). Keep in mind that benzodiazepines can sometimes have a paradoxical effect, worsening confusion and agitation in delirium.

Spiritual and Existential Suffering

Spiritual and existential distress is prevalent in patients and families with serious illness, especially at the end of life. Spirituality is about one's relationship with and responses to transcendent questions that confront one as a human being (e.g., search for meaning and purpose in life). Religion is a set of texts, practices, and beliefs about the transcendence shared by a community. Spirituality is broader than religion. The spiritual issues of seriously ill and dying patients often center on questions of meaning, value, and relationships. Dying patients want to be assured of their value in the face of actual or perceived threats to their intactness as a human being (e.g., physical and cognitive declines, altered appearances). Spirituality can help people find hope in despair and can help restore purpose.

One of the goals of palliative care is to relieve spiritual and existential distress. Patients and families often welcome such discussions. Examples of open-ended questions to facilitate this dialogue include: "*Are you at peace with all of this?*" and "*Is faith (religion, spirituality) important to you?*" Acknowledgement and empathetic listening are the most important responses for most clinicians, as opposed to trying to provide "correct answers."

Other strategies for fostering hope and meaning include developing caring relationships, setting attainable goals, involving the patient in the decision-making process, affirming the patient's worth, using lighthearted humor (when appropriate), and reminiscing with life review. It is important, however, to know one's professional boundaries and refer to chaplains or clergy from the patient's faith traditions if questions move beyond the realm of general exploration (e.g., "*It sounds like it would be good to explore this with someone with more experience than I have. Would it be okay for me to send our chaplain in to discuss this with you?*").

COMMUNICATION AND CARE COORDINATION

Excellent communication skills are central to palliative care, including communication with patients, family members, other physicians, nurses, and other members of the health care team. The overarching aim is to assist the patient and family in establishing the goals of current and future treatment in a shared decision-making process.

Negotiating Goals of Care

When negotiating goals of treatment in palliative care, the focus is often to assist with the following decisions: to help decide types and aggressiveness of disease-directed therapies; to ensure optimum palliation of symptoms; to assist in hospice determinations; to discuss initiating, withholding or withdrawing therapies; to facilitate advance care planning; and to initiate surrogate decision making if the patient lacks capacity. These discussions occur at various time points in the course of advancing illness when new and important information is learned and needs to be communicated to the patient and family. The need to renegotiate goals should also be anticipated when triggers of advancing disease suggest limited life expectancy or excessive suffering. These discussions are almost always variants of "bad news" discussions.

The overall approach to communication and negotiating goals of care is standard among all patients, illnesses, and situations (Table 127.2). This includes running an effective family meeting, with or without the patient present. Initial elements include establishing the proper setting, identifying key stakeholders, and "doing your homework" (i.e., discussing potential plans with all relevant subspecialties who may have communicated with the patient and family). When the meeting begins, find out what the patient and family understand about the medical condition and ask what additional information they want to know. Keep an open mind and try to hold back on a fixed agenda (e.g., to "get the DNR" or to "stop futile care"). This allows patients and family members sufficient time to "tell their stories" and provides the context within which effective decision making can occur. In general, the more patients and families speak in the early parts of such meetings, the better.

The provider then needs to share prognostic information and discuss the benefits and burdens of the available treatment options. Alerting the patient or family of impending bad news with a warning shot (e.g., "*I am afraid I have some difficult news to share with you*") is a useful initial communication strategy. The amount of information should be paced with frequent pauses to allow time for emotional responses. Comprehension should be frequently checked, and questions should be encouraged using an "ask-tell-ask" strategy. The skilled clinician can flexibly assess, probe, and pace the content and depth of the discussion in an emotionally responsive (acknowledge, explore, empathize, and legitimize) and culturally competent manner. This includes the ability to understand and respect diverse religious practices and differing preferences about degree of truth telling. When appropriate, the clinician should make recommendations based on scientific knowledge as well as awareness of a patient's values and preferences and be prepared to help resolve conflicts among the patient, family members, and providers. Finally, providers need to develop strategies to preserve and potentially reframe hope, including ways to "*hope for the best*" and simultaneously "*prepare for the worst.*" Commitments to minimize suffering and to not abandon the patient and family are essential. At the end of the discussions, the provider should summarize key aspects of what was reviewed and establish a follow-up plan for future communications and treatments.

Estimating and Communicating Prognosis

A core component of information shared in the palliative care setting is prognosis. Understanding prognosis is central to making decisions (e.g., treatment, comfort measures, hospice). Prognosis is a prediction of possible future outcomes of a disease (e.g., survival, symptoms, function, quality of life, family and financial impact) with or without treatment. Most patients and families want to know prognosis. Since

TABLE 127.2 General Strategy for Communicating and Negotiating Goals of Care in Common Palliative Care Settings

Step 1	Prepare and establish setting
	Do not have a rigid preset agenda
Step 2	Ask patient and family what they know and understand
	Provide sufficient time for patients and families to "tell their story"
	Active listening skills
Step 3	Find out how much patient and family want to know
	Acknowledge and explore emotions
Step 4	Give information in small amounts, and frequently check understanding
	Discuss prognosis and benefits and burdens of treatment options
	Be mindful of overly optimistic and pessimistic predictions
	Be prepared to make recommendations
Step 5	Respond to emotions and empathetic response
	Convey honesty and reframe hope
	Use "I wish" statements
Step 6	Summarize, establish and implement plan, follow-up
	Possible time-limited trial

there are some patients and families that may not want to know prognosis or may want it communicated in a particular way, it is essential to begin by finding out what the patient and family knows and wants to know.

Inaccurate predictions may lead to poor decision making. Physicians tend to overestimate survival in patients with advanced cancer by about 30%, and the bias is more pronounced the longer the physician-patient relationship. Overly optimistic predictions can lead to overuse of ineffective or unwanted disease-directed treatment, delay in hospice referrals, false expectations, unnecessary tests and procedures, and poor symptom control. Therefore, accurately estimating and communicating prognosis is central to optimal decision making in advanced illness and at the end of life.

In advanced illnesses, common factors found to be predictive of short-term survival (i.e., less than 6 months) include performance status, anorexia-cachexia syndrome, delirium, and dyspnea. The Palliative Performance Scale can be used to measure and track a patient's functional status. It is available in a variety of websites and books. In addition to a physician's subjective predictions of survival, there exist models to assist with prognostic estimates, including generic models for particular populations (e.g., hospice enrollees) as well as disease-specific models (e.g., cancers, heart failure, liver disease, stroke, AIDS, spinal cord compression). Hospice eligibility criteria also differ for specific diseases. While not uniformly reliable, these criteria can be useful in formulating estimates where prognosis might be 6 months or less if the disease is allowed to run its natural course (a prognostic criterion). One example of this is the Functional Assessment Staging (FAST) scale used to determine hospice eligibility for Alzheimer's/dementia patients.

For an individual patient, however, prognostic uncertainty remains the rule. Therefore, it is important to integrate both evidence and experience-based medicine and present the information in formats tailored to the particular patient (verbal descriptions, numeric, frequencies, or graphics). Prognostic estimates should be bounded with ranges to convey realistic uncertainty, being sure to allow for exceptions in both directions. For example, "*in my experience, patients with your condition live on average a few weeks to a few months. It could be longer, but*

it could also be shorter." For survival-oriented prognoses (e.g., "*How long do I have?*"), be mindful of overly optimistic prognoses, remembering to think of and convey the lower bound (e.g., "*some may live longer, but others may, unfortunately, live shorter*"). For quality of life-oriented prognoses (e.g., "*What will life be like?*"), be mindful of overly pessimistic predictions, remembering the power of adaptation and engendering hope by helping patients and families find new meaning.

END-OF-LIFE CARE

The Role of Diagnostic Tests and Invasive Procedures

Several questions should be considered in determining the appropriateness of aggressive medical or palliative interventions near the end of life: What is the goal or expected outcome of the proposed intervention? What is the probable efficacy of the intervention? What is the patient's baseline level of function and life expectancy? What are the potential side effects and burdens of the intervention? What are the patient's and family's wishes, values, and preferences?

The range of medical and palliative options available is huge, so the challenge is to determine what makes sense to enhance the well-being of each patient at their particular stage of illness. Palliative interventions range from pure symptom management and support to invasive options, such as chemotherapy, radiotherapy, surgical/endoscopic interventions, stenting procedures, thoracentesis, paracentesis, pericardiocentesis, home inotropic therapy, noninvasive ventilation, antibiotics, or transfusions. The challenge is to individualize discussions, so that patients can take full advantage of treatments that will help them meet their goals without having their experience dominated by near futile invasive treatments.

Role of Hospice

Hospice care is a specialized form of palliative care aimed at those patients and families in the terminal stages of illness. The National Hospice and Palliative Care Organization defines hospice as follows: *Considered to be the model for quality, compassionate care for people facing a life-limiting illness or injury, hospice and palliative care involve a team-oriented approach to expert medical care, pain management, and emotional and spiritual support expressly tailored to the person's needs and wishes. Support is provided to the person's loved ones as well. The focus of hospice relies on the belief that each of us has the right to die pain free and with dignity, and that our loved ones will receive the necessary support to allow us to do so.*

Since the establishment of the Medicare Hospice Benefit in 1982, use of hospice for end-of-life care has grown steadily. In 2015, more than 1.6 million patients were served by hospice programs in the United States. Cancer used to be the most common diagnosis for patients dying in hospice programs. However, in 2017, Alzheimer's disease was reported as the top principal diagnosis for hospice patients. COPD, heart failure and cancer were listed among the top five. In 2015, the median length of stay for patients in hospice was 23 days.

In most cases, hospice care is provided in the person's home. Hospice care can also be provided in freestanding hospice centers, hospitals, and nursing homes or other long-term care facilities. In order to qualify for the Medicare Hospice Benefit, two physicians must sign a statement certifying that the patient's prognosis for survival, if the disease runs its natural course, is likely to be 6 months or less. Hospice criteria exist to assist in making these determinations for common medical conditions (see section, Estimating and Communicating Prognosis). The Medicare Hospice Benefit covers most costs related to terminal care without a deductible, which includes palliative medications, nursing oversight, supplies, and bereavement care. Hospice also covers up to 2 to 4 hours of custodial caregiver services per day;

however, family and/or friends must provide the remaining care if the patient is to stay at home. Hospice can supplement care in a skilled nursing facility, but patients themselves or their insurance would be responsible for the nursing home room and board charges. The hospice benefit includes bereavement care for the family after the patient's death.

Discussing hospice with patients and families can be challenging. First, some may view the transition to hospice as a way of "giving up" or "giving in to death." It is often initially viewed as a "bad news" discussion given that patients and families need to confront the fact that disease-directed treatment is no longer effective and that prognosis is likely to be 6 months or less. Second, given the reimbursement restrictions, patients may also need to forgo particular types of treatment that are important to them (e.g., acute hospital or ICU-level care, dialysis, chemotherapy, milrinone for heart failure).

Last Hours and Days of Living

An integral aspect of palliative care is preparing and guiding the patient and caregivers through the dying process. When prognosis is measured in hours to days there are typical signs and symptoms that usually occur. Patients become weak and fatigued and gradually lose mobility. There is also a gradual and predictable decrease in food and fluid intake. Most patients do not experience hunger and thirst, and the associated mouth dryness that occurs is easily palliated with small sips or sponges of cold water. Caregivers will frequently ask about intravenous hydration. In rare instances, intravenous or subcutaneous fluids may temporarily improve mental status and energy in the final days of life. Most of the time, however, the benefits are difficult to discern and the excessive fluids may contribute to end-of-life physiologic conditions (edema, ascites, effusions, and pulmonary secretions) that do not improve longevity and may worsen comfort.

As patients become weaker, there is a predictable decrease in the level of consciousness with increasing periods of somnolence, eventually giving way to a comatose state. Education about this process should include associated changes in respiratory patterns, including prolonging periods of apnea, interspersed with episodes of hyperpnea and deep breathing (Cheyne-Stokes respirations). During this process caregivers often feel they are on a "roller-coaster ride," and gentle guidance on what to expect can allay concerns. As consciousness wanes, swallowing slows and the cough reflex weakens. As a result, saliva pools in the oropharynx and can result in noisy respiration ("death rattle"), which can usually be palliated to some degree with scopolamine (transdermal), glycopyrrolate (PO, IV, SC) or hyoscyamine (PO disintegrating tablets or sublingual solution). Families should be reminded that these symptoms are a natural part of the dying process and that persistent shortness of breath is relatively uncommon but can be treated with opiates and benzodiazepines, if needed.

As death approaches, reduced perfusion causes cooling and cyanosis of the extremities, as well as a reduced volume and darkening of the urine. Most deaths are relatively peaceful, but a few can be preceded by periods of intense agitation and restlessness (hyperactive terminal delirium). Antipsychotic medications and conventional doses of benzodiazepines can usually treat terminal delirium. Prior to and when death occurs, families should be encouraged to carry out cultural or religious rituals that are important to them. Providers should express condolences, be available for questions and responsive to intense emotional reactions that sometimes occur. A short condolence card or letter is almost always appreciated. If possible, efforts should be made to follow up with family members and caregivers deemed at risk for complicated bereavement and grief.

COMMON ETHICAL CHALLENGES IN PALLIATIVE CARE

Patient Capacity and Surrogate Decision Making

When discussing goals of care, it is essential to determine if a patient has capacity to make medical decisions. Adults are presumed to have capacity, unless determined by the court. However, many medical conditions can alter a patient's ability to make decisions for themselves (e.g., delirium, dementia, sedation). As many as 25% of adult inpatients are found to lack capacity. In order to be found to have capacity, a patient must (1) be able to comprehend the factual information about their medical condition and treatment options, (2) understand the risks and benefits of the treatment options and the consequences of that decision, (3) be able to accept or reject the proposed treatment voluntarily, and (4) provide reliable choice over time. A physician, psychiatrist, or ethics consultant may determine a patient's capacity to make a medical decision. Only a court can determine legal competence. In the event that the patient lacks capacity, a surrogate decision-maker must be consulted. This could be a health care proxy (legally designated by the patient when he/she did have capacity), a legal next-of-kin, or a court-appointed guardian. When there is question about a patient's capacity, which surrogate decision-maker is legally appropriate, or if the surrogate appears to be making decisions contrary to the patient's best interests, an ethics consultation should be obtained.

When Patients and Families Want Near Futile Treatment

The patient autonomy movement in medicine has led to patients and families taking an active role in their own medical decision making. This is generally a positive development except in two circumstances: (1) when physicians stop taking an active role using their expertise to guide patients in their decision making, thereby abdicating their professional responsibility of advocating for the best possible treatment based on the patient's medical condition and personal values, and (2) when patients or their families want and even demand near futile treatment toward the end of their lives despite physician's advice that treatment has much more burden than benefit. Physicians might try to respond to patients who want "everything" by suggesting that they want to try everything that is "more likely to help than harm," but avoid any treatment that is most likely to "do more harm than good." However, some patients and families will accept no limits on treatment no matter what the burden and the improbability of success. Of course, truly futile treatment should not be offered or provided upon request, but absolute futility has been difficult to define in many cases.

Feeding Tube Questions

Many patients gradually stop eating and drinking as a natural part of the dying process, but this can be very hard for patients and families to accept in light of fears about "starving to death" and in view of seemingly simple technologies that can potentially combat and even reverse the problem. In fact, with few exceptions, feeding tubes have not been shown to prolong life in most advanced illnesses such as metastatic cancer or advanced Alzheimer's disease. It is important to know about the exceptions (e.g., esophageal and oropharyngeal cancers, amyotrophic lateral sclerosis, acute stroke) but also to have an open discussion about the natural progression of diminished eating and drinking as many illnesses advance. If there is uncertainty about whether a particular patient might benefit from a feeding tube, and patient and family are clear about wanting to give it a try, the clinician can frame the decision as a "time-limited trial" to see how the patient tolerates tube feeding psychologically as well as physiologically in a specified timeframe. A potential framework for such a trial is that a nasogastric tube has a built-in time limit of about a month before a PEG tube needs to be inserted. Explaining to patients and families about the positive aspects (smell, taste, and enjoyment) of natural feeding of real food, even in small amounts, may help focus the decision on important quality of life issues, rather than more technical, physiological issues.

Proportionate Palliative Sedation

Proportionate palliative sedation is the use of gradually escalating levels of sedation to help relieve intractable and distressing physical symptoms at the end of a patient's life. The goal is to achieve the lowest level of sedation that adequately relieves the patient's uncontrolled suffering, not to intentionally end a patient's life or hasten a patient's death. Although unconsciousness may eventually be the outcome of proportionate palliative sedation, this is not the intended aim.

Terminally ill patients receiving proportionate palliative sedation should have do-not-resuscitate (DNR) and do-not-intubate (DNI) orders before the treatment is initiated. Patients with capacity should provide verbal or written consent prior to initiating the process because capacity usually will be compromised once it is started. If the patient lacks capacity, the decision to initiate proportionate palliative sedation would be made by the patient's surrogate decision maker.

Medications used to achieve adequate symptom control include sedatives (lorazepam, midazolam, and phenobarbital) in the form of continuous IV infusions. Careful monitoring of the patient's level of sedation/agitation is very important in order to determine need for additional bolus doses or titration of infusion rate. A formal palliative care consult is strongly recommended to help guide this process.

Examples of conditions when proportionate palliative sedation might be initiated include agitated terminal delirium, unrelenting nausea and vomiting, intractable pain, and unrelenting dyspnea in actively dying patients who do not respond to the usual palliative treatments.

Request for Hastened Death

The prevalence of suicidal ideation and suicide attempts is higher in patients with advanced life-limiting illness compared to those without serious disease. In Oregon, where physician-assisted suicide is legally permitted (subject to safeguards), the prevalence of a patient wanting to explore a health care professional's willingness to help hasten death is about 1/50, whereas only about 1/500 die using physician-assisted suicide. The motivation behind such initial explorations may relate to relentless physical suffering, disfigurement, hopelessness, loss of dignity, fear of being a burden, or a "cry for help." Most enduring requests from patients with progressive medical illnesses, however, arise not from inadequate symptom control, but from a patient's belief about dignity, meaning, and control over the circumstances of death. Although some providers might be uncomfortable exploring such requests, before responding, a systematic approach should be used to evaluate and understand the root causes of these requests. A careful evaluation includes a precise clarification and exploration as to exactly what the patient is asking and why. Is the request based on transient thoughts about ending life (common) or a serious appeal for assistance (relatively rare)? Does the request occur in the context of intense physical suffering, psychological despair, an existential crisis, or a combination of factors? Does the patient have full decision-making capacity? Is the request proportionate to the level of suffering? Evaluating such requests can be emotionally fatiguing and conflicting, and clinicians need self-awareness in distinguishing their emotions from the patient's, including tending to one's own support by sharing the burden of such requests with trusted colleagues.

Responding to such a request should first include evaluation for potentially reversible contributions to suffering. This will often include treating physical and psychological symptoms, aggressive attempts to foster hope, consulting psychiatrists or spiritual counselors, and creative brainstorming with trusted colleagues and team members. Some requests for hastened death persist, despite optimal palliative care. In such circumstances, the clinician should seek out a second opinion and confront the possibilities. These possibilities include withdrawal of life-sustaining interventions, palliative sedation, voluntary cessation of oral intake, and assisted suicide. As of publication, it is legal in nine jurisdictions: California, Colorado, District of Columbia, Hawaii, Montana, Maine [starting January 1, 2020], New Jersey, Oregon, Vermont, and Washington. While it is important to support the patient, the clinician must balance integrity and non-abandonment. This may include drawing specific boundaries of what the clinician can and cannot do, while still searching in earnest for a mutually acceptable solution.

PROSPECTUS FOR THE FUTURE

Palliative care became an officially recognized subspecialty within the United States in 2006. Physicians from 10 specialties can be board certified in hospice and palliative medicine, following completion of a fellowship. These specialties include: family medicine, internal medicine, emergency medicine, pediatrics, physical medicine and rehabilitation, anesthesiology, psychiatry, neurology, radiology, and surgery. As patients live longer with chronic illness, there will be an increasing need to fully integrate palliative care providers and programs within hospitals, nursing homes, and the outpatient setting; and to ensure that all primary care providers and non-palliative specialists develop the skill sets needed to provide basic palliative care. There is a compelling need for continued education and research to improve the overall palliative approach to care for everyone and to better define the optimal timing, setting, and delivery of palliative care to improve the quality of life and lessen the suffering of patients and families with advanced illness.

SUGGESTED READINGS

Ben Amar M: Cannabinoids in medicine: a review of their therapeutic potential, J Ethnopharmacol (Review) 105(1-2):1–25, 2006.

Buss MK, Rock LK, McCarthy EP: Understanding palliative care and hospice: a review for primary care providers, Mayo Clin Proc 92(2):280–286, 2017.

Ebbert JO, Scharf EL, Hurt RT: Medical Cannabis, Mayo Clinic Proc 93(12):1842–1847, 2018.

Ferrell B, Twaddle M, Melnick A, Meier DE: National consensus project clinical practice guidelines for quality palliative care guidelines, 4th edition, J Palliat Med 21(12):1684–1689, 2018.

Goldstein NE, Morrison RS, editors: Evidence-Based Practice of Palliative Medicine, Philadelphia, 2013, Elsevier.

Harris PS, Stalam T, Ache KA, et al: Can hospices predict which patients will die within six months? J Palliat Med 17:894–898, 2014.

Moryl N, Coyle N, Foley KM: Managing an acute pain crisis in a patient with advanced cancer: "This is as much of a crisis as a code", JAMA 299:1457–1467, 2008.

Mouhamed Y, Vishnyakov A, Qorri B, et al: Therapeutic potential of medicinal marijuana: an educational primer for health care professionals, Drug Healthc Patient Saf 10:45–66, 2018.

National Institute on Drug Abuse, National Institute of Health: Opioid Overdose Crisis, 2019, Retrieved from https://www.drugabuse.gov/drugs-abuse/opioids/opioid-overdose-crisis.

Quill TE, Abernethy AP: Generalist plus specialist palliative care–creating a more sustainable model, N Engl J Med 368:1173–1175, 2013.

Quill TE, Periyakoil V, Denney-Koelsch E, et al: Primer of palliative care, ed 7, Illinois, 2019, American Academy of Hospice and Palliative Medicine.

Temel JS, Greer JA, El-Jawahri A, et al: Effects of early integrated palliative care in patients with lung and GI cancer: a randomized clinical trial, J Clin Oncol 35(8):834–841, 2017.

Trecki J. A perspective regarding the current state of the opioid epidemic. JAMA Netw Open. Published online January 18, 20192(1):e187104.

Alcohol and Substance Use

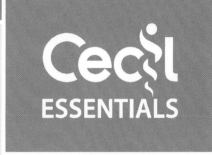
Alcohol and Substance Use

Richard A. Lange, Joaquin E. Cigarroa

ALCOHOL USE

Alcohol use is a major public health problem worldwide, accounting for 3 million deaths (5.3% of all deaths) annually. One in six US adults binge drinks (i.e., a pattern of drinking that brings a person's blood alcohol concentration to 0.08 g percent [80 mg/dL] or above, which typically happens when men consume five or more drinks or women consume four or more drinks in about 2 hours) about four times a month, consuming about seven drinks per binge. Alcohol use is the third leading preventable cause of death in the United States (exceeded only by cigarette smoking and hypertension) and claims over 88,000 lives annually, or 9.8% of all US deaths. Alcohol use accounts for 28% of all traffic-related deaths in the United States, or approximately 10,500 vehicular deaths annually, and is a major contributor to risky sexual behavior, domestic violence, homicide, and suicide. In 2010, the estimated alcohol-related costs in the United States were $249 billion, 77% of which was attributable to binge drinking. These costs resulted from losses in workplace productivity, health care expenditures, criminal justice costs, and other expenses.

DEFINITION AND EPIDEMIOLOGY

The American Psychiatric Association has specific criteria for the diagnosis of *alcohol use disorder*; these 11 criteria are described in the *Diagnostic and Statistical Manual of Mental Disorders*, Fifth Edition, and are listed in Table 128.1. Alcohol use disorder is further characterized as mild, moderate, or severe, based on the number of criteria the individual meets; two to three criteria indicate a mild disorder, four to five criteria a moderate disorder, and six or more a severe disorder. The so-called *binge drinker* is defined as a man who typically consumes five or more drinks or a women who consumes four or more drinks on a single occasion. Nearly 50% of alcohol use disorder risk is heritable (i.e., transmissible from parent to offspring), with the other 50% attributable to environmental factors.

In 2016, 136.7 million Americans aged 12 or older reported current use of alcohol and 65.3 million reported binge alcohol use in the past month (Fig. 128.1). This number of people who were current binge drinkers corresponds to about 1 in 4 people aged 12 or older (Fig. 128.2) and nearly half of current alcohol users. Additionally, 16.3 million reported heavy alcohol use in the past month (see Fig. 128.1), which means that 1 in 8 (12%) current alcohol users or 1 in 4 (25%) binge drinkers reported heavy alcohol use. Although the prevalence of ethanol use is highest in individuals younger than 30 years of age, survey data suggest that about two thirds of persons over age 30 consume it.

In 2016, 73% of men and 66% of women aged 18 years or older reported drinking in the past year, and 7.8% of men and 4.2% of women were diagnosed with an alcohol use disorder. Native American individuals had the highest prevalence of alcohol use disorder (9.2%), followed by non-Hispanic white (5.9%), black (5.6%), Hispanic (5.1%), Pacific Islander (3.5%), and Asian (3.0%) individuals. Alcohol use peaks in younger adults, with those aged 21 through 25 years having the highest prevalence of past-year drinking (83%) and those aged 18 through 25 years having the highest prevalence of alcohol use disorder (11%).

PHARMACOLOGIC AND METABOLIC FACTORS

After oral ingestion, alcohol is absorbed predominantly in the small intestine, and its rate of intestinal absorption is accelerated by the simultaneous ingestion of carbohydrates and carbonated beverages. Prolonged retention of alcohol in the stomach, as occurs when food is consumed before drinking, delays alcohol absorption because absorption in the stomach is considerably slower than in the duodenum. Once in the blood, alcohol equilibrates rapidly across all membranes, including the blood-brain barrier, thereby accounting for the prompt onset of its euphoric effects. Maximal blood alcohol concentrations are reached 45 to 75 minutes after alcohol is ingested.

The liver metabolizes approximately 90% of ethanol to acetaldehyde via the alcohol dehydrogenase pathway; subsequently, acetaldehyde is converted by aldehyde dehydrogenase to acetate, which enters the Krebs cycle. At low or moderate serum concentrations of ethanol, the alcohol dehydrogenase pathway functions almost exclusively in metabolizing ethanol. At high concentrations, the microsomal ethanol oxidizing system (CYP2E1) contributes to metabolism. Less than 10% of ethanol is excreted unchanged through the skin, kidneys, and lungs. Elimination of alcohol from the body is affected by obesity, food intake, previous exposure to alcohol, and variability among individuals in the efficiency of the alcohol and aldehyde dehydrogenase systems. These enzymatic variations also influence a person's risk of developing an alcohol use disorder. The mechanism is thought to involve elevated acetaldehyde levels resulting from a more rapid conversion of ethanol (in cases of alcohol dehydrogenase variants with higher enzymatic activity) or slower elimination of acetaldehyde oxidation (in cases of aldehyde dehydrogenase variants with reduced enzymatic activity). Acetaldehyde causes facial flushing, nausea, and tachycardia, which make individuals reduce their intake of alcohol.

MECHANISMS OF ALCOHOL-INDUCED ORGAN DAMAGE

The major organs that are susceptible to damage by alcohol are the liver, pancreas, heart, brain, and bone (Table 128.2). Several alcohol-related

TABLE 128.1   Criteria for the Diagnosis of Alcohol Use Disorder

Two or More of the Following in the Previous 12 Months

1. Recurrent alcohol use resulting in a **failure to fulfill major** obligations at work, school, or home
2. Recurrent alcohol use in situations in which it is physically **hazardous**
3. Continued alcohol use despite having persistent or **recurrent social or interpersonal problems** caused or exacerbated by the effects of alcohol
4. **Tolerance**, as defined by:
   - need for markedly increased amounts of alcohol to achieve intoxication or desired effect; and/or
   - markedly diminished effect with continued use of the same amount of alcohol
5. **Withdrawal**, as manifested by:
   - characteristic alcohol withdrawal syndrome; and/or
   - alcohol is taken to relieve or avoid withdrawal symptoms
6. Alcohol is often taken in **larger amounts** or over a longer period than was intended
7. Persistent desire or **unsuccessful efforts to diminish** or to control alcohol use
8. A great deal of **time** is spent in activities necessary to obtain, use, or recover from the effects of alcohol
9. Important social, occupational, or recreational **activities are relinquished or reduced** because of alcohol use
10. Alcohol use is **continued despite knowledge** of having a persistent or recurrent physical or psychological problem that is likely to have been caused or exacerbated by alcohol use
11. **Craving** or a strong desire or urge to use a specific type of alcohol

Modified from the American Psychiatric Association: Diagnostic and statistical manual of mental disorders, ed 5, Washington, D.C., 2013, American Psychiatric Press.

medical disorders are caused by various nutritional deficiencies; ethanol is deficient in proteins, minerals, and vitamins. Therefore, the initial management of the alcoholic patient must attend to suggested dietary deficiencies (e.g., thiamine) and electrolyte deficiencies, including potassium, magnesium, calcium, and zinc.

Alcohol-related liver disease is the leading preventable cause of hepatic failure in the industrialized world. Genetic factors are thought to play a role in susceptibility to this disorder, since alcoholic liver disease is more prevalent in white individuals than in other ethnic groups (despite a similar magnitude of ethanol consumption). The histopathologic features of alcoholic liver disease include fatty infiltration, hepatitis, fibrosis, and end-stage cirrhosis.

CLINICAL PRESENTATION

Acute Alcohol Intoxication

Mild ethanol intoxication produces slurred speech, ataxia, irregular eye movements, and poor coordination. Signs of central nervous system (CNS) depression and associated cerebellar or vestibular dysfunction include dysarthria, ataxia, and nystagmus. Although blood alcohol concentrations are not precisely correlated with the degree of intoxication and the clinical effect of ethanol widely varies among individuals, stupor and coma usually develop at blood concentrations approaching 400 mg/dL. Blood levels of 500 mg/dL often are fatal; however, it is important to understand that death may occur even when the blood alcohol concentration is as low as 300 mg/dL.

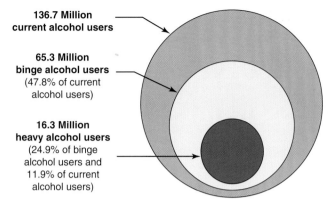

Fig. 128.1 Current, binge, and heavy alcohol use among persons aged 12 years or older according to the National Survey on Drug Use and Health (2016). Binge drinking is defined as males consuming five or more drinks on an occasion and for females consuming four or more drinks on an occasion. Heavy alcohol use is defined as binge drinking on 5 or more days in the past 30 days. (Substance Abuse and Mental Health Services Administration. [2017]. Key substance use and mental health indicators in the United States: Results from the 2016 National Survey on Drug Use and Health [HHS Publication No. SMA 17-5044, NSDUH Series H-52]. Rockville, MD: Center for Behavioral Health Statistics and Quality, Substance Abuse and Mental Health Services Administration.)

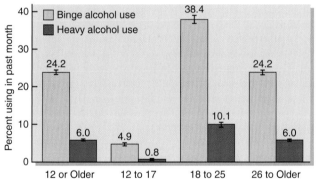

Fig. 128.2 Past month binge and heavy alcohol use among persons aged 12 years or older, by age group, according to the National Survey on Drug Use and Health (2016). Binge drinking is defined as males consuming five or more drinks on an occasion and for females consuming four or more drinks on an occasion. Heavy alcohol use is defined as having had five or more drinks on the same occasion on each of 5 or more days in the previous 30 days. (Substance Abuse and Mental Health Services Administration. [2017]. Key substance use and mental health indicators in the United States: Results from the 2016 National Survey on Drug Use and Health [HHS Publication No. SMA 17-5044, NSDUH Series H-52]. Rockville, MD: Center for Behavioral Health Statistics and Quality, Substance Abuse and Mental Health Services Administration. Retrieved from https://www.samhsa.gov/data.)

Withdrawal Syndrome (Convulsions)

Alcohol withdrawal occurs in three stages. The signs of minor withdrawal usually appear 6 to 12 hours after the discontinuation of ethanol and are caused by central adrenergic hyperexcitability; they consist of anxiety, tremors, sweating, tachycardia, diarrhea, and insomnia. Additional evidence of autonomic nervous system hyperactivity often appears within 12 to 24 hours and includes increased startle response, nightmares, and visual hallucinations. Alcohol withdrawal seizures (so-called *rum fits*) are generalized clonic-tonic convulsions that occur

TABLE 128.2   Medical Complications of Alcohol Use

Neurologic
Encephalopathy (Wernicke, with oculomotor dysfunction; gait ataxia)
Marchiafava-Bignami disease (demyelination of corpus callosum)
Central pontine myelinosis
Cognitive dysfunction
Amnesia (i.e., Korsakoff syndrome)
Dementia
Cerebellar degeneration
Peripheral neuropathy
Seizures

Hematologic
Anemia (often with macrocytosis)
Leukopenia
Thrombocytopenia

Gastrointestinal
Esophagitis
Esophageal varices
Gastritis
Gastrointestinal bleeding
Pancreatitis
Hepatitis
Cirrhosis
Splenomegaly

Cardiovascular
Hypertension
Cardiomyopathy
Stroke
Arrhythmias (especially atrial fibrillation)

Electrolyte or Nutritional
Thiamine deficiency
Niacin deficiency
Folate deficiency
Vitamin B_{12} deficiency
Vitamin D deficiency
Zinc deficiency
Hypokalemia
Hypomagnesaemia
Hypocalcaemia
Ketoacidosis
Hypoglycemia
Hypertriglyceridemia
Malnutrition

Endocrine
Diabetes mellitus
Gynecomastia

Musculoskeletal
Myopathy
Osteoporosis
Testicular atrophy
Amenorrhea
Infertility

Miscellaneous
Spontaneous abortion
Fetal alcohol syndrome
Increased risk of cancer (breast, oropharyngeal, esophageal, hepatocellular, colorectal)
Accidents, trauma, violence, suicide

TABLE 128.3   CAGE: An Alcoholism Screening Test

1. Have you ever felt you should *cut down* on your drinking?
2. Have people *annoyed* you by criticizing your drinking?
3. Have you felt *guilty* about your drinking?
4. Have you ever had a drink first thing in the morning to steady your nerves or to get rid of a hangover (i.e., as an *eye-opener*)?

12 to 48 hours after the discontinuation of ethanol and are estimated to occur in 2% to 5% of alcoholics.

Delirium Tremens

Delirium tremens (DTs) is characterized by delirium (a confused state with varying levels of consciousness), hallucinations, disorientation, agitation, tremor (caused by marked autonomic nervous system over activity), tachycardia, hypertension, fever, and diaphoresis. It occurs in approximately 5% of alcoholics who discontinue or decrease their alcohol use, most often in chronic heavy users with underlying neurologic damage. If unrecognized and untreated, the in-hospital mortality rate of DTs approaches 25%; with early recognition and treatment the mortality is only 1% to 4%.

TREATMENT

Intervention strategies in alcohol users are designed to modify the individual's attitudes, knowledge, and skills to prevent alcohol misuse. In the outpatient setting, increased frequency of contact between the primary care physician and the patient increases the likelihood of

detection, intervention, and prevention of heavy alcohol consumption. All scheduled office visits should include alcohol screening, assessment, and brief attempts at intervention (one or more discussions lasting 10 to 15 minutes), if indicated, as studies show that this approach decreases alcohol intake and its consequences. Behavioral or pharmacologic treatment should be considered because two thirds of treated patients have a reduction in the amount of consumption (by more than 50%) as well as the consequences of consumption (e.g., alcohol-related injury or job loss). A year after treatment, one third of patients are either abstinent or drink moderately without consequences.

Screening and Intervention Strategies

The National Institute on Alcohol Abuse and Alcoholism (NIAAA) provides several web-based guidelines for alcohol screening during the routine health examination (www.niaaa.nih.gov). A four-step plan exists with which physicians can (1) screen patients for alcohol use, (2) assess for the presence of alcohol-related problems, (3) provide advice concerning appropriate action, and (4) monitor the patient's progress. For the current drinker, the physician should inquire about the number of drinks consumed per day, number of days per week on which ethanol is consumed, and total number of drinks consumed per month. Alcohol consumption that exceeds 14 drinks per week or three drinks per day should trigger an in-depth assessment of alcohol-related problems. The physician should ascertain if the individual is at risk for alcohol-related problems, has an existing problem, or may be alcohol-dependent. Difficulties with work-related, interpersonal, or family relationships and/or evidence of high-risk behavior despite self-reported low-risk consumption indicate that the individual is at risk for alcohol use disorder.

The CAGE questionnaire (each of the letters in the acronym refers to one of the questions) (Table 128.3) is a useful screening tool for identifying *alcohol-dependent individuals*. A positive response to two or more of the four questions is indicative of a potential alcohol problem and should prompt questions regarding the quantity and frequency of consumption.

The 2013 US Preventive Services Task Force (USPSTF) recommendation identified one-item screeners such as the Single Item Alcohol Screening Questionnaire (SASQ) and the Alcohol Use Disorders Identification Test (AUDIT) as having the best accuracy to screen for any level of *unhealthy alcohol use* among adults. The SASQ asks, "How many times in the past year have you had 5 [for men]/4 [for women] or more drinks in a day?", where one or more occasions in the previous year constitutes a positive screen. AUDIT (Table 128.4) is the most widely validated instrument for use in primary care settings. Utilizing 10 items and taking 2 to 3 minutes to complete, it is better suited to settings where visit times are longer or when it can be completed and scored before a clinician visit. Evidence supports the use of brief (1-item) instruments as initial screeners, where high sensitivity and lower specificity would be desirable, followed by a longer instrument, such as AUDIT, with greater specificity.

TABLE 128.4   Alcohol Use Disorders Identification Test (AUDIT)

Questions	No. Items/Time to Administer	Scoring Notes

1. How often do you have a drink containing alcohol?
  0. Never
  1. Monthly or less
  2. Two to four times a month
  3. Two so three times a week
  4. Four or more times a week
2. How many drinks containing alcohol do you have on a typical day when you are drinking?
  0. 1 or 2
  1. 3 or 4
  2. 5 or 6
  3. 7 to 9
  4. 10 or more
3. How often do you have six[a] or more drinks on one occasion?
  0. Never
  1. Less than monthly
  2. Monthly
  3. Weekly
  4. Daily or almost daily
4. How often during the last year have you found that you were not able to stop drinking once you had started? *(same options as #3)*
5. How often during the last year have you failed to do what was normally expected from you because of drinking? *(same options as #3)*
6. How often during the last year have you needed a first drink in the morning to get yourself going after a heavy drinking session? *(same options as #3)*
7. How often during the last year have you had a feeling of guilt or remorse after drinking? *(same options as #3)*
8. How often during the last year have you been unable to remember what happened the night before because you have been drinking? *(same options as #3)*
9. Have you or someone else been injured as a result of your drinking?
  0. No
  1. Yes, but not in the last year
  2. Yes, during the last year
10. Has a relative or friend or a doctor or other health worker been concerned about your drinking or suggested you cut down? *(same options as #9)*
	10 items
	2–5 min
		Scoring: ≥8 considered a positive screen for hazardous or harmful drinking.
		In general:
		Scores between 8 and 15 are most appropriate for simple advice focused on the reduction of hazardous drinking
		Scores between 16 and 19 suggest brief counseling and continued monitoring
		Scores of 20 and above clearly warrant further diagnostic evaluation for alcohol dependence

[a]The US version asks about five or more drinks, reflecting standard drink sizes in the United States.

On physical examination, evidence of alcoholic liver disease may be exhibited as jaundice, hepatomegaly, palmar erythema, male gynecomastia, spider angiomata, and ascites. The serum γ-glutamyltransferase concentration typically is elevated in individuals who drink excessively.

Low-Risk Drinking

A standard drink contains 12 g of alcohol, an amount similar to that found in one 12-oz bottle of beer or wine cooler, one 5-oz glass of wine, or 1.5 oz. of distilled (e.g., 80 proof) spirits. In men older than age 64 years and in women older than 21 years, the limit for moderate drinking is one drink per day. For younger men, moderate drinking is defined as no more than two drinks per day. For the same amount of ingested ethanol, women and older adult men achieve a higher blood concentration of ethanol than younger men owing to their smaller volume of body water. A reasonable blood alcohol level should not exceed 50 mg/dL.

A blood-alcohol level as low as 80 mg/dL may exceed the legal definition for driving under the influence (DUI) or driving while intoxicated (DWI). In national surveys, the strategy of the *designated driver*

appears to be effective at preventing unsafe driving by drinkers at risk for DWI. Complete abstinence is recommended for people with a history of alcohol use disorder, other serious medical conditions (e.g., liver disease), and pregnancy.

Nonpharmacologic Therapies

Psychosocial interventions efficacious in treating heavy alcohol use or alcohol use disorder include brief interventions, motivational enhancement therapy, cognitive-behavioral therapy, behavioral approaches, family therapies, and 12-step programs (the recovering alcoholic moves through 12 specific steps aided by his or her attendance at regular meetings within a self-help peer group). Although these therapies provide similar efficacy, brief interventions—which are commonly 15 to 20 minutes long—are most practical in outpatient medical settings. When more intensive psychosocial therapy is needed, it may be most feasible for a therapist trained in the specific method to provide it in concert with a medical practitioner who can prescribe an alcohol treatment medication.

Considerations for Drug Interventions

Three medications are approved by the US Food and Drug Administration (FDA) to treat alcohol use disorders: disulfiram, naltrexone (oral and long-acting injectable formulations), and acamprosate. Medications are prescribed to less than 9% of patients who are likely to benefit from them, despite their inclusion in clinical practice guidelines as first-line treatments for moderate to severe alcohol use disorder. Medications should be administered in conjunction with psychosocial interventions to enhance treatment adherence.

Disulfiram (Antabuse) inhibits aldehyde dehydrogenase (i.e., the enzyme that converts acetaldehyde to acetate), resulting in a 5- to 10-fold increase in serum acetaldehyde concentrations when alcohol is consumed. This produces uncomfortable symptoms (e.g., facial flushing, tachycardia, nausea, vomiting, and headache), which act to deter alcohol consumption. Because of low medication compliance and limited efficacy, disulfiram is rarely prescribed.

Naltrexone is an opioid receptor antagonist. In clinical trials, a combination of naltrexone and psychosocial intervention reduced the number of drinking days, induced a longer period of abstinence from ethanol, and decreased the relapse rate in heavy drinkers when compared with psychosocial intervention alone: it reduced the likelihood of a return to any drinking by 5% and binge-drinking risk by 10%. Naltrexone is administered orally in a dose of 50 mg daily for 12 weeks, although larger doses (i.e., 100 to 150 mg daily) and a longer duration of administration may improve its success in preventing relapse. In 2006, the FDA approved a once-a-month injectable form of naltrexone (380 mg intramuscular) for the treatment of alcohol use disorders; this form appears to be more effective than the pill form at maintaining abstinence, since it eliminates the problem of medication compliance.

Naltrexone can be initiated while the individual is still drinking, thereby permitting treatment to be provided in a community-based setting without the need for enforced abstinence or detoxification. Some recovering alcoholics develop somnolence, nausea or vomiting when naltrexone is initiated. Because hepatic toxicity may occur at high doses (≥300 mg), periodic testing of liver function is recommended. Naltrexone is contraindicated in subjects receiving opioids, given that opiate withdrawal is an unintended adverse effect of the drug.

Acamprosate (Campral), a structural analog of γ-amino butyric acid (GABA), decreases excitatory glutamatergic neurotransmission during alcohol withdrawal. The recommended dosage is 666 to 1000 mg 3 times daily, and its most common side effects are diarrhea and intestinal cramping. In placebo-controlled trials, acamprosate reduced relapse rates and increased abstinence from ethanol. In comparative trials, it did not appear to be as efficacious as naltrexone. Acamprosate should be used once abstinence is achieved; since it is not metabolized by the liver, it can be given safely to individuals with alcoholic liver disease.

The use of several other pharmacologic agents has been associated with a reduction in alcohol consumption, including ondansetron (a selective serotonin reuptake inhibitor), topiramate (an anticonvulsant), baclofen (a GABA agonist), sodium oxybate (the sodium salt of gamma-hydroxybutyrate), nalmefene (an opioid antagonist), and varenicline (a nicotinic acetylcholine-receptor and dopamine partial agonist), but none of these agents has been approved by the FDA for treatment of alcohol dependence.

Fetal Alcohol Spectrum Disorders

Alcohol freely crosses the placenta and is teratogenic. It is a leading preventable cause of birth defects with mental deficiency, with up to 1 in 100 children in the United States being born with fetal alcohol spectrum disorders (FASDs). The scope of disabilities and malformations varies and depends on the amount of alcohol consumed, the frequency of exposure, the stage of fetal development when alcohol is present, maternal parity, nutrition, genetic susceptibility, and individual variation in maternal and fetal alcohol metabolism.

The term FASD is used to characterize the full range of prenatal alcohol damage, varying from mild to severe and encompassing a broad array of physical defects and cognitive, behavioral, and emotional deficits. It includes conditions such as fetal alcohol syndrome (FAS), alcohol-related neurodevelopmental disorder (ARND), and alcohol-related birth defects (ARBDs).

FAS, the most severe form of FASD, is characterized by (a) growth retardation (i.e., height or weight ≥10th percentile); (b) neurodevelopmental abnormalities (i.e., microcephaly, hyperactivity, irritability, altered motor skills, learning disabilities, seizure disorders, and mental retardation); and (c) dysmorphic facial features (i.e., short palpebral fissures, smooth philtrum, and a thin upper lip). Children with typical dysmorphic facial features who lack the other features have partial FAS. Children with ARBDs have typical facies associated with FAS as well as anomalies in other organs (i.e., cardiac, renal, skeletal, auditory) but no growth retardation or neurodevelopmental abnormalities. Children with ARND exhibit behavioral or cognitive abnormalities in the absence of dysmorphic facial features.

Although the damage from prenatal exposure to alcohol cannot be reversed, children with FASDs benefit from early diagnosis and aggressive intervention with physical, occupational, speech and language, and educational therapies. Early recognition can also benefit the impaired mother, resulting in access to alcohol treatment and a better social situation for the entire family.

Although the recognition of FASD is important, its prevention is essential. Given that no safely established level of alcohol consumption in pregnancy exists, recommendations suggest that pregnant women maintain abstinence. In addition, women who are considering pregnancy or are already pregnant must be counseled about the effects of alcohol on the fetus.

Medical Management of Alcohol Withdrawal and Delirium Tremens

Patients admitted to a general medical hospital who have a history of heavy alcohol use have an approximately 2% to 7% chance of developing severe alcohol withdrawal syndrome (SAWS). Appropriate identification, prophylaxis, and treatment of withdrawal are essential in reducing morbidity and mortality associated with this disorder. Unfortunately, individual symptoms or signs do not effectively predict or exclude SAWS. The most effective method for predicting SAWS in acute care settings is use of a risk assessment tool that combines findings from a patient's history and clinical examination. The Prediction of Alcohol Withdrawal Severity Scale (Table 128.5) performs best for predicting the development of SAWS and requires an interview, examination (heart rate), and testing (blood alcohol).

For the patient with probable alcohol withdrawal, comorbid conditions that may coexist or mimic the symptoms of withdrawal (e.g., infection, trauma, hepatic encephalopathy, drug overdose, gastrointestinal bleeding, and metabolic derangements) should be excluded. Once this has been accomplished, the patient should be placed in a quiet and protective environment and should receive parenteral thiamine and multivitamins to decrease the risk of Wernicke encephalopathy or Korsakoff amnestic syndrome.

The Revised Clinical Institute for Withdrawal Assessment for Alcohol (CIWA-Ar) scale (available at https://umem.org/files/uploads/1104212257_CIWA-Ar.pdf), a measure of withdrawal severity, is useful in guiding symptom-triggered therapy in medically stable (i.e., non-ICU or postoperative) patients. Benzodiazepines are the only medications proved to ameliorate symptoms and to decrease the risk of

TABLE 128.5   The Prediction of Alcohol Withdrawal Severity (AW) Scale

Part A: Threshold Criteria (yes or no; no point):

Have you consumed any amount of alcohol (i.e., been drinking) within the last 30 days? OR did the patient have a "+" BAL upon admission? IF the answer to either is YES, proceed with test:

Part B: Based on Patient Interview (1 point each):

1. Have you been intoxicated or drunk within the last 30 days?
2. Have you ever undergone alcohol use disorder rehabilitation treatment or treatment for alcoholism (i.e., inpatient or outpatient treatment programs or AA attendance)?
3. Have you ever experienced previous episodes of alcohol withdrawal, regardless of severity?
4. Have you ever experienced blackouts?
5. Have you ever experienced alcohol withdrawal seizures?
6. Have you ever experienced delirium tremens or DTs?
7. Have you combined alcohol with other "downers" like benzodiazepines or barbiturates during the last 90 days?
8. Have you combined alcohol with any other substance of abuse during the last 90 days?

Part C: Based on Clinical Evidence (1 point each):

1. Was the patient's BAL on presentation ≥200 mg/dL?
2. Is there evidence of increased autonomic activity (i.e., HR >120/min, tremor, sweating, agitation, nausea)?

Maximum score = 10 points.

This instrument is intended as a **SCREENING TOOL**. The greater the number of positive findings, the higher the risk for the development of AWS.

A score of **>4 suggests HIGH RISK** for moderate to severe (complicated) AWS; prophylaxis and/or treatment may be indicated.

AA, Alcoholics Anonymous; *AWS,* alcohol withdrawal syndrome; *BAL,* blood alcohol level; *DT,* delirium tremens

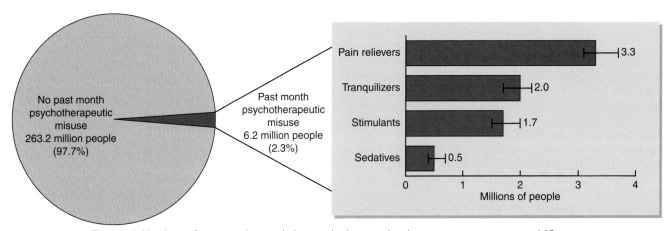

Fig. 128.3 Numbers of past month prescription psychotherapeutic misusers among persons aged 12 years or older according to the National Survey on Drug Use and Health (2016). (Substance Abuse and Mental Health Services Administration. [2017]. Key substance use and mental health indicators in the United States: Results from the 2016 National Survey on Drug Use and Health [HHS Publication No. SMA 17-5044, NSDUH Series H-52]. Rockville, MD: Center for Behavioral Health Statistics and Quality, Substance Abuse and Mental Health Services Administration. Retrieved from https://www.samhsa.gov/data.)

seizures and DTs in patients with alcohol withdrawal. Typically, diazepam (5 to 20 mg), chlordiazepoxide (50 to 100 mg), or lorazepam (1 to 4 mg) is administered intravenously every 5 to 10 minutes until symptoms subside, with the last of these medications preferred in patients with advanced cirrhosis, considering that the liver minimally metabolizes it. All benzodiazepines appear to be similarly efficacious in treating alcohol withdrawal, but long-acting agents may be more effective in preventing withdrawal seizures and are associated with fewer rebound symptoms. Conversely, short-acting agents may offer a lower risk of oversedation. For the patient who is resistant to benzodiazepines, intravenous phenobarbital (130 to 260 mg administered intravenously every 15 minutes until symptoms are controlled) may be given. If the agitation is not controlled by phenobarbital, propofol (0.3 to 1.25 mcg/kg/hr for maximum 48-hour infusion) can be tried, with intubation strongly recommended.

PRESCRIPTION DRUG ABUSE

According to the 2016 National Survey on Drug Use and Health, an estimated 6.2 million Americans aged 12 years or older used prescription-type psychotherapeutic drugs nonmedically in the past month (Fig. 128.3). This estimate represents 2.3% of the population aged 12 years or older. More people in the United States now die of prescription drug overdose (i.e., the nonmedical use of prescription-type pain relievers, tranquilizers, stimulants, and sedatives) than accidental vehicular trauma.

Sedatives and Hypnotics

Benzodiazepines and barbiturates are the major sedative-hypnotic drugs among the commonly abused agents that are listed in Table 128.6. The patient with sedative-hypnotic intoxication may have slurred speech,

TABLE 128.6 Commonly Abused Drugs

Substance: Category and Name	Examples of Commercial and Street Names	How Administered[a]	Intoxication Effects and Potential Health Consequences
Cannabinoids			Euphoria, slowed thinking and reaction time, drowsiness, inattention, confusion, impaired balance and coordination, enhanced perception, cough, frequent respiratory infections, impaired memory and learning, increased heart rate, anxiety, panic attacks, tolerance, addiction
Hashish	Boom, gangster, hash, hash oil, hemp	Smoked, swallowed	
Marijuana	Blunt, dope, ganja, grass, herb, joint, bud, Mary Jane, pot, reefer, green trees, smoke, sinsemilla, skunk, weed	Smoked, swallowed	
K2/Synthetic Marijuana	Spice, K2, fake weed, Yucatan fire, skunk, moon rocks	Smoked, swallowed	Vomiting, agitation, hallucinations, hypertension, myocardial infarction, death, withdrawal and addiction symptoms
Sedative-Hypnotics (CNS Depressants)			Reduced pain and anxiety, feeling of well-being, lowered inhibitions, labile mood, impaired judgment, poor concentration, fatigue, confusion, impaired coordination and memory, respiratory depression and arrest, addiction
Benzodiazepines (Other Than Flunitrazepam)	Ativan, Halcion, Klonopin, Librium, Pro-Som, Restoril, Serax, Tranxene, Valium, Xanax, Doral; candy, downers, sleeping pills, tranks	Swallowed	Sedation, drowsiness, dizziness
Flunitrazepam[b]	Rohypnol; forget-me pill, Mexican Valium, R2, roach, Roche, roofies, roofinol, rope, rophies, woolfies	Swallowed, snorted	Visual and gastrointestinal disturbances, urinary retention, amnesia while under drug's effects
Sleep Medications	Ambien (zolpidem), Sonata (zaleplon), Lunesta (eszopiclone)	Swallowed	Sedation, drowsiness, dizziness
Barbiturates	Amytal, Nembutal, phenobarbital, Seconal; barbs, reds, red birds, phennies, tooies, yellows, yellow jackets	Injected, swallowed	Sedation, drowsiness, depression, unusual excitement, fever, irritability, poor judgment, slurred speech, dizziness
GHB[b]	γ-hydroxybutyrate; G, Georgia home boy, grievous bodily harm, liquid ecstasy, soap, scoop, goop, liquid X, geeb, Gina	Swallowed	Drowsiness, dizziness, nausea and vomiting, headache, loss of consciousness, hallucinations, peripheral vision loss, nystagmus, loss of reflexes, seizures, coma, death
Dissociative Drugs			Increased heart rate and blood pressure, impaired function, memory motor loss, numbness, nausea and vomiting
PCP and Analogues	Phencyclidine; angel dust, boat, hog, love boat, peace pill	Injected, smoked, swallowed	Possible decrease in blood pressure and heart rate, panic, aggression, violence, suicidal ideation; loss of appetite, depression
Ketamine[a]	Ketalar SV; cat Valiums, K, Special K, vitamin K	Injected, smoked, snorted	At high doses: delirium, depression, respiratory depression and arrest, amnesia while under drug's effects
Salvia Divinorum	Salvia, shepherdess's herb, maria pastora, magic mint, sally-d	Chewed, smoked swallowed	
Dextromethorphan (DXM)	Found in some cough and cold medications: Robo, Robotripping, Triple C	Swallowed	Euphoria, slurred speech, confusion, dizziness, distorted visual perceptions
Hallucinogens			Altered states of perception and feeling, nausea, chronic mental disorders, persisting perception disorder (flashbacks)
LSD	Lysergic acid diethylamide; acid, blotter, cubes, microdot, yellow sunshines, blue heaven	Swallowed, absorbed through mouth tissues	LSD: flashbacks, hallucinogen persisting perception disorder. LSD and mescaline: increased body temperature, heart rate, blood pressure, loss of appetite, sleeplessness, numbness, weakness, tremors, impulsive behavior, rapid shift in emotion
Mescaline	Buttons, cactus, mesc, peyote	Smoked, swallowed	

Continued

TABLE 128.6   Commonly Abused Drugs—cont'd

Substance: Category and Name	Examples of Commercial and Street Names	How Administered[a]	Intoxication Effects and Potential Health Consequences
Psilocybin	Magic mushrooms, purple passion, shrooms, little smoke	Swallowed	Nervousness, paranoia, panic
Opioids and Morphine Derivatives			Pain relief, euphoria, drowsiness, respiratory depression and arrest, pinpoint pupils, nausea, confusion, constipation, sedation, unconsciousness, seizures, coma, tolerance, addiction
Codeine	Empirin with Codeine, Fiorinal with Codeine, Robitussin A-C, Tylenol with Codeine, OxyContin, Roxicodone, Vicodin; Captain Cody, Cody, schoolboy (with glutethimide: doors and fours, loads, pancakes and syrup)	Injected, swallowed	Less analgesia, sedation, and respiratory depression than morphine
Other Opioid Pain Relievers			
Oxycodone, hydrocodone bitartrate hydromorphone, oxymorphone, meperidine, propoxyphene	Tylox, OxyContin, Percodan, Percocet; Oxy, O.C., oxycotton, oxycet, hillbilly, heroin, percs	Chewed, injected, snorted, suppositories, swallowed	For oxycodone—muscle relaxation/twice as potent an analgesic as morphine; high abuse potential
	Vicodin, Lortab, Lorcet; vike, Watson-387		
	Dilaudid; juice, smack, D, footballs, dillies		
	Opana, Numorphan, Numorphone; biscuits, blue heaven, blues, Mrs. O, octagons, stop signs, O bomb		
	Demerol, meperidine hydrochloride; demmies, pain killer		
	Darvon, Darvocet		
Fentanyl	Actiq, Duragesic, Sublimaze; apache, China girl, China white, dance fever, friend, goodfella, jackpot, murder 8, TNT, Tango and Cash	Injected, smoked, snorted	80–100 times more potent an analgesic than morphine
Heroin	Diacetylmorphine; brown sugar, dope, H, horse, junk, skag, skunk, smack, white horse, China white, cheese (with OTC cold medicine and antihistamine)	Injected, smoked, snorted	Staggering gait
Morphine	Roxanol, Duramorph, M, Miss Emma, monkey, white stuff	Injected, smoked, swallowed	
Opium	Laudanum, paregoric; big O, black stuff, block, gum, hop	Smoked, swallowed	
Stimulants			Increased heart rate, blood pressure, body temperature; feelings of exhilaration, increased energy and mental alertness, tremors, rapid or irregular heart beat; reduced appetite, irritability, anxiety, panic, paranoia, violent behavior, psychosis, weight loss, insomnia, heart failure, seizures, coma
Amphetamine	Adderall, Biphetamine, Dexedrine; bennies, black beauties, crosses, hearts, LA turnaround, speed, truck drivers, uppers	Injected, smoked, snorted, swallowed	Rapid breathing, hallucinations, loss of coordination, restlessness, delirium, panic, impulsive behavior, Parkinson's disease, tolerance, addiction
Methamphetamine	Desoxyn; chalk, christina, cookies, cotton candy, crank, crystal, dunk, fire, gat, garbage, glass, go fast, go-go, ice, meth, no doze, no stop, pookie, rocket fuel, scooby snacks, speed, tina, trash, tweak, uppers, wash, white cross, yaba, yellow barn	Injected, smoked, snorted, swallowed	Memory loss, cardiac and neurologic damage, impaired memory and learning, tolerance, addiction, severe dental problems
Methylphenidate	Ritalin, Concerta; JIF, MPH, R-ball, Skippy, the smart drug, vitamin R	Injected, snorted swallowed	Increase or decrease in blood pressure, psychotic episodes, digestive problems,

TABLE 128.6   Commonly Abused Drugs—cont'd

Substance: Category and Name	Examples of Commercial and Street Names	How Administered[a]	Intoxication Effects and Potential Health Consequences
Cocaine	Cocaine hydrochloride; blow, bump, C, candy, Charlie, coke, crack, flake, rock, snow, toot	Injected, smoked, snorted	Chest pain, respiratory failure, nausea, abdominal pain, stroke, malnutrition, nasal damage from snorting
MDMA[b] (Methylenedioxymethamphetamine)	Adam, clarity, ecstasy, Eve, lover's speed, peace, uppers, Molly	Injected, snorted, swallowed	Mild hallucinogenic effects, increased tactile sensitivity, empathic feelings, chills, sweating, nystagmus, ataxia, teeth clenching, muscle cramping, impaired memory and learning, lowered inhibition
Synthetic Cathinone (Methylenedioxypyrovalerone (MDPV), Mephedrone ("Drone," "Meph," or "Meow Meow"), and Methylone)	Bath salts, drone, meph, meow meow, ivory wave, bloom, cloud nine, lunar wave, vanilla sky, white lightning, scarface	Injected, smoked, swallowed	Chest pain, paranoia, hallucinations, panic attacks, excited delirium, rhabdomyolysis, renal failure, high abuse and addiction potential
Other Compounds			
Inhalants	Solvents (paint thinners, gasoline), glues, gases (butane, propane, aerosol propellants, nitrous oxide), nitrites (isoamyl, isobutyl, cyclohexyl); laughing gas, poppers, snappers, whippets	Inhaled through nose or mouth	Stimulation, loss of inhibition, headache, nausea or vomiting, slurred speech, loss of motor coordination, wheezing, unconsciousness, cramps, weight loss, muscle weakness, depression, memory impairment, damage to cardiovascular and nervous systems, sudden death
Anabolic Steroids	Anadrol, Oxandrin, Durabolin, Depo-Testosterone, Equipoise; roids, juice, gym candy, pumpers	Injected, swallowed, topical	No intoxication effects. Hypertension, blood clotting and cholesterol changes, hostility and aggression, acne, prostate cancer, reduced sperm production, shrunken testicles, breast enlargement. In females: menstrual irregularities, beard development, and other masculine characteristics.

CNS, Central nervous system.

[a]Taking drugs by injection can increase the risk of infection through needle contamination with staphylococci, human immunodeficiency virus, hepatitis, and other organisms.

[b]Associated with sexual assaults (e.g., date rape).

incoordination, unsteady gait, impaired attention or memory, stupor, and coma. The psychiatric manifestations of intoxication include inappropriate behavior, labile mood, and impaired judgment and social functioning. On physical examination, the person may have respiratory depression or even arrest, nystagmus, and hyperreflexia. Although benzodiazepines rarely depress respiration to the extent that barbiturates do (and, as a result, have a much wider margin of safety), the effects of these drugs are additive with those of other CNS depressants, such as ethanol. Chronic use may produce physical and psychological dependence and a potentially dangerous withdrawal syndrome.

Benzodiazepines potentiate the effects of GABA, which inhibits neurotransmission. They are available as short-acting agents (temazepam [Restoril] and triazolam [Halcion]), intermediate-acting agents (alprazolam [Xanax], chlordiazepoxide [Librium], estazolam [ProSom], lorazepam [Ativan], and oxazepam [Serax]), and long-acting agents (clorazepate [Tranxene], clonazepam [Klonopin], diazepam [Valium], flurazepam [Dalmane], halazepam [Paxipam], Prazepam [Centrax], and quazepam [Doral]). Flunitrazepam (Rohypnol, also known as *roach, rophies, circles, Mexican valium, forget me pill, wolfies,* or *rope*) is a popularly abused benzodiazepine that is not legally available in the United States but is often smuggled here from other countries. It has been implicated in cases of date rape and is known as a club drug because adolescents and young adults often use it at nightclubs and bars or during all-night dance parties called raves.

In persons with an acute benzodiazepine overdose, respiratory depression is the major danger. Flumazenil (Romazicon), a competitive antagonist of benzodiazepines, can be given intravenously for acute overdose. Although it reverses the sedative effects of benzodiazepines, flumazenil may not completely reverse respiratory depression, and it may cause seizures in patients with physical dependence or concurrent tricyclic antidepressant poisoning.

Benzodiazepine cessation may precipitate withdrawal symptoms, depending on the half-life of the specific agent, the duration of use, and the dose. Such withdrawal is characterized by intense anxiety, insomnia, irritability, perceptual changes, hypersensitivity to light and sound, psychosis, hallucinations, palpitations, hyperthermia, tachypnea, diarrhea, muscle spasms, tremors, and seizures. Withdrawal symptoms usually peak 2 to 3 days after the discontinuation of a short-acting agent and 5 to 10 days after discontinuation of a longer-acting one; however, panic attacks and nightmares may recur for months. In general, agents with shorter half-lives produce more intense withdrawal symptoms compared with agents with longer half-lives. Benzodiazepines should be discontinued gradually over a period of several weeks (e.g., 4 to 8 weeks) to prevent seizures and avoid severe withdrawal symptoms. Whether switching to a long-acting agent such as diazepam improves detoxification is unclear. Few evidence-based treatment recommendations for pharmacotherapy of benzodiazepine withdrawal are available but include antidepressant agents for depression and sleep problems, as well as mood stabilizers, especially carbamazepine (200 mg twice per day), although empirical evidence for these approaches is limited. Propranolol can be given to decrease tachycardia, hypertension, and anxiety.

Barbiturates may be short acting (pentobarbital and secobarbital), intermediate acting (amobarbital, aprobarbital, and butabarbital), or long acting (mephobarbital and phenobarbital). The symptoms of acute intoxication with the withdrawal from barbiturates are similar to those of benzodiazepines. For acute barbiturate overdose, oral charcoal and alkalinization of the urine (to a pH >7.5) with forced diuresis are effective in lowering the blood concentration. For patients with hemodynamic compromise refractory to aggressive supportive therapy, barbiturate elimination can be increased by hemodialysis or charcoal hemoperfusion. The effective treatment of withdrawal symptoms requires estimating the daily dose of the abused drug and substituting an equivalent phenobarbital dose to stabilize the patient, after which the dose of phenobarbital is tapered over 4 to 14 days, depending on the half-life of the abused drug. Benzodiazepines may also be used for detoxification, and propranolol and clonidine may help reduce symptoms.

Abuse of γ-hydroxybutyrate (GHB) has increased substantially over the last decade in the United States. This drug is abused for its sedative, euphoric, and bodybuilding effects. GHB is a metabolite of the neurotransmitter GABA, and it also influences the dopaminergic system. It potentiates the effects of endogenous or exogenous opiates. The ingestion of GHB results in immediate drowsiness and dizziness, with the feeling of a *high*. These effects can be potentiated by the concomitant use of alcohol or benzodiazepines. Similar to flunitrazepam and ketamine, GHB is a popular club drug, and it has been implicated in cases of date rape. Its street names include *G, liquid E, liquid X, fantasy, geeb, Georgia home boy, scoop,* and *grievous bodily harm.* Adverse effects that may occur within 15 to 60 minutes of its ingestion include headache, nausea, vomiting, hallucinations, loss of peripheral vision, nystagmus, hypoventilation, cardiac dysrhythmias, seizures, and coma. In rare instances, these adverse effects have led to death. The withdrawal from GHB becomes clinically apparent within 12 hours and may last up to 12 days.

Opioids

Opioids include the natural and semisynthetic alkaloid derivatives of opium as well as the purely synthetic drugs that mimic heroin. They bind to opioid receptors in the brain, spinal cord, and gastrointestinal tract; in addition, they act on several other CNS neurotransmitter systems, including dopamine, GABA, and glutamate, to produce analgesia, CNS depression, and euphoria. With continued opioid use, tolerance and physical dependence develop. As a result, the user must use larger amounts of the drug to obtain the desired effect, and withdrawal symptoms may occur if use is discontinued. Opioid misuse includes the misuse of prescription opioid pain relievers or the use of heroin. The commonly abused opioids include heroin, morphine, codeine, oxycodone (OxyContin, OxyIR, Oxecta, Roxicodone, or combination products, such as Percocet, Percodan, Tylox, Combunox), meperidine (Demerol), propoxyphene (Darvon), hydrocodone (Vicodin, Lortab, Lorcet), hydromorphone (Dilaudid), buprenorphine (Temgesic), and fentanyl (Sublimaze).

In 2016, there were 11.8 million past-year opioid misusers aged 12 or older in the United States, the vast majority of whom (97%) misused prescription pain relievers. The 2016 National Survey on Drug Use and Health reported that 53% of subjects who abused prescription pain relievers obtained them from friends or relatives (40% were given, 9% bought, and 4% stolen), and about one third (35%) indicated that they obtained pain relievers through prescription(s); only 6% were bought from a drug dealer.

Deaths from opioid overdoses have increased dramatically over the last decade. Opioids were involved in 47,600 overdose deaths in 2017

(68% of all drug overdose deaths), with synthetic opioids (other than methadone) the main driver of drug overdose deaths. Deaths involving synthetic opioids in the United States increased from roughly 3000 in 2013 to more than 30,000 in 2018. Synthetic opioids like fentanyl—which is 50 times more potent than heroin and 100 times more potent than morphine—are now involved in twice as many deaths as heroin.

Acute opioid overdose produces pulmonary congestion, with resultant cyanosis and respiratory distress, and changes in mental status that may progress to coma. Other manifestations include fever, pinpoint pupils, and seizures. Unsterile intravenous practices can lead to skin abscesses, cellulitis, thrombophlebitis, wound botulism, meningitis, rhabdomyolysis, endocarditis, hepatitis, or human immunodeficiency virus (HIV) infection. Neurologic complications from intravenous heroin use include transverse myelitis, inflammatory polyneuropathy, and peripheral nerve lesions.

For acute opioid overdose, the patient's respiratory status must be assessed and supported. Naloxone should be administered intravenously and repeated at 2- to 3-minute intervals, often in escalating doses; the patient should respond within minutes with increases in pupil size, respiratory rate, and level of alertness. If no response occurs, opioid overdose is excluded, and other causes of somnolence and respiratory depression must be considered. Naloxone should be titrated carefully, since it may precipitate acute withdrawal symptoms in opioid-dependent patients.

Withdrawal symptoms may appear as early as 6 to 10 hours after the last injection of heroin. Initially the individual often has feelings of drug craving, anxiety, restlessness, irritability, rhinorrhea, lacrimation, diaphoresis, and yawning; these signs are followed by dilated pupils, piloerection, anorexia, nausea, vomiting, diarrhea, abdominal cramps, bone pain, myalgia, tremors, muscle spasms, and, in rare cases, seizures. These symptoms and signs peak at 36 to 48 hours and then subside over 5 to 10 days, if untreated. A protracted abstinence syndrome characterized by bradycardia, hypotension, mild anxiety, sleep disturbance, and decreased responsiveness may occur for up to 5 months.

Treatment for opioid use disorder combines medication with behavioral health services, which is associated with a reduction in deaths from overdose, less opioid use and relapse, and prevention of infectious diseases. Several drugs that target the μ-opioid receptor can be used to manage opioid withdrawal: the full agonist methadone, the partial agonist buprenorphine, and the antagonist naltrexone.

Withdrawal from opioids can be managed with methadone, a long-acting synthetic agonist drug, as withdrawal symptoms of methadone develop more slowly and are less severe than those caused by heroin. Methadone is more highly regulated than the other opioid treatment drugs (i.e., classified as a schedule II substance in the United States) and is usually administered to patients via observed dosing in specialized clinics since it may be abused, diverted, or misused. Methadone can be given twice daily and tapered over 7 to 10 days. Methadone use, in both therapeutic doses and overdoses, has been associated with QTc interval prolongation and torsade de pointes, which, in some cases, has been fatal.

Buprenorphine can alleviate opioid withdrawal signs and symptoms, reduce craving, and block the subjective effects (e.g., so-called drug-liking) of other opioids. Accordingly, treatment with buprenorphine can be titrated to patients' withdrawal symptoms, yielding a well-tolerated transition to treatment. It is available in a daily mucosal formulation (which is also subject to diversion and misuse), as a subdermal implant administered every 6 months, or a monthly subcutaneously injected, extended-release formulation. It is also combined with naloxone in a formulation (Suboxone) developed to decrease the potential for abuse. This combination is available for use in two different forms—under the tongue or in the cheek—and decreases withdrawal symptoms for about 24 hours.

Naltrexone, a long-acting opioid antagonist that blocks impulsive opioid use, is an option for maintenance treatment to prevent relapse. It can be given orally daily or via injectable depot and implantable formulations every 60 to 90 days. It should only be administered after the patient is thoroughly detoxified because it may precipitate withdrawal. Pharmacotherapy must be combined with psychotherapy and structured rehabilitation to achieve an optimal outcome.

Finally, clonidine reduces autonomic hyperactivity and is particularly effective if combined with a benzodiazepine.

Amphetamines

Amphetamines have been used therapeutically for weight reduction and treatment of attention-deficit disorder and narcolepsy. Similar to cocaine, they cause a release of monoamine neurotransmitters (dopamine, norepinephrine, and serotonin) from presynaptic neurons. In addition, however, they have neurotoxic effects on dopaminergic and serotonergic neurons. Their euphoric and reinforcing effects are mediated through dopamine and the mesolimbic system, whereas their cardiovascular effects are caused by the release of norepinephrine. Chronic use leads to neuronal degeneration in dopamine-rich areas of the brain, which may increase the risk for the eventual development of Parkinson's disease.

Amphetamines can be abused orally, intranasally, intravenously, or by smoking. The most frequently used drugs are dextroamphetamine (Dexedrine), methamphetamine (Desoxyn), and methylphenidate (Ritalin). Illicit use of amphetamines has increased substantially, in part because (a) they are easily and quickly synthesized from ephedrine or pseudoephedrine and (b) their psychotropic effects may persist for up to 24 hours. The anorexiants, phenmetrazine and phentermine, which are structurally and pharmacologically similar to amphetamine, also have been used illicitly.

Tolerance to the stimulant effects of amphetamines develops rapidly, and toxic effects can occur with higher doses. Acute amphetamine toxicity is characterized by excessive sympathomimetic effects, including tachycardia, hypertension, hyperthermia, cardiac tachyarrhythmia, tremors, seizures, and coma. The patient may experience irritability, hypervigilance, paranoia, stereotyped compulsive behavior, and tactile, visual, or auditory hallucinations. The clinical picture may simulate an acute schizophrenic psychosis. The symptoms of withdrawal are similar to those seen with cocaine (see discussion of cocaine), but the acute psychosis and paranoia are often pronounced.

The treatment of amphetamine abuse centers on a quiet environment, benzodiazepines for anxiety, and sodium nitroprusside for severe hypertension. Antipsychotics, such as haloperidol, can reduce the agitation and psychosis by blocking the effect of dopamine on the CNS receptor. Urine acidification with ammonium chloride accelerates amphetamine excretion.

ILLICIT DRUG ABUSE

Cocaine

Among individuals 12 years old or older in 2016, 1.9 million had used cocaine within the previous month, including 432,00 users of crack. Cocaine can be taken orally or intravenously; alternatively, because it is well absorbed through all mucous membranes, abusers may achieve a high blood concentration after intranasal, sublingual, vaginal, or rectal administration. Its freebase form (called *crack* because of the popping sound it makes when heated) is heat stable, and it can be smoked. Crack cocaine is considered to be the most potent and addictive form of the drug. Euphoria occurs within seconds after crack cocaine is smoked, and is short lived. Compared with smoking crack cocaine or intravenous injection of the drug, mucosal administration results in a slower onset of action, a later peak effect, and a longer duration of action. The blood half-life is approximately 1 hour. The drug's major metabolite is benzoylecgonine, which can be detected in the urine for 2 to 3 days after a single dose.

An intense, pleasurable reaction lasting 20 to 30 minutes occurs after cocaine use, after which rebound depression, agitation, insomnia, and anorexia occur, which are then followed by fatigue, hypersomnolence, and hyperphagia (the *crash*). This crash usually lasts 9 to 12 hours but occasionally may last up to 4 days. Users often ingest the drug repetitively at relatively short intervals to recapture the euphoric state and to avoid the crash. On occasion, sedatives or alcohol are ingested concomitantly to reduce the intensity of anxiety and irritability associated with the crash. The combination of cocaine and intravenously administered heroin (so-called *speedball, snowball, blanco, boy-girl, Bombita, Belushi,* or *dynamite*) is often used so that the abuser can experience the cocaine-induced euphoria and then *float* down on the opiate. Unfortunately, this combination has been reported to cause sudden death. People who use cocaine in temporal proximity to the ingestion of ethanol produce the metabolite cocaethylene, which has also been implicated in cocaine-related deaths.

Cocaine blocks the presynaptic reuptake of norepinephrine and dopamine, producing an excess of these neurotransmitters at the site of the postsynaptic receptor. Thus, cocaine acts as a powerful sympathomimetic agent, resulting in tachycardia, hypertension, tachypnea, hyperthermia, agitation, pupillary dilation, peripheral vasoconstriction, and seizures. Cocaine causes potent vasoconstriction of cerebral arteries and, therefore, may result in a stroke. It is associated with myocardial ischemia and arrhythmias and, in rare cases, with myocardial infarction in young persons with normal or only minimally diseased coronary arteries. The principal mechanisms of ischemia and infarction are coronary arterial vasoconstriction, thrombosis, platelet aggregation, tissue plasminogen activator inhibition, increased myocardial oxygen demand, and accelerated atherosclerosis (Fig. 128.4).

For patients with cocaine-induced hypertension or tachycardia, labetalol and benzodiazepines are usually effective in lowering systemic arterial pressure and heart rate. Patients with acute cocaine-related myocardial infarction should receive aspirin, heparin, nitroglycerin, and, if indicated, reperfusion therapy (with a thrombolytic agent or primary coronary intervention). The use of β-adrenergic blockers should be avoided when possible, since ischemia may be worsened by unopposed α-adrenergically mediated coronary arterial vasoconstriction. Patients with a normal electrocardiogram or nonspecific changes can be managed safely with observation.

The immediate treatment of acute cocaine intoxication includes obtaining vascular and airway access, if needed, and careful electrocardiographic monitoring. Benzodiazepines can be given to control CNS agitation; haloperidol or risperidone can be used in the severely agitated patient. A supportive environment is needed, but detoxification is not required, given that few physical signs of true dependence are present.

Most chronic cocaine abusers have psychological dependence and an intense craving for cocaine. Personal and group therapies are important adjuncts to pharmacologic treatment, but relapse is common and is difficult to manage. Although no medication is FDA approved for treatment of cocaine addiction, disulfiram, modafinil, anticonvulsants (e.g., topiramate and tiagabine), serotonin reuptake inhibitors (e.g., citalopram), serotonin receptor antagonists (e.g., ondansetron), and GABA receptor agonists (e.g., baclofen) have shown some promise in promoting cocaine abstinence.

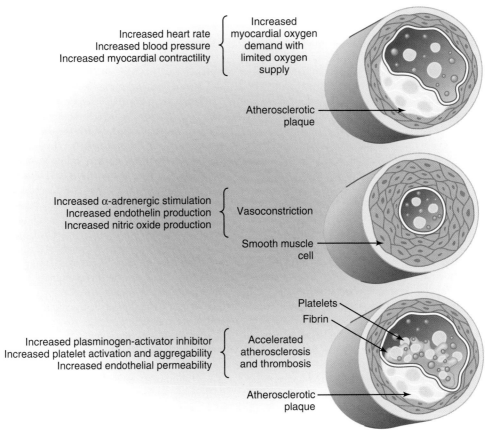

Fig. 128.4 The mechanisms by which cocaine may induce myocardial ischemia or infarction. Cocaine may cause increases in the determinants of myocardial oxygen demand when oxygen supply is limited *(top),* when intense vasoconstriction of the coronary arteries occurs *(middle),* or when accelerated atherosclerosis and thrombosis are present *(bottom).*

Cannabis

The cannabinoid drugs include marijuana (the dried flowering tops and stems of the hemp plant) and hashish (a resinous extract of the hemp plant). Marijuana is the most commonly used "illicit" drug in the United States, recognizing that it is now legalized for recreational use in many states and for medical indications in most states. In 2016, an estimated 24 million Americans had used it in the past month. Between 2007 and 2016, the rate of use increased from 5.8% to 8.9% of the U.S. population, and the number of users increased from 14.5 million to 24 million. This increase reflects the increase in marijuana use by adults aged 26 years or older and, to a lesser extent, the increase in marijuana use among young adults aged 18 to 25 years (Fig. 128.5). In 2018 about 1 in every 13 young adults (8%) aged 19 to 28 was a daily or near daily marijuana user.

Marijuana use disorder occurs when someone experiences clinically significant impairment caused by the recurrent use of marijuana, including health problems, persistent or increasing use, and failure to meet major responsibilities at work, school, or home. Approximately 4.0 million people aged 12 or older in 2016 had a marijuana use disorder in the past year, which represents 1.5% of persons aged 12 years or older.

Marijuana and hashish are among the drugs most commonly used by adolescents, with approximately one third (36%) of 12th graders admitting use at least once and 5.8% reporting that they are daily or nearly daily users. Most of their pharmacologic effects come from metabolites of δ-9-tetrahydrocannabinol, which bind to specific cannabinoid receptors located in the CNS, spinal cord, and peripheral

nervous system. The primary mode of use is smoking, with mood-altering and intoxicating effects noted within 3 minutes and peak effects in approximately 1 hour. However, vaping cannabis extracts and synthetic cannabinoids ("fake marijuana") in electronic cigarette devices has become increasingly popular. The acute physiologic effects are dose-related and often include increased heart rate, conjunctival congestion, dry mouth, fine tremor, muscle weakness, and ataxia. Psychoactive effects include euphoria, enhanced perception of colors and sounds, drowsiness, inattentiveness, and inability to learn new facts. Tolerance and physical dependence occur, and chronic users may experience mild withdrawal symptoms of irritability, restlessness, anorexia, insomnia, or mild hyperthermia. Rarely, acute psychosis with panic reactions occurs. The treatment of withdrawal is supportive and includes reassurance; benzodiazepines may be used in severely agitated patients. Cannabinoids have been used as antiemetic agents in patients with cancer receiving chemotherapy, for weight stimulation (in patients with cancer or HIV infection), and in the treatment of glaucoma.

Severe pulmonary illnesses have been reported in hundreds of otherwise healthy young persons who have "vaped" cannabis extracts (i.e., tetrahydrocannabinol products) in e-cigarettes, with one third requiring mechanical ventilation and some experiencing death. Initial symptoms include shortness of breath, cough, chest pain fever, gastrointestinal issues (i.e., nausea, vomiting, diarrhea, and abdominal pain), and weight loss, which occurs days or weeks after vaping. Bilateral infiltrates are present on chest imaging. Although most patients (>80%) reported having used tetrahydrocannabinol products in e-cigarette

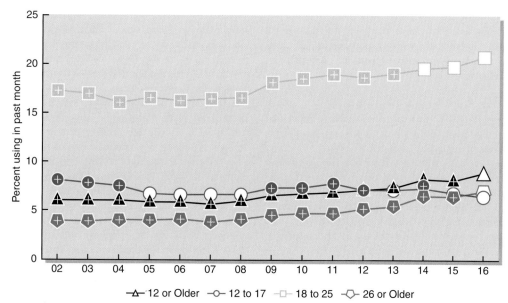

12 or Older **12 to 17** **18 to 25** **26 or Older**

+Difference between this estimate and the 2016 estimate is statistically significant at athe .05 level.

Fig. 128.5 Past-month marijuana use among persons aged 12 years or older, by age group according to the National Survey on Drug Use and Health (2016). (Substance Abuse and Mental Health Services Administration. [2017]. Key substance use and mental health indicators in the United States: Results from the 2016 National Survey on Drug Use and Health [HHS Publication No. SMA 17-5044, NSDUH Series H-52]. Rockville, MD: Center for Behavioral Health Statistics and Quality, Substance Abuse and Mental Health Services Administration. Retrieved from https://www.samhsa.gov/data.)

devices prior to the development of their severe pulmonary symptoms, a wide variety of products and devices have been reported. E-cigarette liquids and aerosols contain a variety of chemical constituents that may have adverse health effects, including propylene glycol, glycerin, hydrocarbons, nitrosamines, volatile organic chemicals, and toxic metals, flavoring compounds (i.e., diacetyl and 2,3-pentanedione), and THC-based oils and vitamin E acetate.

Synthetic marijuana is a psychoactive designer drug composed of a mixture of herbs, spices, or shredded plant material that is sprayed with synthetic chemicals that mimic the effects of cannabis when smoked or prepared as a tea. They have been sold widely in "head shops" as well as through the internet and are best known by the brand names K2 and Spice. Spice products are popular among young people; of the illicit drugs most used by high school seniors, they are second only to marijuana. Synthetic cannabis can precipitate acute psychosis or a worsening of previously stable psychotic disorders; they also may trigger a chronic (long-term) psychotic disorder among vulnerable individuals, such as those with a family history of mental illness. K2 ingestion has been associated with myocardial infarction and death. Regular users may experience withdrawal and addiction symptoms.

Hallucinogens and Dissociative Drugs

Hallucinogens (drugs that cause hallucinations) include lysergic acid diethylamide (LSD), mescaline, psilocybin, and ibogaine. *Dissociative drugs* distort perceptions of sight and sound and produce feelings of detachment (dissociation) without causing hallucinations. They include phencyclidine (PCP), ketamine, salvia, and dextromethorphan (a widely available cough suppressant).

LSD is the most potent of the hallucinogenic drugs. Although it is known to interact with serotonin receptors in the cerebral cortex and *locus ceruleus,* its precise psychoactive mechanism is unknown. Within 30 minutes of its oral ingestion, sympathomimetic effects appear,

including mydriasis, hyperthermia, tachycardia, elevated blood pressure, diaphoresis, dry mouth, increased alertness, tremors, and nausea. Within 2 hours, the psychoactive effects become apparent, with heightened perceptions (highly intensified colors, smells, sounds, and other sensations), body distortions, mood variations, and visual hallucinations. An acute panic reaction may occur, sometimes leading to self-injury or suicide. After approximately 12 hours, the syndrome begins to subside, but fatigue and tension may persist for another day. Flashbacks (brief recurrences of the hallucinations) may occur days or even weeks after the last dose but tend to disappear without treatment. Acute panic reactions are best treated in a supportive environment; benzodiazepines can be given to severely agitated patients.

PCP is a potent, addictive hallucinogen that produces a prompt stimulant effect similar to that of amphetamines, with feelings of euphoria, power, and invincibility. Patients may have hypertension, tachycardia, hyperthermia, bidirectional nystagmus, slurred speech, ataxia, hallucinations, extreme agitation, and rhabdomyolysis. With more severe reactions, patients may be brought to medical attention in a coma-like state, with open eyes and pupils that are partially dilated, a decreased pain response, brief periods of excitation, and muscle rigidity. On occasion, PCP users may have hypertensive urgency, seizures, and bizarre (often violent) behavior, which lead to suicide or extreme violence toward others. Tolerance and mild withdrawal symptoms have been seen in daily users, but the major problem is drug craving. Treatment entails a quiet environment, sedation with benzodiazepines, hydration, haloperidol for terrifying hallucinations, and suicide precautions. Continuous gastric suction and acidification of the urine with intravenous ammonium chloride or ascorbic acid may aid in the drug's excretion, but acidification may increase the risk of renal failure if rhabdomyolysis is present.

Ketamine is a rapidly acting general anesthetic; unlike most anesthetics, it produces only mild respiratory depression and appears to stimulate the cardiovascular system. Adverse effects, including delirium and hallucinations, limit its use as a general anesthetic in humans. Similar to PCP, ketamine is a dissociative anesthetic. In addition, it has both analgesic and amnestic properties and is associated with less confusion, irrationality, and violent behavior than PCP. Ketamine is one of the club drugs that have been implicated in date rape.

Inhalants

Of the 1.8 million people aged 12 years or older who used inhalants in the past year to get high, about 684,000 were adolescents aged 12 to 17. Because they are readily available, inhalants are often among the first drugs that adolescents use, with felt-tip pens/markers or magic markers the most common agents. The inhalants may be classified as (1) *organic solvents,* including toluene (airplane glue and spray paint), paint thinners, kerosene, gasoline, carbon tetrachloride, shoe polish, acetone (nail polish removers and Liquid Paper), xylene (permanent markers), and degreasers (dry cleaning fluids); (2) *gases,* such as butane, propane, aerosol propellants, and anesthetics (ether, chloroform, halothane, and nitrous oxide); and (3) *nitrites,* such as cyclohexyl nitrite, amyl nitrite, and butyl nitrite (room deodorizer). These substances are most often inhaled by children or young adolescents, after which they produce dizziness and intoxication within minutes. Prolonged exposure or daily use may lead to hearing loss, bone marrow depression, cardiac arrhythmias, cerebral degeneration, peripheral neuropathies, and damage to the liver, kidneys, or lungs. A characteristic "glue sniffer's rash" around the nose and mouth is sometimes seen after prolonged use. In rare instances, death may occur, most likely from hypoxemia, cardiac arrhythmias, pneumonia, or aspiration of vomit while unconscious. Detoxification is rarely required for the patient who has abused these substances, but psychiatric treatment may be needed to prevent relapse.

Designer Drugs

The term *designer drug* refers to illicit synthetic drugs, many of which have increased potency in comparison with their parent compounds. The most common designer drugs include analogs of fentanyl, meperidine, piperazine, and methamphetamines. Several fentanyl derivatives, initially sufentanil, alfentanil, remifentanil, carfentanil and, more recently, acetylfentanyl, 6-butyrfentanyl, 4-MeO-butyrfentanyl, isobutyrylfentanyl, furanylfentanyl, α-methylfentanyl (China white), 3-methylfentanyl or TMF, p-methylfentanyl, methylacetylfentanyl, acrylfentanyl, 2-fluorofentanyl, fluoroacetylfentanyl, ocfentanil are illegally manufactured. These derivatives do not have recognized medical uses, are often not detected by routine drug testing, and have worsened the opioid crisis and number of drug-related deaths. Because these drugs are approximately 1000 times as potent as heroin, it is not surprising that fatal overdoses from respiratory depression have been reported.

The major meperidine derivatives are 1-methyl-4-phenyl-4-propionoxypiperidene (MPPP) and 1-methyl-4-phenyl-1, 2, 3, 6-tetrahydropyridine (MPTP), each of which produces euphoria similar to that caused by heroin. In some users, MPTP causes neuronal degeneration in the substantia nigra, which produces an irreversible form of Parkinson's disease.

Piperazines, a new class of designer drugs of abuse, are commonly sold as party pills in the form of tablets, capsules, or powders on the drug black market and in so-called head shops or over the internet under the names of Frenzy, Bliss, Charge, Herbal ecstasy, A2, Legal X, and Legal E. 1-Benzylpiperazine (BZP) is the most prevalent of these compounds. Aside from BZP and 1-(3,4-methylenedioxybenzyl) piperazine (MDBP), the phenylpiperazine derivatives 1-(3-trifluoromethylphenyl) piperazine (TFMPP), 1-(3-chloro phenyl) piperazine (mCPP), and 1-(4-methoxyphenyl)

piperazine (MeOPP) are often abused. Because piperazines and amphetamines cause similar pharmacologic symptoms, piperazine poisoning can easily be wrongly diagnosed as amphetamine poisoning. Furthermore, piperazines are not detected by routinely used immunochemical screening procedures for drugs of abuse, but they require an appropriate toxicologic analysis (e.g., by gas chromatography-mass spectrometry). The methylenedioxy synthetic derivatives of amphetamine and methamphetamine are generally referred to as *ecstasy* and include 3, 4-methylenedioxy methamphetamine (MDMA, also known as *Adam*); 3, 4-methylenedioxy-ethylamphetamine (MDEA, also known as *Eve*); and N-methyl-1-(3, 4-methylenedioxyphenyl)-2-butanamine (MBDB, also known as *Methyl-J* or *Eden*). These drugs have CNS stimulant and hallucinogenic properties. They produce elevated mood and increased self-esteem and may cause acute panic, anxiety, paranoia, hallucinations, tachycardia, nystagmus, ataxia, and tremor. Deaths in some users have been attributed to cardiac arrhythmias, hyperthermia with seizures, and intracranial hemorrhage.

PROSPECTUS FOR THE FUTURE

Immunotherapy (i.e., vaccine development) has emerged as a promising approach to treat abuse of drugs like methamphetamine, heroin, and cocaine. By sequestering the drugs in the periphery without allowing the drug to cross the blood-brain barrier, the toxic and rewarding effects of the drugs are reduced. A novel pharmacokinetic approach to the treatment of drug toxicity involves the development of compounds that can be administered safely to humans and that accelerate the metabolism of the drug to inactive components. For example, catalytic antibodies have been developed to accelerate cocaine metabolism and are administered parentally. In experimental animals, mutations of human butyrylcholinesterase (one of the enzymes responsible for the metabolism of cocaine) accelerate cocaine metabolism and antagonize cocaine's behavioral and toxic effects.

SUGGESTED READINGS

Edenberg HJ, McClintick JN: Alcohol dehydrogenases, aldehyde dehydrogenases, and alcohol use disorders: a critical review, Alcohol Clin Exp Re 42:2281–2297, 2018.

Haight BR, Learned SM, Laffont CM, et al: For the RB-US-13-0001 Study Investigators. Efficacy and safety of a monthly buprenorphine depot injection for opioid use disorder: a multicentre, randomised, double-blind, placebo-controlled, phase 3 trial, Lancet 393:778–790, 2019.

Jonas DE, Amick HR, Feltner C, et al: Pharmacotherapy for adults with alcohol use disorders in outpatient settings: a systematic review and meta-analysis, J Am Med Assoc 311:889–1900, 2014.

Kaner EFS, Beyer FR, Muirhead C, et al: Effectiveness of brief alcohol interventions in primary care populations, Cochrane Database Syst Rev 2, 2018, Art.No.: CD004148, 2018.

Kranzler HR, Soyka: Diagnosis and pharmacotherapy of alcohol use disorder: a review, J Am Med Assoc 320:815–824, 2018.

O'Connor EA, Perdue LA, Senger CA, et al. Screening and behavioral counseling interventions to reduce unhealthy alcohol use in adolescents and adults: an updated systematic review for the U.S. Preventive Services Task Force. Evidence Synthesis No. 171. AHRQ Publication No. 18-05242-EF-1. Rockville, MD: Agency for Healthcare Research and Quality, 2018.

Peacock A, Leung J, Larney S, et al: Global statistics on alcohol, tobacco and illicit drug use: 2017 status report, Addiction 113:1905–1926, 2018.

Schulenberg JE, Johnston LD, O'Malley PM, Bachman JG, Miech RA, Patrick ME: Monitoring the Future national survey results on drug use, 1975–2018: volume II, College students and adults ages 19–60, Ann Arbor, 2019, Institute for Social Research, The University of Michigan, Available at http://monitoringthefuture.org/pubs.html#monographs. Accessed September 2019.

Soyka M: Treatment of benzodiazepine dependence, N Engl J Med 376:1147–1157, 2017.

Substance Abuse and Mental Health Services Administration. (2017). Key substance use and mental health indicators in the United States: Results from the 2016 National Survey on Drug Use and Health (HHS Publication No. SMA 17-5044, NSDUH Series H-52). Rockville, MD: Center for Behavioral Health Statistics and Quality, Substance Abuse and Mental Health Services Administration. Available at https://www.samhsa.gov/data/sites/default/files/NSDUH-FFR1-2016/NSDUH-FFR1-2016.pdf. Accessed September 2019.

Wood E, Albarqouni L, Tkachuk S, et al: Will this hospitalized patient develop severe alcohol withdrawal syndrome? The rational clinical examination systematic review, J Am Med Assoc 320:825–833, 2018.

Wozniak JR, Riley EP, Charness ME: Clinical presentation, diagnosis, and management of fetal alcohol spectrum disorder, Lancet Neurol 18:760–770, 2019.

Coronavirus Disease 2019 (COVID-19)

Edward J. Wing

The Coronavirus Disease 2019 (COVID-19) pandemic occurred after the initial deadline for this book had passed, and as a result I have written this appendix to reflect our knowledge of COVID-19 as of October 2020. The COVID-19 pandemic burst on the world as a totally new viral respiratory infection at the end of 2019 and the beginning of 2020. Initially the virology, epidemiology, transmission, diagnosis, clinical aspects, treatment, and prevention were largely unknown. Since then the amount of scientific focus and effort on all aspects of the disease from its molecular virology to clinical understanding to vaccine and drug development has been extraordinary.

While we know much more now about the infection than initially, our knowledge and hence this appendix is still largely incomplete. The ability to recognize, diagnose, care for our patients, and prevent this virus will undoubtedly change and evolve over time. Therefore, all physicians and health care workers need to continue to update their knowledge of COVID-19 to become long-term learners concerning all aspects of the infection.

COVID-19 PANDEMIC

Infectious pandemics, usually associated with animal–human contact, have afflicted mankind for millennia. Although some infections such as malaria have probably infected primates for millions of years, most pandemic infections have occurred since the beginning of agriculture. Pandemics such as the bubonic plague, which killed from one third to one half of the population of Europe and devastated other parts of the world, and the 1918 to 1919 influenza H1N1 pandemic that killed 675,000 people in the United States and at least 50 million people worldwide, have been catastrophic. More recent pandemics have included HIV, cholera, Zika virus and other influenza strains (1957, H2N2; 1968, H3N2; 2009, H1N1pdm09). The majority of recent pandemics in this century have been due to viral infections in which animals have been either the primary or intermediate host or the vectors of the diseases. RNA viruses such as the influenza and coronaviruses that have inherent genetic instability have been particularly prominent.

Coronaviruses have been known to have natural animal reservoirs, particularly in bat populations, and to cause mild, seasonal upper respiratory disease. Four human coronaviruses—OC43, 229E, HKU1 and NL63 viral strains—have been shown to have a predilection for children under the age of 5, to cause respiratory illness, and to be transmitted similarly to influenza virus. In 2002 to 2003, a new coronavirus, SARS-CoV, derived from bat strains, was identified in China. It caused severe respiratory infection infecting more than 8000 people in 29 countries with a mortality of approximately 10%. Because of limited transmissibility, the pandemic was controlled and then eliminated with strict public health measures. In 2012, a second coronavirus, Middle East respiratory syndrome (MERS-CoV), was first recognized in Saudi Arabia and subsequently in other Middle Eastern countries. Evidence indicates that its source is camels and that close contact with these animals is a risk for contracting the disease. Gastrointestinal and pulmonary symptoms occur. To date there have been approximately 2500 cases with a mortality rate of 34%.

In early December 2019, cases of pneumonia of unknown cause were identified in the city of Wuhan, capital city of Hubei province, China. Many of the initial cases had worked in or had close contact with wet markets that sell fresh meat, fish, and other perishable produce. The outbreak increased during December, and on December 31 the WHO was informed of an outbreak of a new cause of pneumonia. With remarkable speed, the cause was identified as a new coronavirus and the gene sequence reported from China and the WHO on January 9, 2020. The virus was named SARS-CoV-2, and the infection is referred to as COVID-19. The epidemic continued to increase in Wuhan during January 2020 and peaked in late January and early February. The high population density in Wuhan, population movements, and the lack of clarity regarding human-to-human transmission drove the epidemic. Severe overcrowding of medical facilities occurred, prompting draconian public health measures including the imposition of a *cordon sanitaire* that prevented movement in or out of Wuhan, universal and compulsory home restriction with drastic penalties for violations, suspension of public transportation, closure of entertainment venues, closure of the implicated wet markets, and compulsory mask wearing. Subsequently, the number of new cases decreased steadily so that few cases were reported after March 1 in Wuhan although cases continued to be reported in other areas of China including Beijing. The total number of confirmed cases in Mainland China as of February 11 was reported as over 72,000 although this may represent a low estimate. The overall fatality rate was reported as 2.3%, but it was soon understood that mortality rate varies based on age group, testing availability, and other factors. Vigorous public health measures as described appear to have been effective in at least limiting the number of cases in China.

Cases of COVID-19 were reported outside of China as early as January 13 in persons who had traveled from Wuhan. The first case in the United States occurred on January 19, 2020, in Snohomish County, Washington, in an individual who had recently returned from visiting family in Wuhan. The patient had gastrointestinal and respiratory symptoms with fever that persisted for 8 days, requiring treatment with oxygen and remdesivir, an experimental antiviral agent. The patient recovered without incidence. Notably, future studies demonstrated that the virus circulated on both coasts for many weeks before it was recognized.

On January 30 with cases in Asia including Japan, South Korea, Vietnam, and Singapore; in Europe including France; and in the United States, the WHO declared a global emergency. Cases were reported from Africa (first in Egypt) but remained relatively low. By March the number of cases in Europe exploded, with particularly devastating effects in Italy, Spain, France, and the United Kingdom, and the WHO labeled COVID-19 a pandemic. Health care systems were overwhelmed in northern Italy as well as other areas, and mortality was particularly high among the elderly. By June 29 COVID-19 had occurred in over 200 countries with 10 million cases and over 500,000 confirmed deaths. By the fall of 2020 it was estimated that more than 30 million cases of COVID-19, with more than 1 million deaths, had occurred worldwide.

By the end of April 2020, the number of cases in the Americas, primarily the United States, had skyrocketed, reaching over 1 million cases with 58,000 deaths. As an early example in the United States, an outbreak of COVID-19 was identified in February 2020 in a long-term care skilled nursing facility in King County, Washington State. In the facility, 81 residents (median age 81), 48 health care workers (median age 42.5 years), and 14 visitors (median age 42.5 years) were infected. Twenty-two of the 81 residents (27%), 0 of the 48 (0%) health care workers, and 1 of the 14 visitors (7.1%) died. In addition to age and residence in a nursing home, residents had a high rate of chronic underlying conditions, including cardiovascular disease (including hypertension), renal disease, diabetes mellitus/obesity, and pulmonary disease.

By March, the epicenter in the United States was New York City and the surrounding counties where the number of cases exploded, overwhelming some medical centers and devastating nursing homes and their residents where the mortality was the greatest. By May widespread outbreaks were noted in Mid-Atlantic and New England states, Louisiana, Florida, and in West Coast states. The number of cases fell in May in the United States, most likely due to restrictive measures including school and business closings, restrictions on public events, quarantine regulations, and wearing masks. The incidence of COVID-19 began to rise again in June with outbreaks in states such as Florida and Arizona, perhaps due to relaxation of earlier restrictive public health measures. Unfortunately, in late August and September the number of deaths continued at greater than 1000/day and the number of deaths directly associated with COVID-19 in the United States reached 200,000. In the fall, with reopening schools, particularly colleges and universities, and relaxation of restrictions on businesses and entertainment venues such as restaurants and bars, the number of new cases continued to rise as did the rates of hospitalizations. Early data indicate that the age of persons infected has decreased and the severity and mortality is lower. The rise in rates among those 18 to 24 years old was particularly striking. In addition, the disproportionate impact of the pandemic on the Black and Latinx communities became apparent. As of October 15, 2020, 216,035 deaths were reported in the United States, although excess deaths possibly related to the effects of COVID-19 have been estimated to be higher.

Finally, the 2020 to 2021 influenza season will intersect with the COVID-19 pandemic in the United States this winter and spring with unknown severity. The effects of COVID-19 public health measures, vaccination rates for influenza, and the already devastating effects of COVID-19 on vulnerable populations will all influence the morbidity and mortality of the influenza season.

VIROLOGY

The COVID-19 virus is an enveloped single-stranded RNA virus with surface spike proteins, like other coronaviruses, that give the group its distinctive contour under electron microscope, hence its name "coronavirus" ("corona" means crown). COVID-19 has 79% similarity to SARS-CoV and 50% similarity to MERS-CoV based on genetic analysis. Bats are believed to be the original source of COVID-19 with perhaps an intermediate host such as the pangolin, sometimes called the spiny anteater, which is regarded as a delicacy in parts of China and sold in wet markets. Genetic mutations presumably allowed the virus to cross species and cause disease. However, the origins of the virus are not completely understood at this point.

The 180-kDa spike (S) protein binds to the peptidase angiotensin-converting enzyme 2 receptor (ACE2) on cell surfaces and mediates viral and cell membrane fusion for entry into cells. Membrane fusion also requires the interaction of other proteases, particularly transmembrane protease serine 2 (TMPRSS2), on cell surfaces. The presence of ACE2 determines cell tropism of COVID-19 and is found on epithelial cells of both the upper and lower respiratory tract. ACE2 also has a wide distribution in other tissues including vascular endothelial cells, the gastrointestinal tract, and kidney. SARS-CoV-2 virus enters cells by endocytosis, uses the cells' own machinery to reproduce, and then is released to infect other cells. Nasal epithelial cells are infected, which in early infection may result in initial upper respiratory symptoms and anosmia. Bronchial, alveolar, and endovascular epithelial cells are also infected early, causing an inflammatory response consisting of neutrophils, T lymphocytes, macrophages and the release of cytokines including TNF-α, and IL-6. As the infection and inflammation progresses in the lungs there is interstitial thickening, pulmonary edema, activation of the coagulation pathway, and lymphocyte depletion. Further inflammation can result in fibrosis with marked compromise of pulmonary function.

PATHOLOGY

Autopsy findings demonstrate high SARS-CoV-19 titers particularly in the lung, but also in blood, liver, kidney, brain, and heart. In individuals who died of COVID-19, autopsy shows diffuse alveolar damage in all lobes but with more pronounced findings in the lower lobes. During the early phase, signs of acute alveolar damage include edema, hyaline membrane formation, and thickened alveolar septa with perivascular lymphocytic infiltration. There is severe endothelial injury associated with disrupted cell membranes and the presence of virus. Pulmonary vessels including alveolar capillaries show widespread microthrombi and vascular angiogenesis, both of which distinguish it from the pathology of severe influenza infection. In later stages there is diffuse alveolar damage, fibroblastic proliferation leading to fibrosis, pneumocyte hyperplasia and interstitial thickening, and collapsed alveoli. In some areas of diffuse alveolar damage, metaplasia or widespread fibrosis is observed.

Other findings have included bronchopneumonia; lymphocytic myocarditis and epicarditis; periportal lymphocytic infiltration with hepatic congestion and steatosis, hepatic cell necrosis, and central vein thrombosis; acute tubular injury; and thrombotic features in multiple organs including lung, heart, and kidney. Also noted are focal pancreatitis, adrenocortical hyperplasia, and lymphocyte depletion in spleen and lymph nodes. In the brain, extensive inflammation has been noted in the olfactory bulbs and medulla oblongata. It was recognized early on that severe COVID-19 could result in activation of coagulation and consumption of clotting factors resulting in diffuse intravascular coagulation. Increased coagulation can result in deep venous thrombosis and unsuspected pulmonary embolism, myocardial infarction, stroke, and vascular compromise in other organs. Thrombosis of small and mid-sized pulmonary arteries with associated infarction is found in a high percentage of cases. In addition, neutrophilic plugs have been observed composed of neutrophil extracellular traps (NETS). NETS are composed of extracellular strands of DNA from neutrophils that trap pathogens. In an autopsy series NETS have been observed with platelets, which may induce thrombus formation.

HOST DEFENSES

Host defenses against coronaviruses consist of both innate and specific immunity, but the specific mechanisms and their relative importance have yet to be clarified. Sites of infection, particularly the lung with endothelial damage, attract immune cells including T and B lymphocytes, macrophages, and neutrophils. The immune response includes release of cytokines and inflammatory molecules including interleukins 1 and 6, interferons, TNF-α as well as antibody production of IgM and IgG, and activation of the coagulation system with increases in D-dimer and micro- and macro-thrombosis. Inflammatory markers include elevated erythrocyte sedimentation rate, C-reactive protein, ferritin, and lactic dehydrogenase. A characteristic of the inflammatory process is the destruction and apoptosis of both CD4 and CD8 T lymphocytes with resulting lymphopenia. Experimental data suggest that neutralizing antibodies directed towards the S protein afford protection after infection; thus, vaccine development has targeted the response against this protein. Recent data suggest that the specific immune response to SARS-CoV-2 consists of CD4, CD8, and antibody in a coordinated response. Lack of such a response and decreased number of T cells occur in persons over 65 and may account for greater susceptibility to the virus. It is not clear, however, whether infection itself provides long-lasting immunity, whether the presence of antibody after infection protects, whether antibody persists after infections, or what the relative importance of T-cell immunity is.

TRANSMISSION

Transmission of COVID-19 is an essential issue in determining risk for acquiring the virus. At the beginning of the pandemic, it was unclear whether transmission was airborne, through contact with infected animals or material in the wet markets of Wuhan, or by some other mechanism. The rapid spread of the infection within households, among health care workers, and the spread of the disease outside of Wuhan quickly indicated that human-to-human contact was the primary mode of transmission. It is apparent now that most transmission occurs within households, nursing homes, and other congregate settings. Within households, the greatest risk is among the elderly and spouses. Infected individuals appear to be most infectious just before or for several days after the beginning of symptoms when viral loads peak. However, patients who remain asymptomatic can also transmit the infection.

A major question has centered on the infectivity of individuals after contracting COVID-19. Reverse transcriptase-polymerase reaction (RT-PCR) tests usually become negative when an individual recovers from COVID-19 infection but may remain positive for prolonged periods. However, in the majority of cases recovery of viable virus has been shown to disappear 8 days after the onset of symptoms. Thus, in most protocols, the quarantine is stopped 10 to 14 days after the onset of symptoms.

Airborne transmission occurs when viable virus becomes airborne after an infected individual exhales, speaks, particularly in a loud voice, sings, coughs or sneezes. Infectious particles can be broadly classified as either large droplets, which are usually defined as larger than 5 micrometers, or aerosols, which are smaller particles of less than 5 micrometers. A mixture of large particles and aerosols are generated after a person coughs or sneezes. Certain medical procedures such as intubation or noninvasive positive-pressure ventilation potentially cause aerosol formation. After leaving the respiratory tract, large droplets rapidly fall to the ground—usually within 6 feet of an infected individual. Influenza is a typical pathogen transmitted primarily by large droplets. Close contact with someone who is coughing or sneezing maximizes the risk for acquiring influenza. The CDC has recently defined a close contact as "someone who was within six feet of an infected person for a cumulative time of 15 minutes or more over a 24-hour period starting from 2 days before illness onset (or for

asymptomatic patients, 2 days prior to test specimen collection) until the time the patient is isolated."

In contrast, aerosols evaporate quickly, leaving infectious particles suspended in the air for a considerable period of time—usually hours—in closed and particularly in poorly ventilated spaces. Microbial pathogens such as tuberculosis or measles are typically spread by aerosol. These pathogens can potentially infect large numbers of people because of the airborne suspension of infectious particles. The difference between large droplet spread, such as found with influenza, and aerosols, such as found with measles, is indicated by the average number of people who are infected by an index case, which is termed the reproduction number. For COVID-19 the average reproduction number is 2 to 3, similar to influenza. Risk of transmission does vary with the type of exposure. For example, close contact exposure gives a risk of perhaps 5% whereas household contact can be as high as 40%. But brief interactions, such as while shopping, have a risk of less than 1%. For aerosol transmission, the reproduction number can be as high as 18. Thus, in an epidemic, each active measles case infects on average of 18 other individuals. Because the reproduction number for COVID-19 is low, as is the secondary attack rate, and because the evidence that masks and social distancing of 6 feet reduces incidence of disease, large droplet transmission seems the likely mode of most transmission. Also, a potential association between the size of the inoculum and the clinical presentations and outcome has been proposed and is under investigation.

Nonetheless, some data do support the possibility of aerosol transmission of SARS-CoV-2. Aerosols with SARS-CoV-2 RNA have been demonstrated experimentally and in hospitals. In addition, viable virus has been demonstrated in hospital settings. Furthermore, aerosol transmission has been suggested epidemiologically in certain situations. An outbreak in a nursing home in the Netherlands in June and July 2020 suggested aerosol transmission. In this outbreak 17 (81%) residents and 17 (50%) health care workers (who wore masks) from one of seven wards in a psychogeriatric nursing home were diagnosed with COVID-19 as confirmed by RT-PCR. All residents were diagnosed within 4 days of each other. None of the 95 residents or 106 health care workers in the six other wards was infected. Investigation of the ventilation system in this ward revealed the possibility that air was recirculated, rather than circulated to the outside, due to a recent renovation of the system. Thus, circumstantial evidence in this widespread, ward-specific outbreak over a short time suggests aerosol transmission. Other reports of short-term, extensive outbreaks in poorly ventilated venues suggest the possibility of occasional aerosol transmission. Finally, transmission by "super transmitters" has occurred when a single individual appears to infect a large number of people, well beyond the expected number of two (discussed previously). The frequency and the mechanism for transmission from these individuals remains to be clarified.

Therefore, at the time of this writing, the major route of transmission of COVID-19 during the pandemic appears to be by large droplets in situations where there is close contact without the protection of masks (see later) and over a sustained period, and not by aerosol. In certain circumstances, however, usually indoors in poorly ventilated venues, transmission by aerosols may occur.

Experimental conditions with large inocula of SARS-CoV-2 have demonstrated persistence of the virus on fomites for periods of up to 72 hours, depending on the surface and the conditions. Virus persists longer on impermeable surfaces such as steel or plastic than on permeable surfaces such as paper. More realistic conditions with lower inocula suggest survival of the viable virus for several hours. Virus has been found on numerous surfaces in hospital rooms of infected patients, although data from the United Kingdom indicate that the presence of virus as detected by RT-PCR in the air and on surfaces is low, particularly after cleaning, and that recovery of viable virus is very low. There is little epidemiologic or clinical data at this point suggesting significant transmission through fomites, although it is certainly reasonable to keep open the possibility and act on that assumption.

SARS-CoV-2 RNA has been found in stool as might be expected with a gastrointestinal tropic virus, but there is no evidence that transmission results from contaminated water or food.

COVID-19 is much less likely to be transmitted in outside venues because of rapid dispersal of droplets and aerosols. Sunlight and ultraviolet light have been shown to rapidly inactivate the virus.

Finally, epidemiologic data suggest that masks and social distancing reduce the risk of transmission. N-95 masks provide protection for both aerosols and large droplets. Surgical masks in hospital settings have been shown to reduce the risk of transmission. Experimental data showed that surgical masks and well-fitted homemade masks with multiple layers of quilting fabric were most effective in preventing droplet and even aerosol dispersal after a cough or loud singing. Bandana and folded handkerchief masks were less effective. Although epidemiologic and experimental data support mask wearing, to date, there are very limited controlled clinical data supporting the effectiveness of masks for COVID-2.

DIAGNOSIS

To date, RT-PCR testing for COVID-19 in nasopharyngeal swabs or nasal swabs is the most common diagnostic test. Samples from saliva may be as accurate. Different gene targets are used by different manufacturers. Viral RNA is measured by the number of polymerase chain reproductive cycles and expressed as threshold (Ct). Ct values less than 40 cycles indicate that a higher number of RNA copies are in the original sample and are regarded as positive. Specificity for most tests approaches 100%. RT-PCR positivity is highest for bronchoalveolar lavage specimens followed by nasopharyngeal, nasal, and oral specimens. False-negative results may occur due to improper specimen collection or due to collection too long before or after the onset of symptoms. RT-PCR may remain positive in some patients for 6 weeks or more. However, viable SARS-CoV-2 can be detected only for the first 8 days after symptoms begin. Therefore, infectivity is presumed to be low after that point. RT-PCR may remain positive in other sites such as sputum and stool for more prolonged periods but does not seem to have clinical relevance.

One important point to remember for any test is that accuracy depends on both the pretest probability, taking into account the symptomatology, history, and local infection rates of a patient, as well as the sensitivity and specificity of a test. The sensitivity for many of the available RT-PCR tests for COVID-19 varies from 71% to 98% and depends on a number of factors, including how the specimen was collected. With a low pretest probability that a patient has COVID-19 and with a relatively low-sensitivity test, a negative result would not assure lack of disease. Thus, depending on the clinical scenario, it is important not to rule out disease if the RT-PCR is negative.

In addition to RT-PCR technology, diagnostic tests are being rapidly developed and tested. They include assays based on the following technology: antigen based, isothermal amplification (LAMP), sequencing, and CRISPR/Cas. Potential advantages of these methodologies include reduced time for results, reduced resources necessary for the test, use of saliva rather than nasopharyngeal or nasal specimens, and more accuracy.

The antibody response of infected persons is usually measured by an ELISA (enzyme-linked immunoassay) test that detects the host's specific IgM and IgG antibodies to COVID-19 virus. Uses for antibody testing include aid in diagnosing acute disease and determining immunity after infection. Antibodies to the receptor-binding domain of S protein are the most specific and are expected to be a neutralizing antibody. IgM and IgG antibodies are usually not detected until the second or third week of illness, and conversion for most patients occurs by the third to fourth week. After that IgM antibodies begin to decline, usually disappearing by week 7, whereas IgG antibodies persist. The specificity of antibody testing may be compromised by immune responses to other coronaviruses that cause common respiratory illness. Although many serodiagnostic tests have been developed by different manufacturers, most have not undergone appropriate external validation. Therefore, the persistence of the antibody response and whether neutralizing antibodies protect and for how long are unknown at this point.

Most of the data on diagnostic tests for COVID-19 have derived from adults with symptomatic disease. It is not clear whether a similar pattern of RT-PCR and antigen positivity and antibody response will be found in other populations including immunocompromised patients, children, and asymptomatic patients.

CLINICAL ASPECTS

We don't know what percentage of patients who are infected with COVID-19 are asymptomatic. Numerous studies have suggested that a significant percentage of infected people remain asymptomatic. For example, all 217 passengers and crew members on an isolated cruise ship sailing in the South Atlantic Ocean were tested for COVID-19 and 128 (59%) tested positive. Of the positive patients, 24 (19%) were symptomatic, 8 (6%) required evacuation, and 1 patient died. The remaining 104 patients were asymptomatic. Similar data were obtained from analysis of asymptomatic infected patients in a well-publicized outbreak on a cruise ship named *Diamond Princess*. In another remarkable report in September 2020, point prevalence surveys in 33 nursing homes across Connecticut were done on 2117 residents. Six hundred and one were positive and of those 530 (88.2%) were asymptomatic at the time of testing. Sixty-two of 530 developed symptoms within 14 days of testing, and thus 468 of 601(78%) patients with positive tests remained asymptomatic. Furthermore, population-based antibody testing suggests that a significant percentage of patients who test positive for SARS-CoV-2 antibodies were asymptomatic.

A narrative review published in the *Annals of Internal Medicine* concluded that the asymptomatic rate may be as high as 40% to 45%, and a conservative estimate may be closer to 30%. CDC estimates of asymptomatic rates have been even higher. Similar to most clinical aspects of the infection, these numbers depend on the age and comorbidities of the population. Overall, the data are preliminary; however, since reports have been retrospective, presymptomatic or minimally symptomatic disease may have been underestimated, and patient selection was not random.

Initial studies from China indicate that of the symptomatic patients, 81% had mild symptoms, 14% had severe manifestations, and 5% were critically ill. Studies on COVID-19 symptoms initially focused on hospitalized patients, although most of these findings apply to patients with mild disease as well. The incubation period for COVID-19 averages 5 days but can range from 2 to 11 days. Rarely, the incubation period can extend to 14 days or even longer. For symptomatic patients early in the disease, upper respiratory tract symptoms including rhinorrhea and nasal congestion are frequent. Initial symptoms noted in hospitalized patients are fever (initially 50% but up to 90% later), dry cough (60% to 86%) and dyspnea (53% to 80%). Other common symptoms are fatigue, myalgias, and headache. Some patients initially have gastrointestinal symptoms including nausea and vomiting and/or diarrhea (15% to 39%). As in other respiratory viruses, anosmia is frequently reported by patients with COVID-19 (up to 64%), although it is not often the presenting symptom.

Respiratory symptoms predominate in most patients with COVID-19. Nonproductive cough, dyspnea, and at times chest pain predominate. Peripheral pulse oxygen levels are used to determine the degree of pulmonary involvement and the need for hospitalization. One phenomenon noted with some patients is lack of dyspnea despite low peripheral oxygen levels (<90). The respiratory symptoms are progressive, resulting in 17% to 35% of hospitalized patients requiring ICU care. In severe cases hypoxemia may increase in severity, requiring sequentially supplemental oxygen, noninvasive respiratory support (for example noninvasive high-flow nasal cannulas), invasive respiratory support with intubation, and in extreme cases extracorporeal membrane oxygenation (ECMO). The great majority of patients do not progress to invasive respiratory support. The entire topic of respiratory support has undergone re-evaluation and change and remains controversial.

Cough is usually nonproductive; the occurrence of productive cough, worsening respiratory function, and signs of localized pulmonary infection may indicate the onset of bacterial or in some cases fungal superinfection. However, the preemptive use of antimicrobial agents has not improved outcomes.

Chest imaging by plain radiographs and particularly chest CT typically show bilateral ground-glass opacification, consolidation, and peripheral distribution in the lower lobes that are characteristic of viral pneumonia. Plain chest films will often miss disease early. Of note, even patients with no symptoms but positive COVID-19 testing may have characteristic findings on chest CT. Laboratory investigations show blood lymphopenia and elevated erythrocyte sedimentation rate, C-reactive protein, D-dimer, lactate dehydrogenase, and ferritin. Elevated blood sugar, creatinine, and hepatic enzymes are common.

EXTRAPULMONARY MANIFESTATIONS

COVID-19 infection in severely ill patients may have protean extrapulmonary manifestations including cardiovascular, renal, gastrointestinal, neurologic, thromboembolic, and endocrine. Myocarditis, cardiomyopathy, and acute coronary syndrome with cardiac injury as detected by elevated troponin levels have been reported in as high as 20% to 30% of hospitalized patients, particularly critically ill patients. Cardiac injury may occur by direct infection of cardiac myocytes by the virus or by the inflammatory response, which can cause thrombosis and endothelialitis. Cardiac arrhythmias including new-onset atrial fibrillation and heart block have been reported in up to 17% of hospitalized patients. Congestive heart failure, especially with preserved ejection fraction and right ventricular dilation, occurs frequently in critically ill patients, complicating the interpretation of chest radiographs. Vascular instability, sepsis-like picture, and bleeding and coagulation abnormalities are also common in ICU patients. Thrombosis of both the venous and arterial systems occurs in up to one quarter of hospitalized patients and greater than one half in ICU patients.

Acute kidney injury (AKI) occurs in up to 37% of severely ill hospitalized patients with up to 14% requiring dialysis. Hematuria and proteinuria are common in severely ill patients. Pathologic studies have shown high rates of viral infection of kidney cells, presumably due to the high distribution of ACE2 in the kidney. In addition, high rates of microvascular and tubular dysfunction may contribute to AKI and impact the prognosis. Careful fluid management and use of scarce dialysis resources are particularly important. Patients who are already on dialysis before acquiring COVID-19 have a very high mortality rate.

Gastrointestinal symptoms including anorexia, diarrhea, and nausea can occur in up to one third of patients and range in series from 12% to 61%. A smaller percentage will develop vomiting and abdominal pain. Gastrointestinal manifestations including transaminitis, ileus, and mesenteric ischemia are more common in critically ill intubated patients with COVID-19 compared to matched uninfected patients.

In some patients, gastrointestinal symptoms may be the initial indications of COVID-19 and should prompt testing for the virus since delays in diagnosis have been reported. Although the virus infects gastric epithelial cells and glandular cells, which have ACE2 present, and viral shedding can be demonstrated, gastrointestinal bleeding is not common, and endoscopy should be avoided if possible in infected patients because of the risk of aerosolization of the virus.

Hepatocellular injury may occur in up to 20% of patients with severe COVID-19 but rarely results in significant hepatitis. Liver function abnormalities including bilirubin have been associated with disease severity. Abnormal liver studies may also be related to drugs, particularly certain antiviral medications, as well as severe disease-causing cytokine release and with vascular compromise. Diagnostic studies are not indicated in most cases.

Neurologic manifestations are common in hospitalized patients, including headache, dizziness, and anosmia. The nasal epithelium has a high frequency of ACE2 and is an early target for COVID-19, probably contributing to anosmia. Delirium occurs frequently, particularly in ICU patients. Acute vascular stroke, encephalopathy, and encephalitis occur in up to 8% of severely ill patients. The extent of direct viral tropism for the central nervous system has yet to be fully defined.

Endocrine abnormalities in COVID-19 center around glycemic control. Hyperglycemia is common in hospitalized patients. Patients with undiagnosed diabetes mellitus often present with hyperglycemia alone or ketoacidosis. Patients who have preexisting diabetes mellitus or obesity are at greater risk for severe disease.

Preliminary data indicate that many patients continue to have symptoms 2 to 3 months after acute infection and a syndrome of "long COVID" has been described. More recently, post-acute COVID-19 has been defined as symptoms extending beyond 3 weeks and chronic COVID-19 beyond 12 weeks. Fatigue, dyspnea, and joint and chest pain are common. Risk factors include age greater than 50 and three or more chronic medical conditions. In one study of hospitalized patients from the United Kingdom who had been discharged at least 2 to 3 months previously, 74% reported at least one symptom, including dyspnea, fatigue, and insomnia. Approximately 14% continued to have abnormal chest radiographs. Some patients who had had more severe disease continued to have abnormal pulmonary function tests. In other studies, myocarditis and myocardial injury by MRI have been described. Significant emotional health issues are not unusual.

RISK FACTORS FOR SEVERE DISEASE AND MORTALITY

Mortality rates for COVID-19 infection vary based on population characteristics, are impacted by testing availability, and have ranged from 0.1% to 2% to 3%. Calculations are complicated by estimating the number of asymptomatic infected individuals, the normal expected death rate, and the deaths due to COVID-19 not recorded. A more meaningful expression of mortality is the excess number of expected deaths, because the individuals most at risk for COVID-19 (elderly, frail, nursing home residents) have a high baseline mortality rate.

The major risk factors for acquisition of symptomatic disease, hospitalization, and mortality are advanced age, frailty, and residing in a nursing home or congregate living facility. In some series more than 90% of deaths occur in patients over the age of 65, particularly those who are frail and those living in nursing homes or the equivalent. Early

TABLE A.1   Hospitalization, Intensive Care Unit (ICU) Admission, and Case Fatality Percentages for COVID-19 Cases by Age Group of 2499 Cases: United States, February 12–March 16, 2020[a]

Age	Hospitalization	ICU Admission	Case-Fatality
0–19 (123)	1.6–2.5	0	0
20–44 (705)	14.3–20.8	2.0–4.2	0.1–0.2
45–54 (429)	21.2–28.3	5.4–10.4	0.5–0.8
55–64 (429)	20.5–30.1	4.7–11.2	1.4–2.6
65–74 (409)	28.6–43.5	8.1–18.8	2.7–4.9
75–84 (201)	30.5–58.7	10.5–31.0	4.3–10.5
>85 (144)	31.3–70.3	6.3–29	10.4–27.3
Total (2449)	20.7–31.4	4.9–11.5	1.8–3.4

[a]Lower bound of range = number of persons hospitalized, admitted to ICU, or who died among the total in the age group. Upper bound of range = number of persons hospitalized admitted to ICU, or who died among the total in age group.

data from the CDC in Table A.1 show the striking risk that age has for hospitalization, ICU admission, and fatality.

Large outbreaks of COVID-19 have occurred in nursing homes in which both staff and residents have been infected. In one CDC study from West Virginia, nursing homes with low quality ratings from Center for Medicare and Medicaid Services (CMS) were more at risk for outbreaks of COVID-19 than those with high ratings.

Early data from the CDC indicated that 37% of patients diagnosed with COVID-19 had at least one underlying health condition. In addition to age, frailty, and nursing home residence, the most common risk factors for severity and hospitalization are diabetes mellitus and obesity, cardiovascular disease (including hypertension), and chronic lung disease. Risk increases with established diabetes mellitus and increasing BMI and is also related to central obesity and metabolic syndrome. Undiagnosed diabetes mellitus is frequently uncovered and diagnosed when patients are hospitalized for COVID-19. Other chronic diseases associated with COVID-19 include immunocompromised conditions, chronic renal disease, and chronic neurologic and psychiatric disorders. Very weak data have suggested an increased risk for patients with type A blood type although this is controversial. There was initial concern that angiotensin-converting enzyme inhibitors or angiotensin-receptor blockers would increase susceptibility to COVID-19, but subsequent data indicate that use of these agents is not associated with more disease.

Minority populations in the United States have significantly greater risk for mortality from COVID-19 than other populations. For example, the age-adjusted rate for mortality for the Black population is 3.4 times and for the Latinx population is 3.3 times that of the white population. Minority populations also have increased rates of disease and hospitalization. There are multiple causes for this discrepancy including (1) workplace exposure; (2) use of public transportation; (3) poor and crowded housing; (4) underlying diabetes mellitus, obesity, and asthma; (5) congregate living settings; (6) delayed health care and lack of access to health care; and (7) distrust of the health care system. Addressing these issues is a critical priority for the equal care of all patients and for controlling the epidemic.

In addition, there is evidence that COVID-19 affects other populations at a greater rate, including those in prisons (people in prisons have 5.5 times the case rate of the general population), group homes, and those with HIV.

TREATMENT

Treatment for COVID-19 for the vast majority of patients is supportive, similar to other respiratory viral illnesses. For hospitalized patients the primary therapy is respiratory, consisting of conventional supplemental oxygen support. Heated, humidified, high-flow nasal canula oxygen treatment or other oxygen supplementation may be necessary if standard oxygen is inadequate. If invasive ventilation is necessary, low tidal volumes and low plateau pressure are recommended. One lesson from COVID-19 is that hypoxemia is often tolerated well with various modes of supplemental oxygen and without invasive endotracheal ventilation. ECMO has been used in patients who have progressive respiratory and/or cardiovascular failure, but its effectiveness is unknown at this point. Details of ICU care and further goals of ICU care are outlined in guidelines from the Society of Critical Care Medicine, the CDC, and the National Institutes of Health.

A number of drugs in different classes are in clinical trial at this point but few at this time have been shown to be effective. The only one on which there is persuasive data from prospective randomized clinical trials (RCT) is the anti-inflammatory drug dexamethasone. It was shown to reduce mortality in the Randomized Evaluation of COVID-19 Therapy (RECOVERY) trial. Compared to control patients, a significant decrease in mortality was noted in patients on mechanical ventilation (41% vs. 29%) and those on oxygen supplementation (26% vs. 23%). Those without oxygen requirement had no benefit, but even in this situation there could be a subgroup that would benefit, and further studies are ongoing.

Antiviral drugs including remdesivir, hydroxychloroquine, azithromycin, and lopinavir are being studied but none have shown a reduction in mortality. Remdesivir was recently approved by the FDA on the basis of a study in which patients assigned to a 10-day course of remdesivir had a recovery time that was 4 days shorter compared with placebo (median, 11 vs. 15 days).

Other therapies being actively investigated in clinical trials include anti–COVID-19 antibodies, such as convalescent plasma and monoclonal antibodies, and targeted immunomodulatory drugs such as anti-IL-6 (tocilizumab), anti-IL-1, JAK inhibitors, and tyrosine kinase inhibitors. Some of these immunomodulatory drugs may have antiviral properties as well. Likewise, antiviral interferon alpha2b therapy is under active investigation. Chloroquine/hydroxychloroquine has been controversial. A systemic review in August 2020 concluded that the evidence on the benefits and harms of this drug is very weak and conflicting. Future studies should clarify what if any drugs have a significant effect on morbidity and mortality.

It is recommended that all hospitalized patients receive subcutaneous low-molecular-weight heparin to prevent thrombotic complications. Which patients need therapeutic anticoagulation is under study, but in most centers use is based on clinical presentation, comorbidities, and D-dimer level.

Most patients hospitalized with COVID-19 have evidence of viral pneumonia but not bacterial superinfection and thus do not benefit from routine antimicrobial therapy that predisposes to bacterial and fungal superinfection from resistant pathogens.

Standard therapy for cardiac, renal, endocrinologic, hematologic, and neurologic complications is detailed in subspecialty guidelines.

VACCINES

Vaccine development is one of the highest priorities in COVID-19 research. Traditional vaccine development typically takes more than a decade to complete. The traditional process includes: discovery (2 to 5 years); preclinical including animal studies (2 years); clinical (phase 1: 2 years involving 10 to 50 people, phase 2: 2 to 3 years involving hundreds of people, and phase 3: protection studies involving thousands of subjects taking years); regulatory phase of 2 years; and manufacturing and delivery, which takes 1 to 2 years. With the COVID-19 pandemic the process was streamlined with rapid early phases producing as many candidates as possible, then clinical studies using sites across the globe, and eventually building global manufacturing capacity.

Vaccines have in general targeted the spike protein, but it is not clear what site on the molecule will be the most effective target. Types of vaccines include RNA/DNA, inactivated virus, live attenuated virus, nonreplicating vector, protein subunit, and replicating viral vector. Much attention and preliminary findings have focused on mRNA vaccines. At this writing at least eight potential vaccines are in phase 3 trials in various countries around the world.

Concerns about vaccines include the following:

1. Will the vaccine produce lasting immunity in all populations including those most at risk such as the elderly?
2. Are studies adequately addressing both short-term and long-term adverse effects?
3. Vaccines produced for other coronaviruses have shown lung toxicity, and therefore toxicity must be investigated first in animal models.
4. Will manufacturing capacity and clinical capacity be adequate and will distribution of the vaccine be equitable and target the most vulnerable populations?
5. Will people be willing to take the vaccine?
6. What will be the immune response of the vulnerable population to the vaccine? It is important to recognize that vaccines for respiratory illnesses such as influenza are only 40% to 80% effective at most.

Information about vaccines and their effectiveness and safety will be forthcoming rapidly in the next several years. Preliminary data from two phase 3 trials indicate remarkable efficacy and safety for two mRNA vaccines.

PREGNANCY AND CHILDREN

Preliminary experience from China indicated that pregnant women did not have increased risk from COVID-19 during the third trimester of pregnancy and that newborns were not at risk for infection. Data from the United States are accumulating but remain preliminary. Data from the CDC early in the epidemic indicate that pregnant women with COVID-19 may have fewer symptoms but are more likely to be hospitalized and have severe disease than pregnant women who are not infected. In a study among 598 hospitalized pregnant women with COVID-19, 55% were asymptomatic at admission. Severe illness occurred among symptomatic pregnant women including ICU admissions (16%), mechanical ventilation (8%), and death (1%). Pregnancy losses occurred for 2% of pregnancies completed during COVID-19–associated hospitalizations and were experienced by both symptomatic and asymptomatic women. Of concern, however, are women with increased risk factors in the United States, such as glucose intolerance, diabetes mellitus, obesity, hypertension, and minority status. Data from the CDC showed that women with obesity and/or gestational diabetes were at higher risk for severe disease. A later study (PRIORITY study) compared women who tested positive for COVID-19 0 to 14 days before delivery versus those who tested negative. COVID-19 was not associated with a difference in birthweight, difficulty breathing, apnea, or respiratory infection in the first 8 weeks of life. Women infected with COVID-19 delivered 1.5 weeks earlier on average. Guidelines for the care of pregnant women and delivery have been published by the CDC and the American Academy of Pediatrics, the American College of Obstetricians and Gynecologists and the Society for Maternal-Fetal Medicine, and the Society for Obstetric Anesthesia and Perinatology.

Data from the early phase of the pandemic indicate that children account for only a small portion of confirmed cases and that most cases of clinical COVID-19 in children are mild and self-limiting. Subsequent data indicate that a percentage of pediatric patients are asymptomatic. Symptomatic patients have fever and cough; a lower percentage have typical viral respiratory symptoms including nasal congestion, myalgia, fatigue, and sore throat. Less than 10% presented with gastrointestinal symptoms. Case fatality rates in children are less than 0.5% and are lower than those of seasonal influenza. Children with underlying respiratory/cardiac disease are most at risk.

Childhood multisystem inflammatory syndrome (MIS-C) was initially described in the United Kingdom as a disease having some characteristics of Kawasaki disease, a rare vasculitis of childhood that can cause coronary aneurysms, and subsequently was reported worldwide. As of mid-July 2020, approximately 1000 cases had been reported. The pathophysiology is still being defined, but most definitions include an inflammatory illness with fever and increased inflammatory markers that involve at least four organ systems including the gastrointestinal, cardiovascular, hematologic, skin, and respiratory systems and in most patients evidence of COVID-19 infection. The disease typically begins 2 to 4 weeks after COVID-19 symptoms. It occurs in previously healthy children who are older than 5 years of age, including adolescents, compared to patients with Kawasaki disease who are usually younger than 5 years. A relatively high percentage (10% to 20%) have evidence of cardiovascular involvement and coronary artery aneurysms. Treatment is anti-inflammatory agents. Most patients recover but mortality ranges as high as 2%. Further data on the epidemiology, clinical characteristics, and treatment of this rare condition are needed.

PREVENTION

It is beyond this Appendix to review the complex epidemiology and public health efforts to prevent and mitigate the COVID-19 pandemic. It was clear from the experience in Wuhan that draconian governmental action including preventing travel in and out of Wuhan, strict quarantine, wearing face masks, shutting down public transportation and public gatherings, closing businesses, and increasing medical care capacity halted the epidemic over several months. Less stringent measures have been instituted in Europe, the United States, and other parts of the world, although there has been wide variation in the extent of restrictions. Contact tracing has been practiced effectively in some countries such as South Korea, but lack of adequate testing and the high percentage of asymptomatic patients has made that impractical in many settings. What have become generally accepted as effective measures include face masks, social distancing, and restricting social gatherings.

Many countries have seen a marked reduction in cases due to initial public health measures and have begun loosening restrictions with a resultant increase in the number of cases. Early data on resurgent COVID-19 indicate that younger age groups are more affected and that the severity and mortality are less. It is possible, however, that the infection will spread to vulnerable populations, resulting in additional waves of the pandemic that need to be addressed and controlled. Mitigation efforts do not eliminate the virus and until herd immunity is widespread (presumably higher than 40%) and effective vaccines are available, viral transmission and infection will continue.

The downside of public health restrictions has included major negative effects on people. There has been an increase in stress, mental health issues such as depression and anxiety, and unfortunately increases in drug use including alcohol. In one survey, frequency of alcohol use increased 14% overall in 2020 compared to 2019 and affected women more than men. Many patients have avoided the medical care system for acute and routine care out of fear of catching COVID-19. According to a CDC survey early in June 2020, 41% of the US population had delayed or avoided medical care during the pandemic. Care for conditions such as acute infection, acute cardiac disease, and injuries has often not been readily accessible in many locations and as a result mortality has increased for some of these conditions. Routine care including elective surgery, vaccinations, and regular medical visits have been put on hold. Economic disruption with unprecedented economic contraction, massive worldwide unemployment, supply chain disruption, business failures, and food insecurity has wreaked havoc on all countries but has disproportionally affected the poorest and most vulnerable populations. One estimate of the total cost for the United States is $16 trillion resulting from economic disruption and medical costs. School closings and reopenings have been an extremely important issue that continues to be debated, but the downside of school closings has been enormous, particularly for children in minority populations. The balance between restrictions for the pandemic and opening society will be an ongoing issue for the foreseeable future.

SUGGESTED READINGS

Brooks JT, Butler JC, Redfield RR: Universal masking to prevent SARS-CoV-2 transmission—the time is now, JAMA 324(7):635–637, 2020.

Chou R, Dana T, Jungbauer R, Weeks C, McDonagh MS: Masks for prevention of respiratory virus infections, including SARS-CoV-2, in health care and community settings—a living rapid review, Annal Int Med 173(7): 542–555, 2020.

Fineberg HV: The toll of COVID-19, JAMA 324(15):1502–1503, 2020.

Fontanet A, Couchemez S: COVID-19 herd immunity: Where are we? Nature Reviews 20(10):583–584, 2020.

Gupta A, Madhavan MV, Sehgal K, et al: Extrapulmonary manifestations of COVID 19, Nat Med 26:1017–1032, 2020.

MMWR, CDC, March 27, 2020 Severe Outcomes among Patients with Coronavirus Disease 2019 (COVID 19)—United States, February 12-March 16, 2020 page 343.

MMWR, CDC, October 2, 2020 Changing Age Distribution of the COVID-19 Pandemic—United States, May-August 2020, page 1404.

MMWR, CDC, October 23, 2020 Mortality due to COVID-19, page 1522.

Oran DP, Topol EJ: Prevalence of asymptomatic SARS-CoV-2 infection—a narrative review, Annal Int Med 173:362–367, 2020.

Sethuraman N, Jeremiah SS, Ryo A: Interpreting diagnostic tests for SARS-CoV-2, JAMA 323(22):2249–2251, 2020.

The WHO Rapid Evidence Appraisal for COVID-19 Therapies (REACT) Working Group: Association between administration of systemic corticosteroids and mortality among critically Ill patients with COVID-19 a meta-analysis, JAMA 324(13):1330–1341, 2020.

Wiersinga WJ, Rhodes A, Cheng AC, Peacock SJ, Prescott HC: Pathophysiology, transmission, diagnosis, and treatment of coronavirus disease 2019 (COVID 19) a review, JAMA 324(8):782–793, 2020.

INDEX

Page numbers followed by "f" indicate figures, "t" indicate tables, and "b" indicate boxes.